The American Psychiatric Publishing Textbook of Consultation-Liaison Psychiatry

Psychiatry in the Medically Ill

Second Edition

Editorial Board

The American Psychiatric Publishing Textbook of Consultation-Liaison Psychiatry

Psychiatry in the Medically Ill

Second Edition

Edited by

Michael G. Wise, M.D.
James R. Rundell, M.D.

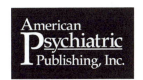

Washington, DC
London, England

Note: The authors have worked to ensure that all information in this book concerning drug dosages, schedules, and routes of administration is accurate as of the time of publication and consistent with standards set by the U.S. Food and Drug Administration and the general medical community. As medical research and practice advance, however, therapeutic standards may change. For this reason and because human and mechanical errors sometimes occur, we recommend that readers follow the advice of a physician who is directly involved in their care or the care of a member of their family. A product's current package insert should be consulted for full prescribing and safety information.

Manufactured in the United States of America on acid-free paper
06 05 04 03 02   5 4 3 2 1
Second Edition

American Psychiatric Publishing, Inc.
1400 K Street, N.W.
Washington, DC 20005
www.appi.org

Library of Congress Cataloging-in-Publication Data
The American Psychiatric Publishing textbook of consultation-liaison psychiatry :
psychiatry in the medically ill / edited by Michael G. Wise, James R. Rundell.—2nd ed.
     p. ; cm.
   Rev. ed. of: The American Psychiatric Press textbook of consultation-liaison psychiatry.
   Includes bibliographical references and index.
   ISBN 0-88048-393-8 (alk. paper)
   1. Consultation-liaison psychiatry. I. Title: Textbook of consultation-liaison
psychiatry. II. Title: Consultation-liaison psychiatry. III. Title: Psychiatry in the
medically ill. IV. Wise, Michael G., 1944- V. Rundell, James R., 1957- VI. American
Psychiatric Publishing. VII. American Psychiatric Publishing textbook of consultation-liaison
psychiatry.
  [DNLM: 1. Mental Disorders—therapy. 2. Mental Disorders—diagnosis. 3. Psychiatry.
4. Referral and Consultation. WM 140 A5127 2002]
  RC455.2.C65 A44 2001
  616.89'14—dc21

British Library Cataloguing in Publication Data
A CIP record is available from the British Library.

Contents

Contributors ix

Preface xv

Dedication xvii

Introduction xix

I

General Principles

1 History of Consultation-Liaison Psychiatry. 3
   Zbigniew J. Lipowski, M.D., F.R.C.P.C., and Thomas N. Wise, M.D.

2 Consultation, Liaison, and Administration of a Consultation-Liaison Psychiatry Service. 13
   Elisabeth J. Shakin Kunkel, M.D., Daniel A. Monti, M.D., and Troy L. Thompson II, M.D.

3 Cost-Effectiveness of the Consultation-Liaison Service 25
   Richard C. W. Hall, M.D., James R. Rundell, M.D., and Michael K. Popkin, M.D., F.A.P.M.

4 Liaison Psychiatry 33
   James J. Strain, M.D.

5 Basic Science of Neuroimaging and Potential Applications for Consultation-Liaison Psychiatry . . . 49
   Peter F. Goyer, M.D.

6 Mental Status Examination and Diagnosis 61
   Michael G. Wise, M.D., and Mark E. Servis, M.D.

7 Neuropsychological and Psychological Assessment 77
   Robert L. Mapou, Ph.D., Wendy A. Law, Ph.D., Jack Spector, Ph.D., and Gary G. Kay, Ph.D.

8 Behavioral Responses to Illness: Personality and Personality Disorders. 107
   Robert J. Ursano, M.D., Richard S. Epstein, M.D., and Susan G. Lazar, M.D.

9 Suicidality. 127
   John Michael Bostwick, M.D.

10 Aggression and Agitation 149
   Robert E. Hales, M.D., M.B.A., Jonathan M. Silver, M.D., Stuart C. Yudofsky, M.D., Mark E. Servis, M.D., and
   Donald M. Hilty, M.D.

11 Legal and Ethical Issues 167
   Robert I. Simon, M.D.

12 Consultation-Liaison Psychiatry Research 191
James R. Rundell, M.D. and Thomas N. Wise, M.D.

13 International Perspectives on Consultation-Liaison Psychiatry 203
Chapter Editors:
Frits J. Huyse, M.D., Thomas Herzog, M.D., and Ulrik F. Malt, M.D.

Contributors:
Ruben Cesarco, M.D., Francis Creed, M.D., Peter de Jonge, Ph.D., Trevor Friedman, M.D., Thomas Herzog, M.D.,
Takashi Hosaka, M.D., Frits J. Huyse, M.D., Yasutaka Iwasaki, M.D., Antonio Lobo, M.D., Ulrik F. Malt, M.D.,
Marco Rigatelli, M.D., Graeme C. Smith, M.D., Wolfgang Söllner, M.D., Barbara Stein, Ph.D., Fritz Stiefel, M.D.,
James J. Strain, M.D., and Paulo R. Zimmermann, M.D.

II
Psychiatric Disorders in General Hospital Patients

14 Epidemiology of Psychiatric Disorders in Medically Ill Patients 237
William R. Yates, M.D.

15 Delirium (Confusional States) 257
Michael G. Wise, M.D., Donald M. Hilty, M.D., Gabrielle M. Cerda, M.D., and Paula T. Trzepacz, M.D.

16 Dementia 273
Kevin F. Gray, M.D., and Jeffrey L. Cummings, M.D.

17 Depression 307
Alvin M. Rouchell, M.D., Richard Pounds, M.D., and John G. Tierney, M.D.

18 Mania 339
J. Stephen McDaniel, M.D., and Sanjay M. Sharma, M.D.

19 Somatization and Somatoform Disorders 361
Susan E. Abbey, M.D., F.R.C.P.C.

20 Anxiety and Panic 393
Eduardo A. Colón, M.D., and Michael K. Popkin, M.D., F.A.P.M.

21 Substance-Related Disorders 417
John E. Franklin Jr., M.D., Martin H. Leamon, M.D., and Richard J. Frances, M.D.

22 Sexual Disorders and Dysfunctions 455
George R. Brown, M.D., Gregory Gass, M.D., and Kemuel Philbrick, M.D.

23 Eating Disorders 477
Richard C. W. Hall, M.D., and James R. Rundell, M.D.

24 Sleep Disorders 495
Jeffrey B. Weilburg, M.D., and John W. Winkelman, M.D., Ph.D.

25 Factitious Disorders and Malingering 519
Charles V. Ford, M.D., and Marc D. Feldman, M.D.

III
Clinical Consultation-Liaison Settings

26 Internal Medicine and Medical Subspecialties 535
Chapter Editor:
Donna B. Greenberg, M.D.

Contributors:
Lewis M. Cohen, M.D., Donna B. Greenberg, M.D., Peter Halperin, M.D., Roger Kathol, M.D., C.P.E.,
Richard L. Kradin, M.D., R. Bruce Lydiard, M.D., Ph.D., and Kevin W. Olden, M.D., F.A.C.G.

27 Surgery and Surgical Subspecialties 593
Charles L. Raison, M.D., Robert O. Pasnau, M.D., Fawzy I. Fawzy, M.D., Christine E. Skotzko, M.D.,
Thomas B. Strouse, M.D., David K. Wellisch, Ph.D., and Alisa K. Hoffman, Ph.D.

28 Solid Organ Transplantation 623
Christine E. Skotzko, M.D., and Thomas B. Strouse, M.D.

29 Oncology and Psychooncology 657
Fawzy I. Fawzy, M.D., Mark E. Servis, M.D., and Donna B. Greenberg, M.D.

30 Neurology and Neurosurgery 679
Gregory Fricchione, M.D., Zeina el-Chemali, M.D., Jeffrey B. Weilburg, M.D., and George B. Murray, M.D.

31 Obstetrics and Gynecology 701
Nada L. Stotland, M.D., M.P.H.

32 Pediatrics 717
Gregory K. Fritz, M.D., and Larry K. Brown, M.D.

33 Physical Medicine and Rehabilitation 729
Duane S. Bishop, M.D., and L. Russell Pet, M.D.

34 Intensive Care Units 753
John L. Shuster Jr., M.D., and Theodore A. Stern, M.D.

35 Psychiatric Issues in the Care of Dying Patients 771
William Breitbart, M.D., and Kathleen Lintz, B.A.

36 HIV Disease/AIDS 807
Mark H. Halman, M.D., F.R.C.P.C., Philip Bialer, M.D., Jonathan L. Worth, M.D., and
Sean B. Rourke, Ph.D., C.Psych.

37 Geriatric Medicine 853
Jürgen Unützer, M.D., M.P.H., Gary W. Small, M.D., and Ibrahim Gunay, M.D.

38 Strategic Integration of Inpatient and Outpatient Medical-Psychiatry Services 871
Roger G. Kathol, M.D., C.P.E., and Alan Stoudemire, M.D.

39 The Emergency Department 889
George E. Tesar, M.D., and Joseph A. Locala, M.D.

40 The Primary Care Clinic 917
Gregory E. Simon, M.D., M.P.H., and Edward A. Walker, M.D.

41 Telepsychiatry 927
Brian J. Grady, M.D.

IV
Treatment

42 **Psychopharmacology** **939**
Martina L. Fait, M.D., Michael G. Wise, M.D., John S. Jachna, M.D., Richard D. Lane, M.D., Ph.D., and
Alan J. Gelenberg, M.D.

43 **Pain Management** **989**
Anna Holmgren, M.D., Michael G. Wise, M.D., and Anthony J. Bouckoms, M.D.

44 **Electroconvulsive Therapy: An Overview** **1015**
Charles H. Kellner, M.D., and Mark D. Beale, M.D.

45 **Psychotherapy** **1027**
Don R. Lipsitt, M.D.

46 **Behavioral Medicine** **1053**
Andrew B. Littman, M.D., and Mark W. Ketterer, Ph.D.

Index. **1081**

Contributors

Susan E. Abbey, M.D., F.R.C.P.C.
Director, Program in Medical Psychiatry, Department of Psychiatry, University Health Network; Associate Professor, University of Toronto, Toronto, Ontario, Canada

Mark D. Beale, M.D.
Clinical Assistant Professor, Department of Psychiatry and Behavioral Sciences, Medical University of South Carolina, Charleston, South Carolina

Philip Bialer, M.D.
Chief, Division of Consultation-Liaison Psychiatry, Beth Israel Medical Center; Associate Professor of Clinical Psychiatry, Albert Einstein College of Medicine, New York, New York

Duane S. Bishop, M.D.
Associate Professor of Psychiatry and Human Behavior, Brown University and Rhode Island Hospital, Providence, Rhode Island; Chairman, Department of Psychiatry, St. Luke's Hospital, New Bedford, Massachusetts

John Michael Bostwick, M.D.
Consultant, Department of Psychiatry and Psychology, Mayo Clinic, Rochester, Minnesota

Anthony J. Bouckoms, M.D.[†]
Assistant Professor of Psychiatry, Harvard Medical School, Boston, Massachusetts

William Breitbart, M.D.
Attending Psychiatrist, Pain and Palliative Care Service, Memorial Sloan-Kettering Cancer Center, New York, New York

George R. Brown, M.D.
Professor and Associate Chairman, Department of Psychiatry, East Tennessee State University; Chief of Psychiatry and Director of Psychiatric Research, James H. Quillen VAMC, Johnson City (Mountain Home), Tennessee

Larry K. Brown, M.D.
Director, Child and Adolescent Psychiatry Outpatient Services, Rhode Island Hospital; Associate Professor, Department of Psychiatry and Human Behavior, Brown University Medical School, Providence, Rhode Island

Gabrielle M. Cerda, M.D.
Clinical Director, Children's Outpatient Psychiatry, Children's Hospital of San Diego; Assistant Clinical Professor of Psychiatry, University of California, San Diego, San Diego, California

Ruben Cesarco, M.D.
Associate Professor of Medical Psychology, Medical School, University of Montevideo; Chief, Psychosocial Medicine Unit, Hospital Maciel, Montevideo, Uruguay

Lewis M. Cohen, M.D.
Co-Director, Psychiatric Consultation Service, Baystate Medical Center, Springfield, Massachusetts; Associate Professor of Psychiatry, Tufts Medical School, Boston, Massachusetts

Eduardo A. Colón, M.D.
Vice-Chief, Department of Psychiatry, Hennepin County Medical Center; Associate Professor of Psychiatry, University of Minnesota Medical School, Minneapolis, Minnesota

[†] Deceased.

Francis Creed, M.D.
Professor of Psychological Medicine and Honorary
Consultant Psychiatrist, Psychological Research Group,
School of Psychiatry and Behavioural Science, University
of Manchester, Manchester, United Kingdom

Jeffrey L. Cummings, M.D.
The Augustus S. Rose Professor of Neurology, Professor
of Psychiatry and Biobehavioral Sciences, and Director,
UCLA Alzheimer's Disease Research Center, University
of California at Los Angeles School of Medicine, Los
Angeles, California

Peter de Jonge, Ph.D.
Senior Researcher, Consultation-Liaison Psychiatry,
VU University Medical Centre, Amsterdam,
The Netherlands

Zeina el-Chemali, M.D.
Instructor in Neurology and Psychiatry, Harvard Medical
School; Brigham Behavioral Neurology Group, Brigham
and Women's Hospital, Boston, Massachusetts

Richard S. Epstein, M.D.
Clinical Professor, Department of Psychiatry,
Uniformed Services University of the Health Sciences,
F. Edward Hébert School of Medicine, Bethesda,
Maryland

Martina L. Fait, M.D.
Clinical Director, Consultation-Liaison Services,
Alvarado Parkway Institute, La Mesa, California

Fawzy I. Fawzy, M.D.
Professor and Executive Vice Chair, Department of
Psychiatry and Biobehavioral Sciences; Medical Director,
Neuropsychiatric Hospital; Associate Director,
Neuropsychiatric Institute, University of California at
Los Angeles School of Medicine, Los Angeles, California

Marc D. Feldman, M.D.
Professor of Psychiatry; Vice Chairman for Clinical
Services, Department of Psychiatry and Behavioral
Neurobiology, University of Alabama at Birmingham,
Birmingham, Alabama

Charles V. Ford, M.D.
Professor of Psychiatry; Director of the UAB
Neuropsychiatry Clinic, University of Alabama at
Birmingham, Birmingham, Alabama

Richard J. Frances, M.D.
President and Medical Director, Silver Hill Hospital,
New Canaan, Connecticut; Clinical Professor of
Psychiatry, New York University School of Medicine,
New York, New York

John E. Franklin Jr., M.D.
Associate Professor of Psychiatry and Division Chief,
Addiction Psychiatry, Department of Psychiatry and
Behavioral Sciences, Northwestern University Medical
School, Chicago, Illinois

Gregory Fricchione, M.D.
Associate Professor of Psychiatry, Harvard Medical
School; Director, Medical Psychiatry Services,
Department of Psychiatry, Brigham and Women's
Hospital, Boston, Massachusetts

Trevor Friedman, M.D.
Consultant Liaison Psychiatrist, Brandon Mental Health
Unit, Leicester, United Kingdom

Gregory K. Fritz, M.D.
Professor and Director, Division of Child and Adolescent
Psychiatry, Department of Psychiatry and Human
Behavior, Brown University Medical School; Director,
Child and Family Psychiatry, Rhode Island Hospital;
Medical Director, E.P. Bradley Hospital, Providence,
Rhode Island

Gregory Gass, M.D.
Staff Psychiatrist, Peninsula Village, Louisville,
Tennessee

Alan J. Gelenberg, M.D.
Professor and Head, Department of Psychiatry, Arizona
Health Sciences Center, Tucson, Arizona

Peter F. Goyer, M.D.
Chief of Staff, Cleveland Veterans Affairs Medical
Center, Cleveland, Ohio; and Associate Professor of
Psychiatry and of Radiology, Case Western Reserve
University School of Medicine, Cleveland, Ohio

Brian J. Grady, M.D.
Lieutenant Commander, U.S. Navy; Head, Primary
Behavioral Healthcare Service, and Clinical Director,
TeleMedicine, National Naval Medical Center,
Bethesda, Maryland

Kevin F. Gray, M.D.
Geriatric Neuropsychiatry, Mental Health Service, VA
Medical Center; Assistant Professor, Departments of
Psychiatry and Neurology, University of Texas,
Southwestern Medical Center, Dallas, Texas

Donna B. Greenberg, M.D.
Associate Psychiatrist, Massachusetts General Hospital,
Boston, Massachusetts

Ibrahim Gunay, M.D.
Assistant Clinical Professor of Psychiatry and
Biobehavioral Sciences, UCLA Neuropsychiatric
Institute, Los Angeles, California

Robert E. Hales, M.D., M.B.A.
Professor and Chair, Department of Psychiatry, University of California, Davis, School of Medicine, Sacramento, California

Richard C. W. Hall, M.D.
Courtesy Clinical Professor of Psychiatry, University of Florida, Gainesville, Florida

Mark H. Halman, M.D., F.R.C.P.C.
Director, HIV Psychiatry Program, St. Michael's Hospital; Assistant Professor of Psychiatry, University of Toronto, Toronto, Ontario, Canada

Peter Halperin, M.D.
Clinical Associate Professor, Department of Psychiatry; Director, Behavioral Medicine Division; Director, Medical Student Education in Psychiatry, State University of New York at Stony Brook Medical School, Stony Brook, New York

Thomas Herzog, M.D.
Chairman and Head, Department of Psychosomatics and Psychological Medicine, Christophsbad, Göppingen; Associate Professor, Albert Ludwigs University, Freiburg, Germany

Donald M. Hilty, M.D.
Assistant Professor of Clinical Psychiatry, University of California, Davis, School of Medicine, Sacramento, California

Alisa K. Hoffman, Ph.D.
Staff Psychologist, Department of Psychiatry, University of California School of Medicine, Los Angeles, California

Anna Holmgren, M.D.
Assistant Professor of Psychiatry, University of California, Davis, Sacramento, California

Takashi Hosaka, M.D.
Professor, Department of Psychiatry and Behavioral Science, Tokai University School of Medicine, Kanagawa, Japan

Frits J. Huyse, M.D.
Director, Consultation-Liaison Service, and Associate Professor of Psychiatry, VU University Medical Centre, Amsterdam, The Netherlands

Yasutaka Iwasaki, M.D.
Associate Director, Medical Economics Division, Health Insurance Bureau, Ministry of Health, Labour and Welfare, Tokyo, Japan

John S. Jachna, M.D.
Assistant Professor of Clinical Psychiatry, Southern Arizona Health Care System, Tucson, Arizona

Roger G. Kathol, M.D., C.P.E.
Adjunct Clinical Professor of Internal Medicine and Psychiatry, Oregon Health Sciences University; President and CEO, Cartesian Solutions, Portland, Oregon

Gary G. Kay, Ph.D.
Director, Washington Neuropsychological Institute; Associate Clinical Professor of Neurology, Georgetown University School of Medicine, Washington, D.C.

Charles H. Kellner, M.D.
Professor, Department of Psychiatry and Behavioral Sciences and Department of Neurology, Medical University of South Carolina, Charleston, South Carolina

Mark W. Ketterer, Ph.D.
Senior Bioscientific Staff, Henry Ford Hospital, Detroit, Michigan

Richard L. Kradin, M.D.
Assistant Physician, Department of Medicine, Massachusetts General Hospital; Research Director, Mind/Body Medical Institute, Beth Israel Deaconess Medical Center; Member, MGH Center for Psychoanalytic Studies; Associate Professor of Pathology, Harvard Medical School, Boston, Massachusetts

Elisabeth J. Shakin Kunkel, M.D.
Professor of Psychiatry and Human Behavior and Director, Consultation-Liaison Psychiatry, Jefferson Medical College, Philadelphia, Pennsylvania

Richard D. Lane, M.D., Ph.D.
Associate Professor, Department of Psychiatry, Arizona Health Sciences Center, Tucson, Arizona

Wendy A. Law, Ph.D.
Assistant Professor, Department of Medical and Clinical Psychology and Department of Psychiatry, Uniformed Services University of the Health Sciences, Bethesda, Maryland

Susan G. Lazar, M.D.
Clinical Professor of Psychiatry and Behavioral Sciences, Georgetown University School of Medicine, Washington, D.C.; Clinical Professor of Psychiatry, Uniformed Services University of the Health Sciences, F. Edward Hébert School of Medicine, Bethesda, Maryland; and Teaching Analyst, Washington Psychoanalytic Institute, Washington, D.C.

Martin H. Leamon, M.D.
Assistant Professor of Clinical Psychiatry, Department of Psychiatry, University of California, Davis, Sacramento, California

Kathleen Lintz, B.A.
Medical Student (Fourth Year), Mount Sinai School of Medicine, New York, New York

Zbigniew J. Lipowski, M.D., F.R.C.P.C.[†]
Professor Emeritus of Psychiatry, University of Toronto, Toronto, Ontario, Canada

Don R. Lipsitt, M.D.
Chairman Emeritus, Department of Psychiatry, Mount Auburn Hospital, Cambridge, Massachusetts

Andrew B. Littman, M.D.
Director of Behavioral Medicine Division of Preventive Cardiology, Department of Psychiatry, Massachusetts General Hospital; Instructor in Psychiatry, Harvard Medical School, Boston, Massachusetts

Antonio Lobo, M.D.
Professor of Psychiatry; Chief, Psychosomatics and Liaison Psychiatry Service, Hospital Clínico Universitario, Zaragoza, Spain

Joseph A. Locala, M.D.
Associate Staff, Department of Psychiatry and Psychology, Cleveland Clinic Foundation, Cleveland, Ohio

R. Bruce Lydiard, M.D., Ph.D.
Professor of Psychiatry, Department of Psychiatry and Behavioral Sciences, Medical University of South Carolina, Charleston, South Carolina

Ulrik F. Malt, M.D.
Professor and Clinical Director, Department of Psychosomatic and Behavioural Medicine, University of Oslo, Rikshospitalet, Oslo, Norway

Robert L. Mapou, Ph.D.
Clinical Associate Professor of Neurology (Psychology), Georgetown University School of Medicine, Washington, D.C.; Research Associate Professor of Psychiatry and Research Assistant Professor of Neurology, Uniformed Services University of the Health Sciences, Bethesda, Maryland

J. Stephen McDaniel, M.D.
Professor of Psychiatry and Behavioral Sciences and Family and Preventive Medicine, Emory University School of Medicine, Atlanta, Georgia

Daniel A. Monti, M.D.
Assistant Professor of Psychiatry and Human Behavior, Jefferson Medical College, Philadelphia, Pennsylvania

George B. Murray, M.D.
Associate Professor of Psychiatry, Harvard Medical School; Director, Consultation Psychiatry Fellowship, Massachusetts General Hospital, Boston, Massachusetts

Kevin W. Olden, M.D., F.A.C.G.
Associate Chair, Department of Medicine, Mayo Clinic Scottsdale; Associate Professor of Medicine and Psychiatry, Mayo Medical School, Scottsdale, Arizona

Robert O. Pasnau, M.D.
Professor Emeritus, Department of Psychiatry and Biobehavioral Sciences, UCLA School of Medicine, Los Angeles, California

L. Russell Pet, M.D.
Chairman, Department of Psychiatry, Charlton Hospital, Fall River, Massachusetts

Kemuel Philbrick, M.D.
Consultant, Department of Psychiatry and Psychology, Mayo Clinic, Rochester, Minnesota

Michael K. Popkin, M.D., F.A.P.M.
Chief of Psychiatry, Hennepin County Medical Center; Professor of Psychiatry and Medicine, University of Minnesota Medical School, Minneapolis, Minnesota

Richard Pounds, M.D.
Medical Director, Spanish Peaks Mental Health Center, Pueblo, Colorado

Charles L. Raison, M.D.
Director, Psychiatric Consultation Liaison Services, Grady Health System; Assistant Professor, Department of Psychiatry and Behavioral Sciences, Emory University School of Medicine, Atlanta, Georgia

Marco Rigatelli, M.D.
Professor of Psychiatry, Chief of C-L Psychiatry Service, University of Modena and Reggio Emilia, Modena, Italy

Alvin M. Rouchell, M.D.
Head, Consultation-Liaison Service, and Chairman, Department of Psychiatry, Ochsner Clinic; Clinical Professor of Psychiatry, Tulane University School of Medicine and Louisiana State University School of Medicine, New Orleans, Louisiana

Sean B. Rourke, Ph.D., C.Psych.
Neuropsychologist, HIV Psychiatry Program, St. Michael's Hospital; Assistant Professor of Psychiatry, University of Toronto, Toronto, Ontario, Canada

---

[†] Deceased.

James R. Rundell, M.D.
Professor of Psychiatry, Uniformed Services University of the Health Sciences, Bethesda, Maryland; Deputy Commander for Clinical Services, Landstuhl Regional Medical Center, Germany

Mark E. Servis, M.D.
Associate Professor of Clinical Psychiatry, University of California, Davis, Medical Center, Sacramento, California

Sanjay M. Sharma, M.D.
Assistant Professor of Psychiatry and Behavioral Sciences, Emory University School of Medicine, Atlanta, Georgia

John L. Shuster Jr., M.D.
Director, UAB Center for Palliative Care, and Associate Professor of Psychiatry and Medicine, University of Alabama at Birmingham School of Medicine, Birmingham, Alabama

Jonathan M. Silver, M.D.
Clinical Professor of Psychiatry, New York University School of Medicine; Assistant Director for Clinical Services and Research, Department of Psychiatry, Lenox Hill Hospital, New York, New York

Gregory E. Simon, M.D., M.P.H.
Investigator, Center for Health Studies, Group Health Cooperative, Seattle, Washington

Robert I. Simon, M.D.
Clinical Professor of Psychiatry and Director, Program in Psychiatry and Law, Georgetown University School of Medicine, Washington, D.C.

Christine E. Skotzko, M.D.
Director of Consultation-Liaison Psychiatry, Robert Wood Johnson Medical School, University of Medicine and Dentistry of New Jersey, New Brunswick, New Jersey

Gary W. Small, M.D.
Professor of Psychiatry and Biobehavioral Sciences, Parlow-Solomon Professor on Aging, and Director, Center on Aging, UCLA Neuropsychiatric Institute, Los Angeles, California

Graeme C. Smith, M.D.
Professor, Department of Psychological Medicine, Monash University, Melbourne, Australia

Wolfgang Söllner, M.D.
Associate Professor, Department of Medical Psychology and Psychotherapy; Head, Psychotherapeutic C-L Service, University Hospital, Innsbruck, Austria

Jack Spector, Ph.D.
Clinical Associate Professor of Neurology (Psychology), Georgetown University School of Medicine, Washington, D.C.

Barbara Stein, Ph.D.
Head, Psychooncological Liaison Service, Department of Psychosomatic Medicine, University Hospital, Freiburg, Germany

Theodore A. Stern, M.D.
Psychiatrist and Chief, The Avery D. Weisman, M.D., Psychiatry Consultation Service, Massachusetts General Hospital; Associate Professor of Psychiatry, Harvard Medical School, Boston, Massachusetts

Fritz Stiefel, M.D.
Associate Professor, Psychiatry Service, University Hospital, Lausanne, Switzerland

Nada L. Stotland, M.D., M.P.H.
Professor, Departments of Psychiatry and Obstetrics and Gynecology, Rush Medical College, Chicago, Illinois

Alan Stoudemire, M.D.[†]
Professor of Psychiatry, Emory University School of Medicine, Atlanta, Georgia

James J. Strain, M.D.
Professor of Consultation-Liaison Psychiatry and Behavioral Medicine, Mount Sinai School of Medicine; Division of Behavioral Medicine, Mount Sinai–NYU Medical Center and Health Service, New York, New York

Thomas B. Strouse, M.D.
Director of Psychosocial Services, Cedars-Sinai Comprehensive Cancer Center, Los Angeles, California

George E. Tesar, M.D.
Chairman, Department of Psychiatry and Psychology, Cleveland Clinic Foundation, Cleveland, Ohio

Troy L. Thompson II, M.D.
Professor of Psychiatry and Human Behavior, Jefferson Medical College, Philadelphia, Pennsylvania

[†] Deceased.

John G. Tierney, M.D.
Clinical Assistant Professor of Psychiatry, University of Texas Health Science Center in San Antonio, San Antonio, Texas

Paula T. Trzepacz, M.D.
Clinical Professor of Psychiatry and Neurology, University of Mississippi Medical School, Jackson, Mississippi; Adjunct Professor of Psychiatry, Tufts University School of Medicine, Boston, Massachusetts; Medical Director, U.S. Neurosciences, Eli Lilly and Company, Indianapolis, Indiana

Jürgen Unützer, M.D., M.P.H.
Associate Professor of Psychiatry and Biobehavioral Sciences, Center for Health Services Research, UCLA Neuropsychiatric Institute, Los Angeles, California

Robert J. Ursano, M.D.
Professor of Psychiatry and Neuroscience and Chairman, Department of Psychiatry, Uniformed Services University of the Health Sciences, F. Edward Hébert School of Medicine, Bethesda, Maryland

Edward A. Walker, M.D.
Professor and Vice Chair, Department of Psychiatry and Behavioral Sciences, University of Washington, Seattle, Washington

Jeffrey B. Weilburg, M.D.
Assistant Professor of Psychiatry, Harvard Medical School; Associate Psychiatrist, Massachusetts General Hospital, Boston, Massachusetts

David K. Wellisch, Ph.D.
Professor-in-Residence and Chief Psychologist/Adult Division, Department of Psychiatry, UCLA School of Medicine, Los Angeles, California

John W. Winkelman, M.D., Ph.D.
Medical Director, Sleep Health Center, Brigham and Women's Hospital; Assistant Professor of Psychiatry, Harvard Medical School, Boston, Massachusetts

Michael G. Wise, M.D.
Clinical Professor of Psychiatry, University of California, Davis, Sacramento, California; Adjunct Professor of Psychiatry, Uniformed Services University of the Health Sciences, F. Edward Hébert School of Medicine, Bethesda, Maryland

Thomas N. Wise, M.D.
Medical Director, Behavioral Health Services, and Chairman, Department of Psychiatry, Inova Fairfax Hospital, Falls Church, Virginia; Professor and Vice Chair, Department of Psychiatry, Georgetown University School of Medicine, Washington, D.C.

Jonathan L. Worth, M.D.
Director, Adult Outpatient Department, Department of Psychiatry, Massachusetts General Hospital; Instructor in Psychiatry, Harvard Medical School, Boston, Massachusetts

William R. Yates, M.D.
Professor of Psychiatry and Family Medicine, and Chairman, Department of Psychiatry, University of Oklahoma College of Medicine, Tulsa, Oklahoma

Stuart C. Yudofsky, M.D.
D.C. and Irene Ellwood Professor and Chairman, Department of Psychiatry and Behavioral Sciences, Baylor College of Medicine; and Psychiatrist-in-Chief, The Methodist Hospital, Houston, Texas

Paulo R. Zimmermann, M.D.
Adjunct Professor, School of Medicine, PUCRS; Chief of C-L Psychiatry, Hospital São Lucas da PUCRS, Porto Alegre, Brazil

Preface

In 1987 we wrote the first edition of the *Concise Guide to Consultation Psychiatry*, in 1994 the second edition, and in 2000 the third edition. We endeavored to make those books practical and clinically focused. These three *Concise Guides to Consultation Psychiatry* were some of the most popular in the Concise Guide series, finding their way into the lab coat pockets of many psychiatrists, psychiatric fellows and residents, nonpsychiatric physician colleagues, and medical students. Following the success of the first two editions of the *Concise Guide*, American Psychiatric Press (now American Psychiatric Publishing) agreed to publish a comprehensive textbook of consultation-liaison (C-L) psychiatry, employing the practical, clinical approach used in the *Concise Guide*. The first edition of the textbook was published in 1996. This edition, the second, updates material, adds new material, and has two new chapters—Chapter 14, "Epidemiology of Psychiatric Disorders in Medically Ill Patients," and Chapter 41, "Telepsychiatry."

This textbook is a unifying, comprehensive, and practical textbook for clinicians who evaluate and treat medically ill patients who have psychiatric disorders. The demand for such a comprehensive text has increased with efforts to attain added qualification status for the practice of psychiatry in the medically ill. That endeavor must have a textbook that coalesces the body of knowledge essential to the field.

The American Psychiatric Publishing Textbook of Consultation-Liaison Psychiatry: The Practice of Psychiatry in the Medically Ill, Second Edition, brings together clinical and academic leaders in the C-L field to share their knowledge, expertise, and research. More than 100 authors describe in a user-friendly way their clinical experience in the evaluation and treatment of psychiatric disorders in patients who have concomitant medical or surgical illnesses.

The textbook is a primary resource for psychiatrists who perform consultation and liaison work, see patients with concurrent psychiatric and medical-surgical conditions, or use a medical model in their psychiatry practice. It is also designed as a reference book for C-L fellows, psychiatry residents rotating on consultation-liaison services, physicians and professionals in related fields—such as internal medicine, neurology, family practice, neuropsychology, and behavioral health psychology—and medical health and mental health colleagues who have a strong interest in neurobehavioral syndromes that occur in medical and surgical patients.

Psychiatrists who consult on medical-surgical patients with psychiatric symptoms must understand unique aspects of evaluation and treatment performed in a variety of clinical settings. To aid in this process, the textbook is organized into four parts: "General Principles," "Psychiatric Disorders in General Hospital Patients," "Clinical Consultation-Liaison Settings," and "Treatment." We believe that this organization (although it occasionally results in overlap among chapters) provides the best approach for learning about consultation and liaison work. Knowledge about the diagnosis and differential diagnosis of psychiatric disorders, as well as about the context of care delivery, improves the psychiatrist's ability to provide effective recommendations in a language and manner relevant to the clinical setting. For example, a clinician who consults on a disoriented posttransplant patient may refer to chapters on mental status examination, delirium, and transplantation. In addition, the book is applicable to both outpatient and inpatient medical-surgical settings. Psychiatrists working in primary care will find this textbook as useful as psychiatrists consulting on or managing patients in tertiary care subspecialty settings.

We believe that long-established principles of C-L psychiatry hold the key to psychiatrists' continued status as physicians and as a part of the medical field. These principles view the psychiatrist as 1) an expert in the mental status examination, 2) knowledgeable about medical conditions and treatments, 3) able to communicate with other physicians in the vocabulary and metaphors of medicine, 4) skilled at forming a comprehensive biopsychosocial differential diagnosis, 5) comfortable in working with medical-surgical colleagues, 6) skilled in both psychopharmacology and psychotherapy, 7) cost-effective, and 8) able to work in a variety of different and even unique medical and surgical settings.

The second edition of this textbook would not have been completed without the support and efforts of many people. We thank the chapter authors for their outstanding work and scholarly manuscripts and for their patience. We frequently asked authors to add tables where we thought they were appropriate and possible. Although a useful table is not easy to construct, authors produced tables with clinically relevant material that are amenable to copying, putting on note cards, and carrying in lab coat pockets. We thank them.

We also want to express our gratitude to the textbook's editorial board. Members were often asked to review chapters and to provide vision, guidance, and focus. We also want to thank individuals who reviewed chapters but were not part of the editorial board. The outstanding staff at American Psychiatric Publishing also deserve praise for their hard work on this textbook.

A special thanks goes to Tina Coltri-Marshall, who kept us organized and kept track of more than 100 authors. At any point in time, the 46 chapters in this textbook were at different stages of review, rewriting, and editing. She was a patient and persistent organizer of this effort.

Finally, we thank our families for their patience and forbearance during the years of hard work this textbook required. They understood that the textbook was an effort to do the right thing for all the medical and surgical patients we see who experience undiagnosed psychiatric conditions and untreated or inappropriately treated psychiatric illnesses.

Michael G. Wise, M.D.
James R. Rundell, M.D.

Dedication

First and foremost, I dedicate this textbook to my wife of 35 years, Buffie. She has tolerated the hours, days, and weekends necessary for completion of this work. Without her support, this textbook would not exist.

I also dedicate this book to three consultation-liaison psychiatrists. They are no longer living, and all have made lasting contributions to the field. They are Drs. Tom Hackett, Anthony Bouckoms, and Alan Stoudemire. Tom Hackett was an unassumingly brilliant, dedicated, always curious, kind man. Although it has been many years since his death, memories of him and his abilities as a teacher and clinician still set the standard for me. He was the finest physician and mentor I have known. Anthony Bouckoms was a friend, and we went through C-L fellowship together. He died tragically in an accident, along with his son; his wife was seriously injured in the accident and is paraplegic. He amazed me with his skills, kindness, quirkiness, and knowledge. Many of Anthony Bouckoms' contributions to the first edition of this textbook appear in this edition (see Chapter 43). Alan Stoudemire was a hard-working clinical and academic consultation-liaison psychiatrist who loved the field and argued passionately for his views. He made significant contributions to consultation-liaison psychiatry (see Chapter 38) up until the time of his death, despite a long battle with cancer.

Michael G. Wise, M.D.

I would like to dedicate this textbook to the mentors I have had the honor to know over the years: Michael Wise, M.D., the coeditor of this book, George Murray, M.D., Robert Ursano, M.D., Ned Cassem, M.D., and Elder Granger, M.D. All these physicians have one trait in common—they went above and beyond their job descriptions to spend time and energy on a young doctor who didn't quite know what he wanted to do professionally. Without their guidance and investment, I would not ever have reached the point where I could edit a textbook like this. It is their professional and personal caring I try to hold up as an ideal for myself and those around me.

James R. Rundell, M.D.

Introduction

George Henry's paper published by the *American Journal of Psychiatry* in 1929 marks the beginning of consultation-liaison psychiatry as we know it today (Lipowski 1992). From these origins, almost 3,000 American psychiatrists now devote at least 25% of their professional time to consultation-liaison activities (Noyes et al. 1992). The years since that 1929 beginning have provided fertile soil for the intellectual growth of psychosomatic medicine, somatopsychic medicine, the roles of stress in the etiology of disease states, and the beneficial effects of social support systems. These important ideas have found wide support among medical professionals and the general public (Lipowski 1987). As a result, and because of the pioneering work of persons such as Eugene Meyer, George Henry, Helen Flanders Dunbar, and Edward Billings, consultation-liaison psychiatrists have been at the forefront of the progressive incorporation of psychiatry into the mainstream of modern medicine.

Consultation-liaison psychiatry is by no means limited to the United States. Consultation-liaison services are now extant in numerous countries, including Australia, the Middle East, Asia, South America, and Europe (Kurosawa et al. 1993; Smith et al. 1994; also see Chapter 13 in this book). European consultation-liaison psychiatry has developed to include research consortium and biannual meetings with representation from numerous countries (Huyse et al. 2000; also see Chapter 13 in this book).

Consultation-liaison psychiatry is increasingly accepted as an important part of psychiatric education. The American Council on Graduate Medical Education requires clinical experience in consultation-liaison psychiatry for all general psychiatry residents. Standards for consultation-liaison training in general psychiatry residency and also for fellowship training programs have been established (Ford et al. 1994; Gitlin et al. 1996).

The growing body of systematically collected medical-scientific knowledge, as well as the efforts of a number of national leaders, led to the recommendation by the American Psychiatric Association that consultation-liaison psychiatry be formally recognized as a subspecialty of the American Board of Psychiatry and Neurology. The evolution of consultation-liaison psychiatry as a defined and recognized subspecialty has driven an often vigorous debate about the goals and limits of the field of psychiatry (Wise and Ford 1991). There has been, however, a long-standing debate concerning the appropriate name for the subspecialty; the most recently proposed name is *psychiatry for the medically ill*. Irrespective of the ultimate outcome, there is little question that, by whichever name it is called, consultation-liaison psychiatry does meet the criteria for a subspecialty as defined by the American Psychiatric Association (Lipowski 1992). The most clinically relevant of these subspecialty criteria form the four parts of this textbook: clinical skills, a knowledge base about specific medical and psychiatric disorders, defined patient-based clinical settings, and specific treatment modalities.

The specific skills required of the consultation-liaison psychiatrist include 1) the ability to conduct detailed mental status examinations and to interpret findings in conjunction with modern technological tests such as neuroimaging, 2) the capacity to assess the potential for suicidality, aggression, and agitation within a medical-surgical setting, 3) the capacity to apply medical, legal, and ethical principles in the psychiatric management of physically ill patients, and 4) the ability to work with and clearly communicate findings and recommendations to nonpsychiatric physicians, other health care workers, and families. The consultation-liaison psychiatrist must also be knowledgeable about psychiatric and medical comorbidity, the various psychiatric presentations of medical illnesses, and the use of medical symptoms or simulated physical disease to communicate psychosocial distress. In addition, expertise in the diagnosis and management of delirium, dementia, depression, anxiety, and the effects of toxic substances is essential in the medical setting.

The traditional setting for the practice of consultation-liaison psychiatry is the general hospital. Within this medical environment, especially in highly specialized areas such as transplantation, psychiatrists increasingly function as integral parts of medical care teams. As general medicine has become less hospital based and more outpatient oriented, consultation-liaison psychiatrists have also made the shift, and outpatient consultation-liaison services are increasingly common (Epstein et al. 1996; Steinberg et al. 1996).

In the past, the liaison psychiatrist was at times stereotypically depicted as a pleasant, pipe-smoking gentleman wearing a tweed jacket who, with much time on his hands, proselytized for the psychosocial model. Assuming that that was ever an accurate description, it can be confidently said that the stereotype has changed. Present-day consultation-liaison psychiatrists, both men and women, must possess a fund of knowledge about physiological and psychological responses to advanced technologies and high-stress medical settings, the interactions and psychotropic effects of a wide variety of medications, and emotional responses to advanced therapies such as in vitro fertilization and organ transplantation. With effective integration of the consultation-liaison psychiatrist into the treatment team, the components of psychiatric liaison and consultation merge. The results include education of health care personnel about psychological issues, improvements in patient care, and attention to systemic issues that influence the quality of life for both patients and care providers. Each medical care setting has its own micro-ecological characteristics; the consultation-liaison psychiatrist must know how to best meet the needs of specific programs and providers. For example, the characteristics and psychiatric issues of an intensive care unit differ greatly from those of a physical medicine and rehabilitation center.

The value of a psychiatric consultation to the patient, to the physician seeking consultation, or to a system depends on the success of recommendations made. Philosophical formulations, regardless of how accurate, are useless unless they positively influence diagnosis, management, or treatment of the patient. To do this, the consultation-liaison psychiatrist must communicate clearly and know psychiatric medications and their interactions with medications used for medical-surgical illness. This textbook contains a detailed discussion of psychopharmacology. Nonpharmacological interventions are also important. Behavioral techniques, particularly cognitive-behavioral therapy, are invaluable in the treatment of patients with somatization syndromes, including chronic pain. Psychotherapy, particularly that which is focused on acute problems, is an essential treatment for many medically ill patients. Early psychiatric consultation, with diagnosis and treatment of psychiatric comorbidity, not only improves the quality of life for the medical patient but, as research described in this textbook demonstrates, often results in shorter hospitalizations and reduced costs and resource utilization.

This textbook brings together the body of knowledge and skills that defines the subspecialty of consultation-liaison psychiatry. During the past 70-plus years, scientific knowledge about relations between psychological factors and medical illness has greatly advanced. Yet past publications of consultation-liaison pioneers make it obvious that many issues remain remarkably unchanged. Among these issues are the personal motivations and enthusiasm of consultation-liaison psychiatrists, which are qualities possessed by all great clinicians. I believe that most consultation-liaison psychiatrists would endorse the words of orthopedic surgeon Lorin Stephens in an address he made to a graduating medical school class: "to be a physician, to be permitted to be invited by another human being into his life in the circumstances of the crucible which is illness, to be a trusted participant in the highest of dramas, for these privileges I am grateful beyond my ability to express. . . . " (Werner and Korsch 1976, p. 327).

Although later twenty-first-century consultation-liaison psychiatrists (or whatever other term is used for them at that time) will use knowledge and skills that we cannot envision, they must retain a commitment to medical excellence, a respect for patients, and a love of medicine. Consultation-liaison psychiatrists exemplify these qualities and will remain "real doctors" who are participants in the high dramas of birth, illness, and death.

Charles V. Ford, M.D.

REFERENCES

Epstein SA, Gonzales JS, Stockton P, et al: Functioning and well-being of patients in a consultation-liaison psychiatry clinic. Gen Hosp Psychiatry 18: 3–7, 1996

Ford CV, Fawzy FI, Frankel BL, et al: Fellowship training in consultation-liaison psychiatry. Psychosomatics 35:118–124, 1994

Gitlin DF, Schindler BA, Stein TA, et al: Recommended guidelines for consultation-liaison psychiatric training in psychiatry residency programs. Psychosomatics 37:3–11, 1996

Huyse FJ, Herzog T, Lobo A, et al: European consultation-liaison psychiatric services: the ECLW Collaborative Study. Acta Psychiatrica Scand 101:360–366, 2000

Kurosawa H, Iwasaki Y, Watanabe N, et al: The practice of consultation-liaison psychiatry in Japan. Gen Hosp Psychiatry 15:160–165, 1993

Lipowski ZJ: The interface of psychiatry and medicine: toward integrated health care. Can J Psychiatry 32:743–748, 1987

Lipowski ZJ: Consultation-liaison psychiatry at century's end. Psychosomatics 33:128–133, 1992

Noyes R, Wise TN, Hayes JR: Consultation-liaison psychiatrists: how many are there and how are they funded? Psychosomatics 33:123–127, 1992

Smith GC, Ellis PM, Carr VJ, et al: Staffing and funding: consultation-liaison psychiatry services in Australia and New Zealand. Aust N Z J Psychiatry 28:398–404, 1994

Steinberg MD, Cole SA, Saravay SM: Consultation-liaison psychiatry fellowship in primary care. Int J Psychiatry Med 26:135–143, 1996

Werner ER, Korsch BM: The vulnerability of the medical student: posthumous presentation of L. L. Stephens' ideas. Pediatrics 57:321–328, 1976

Wise TN, Ford CV: Subspecialization at the crossroads. Psychosomatics 32:121–123, 1991

General Principles

History of Consultation-Liaison Psychiatry

Zbigniew J. Lipowski, M.D., F.R.C.P.C.[†]

Thomas N. Wise, M.D.

Consultation-liaison psychiatry is a clinical field that has developed over time, and hence one can speak of its history as a train of events involving the development of organizational structures, clinical services, teaching, relevant literature, and specific investigative endeavors. The discipline has developed out of two broad movements, one organizational and the other theoretical. First, its early origins reflect the emergence of general hospital psychiatry. Beginning in the 1920s, general hospitals began to establish psychiatric units that brought psychiatry closer to medicine in clinical activities, research, and education. No longer were psychiatrists isolated in asylum settings, separate from other physicians. Within general hospital settings, they could conveniently see medical and surgical patients in consultation. Second, consultation psychiatry also developed at a time when the concept of psychosomatic relationships was capturing both the public and professional imagination (Alexander 1950). The focus of psychosomatic theories was on the role of emotions and psychological states in the genesis and maintenance of organic diseases. In this context, consultation-liaison psychiatry became an applied form of psychosomatic medicine.

In the United States, the earliest advocate for integration of psychiatry and medicine was Benjamin Rush, a professor of medicine at the University of Pennsylvania and a clinician associated with the Pennsylvania Hospital (Lipowski 1986). He stressed in his lectures the importance of the physician's knowledge of mental functions. He spoke about the knowledge of the human mind and

observed that diseases of the mind are as certainly objects of medicine as those of the body (Rush 1811). In another lecture, he spelled out a unified view of medicine:

> Man is said to be a compound of soul and body. However proper this language may be in religion, it is not so in medicine. He is, in the eye of a physician, a single and indivisible being, for so intimately united are his soul and body, that one cannot be moved without the other. The actions of the former upon the latter are numerous and important. They influence many of the functions of the body in health. They are the causes of many diseases; and if properly directed, they may easily be made to afford many useful remedies. (Rush 1811, p. 256)

Rush's views were typical of many of his contemporaries, who linked emotional events with disease onset and maintenance (Brown 1985). As medicine became more scientifically based, however, the role of psychological factors in medical practice became less an object of study or clinical attention and the two areas drifted apart (Brown 1989). Throughout the nineteenth century, psychiatry was confined to the asylums, whereas medicine became increasingly biomedical in its orientation. Until 1867, no systematic course on mental diseases was given as part of American medical education (Ebaugh 1944). There were isolated calls for integration of medicine and psychiatry (Lipowski 1981). Between 1867 and 1873, several clinics for the treatment of nervous and mental disorders were opened in Philadelphia, New York, St. Louis, and Boston (Hall 1944). Gray (1868), the editor

---

†Deceased.

of the *American Journal of Insanity*, appealed that psychological medicine be made a required part of medical teaching and practice. Other writers called for the establishment of psychiatric wards in general hospitals (Sweeney 1962). The first such ward was organized by George Mosher at the Albany Hospital in Albany, New York, in 1902 (Sweeney 1962). This set the stage for the growth of consultation psychiatry.

Concurrent with the growth of general hospital psychiatry, psychobiological theories espoused by Adolf Meyer (1957) gave a pragmatic underpinning to American psychiatry in contradistinction to the theory-laden approach of European psychiatry. Meyer advocated the study of humans as people who experience health and disease and spoke of the medically useless contrast of mental and physical disorders (Winters 1951). The focus on the scientific study of the person as a unique biological unit capable of symbolization or mentation was the hallmark of psychobiology. His emphasis on understanding each individual in the context of carefully detailed life events (physical, social, or psychological) paralleled the emphasis on medical history in traditional physical diagnosis. Meyer's teachings had a profound impact on all major aspects of American psychiatry. He and other psychobiologists laid the groundwork for the development of general hospital psychiatry and consultation-liaison psychiatry. Meyer trained a group of psychiatrists who were comfortable in general hospital settings and interested in collaboration with other specialists (Rennie 1927). From these psychiatrists arose a cadre of early consultation psychiatrists.

The development and growth of psychoanalysis also fostered an interest in relationships between mind and body. Early psychoanalysts developed theories about such relationships (Deutsch 1948). Franz Alexander and colleagues at the Chicago Psychoanalytic Institute developed theoretical models for unconscious conflicts that appeared to potentiate classic psychosomatic disorders such as peptic ulcer disease, hypertension, and asthma (Alexander 1950). Their theories were based on their psychoanalytic treatment observations. Unfortunately, such work was office based and involved the use of a language that differed from that of their medical colleagues. This further estranged such psychoanalysts from general medicine but at the same time fostered great public interest in the importance of psychological issues in physical illness (Brown 1985).

DEFINITIONS

Consultation-liaison psychiatry is a subspecialty of psychiatry that incorporates clinical service, teaching, and

research at the borderland of psychiatry and medicine (Lipowski 1983). The clinical service includes provision of psychiatric consultations to nonpsychiatrist physicians, as well as ongoing interactions for teaching psychosocial aspects of medical care. The term *liaison* refers to such interactions (Lipowski 1986). The educational function of consultation-liaison psychiatry involves teaching psychiatric and psychosocial aspects of medical care to medical students, residents, and fellows. Finally, research in this context involves matters such as psychosocial reactions to physical illness and injury, psychiatric complications of such illness, abnormal illness behavior, somatoform and factitious disorders, prevalence of psychiatric morbidity in medical settings, and assessment of the effectiveness of consultation-liaison clinical and teaching activities (Lipowski 1986).

This definition outlines the scope of consultation-liaison psychiatry in terms of its functions, areas of work, patient population, and educational and investigative activities (Lipowski 1986). Defining psychosomatic medicine is also useful, because it may be confused with consultation psychiatry. *Psychosomatic medicine* is a discipline concerned with 1) the study of the correlations of psychological and social phenomena with physiological functions (normal or pathological) and the interplay of biological and psychosocial factors in the development, course, and outcome of all diseases and 2) advocacy of a biopsychosocial approach to patient care (Lipowski 1984). However, psychosomatic medicine is not an organized specialty of medical care, whereas consultation psychiatry is such a subspecialty.

HISTORY OF CONSULTATION-LIAISON PSYCHIATRY

The development of general hospital psychiatric units and psychosomatic medicine led to the emergence of consultation-liaison psychiatry. Initially, psychiatrists from freestanding psychiatric hospitals regularly attended outpatient clinics. Thus were forged the early links between general hospitals, such as the Radcliffe Infirmary in Oxford and Massachusetts General Hospital (Mayou 1989; Tillotson 1932). By 1923, general hospital psychiatric units finally began to flourish. In that year, Thomas J. Heldt, M.D. (1927), the director of the Henry Ford Hospital psychiatry department, reported that medical patients were referred for psychiatric consultation. He estimated that about 30% of all hospital admissions were for primary or secondary psychiatric disorders. His estimate was supported by Moersch (1932), who reported on a study of 500 consecutive admissions to the Mayo Clinic in which 40% of patients had some type of psychiatric problem. These two studies highlighted the need for the development of consultation-liaison psychiatry.

A seminal article devoted to consultation-liaison psychiatry was written by George W. Henry (1929–1930), a student of Adolph Meyer. He reflected on his several years of consulting in general hospitals and his experience with medical and surgical patients. He noted that nonpsychiatric physicians tended to request psychiatric consultations only as a last resort, after they were unable to diagnose a physical illness. He observed that the psychiatric consultant often felt insecure in a medical setting and might resort to using professional jargon. He stressed that the consultant must interview every patient in depth, report his or her findings in plain English, and remain close to the facts. He argued that "in no psychiatric work is it so necessary to determine the facts, and the less the psychiatrist is influenced by theories the more accurate are his observations likely to be" (Henry 1929–1930, p. 494). Henry recommended that at least one psychiatrist be available in every general hospital to perform consultations and to participate in medical staff conferences. He also championed the general hospital setting as an arena for teaching medical students psychiatry that they could use during their medical careers.

Henry's was a landmark paper that launched consultation-liaison psychiatry as a distinct area of clinical work and teaching at the borderland between medicine and psychiatry. A few years later, Helen Flanders Dunbar, one of the pioneers of psychosomatic medicine, began to work at the Columbia-Presbyterian Hospital as a psychiatrist on assignment to the department of medicine. She began an ambitious study involving about 600 patients with cardiovascular diseases, diabetes, or fractures, and in 1936, she and her co-workers reported their findings (Dunbar et al. 1936). They concluded that psychological factors appeared to influence both the etiology and the course of the illnesses in a substantial proportion of these patients. Dunbar and her colleagues predicted that before long, psychiatrists would be required to work on all medical and surgical wards, as well as in medical and surgical clinics. This prediction has never been fulfilled.

There are three phases in the history of consultation-liaison psychiatry: 1) the organizational phase, 2) the conceptual-development phase, and 3) the rapid-growth phase (Lipowski 1986).

Organizational Phase: Circa 1935–1960

The chief features of the organizational phase included the formation of consultation-liaison services, develop-ment of modes of operation, evaluation of consultation-liaison activities, and expansion of teaching (Lipowski 1986).

A major event in the early history of consultation-liaison psychiatry was the provision of grants in 1934–1935 by the Rockefeller Foundation to five general hospitals to establish psychiatric divisions and to stimulate closer collaboration between psychiatrists and other physicians (Billings 1966). One of the hospitals to receive a grant was the Colorado Hospital in Denver. Edward G. Billings was appointed director of that division and reported on its activities between 1936 and 1942 (Billings 1936, 1939, 1941). The psychiatric division in Denver had no beds; it consisted entirely of a consultation-liaison service that was called the "psychiatric liaison department" (Billings 1966). In this department, the main activities involved providing consultations to all hospital wards, teaching psychiatry and psychosocial aspects of medicine to medical students and interns, and performing collaborative research. Billings considered the main goals of the department to include the integration of the principles of psychobiology and psychiatry with those of general medicine and the sensitization of physicians and trainees to the psychosocial aspects of medical practice. Billings was the first writer to use the term *liaison psychiatry* (Billings 1939). He asserted that "the integration of the principles of psychiatry with those of the other branches of medicine reduces diagnostic and therapeutic floundering, shortens the hospital stay for the patient and thereby saves the hospital, patient, and community money" (Billings 1941, p. 34).

There is no doubt that the model of consultation-liaison psychiatry provided by Billings is still valid. This model included clinical service, teaching, and research. The consultation-liaison service at the Mount Sinai Hospital in New York City, which was organized in 1939, was based on a different model (Kubie 1944). Kaufman expanded the Mount Sinai service in 1946, and he and his colleagues reported on it in several seminal papers (Bernstein and Kaufman 1962; Kaufman 1953, 1957; Kaufman and Margolin 1948). All these authors maintained that a liaison psychiatrist should play a key role in the development of collaboration between the psychiatric unit and the rest of the hospital. To this end, Kaufman drew on the large cadre of practicing psychiatrists in Manhattan, who volunteered their services to teach and do consultations on Mount Sinai's medical wards. This service also benefited the psychiatrists who got to know the nonpsychiatric physicians. Kaufman's approach infused the hospital with psychiatric personnel and thereby increased the psychiatric knowledge base and options for clinical care.

A different model of a consultation-liaison service was established at the University of Rochester Medical School in 1946. It was called the "medical liaison group" (Engel et al. 1957). A department of psychiatry was organized in Rochester by John Romano in 1946, and liaison services were directed by George Engel, an internist with psychoanalytic training. Similar projects were organized by Romano at the University of Cincinnati College of Medicine and by Franz Reichsman, an internist, at the Downstate Medical Center in Brooklyn, New York. Both consultation-liaison services were staffed by physicians who were trained as internists and subsequently received psychological training (Engel et al. 1957). Education (i.e., promotion of knowledge of psychosocial aspects of health and disease) was the main objective. In each of these institutions, liaison fellows taught physical diagnosis and interviewing within the department of medicine and were viewed as not purely psychiatric educators. These liaison services generally depended on the beneficence of the department of medicine. When such unique leaders as Engel and Reichsman retired, the services disbanded and more typical psychiatric consultation groups took their place. Thus, the Rochester-Downstate model of liaison differed from that described by Strain and Grossman (1975) in that the latter was a purely psychiatric endeavor, to teach nonpsychiatric physicians the biopsychosocial model, whereas the former involved a staff primarily of internists within a division of internal medicine.

Between 1935 and 1960, consultation-liaison services were established in many American teaching hospitals (Greenhill 1977). As was described earlier in this chapter, more than one organizational model could be identified in those early years of consultation-liaison psychiatry. In some consultation-liaison services, the focus was on consultations (i.e., clinical service), whereas in others, the importance of liaison was emphasized. Which model was followed depended largely on the preference of the service's leader. This issue was discussed in detail by Greenhill (1977).

During this time, some writers on consultation-liaison psychiatry stressed the role of the consultation-liaison psychiatrist as a therapist, an issue that was conspicuously absent in early writings. Grinker (1952) and Bibring (1956) offered practical suggestions regarding how consultation-liaison psychiatrists could apply psychotherapy in their work. Bibring (1956) provided a description of several personality profiles that tended to influence a patient's reaction to illness and behavior. She argued persuasively that evaluation of patient personality should be part of medical management in every case and should influence the manner of therapeutic intervention.

From the beginning of consultation-liaison psychiatry, the teaching of psychosocial and psychiatric aspects of medical care was one of the main tasks of consultation-liaison psychiatrists. Ebaugh and Rymer, in a book published in 1942, addressed this issue in some detail. They pointed out that psychiatric liaison teaching was "one of the most valuable means of emphasizing the total aspect of the patient and of breaking down the barriers between psychiatry and other clinical subjects" (Ebaugh and Rymer, p. 229).

By 1960, consultation-liaison programs had been organized in the majority of teaching hospitals in the United States, but fellowship training in consultation-liaison psychiatry was offered in only a few centers. The literature on consultation-liaison psychiatry was sparse, and the term *liaison psychiatry* was hardly a household word. During the 1960s, the community mental health movement was dominant; psychiatry drifted away from medicine once more. That climate was rather unfavorable for consultation-liaison psychiatry, which entered the second phase—that of consolidation and conceptual development.

Conceptual-Development Phase: Circa 1960–1975

As the number of consultation-liaison services grew, more attention was paid to their methods of operation, particularly strategies and procedures used to attain specific objectives. The process and conduct of psychiatric consultation in a medical setting became a major focus. The five models for consultation that were proposed are described in Table 1–1.

TABLE 1–1.   Models for consultation

1. *Patient-oriented* consultation included not only a diagnostic interview and assessment but also a psychodynamic evaluation of the patient's personality and reaction to illness (Lipowski 1967).
2. *Crisis-oriented, therapeutic* consultation involved a rapid assessment of the patient's problems and coping style, as well as incisive therapeutic intervention by the consultant (Weisman and Hackett 1960); this model was inspired by Lindemann's crisis theory (Satin 1982).
3. *Consultee-oriented* consultation focused on the consultee's problem with a given patient (Schiff and Pilot 1959).
4. *Situation-oriented* consultation was concerned with the interaction between the patient and the clinical team (Greenberg 1960).
5. *Expanded psychiatric* consultation involved the patient as a central figure in an operational group that included the patient, the clinical staff, other patients, and the patient's family (E. Meyer and Mendelson 1961).

All the relevant articles during the phase of conceptual development were published between 1959 and 1964, and in them was underscored the multifaceted and interactional character of psychiatric consultations to medicine and surgery. Moreover, the communications aspects, as well as the distinct phases of the consultation process, became the primary concern of a number of writers. These new approaches to consultation went far beyond a traditional medical model, which consisted only of diagnostic assessment and advice on management of the patient (Lipowski 1967).

Another feature of this phase was the focus on specific problems encountered by consultants in a variety of specialized clinical settings, such as intensive care, oncology, hemodialysis, cardiac rehabilitation, and pediatric units (Lipowski 1986). This development paralleled the marked development of medical technology and the increase in emotionally arduous requirements of medical care that taxed the emotional equilibrium of patients. Consultation-liaison psychiatrists developed special interests in and initiated research projects on psychosocial and psychiatric problems found in these specialized areas of health care. Examples of the writings on those subjects include the work of Levy (1974) in psychonephrology, of Cassem and Hackett (1971) in coronary care units, and of Titchener and Levine (1960) in surgery.

Still another important feature of this phase of conceptual development was the growth of relevant literature. Before the mid-1960s, no book or comprehensive review on consultation-liaison psychiatry had been published. In this second phase, the literature became enriched by three books (Pasnau 1975; Schwab 1968; Strain and Grossman 1975) and two overviews (Lipowski 1967, 1974). Journals in the field flourished. *Psychosomatic Medicine* published papers on consultation psychiatry, as well as on more basic research topics germane to psychosomatic theory. *Psychosomatics*, founded in 1959, focused on clinical issues. The *Journal of Psychosomatic Research* featured contributions from England as well as North America, whereas *Psychotherapy and Psychosomatics* drew authors from continental Europe and elsewhere. *Psychiatry in Medicine*, which was largely devoted to consultation-liaison psychiatry, began publication in 1970, under the editorship of D. R. Lipsitt, M.D. *General Hospital Psychiatry*, which also focused on consultation-liaison topics, was established in 1979 under the aegis of Lipsitt.

A number of other important publications during this phase include a discussion of consultation-liaison teaching (McKegney 1972), a survey of education in consultation-liaison psychiatry in American medical schools (Mendel 1966), a survey of referral patterns for consultation (Kligerman and McKegney 1971), and observations on countertransference problems of consultation-liaison psychiatrists (Mendelson and Meyer 1961). Furthermore, several books dealt with psychosocial and psychiatric aspects of medicine and thus expanded the knowledge base of consultation-liaison psychiatry (Lief et al. 1963; Lipowski 1972; Zinberg 1964).

Organizations devoted to consultation-liaison psychiatry were established. The American Psychosomatic Society, founded in 1939, included many consultation psychiatrists in its membership, and consultation-liaison topics were frequently discussed at its meetings. Started in 1955, the Academy of Psychosomatic Medicine has established itself as the national organization of the subspecialty; full membership is limited to psychiatrists, and the focus of its annual meeting is on emerging research within the consultation-liaison field.

Consultation-liaison psychiatry became a recognized subspecialty of psychiatry, and thus proper training of its practitioners was called for. However, serious financial obstacles hindered the further development of consultation-liaison psychiatry during the 1960s, when the major influence of community psychiatry caused psychiatry and medicine to drift apart. This gap was firmly established when the requirement for the medical internship was abolished and psychiatric residents could train without any significant postgraduate experience in a medical setting.

Rapid-Growth Phase: 1975–1980s

In 1974, the Psychiatry Education Branch of the National Institute of Mental Health (NIMH) decided to support the development and expansion of consultation-liaison services throughout the United States (Eaton et al. 1977). The director of the branch was James Eaton, M.D., who had led the consultation service at the department of psychiatry of Tulane University. Eaton recognized the need for better integration of psychiatry into medicine and took the opportunity to launch this initiative. This decision was based on the assumption that the focus of health care delivery should be on primary care; it was clear that psychosocial and psychiatric problems were an important aspect of primary practice. It followed that primary care physicians needed proper training to deal effectively with such problems, and consultation-liaison psychiatrists were the most appropriate teachers. In 1975, NIMH provided grants for 31 consultation-liaison programs (Eaton et al. 1977). In 1979–1980, it supported 130 programs and awarded 60 stipends, for a total of $5.3 million (A. S. Abraham, personal communication, September 20, 1979). The stipends led to the establishment of fellowships in consultation-liaison psychiatry, and by 1980, more than 300 fellows had received financial support. However, budgetary cuts during the 1980s resulted in a dramatic decrease in the number of stipends awarded. It was hoped that institutions might continue these fellowships, but this did not always happen. Interestingly, the residency programs again required each of their trainees to spend a postgraduate year in a medical setting. Several books (Faguet et al. 1978; Glickman 1980; Lewis and Levy 1982; Lipowski 1985) and reviews (Greenhill 1977; Lipowski 1983; Psychiatry Update 1984) on consultation-liaison psychiatry were published. In 1984, the American Hospital Association reported that 869 hospitals had consultation-liaison services (J. Stewart, personal communication, November 4, 1985).

Apart from government grants, several other factors between 1975 and 1985 contributed to the rapid growth of consultation-liaison psychiatry. As more sophisticated medical treatments prolonged the lives of individuals whose conditions had previously been considered terminal, quality of life became an important focus. Biomedical researchers needed to collaborate with psychiatrists when conducting clinical studies of cancer, cardiovascular disease, and other serious disorders. The number of general hospital psychiatric units continued to grow: there were 1,358 in 1984. Primary care expanded as planned, and consultation-liaison psychiatrists were considered well suited to teach primary care physicians. In behavioral medicine, treatments for chronic pain states and techniques for improving compliance were developed, based largely on learning theory; both have augmented the consultation psychiatrist's armamentarium. As the field grew, differences of opinion emerged about the primary goal of its endeavors (Pasnau 1988). In the consultation model, psychiatrists taught psychiatry by being role models of active, useful clinicians, whereas liaison psychiatry was more directly didactic (Hackett 1982; Strain 1983). Debates were held at national meetings in an attempt to resolve these issues (Pasnau et al. 1986). Financial difficulties helped resolve the problem, because liaison psychiatry was difficult to fund. Consultation programs predominated, and liaison activities were important training elements for both psychiatrists and other specialists. Finally, the growth of consultation-liaison research enhanced the prestige of consultation-liaison psychiatry.

AREAS OF CONSULTATION-LIAISON RESEARCH

Research at the interface of medicine and psychiatry is one of the main tasks of consultation-liaison psychiatrists

(Wise 1995). Early research consisted primarily of case reports, with observations framed in psychoanalytic theory. This form of research was followed by case series and the development of experimental models in patient populations with homogeneous disease states. Animal research also made important basic contributions, demonstrating psychosocial variables that affect disease states (Weiner 1996). Such research developed slowly at first but expanded considerably in the 1990s. The first Consultation-Liaison Research Forum took place in New York on May 12, 1990, and abstracts of the presented papers were published (Strain and Holland 1991). The range of the presented studies was quite remarkable. Referring to the forum, Pasnau (1990) observed that the opportunities for consultation-liaison research in the 1990s were enormous. Consultation-liaison research has grown considerably in both quantity and scope in recent years. Three reviews of consultation-liaison research have been published (Cohen-Cole et al. 1986; McKegney and Beckhardt 1982; Wise 1995).

Two main areas of contemporary research by consultation-liaison psychiatrists may be distinguished: 1) evaluative studies of consultation-liaison work and 2) studies of a wide range of clinical problems at the interface of medicine and psychiatry (Lipowski 1983). Evaluative research includes topics such as patterns of referral for psychiatric consultation in various types of medical settings; demographic, diagnostic, and other characteristics of the referred patients; modes of intervention by consultation-liaison psychiatrists; and outcomes of consultations (McKegney and Beckhardt 1982). Outcome studies comprise issues such as the cost-effectiveness of consultation-liaison psychiatry and consultation-liaison intervention (Lyons et al. 1985; Strain et al. 1991), the impact of liaison work on the rate of referrals and on attitudes toward psychiatry (Schubert et al. 1989), the degree of physicians' compliance with consultants' recommendations (Mackenzie et al. 1983), and patients' perceptions of psychiatric consultations (Wise et al. 1985).

Clinical research at the interface of psychiatry and medicine covers a wide range of subjects (Lipowski 1983). Investigations in this area are influenced by the nature of the patient populations to which consultation-liaison psychiatrists have direct access, as well as by the types of clinical settings in which they work. The clinical setting may be a coronary care unit, an oncology hospital, a neurological division, or a primary care setting. The two main patient groups with whom consultation-liaison psychiatrists have direct contact include patients with physical illness and patients with somatizing disorders who use somatic symptoms to enter the health care setting. A particularly important area of research is that of the prevalence of comorbidity among hospitalized medical patients. Cavanaugh (1983) reported that only about one-third of 335 randomly selected medical inpatients showed no evidence of emotional or cognitive dysfunction. Psychiatric disorders were relatively mild and transient in this patient population, yet in some of the patients, these disorders were chronic, severe, and associated with a poor prognosis for the comorbid medical condition (Dvoredsky and Cooley 1986). Moreover, patients with comorbidity often had prolonged hospital stays, and hence their psychological dysfunction contributed to the higher cost of hospitalization (Fulop et al. 1989). As an aside, a survey of 327 hospitals found that only 0.9% of medical patients are referred for psychiatric consultation (Wallen et al. 1987). A much higher percentage of patients should be referred to reduce their suffering and to reduce the cost of hospitalization.

Other areas of consultation-liaison research include psychosocial reactions to and psychiatric complications of a wide range of physical illnesses and injuries and medical treatments; somatization; and the effectiveness of psychological and psychopharmacological therapies for medical problems (Lipowski 1983, 1985). Somatization is an important subject because of its high prevalence and cost (Barsky and Klerman 1983; Kellner 1985; Lipowski 1988). Consultation-liaison psychiatrists are strategically placed to diagnose and treat somatization in medical patients.

It is beyond the scope of this chapter to review the various aspects of consultation-liaison research involving psychosocial reactions to and psychiatric complications of physical illnesses. An area of major importance is oncology, in which consultation-liaison psychiatrists are considerably involved (Massie and Holland 1987; McCartney et al. 1985; Redd et al. 1991). One of the more common reasons for referral of a patient to consultation-liaison psychiatry is delirium. This common complication of a variety of physical illnesses and their treatments was neglected by researchers for decades, but its growing incidence in elderly medically ill patients has stimulated research more recently (Lipowski 1990; Miller and Lipowski 1991). Consultation psychiatrists are also leading the way toward a better understanding of the ethics of new medical technologies. A final area of consultation research is transplantation psychiatric research. Issues such as the selection of proper organ recipients and reactions to various immunosuppressants make this a growing area for clinical practice and research.

FUTURE TRENDS IN CONSULTATION-LIAISON PSYCHIATRY

Several issues face consultation-liaison psychiatry in the near future. First, the time has come for it to be formally recognized as a subspecialty of psychiatry (Lipowski 1992; Wise and Ford 1991). Such recognition would strengthen the teaching of the subject and the training of consultation-liaison psychiatrists. Formal designation of added qualifications by the American Board of Psychiatry and Neurology would allow the acquisition of much-needed federal educational stipends for consultation fellowships. Second, given the high prevalence of psychiatric disorders in primary care (Schulberg and Burns 1988), it is clear that consultation-liaison psychiatry needs to extend its services to primary care physicians and to be actively involved in their training. Third, the aging of the population and the growing proportion of elderly patients admitted to medical and surgical services calls for a close collaboration between consultation-liaison psychiatrists and gerontologists (Lipowski 1991). About one-third of medical patients referred for psychiatric consultation are age 65 years and older. Depression, dementia, and delirium predominate among those patients and are the main reasons for their referral to consultation-liaison psychiatrists. Fourth, consultation-liaison research is growing and has become increasingly diversified and methodologically sophisticated. Studies evaluating the effectiveness of consultation-liaison work should have high priority.

In summary, consultation-liaison psychiatry has grown considerably during the past 60 years, especially in the last two decades. It has become an integral part of psychosomatic medicine and general hospital psychiatry and represents the application of the biopsychosocial model to medical practice (Engel 1977). It is in the interest of patients that it continue to grow in all of its aspects.

REFERENCES

Alexander F: Psychosomatic Medicine. New York, Norton, 1950

Barsky AJ, Klerman GL: Overview: hypochondriasis, bodily complaints, and somatic styles. Am J Psychiatry 140:273–283, 1983

Bernstein S, Kaufman MR: The psychiatrist in a general hospital. Journal of Mount Sinai Hospital 29:385–394, 1962

Bibring GL: Psychiatry and medical practice in a general hospital. N Engl J Med 254:366–372, 1956

Billings EG: Teaching psychiatry in the medical school general hospital. JAMA 107:635–639, 1936

Billings EG: Liaison psychiatry and intern instruction. Journal of the Association of American Medical Colleges 14:375–385, 1939

Billings EG: Value of psychiatry to the general hospital. Hospitals 15:30–34, 1941

Billings EG: The psychiatric liaison department of the University of Colorado Medical School and Hospitals. Am J Psychiatry 122 (suppl):28–33, 1966

Brown TM: Descartes, dualism and psychosomatic medicine, in The Anatomy of Madness: Essays in the History of Psychiatry, Vol 1. Edited by Bynum WF, Porter R, Shepard M. London, Tavistock, 1985, pp 40–62

Brown TM: Cartesian dualism and psychosomatics. Psychosomatics 30:322–331, 1989

Cassem NH, Hackett TP: Psychiatric consultation in a coronary care unit. Ann Intern Med 75:9–14, 1971

Cavanaugh S: The prevalence of emotional and cognitive dysfunction in a general medical population: using the MMSE, GHQ, and BDI. Gen Hosp Psychiatry 5:15–24, 1983

Cohen-Cole SA, Pincas HA, Stoudemire A, et al: Recent research developments in consultation-liaison psychiatry. Gen Hosp Psychiatry 8:316–329, 1986

Deutsch F: The psychosomatic concept. Acta Medica Orient 10:67–86, 1948

Dunbar FH, Wolfe TP, Rioch JM: Psychiatric aspects of medical problems. Am J Psychiatry 93:649–679, 1936

Dvoredsky AE, Cooley HW: Comparative severity of illness in patients with combined medical and psychiatric diagnoses. Psychosomatics 27:625–630, 1986

Eaton JS Jr, Goldberg R, Rosinski E, et al: The educational challenge of consultation-liaison psychiatry. Am J Psychiatry 134 (suppl):20–23, 1977

Ebaugh FG: The history of psychiatric education in the United States from 1844 to 1944. Am J Psychiatry 100:151–160, 1944

Ebaugh FG, Rymer CA: Psychiatry in Medical Education. New York, Commonwealth Fund, 1942

Engel GL: The need for a new medical model: a challenge for biomedicine. Science 196:129–136, 1977

Engel GL, Greene WA, Reichsman F, et al: A graduate and undergraduate teaching program on the psychological aspects of medicine. Journal of Medical Education 32:859–870, 1957

Faguet RA, Fawzy FL, Wellisch DK, et al (eds): Contemporary Models in Liaison Psychiatry. New York, SP Medical & Scientific Books, 1978

Fulop G, Strain JJ, Fahs MC, et al: Medical disorders associated with psychiatric comorbidity and prolonged hospital stay. Hosp Community Psychiatry 40:80–82, 1989

Glickman LS: Psychiatric Consultation in the General Hospital. New York, Marcel Dekker, 1980

Gray JP: Insanity and its relations to medicine. American Journal of Insanity 25:145–172, 1868

Greenberg IM: Approaches to psychiatric consultation in a research hospital setting. Arch Gen Psychiatry 3:691–697, 1960

Greenhill MH: The development of liaison programs, in Psychiatric Medicine. Edited by Usdin G. New York, Brunner/Mazel, 1977, pp 115–191

Grinker RR: Psychotherapy in medical and surgical hospitals. Diseases of the Nervous System 13:269–273, 1952

Hackett TP: Consultation psychiatry held valid, liaison held invalid. Clinical Psychiatry News, January 1982, p 36

Hall JK (ed): One Hundred Years of American Psychiatry. New York, Columbia University Press, 1944

Heldt TJ: Functioning of a division of psychiatry in a general hospital. Am J Psychiatry 84:459–476, 1927

Henry GW: Some modern aspects of psychiatry in general hospital practice. Am J Psychiatry 86:481–499, 1929–1930

Kaufman MR: The role of the psychiatrist in a general hospital. Psychiatr Q 27:367–381, 1953

Kaufman MR: A psychiatric unit in a general hospital. Journal of Mount Sinai Hospital 29:385–394, 1957

Kaufman MR, Margolin SG: Theory and practice of psychosomatic medicine in a general hospital. Med Clin North Am 32:611–616, 1948

Kellner R: Functional somatic symptoms and hypochondriasis. Arch Gen Psychiatry 42:821–833, 1985

Kligerman MJ, McKegney FP: Patterns of psychiatric consultation in two general hospitals. Psychiatr Med 6:126–132, 1971

Kubie LS: The organization of a psychiatric service for a general hospital. Psychosom Med 6:252–272, 1944

Levy NB (ed): Living or Dying: Adaptation to Hemodialysis. Springfield, IL, Charles C Thomas, 1974

Lewis A, Levy J: Psychiatric Liaison Nursing. Reston, VA, Reston Publishers, 1982

Lief HI, Lief VF, Lief NR (eds): The Psychological Basis of Medical Practice. New York, Harper & Row, 1963

Lipowski ZJ: Review of consultation psychiatry and psychosomatic medicine, 1: general principles. Psychosom Med 29:153–171, 1967

Lipowski ZJ (ed): Psychosocial Aspects of Physical Illness. Basel, Karger, 1972

Lipowski ZJ: Consultation-liaison psychiatry: an overview. Am J Psychiatry 131:623–630, 1974

Lipowski ZJ: Holistic-medical foundations of American psychiatry: a bicentennial. Am J Psychiatry 138:888–895, 1981

Lipowski ZJ: Current trends in consultation-liaison psychiatry. Can J Psychiatry 28:329–338, 1983

Lipowski ZJ: What does the word "psychosomatic" really mean? A historical and semantic inquiry. Psychosom Med 46:153–171, 1984

Lipowski ZJ: Psychosomatic Medicine and Liaison Psychiatry: Selected Papers. New York, Plenum, 1985

Lipowski ZJ: Consultation-liaison psychiatry: the first half century. Gen Hosp Psychiatry 8:305–315, 1986

Lipowski ZJ: Somatization: the concept and its clinical application. Am J Psychiatry 145:1358–1368, 1988

Lipowski ZJ: Delirium: Acute Confusional States. New York, Oxford University Press, 1990

Lipowski ZJ: Consultation-liaison psychiatry 1990. Psychother Psychosom 55:62–68, 1991

Lipowski ZJ: Consultation-liaison psychiatry at century's end. Psychosomatics 33:128–133, 1992

Lyons JS, Hammer JS, Wise TN, et al: Consultation-liaison psychiatry and cost-effectiveness research. Gen Hosp Psychiatry 7:302–308, 1985

Mackenzie TB, Popkin MK, Callies AG, et al: Consultation outcomes. Arch Gen Psychiatry 40:1211–1214, 1983

Massie MJ, Holland JC: Consultation and liaison issues in cancer care. Psychiatr Med 5:343–359, 1987

Mayou R: The history of general hospital psychiatry. Br J Psychiatry 155:764–776, 1989

McCartney CF, Evans DL, Richardson W: Library collection of the psychosocial publications in consultation-liaison psychiatry. Gen Hosp Psychiatry 7:73–82, 1985

McKegney FP: Consultation-liaison teaching of psychosomatic medicine: opportunities and obstacles. J Nerv Ment Dis 154:198–205, 1972

McKegney FP, Beckhardt RM: Evaluative research in consultation-liaison psychiatry. Gen Hosp Psychiatry 4:197–218, 1982

Mendel WM: Psychiatric consultation education: 1966. Am J Psychiatry 123:150–155, 1966

Mendelson M, Meyer E: Countertransference problems of the liaison psychiatrist. Psychosom Med 23:115–122, 1961

Meyer A: Psychobiology: A Science of Man. Springfield, IL, Charles C Thomas, 1957

Meyer E, Mendelson M: Psychiatric consultations with patients on medical and surgical wards: patterns and processes. Psychiatry 24:197–220, 1961

Miller NE, Lipowski ZJ (eds): Advancing age and the syndrome of delirium; ancient conondrums and modern research advances. Int Psychogeriatr 3:103–113, 1991

Moersch FP: Psychiatry in medicine. Am J Psychiatry 11:831–843, 1932

Pasnau RO (ed): Consultation-Liaison Psychiatry. New York, Grune & Stratton, 1975

Pasnau RO: Consultation-liaison psychiatry: progress, problems, and prospects. Psychosomatics 29:4–15, 1988

Pasnau RO: Opportunities for consultation-liaison research in the 1990s (comment). Gen Hosp Psychiatry 12:353–354, 1990

Pasnau RO, Hackett TP, Wise TN, et al: Resolved: liaison psychiatry's relationship with the other medical specialties. In Continuing Medical Educations Syllabus, annual meeting of the American Psychiatric Association, Washington, DC, May 1986

Psychiatry Update: The American Psychiatric Association Annual Review, Vol 3. Edited by Grinspoon L. Washington, DC, American Psychiatric Press, 1984

Redd WH, Silberfarb PM, Andersen BL, et al: Physiologic and psychobehavioral research in oncology. Cancer 67:813–822, 1991

Rennie TAC: Psychiatric service to a general hospital. N Engl J Med 217:346–351, 1927

Rush B: Sixteen Introductory Lectures. Philadelphia, PA, Bradford & Innskeep, 1811

Satin DG: Erich Lindemann: the humanist and the era of community mental health. Proceedings of the American Philosophical Society 126:229–248, 1982

Schiff SK, Pilot ML: An approach to psychiatric consultation in the general hospital. Arch Gen Psychiatry 1:349–357, 1959

Schubert DSP, Billowitz A, Gabinet L, et al: Effect of liaison psychiatry on attitudes toward psychiatry, rate of consultation, and psychosocial documentation. Gen Hosp Psychiatry 11:77–87, 1989

Schulberg HC, Burns BJ: Mental disorders in primary care: epidemiologic, diagnostic, and treatment research directions. Gen Hosp Psychiatry 10:79–87, 1988

Schwab JJ: Handbook of Psychiatric Consultation. New York, Appleton-Century-Crofts, 1968

Strain JJ: Liaison psychiatry and its dilemmas. Gen Hospital Psychiatry 5:209–212, 1983

Strain JJ, Grossman S: Psychological Care of the Medically Ill: A Primer in Liaison Psychiatry. New York, Appleton-Century-Crofts, 1975

Strain JJ, Holland JCB: Abstracts from the First Consultation-Liaison Research Forum. Gen Hosp Psychiatry 13:359–384, 1991

Strain JJ, Lyons JS, Hammer JS, et al: Cost offset from a psychiatric consultation-liaison intervention with elderly hip fracture patients. Am J Psychiatry 148:1044–1049, 1991

Sweeney GH: Pioneering general hospital psychiatry. Psychiatr Q 36 (suppl):209–268, 1962

Tillotson KJ: Comments on Dr. Moersch's paper. Am J Psychiatry 5:841–842, 1932

Titchener JL, Levine M: Surgery as a Human Experience. New York, Oxford University Press, 1960

Wallen J, Pincus HA, Goldman HH, et al: Psychiatric consultations in short term general hospitals. Arch Gen Psychiatry 44:163–168, 1987

Weiner H: Use of animal models in peptic ulcer disease. Psychom Med

Weisman AD, Hackett TP: Organization and function of a psychiatric consultation service. International Record of Medicine 173:306–311, 1960

Winters EE (ed): The Collected Papers of Adolf Meyer, Vol 3. Baltimore, MD, Johns Hopkins University Press, 1951

Wise TN: Consultation-liaison research: the use of different perspectives. Psychother Psychosom 63:9–21, 1995

Wise TN, Ford CV: Subspecialization at the crossroads. Psychosomatics 32:121–123, 1991

Wise TN, Mann LS, Dove HW, et al: Patients' perceptions of psychiatric consultations. Compr Psychiatry 26:554–557, 1985

Zinberg N (ed): Psychiatry and Medical Practice in a General Hospital. New York, International Universities Press, 1964

2

Consultation, Liaison, and Administration of a Consultation-Liaison Psychiatry Service

Elisabeth J. Shakin Kunkel, M.D.

Daniel A. Monti, M.D.

Troy L. Thompson II, M.D.

In this chapter we outline key factors contributing to the effectiveness of psychiatric consultants to medical and surgical units and clinics. We then address the organizational elements necessary for the day-to-day functioning and subsequent expansion of a consultation-liaison psychiatry service.

THE PSYCHIATRIC CONSULTANT

Qualities of an Effective and Competent Psychiatric Consultant

Good consultation and liaison psychiatry practice begins with the acquisition of basic psychiatric and medical-surgical knowledge and skills. The basic body of knowledge and skills needed for performing consultation and liaison activities includes an understanding of psychopathology, psychiatric differential diagnosis, psychotherapy (psychodynamic, cognitive, and behavioral), administrative management of systems problems, medical economics, geriatrics, and forensics. Some knowledge of how such psychiatric comorbidity varies and interplays with differ-

ent illnesses, ages, socioeconomic statuses, and other factors also is important for consultation-liaison psychiatrists.

Although a large number of psychiatrists perform psychiatric consultations as part of their clinical practices, there is a wide range of expertise at different levels of education and clinical experience (e.g., resident, fellow, and faculty levels) (Bronheim et al. 1998). The need for qualified psychiatric consultants is highlighted by the significant underdetection of major psychiatric illness in patients in primary care settings (Cole et al. 1998; D. Goldberg et al. 1982; Strain et al. 1991). By effectively treating psychiatric disorders in medical patients, consultation-liaison psychiatry consultants improve compliance, shorten lengths of stay, and reduce use of medical resources (Fulop et al. 1998; Saravay and Lavin 1994; Strain et al. 1994).

An effective psychiatric consultant comprehensively reviews the patient's clinical data to make a reasonable differential diagnosis and treatment recommendations (Stotland and Garrick 1990). Detailed psychodynamic formulations with psychiatric jargon usually are not useful to the consulting physician. Rather, a concise impression with standard psychiatric diagnoses and clear treat-

The authors appreciate the technical assistance of Edwina Benson in the preparation of this manuscript.

ment recommendations is most useful. Availability, flexibility, clarity of thought, and a natural curiosity about new phenomena enhance the consultation process (see Table 2–1) (Pasnau 1985; M. G. Wise and Rundell 1994). The consultant should be willing to tap outside resources when confronted with clinical problems beyond his or her scope of knowledge and abilities.

What Other Physicians Expect

Consulting physicians expect the consultant to help clarify the diagnosis, treat the symptoms, and assist the medical and surgical staff in treating the patient, with the consultant sometimes assuming some or all responsibility for the patient. The priorities of the consulting service will vary (Karasu et al. 1977), so it is important that the consultant assess the specific needs of the consulting service. For example, a surgeon who wants to know whether his or her patient can provide informed consent for an operation is often not particularly interested in the psychological aspects of the surgical problem. Tailoring one's consultations to the needs of the referring service helps increase the number of referrals (Schubert et al. 1989). For all physicians, the most important aspect of the psy-

chiatric consultation is dealing with patient disposition problems (e.g., transferring a patient to the psychiatry ward or making outpatient psychiatric referrals) (Cohen-Cole and Friedman 1982).

APPROACH TO THE CONSULTATION

Examination Style

There has been much debate about the best way to conduct a psychiatric examination of the medical or surgical patient. Although a psychodynamic understanding of the patient's personality, especially an understanding of the meaning that illness and hospitalization have for the patient, is often quite helpful, psychoanalytic techniques, such as lengthy free associations and silence, are rarely appropriate with the consultation patient. Most of these patients have had no experience with psychiatry or psychotherapy, many are psychologically regressed in the context of the patient experience and usually did not request psychiatric consultations. Some have cognitive impairments that would interfere with this approach.

TABLE 2–1. Characteristics of an effective psychiatric consultant

1. Talks with the referring physician, nursing staff, and other staff (e.g., social workers) before and after the consultation. Clarifies the reason for the consultation.
2. Establishes urgency—emergent, urgent, or routine.
3. Reviews the chart and data thoroughly and collects new information as needed.
4. Performs a complete mental status examination, obtains relevant history, and performs relevant portions of a physical examination.
5. Talks with the patient's family and friends as indicated.
6. Makes notes as brief as appropriate (i.e., no need to repeat in full detail the data already recorded in the chart).
7. Arrives at a tentative diagnosis based on signs, symptoms, laboratory values, and epidemiology.
8. Formulates a differential diagnosis among medical, neurological, and psychiatric disorders.
9. Recommends diagnostically helpful radiological and laboratory tests.
10. Has the knowledge to prescribe psychotropic drugs in patients with medical and surgical conditions and is aware of interactions with nonpsychotropic medications.
11. Makes treatment recommendations: medications, electroconvulsive therapy, psychotherapy, and elimination of possible medical or iatrogenic cause of the symptoms.
12. Is specific (i.e., brief and goal oriented). Provides contingency plans and anticipates potential problems. Makes direct personal contact—especially if recommendations are crucial or potentially controversial. Does not take over the patient's care, and teaches with tact (cites references, uses personal communication).
13. Conducts appropriate patient education and psychotherapy, when indicated.
14. Follows the patient during the entire hospitalization.
15. Makes appropriate postdischarge recommendations, including outpatient care. Helps arrange postdischarge referrals.
16. Follows advances in other medical fields and is not isolated from the rest of the medical community.

Source. Adapted from Goldman L, Lee T, Rudd P: "Ten Commandments for Effective Consultation." *Archives of Internal Medicine* 143:1753-1755, 1983. Copyright 1983, American Medical Association. Used with permission. Subsequently reprinted and adapted from Wise MG, Rundell JR: *Concise Guide to Consultation Psychiatry*, 2nd Edition. Washington, DC, American Psychiatric Press, 1994. Used with permission.

Maintaining absolute doctor-patient confidentiality is not possible for a psychiatric consultant, because the patient's primary doctor expects an answer from the consultant. In addition, it is sometimes necessary to speak with family members or friends to make a full assessment. This process should be clarified for the patient (e.g., "I will be providing a summary of my findings and recommendations to your doctor" and "It would be helpful for me to talk with your wife to get her perspective"). If the patient wants to tell the consultant a "secret," the consultant should explain that sharing the "secret" with the patient's physician may improve the physician's understanding of the patient's perspective and may result in better medical care. This approach decreases the possibility of patient-related splitting in the treatment team.

It is important to obtain a thorough history and perform a complete mental status examination, because the data gained serve as the basis for developing an accurate differential diagnosis and treatment plan. Obtaining this information is best accomplished by establishing rapport with the patient as quickly as possible. Some guidelines for setting the stage for a meaningful interaction follow.

1. Greet the patient in a friendly and genuine manner, making a caring gesture such as shaking the patient's hand or adjusting a pillow. If there is a personal item, such as a photo or a book, in the patient's room, comment on it in a complimentary or interested way. Such warmth makes the patient feel cared for.
2. Put the patient at ease by sitting down and not appearing rushed. A patient is not going to attribute interest and concern to a doctor who looks anxious to leave.
3. Maintain good eye contact and lean slightly toward the patient. While interviewing, do not write intensely or spend an excessive amount of time looking through the patient's records or laboratory reports; you will be better able to remember key points and gain valuable information by observing the patient's reactions during the interview.

To establish an alliance with the patient, the consultant should open with statements that help ease the patient's discomfort, such as "Being in the hospital is distressing for anyone. It is bad enough to be sick, but to also have to be in a strange place with unfamiliar people all around can be very difficult. How has it been for you?" Using a combination of open-ended questions (e.g., "Would you tell me more about that?") and close-ended questions (e.g., "What is your job?") will be the most effective. In general, it is best to proceed from more open-ended to more focused questions during the interview. Formulations should be translated into jargon-free impressions and recommendations in the written report and in discussions with the consulting physician and staff. A concise, well-written report usually improves the team's understanding of the patient. A DSM-IV-TR diagnosis, including Axes I–V, is often necessary for reimbursement purposes.

Tools of the Trade

The psychiatric consultant uses information from his or her fund of knowledge, the hospital chart and old records, the medical-surgical staff, the examination of the patient and/or the patient's family, and various reference sources. The patient's medical records and findings from the examination are summarized in the initial consultation note (see Table 2–2). In an academic setting, the physician needs to document that he or she has personally interviewed the patient and reviewed the history (including the past medical history), family history, and social history with the resident. All consultation-liaison psychiatrists need to be familiar with Medicare documentation guidelines, to assure ongoing compliance and to maximize service revenues (Kunkel et al. 1999; Worley et al. 1998).

Medical students and residents often find that learning consultation-liaison psychiatry is easier if they initially use a standardized assessment format. Bedside examination can include clock drawing or drawing of another figure, a Mini-Mental State Exam (MMSE) (Folstein et al. 1975), the Taylor Equivalent Drawing (Nelson et al. 1986), and other neuropsychological tools (M. G. Wise and Rundell 1994; see also Chapter 7, this volume). Biological, psychotherapeutic, psychosocial, and systems interventions are all used by practicing consultation-liaison psychiatrists (Fulop and Strain 1991; Huyse et al. 1988, 1990).

The Process of the Consultation

An initial visit by a psychiatrist may be quite frightening to many patients. Their defenses, including denial, minimization, and being on their best behavior, may color the psychiatric consultant's initial impressions. Therefore, the "real" reason for the consultation may not be apparent to the consulting psychiatrist on the first visit; repeated visits are often necessary to better understand the factors that triggered the initial consultation. Follow-up visits also allow the patient and his or her family and friends to become more comfortable with the psychiatrist; this facilitates a positive, therapeutic alliance.

Table 2–2.   Elements of the initial consultation note

1. **Date** and **time** of visit—write *psychiatry* at the top
2. Name of **doctor** who requested consultation and the ***reason*** for the request
3. Summary of the patient's **medical history** relevant to the current psychiatric situation; do not just duplicate the medical record and problem list
4. **Present psychiatric symptoms** (or events leading up to psychiatric consultation)
5. **Psychiatric history**—be specific about medication and other treatment effects and adverse reactions
6. **Family psychiatric history** (including drug/alcohol use)—family members with same illnesses/problems as patient's; medication and other treatment responses in family members
7. **Social history**—work and school history, sexual history, drug and alcohol use history, legal history, social supports, current living arrangements
8. **Past medical history**
9. **Review of systems**
10. Complete **mental status examination**—appearance; behavior; speech; affect/mood; thought process/form; thought content (suicidal, homicidal, delusions, hallucinations); orientation; memory, concentration, attention, and other cognitive tests; language; fund of knowledge; insight; judgment
11. **Current medications**—review hospital medication records as well as doctors' orders
12. Recent and pertinent **tests and procedures**—e.g., laboratory studies, roentgenography, computed tomography, magnetic resonance imaging, electrocardiography, electroencephalography
13. Pertinent aspects of the **physical examination**—e.g., vital signs, neurological examination findings, abnormal movements
14. **Impression**—Use DSM-IV (American Psychiatric Association 1994) diagnosis and readily understandable terminology; avoid psychiatric jargon and psychodynamic formulations
15. **Recommendations**—be clear and concise; list medications exactly as you wish them given; include suicide precautions, recommendations for restraints or other consultations, and so on; medication recommendations made by M.D.'s only
16. All notes from consultations and follow-up written with **discretion**—keep in mind that medical-surgical charts frequently are read by hospital staff and sometimes by patients and their families
17. Date of next **follow-up** visit and planned frequency of visits
18. Signed and printed **consultant's name,** along with telephone and/or beeper number

Source. Adapted from Cohen-Cole 1988; Garrick and Stotland 1982; Stotland and Garrick 1990.

Psychiatric consultations may be precipitated when the consulting physician and staff are unable to establish trusting doctor-patient and staff-patient relationships or when the consulting physician feels uncomfortable or unqualified to manage particular patients' problems. With this in mind, the psychiatric consultant should avoid asking overly confrontational questions. (For example, the consultant should not ask the patient, "Why aren't you cooperating with your medical team?" nor should he or she ask the consulting physician, "Why did you tell the patient that he had to have this test or you wouldn't help him anymore?") Such tactics only worsen the situation. In addition, the consulting physician and staff are often concerned that the consultant will be critical of them for overlooking something "obvious." When making suggestions to the consulting team for improving their relationship with their patient, the consultant should communicate in a supportive, nonaccusatory manner. He or she must strive to establish a trusting doctor-patient relationship. The consultant can address issues that stem from problems in the doctor-patient and staff-patient relationships more directly during subsequent visits, when the highly emotional states that may have triggered the consultation request have diminished or passed.

As the process of the consultation continues through repeated follow-up visits, the consultation-liaison psychiatrist conducts more interviews and gathers more data from the patient, the patient's family and friends, the consulting physician, nursing staff, social workers, and other health care professionals. The psychiatrist must tailor his or her discussions with each of these individuals and groups so that they understand the evolving clinical situation. Systems interventions should occur in the consulting health care unit (e.g., a joint discussion with the psychiatrist, consulting physician, nurses, and social worker about how to provide structure, set consistent limits, and decrease staff splitting in difficult patients).

Follow-up visits allow the psychiatrist to observe the patient's mental status over time and to establish the patient's premorbid mental status based on information from the patient, family, and friends. Follow-up visits are also necessary to monitor the dosages, effects, and side effects of psychopharmacological drugs that are recommended. Especially in medically and surgically ill patients, who are almost always taking other medications, several visits and laboratory monitoring are often required to achieve optimal therapeutic drug levels and effects. The consultant must minimize potential side effects, which often lead to noncompliance.

T. N. Wise et al. (1987) suggested that concordance with consultant suggestions regarding diagnostic tests and medications is increased if the consultant, with the sanction of the patient's attending physician, personally writes the order. However, many consultation-liaison psychiatrists believe that this approach is problematic. The consultant must ensure that his or her orders are not medically contraindicated and do not conflict with orders written by the primary physician. Consultants who choose to write such orders may increase their own liability. Also, once a consultant writes an order, he or she is considered a treating physician by insurance companies, and evaluation and management codes for psychiatric consultation cannot be used on billing forms. Finally, hospital policy at some facilities prohibits consultants from writing orders.

Psychiatric consultants should generally follow patients until they are discharged. One reason for doing so is that urges to "sign off" on patients are frequently more related to negative or overly positive reactions toward patients than to permanent resolution of the presenting symptoms. A second reason is that patients who have neuropsychiatric signs and symptoms are at risk for recurrence of such syndromes. Finally, persistent follow-up helps to instill confidence in the consultation-liaison psychiatrist and reinforces that the psychiatrist is always available and willing to help in any clinical situation.

ORGANIZATIONAL STRUCTURE OF A CONSULTATION-LIAISON SERVICE

General Administrative Concerns

Consultation-liaison program directors often acquire the administrative skills required to organize a consultation-liaison psychiatry service by trial and error and on-the-job training. In a survey of general psychiatry residency programs, 30.5% of programs did not provide formal education in administrative psychiatry (Arnold et al. 1991). The new consultation-liaison psychiatrist who must establish or modify a consultation-liaison service should conduct advance investigation and planning about the specific hospital and clinic environment. A consultation-liaison psychiatrist must learn as much as possible about the need and potential resources for establishing the new

consultation-liaison service (Holtz 1992). This means selecting which services to target (e.g., services for inpatient versus outpatient populations, oncology, trauma, transplantation, obstetrics); obtaining annual statistics for the hospital and specific services; meeting potential faculty, fellows, and staff; and assessing the availability of resources at the targeted locale and comparing numbers of local staff with national staffing averages (see Table 2–3) (Hammer et al. 1985; Noyes et al. 1992). By focusing on the most cost-effective and needed clinical efforts, the consultation-liaison psychiatrist can provide care commensurate with resources and then expand the services into other general and focused areas of need and interest. In addition, the modern consultation-liaison psychiatry service director must familiarize himself or herself with regional billing practices, reimbursement issues, and strategic planning (Goldberg 2001) to increase service revenues in times of lower reimbursements (Hall and Frankel 1996; Kunkel et al. 1999; Worley et al. 1998).

TABLE 2–3. Information needed to establish or enhance a consultation-liaison service

Where to establish the service(s)
General medical and surgical hospitals
Specialized inpatient facilities and units, such as
    Oncology
    Rehabilitation
    Pain
    Dialysis
    Burns
    Transplantation
    Acquired immunodeficiency syndrome
    Neuropsychiatry
    Obstetrics and gynecology
    Pediatrics
Outpatient clinics and specialized centers, as above
Demographics of the site
Centralized versus scattered beds
Medical-surgical and psychiatric admissions in recent years
    Total population
    Population of specific diagnoses
Psychiatric consultations in recent years
    Total population
    Population of specific diagnoses
Psychiatry inpatient and outpatient resources
Financial resources and payer mix of locale, institution, and specialized units
Staffing and available personnel in related disciplines (e.g., social work)
Number of transfers to inpatient psychiatry units or outpatient psychiatric clinics

General Medical-Surgical Hospitals With Teaching Programs

It is important for a new consultation-liaison psychiatrist to make courtesy visits to key hospital personnel after obtaining the essential information described in the previous section. These visits increase the visibility of the service, allow the consultation-liaison psychiatrist to identify potential problems, and communicate a willingness to consider the concerns of nonpsychiatric departments in providing services for their patients. The consultant should visit important personnel early on and periodically reconsult with them to assess how the service is progressing. Courtesy visits should include visits to the chairpersons and residency directors of medicine, surgery, and any other departments or subspecialty programs that request consultations from the consultation-liaison psychiatry service. In addition, visits to the directors of nursing, social work, pastoral care, volunteer services, and security may be advantageous when problems arise. Such courtesy calls also may allow the consultation-liaison psychiatrist to identify other personnel (and/or other services) with useful interests and qualifications who can support and extend the resources of the service.

Medical Students

Personnel on the consultation-liaison service have defined needs. Third- and fourth-year medical students often complete a portion of their psychiatry clerkships on the consultation-liaison service. They need to integrate their knowledge of normal human development, ethics, interviewing, and basic psychopathology with the new skills and knowledge required of a consultant. Under supervision, they should refine their interviewing skills, learn the techniques of performing a good mental status examination, and come to understand some aspects of psychopathology and the psychological problems of medically and surgically ill patients (Stoudemire 1990). In general, most medical students enjoy the consultation-liaison portion of their psychiatry clerkships and can gradually take on increased responsibility for patients if the consultation-liaison psychiatry portion is integrated into the clinical teaching process (Engel 1978; Orleans et al. 1981). The Health Care Financing Administration (HCFA) has strict limitations on which parts of the history students are allowed to document. Students can document the past medical history, personal/social history, past psychiatric history, and review of systems (Chappelle et al. 200; Kunkel et al. 1999; Worley et al. 1998). In addition, exposure to consultation-liaison psychiatry may be a useful recruiting strategy for psychiatry residency programs; many medical students with potential interests in psychiatry are interested in how medical-surgical specialties interface with psychiatry.

Residents

Psychiatric residents must acquire knowledge of the consultation process, the biopsychosocial model, specific clinical syndromes, and available treatments (Cohen-Cole et al. 1982; Gallagher et al. 1990). They must also gain or extend their confidence in working with and around medically ill patients and with other medical specialties. Educational programs must address issues in psychopathology, forensics, and biological and nonbiological interventions and must also address how to deal with nonpsychiatric physicians and staff in the general hospital (Cassem 1991; Frankel et al. 1986; Perry and Viederman 1981; M. G. Wise and Rundell 1994). The program director should be aware of the Academy of Psychosomatic Medicine guidelines for consultation-liaison psychiatry training, which were published in 1996 (Gitlin et al. 1996), as well as earlier National Institute of Mental Health training objectives (Saravay et al. 1984).

The Accreditation Council for Graduate Medical Education makes both general and specific references to consultation-liaison psychiatry in their special requirements for residency training in psychiatry. In the first postgraduate year, the trainee is expected to acquire the medical skills necessary to make diagnoses in, treat, and refer patients with medical and surgical disorders; to become familiar with medical disorders that present with psychiatric symptoms and psychiatric disorders that present with medical symptoms; and to be cognizant of the interaction between psychiatric treatments and medical or surgical treatments. In postgraduate years 2–4, knowledge, skills, and clinical experience must be expanded. Knowledge requirements include the diagnosis and treatment of many specific neurological disorders and diseases. The resident is expected to be skilled in psychiatric consultation on both the medical and surgical units; the resident's clinical experience must include at least 2 months of supervision on the diagnosis and management of medical and neurological problems germane to psychiatric practice, general consultation-liaison psychiatry, and acute and chronic drug and alcohol problems (Accreditation Council for Graduate Medical Education 1993–1994, 1998).

Fellows

Consultation-liaison fellows must further refine, expand, and focus the consultation-liaison skills and knowledge acquired during residency education. Fellows often deal with more complicated clinical, legal, and administrative problems. Ideally, a consultation-liaison fellowship also provides an opportunity to specialize in one or more specific clinical areas of interest (Table 2–4). The emphasis on clinical care versus research and service responsibilities versus academic productivity varies substantially among current consultation-liaison fellowship programs in the United States. Specialized experience with one consultation-liaison psychiatry subspecialty (e.g., pain) often serves as a training model that allows the fellow then to generalize his or her skills, training, and knowledge to more varied and more general consultation-liaison psychiatry activities (Table 2–5) (Stoudemire and Fogel 1987, 1991, 1993).

According to a national survey of 45 consultation-liaison psychiatry programs, most fellowships involve training of one or two half- or full-time fellows for 1 or 2 years. Teaching and supervision (e.g., conferences and rounds) consume 2–20 hours per week. Fellows typically supervise both psychiatry residents and medical students on the service. In only 29% of clinical consultation-liaison fellowships is completion of a specific research project required, but in 90% of such fellowships, completion of some type of academic project is mandated (Academy of Psychosomatic Medicine 1992; Ford et al. 1994). Fellowships may be funded directly by hospitals, or through Medicare or grants (Magen and Banazek 1995).

TABLE 2–4. Specialized consultation-liaison psychiatry fellowships and liaison opportunities within general consultation-liaison programs

Acquired immunodeficiency syndrome
Burns
Cardiology
Consultation-liaison psychiatry service administration
Dermatology
Dialysis
Ethics
Hematology
Intensive care
Medical economics
Neuropsychiatry
Obstetrics and gynecology
Oncology
Pain
Pediatrics
Pulmonary
Rehabilitation
Research projects and fellowships
Spinal cord injury
Transplantation
Traumatic brain injury
Other clinical programs

Source. Adapted from Academy of Psychosomatic Medicine 1992.

TABLE 2–5. Suggested curriculum topics for consultation-liaison psychiatry fellows

1. Psychopharmacology and pharmacokinetics for patients with concurrent medical-surgical illness and/or pregnancy
2. Psychiatric symptoms caused by nonpsychiatric pharmacological agents (e.g., depression caused by β-blockers)
3. Psychiatric manifestations of diseases (e.g., pancreatic cancer and depression)
4. Diagnosis and treatment of depression and anxiety in medically ill patients
5. Psychiatric syndromes associated with high-stress procedures (e.g., cardiac transplantation)
6. Characteristics of the somatoform and factitious disorders
7. Techniques of consultation that emphasize different models of consultation and mechanisms by which to communicate findings
8. Sex-specific disorders, including syndromes and disorders related to menstruation, pregnancy, menopause, and sexual dysfunction
9. Behavioral modification and psychotherapeutic techniques for the medically ill
10. Legal principles related to issues such as the right to refuse treatment, decision-making capacity, and living wills
11. Knowledge concerning major ethical issues in medicine such as abortion, euthanasia, and genetic counseling
12. The sociology of the medical system and general hospital
13. A history and past research findings of psychosomatic medicine and psychophysiology
14. Current research topics and techniques in consultation-liaison psychiatry
15. Knowledge of consultation-liaison administration, which includes such issues as quality assurance, insurance billing, hospital procedures manuals, and medical and legal issues
16. Conducting outpatient consultation-liaison clinical activities with other medical and surgical services

Source. Adapted from Ford CV, Fawzy FI, Frankel BL, et al: "Fellowship Training in Consultation-Liaison Psychiatry: Education Goals and Standards." *Psychosomatics* 35:118–124, 1994. Copyright 1992, Academy of Psychosomatic Medicine. Used with permission.

Other Staff

Nonpsychiatric house staff and attending physicians often appreciate lectures, discussions, and consultation-liaison rounds that focus on a variety of topics (Table 2–6). They interact with the consultation-liaison psychiatrists during psychiatric consultations, during liaison activities, and during the portion of their educations on the consultation psychiatry service (Fuller et al. 1980).

A consultation-liaison service may also have social workers, nurse specialists, clinical psychologists, and other nonphysicians as part of the staff. Such personnel come from diverse backgrounds and bring their own educational perspectives and orientations to their work (R. J. Goldberg et al. 1984). Nurse specialists, for example, may have more training than most psychiatrists in teaching relaxation techniques, leading patient education groups, and teaching patients and the lay population about preventive measures or improving compliance. Although nonphysician personnel are often helpful in solidifying liaison relationships and extending physician services, it is important to supplement their skills and knowledge regarding medical problems and the biopsychosocial model, usually by direct supervision during psychiatric consultations and follow-up.

Group Practice

A consultation-liaison psychiatrist may function as part of a multidisciplinary group (e.g., a pain center) or may share a clinical practice with other consultation-liaison psychiatrists (Schwab 1968). In a pain center, expertise from neurology, neurosurgery, rehabilitation medicine, anesthesiology, psychiatry, physical therapy, and other disciplines may be consolidated to evaluate and treat patients. A consultation-liaison psychiatrist must not only provide useful consultation but also be ready to serve as a liaison for staff stress management and education and as a public relations representative for the importance and relevance of psychiatry.

Consultation-liaison psychiatrists in a group practice can provide night and weekend coverage for one another and can consolidate their subspecialty expertise to provide a wider spectrum of consultations (e.g., regarding palliative care and transplantation). Establishing outpatient consultation-liaison clinics allows the consultation-liaison psychiatrist to provide continuity of care and follow-up for problems initially identified in the hospital (Wolcott et al. 1984). These clinics sometimes also provide service to patients treated in outpatient and day-hospital settings.

TABLE 2–6. Potential topics for consultation-liaison psychiatry teaching programs to nonpsychiatric physicians (e.g., family practice residents)

Making appropriate psychiatric consultations and referrals

Improving identification of anxiety and depression in patients with physical problems

Early identification of organic mental syndromes, especially those of mild to moderate severity

Psychiatric and psychological symptoms and syndromes frequently associated with various diseases (e.g., cancer) and various treatment modalities (e.g., radiation therapy)

Pain management

Somatizing patients

Medication issues (e.g., psychiatric symptoms produced by nonpsychotropic medications; drug-drug interactions; modifications of psychotropic drug use in medical illnesses)

Discussions with patients and families about do-not-resuscitate (DNR) orders

Death and dying issues

Conferences, lectures, and support groups for the management of stress and burnout in caregivers

Competency assessment and other medicolegal issues

Private Practice

Psychiatrists in private practice who have consultation-liaison psychiatry interests must maintain their visibility among nonpsychiatric colleagues while providing timely and practical advice for their patients. Relationships with both psychiatric and nonpsychiatric physicians are reinforced by the solo psychiatrist's being available for emergencies and pressing problems throughout the patient's hospitalization, by his or her providing straightforward written and oral feedback to the consulting physician, and by his or her becoming familiar with referring physicians at their professional and hospital meetings and at social gatherings.

Liaison With Other Specialties

Providing good consultations to other physicians is only the beginning of establishing solid liaison relationships (Gomez 1987). The psychiatric consultant must develop expertise and experience in the problems germane to the specific liaison service. Attempting to integrate one's psychiatric services and teaching into the day-to-day routine of a medical or surgical service is usually challenging and tests one's skills and commitment (see also Chapter 4; Gise et al. 1978; Kates et al. 1992).

KEYS TO ESTABLISHING A SUCCESSFUL CONSULTATION-LIAISON SERVICE

The effective psychiatric consultant uses clinical, educational, administrative, financial, scholarly, and research knowledge and skills to establish and expand a successful consultation-liaison service (Table 2–7) (Cohen-Cole et al. 1986; Dimsdale 1991; Hall and Frankel 1996; Lipowski 1974). The relative priorities of these tasks vary according to the setting of the consultation-liaison service. For example, in an academic setting, virtually all of the previously mentioned skills are necessary elements for success; the consultation-liaison faculty member must juggle multiple competing responsibilities to excel. Good communication, conscientious follow-up during hospitalization, practical recommendations, and outpatient follow-up, when indicated, are fundamental elements in expanding one's referral base from other services and practitioners (Strain et al. 1990; Thompson et al. 1990).

Appropriate psychiatric consultation, liaison, and follow-up visits will improve the quality of care of many medical and surgical patients with psychiatric comorbidity. With increased physician understanding of the role of psychiatric comorbidity, the patient's hospital course will be smoother, more effective, and often shorter. Improved recognition of psychiatric conditions by nonpsychiatric physicians and other health care professionals will lead to more psychiatric consultations and increased opportunities for effective psychiatric interventions. The psychiatric consultant who sees all referred patients promptly, follows patients throughout their hospital stays, arranges for outpatient psychiatric follow-up, and provides succinct, practical, and diplomatic recommendations will be busy and well respected in the general hospital.

POSSIBLE SUBSPECIALIZATION

Many consultation-liaison psychiatrists believe that criteria for added-qualifications status for consultation-liaison psychiatry have been met. Several journals and textbooks focus on consultation-liaison psychiatry. This body of scientific knowledge is large and rapidly expanding as procedures and technologies are developed or become refined in the complex care of medical and surgical patients. There are many fellowship training programs in consultation-liaison psychiatry, and many members of

TABLE 2–7. Keys to establishing a successful consultation-liaison service

1. Prompt response to consultation requests
2. Useful evaluations and practical recommendations
3. Effective communication (written and oral) with consulting physicians and others involved in the patient's care
4. Available and reliable follow-up care during hospitalization
5. Arrangement of outpatient referrals after discharge
6. Establishment of effective teaching and education programs, including concise and relevant written handouts, clinical supervision, and formal and informal lectures
7. Public relations efforts directed toward relevant services and institutions, as well as marketing to other physicians and health care organizations to increase the referral base of the service
8. Acquisition of administrative/decision-making roles with high involvement and visibility within the general hospital (e.g., ethics, medical staff, pharmacy and therapeutics, student curriculum, promotions committee assignments)
9. Working with the business office and administrative staff to maximize economic viability
10. Professional dress (e.g., wearing white coats in clinical settings)
11. Establishing rotations for residents, fellows, and medical students from other disciplines, which helps to establish and expand the consultation-liaison service and improve its credibility[a]
12. Academic productivity (e.g., research publications, presentations at regional and national meetings) to stimulate intellectual growth and academic advancement and to increase the regional, national, and international visibility as well as prestige of the service and institution[a]
13. Networking, collaboration, and solicitation of funds (grantsmanship) for expansion of the consultation-liaison service, related research, and educational endeavors[a]

[a]Primarily for academic consultation-liaison services.

the American Psychiatric Association believe that the field of consultation-liaison psychiatry meets the criteria for a certificate of added qualifications. The existence of many advantages suggests that medical students, residents, psychiatrists, and other medical specialists and health care personnel involved in the field should continue their attempts to make consultation-liaison psychiatry a well-organized and recognized added-qualifications subspecialty (Thompson 1993). Starting in 1999, the academy of Psychosomatic Medicine spearheaded a task force to pursue the issue of added qualifications. In 2001, the APA's joint reference committee recommended that the APA Board of Trustees approve this application for added qualifications (C. Lyketsos, personal communication, 2001).

REFERENCES

Academy of Psychosomatic Medicine: Directory of U.S. Consultation-Liaison Fellowship Training Programs. Chicago, IL, Academy of Psychosomatic Medicine, 1992

Accreditation Council for Graduate Medical Education: Special requirements for residency training in psychiatry, in Graduate Medical Education Directory 1993–1994. Essentials and Information Items From Graduate Medical Education Directory 1993–1994. Chicago, IL, American Medical Association, 1993–1994, pp 121–126

Accreditation Council for Graduate Medical Education: Program requirements for residency training in psychiatry. Chicago, IL, Residency Review Committee for Psychiatry, 1998

American Psychiatric Association: Diagnostic and Statistical Manual of Mental Disorders, 4th Edition. Washington, DC, American Psychiatric Association, 1994

Arnold W, Rodenhauser P, Greenblatt M: Residency education in administrative psychiatry: a national survey. Academic Psychiatry 15:188–194, 1991

Bronheim HE, Fulop G, Kunkel EJ, et al: The Academy of Psychosomatic Medicine practice guidelines for psychiatric consultation in the general medical setting. Psychosomatics 39:S8–S30, 1998

Cassem NH (ed): Massachusetts General Hospital Handbook of General Hospital Psychiatry, 3rd Edition. St. Louis, MO, Mosby Year–Book, 1991

Chappelle KG, Blanchard SH, Ramirez-Williams MF, et al: Medical students and Health Care Financing Administration documentation guidelines. Fam Med 32(8):459–461, 2000

Cohen-Cole SA: Consultation psychiatry: a practical guide, in Psychiatry, Vol 2. Edited by Michels R, Cavenar JO, Cooper AM, et al. Philadelphia, PA, JB Lippincott, 1988, pp 1–9

Cohen-Cole SA, Friedman CP: Attitudes of non-psychiatric physicians toward psychiatric consultation. Hosp Community Psychiatry 33:1002–1005, 1982

Cohen-Cole SA, Haggerty J, Raft D: Objectives for residents in consultation psychiatry: recommendations of a task force. Psychosomatics 23:699–702, 1982

Cohen-Cole SA, Pincus HA, Stoudemire A, et al: Recent research developments in consultation-liaison psychiatry. Gen Hosp Psychiatry 8:316–329, 1986

Cole S, Saravay S, Hall R, et al: Mental Disorders in General Medical Practice: Adding Value to Healthcare Through Consultation-Liaison Psychiatry. (Task Force on Healthcare Value Enhancement, Academy of Psychosomatic Medicine.) Dubuque, IA, Kendall/Hunt Publishing, 1998

Dimsdale JE: Challenges, problems and opportunities in consultation-liaison psychiatry research. Psychiatr Med 9:641–648, 1991

Engel GL: The biopsychosocial model and the education of health professionals. Ann N Y Acad Sci 310:169–181, 1978

Folstein MF, Folstein SE, McHugh PR: Mini-Mental State: a practical method for grading the cognitive state of patients for the clinician. J Psychiatr Res 12:189–198, 1975

Ford CV, Fawzy FI, Frankel BL, et al: Fellowship training in consultation-liaison psychiatry: education goals and standards. Psychosomatics 35:118–124, 1994

Frankel BL, Cohen-Cole SA, Milne J, et al: A pilot program for assigned reading by residents in consultation psychiatry. Psychosomatics 27:644–653, 1986

Fuller WC, Roberts CM, Gulledge AD, et al: Liaison psychiatry: approach to curriculum development. Journal of Psychiatric Education 4:14–24, 1980

Fulop G, Strain JJ: Diagnosis and treatment of psychiatric disorders in medically ill inpatients. Hosp Community Psychiatry 42:389–394, 1991

Fulop G, Strain JJ, Fahs MC, et al: A prospective study of the impact of psychiatric comorbidity on length of hospital stays of elderly medical-surgical inpatients. Psychosomatics 39:273–280, 1998

Gallagher RM, McCann WJ, Jerman A, et al: The behavioral medicine service: an administrative model for biopsychosocial medical care, teaching, and research. Gen Hosp Psychiatry 12:283–295, 1990

Garrick TR, Stotland NL: How to write a psychiatric consultation. Am J Psychiatry 139:849–855, 1982

Gise LH, Strain JJ, Manne S, et al: An instrument for evaluating liaison teaching in the primary care setting. Journal of Psychiatric Education 2:215–221, 1978

Gitlin DF, Schindler BA, Stern TA, et al: Recommended guidelines for consultation-liaison psychiatric training in psychiatry residency programs. A report from the Academy of Psychosomatic Medicine Task Force on Psychiatric Resident Training in Consultation-Liaison Psychiatry. Psychosomatics 37:3–11, 1996

Goldberg D, Steele JJ, Johnson A, et al: Ability of primary care physicians to make accurate ratings of psychiatric symptoms. Arch Gen Psychiatry 39:829–833, 1982

Goldberg RJ: financial management challenges for general hospital psychiatry 2001. Gen Hosp Psychiatry 23:67–72, 2001

Goldberg RJ, Tull R, Sullivan N, et al: Defining discipline roles in consultation psychiatry: the multidisciplinary team approach to psychosocial oncology. Gen Hosp Psychiatry 6:17–23, 1984

Goldman L, Lee T, Rudd P: Ten commandments for effective consultation. Arch Intern Med 143:1753–1755, 1983

Gomez J: Liaison Psychiatry: Mental Health Problems in the General Hospital. New York, Free Press, 1987

Hall RCW, Frankel BL: The value of consultation-liaison interventions to the general hospital. Psychiatr Serv 47:418–420, 1996

Hammer JS, Lyons JS, Bellina BA, et al: Toward the integration of psychosocial services in the general hospital. Gen Hosp Psychiatry 7:189–194, 1985

Holtz JL: Making a consultation service work: an organizational commentary. Psychosomatics 33:324–328, 1992

Huyse FJ, Strain JJ, Hengeveld MW, et al: Interventions in consultation-liaison psychiatry: the development of a schema and a checklist for operationalized interventions. Gen Hosp Psychiatry 10:88–101, 1988

Huyse FJ, Strain DG, Hammer JS: Interventions in consultation-liaison psychiatry, part I: patterns of recommendations. Gen Hosp Psychiatry 12:213–220, 1990

Karasu TB, Plutchik R, Conte H, et al: What do physicians want from a psychiatric consultation service? Compr Psychiatry 18:73–81, 1977

Kates N, Craven M, Webb S, et al: Case reviews in the family physician's office. Can J Psychiatry 37:2–6, 1992

Kunkel EJS, Worley LL, Monti DA, et al: Follow-up consultation documentation and billing. Gen Hosp Psychiatry 21:197–208, 1999

Lipowski ZJ: Consultation-liaison psychiatry: an overview. Am J Psychiatry 131:623–630, 1974

Magen JG, Banazek DA: Graduate medical education financing in psychiatry. Academic Psychiatry 19:6–11, 1995

Nelson A, Fogel BS, Faust D: Bedside cognitive screening instruments: a critical assessment. J Nerv Ment Dis 174:73–83, 1986

Noyes R, Wise TN, Hayes JR: Consultation-liaison psychiatrists: how many are there and how are they funded? Psychosomatics 33:123–127, 1992

Orleans CS, Houpt JL, Larson DB, et al: Traditional vs. consultation-liaison psychiatry clerkships: a closer look. Journal of Psychiatric Education 5:306–315, 1981

Pasnau RO: Ten commandments of medical etiquette for psychiatrists. Psychosomatics 26:128–132, 1985

Perry S, Viederman M: Adaption of residents to consultation-liaison psychiatry, II: working with the non-psychiatric staff. Gen Hosp Psychiatry 3:149–156, 1981

Saravay SM, Lavin M: Psychiatric comorbidity and length of stay in the general hospital: a critical review of outcome studies. Psychosomatics 35:233–252, 1994

Saravay SM, Steinberg H, Solomon SP, et al: A confirmation of NIMH training objectives for consultation-liaison residents. Am J Psychiatry 141:1437–1440, 1984

Schubert DSP, Billowitz A, Gabinet L, et al: Effect of liaison psychiatry on attitudes toward psychiatry, rate of consultation, and psychosocial documentation. Gen Hosp Psychiatry 11:77–87, 1989

Schwab JJ: Handbook of Psychiatric Consultation. New York, Appleton-Century-Crofts, 1968

Stotland NL, Garrick TR: Manual of Psychiatric Consultation. Washington, DC, American Psychiatric Press, 1990

Stoudemire A (ed): Clinical Psychiatry for Medical Students. Philadelphia, PA, JB Lippincott, 1990

Stoudemire A, Fogel BS (eds): Principles of Medical Psychiatry. Orlando, FL, Grune & Stratton, 1987

Stoudemire A, Fogel BS (eds): Medical Psychiatric Practice, Vol 1. Washington, DC, American Psychiatric Press, 1991

Stoudemire A, Fogel BS (eds): Psychiatric Care of the Medical Patient. New York, Oxford University Press, 1993

Strain JJ, Ginsburg J, Fulop G: Follow-up of psychiatric comorbidity in the general hospital. Int J Psychiatry Med 20:227–234, 1990

Strain JJ, Lyons JS, Hammer JS, et al: Cost offset from a psychiatric consultation-liaison intervention with elderly hip fracture patients. Am J Psychiatry 148:1044–1049, 1991

Strain JJ, Hammer JS, Fulop G: APM task force on psychosocial interventions in the general hospital inpatient setting: a review of cost-offset studies. Psychosomatics 35:253–262, 1994

Thompson TL II: Some advantages of consultation-liaison (medical-surgical) psychiatry becoming an added qualification subspecialty. Psychosomatics 34:343–349, 1993

Thompson TL II, Wise TN, Kelley AB, et al: Improving psychiatric consultation to non-psychiatric physicians. Psychosomatics 31:80–84, 1990

Wise MG, Rundell JR: Concise Guide to Consultation Psychiatry, 2nd Edition. Washington, DC, American Psychiatric Press, 1994

Wise TN, Mann LS, Silverstein R, et al: Consultation-liaison outcome evaluation system (CLOES): resident or private attending physicians' concordance with consultants' recommendations. Compr Psychiatry 28:430–436, 1987

Wolcott DL, Fawzy FI, Pasnau RO: Consultation-liaison outpatient clinics. Gen Hosp Psychiatry 6:153–161, 1984

Worley LM, Kunkel EJS, Hilty DM: How consultation-liaison services can comply with new HCFA guidelines. Gen Hosp Psychiatry 20:160–169, 1998

3

Cost-Effectiveness of the Consultation-Liaison Service

Richard C. W. Hall, M.D.

James R. Rundell, M.D.

Michael K. Popkin, M.D., F.A.P.M.

At a time when funding for health care is under serious scrutiny, consultation-liaison services throughout the United States have experienced increasing pressure to justify their existence. Although making money is not the raison d'être of many consultation-liaison services, several departments of psychiatry have recently curtailed their consultation-liaison services because of suboptimal financial viability. In this chapter, we provide the reader with a review of the pertinent literature on cost-effectiveness of consultation-liaison interventions and describe a realistic method to evaluate the cost-effectiveness of the consultation-liaison service that considers not only direct reimbursements but also secondary reimbursements and cost savings.

VALUE OF A CONSULTATION-LIAISON SERVICE TO A CLINIC OR HOSPITAL: REVIEW OF THE LITERATURE

Effect of Psychiatric Illness on Medical Outcome and Health Care Costs

Third-party payment restrictions on psychiatric treatment (Olfson et al. 1999; Villani and Sharfstein 1999) are increasing the importance of consultation-liaison services. Thirty percent to 60% of all hospitalized medically ill patients manifest some psychiatric syndrome associated with their medical illness; these problems often detract from the total quality of their care (Borus et al. 2000; Lipowski 1967; McGuire et al. 1974; Saravay et al. 1991; Strain 1982; von Ammon Cavanaugh and Wettstein 1989). Epidemiologic surveys typically find that 10%–15% of primary care outpatients have well-defined anxiety or depressive disorders (Eisenberg 1992). Fewer than 25% of patients with psychiatric disorders are seen by mental health care providers; the majority are seen by primary care providers (Simon and Walker 1999).

Depression, anxiety, and cognitive dysfunction have each been shown to predict longer hospital stays and greater medical costs, even after accounting for demographics, degree of physical impairment, type of hospital unit, medical diagnosis, and circumstances of admission (Druss et al. 1999; Kales et al. 1999; Levenson et al. 1990; Saravay et al. 1991). Saravay et al. (1991) studied patients during hospital days 3–5 using the Mini-Mental State Exam, Zung Self-Rating Depression Scale, and Hopkins Symptom Checklist–90. They also rated physical impairment using the Karnofsky scale. They then correlated length of stay, rating scale scores, demographics, and discharge diagnoses. Of 424 patients surveyed, 321 (76%) agreed to participate in the study, and 65.6% completed the test battery. Depression, anxiety, and "organicity" as measured by rating scales were each significantly correlated with longer hospital stays, even after correction was made for degree of physical impairment, emergency versus elective admission status, and whether a patient was admitted to a medical or surgical service. Previous studies had defined this association (Billings 1941; Cushman 1988; Dvoredsky and Cooley 1986; Fulop et al. 1987; Levenson et al. 1986–1987; Lyons et al. 1988; Rogers et al. 1989), but the study by Saravay et al. (1991) is particularly important because its methodological design addressed design faults, which clouded the results of other studies.

In a carefully controlled study analyzing the severity of psychopathology in medical inpatients and their subsequent use of and the cost of medical services, Levenson et al. (1990) showed that patients with high levels of psychopathology had a 40% longer median hospital stay and a 35% greater mean hospital cost than did patients with low levels of psychopathology. Psychiatrically sicker patients incurred higher hospital costs, had more diagnostic procedures, and received more discharge diagnoses but showed no differences in sex, age, race, diagnosis-related group (DRG) classification, or DRG-weighted diagnoses.

Dvoredsky and Cooley (1986) reviewed the records of 37,000 patients discharged from Veterans Administration hospitals and documented a significant correlation between psychiatric comorbidity and length of hospital stay. Fulop et al. (1987), in a review of 59,000 charts, showed that general hospital patients who met strict criteria for comorbid psychiatric diagnoses had significantly longer lengths of stay than did matched control subjects with similar medical illnesses but without psychiatric comorbidity. Lyons et al. (1988) reported similar findings for patients with head and spinal cord trauma during both the acute and the rehabilitative-convalescent phases of hospitalization. Cushman (1988) documented significantly longer hospital stays among psychiatrically ill stroke patients compared with stroke patients without psychiatric comorbidity. Brezel et al. (1988) demonstrated similar findings in burn patients.

Having multiple psychiatric diagnoses appears to magnify the effects of psychiatric illness on health care costs (Kessler et al. 1999). Kales et al. (1999) studied 7,115 elderly veterans with diagnoses of major depressive disorder, dementia, or both. Patients with coexisting dementia and depression had significantly more psychiatric inpatient days, medical inpatient days, and nursing home readmissions than did the other two study groups. The incidence and prevalence of these complex comorbid conditions will increase in coming decades with the aging of the population (Jeste et al. 1999).

Effect of Consultation-Liaison Services on Clinical Outcome and Health Care Costs

Studies have repeatedly demonstrated that a well-staffed and readily available (i.e., with consultations being done on the date of referral during a regular workweek) consultation-liaison service can significantly lower health care costs and at the same time improve the quality of medical care for medically ill patients with psychiatric symptoms (Beresford et al. 1985; Cohen-Cole and Stoudemire 1987; Dewan 1999; Fulop et al. 1987; Hall 1980, 1985; Hall and Beresford 1984; Lyons et al. 1988; Mumford et al. 1984; Pasnau 1975; Popkin et al. 1982; Schwab et al. 1967; Strain 1999; von Ammon Cavanaugh 1983; Wallen et al. 1987). Rundell and Hall (1993) reviewed outcomes of 135 consecutive inpatient consultations at Florida Hospital in Orlando and found that patients referred for psychiatric consultation were discharged from the hospital 1.5 days earlier than were matched patients with similar medical diagnoses who were not referred for consultation. Psychiatric consultation reduced the total cost of the average hospital stay by almost $2,000.

Strain et al. (1991) studied 452 consecutively admitted patients age 65 years or older who were hospitalized for surgical repair of fractured hips at Mount Sinai Medical Center in New York City and Northwestern Memorial Hospital in Chicago. During the baseline year, patients had traditional physician-based referral for psychiatric consultation, whereas during the experimental year, all patients at Mount Sinai and patients at one Northwestern unit were screened for possible psychiatric consultation and were referred for consultation. Patients who underwent psychiatric liaison screening had a higher consultation rate than did patients on units where no such programs were available. The incidence of DSM-III (American Psychiatric Association 1980) psychiatric disorders during the experimental year was 56% for the patients at Mount Sinai and 60% for those at Northwestern. During the year with liaison screening, mean length of stay decreased from 20.7 to 18.5 days at Mount Sinai and from 15.5 to 13.8 days at Northwestern, resulting in reductions in hospital costs of $166,926 at Mount Sinai and $97,361 at Northwestern. Screening elderly patients on admission resulted in early detection of psychiatric morbidity, better psychiatric care, and earlier discharge from the hospital. In addition, the hospital realized substantial cost savings.

The findings of Strain et al. (1991) closely parallel those of Rundell and Hall (1993). The former study also confirmed the earlier work of Levitan and Kornfeld (1981), who studied elderly patients with hip fractures and showed that early psychiatric consultation resulted in shortened hospital stays. Lyons and co-workers (1986) found in two separate studies that the earlier psychiatric consultation was initiated during a patient's hospital stay, the greater the reduction was in length of hospital stay.

There is increasing emphasis on shifting as much mental health treatment as possible from specialty mental health care settings to the general medical setting. Costs for treatment of depression are considerably less in the general medical setting (Zhang et al. 1999). However, treatment costs account for only one-quarter of the total cost of depression (Greenberg et al. 1993); lost earnings because of missed workdays and other societal costs account for the remainder. Specialty treatment for depression, though more expensive than general medical treatment for depression, is twice as likely (48% vs. 21%) to meet rigid clinical practice guidelines and more than pays for itself in faster returns to work (Zhang et al. 1999). Treatment for depression costs $1,200 more per year in the mental health care setting than in the general medical setting, but lost earnings average $2,000 less annually.

Psychiatrists with consultation-liaison experience bring the unique combination of medical background and mental health specialty training to the general medical setting. Health services research suggests that when integrated treatment (e.g., medication treatment combined with psychotherapy) is necessary, the use of a psychiatrist, rather than a physician plus a psychologist, is most cost-effective (De Jonge 2000; Dewan 1999).

OPTIMIZATION OF THE FINANCIAL VIABILITY OF CONSULTATION-LIAISON SERVICES

Psychiatric consultation-liaison services conserve hospital resources by providing for more timely discharge from inpatient settings, conserve clinic resources by decreasing outpatient health care utilization, improve collection of hospital revenues by upgrading DRGs with appropriate psychiatric comorbidities, and generate specific direct charges for services rendered. Nonetheless, many excellent consultation-liaison psychiatry services have had serious staff setbacks or are no longer available because of their inability to document their financial viability for their health care systems. To avoid common pitfalls that may financially cripple a consultation-liaison service, we suggest the following strategies (summarized in Table 3–1).

1. *Be an advocate.* Consultation-liaison psychiatrists work in an environment that is more competitive than that of 10 years ago (Alter et al. 1997; Gonzalez and Randel 1996; Schreter 1998; Thompson et al. 1997). Whereas psychiatrists' numbers and incomes have remained fairly unchanged, the num-

TABLE 3–1. Strategies for improving financial viability of consultation-liaison services

1. Be an advocate.
2. Maintain a proper information management system.
3. Target services to maximize payment.
4. Be a regular visitor to the business office.
5. Train consultation-liaison service staff in coding procedures.
6. Record each diagnosis and its complexity.
7. Ensure that diagnosis-related group upgrades are performed and the consultation-liaison service is credited.
8. Ensure that patients sign payment authorization forms.
9. Bill for follow-up visits.
10. Appeal all insurance disallowals.
11. Optimize tax benefits when payment is not received.
12. Ensure that the head of the psychiatry department understands the value of the consultation-liaison service.
13. Become an outpatient consultation-liaison service.
14. Target consultation-liaison services to patients who may be referred for consultation.
15. Integrate a neuropsychologist into the service.
16. Work closely with social workers and case managers.
17. Consider seeking research monies.
18. In academic centers, consider a consultation-liaison psychiatry fellowship.
19. Invest time to demonstrate cost-effectiveness.

bers and incomes of psychologists, social workers, and nurses have increased significantly (Scheffler and Ivey 1998; Scheffler et al. 1998). To establish fair remuneration for their members, consultation-liaison services must continually highlight the value of their services. All consultation-liaison service staff must continually point out the power of the service to save the health care system money and emphasize that this is at least as important, if not more financially important, than reimbursements received. However, as long as billings and reimbursements exist, it is important to maximize them. A general hospital or health care system consultation service must have direct and ongoing input into its billing process.

In consultation to a major university hospital, a consultation-liaison service with five full-time attending physicians, three residents, one fellow, two nurses, and one psychologist was credited with having collected only $68,000 during a calendar year. The service estimated that it had billed more than $600,000. In an attempt to understand why the service had collected so little, a review was conducted. The faculty practice coders found it tedious and tiresome to bill for consultations costing small amounts of money when they could use the same amount of time to generate considerably larger bills for other departments, such as surgery and cardiology, that brought more revenue to the hospital. As a result, the consultation service billings were never appropriately filed. The service worked diligently, provided excellent service, and generated enough billings to be self-sufficient; however, practically no money was collected, and the service faced extinction because of the lack of a dedicated billing clerk. The lesson was clear: this consultation-liaison service needed to collect its own data and hire a billing clerk to expedite the coding and filing of appropriate bills.

The chief of the consultation service must review collections and work closely with the hospital administration to ensure that services are appropriately billed for and revenues are collected and *posted* to the service. It is best for the consultation service to control its own billing and accounting. Cost savings and revenues generated from consultations should be credited to the consultation-liaison service, *not* the consulting service or the overall psychiatry department.

2. *Maintain a proper information management system.* Consultation-liaison services must be regarded as business entities. Few services can prosper, expand, and have the teaching and training resources necessary to remain state of the art if there is not adequate information management. This simple point is well understood in the private sector but often missed or ignored in the academic and governmental sectors. At a time when institutions are trying to tighten budgets wherever possible, consultation-liaison service directors must have or obtain viable medical information and management systems to demonstrate their services' efficacy. All initial consultations and subsequent follow-up visits, both billable and nonbillable, must be carefully recorded. For each patient, the referring physician, reason for consultation, diagnosis, clinical complexity, clinical outcomes, psychotherapeutic interventions received, medications prescribed, payer status, and whether the payer is DRG regulated must be carefully noted. In addition, each consultation-liaison–credentialed provider should document the amount of time spent discussing care with patients, their physicians and other hospital staff, and their families, as well as time needed to review records, deal with managed care reviewers, and answer telephone calls.

3. *Target services to maximize payment.* Treatment of psychiatric disorders early in their courses is associated with good outcome in the long term, as well as cost savings (Rabinowitz et al. 1998). Unfortunately, many people lack any type of health insurance and receive no treatment until late in the disease course. In a consultation-liaison service that provides services (to indigent patients and other groups) not likely to be sufficiently reimbursed, the director must identify areas for cost reduction, high productivity, and financial reward. The service should direct particularly strong clinical efforts toward helping patients who are most likely to benefit from intervention, focusing on areas where the parent facility has its greatest needs, enabling outcome (especially cost-saving) research to be appropriately accomplished, and ensuring that the service is compensated for its time. This is not to say that other areas of the hospital should not be served; rather, they will not be served if the consultation-liaison service is eliminated or scaled back.

4. *Be a regular visitor to the business office.* The consultation-liaison service chief should meet with business office personnel on a regular basis to review the following:
   Intake data. These data include insurance (primary and secondary), patients' patterns of use of psychiatric services, evaluation of the types of consultations generated, psychological tests provided, and diagnostic studies completed.
   Coded diagnoses. All diagnoses relevant to a patient's case should be coded when a request for reimbursement is made. Coders often object, but a full listing defines complexity and often results in increased revenue and, in disputed cases, may result in a payment that would otherwise be withheld.
   Bills. Bills should be posted in a timely fashion. A consultation-liaison service should post its billings no later than 7 days after providing services. Optimally, bills are posted within 48 hours of service.
   Delinquent bills. All delinquent bills should be reviewed and a decision should be made about which should be turned over for collection. Administrative personnel should be trained to work with patients on accounts that are delinquent before turning these accounts over for collection. All unpaid accounts should be reviewed for collection at 30, 60, and 90 days. During a systems consultation at one large county hospital, it became clear that the hospital had never attempted to collect on the consultation-liaison service's unpaid bills. The insti-

tution had a policy that after an initial letter requesting payment, all bills less than $500 were written off. Accounts receivable totaled more than $500,000.

5. *Train consultation-liaison service staff in coding procedures.* Proper coding is essential for payment and accounting of cost-effectiveness. In a small consultation service, suicide attempts resulting in emergency room visits were often being coded as "adult situational adjustment reaction." Collection was not forthcoming. Many of these patients' conditions could have appropriately been diagnosed as depression not otherwise specified, major depression with suicide attempt, or medicinal poisoning, resulting in a much higher likelihood of reimbursement. Providing accurate diagnoses is crucial. Diagnoses should never be altered or falsified, but well-trained coders understand how to code in an appropriate fashion to obtain fair reimbursements.

6. *Record each diagnosis and its complexity.* The consultant should list all appropriate medical and psychiatric diagnoses and provide specific diagnostic criteria for each major psychiatric diagnosis. In addition, he or she should rate the level of complexity of the case. The consultant should record the time spent in consultation with other physicians, with the patient and the family, reviewing laboratory and X-ray data, discussing the case with the nursing staff, physically examining the patient, and obtaining a psychiatric anamnesis. The complexity of the case, number of different diagnoses, and time spent may all significantly alter the level of billing for an initial consultation. Although faculty and residents may spend an hour or two in an initial consultation, notes are often too brief and lack documentation of actual time spent in rendering the service. In addition, the nature of services rendered is sometimes absent from the consultation report. *Lack of proper documentation hinders fair billing, reimbursement, and financial accounting.* Elements necessary for appropriate billing are shown in Table 3–2.

7. *Ensure that DRG upgrades are performed and the consultation-liaison service is credited.* Psychiatric consultation that defines psychiatric comorbidity may significantly increase the DRG reimbursement made to the hospital (Hall et al. 1996). The director of the consultation-liaison service should have quarterly updates on reviews collected from the DRG upgrade process: these reviews strengthen the consultation-liaison service's position with the general hospital administration, which is helpful when

TABLE 3–2. Consultation-liaison data worksheet

1. Patient name, address, telephone number; primary and secondary insurance; date of admission; date of discharge; identification number; date seen; time spent
2. Complexity of consultation, all medical and psychiatric diagnoses, associated stressors
3. Referring physician, referring physician's personal identification number (PIN) or license number, reason for consultation
4. Number of visits, reasons for follow-up visits and services rendered
5. Psychological tests administered by physician and psychologist
6. Medications prescribed, other somatic treatment rendered
7. Psychological therapy provided (e.g., individual psychotherapy, family therapy, group therapy)
8. Patient's diagnosis-related group (DRG); is DRG upgrade indicated and substantiated by patient's diagnosis?
9. Referral to
   (None made)
   Outpatient treatment
   Inpatient unit
   Day hospital
   Other
10. Charges generated—billed, credited to service

requests are being made for additional staff or equipment or for increases in salaries or benefits.

8. *Ensure that patients sign payment authorization forms.* When available, a signed insurance assignment form or authorization for psychiatric treatment should be obtained from the patient or designated approval authority at the time of the first patient visit. Without such forms, billing and collection are often impossible. These forms should be submitted with the consultation report to the appropriate secretary, coder, or billing clerk at the end of each day. Many hospitals have universal forms that patients sign at clinic check-in or admission, which authorize payment to all providers. A copy of these forms should be submitted to the consultation-liaison service's biller.

9. *Bill for follow-up visits.* Each follow-up visit should be defined for content, level of severity, and duration of contact with both patient and staff. For a patient whose case is clinically complex, there should be careful documentation in both the consultation record and on the patient's chart that this patient requires an increased level of care. The note should define what care is necessary and how long psychiatric follow-up or inpatient treatment will be required.

10. *Appeal all insurance disallowals.* The chief of the consultation-liaison service should be notified immediately of any insurance disallowals. These should be appealed immediately, when appropriate. The appeal should note the specific reasons for the consultation and the necessity for specific treatments and follow-up.

11. *Optimize tax benefits when payment is not received.* For accounts in which chances for eventual payment appear remote, the consultation-liaison service should work with the hospital business office to optimize any tax benefits that the hospital may be entitled to because of this revenue loss. Tax savings should be credited to the consultation-liaison service.

12. *Ensure that the head of the psychiatry department understands the value of the consultation-liaison service.* In our experience, consultation-liaison services transfer one in five patients to an inpatient psychiatric unit, medical-psychiatric unit, partial hospital program, or substance use disorder program. The consultation-liaison service therefore is an important source of inpatient psychiatric referrals. This function of the service must be carefully documented so that it can be brought to the attention of the department's or hospital's administration.

13. *Become an outpatient consultation-liaison service.* One of the greatest changes in health care over the past decade has been the shift to outpatient medical care. Hospital censuses are a fraction of what they once were. Short hospitalizations mean fewer days of practice for consultation-liaison psychiatrists who work solely with inpatients, as well as less time for psychiatric interventions. Psychiatric treatment has been shown to be as valuable in outpatient medical settings as on inpatient wards (Simon and Walker 1999). Consultation-liaison services should aggressively pursue avenues for outpatient consultation.

14. *Target consultation-liaison services to patients who may be referred for consultation.* Several consultation-liaison services have developed consultation-liaison, psychosomatic, or psychiatric medicine outpatient clinics where faculty and residents can manage outpatient groups and conduct individual therapy and diagnostic evaluations. Subspecialty clinical consultation in an outpatient mode to rheumatology services, diabetic clinics, transplant services, dialysis clinics, oncology clinics, and other services can improve the quality of care delivered to the target population, dramatically decrease health care utilization and costs, and supply important sources of revenue to the consultation-liaison service by providing postdischarge follow-up.

15. *Integrate a neuropsychologist into the service.* Neuropsychodiagnostic testing by a neuropsychologist who is a member of the consultation-liaison service can provide important and useful information for patient management and can represent an additional revenue base for the service. This is particularly true in an outpatient setting, where neurological impacts of acute medical events and treatments are less likely than in a hospital setting to detract from neuropsychological and psychological assessment findings.

16. *Work closely with social workers and case managers.* Nurses and social workers who conduct case management are aware, perhaps more than anyone, of the improvements and cost savings that result when there is effective psychiatric inpatient and outpatient consultation. Working closely with these professionals often pays dividends in terms of maintaining institutional support for the consultation-liaison service and demonstrating its effectiveness.

17. *Consider seeking research monies.* Consultation-liaison psychiatry research is important for clinical reasons and to demonstrate the financial benefit of a consultation-liaison service. In addition, research grant monies brought in by the consultation-liaison service will significantly help the financial viability of the service. Similarly, the consultation-liaison service can provide psychiatric services to patients who are participating in various medication, cost-offset, or other outcome studies. Fostering working relationships with the chiefs of various services who are developing grants permits involvement by the consultation-liaison service in the grant progress. This may generate funding for psychiatric consultations to evaluate behavioral and cognitive effects of new medications and medical treatments.

18. *In academic centers, consider a consultation-liaison psychiatry fellowship.* Consultation-liaison fellows add an academic touch to a consultation-liaison service. Having a training program helps a service recruit the most experienced and seasoned consultation-liaison staff psychiatrists. Consultation-liaison outcome research is also facilitated when there is a fellowship. External financial support may be obtained for training consultation-liaison psychiatry fellows and residents and fellows from other hospital services.

19. *Invest time to demonstrate cost-effectiveness.* In capitated, government-run, and other types of managed

care systems, reducing overall medical costs is more important than generating reimbursements. Consultation-liaison research (see Chapter 12) will help demonstrate the value of the consultation-liaison service within the organization. Preconsultation health care utilization should be compared with postconsultation clinic visits, emergency room visits, pharmacy costs, laboratory costs, and hospitalization days. Case manager nurses and social workers can be of significant help in this regard, and pharmacy, medical records, and laboratory personnel are typically willing to assist with these reviews. Most data necessary for such reviews are readily available in computerized databases. Experts in the business offices of health care organizations may help with data collection and conduct data analyses.

CONCLUSION

A well-run consultation-liaison service is cost-effective for the general hospital and for the larger department of psychiatry. However, this is true only if adequate medical information systems, administrative personnel, and control of billing functions are centralized in the consultation-liaison service. We believe that during the next decade, as revenues for health care diminish and health care continues to shift to the outpatient setting, the value of consultation-liaison services to general hospitals and clinics will increase. These services will become increasingly outpatient and data driven, and the focus will be more on quality improvement and cost saving than on reimbursement. Today more than ever, a research agenda is necessary to make the case for complete and fair coverage of psychiatric illness (Sharfstein et al. 1993), especially in the general hospital and outpatient medical-surgical clinic settings.

REFERENCES

Alter CL, Schindler BA, Hails K, et al: Funding for consultation-liaison services in public sector-managed care plans: the experience of the Consultation-Liaison Association of Philadelphia. Psychosomatics 38:93–97, 1997

American Psychiatric Association: Diagnostic and Statistical Manual of Mental Disorders, 3rd Edition. Washington, DC, American Psychiatric Association, 1980

Beresford TP, Holt RE, Hall RCW, et al: Cognitive screening at the bedside: usefulness of a structured examination. Psychosomatics 26:319–324, 1985

Billings EG: Value of psychiatry to the general hospital. Hospitals 15:30–34, 1941

Borus JF, Barsky AJ, Carbone LA, et al: Consultation-liaison cost offset: searching the wrong grail (editorial). Psychosomatics 41:285–288, 2000

Brezel BS, Kassenbrock JM, Stein JM: Burns in substance abusers and neurologically and mentally impaired patients. J Burn Care Rehabil 9:169–171, 1988

Cohen-Cole SA, Stoudemire A: Major depression in physical illness: special considerations in diagnosis and biological treatment. Psychiatr Clin North Am 10:1–17, 1987

Cushman LA: Secondary neuropsychiatric complications in stroke: implications for acute care. Arch Phys Med Rehabil 69:877–879, 1988

De Jonge P, Huyse FJ, Ruinemans G, et al: Timing of psychiatric consultations: the impact of social vulnerability and level of psychiatric dysfunction. Psychosomatics 41:505–511, 2000

Dewan M: Are psychiatrists cost-effective? An analysis of integrated versus split treatment. Am J Psychiatry 156:324–326, 1999

Druss B, Schlesinger M, Thomas T, et al: Depressive symptoms and plan switching under managed care. Am J Psychiatry 156:697–701, 1999

Dvoredsky AE, Cooley WH: Comparative severity of illness in patients with combined medical and psychiatric diagnoses. Psychosomatics 27:625–630, 1986

Eisenberg L: Treating depression and anxiety in primary care: closing the gap between knowledge and practice. N Engl J Med 326:1080–1084, 1992

Fulop G, Strain JJ, Vita J, et al: Impact of psychiatric comorbidity on length of hospital stay for medical/surgical patients: a preliminary report. Am J Psychiatry 144:878–882, 1987

Gonzalez JJ, Randel L: Consultation-liaison psychiatry in the managed care arena. Psychiatr Clin North Am 19:449–466, 1996

Greenberg PE, Stiglin LE, Finkelstein SN, et al: The economic burden of depression in 1990. J Clin Psychiatry 54:405–418, 1993

Hall RCW (ed): Psychiatric Manifestations of Medical Illness: Somatopsychic Disorders. New York, Spectrum, 1980

Hall RCW: Psychiatric effects of thyroid hormone disturbance, in Psychosomatic Illness Review. Edited by Dorfman W, Cristofar L. New York, Macmillan, 1985, pp 107–123

Hall RCW, Beresford TP: Psychological aspects of physical illness, in Current Themes in Psychiatry. Edited by Gaind RN, Hudson BL: New York, Spectrum, 1984, pp 1–11

Hall RCW, Rundell JR, Hirsch T: Economic issues in consultation-liaison psychiatry, in The American Psychiatric Press Textbook of Consultation-Liaison Psychiatry. Edited by Rundell JR, Wise MG. Washington DC, American Psychiatric Press, 1996, pp 31–34

Jeste DV, Alexopoulos GS, Bartels SJ, et al: Consensus statement on the upcoming crisis in geriatric mental health: research agenda for the next two decades. Arch Gen Psychiatry 56:848–853, 1999

Kales HC, Blow FC, Copeland LA, et al: Health care utilization by older patients with coexisting dementia and depression. Am J Psychiatry 156:550–556, 1999

Kessler RC, Zhao S, Katz SJ, et al: Past-year use of outpatient services for psychiatric problems in the National Comorbidity Survey. Am J Psychiatry 156:115–123, 1999

Levenson JL, Hamer RM, Silverman JJ, et al: Psychopathology in medical inpatients and its relationship to length of hospital stay: a pilot study. Int J Psychiatry Med 16:231–236, 1986–1987

Levenson JL, Hamer RM, Rossiter LD: Relation of psychopathology in general medical inpatients to use and cost of services. Am J Psychiatry 47:1498–1503, 1990

Levitan SJ, Kornfeld DS: Clinical and cost benefits of liaison psychiatry. Am J Psychiatry 138:790–793, 1981

Lipowski Z: Review of consultation psychiatry and psychosomatic medicine, 1: general principles. Psychosom Med 29:153–171, 1967

Lyons JS, Hammer JS, Strain JJ, et al: The timing of psychiatric consultation in the general hospital stay. Gen Hosp Psychiatry 8:159–186, 1986

Lyons JS, Larson DB, Burns BJ, et al: Psychiatric co-morbidities and patients with head and spinal cord trauma: effects on acute hospital care. Gen Hosp Psychiatry 10:292–297, 1988

McGuire GP, Julier DL, Hawton KE, et al: Psychiatric morbidity and referral on two general medical wards. BMJ 1:268–270, 1974

Mumford E, Schlesinger HJ, Glass GV, et al: A new look at evidence about reduced cost of medical utilization following mental health treatment. Am J Psychiatry 141:1145–1158, 1984

Olfson M, Marcus SC, Pincus HA: Trends in office-based psychiatric practice. Am J Psychiatry 156:451–457, 1999

Pasnau RO (ed): Consultation-Liaison Psychiatry. New York, Grune & Stratton, 1975

Popkin MK, Mackenzie TB, Hall RCW, et al: The yield of psychiatric consultants' recommendations for diagnostic action. Arch Gen Psychiatry 39:843–845, 1982

Rabinowitz J, Bromet EJ, Lavelle J, et al: Relationship between type of insurance and care during the early course of psychosis. Am J Psychiatry 155:1392–1397, 1998

Rogers MP, Liang MH, Daltroy LH, et al: Delirium after elective orthopedic surgery: risk factors and natural history. Int J Psychiatry Med 19:109–121, 1989

Rundell JR, Hall RCW: Psychiatric consultation in general hospital medical-surgical inpatients: impact of consultation on cognitive function and psychiatric status—results from a pilot study. Paper presented at the 40th annual meeting of the Academy of Psychosomatic Medicine, New Orleans, LA, November 1993

Saravay SM, Steinberg MD, Weinschel B, et al: Psychological comorbidity and length of stay in the general hospital. Am J Psychiatry 148:324–329, 1991

Scheffler R, Ivey SL: Mental health staffing in managed care organizations: a case study. Psychiatr Serv 49:1303–1308, 1998

Scheffler R, Ivey SL, Garrett AB: Changing supply and earning patterns of the mental health workforce. Adm Policy Ment Health 26:85–99, 1998

Schreter RK: Reorganizing departments of psychiatry, hospitals, and medical centers for the 21st century. Psychiatr Serv 49:1429–1433, 1998

Schwab JJ, Bialow M, Brown JM, et al: Diagnosing depression in medical inpatients. Ann Intern Med 67:695–707, 1967

Sharfstein SS, Stoline AM, Goldman HH: Psychiatric care and health insurance reform. Am J Psychiatry 150:7–18, 1993

Simon GE, Walker EA: The consultation-liaison psychiatrist in the primary care clinic, in Essentials of Consultation-Liaison Psychiatry. Edited by Rundell JR, Wise MG. Washington, DC, American Psychiatric Press, 1999, pp 513–520

Strain JJ: Needs for psychiatry in the general hospital. Hosp Community Psychiatry 33:996–1001, 1982

Strain JJ: Liaison psychiatry, in Essentials of Consultation-Liaison Psychiatry. Edited by Rundell JR, Wise MG. Washington DC, American Psychiatric Press, 1999, pp 3–11

Strain JJ, Lyons JS, Hammer JS, et al: Cost offset from a psychiatric consultation-liaison intervention with elderly hip fracture patients. Am J Psychiatry 148:1044–1049, 1991

Thompson TL 2nd, Folks DG, Silverman JJ: Challenges and opportunities for consultation-liaison psychiatry in the managed care environment. Psychosomatics 38:70–75, 1997

Villani S, Sharfstein SS: Evaluating and treating violent adolescents in the managed care era. Am J Psychiatry 156:458–464, 1999

von Ammon Cavanaugh S: The prevalence of emotional and cognitive dysfunction in a general medical population: using the MMSE, GHQ, and BDI. Gen Hosp Psychiatry 5:15–24, 1983

von Ammon Cavanaugh S, Wettstein RM: Emotional and cognitive dysfunction associated with medical disorders. J Psychosom Res 33:505–514, 1989

Wallen J, Pincus HA, Goldman HH, et al: Psychiatric consultations in short-term general hospitals. Arch Gen Psychiatry 44:163–168, 1987

Zhang M, Rost KM, Fortney JC: Earnings changes for depressed individuals treated by mental health specialists. Am J Psychiatry 156:108–114, 1999

4

Liaison Psychiatry

James J. Strain, M.D.

The liaison psychiatrist (who studies, deals with, and teaches about medical and psychiatric comorbidity) may encounter any illness listed in *International Statistical Classification of Diseases and Related Health Problems*, 10th Revision (World Health Organization 1992) and must understand the end-organ dysfunction of that medical or surgical disorder. He or she must also be aware of the effects of medical drugs and the interaction between medical and psychotropic drugs and must know how to stay abreast of these interactions. Consequently, liaison psychiatrists must possess or have access to a monumental database if they are to manage their patients safely and effectively. This knowledge base is essential for one of the major functions of the liaison psychiatrist—teacher of other physicians, nurses, social workers, and patients. The knowledge base is doubling every 5–6 years. It is estimated that as many as 6,000–7,000 new scientific publications appear each day; often these publications pertain to medicine (Piemme 1988). The liaison psychiatrist must develop methods to process this plethora of new knowledge. Medical informatics—which includes artificial intelligence, archives of clinically relevant information, and software to codify large data pools—provides mechanisms that will enable the liaison psychiatrist to have relevant information at the point of clinical decision making—at the patient's side (Hammer et al. 1995).

This database is essential for the discipline of liaison psychiatry, which involves or focuses on screening, problem level diagnosis, disorder level diagnosis, interventions, outcomes, randomized controlled trials, costs, and finally, product substitution; this last relates to the choice of the profession to provide mental health care. The flowchart in Figure 4–1 will help the liaison psychiatrist develop a systems approach to the patient, and to the unit and even the institution where he or she works. This systems approach to information management by the

psychiatrist on the medical or surgical ward includes randomized controlled trials, critical laboratory studies, technical reports, compliance with medical and psychiatric recommendations, and determination of patient outcome using standardized instruments. The systems approach not only helps the liaison psychiatrist make clinical decisions but also serves as a teaching model for the kinds of information the primary care physician or other mental health care providers need with regard to psychiatric comorbidity in physically ill patients. As each step of the mental health assessment is completed, reminders (alerts) are provided to underscore certain key domains (e.g., medical drug–psychotropic drug interactions, patient or consultee noncompliance with psychiatric recommendations, or laboratory abnormalities) (Strain et al. 1996b).

The liaison psychiatrist focuses not only on the patient but on the system that cares for the patient. Therefore, the pedagogical function is primary. The liaison psychiatrist's role as a teacher of psychiatric skills and information in the medical setting also underscores the fact that psychiatrists assist others in dealing with psychological, psychiatric, and psychophysiological morbidity in the medical setting. Whether nonpsychiatric physicians consult with psychiatrists depends on the abilities of psychiatrists as teachers during the nonpsychiatrists' training years. This is also why it is important to point out the differences between consultation and liaison psychiatry. As Hackett and Cassem so aptly said:

> A distinction must be made between a consultation service and a consultation liaison service. A consultation service is a rescue squad. It responds to requests from other services for help with the diagnosis, treatment, or disposition of perplexing patients. At worst, consultation work is nothing more than a brief foray into the territory of another service, usually ending

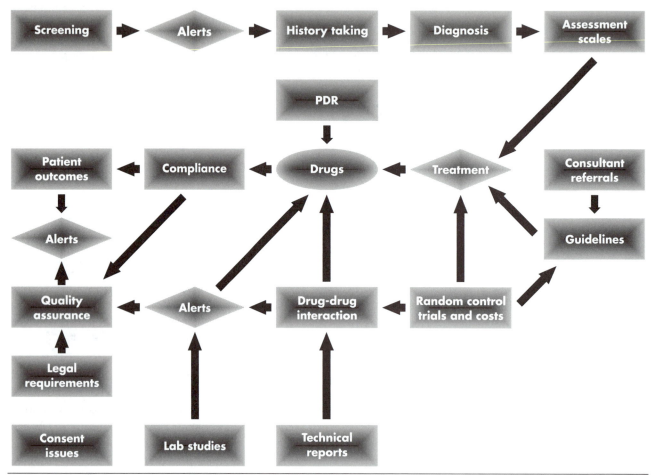

FIGURE 4–1.   Computer-assisted physician management system.

Source.   Reprinted from Strain JJ, Hammer JS, Himelein C, et al: "Further Evolution of a Literature Database: Content and Software." *Gen Hosp Psychiatry* 18(5):296, 1996. Copyright 1996, Elsevier Science. Used with permission.

with a note written in the chart outlining a plan of action. The actual intervention is left to the consultee. Like a volunteer firefighter, a consultant puts out the blaze and then returns home. Like a volunteer fire brigade, a consultation service seldom has the time or manpower to set up fire prevention programs or to educate the citizenry about fireproofing. A consultation service is the most common type of psychiatric-medical interface found in the departments of psychiatry around the United States today.

A liaison service requires manpower, money and motivation. Sufficient personnel are necessary to allow the psychiatric consultant time to perform services other than simply interviewing troublesome patients in the area assigned to him. He must be able to attend rounds, discuss patients individually with house officers, and hold teaching sessions for nurses. Liaison work is further distinguished from consultation activity in that patients are seen at the discretion of the psychiatric consultant as well as the referring physicians. Because the consultant attends social service rounds with the house officers, he is able to spot potential psychiatric problems. (Hackett and Cassem 1979, p. 5)

Liaison psychiatry is positioned at the interface of psychiatry and medicine. It includes not only the traditional psychiatric consultation on an individual patient, but going beyond this essential task to establish the psychiatrist as a bona fide member of the medical-surgical team. Establishing a liaison relationship means that the psychiatrist will be in contact with all the psychiatric and medical comorbidity on a unit or ward, and not just consultant to those referred. In epidemiological terms liaison psychiatry attempts to interact with the **denominator** of the prevalence of psychiatric morbidity in the medical setting, whereas consultation psychiatry, by the very nature of the referral process, is involved only with the **numerator.** (Strain and Strain 1988, p. 76)

Historically, consultation has been the method by which one medical discipline interacts with another. It requires that one discipline discern when needs in another discipline are extant. However, at least with regard to psychiatry, physicians in the medical-surgical specialties recognize relatively few patients with psychiatric morbidity, and when they do, relatively few are referred (Fulop and Strain 1985; Strain et al. 1991; Wallen et al. 1987). There is a great disparity between the amount of psychiatric pathology that exists in the medical-surgical setting and that which is identified by medical-surgical staff and/or the focus of referral to psychiatrists. The patients who are referred to consultation-liaison psychiatrists represent only the tip of a very large iceberg. The traditional consultation process imposes a sampling bias for establishing clinical needs; that process also impedes research on prevalence, mind-body interactions, outcome of interventions, cost offset, and mechanism issues in the medical setting. In the majority of patients with psychiatric and medical comorbidity in the medical setting, psychiatric pathology remains undetected, and these patients remain untreated and unreferred (Strain et al. 1986).

Consequently, the consultation methodology limits needed psychiatric, biopsychosocial, and behavioral assessments and interventions that have been demonstrated to affect not only mental health but also general health. The conceptual framework of liaison psychiatry is to enter the system of the medical-surgical setting to have access to the denominator—the entire patient cohort—and not be restricted to the numerator—the limited referred patient population. It is further designed for interaction with the other disciplines (such as medical specialties, nursing, or social work) to expand the abilities of practitioners of those disciplines to detect psychiatric disorders and to treat and/or refer patients with psychiatric disorders (and to assist caregivers in dealing with patients); to affect systems of medical care; to involve patients' support systems; and for conducting research on medical and psychiatric comorbidity.

On the liver transplantation service at one major teaching hospital, the psychiatrists who are part of the transplantation team are asked their opinions on patients' psychological capacities to maintain a scarce resource—the liver. At times, it will be the psychiatrist who will state that a patient does not have the psychological capacity to maintain the organ. The scarce resource will then be given to an alternate and the patient so assessed will be left to die. To offer such a clinical opinion and have it accepted by the other caregivers requires knowing not only the patient but also the process of liver transplantation, the team, and the patient's significant others. It is unlikely that a consultation psychiatrist "dropping in" for a consultation with an unknown patient and an unknown medical professional could make this decision, and if he or she did, it is unlikely that such a decision would be accepted.

In this chapter, I review 1) studies on the incidence of psychiatric and medical comorbidity in general medical-surgical inpatient settings; 2) psychiatric interventions in general medical-surgical inpatient settings; 3) the conceptual framework of liaison psychiatry and how this framework differs from traditional consultation methodology; 4) models of liaison psychiatry mental health training for primary care physicians; and 5) the importance of guidelines for clinical practice and their implications for liaison psychiatry. All these issues underscore the need to deal with the referred and unreferred medically ill population, rather than merely with the referred population—a need that justifies the mandate to use methods beyond the limits of referral.

PSYCHIATRIC AND MEDICAL COMORBIDITY IN THE GENERAL HOSPITAL

Saravay and Lavin (1994) described psychiatric comorbidity and length of stay (LOS) in the general hospital and reviewed several outcome studies. A critical element in such studies is whether the research is prospective (Ford 1988) and whether potentially confounding factors are controlled for. Saravay et al. (1991, p. 324) noted that "a study design that is not prospective cannot usually determine whether psychiatric morbidity precedes, and may therefore contribute to extended hospital stays, or whether it arises later in the hospital course as a consequence of a stay prolonged by medical factors." It is also important to take into account the number of subjects in the study, to avoid a type II error.

Saravay and Lavin (1994) reviewed 21 studies: 7 international (1 retrospective, 2 cross-sectional, and 4 prospective) and 14 in the United States (7 retrospective and 7 prospective [with no control for severity of illness in 4]). Of the 21 studies described, 16 (76%) found a significant association between psychiatric or psychological and medical comorbidity and increased LOS. Of the studies with more than 110 subjects (to avoid a type II error), 87% demonstrated statistically significant results. Geriatric patients were studied in 12 of the 21 studies. Depending on the kind of psychiatric morbidity seen, indicators varied among the studies: cognitive disturbance, affective disorder, alcohol use, anxiety, and LOS. Mayou et al. (1991) observed that cognitive disturbance and affective disorder predicted a greater likelihood of rehospitalization during the year after discharge from a British general hospital. Narain et al. (1988) noted that cognitive disturbance predicted nursing home placement but not rehospitalization among Veterans Administration patients 6 months after discharge. Rogers et al.

(1989) found that postoperative delirium was associated with worse physical outcomes at 6-month follow-up among orthopedic patients older than 60 years, even when preoperative neuropsychological status was controlled for. Also, Francis et al. (1990) observed that patients with delirium were less likely to be discharged to their homes, with twice as many institutionalized at 6-month follow-up.

Saravay and Lavin (1994) described three generations of United States studies. The retrospective studies all found significant correlations between psychiatric and psychological comorbidity and LOS (Ackerman et al. 1988; Billings 1941; Brezel et al. 1988; Cushman 1988; Dvoredsky and Cooley 1986; Fulop et al. 1987; Lyons et al. 1988). Of the three prospective studies that did control for severity of illness or other confounding variables (the second-generation studies), the two that failed to show significance had small samples (Levenson et al. 1986; Rogers et al. 1989).

Three of the four third-generation studies (prospective and with severity of illness, degree of functional impairment, and other potentially confounding variables controlled for) had significant results. Narain et al. (1988) observed that cognitive impairment predicted nursing home placement within 6 months after discharge. Francis et al. (1990) found a significant positive association in geriatric patients between delirium and LOS. Levenson et al. (1990) noted significant positive associations between depression, anxiety, cognitive impairment, and pain on the one hand and LOS and expenses on the other. Saravay et al. (1991) also demonstrated an association between cognitive impairment, depression, and psychopathology on the Symptom Checklist—90 (SCL-90; Derogatis et al. 1974) and increased LOS, more frequent hospitalization, and more days spent hospitalized during a 4-year period. These studies were denominator based (i.e., involved the entire patient cohort). Examining the inpatient phase only, and not taking into account severity of illness, reduces the value of research findings. Using only patients referred for consultation limits the conclusions that can be drawn.

PSYCHIATRIC INTERVENTIONS IN THE INPATIENT MEDICAL SETTING

Inpatient hospital care remains the most expensive form of care. Interventions to identify hospitalized patients' psychiatric and psychosocial needs, to treat them, to reduce physical morbidity, and to decrease LOS are crucial to the maintenance of a viable, affordable health care system.

In fact, several variables other than the patient's medical condition contribute to LOS. Zimmer (1974) observed that for more than 2,500 patients, 11.8% of all hospital days could not be accounted for by physical needs. Glass et al. (1977) reported that for 363 hospitalized medical-surgical inpatients, 18% of the hospital days were due to social rather than physical factors. Mason et al. (1980) described many reasons that patients are admitted to the hospital and preventable factors leading to admission for a physical illness. They reported that social factors were critical in the decision to admit 21% of patients to a metropolitan hospital. Boaz (1979) described how utilization review could help contain hospital costs; for patients admitted on an emergency basis, LOS was strongly affected by social factors.

Therefore, psychiatric and psychosocial factors are operative at every phase of an illness episode: before admission, as reasons or "pressures" for admission; during hospitalization; and when decisions are made that influence discharge and aftercare placement. Decisions made at any of these phases will affect detection and treatment of psychiatric comorbidity and LOS and will therefore affect outcome and costs. Thus, interventions must be designed to address the biopsychosocial issues that affect decisions to admit and retain patients who have no medical reasons for admission or for prolonged LOS. Aftercare and discharge planning ultimately affect LOS, and these are often dependent on biopsychosocial factors.

In the early 1970s, Berkman and Rehr (1972, 1973) reported that biopsychosocial needs were typically identified only late in the hospitalization (if at all), by social workers. Decreasing the lag time (i.e., timing the psychosocial intervention so that it occurred as early as possible in the hospitalization) was hypothesized to enhance patient care and decrease LOS. Currently, social workers are part of the medical-surgical team, do not wait for referrals, and are involved with the entire ward population (the denominator); they have moved from the referral to the liaison model. In so doing, they have become the primary mental health professionals on medical or surgical wards.

Most studies involving inpatient medical populations are flawed because of one or more confounding factors, including measurement and instrumentation problems; a lack of randomization of control and experimental samples; the transfer from experimental to control environments (i.e., extending the intervention to the control setting); the failure to consider the seriousness of the medical illness, the number of medical and psychiatric diagnoses, and the complexity of medical and surgical interventions; and poor statistical management of physiologic and psychosocial data. More than 60 years ago, Billings (1936) described improved biopsychosocial status and earlier hospital discharge after a psychiatric intervention. Bonilla et al. (1961) noted improved well-being and reduced complaints of pain on a surgical service after hypnosis. Boone et al. (1981) reported that early and comprehensive intervention by social workers improved psychosocial well-being and reduced LOS by 1.25 days ($P = 0.001$, F $= 10.10$, $df = 1,362$) in an experimental group compared with a control cohort. However, the investigators did not control for transfer effect (the control group thereby mitigated the difference in the intervention). The intervention permitted early access to every patient (the liaison method) without a wait for referral (i.e., a consultation request) and resulted in a cost-offset effect.

Levitan and Kornfeld (1981) documented in orthopedic patients that a psychiatric liaison service, in contrast to the traditional consultation approach, resulted in a cost offset—earlier discharge and more discharges to home than to a nursing home (LOS was 30 vs. 42 days, and discharge to home was 16 vs. 8 patients, respectively, for the experimental and control cohorts [$P < 0.05$]).

Ackerman et al. (1988) described the effect of coexisting depression and the timing of psychiatric consultation on medical inpatients' LOSs. They found that 11% of the variance in LOS in the control and experimental populations was accounted for by the timing of the consultation. Specifically, psychiatric consultations that occurred earlier in the hospital stay were associated with an LOS closer to that expected for the diagnosis-related group system. Therefore, early detection and treatment, when necessary, may significantly decrease LOS and the expenditure of medical resources.

Levenson et al. (1992) examined the psychiatric and economic outcomes of psychiatric consultation guided by screening in general medical patients. Although they found neither psychosocial improvement nor earlier discharge—hospital stays were quite short to begin with—these results may have been due to the use of heterogeneous medical populations; the fact that each patient had only one visit by the psychiatrist; the use of "indirect" interventions implemented through the consultee, with less than 50% concordance with the consultant's recommendations; the use of an inner-city disadvantaged population; and the examination of patients whose preintervention LOSs were already short.

Strain et al. (1991) compared liaison psychiatry interventions and the traditional consultation approach in elderly hip-fracture patients at two sites—Mount Sinai Hospital (MSH) in New York City and Northwestern Memorial Hospital (NMH) in Chicago—using identical assessment and intervention designs. All patients were assessed by the psychiatrist at the time of admission and were treated as needed with psychological therapy and/or pharmacotherapy after a review of all medications. Cases were discussed in weekly multidisciplinary ombudsman rounds (Strain and Hamerman 1978), and psychosocial or psychological issues were reviewed and dealt with (e.g., appropriate follow-up care was arranged) during discharge planning. Treatment was coordinated with the social worker, the patient's significant others and caretakers (including nursing home personnel), and the treatment team. In the comparison (traditional consultation) group, less than 10% (MSH) and 3% (NMH) were referred for consultation, whereas in the experimental (liaison) cohort, 70%–80% underwent assessment and intervention when indicated. (The remaining patients refused to give informed consent and therefore had to be excluded.)

The liaison intervention, in contrast to the consultation approach, detected significant DSM-III-R (American Psychiatric Association 1987) psychiatric morbidity (56%), resulted in less depression and cognitive impairment at the time of discharge, decreased LOS by 2 days, led to fewer rehabilitation days, and resulted in no rehospitalizations within a 12-week follow-up period. The confounds of age, sex, severity of illness, number of psychiatric diagnoses, bone density, complexity of orthopedic procedures, stability of fracture, socioeconomic class, study site, and year of study were all taken into account in the regression analysis, which revealed that 11% of the variance in the difference in cost could be explained by assessment and intervention. There was no transfer of cost from the inpatient to the outpatient phase. In fact, not only were inpatient costs reduced, but postdischarge costs—12-week ambulatory costs—were diminished as well. In conclusion, the liaison approach resulted in increased psychiatric well-being and significant cost offset at both hospitals (e.g., at MSH, the $20,000 cost of intervention resulted in a $167,000 savings—a 1:8 cost-offset ratio).

Other studies have shown the importance of addressing the biopsychosocial needs of all patients at or near the time of admission to enhance screening of the patients' status and to conserve health care costs. Hammer and colleagues (J.S. Hammer, H.T.C. Lam, and J.J. Strain, unpublished data, September 1993) used a high-risk screening approach in the admission office to evaluate the denominator (i.e., every admission to a large municipal general hospital) and observed that when the time between psychosocial assessment and treatment was shortened, patients with psychiatric and medical comorbidity were discharged earlier. For each dollar spent on the social-risk screening program, the study hospital saved \$48 (a 1:48 cost-offset ratio).

The mechanisms that underlie the liaison intervention and the effects of its components are not fully understood. As they are discovered, the liaison model can be tailored to achieve the maximum effect: For example, early discharge planning, working with the nursing staff, decreasing the use of unnecessary sleep medication, early treatment of delirium, and encouragement of compliance may be key to the effectiveness of a liaison intervention. Results of one study indicated that patients with less serious psychiatric disorders, or none at all, may benefit most from a liaison intervention (A. Diefenbacher, J. J. Strain, and G. Fulop, "Comparison of consultation-liaison psychiatry units in two university teaching hospitals: Free University of Berlin and Mount Sinai Medical Center (New York City)," unpublished data, December 1999). The study patients' compliance was enhanced, physical therapists were encouraged to "push" recalcitrant elderly patients, family members and nursing home staff were counseled about managing psychotic states, and the use of neuroleptics allowed earlier discharge of patients who had previously been frightening to significant others.

CONCEPTUAL FRAMEWORK OF LIAISON PSYCHIATRY

Although consultation remains the cornerstone of the liaison process, the emphasis of liaison differentiates these two models of psychiatric intervention. The pedagogical thrust of liaison psychiatry and the attempt to formalize patient care—in contrast to the catch-as-catch-can format of the consultation intervention—are underscored by the aims of liaison psychiatry (Strain and Grossman 1975): to

- Practice primary, secondary, and tertiary prevention
- Foster case detection and triage methodologies
- Provide continuing education to nonpsychiatric staff to promote assessment, treatment, and/or referral of patients with psychiatric disorders
- Develop basic biopsychosocial knowledge
- Promote structural or methodological changes in the medical setting to enhance detection and treatment of psychiatric disorders

Liaison psychiatry differs from consultation in yet another way: liaison psychiatrists cannot charge third-

party payers for their nondirect patient encounters and instead depend on support from host departments, hospital administrations, federal grants, or innovative forms of funding. Finally, a systematic attempt at "liaison" occurs in no other specialty of medicine. For example, radiology, surgery, and internal medicine all rely on the consultation method for the primary exchange of information and patient care on a host service. What makes the liaison model particularly appropriate in the medical setting is that the biopsychosocial model dictates that for every illness and every patient, psychological, social, and psychiatric considerations for assessment, treatment, and follow-up should be considered (Engel 1977).

Primary, Secondary, and Tertiary Prevention

Using Caplan's (1964) model of prevention—that is, anticipating and preventing the development of psychiatric or psychological symptoms (primary prevention), treating such symptoms when they are manifested (secondary prevention), and forestalling their recurrence or ensuring early treatment (tertiary prevention)—enhances the quality of psychological and medical care when liaison principles are applied.

The goal of primary prevention is to prevent psychiatric disorders through early intervention. An example of primary prevention would be conducting psychiatric interviews of all patients before cardiotomy. This intervention might prevent the occurrence of delirium (Surman 1974). Frasure-Smith et al. (1993) demonstrated that myocardial infarction patients who are depressed have a three times greater chance of dying than myocardial infarction patients who do not have a mood disorder. This chance is even greater among depressed patients with non–Q-wave infarction (Frasure-Smith et al. 1993). The occurrence of black patch psychosis has taught us to operate on only one eye at a time.

In secondary prevention, the clinician uses tactics to attempt to reduce the factors—biological, psychological, and social—that have initiated disease; attend to the stress of illness; and manage acute symptoms such as anxiety, depression, and exaggeration of character traits that may worsen stress and impede recovery. As Hackett and Cassem (1979) stated, consultation psychiatry is primarily a secondary prevention effort.

In tertiary prevention, the liaison psychiatrist strives to alter the psychological sequelae that may follow an acute episode (e.g., psychological conflicts that result in mood disturbances, anxiety, and inhibitions and phobias about returning to work or resuming sexual activity despite physiologic competence to do so). Frasure-Smith et al. (1992, 1993) determined that patients with myocardial infarction should be screened for depressive mood disorders, which, if present, should then be treated. Such screening may be lifesaving. Psychiatric tertiary intervention facilitates patients' adaptation to their physiologic limitations, thereby lessening the possibility of recurrent illness. Preventing recurrence of illness frequently requires skilled outpatient follow-up after discharge from the general hospital (Rowan et al. 1984).

Detection and Diagnosis

Case detection in the medical setting is a skill possessed by the liaison psychiatrist that often goes well beyond the skill of the consultation psychiatrist, who waits to be called by colleagues. Consultation psychiatrists typically have difficulties in detecting psychosocial dysfunction. These difficulties may be due to interrelationships with staff, or they may occur either because the dysfunction is not readily apparent or because the patient or the staff do not reveal the conflict. The liaison method encourages staff to verbalize their frustrations with a patient, and often staff feelings should be the focus of the consultation. Some interventions with staff require a special relationship that allows the verbalization of intense feelings and conflicts (e.g., anger toward the patient, wishing that the patient would die, or not wanting to give the patient a scarce donor organ). In fact, because consultation psychiatry must depend on referral from poorly motivated or poorly informed consultees, it remains a secondary prevention intervention, and often the relationship between consultee and consultant is tenuous.

The liaison psychiatrist teaches prospective consultees to acquire and synthesize data, which enhances awareness, detection, diagnosis, and/or referral of psychiatric morbidity, in contrast to the consultant psychiatrist, who waits for the consultee to seek him or her out. Psychiatric disorders due to a medical illness and substance-induced psychiatric disorders are the prototype of the psychophysiological disorders frequently present, but often undetected, in the medical-surgical setting (Engel 1967).

If potential consultees are unaware that their patients have a dysfunction, why would they request a consultation? Strategies and tactics for case detection and triage are essential in the medical-surgical setting and constitute hallmarks of liaison psychiatry. Diagnostic screening devices for the disorders of cognitive function (Folstein et al. 1975; Jacobs et al. 1977), depression, anxiety, and substance abuse are currently available if the structure is altered from a consultation model to one that incorporates triage methodology (Gehi et al. 1980).

Appropriately trained physicians are the best screening tools for psychiatric morbidity in medically ill patients; however, easily used screening devices are available for primary care providers. One such device, the Symptom-Driven Diagnostic System (Broadhead et al. 1995), can also be used in the following way: A telephone admission screen report of potential psychiatric morbidity is provided to the physician at the time of evaluation. An alert is then forwarded regarding the potential risk of depression, panic, obsessive-compulsive disorder, anxiety, and suicide. Such an alert helps focus the history taking to confirm the suspicion of a psychiatric disorder. The Symptom-Driven Diagnostic System can also be used for follow-up evaluation of psychiatric morbidity during and after a course of treatment. The Primary Care Evaluation of Mental Disorders (PRIME-MD; Spitzer et al. 1994) is another important screening device used in the general medical or surgical setting to improve detection of psychiatric morbidity.

The liaison psychiatrist must caution that these screening devices may produce false-negative and false-positive results. Liaison psychiatry attempts to develop reliable, valid, cost-effective structures to identify psychiatric mobidity. These structures then require further validation by clinical assessment and verification against clinical algorithms (e.g., DSM-IV-TR [American Psychiatric Association 2000]). The liaison psychiatrist strives to improve detection, avoiding false-negative and false-positive screening assessments, and to offer guidelines for clinical assessment and necessary treatment. To do this, the liaison psychiatrist must first develop mechanisms to screen at-risk patient groups entering the health care system for psychosocial and psychiatric morbidity and must also develop appropriate alert systems for the primary care physician or case manager. Second, the liaison psychiatrist must help establish protocols to confirm or rule out these suspicions. Third, the liaison psychiatrist must establish diagnostic and treatment plans for patients found to have psychiatric morbidity.

Assessment of Medical Care Providers

The alliance model of liaison psychiatry incorporates the proposition that psychiatric care of medically ill patients is not solely the responsibility of the psychiatrist. Rather, the responsibility is shared by doctors, nurses, social workers, important family members, and others who create the psychological climate of the ward.

The crucial function of the consultation-liaison psychiatrist is to assess the degree of stress that patients produce in their medical care providers and in their families, the capacity of hospital staff and family members to adapt to patients and to their illnesses (and to the interventions of psychological care), and, above all, the ability of staff and family to conduct or at least support psychiatric or psychological care. In liaison psychiatry, the goals of consultation-liaison psychiatry are expanded to include teaching awareness, interviewing, and knowledge of simple psychiatric interventions. These liaison goals are based on the fact that the majority of mentally ill individuals are seen as outpatients in the general medical setting, where a consulting psychiatrist is not always available to take over a patient's mental health care. Katon and Gonzales (1994) reviewed randomized controlled trials and determined that merely telling the primary care physician about the existence of psychiatric morbidity, or even giving diagnostic and treatment advice, is not sufficient to alter patient outcome. The psychiatrist must examine the patient with his or her primary care physician, and information must be provided to both the patient and the doctor. Two or three follow-up visits should be conducted with the psychiatrist in attendance. In the trials reviewed by Katon and Gonzales (1994), less effort than this liaison involvement did not result in a difference in patient outcome.

Development of Autonomy in Nonpsychiatric Staff

Burns et al. (1983) described several domains of mental health knowledge and skills used as a schema for teaching and assessment. This grid allows educators and evaluators to establish goals for their training programs or for particular disciplines: psychiatry, primary care, psychology, social work, clinical nursing, pastoral counseling, discharge planning, patient advocacy, and even village health care in developing countries (Strain et al. 1985b) (Figure 4–2).

The development and distribution of guidelines by the liaison psychiatrist enhances the competence of the medical and nursing staff. Such guidelines are regarded as important tools for teaching and enhancing clinical care. The Institute of Medicine described eight attributes of a guideline: 1) validity (including the strength of the evidence and estimated outcomes), 2) reliability and reproducibility, 3) clinical applicability, 4) clinical flexibility, 5) clarity, 6) multidisciplinary process, 7) scheduled review, and 8) documentation (Field and Lohr 1990, 1992). The Agency for Health Care Policy and Research's publication *Depression in Primary Care* incorporates these attributes and is a primer for teaching about, diagnosing, and treating depression in the medical setting (Rush et al. 1993). One of the first guidelines is for depression in primary care (Depression Guideline Panel 1993a, 1993b). This guideline (published in two vol-

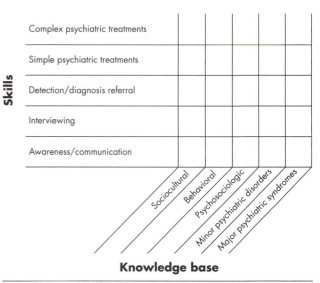

FIGURE 4–2.   Domains of knowledge and skills.

Source. Reprinted from Strain JJ, Pincus HA, Gise LH, et al: "The Role of Psychiatry in the Training of Primary Care Physicians." *Gen Hosp Psychiatry* 8:372–385, 1986. Copyright 1986, Elsevier Science. Used with permission.

umes: *Detection and Diagnosis* and *Treatment of Major Depression)* carefully details how to manage depression in primary care and when to refer patients to other mental health specialists. The American Psychiatric Association (1999) recently published its guideline for the diagnosis and management of delirium. Such guidelines are an important adjunct to the teaching function of the liaison psychiatrist.

To improve the national level of health care and cost controls, the Agency for Health Care Policy and Research formulated guidelines to describe parameters of clinical care that will set the stage for Health Care Financing Agency reimbursement of Medicare claims:

> Practice guidelines are "systematically developed statements to assist practitioner and patient decisions about appropriate health care for specific clinical circumstances....Practice guidelines focus...on assisting patients and practitioners in making decisions, but this defining characteristic does not and should not preclude their use for other purposes including quality improvement and payment policymaking (Field and Lohr 1992, p. 27).

Development of New Knowledge

Until recently, consultation-liaison psychiatry lacked both a systematic method for accumulating a clinical database and suitable models for processing data. In addition, very few randomized controlled trials had been undertaken regarding psychiatric morbidity in the medical setting (Katon et al. 1995, 1996). There is available an optically scanned computerized clinical database schema for needs assessment, learner appraisal, systems analysis, and measurement of the impact of liaison teaching on the consultation-referral process. With MICROCARES (Hammer et al. 1985a, 1995), which currently uses Windows 95/98 technology, data may be entered on a computerized notepad with an electronic pen while at the patient's side. This program allows the user to develop and print the medical chart note from the computerized record, create a letter to the referring physician, print out the patient's Current Procedural Terminology (CPT) treatment codes, and create a diskette with the patient's data that can be read by another physician as a text file. The program automatically constructs a case profile of every consulting physician—a portfolio of the physician's caseload—and allows the study of specific subsets of patients, whose data can be exported to statistical programs for analyses. Thus, important liaison functions can flow directly from the pen entry dataset to clinical, administrative, research, and education (CARE) pursuits.

Using this system, Strain et al. (1998) were able to study adjustment disorders in the general medical setting. New information became available through observation of patients at multiple teaching hospitals. Adjustment disorders took as much clinical and supervisory time as major psychiatric disorders. The percentage of patients prescribed psychotropic drugs was the same for those with adjustment disorders as for those with major psychiatric disorders (Smith et al. 1998). When patients with "organic mental disorders" (a term eliminated in DSM-IV [American Psychiatric Association 1994]) were studied at multiple sites, personality disorder was found to be a common comorbidity (Smith et al. 1997).

Administrative uses include tracking the compliance with recommendations from consultations over time (Popkin et al. 1983). Patterns of consultation use and misuse may be studied along with over- or underutilization of services. Workloads of staff can also be monitored. By noting the problem stated by the consultee and comparing it with the problem assessed by the consultant, it is possible to detect the nonpsychiatric physician's view of "labeling" of the patient and the need for enhanced teaching (Strain et al. 1985a). The clinical database and optiscan software management system permit a comparison of a liaison ward and a nonliaison ward. For example, Strain et al. (1985b) found that liaison ward consultees were more likely to detect cognitive dysfunction than were those from nonliaison wards and that there was less mislabeling (*P* < 0.01).

Because the literature database is burgeoning, there must be some system to sift this enormous data set for information important to psychiatric care in the medical

setting. By using 100 experts to sort through thousands of studies, select the crème de la crème, and describe why the selections are important, it is possible to have a database at the patient's side to enhance clinical decision making. The liaison psychiatrist can also print a computerized summary of the scientific report to accompany the computer-generated medical chart note, both of which serve as pedagogical instruments for the consultant and the consultee (Strain et al. 1996b, 1999b).

With these technological advances, the liaison psychiatrist can study and record the system of the ward, teach the medical, nursing, and social worker caretakers, and develop important observations and access a literature database for the subspecialty.

Structural Changes in the Medical Setting

Liaison psychiatry strives to effect structural changes in the department of psychiatry and in other departments throughout the hospital (e.g., psychiatric-medical units, pain clinics, postpartum assessment units, and orthopedic departments) that will endure beyond the tenure of a given individual (Strain et al. 1991). The psychiatric-medical unit (in the department of medicine) and the medical-psychiatric unit (in the department of psychiatry) manage medically ill patients too psychiatrically disturbed to be on a medical ward and too medically ill to be on a psychiatry ward. This approach offers a way to deal with serious medical and psychiatric comorbidity (Kathol 1994; Kathol et al. 1992). In such units, the psychiatrist has a special opportunity to work with the medical nursing staff in the diagnosis and treatment of complex and at times intractable comorbid conditions (e.g., pain syndromes).

The liaison clinic permits follow-up of consultations after hospitalization, of patients discharged from the psychiatric-medical unit, and of ambulatory patients from the medical and surgical clinics who have psychological dysfunction (Rowan et al. 1984). Because psychiatric outpatient departments in most hospitals are often unable to accommodate psychologically dysfunctional medically ill patients, an outpatient clinic under liaison psychiatry auspices offers an important addition to the psychiatric armamentarium in the general hospital. Another model is to attach a liaison psychiatrist to a clinic as part of the team. In such a role, the psychiatrist not only assists in the diagnosis and management of patients but also serves as teacher, advisor, and collaborator in the clinic team.

In many hospitals, psychiatric clearance is now standard for all drug overdose patients before they are discharged from the intensive care unit or medical wards. The next logical step is to make psychiatric clearance mandatory for all high-risk or difficult patients, such as candidates for open-heart surgery who have affective disorders; patients with recent myocardial infarction (in particular, those with non–Q-wave infarction), who may be at greater risk of dying if they are also depressed (Frasure-Smith et al. 1992, 1993); liver transplant candidates whose need for surgery is in doubt; and patients whose repeated hospital admissions appear to be the result of self-abuse or self-neglect. Psychiatric assessment of these patients and other groups yet to be identified should be regarded as an intrinsic part of liaison psychiatry patient evaluation and management in the contemporary teaching hospital. Administrative changes are needed to ensure that these at-risk cohorts are screened and evaluated for life-threatening psychiatric morbidity (Frasure-Smith et al. 1993). Yet one of the most important steps toward implementing liaison psychiatry is through the mental health training of primary care physicians.

MODELS OF PSYCHIATRIC TRAINING FOR PRIMARY CARE PHYSICIANS

One of the most important functions of liaison psychiatry is to teach certain mental health concepts to primary care physicians, who see the majority of patients with mental health morbidity in the United States. The issue in such teaching is not involving a patient in consultation, but forming a relationship founded on the pedagogic needs of the primary care physician to detect, diagnose, refer, or treat his or her patient who has primary psychiatric disorders or psychiatric sequelae to physical dysfunction (Strain and Grossman 1975).

To elucidate the models of mental health training employed for residents in three primary care specialties—internal medicine (7,000 trainees), family practice (4,000 trainees), and general primary care (1,000 trainees)—three research contracts were awarded to me by the National Institute of Mental Health (NIMH). Strain et al. (1985b) and Pincus et al. (1983) reviewed the literature, examined NIMH training grant proposals, interviewed funding agency personnel, and made 35 site visits to internal medicine, general primary care medicine, and family practice residency training programs supported by NIMH and the Health Resources Services Administration. On the basis of this multifaceted survey, we described six models of mental health training for the nonpsychiatric physician (Figure 4–3) (Strain et al. 1987). A seventh model has also been added below, following the six described in the survey.

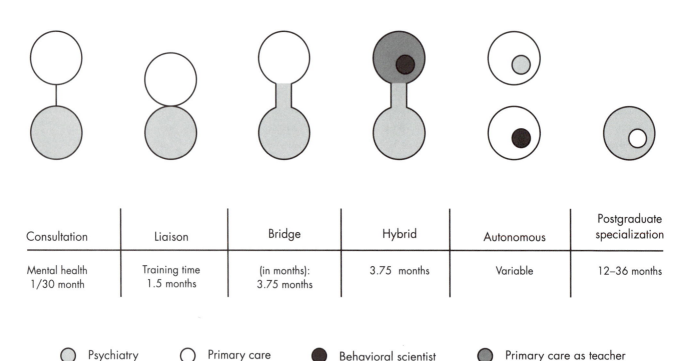

Consultation	Liaison	Bridge	Hybrid	Autonomous	Postgraduate specialization
Mental health 1/30 month	Training time 1.5 months	(in months): 3.75 months	3.75 months	Variable	12–36 months

○ Psychiatry   ○ Primary care   ● Behavioral scientist   ● Primary care as teacher

FIGURE 4–3. Models of primary care training in mental health.

Source. Reprinted from Strain JJ, Pincus HA, Gise LH, et al: "The Role of Psychiatry in the "Training of Primary Care Physicians." *Gen Hosp Psychiatry* 8:372–385, 1986. Copyright 1986, Elsevier Science. Used with permission.

1. **Consultation model.** The standard medical consultation approach is based on the case method (i.e., the consultee initiates the consultation and undergoes no formal, structured teaching such as didactic sessions, seminars, and precepting). The psychiatrist acts as a consultant and may teach the staff in the context of an individual case but by and large takes over the mental health aspects of the patient's care. Some teaching may take place through the psychiatrist's consultation note or spoken exchanges with the medical staff.

2. **Liaison model.** In addition to the elements of the consultation model, formal, structured, pedagogical exercises are used to teach basic information and skills. A teaching structure is established (e.g., weekly medical-psychiatric rounds, monthly lunch teaching sessions with residents, and monthly meetings with attending physicians). Teaching conferences led by prominent and respected teachers from the fields of medicine and psychiatry are presented, with residents, medical students, fellows, nurses, and social workers in attendance. A psychiatrist-teacher often becomes a continuing member of a medical or surgical unit or team. The liaison psychiatrist imparts psychiatric information to medical and surgical residents, which is important because mental health education is at a minimum during most medical and surgical residencies.

3. **Bridge model.** A psychiatrist-teacher, affiliated with a department of psychiatry, is assigned to one primary care teaching site (often an ambulatory training site) for a major portion of his or her time; teaching is structured. The host medical service pays for the psychiatrist and "employs" him or her as a teacher for the staff and, in particular, for house staff. The teaching sessions are required, and the availability of the psychiatrist allows constant dissemination of information about mental health issues.

4. **Hybrid model.** Mental health teaching is done by a psychiatrist, a behavioral scientist (e.g., psychologist, social worker, or sociologist) who is part of a multidisciplinary team, and the primary care faculty. The focus of the teaching depends on the discipline of the teacher. Communication skills, doctor-patient relationship issues, family conflicts, adaptation to medical illness, and compliance are often emphasized by nonpsychiatric teachers.

5. **Autonomous, psychiatric model.** The psychiatrist is hired by the primary care group and has no formal connection with a department of psychiatry or teaching service, or psychosocial teaching is done exclusively by a nonpsychiatrist behavioral scientist (e.g., psychologist, social worker, or sociologist) not affiliated with a department of psychiatry.

6. **Postgraduate specialty training model.** The primary care physician is trained in a mental health setting for 1 or 2 years, gaining considerable expertise in detecting, diagnosing, and treating mental health disorders. In essence, the primary care physician has had a fellowship in medical psychiatry. With the exception of the most complicated and difficult patients, this model trains a primary care physician in the majority of interventions for the psychiatric morbidity of medically ill patients.

7. **Double-board training model.** The primary care physician is trained in psychiatry as well as his or her medical or surgical specialty. In essence, the primary care physician should have the full range of competencies expected of a resident completing psychiatric training. This training is very expensive, takes several years to complete, and often results in a physician whose primary focus is psychiatry. The outcome of such training needs to be more carefully studied with regard to career choices and the types of patients such physicians eventually treat.

Several methods for teaching mental health information, skills, and attitudes were reported. Internal medicine employed the formal psychiatric consultation model for 68% of its mental health training, in contrast to 30% and 22.5% for family practice and general primary care, respectively. Internal medicine rarely used a psychiatric rotation but relied on the medical inpatient setting for 80% of its mental health training. The modal internal medicine resident requested three or four psychiatric consultations per year and spent an average of less than 15 minutes per patient with the consultant. Consequently, with the psychiatric consultation model, internal medicine residents inclined to initiate consultations received a total of 3–4 hours of instruction in mental health.

Furthermore, internal medicine, which relied on the consultation for teaching, was less likely than general primary care or family practice to emphasize sociocultural issues, focus on communication skills, use complex psychosocial management or simple pharmacotherapy, evaluate trainees' performance as a result of pedagogical efforts, or pay for the mental health instruction of their trainees. Seventy-one percent of the funds for mental health training in internal medicine programs came exclusively from psychiatry departments, in contrast to 15% in primary care programs and 1.6% in family practice programs.

Overall, the consultation method of relating with medicine was the weakest model that psychiatry offered. When the consultation model was used in primary care and family practice, it was relegated to a minor role because these specialties relied primarily on nonpsychiatric behavioral scientists for most of their teaching. They preferred a liaison relationship with the teacher rather than with an intermittent, itinerant consultant. These teaching models will have enhanced importance with the advent of health care reform, which projects that the majority of mental health care will be delivered in primary care settings (see guidelines in "Conclusion"). In addition, randomized controlled trials reviewed by Katon and his group (Katon and Gonzalez 1994) demonstrated a need for a structured teaching relationship with primary care to improve outcome of patients with depressive disorders. This training experience needs to be sufficiently intense and repeated sufficiently over time to obtain a significant difference in patient outcomes, compared to outcomes for patients treated for a similar depressive disorder by an untrained or less trained primary care physician. The intensity of mental health training required for improving patient outcome is an important lesson for medicine and psychiatry to observe. If we are to expect that primary care physicians take a major role in the treatment of major mental disorder, such as major depressive disorders, single consultations are not sufficient to deliver this competency.

Another classification program was presented by Greenhill (1977), who conceptualized five variations of liaison psychiatry on methods of practice rather than pedagogical relationships between psychiatry and medicine:

1. **Basic liaison model.** The basic liaison model typically involves a psychiatrist from a department of psychiatry who is assigned to a medical-surgical unit for the express purpose of teaching.
2. **Critical care model.** The critical care model provides for the assignment of mental health care providers to critical care units rather than to clinical departments. The goals are patient care and staff consultation. The psychiatrist is a member of the unit team. Teaching combines behavioral and psychodynamic models as well as the model of biological psychiatry, including focus on topics such as the use of psychopharmacological agents in patients who are seriously medically ill and the effects of drug interactions and end-organ dysfunction on assessment and choice of treatment.
3. **Biological model.** The biological model is a more exacting variation of the critical care model that emphasizes neuroscience, psychopharmacology, and psychological management. The psychiatrist acts as a member of diagnosis-centered treatment units (e.g., dysphoria clinic, pain center, psychopharmacology clinic) and, through psychiatric, psychological, psychopharmacological, and environmental manipulation, serves as a member of the team. Biological measures are important to diagnosis and treatment interventions.
4. **Milieu model.** The milieu model emphasizes the group aspects of the patient care–group process, staff reactions and interactions, interpersonal theory, and creation of a therapeutic environment on the ward. This model was formulated before psychiatry-medicine units were described.
5. **Integral model.** The integral model is emerging as a result of social pressure on medicine. It relies more on hospital governance than on triage by physicians. The aforementioned models of liaison programs depend on consultation with patients and staff and on working relationships with physicians. This model is based, in addition, on the inclusion of psychological care.

Hammer et al. (1985b), at Northwestern University, took the integral model of liaison psychiatry to its most developed form in an innovative human services department (Strain and Grossman 1975). Moving well beyond the consultation and referral model, Hammer and colleagues (1985b) established an administrative organization for the delivery of biopsychosocial care in the contemporary teaching hospital. This model takes an evolutionary step beyond multidisciplinary team approaches by combining core psychosocial service delivery disciplines under centralized medical leadership: consultation-liaison psychiatry, social work services, pastoral care, home care, supportive care, and patient representatives. Thus, these investigators asserted that "the long range goal of this organization is to provide cost-effective psychosocial services . . . while maintaining the unique role contributions of the participating disciplines" (Hammer et al. 1985b, p. 189).

The integrated human services model of consultation-liaison psychiatry remedies the isolation among mental health disciplines in the medical setting and the lack of integrated formal structure that characterize the traditional consultation model. Unfortunately, this model of central triage of requests for mental health services, assignment to the appropriate disciplines, unified record keeping, and evaluation of consultation and treatment outcomes was not continued after Hammer left Northwestern University. It was proposed that such an integrated model would affect the structure of the hospital at the highest level, and, as with the role taken by infectious-disease personnel, the identification and treatment of psychiatric and psychosocial needs would be part of the warp and woof of the general hospital. There would be a concerted effort to measure the effect of addressing the psychological care of the medical ill regarding 1) medical outcome, 2) psychiatric morbidity, 3) hospital costs (primarily length of hospital stay), 4) placement after discharge (e.g., health-related facility or home), 5) quality of life and satisfaction of care. If it can be shown that global attention to psychiatric needs, as now practiced for infection control, leads to significant improvement in the majority of the five outcome measures described, and that the cost of interventions is more than compensated by cost-effectiveness and cost savings, then addressing the psychiatric and psychosocial needs of medically ill patients in the general hospital should be universal.

CONCLUSION

Physicians in the medical specialties increasingly have been turning to mental health disciplines other than psychiatry for training and collaborative care of their patients. Many reasons have been postulated. Nonpsychiatric mental health care workers charge less, are easier to incorporate into the medical-surgical team (consider, for example, a social worker's daily presence on the ward and his or her participation in team rounds, knowledge about the majority of patients and multidisciplines, and willingness to interact with families), are comfortable using the problem level of diagnosis rather than a formal psychiatric taxonomy, and are willing to provide postdischarge ambulatory care for probands identified during hospitalization (e.g., to follow patients through an episode of illness). Liaison psychiatry has attempted to address these mandates prescribed by the medical-surgical specialties.

Internal medicine uses psychiatry to "educate" through the consultation but usually pays nothing for mental health training. The number of nonpsychiatric behavioral science teachers will continue to increase, because primary care specialists, other than those who practice internal medicine, want a liaison presence and want their teachers to be team members. As long as psychiatry's relationship with the other specialties of medicine is formulated on the consultation model (and consultation psychiatry's reliance on the medical inpatient), the ability of primary care physicians to adequately meet the needs of the de facto mental health service (Regier et al. 1978) will become even more attenuated. With the current health care revolution that often mandates primary care providers as gatekeepers for health care, initial assessment and treatment of psychiatric disorders often occur in the primary care setting.

However, not having a psychiatrist as a teacher for primary care presents a problem in the area of interactions between psychotropic agents and medical drugs (Strain et al. 1996a, 1999b). The psychiatrist teacher also understands pharmacokinetics as it relates to end-organ dysfunction (e.g., kidney, liver, lung, heart, the aging process). Furthermore, because most medically ill patients are receiving drug therapy, the liaison psychiatrist must develop methods to review, codify, and describe the most important interactions and must be able to obtain adequate information to update his or her knowledge about these interactions.

Because many psychotropic drugs have not been tested in conjunction with medical drugs (e.g., protease inhibitors), the psychiatrist must have access to technical reports and materials that highlight drug interactions. Important information may be obtained from the F-D-C Reports' "Pink Sheets" and the Micromedex Drug-Reax database. In addition, it may be important for the psychiatrist working with medically ill patients to consult the journals *Pharmacotherapy, Annals of Pharmacotherapy, Clinical Pharmacology and Therapeutics, Drug Safety,* and *Drugs.* Other sources of information on drug interactions are Clin-Alert, Reactions, Clinical Abstracts/Current Therapeutic Findings, Current Contents/Adverse Reactions, Excerpta Medica/Adverse Reactions, *American Journal of Health-System Pharmacy,* and Current Literature. Stoudemire and Brown (1998) wrote an excellent volume entitled *Psychiatric Side Effects of Prescription and Over the Counter Medications,* but this work does not cover interactions in detail. Ciraulo et al. (1995) developed an important work on drug-drug interactions, but at the time of writing this chapter, they do not plan to bring out an updated edition. Goldman has developed a software package dealing with psychotropic drug interactions, *Interact,* available on CD (Goldman 1999).

Liaison psychiatrists must keep up with this important information, which can be lifesaving, and share it in understandable forms with primary care providers. Mastering information about psychotropic–medical drug interactions will only become more difficult and time-consuming. No other mental health discipline has the training to do so, nor the conceptual framework to apply this knowledge in the medical setting to patients with psychiatric and medical comorbidity.

Primary care must have bridges to psychiatry that far exceed the bridge to psychiatry provided by the consultation model if primary care providers are to effectively diagnose and treat depression, deal with psychotropic–medical drug interactions, and continually access mechanisms for updating recent adverse drug interactions. The limited training received through use of the consultation model is not sufficient, nor is the liaison model commonly applied in the inpatient setting. Rather, a pedagogical relationship between psychiatry and primary care is needed, to transmit knowledge and skills so that primary care physicians can adequately assess, treat, and/or refer patients. As described previously, Katon and Gonzales (1994) showed that an extended relationship with primary care is needed to improve outcome in depressed patients.

In liaison psychiatry, which targets all individuals, the conceptual framework includes the goal of early detection and treatment of many disorders. Liaison psychiatry will have even greater importance in this era of national health care reform, improved standards of care, and cost containment. Wells (1994), reporting findings of three health policy studies, noted that 1) in the general medical sector, prepaid care is associated with lower rates of detection of depression and psychosocial counseling of depressed patients; 2) across types of payment in the general medical sector, quality of care for depressed patients is moderate to low; and 3) in acute care general medical hospitals, depressed elderly patients receive better psychological care in psychiatric units but better medical care in general medical wards. The findings emphasize "the role of the consultation-liaison psychiatrist in educating general medical providers about treatment of depression, regardless of system of care, but giving special emphasis to improving outcomes for the sickest patients and improving detection of depression and psychosocial counseling in prepaid practices" (Wells 1994, p. 279). Liaison psychiatry defines the next generation of interaction with other medical disciplines and is positioned to move well beyond the traditional consultation model.

REFERENCES

Ackerman AD, Lyons JS, Hammer JS, et al: The impact of co-existing depression and timing of psychiatric consultation on medical patients' length of stay. Hospital and Community Psychiatry 39:173–176, 1988

American Psychiatric Association: Diagnostic and Statistical Manual of Mental Disorders, 3rd Edition, Revised. Washington, DC, American Psychiatric Association, 1987

American Psychiatric Association: Diagnostic and Statistical Manual of Mental Disorders, 4th Edition. Washington, DC, American Psychiatric Association, 1994

American Psychiatric Association: Practice Guideline for the Treatment of Patients With Delirium. Edited by Work Group on Delirium (Trzepacz P, Breitbart W, Frankline J, et al). Washington, DC, American Psychiatric Association, 1999

American Psychiatric Association: Diagnostic and Statistical Manual of Mental Disorders, 4th Edition, Text Revision. Washington, DC, American Psychiatric Association, 2000

Berkman BG, Rehr H: The sick role cycle and the timing of social work intervention. Social Service Review 46:567–580, 1972

Berkman BG, Rehr H: Early social service case finding for hospitalized patients: an experiment. Social Service Review 47:256–265, 1973

Billings EG: Teaching psychiatry in a general hospital. JAMA 107:635–639, 1936

Billings EG: Value of psychiatry to the general hospital. Hospitals 15:30–34, 1941

Boaz R: Utilization review and containment of hospital utilization. Med Care 17:315–330, 1979

Bonilla K, Quigley W, Bowers W: Experiences with hypnosis on a surgical service. Mil Med 126:364–370, 1961

Boone CR, Coulton CJ, Keller SM: The impact of early and comprehensive social work services on length of stay. Soc Work Health Care 7:1–9, 1981

Brezel BS, Kassenbrock JM, Stein JM: Burns in substance abusers and in neurologically and mentally impaired patients. J Burn Care Rehabil 9:169–171, 1988

Broadhead WE, Leon AC, Weissman MM, et al: Development and validation of the SDDS-PC screen for multiple mental disorders in primary care. Arch Fam Med 4:211–219, 1995

Burns B, Scott J, Burke J, et al: Mental health training of primary care residents: a review of recent literature (1974–1981). Gen Hosp Psychiatry 5:157–169, 1983

Caplan C: Principles of Preventive Psychiatry. New York, Basic Books, 1964

Ciraulo DA, Shader RI, Greenblatt DJ, et al: Drug Interactions in Psychiatry, 2nd Edition. Baltimore, MD, Williams & Wilkins, 1995

Cushman LA: Secondary neuropsychiatric complications in stroke: implications for acute care. Arch Phys Med Rehabil 69:877–879, 1988

Depression Guideline Panel: Depression in Primary Care, Vol 1: Detection and Diagnosis. Clinical Practice Guideline, No 5 (AHCPR Publ No 93-0050). Rockville, MD, U.S. Department of Health and Human Services, Public Health Service, Agency for Health Care Policy Research, 1993a

Depression Guideline Panel: Depression in Primary Care, Vol 2: Treatment of Major Depression. Clinical Practice Guideline, No 5 (AHCPR Publ No 93-0051). Rockville, MD, U.S. Department of Health and Human Services, Public Health Service, Agency for Health Care Policy Research, 1993b

Derogatis LR, Lipman RS, Rickels K, et al: The Hopkins Symptom Checklist (HSCL): a self-report symptom inventory. Behav Sci 19:1–15, 1974

Dvoredsky AE, Cooley HW: Comparative severity of illness in patients with combined medical and psychiatric diagnoses. Psychosomatics 27:625–630, 1986

Engel G[L]: Delirium, in The Comprehensive Textbook of Psychiatry. Edited by Freedman MA, Kaplan HI. Baltimore, MD, Williams & Wilkins, 1967, pp 711–716

Engel GL: The need for a new medical model: a challenge for biomedicine. Science 196:129–136, 1977

Field MJ, Lohr KN (eds): Clinical Practice Guidelines: Directions for a New Program. Washington, DC, National Academy Press, 1990

Field MJ, Lohr KN (eds): Guidelines for Clinical Practice: From Development to Use. Washington, DC, National Academy Press, 1992

Folstein MF, Folstein SE, McHugh PRH: "Mini-mental state": a practical method for grading the cognitive state of patients for the clinician. J Psychiatr Res 12:189–198, 1975

Ford DE: Principles of screening applied to psychiatric disorders. Gen Hosp Psychiatry 10:177–188, 1988

Francis J, Martin D, Kapoor WN: A prospective study of delirium in hospitalized elderly. JAMA 263:1097–1101, 1990

Frasure-Smith N, Lesperance F, Juneau M: Differential long-term impact of in-hospital symptoms of psychological distress after non-Q-wave and Q-wave acute myocardial infarction. Am J Cardiol 69:1128–1134, 1992

Frasure-Smith N, Lesperance F, Talajic M: Depression following myocardial infarction: impact on 6-month survival. JAMA 270:1819–1825, 1993

Fulop G, Strain JJ: Patients who self-initiate a psychiatric consultation. Gen Hosp Psychiatry 7:267–271, 1985

Fulop G, Strain JJ, Vita J, et al: Impact of psychiatric comorbidity on length of hospital stay for medical/surgical patients: a preliminary report. Am J Psychiatry 144:878–882, 1987

Gehi M, Strain JJ, Weltz N, et al: Is there a need for admission and discharge cognitive screening for the medically ill? Gen Hosp Psychiatry 2:186–191, 1980

Glass RI, Mulvihill MN, Smith H, et al: The 4 score: an index for predicting a patient's non-medical hospital days. Am J Public Health 67:751–755, 1977

Goldman LS: Psychotropic Drug Interactions: Interact. Washington, DC, American Psychiatric Press, 1999 (CD-ROM)

Greenhill MH: The development of liaison programs, in Psychiatric Medicine. Edited by Usdin G. New York, Brunner/Mazel, 1977, pp 115–191

Hackett T, Cassem N: The Massachusetts General Hospital Handbook of Psychiatry. St. Louis, MO, Mosby, 1979

Hammer JS, Lyons JS, Strain JJ: Microcomputers and consultation psychiatry in the general hospital. Gen Hosp Psychiatry 7:119–127, 1985a

Hammer JS, Lyons JS, Bellina BA, et al: Toward the integration of psychosocial services in the general hospital: the human services department. Gen Hosp Psychiatry 7:189–194, 1985b

Hammer JS, Strain JJ, Friedberg A, et al: Operationalizing a bedside pen entry notebook clinical database system in consultation-liaison psychiatry. Gen Hosp Psychiatry 17:165–172, 1995

Jacobs J, Bernhard MR, Delgado A, et al: Screening for organic mental syndromes in the medically ill. Ann Intern Med 86:40–46, 1977

Kathol RG: Medical psychiatry units: the wave of the future. Gen Hosp Psychiatry 16:1–3, 1994

Kathol RG, Harsch HH, Shakespeare A, et al: Categorization of types of medical psychiatric units based on level of acuity. Psychosomatics 33:376–386, 1992

Katon W, Gonzales J: A review of randomized trials of psychiatric consultation-liaison studies in primary care. Psychosomatics 35:268–278, 1994

Katon W, Von Korff M, Lin E, et al: Collaborative management to achieve treatment guidelines: Impact on depression in primary care. JAMA 273:1026–1031, 1995

Katon W, Robinson P, Von Korff M, et al: A multifaceted intervention to improve treatment of depression in primary care. Arch Gen Psychiatry 53:924–932, 1996

Levenson JL, Hamer R, Silverman JJ, et al: Psychopathology in medical inpatients and its relationship to length of hospital stay: a pilot study. Int J Psychiatry Med 16:231–236, 1986

Levenson JL, Colenda CC, Larson DB, et al: Methodology in consultation-liaison research: a classification of biases. Psychosomatics 31:367–376, 1990

Levenson JL, Hamer RM, Rossiter LF: A randomized controlled study of psychiatric consultation guided by screening in general medical inpatients. Am J Psychiatry 149:631–637, 1992

Levitan S, Kornfeld D: Clinical and cost benefits of liaison psychiatry. Am J Psychiatry 138:790–793, 1981

Lyons JS, Larson DB, Burns BJ, et al: Psychiatric comorbidities and patients with head and spinal cord trauma: effects on acute hospital care. Gen Hosp Psychiatry 10:292–297, 1988

Mason W, Bedwell C, Zwaag R, et al: Why people are hospitalized: a description of preventable factors leading to admission for medical illness. Med Care 18:147–163, 1980

Mayou R, Hawton K, Feldman E, et al: Psychiatric problems among medical admissions. Int J Psychiatry Med 21:71–84, 1991

Narain P, Rubenstein LZ, Wieland GD, et al: Predictors of immediate and 6 month outcomes in hospitalized elderly patients: the importance of functional status. J Am Geriatr Soc 36:775–783, 1988

Piemme TE: Computer-assisted learning and evaluation in medicine. JAMA 260:367–372, 1988

Pincus HA, Strain JJ, Houpt JL, et al: Models of mental health training in primary care. JAMA 249:3065–3068, 1983

Popkin M, MacKenzie T, Callies A: Consultation liaison outcome evaluation system. Arch Gen Psychiatry 40:215–219, 1983

Regier DA, Goldberg ID, Taube CA: The de-facto US mental health services system: a public health perspective. Arch Gen Psychiatry 35:685–693, 1978

Rogers MP, Liang MH, Daltroy LH, et al: Delirium after elective orthopedic surgery: risk factors and natural history. Int J Psychiatry Med 19:109–121, 1989

Rowan G, Strain JJ, Gise LH: The liaison clinic: a model for liaison psychiatry funding, training and research. Gen Hosp Psychiatry 6:109–115, 1984

Rush AJ, Golden WE, Hall GE, et al: Depression in Primary Care. Clinical Practice Guideline 5 (AHCPR Publ No 93-0550). Rockville, MD, U.S. Department of Health and Human Services, Public Health Service, Agency for Health Care Policy and Research, 1993

Saravay SM, Lavin M: Psychiatric comorbidity and length of stay in the general hospital: a review of outcome studies. Psychosomatics 35:233–252, 1994

Saravay SM, Steinberg MD, Weinschel B, et al: Psychological comorbidity and length of stay in the general hospital. Am J Psychiatry 148:324–329, 1991

Smith GC, Strain JJ, Hammer JS, et al: Organic mental disorders in the consultation-liaison psychiatry setting: a multisite study. Psychosomatics 38:363–373, 1997

Smith GC, Clarke DM, Handrinos D, et al: Consultation-liaison psychiatrist's management of depression. Psychosomatics 39:244–252, 1998

Spitzer RL, Williams JBW, Kroenke K, et al: Utility of a new procedure for diagnosing mental disorders in primary care: the PRIME-MD 1000 study. JAMA 272:1749–1756, 1994

Stoudemire A, Brown TM: Psychiatric Side Effects of Prescription and Over the Counter Medications. Washington, DC, American Psychiatric Press, 1998

Strain JJ, Grossman S: Psychological Care of the Medically Ill: A Primer in Liaison Psychiatry. New York, Appleton-Century-Crofts, 1975

Strain JJ, Hamerman D: Ombudsmen (medical psychiatric) rounds: an approach to meeting patient-staff needs. Ann Intern Med 88:550–555, 1978

Strain JJ, Strain JW: Liaison psychiatry, in Modern Perspectives in Clinical Psychiatry. Edited by Howells JG. New York, Brunner/Mazel, 1988, pp 76–101

Strain JJ, Norvell CM, Strain JJ, et al: A minicomputer approach to consultation-liaison data basing: Pedagog-Admin-CLINFO. Gen Hosp Psychiatry 7:113–118, 1985a

Strain JJ, Gise LH, Houpt JL, et al: Models of mental health training in primary care. Psychosom Med 47:95–110, 1985b

Strain JJ, Fulop G, Strain JJ, et al: Use of the computer for teaching in the psychiatric residency. Journal of Psychiatric Education 10:178–186, 1986

Strain JJ, George LK, Pincus HA, et al: Models of mental health training for primary care. Psychosom Med 49:88–98, 1987

Strain JJ, Lyons JS, Hammer JS, et al: Cost offset from a psychiatric consultation-liaison intervention with elderly hip fracture patients. Am J Psychiatry 148:1044–1049, 1991

Strain JJ, Caliendo G, Himelein C: Drug-psychotropic drug interactions and end organ dysfunction: clinical management recommendations, selected bibliography, and updating strategies. Gen Hosp Psychiatry 18:300, 1996a, pp 300–313

Strain JJ, Hammer JS, Himelein C, et al: Further evolution of a literature database: content and software. Gen Hosp Psychiatry 18:294–299, 1996b

Strain JJ, Smith GC, Hammer JS, et al: Adjustment disorder: a multisite study of its utilization and interventions in the consultation-liaison psychiatry setting. Gen Hosp Psychiatry 20:139–149, 1998

Strain JJ, Caliendo G, Alexis JD, et al: Cardiac drug and psychotropic drug interactions: significance and recommendations. Gen Hosp Psychiatry 21:408–429, 1999a

Strain JJ, Campos-Rodenas R, Carvalho S, et al: Further evolution of a literature database: the international use of common software structure and methodology for the establishment of national consultation/liaison databases. Gen Hosp Psychiatry 21:402–407, 1999b

Surman OS: Usefulness of psychiatric intervention in patients undergoing cardiac surgery. Arch Gen Psychiatry 30:830–835, 1974

Wallen J, Pincus HA, Goldman HH, et al: Psychiatric consultations in short term hospitals. Arch Gen Psychiatry 44:163–168, 1987

Wells KB: Depression in general medical settings: implications of three health policy studies for consultation-liaison psychiatry. Psychosomatics 35:279–296, 1994

World Health Organization: International Statistical Classification of Diseases and Related Health Problems, 10th Revision. Geneva, World Health Organization, 1992

Zimmer J: Length of stay and hospital bed misutilization. Med Care 14:453–462, 1974

5

Basic Science of Neuroimaging and Potential Applications for Consultation-Liaison Psychiatry

Peter F. Goyer, M.D.

The purpose of this chapter is to provide an introduction to the basic science underlying various neuroimaging modalities. Although this may at first seem of uncertain relevance in a clinically oriented book, many current and future neuroimaging research findings may eventually become clinical tools in consultation-liaison psychiatry. An understanding of what different neuroimaging modalities can and cannot do and how they do it is also essential for the consultation-liaison psychiatrist to appropriately evaluate the increasing number of scientific publications and presentations on neuroimaging.

BACKGROUND

All current neuroimaging modalities are based on detection of electromagnetic (EM) radiation. Visible light is, of course, EM radiation; in this sense, neuroimaging detectors have the same function as the human eye. The human eye detects EM radiation with energies around 2 electron volts (ev). Energy of EM radiation is directly proportional to its frequency. EM radiation is thus sometimes described in terms of its frequency. Although I do not often refer to wavelength in this chapter, EM radiation may also be described by its wavelength, which varies inversely with its frequency.

Some neuroimaging modalities, such as computed tomography (CT), detect EM radiation with energies above what the human eye can detect. Others, such as

magnetic resonance imaging (MRI), detect EM radiation with energies lower than the human eye can detect. EM radiation with energy levels considerably lower than those detected by MRI is often described in terms of its field strength. Electroencephalography, for example, detects EM radiation at these very low energy levels. Changes in EM fields, as measured with EEG, can be localized in three-dimensional space with computerized electroencephalography (CEEG) and schematically mapped as an "image." Neuroimaging detectors thus extend the ability of the human eye to visualize EM radiation considerably above or below the visual range of energies.

Although all neuroimaging modalities are designed to detect EM radiation, there are variations not only in the energy of the EM radiation but also in the source of the EM radiation. Outside on a clear summer day, for example, the human eye can appreciate the shape and color of a deciduous tree. The tree is the object visualized, but the sun, not the tree, is the source of the EM radiation. In contrast, on a summer night, a firefly would be detected by the human eye from the EM radiation intrinsic to the firefly.

Neuroimaging modalities such as CT and MRI depend on a source of EM radiation that is extrinsic to the object being imaged. Extrinsic radiation is used for a transmission scan. In a CT scan, X rays are directed toward the brain from an extrinsic X-ray source outside the brain, and those rays that transmit through the brain are imaged as a transmission scan. In single photon emission computed tomography (SPECT), a radiopharmaceutical agent is injected intravenously. EM radiation is emitted from the radiopharmaceutical agent in the brain and is imaged as an emission scan. Other imaging modalities such as electroencephalography and CEEG are designed to detect EM radiation intrinsic to and generated by the brain itself.

BASIC SCIENCE OF NEUROIMAGING MODALITIES

Structural Imaging

Computed Tomography

CT was one of the seminal developments in high-resolution structural brain imaging. The technique of computerized reconstruction of image data was perfected by Kuhl and Edwards (1963) with nuclear medicine emission scans. Hounsfield (1973) and Ambrose (1973) used that and other work to develop computerized reconstruction of tomographic transmission scans. Without this concurrent development of sophisticated computer hardware and software, CT and other neuroimaging modalities would not exist. The computer is to EM radiation detectors what the brain is to the human eye.

CT uses X-ray tube radiation with energies around 70,000–140,000 ev (70–140 kilo electron volts [kev]). Using multiple extrinsic X-ray sources, EM radiation beams are focused on the brain at numerous angles throughout 360 degrees. Because X rays have higher energy than visible light, some will pass through the brain. The amount of transmission depends on many factors, one of which is the density of the material traversed. Rings of detectors sense differences in the transmission attenuation of the X rays. These differences provide mathematical data that are related to regional tissue densities. Computerized reconstruction is then used to translate the mathematical data into a transmission image. Current CT scanners have a relative in-plane spatial resolution of about 1 mm or less.

Magnetic Resonance Imaging

MRI, an application of nuclear magnetic resonance, offers the highest available contrast resolution for structural brain imaging. Although the word *magnetic* is used, the magnetic field is not what is directly imaged. The brain is placed in a magnetic field to align the nuclear magnetic dipoles of atoms with an odd number of protons. In the absence of an external magnetic field, these dipoles are randomly distributed and hence not aligned. Once aligned in a magnetic field, the magnetic dipoles precess around a central axis. An analogy for this is a top or a toy gyroscope that has a metal rod protruding through its center and is spinning on a flat surface. The metal rod or axis of the spinning top is at an angle to an axis perpendicular to the flat surface. As the top spins, the axis of the spinning top rotates or precesses around the central axis.

In MRI, EM radiation from an extrinsic source is focused into the brain in a brief series of bursts. The frequency of the EM radiation must match the frequency with which the magnetic dipole precesses; this frequency is in the radiofrequency (RF) range and is called the Larmor frequency or resonance of the atomic nuclei. This frequency is the source of the word *resonance* in the terms *magnetic resonance imaging* and *nuclear magnetic resonance*. Nuclei with different atomic numbers have differing Larmor frequencies. Currently, most magnetic resonance scanners image at the Larmor frequency of the hydrogen atom, so I focus on hydrogen nuclei in this chapter.

When the burst of EM energy interacts with the magnetic dipoles, the angle at which the dipole precesses is changed. The intensity and timing of these bursts affect the degree of perturbation of the magnetic dipole axis relative to the central axis. After the burst stops, the magnetic dipole returns to its original angle relative to the central axis and continues its resonance. As the magnetic dipole returns to its original position, EM radiation in the RF range is generated and is detected by an RF receiver in the magnetic resonance scanner. The intensity of the RF signal varies in stationary brain tissue depending on several factors, including the hydrogen nuclei concentration in specific tissue regions. Data obtained from these several factors are reconstructed by the computer to provide a transmission image.

Although MRI is grouped here under its historical classification as primarily a structural imaging modality, rapid advances in magnetic resonance angiography have led to high spatial and temporal resolution for imaging regional cerebral blood flow (rCBF). Magnetic spectroscopy is also undergoing rapid development; as spatial resolution is improved, magnetic spectroscopy may become another application of magnetic resonance as a functional imaging modality.

Functional Imaging

Single Photon Emission Computed Tomography

SPECT uses a radiation source that is injected intravenously. EM radiation is subsequently emitted from the brain, and detectors rotating in a 360-degree ring provide tomographic data. A computer reconstructs these data into an emission image. SPECT, like other nuclear medicine techniques, images emission data from a variety of radiopharmaceuticals. The radioactive nuclei in these pharmaceuticals emit EM radiation, called γ rays. Each half-life represents decay of half of the parent radionuclide. Some radioactive decay processes result in the emission of single photons, whereas others result in the simultaneous emission of dual photons. As would be expected from its name, SPECT images γ rays from radiopharmaceuticals with single photon emission. The energy of the EM radiation imaged in nuclear medicine is usually in the range of 50–500 kev. The most technically ideal energy for SPECT imaging with current cameras is approximately 150 kev.

A discussion of the many radiopharmaceuticals used for brain imaging in nuclear medicine is beyond the scope of this chapter; thus, I present only a few illustrative examples of single photon emitters. Xenon (Xe) is a lipophilic inert gas with high first-pass uptake across the blood-brain barrier; thus, the physiologic properties of ^{133}Xe and ^{127}Xe make them well suited as CBF imaging agents, and quantitation is possible. Although neither ^{133}Xe nor ^{127}Xe can be generated on site, their long half-lives (about 5.3 and 36 days, respectively) are suitable for external purchase and on-site storage. If Xe is used in gaseous form, a special inhalation apparatus and negative-pressure room are necessary. The low energy of the γ rays from ^{133}Xe (about 80 kev) results in poor resolution. Differentiation between caudate and putamen, for example, is not likely even with the most current cameras. ^{127}Xe is a preferred substitute because better resolution is obtained with appropriate collimation of its higher-energy γ rays (about 200 kev). However, because facilities in the United States no longer manufacture ^{127}Xe on a consistent basis, it is not reliably available.

A more widely available brain imaging agent with energy greater than 100 kev is technetium Tc 99m exametazime, previously called technetium Tc 99m hexamethyl-propyleneamine-oxime (HMPAO). The half-life of technetium 99m (a metastable state of technetium 99) is about 6 hours, and the predominant emission energy is about 140 kev. Because exametazime is available in kit form, the radiopharmaceutical can be prepared on demand and on site. Technetium Tc 99m exametazime is primarily a CBF imaging agent, but there is also a component of metabolic transport into neural tissue. These combined properties and a less clear relationship between technetium Tc 99m exametazime and brain physiology result in difficulties in constructing a modeling equation to convert reconstructed image data into quantified physiologic units. Although quantitation with technetium Tc 99m exametazime is problematic at present, current three-headed whole-body cameras or dedicated head cameras do allow state-of-the-art spatial image resolution of 6 mm or less. At this resolution, some differentiation between caudate and putamen is possible.

In addition to its functional capabilities for CBF imaging, SPECT may become extremely useful for receptor imaging. A number of SPECT radiopharmaceuticals are under development for imaging brain neuroreceptors.

Positron-Emission Tomography

The term *positron-emisson tomography* (PET) is something of a misnomer. The name is derived from a nuclear radioactive decay process called β-positive decay. In this process, a β-positive particle or positron is emitted from the nucleus. The positron has rest mass and is not EM radiation. After traveling a few millimeters at most, the positron combines with a negative electron; the two annihilate each other and produce EM radiation in the form of two γ rays. Each γ ray travels approximately 180 degrees away from the other. A ring of detectors records the essentially simultaneous coincidence of each γ ray impinging on detectors separated by 180 degrees. Computer reconstruction of these tomographic data results in an emission image. PET is therefore more accurately conceptualized as dual photon emission computed tomography. The positron itself is neither emitted from the brain nor imaged by the PET camera. *Positron-emission tomography* is, however, a useful term to describe the initial nuclear event of positron emission.

Although any radionuclide that undergoes β-positive decay is theoretically capable of being utilized for PET, four of the more commonly used radionuclides are carbon 11 (^{11}C), nitrogen 13 (^{13}N), oxygen 15 (^{15}O), and fluorine 18 (^{18}F). The physiologic significance of the first three is obvious. With ^{18}F, substitution for a hydrogen atom is sometimes possible with only minimal disruption of the biochemistry of the molecule. Although the physiologic chemistry of these four radionuclides is an advantage, their short half-lives (^{11}C, 20 minutes; ^{13}N, 10 minutes; ^{15}O, 2 minutes; and ^{18}F, 118 minutes) are an economic disadvantage. With the possible exception of ^{18}F, all must be generated on site in a cyclotron and robotically transferred to a hot cell for rapid conversion to an injectable or inhalable radiopharmaceutical. On-site cyclotrons and sophisticated hot cells increase equipment and personnel costs, making PET one of the more expensive neuroimaging modalities.

In general, PET has better spatial resolution than SPECT, with a full-width half-maximum resolution in the newer scanners of 4–6 mm. This does not match the spatial resolution of CT or MRI, but functional data obtained with PET cannot currently be obtained in the same quantified units with any other neuroimaging modality. Some imaging centers improve the spatial display resolution of PET or SPECT by coregistering PET or SPECT images with magnetic resonance images so that the more desirable features of each are available in the same superimposed image.

Because the corresponding radioactive isotopes can be substituted for the carbon, nitrogen, oxygen, and fluorine atoms in known pharmacological agents, neuroreceptor imaging is perhaps more fully developed in PET than in SPECT. For example, ^{11}C and ^{18}F substitutions in spiperone and its analogues have contributed to studies of receptor density and receptor occupancy for dopamine and serotonin (5-HT) receptors (Goyer et al. 1996).

Topographical Brain Mapping

Propagation of a signal along a brain neuron generates an EM field. If an adequate number of brain neurons in sufficiently close proximity are contributing to this field, it is possible to detect changes in these internal EM fields using detectors placed on the skull surface. These EM fields have both an electrical component and a magnetic component. An electroencephalographic detector is designed to detect primarily the electrical component. A magnetoencephalographic detector is designed to detect primarily the magnetic component. Currently, magnetoencephalography is used mostly in research, so I concentrate on electroencephalography in this chapter.

The electroencephalographic computer uses information from each detector or channel to translate the timing and magnitude of changes in the electrical component of these intrinsic EM fields into an oscillating graphic display. The number of electroencephalographic detectors placed at defined grid locations over the skull curvature may vary. Because classic electroencephalographic recordings are displayed in graphic form, it is necessary to computer-model, or "computerize," the EEG (CEEG) to perform topographical brain mapping (TBM). This is accomplished by a complex data reduction and statistical analysis. The results of this process are color coded and projected or mapped onto a schematic plane for visual display.

Although some may argue that TBM is not an imaging modality, I have included it for the following reasons. On the basis of spatial resolution, projecting cortical electroencephalographic contours onto a single plane would suggest a relative Z-axis "resolution" of about 6 cm. Ongoing work in dipole localization may result in reproducible projections onto more than one XY plane and hence increased Z-axis resolution. Within a given schematically mapped XY plane, projection may be possible to within millimeters, depending on the number of detectors. Regardless of the difficulties involved in projecting spatial schematics, I believe TBM can be considered a functional imaging modality on the basis of its temporal resolution of functional events. The ability to image or condense functional changes in electric-field strength within a few milliseconds exceeds the ability, in terms of temporal resolution, of PET or SPECT.

POTENTIAL APPLICATIONS

Structural Brain Imaging: CT and MRI

In this chapter, *structural brain imaging* refers to CT and MRI. Presumably, the discussion would remain applicable if additional techniques became available for structural brain imaging. Although structural brain imaging is an important investigative tool in primary and secondary psychiatric disorders, its day-to-day clinical role in assessment and treatment of patients with primary psychiatric disorders such as schizophrenia, mood disorder, anxiety disorder, and personality disorder is most often related to ruling out structural neurological lesions.

Structural brain imaging, like functional brain imaging, is expensive, and its use is frequently the subject of third-party utilization review and management. Although MRI is generally more expensive than CT, it is usually the initial choice for structural brain tissue imaging. The consultant psychiatrist needs to be aware of institutional constraints and policies before recommending or ordering MRI or CT studies. For example, some third-party payers may not reimburse if the patient undergoes MRI within 1 year of undergoing CT. Therefore, use of CT as a screening technique would not be in the economic interest of the patient when an initial CT scan suggested the need for MRI follow-up. Various neuroimaging techniques may also be the subject of local or outside utilization review studies. In a study by Olfson (1992), hospital size and location had a modest influence on the likelihood of performance of CT, but the ownership of the hospital and the patient's source of payment were not significant influences. Despite constraints, the decision to perform CT or MRI should be made based on clinical variables rather than institutional or financial variables.

Olfson (1992) analyzed data from the 1989 National Hospital Discharge Survey to determine the number, proportion, and general characteristics of 11,628 discharged patients with primary diagnoses of mental disorders who underwent CT or MRI. Olfson (1992) found that 5.1% of patients underwent CT brain scans and 0.7% of patients underwent MRI brain scans. These rates are lower than the rates among patients discharged with primary diagnoses of neurological disorders but higher than the rates among patients discharged with primary diagnoses of other medical disorders. In the group of patients with psychiatric disorder diagnoses, the likelihood of undergoing a structural brain scan was greater if the primary diagnosis was an organic disorder or if the secondary diagnosis was a medical disorder. Patients older than 65 years were also more likely to undergo structural imaging.

In a study of CT scans in a psychiatric center, head CT was ordered for 13.5% of admissions (Berk 1992). The group of patients who underwent CT had a significantly higher incidence of delirium and dementia on Axis I of DSM-III-R (American Psychiatric Association 1987) and a much higher rate of medical illness on Axis III. The rate of CT-detected abnormality was 45.2%. A head CT scan indicating abnormalities was associated with the diagnosis of dementia, the presence of other deficiencies in cognition, or an abnormality found during a neurological examination (Berk 1992). Head CT scans showing abnormalities were also associated with focal electroencephalograms (EEGs) showing abnormalities in a significant number of patients.

General hospital patients with psychiatric syndromes may selectively require neuroimaging diagnostic tests in the course of routine evaluation. Structural brain imaging, for example, may be clinically important in the evaluation of primary neurological disorders (Table 5–1).

TABLE 5–1. Sample indications for using magnetic resonance imaging to rule out structural brain lesions in patients with primary neurological disorders

Brain edema
Central nervous system infections
Concussive-contusive injuries
Connective tissue diseases
Delirium
Dementia
Focal neurological deficits
Hemorrhage
Increased intracranial pressure
Movement disorders
Prolonged catatonia
Seizure disorders
Toxic encephalopathies

Medical-surgical workups for illnesses with potential central nervous system (CNS) effects on cognition or behavior may include requests for psychiatric consultation in cases of neurological disorders other than those listed in Table 5–1. An extensive review of neurological indications for MRI is beyond the scope of this chapter; thus, I will briefly discuss only a few of them as illustrative examples.

When a consultation-liaison psychiatrist is asked to evaluate a patient with dementia, CT or MRI may be needed to exclude focal pathology. Roberts and Caird (1990), for example, found that approximately 20% (32 of 155) of their patients who had dementia for less than a year had space-occupying lesions (tumor or subdural hematoma). Leuchter and Jacobson (1991) reported similar findings in 10% of their patients with acute dementia. Although CT scans have been used to document increased ventricular size and brain atrophy in dementia of the Alzheimer's type, MRI has been shown in more recent studies to be technically superior (Tanna et al. 1991), and some authors (Bondareff et al. 1990) have suggested that MRI is more useful than CT for monitoring dementia.

During a dementia workup, white matter changes can be detected more readily on magnetic resonance images than on CT scans. The interpretation of these changes, however, is problematic, and interpretations may differ. Hachinski et al. (1987) suggested the term *leuko-araiosis* as a general description of patchy or diffuse lucent areas in the white matter. They further suggested that white matter changes noted on CT scans may or may not represent the same physiologic events as lesions noted on magnetic resonance images. The group also wondered whether the term *leuko-araiosis* was often being used in place of *Binswanger's disease* (subcortical arteriosclerotic encephalopathy). Leuko-araiosis as a general description is not limited to patients with dementia; it is also associated with increased age, hypertension, limb weakness, and extension-plantar responses (Steingart et al. 1987).

Other authors describe white matter changes in terms of their location (e.g., periventricular, subcortical [deep], or cortical). Gupta et al. (1988) investigated leuko-araiosis–type lesions in the periventricular white matter and found that 84% of patients with these lesions had hypertension. Ninety-five percent had hypertension when the additional cerebrovascular risk factor of diabetes mellitus or coronary artery disease was also present. Noting the presence of deep white matter hyperintense lesions may not be particularly useful in distinguishing patients with dementia of the Alzheimer's type from healthy elderly people (Fazekas et al. 1987). However, Bowen et al. (1990) found that the taking into account of higher severity scores for subcortical white matter lesions was helpful in distinguishing multi-infarct dementia from dementia of the Alzheimer's type and that "a patient with prominent subcortical white-matter abnormalities is more likely to have a diagnosis of vascular than degenerative dementia" (p. 1288). Noting periventricular signal hyperintensity (halos) rather than the existence of subcortical lesions may be useful in distinguishing elderly patients with dementia from healthy elderly people, because halos correlate significantly with dementia severity (Bondareff et al. 1990; Roberts and Caird 1990).

Delirium may have a multifactorial etiology, especially in geriatric patients. Metabolic aberrations, infections, alcoholism, medications, hypoxia, cardiovascular disorders, and nutritional deficiency may all cause delirium (American Psychiatric Association 1999; Francis et al. 1990; Golinger et al. 1987; Levkoff et al. 1988). These same predisposing factors may also result in psychiatric findings with or without delirium (e.g., CNS infections such as herpes simplex or human immunodeficiency virus infection). MRI, which is calibrated to the Larmor frequency of hydrogen nuclei, has a high sensitivity for changes in water content, and therefore MRI is useful for detecting inflammation-induced edema. MRI localizes infectious lesions more precisely than does CT and may show more extensive involvement than is suspected clinically (Albertyn 1990; Schroth et al. 1987). Because structural brain disease predisposes patients to delirium, structural brain imaging may be indicated in the case of a delirious patient (Koponen et al. 1987). This is especially true when the cause of delirium in a patient is not readily evident or when diagnostic uncertainty exists.

Consultation-liaison psychiatrists are also sometimes asked to evaluate the psychological and behavioral sequelae in patients with medical illnesses that are known to have potential CNS effects. For example, in patients with systemic lupus erythematosus and clinical evidence of CNS involvement, MRI is far superior to CT in detecting atrophy or focal pathology such as edema, infarct, hemorrhage, or sinusitis. Additionally, sequential MRI is useful for monitoring the effects of corticosteroids on brain edema (Sibbitt et al. 1989). MRI can also be useful for detecting focal cerebral lesions in Sjögren's syndrome patients with focal neurological deficits and in Sjögren's syndrome patients who have only psychiatric or cognitive brain dysfunction (Alexander et al. 1988).

The neurological indications for MRI may overlap with some DSM-IV-TR (American Psychiatric Associa-

tion 2000) psychiatric diagnoses (e.g., dementia, delirium, and other secondary brain syndromes); however, the use of MRI in the evaluation of patients with primary DSM-IV-TR psychiatric diagnoses may be more controversial. As early as the mid-1980s, Weinberger (1984) included both primary and secondary psychiatric diagnoses in his clinical indications for CT in psychiatric patients—specifically, confusion and/or dementia of unknown etiology, movement disorder of unknown etiology, prolonged catatonia, the first episode of psychosis of unknown etiology, and the first episode of a major mood disorder or personality change after age 50 years. Given the significant improvements in structural brain imaging with MRI relative to CT, I suggest that the indications for structural brain imaging with MRI be expanded to include any acute episode of psychosis or severe mood disorder on initial presentation, regardless of whether the etiology is known or whether the patient is older than 50 years. I also believe that MRI has a role in the primary psychiatric disorders of chronic psychosis or chronic severe mood disorder. In these cases of chronicity, I suggest that MRI may be useful in the following instances: 1) when a magnetic resonance image has not been previously obtained, 2) when the illness remains refractory to pharmacological intervention, 3) when a patient with pharmacological compliance experiences a marked change in the previous symptom pattern, and 4) when pharmacological treatment is changed to treatment with an agent with an increased risk of seizure or other CNS side effects. These suggestions are summarized in Table 5–2. In addition, individual practitioners may sometimes choose to obtain a magnetic resonance image before electroconvulsive therapy or after electroconvulsive therapy that is not efficacious.

TABLE 5–2. Sample indications for using magnetic resonance imaging to rule out structural brain lesions in patients with primary psychiatric disorders

Abrupt personality change

Acute psychosis or severe mood disorder on initial presentation

Chronic psychosis or severe mood disorder, if

    A magnetic resonance image has not been previously obtained or

    The illness remains refractory to pharmacological intervention or

    A patient with pharmacological compliance has a marked change in the previous symptom pattern or

    Pharmacological treatment is changed to treatment with an agent with an increased risk of seizure or other central nervous system side effects

Functional Imaging: SPECT and PET

With the development of SPECT and PET cameras capable of three-dimensional versus planar imaging and the development of radiopharmaceuticals that readily cross an intact blood-brain barrier (such crossing has historically been more difficult in SPECT than in PET), functional brain imaging in psychiatry not only is possible but is in fact occurring. Measurement of regional cerebral metabolic rate of glucose (rCMRG) and rCBF is considered useful in studying the pathophysiology and pharmacological treatment of psychiatric illness, the assumption being that energy use associated with increased or decreased neuronal activity is directly related to increased or decreased rCMRG and that rCMRG is directly related to or coupled with rCBF.

Differences in rCMRG and rCBF among diagnostic groups have been examined for a variety of psychiatric illnesses. Unfortunately, these differences are currently so subtle that computerized image analyses of group comparisons are usually necessary for their detection. Consequently, diagnostic sensitivity and specificity, based on visual interpretation of individual patients' functional imaging scans, are not well established. Although functional brain imaging studies have found statistical differences in rCMRG and rCBF between diagnostic groups or between psychiatric symptom groupings, these group findings cannot automatically be applied to an individual patient. Such scans may, however, be clinically useful in providing adjunctive diagnostic information. This diagnostic information may or may not correspond to our current symptom-based classification system. In clinical diagnosis, measurement of rCMRG and rCBF might also be useful in predicting treatment response to specific pharmacological agents. At present, however, group comparisons of rCMRG and rCBF are primarily useful in research studies of primary and secondary psychiatric illnesses.

In these studies, diagnostic comparisons with functional imaging may be sensitive for psychiatric illness but lack specificity for DSM-IV-TR symptom-based diagnoses. For example, PET findings in patients with mood disorders resemble those in patients with schizophrenia (Baxter et al. 1985, 1989; Buchsbaum et al. 1984, 1986; Cohen et al. 1989; Hurwitz et al. 1990; Martinot et al. 1990; Sackeim et al. 1990). Additionally, in depression but not in mania, cortical CMRG is globally decreased. In a study of depressed patients with summer seasonal affective disorder (SSAD), Goyer et al. (1992) also found globally decreased cortical CMRG. However, specific differences in rCMRG did not match those reported for other types of depressive illness. This finding is consistent with the concept that, physiologically, SSAD is different from bipolar or unipolar depression.

In contrast to findings of hypofrontality in schizophrenia and mood disorders, patients with obsessive-compulsive disorder (OCD) appear to have *increased* metabolism in the orbital frontal and/or prefrontal cortex (Baxter et al. 1987, 1988, 1989; Benkelfat et al. 1990; Machlin et al. 1991; Nordahl et al. 1989; Rubin et al. 1992; Swedo et al. 1989). The rCMRG findings reported by Goyer et al. (1992) for SSAD resemble in part the orbital frontal findings reported for OCD. However, none of the patients in the SSAD study received a diagnosis of OCD, and nondepressed patients with OCD do not exhibit global decreases in cortical CMRG.

Other psychiatric disorders that have been studied with functional brain imaging include panic disorder (Gur et al. 1987; Nordahl et al. 1990; Reiman et al. 1984, 1986, 1989), eating disorders (Emrich et al. 1984; Herholz et al. 1987), substance use disorders (London et al. 1990a, 1990b; Tumeh et al. 1990; Volkow et al. 1988, 1991, 1992), posttraumatic stress disorder (Semple et al. 1993, 1996), antisocial personality disorder (Raine et al. 1992), and borderline personality disorder (Goyer et al. 1991, 1994). In addition to examining borderline personality disorder as a cluster of symptoms, Goyer et al. (1991, 1994) examined the specific symptom of aggressive impulse control difficulty within a larger group of patients with various personality disorders. They found an inverse correlation with rCMRG in the orbital frontal cortex (Goyer et al. 1994; Goyer and Semple 1996).

As interesting as these findings are for differences in rCMRG and rCBF between diagnostic groups, the earliest possible application to individual patients may be imaging of neuroreceptor density and of relative neuroreceptor occupancy. Numerous investigators have used a wide variety of receptor tracers with both PET and SPECT scanners, and a review of this field is beyond the scope of this chapter. A noninclusive sampling limited to dopamine and/or 5-HT receptor antagonists includes [^{11}C]-*N*-methylspiperone (Goyer et al. 1993a, 1996a; Wagner et al. 1983; Wong et al. 1984, 1985, 1986a, 1986b), [^{11}C]raclopride (Farde and Nordstrom 1992; Farde et al. 1988, 1989, 1992; Nordstrom et al. 1993), [^{76}Br]bromolisuride (Martinot et al. 1991), [^{76}Br]spiperone (Arnett et al. 1986), [^{18}F]-*N*-methylspiperone (Smith et al. 1988; Wolkin et al. 1989), and [^{18}F]setoperone (Blin et al. 1989, 1990). PET may also be used to study receptor agonists through examination of the changes in rCBF induced by these agents (Goyer et al. 1993b), but the applicability of this technique to individual patients is not as developed.

Although the usefulness of PET and SPECT in diagnosing primary psychiatric disorders is currently related to group comparisons in research studies, functional imaging with PET or SPECT may be helpful to the consultation-liaison psychiatrist in ruling out neurological illness in individual patients. In the early phases of dementia, for example, PET and SPECT are more sensitive than structural brain imaging. PET reveals changes in parietotemporal metabolism that differentiate patients with dementia of the Alzheimer's type or multi-infarct dementia from healthy elderly people (Fazekas et al. 1989). Hypometabolism may be present even when there is no evidence of atrophy on anatomic images. PET reveals several abnormalities in patients with dementia of the Alzheimer's type: 1) reductions in whole-brain metabolism parallel increases in dementia severity, 2) metabolism is decreased more in the association cortex than in the primary sensorimotor cortex, and 3) metabolic asymmetry in cortical areas correlates with neuropsychological deficits (Haxby and Rapoport 1986). In less severe cases of dementia of the Alzheimer's type, metabolic deficits were present in the parietotemporal cortex. In more severe cases of dementia of the Alzheimer's type, frontal metabolism was also decreased. Dementia of the Alzheimer's type spares the primary sensorimotor cortex (Frackowiak et al. 1981).

Multi-infarct dementia produces focal areas of hypometabolism. However, global reductions in cerebral metabolism also occur. Imaging patterns are distinct from those in patients with dementia of the Alzheimer's type. PET imaging of rCMRG in patients with multi-infarct dementia reveals multiple defects in the cortex, deep nuclei, subcortical white matter, and cerebellum (Kuhl et al. 1985). The presence of parietal deficits on SPECT images can also be used to distinguish dementia of the Alzheimer's type from multi-infarct dementia (Ebmeier et al. 1987). Dementia increases as global and frontal hypometabolism develop. Differences in 5-HT receptor function have also been noted in the nonsensorimotor cortex of patients with dementia of the Alzheimer's type (Blin et al. 1993).

Sometimes structural brain imaging cannot differentiate between brain tumor recurrence and radiation necrosis. One of the most clinically useful applications of functional brain imaging with PET may be its ability to assist in this differential diagnosis. Although the only other approach, repeat craniotomy, is associated with greater economic costs and greater patient morbidity, local standards and third-party reimbursement may nonetheless favor repeat craniotomy. Again, the consultation-liaison psychiatrist must be familiar with local standards of practice.

TBM From CEEG

CEEG brain mapping involves several quantitative electroencephalographic techniques. CEEG permits spatial analysis of electrical activity recorded from the scalp. The display may include electroencephalographic frequency analysis, statistical comparison with a database, or other calculations. CEEG records electrical changes intrinsic to the brain, but the data must be color coded and mapped onto a schematic for visual display. The spatial resolution of the projected EEG increases as the number of electrodes increases, but attenuation and filtering from tissues of the head limit localization. Choice of the reference will alter the visual display, and common electroencephalographic artifacts or variants may distort the maps. The physiologic state of arousal, the degree of cooperation, and other patient-related factors are also important. The main advantage of CEEG is its temporal resolution of functional events. As noted earlier in this chapter, the ability to image or condense functional changes in electric-field strength within a few milliseconds exceeds the ability, with regard to temporal resolution, of PET or SPECT.

Consultation psychiatrists will be familiar with the use of electroencephalography in evaluating patients with seizure disorders. Characteristic electrical patterns also distinguish other CNS disorders such as Creutzfeldt-Jakob disease and herpes simplex, but the EEG is usually nonspecific in the encephalopathies most frequently encountered by consultation psychiatrists. Nonetheless, electroencephalographic changes regularly accompany diffuse disturbances in brain function. The most common finding is symmetrical slowing. The EEG frequency becomes slower as the encephalopathy intensifies. CEEG can quantitate the degree of electroencephalographic slowing. However, this data analysis may not detect features such as paradoxical arousal responses, frontal intermittent delta activity, triphasic waves, or epileptic spikes. Because the computerized electroencephalograph can obtain data and analyze them over long periods, CEEG can add to the management of patients in the intensive care unit setting (K. G. Jordan 1993). In the intensive care unit, data can be analyzed for frequency trends, variability, and other parameters. In addition, CEEG techniques can help to identify subclinical seizures and seizures in paralyzed patients. Because CEEG records events related to cerebral metabolism, it is sensitive to ischemia and hypoxemia.

Compared with electroencephalography, CEEG may be better able to detect abnormalities in patients with dementia. CEEG and evoked potentials may aid in differentiating depression, multi-infarct dementia, and

Alzheimer's disease. In the case of depressed patients who have not begun taking psychotropic drugs, EEGs usually show no abnormalities; therefore, an abnormality should lead to neurological investigation. The computerized EEG more frequently shows abnormalities in non-Alzheimer's dementia, particularly in multi-infarct dementia (S. E. Jordan et al. 1989). In Alzheimer's disease, CEEG may detect abnormalities in the parietal and/or temporal regions. Such findings are consistent with PET and SPECT findings of function abnormalities. In addition, P300 may show delay, asymmetry, or parietal attenuation in patients with dementia. This finding is more prominent in patients with Alzheimer's disease.

An extensive amount of literature exists on the use of CEEG and evoked potentials in differentiating a variety of psychiatric illnesses. It is unfortunate that data acquisition and interpretation lack standardization. Results often are not reproducible. Nonetheless, several companies have produced machinery that provides automated interpretation of computerized EEGs. To the uninitiated, this simplistic approach is misleading. The attractive maps and printed interpretations may also be misleading. Although some clinicians overuse unsubstantiated techniques, sufficient scientific literature supports the contention that CEEG may reveal distinct profiles of abnormal brain electrical features (John et al. 1988). In the future, these methods may be relevant for diagnostic validation or more individualized therapy.

SUMMARY

Neuroimaging research with both structural and functional brain imaging has resulted in extremely interesting findings for psychiatry and neurology. In psychiatric research, the coregistration of structural and functional imaging can provide superb anatomic resolution concomitant with quantified physiologic data. The transfer of functional imaging research into clinical psychiatry is expected to continue and may result in an increase in diagnostic sensitivity and specificity for individual patients. At present, clinical applicability to individual psychiatric patients appears to be restricted primarily to neuroreceptor imaging and to imaging that helps rule out structural neurological lesions.

REFERENCES

Albertyn LE: Magnetic resonance imaging in herpes simplex encephalitis. Australas Radiol 34:117–121, 1990

Alexander EL, Beall SS, Gordon B, et al: Magnetic resonance imaging of cerebral lesions in patients with the Sjögren syndrome. Ann Intern Med 108:815–823, 1988

Ambrose J: Computerized transverse axial scanning (tomography), part 2: clinical application. Br J Radiol 46:1023–1047, 1973

American Psychiatric Association: Diagnostic and Statistical Manual of Mental Disorders, 3rd Edition, Revised. Washington, DC, American Psychiatric Association, 1987

American Psychiatric Association: Diagnostic and Statistical Manual of Mental Disorders, 4th Edition, Text Revision. Washington, DC, American Psychiatric Association, 2000

American Psychiatric Association: Practice Guideline for the Treatment of Patients With Delirium. Washington, DC, American Psychiatric Association, 1999

Arnett CD, Wolf AP, Shiue C-Y, et al: Improved delineation of human dopamine receptors using [^{18}F]-N-methylspiroperidol and PET. J Nucl Med 27:1878–1882, 1986

Baxter LR, Phelps ME, Mazziotta JC, et al: Cerebral metabolic rates for glucose in mood disorders: studies with positron emission tomography and fluorodeoxyglucose F18. Arch Gen Psychiatry 42:441–447, 1985

Baxter LR, Phelps ME, Mazziotta JC, et al: Local cerebral glucose metabolic rates in obsessive-compulsive disorder: a comparison with rates in unipolar depression and in normal controls. Arch Gen Psychiatry 44:211–218, 1987

Baxter LR, Schwartz JM, Mazziotta JC, et al: Cerebral glucose metabolic rates in nondepressed patients with obsessive-compulsive disorder. Am J Psychiatry 145:1560–1563, 1988

Baxter LR, Schwartz JM, Phelps ME, et al: Reduction of prefrontal cortex glucose metabolism common to three types of depression. Arch Gen Psychiatry 46:243–250, 1989

Benkelfat C, Nordahl TE, Semple WE, et al: Local cerebral glucose metabolic rates in obsessive-compulsive disorder: patients treated with clomipramine. Arch Gen Psychiatry 47:840–848, 1990

Berk M: Indications for computed tomographic brain scanning in psychiatric inpatients. S Afr Med J 82:338–340, 1992

Blin J, Baron JC, Cambon H, et al: Striatal dopamine D2 receptors in tardive dyskinesia: PET study. J Neurol Neurosurg Psychiatry 52:1248–1252, 1989

Blin J, Sette G, Fiorelli M, et al: A method for the in vivo investigation of the serotonergic 5-HT$_2$ receptors in the human cerebral cortex using positron emission tomography and ^{18}F-labeled setoperone. J Neurochem 54:1744–1754, 1990

Blin J, Baron JC, Budois B, et al: Loss of brain 5-HT2 receptors in Alzheimer's disease: in vivo assessment with positron emission tomography and [18F] setoperone. Brain 116:497–510, 1993

Bondareff W, Raval J, Woo B, et al: Magnetic resonance imaging and the severity of dementia in older adults. Arch Gen Psychiatry 47:47–51, 1990

Bowen BC, Barker WW, Loewenstein DA, et al: MR signal abnormalities in memory disorder and dementia. AJR Am J Roentgenol 154:1285–1292, 1990

Buchsbaum MS, DeLisi LE, Holcomb HH, et al: Anteroposterior gradients in cerebral glucose use in schizophrenia and affective disorders. Arch Gen Psychiatry 41:1159–1166, 1984

Buchsbaum MS, Wu J, DeLisi LE, et al: Frontal cortex and basal ganglia metabolic rates assessed by positron emission tomography with [¹⁸F]2-deoxyglucose in affective illness. J Affect Disord 10:137–152, 1986

Cohen RM, Semple WE, Gross M, et al: Evidence for common alterations in cerebral glucose metabolism in major affective disorders and schizophrenia. Neuropsychopharmacology 2:241–254, 1989

Ebmeier KP, Besson JAO, Crawford JR, et al: Nuclear magnetic resonance imaging and single photon emission tomography with radio-iodine labeled compounds in the diagnosis of dementia. Acta Psychiatr Scand 75:549–556, 1987

Emrich HM, Pahl JJ, Herholz K, et al: PET investigation in anorexia nervosa: normal glucose metabolism during pseudoatrophy of the brain, in The Psychobiology of Anorexia Nervosa. Edited by Pirke KM, Ploog D. Berlin, Springer-Verlag New York, 1984, pp 172–178

Farde L, Nordstrom A-L: PET analysis indicates atypical central dopamine receptor occupancy in clozapine-treated patients. Br J Psychiatry 160:30–33, 1992

Farde L, Wiesel FA, Halldin C, et al: Central D2-dopamine receptor occupancy in schizophrenic patients treated with antipsychotic drugs. Arch Gen Psychiatry 45:71–76, 1988

Farde L, Wiesel FA, Nordstrom A-L, et al: D1- and D2-dopamine receptor occupancy during treatment with conventional and atypical neuroleptics. Psychopharmacology 99 (suppl):28–31, 1989

Farde L, Nordstrom A-L, Wiesel FA, et al: Positron emission tomographic analysis of central D_1 and D_2 dopamine receptor occupancy in patients treated with classical neuroleptics and clozapine: relation to extrapyramidal side effects. Arch Gen Psychiatry 49:538–544, 1992

Fazekas F, Chawluk JB, Alavi A, et al: MR signal abnormalities at 1.5 T in Alzheimer's dementia and normal aging. AJR Am J Roentgenol 149:351–356, 1987

Fazekas F, Alavi A, Chawluk JB, et al: Comparison of CT, MR, and PET in Alzheimer's dementia and normal aging. J Nucl Med 30:1607–1615, 1989

Frackowiak RSJ, Pozzilli C, Legg NJ, et al: Regional cerebral oxygen supply and utilization in dementia: a clinical and physiological study with oxygen-15 and positron tomography. Brain 104:753–778, 1981

Francis J, Martin D, Kapoor WN: A prospective study of delirium in hospitalized elderly. JAMA 263:1097–1101, 1990

Golinger RC, Peet T, Tune LE: Association of elevated plasma anticholinergic activity with delirium in surgical patients. Am J Psychiatry 144:1218–1220, 1987

Goyer PF, Semple WE: PET studies of aggression in personality disorder and other non-psychotic patients, in Aggression and Violence: Genetic, Neurobiological, and Biosocial Perspectives. Edited by Stoff DM, Cairns RB. Hillsdale, NJ, Erlbaum, 1996, pp 219–235

Goyer PF, Andreason PJ, Semple WE, et al: PET and personality disorders (abstract). Biol Psychiatry 29:94A, 1991

Goyer PF, Schulz PM, Semple WE, et al: Cerebral glucose metabolism in patients with summer seasonal affective disorder. Neuropsychopharmacology 7:233–240, 1992

Goyer PF, Berridge MS, Semple WE, et al: Dopamine-2 and serotonin-2 receptor indices in clozapine treated schizophrenic patients (abstract). Schizophr Res 9:199, 1993a

Goyer PF, Semple WE, Morris ED, et al: Effects of MK-212 on regional cerebral blood flow in humans (abstract). Schizophr Res 9:199, 1993b

Goyer PF, Andreason PJ, Semple WE, et al: Positron-emission tomography and personality disorders. Neuropsychopharmacology 10:21–28, 1994

Goyer PF, Berridge MS, Morris ED, et al: PET measurement of neuroreceptor occupancy by typical and atypical neuroleptics. J Nucl Med 37:1122–1127, 1996

Gupta RS, Naheedy MH, Young JC, et al: Periventricular white matter changes and dementia. Arch Neurol 45:637–641, 1988

Gur RC, Gur RE, Resnick SM, et al: The effect of anxiety on cortical cerebral blood flow and metabolism. J Cereb Blood Flow Metab 7:173–177, 1987

Hachinski VC, Potter P, Merskey H: Leuko-araiosis. Arch Neurol 44:21–23, 1987

Haxby JV, Rapoport SI: Abnormalities of regional brain metabolism in Alzheimer's disease and their relation to functional impairment. Prog Neuropsychopharmacol Biol Psychiatry 10:427–438, 1986

Herholz K, Krieg JC, Emrich HM, et al: Regional cerebral glucose metabolism in anorexia nervosa measured by positron emission tomography. Biol Psychiatry 22:43–51, 1987

Hounsfield GN: Computerized transverse axial scanning (tomography), I: description of system. Br J Radiol 46:1016–1022, 1973

Hurwitz TA, Clark C, Murphy E, et al: Regional cerebral glucose metabolism in major depressive disorder. Can J Psychiatry 35:684–688, 1990

John ER, Prichep LS, Fridman J, et al: Neurometrics: computer-assisted differential diagnosis of brain dysfunctions. Science 239:162–169, 1988

Jordan KG: Continuous EEG and evoked potential monitoring in the neuroscience intensive care unit. J Clin Neurophysiol 10:445–475, 1993

Jordan SE, Nowacki R, Newer M: Computerized electroencephalography in the evaluation of early dementia. Brain Topogr 1:271–282, 1989

Koponen H, Hurri L, Stenback U, et al: Acute confusional states in the elderly: a radiological evaluation. Acta Psychiatr Scand 76:726–731, 1987

Kuhl DE, Edwards RQ: Image separation isotope scanning. Radiology 80:653–661, 1963

Kuhl DE, Metter EJ, Riege WH, et al: Determination of cerebral glucose utilization in dementia using positron emission tomography. Dan Med Bull 32 (suppl 1):51–55, 1985

Leuchter AF, Jacobson SA: Quantitative measurement of brain electrical activity in delirium. Int Psychogeriatr 3:231–247, 1991

Levkoff SE, Safran C, Cleary PD, et al: Identification of factors associated with the diagnosis of delirium in elderly hospitalized patients. J Am Geriatr Soc 36:1099–1104, 1988

London ED, Wilkerson G, Ori C, et al: Central action of psychomotor stimulants on glucose utilization in extrapyramidal motor areas of the rat brain. Brain Res 512:155–158, 1990a

London ED, Cascella NG, Wong DF, et al: Cocaine-induced reduction of glucose utilization in human brain: a study using positron emission tomography and [fluorine18]-fluorodeoxyglucose. Arch Gen Psychiatry 47:567–574, 1990b

Machlin SR, Harris GJ, Pearlson GD, et al: Elevated medial-frontal cerebral blood flow in obsessive-compulsive patients: a SPECT study. Am J Psychiatry 148:1240–1242, 1991

Martinot JL, Hardy P, Feline A, et al: Left prefrontal glucose hypometabolism in the depressed state: a confirmation. Am J Psychiatry 147:1313–1317, 1990

Martinot JL, Paillere-Martinot ML, Loc'h C, et al: The estimated density of D_2 striatal receptors in schizophrenia: a study with positron emission tomography and ^{76}Br-bromolisuride. Br J Psychiatry 158:346–350, 1991

Nordahl TE, Benkelfat C, Semple WE, et al: Cerebral glucose metabolic rates in obsessive compulsive disorder. Neuropsychopharmacology 2:23–28, 1989

Nordahl TE, Semple WE, Gross M, et al: Cerebral glucose metabolic differences in patients with panic disorder. Neuropsychopharmacology 3:261–272, 1990

Nordstrom A-L, Farde L, Wiesel F-A, et al: Central D2-dopamine receptor occupancy in relation to antipsychotic drug effects: a double-blind PET study of schizophrenic patients. Biol Psychiatry 33:227–235, 1993

Olfson M: Utilization of neuropsychiatric diagnostic tests for general hospital patients with mental disorders. Am J Psychiatry 149:1711–1717, 1992

Raine A, Buchsbaum MS, Stanley J, et al: Selective reduction in pre-frontal glucose metabolism in murderers assessed with positron emission tomography. Psychophysiology 29 (suppl 4A):58–63, 1992

Reiman EM, Raichle ME, Butler FK, et al: A focal brain abnormality in panic disorder, a severe form of anxiety. Nature 310:683–685, 1984

Reiman EM, Raichle ME, Robins E, et al: The application of positron emission tomography to the study of panic disorder. Am J Psychiatry 143:469–477, 1986

Reiman EM, Fusselman MJ, Fox PT, et al: Neuroanatomical correlates of anticipatory anxiety. Science 243:1071–1074, 1989

Roberts MA, Caird FI: The contribution of computerized tomography to the differential diagnosis of confusion in elderly patients. Age Ageing 19:50–56, 1990

Rubin RT, Villanueva-Meyer J, Ananth J, et al: Regional xenon 133 cerebral blood flow and cerebral technetium 99m HMPAO uptake in unmedicated patients with obsessive-compulsive disorder and matched normal control subjects: determination by high-resolution single-photon emission computed tomography. Arch Gen Psychiatry 49:695–702, 1992

Sackeim HA, Prohovnik I, Moeller JR, et al: Regional cerebral blood flow in mood disorders, I: comparison of major depressives and normal controls at rest. Arch Gen Psychiatry 47:60–70, 1990

Schroth G, Gawehn J, Thron A, et al: Early diagnosis of herpes simplex encephalitis by MRI. Neurology 37:179–183, 1987

Semple WE, Goyer P, McCormick R, et al: Preliminary report: brain blood flow using PET in patients with posttraumatic stress disorder and substance-abuse histories. Biol Psychiatry 34:115–118, 1993

Semple WE, Goyer PF, McCormick R: Attention and regional cerebral blood flow in posttraumatic stress disorder patients with substance abuse histories. Psychiatry Res 67:17–28, 1996

Sibbitt WL Jr, Sibbitt RR, Griffey RH, et al: Magnetic resonance and computed tomographic imaging in the evaluation of acute neuropsychiatric disease in systemic lupus erythematosus. Ann Rheum Dis 48:1014–1022, 1989

Smith M, Wolf AP, Brodie JD, et al: Serial [^{18}F]N-methylspiroperidol PET studies to measure changes in antipsychotic drug D-2 receptor occupancy in schizophrenic patients. Biol Psychiatry 23:653–663, 1988

Steingart A, Hachinski VC, Lau C, et al: Cognitive and neurologic findings in demented patients with diffuse white matter lucencies on computed tomographic scan (leukoaraiosis). Arch Neurol 44:36–39, 1987

Swedo SE, Schapiro MB, Grady CL, et al: Cerebral glucose metabolism in childhood-onset obsessive-compulsive disorder. Arch Gen Psychiatry 46:518–523, 1989

Tanna NK, Kohn MI, Horwich DN, et al: Analysis of brain and cerebrospinal fluid volumes with MR imaging: impact on PET data correction for atrophy, part II: aging and Alzheimer dementia. Radiology 178:123–130, 1991

Tumeh SS, Nagel JS, English RJ, et al: Cerebral abnormalities in cocaine abusers: demonstration by SPECT perfusion brain scintigraphy. Work in progress. Radiology 176:821–824, 1990

Volkow ND, Mullani N, Gould L, et al: Effects of acute alcohol intoxication on cerebral blood flow measured with PET. Psychiatry Res 24:201–209, 1988

Volkow ND, Fowler JS, Wolf AP, et al: Changes in brain glucose metabolism in cocaine dependence and withdrawal. Am J Psychiatry 148:621–626, 1991

Volkow ND, Hitzemann R, Wang G-J, et al: Decreased brain metabolism in neurologically intact healthy alcoholics. Am J Psychiatry 149:1016–1022, 1992

Wagner HN, Burns HD, Dannals RF, et al: Imaging dopamine receptors in the human brain by positron tomography. Science 221:1264–1266, 1983

Weinberger DR: Brain disease and psychiatric illness: when should a psychiatrist order a CAT scan? Am J Psychiatry 141:1521–1527, 1984

Wolkin A, Barouche F, Wolf AP, et al: Dopamine blockade and clinical response: evidence for two biological subgroups of schizophrenia. Am J Psychiatry 146:905–908, 1989

Wong DF, Wagner HN, Dannals RF, et al: Effects of age on dopamine and serotonin receptors measured by positron tomography in the living human brain. Science 226:1393–1396, 1984

Wong DF, Wagner HN, Coyle J, et al: Assessment of dopamine receptor blockade by neuroleptic drugs in the living human brain (abstract). J Nucl Med 26:52–53, 1985

Wong DF, Gjedde A, Wagner HN: Quantification of neuroreceptors in the living human brain, I: irreversible binding of ligands. J Cereb Blood Flow Metab 6:137–146, 1986a

Wong DF, Gjedde A, Wagner HN, et al: Quantification of neuroreceptors in the living human brain, II: inhibition studies of receptor density and affinity. J Cereb Blood Flow Metab 6:147–153, 1986b

6

Mental Status Examination and Diagnosis

Michael G. Wise, M.D.

Mark E. Servis, M.D.

The mental status examination (MSE) is to the consultation-liaison psychiatrist what the cardiac examination is to the cardiologist or the neurological examination is to the neurologist. To perform effective psychiatric consultation, one must be able to perform a complete MSE and integrate the findings with historical and behavioral information, as well as psychological, neurological, physical, and laboratory information, to arrive at a final diagnosis. The components of the MSE include assessments of general appearance and behavior, affect and mood, thought processes and content, perceptions (delusions, hallucinations), judgment, and insight. In addition, it is essential to assess cognitive function, such as level of consciousness or awareness, attention, speech, orientation and memory, and abstracting ability.

MSE findings reflect mental and psychological function at a particular time and are fully appreciated only when placed in the context of the patient's history. For example, the rapidity of mental status changes is an important element in the history that helps to establish the differential diagnosis. Changes can occur acutely as in a stroke or delirium, subacutely as in some types of delirium, or chronically as in dementia. An inexperienced examiner sometimes moves too quickly from a few symptoms and a brief history to a clinical diagnosis. Even for the seasoned consultation-liaison psychiatrist, there is no substitute for a complete history with a mental status and neurological examination.

Integration of the history and results of the MSE is especially important for the consultation-liaison psychiatrist, because neurological, medical, and substance-induced neuropsychiatric disorders—referred to in this chapter as secondary disorders—are found frequently among medically ill hospitalized patients. For example, Anthony and colleagues (1982) examined all patients admitted to a general medical ward and found that 23 (24%) of 97 patients had dementia or delirium, and Jacobs et al. (1977) found significant cognitive dysfunction in 37% of consecutive medical admissions. Therefore, the consultation-liaison psychiatrist must be an expert in identifying and documenting cognitive impairment.

It is unfortunate that cognitive impairment is not always recognized by nonpsychiatric medical personnel. In one study, 37% of nonpsychiatric ward physicians, 55% of nurses, and 46% of medical students did not identify cognitively impaired patients who were hospitalized on a general medical service (Knights and Folstein 1977). In a study involving elderly patients referred for evaluation, substantial cognitive dysfunction went unrecognized by the referring physician in 73% of the patients; cognitive dysfunction was related to pharmacotherapy 75% of the time (Kallman and May 1989).

Psychiatrists often depend too heavily on verbal communication and testing to exclude a secondary psychiatric diagnosis. For that reason, psychiatrists will miss nonverbal cognitive impairment if the patient's ability to communicate is reasonably good. Formal tests of right-hemisphere, or nondominant, brain function are as important as the more traditional tests of verbal function, the domain of the left hemisphere. The psychiatrist who asks the patient to remember three verbal items but does not have the patient recall three shapes succumbs to this pitfall and essentially does not test a major part of the brain's function (Ovsiew 1992).

Finally, mental status testing in a general hospital environment is difficult. Hospital rooms are noisy, and there are many distractions, such as intravenous alarms, a roommate who is groaning or loudly conversing with visitors, or a harried nurse or phlebotomist who must have immediate access to the patient. In addition, the patient being examined is sick, often frightened, and sleep deprived. As a result, the consultation-liaison psychiatrist can identify gross deficits much more readily than subtle abnormalities. Before testing, the psychiatrist should always ensure that the patient has his or her usual sensory aids (e.g., hearing aid or glasses).

In this chapter, we discuss the patient's history and performance on the MSE. The mental status test is separated into two categories: noncognitive and cognitive (Table 6–1).

NONCOGNITIVE COMPONENTS OF THE MENTAL STATUS EXAMINATION

Evaluating a patient with changes in noncognitive abilities is often more difficult than evaluating a patient who has abnormalities in cognitive function. Noncognitive changes are more subjective and are more often symptomatic of a primary psychiatric disorder. Certain features help the clinician to identify patients who have noncognitive changes secondary to medical illness (e.g., brain pathology) or medications (substance induced). First, the clinician must know the epidemiology of common psychiatric disorders (Figure 6–1). For example, a 60-year-old man with no prior psychiatric problems who is referred for evaluation of new-onset "schizophrenia" virtually never has schizophrenia. Typically, this patient's mental status changes are due to a medical condition or are substance induced.

Appearance and Behavior

The MSE begins the instant the psychiatrist sees the patient. From that moment on, information is collected and hypotheses are formulated about the patient's diagnosis. In the written consultation report, these findings should be summarized in a straightforward manner. The patient's physical appearance, attitude, and behavior should be described without the use of jargon, and judgmental terms that imply a diagnosis—for example, "She acted hysterically" or "He exhibited borderline characteristics"—should be avoided. Such terms are not helpful, and are usually wrong. How the patient looks and

TABLE 6–1.   Components of a mental status examination

Noncognitive
  Appearance and behavior
  Affect and mood
  Thought process and content
  Perceptions
  Abstracting abilities
  Judgment
  Insight
Cognitive
  Level of consciousness and awareness
  Attention
  Speech and language
  Orientation
  Memory

Source.   Reprinted from Strub RL, Wise MG: "Differential Diagnosis in Neuropsychiatry," in *The American Psychiatric Press Textbook of Neuropsychiatry*, 2nd Edition. Edited by Yudofsky SC, Hales RE. Washington, DC, American Psychiatric Press, 1992, p. 231. Used with permission.

behaves during the examination should be reported, and behavior such as increased or decreased body movements, posturing, pacing, tremor, and choreiform or dyskinetic movements should be described. In the case of patients who appear ill, depressed, angry, distractible, anxious, or disheveled, the clinician should state specific aspects of the patients' appearance or behavior that led to these conclusions. An accurate, unbiased description of behavior and appearance aids diagnosis. This information is also useful to other physicians who read the consultation report.

Affect and Mood

Mood is the patient's pervasive and sustained emotional state. Terms used to describe mood are *dysphoric, elevated, euthymic, expansive,* and *irritable.* The word *affect* refers to more rapid fluctuations in the patient's emotional state. If the patient's affect does not change during the interview (e.g., the patient is constantly depressed, emotionless, or elated), that would, in all likelihood, represent the patient's mood. When reporting affect, the clinician considers range, intensity, lability, and appropriateness. Affective range may be full (e.g., the patient shows a wide range of emotional states during the interview), or affect may be restricted to a particular affective state (e.g., depressed). Affective intensity among patients can also vary greatly (e.g., from the extreme rage seen in a borderline patient to the flat or affectless expression typically observed in a patient with Parkinson's disease). The patient who fluctuates rapidly from one affective state to

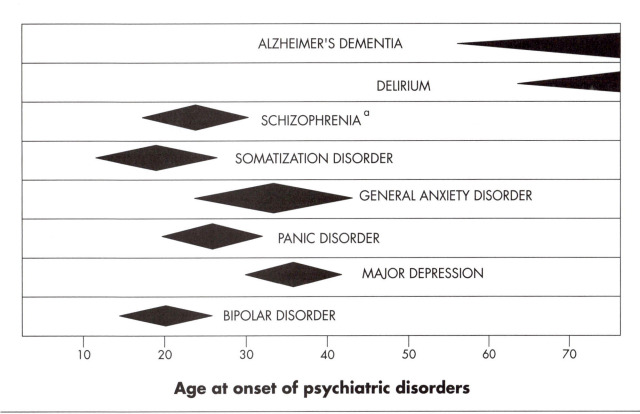

Age at onset of psychiatric disorders

FIGURE 6–1. Epidemiology of common psychiatric disorders.
[a]Earlier onset in males.
Source. Reprinted from Strub RL, Wise MG: "Differential Diagnosis in Neuropsychiatry," in *The American Psychiatric Press Textbook of Neuropsychiatry*, 2nd Edition. Edited by Yudofsky SC, Hales RE. Washington, DC, American Psychiatric Press, 1992, p. 231. Used with permission.

another demonstrates affective lability, which often indicates a toxic or medical etiology. Affect is also described as either appropriate or inappropriate to the topic under discussion. For example, a patient who describes the recent traumatic death of a loved one appears sad (appropriate expression of affect); however, another patient during a similar discussion appears elated and laughs (inappropriate expression of affect).

Mood disorders are commonly seen among patients who are medically ill (Silverstone 1996; Wise and Taylor 1990). When a medical disorder or a substance causes a clinically significant change in mood, the DSM-IV (American Psychiatric Association 1994) psychiatric diagnosis is mood disorder due to a general medical condition (the medical condition is specifically named) or substance-induced mood disorder.

Consultation-liaison psychiatrists frequently see patients with medical or substance-induced mood disorders. In a study involving 755 hospitalized patients consecutively seen in psychiatric consultation (Rundell and Wise 1989), the conditions of 87% of patients with mania and 38% of patients with depression warranted diagnoses of medical or substance-induced mood disorders. Medical illness, especially subcortical neurological disease, and medications can cause major depression.

Patients who have had strokes, for example, are at high risk for depression. Factors that influence the likelihood of developing a mood disorder include the location of the stroke and, possibly, the presence of preexisting central nervous system (CNS) pathology (Robinson and Starkstein 1990). Failure to recognize and treat poststroke depression can affect long-term recovery (Parikh et al. 1990). Neurological lesions can also cause anxiety disorders (Wise and Rundell 1999). Thyroid disease and other medical illnesses can markedly alter mood. A patient with hyperthyroidism can become manic (Lishman 1998) or depressed (Gold et al. 1981). Other medical illnesses commonly associated with mood disorders include human immunodeficiency virus infection, cancer, multiple sclerosis, Parkinson's disease, and chronic renal failure.

Medications can also cause depression, and numerous medications are reported to cause mania (Krauthammer and Klerman 1978). However, the cause-and-effect connection between medications and mood changes is based largely on anecdotal reports, not prospective data. More research is required to investigate the relationship between medications and mood disorders. Two classic examples of medications that cause depression are reserpine and α-methyldopa (Benson et al. 1983). On the other hand, corticosteroids, particularly when given in high doses such as after organ transplantation, commonly cause mood elevation and may cause a manic episode (Rundell and Wise 1989; Wise et al. 1988). If no medical condition or substance causes the mood alteration, the correct diagnosis is a primary mood disorder (i.e., major depressive disorder, bipolar disorder, dysthymic disorder, or adjustment disorder with depressed mood).

Thought Processes and Content

Thought processes and thought content are judged by the patient's quality and quantity of speech and behavior. How does the patient respond to a question? Is his or her answer responsive to the question asked (goal directed), or does he or she ramble purposelessly (tangential)? The pattern of thoughts is also an important measure of thought processes. The patient's thoughts may move extremely rapidly from one idea to another (flight of ideas), may not relate in an understandable way (loose associations), or may stop suddenly (thought blocking). The patient's thought content or major themes reflect the patient's concerns, including obsessional preoccupation, suicidal or homicidal ideation, and irrational beliefs.

The division of thought disorders into a functional-versus-organic dichotomy is no longer appropriate, because all observed psychiatric symptomatology is linked to biological activity in the brain. Therefore, *primary thought disorders* (e.g., manic episode due to bipolar I disorder) and *secondary thought disorders* (e.g., substance-induced mania due to steroids) are the terms used in this chapter. Disordered thinking is seen in secondary thought disorders, such as delirium, dementia, and substance-induced disorders, and in primary thought disorders, such as schizophrenia, mania, and psychotic depression (D. W. Black and Andreasen 1999). Several clinical characteristics differentiate primary and secondary thought disorders. Patients with primary thought disorders are usually younger and have no related medical illness, no clouding of consciousness, and no disorientation, but they do have a psychiatric history and predominantly auditory hallucinations. Patients with secondary thought disorders usually are older at the time of onset, have associated medical illness(es), are taking associated medication(s), and have fluctuating consciousness, disorientation, nonauditory hallucinations, and fleeting, poorly systematized delusional beliefs but no prior psychiatric history.

The clinician must use his or her knowledge and collective experience about psychiatric disorders to recognize secondary thought disorders. An obvious example would be an 82-year-old woman referred for evaluation of new-onset schizophrenia. She would most likely have

a delirium or dementia or possibly some other medically induced or medication-induced alteration in mental status. In cases of newly diagnosed thought disorder, the clinician should obtain a thorough history and perform a thorough examination and laboratory investigation.

A patient's behavior may also reflect abnormal thought content. A patient who is reluctant to talk and leers suspiciously at the examiner is displaying paranoid behavior, even if he or she denies it. A patient who is oriented and alert during an examination but who was combative and urinated in the corner of his or her hospital room the previous night is, or at least was, delirious.

Perceptions

Disorders of perception include illusions (misinterpretation of a real sensory experience), hallucinations (sensory perception in the absence of an external stimulus), delusions (false beliefs), and ideas of reference (incorrect interpretations that events have direct reference to oneself). In addition to questioning the patient about misperceptions, the physician should ask nurses and family members whether the patient attends to nonapparent stimuli, mentions hallucinations, makes bizarre comments, or behaves inappropriately. The patient who denies misperceptions but responds to hallucinations illustrates the importance of observing behavior during assessment.

Hallucinatory perception can be visual, auditory, tactile, olfactory (smell), gustatory (taste), or kinesthetic (body movement). Although cultural variations are important, hallucinations that occur in an awake individual are almost always symptomatic of a pathological process. Auditory hallucinations are more typical of primary psychiatric disorders, such as schizophrenia, mania, or psychotic depression; one notable exception is alcoholic hallucinosis, in which vivid auditory hallucinations occur in a fully oriented alcoholic patient (Victor and Hope 1958). Hallucinations that involve other sensory modalities are more typically associated with secondary disorders. (For a more detailed discussion, see Cummings 1995.)

Of patients with schizophrenia, 28%–72% have auditory hallucinations (D. W. Black and Andreasen 1999). Determining the quality and quantity of the auditory hallucinations may help the clinician diagnostically. Patients with primary psychiatric disorders often report clearly audible voices that comment on their actions, argue, repeat thoughts, or deprecate. A patient who only reports hearing his or her name called or other brief, repetitive auditory hallucinations may have CNS pathology or a nonpsychotic psychiatric disorder such as borderline personality disorder, somatization disorder, or dissociative identity disorder.

Visual hallucinations are more typically associated with brain disease, although they also occur in nonpsychiatric patients with severe, recent visual loss and in some patients with schizophrenia (Bracha et al. 1989). Visual hallucinations occur with delirium, narcolepsy, epilepsy, migraine, brain stem lesions, optic nerve disease, postocular surgery, vitreous detachment, stimulant and hallucinogen intoxication, and withdrawal syndromes. Visual hallucinations can also occur in healthy individuals during sensory or sleep deprivation, hypnosis, or sleep (dreams). Individuals who have a mood syndrome, such as a manic or depressive episode, sometimes report visual hallucinations. For example, a psychotically depressed patient may see the "face of the devil," or a manic patient may see the "face of God smiling at me." Patients with other psychiatric disorders such as conversion disorder, somatization disorder, or borderline personality disorder occasionally report visual hallucinations.

Tactile hallucinations occur commonly in patients who have undergone limb amputation or have substance-induced withdrawal delirium. Phantom limb—the feeling that the amputated limb is still present—occurs in a majority of patients who undergo amputation. Over time, the tactile hallucinations diminish and usually disappear (Frederiks 1969). Tactile hallucinations also occur in primary psychiatric disorders, such as schizophrenia, or in secondary psychiatric disorders, such as delirium, complex partial seizures, or substance-induced psychosis (e.g., hallucinogen-induced psychosis).

Olfactory, gustatory, or kinesthetic hallucinations are rare and are most commonly experienced by patients with partial seizures (Lishman 1998). However, these hallucinations can occur in patients with primary psychiatric disorders. For example, patients with somatization disorder or psychotic disorders occasionally report all three types of hallucinations. Patients with monosymptomatic hypochondriasis sometimes experience olfactory, tactile, or gustatory hallucinations.

Abstracting Abilities

Educational level is a strong determinant of the ability to abstract. Bedside testing is usually done by asking the patient to interpret simple proverbs, such as "People who live in glass houses should not throw stones." The patient who replies "Because the glass will break" has given a concrete answer. Concrete interpretations are commonly found in three groups: 1) individuals with less than a high school education, 2) patients with schizophrenia, and 3) patients with dementia. Proverbs are also diagnosti-

cally helpful when the patient gives a bizarre and personalized reply such as "That's what they do to crack people like me." Bizarre interpretation of proverbs almost always signifies an underlying psychosis.

Judgment

Judgment is the ability to anticipate the consequences of one's behavior and to behave in a culturally acceptable way. Recent behavior is the best indicator of a patient's judgment. For example, the confused, paranoid man with an acute myocardial infarction who believes he is about to be killed in the hospital, spits out his medications, and states "I'm leaving here now!" has very poor judgment. Examiners will sometimes ask the same patient questions like "What would you do if you found a stamped, sealed, addressed envelope in the street?" to assess judgment. If the patient replies that he or she would drop it in the nearest mailbox, sound judgment is supposedly implied. These types of questions are less adequate than the commonsense standard of recent behavior.

Insight

The term *insight* can have a wide range of meanings, including a simple awareness of one's own symptoms or a complex psychological awareness of conscious and unconscious determinants of one's behavior (Feher et al. 1989). In general, insight is present if the patient realizes that a problem exists, that his or her thinking and behavior may contribute to that problem, and that he or she may need assistance.

COGNITIVE COMPONENTS OF THE MENTAL STATUS EXAMINATION

Psychiatric residents and medical students who rotate on psychiatric consultation-liaison services, as well as some experienced psychiatrists, fall prey to two *fallacies* about testing cognitive function:

1. *Cognitive deficits are obvious during an interview or lengthy conversation.* Although this statement is true for patients with substantial cognitive dysfunction such as severe dementia or delirium, cognitive deficits are not obvious in most patients with mild to moderate global deficits or in many patients with focal neuropsychiatric deficits. Psychiatrists tend to rely heavily on the verbal output of patients to determine whether cognitive function is normal. Consequently, psychiatrists will not detect injury to brain areas that

do not influence verbal communications or deficits that may have been compensated for by the patient.

2. *Screening MSEs, such as those described later in this chapter, are sufficient to detect severe, global cognitive deficits.* Ideally, screening examinations should be both highly sensitive and specific enough to identify patients with cognitive impairments. Unfortunately, neither is the case, particularly in patients with focal deficits. Two frequently used examinations—the Mini-Mental State Exam (MMSE; Folstein et al. 1975) and the Cognitive Capacity Screening Examination (CCSE; Jacobs et al. 1977)—do not identify many patients who have cognitive deficits. In a neurosurgical population with known brain lesions, Schwamm et al. (1987) reported a false-negative rate of 43% with the MMSE and 53% with the CCSE.

Level of Consciousness

Psychiatric consultation is often requested for patients with a rapid or recent change in mental status. In most instances, the patient is either lethargic (not as alert as expected) or agitated and disruptive after surgery or some medical intervention. In addition to changes in arousal, such patients often exhibit altered thought content. This change in both alertness and thought content produces the clouded consciousness that typifies the confusional behavior seen in delirium (Lipowski 1990).

Any patient who is difficult to arouse or who will not remain alert without constant stimulation is usually physically ill. However, other clinical situations may produce or mimic a decreased level of consciousness. For example, sleepiness, boredom, simple intoxication, or a primary sleep disorder may produce lethargy. In addition, depressed patients with significant psychomotor retardation are sometimes withdrawn and very slow to respond. They are, however, rarely confused or lethargic in the sense used here. Also, a few patients will actually feign unconsciousness (so-called psychogenic unresponsiveness). One should consider this diagnosis only after a complete medical and neurological evaluation has failed to yield a more plausible explanation. Such patients usually have a psychiatric history and/or significant current environmental chaos to explain their behavior.

In the case of a patient with a decrease in level of consciousness, the clinician begins with an assessment for causes of a delirium or coma. The most common causes include toxic (medications, alcohol, illicit drugs, and withdrawal syndromes) and metabolic disturbances; these patients undergo a nonlocalizing neurological examination. Destructive cerebral lesions such as stroke, subdural hematoma, tumor, or abscess will also cause a decreased level of consciousness (Magoun 1963) but characteristically are associated with focal neurological findings. Meningitis, head trauma, seizures, and subarachnoid hemorrhage are also diagnostic possibilities. (For a more extensive discussion of this topic, please refer to Chapters 15 and 16 in this volume.)

Attention

The capacity to direct and maintain one's attention while screening out extraneous and irrelevant stimuli is a fundamental yet highly complex cognitive function (Berlucchi and Rizzolatti 1987; McGhie 1969). Inattention (the breakdown of selective attention) and distractibility are common and clinically significant neuropsychiatric symptoms. Inattention can also complicate the entire evaluation process (Mesulam 1985; Pribram and McGuinness 1975). For example, an inattentive patient will frequently fail tests of memory or calculation on the basis of inattention alone. Therefore, the clinician must use caution in the interpretation of cognitive failure in an inattentive patient.

Tests of attention include Forward Digit Span and the *A* Test for Vigilance (Strub and Black 1985). Digit span is a standard psychological test for attention. The patient must immediately repeat a series of numbers that are read to him or her in a slow, clear fashion. Five digits forward is the minimum required for a rating of normal attention. Backward digit span may depend on visuospatial processing as well as attention (F. W. Black 1986). In the vigilance test, the patient is presented letters at a rate of one per second and is asked to signal each time the letter *A* is said. A single error is considered indicative of an abnormal inability to sustain attention.

As important as it is to recognize that inattention can adversely affect performance on the MSE, it is equally important to realize that inattention is one of the least specific symptoms in psychiatry. Inattention is seen in conditions as diverse as simple anxiety or fatigue, delirium, dementia, schizophrenia, mania, and focal brain lesions, particularly those localized in the inferior frontal or parietal lobes.

In addition to conditions in which patients display global inattention, there is a special type of inattention called hemiattention or hemineglect (Kinsbourne 1970). In this condition, the patient is attentive to only half of his or her body and the extrapersonal space on that side and neglects the other half. This syndrome is most frequently manifested as a left hemiattention in a patient who has had a right-hemisphere brain lesion (Weinstein and Friedland 1977). Because it is nonspecific, inattention indicates only the presence of a problem. For the consultation-liaison psychiatrist, inattention is equivalent to the sedimentation rate for the internist. Its clinical significance is more fully appreciated when the inattention is combined with more specific symptoms.

Speech and Language

Brain disease, particularly dominant-hemisphere insults, frequently disrupts a patient's speech and language. Speech defects include the slurred speech of the intoxicated patient, the soft, trailing speech of the patient with Parkinson's disease, and the dysphonia and dysarthria of the patient with amyotrophic lateral sclerosis. Language disturbances, specifically aphasias, are defects in word choice, comprehension, and syntax seen when language areas of the brain are affected.

The consultation-liaison psychiatrist must develop a systematic way to screen for aphasia. A simple way to screen is to administer a bedside test, such as the pocket-size Reitan-Indiana Aphasia Screening Test (Reitan 1984). The clinical characteristics of aphasia syndromes are listed in Table 6–2.

First, the patient's spontaneous speech should be observed, and its rate, rhythm, and fluency should be described. Is speech fluent, and does the patient make sense? Speech content mirrors thought content. If speech is disorganized, absent, or bizarre, the clinician should suspect a psychotic process and must rule out an organic etiology. Next, comprehension must be tested. This is particularly important when the patient is on a respirator and normal speech is not possible. Yes-or-no questions should be asked. Examples include "Do you put on your socks before your shoes?" "Is there a tree in the room?" and "Can an elephant ride a tricycle?" (The psychiatrist should also note whether the patient smiles when asked absurd questions.) If the patient misses the humorous aspect of these questions, it usually means significant cognitive impairment, severe fear (terror), or depression.

Other aspects of speech that are tested include repetition (e.g., the patient is asked to repeat "no ifs, ands, or buts"), naming (the patient is asked to name both common and less frequently used items), reading, and writing. Agraphia accompanies aphasia and is also very frequently seen in patients with delirium (Chedru and Geschwind 1972).

In a practical sense, making the correct diagnosis in a patient with cognitive dysfunction is potentially lifesaving. For example, if an examiner cannot differentiate the fluent aphasia of a patient with a temporal lobe mass from the psychotic language of a decompensated patient with schizophrenia, he or she is likely to make a serious misdiagnosis. Patients with different disorders require different plans of management. The patient with an aphasia or parietal lobe syndrome caused by a focal brain lesion is referred to a neurologist or neurosurgeon. These examples underscore the tremendous practical importance of proper diagnosis in the emergency room or at the bedside on the acute medical ward.

TABLE 6–2.   Clinical characteristics of aphasia

Type	Speech	Comprehension	Repetition	Naming	Writing	Reading	Associated deficits	Emotional reaction
Broca's	Nonfluent	Intact	Impaired	Impaired	Impaired	Impaired	Right hemiparesis	Despair
(Patient cannot articulate and is frustrated; speech is sparse [or absent] and telegraphic.)								
Wernicke's	Fluent	Impaired	Impaired	Impaired	Impaired	Impaired	Hemianopsia ± hemisensory loss	Unaware
(Patient articulates well but speaks nonsense and does not understand.)								
Conduction	Fluent	Intact	Impaired	Impaired	± Impaired	Intact	± Hemisensory loss	Frustration
(Like Wernicke's aphasia except patient can understand and is aware of deficits.)								
Anomic	Fluent	Intact	Intact	Impaired	± Impaired	Intact	Varies	± Aware
(Patient cannot name objects but describes their use; makes lame excuses for deficit.)								
Global	Nonfluent	Impaired	Impaired	Impaired	Impaired	Impaired	Right hemiparesis, hemisensory loss, hemianopsia	Unaware
(Very large lesion, marked impairment.)								

Source.   Reprinted from Wise MG, Rundell JR: *Concise Guide to Consultation Psychiatry,* 2nd Edition. Washington, DC, American Psychiatric Press, 1994, p. 13. Used with permission.

Orientation

When the patient correctly answers questions about orientation to self, time (year, month, day, and time of day), location, and circumstance, this fact is usually recorded in the medical chart as "oriented×4." An oriented×4 entry in the chart can lead to diagnostic errors. First, the phrase is used loosely by nonpsychiatric physicians, surgeons, and nurses. It typically means that the patient is not obviously confused. Oriented×4 does not mean that the patient was formally tested. Second, some clinicians equate disorientation with brain dysfunction or, conversely, believe that accurate orientation implies normal brain function. Clinicians who adopt this way of thinking are prone to making diagnostic errors. For example, in patients with focal CNS lesions, mild delirium, or early dementia, orientation is often normal. In addition, disorientation to self is rarely exhibited by patients with neurological dysfunction other than patients with severe dementia or aphasias. Disorientation to self is almost always due to a primary psychiatric disorder, especially dissociative disorders such as dissociative identity disorder, dissociative amnesia, and dissociative fugue. Even when global cognitive dysfunction such as dementia or delirium is present, disorientation is not found as frequently as one might suspect. In one study, for example, only 36% of patients with acute delirium were disoriented to year, 43% to month, and 34% to location (Cutting 1980).

Disorientation in space is potentially a very frightening experience for patients. Driving to the store and becoming hopelessly lost, being unable to find one's car in a shopping center parking lot, and losing one's way to the bathroom in one's own home are common clinical examples of geographic disorientation or disorientation in space. Several neuropsychological mechanisms can impair spatial orientation. For example, a person who loses his or her car in a large parking lot may have normal brain function but may have been preoccupied at the time the car was parked and thus may have failed to note its location. In other circumstances, the symptom is not so innocent. For example, a patient with mild delirium may, because of clouded consciousness and muddled thinking, become disoriented and lose his or her car. In addition, patients with dementia or amnesia may not remember the car's location because of deficits in recent memory function.

A different type of spatial disorientation occurs in patients with parietal lobe damage (DeRenzi 1985). Such patients have a true geographic disorientation and fail to find their cars because of visual-spatial disorientation. These patients have visual perception deficits and cannot integrate that information with the location of objects in extrapersonal space. True spatial disorientation occurs more commonly in patients with right parietal lesions but can occur in patients with lesions in other areas of the brain. Spatial disorientation also is seen in patients with hemineglect or hemiattention. These patients usually have right parietal lesions and neglect events that occur in the left side of their environment. Geographic disorientation is caused by various neuropsychological mechanisms and disease processes. The ability to recognize a specific symptom and connect it with brain dysfunction is an important diagnostic skill for the consultation-liaison psychiatrist to develop.

Memory

Memory loss is a common symptom seen by the consultation-liaison psychiatrist and has many different causes. Memory loss can be symptomatic of either a primary or secondary psychiatric disorder. The patient's history is very useful in sorting through the differential diagnosis of memory dysfunction. In general, in patients younger than 40 years, especially those with a history of previous or concomitant emotional problems, a psychiatric disorder is the most likely explanation for their amnesia; however, elderly people with progressive memory loss more frequently have a type of dementia.

The ability to assess memory function is a crucial clinical skill. Haphazard testing leads to erroneous findings. For example, a patient may be given a diagnosis of dementia when the memory problem is actually due to anxiety or depression. This is especially true in elderly patients. A diagnosis is only as good as the data used to formulate it. More detailed discussions of memory testing are found in works by Strub and Black (1985, 1988), Squire and Butters (1984), and Victor et al. (1989).

Questions about orientation serve as a basic test of recent memory. In addition, the patient should be asked to remember four unrelated objects, such as tulip, eyedropper, car, and ball. The patient should immediately repeat them to ensure that he or she has properly heard and understood the words. After conversing with the patient about other things for about 3 minutes, the psychiatrist should ask the patient to repeat the words. If the patient cannot recall the words, the psychiatrist should determine whether the words were not encoded into memory or were encoded but cannot be retrieved. Such differentiation can be made by giving the patient clues. Patients who did not learn the words will not be aided by prompting, whereas patients who learned the words but cannot access them quickly will recall with prompting. These two patterns imply possible damage to different anatomic structures: medial hemispheric structures (hippocampus, fornix, and mammillary bodies) in the case of amnesia and frontal-subcortical structures in the case of poor retrieval

(Cummings 1993). Testing memory for designs is also easy. The patient should be asked to replicate designs used to test constructional praxis. The examiner can use a three-word/three-shape test, such as that described by Weintraub and Mesulam (1985).

It is more difficult to test remote memory, because the examiner must know whether the information given by the patient is correct or confabulated. The clinician can ask the patient to name the last five presidents or, better yet, ask about important world events that almost everyone knows. A good subject for memory testing, possibly for many years to come, is the O. J. Simpson trial.

SCREENING MENTAL STATUS EXAMINATIONS

A number of bedside examinations can be used to screen patients for cognitive dysfunction (Borson et al. 2000; Folstein et al. 1975; Isaacs and Kennie 1973; Jacobs et al. 1977; Katzman et al. 1983; Kiernan et al. 1987; Reitan 1958; M. A. Taylor et al. 1987) (Table 6–3). These screening examinations have advantages and disadvantages (Table 6–4). Screening MSEs are very useful for physicians who do not normally include an MSE in their examinations. For the consultation-liaison psychiatrist, who is an expert in cognition and its measurement, screening MSEs are only one part of a more extensive examination of cognitive function. Sometimes the score on an MSE such as the MMSE will influence a physician who doubts a psychiatrist's opinion but who believes "hard data." In addition, serial screening MSEs are useful when the clinical course of a patient with delirium or dementia is being followed.

The MMSE is probably the most widely used and best-known screening MSE. The MMSE (Figure 6–2) tests orientation, memory (registration and recall), attention, calculation, language (naming, repetition, ability to follow complicated commands, reading, and writing), and constructional ability. The test takes about 5 minutes to administer, can be administered serially to follow a patient's clinical course, and is a reliable and valid test in medical patients (Anthony et al. 1982; Nelson et al. 1986; Strub and Black 1977).

Various MMSE cutoff scores are proposed to indicate delirium or dementia. A score of 20 or less may indicate impairment (Folstein et al. 1975); however, Mungas (1991) proposed that a score of 0–10 corresponds to severe cognitive impairment, 11–20 to moderate impairment, 20–25 to mild impairment, and 25–30 to questionable impairment or intact function. Delirium and demen-

TABLE 6–3. Screening mental status examinations

A Test for Vigilance
Bender Gestalt Test
Blessed Dementia Scale
Draw a clock face
Frank Jones story
Marie Three Paper Test
Mini-Cog (Borson et al. 2000)
Mini-Mental State Exam
Modified Mini-Mental State Exam
Neurobehavioral Cognitive Status Examination
Reitan-Indiana Aphasia Screening Test
Set Test
Taylor Equivalent Test
Trail Making Test (Trail Parts A and B)

TABLE 6–4. Screening mental status examinations (MSEs): advantages and disadvantages

Advantages
Brief (usually take only 5–10 minutes)
Structures format (ensures consistent examination of cognitive functions)
Single score (uncomplicated)
Face validity (questions from traditional MSE)
Familiar (questions from traditional MSE)
Less fatiguing for medically ill patients
Used repeatedly to follow course of cognitive dysfunction

Disadvantages
Does not identify people with focal deficits (high false-negative rate)
Does not identify mild global deficits (low sensitivity)
Does not identify well-educated patient with significant deficits
May create false sense of security when score indicates "normal" function
Education dependent (score likely to be lower with less than an eighth-grade education)
Few validation studies with outpatients
Few studies on the effect of sociodemographic factors

Source. Reprinted from Wise MG, Rundell JR: *Concise Guide to Consultation Psychiatry,* 2nd Edition. Washington, DC, American Psychiatric Press, 1994, p. 18. Used with permission.

tia are not the only reasons for a low score on the MMSE. Other reasons include deafness, blindness, mutism, inability to understand English, aphasia, mental retardation, lack of cooperation, and an educational level of less than eighth grade. The clinician can adjust MMSE cutoff scores for age and educational level (Bravo and Hebert 1997). A cutoff score of 17 yields a sensitivity of 81% and a specificity of 100% for dementia in geriatric patients with

Patient _____

Examiner _____

Date _____

Maximum score	Score	
		Orientation
5	( )	What is the (year) (season) (date) (day) (month)?
5	( )	Where are we: (state) (country) (town) (hospital) (floor)?
		Registration
3	( )	Name 3 objects; 1 second to say each. Then ask the patient all 3 after you have said them. Give 1 point for each correct answer. Then repeat them until he learns all 3. Count trials and record.

Trials _____

Attention and Calculation

5	( )	Serial 7's. 1 point for each correct. Stop after 5 answers. Alternatively spell "world" backwards.

Recall

3	( )	Ask for the 3 objects repeated above. Give 1 point for each correct.

Language

9	( )	Name a pencil, and watch (2 points)
		Repeat the following "No ifs ands or buts." (1 point)
		Follow a 3-stage command:

"Take a paper in your right hand, fold it in half, and put it on the floor" (3 points)

Read and obey the following:

Close YOUR eyes (1 point)

Write a sentence (1 point)
Copy design (1 point)
Total score
ASSESS level of consciousness
   along a continuum _____

Alert   Drowsy   Stupor   Coma

FIGURE 6–2. Mini-Mental State Exam with instructions for its administration.

Source. Reprinted from Folstein MF, Folstein SE, McHugh PR: "Mini-Mental State, a Practical Method for Grading the Cognitive State of Patients for the Clinician." *Journal of Psychiatric Research* 12:189–198, 1975. Copyright 1975, MF Folstein. Used with permission.

INSTRUCTIONS FOR ADMINISTRATION
OF MINI-MENTAL STATE EXAM

Orientation

(1)   Ask for the date. Then ask specifically for parts omitted, e.g., "Can you also tell me what season it is?" One point for each correct.

(2)   Ask in turn "Can you tell me the name of this hospital?" (town, county, etc.). One point for each correct.

Registration

Ask the patient if you may test his memory. Then say the names of 3 unrelated objects, clearly and slowly, about 1 second for each. After you have said all 3, ask him to repeat them. This first repetition determines his score (0–3) but keep saying them until he can repeat all 3, up to 6 trials. If he does not eventually learn all 3, recall cannot be meaningfully tested.

Attention and Calculation

Ask the patient to begin with 100 and count backwards by 7. Stop after 5 subtractions (93, 86, 79, 72, 65). Score the total number of correct answers.

If the patient cannot or will not perform this task, ask him to spell the word "world" backwards. The score is the number of letters in correct order. E.g., dlrow = 5, dlorw = 3.

Recall

Ask the patient if he can recall the 3 words you previously asked him to remember. Score 0–3.

Language

Naming: Show the patient a wrist watch and ask him what it is. Repeat for pencil. Score 0–2.

Repetition: Ask the patient to repeat the sentence after you. allow only one trial. Score 0 or 1.

3-Stage command: give the patient a piece of plain blank paper and repeat the command. Score 1 point for each part correctly executed.

Reading: On a blank piece of paper print the sentence "Close your eyes," in letters large enough for the patient to see clearly. Ask him to read it and do what it says. Score 1 point only if he actually closes his eyes.

Writing: Give the patient a blank piece of paper and ask him or her to write a sentence for you. Do not dictate a sentence, it is to be written spontaneously. It must contain a subject and verb and be sensible. Correct grammar and punctuation are not necessary.

Copying: On a clean piece of paper, draw intersecting pentagons, each side about 1 in., and ask him to copy it exactly as it is. All 10 angles must be present and 2 must intersect to score 1 point. Tremor and rotation are ignored.

Estimate the patient's level of sensorium along a continuum, from alert on the left to coma on the right.

FIGURE 6–2.   Mini-Mental State Exam with instructions for its administration. *(continued)*

---

8 years of education or less. A more standard cutoff score of 23 yielded a sensitivity of 93% and a specificity of 100% in geriatric patients with more than 8 years of education (Murden et al. 1991). A number of MMSE modifications are available to address cultural and language differences, increase sensitivity and specificity, and ease administration (Koenig 1996; Shadlen et al. 1999; Teng and Chui 1987; Wang and Starren 1999; Yaffe et al. 1999).

The clinician must ensure that the patient has his or her usual sensory aids before testing, such as a hearing aid or glasses. Regardless of the reason for a low score on the MMSE, the information has clinical relevance. For example, if the patient cannot understand questions because of a language barrier, he or she will not understand his or her treatment or discharge medications and instructions. When alternative explanations for poor MMSE performance are ruled out, the disturbance is most likely caused by delirium, dementia, or dementia with a superimposed delirium. Chapters 15 and 16 contain detailed discussions of delirium (confusional states) and dementia.

Kiernan et al. (1987) developed the Neurobehavioral Cognitive Status Examination (NCSE), which is another approach to cognitive function assessment. The NCSE independently profiles multiple areas of cognitive function, takes about 20 minutes to administer in impaired patients, and has a lower false-negative rate than the MMSE.

Other Useful Tests of Cognitive Function

The consultation-liaison psychiatrist must have expertise in administering several tests, even to patients who are bedridden or on a respirator. In this section, we describe a few tests that are clinically useful. Lishman's classic text, *Organic Psychiatry* (Lishman 1998), has an excellent detailed discussion of cognitive function and psychometric tests.

The A *Test for Vigilance* measures the ability to sustain attention. For example, a series of letters is read at a rate of one per second, and the patient is asked to raise his or her hand each time the letter *A* is read.

The *Bender Gestalt Test* (Bender 1938) examines the patient's ability to copy designs. Nine designs are presented to the patient, one at a time, and he or she is asked to copy them. Errors suggest brain dysfunction, and error-free performance strongly supports the absence of brain disease. Memory for designs can be tested by asking the patient to reproduce the figures after a brief period.

The *Blessed Dementia Scale* consists of two parts, which can be used separately or together (Blessed et al. 1968). One part measures the patient's ability to perform everyday activities, and the second part measures the patient's ability to complete an information-memory-concentration test. Information about daily activities is provided by a knowledgeable family member or close friend. The Blessed Dementia Scale does not have a cutoff score to establish the diagnosis of dementia. Instead, an increasing score correlates with worsening dementia.

Draw a clock face is another useful bedside test that should be part of the core MSE (Lishman 1987). This task is easy to administer and is very instructive, particularly with regard to constructional apraxia and therefore early dementia (Esteban-Santillan et al. 1998) or delirium (Wise and Rundell 1999). (See Figure 16–3 in this volume for a further explanation of this test.)

The *Frank Jones story* tests the patient's ability to conceptualize a situation and to solve a problem (Wise and Rundell 1994). The patient is asked to explain the following story: "I have a friend by the name of Frank Jones whose feet are so big that he has to put on his pants by pulling them over his head. Can Mr. Jones do that?" A patient with normal cognitive function will typically laugh and then explain in an understandable way why it is impossible. When a patient with dementia hears the story, he or she usually will not laugh, because he or she does not understand the problem. The patient is also unable to rationally explain his or her response. A patient

with delirium usually will laugh because he or she finds the situation humorous. However, regardless of his or her answer, the patient usually gives a bizarre or extremely inadequate explanation for that answer. For example, "He can't...well, maybe he can if he unzips his fly," "He just can't," or "I guess so if he takes off his shoes."

The *Marie Three Paper Test* permits a quick assessment for comprehension problems and receptive aphasia (Lishman 1987). Three different-sized pieces of paper are placed in front of the patient. The patient is then told to take the biggest piece and hand it to the examiner, take the smallest piece and throw it to the ground, and take the middle-sized one and place it in his or her pocket.

The *Reitan-Indiana Aphasia Screening Test* is a pocket-size, easily administered, brief aphasia screen (Reitan 1984). This test permits a reasonable survey of aphasic symptoms, including the ability to copy, name, spell, write, read, calculate, and demonstrate the use of an object (ideomotor praxis).

The *Set Test* is a test of verbal fluency designed to screen elderly patients for dementia (Isaacs and Kennie 1973). The patient is asked to name 10 items from each of four categories. A useful mnemonic to recall the categories is *FACT*—fruits, animals, colors, towns. The patient is asked to name 10 fruits, then to name 10 animals, and so on. The score is the total number of items named, with a maximum score of 40. In patients age 65 or older, scores below 15 are clearly abnormal and indicate impairment. (Note: This is not a timed test. It is an excellent test for frontal lobe dysfunction and is a great distraction after presentation of four words to remember.)

The *Taylor Equivalent Test* (Figure 6–3) is a test of constructional ability (L. B. Taylor 1979). The patient is asked to draw the figure and is then asked to draw the picture from memory several minutes later. A standard scoring system is used for this test.

The *Trail Making Test (Trail Parts A and B)* consists of several circles distributed on a sheet of paper (Reitan 1958). In Part A, the circles contain numbers, and the patient is asked to connect the numbers in sequence by drawing a line as quickly as possible from one circle to the next. In Part B, each circle contains either a number or a letter. The patient is asked to alternate between numbers and letters (1, then *A*, then 2, then *B*, and so on). Both Trail Part A and Trail Part B are timed tests, and age-corrected norms are available. More than one error on either test is usually significant.

Other bedside tests that are particularly useful include a sheet of paper with a drawing on one side for the patient to copy and a series of mathematical problems on the other side. The problems should vary from simple (e.g., $1 + 7 = \_$) to more complex (e.g., $9,798 \div 23 = \_$). Observing the patient while he or she

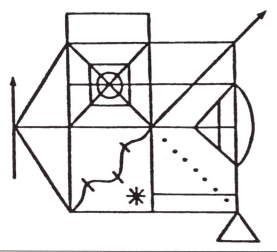

FIGURE 6–3. The Taylor Equivalent Test.

Source. Reprinted from Taylor LB: "Psychological Assessment of Neurosurgical Patients," in *Functional Neurosurgery.* Edited by Rasmusen TB, Marino R. New York, Raven, 1979, pp. 165–180. Used with permission.

attempts to draw and calculate is quite revealing, both about possible brain dysfunction and about the patient's personality style.

THE CONSULTATION-LIAISON PSYCHIATRIST AS NEUROPSYCHIATRIST

The consultation-liaison psychiatrist who can administer a variety of tests of cognitive function and perform a brief neurological examination is able to identify cognitive and neurological deficits. If the psychiatrist also has a knowledge of neuropsychiatry, he or she can organize and understand symptoms within the context of brain-behavior relationships and identify specific clinical syndromes, such as dementia, left-hemisphere lesions, and delirium.

Neurological Examination

During a consultation, the consultation-liaison psychiatrist will often need to perform a basic neurological examination. A neurological examination is essential in any patient with cognitive dysfunction, suspected somatoform or conversion disorder with neurological complaints, or malingering. The examination does not have to be time-consuming. The patient's history may also suggest deficits. A spouse may state, "He only writes on the right side of the paper and never on the left side." This patient probably has nondominant (right-sided) brain dysfunction with associated left-sided neglect.

In a basic bedside neurological examination, the clinician should do the following:

1. Check deep tendon reflexes for symmetry. Check for the presence of a Babinski reflex. Some clinicians also check for primitive reflexes (snout, grasp, glabellar, and palmomental), although the usefulness of frontal release signs has been challenged (Fogel and Eslinger 1991; Ovsiew 1992). The presence of two or three primitive reflexes often indicates dementia (Ovsiew 1992).
2. Check muscle strength for asymmetry, weakness, tone, or embellishment.
3. Observe the gait and associated arm movements.
4. Examine cranial nerve function.
5. Check the distribution of any sensory complaints.
6. Check for signs of meningeal irritation, such as neck stiffness, headache, or Kernig and Brudzinski signs.

Knowledge of brain-behavior relationships is important for psychiatrists to function well as consultants in the hospital setting. The consultation-liaison psychiatrist must understand neurological terminology. The following list contains a few commonly used neurological terms. The prefix *a-* means complete loss of ability (e.g., aphasia is the loss of ability to comprehend or produce speech), and the prefix *dys-* means an impaired ability (e.g., dysphasia is an impairment in the ability to comprehend or produce speech).

- *Abulia*—loss of willpower
- *Acalculia*—loss of the ability to do mathematical calculations
- *Agnosia*—loss or diminution of the ability to recognize familiar objects
- *Agraphia*—loss of the ability to express thought in writing
- *Alexia*—loss of the ability to read (acquired)
- *Apraxia*—loss or impairment of the ability to use objects correctly
- *Ataxia*—impaired motor coordination
- *Dysarthria*—disturbance of articulation of speech caused by muscle dysfunction
- *Dyslexia*—disturbance of the ability to read
- *Dysphasia*—impaired ability to comprehend, elaborate, or produce speech
- *Dysprosody*—disturbance of pitch, rhythm, and variation of speech

Correlating neuropsychiatric or behavioral dysfunction with cortical anatomy is difficult. It requires effort and practice, and it is not an exact science. Approximate cortical localization of various cognitive and behavioral functions is summarized in Table 6–5.

TABLE 6–5. Cortical mapping of brain dysfunction

Abnormality	Frontal	Dominant temporoparietal	Dominant parietal	Nondominant parietal	Nondominant temporoparietal	Occipital	Corpus callosum
Motor	Motor impersistence Inertia Impaired rapid sequential movements Stimulus-bound behavior (e.g., echopraxia)	Dysgraphia	Ideokinetic (ideomotor) dyspraxia Kinesthetic dyspraxia	Constructional dyspraxia Dressing dyspraxia Kinesthetic dyspraxia			Inability to tie shoes with eyes closed Ideokinetic dyspraxia in hand ipsilateral to dominant hemisphere Constructional dyspraxia in hand contralateral to dominant hemisphere Alexia without agraphia
Language	Broca's aphasia Transcortical aphasia Motor aprosodia[a] Verbigeration	Wernicke's aphasia Driveling, word approximations, neologisms Pure word deafness Dysgraphia Dyslexia Dysnomia Letter and number agnosia Sensory aprosodia	Dyslexia Dysnomia				
Memory	Impaired short-term memory store	Impairment of rehearsed consolidated memory			Impaired musical memory	Impaired visual memory	
Other	Impaired concentration Global disorientation Impaired judgment Impaired problem solving Impaired abstraction Right spatial neglect		Finger agnosia Dyscalculia Right-left and east-west disorientation Dysstereognosis Dysgraphesthesis Impaired symbolic categorization	Dysstereognosis Dysgraphesthesis Anosognosia Prosopagnosia Reduplicative paramnesia Left spatial neglect			Dysstereognosis of hand ipsilateral to dominant hemisphere Dysgraphesthesis of hand ipsilateral to dominant hemisphere

[a]Nondominant frontal lobe.

Source. Adapted from Hales RE, Yudofsky SC: *The American Psychiatric Press Textbook of Neuropsychiatry.* Washington, DC, American Psychiatric Press, 1987, p. 6. Copyright 1987, American Psychiatric Press. Used with permission.

SUMMARY

Effective psychiatric consultation in patients who are medically ill requires many clinical skills and the ability to integrate diverse pieces of information into a diagnosis. Essential skills for the consultation-liaison psychiatrist are the ability to perform a comprehensive MSE—especially the ability to test cognitive functions at the patient's bedside—and the ability to perform a brief neurological and focused physical examination. These data are combined with historical information (e.g., the patient's medical and psychiatric history, medications, and laboratory results) and the clinician's knowledge of medicine, psychiatric disorders, defense mechanisms, characterology, and brain-behavior relationships to formulate a diagnosis. This sophisticated process is essential to the proper diagnosis and treatment of medically ill patients who develop psychiatric symptoms.

REFERENCES

American Psychiatric Association: Diagnostic and Statistical Manual of Mental Disorders, 4th Edition. Washington, DC, American Psychiatric Association, 1994

Anthony JC, LeResche L, Niaz U, et al: Limits of the 'Mini-Mental State' as a screening test for dementia and delirium among hospital patients. Psychol Med 12:397–408, 1982

Bender L: A Visual Motor Gestalt Test and Its Clinical Use. New York, American Orthopsychiatric Association, 1938

Benson D, Peterson LG, Bartay J: Neuropsychiatric manifestations of antihypertensive medications. Psychiatr Med 1:205–214, 1983

Berlucchi G, Rizzolatti G: Selective visual attention. Neuropsychologia 25:1–3, 1987

Black DW, Andreasen NC: Schizophrenia, schizophreniform disorder, and delusional (paranoid) disorders, in The American Psychiatric Press Textbook of Psychiatry, 3rd Edition. Edited by Hales RE, Yudofsky SC, Talbott JA. Washington, DC, American Psychiatric Press, 1999, pp 425–477

Black FW: Digit repetition in brain-damaged adults: clinical and theoretical implications. J Clin Psychol 42:770–782, 1986

Blessed G, Tomlinson BE, Roth M: The association between quantitative measures of dementia and of senile changes in the cerebral gray matter of elderly subjects. Br J Psychiatry 114:797–811, 1968

Borson S., Scanlan J, Brush M, et al: The mini-cog: a cognitive "vital signs" mesure for dementia screening in multi-lingual elderly. International Journal of Geriatric Psychiatry 15:1021–1027, 2000

Bracha HS, Wolkowitz OM, Lohr JB, et al: High prevalence of visual hallucination in research subjects with chronic schizophrenia. Am J Psychiatry 146:526–528, 1989

Bravo G, Hebert R: Age- and education-specific reference values for the Mini-Mental and modified Mini-Mental State Examinations derived from a non-demented elderly population. Int J Geriatr Psychiatry 12:1008-1018, 1997

Chedru F, Geschwind N: Writing disturbances in acute confusional states. Neuropsychologia 10:343–353, 1972

Cummings JL: The mental status examination. Hosp Pract (Off Ed) 28:56–58, 60, 65–68, 1993

Cummings JL: Concise Guide to Neuropsychiatry and Behavioral Neurology. Washington, DC, American Psychiatric Press, 1995

Cutting J: Physical illness and psychosis. Br J Psychiatry 136: 109–119, 1980

DeRenzi E: Disorders of spatial orientation, in Handbook of Clinical Neurology, Vol 1: Clinical Neuropsychology. Edited by Frederiks JAM. Amsterdam, Elsevier, 1985, pp 405–422

Esteban-Santillan C, Praditsuwan R, Ueda H, et al: Clock drawing test in very mild Alzheimer's disease. J Am Geriatr Soc 46:1266-1269, 1998

Feher EP, Doody R, Pirozzolo FJ, et al: Mental status assessment of insight and judgment. Clin Geriatr Med 5:477–498, 1989

Fogel BS, Eslinger PJ: Diagnosis and management of patients with frontal lobe syndromes, in Medical-Psychiatric Practice, Vol 1. Edited by Stoudemire A, Fogel BS. Washington, DC, American Psychiatric Press, 1991, pp 349–392

Folstein MF, Folstein SE, McHugh PR: Mini-Mental State: a practical method for grading the cognitive state of patients for the clinician. J Psychiatr Res 12:189–198, 1975

Frederiks JAM: Disorders of the body schema, in Handbook of Clinical Neurology, Vol 4. Edited by Vinken PJ, Bruyn GW. Amsterdam, North-Holland, 1969, pp 207–240

Gold MS, Pottash ALC, Extein I: Hypothyroidism and depression: evidence from complete thyroid function evaluation. JAMA 245:1919–1922, 1981

Isaacs B, Kennie AT: The Set Test as an aid to the detection of dementia in old people. Br J Psychiatry 123:467–470, 1973

Jacobs JW, Bernhard MR, Delgado A, et al: Screening for organic mental syndromes in the medically ill. Ann Intern Med 86:40–46, 1977

Kallman H, May HJ: Mental status assessment in the elderly. Prim Care 16:329–347, 1989

Katzman R, Brown T, Fuld P: Validation of a short orientation-memory-concentration test of cognitive impairment. Am J Psychiatry 140:734–739, 1983

Kiernan RJ, Mueller J, Langston JW, et al: The Neurobehavioral Cognitive Status Examination: a brief but quantitative approach to cognitive assessment. Ann Intern Med 107:481–485, 1987

Kinsbourne M: The cerebral basis of lateral asymmetries in attention. Acta Psychol (Amst) 33:193–201, 1970

Knights EB, Folstein MF: Unsuspected emotional and cognitive disturbance in medical patients. Ann Intern Med 87:723–724, 1977

Koenig HG: An abbreviated Mini-Mental State Exam for medically ill older adults (letter). J Am Geriatr Soc 44:215-216, 1996

Krauthammer C, Klerman GL: Secondary mania. Arch Gen Psychiatry 35:1333–1339, 1978

Lipowski ZJ: Delirium: Acute Confusional States. New York, Oxford University Press, 1990

Lishman WA: Organic Psychiatry: The Psychological Consequences of Cerebral Disorder, 2nd Edition. Oxford, Blackwell Scientific, 1987

Lishman WA: Organic Psychiatry: The Psychological Consequences of Cerebral Disorder, 3rd Edition. Oxford, Blackwell Scientific, 1998, pp 68-121

Magoun HW: The Waking Brain. Springfield, IL, Charles C Thomas, 1963

McGhie A: Pathology of Attention. Middlesex, UK, Penguin, 1969

Mesulam M-M: Attention, confusional states, and neglect, in Principles of Behavioral Neurology. Edited by Mesulam M-M. Philadelphia, PA, FA Davis, 1985, pp 125–140

Mungas D: In-office mental status testing: a practical guide. Geriatrics 46:54–66, 1991

Murden R, McRae T, Kaner S, et al: Mini-Mental State Exam scores vary with education in blacks and whites. J Am Geriatr Soc 117:326-328, 1991

Nelson A, Fogel BS, Faust D: Bedside cognitive screening instruments: a critical assessment. J Nerv Ment Dis 174:73–83, 1986

Ovsiew F: Bedside neuropsychiatry: eliciting the clinical phenomena of neuropsychiatric illness, in The American Psychiatric Press Textbook of Neuropsychiatry, 2nd Edition. Edited by Yudofsky SC, Hales RE. Washington, DC, American Psychiatric Press, 1992, pp 89–126

Parikh RM, Robinson RG, Lipsey JR, et al: The impact of poststroke depression on recovery in activities of daily living over a 2-year follow-up. Arch Neurol 47:785–789, 1990

Pribram KH, McGuinness P: Arousal, activation and effort in the control of attention. Psychol Rev 82:116–149, 1975

Reitan RM: Validity of the Trail Making Test as an indicator of organic brain damage. Percept Mot Skills 8:271–276, 1958

Reitan RM: Aphasia and Sensory-Perceptual Deficits in Adults. Tucson, AZ, Neuropsychology Press, 1984

Robinson RG, Starkstein SE: Current research in affective disorders following stroke. J Neuropsychiatry Clin Neurosci 2:1–14, 1990

Rundell JR, Wise MG: Causes of organic mood disorder. J Neuropsychiatry Clin Neurosci 1:398–400, 1989

Schwamm LH, Van Dyke C, Kiernan RJ, et al: The Neurobehavioral Cognitive Status Examination: comparison with the Cognitive Capacity Screening Examination and the Mini-Mental State Examination in a neurosurgical population. Ann Intern Med 107:486–491, 1987

Shadlen MF, Larson EB, Gibbons L, et al: Alzheimer's disease symptom severity in blacks and whites. J Am Geriatr Soc 47:482-486, 1999

Silverstone PH: Prevalence of psychiatric disorders in medical inpatients. J Nerv Ment Dis 184:43-51, 1996

Squire LR, Butters N (eds): Neuropsychology of Memory. New York, Guilford, 1984

Strub RL, Black FW: The Mental Status Examination in Neurology. Philadelphia, PA, FA Davis, 1977

Strub RL, Black FW: The Mental Status Examination in Neurology, 2nd Edition. Philadelphia, PA, FA Davis, 1985

Strub RL, Black FW: Neurobehavioral Disorders: A Clinical Approach. Philadelphia, PA, FA Davis, 1988

Taylor LB: Psychological assessment of neurosurgical patients, in Functional Neurosurgery. Edited by Rasmussen TB, Marino R. New York, Raven, 1979, pp 165–180

Taylor MA, Sierles FS, Abrams R: The neuropsychiatric evaluation, in The American Psychiatric Press Textbook of Neuropsychiatry. Edited by Hales RE, Yudofsky SC. Washington, DC, American Psychiatric Press, 1987, pp 3–16

Teng EL, Chui HC: The Modified Mini-Mental State (3MS) Examination. J Clin Psychiatry 48:314-318, 1987

Victor M, Hope JM: The phenomenon of auditory hallucinations in chronic alcoholism: a critical evaluation of the status of alcoholic hallucinosis. J Nerv Ment Dis 126:451–481, 1958

Victor M, Adams RD, Collins GH: The Wernicke-Korsakoff Syndrome and Related Neurologic Disorders Due to Alcoholism and Malnutrition, 2nd Edition. Philadelphia, PA, FA Davis, 1989

Wang SS, Starren J: A Java speech implementation of the Mini Mental State Exam. Proceedings of the Amia Symposium, 1999, pp 435–439

Weinstein EA, Friedland RP (eds): Hemi-Inattention and Hemispheric Specialization (Advances in Neurology Series, Vol 18). New York, Raven, 1977

Weintraub S, Mesulam M-M: Mental state assessment of young and elderly adults in behavioral neurology, in Principles of Behavioral Neurology. Edited by Mesulam M-M. Philadelphia, PA, FA Davis, 1985, pp 71–123

Wise MG, Rundell JR: Concise Guide to Consultation Psychiatry, 2nd Edition. Washington, DC, American Psychiatric Press, 1994, pp 11-30

Wise MG, Rundell JR: Concise Guide to Consultation Psychiatry, 3rd Edition. Washington, DC, American Psychiatric Press, 1999

Wise MG, Taylor SE: Anxiety and mood disorders in medically ill patients. J Clin Psychiatry 51 (suppl):27–32, 1990

Wise MG, Brannan SK, Shanfield SB, et al: Psychiatry aspects of organ transplantation (letter). JAMA 260:3437, 1988

Yaffe K, Blackwell T, Gore R, et al: Depressive symptoms and cognitive decline in nondemented elderly women: a prospective study. Arch Gen Psychiatry 56:425–430, 1999

7

Neuropsychological and Psychological Assessment

Robert L. Mapou, Ph.D.

Wendy A. Law, Ph.D.

Jack Spector, Ph.D.

Gary G. Kay, Ph.D.

Over the past 15 years, advances in neurodiagnostic technology have revolutionized how medical professionals diagnose and treat neuropsychiatric disorders. Refinement of magnetic resonance imaging (MRI) has facilitated examination of structural brain abnormalities, and the newer functional MRI enables researchers to examine brain functioning during cognitive task performance. The advent of computerized electroencephalography, including spectral analysis and topographic brain mapping, has increased the precision of electrophysiological measurement. Evoked and cognitive event-related potential studies, such as the P300, are being used increasingly in diagnosis. Brain metabolic function can now be elucidated using positron-emission tomography or single photon emission computed tomography.

Although one can learn much about brain structure and function using these neurodiagnostic modalities, they provide no information about a patient's everyday functioning. They do not tell clinicians anything about whether a patient can work, can perform basic activities of daily living, has independent living skills, or will require supervised care throughout the day. To address these issues, one must turn to other objective measures of actual functioning and behavior, such as clinical neuropsychological and psychological assessment.

Neuropsychology is the study of brain-behavior relationships; clinical neuropsychology is the application of this knowledge to the assessment of individuals who have or who are suspected of having brain dysfunction due to illness, trauma, or developmental abnormality. Over the years, relationships between neuropsychological performance and brain functioning have been well established (Kolb and Whishaw 1996; Lezak 1995; Mapou and Spector 1995), and much is now known about how different structures of the brain mediate cognitive, motor, and affective functioning.

Although sometimes considered only a diagnostic tool, neuropsychological assessment has a much wider application, for several reasons. First, the development of neurodiagnostic technologies has reduced the need for neuropsychological assessment simply to detect and localize brain dysfunction (Mapou 1988). Second, attempting to localize function solely through neuropsychological testing has drawbacks in the absence of corroborating clinical data. Third, because neuropsychologists have a background in understanding human behavior, they are in an excellent position to integrate clinical and psychometric findings from the evaluation into a view of the whole patient. Such an approach goes beyond simply testing for and diagnosing a disorder. Thus, neuropsychological assessment should be focused on its strength: describing a

The views and opinions expressed herein are the private views of the authors and are not to be considered as official or as reflecting the views of the U.S. Department of Defense.

patient's neurobehavioral competencies (Mapou 1995). In addition to contributing to diagnosis, neuropsychologists can use their evaluations to 1) describe current daily functioning, including medicolegal competence, 2) predict future cognitive or daily functioning, 3) develop a treatment plan to address difficulties, and 4) with repeated testing, monitor a patient's progress (or decline, in the case of progressive conditions) and identify new areas for intervention. The ability to address these issues makes neuropsychological assessment a valuable tool for patient care within consultation-liaison settings.

Psychological assessment provides objective information about a patient's emotional functioning and personality style; a cognitive evaluation is incomplete without consideration of these factors. Psychiatric disorders often affect neuropsychological performance. Even when a patient does not have a diagnosable psychiatric disorder, his or her psychological state at the time of the evaluation can determine whether the clinician achieves an accurate picture of the patient's functioning. In addition, some patients exaggerate or emphasize difficulties for primary or secondary gain. Thus, in addition to cognitive and motor measures, psychological assessment must be included in neuropsychological assessment.

Meyer et al. (2001) summarized evidence and issues associated with neuropsychological and psychological assessment. They demonstrated that psychological test validity is strong and comparable to medical test validity. The authors concluded that a multimethod assessment is the best way for trained clinicians to maximize diagnostic accuracy; single tests or interviews alone are insufficient to answer referral questions adequately. In this chapter, we review methods and applications of neuropsychological and psychological assessment in the consultation-liaison psychiatry setting. We begin with an overview of Luria's theory of brain functioning. We then review neuropsychological assessment techniques, including the most frequently used approaches, along with their application to the differential diagnosis of common disorders. An overview of psychological assessment techniques follows, with illustrations of application to both neurological and psychiatric disorders. We then discuss special issues in assessment and conclude with some guidelines for referring patients for neuropsychological evaluation.

LURIA'S FRAMEWORK OF BRAIN FUNCTIONING

A.R. Luria, the Russian neurologist and neuropsychologist, provided a framework to understand brain function-

ing and to guide neuropsychological assessment. Luria (1973, 1980) developed the concept of *functional systems*. He proposed that complex cognitive and motor functions were not localized to a specific region of the brain but rather reflected the integrated functioning of multiple systems located throughout the brain. Thus, in different patients, the same behavioral deficit could reflect very different sources of underlying dysfunction. In contrast, the same lesion could have different effects in different patients.

Luria (1973, 1980) described three principal functional units of the brain (Table 7–1). Each unit has a role in one aspect of brain functioning.

1. *Unit 1* regulates sleep and wakefulness and contributes to the overall ability of the brain to function efficiently.
2. *Unit 2* is the input unit, which registers, integrates, and stores sensory information from the visual, auditory, and somatosensory modalities.
3. *Unit 3* is the output unit, which generates and controls behavior and motor functioning.

Within Units 2 and 3, organization was hypothesized to be hierarchical, consisting of primary, secondary, and tertiary regions. The primary (projection) regions receive (Unit 2) or send (Unit 3) information to and from the peripheral sense organs and the extremities. The secondary (projection-association) regions process information within a single modality (Unit 2) or prepare a program of action for execution (Unit 3). Finally, the tertiary (zones of overlapping) regions reflect the most complex regions of processing (Unit 2) and programming of action (Unit 3) and integrate information across modalities. In the following sections, we describe units and associated regions in more detail.

Each unit is defined by neuroanatomy and function. Unit 1, which regulates cortical tone, sleep, and wakefulness, controls functions related to the deployment of attention, including level of arousal, orienting, focused attention, and sustained attention. Neuroanatomically, Unit 1 includes portions of the brain stem, the ascending reticular activating system, and subcortical structures to which the reticular activating system projects. Furthermore, there are feedback loops from higher cortical structures (e.g., frontal cortex) to this unit, via which these structures can influence the functioning of Unit 1. Because the role of Unit 1 is relatively nonspecific, dysfunction of Unit 1 will affect the efficient functioning of Units 2 and 3. Lesions in Unit 1 do not produce focal disturbances in function, such as aphasia, agnosia, or apraxia. Instead, they result in a general lowering of arousal, with

TABLE 7–1. Luria's model of brain functioning

Unit	Unit role	Neuroanatomy	Region	Region functions
Unit 1	Regulation of sleep and wakefulness Deployment of attention	Brain stem Ascending reticular activating system Subcortical structures	No differentiation	
Unit 2	Registration, integration, and storage of sensory information (input)	Occipital lobes	Primary (projection)	Initial processing of visual information
			Secondary (projection-association)	Integration of visual information
		Temporal lobes	Primary (projection)	Initial processing of auditory information
			Secondary (projection-association)	Integration of auditory information
		Parietal lobes	Primary (projection)	Initial processing of somatosensory information
			Secondary (projection-association)	Integration of somatosensory information
		Occipito-parieto-temporal	Tertiary (association)	Integration and storage of information from the visual, auditory, and somatosensory modalities
Unit 3	Production and control of behavior and motor functioning	Frontal lobes	Primary	Output of individual motor movements
			Secondary	Preparation of motor programs ("kinetic melodies")
			Tertiary (prefrontal)	Executive functions (planning, monitoring, and correcting behavior)

concomitant difficulty in responding to the environment. Patients with lesions in Unit 1 will manifest cognitive and motor slowing, affective changes, impaired orientation, and certain types of memory disturbance (e.g., reduced learning efficiency due to impaired attention and retrieval). Patients with subcortical dementias or diseases (e.g., Parkinson's disease, progressive supranuclear palsy, Huntington's disease) (J.L. Cummings 1990), delirium, or cerebrovascular accidents (CVAs) in the brain stem and subcortical regions frequently have dysfunction of Unit 1.

Unit 2 receives, integrates, and stores sensory information and manages the familiar focal and modality-specific functions of the brain (i.e., language and visuospatial skills). Neuroanatomically, Unit 2 subsumes most of the posterior cortex, including the occipital lobes, which process visual information; the temporal lobes, which process auditory information; and the parietal lobes, which process somatosensory information. Within each modality, these regions receive information from the sense organs and extremities (primary projection region), pro-

cess the information within that modality (secondary projection-association region), and integrate information among modalities and store it (tertiary association region). Luria also proposed that progressive lateralization of function occurs as one proceeds from the primary to the tertiary regions. For example, although both temporal lobes can process auditory sensory information (primary region), only the left hemisphere can process language (tertiary region) in most individuals.

Lesions in Unit 2 can produce focal brain disturbances. However, the type of deficit will be influenced by whether the lesion occurs in the primary, secondary, or tertiary region and by whether one or both hemispheres are involved. For example, within the auditory system, a unilateral lesion in the primary area can produce subtle deficits in acoustic processing. Central deafness will occur only if the primary auditory regions of *both* hemispheres are damaged—an extremely rare condition. In most instances, the contralateral hemisphere can compensate for lesions of the primary auditory system, and the impact on functioning is minimal. Lesions in the secondary auditory region, in contrast, can produce difficulty with phonemic discrimination (left hemisphere), which can affect language comprehension. Finally, lesions in the tertiary region of the auditory system can produce aphasia, alexia, agraphia, and/or anomia as a result of loss of integration between word forms and visual images. Similar analyses can be used to understand the effects of lesions in the visual and somatosensory systems. These types of deficits are most frequently seen in patients with cortical dementias, such as Alzheimer's disease, cortical CVAs, and focal cortical brain injury due to trauma.

Unit 3, which programs, regulates, and verifies motor output and behavior, is linked predominantly to the frontal lobes and their projections to other cortical and subcortical brain structures. Unit 3 allows an individual to plan, initiate, execute, monitor, and correct goal-directed behavior. Unit 3 also includes cortical structures associated with motor functioning. Because Unit 3 is the output unit, its organization is different from that of Unit 2. The tertiary region of Unit 3 performs the most complex functions, which include the overall planning and monitoring of goal-directed behavior. The secondary region then generates the action sequences or movements needed to carry out the behavior. Finally, the primary region, comprising the motor cortex, controls the specific individual motor movements.

Lesions in the tertiary region of Unit 3 produce deficits in the so-called executive functions—the basic behavioral control functions associated with planning and initiating behavior—and can also produce deficits in aspects of complex, directed attention. Lesions in the secondary region can impair the ability to execute sequences of skilled movements. Finally, lesions in the primary region produce paresis and impaired ability to execute simple movements. Patients with cortical dementias and CVAs affecting the frontal lobes manifest these types of deficits. In addition, because the tertiary regions of Unit 3 are connected with most other brain regions, conditions or disorders that affect the brain diffusely (e.g., traumatic brain injury, early dementia, psychiatric disorders) or that affect subcortical regions (e.g., Parkinson's disease, Huntington's disease) frequently produce deficits in executive functions and complex attention.

The integrated operation of the three functional units results in effective cognitive and motor functioning. Thus, attention, movement and action, language, perception, and memory can be impaired by lesions in any of the functional systems. Manifestations of impairment, however, will depend on the location of the lesion and its effect on a functional system. For example, impairment of verbal learning and memory can result from a lesion in Unit 1, 2, or 3. A lesion in Unit 1 can impair verbal learning and memory by reducing an individual's ability to attend adequately to presented stimuli. In contrast, a lesion within the secondary auditory region of Unit 2 can disrupt auditory-verbal processes necessary for initial comprehension and processing of words. Finally, a lesion in the tertiary region of Unit 3 can produce a deficit in an individual's ability to organize verbal information and store that information in a manner that will facilitate recall. Thus, the same symptom (impaired verbal learning and memory) can be due to vastly different underlying lesions and deficits.

Luria's framework provides an excellent background for understanding the types of problems in patients and for appreciating the interrelation between different cognitive and motor functions. Although many neuropsychological procedures were developed independently of Luria's work, his work has significantly influenced the practice of neuropsychology today.

NEUROPSYCHOLOGICAL ASSESSMENT

Although there are different schools of neuropsychological assessment, all have the goals of 1) describing cognitive, motor, and affective functioning in a patient who has or is suspected of having brain dysfunction; 2) helping diagnose the cause of the problems; and 3) elucidating how difficulties affect a patient's everyday functioning. Despite differences among schools, much overlap exists in terms of test use. For example, a proponent of the Halstead-Reitan Neuropsychological Test Battery (HRNTB; Reitan and Wolfson 1985) is likely to supplement the battery with other measures. Someone who applies the Boston Process Approach (E. Kaplan 1988, 1990; Milberg et al. 1996) to neuropsychological assessment is likely to use some measures from the HRNTB as well. Each approach has particular advantages and disadvantages within the consultation-liaison setting (Table 7–2). All approaches, however, have been applied to a range of patients, including medical-surgical patients (see, for example, Tarter et al. 1988), and are appropriate for use with the types of patients seen in consultation-liaison settings.

Patient-Centered and Process-Oriented Approaches

In patient-centered and process-oriented approaches, neuropsychological assessment is centered around the

TABLE 7–2. Advantages and disadvantages of neuropsychological assessment methods for the consultation-liaison setting

Method	Advantages	Disadvantages
Patient-centered and process approaches	Comprehensive assessment	Methods not validated together
	Can be tailored to answer the referral question	Can be time-consuming if not applied selectively
Battery-based approaches	Highly standardized and quantified	Require special equipment
	Very sensitive to neurological dysfunction	Limited assessment of certain cognitive realms
Halstead-Reitan Neuropsychological Test Battery	Large body of supporting research	Always time-consuming
Luria-Nebraska Neuropsychological Battery	Relatively brief	Criticized for problems with design and validity
Mental status assessment and screening instruments (e.g., MMSE)	Brief	Not comprehensive
	Can be done anywhere	Limited sensitivity and specificity
	Used frequently in consultation-liaison settings	

Note. MMSE = Mini-Mental State Exam.

referral question. Although a core set of measures is used, supplementary measures are added selectively, depending on the referral question. In addition, some procedures are modified to test limits, and qualitative data supplement test scores. The advantage of this type of approach in the consultation-liaison setting is that assessment can be limited to those measures likely to be most effective for answering the referral question. The disadvantage is that some scores (e.g., IQ, impairment index) cannot be computed when more limited sets of measures are used, and these scores are sometimes required by the referral source.

Assessment using Luria's techniques. Luria's approach to assessment involves progressive hypothesis testing, based on his framework (Table 7–1), to determine the structural basis for cognitive or motor difficulty (Jørgensen and Christensen 1995; Luria 1973, 1980). His measures are oriented toward a qualitative evaluation of the patient's difficulties but provide little or no quantitative information. Furthermore, the full method can be very time-consuming, a definite limitation in consultation-liaison settings. Nevertheless, many neuropsychologists use some of Luria's methods, described by Christensen (1979), as part of a battery of standardized measures.

Flexible battery approach (Lezak). Lezak (1983) described a flexible battery approach to assessment in which the neuropsychologist "tailor[s] the examination to the patient's needs, abilities, and limitations" (p. 98). Lezak advocated choosing instruments that would be most relevant for answering the referral question. She also advocated adapting instruments, as necessary, "to suit the patient's condition and enlarging upon them to gain a full measure of information" (Lezak 1983, p. 98).

Hypothesis testing is used to rule in or rule out diagnostic possibilities. Lezak (1983, 1995) provided details of her approach, including a basic test battery, general testing issues, methods for modifying measures in special populations (e.g., individuals with severe handicaps), and interpretation of findings.

Boston Process Approach (E. Kaplan). Perhaps the most well-known non–battery-based approach to assessment is the Boston Process Approach. In this approach, the evaluation is centered around the referral question, and hypothesis testing is used. E. Kaplan's emphasis, however, is on observing and understanding the *process* by which a patient completes tasks during testing, rather than on the absolute level of achievement obtained. That is, E. Kaplan (1988) argued that understanding how a patient completes a task is much more important than his or her final score on the measure. For example, E. Kaplan (1993) noted that a patient could fail an item on the Block Design subtest of the Wechsler Adult Intelligence Scale—Revised (WAIS-R; Wechsler 1981), a measure of visuospatial constructional skills, for a variety of reasons: a lack of motor skills needed to manipulate the blocks, an inability to see or perceive the model accurately, an inability to plan an organized approach to the task, or an inability to comprehend or to cooperate with the procedure (e.g., the patient eats the blocks or throws them at the examiner). Each of these reasons for failure, consistent with Luria's (1980) framework of functional systems, reflects a different type of breakdown in brain functioning.

E. Kaplan (1988, 1990, 1993) outlined a core set of measures for assessment that can be supplemented with additional measures to test specific hypotheses. She also illustrated how modifying data collection procedures, including suspending time limits on timed tasks, observing errors made en route to solutions, testing limits, and quantifying observed performance information, can provide additional information on the pattern of spared and impaired cognitive functions. These techniques are flexible and can be applied to many different instruments.

Kaplan's work has resulted in a number of new neuropsychological measures and modifications to existing measures. Among them are the WAIS-R as a Neuropsychological Instrument (E. Kaplan et al. 1991), portions of which are included in the Wechsler Adult Intelligence Scale—Third Edition (WAIS-III; Wechsler 1997); the California Verbal Learning Test—Second Edition (Delis et al. 2000), the Delis-Kaplan Executive Function Sequence (Delis et al. 2001), the Kaplan Baycrest Neurocognitive Assessment (Leach et al. 2000), the Boston Naming Test—Third Edition (E. Kaplan et al. 2001), and the Boston Diagnostic Aphasia Examination (Goodglass et al. 2001). In addition, new measures are being developed.

Battery-Based Approaches

Battery-based approaches to assessment are probably more familiar to physicians than non–battery-based approaches. A fixed neuropsychological battery consists of a group of tests that have been standardized and validated together and that have established sensitivity to brain dysfunction as a group. Patient-centered approaches, by contrast, involve a core set of measures, and supplementary measures used differ depending on the referral question. In addition, although individual measures in patient-centered approaches have established reliability, validity, and sensitivity to brain dysfunction, these characteristics have not been evaluated in the measures as a group. When a standardized group of measures is required (e.g., for litigation), a battery has an advantage.

Interpretation of findings of a battery is based on the level and pattern of subtest performance, as indicated by subtest scores. In practice, however, most clinicians use standardized test batteries in a flexible manner. Because most batteries do not provide a comprehensive assessment of cognitive function, additional measures are generally used (Heaton et al. 1991). Clinicians also are likely to observe qualitative aspects of performance and may use subtests selectively. The advantages of neuropsychological test batteries include a standard administration that facilitates comparison of findings across different sites and examiners and a wealth of empirical data that have been collected using a fixed group of neuropsychological measures.

Halstead-Reitan Neuropsychological Test Battery (Reitan).   The HRNTB is the most frequently used battery in clinical practice. Since its initial development by Halstead in the 1940s, the battery has been refined and has been administered to thousands of patients with different neurological and psychiatric disorders. Extensive normative data have been obtained. The battery consists of five types of measures: "1) input measures; 2) tests of verbal abilities; 3) measures of spatial, sequential, and manipulative abilities; 4) tests of abstraction, reasoning, logical analysis, and concept formation; and 5) output measures" (Reitan and Wolfson 1986, p. 136). Strict interpretation emphasizes the pattern and level of performance on individual measures and on computed summary indices, including a measure of overall impairment.

The HRNTB has been extensively researched and standardized. Normative data stratified by age, education, and gender are available (Heaton et al. 1991). When strictly standardized testing procedures are necessary (e.g., in forensic settings), the HRNTB is recommended. However, when time is limited (the full battery requires 6–7 hours), as in consultation-liaison settings, or when more in-depth assessment of particular functions such as learning and memory is necessary, the complete HRNTB is less useful. Just as Luria's measures are applied selectively, many clinicians use portions of the HRNTB, to take advantage of its standardization, and they supplement these with other measures as time permits.

Luria-Nebraska Neuropsychological Battery (LNNB; Golden).   Using Luria's (1980) theory of brain functioning and organization, Golden et al. (1985) attempted to standardize the administration and interpretation of Luria's procedures, as described by Christensen (1979). Form I of the LNNB (Golden et al. 1985) consists of 269 items, organized into 11 ability scales, and requires approximately 2.5 hours for administration. Form II of the LNNB is an alternate form with 279 items, 12 ability scales, and improved stimulus cards. As in the case of the HRNTB, interpretation is based on the level and pattern of performance on the different scales and on several summary impairment indices.

The LNNB has been administered to patients with different neurological and psychiatric disorders, and data from these groups have been compared with those from control subjects (Golden and Maruish 1986). The LNNB also is as sensitive to the presence of brain dysfunction as the HRNTB (Kane et al. 1985). Compared with the HRNTB, the LNNB samples a wider range of cognitive skills and requires considerably less administration time. Nevertheless, concerns have been raised about the statistical characteristics of the LNNB (Adams 1980, 1984;

Stambrook 1983) and the content validity of its clinical scales (Delis and Kaplan 1983; Klein 1993; Spiers 1984). Although the LNNB has utility as an instrument for screening for cognitive dysfunction, it is limited as an in-depth measure of cognitive and motor function. Because of these difficulties, the LNNB must be used with caution and should always be supplemented with other measures.

Bedside Screening and Extended Mental Status Examinations

The mental status examination has a long history in psychiatry and neurology and is always included in a standard psychiatric or neurological examination. Physicians perform cognitive screening to determine whether cognitive impairment is present and to develop initial hypotheses about diagnosis. Hodges (1994) outlined an approach to cognitive screening and summarized available measures. Mental status tests run the gamut from informal and idiosyncratic measures of cognitive and motor function to the brief but standardized Mini-Mental State Exam (MMSE; Folstein et al. 1975, 2001), to more comprehensive screening tests such as the Dementia Rating Scale (Mattis 1988) and the Neurobehavioral Cognitive Status Examination (Schwamm et al. 1987), now known as COGNISTAT (Northern California Neurobehavioral Group 1995). All screening measures, however, require little time for administration (5–45 minutes), do not require the use of specialized equipment (although some measures use stimuli on printed cards), and are easily administered in the office, in the clinic, or at the bedside. Thus, in contrast to more extensive neuropsychological testing, extended mental status examinations have the advantages of brevity and flexibility of administration.

Most mental status examinations assess the following areas of function: orientation, simple attention, short-term memory, comprehension, repetition, naming, construction, and abstraction skills. Within each area, however, the assessment is necessarily brief. Thus, what is gained in time and flexibility is lost in sensitivity and specificity. Although brief mental status examinations, such as the MMSE, can detect gross changes in cognitive function and provide a baseline for follow-up assessment, they are likely to miss subtle cognitive deficits (Stokes et al. 1991).

Nelson et al. (1986) reviewed five frequently used bedside screening examinations: the MMSE, the Dementia Rating Scale, the Cognitive Capacity Screening Examination (Jacobs et al. 1977), the Mental Status Questionnaire (Montgomery and Costa 1983), and the Short Portable Mental Status Questionnaire (Omer et al. 1983). They found all of the tests to be useful for diagnosis of dementia and delirium but questioned whether these measures substantially improved diagnostic accuracy beyond that of clinical examinations. They expressed concern that these measures were likely to miss subtle cognitive deficits and recommended further development of new screening tests that would be applicable to a broader range of clinical problems.

A new measure, the Repeatable Battery for the Assessment of Neuropsychological Status (Randolph 1998), was designed to address shortcomings of past measures but retain brevity of testing time. This measure has 12 subtests that evaluate immediate memory, visuospatial and constructional skills, attention, language, and delayed memory. It takes 30 minutes to administer; has two parallel forms specifically designed to permit repeated testing, with an emphasis on detection of dementia; and has normative data for individuals ages 20–89 years.

Bedside screening and extended mental status examinations are important tasks for the consultation-liaison psychiatrist at the initial stages of evaluation. Such brief examinations, however, may or may not contribute to clinical diagnostic assessment. It is important to recognize the trade-off between the amount of information obtained using a test and the diagnostic utility of the test in the consultation-liaison setting. For example, an examination that is too brief and too restricted in scope will assess a limited range of functions and, because of its simplicity, is unlikely to be sensitive to subtle deficits. In contrast, a full neuropsychological evaluation that provides more specific data is likely to be lengthy (a problem in the inpatient setting) and more difficult (a problem for patients with limited cognitive or physical skills). (A more in-depth discussion of the clinical use of screening tests can be found in Chapter 6.)

Summary of Neuropsychological Assessment Methods

A variety of neuropsychological assessment methods are available for use in the consultation-liaison setting (Table 7–2). The method chosen depends on the referral question and on the available time, equipment, and personnel. In the consultation-liaison setting, a two-tiered assessment approach is recommended. Patients with complex neurobehavioral disorders can first be seen in a clinic or on a medical ward, at which time a 20- to 45-minute cognitive screening is conducted. In many instances, this first-tier screening examination will indicate the need for more detailed, formal neuropsychological testing with one of the approaches described here. In other instances, the findings of the initial screening will be sufficient to answer the referral question.

Applications to Neuropsychiatric Diagnosis

Within consultation-liaison settings, neuropsychologists are most frequently consulted to help with differential diagnosis of neuropsychiatric disorders. Although some referrals may still be requests to "rule out organicity," we believe that advancing knowledge of brain-behavior relationships has rendered such referrals things of the past (Leonberger 1989; Mapou 1988, 1993; Miller 1986). DSM-IV-TR (American Psychiatric Association 2000), for example, includes several categories for cognitive disorders associated with central nervous system disease and specific medical conditions. Table 7–3 lists some common patient presentations that warrant referral for neuropsychological assessment. Table 7–4 lists the typical applications of assessment associated with these presentations.

In the following sections, we describe, with case examples, several of the more common applications of neuropsychological assessment in the consultation-liaison setting.

Dementia. Neuropsychological assessment is an essential component of the clinical evaluation of patients suspected of having dementing conditions. Patients with cortical dementias, such as Alzheimer's disease, have memory deficits, language dysfunction or visuospatial impairment, executive functioning deficits, and diminished self-awareness, typically observed in the context of normal psychomotor abilities and near-normal attentional function (J.L. Cummings 1985). In contrast, subcortical dementias, such as those associated with Parkinson's disease or progressive supranuclear palsy, are marked by psychomotor retardation, attentional impairment, and emotional lability, typically in the context of intact language and visuospatial skills and recognition memory (J.L. Cummings 1985, 1990). When changes in demented patients are being tracked over time, neuropsychological evaluation also can be useful to provide objective assessment of the deficit, periodic evaluation of competency, and indications of response to treatment.

Case Example 1

Dr. A, a 73-year-old male retired Ph.D. engineer, was admitted to the neuropsychiatric evaluation unit of a psychiatric hospital because of confusion and agitation while visiting relatives. Three months before admission, he had apparently developed language problems

TABLE 7–3. Patient presentations appropriate for neuropsychological assessment referral

Decreasing memory or general cognitive functioning beyond the expectations for age

Cognitive or behavioral changes after a traumatic brain injury

Cognitive or behavioral changes without obvious cause

Complaints of cognitive difficulties after exposure to toxic agents

Unexpected or initial difficulties in primary or secondary school

Unexpected difficulties in college, graduate, or professional school

Unusual findings on mental status examination that are not consistent with apparent medical, psychiatric, or neurological condition

TABLE 7–4. Applications of neuropsychological assessment

Differentiate among disorders that can be the cause of progressive dementia, including Alzheimer's disease, Parkinson's disease, multiple sclerosis, human immunodeficiency virus disease or acquired immunodeficiency syndrome, Huntington's disease, or multiple cerebral infarctions

Differentiate between a dementia or other central nervous system disorder and psychiatric disorders

Document the cognitive and motor sequelae of stroke, traumatic brain injury, hypoxic brain injury, or seizure disorders, and apply information to prognosis and treatment

Differentiate relatively static amnestic disorders, as might be associated with Korsakoff's syndrome or certain types of strokes, from progressive dementias

Assess the cognitive sequelae of systemic illness, such as systemic lupus erythematosus, end-stage renal disease, cardiac disease, or liver disease

Document the presence of a specific learning disability or attention-deficit/hyperactivity disorder, and make recommendations for accommodations, compensation, and remediation

Assess the ability of a neuropsychologically impaired individual to return to work or school or to perform independent living skills such as driving or managing finances

Assess the competence of a neuropsychologically impaired individual to make medical, legal, or financial decisions

Provide longitudinal evaluation to assess level of functioning

after prostate surgery; 1 month before admission, he had become increasingly disorganized, confused, and agitated. His judgment became quite poor. His medical history was notable for hypertension, for which he was taking medication. A magnetic resonance image was less than optimal because of motion artifact but was read as showing infarction of the right occipital lobe and left frontal lobe near the caudate nucleus. Although one electroencephalogram (EEG) was described in the record as mildly abnormal due to localized bitemporal slow-wave activity, a second EEG was described as normal.

During evaluation, Dr. A was cooperative but had great difficulty completing what was asked of him. On several occasions, he became frustrated when unable to complete a task but could not explain why he was feeling upset. Despite these episodes, he lacked insight into his deficits. Neuropsychological evaluation revealed impairment in all cognitive realms, with the exception of spoken language. Dr. A had particularly notable deficits in executive function. He was perseverative, could not establish and shift response set, had difficulty with initiation, and was stimulus bound. He also had noteworthy deficits in visuospatial perceptual and constructional skills. Findings were consistent with dementia secondary to multiple infarctions. Dr. A was judged unable to live independently, and placement in a structured living situation was recommended.

Cerebrovascular accident (CVA). Neuropsychological evaluation is an essential component of the treatment planning process for numerous CVA survivors (Tupper 1991). Although clinical and speech-language evaluation can suffice for patients with large dominant-hemisphere lesions, careful evaluation of higher cognitive functioning can identify more unusual or subtle deficits in memory, attention, or judgment (Brown et al. 1996; Lishman 1998). For example, patients with right-hemisphere or frontal lobe CVA may not acknowledge their deficits or even note obvious motor or sensory disabilities (McGlynn and Schacter 1989). These patients often want to drive or return to the workplace, despite potential risk to themselves or others. Neuropsychological assessment can contribute to evaluation of competency in such patients.

CVA syndromes can change rapidly in the weeks after occurrence of CVA (Meier and Strauman 1991). Therefore, shortly after CVA, cognitive testing should be relatively brief but repeated frequently; later, a more thorough evaluation can establish a baseline against which to compare recovery and ongoing therapeutic needs. The following two cases show the contrasting effects of right- and left-hemisphere CVAs, respectively.

Case Example 2

Ms. B, a 51-year-old bank customer service representative, was undergoing outpatient rehabilitative treatment 2 months after a right-hemisphere CVA. Her medical history was notable for systemic lupus erythematosus and cardiac disease; her CVA was believed to have been caused by an embolus from a replaced heart valve, but this was never established. During evaluation, she became teary when discussing her deficits and performing tasks that were difficult for her; she acknowledged a moderate degree of depression. These episodes were brief, however, and she easily regained composure. Between these episodes, her affect was

flattened, with little change observed in facial expression and prosody. Ms. B was aware of her physical limitations but seemed unaware of the extent of her cognitive deficits. Neuropsychological evaluation revealed deficits in attention, visual scanning, executive functions, visuospatial constructional skills, nonverbal learning and memory, and nonverbal intellectual skills. In contrast, her language functions, visuospatial perceptual skills, verbal learning and memory, and verbal intellectual skills were relatively preserved. Clinical findings were consistent with a classic right-hemisphere syndrome. Rehabilitation was recommended, with an emphasis on functional skills and on using language to help her compensate for her deficits.

When seen for reevaluation 7 months later, Ms. B showed considerable progress in walking and in a variety of independent living skills. Nevertheless, she remained highly dependent on her family and was unable to work. Neuropsychological evaluation revealed little change in her cognitive and motor functioning, indicating that most improvement had occurred through compensatory mechanisms.

Case Example 3

Ms. C, a 37-year-old nursing supervisor, was initially admitted to a psychiatric unit because of acute behavioral changes, including muteness and refusal to cooperate with her husband with regard to treatment for her difficulties. Findings of the initial neurodiagnostic workup, including MRI, were unremarkable. While hospitalized, she had a generalized seizure and was transferred to a neurology ward. A left-hemisphere CVA, secondary to mitochondrial encephalopathy, lactic acidosis, and strokelike syndrome (MELAS), was diagnosed. She was cooperative during neuropsychological evaluation, which occurred 1 month after the initial event, but her significant language difficulties interfered with her performance. She was distressed and frustrated by her deficits and cried many times. She also had difficulty responding to nonverbal cues from the examiner; for example, she did not pick up cues indicating the end of a conversation. Evaluation revealed significant aphasia, characterized by relatively fluent speech, phonemic paraphasic errors, and word-finding difficulties. Her prosody was normal. Deficits in executive functioning, problem solving, and reasoning were also noted; she was impulsive, perseverative, and stimulus bound on a variety of tasks. In contrast, her visuospatial skills, simple verbal learning and memory, and nonverbal learning and memory were relatively intact. The pattern was consistent with the effects of a posterior left-hemisphere CVA.

Ms. C was referred for outpatient rehabilitation and also participated in an adjustment-to-disability group. Her insight improved; she was aware of her language problems, once stating to group members: "I have apheesia," and was appropriately sad. Her sadness lifted, however, and she rapidly engaged in the rehabilitation program, where she regained her basic independent living skills. Furthermore, she was a constant source of help and encouragement to other program participants.

Traumatic brain injury (TBI).   Although the utility of neuropsychological assessment while a patient is still experiencing posttraumatic amnesia is questionable, subsequent evaluation is essential to assess the presence, extent, and effect of brain injury–related difficulties. Moderate to severe closed-head injuries typically produce deficits in attention, memory, and executive skills (Brooks 1984; Levin et al. 1982, 1987). Judgment and reasoning can be impaired and can affect willingness to participate in treatment. Although subtle naming and perceptual deficits can occur, more severe impairment in these areas is rare, in the absence of focal damage.

Preexisting learning disabilities, a history of attention-deficit/hyperactivity disorder (ADHD), prior substance abuse, and prior head injuries are frequent in TBI survivors; their contributions to the patient's postinjury status must always be carefully considered (Dikmen and Levin 1993). Depression, anxiety, rage, and regret are common, especially months to years after injury; careful assessment of the head-injured patient's emotional status and personality structure before and after injury are essential for evaluation of functional deficit and prediction of outcome (Prigatano 1991; Prigatano et al. 1986).

Case Example 4

Mr. D, a 33-year-old carpenter, sustained a severe head injury in a motor vehicle accident. He was followed through inpatient, outpatient, and vocational rehabilitation and in psychotherapy. Neuropsychological evaluations were performed 3 months, 18 months, and 3 years after injury. Initial evaluation revealed right-sided motor deficits, language deficits, and a moderate loss of intellectual efficiency compared with estimated preinjury functioning. The pattern of deficits was consistent with diffuse damage and focal left-hemisphere injury. Mr. D's cognitive deficits were accompanied by impulsivity, diminished interpersonal judgment, and denial of deficit, which were also attributed to his injury. Mr. D's deficits stabilized within 18 months of injury. Three years after injury, problems with complex verbal memory and attention persisted, along with right-sided weakness and dysphasia. His emotional and interpersonal difficulties, however, affected his recovery as much as, if not more than, his cognitive deficits alone. His psychosocial difficulties were a focus of psychotherapy.

Amnestic syndromes.   Memory deficits are common sequelae of brain disease and injury, but true amnestic disorders are relatively rare. DSM-IV-TR criteria for amnestic disorder due to a general medical condition are presented in Table 7–5. Criteria for substance-induced

TABLE 7–5.   DSM-IV-TR criteria for amnestic disorder due to a general medical condition

A. The development of memory impairment as manifested by impairment in the ability to learn new information or the inability to recall previously learned information.

B. The memory disturbance causes significant impairment in social or occupational functioning and represents a significant decline from a previous level of functioning.

C. The memory disturbance does not occur exclusively during the course of a delirium or a dementia.

D. There is evidence from the history, physical examination, or laboratory findings that the disturbance is the direct physiological consequence of a general medical condition (including physical trauma).

Specify if:

Transient: if memory impairment lasts for 1 month or less

Chronic: if memory impairment lasts for more than 1 month

persisting amnestic disorder are similar but include evidence of a causal relationship between substance use or toxin exposure and the disorder (American Psychiatric Association 2000). Neuropsychological evaluation of memory processes forms the basis for diagnosis of the amnesia. At minimum, neuropsychological evaluation should assess attentional functioning; immediate, delayed, and remote memory; single- and repeated-trial learning; free recall and recognition memory; and implicit or procedural learning.

Amnesia can be a result of discrete frontal lobe injuries, such as rupture of anterior communicating artery aneurysms (DeLuca 1992), or certain neurosurgical procedures, such as resections of third-ventricle cysts (Gaffan and Gaffan 1991). Diencephalic lesions can produce severe and lasting amnesias; Korsakoff's amnesia is believed to result from chronic alcohol-related thiamine deficiency and is related to deterioration in certain thalamic and hypothalamic structures (Butters 1984). Hippocampal damage can also produce amnestic conditions, such as those that occur in cases of herpes simplex encephalitis or after posterior temporal lobe CVA (Butters 1984).

Depression versus dementia.   High-functioning patients who are knowledgeable about Alzheimer's disease and related disorders and are having difficulties with attention, memory, and word finding may believe that they are in the early stages of a dementing disorder. After they initiate a consultation, the clinician must always consider the possibility that depression (or another psychiatric disorder) is the cause of their complaints.

Major depression is often accompanied by impairment in attention and in the ability to encode information actively, with associated reduction in learning and memory (Burt et al. 1995; Cassens et al. 1990; Sweeney et al. 1989; Veiel 1997). Psychomotor slowing is also frequently present. Reductions in Performance IQ (nonverbal intelligence) and in visuospatial skills may be observed. In contrast, focal language deficits are unlikely in depressed patients, and difficulties with memory tend to reflect inadequate encoding rather than the forgetting that is more typical of dementia. In fact, despite the frequency of word-finding complaints, formal tests of naming often help differentiate depression from dementia; naming deficits are much less common in depressed individuals (Hill et al. 1992). Furthermore, although some depressed individuals show no cognitive deficits on formal testing, others manifest a neuropsychological pattern similar to that associated with subcortical dementia (Massman et al. 1992). In the absence of any etiological factors related to subcortical dementia (e.g., Parkinson's disease, Huntington's disease, and multiple, small subcortical infarctions secondary to hypertension), the differential diagnosis becomes relatively straightforward. However, researchers have seen small, subcortical lesions on magnetic resonance images obtained from elderly depressed individuals, but not on images from elderly control subjects (Coffey et al. 1989). Thus, cognitive deficits in elderly depressed patients may ultimately be linked to structural brain changes.

Case Example 5

Ms. E, an elderly patient, was self-referred to a neuropsychiatry clinic for evaluation of memory and attention complaints. She was referred subsequently for neuropsychological assessment as part of her evaluation. She had no history of psychiatric disorder or treatment. Ms. E indicated that her symptoms had begun and had rapidly worsened after the death of her husband several months earlier. Neuropsychological assessment revealed that Ms. E was slower in thinking and behavior than was expected for her age, but other skills (language proficiency, visual-perceptual skills, recognition memory, and executive function reasoning) were normal. Her affect was shallow, and her mood was stoic and sad. Several measures of personality and emotional functioning revealed significant depression and anxiety, self-deprecating thoughts, feelings of interpersonal estrangement, and vegetative changes in sleep, appetite, energy, and interest. The evaluation indicated that Ms. E's cognitive complaints were consistent with a primary mood disorder. She was treated with antidepressant medication and psychotherapy. At 6-month follow-up, her cognitive complaints had resolved and she appeared more attentive, responsive, and energetic.

Developmental learning disorders in adults. Researchers and clinicians have come to recognize that developmental learning disorders—which include specific learning disabilities, such as dyslexia, and disorders that broadly affect learning, such as ADHD—do not disappear when children grow up (Mapou, in press). If these disorders are not diagnosed and treated effectively, they can have profound effects on academic and vocational achievement and on psychosocial functioning. Because of the Americans With Disabilities Act of 1990 (U.S. Code, vol. 42, secs. 12101–12213; P.L. 101-336), clinicians are increasingly being referred adults who believe they may have one of these disorders. Indeed, ADHD has become a "diagnosis du jour," with many adults seeking evaluation and treatment for long-standing difficulties that they believe are caused by this disorder (Shaffer 1994). A comprehensive neuropsychological assessment, including a diagnostic interview and complete history, can help the clinician diagnose the cause of problems in an adult presenting for evaluation. Although the gold standard for diagnosis of ADHD is the diagnostic interview (Barkley 1998), neuropsychological assessment plays a significant role in differential diagnosis. Data obtained through neuropsychological assessment can help the clinician 1) diagnose a specific learning disability, 2) determine whether that disability or another disorder accounts for the symptoms of ADHD, and 3) direct treatment efforts. Historical data are critical for diagnosis, particularly in the case of patients whose disorders have never been previously diagnosed. Individuals with developmental learning problems typically report some type of academic difficulty dating to childhood, even if they successfully compensated for the problem through high school. However, the decreased structure and increased amount of reading and writing in college, graduate school, or professional school can present great difficulties for these individuals. Their grades may decrease dramatically, and they may have problems keeping up with academic work. Certainly, a few individuals who come for evaluation want to be accommodated for disabilities that are not in fact present. Most, however, are accurately reporting long-standing problems that can be quantified by neuropsychological assessment.

Many persons with learning disabilities or ADHD who are in postsecondary education programs can benefit from accommodations, tutoring and other interventions designed to help individuals compensate for weaknesses and improve learning skills. These interventions level the playing field and do not give an unfair advantage (Mapou, in press). Guidelines for documenting these disorders in adults in postsecondary education have been published and should be followed (Association on Higher Education and Disability 1997; Educational Testing Service 1998a, 1998b).

Case Example 6

Ms. F, a 47-year-old woman, was referred for evaluation by her psychiatrist. Ms. F, who was in the process of separating from her husband, was thinking of returning to school to further her career; she had been working as an assistant librarian in a middle school. However, she had a long history of difficulties with reading comprehension and attention. Her high school grades had been mediocre, and, as a younger woman, she had dropped out of a teacher's college because of academic difficulties. More recently, she had taken two college courses and had done well in them. Nonetheless, Ms. F was concerned that her cognitive problems would make handling a full college load difficult. Testing revealed intellectual skills that were above average but clear weaknesses in reading speed, reading comprehension, spelling, holding verbal information in mind, verbal organizational skills, and verbal learning and memory. When spelling, Ms. F made errors that showed problems with sounding out words. She also had weaknesses in focused and sustained attention; however, she did not meet criteria for ADHD. In contrast, her visuospatial skills and visual learning and memory skills were very strong. Symptoms of anxiety and depression were evident on psychological testing but could not account for her cognitive problems. Ms. F received a diagnosis of mild dyslexia. Recommendations were made for accommodations in college, including extra time on examinations, individual testing, access to textbooks on tape, use of a personal note-taker, taping of lectures, and a reduced course load. Individual tutoring was also recommended, to help her learn to compensate for her weaknesses and improve her skills.

Case Example 7

Mr. G, a 48-year-old man with a history of bipolar disorder, was referred for a evaluation by his psychiatrist. He reported a long history of problems with reading comprehension and retention, attention, and impulsivity. Despite successful treatment of bipolar disorder, his cognitive symptoms persisted, and he was having difficulty passing the bar examination. Mr. G had done well in high school and college, despite early problems with attention. Rating scales completed by him and his sister showed evidence of ADHD symptoms in childhood, and there was continued evidence of ADHD symptoms on a current rating scale and in the diagnostic interview. Mr. G had worked successfully, first as a teacher, then as an educational tester, and finally as a lobbyist. However, law school had been much for more difficult for him. While there, he had been permitted to take examinations on a computer. Neuropsychological testing revealed that his intellectual and academic skills were far above average, as were his language and visuospatial skills. In contrast, he showed significant weaknesses in focused and sustained attention, organizational skills, and planning. He was impulsive throughout the evaluation. Evidence of hyperactive, impulsive, and unpredictable behavior was noted in his profile on psychological testing. However, Mr. G showed no acute symptoms of bipolar disorder, and his life was very stable. A diagnosis of ADHD, combined type, was made, and psychostimulant treatment was recommended. In addition, accommodations for the bar examination were recommended, including 50% more time, individual testing, breaks during testing, and use of a laptop computer to complete the essay portion of the examination. Ways to compensate for his weaknesses and improve his skills were also recommended.

PSYCHOLOGICAL ASSESSMENT

Psychological assessment integrates objective and projective test results, behavioral observations, and a patient's self-report with professional clinical knowledge and expertise, providing a means of evaluating a patient's emotional status, personality structure, psychological symptoms, and motivational state. It can supplement standard clinical assessment because

> clinicians often see what they anticipate…questions likely to elicit unanticipated information are rarely asked. It is in this regard that objective psychological assessment is so important; these tools serve to standardize clinical evaluations and ensure comprehensive coverage. Moreover, it seeks to appraise the patient's present status within the context of the past and within his or her larger social environment, including both current physical and psychosocial stressors. (Green 1982, p. 340)

In a consultation-liaison setting, psychological assessment can help to 1) generate diagnostic considerations, 2) assess a patient's general resistance to treatment and resistance to specific treatment approaches, 3) evaluate the role of psychological factors in a patient's medical condition, 4) determine the need for psychosocial interventions to improve outcomes of medical or surgical treatments (e.g., stress management in anxious individuals before a medical procedure), and 5) predict outcomes of surgical, medical, or psychiatric treatments. Psychological assessment is also a requisite portion of any neuropsychological evaluation.

Psychological assessment typically involves combining information obtained through psychological tests, interviews, and other clinical evaluations. Although a range of tests and approaches to testing are available, most instruments have common qualities of standardization, reliability, and validity (Anastasi and Urbina 1997). A *standardized* test has explicit instructions for administration and scoring, which guarantees reasonable constancy regardless of when, where, or by whom the test is administered. *Reliability* refers to test stability and consistency within and between administrations and consistency across raters or scorers. Thus, the reliability of a test may be its stability in identifying a stable nonchanging characteristic of an individual over time, or its stability in identifying consistent changes in test scores over time, across individuals with similar medical or psychiatric features. *Validity* refers to the usefulness of a test and provides an estimate of the extent to which a test measures the skills or qualities it purports to measure. Validity also refers to the accuracy with which a test classifies patients according to diagnostic groups, treatment outcomes, or levels of severity. Reliability and validity are distinct but related psychometric features for evaluating the usefulness and relevance of psychological tests for specific purposes.

Objective Personality Measures

In this section, we discuss the most frequently used instruments with demonstrated reliability and validity. These objective personality instruments are self-report measures, in which the patient responds to a series of statements or questions relating to attitudes, beliefs, symptoms, and experiences. On some tests, patients simply agree or disagree with target statements; on other tests, they report a degree of endorsement on a scale. Typically, the patient's responses are aggregated, scaled, and compared with data from normative groups.

However, general cautions should be followed when using self-report instruments with medical or surgical patients. Instruments that are reliable and valid for identification of psychopathology in psychiatric patients may be inappropriate for use with medical patients, because somatic items on these instruments will be endorsed by medical patients based on symptoms of their illness; thus, endorsement cannot be automatically attributed to psychiatric causes. For example, self-report depression scales typically include items on fatigue, pain, and consequences of illness such as the inability to work. Although these items reflect the presence and severity of depression in patients without medical illness, their endorsement by medical patients may reflect disease severity

rather than depression. Conversely, somatic symptoms in medical patients also can be a manifestation of depression, independent of physical symptoms associated with the medical illness. A differentiation between these possibilities can sometimes be made by comparing the individual's score on a measure with the standard scores of a sample of subjects who also have that medical condition. Thus, selection of the appropriate comparison group will vary in relation to the specific question addressed. Here we discuss issues with regard to use of specific instruments in medical settings.

Minnesota Multiphasic Personality Inventory (MMPI/ MMPI-2). The MMPI was developed by Hathaway and McKinley (1967) in the early 1940s and is the most widely used and researched objective personality measure. It has demonstrated sensitivity to many psychiatric disorders. The MMPI was restandardized (Butcher et al. 1989), and debate continues regarding the comparability of the two forms (Helmes and Reddon 1993). The MMPI-2 consists of 567 true-false items. It yields scores on 3 major validity indices and 10 major clinical scales. In addition to these scales, many specific content scales are sensitive to health concerns, neurological disorders, affective symptoms, thought disturbance, and ego strength, among other factors. Other scales also permit assessment of response bias and potential symptom embellishment. Test results are interpreted in terms of the profile of elevated scores on the major clinical scales relative to census-based normative data. Additional information is added by reviewing a patient's responses to critical items. A vast body of literature exists on the interpretation of MMPI results in mental health settings.

It may be inappropriate, however, to apply these interpretations to general medical patients, given the sensitivity of the MMPI to the "normal" experiences and symptoms of patients with well-defined medical conditions (Cripe 1989). Pincus and Callahan (1993), for example, studied MMPI use in patients with rheumatoid arthritis. They asked rheumatologists to identify the test items that were expected to differ between rheumatoid arthritis patients and matched individuals without arthritis, based on rheumatoid arthritis symptoms and not psychological state. They also compared MMPI results from rheumatoid arthritis patients with those from control subjects without medical or psychiatric illness. Using these criteria, the authors identified five MMPI items that were clearly related to rheumatoid arthritis (Table 7–6; equivalent MMPI-2 items are listed). These items appeared to account for the higher scores of rheumatoid arthritis patients on the hypochondriasis (Hs), depression (D), and hysteria (Hy) scales.

TABLE 7–6.   MMPI-2 items likely to be endorsed by patients with rheumatoid arthritis

Item no.	Item
9	I am about as able to work as I ever was.
51	I am in just as good physical health as most of my friends.
153	During the past few years, I have been well most of the time.
163	I do not tire quickly.
243	I have few or no pains.

Note.   MMPI-2 = Minnesota Multiphasic Personality Inventory—2.
Source.   Adapted from Pincus and Callahan 1993.

Other MMPI items are frequently endorsed by patients with neuropsychiatric disorders. Specifically, patients with seizure disorders, TBI, and CVA often have elevated scores, in the clinical range, on scales designed to measure somatic preoccupation (Hs), conversion (Hy), depression (D), and thought disorder (schizophrenia, Sc) (Alfano et al. 1992; Bornstein and Kozora 1990; Gass and Russell 1986; Wooten 1983). For this reason, Alfano and colleagues (1992) and Gass and Russell (1986) recommended computing "neurocorrected" scores on these scales by eliminating specific items when determining the total scale score, to separate the effects of neurological disorder. The resulting MMPI/MMPI-2 profile would then, presumably, reflect only the "pure" psychiatric symptoms experienced by the patient. A competing view, however, is that a neuropsychiatric patient's report of atypical experiences is due to the actual cognitive deficits, affective reactions, and personality changes associated with these disorders. Therefore, increased scores on scales that assess these symptoms accurately reflect a patient's experience of his or her disorder, but results do need to be interpreted differently than results from psychiatric patients (Mack 1979).

In general, because somatic items are prevalent in MMPI/MMPI-2 scales used to identify depression, conversion, somatization, and somatoform disorders, scores on these scales can be increased among medical and surgical patients. For example, Mayo Clinic data on the MMPI for general medical outpatients showed that 32.4% of females and 24.5% of males had significantly increased scores on the Hs and Hy scales compared with the original MMPI normative data (Osborne et al. 1983). In a parallel study, new MMPI normative data were collected, data considered more comparable to MMPI-2 normative data than the original MMPI data (Colligan et al. 1983). Investigators who used these normative data found that 37.8% of females and 30.6% of males in a general medical outpatient sample had elevated scores on the same two scales (Osborne et al. 1983). It is clear that caution must be exercised when interpreting elevated scores of medical or surgical patients on the Hs and Hy scales.

An elevation in scores on the Hs and Hy scales, with a significantly lower score on the D scale, is often referred to as the classic "conversion V" configuration. In psychiatric patients, this pattern is interpreted as showing that the "client is using somatic symptoms to avoid thinking about or dealing with psychological problems…[and is] converting personally distressing troubles into more rational or socially acceptable problems" (Greene 1991, p. 148). Patients with this profile are described as lacking insight, being very resistant to psychological interpretations of their problems, and presenting bizarre somatic complaints. However, these interpretations may not apply to medical patients, whose scores on these scales may be elevated to a level approximately equivalent to that among patients with conversion disorders (Fricke 1956; Lair and Trapp 1962). Not surprisingly, somatic complaints without immediate medical explanation in medical settings are very frequent (noted at up to 60% of physician office visits) and, in the absence of firm medical findings, are frequently interpreted as somatizing (N.A. Cummings 1998). However, caution should be exercised with regard to accepting such statements at face value, if the base rates of complaints were established using objective measures that are (unavoidably) biased against detecting medical causes of symptomatology. Again, studies have shown significant overlap between symptoms of physical diseases (e.g., multiple sclerosis, pulmonary disease) and MMPI/MMPI-2 items that lead to clinically significant increases in scale scores (Labott et al. 1996; Meyerink et al. 1988; Mueller and Girace 1988). Moreover, as medical diagnostic technology advances, many of these somatizing patients may be identified as having recognizable medical conditions. Thus, the presence of a "conversion V" in a medically ill patient or a patient presenting to a physician should not be interpreted as indicating a conversion disorder without careful review of endorsed items and the patient's medical symptoms and signs.

In summary, the MMPI-2 and its predecessor are powerful tools that can help clinicians understand the effects and prognosis of invasive treatments for many medical illnesses. However, the clinician must take the patient's medical condition into consideration and should not blindly attempt a standard psychiatric interpretation in the absence of other findings of psychiatric illness. When included as one component of a comprehensive psychological assessment, MMPI/MMPI-2 results can help the clinician understand a medical or surgical patient's ongoing symptoms and his or her experience of disorder. In addition, the MMPI can help to predict outcome and identify treatment modalities for some specific medical conditions (e.g., headache [Kudrow and Sutkers 1979] and impotence [Beutler et al. 1975]) and for some specific patients (e.g., candidates for cardiac surgery [Henrichs and Waters 1972] or laminectomy [Long 1981] and patients with intractable seizures who are candidates for surgery [Dodrill et al. 1986]). However, because of the frequent misuse of MMPI results by health care providers who have little knowledge of or expertise in the application of the results to patients with medical conditions, others have been more circumspect about use of the MMPI in medical patients when psychiatric disorder is not present (Green 1982).

Millon Clinical Multiaxial Inventory (MCMI/MCMI-II/MCMI-III). The MCMI-II and MCMI-III address psychopathology according to DSM-III-R (American Psychiatric Association 1987) and DSM-IV diagnostic categories, respectively (Davis et al. 1999; Goncalves and Woodward 1994; Groth-Marnat 1997; Millon 1987, 1994). The MCMI-III consists of 175 true-false questions about basic personality patterns, severe personality disorders, and clinical syndromes. The test is computer scored; specific normative data, such as the distribution of scores on specific scales, are treated as proprietary and generally are not available to the user. The MCMI-III generates a narrative report and a score profile. The test is designed for use in mental health settings and assumes that the examinee is seeking assistance. The explicit purpose of the MCMI-III is to determine personality and characterological contributions to behavioral difficulties in individuals with confirmed Axis I psychopathology. To our knowledge (based on a July 1999 literature search), there are no published studies on the use of the MCMI-III or its predecessors in medical or surgical populations, in which the profiles have been established by comparing performance of research study samples with that of non-psychiatric samples. Thus, all published findings of studies evaluating MCMI/MCMI-II/MCMI-III profiles and score elevations in medical and surgical populations must be interpreted with caution.

Personality Assessment Inventory (PAI). The PAI (Morey 1991) is an instrument with psychometric properties that is intended to be an advance over the MMPI. The PAI consists of 344 items, yielding standard scores on 4 validity scales, 11 clinical scales, 5 treatment scales, and 2 interpersonal scales. The test can be completed by persons able to read at the fourth-grade level, requires

approximately 45 minutes to complete, and is easily scored by hand or by computer. The patient's responses are plotted and compared with data from a large, census-based psychiatrically healthy population and from a large, community-based sample of psychiatric patients. In addition to measures of type and severity of psychopathology, the test yields measures of suicidality, aggression, perception of social support, level of recent stress, and resistance to psychological treatment. As with the MMPI tests, one must be careful interpreting PAI findings obtained from medically ill patients. Medical symptoms elevate scores on clinical scales, leading to a risk of overdiagnosis of conversion or other somatization disorders. Therefore, the same caveats mentioned regarding the MMPI and MCMI tests must also be considered when the PAI is used in clinical settings.

Millon Behavioral Health Inventory (MBHI). The MBHI (Millon et al. 1982) was designed specifically to assess personality traits, interpersonal style, the impact of stress, motivation for change, and compliance with care in medical settings. The test provides specific predictions for patients with cardiac, gastrointestinal, genitourinary, or orthopedic disease, as well as predictions about compliance with treatment. Our experience with the test, however, suggests that it is somewhat lacking in terms of assessment of personality traits and that content is too obvious to many patients.

Projective Personality Measures

Among the best-known and least-understood psychological tests are the projective measures. These tests employ less structure and more ambiguous stimuli and task demands than the objective measures, elicit responses rich enough to permit psychodiagnostic inference, and can detect disorders of reality testing and thought processes (Anastasi and Urbina 1997). Although many clinicians rely on qualitative analysis of responses, some of these measures are as reliable, valid, and objective as the personality inventories described earlier in this chapter. Data on medically ill populations are available for few of the tests, however, and caution must be exercised when using these instruments with cognitively impaired patients. Deficits in attention, executive functioning, language, and visuospatial skills can render a patient's responses on these instruments unsuitable for measuring psychopathology. Nonetheless, extensive information on how the individual's medical condition affects his or her perceptual processing often can be obtained and, when applied appropriately, may be useful for treatment planning.

Rorschach inkblot test. The best-known projective test—the Rorschach inkblot test—was developed by Hermann Rorschach (1921). However, Exner (1993) applied psychometric principles of reliability and validity to the Rorschach test and developed the Comprehensive System. This is the most popular scoring system currently in use. Now characterized as a perceptual-cognitive measure rather than strictly as a personality measure, the test yields a wealth of information regarding the patient's perceptual processing and inferential reasoning about the world. This information is interpreted as reflecting current and long-standing personality structure and functioning and can be very useful in psychiatric diagnosis. Although Exner (1993) provided an example of the use of the Comprehensive System in the evaluation of a medical patient, no empirical data on medical patients were supplied, and interpretations appear to be similar to those made in the evaluation of psychiatric patients. Once again, the psychologist's expertise and knowledge about this test are key to its appropriate clinical use in other than strictly psychiatric patient populations. If such expertise and knowledge are lacking both when the Rorschach test is administered to a patient with a medical or neuropsychological disorder and when the results are interpreted, the diagnosis is likely to be inaccurate, and the patient could be seriously harmed.

Thematic Apperception Test (TAT). The TAT (Bellak 1986; Murray 1943) consists of 31 pictures of ambiguous (primarily social) situations, of which 10 are used in any given test administration. The patient is instructed to tell a story about each picture (a story with a beginning, middle, and end) and is asked to include information about the feelings, thoughts, and actions of the story's protagonists. Scoring systems for the TAT are designed to describe the patient's mood states, drives, attitudes, and conflicts. Despite the more highly structured and more obvious nature of the stimuli, compared with the ambiguous stimuli of the inkblot technique, the reliability and validity of the TAT for determining enduring personality style are a source of professional debate, because state characteristics of the individual affect the consistency of TAT responses (Anastasi and Urbina 1997). Some investigators are concerned that the richness of information yielded by this technique does not adequately compensate for the lack of demonstrated psychometric power. Methods such as the TAT might be better described as interview procedures rather than tests.

Rotter Incomplete Sentences Blank. The Rotter Incomplete Sentences Blank (Rotter et al. 1992) is the best known of the instruments that use incomplete sentences. It consists of a series of sentence stems (e.g., "I think fathers should _____"); the patient must finish the sentences. Although a qualitative approach has been used in the past, the new version of the Rotter instrument includes scoring criteria and normative data. The reliability and validity of qualitative approaches to this procedure have been questioned, and the test depends on the overall verbal ability of the patient. Like the TAT, most tests involving incomplete sentences might best be considered interview techniques.

Self-Rating Scales

Specific self-rating scales have been developed to measure anxiety, depression, life-event stress, and other symptoms. New instruments have been designed to measure health-related quality of life and well-being in medical patients, with less emphasis placed on diagnosing psychiatric disorders. Self-rating scales have the advantage of permitting a relatively brief and objective assessment of current emotional functioning and are sensitive to factors that can affect neuropsychological functioning. Because their purpose is usually obvious, however, patients are prone to under- or overreport difficulties. Furthermore, these measures provide little information about personality structure or typical coping style, and their psychometric properties are sometimes questionable (Green 1982). If more extensive information is needed, objective or projective personality inventories should be used. Finally, because many of these instruments include somatic content, results should also be interpreted with caution when scores in the clinical range occur in patients with medical illness; few data are available to guide interpretation of these measures in medical patients (Green 1982).

Depression scales. One of the best-known scales for measuring depression is the Beck Depression Inventory (BDI; Beck and Steer 1987) and its revision, the BDI-II (Beck et al. 1996), a 21-item scale on which a patient rates the severity of current affective and somatic symptoms. Although the BDI is sensitive to depressive symptoms, its use among patients with medical illness has been criticized because of the scale's somatic content (Cavanaugh et al. 1983; Emmons et al. 1987; Schulberg et al. 1985). For this reason, Cavanaugh and co-workers (1983) recommended using only affective items on the BDI when evaluating general medical patients. Similarly, Pincus and Callahan (1993), in the study described earlier in this chapter, found that six BDI items were likely to be endorsed by rheumatoid arthritis patients (Table 7–7). Thus, clinicians using the BDI or the newer BDI-II (Beck

TABLE 7–7. Beck Depression Inventory items likely to be endorsed by patients with rheumatoid arthritis

Item no.	Item
15	I can work about as well as before.
16	I can sleep as well as usual.
17	I don't get more tired than usual.
18	My appetite is no worse than usual.
20	I am no more worried about my health than usual.
21	I have not noticed any recent changes in my interest in sex.

Source. Adapted from Pincus and Callahan 1993.

et al. 1996) with medical and surgical patients should examine the pattern and level of item endorsement before interpreting a total score that is in the clinical range.

The Zung Self-Rating Depression Scale (Zung 1965), also known as the Zung Depression Scale, is frequently used in consultation-liaison settings. It is a 20-item scale that measures severity of affective and physiologic symptoms of depression. The Zung Depression Scale is less highly standardized than the BDI (Green 1982). As with the BDI, the total score must be interpreted judiciously in patients with medical illness. Another popular depression inventory is the Geriatric Depression Scale (Gallagher 1986; Yesavage et al. 1983). However, the validity of this scale in patients with dementia is questionable (Feher et al. 1992). In general, objective self-report measures of depression yield relatively lower scores regarding changes due to treatment compared with assessment scales of depression in which professional expertise must be integrated with patient-reported information (e.g., Hamilton Rating Scale for Depression [Hamilton 1960]). Furthermore, analysis of specific symptoms addressed in these scales tends to reveal less change in response to treatment in comparison with overall summary scores (Lambert and Lambert 1999).

Anxiety scales.   The best-known anxiety scale is the State-Trait Anxiety Inventory (STAI; Spielberger et al. 1983). It consists of two sections: 20 items that assess the patient's anxiety at the time of evaluation (state) and 20 items that evaluate the patient's long-standing, characteristic level of anxiety (trait). Unfortunately, if patients do not read the instructions for each section carefully, the distinction between state and trait measures can be minimal. The STAI was designed as a research instrument, and normative data are limited (Spielberger et al. 1983). Because normative data for medical patients are especially limited, results from these

individuals must be interpreted with caution (Green 1982).

The Beck Anxiety Inventory (Beck 1993) is an alternative to the STAI and is reportedly more effective in differentiating individuals with anxiety from those with depression. However, the extensive overlap between these two disorders complicates differential diagnosis, and reliance should not be placed solely on summary scores of self-report measures (Wilson et al. 1999).

General distress and life-event scales.   A more general instrument that surveys psychiatric and medical symptoms as well as general level of distress is the Symptom Checklist–90—Revised (SCL-90-R; Derogatis 1992); the abbreviated version of this measure is the Brief Symptom Inventory (Derogatis 1993). The SCL-90-R includes 90 items, which patients are asked to rate in terms of severity, and provides results on several psychiatric symptom scales. Its utility in both psychiatric and medical populations has been criticized (Green 1982). However, when this type of self-report measure is included as part of a comprehensive assessment, it can provide useful information about specific symptoms experienced by the patient (Anastasi and Urbina 1997).

Another popular measure, particularly in consultation-liaison settings, is the Profile of Mood States (McNair et al. 1981). Patients rate a series of words that are specific to affective state, and results are reported on several different scales. Because this measure includes few somatic items, it can be used for the assessment of medically ill patients. For measurement of life-event stress, the Schedule of Recent Experience (Casey et al. 1967) and the Social Readjustment Rating Scale (Holmes and Rahe 1967) are particularly well established.

Health-related quality-of-life and well-being scales.   Self-report questionnaires addressing quality of life have been developed with medical patients in mind. These scales evaluate well-being, distress, and life events that can affect coping and psychological response to medical conditions. They either target behavioral characteristics and complaints associated with an illness or survey multiple attributes that are prevalent features of an illness. Well-being and quality of life are subjective individual characteristics measured best by self-report. Effective treatment of symptoms (psychological or medical) does not always improve subjective satisfaction or perceived quality of life. Conversely, quality of life can sometimes be improved with treatment, without a corresponding change in medical symptoms (Frisch 1999). The importance of measuring quality of life through patient self-report, rather than through physician observation, has been emphasized in at least one review (Gill and Feinstein 1994). Some have even argued that behavioral outcomes are even more important measures of health outcomes than are indices of symptoms (R.M. Kaplan 1990). Consequently, these measures can be useful supplements to more traditional measures of psychiatric symptoms.

The Quality of Life Inventory (Frisch 1994) is a brief and objective self-report measure that assesses satisfaction and perceived importance of basic life pursuits in 16 domains (e.g., personal health, relationship status). The measure's psychometric properties have been well established and have contributed to its frequent description as one of the best of the available measures of health-related quality of life (Frisch 1999). Another well-known measure was developed by the Rand Corporation for the Medical Outcomes Study (Tarlov et al. 1989). This instrument, too, has been used frequently in research, and an abbreviated version has been developed (Hays 1998; Ware and Sherbourne 1992). The Functional Assessment of Cancer Therapy Scale (Cella et al. 1993) was designed to measure quality of life in cancer patients. The scale contains questions for all cancer patients, and additional scales have been designed to measure symptoms of specific cancers and of human immunodeficiency virus infection and acquired immunodeficiency syndrome (Cella 1994). All these measures of patients' subjective status can provide useful indications of the need for psychological intervention or the effectiveness of a medical treatment regimen, even in the absence of a reduction in primary symptoms. With any of these measures, however, the selection of the appropriate normative comparison group is still of paramount importance when making a diagnosis and planning treatment for medically ill patients with psychiatric symptoms (Derogatis et al. 1995).

Summary of Psychological Assessment Instruments

Objective and projective personality measures and symptom rating scales can supplement information provided by clinical interviews. In the consultation-liaison setting, findings obtained with these instruments can contribute to establishing a diagnosis, predicting outcome, and planning treatment. Advantages and disadvantages of the different types of measures are listed in Table 7–8. As noted previously, caution must always be exercised when interpreting elevations in scale scores or total scores of patients with medical illness, in the absence of converg-

ing information from a variety of sources, because normative data established for psychiatric patients are less directly applicable. This is especially true when using computer-generated interpretations of objective measures, such as the MMPI/MMPI-2, which do not take medical illness or other unique factors about the patient into account. In addition, cognitive disorders can make it difficult for a patient to complete a measure and can render results invalid. However, when results are interpreted in the context of the patient's history, presenting symptoms, and specific medical condition, findings can provide information on the patient's current coping style, emotional state, reactions to illness, quality of life, and general well-being. (For more detailed information on factors that must be considered when administering psychological tests to general medical patients, please refer to Green 1982.)

Applications to Neuropsychiatric Diagnosis

In a variety of circumstances, psychological testing can be useful in the consultation-liaison setting. Table 7–9 lists some applications of psychological assessment. In the following sections, we describe several of these applications in more detail.

Differential diagnosis of psychiatric disorder. Psychological testing, when integrated with clinical information from other sources, is useful to evaluate an individual for the presence of significant psychopathology and psychiatric disorder. For example, the Comprehensive System for the Rorschach inkblot test (Exner 1993) can assess an individual's perceptual accuracy and reality testing. This assessment can help to establish the presence of a formal thought disorder. Similarly, elevated scores on selected MMPI/MMPI-2 scales indicate the degree to which an individual reports symptoms associated with specific psychopathological conditions, such as depression, anxiety, conversion, or somatization disorders.

Emotional factors and physical symptoms. Psychological tests can help to determine how emotional factors contribute to a patient's physical symptoms. A patient's current and chronic levels of stress can be evaluated with instruments such as the PAI, the STAI, and specific Rorschach indices. These instruments assess tendencies toward repression and denial, coping resources, and personal reaction to illness, among other factors. These factors affect the development, maintenance, and progression of a disorder, as well as success or failure of

TABLE 7–8. Advantages and disadvantages of psychological assessment methods in the consultation-liaison setting

Method	Advantages	Disadvantages
Objective personality measures	Standardized, reliable, and valid for psychiatric diagnosis Large body of supporting data Quantitative indices of distress, coping, and personality style	Time-consuming (30–45 minutes) Results must be interpreted with caution in the case of patients with medical conditions Can be difficult for patients with neuropsychological deficits to complete
Projective personality measures	Qualitative information on personality structure Sensitive to thought disorder Rich psychodiagnostic information Less vulnerable to self-report bias	Time-consuming (45–60 minutes) Few data on profiles of medical patients Results are difficult to interpret when cognitive dysfunction is present
Self-rating symptom scales	Standardized, reliable, and valid for psychiatric diagnosis Brief (5–15 minutes) Easily administered at bedside	Results must be interpreted with caution in the case of patients with medical conditions Prone to under- or overreporting of symptoms Do not provide comprehensive assessment of psychopathology
Health-related quality-of-life scales	Standardized, reliable, and valid Brief (5–15 minutes) Easily administered at bedside Supplement traditional measures of psychopathology Evaluate issues important to recovery from illness	Must be selected with reference to a specific medical condition Prone to under- or overreporting of symptoms Do not assess psychopathology

TABLE 7–9. Applications of psychological assessment

Contribute to differential diagnosis of medical, psychiatric, and neurological disorders

Differentiate among psychiatric conditions, including major affective disorders, anxiety disorders, and personality disorders

Evaluate the role of psychological factors in a patient's physical or cognitive symptoms

Evaluate the source of resistance to psychotherapeutic treatment

Determine the patient's adjustment to medical or neurological illness

Determine the personality characteristics or psychopathological conditions affecting a patient's medical condition and response to treatment

Determine a patient's well-being and quality of life, independent of specific medical or psychiatric symptoms

treatment programs. The MMPI/MMPI-2 and PAI provide measures of guardedness, willingness to address psychological conflicts, and ability to admit directly to experiencing distress.

Case Example 8

Mr. H, an adolescent male, was admitted to a neurology ward for evaluation of atypical dystonias. While hospitalized, he experienced prolonged periods of tonic-clonic movements, head thrashing, and pelvic thrusting. These events almost always occurred during mental status examinations or psychiatric interviews.

They were not accompanied by incontinence, postictal confusion, or interictal cognitive deficit. The patient's approach to the MMPI-2 was guarded and defensive. He denied common shortcomings and presented himself in an unusually positive light. He expressed no psychological concerns. The clinical scale profile revealed a tendency to emphasize physical symptoms as a defense against emotional discomfort. Naive, immature, and demanding, such patients typically employ repression and denial as defenses against psychological stress or conflict. The consultation-liaison psychiatry resident was able to alternately provoke and terminate the patient's attacks in an amobarbital interview. Eventually, suggestion-based intervention resulted in remission of the events, and the dystonic posturing resolved.

Adjustment to medical illness. Interpersonal style, psychosocial competencies, and character structure can interact with physical illness and can determine a patient's ability to cope with illness, deal with health care providers, and respond to intervention. Psychological and personality testing are essential components of the psychiatric assessment of patients whose physical conditions force them into regressed and intense relationships with their care providers. In some patients, severe character pathology may manifest as unusual physical symptoms or as pathological interactions with the treatment team. Careful assessment of personality variables can protect patient and provider alike from maladaptive or destructive interactions.

Case Example 9

Ms. I, a 35-year-old licensed practical nurse, was referred for testing by a defense law firm; she presented with severe cognitive and emotional difficulties after a very mild head injury sustained in a fall from a chair. Clinical interview, projective testing, and responses on personality inventories revealed chronic impairment in emotionality, judgment, impulse control, and interpersonal relationships. Her interpersonal boundaries were rather weak, with marked evidence of a pattern of chronic overidealization and undervaluation of those close to her. Symptom inventories and a review of records revealed impulsive behaviors extending to buying sprees, sexual improprieties, and substance abuse. Her relationships were typically intense and short-lived. On self-report checklists and on structured interviews, Ms. I reported many inconsistent and incompatible symptoms and could be led to endorse vague, unusual, and nonanatomical complaints. A review of the patient's record revealed marked inconsistencies and outright fabrications in her medical and psychosocial history. Evidence suggested that she may have misrepresented her symptoms in the past, which caused her to undergo a number of painful and invasive procedures. Psychological testing supported the diagnostic impression of borderline personality disorder and a factitious disorder. It was later discovered that the patient had been pursuing treatment for other medical problems acquired in equally unlikely ways. She had, in fact, had nearly 140 diagnostic and treatment appointments in the 90 days before her psychological evaluation.

Emotional sequelae of neurological disorders. A number of neurological and medical disorders are associated with cognitive and emotional sequelae. At times, central nervous system manifestations of a patient's disorder are difficult to discriminate from emotional reactions to the disorder. Psychological testing can help to determine how the psychomotor retardation, agitation, cognitive inefficiency, and/or emotional lability of patients with brain disease are related to illness.

Case Example 10

Mr. J was referred for neuropsychiatric evaluation during his third admission for exacerbation of symptoms of multiple sclerosis. Neuroimaging studies revealed relatively few cerebral lesions, but the patient appeared cognitively slowed, amnestic, and mentally impersistent at bedside. Neuropsychological testing revealed evidence of psychomotor slowing; memory and attention lapses; and difficulties establishing, maintaining, and shifting mental set. Psychological testing further revealed that the patient had significant emotional distress, marked by anxiety, depression, and ruminative concern. Vegetative symptoms of depression thwarted his intellectual efficiency and interfered with memory and attention on neuropsychological testing and in everyday life. The diagnostic impression was pseudodementia of depression, although the possibility of a subcortical dementing process was also considered. Treatment with antidepressant medication was started, and Mr. J's cognitive functioning and psychomotor performance significantly improved.

SPECIAL TOPICS

Medicolegal Competence

Neuropsychological and psychological testing can provide objective data on cognitive or emotional factors that affect a patient's ability to appreciate his or her circumstances, to access cognitive and emotional resources needed for daily functioning, and to respond to environmental demands in an appropriate manner. Decisions regarding competence and the ability to function independently are frequently assisted by objective data (see Chapter 11 for an in-depth discussion).

The concept of competence can be better addressed as a constellation of cognitive and emotional competencies rather than as an aggregate whole (Alexander 1988). Grossberg (1998) suggested a "sliding scale" of competencies, in which a patient's ability to decide is weighed against the risk associated with the treatment decision in question. For example, a person can be competent to make decisions about where to live but not about whether he or she can drive. Deficits in language, memory, or perceptual skills can limit competency for some decisions but not others. Because compensation can occur across cognitive domains, the examiner is obligated to evaluate a range of skills and to permit the patient to use alternative strategies for completing tasks. A thorough evaluation of the patient's decision making, judgment, insight, cognitive strengths, and vulnerabilities requires a more extensive evaluation than that which typically occurs during screening examinations conducted at bedside or in the office. Specialized interview or vignette techniques, such as the Cambridge Examination for Mental Disorders of the Elderly (Schmand et al. 1999), have shown promise for the behavioral assessment of medicolegal competence and complement direct assessment of cognitive proficiencies through neuropsychological testing.

Case Example 11

Mr. K, a 67-year-old resident of a senior citizen apartment complex, sustained a left middle cerebral artery infarction, which initially left him globally aphasic, emotionally labile, and hemiparetic. Immediately after the CVA, he was not competent to make decisions on his own behalf, and plans were made to have him transferred on discharge from the hospital to a nursing home near his eldest daughter, hundreds of miles from his home and friends. Mr. K grew increasingly alert, oriented, and engaged as he recovered from his CVA and was markedly upset by the decision to move him to a nursing home.

Neuropsychological testing revealed that Mr. K had relatively intact intellectual resources. Despite language difficulties, his nonverbal processing skills, memory, and reasoning abilities were near normal for his age and education. He became facile at using gesture and other forms of nonverbal communication to overcome his expressive language problems and could apparently understand most of what he heard. Mr. K expressed his desire to remain in his home and to receive additional rehabilitation services on a home-care and outpatient basis. He formulated a plan to receive these services and demonstrated the planning skills necessary to manage the social and financial resources needed to remain in his home. The family's initial reticence was overcome as Mr. K demonstrated his competencies in a number of areas.

Malingering

A patient may intentionally misrepresent or exaggerate his or her symptoms. Even the most senior or experienced clinicians may be far less capable than they suspect of determining when patients are feigning psychological or cognitive deficits (Bernard 1990; Faust et al. 1988; Heaton et al. 1978). Psychological testing can help clinicians detect feigning of neuropsychiatric symptoms. The MMPI/MMPI-2 and PAI both contain scales sensitive to intentional efforts to misrepresent symptoms. The Structured Interview of Reported Symptoms (Rogers et al. 1992) is a "rare symptom" inventory that is sensitive to inconsistent or unusual complaints not associated with known clinical entities. Careful analysis of neuropsychological test performance also helps to identify patients whose neuropsychological deficits are inconsistent with or disproportionate to their complaints (Ruff et al. 1993; Trueblood and Schmidt 1993).

Symptom validity testing refers to the process of repeatedly administering a simple forced-choice task to assess possible malingering (Bianchini et al. 2001; Pankrantz 1979, 1983). Trials with longer interresponse intervals and more complex interresponse tasks are described to the patient as "harder," and a large number of such trials are used. Malingering patients frequently deviate from the standard normal distribution, perform significantly worse than chance (a patient responding randomly is expected to respond correctly 50% of the time), and often perform far worse than genuinely brain-injured

patients (Binder 1993). One can generate statistical probabilities that a patient's performance on this deceptively easy procedure reflects a conscious effort to perform poorly. The Portland Digit Recognition Test (PDRT; Binder 1993; Binder and Willis 1991) is a frequently used version of this procedure. Computerized versions of the PDRT and other forced-choice procedures have been developed and are seeing increased clinical use (Bianchini et al. 2001; Gutierrez and Gur 1998).

Case Example 12

Ms. L, a 30-year-old woman, was tested 2 years after she sustained a mild head injury in a motor vehicle accident. Her injury was unaccompanied by loss of consciousness, and she had had less than 30 minutes of posttraumatic amnesia. However, in the ensuing months, her descriptions of her injury worsened. She reported retrograde memory loss of more than 2 years and scattered loss of overlearned job skills and autobiographical information. She gradually developed a dense anterograde amnesia that lasted for more than a year after her accident.

Testing indicated that Ms. L was of average intelligence. Her only deficit on intellectual testing was on a simple auditory attention task, even though her performances on more complex measures of attention were normal. She exhibited markedly impaired performance on most memory tasks, with little improvement in performance even when she was provided with prompts, cues, and recognition trials. Her profile on the MMPI-2 revealed a conscious effort to overreport symptoms and an apparent effort to present her circumstances in the worst possible light. Performance on the PDRT was so poor that there was less than a 1% probability that she had a genuine memory deficit or that her answers had occurred by chance. On this and other measures, she could have produced errors only by knowing the correct answer and intentionally and repeatedly giving the wrong one. Ms. L claimed to be totally disabled because of her injury, but she was tracked by subsequent videotape surveillance to her job as a tax preparer and to a farm where she continued to provide horseback-riding lessons.

Computerized Testing

Computers have been used to score and interpret neuropsychological and psychological test results for many years. More recently, computers have been used to administer neuropsychological and psychological measures. Computerized assessment offers a number of advantages over traditional assessment methods. First, a computer can administer tests in a strictly standardized, objective manner; subtle differences in how examiners administer tests can be eliminated. Second, computers allow flexibility in the presentation of test stimuli, facilitating changes in such characteristics as the type, location, color, and presentation time. Third, computers can easily collect a wealth of information about an individual's test performance, including accuracy and reaction time. Fourth, the computer can store, sort, and retrieve enormous amounts of information. Finally, computerized tests can be designed to permit repeated testing and are therefore suitable for tracking a patient's status over time, including response to treatment. Several familiar neuropsychological measures have been adapted for computerized administration, and new computerized neuropsychological tests have also been developed.

Computerized cognitive screening tests represent some of the recent innovations in computerized testing. Computers offer a way to administer brief cognitive function tests; laptop computers enable bedside administration. Two batteries have been available for several years. CogScreen (Kay 1995), a group of 11 tests, requires approximately 30 minutes for administration. CogScreen was designed to detect subtle cognitive deficits that could affect aviation performance and is sensitive to mild neuropsychiatric disorder in general. MicroCog (Powell et al. 1996) was designed to assess mild cognitive decline in physicians. MicroCog has been applied to cognitive screening of a wide range of patients, particularly older adults. The Cambridge Neuropsychological Test Automated Battery (Sahakian and Owen 1992) includes computerized versions of several common neuropsychological tasks, accompanied by novel measures of reaction time and executive problem solving, and has been used extensively in dementia, pharmacology, and neurotoxicology research. However, it is our impression that these computerized batteries have not seen widespread clinical use.

Computerized continuous performance tests (CPTs), however, have been used increasingly as part of a more comprehensive neuropsychological assessment battery. These measures of sustained attention require a client to respond to a specific, but infrequent, stimulus (e.g., the number 1 presented among many 2s, an X presented among many different letters) for a lengthy period (Rosvold et al. 1956). Examples of these instruments include the Test of Variables of Attention (Leark et al. 1996), the Integrated Auditory and Visual Continuous Performance Test (Sandford and Turner 1999), and Conners' Continuous Performance Test (Conners 1994). The most common application of these measures has been to diagnose ADHD. Unfortunately, because of their ease of administration, they have come to be used in isolation, with some psychiatrists or psychologists making a diagnosis of ADHD solely on the basis of an abnormal CPT result. However, it has been well established that there is

no single cognitive test, the CPT included, that is sensitive to and specific for diagnosing ADHD (Barkley 1998). Consequently, with regard to diagnosing ADHD, these measures should be used only as a part of a comprehensive assessment that includes a thorough diagnostic interview and, if desired, additional psychological and neuropsychological tests.

Although computerized cognitive screening measures offer advantages over more traditional screening measures, cautions apply. Computerized measures provide initial hypotheses for further exploration. This is especially the case for single cognitive measures, such as the CPT. In some instances, a diagnosis can be made or ruled out based on initial findings. In other instances, screening will indicate the need for more comprehensive assessment. Results must never be interpreted in isolation from the patient's history and other medical findings. Guidelines for computer-assisted evaluation, reflecting these and other issues, have been published by the American Psychological Association and apply to neuropsychological and psychological tests (Committee on Professional Standards and Committee on Psychological Tests and Assessment 1986). A comprehensive review of computerized assessment in neuropsychology is found in Kane and Kay 1992.

STEPS FOR MAKING A REFERRAL

Selecting a Neuropsychologist

Clinical neuropsychology is a specialized area of practice within clinical psychology. It is unfortunate that no formal regulations exist regarding use of the title of neuropsychologist. Although guidelines for training and continuing education in neuropsychology have been published (Bornstein 1988b; Hannay et al. 1998; "Reports of the INS–Division 40 Task Force" 1987), adherence to these guidelines is not yet required. Neuropsychology has now been recognized as a specialty by the American Psychological Association, which is responsible for credentialing psychological training programs in the United States, but it will be several years before graduates begin emerging from accredited programs. Hence, consultation-liaison psychiatrists should ensure that the credentials of someone presenting himself or herself as a neuropsychologist meet certain criteria.

One indicator of competence is board certification in Clinical Neuropsychology by the American Board of Professional Psychology (ABPP). The ABPP is recognized by state licensing boards, Department of Veterans Affairs medical centers, and other organizations as the primary credentialing body for certifying specialized skills in psychology, in general. Being board certified in clinical neuropsychology is recognized as the "clearest evidence of competence as a Clinical Neuropsychologist" by the Clinical Neuropsychology Division of the American Psychological Association ("Definition of a Clinical Neuropsychologist" 1989, p. 22). Candidates for board certification must meet specific requirements for training and must pass oral and written examinations, similar to board examinations in medical specialties.[1] The American Board of Professional Neuropsychology, a second neuropsychological credentialing organization, also has formal examination procedures.

Because the ABPP board certification in Clinical Neuropsychology is relatively new, and because there are no legal requirements for certification, some excellent neuropsychologists are not board certified. Many started their careers as clinical psychologists but chose to specialize. Others began careers as experimental psychologists but retrained as clinical psychologists or clinical neuropsychologists. Criteria for judging the training and experience of a clinical neuropsychologist are listed in Table 7–10. The neuropsychologist should, of course, be licensed or certified (or should be eligible for licensure or certification) as a psychologist in the state where he or she practices. Well-trained neuropsychologists typically have completed course work in basic and applied neuropsychology at the graduate level and have completed at least a year of full-time supervised training in an inpatient neuropsychology setting. Most well-trained neuropsychologists devote 50% or more of their practice to clinical neuropsychology and identify themselves as clinical neuropsychologists rather than clinical psychologists. A workshop or the individual supervision of outpatient cases, without formal intensive training, is considered insufficient training for neuropsychological practice (Bornstein 1988a; Hannay et al. 1998; "Reports of the INS-Division 40 Task Force" 1987).

Well-trained neuropsychologists have experience working with a wide range of patients with different neurobehavioral disorders in neurological, neurosurgical, psychiatric, rehabilitative, and general medical settings. Although some neuropsychologists specialize in particular disorders (e.g., epilepsy, TBI, psychiatric disorder), most work with all types of patients. Some neuropsychologists work only with children or only with adults, but others see patients across the life span. Unless the referral is extremely complex or involves litigation, spe-

TABLE 7–10. Criteria for competence in clinical neuropsychology (adopted by the Clinical Neuropsychology Division of the American Psychological Association, August 1988)

Successful completion of systematic didactic and experiential training in neuropsychology and neuroscience at a regionally accredited university

Two or more years of appropriate supervised training applying neuropsychological services in a clinical setting

Licensing and certification to provide psychological services to the public by the laws of the state or province in which the neuropsychologist practices

Source. Reprinted from "Definition of a Clinical Neuropsychologist." *The Clinical Neuropsychologist* 3:22, 1989. Used with permission.

cialized expertise in a particular disorder is usually not essential, although some familiarity with the disorder is important. If the consultation-liaison psychiatrist has questions about a neuropsychologist's specialty or area of expertise, he or she should ask the neuropsychologist or request a curriculum vitae.

Finally, although some neuropsychologists complete evaluations themselves, many use specially trained technicians to complete most of the testing. This is a fully accepted practice (Brandt and van Gorp 1999; "Guidelines Regarding the Use of Nondoctoral Personnel" 1989) and does not detract from the quality of evaluations.

Writing a Referral Request

When requesting an evaluation, the consultation-liaison psychiatrist should be as specific as possible. He or she should provide a summary sketch of the patient, including age, gender, ethnicity, educational background, and presenting signs and symptoms, as well as the specific question he or she wants the neuropsychologist to answer. Some suggested questions, based on applications of assessment in Tables 7–4 and 7–9, are listed in Table 7–11. Using these types of specific referral questions will ensure that the consultation-liaison psychiatrist receives the information that he or she needs.

Preparing a Patient for Evaluation

Neuropsychological assessment can be stressful and anxiety provoking, especially when a patient is concerned that he or she has a brain-based disorder. Preparing the

[1]A directory of diplomates in clinical neuropsychology, listed alphabetically and geographically, is available from the American Academy of Clinical Neuropsychology, Department of Psychiatry (B2954, CFOB), University of Michigan Health Systems, 1500 East Medical Center Drive, Ann Arbor, MI 48109-0704.

TABLE 7–11.   Examples of specific referral questions for neuropsychological and psychological assessment

Rule out progressive dementia

Differentiate cortical from subcortical dementia

Document cognitive and emotional status following traumatic brain injury or stroke

Evaluate for objective evidence of a memory disorder

Determine whether the patient is competent to return to work, drive, handle finances, or make medical decisions

Rule out cognitive impairment associated with human immunodeficiency virus disease, multiple sclerosis, systemic lupus erythematosus, or other medical illness

Determine whether a change in functioning has occurred since prior evaluation

Evaluate for the possibility of a specific learning disability or attention-deficit/hyperactivity disorder

Determine the contribution of emotional factors to the patient's recovery from illness, surgery, injury, or neurological disorder

Evaluate for possible thought disorder, major affective disorder, or anxiety disorder

Determine the contribution of motivational factors to the patient's presentation

Note.   All assume that recommendations for further evaluation and/or treatment will be included in the report.

patient for evaluation can ease these anxieties and ensure that the patient gives his or her best effort. The neuropsychologist is also helped when the patient has some sense of why he or she has been referred, because less time must be spent explaining the evaluation to the patient. When referring a patient for evaluation, the consultation-liaison psychiatrist should always tell the patient why he or she is being referred, while being sensitive to the patient's anxieties. For example, a patient with possible dementia could be told: "You've been having some problems with your memory. We want to figure out exactly what's causing the problem and what we can do about it. These tests will help us do that." It can also help to tell the patient something about the evaluation. For example, the consultation-liaison psychiatrist can say: "You will be completing a neuropsychological evaluation. These are tests of your skills in attention and concentration, language, visual processing, problem solving, reasoning, learning, and memory. These tests will also tell us how stressed you are and how that might be affecting your thinking. You will not be getting a grade on any of these tests, but it is important for you to do your very best." If the patient has additional questions about the evaluation, he or she can be encouraged to ask the neuropsychologist directly or to call the neuropsychologist before the evaluation.

CONCLUSION

Within consultation-liaison psychiatry settings, neuropsychological and psychological testing can contribute significantly to the diagnostic process. Evaluation can differentiate among neuropsychiatric syndromes and can establish how cognitive deficits, emotional functioning, and personality style contribute to a patient's difficulties. Various methods are available for assessment, ranging from brief screens and self-rating scales to comprehensive batteries and personality inventories. The method selected depends on the referral question and the availability of time, equipment, and personnel. In almost every instance, however, a method will be available to provide a description of the patient's neurobehavioral competencies, to assist with the diagnostic process, and to contribute to treatment planning. Thus, in cases of complex neuropsychiatric issues, psychiatrists should strongly consider referral for neuropsychological and/or psychological evaluation.

REFERENCES

Adams KM: In search of Luria's battery: a false start. J Consult Clin Psychol 48:511–516, 1980

Adams KM: Luria left in the lurch: unfulfilled promises are not valid tests. Journal of Clinical Neuropsychology 6:455–458, 1984

Alexander MP: Clinical determination of mental competence. Arch Neurol 45:23–26, 1988

Alfano DP, Neilson PM, Paniak CE: The MMPI and closed-head injury. The Clinical Neuropsychologist 6:134–142, 1992

American Psychiatric Association: Diagnostic and Statistical Manual of Mental Disorders, 3rd Edition, Revised. Washington, DC, American Psychiatric Association, 1987

American Psychiatric Association: Diagnostic and Statistical Manual of Mental Disorders, 4th Edition. Washington, DC, American Psychiatric Association, 1994

American Psychiatric Association: Diagnostic and Statistical Manual of Mental Disorders, 4th Edition, Text Revision. Washington, DC, American Psychiatric Association, 2000

Anastasi A, Urbina S: Psychological Testing, 7th Edition. Englewood Cliffs, NJ, Prentice-Hall, 1997

Association on Higher Education and Disability: Guidelines for Documentation of a Learning Disability in Adolescents and Adults. Columbus, OH, Association on Higher Education and Disability, 1997

Barkley RA: Attention Deficit Hyperactivity Disorder: A Handbook for Diagnosis and Treatment, 2nd Edition. New York, Guilford, 1998

Beck AT: Beck Anxiety Inventory. San Antonio, TX, Psychological Corporation, 1993

Beck AT, Steer RA: Beck Depression Inventory Manual. San Antonio, TX, Psychological Corporation, 1987

Beck AT, Steer RA, Brown GK: Beck Depression Inventory–II. San Antonio, TX, Psychological Corporation, 1996

Bellak L: The TAT, CAT, and SAT in Clinical Use, 4th Edition. New York, Grune & Stratton, 1986

Bernard L: Prospects for faking believable memory deficits on neuropsychological tests and the use of incentives in simulation research. J Clin Exp Neuropsychol 12:715–728, 1990

Beutler LE, Karacan I, Anch AM, et al: MMPI and MIT discriminators of biogenic and psychogenic impotence. J Consult Clin Psychol 43:899–903, 1975

Bianchini KJ, Mathias CW, Greve KW: Symptom validity testing: a critical review. Clin Neuropsychol 15:19–45, 2001

Binder LM: Assessment of malingering after mild head trauma with the Portland Digit Recognition Test. J Clin Exp Neuropsychol 15:170–182, 1993

Binder LM, Willis SC: Assessment of motivation after financially compensable minor head trauma. Psychological Assessment: A Journal of Consulting and Clinical Psychology 3:175–181, 1991

Bornstein RA: Entry into clinical neuropsychology: graduate, undergraduate, and beyond. The Clinical Neuropsychologist 2:213–220, 1988a

Bornstein RA: Guidelines for continuing education in clinical neuropsychology. The Clinical Neuropsychologist 2:25–29, 1988b

Bornstein RA, Kozora E: Content bias of the MMPI Sc scale in neurological patients. Neuropsychiatry Neuropsychol Behav Neurol 3:200–205, 1990

Brandt J, van Gorp W: American Academy of Clinical Neuropsychology policy on the use of non-doctoral level personnel in conducting clinical neuropsychological evaluations. J Clin Exp Neuropsychol 21:1, 1999

Brooks N (ed): Closed Head Injury: Psychological, Social, and Family Consequences. New York, Oxford University Press, 1984

Brown GG, Baird AD, Shatz MW, et al: The effects of cerebrovascular disease on neuropsychological functioning, in Neuropsychological Assessment of Neuropsychiatric Disorders, 2nd Edition. Edited by Grant I, Adams KM. New York, Oxford University Press, 1996, pp 342–378

Burt DB, Zembar MJ, Niederehe G: Depression and memory impairment: a meta-analysis of the association, its pattern, and specificity. Psychol Bull 117:285–305, 1995

Butcher JN, Dahlstrom WG, Graham JR, et al: Minnesota Multiphasic Personality Inventory–2 (MMPI-2): Manual for Administration and Scoring. Minneapolis, MN, University of Minnesota Press, 1989

Butters N: The clinical aspects of memory disorders: contributions from experimental studies of amnesia and dementia. Journal of Clinical Neuropsychology 6:17–36, 1984

Casey RL, Masuda M, Holmes TH: Quantitative study of recall of life events. J Psychosom Res 11:239–247, 1967

Cassens G, Wolfe L, Zola M: The neuropsychology of depressions. J Neuropsychiatry Clin Neurosci 2:202–213, 1990

Cavanaugh S, Clark DC, Gibbons RD: Diagnosing depression in the hospitalized medically ill. Psychosomatics 24:809–815, 1983

Cella D[F]: Manual: Functional Assessment of Cancer Therapy (FACT) Scales and the Functional Assessment of HIV Infection (FAHI) Scale (Version 3). Chicago, IL, D Cella, 1994

Cella DF, Tulsky DS, Gray G, et al: The Functional Assessment of Cancer Therapy Scale: development and validation of the general measure. J Clin Oncol 11:570–579, 1993

Christensen A-L: Luria's Neuropsychological Investigation, 2nd Edition. Copenhagen, Munksgaard, 1979

Coffey CE, Figiel GS, Djang WT, et al: White matter hyperintensity on magnetic resonance imaging: clinical and neuroanatomic correlates in the depressed elderly. J Neuropsychiatry Clin Neurosci 1:135–144, 1989

Colligan RC, Osborne D, Swensen WM, et al: The MMPI: a contemporary normative study. Paper presented at the 91st annual convention of the American Psychological Association, Anaheim, CA, August 1983

Committee on Professional Standards and Committee on Psychological Tests and Assessment: Guidelines for Computer-Based Tests and Interpretations. Washington, DC, American Psychological Association, 1986

Conners CK: Conners' Continuous Performance Test Computer Program. Orlando, FL, Psychological Assessment Resources, 1994

Cripe LI: Neuropsychological and psychosocial assessment of the brain-injured person: clinical concepts and guidelines. Rehabilitation Psychology 34:93–100, 1989

Cummings JL: Clinical Neuropsychiatry. Boston, MA, Allyn & Bacon, 1985

Cummings JL (ed): Subcortical Dementia. New York, Oxford University Press, 1990

Cummings NA: The new structure of health care and a role for psychology, in Health Psychology Through the Life Span: Practice and Research Opportunities. Edited by Resnick RJ, Rozensky RH. Washington DC, American Psychological Association, 1998, pp 27–38

Davis RD, Meagher SE, Goncalves A, et al: Treatment planning and outcome in adults: the Millon Clinical Multiaxial Inventory–III, in The Use of Psychological Testing for Treatment Planning and Outcome Assessment, 2nd Edition. Edited by Maruish M. Mahwah, NJ, Erlbaum, 1999, pp 1051–1081

Definition of a clinical neuropsychologist. The Clinical Neuropsychologist 3:22, 1989

Delis DC, Kaplan E: Hazards of a standardized neuropsychological test with low content validity: comment on the Luria-Nebraska Neuropsychological Battery. J Consult Clin Psychol 51:396–398, 1983

Delis DC, Kramer JH, Kaplan E, et al: California Verbal Learning Test, 2nd Edition. San Antonio, TX, Psychological Corporation, 2000

Delis DC, Kaplan E, Kramer J: Delis-Kaplan Executive Function Sequence. San Antonio, TX, Psychological Corporation, 2001

DeLuca J: Cognitive dysfunction after aneurysm of the anterior communicating artery. J Clin Exp Neuropsychol 14:924–934, 1992

Derogatis LR: SCL-90-R: Administration, Scoring, and Procedures Manual. Minneapolis, MN, National Computer Systems, 1994

Derogatis LR: BSI: Administration, Scoring, and Procedures Manual, 3rd Edition. Minneapolis, MN, National Computer Systems, 1993

Derogatis LR, Fleming MP, Sudler NC, et al: Psychological assessment, in Managing Chronic Illness: A Biopsychosocial Perspective. Edited by Nicasio PM, Smith TW. Washington DC, American Psychological Association, 1995, pp 59–116

Dikmen SS, Levin HS: Methodological issues in the study of mild head injury. J Head Trauma Rehabil 8:30–37, 1993

Dodrill CB, Wilkus RJ, Ojemann GA, et al: Multidisciplinary prediction of seizure relief from cortical resection surgery. Ann Neurol 20:2–12, 1986

Educational Testing Service: Policy Statement for Documentation of Attention-Deficit/Hyperactivity Disorder in Adolescents and Adults. Princeton, NJ, Educational Testing Service, 1998a

Educational Testing Service: Policy Statement for Documentation of Learning Disabilities in Adolescents and Adults. Princeton, NJ, Educational Testing Service, 1998b

Emmons CA, Fetting JH, Zonderman AB: A comparison of the symptoms of medical and psychiatric patients matched on the Beck Depression Inventory. Gen Hosp Psychiatry 9:398–404, 1987

Exner JE: The Rorschach: A Comprehensive System, 3rd Edition. Vol 1: Basic Foundations. New York, Wiley, 1993

Faust D, Hart K, Guilmette TJ: Pediatric malingering: the capacity of children to fake believable deficits on neuropsychological testing. J Consult Clin Psychol 56:578–582, 1988

Feher EP, Larrabee GJ, Crook TH: Factors attenuating the validity of the Geriatric Depression Scale in a dementia population. J Am Geriatr Soc 40:906–909, 1992

Folstein MF, Folstein SE, McHugh PR: "Mini-mental state": a practical method for grading the cognitive state of patients for the clinician. J Psychiatr Res 12:189–198, 1975

Folstein MF, Folstein SE, McHugh R: Mini-Mental State Examination. Odessa, FL, Psychological Assessment Resources, 2001

Fricke BG: Conversion hysterics and the MMPI. J Clin Psychol 12:322–326, 1956

Frisch MB: Quality of Life Inventory (QOLI). Minneapolis, MN, National Computer Systems, 1994

Frisch MB: Quality of life assessment/intervention and the Quality of Life Inventory (QOLI), in The Use of Psychological Testing for Treatment Planning and Outcome Assessment, 2nd Edition. Edited by Maruish M. Mahwah, NJ, Erlbaum, 1999, pp 1277–1331

Gaffan D, Gaffan EA: Amnesia in man following transection of the fornix. Brain 114:2611–2618, 1991

Gallagher D: Assessment of depression by interview methods and psychiatric rating scales, in Handbook for Clinical Memory Assessment of Older Adults. Edited by Poon LW. Washington, DC, American Psychological Association, 1986, pp 202–212

Gass CS, Russell EW: Minnesota Multiphasic Personality Inventory correlates of lateralized cerebral lesions and aphasic deficits. J Consult Clin Psychol 54:359–363, 1986

Gill TM, Feinstein AR: A critical appraisal of the quality of quality-of-life measurements. JAMA 272:619–626, 1994

Golden CJ, Maruish M: The Luria-Nebraska Neuropsychological Battery, in The Neuropsychology Handbook. Edited by Wedding DJ, Horton AM, Webster J. New York, Springer, 1986, pp 161–193

Golden CJ, Hammeke TA, Purisch AD: Luria-Nebraska Neuropsychological Battery. Los Angeles, CA, Western Psychological Services, 1985

Goncalves AA, Woodward MJ: Millon Clinical Multiaxial Inventory–II, in The Use of Psychological Testing for Treatment Planning and Outcome Assessment. Edited by Maruish M. Hillsdale, NJ, Erlbaum, 1994, pp 161–184

Goodglass H, Kaplan E, Barresi B: Assessment of Aphasia and Related Disorders, 3rd Edition. Baltimore, MD, Lippincott Williams & Wilkins, 2001

Green CJ: Psychological assessments in medical settings, in Handbook of Clinical Health Psychology. Edited by Millon T, Meagher R. New York, Plenum, 1982, pp 339–375

Greene RL: The MMPI-2/MMPI: An Interpretive Manual. Boston, MA, Allyn & Bacon, 1991

Grossberg GT: Advance directives, competency evaluation, and surrogate management in elderly patients. Am J Geriatr Psychiatry 6:S79–S84, 1998

Groth-Marnat G: Handbook of Psychological Assessment, 3rd Edition. New York, Wiley, 1997

Guidelines regarding the use of nondoctoral personnel in clinical neuropsychological assessment (editorial). The Clinical Neuropsychologist 3:23–24, 1989

Gutierrez JM, Gur RC: Detection of malingering using forced choice techniques, in Detection of Malingering During Head Injury Litigation. Edited by Reynolds CR. New York, Plenum, 1998, pp 81–104

Hamilton M: A rating scale for depression. J Neurol Neurosurg Psychiatry 23:56–62, 1960

Hannay HJ, Bieliauskas LA, Crosson BA, et al: Proceedings of the Houston Conference on Specialty Education Training in Clinical Neuropsychology. Archives of Clinical Neuropsychology 13:157–250, 1998

Hathaway SR, McKinley JC: Minnesota Multiphasic Personality Inventory, Revised Edition. New York, Psychological Corporation, 1967

Hays RD: RAND-36 Health Status Inventory. San Antonio, TX, Psychological Corporation, 1998

Heaton RK, Smith HH, Lehman RAW, et al: Prospects for faking believable deficits on neuropsychological testing. J Consult Clin Psychol 46:892–900, 1978

Heaton RK, Grant I, Matthews CG: Comprehensive Norms for an Expanded Halstead-Reitan Battery. Orlando, FL, Psychological Assessment Resources, 1991

Helmes E, Reddon JR: A perspective on developments in assessing psychopathology: a critical review of the MMPI and MMPI-2. Psychol Bull 113:453–471, 1993

Henrichs TF, Waters WF: Psychological adjustment and response to open-heart surgery: some methodological considerations. Br J Psychiatry 120:491–496, 1972

Hill CD, Stoudemire A, Morris R, et al: Dysnomia in the differential diagnosis of major depression, depression-related cognitive dysfunction, and dementia. J Neuropsychiatry Clin Neurosci 4:64–69, 1992

Hodges JR: Cognitive Assessment for Clinicians. New York, Oxford University Press, 1994

Holmes TH, Rahe RH: The Social Readjustment Rating Scale. J Psychosom Res 11:213–218, 1967

Jacobs JW, Bernhard MR, Delgado A, et al: Screening for organic mental syndromes in the medically ill. Ann Intern Med 86:40–46, 1977

Jørgensen K, Christensen A-L: The approach of A.R. Luria to neuropsychological assessment, in Clinical Neuropsychological Assessment: A Cognitive Approach. Edited by Mapou RL, Spector J. New York, Plenum, 1995, pp 217–236

Kane RL, Kay GG: Computerized assessment in neuropsychology: a review of tests and test batteries. Neuropsychol Rev 3:1–117, 1992

Kane RL, Parsons OA, Goldstein G: Statistical relationships and discriminative accuracy of the Halstead-Reitan, Luria-Nebraska, and Wechsler IQ scores in the identification of brain damage. J Clin Exp Neuropsychol 7:211–223, 1985

Kaplan E: A process approach to neuropsychological assessment, in Clinical Neuropsychology and Brain Function: Research, Measurement, and Practice. Edited by Boll T, Bryant BK. Washington, DC, American Psychological Association, 1988, pp 129–167

Kaplan E: The process approach to neuropsychological assessment of psychiatric patients. J Neuropsychiatry Clin Neurosci 2:72–87, 1990

Kaplan E: The Boston Process Approach to neuropsychological assessment. Workshop presented at Walter Reed Army Medical Center, Washington, DC, March 1993

Kaplan E, Fein D, Morris R, et al: The WAIS-R as a Neuropsychological Instrument. San Antonio, TX, Psychological Corporation, 1991

Kaplan E, Goodglass H, Weintraub S: Boston Naming Test, 3rd Edition. Baltimore, MD, Lippincott Williams & Wilkins, 2001

Kaplan RM: Behavior as the central outcome in health care. American Psychol 45:1211–1220, 1990

Kay GG: CogScreen—Aeromedical Edition: Professional Manual. Odessa, FL, Psychological Assessment Resources, 1995

Klein SH: Misuse of the Luria-Nebraska localization scales—comments on a criminal case study. The Clinical Neuropsychologist 7:297–299, 1993

Kolb B, Whishaw IQ: Fundamentals of Human Neuropsychology, 4th Edition. New York, WH Freeman, 1996

Kudrow L, Sutkers BJ: MMPI pattern specificity in primary headache disorders. Headache 19:18–24, 1979

Labott SM, Preisman RC, Torosian T, et al: Screening for somatizing patients in the pulmonary subspecialty clinic. Psychosomatics 37:327–338, 1996

Lair CV, Trapp EP: The differential diagnostic value of MMPI with somatically disturbed patients. J Clin Psychol 37:744–749, 1962

Lambert MJ, Lambert JM: Use of psychological tests for assessing treatment outcome, in The Use of Psychological Testing for Treatment Planning and Outcome Assessment, 2nd Edition. Edited by Maruish M. Mahwah, NJ, Erlbaum, 1999, pp 115–151

Leach L, Kaplan E, Rewilak D, et al: Kaplan Baycrest Neurocognitive Assessment. San Antonio, TX, Psychological Corporation, 2000

Leark RA, Dupuy TR, Greenberg LM, et al: Test of Variables of Attention Professional Manual, Version 7.0. Los Alamitos, CA, Universal Attention Disorders, Inc, 1996

Leonberger FT: The question of organicity: is it still functional? Professional Psychology: Research and Practice 20:411–414, 1989

Levin HS, Benton AL, Grossman RG: Neurobehavioral Consequences of Closed Head Injury. New York, Oxford University Press, 1982

Levin HS, Grafman J, Eisenberg HM (eds): Neurobehavioral Recovery From Head Injury. New York, Oxford University Press, 1987

Lezak MD: Neuropsychological Assessment, 2nd Edition. New York, Oxford University Press, 1983

Lezak MD: Neuropsychological Assessment, 3rd Edition. New York, Oxford University Press, 1995

Lishman WA: Organic Psychiatry: The Psychological Consequences of Cerebral Disorder, 3rd Edition. Malden, MA, Blackwell Science, 1998

Long CJ: The relationship between surgical outcome and MMPI in chronic pain patients. J Clin Psychol 37:744–749, 1981

Luria AR: The Working Brain: An Introduction to Neuropsychology. New York, Basic Books, 1973

Luria AR: Higher Cortical Functions in Man, 2nd Edition. New York, Basic Books, 1980

Mack JL: The MMPI and neurological dysfunction, in MMPI: Clinical and Research Trends. Edited by Newmark CS. New York, Praeger, 1979, pp 53–79

Mapou RL: Testing to detect brain damage: an alternative to what may no longer be useful. J Clin Exp Neuropsychol 10:271–278, 1988

Mapou RL: DSM-IV "cognitive disorders" (letter). J Neuropsychiatry Clin Neurosci 5:223–224, 1993

Mapou RL: Introduction, in Clinical Neuropsychological Assessment: A Cognitive Approach. Edited by Mapou RL, Spector J. New York, Plenum, 1995, pp 1–13

Mapou RL: Learning disabilities, in Differential Diagnosis in Adult Neuropsychological Assessment. Edited by Ricker J. New York, Springer (in press)

Mapou RL, Spector J (eds): Clinical Neuropsychological Assessment: A Cognitive Approach. New York, Plenum, 1995

Massman PJ, Delis DC, Butters N, et al: The subcortical dysfunction hypothesis of memory deficits in depression: neuropsychological validation in a subgroup of patients. J Clin Exp Neuropsychol 14:687–706, 1992

Mattis S: Dementia Rating Scale. Odessa, FL, Psychological Assessment Resources, 1988

McGlynn SM, Schacter DL: Unawareness of deficits in neuropsychological syndromes. J Clin Exp Neuropsychol 11:143–205, 1989

McNair DM, Lorr M, Droppelman LS: Profile of Mood States Manual. San Diego, CA, Educational & Industrial Testing Service, 1981

Meier M, Strauman SE: Neuropsychological recovery after cerebral infarction, in Neurobehavioral Aspects of Cerebrovascular Disease. Edited by Bornstein RA, Brown G. New York, Oxford University Press, 1991, pp 273–296

Meyer GJ, Finn SE, Eyde LD, et al: Psychological testing and psychological assessment: a review of evidence and issues. Am Psychol 56:128–165, 2001

Meyerink LH, Reitan RM, Selz M: The validity of the MMPI with multiple sclerosis patients. J Clin Psychol 44:764–769, 1988

Milberg WP, Hebben N, Kaplan E: The Boston Process Approach to neuropsychological assessment, in Neuropsychological Assessment of Neuropsychiatric Disorders, 2nd Edition. Edited by Grant I, Adams KM. New York, Oxford University Press, 1996, pp 58–80

Miller L: 'Narrow localizationalism' in psychiatric neuropsychology. Psychol Med 16:729–734, 1986

Millon T: Millon Clinical Multiaxial Inventory–II Manual. Minneapolis, MN, National Computer Systems, 1987

Millon T: MCMI-III Test Manual. Minneapolis, MN, National Computer Systems, 1994

Millon T, Green CJ, Meagher RB: Millon Behavioral Health Inventory Manual, 3rd Edition. Minneapolis, MN, National Computer Systems, 1982

Montgomery K, Costa L: Neuropsychological test performance of a normal elderly sample. Paper presented at the 6th European conference of the International Neuropsychological Society, Lisbon, Portugal, June 1983

Morey LC: The Personality Assessment Inventory Manual. Odessa, FL, Psychological Assessment Resources, 1991

Mueller SR, Girace M: Use and misuse of the MMPI: a reconsideration. Psychol Rep 63:483-491, 1988

Murray HA: Thematic Apperception Test Manual. Cambridge, MA, Harvard University Press, 1943

Nelson A, Fogel BS, Faust D: Bedside cognitive screening instruments: a critical assessment. J Nerv Ment Dis 174:73–83, 1986

Northern California Neurobehavioral Group: Manual for COGNISTAT (The Neurobehavioral Cognitive Status Examination). Fairfax, CA, Northern California Neurobehavioral Group, 1995

Omer H, Foldes J, Toby M, et al: Screening for cognitive deficits in a sample of hospitalized geriatric patients: a re-evaluation of a brief mental status questionnaire. J Am Geriatr Soc 31:266–268, 1983

Osborne D, Colligan RC, Swensen WM, et al: Use of contemporary MMPI norms in a medical population. Paper presented at the 91st annual convention of the American Psychological Association, Anaheim, CA, August 1983

Pankrantz L: Symptom validity testing and symptom retraining: procedures for the assessment and treatment of functional sensory deficits. J Consult Clin Psychol 47:409–410, 1979

Pankrantz L: A new technique for the assessment and modification of feigned memory deficit. Percept Mot Skills 57:367–372, 1983

Pincus T, Callahan LF: Depression scales in rheumatoid arthritis: criterion contamination in interpretation of patient responses. Patient Education and Counseling 20:133–143, 1993

Powell D, Kaplan E, Whitla D, et al: MicroCog: Assessment of Cognitive Functioning, Version 2.4. San Antonio, TX, Psychological Corporation, 1996

Prigatano GP: Disordered mind, wounded soul: the emerging role of psychotherapy in rehabilitation after brain injury. J Head Trauma Rehabil 6:1–10, 1991

Prigatano GP, Fordyce DJ, Zeiwer HK, et al: Neuropsychological Rehabilitation After Brain Injury. Baltimore, MD, Johns Hopkins University Press, 1986

Randolph C: Repeatable Battery for the Assessment of Neuropsychological Status (RBANS). San Antonio, TX, Psychological Corporation, 1998

Reitan RM, Wolfson D: The Halstead-Reitan Neuropsychological Test Battery: Theory and Clinical Interpretation. Tucson, AZ, Neuropsychology Press, 1985

Reitan RM, Wolfson D: The Halstead-Reitan Neuropsychological Test Battery, in The Neuropsychology Handbook. Edited by Wedding DJ, Horton AM, Webster J. New York, Springer, 1986, pp 134–160

Reports of the INS-Division 40 Task Force on Education, Accreditation, and Credentialing. The Clinical Neuropsychologist 1:29–34, 1987

Rogers R, Bagby RM, Dickens SE: SIRS—Structured Interview of Reported Symptoms: Professional Manual. Odessa, FL, Psychological Assessment Resources, 1992

Rorschach H: Psychodiagnostics. Bern, Switzerland, Bircher, 1921

Rosvold HE, Mirksy AF, Sarason I, et al: A continuous performance test of brain damage. Journal of Consulting Psychology 20:343–350, 1956

Rotter JB, Lah MI, Rafferty JE: The Rotter Incomplete Sentences Blank Manual, 2nd Edition. San Antonio, TX, Psychological Corporation, 1992

Ruff RM, Wylie T, Tennant W: Malingering and malingering-like aspects of mild closed head injury. J Head Trauma Rehabil 8:60–73, 1993

Sahakian BJ, Owen AM: Computerized assessment in neuropsychiatry using CANTAB. Journal of Research in Social Medicine 85:399–402, 1992

Sandford JA, Turner A: Integrated Auditory and Visual Continuous Performance Test Manual. Richmond, VA, Braintrain, 1999

Schmand B, Gouwenberg B, Smit JH, et al: Assessment of mental competency in community-dwelling elderly. Alzheimer Dis Assoc Disord 13:80–87, 1999

Schulberg HC, Saul M, McClelland M, et al: Assessing depression in primary medical and psychiatric practices. Arch Gen Psychiatry 42:1164–1170, 1985

Schwamm LH, Van Dyke C, Kiernan RJ: The Neurobehavioral Cognitive Status Examination: comparison with the Cognitive Capacity Screening Examination and the Mini-Mental State Examination in a neurosurgical population. Ann Intern Med 107:486–491, 1987

Shaffer D: Attention deficit hyperactivity disorder in adults (editorial). Am J Psychiatry 151:633–638, 1994

Spielberger CD, Gorsuch RL, Lushene R, et al: Manual for the State-Trait Anxiety Inventory (Form Y). Palo Alto, CA, Consulting Psychologists Press, 1983

Spiers PA: Have they come to praise Luria or to bury him? The Luria-Nebraska Battery controversy. J Consult Clin Psychol 49:331–341, 1984

Stambrook M: The Luria-Nebraska Neuropsychological Battery: a promise that may be partly fulfilled. Journal of Clinical Neuropsychology 5:247–269, 1983

Stokes AF, Banich MT, Elledge VC: Testing the tests—an empirical evaluation of screening tests for the detection of cognitive impairment in aviators. Aviat Space Environ Med 62:783–788, 1991

Sweeney JA, Wetzler S, Stokes P, et al: Cognitive functioning in depression. J Clin Psychol 45:836–842, 1989

Tarlov AR, Ware JE, Greenfield S, et al: The Medical Outcomes Study: an application of methods for monitoring the results of medical care. JAMA 262:925–930, 1989

Tarter RE, van Thiel DH, Edwards KL (eds): Medical Neuropsychology. New York, Plenum, 1988

Trueblood W, Schmidt M: Malingering and other validity considerations in the neuropsychological evaluation of mild head injury. J Clin Exp Neuropsychol 15:578–590, 1993

Tupper D: Rehabilitation of cognitive and neuropsychological deficit following stroke, in Neurobehavioral Aspects of Cerebrovascular Disease. Edited by Bornstein RA, Brown G. New York, Oxford University Press, 1991, pp 273–296

Veiel HOF: A preliminary profile of neuropsychological deficits associated with major depression. J Clin Exp Neuropsychol 19:587–603, 1997

Ware JE, Sherbourne CD: The MOS 36-item short-form health survey (SF-36), I: conceptual framework and item selection. Med Care 30:473–483, 1992

Wechsler D: Wechsler Adult Intelligence Scale—Revised. San Antonio, TX, Psychological Corporation, 1981

Wechsler D: Wechsler Adult Intelligence Scale—3rd Edition. San Antonio, TX, Psychological Corporation, 1997

Wilson KA, de Beurs E, Palmer CA, et al: Beck Anxiety Inventory, in The Use of Psychological Testing for Treatment Planning and Outcome Assessment, 2nd Edition. Edited by Maruish M. Mahwah, NJ, Erlbaum, 1999, pp 971–992

Wooten A: MMPI profiles among neuropsychology patients. J Clin Psychol 39:392–406, 1983

Yesavage J, Brink T, Rose T, et al: Development and validation of a geriatric depression screening scale: a preliminary report. J Psychiatr Res 17:37–49, 1983

Zung WK: A self-rating depression scale. Arch Gen Psychiatry 12:63–70, 1965

8

Behavioral Responses to Illness

Personality and Personality Disorders

Robert J. Ursano, M.D.

Richard S. Epstein, M.D.

Susan G. Lazar, M.D.

What is personality? How is it related to medical illness? These challenging questions are stimuli to much science and to much ancient and modern intellectual thought. The consultation-liaison psychiatrist is constantly involved in understanding the interaction between personality and disease.

Personality may be understood as a cluster of characteristic behavioral responses that depend on a person's past experiences, biological propensities, social context, and view of the future. The patient's past experiences form the lenses through which the patient looks at the present world and, in this way, directs the pattern of future behaviors. Although we are still only beginning to understand the contributions of biology to behavior, we know that biology is the underpinning of basic human feelings such as anxiety and excitement and therefore, from infancy, directs individuals' needs for security, novelty, and avoidance. Social context is measured in gross form by questions such as "Living alone or with family?" But we also measure our social context by the complex web of interpersonal relationships that make up our world and influence our behavior.

The patient's view of the future is often overlooked as a major organizer of behavior. Perhaps it is most noticed with the dying patient; too often, physicians and other providers assume the patient "has no future." The patient's behavior, however, may become organized by his or her own notion of the future. For example, the future may be the issue of who will come to visit today or whether remaining tasks can be accomplished—including saying good-bye (Ursano and Fullerton 1991).

Personality is not static. It changes throughout the life cycle, from childhood to adulthood to old age (Colarusso and Nemiroff 1981). A patient's particular illness, developmental stage, interpersonal resources, and unique past and present life events all influence the feelings, thoughts, and behaviors (observable data of personality) that occur in response to an acute illness or a chronic disease.

The patient's personality interacts with and is reactive to the individuals on the treatment team. These interactions may be realistic or influenced by past interpersonal relationships (e.g., transference and countertransference). One of the consultation-liaison psychiatrist's goals is to understand how the patient's personality contributes to the patient's illness, treatment, and adaptation. With this understanding, the consultation-liaison psychiatrist can recommend interventions that will maximize good medical treatment, healthy behaviors, and the patient's sense of hope and realistic expectations for the future.

In this chapter, we review the contributions of personality to medical illness. First, we review the relationship between personality and illness in the light of the most common patient experiences: feelings of helplessness, lack of control, shame, and guilt. We then examine how the doctor-patient relationship affects disease and treatment outcome. The doctor-patient relationship is central to the patient's illness response and to the physician's response to the patient. We then address the relationship between personality disorders and medical illnesses. Little systematic study has been done in this area, and much of the literature on personality and personality disorders overlaps. This overlap reflects the difficulties in diagnosing personality disorders, particularly in medically ill patients. The consultation-liaison psychiatrist is often more interested in detecting adaptive and maladaptive behavioral response patterns than in making the distinction between a personality style and a disorder, which is difficult at best and often impossible in the hospital.

PATIENT'S RESPONSE TO ILLNESS

Most individuals are highly resilient and cope well with illnesses or injuries. The consultation-liaison psychiatrist is usually consulted when personality issues complicate the treatment of an illness or hinder the patient's cooperation with the medical or nursing staff. Anxiety, agitation, depression, hostility, uncooperativeness, or even psychosis may reflect an adverse interaction between the patient's personality and the illness, which requires psychiatric consultation. The patient may or may not have a diagnosable psychiatric disorder, but the patient's personality structure (i.e., cluster of behavioral response tendencies) may increase morbidity or even mortality related to his or her disease. Feelings of helplessness, loss of control, shame, guilt, and negative responses to the doctor-patient relationship underlie many of these adverse reactions to illness.

The subtle and complex interrelation between psyche and soma requires a thorough assessment to identify and clarify illness-personality relationships. For instance, chronically dysthymic individuals may be more vulnerable to a number of medical illnesses including cancer. Similarly, individuals with type A behavior, especially the hostility and cynical components, are at increased risk for coronary artery disease. Chronic nervous tension, recent stress, and pessimism appear to contribute to irritable bowel syndrome (Richter et al. 1986). Depression, anxiety, and somatization are associated with esophageal motility disorders (Richter et al. 1986). Personality disorders may also predispose patients to some chronic dermatoses (Laihinen 1991). Given the complex relationship between personality and illness, the consultation-liaison psychiatrist must have considerable skill in patient assess-

ment if he or she is to provide effective and helpful consultation to both the patient and the referring physician.

Defense Mechanisms

Understanding the patient's defense mechanisms is one way to identify the patient's behavioral tendencies both during times of acute stress and throughout the life cycle. DSM-IV-TR (American Psychiatric Association 2000) contains a proposed axis for further study that assesses defense mechanisms and coping styles—the Defensive Functioning Scale (see Table 8–1 for defense mechanism information from DSM-IV-TR associated with the scale; see DSM-IV-TR, Appendix B, for the proposed scale). Characteristic defense mechanisms are identified from the present and past history of the patient, the mental status examination, and observations of how the patient relates to others. The Defensive Functioning Scale organizes defense mechanisms into defense levels: high adaptive level, mental inhibitions (compromise formation) level, minor image-distorting level, disavowal level, major image-distorting level, action level, and level of defensive dysregulation. Denial is a disavowal-level defense mechanism sometimes seen in consultation-liaison patients. Denial may be identified in the patient who avoids any expression of fear or depression about a serious prognosis. A patient in denial who avoids painful conflicts or illness-related life issues may further complicate the course of a chronic medical illness. A patient who shortly after being told he or she has cancer talks of fears of his or her cat's not being fed is likely to be using displacement, a mental inhibitions (compromise formation)–level defense. Some degree of regression is commonly seen in frightened patients, who may become extremely dependent on and demanding of the medical staff. These patients often give mixed and conflicting calls for help that are impossible to satisfy.

Patients with borderline, schizoid, paranoid, schizotypal, antisocial, or dependent personality disorders often display a spectrum of less mature defense mechanisms. These patients are especially vulnerable to more pronounced regression leading to poor cooperation with the medical team. Patients who try to pit members of the medical staff against one another and attribute blame and evil intent to their caregivers are exhibiting splitting. The consultation-liaison psychiatrist, called to intervene in such situations, must try to be empathic and accepting even in the face of a hostile, accusatory patient. Simultaneously, the psychiatrist may need to encourage an alienated, divided, and sometimes overtly hostile medical staff to present a united front to the patient and correct any actual lapses in empathy. Reestablishing empathy, responsiveness, and respect toward the patient, regard-

TABLE 8–1.   Common responses to illness

Individual defense mechanisms

High adaptive level: maximize gratification and promote optimum balance between conflicting motives
  Affiliation
  Altruism
  Anticipation
  Humor
  Self-assertion
  Self-observation
  Sublimation
  Suppression

Mental inhibitions (compromise formation) level: keep threats out of awareness
  Displacement
  Dissociation
  Intellectualization
  Isolation of affect
  Reaction formation
  Repression
  Undoing

Minor image-distorting level: distortions used to regulate self-esteem
  Devaluation
  Idealization
  Omnipotence

Disavowal level: removal from awareness or misattribution to external causes
  Denial
  Projection
  Rationalization

Major image-distorting level: gross distortion or misattribution of the image of self or others
  Autistic fantasy
  Projective identification
  Splitting of self-image or image of others

Action level: action or withdrawal
  Acting out
  Apathetic withdrawal
  Complaining
  Help-rejecting
  Passive aggression

Level of defensive dysregulation: pronounced break with objective reality
  Delusional projection
  Psychotic denial
  Psychotic distortion
  Exaggerated character defense mechanisms

Particularly the defenses of
  Denial
  Displacement
  Regression
  Reversal
  Splitting

Reactions to feelings of helplessness and lack of control

Reactions to feelings of shame and guilt

Transference reactions

---

less of how irrational the patient's complaints may have been, is one of the most difficult tasks of the consultant.

A patient's characteristic defense mechanisms can stir powerful feelings in his or her primary physician and treatment team. These feelings are often the focus of the psychiatric consultation. The consultation-liaison psychiatrist's feelings toward the patient are important data. If the patient stimulates dislike, hate, strong attraction, or sexual thoughts, the physician or others on the treatment team may want to ignore or disown these feelings. However, these feelings can profoundly influence the primary physician's responses to the patient.

Groves (1978) identified four types of patients who stir dislike and hate in physicians: 1) dependent clingers, 2) entitled demanders, 3) manipulative help rejecters, and 4) self-destructive deniers. All manifest an insatiable dependency that may evoke hate, avoidance, and distrust in caregivers. All of these patients may have an atypical, agitated depression or another underlying psychiatric disorder (or disorders); thus, it is critical to consider such conditions and treat them if present.

The *dependent clinger* is usually demanding and prone to rejection. Often, because the staff feel idealized, they begin to like the patient, but eventually the staff see the patient as "sticky" and unable to be left alone. For "sticky" patients, clinicians must make time limits clear in advance and schedule appointments so that patients know when their next contacts will be. Ensuring consistency in staff-patient interactions may decrease the aversion these patients stimulate in staff.

The *entitled demander*, who is also profoundly needy, is overtly hostile and belittling in an unconscious attempt to avoid feelings of helplessness and overwhelming fear of the illness situation. The treatment team or primary physician often wants to, and in subtle ways does, counterattack. The counterattack is usually hidden in the language of caring (e.g., "we should set limits on him"). What starts as a reasonable response can easily become vindictive and meant to punish rather than to help. In such cases, the medical staff should be encouraged to accept the patient's angry sense of entitlement and redirect the entitlement to an expectation of appropriate medical attention. Most important, the clinician must not challenge the entitlement. The consultation-liaison psychiatrist can be especially helpful to both the patient and the treatment team by recognizing and decreasing the terror of abandonment and mistreatment that often fuels this type of patient's angry demands.

Manipulative help rejecters are pessimistic, undermine treatment, and are usually negative about their care. They are very dependent and seemingly inexhaustible in their demands. They typically defeat all attempts to satisfy their needs. Their doctors feel anxious, irritated, frustrated, and depressed and eventually may even doubt their own skills. These patients want to be close to their doctors and nurses while keeping them at a safe distance. The consultation-liaison psychiatrist must help the patient limit demands and hostility by reassuring him or her that good care will be provided, while encouraging the treatment team to help the patient maintain a sense of separateness and autonomy.

The *self-destructive denier* is perhaps the most difficult of the four types of patients. These patients believe that there is no hope, and they are simultaneously uncooperative and dependent. They may appear to desire self-destruction by continuing to engage in self-injurious behaviors, such as drinking or smoking, after developing repeated serious medical complications caused by these behaviors. These patients may stimulate the wish by their treatment teams that they would "just die." Groves (1978) recommends an attitude of diligence and compassion. Treating any underlying depression is especially important in this subgroup of patients. The physician must lower his or her expectations and accept the limits the patient places on the treatment and on the physician. The physician often feels angry and must grapple with his or her ongoing feeling of loss of power and competence. Recognizing these limits and still not abandoning the patient are a major treatment challenge, as seen in the following case.

Case Example 1

Psychiatry was asked to consult on Ms. A, a 29-year-old woman admitted with fever, chills, and right-upper-quadrant pain. A workup had revealed pyelonephritis and a right renal abscess. The patient was hostile and uncooperative about receiving intravenous medications and undergoing other procedures. Given her belligerence, the medical staff was concerned about the potential for medication noncompliance after discharge. They reacted to this difficult patient with frustration and anger. During the consultation-liaison psychiatrist's interview with her, Ms. A expressed anger and frustration that the house staff did not answer her questions or explain what was

being done or why. Most important, she acknowledged her fear of how sick she was. The consultation-liaison psychiatrist empathized with her fear and encouraged her to tell the staff about her anxieties and to more directly raise questions about her care. In turn, the staff was informed of Ms. A's fear and sense of helplessness and ignorance. The psychiatrist recommended that the staff explain each step of the treatment to the patient and acknowledge her anxiety and frustration. This intervention altered the patient's primitive reaction to the staff, which was shaped by denial of her fears and projection of blame. The patient was thereby able to shift from largely passive-dependent and passive-aggressive behavior to a more collaborative relationship with the medical staff. (C. Stevens, personal communication, August 1993)

Helplessness and Control

Patients with acute, life-threatening medical illnesses frequently experience fear and feelings of helplessness. Not knowing enough facts about their illness and treatment increases their sense of helplessness. A monitor- and machine-laden intensive care unit, critical care unit, or recovery room may heighten a patient's sense of isolation and fear. When a critical care patient is oriented and attentive, his or her anxiety usually decreases when information is provided about the realities of his or her condition and what he or she can do to actively exert some control over his or her situation and recovery. At the same time, consultation-liaison psychiatrists can also help medically ill patients accept the inevitable demands of the hospital, their loss of autonomy, and their dependency on the treatment team (Perry and Viederman 1981a, 1981b). For type A cardiac patients, information that provides an opportunity for more control over their illness can greatly enhance the doctor-patient relationship and reduce fears and uncooperativeness. A sense of control over his or her illness can also empower the cancer patient who experiences pessimism and depression (Lederberg et al. 1990). Similarly, an aggressive, uncooperative middle-aged male executive may decide not to sign out against medical advice if he is given more authority and access to his business affairs (Perry and Viederman 1981a, 1981b).

Personality characteristics that are adaptive in the face of illness have recently been explored. Grossarth-Maticek and Eysenck (1995) introduced a new personality inventory dealing with self-regulation (which is, in some ways, the opposite of neuroticism) that measures personal autonomy. They detected a correlation between self-regulation and health, independent of physical risk factors. Those with high degrees of self-regulation actively regulate their own lives, without a degree of emotional dependence on others that thwarts their own needs. Those with low degrees of self-regulation have higher blood pressure, are more likely to have diabetes, exercise less, are more overweight, smoke and drink more, have more accidents, have poorer diets, and are more frequently ill and spend more time in the hospital. The investigators also showed that altering psychological risk factors with cognitive behavioral treatment reduced mortality.

Geyer (1997) elaborated the concept of *sense of coherence*. Those with a strong sense of coherence see the world as comprehensible, manageable, and meaningful. A strong sense of coherence is correlated with better health.

Heszen-Niejodek (1997) investigated various coping strategies and was able to distinguish different patient attitudes toward information about their illnesses. *Monitoring* is a tendency to focus attention on a stressor and one's responses to it. Monitoring includes gathering and applying relevant information. *Blunting*, on the other hand, consists of focusing attention away from the stressor and one's own reactions and thus avoiding, rejecting, and denying the existence of relevant information. The controllability of a given illness is a crucial variable in coping behavior. In controllable conditions, for example, monitoring information is adaptive, whereas in uncontrollable conditions (such as terminal illnesses), avoiding distressing information and blunting may be more adaptive.

Shame and Guilt

Patients often react with shame and guilt if their lifestyles have contributed to their illnesses. This is especially true for illnesses that result from smoking, substance abuse, and risky sexual behaviors. A nonjudgmental, empathic, and supportive stance by the consultation-liaison psychiatrist is important with these patients. Encouraging ventilation of self-criticism and guilty ruminations can increase cooperativeness, improve the patient's mood, and strengthen the doctor-patient relationship. Some of these features are shown in the following case example.

Case Example 2

Mr. B, a 76-year-old man, experienced a right-sided cerebrovascular accident (CVA) and a residual left hemiparesis. He was referred for psychiatric consultation because of "possible depression and incessant talking." The psychiatrist learned that the patient had led an active and independent life before his CVA. He was frustrated, embarrassed, and upset because he was unable to care for himself and had to relearn basic

living skills. Mr. B was aware that he talked a lot, especially at night. He talked about whatever came to mind and had to struggle to stop talking. He noticed that the house staff's visits were becoming briefer and less frequent during afternoon and evening rounds. On mental status examination, the patient had several neurovegetative signs of depression. He also had significant difficulty with recall and concentration. The consultation-liaison psychiatrist learned that the medical staff did not fully appreciate the devastating changes that had recently occurred in Mr. B's life because of the stroke. They said that they avoided the patient in the evenings because that was when he was most talkative and controlling. The consulting psychiatrist encouraged the medical staff to provide consistent attention at predictable intervals and helped the treatment team to better understand Mr. B's feelings of loss and shame about his condition. The psychiatrist also helped Mr. B understand his response to the injury to his self-esteem. After the psychiatric consultation, Mr. B could more directly express his grief over his lost functioning. The intervention decreased Mr. B's dependent, clinging, and controlling behaviors. In turn, the house staff's avoidant behaviors changed. The patient and staff forged a more collaborative relationship. (C. Stevens, personal communication, August 1993)

DOCTOR-PATIENT RELATIONSHIP: WORKING ALLIANCE AND SUPPORTIVE INTERVENTIONS

As with all patients, clinicians doing a psychiatric consultation should avoid both the pseudoanalytic, unresponsive posture and the rigidly "biological" impersonal approach (Perry and Viederman 1981a, 1981b). On the other hand, an overly sympathetic stance, which overidentifies with the patient's problems, may leave the patient wondering "Where is the doctor?" and diminish the patient's feelings of hope. Davis (1968) used tape-recorded evaluations of 154 new patients at a general medicine clinic to study how various combinations of patient and physician interactive styles affected treatment compliance. He found that compliance was significantly reduced if both patient and doctor had a formal relationship and rejected or withheld help from each other. Patients in this situation became antagonistic and withdrew. Patients who were very active and authoritative with a physician who passively acquiesced were even more noncompliant with the doctor's recommendations. Davis (1968) concluded that the physician, including the consultation-liaison psychiatrist, is best served by a style that can engage the patient with "a spontaneity tempered by rational control and intent" (p. 276).

One goal of most psychiatric consultations with medically ill patients is improved adaptation and mastery of the illness situation and treatment. Unlike traditional outpatient psychotherapy, the goal is not primarily psychological growth. The patient is truly dependent on the physician, and the physician and other care providers must comfortably accept this burden and opportunity. In brief psychotherapy in hospitalized patients, the consultation-liaison psychiatrist usually will strengthen the patient's defenses rather than explore them (see Chapter 45). For example, a regressed and dependent patient who normally manages his or her own business may respond to active encouragement to participate in the treatment regimen. In this case, the consultation-liaison psychiatrist should use the skills of supportive psychotherapy to strengthen the patient's adaptive defenses and healthy responses. The patient may need no further psychiatric treatment after adapting to the medical situation.

Obtaining a patient's psychodynamic life narrative (Viederman and Perry 1980) may help the consultation-liaison psychiatrist identify adaptive coping mechanisms. In this process, the psychiatrist obtains a detailed psychiatric history and performs a careful psychodynamic evaluation to help the patient develop a new understanding of his or her illness in the context of his or her unique history, character, life situation, and personal goals.

For example, consider a depressed renal patient with obsessional features and well-defined personal and professional goals who is unwilling to accept a kidney from a sibling. With the life narrative approach, the consultation-liaison psychiatrist can identify the patient's take-charge attitude and natural reluctance to be indebted. Sympathetically reflecting the patient's experience of having his or her goals derailed can be very supportive. Such an in-depth "taking stock" of the meaning of the illness in the context of the patient's life can provide great relief to the patient. The life narrative can also increase the patient's flexibility in coping with the illness and necessary medical care (Viederman and Perry 1980).

Studies demonstrate that people normally seek to distance themselves both physically and psychologically from individuals with serious illnesses. This defensiveness presumably aids in denying vulnerability to a similar fate. The tendency to distance may appear both in medical and in surgical caregivers, who may need clarification and support to counter this tendency. The psychiatric consultant can also experience a need to distance and should be alert to this reaction and use it as a possible guide to the reaction of others around the patient (Pyszczynski et al. 1999).

Transference and Countertransference

All patients have positive and negative reactions to their physicians. Many patients have dramatic transference reactions to their physicians and other caregivers. Illness, hospitalization, pain, and fear increase the frequency and intensity of transference reactions. The physician is often seen as a reliable parent or an authority figure from the past. Alternatively, the physician is sometimes viewed with fear and suspicion as a disappointing figure from the past (Ursano et al. 1998). Manifestations of the transference to the physician and the medical staff often prompt the request for a psychiatric consultation. During the assessment, the patient may also have similar transference feelings toward the consultation-liaison psychiatrist. Often, however, the patient's transference feelings toward the consultation-liaison psychiatrist are less intense because the consultant has had less contact with the patient. Therefore, these distortions of the patient–treatment team relationship can perhaps be worked out with the consultation-liaison psychiatrist's help. It is helpful for the consultation-liaison psychiatrist to remember: "There but for the grace of God go I." This reminder that the patient and the treating physician are caught in this web of the past helps the psychiatrist to see the situation more clearly.

Similarly, all patients elicit in their physicians—both in their primary physicians and in consultation-liaison psychiatrists—positive or negative reactions (countertransference responses). Countertransference can be in either of two forms: a response to the patient or an identification with the patient's feelings and beliefs. In the first case, an older patient may remind the physician of a paternal figure. Such a patient who is hostile, suspicious, and demanding and subtly or overtly blames the physician might make the physician feel too defensive and rejecting. The consultant might find himself or herself forgetting to see the patient on rounds or making pointed and angry jokes about the patient. This overreaction is the physician's countertransference. The physician might then realize that his or her reaction was similar to the reaction he or she had to a past figure who was demeaning and belittling. Alternatively, the countertransference may show up as an identification: the physician might agree with the patient's views of the world without verifying them, perhaps assuming that the patient's treatment staff were really evil or not caring. In both situations, the consultation-liaison psychiatrist should perform a thorough evaluation and obtain information from the treatment team. Using one's reactions to a patient as information to help understand what the treatment team experiences can help the consultation-liaison psychiatrist recommend effective interventions.

A major task for the consultation-liaison psychiatrist is to forge a therapeutic alliance with the patient and to help the patient form an alliance with the medical and surgical treatment team. To do this, the consultation-liaison psychiatrist may need to address the patient's transference and/or the countertransference of the staff. The psychiatrist should empathize with the patient's specific fears and foster a sense of mastery and control. This may alleviate anxiety and regression and reinforce more mature cooperation. The psychiatrist often must help other physicians and staff to avoid defensive postures that are stimulated by countertransference responses such as being too competitive, solicitous, or detached. When the consultation-liaison psychiatrist can convey to the house staff and the nurses an understanding of the patient's behaviors based on present and past events in the patient's life, the treatment team's reactions to the patient may change substantially. Helping physicians and staff understand what it is about a particular patient that makes them feel uncomfortable can help the staff better tolerate strong affect. When the caregivers can understand the patient's concerns, they often can return to their usual role of attempting to alleviate the patient's suffering. The consultation-liaison psychiatrist facilitates this process by both modeling and explaining how best to react supportively in the face of the patient's regressive behavior and defenses (Perry and Viederman 1981a, 1981b), as shown in the following case example.

Case Example 3

Mr. C, a 35-year-old white, homosexual man, was admitted to the hospital with dysphagia and abdominal pain. When fungal esophagitis was diagnosed, a human immunodeficiency virus (HIV) test was ordered. On hearing that the results were positive, the patient became tearful, angry, and depressed. Psychiatric consultation was requested. On initial interview, Mr. C asked that his HIV-negative life partner be present. Together, they described a mutually supportive 11-year monogamous relationship. At first, the consultation-liaison psychiatrist felt both extremely sympathetic and confused. He was reluctant to interview each partner separately to press for a careful history of other sexual relationships. However, he managed to establish enough emotional distance to conduct the separate interviews. In these interviews, he learned that Mr. C had had a brief sexual encounter several years earlier. He helped the patient express and ventilate his own intense guilt and then supported him during a meeting in which he relayed this history to his partner. When Mr. C faced and explored his sense of guilt, he felt relief, especially when the consultation-liaison psychiatrist supported the couple in their adjustment to the situation. (C. Stevens, personal communication, August 1993)

SPECIFIC ILLNESSES, PERSONALITY, AND BEHAVIOR

Many diseases are associated with characteristic behavioral patterns. In this section, we briefly identify and describe four examples of disease-personality interactions. Personality is a collection of behavioral response probabilities. That is, personality is a way to say that an individual has a high likelihood of certain affective, cognitive, or behavioral responses to life events. These expectable responses result from biological predispositions, past learned behavioral propensities, and the similarities of present to past stressors. The disease-personality interaction has predictable patterns because 1) individuals who develop a disease have similar personality or behavioral response styles (e.g., type A behavior), 2) the underlying causes of the medical disease lead to personality or behavioral responses in common directions (e.g., hyperthyroidism and anxiety), 3) the chronic illness directs certain personality or behavioral responses (e.g., chronic pain and depression), and 4) the stressors of a particular medical disease are highly predictable and sufficiently severe to elicit similar responses in patients (e.g., cancer and the expectation of death).

Cardiac Disease

Consultation-liaison psychiatrists are frequently called on to assess patients with cardiac disease. Many studies have found a high rate of major depression after myocardial infarction (Fielding 1991) and that depression is an independent risk factor affecting mortality at 6 months (Frasure-Smith et al. 1993). Subjective complaints after cardiac surgery are predicted by neuroticism, self-reported depression, and anxiety (Vingerhoets 1998). Patients with cardiac disease are often referred for consultation when they are agitated, hostile, or uncooperative. The assessment and treatment of patients with cardiac disease benefit from an understanding of the type A personality often found in patients with cardiac disease.

Examination of the personality and behavioral style in patients with cardiac disease includes an assessment for a type A behavior pattern, which is a risk factor for myocardial infarction (Rosenman 1990). The type A behavior pattern includes ambitiousness, aggressiveness, competitiveness, impatience, muscle tenseness, alertness, rapid and emphatic vocal style, irritation, cynicism, hostility, and increased potential for anger (see also Chapter 46 in this volume). Frequently, such patients are also workaholic people who deny any physical or emotional vulnerability. Their self-esteem is often dependent on constant achievement, to which an unstable cardiac status poses an immediate and ongoing threat. They may also be mistrustful and need to feel they are in control of their environment.

Recent studies have continued to show correlations between type A behavior patterns and cardiac disease. For example, Jenkins et al. (1996) found that absence of type A behavior was a predictor of lower likelihood of bed rest 6 months after coronary artery bypass surgery. Fukunishi and Hattori (1997) conducted a 5-year prospective study involving men who had had myocardial infarction. They found that depression was significantly correlated with type A behavior.

An acute cardiac episode and the critical care unit itself may heighten the anxiety of such a patient or be experienced as a defeat. The consulting psychiatrist may encounter a patient with a normally hostile, abrasive personality whose aggressiveness is further increased by his or her attempt to try to control the anxiety of the acute emergency and the fears of the threat to his or her life. Such a patient may feel insulted by the request for psychiatric consultation. The consultation-liaison psychiatrist should expect the patient's hostile or rude behavior and not take it personally. The psychiatrist should initially focus on identifying the patient's underlying anxiety and shoring up the patient's defenses. Facilitating expression of or at least acknowledging the patient's fears may relieve some of the anxiety and sense of personal failure. However, this is often difficult to achieve and, even when accomplished, may not be acknowledged by the patient. The best approach to this type of patient is to be respectful and reassuring (Ursano and Silberman 1999). By not taking offense at the abrasive behavior and by speaking calmly, firmly, and reassuringly to the patient's intense underlying fear about loss of function, self-esteem, and life itself, the consultation-liaison psychiatrist is in a good position to forge a therapeutic alliance. The psychiatrist should encourage the patient to ask questions about his or her illness and treatment and to involve himself or herself actively in recuperation. In this way, the psychiatrist channels the patient's characterological assertiveness in positive directions.

Case Example 4

Mr. D, a 62-year-old man, developed chest pain during a dispute with his business partner. Although he was concerned about the pain, he ran up the stairs of his office building to prove that he was not having a heart attack. After a short sprint up one flight, he collapsed because of crushing substernal pain. Mr. D was rushed to the hospital, and a diagnosis of massive myocardial infarction was made. Psychiatric examina-

tion revealed several features of a narcissistic personality disorder: aggressiveness, marked competitiveness, an unremitting need to prove his prowess and masculinity through monetary acquisition, public display of his many material possessions, and efforts to dominate others. Although Mr. D was quite ill, he was very resistant to medical recommendations, because that would mean admitting that he was ill. He saw any illness as a sign of weakness. He was also extremely distressed that his heart attack would cause him to lose face with his younger business partner, whom he had always been able to dominate. With frequent, brief meetings with the consulting psychiatrist, Mr. D decreased his resistance to medical treatment. He began to see his heart attack as a sign of how much harder he worked than his colleagues and as a medal rather than a scar.

Acquired Immunodeficiency Syndrome (AIDS)

AIDS is often associated with psychiatric symptoms and syndromes. Careful neuropsychiatric differential diagnosis to identify central nervous system complications is important (see Chapter 36). Anxiety, depression, and psychotic syndromes can complicate the course of AIDS. Patients who have contracted HIV by high-risk sexual behaviors or intravenous drug use may struggle with guilt, shame, and self-blame that exacerbate depression or even induce paranoid delusions. If the patient has also been rejected by family or has lost other social supports, the depression is often quite severe. Patients who are unwittingly infected by a transfusion or a sexual partner may struggle with feelings of rage and betrayal in addition to the emotional burden of their illness and their prognosis. Patients with AIDS require careful ongoing history and psychosocial assessments to facilitate the mourning of losses and the marshaling of personality strengths.

Gastrointestinal Disease

The bowel is highly reactive to emotional distress. Many patients with gastrointestinal illness report anxiety and depression (Richter et al. 1986). Patients with irritable bowel syndrome often have pervasive psychological disturbances in several areas of their lives. In a study of irritable bowel syndrome and esophageal motility disorders, 84% of patients with esophageal motility disorders ("nutcracker esophagus") had psychiatric illness, primarily depression, anxiety, and somatization disorders. In a study involving 206 consecutive female patients presenting to a university-based gastroenterology practice, 44% reported a history of sexual and/or physical abuse either in childhood or later in life. Patients with functional gastrointestinal disorders were more likely to report a history of abuse, and the patients who reported abuse were more likely to have a history of pelvic pain, multiple somatic symptoms, and multiple lifetime surgeries (Drossman et al. 1990). Given these findings, the consultation-liaison psychiatrist should obtain a careful history from patients with gastrointestinal disorders, because most of these patients do not inform their physicians of their history of abuse. Psychological exploration and ventilation of traumatic histories can lead to symptom relief and better compliance. The severity of any accompanying emotional illness often warrants evaluation for psychotherapy.

Somatization and Somatization Disorder

Consultation-liaison psychiatrists are frequently called on to consult with patients who present with multiple somatic complaints and who may have a somatoform disorder (see also Chapter 19). In one study, 38% of patients referred for psychiatric consultation had somatization symptoms (Katon et al. 1984). Patients with multiple somatic complaints who present in a dramatic or unusual manner are often focusing on somatic symptoms to defend against dysphoria and intrapsychic conflict. They may also minimize life stresses that have precipitated their illness. Among these patients—some of whom meet diagnostic criteria for somatization disorder (Briquet's syndrome)—major depression, generalized anxiety disorder, and specific phobias are frequent diagnoses (Brown et al. 1990). In addition, patients with somatoform disorder often have personality disorders. Rost and colleagues (1992) examined a group of patients with somatization disorder and found that 24.3% had one personality disorder and 37.2% had two or more. The four most common personality disorders were avoidant (26.7%), paranoid (21.3%), self-defeating (19.1%), and obsessive-compulsive (17.1%) disorders. Despite some historical expectations to the contrary, histrionic and antisocial personality disorders were not among the most common types found.

Somatization disorder itself has received increasing attention. Patients with somatization disorder are typically not very psychologically minded. Therefore, the consultation-liaison psychiatrist must empathize with and take at face value their bodily complaints while assessing for psychiatric disorders. In the history, the consultant must search carefully for psychodynamic factors and acute life stressors that may have precipitated or exacerbated the somatic preoccupation. The psychiatrist may help these patients reframe and refocus their distress in terms of their upsetting life events and refer them for ongoing psychiatric care when appropriate. One

study showed a 53% decrease in total health care charges incurred by patients with somatization disorder after an intervention consisting of psychiatric consultation and management advice for the primary physicians (G. Smith et al. 1986).

Seagal and Pennebaker (1998) discussed patients at higher risk for somatization disorder. These patients include those high in hypnotic ability who suppress emotion and are hypersensitive in certain situations. The authors also described a very different group, patients who are low in hypnotic ability, rational and analytical, and out of touch with their feelings. A third group includes patients who score high on the Marlowe-Crowne Social Desirability Scale. These patients repress unpleasant emotional experiences, are concerned with their social acceptability, and avoid reporting and feeling negative emotions. The authors speculated on possible biological mediators between coping styles and autonomic nervous system activity (e.g., several studies have found associations between high scores on the Marlowe-Crowne Social Desirability Scale and asthma and irritable bowel syndrome).

Fogel and Sadavoy (1996) reviewed somatoform illness and personality disorders in geriatric patients. They reported that neuroticism is a stronger predictor of somatic complaints than age. Therefore, hypochondriacal behavior is not a normal part of aging. In studies of health care utilization, older patients do not differ from younger patients in terms of obtaining health care for illnesses considered serious by physicians. Active management of anxiety-based somatic complaints and aggressive treatment of depressive and dysthymic disorders are particularly important in treating somatization in geriatric patients.

A related but more extreme and much rarer disorder related to the somatoform disorders and the somatizing patient is factitious disorder, or Munchausen syndrome (see also Chapter 25). In this disorder, severely emotionally ill patients present to hospitals with somatic signs and symptoms that are dramatic and self-induced. Patients with factitious disorder often complain of acute abdominal pain, fever, or blood in sputum, feces, or urine. These patients frequently have a history of emotional deprivation and severe personality disorders. They have a primitive capacity for interpersonal relationships, a fragile sense of identity, and a profound sense of helplessness. They have difficulty verbally expressing feelings, which are expressed instead through factitious symptoms (Fink and Tensen 1989; Ronen et al. 1980). Patients with factitious disorder inevitably require complicated management and often prompt splitting and hostility among the medical staff, leading to prompt psychiatric consultation. The consultation-liaison psychiatrist is often in the position to make the diagnosis and to help the staff better understand and therefore tolerate the patient's behavior. Such patients are usually highly resistant to treatment, but educational interventions and psychiatric referral can often decrease the inappropriate, costly, and sometimes life-threatening treatment in the hospital.

PERSONALITY DISORDERS AND SOMATIC ILLNESS

Classification and Assessment

Personality traits—characteristic behavioral response patterns—are the typical ways that an individual thinks, feels, and relates to others. These traits are often called chronic or severe. When these patterns are fixed, inflexible, unresponsive to changes in the environment, and maladaptive, they can result in psychological and social dysfunction and may constitute a personality disorder.

The psychiatric diagnostic classification system (DSM-IV-TR) causes some major problems for the study of the personality disorders because the clinically recognized dysfunctional personalities are not limited to the types listed in that classification system (see Table 8–2).

The various taxonomic systems for classifying characterological features, including Hippocrates' four humors and Fourier's 810 character types, were thoroughly discussed by Frances and Widiger (1986). There is considerable overlap between the various systems, although different terms are often used for the same idea (McCrae and Costa 1990).

By studying the problems of distinguishing between pairs of personality disorders, Blashfield et al. (1985) found they could scale diagnoses along a two-dimensional continuum. Each Axis II disorder could be defined and distinguished by two dimensions: 1) acting out (highest in antisocial and lowest in dependent personality disorders) and 2) interpersonal involvement (highest in histrionic and borderline and lowest in paranoid and compulsive personality disorders). Widiger et al. (1987) used a similar multidimensional scaling method to assess the DSM-III (American Psychiatric Association 1980) Axis II symptoms of 84 state hospital patients. They found that personality disorders could be separated using three dimensions: social involvement, assertion or dominance, and activity (anxious rumination versus acting out).

A five-factor model of personality (Dembrowski and Costa 1987; T. W. Smith and Williams 1992; Wise 1992) has been used to study the relationship between individual traits and somatic diseases. This system of classifying personality traits was derived from a factor analysis of approximately 18,000 adjectives in the English language used to describe personality characteristics (McCrae and Costa 1990). The five factors McCrae and Costa found included neuroticism, extroversion, openness, agreeableness, and conscientiousness (see Table 8–3).

Cloninger (1987, 1988) proposed a classification system that attempts to integrate knowledge of the major neurotransmitter systems (dopaminergic, serotonergic, and noradrenergic) with a tridimensional description of personality traits (novelty seeking, harm avoidance, and reward dependence). The results of a study involving a probability sample of 1,000 people provided some support for Cloninger's hypotheses (Cloninger 1988) (see Table 8–4).

TABLE 8–2.   DSM-IV-TR Axis II disorders

Cluster A: odd or eccentric characteristics
Paranoid personality disorder
Schizoid personality disorder
Schizotypal personality disorder

Cluster B: dramatic, emotional, or erratic characteristics
Antisocial personality disorder
Borderline personality disorder
Histrionic personality disorder
Narcissistic personality disorder

Cluster C: anxious or fearful characteristics
Avoidant personality disorder
Dependent personality disorder
Obsessive-compulsive personality disorder

TABLE 8–3.   Five-factor system of personality traits

Neuroticism
Tendency toward negative affects (e.g., anxiety, depression, self-consciousness, poor impulse control, and angry or hostile thoughts)

Extroversion
Tendency to be outgoing and talkative

Openness to experience
Tendency to be curious, interested, and creative

Agreeableness
Tendency to be good-natured and trusting; a negative score on this dimension indicates an antagonistic, rude, and behaviorally aggressive style

Conscientiousness
Tendency to be ambitious and goal directed

TABLE 8–4. Cloninger's neurotransmitter–personality trait classification system

Behavioral activation (novelty seeking)
High activity in the dopaminergic system

Behavioral inhibition (harm avoidance)
High activity in the serotonergic system

Behavioral maintenance (reward dependence)
High activity in the noradrenergic system

Cloninger (1987) reasoned that DSM-III personality disorders could be defined in terms of abnormally high or low activity along each of the three personality dimensions. For example, antisocial personality disorder would reflect very high novelty seeking with very low harm avoidance and reward dependence. Obsessive-compulsive personality disorder would combine very high harm avoidance with very low novelty seeking and reward dependence. More recently, Cloninger et al. (1998) found a significant linkage between the harm avoidance trait and a specific locus on chromosome 8p21-23 in 758 pairs of siblings from families of alcoholic patients. This linkage explained 38% of the trait variance. The strength of the system presented by Cloninger (1987) lies in its attempt to assess basic temperament constructs rather than interpersonal dynamics.

The American Psychiatric Association's classification of personality disorders has evolved through an interesting series of revisions of the *Diagnostic and Statistical Manual of Mental Disorders* (Blashfield and McElroy 1989). The current version, DSM-IV-TR, relies on a nontheoretical set of categories. Diagnosis is based on meeting a threshold number of symptoms. Because of considerable symptom overlap among the various Axis II conditions, personality disorders have been described as "fuzzy sets" (Livesley 1986). Although the personality disorders are divided into A, B, and C clusters in DSM-IV-TR (see Table 8–2), this grouping has not received much support from a clinical or practical standpoint (Widiger and Rogers 1989).

Axis II diagnoses are defined by symptom "menus" that range from 7 to 10 items. Depending on the disorder, at least 4 or 5 symptoms are necessary before a specific Axis II diagnosis can be made. This results in a numerical anomaly that can bias the prevalence of the different disorders in epidemiological studies. For example, there are 210 possible combinations of symptoms by which an individual can meet criteria for the diagnosis of antisocial personality disorder (4 symptoms out of 10) but only 35 ways that a person could receive a diagnosis of avoidant personality disorder (4 symptoms out of 7). Humorists might conclude that it is more difficult to be shy than to be psychopathic.

Some investigators have criticized the diagnostic reliance on behavioral checklists. Although diagnosis based on discrete behavior has relatively high reliability, it does not address personality traits detected by studying the patient's characteristic defense mechanisms (Grossman 1982), psychometric test results, or longitudinal clinical observations. Because of these shortcomings, many aspects of a patient's personality dysfunction are overlooked in the DSM-IV classification system. For example, Lilienfeld (1992) noted that individuals manifesting typical psychopathic traits such as superficial charm, lack of guilt or anxiety, impaired ability to plan, failure to learn from experience, and egocentricity may not necessarily meet the criteria for antisocial personality disorder. This is a major problem in diagnosing a condition that appears to have significant genetic determinants. On the other hand, Livesley (1986) compared the way that American and Canadian psychiatrists actually diagnosed personality disorders and found that a method based on behaviors was as reliable as one based on traits. For borderline and paranoid personality disorders, however, behavioral ratings were not quite as successful as ratings based on psychological traits.

Westen and Shedler (1999a, 1999b) devised and validated a personality assessment method (the Shedler-Westen Assessment Procedure [SWAP-200]) that may prove to be more psychometrically sound and clinically useful than the current DSM-IV-TR criteria. The SWAP-200 relies on 200 personality descriptor statements regarding aspects of functioning, affect-regulation strategies, motives, and conflicts that were never included in the DSM-IV-TR criteria because they were thought to be unmeasurable. The clinician is required to sort a specified number of the 200 statements into each of 8 categories from 0 to 7 according to the degree to which each statement is considered clinically applicable or inapplicable to a patient. Much more research is required to solidify our classification of personality disorders.

Clinical observational studies have shown that other characterological disturbances exist in addition to the official list of Axis II conditions that qualify as personality disorders (see Table 8–5). Many of these conditions, such as alexithymia and type A behavior pattern, have been of great interest to consultation-liaison psychiatrists. Some conditions such as dysthymia, cyclothymia, and multiple personality disorder are categorized by the DSM classification committee as Axis I disorders, although they are more characteristic of the usual understanding of a personality disorder. In the case of sadistic personality disorder and self-defeating (masochistic) personality disorder, controversy about the potential "misuse" of the diagnoses led to their placement in an appen-

TABLE 8–5.   Personality disturbances not included in the official list of Axis II conditions

DSM-IV-TR criteria sets provided for further study

Depressive personality disorder

A. A pervasive pattern of depressive cognitions and behaviors beginning by early adulthood and present in a variety of contexts, as indicated by five (or more) of the following:

　(1) usual mood is dominated by dejection, gloominess, cheerlessness, joylessness, unhappiness

　(2) self-concept centers around beliefs of inadequacy, worthlessness, and low self-esteem

　(3) is critical, blaming, and derogatory toward self

　(4) is brooding and given to worry

　(5) is negativistic, critical, and judgmental toward others

　(6) is pessimistic

　(7) is prone to feeling guilty or remorseful

B. Does not occur exclusively during major depressive episodes and is not better accounted for by dysthymic disorder.

Passive-aggressive personality disorder (negativistic personality disorder)

A. A pervasive pattern of negativistic attitudes and passive resistance to demands for adequate performance, beginning by early adulthood and present in a variety of contexts, as indicated by four (or more) of the following:

　(1) passively resists fulfilling routine social and occupational tasks

　(2) complains of being misunderstood and unappreciated by others

　(3) is sullen and argumentative

　(4) unreasonably criticizes and scorns authority

　(5) expresses envy and resentment toward those apparently more fortunate

　(6) voices exaggerated and persistent complaints of personal misfortune

　(7) alternates between hostile defiance and contrition

B. Does not occur exclusively during major depressive episodes and is not better accounted for by dysthymic disorder.

Listed as Axis I disorders

Dysthymia

Cyclothymia

Dissociative identity disorder (formerly multiple personality disorder)

Other personality disturbances

Type A behavior pattern

Alexithymia

Pain-prone disorder (Blumer and Heilbronn 1982)

---

dix in DSM-III-R (American Psychiatric Association 1987) and elimination from DSM-IV. Type A behavior pattern is an important risk factor for coronary artery disease and has received an enormous amount of attention and study (e.g., Costa et al. 1987; Dembrowski and Costa 1987; Rosenman 1990; T. W. Smith and Williams 1992). However, it is not part of the present diagnostic system.

Alexithymia is an impaired ability to perceive or express emotions. In an extreme form, it might qualify as a personality disorder because the individual's characteristic way of dealing with feelings is maladaptive and inflexible. However, based on the operational definition, reliable measurement of alexithymia is difficult. In various studies, alexithymia was highly prevalent in patients with psychosomatic conditions, chronic psychogenic pain, and psychological conditions affecting a physiological disorder (Krystal 1988; Lesser and Lesser 1983; Taylor 1984; Taylor et al. 1990).

Diagnosis

Obtaining the comprehensive history necessary for diagnosing a personality disorder is time-consuming and difficult. This is particularly problematic for consultation-liaison psychiatrists, who must make practical recommendations to the referring physician after a relatively short evaluation. In addition, patients with somatic complaints often have physical pain and are fatigued, distractible, and sometimes not cooperative with extensive diagnostic evaluations. It is also difficult to differentiate a characteristic behavioral pattern from acute stress disorder or typical behavior during a significant illness or hospitalization. In the case of patients with several Axis II conditions, it may take several hours of interviewing, along with collateral information obtained from family members, to establish a reliable diagnosis. For these reasons, consultation-liaison psychiatrists initially tend to focus on the most prominent and remediable psychiatric symptomatology and defer Axis II assessment until the patient is discharged to his or her usual environment.

Several promising standardized assessment instruments are available for diagnosing personality disorders (Dowson 1992; Merikangas and Weissman 1986). Each has flaws, relating to the amount of time needed, the limitation of cross-sectional observation (rather than observation over time), and the lack of collateral information. For example, on a self-report instrument, narcissistic patients are not likely to volunteer information that they are exploitive and heedless of the feelings of others. Therefore, reliable diagnosis of conditions in these individuals is very dependent on direct behavioral observation and family interviews. Some patients' chronic physical disorders or Axis I conditions (e.g., bipolar disorder or posttraumatic stress disorder) are sometimes misdiagnosed as personality disorders because the clinician incorrectly assesses the onset and chronicity of the symptoms. Consequently, it is important during the evaluation to determine whether the personality traits and behaviors observed during the mental status examination are longstanding, stable maladaptations that predate the present stressful clinical situation. Patients may behave much differently in the hospital than they do at home. Obtaining collateral information from family members is a critical part of this process.

The high comorbidity of Axis I and Axis II disorders (Dowson 1992; Goldsmith et al. 1989; Widiger and Rogers 1989) also creates diagnostic difficulties. The inflexible and maladaptive coping behaviors exhibited by patients with personality disorders make them more likely to develop depression and anxiety syndromes (Widiger and Rogers 1989). Subclinical anxiety, depression, or hypomania may be identified as an Axis II condition on some personality assessment instruments (O'Connell et al. 1991). The ideal assessment of personality should combine the patient's self-report, the report of a close family member, the clinician's assessment of the presence or absence of specific behaviors, serial assessments over time, and a diagnostic evaluation of comorbid conditions.

Epidemiology

The epidemiology of personality disorders in medical-surgical patients has been limited by the nosological fuzziness of the personality disorders, the comorbidity of Axis II and Axis I disorders, the difficulty in making cross-sectional assessments at times of great duress, and the fact that epidemiological assessments of Axis II disorders are time-consuming and expensive. Therefore, it is not surprising that present estimates of the prevalence of personality disorders range widely from study to study, even in physically healthy populations. More efficacious and reliable instruments are needed to overcome these problems.

Merikangas and Weissman (1986) reviewed the epidemiological studies of the prevalence of personality disorders in the general population. Four studies conducted between 1951 and 1963, involving a total of 5,471 individuals, suggested that the prevalence of personality disorders ranged from 6% to 9%.

Widiger and Rogers (1989) reviewed eight studies and estimated the prevalences of DSM-III personality disorder diagnoses in different samples of inpatients and outpatients. Listed in Table 8–6 are weighted averages of the prevalences of DSM-III personality disorders calculated from four of the studies of psychiatric patients (N = 1,060) cited by Widiger and Rogers (1989). These figures are presented as a rough estimate. If DSM-IV-TR criteria had been used, some figures probably would have been quite different.

Morey (1988), in his study involving 291 outpatients, used both DSM-III and DSM-III-R criteria and found large discrepancies in several Axis II categories. For example, he found that for narcissistic personality disorder, DSM-III criteria suggested a prevalence of 6.2% whereas DSM-III-R criteria suggested a prevalence of 22.0%. Widiger and Rogers (1989) presented a similar table of relative prevalences and cautioned that these percentages might best be viewed in terms of the relative rank order of occurrence among various Axis II conditions rather than as absolute figures. They also reviewed the high probability (88%–100%) of diagnosing at least a second personality disorder when a first had been diagnosed. Some combinations of Axis II disorders appear to occur more frequently. For example, histrionic personality disorder was comorbid with borderline personality disorder 46% of the time but with schizoid personality disorder only 1% of the time (Widiger and Rogers 1989).

Antisocial personality disorder is the Axis II diagnosis given the most attention in large community samples. In the National Institute of Mental Health Epidemiologic Catchment Area study, Regier et al. (1993) found a point prevalence of antisocial personality disorder of 0.5% and a 1-year prevalence of 1.5%. Similarly, Chen and colleagues (1993) found a lifetime prevalence of antisocial personality disorder of 2.78% in men and 0.53% in women in a population sample of 7,229 residents of the Shatin community in Hong Kong. This compares with an average prevalence of antisocial personality disorder of 6.0% calculated from mental health clinic populations (see Table 8–6).

TABLE 8–6. Prevalences of DSM-III personality disorders in clinical populations of patients with mental illness

Personality disorder	Average prevalence (%)
Borderline	23
Histrionic	15
Dependent	14
Schizotypal	13
Avoidant	10
Passive-aggressive	8
Paranoid	7
Antisocial	6
Narcissistic	5
Obsessive-compulsive	4
Schizoid	2

Note. $N = 1,060$ (outpatients = 976, inpatients = 84). Weighted averages were calculated from four studies: Frances et al. 1984; Kass et al. 1985; Morey 1988; Widiger et al. 1987.

In many inpatients with personality disorders who are referred to consultation-liaison psychiatrists, these conditions are not always recognized and written in the medical record. Personality disorder diagnoses are almost never included in hospitalization discharge summaries. Hales et al. (1986) found that only 4.5% of 1,065 patients referred within a military hospital received an Axis II diagnosis, even though 16.5% of referrals were made because of behavior difficulties (e.g., adjustment difficulties or conflict with physicians and staff). They suggested that military psychiatrists may have been reluctant to diagnose a condition that could lead to the patient's administrative discharge from the military. In contrast, in a prospective study of psychiatric consultations in a family practice clinic, Katon et al. (1981) found that 25% of the patients received a personality disorder diagnosis.

Mounting evidence suggests that somatization is associated with Axis II disorders. In a prospective study involving 100 patients with somatizing illness (not somatization disorder) referred to a hospital-based consultation-liaison psychiatric service, Katon and colleagues (1984) made a definite personality disorder diagnosis in 37%. This rate was significantly higher than the rate in patients without somatizing illness (16%). Histrionic personality disorder was diagnosed in 12% of the patients with somatizing illness but in only 2% of those without somatizing illness.

Rost et al. (1992) found that 37.2% of a series of primary care patients with somatization disorder had one personality disorder, and 23.4% had two or more. The most common diagnoses were avoidant personality disorder (26.7%), paranoid personality disorder (21.3%), self-defeating personality disorder (19.1%), and obsessive-

compulsive personality disorder (17.1%). Histrionic personality disorder was found in only 12.8% of their sample, leading the authors to suggest that patients with somatization disorder present with Cluster A or C traits (odd or anxious characteristics) rather than dramatic characteristics. G. R. Smith et al. (1991) found that 8% of women and 18%–25% of men with somatization disorder also had antisocial personality disorder, depending on the personality assessment instrument used. Similarly, Barsky et al. (1992) diagnosed personality disorder three times more frequently in a group of patients with DSM-III-R hypochondriasis than in a comparable group of control subjects randomly selected from the same clinic setting. It is important to exercise caution when interpreting findings of studies that attempt to correlate the occurrence of personality disorders with other medical and psychiatric conditions, because of the wide variation in prevalence from study to study, the different study populations, and the use of different assessment methods.

Interaction of Personality Disorders and Somatic Illness

The relatively fixed behavioral response patterns found in patients with personality disorders can affect somatic illness in many ways. For example, maladaptive behaviors such as alcohol use can directly increase the risk of diseases such as liver disease, or not using a seat belt can increase the risk of traumatic injury. Alternatively, chronic medical conditions such as chronic pain or life-threatening chronic illness can lead to maladaptive chronic behavioral patterns (e.g., expectation of disappointment and rejection).

The patient's personality greatly influences his or her likelihood of seeking out rather than delaying obtaining appropriate treatment or complying with rather than interfering with needed treatment. This problem may reflect specific "hypertrophied" defenses of the personality disorder (e.g., denial) or may be a specific negative transference reaction. Frances and Widiger (1986) emphasized that character pathology is often at the core of negative transference manifestations that interfere with a patient's ability to seek out and cooperate with treatment. This problem is very important and difficult to manage in patients whose passive-aggressiveness leads them to act out against their treating physicians or family members who are concerned about their health.

Personality disorders per se can be major etiological factors in somatic symptomatology. In most cases of factitious disorder, a personality disorder is at the core of the patient's inappropriate need to be in the patient role.

Many of these patients exhibit borderline, self-defeating, and antisocial features. In a consecutive series of 1,288 patients referred to a consultation-liaison psychiatric service, Sutherland and Rodin (1990) found that 10 patients (0.8%) received a diagnosis of factitious disorder. One patient feigned psychiatric symptoms, and the other patients presented with a variety of somatic symptoms, such as self-inflicted trauma and infections. The conditions of three of these patients were diagnosed as borderline personality disorder, and the condition of one of them was diagnosed as atypical personality disorder. Elliott (1987) reviewed clinical observations of patients with Munchausen syndrome and suggested that masochistic personality features were prominent.

Personality disorders can also influence use of medications, both prescribed and over the counter, particularly use of hypnotic and psychotropic medications. Allgulander et al. (1990) studied a sample of 30,344 Swedish twins. They found that individuals with a diagnosis of neurosis or personality disorder, as defined by *International Classification of Diseases*, 8th Revision (ICD-8) (World Health Organization 1967) criteria, were 11 times more likely to use sedative-hypnotic and other psychotropic drugs than were individuals without such a diagnosis.

Poor health care habits and improper attention to early symptoms of an impending medical condition can lead to exacerbation or early onset of a disease. For example, Small et al. (1970) found that most of their sample of 100 patients with passive-aggressive personality disorder had frequent somatic complaints and neglected their personal hygiene. Failure to maintain good physical hygiene is a way that passive-aggressive patients act out their anger toward individuals they depend on in their lives.

A somatic presentation is also very common in dissociative identity disorder (DID), formerly called multiple personality disorder (Ross et al. 1990), and may be more frequent than in other psychiatric conditions. Ross et al. (1989) found that 35% of patients with DID also met criteria for somatization disorder. In the following case, the appearance of pharyngitis was related to the characteristic dissociative defenses of a patient with DID:

Case Example 5

Mr. E received a diagnosis of DID, with eight distinct personalities identified. Over several days, while attempting to explore his memories of being sexually abused, Mr. E developed severe pharyngitis. Throat cultures were negative, and his psychiatrist was concerned that he might have developed leukopenia in response to one of his psychotropic medications.

Before a white blood cell count could be performed, during a psychotherapeutic trance one of the patient's personalities revealed that "he" had deliberately been coughing and hacking at Mr. E's throat in an effort to "silence" the other personality's efforts to tell the therapist about the episodes of childhood abuse. When the first personality's concerns were addressed, the pharyngitis rapidly cleared.

Stoudemire and Thompson (1983) examined the ways that patients with certain personality disorders become noncompliant with drug therapy. Denial was a characteristic defense mechanism that interfered with the patient's ability to either acknowledge the presence of somatic illness or realistically appraise the risks of refusing treatment. They also noted that patients with borderline personality disorder often experience considerable difficulty trusting their physicians and that their impulsiveness and self-destructive behavior hamper cooperation with medical recommendations. Patients with paranoid or schizoid personality disorders are often highly suspicious of authority figures such as physicians.

Laihinen (1991) reported that dermatological conditions often become chronic because of a personality disorder, emotional immaturity, untreated depression, and pleasure derived from scratching. Kellner (1983) found that patients with DSM-III hypochondriasis who had concurrent personality disorders were less likely to improve with psychotherapy than were patients with hypochondriasis who did not have a personality disorder.

Self-defeating behavior has been implicated frequently in treatment compliance problems. Elliott (1987) reviewed masochistic behavior and some mechanisms by which patients with self-defeating behavior resist their physicians' efforts to treat their somatic conditions. He described self-defeating behavior as 1) an unconscious need to suffer and to be punished, 2) a way to punish the physician, 3) a wish for attention and caring, 4) a way to provoke rejection, 5) an exhibitionistic attempt to parade suffering to ensure lovability and respect, and 6) a way to maintain worthiness to be taken care of.

The following case is an example of a patient with self-defeating personality disorder:

Case Example 6

Ms. F, a 35-year-old woman, had a long-standing history of explosive urinary urgency that seriously interfered with her social and occupational functioning. Despite a thorough urological workup that included repeated cystoscopies, no somatic basis was found for her symptomatology. Psychiatric examination revealed that she had been subjected to repeated sexual abuse as a child. Once, while Ms. F was hospitalized for a workup for these urinary problems, a nurse mistakenly came to her bed to administer a medication meant for another patient. Although she "knew" that it was not her medication, Ms. F "assumed" that her doctor and the nurse knew what was best for her and did not challenge the nurse. She had a severe reaction to this medication. She was later referred for intensive psychoanalytically oriented psychotherapy, which gradually helped to abate her somatic symptoms.

Patients with personality disorders probably constitute the group with the highest likelihood of stimulating countertransference reactions that lead to nontherapeutic staff and physician behaviors. The patient's personality disorder may interfere with the physician's or the medical staff's ability to function and respond as appropriate caregivers. This may lead to avoiding the patient, being unable to notice a change in symptom pattern, or assigning the patient's care to the least skilled member of the medical team. In this way, countertransference problems of caregivers elicited by the patient's personality disorder can influence the patient's clinical outcome.

Patients with borderline, self-defeating, paranoid, passive-aggressive, or antisocial personality disorder are particularly likely to engender anger, confusion, and frustration in their caregivers. When these feelings interfere with the care of the patient or are out of proportion to the events, a countertransference reaction is likely to be present and must be addressed.

The excessive demandingness of masochistic patients with somatic illness can especially irritate the treatment team (Elliott 1987). Patients who "doctor shop" and become labeled as crocks frequently have a masochistic character (Lipsitt 1970). Their self-defeating method of seeking help results in physicians' not taking their complaints seriously because their symptoms appear impervious to relief. These patients may unconsciously request caring rather than cure (Lipsitt 1970). They experience the physician's impatient therapeutic zeal as a rejection because they feel unworthy of care without their suffering. One way of avoiding a sadomasochistic struggle with such patients is to offer them conservative ongoing care that is not predicated on symptomatic results.

Personality disorders also influence the presentation of somatic illness. The patient's personality disorder can distort the presentation of a somatic disorder, emphasizing one symptom (e.g., chest pain) to the exclusion of other symptoms (e.g., difficulty urinating). The patient's characteristic way of experiencing and expressing pain is another important factor in the presentation of somatic

illness. Although some patients present with complaints that appear to be solely psychogenic, many patients' seemingly exaggerated complaints are intermixed with just enough somatic pathology to create confusion in the clinician's mind. Patients who have somatizing illness are not immune to the ordinary diseases that befall other people, but their tendency toward sensory augmentation of perceived physical distress will frequently create considerable doubt, frustration, and worry in their care providers.

Consultation-liaison psychiatrists are sometimes consulted for assessment of an unusual presentation of pain by a patient. Engel (1959) classically described the pain-prone patient. More recently, Blumer and Heilbronn (1982) examined 900 patients with chronic pain that lacked a discernible somatic basis. They identified the "typical" patient with chronic pain as a solid citizen whose prepain adjustment consisted of relentless "ergomania" (workaholism), an idealized image of self and family relationships, a need to please others that may have led to self-defeating behavior, and difficulty feeling or expressing emotion (alexithymia). These patients possessed a consciously idealized image of themselves as independent, active, and needing to care for others, which concealed their hidden core wish to be dependent, to be passive-submissive, to be cared about, and to receive care. Jensen (1988) found a high frequency of personality disorders in patients reporting pain symptoms. Patients with pain were more likely to report hostile feelings, somatic anxiety, and muscular tension than were patients without pain, whereas patients with pain were less likely to report compulsive thoughts.

Patients with alexithymia also use maladaptive ways to deal with emotions, physical stress, pain, and the dysfunction of medical illness. Because of their difficulty in experiencing or expressing emotions, patients with alexithymia are limited in their ability to communicate distress. Therefore, it is easier for them to focus on nonemotional aspects of somatic disease, such as pain or physical dysfunction. They have considerable difficulty perceiving the psychosocial context in which the somatic illness originated, which affects the way they communicate their distress to physicians. Krystal (1988) postulated that the main problem in patients with alexithymia was their internal prohibition against caring for themselves or regulating their own internal state of being. The lack of a reliable measure of alexithymia has been one of the main limiting factors in studying this trait. One instrument, the Toronto Alexithymia Scale developed by Taylor et al. (1992), appears to have overcome many earlier problems.

CONCLUSION

Personality is best thought of as characteristic behavioral response patterns that are formed from past life experiences, biological predispositions, current life events, social contexts, and one's view of the future. Personality disorder is an inflexible pattern of behaviors maintained despite evidence that it is maladaptive. Assessment of the patient's personality is a necessary part of a comprehensive psychiatric consultation. The consultation-liaison psychiatrist observes the patient's present characteristic defense mechanisms and gathers information about previous response patterns. Patterns of relating to the treatment team and the consultation-liaison psychiatrist provide data on the patient's present defense mechanisms, level of psychological defensive functioning, and potential transference reactions. In addition, the consultation-liaison psychiatrist's feelings about the patient can provide valuable clinical information. The issue of helplessness or lack of control and the issue of shame or guilt are often prominent in patients referred for psychiatric consultation.

Personality disorders per se are also common in medically ill patients. As with personality styles, personality disorders influence the medical illness and are influenced by it. The presentation of an illness and styles of relating to the caregivers can be influenced by a personality disorder. The consultation-liaison psychiatrist "translates" the description of the patient's "pain" from the language and behavior of a unique personality to the language of the treating physician and vice versa. Alertness to personality-related behaviors that may put a patient at increased risk can offer new avenues for intervention to alter morbidity and mortality.

REFERENCES

Allgulander C, Nowak J, Rice JP: Psychopathology and treatment of 30,344 twins in Sweden, I: the appropriateness of psychoactive drug treatment. Acta Psychiatr Scand 82: 420–426, 1990

American Psychiatric Association: Diagnostic and Statistical Manual of Mental Disorders, 3rd Edition. Washington, DC, American Psychiatric Association, 1980

American Psychiatric Association: Diagnostic and Statistical Manual of Mental Disorders, 3rd Edition, Revised. Washington, DC, American Psychiatric Association, 1987

American Psychiatric Association: Diagnostic and Statistical Manual of Mental Disorders, 4th Edition. Washington, DC, American Psychiatric Association, 1994

American Psychiatric Association: Diagnostic and Statistical Manual of Mental Disorders, 4th Edition, Text Revision. Washington, DC, American Psychiatric Association, 2000

Barsky AJ, Wyshak G, Klerman GL: Psychiatric comorbidity in DSM-III-R hypochondriasis. Arch Gen Psychiatry 49:101–108, 1992

Blashfield RK, McElroy RA: Ontology of personality disorder categories. Psychiatric Annals 19:126–131, 1989

Blashfield RK, Sprock J, Pinkston K: Exemplar prototypes of personality disorder diagnoses. Compr Psychiatry 26:11–21, 1985

Blumer D, Heilbronn M: Chronic pain as a variant of depressive disease: the pain-prone disorder. J Nerv Ment Dis 170:381–406, 1982

Brown F, Golding J, Smith R: Psychiatric comorbidity in primary care somatization disorder. Psychosom Med 52:445–451, 1990

Chen CH, Wong J, Lee N, et al: The Shatin community mental health survey in Hong Kong. Arch Gen Psychiatry 50:125–133, 1993

Cloninger CR: A systematic method for clinical description and classification of personality variants: a proposal. Arch Gen Psychiatry 44:573–588, 1987

Cloninger CR: A unified biosocial theory of personality and its role in the development of anxiety states: a reply to commentaries. Psychiatric Developments 6:83–120, 1988

Cloninger CR, Van Eerdewegh P, Goate A, et al: Anxiety proneness linked to epistatic loci in genome scan of human personality traits. Am J Med Genet 81:313–317, 1998

Colarusso CA, Nemiroff RA: Adult Development. New York, Plenum, 1981

Costa PT Jr, Krantz DS, Blumenthal JA, et al: Psychological risk factors in coronary artery disease. Circulation 76 (suppl 1 pt 2):I145–I149, 1987

Davis MS: Variations in patients' compliance with doctors' advice: an empirical analysis of patterns of communication. Am J Public Health 58:274–288, 1968

Dembrowski TM, Costa PT: Coronary prone behavior: components of the type A pattern and hostility. J Pers 55:211–235, 1987

Dowson JH: Assessment of DSM-III-R personality disorders by self-report questionnaire: the role of informants and a screening test for co-morbid personality disorders (STCPD). Br J Psychiatry 161:344–352, 1992

Drossman DA, Leserman J, Nachman G, et al: Sexual and physical abuse in women with functional or organic gastrointestinal disorders. Ann Intern Med 113:828–833, 1990

Elliott RL: The masochistic patient in consultation-liaison psychiatry. Gen Hosp Psychiatry 9:241–250, 1987

Engel GL: "Psychogenic" pain and the pain-prone patient. Am J Psychiatry 26:899–918, 1959

Fielding R: Depression and acute myocardial infarction: a review and reinterpretation. Soc Sci Med 32:1017–1027, 1991

Fink P, Tensen S: Clinical characteristics of the Munchausen syndrome: a review and 3 new case histories. Psychother Psychosom 52:164–171, 1989

Fogel BS, Sadavoy J: Somatoform and personality disorders, in Comprehensive Review of Geriatric Psychiatry, 2nd Edition. Edited by Sadavoy J, Lazarus LW, Jarvik LF, et al. Washington, DC, American Psychiatric Press, 1996, pp 637–658

Frances AJ, Widiger T: The classification of personality disorders: an overview of problems and solutions, in Psychiatry Update: American Psychiatric Association Annual Review, Vol 5. Edited by Frances AJ, Hales RE. Washington, DC, American Psychiatric Press, 1986, pp 240–257

Frances A[J], Clarkin JF, Gilmore M, et al: Reliability of criteria for borderline personality disorder: a comparison of DSM-III and the Diagnostic Interview for Borderline Patients. Am J Psychiatry 141:1080–1084, 1984

Frasure-Smith N, Lesperance F, Talajic M: Depression following myocardial infarction: impact on 6-month survival. JAMA 270:1819–1825, 1993

Fukunishi I, Hattori M: Mood states and Type A behavior in Japanese male patients with myocardial infarction. Psychother Psychosom 66:314–318, 1997

Geyer S: Some conceptual considerations on the sense of coherence. Soc Sci Med 44:1771–1779, 1997

Goldsmith SJ, Jacobsberg LB, Bell R: Personality disorder assessment. Psychiatric Annals 19:139–142, 1989

Grossarth-Maticek R, Eysenck HJ: Self-regulation and mortality from cancer, coronary heart disease, and other causes: a prospective study. Personality and Individual Differences 19:781–795, 1995

Grossman S: A psychoanalyst-liaison psychiatrist's overview of DSM III. Gen Hosp Psychiatry 4:291–295, 1982

Groves JE: Taking care of the hateful patient. N Engl J Med 298:883–887, 1978

Hales RE, Polly S, Bridenbaugh H, et al: Psychiatric consultations in a military general hospital. Gen Hosp Psychiatry 8:173–182, 1986

Heszen-Niejodek I: Coping style and its role in coping with stressful encounters. European Psychologist 2:342–351, 1997

Jenkins CD, Jono RT, Stanton BA: Predicting completeness of symptom relief after major heart surgery. Behav Med 22:45–57, 1996

Jensen J: Pain in non-psychotic psychiatric patients: life events, symptomatology and personality traits. Acta Psychiatr Scand 78:201–207, 1988

Kass F, Skodol AE, Charles E, et al: Scaled ratings of DSM-III personality disorders. Am J Psychiatry 142:627–630, 1985

Katon W, Williamson P, Ries R: A prospective study of 60 consecutive psychiatric consultations in a family medicine clinic. J Fam Pract 13:47–56, 1981

Katon W, Ries RK, Kleinman A: A prospective DSM-III study of 100 consecutive somatization patients. Compr Psychiatry 25:305–314, 1984

Kellner R: Prognosis of treated hypochondriasis. Acta Psychiatr Scand 67:69–79, 1983

Krystal H (ed): Integration and Self-Healing: Affect, Trauma, Alexithymia. Hillsdale, NJ, Analytic Press, 1988, pp 144–146

Laihinen A: Assessment of psychiatric and psychosocial factors disposing to chronic outcome of dermatoses. Acta Derm Venereol Suppl (Stockh) 156:46–48, 1991

Lederberg M, Massie MJ, Holland JC: Psychiatric consultation to oncology, in American Psychiatric Press Review of Psychiatry, Vol 9. Edited by Tasman A, Goldfinger SM, Kaufmann C. Washington, DC, American Psychiatric Press, 1990, pp 491–514

Lesser IM, Lesser BZ: Alexithymia: examining the development of a psychological concept. Am J Psychiatry 140:1305–1308, 1983

Lilienfeld SO: The association between antisocial personality and somatization disorders: a review and integration of theoretical models. Clin Psychol Rev 12:641–662, 1992

Lipsitt DR: Medical and psychological characteristics of "crocks." Psychiatry in Medicine 1:15–25, 1970

Livesley WJ: Trait and behavioral prototypes of personality disorder. Am J Psychiatry 143:728–732, 1986

McCrae RR, Costa PT: Personality in Adulthood. New York, Guilford, 1990

Merikangas KR, Weissman MM: Epidemiology of DSM-III Axis II personality disorders, in Psychiatry Update: American Psychiatric Association Annual Review, Vol 5. Edited by Frances AJ, Hales RE. Washington, DC, American Psychiatric Press, 1986, pp 258–278

Morey LC: Personality disorders in DSM-III and DSM-III-R: convergence, coverage, and internal consistency. Am J Psychiatry 145:573–577, 1988

O'Connell RA, Mayo JA, Sciutto MS: PDQ-R personality disorders in bipolar patients. J Affect Disord 23:217–221, 1991

Perry S, Viederman M: Adaptation of residents to consultation/liaison psychiatry, I: working with the physically ill. Gen Hosp Psychiatry 3:141–147, 1981a

Perry S, Viederman M: Adaptation of residents to consultation/liaison psychiatry, II: working with the nonpsychiatric staff. Gen Hosp Psychiatry 3:149–156, 1981b

Pyszczynski T, Greenberg J, Solomon S: A dual-process model of defense against conscious and unconscious death-related thoughts. Psychol Rev 106:835–845, 1999

Regier DA, Narrow WE, Rae DS, et al: The de facto US mental and addictive disorders service system: Epidemiologic Catchment Area prospective 1-year prevalence rates of disorders and services. Arch Gen Psychiatry 50:85–94, 1993

Richter J, Obrecht F, Bradley A: Psychological comparison of patients with nutcracker esophagus and irritable bowel syndrome. Dig Dis Sci 31:131–138, 1986

Ronen R, Kampman R, Ikoven V: Munchausen syndrome: a review and two case reports. Psychother Psychosom 33:185–192, 1980

Rosenman RH: Type A behavior pattern: a personal overview. Journal of Social Behavior and Personality 5:1–24, 1990

Ross CA, Heber S, Norton GR, et al: Somatic symptoms in multiple personality disorder. Psychosomatics 30:154–160, 1989

Ross CA, Miller SD, Reagor P, et al: Structured interview data on 102 cases of multiple personality disorder from four centers. Am J Psychiatry 147:596–601, 1990

Rost KM, Akins RN, Brown FW, et al: The comorbidity of DSM-III-R personality disorders in somatization disorder. Gen Hosp Psychiatry 14:322–326, 1992

Seagal JD, Pennebaker JW: Cognition, personality, and treatment considerations among somatoform patients. Advances in Mind-Body Medicine 14:118–120, 1998

Small IF, Small JG, Alig VB, et al: Passive-aggressive personality disorder: a search for a syndrome. Am J Psychiatry 126:973–983, 1970

Smith GR Jr, Monson RA, Ray DC: Psychiatric consultation in somatization disorder: a randomized controlled study. N Engl J Med 314:1407–1413, 1986

Smith GR Jr, Golding JM, Kashner TM, et al: Antisocial personality disorder in primary care patients with somatization disorder. Compr Psychiatry 32:367–372, 1991

Smith TW, Williams PG: Personality and health: advantages and limitations of the five-factor model. J Pers 60:395–423, 1992

Stoudemire A, Thompson TL II: Medication noncompliance: systematic approaches to evaluation and intervention. Gen Hosp Psychiatry 5:233–239, 1983

Sutherland AJ, Rodin GM: Factitious disorders in a general hospital setting. Psychosomatics 31:392–399, 1990

Taylor GJ: Alexithymia: concept, measurement, and implications for treatment. Am J Psychiatry 141:725–732, 1984

Taylor GJ, Bagby RM, Ryan DP, et al: Validation of the alexithymia construct: a measurement-based approach. Can J Psychiatry 35:290–297, 1990

Taylor GJ, Bagby RM, Parker JD: The Revised Alexithymia Scale: some reliability, validity and normative data. Psychother Psychosom 57:34–41, 1992

Ursano RJ, Fullerton CS: Psychotherapy: medical intervention and the concept of normality, in The Diversity of Normal Behavior. Edited by Offer D, Sabshin M. New York, Basic Books, 1991, pp 39–59

Ursano RJ, Silberman EK: Psychoanalysis, psychoanalytic psychotherapy, and supportive psychotherapy, in The American Psychiatric Press Textbook of Psychiatry, 3rd Edition. Edited by Hales RE, Yudofsky SC, Talbot JA. Washington, DC, American Psychiatric Press, 1999, pp 1157–1183

Ursano RJ, Sonnenberg SM, Lazar SG: Concise Guide to Psychodynamic Psychotherapy: Principles and Techniques in the Era of Managed Care, 2nd Edition. Washington, DC, American Psychiatric Press, 1998

Viederman M, Perry SW 3rd: Use of a psychodynamic life narrative in the treatment of depression in the physically ill. Gen Hosp Psychiatry 2:177–185, 1980

Vingerhoets G: Cognitive, emotional and psychosomatic complaints and their relation to emotional status and personality following cardiac surgery. British Journal of Health Psychology 3:159–169, 1998

Westen D, Shedler J: Revising and assessing Axis II, part I: developing a clinically and empirically valid assessment method. Am J Psychiatry 156:258–272, 1999a

Westen D, Shedler J: Revising and assessing Axis II, part II: toward an empirically based and clinically useful classification of personality disorders. Am J Psychiatry 156:273–285, 1999b

Widiger TA, Rogers JH: Prevalence and comorbidity of personality disorders. Psychiatric Annals 19:132–136, 1989

Widiger TA, Trull TJ, Hurt SW, et al: A multidimensional scaling of the DSM-III personality disorders. Arch Gen Psychiatry 44:557–563, 1987

Wise TN: Psychiatric management of functional gastrointestinal disorders. Psychiatric Annals 22:606–611, 1992

World Health Organization: International Classification of Diseases, 8th Revision. Geneva, World Health Organization, 1967

9

Suicidality

John Michael Bostwick, M.D.

One of the most common questions posed to a consultation-liaison psychiatrist is whether a patient is suicidal. Unlike many medical-surgical patients with psychiatric symptoms, those who talk about killing themselves receive prompt psychiatric attention. Few events arouse more anguish in a physician than loss of a patient to suicide. Suicide attempts are costly financially as well as emotionally. At the Massachusetts General Hospital, 1%–2% of all emergency room visits and up to 5% of medical intensive care unit admissions stem from suicide attempts (Hackett and Stern 1991). Of 164 patients admitted to a burn unit in a year, 15 had attempted suicide. Each of these patients spent an average of 32 days in the hospital, for a total of 482 patient-days at a cost of nearly $1 million in 1983 (Scully and Hutcherson 1983).

Suicide, even in the psychiatric population, is a rare event, and the demographic risk factors alone will identify many more patients potentially at risk than imminently in danger of dying (Goldberg 1987). There is no "suicide test," although hundreds of studies over the last several decades have made dozens of epidemiologic correlations, which are difficult to integrate, that parse out subgroups with a suicide rate higher than that in comparison populations (Pokorny 1983). Unfortunately, no epidemiologic factors represent an individual's suicidal intent—the essential variable in suicide prediction (Davidson 1993). Yet this absence of specific suicide attempt predictors is no cause for therapeutic nihilism. A suicide threat is a statement of ambivalent distress about something of meaning to the patient that must be understood if he or she is to be helped.

In this chapter, I discuss the epidemiology of suicide, exploring why the epidemiologic data alone are inadequate to predict suicide. I describe methods for keeping suicidal patients safe during assessment and discuss diverse approaches to the evaluation of suicidality. I suggest that the purpose of the assessment of suicidality is to identify treatable psychiatric and social contributors to the suicidal state and to propose interventions that reduce the drive toward self-destructive behavior and thoughts.

EPIDEMIOLOGY

General Population

Completed suicide. In 1997, a total of 29,725 Americans were reported to have killed themselves. The actual number is undoubtedly higher, because many suicides are never identified as such or are reported as accidents or as deaths by other causes. At 11.1 deaths per year per 100,000 Americans—1.3% of all deaths in the United States—suicide was the eighth leading cause of death in 1997 (Ventura et al. 1998). The known suicide rate is nearly identical to what it was in 1900 (Monk 1987).

Table 9–1 summarizes relative suicide risk factors for the general population. The suicide rate among men is three times higher than among women, and the rate for whites is almost twice that for blacks (Roy 1989). People who are socially isolated or who are widowed, divorced, or separated have higher rates of suicide than those who have ongoing, supporting relationships with friends and family (Monk 1987).

Suicide assessment begins with epidemiologic analysis. With the first glance at the hospital card or consultation request, the consultant already has many demographic clues to the patient's relative risk of suicide. The consultation-liaison psychiatrist thus begins to build a formulation of suicide risk on an epidemiologic foundation. Traditionally, epidemiologic studies have shown that suicide attempters are more likely to be younger, female, and married and to use pills, whereas completers are more likely to be older, male, and single and to use vio-

TABLE 9–1.   Relative suicide risk factors for the general population

Target group	Incidence per 100,000	Control group	Relative risk (target group/control group)	Source
General population, United States, 1979	11.9			
Men	18.3	Women	3.1	
Women	6.0	Men	0.3	
White (both sexes)	12.4	Black	1.7	Roy 1989
Black (both sexes)	7.5	White	0.6	
Married				
Men	18.0			
Women	5.5			
Widowed				
Men, 1959–1961	78.4	Married men	4.4	
Women, 1959–1961	10.7	Married women	1.9	
Divorced				
Men, 1959–1961	69.4	Married men	3.9	
Women, 1959–1961	18.4	Married women	3.3	Monk 1987
Single				
Men, 1959–1961	33.2	Married men	1.8	
Women, 1959–1961	7.7	Married women	1.4	

lent means (Fawcett and Shaughnessy 1988). However, anyone at any age may contemplate or execute suicide.

The epidemiology of suicide over the last several decades has been shifting. Suicide rates are increasing (they tripled in the last three decades) among young people (ages 15–24 years) and elderly individuals (older than 65 years) (Dorwart and Chartock 1989). Fifteen percent of adolescents who die perish by their own hands, often impulsively, making suicide the second leading cause of death in that population (Shneidman 1989).

Over the course of the life cycle, men and women have different patterns of suicide. For men, suicide rates gradually rise during adolescence, increase sharply in early adulthood, and then decrease before starting an upward trajectory in midlife, increasing into the 75- to 84-year age bracket and beyond (Shneidman 1989). Suicide rates for women peak in midlife and then decrease, in contrast to the bimodal peaks for men. Men's suicide methods tend to be more violent and lethal; men are more likely to die by hanging, drowning, and shooting. Women are less likely to die in suicide attempts, because they are more likely to choose the less lethal methods of wrist cutting and overdose (Kaplan and Klein 1989; A.C. Morgan 1989).

In the general population, psychiatric disorders—particularly depression and alcoholism—are associated with the vast majority of retrospectively studied completed suicides. Of 134 persons who committed suicide in St. Louis County, Missouri, 94% had diagnosable psychiatric disorders and an additional 4% had terminal medical illness. Forty-seven percent of those who died

had major depression, and 24% had alcoholism. Of 100 individuals who committed suicide in West Sussex or Portsmouth, England, 93% were judged to have mental illness, 70% to have depression, and 15% to have alcoholism. In a Seattle, Washington, study, all of 108 patients who had committed suicide were found retrospectively to have at least one psychiatric illness (Roy 1989). It is unfortunate that most of the patients in these studies had not been identified as being psychiatrically ill and, thus, their psychiatric conditions were not treated. In one of the largest epidemiologic studies, in Monroe County, New York, only 133 of 408 individuals who committed suicide in a 7-year period had ever had contact with a psychiatric facility (Babigian and Odoroff 1969).

In a nation with a population approaching 300 million, 30,000 known successful suicides per year constitute statistically rare events and pose particular problems that bedevil those who study infrequent phenomena. In an article addressing psychobiological risk factors for suicide, Mann (1987) stated the problem succinctly: "Thus far, psychopathologic risk indicators have suffered from the same predictive problem that plagues other psychosocial risk factors—low specificity despite high sensitivity" (p. 42). In other words, of the individuals who commit suicide, many fit the epidemiologic risk factor profile. However, many more who never express thoughts of suicide, let alone attempt it, also fit the profile. As a result, with an incidence rate of 1 in 10,000 in the general population and 1 in 80–250 in the psychiatric population, prospective studies would need to prospectively enroll hundreds of thousands of subjects to examine a few dozen persons who commit suicide (Capodanno and Targum 1983).

Attempted suicide.   It is false security to regard attempted suicides as a discrete category from completed ones (Table 9–2). For some reason, many patients who make a potentially lethal suicide attempt survive (Kellner et al. 1985). Nonetheless, some characteristics distinguish surviving attempters from those who die. Although men die as a result of suicide at higher rates than women do, women attempt at higher rates than men. Men tend to use more lethal, less reversible means (e.g., shooting, hanging), whereas women are more likely to attempt suicide by overdosing on medication. Patients who overdose are more likely to survive, because they have time after the act to reconsider (or be found) and undergo medical treatment, an option not so frequently available after a jump or a gunshot wound.

Overdoses are not without significant morbidity. Hackett and Stern (1991) reported that 1%–2% of all patients evaluated in the Massachusetts General Hospital Emergency Ward had overdosed, and 47% of these required inpatient treatment—one-half on medical-surgical wards and one-half on psychiatric units. The drugs they took were commonly available. In the case of 85% of the patients, six classes of drugs were implicated: benzodiazepines, alcohol, nonnarcotic analgesics, antidepressants, barbiturates, and antihistamines/anticholinergics. Overdoses of acetaminophen, with its potential liver toxicity and over-the-counter availability, were particularly likely to result in admission. Twenty-five percent of chronically self-destructive or suicidal patients eventually kill themselves (Litman 1989).

TABLE 9–2.   Attempted versus completed suicide in the general population

Risk category	Attempted	Completed
Male:female ratio	1:3	3:1
Most common methods	Wrist slashing Overdosing	Hanging Jumping Shooting
Most common psychiatric diagnoses	Personality disorder	Depression
Most common affect	Impulsive anger	Hopelessness
Most common precipitant	Acute relationship difficulty or loss	Chronic painful or disfiguring illness
Most common goal	Manipulation of others	Annihilation of self

Medically Ill Patients

Physical disease is an independent suicide risk factor present in a high proportion of people who commit suicide (Kontaxakis et al. 1988). Physical illness is present in 25%–75% of all persons who kill themselves (Roy 1989). Sanders (1988) reviewed six studies of individuals who committed suicide while inpatients at a general hospital. Most of these patients had chronic or terminal illnesses that were painful, debilitating, or both. Some had multiple illnesses. Patients with dyspnea, ostomies, or disfiguring surgery were among those who died (Sanders 1988). Epilepsy, multiple sclerosis, head injury, cardiovascular disease, Huntington's chorea, dementia, acquired immunodeficiency syndrome (AIDS), Cushing's disease, Klinefelter's syndrome, porphyria, prostatic hypertrophy, renal failure, and cancer of the female breast and genitals are all associated with mood disorder and increased suicide risk. Peptic ulcer disease and cirrhosis of the liver are linked to both alcoholism and increased suicide risk. For medical-surgical patients with concurrent depression and alcoholism, precise cause-and-effect relations are difficult to determine.

As in the general population, suicides are usually committed by medically ill patients who have comorbid, often unrecognized, psychiatric or neurological illness (Davidson 1993; Kellner et al. 1985). These neuropsychiatric conditions include depression, substance-related disorders, substance withdrawal, delirium, dementia, and personality disorder (Table 9–3).

The association between characterological factors and suicide among medically ill patients was examined in a postmortem study comparing 45 patients who committed suicide and 45 nonsuicidal control patients. The index patients and control subjects were matched for cardiorespiratory diagnosis, age, sex (all male), race (all white), and religion (Farberow et al. 1966). The authors identified personality styles and behavioral characteristics that they hypothesized might help clinicians to understand and prevent suicide. They identified a "dependent-dissatisfied" behavior pattern among patients who committed suicide. They wrote that "in general the suicides seemed more emotionally disturbed, had poorer relationships with hospital staff and family, and were seen as problem patients because of their provoking, complaining and demanding behavior" (Farberow et al. 1966, p. 426).

It must be emphasized that no matter how horrific the medical condition, significant suicide risk is not the rule. According to Brown et al. (1986), in a study involving 44 terminally ill patients, only 10, all of whom had major depression, were at risk for suicide. The investiga-

TABLE 9–3.   Factors associated with suicide in medical-surgical patients

Completed suicide

Chronic or terminal illness

Painful or disfiguring illness

Dyspnea

Ostomy

Comorbid psychiatric pathology

Depression

Dependent-dissatisfied personality

Agitated delirium

Hopelessness

Attempted suicide

Distinguishing characteristics

Impaired impulse control due to personality disorder, psychosis, functional disorder (schizophrenia or bipolar disorder), organic brain syndrome

Method

Lower lethality, greater reversibility

Affect

Anger, not depression

Precipitant

Loss of emotional support/interpersonal struggles with staff or family

Source.   Adapted from Reich P, Kelly MJ: "Suicide Attempts by Hospitalized Medical and Surgical Patients." *New England Journal of Medicine* 294:298–301, 1976. Copyright 1976, Massachusetts Medical Society. Used with permission.

tors concluded that "the majority of fatally ill people do not develop a severe depression" and "suicidal thoughts and desire for death appear in our patient group to be linked exclusively to the presence of mental disorder" (Brown et al. 1986, p. 210). The consultation-liaison psychiatrist has the dual task of knowing which medical conditions and treatments are associated with mood disorder and identifying the psychiatric syndrome, if present, that increases the suicide risk.

Hospitalized Medical-Surgical Patients

Suicidal hospitalized patients, especially those who are impulsive, harm themselves by the most expedient means available. In modern, multilevel hospitals, the easiest and quickest method has proven to be jumping from a window. In Glickman's (1980) study of 22 completed and 23 attempted suicides in King's County Hospital, Brooklyn, New York, between 1963 and 1978, a total of 19 patients who committed suicide jumped, as did 9 of the 23 patients who attempted suicide. Five additional patients who attempted suicide tried to jump. These findings confirm those of earlier studies by Pollack (1957) and

Farberow and Litman (1970), who found that 10 of 11 patients who committed suicide and 10 of 12 general hospital patients who committed suicide, respectively, jumped to their deaths.

The high lethality of jumping from a significant height makes death usually inevitable regardless of whether the patient actually intends to die. In a sample of medical inpatients at Peter Bent Brigham Hospital, Boston, Massachusetts, between 1967 and 1973, Reich and Kelly (1976) studied 17 patients who attempted suicide and survived. Of these 17 patients, 7 overdosed, 7 cut themselves, 1 hung herself, 1 inhaled a poisonous agent, and only 1 jumped. Reich and Kelly attributed the lack of jumpers to the fact that their hospital consisted of a group of low buildings. It is instructive that the 16-story patient tower that replaced the low facility in the 1980s was designed with thick windows that cannot be opened and stairways that have no wells down which a body could fit and fall (J.M. Bostwick, personal observation, June 1993). They judged 15 of the 17 patients to have mental disorders, but the cardinal suicide characteristics of depression and hopelessness were not present in this sample. "All…were impulsive acts, none of the patients gave warnings, left notes, expressed suicidal thoughts or appeared to be seriously depressed" (Reich and Kelly, p. 973). The investigators linked these 17 attempts to impulsive reactions to loss of emotional support, usually from staff. The primary affect was anger. The authors attributed underlying impaired impulse control to personality disorders in 8 of the patients and to psychosis in 7 patients: 3 with schizophrenia, 1 with bipolar disorder, and 3 with neuropsychiatric syndromes (Table 9–3).

The most recent study of suicide by jumping paints a far different picture of the patient who jumps. White and colleagues (1995) also found impulsivity in many of the 12 patients who jumped from an Australian general hospital during a 12-year period. Only 1 of the 12 had been admitted after a suicide attempt, however. Five patients had been noted to be delirious on the day of the jump, 7 were dyspneic, and 10 were in pain. Ten of the 12 had two of these factors, and 1 had all three. "Agitation," the investigators observed, "should be more closely monitored as an indicator of [both] delirium and suicidality" (White et al. 1995, p. 214).

Impulsivity can be countered. Pisetsky and Brown (1979) calculated a suicide rate of 1.55 per 10,000 patient admissions at the Bronx Veterans Administration Hospital in New York from 1947 to 1958 but found a rate of only 0.32 per 10,000 from 1971 to 1975. Between the two data collection periods, the authors successfully persuaded the hospital to implement programs to secure the windows and have the staff pay more careful attention to disruptions in the doctor-patient relationship. As a result of their recommendations, the suicide rate decreased (Sanders 1988).

Shah and Ganesvaran (1997) found that one-third of 103 suicides committed by inpatients at their hospital involved patients on pass and another third involved patients away from the hospital without permission. Methods included jumping in front of trains, streetcars, and cars that passed near the hospital, as well as leaping from buildings and drowning in nearby bodies of water. The researchers advocated locating psychiatric units away from potentially lethal methods or at least doing everything possible to minimize access.

Providers must think like suicidal patients to identify local dangers. The environment must be safe, and egress must be controlled. The hospital surroundings may provide means for completing suicide (H.G. Morgan and Priest 1991). In the building itself, patients should be prevented access to open stairwells and laundry chutes, upper-story windows should be secured, and sharps and potentially harmful substances should be removed (Berger 1995).

SUICIDE RISK FACTORS AMONG MEDICAL-SURGICAL PATIENTS

Medical Factors

Certain medical disorders that the psychiatric consultant will encounter in both inpatient and outpatient settings are associated with increased suicide risk (Table 9–4). Three of these disorders are discussed in the following sections.

Cancer. Three large studies have found an increased suicide rate among patients with cancer. Luohivuori and Hakama (1979) studied 63 suicides among 28,857 Finnish patients whose cancers were diagnosed in the index years of 1955, 1960, and 1965 and found a relative risk (the rate in a target group versus the rate in a control group) of 1.3 for women and 1.9 for men, with the highest excess mortality associated with gastrointestinal tumors. Fox and co-workers (1982) studied 192 suicides between 1940 and 1973 among 144,530 patients in the Connecticut Tumor Registry and calculated no increased suicide risk for women but a 2.3 relative risk for men. In the most comprehensive study of the relation between cancer and suicide, Allebeck and colleagues (1985) gathered statistics on 963 suicides between 1962 and 1979 among 424,127 Swedes with a diagnosis of cancer and found a 1.9 relative risk for men and a 1.6 relative risk for women. Gas-

trointestinal tumors (excluding colon and rectal tumors) in men (relative risk, 3.1) and lung tumors in either sex (relative risk, 3.1 for men and 3.5 for women) were associated with the highest rate of death due to suicide. Allebeck's group also made the important discovery that the longer the time from diagnosis, the lower the relative risk. In the first year after diagnosis, the relative risk is 16.0 for men and 15.4 for women. From 1 to 2 years, the ratio decreases to 6.5 for men and 7.0 for women. By 3–6 years, the ratio is 2.1 for men and 3.2 for women. By 10 years after diagnosis, the rate, at 0.4, is actually less than one-half that in the general population.

The pain, disfigurement, and loss of function that cancer evokes in the popular imagination can precipitate suicide, especially early in patients' courses. The high relative risk of suicide just after diagnosis corresponds to a time of great fear. However, the data also suggest that as cancer patients live longer with their disease, they become less frightened and less susceptible to suicide as an escape from the terror.

Chronic renal failure. More formidable than the suicide risk among cancer patients is the increase in relative risk of suicide among patients with chronic renal failure. Abrams et al. (1971) reported very high rates of suicide and suicidal behavior among 3,478 renal dialysis patients studied at 127 dialysis centers. In their sample, 20 deaths were a result of suicide; 17 suicide attempts were unsuccessful; 22 patients withdrew from the program, knowing that doing so would hasten their deaths; and 117 deaths were attributed to noncompliance with treatment regimens. Although the authors claim a widely quoted suicide incidence rate of 400 times that in the general population, they do not make clear in their article the time frame during which the dialysis patients committed suicide. Thus, the investigators' suicide figure is a prevalence rate. In arriving at a 5% figure for suicidal behavior in dialysis patients, they also used an extremely broad definition of suicide that encompassed death caused by a wide range of causes, from willful acts of self-destruction to noncompliance. Although the report by Abrams et al. (1971) is widely cited, no other study since (there have been nearly 20) has defined suicide so globally (J.M. Bostwick, unpublished data, November 1999).

In contrast, of 1,766 Minnesota dialysis patients followed for 17 years, only 3 killed themselves (Neu and Kjellstrand 1986). The suicide rate in this sample of dialysis patients is only about 15 times that in the general population. Haenel et al. (1980) also found less dramatic suicide rates among European patients undergoing chronic dialysis between 1965 and 1978. For example, in Switzerland, dialysis patients killed themselves at about

Table 9–4.   Suicide relative risk: medical diagnoses

Target group	Control group	Relative risk (target group/control group)	Source
Cancer			
Men	General population	1.9	
Women	General population	1.6	
0–1 year after diagnosis			
Men	General population	16.0	
Women	General population	15.4	
1–2 years after diagnosis			
Men	General population	6.5	Allebeck et al. 1985
Women	General population	7.0	
3–6 years after diagnosis			
Men	General population	2.1	
Women	General population	3.2	
10 years after diagnosis			
Men and women	General population	0.4	
Chronic renal failure/Dialysis (Switzerland)			
Suicide	General population	10	Haenel et al. 1980
Suicide and refusal of treatment	General population	25	
AIDS (1989)			
Men	Men in general population	7.4	Cote et al. 1991

Note.   AIDS = acquired immunodeficiency syndrome.

10 times the rate in the general population. When patients who refused therapy and died as a result were included in the suicide group, the rate was 25 times higher. Haenel and co-workers (1980) also found no statistically significant difference between suicide rates among patients with functioning cadaveric renal transplants and patients undergoing maintenance dialysis, suggesting that transplantation may not in and of itself be associated with decreased suicide risk. Overall, among European dialysis patients pooled from all countries belonging to the European Dialysis and Transplant Association (Haenel et al. 1980), the suicide rate was 108 per 100,000 per year. Whether compared with the general population suicide rate of 4–5 per 100,000 in Mediterranean countries or 20–25 per 100,000 in central European or Scandinavian countries, the figure of 108 per 100,000 represents a higher suicide rate, although not orders of magnitude greater, than that in the general population.

Acquired immunodeficiency syndrome.   AIDS patients also have a high relative risk of suicide, even though the risk may be decreasing. Marzuk and associates (1988) found a suicide rate 36 times that in an age-matched sample of men without AIDS and 66 times that in the general population in New York City in 1985. In California, in 1986, the rate was 21 times higher than that in the gen-

eral population (Kizer et al. 1988). In the largest study to date, Cote et al. (1991) charted a continuous decrease of suicide rates, year by year, among AIDS patients in 45 states and the District of Columbia. In 1987, 1988, and 1989, a total of 165 suicides among AIDS patients were reported to the National Center for Health Statistics. Of these, 164 were committed by men. The relative suicide risk calculated for AIDS patients was 10.5 in 1987, 7.4 in 1988, and 6.0 in 1989. The authors attributed the decrease to advances in medical care, diminishing social stigma, and improved psychiatric services; they also noted underreporting of deaths due to both AIDS and suicide.

Frierson and Lippman (1988) considered that suicide risk may also be increased among 1) human immunodeficiency virus (HIV)–positive but asymptomatic people who fear the eventual encroachment of the illness, 2) HIV-negative people who are worried about contracting the disease, and 3) people who enter suicide pacts with dying loved ones. Rundell et al. (1992) compared 15 HIV-infected, active-duty members of the Air Force who attempted suicide with 15 who did not and identified several risk factors that parallel risk factors in the general population almost exactly. Definite risk factors included social isolation, perceived lack of social support, adjustment disorder, personality disorder, alcohol abuse, HIV-related interpersonal or occupational problems, and history of depression. Possible contributing factors included current major depression, history of suicide attempts, and history of alcohol abuse.

Psychiatric Risk Factors

If a patient has a long-standing psychiatric diagnosis that predates a medical or surgical condition, the consultant must be more alert to the possibility of suicide (Table 9–5). Patients with psychiatric disorders kill themselves at rates 3–12 times higher than those for other patients (Evenson et al. 1982). Male patients who have ever had a psychiatric admission die as a result of suicide at 5.7 times the rate for men in the general population. For men identified as psychiatric patients but never actually hospitalized, the rate is 3.4 times that in the general population. For women, the respective rates are 10.4 times and 4.0 times those in the general population. Men who have had a psychiatric admission kill themselves at a rate only 1.7 times greater than that for women with similar histories, versus 3 times greater than the rate in the general population.

History of a suicide attempt appears to be an important predictor of future suicide risk (Pokorny 1983). One of every 100 suicide attempt survivors will die by suicide within 1 year of their index attempt, a suicide risk approximately 100 times that for the general population (Hawton 1992). Of those who complete suicide, 25%–50% have tried before (Patterson et al. 1983). Motto (1989) likened this propensity to suicidal behavior to "kindling," leading to decreased ability to withstand self-destructive urges after succumbing to them the first time.

Litman (1989) estimated that based on psychological autopsies, 95% of patients who completed suicide had psychiatric diagnoses, including 40% with mood disorders (bipolar or unipolar), 20%–25% with chronic alcoholism, 10%–15% with schizophrenia, and 20%–25% with severe personality disorder (Table 9–6). Command hallucinations in patients with psychosis or chronic self-destructive acts in patients with personality disorders, particularly acts involving trauma, increase the possibility of suicide (see Tables 9–3 and 9–4).

TABLE 9–5. Suicide relative risk: psychiatric factors

Target group	Incidence per 100,000	Control group	Relative risk (target group/ control group[a]	Source
Patients with history of psychiatric admission				
Men	170	General population	5.7	
Women	100	General population	10.4	
Inpatients				
Depression				
Men	400	General population	13.6	
Women	180	General population	18.4	Evenson et al. 1982
Dysthymia				
Men	190	General population	6.4	
Women	70	General population	7.5	
Schizophrenia				
Men	210	General population	7.2	
Women	90	General population	9.5	
Alcoholism				
Men	180	General Population	5.9	
Women	130	General population	13.4	
Psychiatric outpatients (never admitted)				
Men	100	General population	3.4	
Women	40	General population	4.0	
Insured patients with depression				
History of inpatient treatment	224	General population	21	
Outpatient mental health treatment only	64	General population	6	Simon and VonKorff 1998
Antidepressants through outpatient primary care only	43	General population	4	
Suicide attempters within a year of attempt		General population	100	Hawton 1992

[a]Age adjusted except in the case of insured patients with depression and suicide attempters.

TABLE 9–6. Lifetime suicide risk among patients with history of psychiatric hospitalizations

Diagnosis	Lifetime risk of suicide (%)	Source
Primary mood disorders	4–6	Bostwick and Pankratz 2000
Schizophrenia	6.4	Fenton et al. 1997
Psychopathic personality	5	Miles 1977
Alcoholism	3.4	Murphy and Weitzel 1990

Note. In the United States, the incidence of suicide in the general population in 1997 was 1.3% (Ventura et al. 1998).

An estimated 4%–6% of patients hospitalized with mood disorders eventually commit suicide, with the risk highest early in the illness course (Bostwick and Pankratz 2000). The Epidemiologic Catchment Area study revealed a lifetime suicide attempt rate of 7.0% among patients with uncomplicated panic disorder and 7.9% among patients with uncomplicated major depression. With comorbid panic disorder and depression, the lifetime rate of suicide attempts increased to 19.5% (Johnson et al. 1990). Ten percent of patients with schizophrenia will eventually kill themselves, with the risk greatest early in the illness course (Miles 1977).

One-quarter of all suicides are committed by patients with active alcohol use disorders. Although alcohol abusers may kill themselves at any age, especially when acute intoxication clouds their judgment and disinhibits them, most alcoholic individuals tend to commit suicide decades into their drinking, after family and social relationships have been ravaged and work performance and health adversely affected. Murphy and Weitzel (1990) estimated that 3.4% of alcoholic patients kill themselves, a rate that is nearly three times the lifetime risk in the general population. Klerman (1987) suggested that most of the higher suicide rates among men may be accounted for by the higher rates of alcoholism among men.

Suicide is often committed by alcoholic patients in response to crises in their interpersonal lives. One-third of alcoholic patients who kill themselves have lost a close relationship within the previous 6 weeks, and one-third anticipate experiencing an equally severe interpersonal loss (Murphy 1992). Alcoholic patients frequently have many other suicide risk factors, many of which are a direct result of their substance abuse, including comorbid major depression, estrangement from family and social supports, unemployment, and serious medical illness. Other people who abuse psychoactive substances also

have high suicide rates. For example, opiate-dependent patients kill themselves at 20 times the expected rate (Miles 1977).

Biological and Genetic Risk Factors

The search for possible biological markers for suicide has focused on the brain stem serotonergic system. Several biological findings among individuals who commit suicide, irrespective of psychiatric diagnosis, implicate serotonergic dysfunction (Hawton 1992; Monk 1987; Stanley and Stanley 1989), including low levels of cerebrospinal fluid serotonin, increased levels of cerebrospinal fluid serotonin metabolites, and platelet serotonin abnormalities. A history of child abuse, a familial depression history, substance abuse, and low cholesterol levels are all associated with both lower serotonergic activity and greater suicide risk (Mann 1998). Biochemical vulnerability may be present, but no practical test for use in the clinical setting exists. If a test were available, it would likely provide only one more risk factor in a complex biopsychosocial formulation.

Persons with a family history of suicide also appear to have an increased risk of suicide (Egeland and Sussex 1985). Roy (1983) studied 243 consecutive psychiatric inpatients with a family history of suicide and found that 48.6% of the patients had attempted suicide and 56.4% received a diagnosis of major depression at least once. In a control population of 5,602 psychiatric inpatients without a family history of suicide, only 21.0% had ever attempted suicide and only 26.6% had a history of major depression.

Psychological and Psychosocial Risk Factors

Suicide is frequently a response to a loss, real or imagined. To help assess the meaning of suicidal ideation or behavior, the consultation-liaison psychiatrist must inquire about recent or anticipated losses and coping strategies that the patient has used with past losses (Davidson 1993). Fantasies of revenge, punishment, reconciliation with a rejecting object, relief from the pain of loss, or reunion with a dead loved one may be evident (Furst and Ostow 1979).

A patient's degree of autonomy and extent of dependency on external sources of emotional support will shed light on the level of psychic resilience (Buie and Maltsberger 1989). A recent loss of a loved one or a parental loss during childhood increases suicide risk. Holidays and anniversaries of important days in the life and death of the deceased person, when the loved one's absence is experienced more intensely, also increase suicide risk.

Glickman (1980) believed that a suicidal patient cannot be judged safe until he or she has either regained the lost object, accepted its loss, or replaced it with a new object.

Case Example 1

Mrs. A, an 80-year-old woman, was admitted to the hospital for the second time with delirium from salicylate poisoning. She had a long history of mood disorder, although she had never made a suicide attempt. She also had arthritis, for which she had been advised to take aspirin, and gastrointestinal complaints whose etiology had never been determined. Her social isolation was pronounced. Her husband of 55 years had entered a nursing home several years earlier, and she was estranged from her children. She did not drive but continued to live, unhappily, in the large suburban house she and her husband had shared for many years. She finally admitted that she had recently been awakening in the middle of the night, agitated and unable to return to sleep. She would take aspirin tablets, one after the other, not counting or caring how many she ingested, in hope of relieving the abdominal pain and overwhelming sense of aloneness she felt.

In the general hospital, the consultation-liaison psychiatrist will consult on a wide range of potentially suicidal patients—for example, patients admitted in the aftermath of suicide attempts, patients prone to suicide because of a substance-related disorder, or patients at increased risk for suicide because of painful or disfiguring illnesses. Patients like Mrs. A may even demonstrate masked suicidal behavior. A consultation-liaison psychiatrist's caseload will include psychiatric patients transferred to the general hospital because the psychiatric facilities where they were being treated were ill equipped to manage their medical problems.

SUICIDE RISK FACTOR SCALES

A great deal of research has been done in the attempt to develop clinical predictor scales for suicide risk. Unfortunately, scales developed to date have only been correlational, predicting groups at risk rather than identifying individuals within groups (Pokorny 1983). The main utility of such scales may be in increasing the likelihood that the clinician will ask about suicidal ideation and behaviors and other known risk factors (Davidson 1993). Roy (1985) and Sanders (1988) endorsed risk factor scales for use by nonpsychiatric clinicians, who may be prompted to identify patients at risk and seek psychiatric consultation.

Patterson et al. (1983) devised one of the most popular of these scales, the SAD PERSONS Scale for assessing the risk of suicide; the scale is summarized in Table 9–7.

This 10-point mnemonic includes **s**ex, **a**ge, **d**epression, **p**revious attempt, **e**thanol abuse, **r**ational thinking loss, **s**ocial supports lacking, **o**rganized plan, **n**o spouse, and **s**ickness as categories that should be surveyed. The higher scores on this scale correspond to greater suicide risk. The device, like all mnemonics, is useful to remind the examiner to address pertinent areas in a clinical interview, but the scale has not been demonstrated to have validity in specific assessments (Goldberg 1987). The SAD PERSONS Scale may have both sensitivity and specificity problems. There may be both false-positive and false-negative results. Nevertheless, this scale provides a summary of current knowledge about suicide epidemiology, a body of information that borrows from biological, psychological, and social sources of data in attempting to identify suicide risk.

A state-of-the-art conceptual model is Mann's (1998) stress-diathesis model of suicidal behavior (Figure 9–1). On the basis, in part, of the clinical observation that two groups of patients, each with the same severity of depressive illness, attempt suicide at different rates, Mann proposed a suicide diathesis whose components include genetic predisposition, early life experience, chronic illness, chronic substance abuse, and certain dietary factors. Extreme stress alone, which Mann defined as acute psychiatric illness, intoxication, medical illness, or family/social stress, is not typically enough to invoke suicidal behavior. A suicidal individual already has the predisposition, or diathesis, on which the stress is superimposed, resulting in the suicide attempt (Mann 1998).

TABLE 9–7. The SAD PERSONS Scale for assessing the risk of suicide

Sex

Age

Depression

Previous attempt

Ethanol abuse

Rational thinking loss

Social supports lacking

Organized plan

No spouse

Sickness

One point is scored for each factor deemed present. The total score thus ranges from 0 (very little risk) to 10 (very high risk).

Source. Reprinted from Patterson WM, Dohn HH, Bird J, et al: "Evaluation of Suicidal Patients: The SAD PERSONS Scale." *Psychosomatics* 24:343–349, 1983. Copyright 1983, Academy of Psychosomatic Medicine. Used with permission.

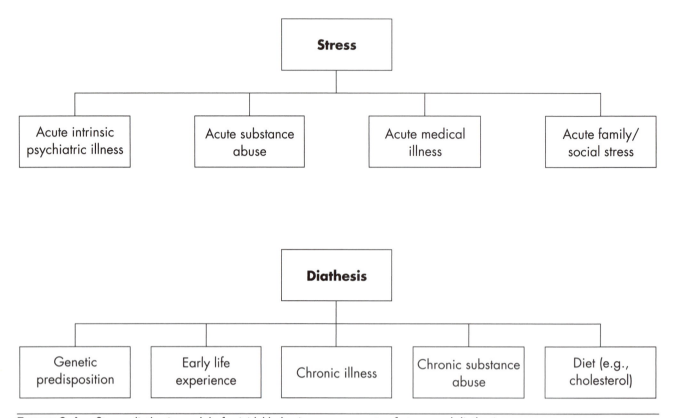

FIGURE 9–1.   Stress-diathesis model of suicidal behavior: components of stress and diathesis.
Source.   Adapted from Mann JJ: "The Neurobiology of Suicide." *Nature Medicine* 4:25–30, 1998. Copyright 1998. Used with permission.

PATIENT ASSESSMENT

The purpose of a suicide evaluation is to integrate an individual's feelings and thoughts in a moment of crisis with the aforementioned demographic and social variables. It is difficult to garner adequate information in enough spheres in a brief interview or two with a complex patient and then contextualize it using unwieldy epidemiologic data fraught with inconsistencies and lacunae. Blumenthal and Kupfer (1986), who envisioned suicide as a final common pathway, proposed a multiaxial, or matrix, approach for organizing and integrating the medical, psychiatric, psychological, social, and demographic risk factors that contribute to the suicidal state. This research model was created to direct clinical investigations toward greater precision and success in early detection and treatment. Matrix approaches such as theirs (Table 9–8) and Yufit's (1991) (Table 9–9) flesh out a stress-diathesis model like Mann's and allow the consultant to organize his or her data and formulate an approach to assigning baseline epidemiologic risk.

Cumbersome complexity notwithstanding, the ultimate problem with sifting through extensive clinical and demographic data is that it does not inform the consultant whether the person is at immediate risk for suicide. Litman (1989) noted that the 95% prevalence of psychiatric illness among individuals who commit suicide is derived from psychological autopsies and retrospective studies, the scientific equivalent of Monday morning quarterbacking. Among dozens of patients who are depressed or psychotic at a given time, depression or psychosis degenerates into suicidality in only an individual or two. At any moment, very few of those who are "at risk" will die by suicide. Once the medical inpatient, outpatient, or emergency room patient at high risk has been identified, the psychiatric consultant must decide what to do based on the clinical examination.

The consultation-liaison psychiatrist's first task is to create a clinical situation in which the patient feels free to reveal the unacceptable thoughts that may be driving his or her present suicidality.

Case Example 2

Mr. B, a 32-year-old man, was brought to the emergency room by police officers. His estranged wife had called the police after he gave her suicide notes to give to their three children "after I'm gone." In the emergency room, he was wild-eyed and pacing; because the emergency room staff were unable to soothe him,

TABLE 9–8. Suicide assessment: a matrix approach

Psychiatric diagnosis and personality style

Affective disorder or schizophrenia, particularly early in its course or with command hallucinations

Alcoholism, particularly late in its course, or other substance abuse

Personality disorder, especially borderline, compulsive, or antisocial

Delirium or organic psychosis

Previous suicide attempt, particularly if serious

Psychosocial factors, life events, chronic medical illness

History of early loss

  Parental loss in childhood

  Childhood abuse or neglect

  Anniversary of loss

Negative life events

  Recent bereavement, separation, or divorce

  Recent loss of job or significant humiliation

  Recent discharge from psychiatric hospital

  Recovery from major depressive episode or schizophrenic break

Decreased social supports

  Increased isolation, alienation, withdrawal

  Family turbulence or limited support

  Family exhaustion with patient's illness

  Sudden life changes

Terminal, chronic, painful, or disfiguring illness, especially causing cognitive change or associated with depression

Recent diagnosis of cancer

Genetics

Family history of suicide

Family history of affective disorder

Biological factors

Decrease in central serotonergic activity

Increased aggression and/or impulsivity

Mental status examination

Lack of rapport with interviewer

Expressions of hopelessness or intolerable pain

Explicit suicide plan with means to carry it out

  Recent history of giving away cherished possessions, putting affairs in order, saying good-byes

  Rehearsal of fatal behavior

Mood nonreactivity

Panic attacks

Psychosis (impaired reality testing)

  Command hallucinations

  Self-destructive delusions

Source. Adapted from Blumenthal SJ, Kupfer DJ: "Generalizable Treatment Strategies for Suicidal Behavior." *Annals of the New York Academy of Sciences* 487:327–340, 1986. Used with permission.

TABLE 9–9. Major variables of focus for the assessment of suicide potential

Vulnerability variables: primary

Hopelessness

Anger (internalized)

Depression

Alcohol or drug abuse

Vulnerability variables: secondary

Rigid/Constricted cognitive style

Primary orientation to past

Lack of belonging

Psychiatric history

Isolation/Loneliness

Major coping abilities that help negate suicide

Trust in self, others

Resiliency in adapting to change or loss

Capacity for intimacy and love

Sense of belonging

Well-developed future time perspective

Continuity of self (identity)

Source. Reprinted from Yufit RI: "American Association of Suicidology. Presidential Address: Suicide Assessment in the 1990's." *Suicide and Life-Threatening Behavior* 21:152–163, 1991. Copyright 1991, Guilford Publications. Used with permission.

they locked him in the observation room by himself. Gradually, during an interview with the psychiatric consultant that lasted more than 2 hours, Mr. B became calm.

The consultation-liaison psychiatrist in the emergency room learned that Mr. B had separated from his wife a year earlier and moved in with his girlfriend, who was now pregnant with their child. He had been fighting with his girlfriend for weeks. The previous night, after a "major blowout," they had agreed to "split." He was feeling as though he had nowhere to go because his girlfriend was still living in the apartment they shared and his wife refused to take him back.

Mr. B had no formal psychiatric or substance abuse history, although a brother was dependent on opiates. Mr. B was a hard-driving perfectionist, and he normally worked an 80-hour week at his own business. However, he had recently reduced his hours, citing burnout. He admitted that he denied problems exist, "until they explode," and added that he was "ashamed at the mess my life is in." Although he denied any intent to harm himself, he appeared too agitated to formulate a reasonable plan for where to stay, even for that night, let alone figure out a way to sort out the various competing entanglements. He could not think of anyone he was willing to call to ask for support. He realized that he was now "utterly alone in the world."

Finally, 2 hours into the interview, Mr. B admitted that he knew his parents would take him in. He hated to trouble them after all his brother had put them through, but he confessed that his father was the one person he trusted to give him sound advice. Yet he flatly refused to call him, because he did not want to burden his parents and he did not want to disclose the embarrassing details of his love life.

When the emergency room psychiatric consultant finally began to discuss admission to a psychiatric hospital, Mr. B agreed to call his father, who said he would be at the hospital within 30 minutes to discuss the situation. After Mr. B heard this, his demeanor changed almost instantly from tense edginess to relaxed calm, and he began to talk about how he would use his "old room" in his parents' house to start rebuilding his life.

All patients seen by consultation-liaison psychiatrists in medical, surgical, and emergency settings should be asked about suicidality. Inquiring about suicidality does not increase suicide risk, whereas not asking may increase both patient mortality and physician liability if the patient commits suicide. The psychiatric consultant must realize that there is something special and salvageable about people who survive their suicidal urges long enough to bring them to medical attention, and the consultant must address the ambivalence that is central to the patient's suicidality. The psychiatrist must ally with the parts of these patients that want to survive.

A psychodynamic formulation weaves together the precipitating events, the conscious and unconscious motives driving the suicidality, and the characteristics of the patient's personality that propel him or her toward acting on suicidal thoughts (Gabbard 1990). Mr. B, in Case Example 2, fought with his pregnant girlfriend and separated from her only hours before being brought to the emergency room. His suicide threats were impulsive. His crisis had urgency, and Mr. B was acting without regard for the future (Pokorny 1983). Mr. B was rigid and obsessional, and he had been using denial to stave off having to face the consequences of leaving his wife and children and impregnating his girlfriend. In the wake of his latest fight with his girlfriend, however, he had crossed a threshold beyond which he could no longer ignore the pain he had caused and that he felt (Motto 1989). The psychiatric consultant elected to conduct a comprehensive interview. The therapeutic value of abreaction was used to clarify the conflict and thus deprive it of its force (Havens 1967).

Mr. B had few traditional epidemiologic features of a suicide-prone patient. In a suicidal crisis, the specific here-and-now events take precedence over social and demographic data. In this short-term time frame, the concept of prediction may not even apply. Formulating the unfolding drama and identifying the crisis draw on a different set of concepts and clinical skills than epidemiologic prediction (Pokorny 1983). Suicidality is a dynamic entity that waxes and wanes with the patient's circumstances. Determining that a patient is a member of a high-risk group is neither necessary nor sufficient to conclude that the patient is in suicidal crisis. The clinician must discern the individual variables that will ultimately determine the time of highest risk (Fawcett et al. 1987). The majority of suicidal episodes occur in patients with psychiatric diagnoses, but the diagnosis itself does not drive suicidality; rather, it is a crisis imposed on the substrate of the diagnosis (Klerman 1987).

Litman (1989) described a *presuicidal syndrome*, which characterizes lethal attempts and completed suicides. The presuicidal patient in crisis has constricted choices, constricted perception, a tunnel vision of life as hopeless, physical tension, and emotional perturbation. The tension and distress may be relieved by a fantasy of death. The hopelessness is combined with help rejection and distrust. Often the patient has, in the background, a long-term disposition toward impulsive action, an all-or-nothing approach to problems, and the characterological attitude "my way or no way."

Klerman (1987) framed the presuicidal crisis in terms of a medical model: there is an underlying condition that intermittently flares. The clinician must look for signs in the mental status examination that the patient has lost the capacity to think rationally. The hopelessness and helplessness of severe depression can reach irrational proportions. Hallucinations may command self-harm. Clouded sensorium; impaired judgment; disinhibition; and misperceptions of delirium, intoxication, or substance withdrawal may all cause a patient to act in self-destructive or dangerous ways. Table 9–9 summarizes key elements of the assessment of the potentially suicidal patient.

Shneidman (1989) identified "10 commonalities of suicide" that may help the consultation-liaison psychiatrist to narrow a broad epidemiologic suicide risk assessment so that it is relevant to an individual patient (Table 9–10). Hopelessness is a common finding by researchers who study psychological factors associated with suicide and suicide attempts (Fawcett et al. 1987; Shneidman 1989; Siomopoulos 1990).

The perspective of time appears to shift significantly among patients in suicidal crisis. Yufit (1991) found that suicidal persons typically have little interest in the future, much involvement in the past, and dissatisfaction with the present, unlike nonsuicidal control subjects, who were focused on the present and the future and had little interest in the past (Table 9–11). Litman (1989) reviewed 1,000 suicide notes from Los Angeles residents who had died and noted recurrent themes of regret over lost lovers or encroaching illness: "Often the communications describe fatigue, exhaustion and a need to escape....The

TABLE 9–10. Ten commonalities of suicide

1. The common purpose of suicide is to seek a solution.
2. The common goal of suicide is cessation of consciousness.
3. The common stimulus in suicide is intolerable psychological pain.
4. The common stressor in suicide is frustrated psychological needs.
5. The common emotion in suicide is hopelessness or helplessness.
6. The common cognitive state in suicide is ambivalence.
7. The common perceptual state in suicide is constriction.
8. The common action in suicide is aggression.
9. The common interpersonal act in suicide is communication of intention.
10. The common consistency in suicide is with life-long coping patterns.

Source. Reprinted from Shneidman ES: "Overview: A Multidimensional Approach to Suicide," in *Suicide: Understanding and Responding.* Edited by Jacobs D, Brown HN. Madison, CT, International Universities Press, 1989, p 16. Used with permission.

TABLE 9–11. Time perspective profiles

Time perspective profile of suicidal person
High in the past (nostalgia, obsessions)
Nominal, negative in the present
Minimal or zero in the future

Time perspective profile of nonsuicidal person
Very low in the past (except anniversaries)
Moderately high in the present
High in the future

Source. Reprinted from Yufit RI: "American Association of Suicidology. Presidential Address: Suicide Assessment in the 1990's." *Suicide and Life-Threatening Behavior* 21:152–163, 1991. Copyright 1991, Guilford Publications. Used with permission.

notes seldom (less than 10%) express anger or reproach. Humor is absent. The general mood of these notes that express feelings is one of hopelessness" (Litman 1989, pp. 149–150).

Consultation-liaison psychiatrists who examine potentially suicidal patients must monitor themselves for reactions and countertransference feelings toward patients. A clinician may sense a patient's hopelessness and feel hopeless about the patient's prospects, identify with a patient's anger and become furious at the patient, or respond to haughty disdain with arrogant dismissal of the patient and his or her complaints. Particularly when evaluating patients with character disorders, the clinician must identify these feelings—what Maltsberger and Buie (1974) called *countertransference hate*—for what they are: something aroused in the consultant by the patient. The clinician must ensure that he or she does not act on

these feelings and must regard them instead as further information about the state of the patient's mind and social relations. The clinician's unrecognized aversion to his or her patient can have dire consequences. If the clinician stops attempting to reach the buried rage and despair because of manifest antagonism, he or she can rationalize a relatively benign mental status examination in order to discharge a potentially lethal patient.

TREATMENT, MANAGEMENT, AND PREVENTION

Identify Risk Level

In one of the most practical approaches to suicide assessment, Goldberg (1987) argued that despite the lack of valid measures for predicting suicide risk, there are "issues that are considered so fundamental for suicide assessment that failure to obtain and record such information would practically constitute inadequate practice" (p. 449). He described the minimum legal requirements for meeting the standard of care and enumerated what should become part of the medical record regardless of the consultant's theoretical stance. His recommendations for the fundamentals of suicide assessment are listed in Table 9–12.

TABLE 9–12. Fundamentals of suicide assessment

1. Determine whether delirium, psychosis, or depression is present.
2. Elicit the patient's statements about his or her suicidality.
3. Elicit the patient's ideas about what would help to mitigate his or her suicidality.
4. Confirm the patient's story with a third party.
5. Make a global formulation that includes acute and chronic management suggestions.
6. Ask a series of escalating questions addressing suicidality in medically hospitalized patients:
   - Are you discouraged about your medical condition?
   - Are there times when you think about your situation and feel like crying?
   - When you feel that way, what sort of thoughts go through your mind?
   - Did you ever feel that if your life were to go on like this, it would not be worth living?
   - Have you gotten to the point at which you've actually thought of a specific plan to end your life?
   - You say you've thought of shooting yourself. Do you have access to a gun?

Source. Adapted from Goldberg RJ: "The Assessment of Suicide Risk in the General Hospital." *General Hospital Psychiatry* 9:446–452, 1987. Copyright 1987, Elsevier Science. Used with permission.

Goldberg's approach is simple as well as sophisticated. The mental status examination, with its search for factors clouding insight, judgment, or consciousness, is the biological state of the art in the absence of any chemical or imaging test to characterize suicidality. Asking the patient to describe his or her ideas for disposition is a psychologically astute projective technique that provides a view of the patient's inner world and degree of hopelessness, which is correlated with self-destructiveness. Encouraging the patient's collaboration in negotiating a follow-up plan increases the chance of compliance after discharge (Hofmann and Dubovsky 1991). Including a third party helps the clinician both to evaluate the veracity of the patient's account and to gain other perspectives on the patient's situation. The responses of both the patient and the third party to the intervention give some indication of the degree of the patient's social isolation and alienation, as well as of the social resources available to aid in recovery from the suicidal crisis. These diverse sources of information help the consultant to produce a global biopsychosocial formulation of risk level.

Siomopoulos (1990) believed that to help a patient overcome the crisis, "every patient who has attempted suicide or who talks about committing suicide should be offered hospitalization" (p. 212). These are the patients at highest risk for completed suicide (Bostwick and Pankratz 2000). Siomopoulos (1990) advocated telling a patient that his or her suffering is temporary and will pass and admitting the patient to a psychiatric unit when medically possible for containment and treatment until he or she has weathered the self-destructive storm.

Case Example 3

Ms. C, a 22-year-old woman addicted to crack cocaine, developed severe cardiomyopathy after the birth of her third child. Four months later, she was admitted to the hospital after telling the emergency room physician that she could no longer climb the two flights of stairs to her apartment without becoming short of breath. Results of toxicology screens performed in the emergency room were positive for alcohol and cocaine.

After she arrived at the medical floor, Ms. C curled up in a fetal position in her room and refused to speak to her nurse until she was found lighting a cigarette while receiving oxygen. When the nurse attempted to stop her, Ms. C immediately began yelling curses and shrieked at the nurse that if she were not allowed to smoke, she intended to overdose on the digitalis she had hidden in the room.

Ms. C refused to submit to a room search. The psychiatrist was consulted emergently and recommended that security be called so that the patient would not leave before emergency evaluation. Ms. C had to be placed in leather restraints when she started swinging at the officers. After the opportunity to speak with the consultation-liaison psychiatrist, Ms. C agreed to take 5 mg of haloperidol and 1 mg of lorazepam. She then consented to a search of her belongings. Her nurse confiscated the bottle of 50 digitalis tablets found in her suitcase. Because of her threats and impulsivity, the psychiatrist recommended close observation with sitters.

As Ms. C's case demonstrates, the psychiatric consultant's initial tasks in assessing suicidality in the hospital, emergency room, or clinic are not primarily diagnostic. Before assessment and formulation, the psychiatrist must first ensure the patient's safety (Gutheil and Appelbaum 2000).

Until determined otherwise, a suicidal person is a patient in crisis from a life-threatening illness. In the absence of medical or surgical complications, such a patient is usually transferred from an emergency room to a secure psychiatric facility. In the general hospital, the patient's medical condition often prevents immediate transfer. Thus, a secure environment must be created within the medical-surgical setting until the patient is stable enough for psychiatric transfer.

The patient's room must be secured—that is, anything that a patient could potentially use to injure himself or herself, such as sharp objects or material that could be fashioned into a noose, must be removed. Luggage and possessions should be searched with a suspicious eye and a morbid imagination. Staff must ferret out sharp objects, lighters, belts, caches of pills—anything that could inflict damage in either an impulsive or carefully planned way. Objects coming into the room (e.g., cutlery on the dinner tray, the pop tops from soft drink cans) must be regarded as potential weapons.

The patient will need a sitter for constant observation, a process that must be truly constant. Social amenities may no longer apply. Patients permitted to use the bathroom unobserved have been known to leap from that window or maim themselves behind the closed door. A moment of privacy granted to the patient out of misplaced civility, or a few minutes of inattention or absence by the sitter, may be all the time a suicidal person needs to execute a suicide plan.

It should never be forgotten that given the right circumstances, any patient can overpower a sitter or staff member. All staff guarding suicidal patients should know how to summon security personnel as reinforcements when they perceive that they have lost control of the patient or the situation. In these days of cost-cutting measures, the consultant may feel pressure to limit the use of constant observation. The decision to employ constant observation must always be made on clinical grounds and must not be affected by fiscal concerns. Economizing on sitters could mean the life of the suicidal patient.

Remove or Treat Risk Factors

Underlying medical problems. The consulting psychiatrist must review the patient's chart to ensure that any underlying medical problem or condition is not contributing to a delirium or other secondary psychiatric disorder. The patient's substance abuse history should be elicited to determine whether the agitation driving the patient's suicidality is the result of substance withdrawal. Using a device such as the WHHHHIMP mnemonic (Wise and Rundell 1994) will help to elicit causes of delirium, which, if found, must be aggressively treated.

Medical illness or medications that may be contributing to mood, anxiety, or psychotic disorders require prompt identification and management. The consultation-liaison psychiatrist must collaborate with medical or surgical colleagues to establish medical and psychiatric treatment regimens that maximize benefits while minimizing deleterious effects on the sensorium. Psychotic depression demands treatment with both an antidepressant and a neuroleptic, or electroconvulsive therapy may be necessary if the patient is too agitated, self-destructive, or catatonic to wait the days to weeks for the antidepressant to take effect.

Withdrawal syndromes, particularly withdrawal from alcohol, benzodiazepines, and barbiturates, can be deadly and must be recognized and treated aggressively with detoxification protocols. The consultant may need to request additional medical treatment if he or she believes the mental status anomalies remain primarily because of medical or toxic etiologies.

One medication that has been implicated as a cause of suicidal states is fluoxetine. In early 1990, Teicher et al. reported the emergence of new-onset intense, violent suicidal preoccupation in six patients within weeks of starting fluoxetine therapy. It appeared that a primary suicide risk factor had been found in the guise of the most widely prescribed and highly touted antidepressant in the world. Further research has not confirmed this fear. Fava and Rosenbaum (1991) surveyed 27 psychiatrists who had treated 1,017 patients with fluoxetine, and the investigators' findings did not corroborate the results of Teicher and colleagues (1990). Fava and Rosenbaum explained the initial report by noting the following:

- Most of the six patients had borderline personality disorder, psychosis, or worsening depression despite treatment.

- Suicidal ideation has been reported after initiation of treatment with any antidepressant, except monoamine oxidase inhibitors.
- The incidence of suicidality emerging during treatment with fluoxetine was not statistically higher than with any other antidepressant.

In a more recent study, involving 654 patients with anxiety disorders, fluoxetine was not associated with a higher incidence of suicidal behavior, and patients treated with the drug had more suicide risk factors than those not prescribed the medication (Warshaw and Keller 1996).

Physical or chemical restraint. Agitation and overt suicidal behavior must be promptly treated with physical restraints, chemical restraints, or both. Neuroleptics should be used in patients with delirium, and neuroleptics and/or benzodiazepines should be given to agitated, anxious, or psychotic patients. Physical restraints may be required if a patient is believed to be unpredictable or impulsive.

Psychotherapy. A flexible approach to psychotherapy in medically ill patients who are potentially suicidal may include supportive therapy for dealing with the ravages of illness on the body or the sense of self. Family therapy should be employed, particularly when it will reinforce the patient's sense of connection to other people.

The medical social worker's assessment and intervention may be critical. Situational factors that contribute, either medically or psychologically, to the hospitalization and concomitant suicidality must be recognized and addressed. These could include broken relationships, financial stresses, and inadequate housing (Lloyd 1995). To combat social isolation, efforts should be made to reestablish or strengthen connections to friends or community social service agencies.

Follow-up. The consultant's chart notes should identify the level of risk, clearly state the plan, and report when the consultant will return to continue the assessment and recommend modifications to the plan. The consultant must discuss his or her recommendations by telephone or in person with the referring physician and maintain close contact with the medical team throughout the hospitalization, to ensure agreement and to minimize potentially life-threatening confusion about or deviation from the plan.

The consultant should also arrange follow-up care for the patient and detail it in the chart so that it becomes part of the inpatient's discharge plan. Making such arrangements is crucial because many general hospital patients who are at risk for suicide have had no previous mental health contact and thus have no health care provider to continue the treatments the consultation-liaison psychiatrist began during hospitalization. On discharge, in keeping with the idea that patients should not unwittingly be provided with the instruments of their own destruction, medication that could be lethal in overdose should be prescribed only in small quantities. The patient should be given only enough to last until the first outpatient appointment, and the consultant should keep in mind that the patient may hoard it anyway if absolutely intent on suicide. *Contracting for safety* refers to the agreement patients make with their psychiatrist that they will not harm themselves before the next session. Although this "contract" probably has no legal merit, the process permits the patient and the consultation-liaison psychiatrist to anticipate dangerous situations and make plans collaboratively for the patient to deal with these situations by seeking help rather than engaging in self-destructive behavior.

Davidson (1993) suggested that in the emergency or outpatient setting, outpatient management may be an acceptable plan if the suicidal patient has 1) satisfactory impulse control, 2) no psychosis or intoxication, 3) no specific plan or easily accessible means, 4) accessible social supports to which he or she is willing to turn, and 5) the capacity for establishing rapport with the consultant. The converse of each of these points—namely, 1) poor impulse control, 2) psychosis, intoxication, or delirium, 3) a plan and the means to execute it, 4) isolation, exhaustion of family or friends, or changes in the network of support services that sustain the patient, and 5) a difficult interview on any grounds—should prompt transfer to a psychiatric facility or medical-psychiatric unit.

Psychiatric hospitalization. If the consultant has any doubts about a potentially suicidal patient in the emergency or outpatient medical setting, he or she should admit first and ask questions later. The potential consequences of undertreating suicidality are deadly. A psychiatric or medical-psychiatric unit admission, even a brief one, may provide the opportunity to observe the patient further and the time and resources to construct the patient's formulation comprehensively enough to make a more appropriate disposition. In an inpatient psychiatric or medical-psychiatric unit, the doctor can learn more about the patient and the patient can demonstrate what kind of care he or she might need. Table 9–13 presents 12 reasons for admitting a suicidal patient to a psychiatric or medical-psychiatric unit.

TABLE 9–13. Twelve reasons to admit a suicidal patient to a psychiatric or medical-psychiatric unit

1. The need to obtain an accurate history from sources other than the patient
2. The need to examine the patient in an undrugged state
3. The need for a period of observation to ascertain suicide risk
4. The patient's need for punishment
5. The patient's need for an external target or rage
6. The patient's need to reestablish an object relationship
7. The need to destroy the patient's or the family's denial that the patient is seriously ill
8. The need to reassess the outpatient psychiatric treatment that the patient has been receiving
9. The patient's need for time to adjust to the loss that precipitated the suicide attempt
10. The patient's need to regress and be cared for
11. The patient's need to be rescued
12. The need to remove the patient from a stressful situation

Source. Reprinted from Glickman LS: "The Suicidal Patient," in *Psychiatric Consultation in the General Hospital.* New York, Marcel Dekker, 1980, pp. 181–202. Copyright 1980, Marcel Dekker. Used with permission.

Prevention

Case Example 4

Mr. D, a 41-year-old married man with no previous psychiatric history, was brought by helicopter to a tertiary medical center from an outlying hospital after he shot off part of the lower left side of his jaw and face. Despite his disfiguring, painful injury, he was awake and alert in the intensive care unit. He said that after a spat with his wife, he had stormed from their second-floor bedroom to the basement, where he shoved the muzzle of a loaded duck-hunting rifle into his mouth and pulled the trigger while his wife, who had raced after him, watched. He survived the blast only because the barrel was too long for him to wedge the muzzle against the roof of his mouth and still reach the trigger with his finger. Instead, the gun blew out his cheek.

During his 10 days in the hospital, Mr. D gradually revealed that he and his wife had always had difficulty communicating, particularly about topics that made them angry, during their 18 years of marriage. He had agreed to quit drinking 6–12 beers a day 2 years previously, when she became concerned about his behavior while drunk. However, he had continued to drink as heavily as before and told his wife that he was imbibing nonalcoholic brews. When he shot himself, he was intoxicated.

While in the hospital, Mr. D revealed his secret to his wife in the presence of the consulting psychiatrist, who had found no psychopathology other than alcoholism. He admitted that his drinking was out of control. He thought that his situation was hopeless. For the first time in their marriage, he agreed to participate in couples counseling. He also welcomed discharge directly from the hospital to a 28-day alcohol treatment program and requested referral for individual outpatient psychotherapy.

With his alcoholism and marital problems, Mr. D is typical of many people at increased risk for suicide. The fact that he actually attempted suicide at that moment was atypical, both in the alcoholic population and the population at large. Psychiatric consultants fortunately have the opportunity to intervene in most instances before the actual suicide attempt. Prevention often means psychiatric hospitalization or transfer.

Potentially suicidal patients require preventive interventions for the biopsychosocial risk factors that originally drove their suicidal ideation. In the general hospital, the preventive medicine interventions may overcome the acute crisis before the suicidal patient is ready for medical discharge, particularly with timely psychiatric intervention. "The suicidal urge is state-dependent, and is thus susceptible to treatments that alter that state," wrote George Murphy (1983, pp. 344–345), a clinician noted for his study of suicide among alcoholic patients. He added that "within high-risk populations…the steps toward prevention of suicide are little steps, taken one or a few at a time, according to the individual case." Within the general hospital, these "little steps" are exactly the type of intervention the consultation-liaison psychiatrist can provide to prevent future suicidal behavior (Table 9–14). The consultation-liaison psychiatrist has the opportunity and advantage of repeated visits to the bedside of medically hospitalized suicidal patients, as well as time to conduct a brief treatment or preventive intervention. Farberow et al. (1966) and Frierson and Lippman (1988) made proactive suggestions about how to make patients and significant others, including family and staff, more comfortable, thereby ameliorating suicide risk factors. Mr. D, with his shattered face, was no longer suicidal after areas of treatment were identified. The consultation-liaison psychiatrist was able to arrange interventions that would help to address the alcoholism and marital difficulties that drove his suicide attempt, and this dealing with his problems would help to prevent future attempts.

Several specific psychiatric interventions can help to prevent suicidal behavior in medical-surgical inpatients and outpatients. These include

- Identifying and eliminating the factors driving an agitated delirium
- Diagnosing and treating alcohol withdrawal

TABLE 9–14. Steps to prevent suicidal behavior

1. *The people who committed suicide were more agitated, depressed, anxious, and distressed than were control subjects.*
   Treat agitation, anxiety, and depression immediately and aggressively.
   Seek psychiatric consultation early for mental status changes or abnormalities.

2. *External support, whether from family or from the hospital personnel, was a distinct deterrent to suicide.*
   Encourage family support and involvement if possible.
   Discourage impersonality, distance, and disinterest in staff, which may serve as "family equivalent."

3. *It is now well known that the suicidal patient gives prior indications of his or her intent by word or behavior.*
   Encourage staff communication.
   Seek psychiatric consultation about patient's suicide potential early.

4. *The suicidal group was more concerned with their body functions and was less able to tolerate pain than were the control subjects.*
   Treat pain aggressively and consider psychiatric overlay when pain seems out of proportion to its cause.

5. *Experience has shown that practical safeguards are effective, especially in deterring impulsive suicides.*
   "Safety-proof" patient rooms and bathrooms (e.g., place stops on windows, eliminate overhead bars, limit time alone in the bathroom).

6. *The most important antisuicidal measures are the sensitivity and alertness of the staff to the suicidal danger and the indication of interest and concern for the patient as a person.*

Source. Adapted from Farberow N[L], McKelligott JW, Cohen S, et al: "Suicide Among Patients With Cardiorespiratory Illness." *Journal of the American Medical Association* 195:422–428, 1966. Copyright 1966, American Medical Association. Used with permission.

- Exploring and neutralizing the rageful affects of a man or woman caught up in a marital crisis
- Offering comfort and support in the face of a life-threatening illness
- Effecting a reunion between the suicidal patient and estranged family members or friends
- Implementing a referral plan for ongoing inpatient or outpatient psychiatric treatment for the major depression or other psychiatric disorders that may have prompted the suicide attempt

In a public health model, the secondary effect of providing appropriate and necessary psychiatric care to high-risk populations should improve the general mental health of the general population while reducing the suicide incidence rate.

Hospitalizing patients to rule out suicide is as defensible as admitting them to rule out myocardial infarction (Hofmann and Dubovsky 1991; Tsuang and Simpson 1984). Another preventive medicine and public health benefit of a suicide assessment is the window it opens on the entire spectrum of psychopathology, because almost any psychiatric illness can present with suicidal ideation or behavior (Shershow 1976). The chief complaint, "I want to kill myself," garners a psychiatric intervention for someone whose underlying disorders might otherwise go unrecognized and untreated. The suicidal statement or act becomes the most urgent manifestation of underlying, usually unaddressed psychopathology.

Patients with HIV disease or AIDS may have several risk factors that predispose them to suicidal behavior. Specific interventions to prevent HIV disease–related or AIDS-related suicide are listed in Table 9–15.

PHYSICIAN-ASSISTED SUICIDE VERSUS AGGRESSIVE PALLIATIVE CARE

In a pair of unanimous 1997 decisions, the U.S. Supreme Court ruled that there is no constitutional right to physician-assisted suicide (PAS) and that states can prohibit physician conduct whose primary purpose is to hasten death (Burt 1997). Only one state, Oregon, has legalized PAS; that legislation was passed in 1997. Terminally ill Oregonians are permitted to ask their physicians for a prescription for a lethal dose of medication, but the patients must be able to administer the killing dose themselves. The law specifically forbids active euthanasia, also known as mercy killing, in which a physician would actively perform the lethal act; PAS is therefore denied to patients who lack motor capacity (e.g., patients with amyotrophic lateral sclerosis) (Rowland 1998).

The safeguards built into the Oregon process closely resemble in many ways the de facto criteria under which euthanasia has been permitted in the Netherlands since 1973. In the Netherlands, the patient must experience his or her situation as intolerable and voluntarily and repeatedly make the request to be euthanized. The physician receiving the request must ask a colleague to "confirm the correctness of diagnosis and prognosis, to support and verify the correct medical performance of euthanasia, and to check if all (legal) requirements are met" (de Wachter 1989, p. 3317).

The Oregon law further specifies that the patient must be able to make health care decisions and must have

TABLE 9–15. Recommendations for decreasing AIDS-related suicides

1. Increase sensitivity to depression and suicidality among AIDS patients and their loved ones. Psychotherapy aimed at facilitation of grief and antidepressant pharmacotherapy are often warranted.
2. Provide patients and families with accurate, up-to-date information about the disease. Topics should include reasonable precautions, modes of transmission, and so-called safe-sex practices. Myths about AIDS should be dispelled.
3. Solicit and respect the wishes of AIDS patients regarding the use of artificial life supports. Such an action gives the patient a semblance of control and relieves the family of a difficult decision.
4. Heighten appreciation of the emotional stress caused by fear of AIDS, especially in persons prone to depression, delusional thinking, or somatization. Treatment should be directed to the underlying diagnosis. Redundant HIV testing should be avoided; however, high-risk persons who have negative test results should refrain from risky behavior and be retested in 6–14 months.
5. Increase pre- and posttest counseling for persons undergoing AIDS antibody screening. Issues such as the meaning of a positive result, advisability of repeat testing, and degree of confidentiality should be addressed.
6. Be aware of the pressure on families and lovers to assist the patient with AIDS in his or her plans for suicide. Frank, open discussion of suicidal thoughts is helpful.
7. Provide patients with a spiritual perspective. Spiritual beliefs are often deterrents to suicide and important components of normal grieving. Pastoral counseling, with the patient's consent, is helpful.
8. Be familiar with community agencies such as crisis hotlines, Narcotics Anonymous, hospice associations, home-visiting nurses, organizations offering psychosocial support services for persons with AIDS and their families, local mental health caregivers, and domiciliaries for HIV-positive individuals.
9. Encourage support groups for family members of patients with AIDS. Loved ones involved in such interactions will realize that their feelings and experiences are not unique.
10. Be aware of the depressant effects of medications and illicit drugs the patient may be taking.
11. Recognize that patients with dementia and delirium are at significant risk for self-harm.

Note. AIDS = acquired immunodeficiency syndrome; HIV = human immunodeficiency virus.
Source. Reprinted from Frierson R, Lippmann S: "Suicide and AIDS." *Psychosomatics* 29:226–231, 1988. Copyright 1988, Academy of Psychosomatic Medicine. Used with permission.

an illness expected to lead to death within 6 months. The requests to the physician must be in the form of one written statement and two oral statements, each of which must be at least 15 days apart. The primary physician and the consultant giving a second opinion must not only agree on capacity, diagnosis, and terminal prognosis but also refer the patient for mental health evaluation if they suspect that depression or some other psychological disorder is affecting the patient's judgment. The primary physician "must also inform the patient of all feasible alternatives, such as comfort care, hospice care, and pain-control options" (Chin et al. 1999, p. 577). Only then can the patient be given a lethal prescription (Chin et al. 1999). Although the Oregon legislation permits PAS under the protection of law, the Oregon situation is far more conservative than the situation in the Netherlands. Euthanasia and PAS are technically illegal in the Netherlands, but both are practiced relatively openly without prosecution (van der Maas et al. 1996). Employing a rationale that has no parallel in the United States, the Supreme Court of the Netherlands even ruled that "unbearable mental suffering can in exceptional cases, justify physician-assisted suicide, even if there is no concurrent medical disease, and that the degree of suffering rather than its cause is decisive" (Groenewoud et al. 1997, p. 1795). Psychiatric patients with nonterminal conditions have been killed.

Although he granted that a request for suicide could be rational, Muskin (1998) advocated a psychodynamic approach to a dialogue between the patient and the physician, a dialogue he believed any such request demands. He saw the query as "an opportunity for patient and physician to more fully understand and know one another" (Muskin 1998, p. 327) and asserted that "every request to die should be subjected to careful scrutiny of its multiple potential meanings" (Muskin 1998, p. 323). Is the patient asking the physician to provide a reason to live? Does the patient harbor revenge fantasies or a wish to kill the split-off sick part of himself or herself, imagining the healthy self will live on once unencumbered with disease? Is the patient driven by inadequately treated pain or depression, by guilt or hopelessness, by feelings of already being dead?

Although the U.S. Supreme Court in its 1997 decisions specifically forbade PAS, it endorsed "requiring states to remove the barriers that their laws and policies impose on the availability of palliative care" (Burt 1997, p. 1236). Alleviating pain and other uncomfortable physical symptoms has assumed top priority, with complicated ethical ramifications. "The Court acknowledged the legal acceptability of providing pain relief, even to the point of hastening death if necessary," wrote Quill and colleagues (1997, p. 2099). Terminal sedation (in which a patient is given narcotics, even to the point of unconsciousness) accompanied by withdrawal or withholding

of life-sustaining therapies (as well as food and water) has become normative end-of-life management.

Some would define the withdrawal or withholding of life-sustaining treatment, an approach that is now firmly grounded in case law, as passive euthanasia (de Wachter 1989). Over the past two decades, courts have gradually broadened the circumstances under which treatment can be withheld, to include not only high technology such as assisted ventilation but also basic needs such as hydration and artificial feeding. Landmark cases such as *In re Quinlan* (1976) have set the precedent for withdrawing treatment from patients who are not brain dead but have irreversible central nervous system injury that consigns them to persistent vegetative states (Wanzer et al. 1989). One investigator wrote that "during the past 15 years we have evolved from situations in which it was a deviation from the medical and ethical standard to withdraw a respirator, nutrition, or intravenous fluid from a non-brain dead patient to the present environment, in which it is accepted practice and becoming the norm to withdraw such medical treatments in certain groups of patients" (Sprung 1990, p. 2214).

Proponents argue that what distinguishes death hastened by aggressive palliative care from death by active euthanasia is the physician's primary intent to relieve suffering rather than to kill. The subject remains controversial. Quill and colleagues (1997) cited the doctrine of double effect, writing: "As long as the physician's intentions are good, it is permissible to perform actions with foreseeable consequences it would be wrong to intend" (p. 2101). Foley (1997), a physician, argued that terminal sedation is grounded in an ethic of caring, not killing: "In the real world in which physicians care for dying patients, withdrawing treatment and aggressively treating pain are acts that respect patients' autonomous decision not to be battered by medical technology and to be relieved of their suffering. The physician's intent is to provide care, not death" (Foley 1997, p. 54).

Critics have failed to accept the distinction the Supreme Court made and Foley defended. According to Orentlicher (1997), a lawyer, "assisted suicide is rejected only by embracing what is essentially euthanasia" (p. 1239). The physicians Billings and Block (1996) agreed, referring to as "ethically problematic" the clinical practice of treating a terminal patient in a fashion that will assuredly lead to a comfortable death, but not too quickly." They termed this practice "slow euthanasia."

Orentlicher's grim pronouncement notwithstanding, an evolution to active euthanasia, as has to some extent already occurred in the Netherlands, has yet to happen anywhere in the United States. In recent years, voters defeated initiatives in California and Washington State, the latter initiative advocating active euthanasia for competent patients. All 50 states outlaw active euthanasia, and the Supreme Court has forbidden PAS.

Many worry that life-terminating choices are being made not by the individual (the patient who is deciding whether his or her life is worth living) but by society— that is, that choices are being made in response to, for example, financial exigencies such as strained health care resources. As an American approach to end-of-life decision-making continues to emerge from competing political, ethical, and financial principles, consultation-liaison psychiatrists will undoubtedly play an important part in its implementation. One role already familiar to psychiatrists, based on evaluating patients who refuse treatment, may be determining the competency of those who request withdrawal of life support. The consultation-liaison psychiatrist will likely be asked whether a psychiatric disorder is clouding the patient's decision. In an examination of 44 terminally ill patients, Brown et al. (1986) noted that only 10 wished for early death; the authors judged all 10 to have severe depression.

Cassem (1991) outlined many factors that must be considered in evaluating a patient who is requesting PAS, potentially life-threatening analgesics, or withdrawal of life support. The attending physician and consulting psychiatrist must each take sufficient time to understand the wishes of the patient. What has the patient pictured his or her clinical course to be? What are his or her values? What notions exist about the end of life? Is the patient clinically depressed? Where does the family stand? Does the family understand the patient's requests, and how is the family affected by them? At what point does the patient specify that the potential for meaning in his or her life has been exhausted? Does the patient fear that he or she will become either a financial burden or a burden to care for, or both? Has any of this been discussed with the family? If the patient considers life devoid of value and meaning for himself or herself, does it have meaning for certain others? Does that affect the patient's thinking? Has the patient made any effort to achieve family consensus so that death could actually be a meaningful shared family experience?

Rather than conforming to regulations formulated to standardize the dying process, the consultation-liaison psychiatrist facilitates an individual's examination of the personal considerations that will help shape a death that is a fitting conclusion to life. In this approach, euthanasia is not the issue. Dying gracefully is.

REFERENCES

Abrams H, Moore GL, Westervelt FB: Suicidal behavior in chronic dialysis patients. Am J Psychiatry 127:1199–1204, 1971

Allebeck P, Bolund C, Ringback F: Increased suicide rate in cancer patients. J Clin Epidemiol 42:611–616, 1985

Babigian HM, Odoroff CL: The mortality experience of a population with psychiatric illness. Am J Psychiatry 126:52–62, 1969

Berger D: Suicide risk in the general hospital. Psychiatry Clin Neurosci 49 (suppl 1):585–589, 1995

Billings JA, Block SD: Slow euthanasia. J Palliat Care 12:21–30, 1996

Blumenthal SJ, Kupfer DJ: Generalizable treatment strategies for suicidal behavior. Ann N Y Acad Sci 487:327–340, 1986

Bostwick JM, Pankratz VS: Affective disorders and suicide risk: a reexaminatin. Am J Psychiatry 157:1925–1932, 2000

Brown J, Henteleff P, Barakat S, et al: Is it normal for terminally ill patients to desire death? Am J Psychiatry 143:208–211, 1986

Buie DH, Maltsberger JT: The psychological vulnerability to suicide, in Suicide: Understanding and Responding. Edited by Jacobs D, Brown HN. Madison, CT, International Universities Press, 1989, pp 59–71

Burt RA: The Supreme Court speaks—not assisted suicide but a constitutional right to palliative care. N Engl J Med 337:1234–1236, 1997

Capodanno AE, Targum SD: Assessment of suicide risk: some limitations in the prediction of infrequent events. Journal of Psychiatric Nursing in Mental Health Services 21:11–14, 1983

Chin AE, Hedberg K, Higginson GK, et al: Legalized physician-assisted suicide in Oregon: the first year's experience. N Engl J Med 340:577–583, 1999

Cote TR, Biggar RJ, Dannenberg AL: Risk of suicide among persons with AIDS: a national assessment. JAMA 268:2066–2068, 1991

Davidson L: Suicide and aggression in the medical setting, in Psychiatric Care of the Medical Patient. Edited by Stoudemire A, Fogel BS. New York, Oxford University Press, 1993, pp 71–86

de Wachter MA: Active euthanasia in the Netherlands. JAMA 262:3316–3319, 1989

Dorwart RA, Chartock L: Suicide: a public health perspective, in Suicide: Understanding and Responding. Edited by Jacobs D, Brown HN. Madison, CT, International Universities Press, 1989, pp 31–55

Egeland JA, Sussex JN: Suicide and family loading for affective disorders. JAMA 254:915–918, 1985

Evenson RC, Wood JB, Nuttall EA, et al: Suicide rates among public mental health patients. Acta Psychiatr Scand 66:254–264, 1982

Farberow NL, Litman RE: Suicide prevention in hospitals, in The Psychology of Suicide. Edited by Shneidman ES, Farberow NL, Litman RE. New York, Science House, 1970, pp 423–458

Farberow N[L], McKelligott JW, Cohen S, et al: Suicide among patients with cardiorespiratory illness. JAMA 195:422–428, 1966

Fava M, Rosenbaum JF: Suicidality and fluoxetine: is there a relationship? J Clin Psychiatry 52:108–111, 1991

Fawcett J, Shaughnessy R (eds): The suicidal patient, in Psychiatry: Diagnosis and Therapy. Edited by Flaherty JA, Channon RA, Davis JM. Norwalk, CT, Appleton & Lange, 1988, pp 49–56

Fawcett J, Scheftner W, Clark D, et al: Clinical predictors of suicide in patients with major affective disorders: a controlled prospective study. Am J Psychiatry 144:35–40, 1987

Fenton WS, McGlashan TH, Victor BJ, et al: Symptoms, subtype, and suicidality in patients with schizophrenia spectrum disorders. Am J Psychiatry 154:199–204, 1997

Foley KM: Competent care for the dying instead of physician-assisted suicide. N Engl J Med 336:54–58, 1997

Fox BH, Stanek EJ, Boyd SC, et al: Suicide rates among cancer patients in Connecticut. Journal of Chronic Disease 35:89–100, 1982

Frierson R, Lippman S: Suicide and AIDS. Psychosomatics 29:226–231, 1988

Furst S, Ostow M: The psychodynamics of suicide, in Suicide: Theory and Clinical Aspects. Edited by Hankoff LD, Einsidler B. Littleton, MA, PSG Publishing, 1979, pp 165–178

Gabbard GO: Affective disorders, in Psychodynamic Psychiatry in Clinical Practice. Washington, DC, American Psychiatric Press, 1990, pp 177–198

Glickman LS: The suicidal patient, in Psychiatric Consultation in the General Hospital. New York, Marcel Dekker, 1980, pp 181–202

Goldberg RJ: The assessment of suicide risk in the general hospital. Gen Hosp Psychiatry 9:446–452, 1987

Groenewoud JH, van der Maas PJ, van der Wal G, et al: Physician-assisted death in psychiatric practice in the Netherlands. N Engl J Med 336:1795–1801, 1997

Gutheil TG, Appelbaum PS: Legal issues in emergency psychiatry, in Clinical Handbook of Psychiatry and the Law, 3rd Edition. Philadelphia, PA, Lippincott Williams & Wilkins, 200, pp 39–82

Hackett TP, Stern TA: Suicide and other disruptive states, in The Massachusetts General Hospital Handbook of General Hospital Psychiatry, 3rd Edition. Edited by Cassem NH. St. Louis, MO, Mosby–Year Book, 1991, pp 281–307

Haenel T, Brunner F, Battegay R: Renal dialysis and suicide: occurrence in Switzerland and Europe. Compr Psychiatry 21:140–145, 1980

Havens L: Recognition of suicidal risk through the psychological examination. N Engl J Med 276:211–215, 1967

Hawton K: Suicide and attempted suicide, in Handbook of Affective Disorders, 2nd Edition. Edited by Paykel ES. New York, Guilford, 1992, pp 635–650

Hofmann D, Dubovsky S: Depression and suicide assessment. Emerg Med Clin North Am 9:107–121, 1991

In re Quinlan, 70 NJ 10, 355 A2d 657, cert denied, 429 US 922 (1976)

Johnson J, Weissman MM, Klerman GL: Panic disorder, comorbidity, and suicide attempts. Arch Gen Psychiatry 47:805–808, 1990

Kaplan A, Klein R: Women and suicide, in Suicide: Understanding and Responding. Edited by Jacobs D, Brown HN. Madison, CT, International Universities Press, 1989, pp 257–282

Kellner CH, Best CL, Roberts JM, et al: Self-destructive behavior in hospitalized medical and surgical patients. Psychiatr Clin North Am 8:279–289, 1985

Kizer KW, Green M, Perkins CI, et al: AIDS and suicide in California (letter). JAMA 260:1881, 1988

Klerman GL: Clinical epidemiology of suicide. J Clin Psychiatry 48 (suppl):33–38, 1987

Kontaxakis VP, Christodoulou GN, Mavreas VG, et al: Attempted suicide in psychiatric outpatients with concurrent physical illness. Psychother Psychosom 50:201–206, 1988

Litman RE: Suicides: what do they have in mind? in Suicide: Understanding and Responding. Edited by Jacobs D, Brown HN. Madison, CT, International Universities Press, 1989, pp 143–154

Lloyd GG: Suicide in hospitals: guidelines for prevention. J R Soc Med 88:344P–346P, 1995

Luohivuori K, Hakama M: Risk of suicide among cancer patients. Am J Epidemiol 109:59–65, 1979

Maltsberger JT, Buie DH: Countertransference hate in the treatment of suicidal patients. Arch Gen Psychiatry 30:625–633, 1974

Mann JJ: Psychobiologic predictors of suicide. J Clin Psychiatry 48 (suppl):39–43, 1987

Mann JJ: The neurobiology of suicide. Nat Medicine 4:25–30, 1998

Marzuk P, Tierney H, Tardiff K, et al: Increased risk of suicide in AIDS. JAMA 259:1333–1337, 1988

Miles CP: Conditions predisposing to suicide: a review. J Nerv Ment Dis 164:231–246, 1977

Monk M: Epidemiology of suicide. Epidemiol Rev 9:51–69, 1987

Morgan AC: Special issues of assessment and treatment of suicide risk in the elderly, in Suicide: Understanding and Responding. Edited by Jacobs D, Brown HN. Madison, CT, International Universities Press, 1989, pp 239–255

Morgan HG, Priest P: Suicide and other unexpected deaths among psychiatric inpatients. Br J Psychiatry 158:368–374, 1991

Motto JA: Problems in suicide risk assessment, in Suicide: Understanding and Responding. Edited by Jacobs D, Brown HN. Madison, CT, International Universities Press, 1989, pp 129–142

Murphy GE: On suicide prediction and prevention. Arch Gen Psychiatry 40:343–344, 1983

Murphy GE: Recognizing the alcoholic at risk for suicide. Lifesavers: Newsletter of the American Suicide Foundation 4:3, 1992

Murphy GE, Weitzel RD: The lifetime risk of suicide in alcoholism. Arch Gen Psychiatry 47:383–392, 1990

Muskin PR: The request to die: role for a psychodynamic perspective on physician-assisted suicide. JAMA 279:323–328, 1998

Neu S, Kjellstrand CM: Stopping long-term dialysis: an empirical study of withdrawal of life-supporting treatment. N Engl J Med 314:14–20, 1986

Orentlicher D: The Supreme Court and physician-assisted suicide: rejecting assisted suicide but embracing euthanasia. N Engl J Med 337:1236–1239, 1997

Patterson WM, Dohn HH, Bird J, et al: Evaluation of suicidal patients: the SAD PERSONS Scale. Psychosomatics 24:343–349, 1983

Pisetsky JE, Brown W: The general hospital patient, in Suicide: Theory and Clinical Aspects. Edited by Hankoff LD, Einsidler B. Littleton, MA, PSG Publishing, 1979, pp 279–290

Pokorny AD: Prediction of suicide in psychiatric patients: report of a prospective study. Arch Gen Psychiatry 40:249–257, 1983

Pollack S: Suicide in a general hospital, in The Psychology of Suicide. Edited by Shneidman ES, Farberow NL. New York, McGraw-Hill, 1957, pp 152–176

Quill TE, Lo B, Brock DW: Palliative options of last resort: a comparison of voluntarily stopping eating and drinking, terminal sedation, physician-assisted suicide, and voluntary active euthanasia. JAMA 278:2099–2104, 1997

Reich P, Kelly MJ: Suicide attempts by hospitalized medical and surgical patients. N Engl J Med 294:298–301, 1976

Rowland L: Assisted suicide and alternatives in amyotrophic lateral sclerosis. N Engl J Med 339:987–989, 1998

Roy A: Family history of suicide. Arch Gen Psychiatry 40:971–974, 1983

Roy A: Suicide: a multi-determined act. Psychiatr Clin North Am 8:243–250, 1985

Roy A: Emergency psychiatry: suicide, in Comprehensive Textbook of Psychiatry/V, 5th Edition. Edited by Kaplan HI, Sadock BJ. Baltimore, MD, Williams and Wilkins, 1989, pp 1414–1427

Rundell JR, Kyle KM, Brown GR, et al: Risk factors for suicide attempts in a human immunodeficiency virus screening program. Psychosomatics 33:24–27, 1992

Sanders R: Suicidal behavior in critical care medicine: conceptual issues and management strategies, in Problems in Critical Care Medicine. Edited by Wise MG. Philadelphia, PA, JB Lippincott, 1988, pp 116–133

Scully JH, Hutcherson R: Suicide by burning. Am J Psychiatry 140:905–909, 1983

Shah AK, Ganesvaran T: Inpatient suicides in an Australian mental hospital. Aust N Z J Psychiatry 31:291–298, 1997

Shershow JC: The sometimes science of suicidology. N Engl J Med 294:332–333, 1976

Shneidman ES: Overview: a multidimensional approach to suicide, in Suicide: Understanding and Responding. Edited by Jacobs D, Brown HN. Madison, CT, International Universities Press, 1989, pp 1–30

Simon GE, VonKorff M: Suicide mortality among patients treated for depression in an insured population. Am J Epidemiol 147:155–160, 1998

Siomopoulos V: When patients consider suicide: risk factors to watch for. Postgrad Med 88:205–206, 209, 212–213, 1990

Sprung CL: Changing attitudes and practices in forgoing life-sustaining treatments. JAMA 263:2211–2215, 1990

Stanley M, Stanley B: Biochemical studies in suicide victims: current findings and future implications. Suicide Life Threat Behav 19:30–42, 1989

Teicher MH, Glod C, Cole JO: Emergence of intense suicidal preoccupation during fluoxetine treatment. Am J Psychiatry 147:207–210, 1990

Tsuang MT, Simpson JC: Mortality studies in psychiatry. Arch Gen Psychiatry 42:98–103, 1984

van der Maas PJ, van der Wal G, Haverkate I, et al: Euthanasia, physician-assisted suicide, and other medical practices involving the end of life in the Netherlands, 1990–1995. N Engl J Med 335:1699–1705, 1996

Ventura SJ, Anderson RN, Martin JA, et al: Births and deaths: preliminary data for 1997. Natl Vital Stat Rep 47:1–41, 1998

Wanzer SH, Federman DL, Adelstein SJ, et al: The physician's responsibility toward hopelessly ill patients. N Engl J Med 320:844–849, 1989

Warshaw MG, Keller MB: The relationship between fluoxetine use and suicidal behavior in 654 subjects with anxiety disorders. J Clin Psychiatry 57:158–166, 1996

White RT, Gribble RJ, Corr MJ, et al: Jumping from a general hospital. Gen Hosp Psychiatry 17:208–215, 1995

Wise MG, Rundell JR: Suicidality and aggression, in the Concise Guide to Consultation Psychiatry, 2nd Edition. Washington, DC, American Psychiatric Press, 1994, pp 211–224

Yufit RI: American Association of Suicidology Presidential Address: suicide assessment in the 1990's. Suicide Life Threat Behav 21:152–163, 1991

10

Aggression and Agitation

Robert E. Hales, M.D., M.B.A.

Jonathan M. Silver, M.D.

Stuart C. Yudofsky, M.D.

Mark E. Servis, M.D.

Donald M. Hilty, M.D.

Consultation-liaison psychiatrists are frequently called on to assess and treat patients with aggression. Overall, approximately 10% of patients admitted to psychiatric units in general hospitals exhibit violence toward others just before admission (Tardiff and Swelliam 1982). Among patients with neuropsychiatric disorders—such as those with posttraumatic brain injury, delirium, Alzheimer's disease, human immunodeficiency virus infection–related dementia, or other dementias—the prevalence of agitation and aggression is much higher than among hospitalized patients with chronic psychiatric disorders (Elliott 1992; Hales et al. 1999). For example, Reisberg and co-workers (1987) reported that 48% of a sample of outpatients with Alzheimer's disease exhibited agitation, 30% exhibited violent behavior, and 24% exhibited verbal outbursts. The most common behavioral problems in a sample of 65 nursing home residents were agitation and aggression, which affected 48% of the sample (Chandler and Chandler 1988).

The consultation-liaison psychiatrist who is asked to evaluate a brain-injured patient should note that aggression is highly prevalent in both the acute and chronic recovery stages (Silver and Yudofsky 1994a). For instance, in one study, 96% of 26 patients were acutely agitated after traumatic brain injury (Rao et al. 1985). In a prospective study in which the Overt Aggression Scale (OAS) (Yudofsky et al. 1986) was used, 11% of 100 patients who experienced acute brain injury were aggressive and agitated, and 35% were restless (Brooke et al.

1992a). Like posttraumatic seizure disorders, aggression may occur in patients months to many years after head injury. Of 44 patients followed for 7 years after severe traumatic brain injury, 31% exhibited agitation and an additional 43% displayed severe irritability, temper outbursts, and aggression (Oddy et al. 1985). The high prevalence of aggression and violence among psychiatric patients is reflected in reports of assaults against psychiatrists and other physicians by patients. Approximately 40% of psychiatrists report being attacked at least once during their careers, and 48% of psychiatric residents acknowledge that they were assaulted at least once during residency training (Tardiff and Swelliam 1982). In Veterans Administration hospitals, 12,000 assaultive incidents were reported over a 5-year period (Lion and Reid 1983). Aggression among psychiatric patients exacts an even greater toll on the family members and other primary caregivers than it does on mental health professionals. In a study of the families and primary caregivers of 55 patients with dementia, the most serious problem faced by the families was the patient's aggressive behavior, which occurred regularly in 28 of the 55 families (Rabins et al. 1982).

The consultation-liaison psychiatrist who works in a general hospital setting often encounters elderly patients whose rageful affects and aggressive behaviors precipitated referral for assessment and management. However, a significant percentage of elderly patients with agitation and aggression are not referred to consultation psychiatrists but are sent to nursing homes or other restrictive institutional environments. Appropriate diagnosis and treatment of the medical disorders underlying aggression (such as delirium secondary to treatment with anticholinergic agents) in addition to the enlightened pharmacological management of aggressive symptoms (such as the use of β-blockers to treat aggression associated with Alzheimer's disease) may help many of these elderly patients. Psychiatrists are far better trained in assessing and treating people who direct aggression toward themselves (suicidal individuals) than in assessing and treating those who are aggressive toward others (violent and homicidal individuals). Given the approximately 30,000 recorded suicides and 22,000–24,000 homicides in the United States each year (Malmquist 1996; Reid et al. 1985), there is great potential for improved preventive and interventional strategies for patients with either type of aggression. In this chapter, we review diagnostic and pathophysiological aspects of aggression and outline a pharmacological treatment approach to aggression for the consultation-liaison psychiatrist.

DIAGNOSIS

Agitation is nearly universally considered a symptom that is the result of a primary medical disorder, whereas aggressive symptoms are assessed in an unusually broad and disparate fashion. Aggressive behavior is sometimes described as a symptom or as the central aspect of a distinct disorder. The DSM-IV-TR (American Psychiatric Association 2000) classification of primary aggressive disorders consists of two diagnoses: intermittent explosive disorder (Table 10–1) and personality change due to a general medical condition, aggressive type (Table 10–2). However, personality change due to a general medical condition, aggressive type, remains a catchall diagnosis that is overinclusive and indiscriminate with regard to the number and types of associated symptoms and does not describe the kinds of dyscontrol due to brain lesions (Silver and Yudofsky 1987a; Silver et al. 1997; Yudofsky et al. 1989). Therefore, we propose an alternative diagnostic category—neuroaggressive disorder (Table 10–3)—to describe the condition of dyscontrol or rage and violence secondary to brain lesions (Ghosh and Victor 1999; Yudofsky et al. 1990).

In animal models, when brain lesions are made in specific brain regions, the animals exhibit increased aggression in response to irritating stimuli (Eichelman 1971; Leavitt et al. 1989) but otherwise behave normally. Furthermore, in reviewing the literature on intermittent explosive disorder for DSM-IV, Wise and Tierney

TABLE 10–1. DSM-IV-TR diagnostic criteria for intermittent explosive disorder

A. Several discrete episodes of failure to resist aggressive impulses that result in serious assaultive acts or destruction of property.
B. The degree of aggressiveness expressed during the episodes is grossly out of proportion to any precipitating psychosocial stressors.
C. The aggressive episodes are not better accounted for by another mental disorder (e.g., antisocial personality disorder, borderline personality disorder, a psychotic disorder, a manic episode, conduct disorder, or attention-deficit/hyperactivity disorder) and are not due to the direct physiological effects of a substance (e.g., a drug of abuse, a medication) or a general medical condition (e.g., head trauma, Alzheimer's disease).

(1999), as well as Hales (1996), have questioned whether the diagnosis, which has so many exclusionary diagnoses, actually exists. According to DSM-IV, this diagnosis does *not* apply if the episodes of aggression are better accounted for by another mental disorder or are due to the direct physiological effects of a substance or a general medical condition. These exclusions are so broad that rarely, if ever, will one encounter a patient who meets criteria for intermittent explosive disorder. Elliott (1976) found that 95% of 286 patients with a history of recurrent uncontrolled rage attacks associated with little or no provocation had objective evidence of developmental or acquired brain deficits. Thus, the nosological imprecision of DSM-IV will continue to contribute to the pervasive failure of clinicians to diagnose and, consequently, to treat aggression in all patients.

Much more attention has been devoted to the neurobiology, neuropathology, and brain pathways involved in aggression than to those involved in agitation (Ovsiew and Yudofsky 1993). Neuropathological details of aggression are included in Table 10–4.

Agitation and aggression most often occur as a result of a variety of neuropsychiatric conditions. Aggressive symptoms are often not considered part of a diagnosed condition and may not be treated at all or may be treated with medications that do not have antiaggressive properties. Alzheimer's disease, for example, should not be considered merely a disorder of memory and cognition; agitation, depression, and anxiety should be recognized as among the most disabling aspects of the disorder. Similarly, Parkinson's disease is primarily considered a movement disorder, but it is well documented that depression, delirium, and dementia occur concomitantly. Because schizophrenia is often considered a psychotic disorder, symptoms of depression and aggression are usually

TABLE 10–2. DSM-IV-TR diagnostic criteria for personality change due to a general medical condition

A. A persistent personality disturbance that represents a change from the individual's previous characteristic personality pattern. (In children, the disturbance involves a marked deviation from normal development or a significant change in the child's usual behavior patterns lasting at least 1 year).

B. There is evidence from the history, physical examination, or laboratory findings that the disturbance is the direct physiological consequence of a general medical condition.

C. The disturbance is not better accounted for by another mental disorder (including other mental disorders due to a general medical condition).

D. The disturbance does not occur exclusively during the course of a delirium.

E. The disturbance causes clinically significant distress or impairment in social, occupational, or other important areas of functioning.

Specify type:

Labile Type: if the predominant feature is affective lability

Disinhibited Type: if the predominant feature is poor impulse control as evidenced by sexual indiscretions, etc.

Aggressive Type: if the predominant feature is aggressive behavior

Apathetic Type: if the predominant feature is marked apathy and indifference

Paranoid Type: if the predominant feature is suspiciousness or paranoid ideation

Other Type: if the presentation is not characterized by any of the above subtypes

Combined Type: if more than one feature predominates in the clinical picture

Unspecified Type

Coding note: Include the name of the general medical condition on Axis I, e.g., 310.1 Personality Change Due to Temporal Lobe Epilepsy; also code the general medical condition on Axis III (see Appendix G for codes).

TABLE 10–3. Diagnostic criteria for proposed neuroaggressive disorder

Persistent or recurrent aggressive outbursts, whether of a verbal or physical nature.

The outbursts are out of proportion to the precipitating stress or provocation.

Evidence from history, physical examination, or laboratory tests of a specific organic factor that is judged to be etiologically related to the disturbance.

The outbursts are not primarily related to the following disorders: paranoia, mania, schizophrenia, narcissistic personality disorder, borderline personality disorder, antisocial personality disorder, or conduct disorder.

Source. Reprinted from Yudofsky SC, Silver J, Yudofsky B: "Organic Personality Disorder, Explosive Type," in *Treatments of Psychiatric Disorders: A Task Force Report of the American Psychiatric Association,* Vol 2. Washington, DC, American Psychiatric Association, 1989, pp. 839–852. Copyright 1989, American Psychiatric Association. Used with permission.

TABLE 10–4. Neuropathology of aggression

Locus	Activity
Hypothalamus	Orchestrates neuroendocrine response via sympathetic arousal
	Monitors and regulates somatic status
Limbic system	
Amygdala	Activates and/or suppresses hypothalamus
	Receives input from neocortex
Temporal cortex	Associated with aggression in both ictal and interictal states; associated with experiential memory for pain and danger
Frontal neocortex	Modulates limbic and hypothalamic states
	Associated with social and judgment aspects of aggression

Source. Adapted from Silver JM, Hales RE, Yudofsky SC: "Neuropsychiatric Aspects of Traumatic Brain Injury," in *The American Psychiatric Press Textbook of Neuropsychiatry,* 2nd Edition. Edited by Yudofsky SC, Hales RE. Washington, DC, American Psychiatric Press, 1997, pp. 363–395. Copyright 1997, American Psychiatric Press. Used with permission.

untreated or mistreated; specifically, neuroleptics are used to treat agitation and aggression that do not stem from psychotic ideation. As a result, patients are oversedated and are unnecessarily placed at risk for numerous other side effects associated with neuroleptic drugs, including tardive dyskinesia and potentially fatal neuroleptic malignant syndrome. In all these cases, accurate classification would aid the clinician in determining specific and effective treatment.

Although several rating scales are available to measure agitation, no existing rating scale is adequate to document and monitor the responses of agitation to intervention. One major problem is that most currently used rating scales blur the boundaries between anxiety, agitation, and aggression; they also depend too heavily on inferences made by the rater.

In the next section of this chapter, we review two rating scales: the Overt Aggression Scale (OAS) (Yudofsky et al. 1986) (Figure 10–1), which encompasses the definition, diagnosis, and treatment of aggression; and the Overt Agitation Severity Scale (OASS) (Kopecky et al. 1998; Yudofsky et al. 1997) (Figure 10–2). These two scales help clinicians differentiate aggression from agitation. Anxiety and neuropsychiatric syndromes or side effects from medication, such as akathisia secondary to neuroleptic therapy, also require differentiation from aggression. Clinicians who confuse akathisia with aggression may increase the neuroleptic dose. Apart from producing increased sedation, the increase in neuroleptic medication ultimately will aggravate the akathisia and may result in a cycle of ever-increasing doses and worsening akathisia.

DOCUMENTATION OF AGGRESSION

Accurate documentation of aggressive episodes is critical to assess the effectiveness of interventions and to conduct outcome research. To assess the effects of pharmacological agents in the treatment of aggressive behaviors, consultation-liaison psychiatrists can use the OAS to document and measure specific aspects of aggressive behavior (Silver and Yudofsky 1991; Yudofsky et al. 1986). The OAS divides aggressive behaviors into four categories: 1) verbal aggression, 2) physical aggression against objects, 3) physical aggression against self, and 4) physical aggression against others. Within each category, descriptive statements define and numerical scores rate four levels of severity. All behaviors exhibited by the patient during an aggressive episode are checked off by an observer (such as a nurse or a family member). Therapeutic interventions used in response to these aggressive episodes are also listed, rated on the OAS, and checked off by the rater. These interventions are documented because they may reflect the observer's interpretation of the severity of the aggressive behaviors. Consulting psychiatrists may want to use the OAS to establish a baseline score for aggression before initiating psychopharmacological intervention and thereafter to document the efficacy, or lack thereof, of any therapeutic intervention.

Each type of aggression and behavior is accorded a weighted score (Table 10–5). Verbal aggression is scored 1–4; physical aggression against objects, 2–5; and physical aggression against self or others, 3–6. We believe that weighing the different categories of behavior as multiples (i.e., weighing physical aggression against objects as twice that of verbal aggression, and weighing physical aggression against others as three or four times that of verbal aggression) would render verbal aggression insignificant and overly weight a single episode of physical aggression. Each type of intervention is also accorded a weighted score from 1 to 5.

Our research, an evaluation of more than 5,000 episodes of aggression in chronically hospitalized psychiatric inpatients, demonstrated that hospital records and other documentation did not include descriptions of the majority of aggressive behaviors that occurred; however, the simultaneous use of the OAS ensured that a significantly greater percentage of aggressive episodes and behaviors were documented (Silver and Yudofsky 1987b).

The documentation of aggression is essential to organize and maintain a treatment plan. For example, the psychiatrist is sometimes consulted by other physicians or family members who contend that prescribed psychopharmacological medication has "stopped working." In these circumstances, the physicians and family members are typically so alarmed by a single episode of violence and its implications that they demand substantial revisions in the treatment plan. In a significant percentage of these patients, the pharmacological agent is at least partially effective; however, for a variety of reasons (e.g., increased stress, significant environmental changes, poor compliance with drug therapy, or concomitant use of alcohol), the aggression has "broken through." The OAS often demonstrates to patients, families, and caregivers that a pharmacological intervention is effective (e.g., it might show that the number of aggressive events has decreased by 80% and the intensity of the events has diminished by 94%). This information may obviate a potentially deleterious overreaction to an aggressive event by caregivers and the discontinuation of an effective pharmacological regimen.

DOCUMENTATION OF AGITATION

The Overt Agitation Severity Scale (OASS) (Kopecky et al. 1998; Yudofsky et al. 1997) includes 47 observable characteristics of agitation that are subcategorized into 12 behaviorally related units. The characteristics were identified as representative of agitation from the clinical and theoretical literature. To make the scale easier to use, characteristics are further grouped into vocalizations and oral or facial movements; upper torso and upper extremity movements; and lower extremity movements.

Each behavioral subgroup is rated with a Likert-type frequency score between 1 (mild signs) and 4 (very severe signs). For each subgroup, a corresponding 5-point Likert-type frequency score between 0 (behavior not present) and 4 (behavior always present) is selected by the rater. The total OASS score is obtained by multiplying each item's frequency response by a weight that corresponds to the intensity of the symptom being measured. The total of the weighted responses indicates the severity of agitation. For patients with neuromuscular

OVERT AGGRESSION SCALE (OAS)

Stuart Yudofsky, M.D., Jonathan Silver, M.D., Wynn Jackson, M.D., and Jean Endicott, Ph.D.

IDENTIFYING DATA

Name of Patient	Name of Rater
Sex of Patient: 1 Male 2 Female	Date / / (month/day/year) Shift: 1 Night 2 Day 3 Evening

❏ No aggressive incidents (verbal or physical) against self, others, or objects during the shift. (check here)

AGGRESSIVE BEHAVIOR (check all that apply)

VERBAL AGGRESSION	PHYSICAL AGGRESSION AGAINST SELF
❏ Makes loud noises, shouts angrily	❏ Picks or scratches skin, hits self, pulls hair (with no or minor injury only)
❏ Yells mild personal insults (e.g., "You're stupid!")	❏ Bangs head, hits fist into objects, throws self onto floor or into objects (hurts self without serious injury)
❏ Curses viciously, uses foul language in anger, makes moderate threats to others or self	❏ Small cuts or bruises, minor burns
❏ Makes clear threats of violence toward others or self (e.g., "I'm going to kill you") or requests to help to control self	❏ Mutilates self, makes deep cuts, bites that bleed, internal injury, fracture, loss of consciousness, loss of teeth

PHYSICAL AGGRESSION AGAINST OBJECTS	PHYSICAL AGGRESSION AGAINST OTHER PEOPLE
❏ Slams door, scatters clothing, makes a mess	❏ Makes threatening gesture, swings at people, grabs at clothes
❏ Throws objects down, kicks furniture without breaking it, marks the wall	❏ Strikes, kicks, pushes, pulls hair (without injury to them)
❏ Breaks objects, smashes windows	❏ Attacks others causing mild–moderate physical injury (bruises, sprains, welts)
❏ Sets fires, throws objects dangerously	❏ Attacks others causing severe physical injury (broken bones, deep lacerations, internal injury)

Time incident began: ____:____ A.M./P.M.	Duration of incident: ____:____ (hours/minutes)

INTERVENTION (check all that apply)

❏ None	❏ Immediate medication given by mouth	❏ Use of restraints
❏ Talking to patient	❏ Immediate medication given by injection	❏ Injury requires immediate medical treatment for patient
❏ Closer observation	❏ Isolation without seclusion (time-out)	❏ Injury requires immediate treatment for another person
❏ Holding patient	❏ Seclusion	

COMMENTS

FIGURE 10–1. Overt Aggression Scale.

Source. Reprinted from Yudofsky SC, Silver JM, Jackson M, et al: "The Overt Aggression Scale: An Operationalized Rating Scale for Verbal and Physical Aggression." *American Journal of Psychiatry* 143:35–39, 1986. Used with permission.

Overt Agitation Severity Scale (OASS)

Intensity (I)	Behavior	Frequency					Severity score (SS) (I x F = SS)
		Not present	Rarely	Some of the time	Most of the time	Always present	
A	**Vocalizations and oral/facial movements**						
1	Whimpering, whining, moaning, grunting, crying	0	1	2	3	4	= _____
2	Smacking or licking of lips, chewing, clenching jaws, licking, grimacing, spitting	0	1	2	3	4	= _____
3	Rocking, twisting, banging of head	0	1	2	3	4	= _____
4	Vocal perseverating, screaming, cursing, threatening, wailing	0	1	2	3	4	= _____
B	**Upper torso and upper extremity movements**						
1	Tapping fingers, fidgeting, wringing of hands, swinging or flailing arms	0	1	2	3	4	= _____
2	Task perseverating (e.g., opening and closing drawers, folding and unfolding clothes, picking at objects, clothes, or self)	0	1	2	3	4	= _____
3	Rocking (back and forth), bobbing (up and down), twisting or writhing of torso, rubbing or masturbating self	0	1	2	3	4	= _____
4	Slapping, swatting, hitting at objects or others	0	1	2	3	4	= _____
C	**Lower extremity movements**						
1	Tapping toes, clenching toes, tapping heel, extending, flexing, or twisting foot	0	1	2	3	4	= _____
2	Shaking legs, tapping knees and/or thighs, thrusting pelvis, stomping	0	1	2	3	4	= _____
3	Pacing, wandering	0	1	2	3	4	= _____
4	Thrashing legs, kicking at objects or others	0	1	2	3	4	= _____

Total OASS   = _____
Subtract baseline OASS   = _____
Revised OASS   = _____

Instructions for Completing Form

Step one: For each behavior, circle the corresponding frequency.

Step two: For every behavior *exhibited*, multiply the intensity score (I) by the frequency (F) and record as the severity score (SS).

Step three: For the Overt Agitation Severity Score (OASS), total all severity scores and record as total OASS.

Step four: Does this patient have a neuromuscular disorder (i.e., Parkinson's disease, tardive dyskinesia) affecting total OASS?
             Yes   No

Step five: If yes, please establish a baseline OASS in nonagitated state and subtract from above total OASS for revised OASS.

Comments: _____

Diagnosis: _____   Name of rater: _____

Sex of patient: Male (1)   Female (2)   Time of observation: _____

Age: _____   Date: _____

Current medication:

Name: Dose: Frequency:
Name: Dose: Frequency:
Name: Dose: Frequency:
Name: Dose: Frequency:

FIGURE 10–2.   Overt Agitation Severity Scale.

Source.   Reprinted from Yudofsky SC, Kopecky HJ, Kunik M, et al: "The Overt Agitation Severity Scale for the Objective Rating of Agitation." *Journal of Neuropsychiatry and Clinical Neurosciences* 9:541–548, 1997. Copyright 1997, American Psychiatric Press. Used with permission.

TABLE 10–5. Weighted scores for aggressive behaviors and interventions for the Overt Aggression Scale

Behavior	Weighted score
Verbal aggression	
Makes loud noises, shouts angrily	1
Yells mild personal insults (e.g., "You're stupid!")	2
Curses viciously, uses foul language in anger, makes moderate threats to others or self	3
Makes clear threats of violence toward others or self (e.g., "I'm going to kill you"), or requests help to control self	4
Physical aggression against objects	
Slams door, scatters clothing, makes a mess	2
Throws objects down, kicks furniture without breaking it, marks the wall	3
Breaks objects, smashes windows	4
Sets fires, throws objects dangerously	5
Physical aggression against self	
Picks or scratches skin, hits self on arms or body, pinches self, pulls hair (without injury or with only minor injury)	3
Bangs head, hits fist into objects, throws self onto floor or into objects (hurts self without serious injury)	4
Small cuts or bruises, minor burns	5
Mutilates self, makes deep cuts, bites that bleed, internal injury, fracture, loss of consciousness, loss of teeth	6
Physical aggression against other people	
Makes threatening gestures, swings at people, grabs at clothes	3
Strikes, kicks, pushes, pulls hair (without injury to them)	4
Attacks others, causing mild to moderate physical injury (bruises, sprains, welts)	5
Attacks others, causing severe physical injury (broken bones, deep lacerations, internal injury)	6
Interventions	
Talking to patient	1
Closer observation	2
Holding patient	3
Isolation without seclusion (time-out)	3
Immediate medication given by mouth	4
Immediate medication given by injection	4
Seclusion	5
Use of restraints	5

disorders (e.g., Parkinson's disease, akathisia, or tardive dyskinesia), in which impaired motor activity can mimic agitation, a baseline nonagitated OASS score is obtained and subtracted from the score obtained during an agitated state.

Consulting psychiatrists may find it useful to obtain a baseline OASS score for agitation before treatment with psychopharmacological agents and then to obtain more scores during treatment to determine the efficacy of that treatment.

NEUROTRANSMITTERS AND AGITATION AND AGGRESSION

Multiple neurotransmitters and neurotransmitter systems mediate aggression. Serotonin, norepinephrine, dopamine, acetylcholine, and γ-aminobutyric acid (GABA) all play important roles. In neuropsychiatric disorders, it is the rule rather than the exception that multiple neurotransmitter systems are involved simultaneously in regions of the brain. In addition, as we have learned about the roles of neurotransmitters in depression, it is likely that neurotransmitters interface with one another to influence aggression. Norepinephrine originates in the locus coeruleus in the lateral tegmental system and follows a course to the forebrain. Damage to the frontal and temporal lobes of the forebrain is frequently associated with rage and violent behavior. β_1-Adrenergic receptors are localized in this region (limbic forebrain and cerebral cortex) and are implicated in the mediation of aggressive behavior (Alexander et al. 1979).

Animal studies have suggested that norepinephrine is involved in many aspects of aggressive behavior, including sham rage, affective aggression, and shock-induced fighting (Eichelman 1987). Other studies documented an association between aggression and cerebrospinal fluid norepinephrine in free-ranging rhesus monkeys (Higley et al. 1992), whereas some investigators reported that humans who exhibit aggressive or impulsive behavior have increased levels of the norepinephrine metabolite 3-methoxy-4-hydroxyphenylglycol (MHPG) (Brown et al. 1979; Victoroff et al. 1996).

Serotonergic neurons originate in the raphe, are located in the pons and upper brain stem, and project to the frontal cortex. Lower levels of serotonergic activity have been found to be associated with increased aggression in a variety of studies, including studies of predatory aggression and shock-induced fighting in rats (Eichelman 1987). Clinical studies have implicated the role of lowered serotonin levels in the central nervous system in the expression of aggression and impulsivity in humans, particularly violent self-destructive acts (Kavoussi et al. 1997; Kruesi et al. 1992; Linnoila and Virkkunen 1992).

Dopamine systems are prominent in both mesolimbic and mesocortical regions of the brain. There is indirect evidence that elevated brain dopamine levels—particularly as a result of the release of dopamine after development of brain lesions—lead, in animal models and in humans, to increased aggression (Bareggi et al. 1975; Hamill et al. 1987). The profound increase in aggressive behavior after severe traumatic brain injury is closely associated with subsequent changes in dopaminergic systems (Eichelman et al. 1972).

DIFFERENTIAL DIAGNOSIS

As with other symptoms or disorders in medicine and psychiatry, proper diagnosis is crucial. A good history is a critical part of the evaluation because many psychiatric disorders are associated with violent behavior (Table 10–6).

TABLE 10–6. DSM-IV diagnoses associated with violent behavior

Violent behavior as an essential feature
Intermittent explosive disorder
Conduct disorder
Oppositional defiant disorder
Antisocial personality disorder
Borderline personality disorder
Sexual sadism

Violent behavior as an associated feature
Substance-related disorders
Delirium, dementia, and other cognitive disorders
Mental retardation
Attention-deficit/hyperactivity disorder
Brief psychotic disorder
Schizoaffective disorder
Delusional disorder
Bipolar disorder
Posttraumatic stress disorder

Violent behavior as an infrequent feature
Atypical psychosis
Major depressive disorder
Dysthymic disorder
Cyclothymic disorder
Atypical depression
Paranoid personality disorder
Histrionic personality disorder
Schizoid personality disorder
Schizotypal personality disorder
Dissociative fugue
Adjustment disorder with disturbance of conduct

Source. Adapted from Reid WH, Balis GU: "Evaluation of the Violent Patient," in *Psychiatry Update: The American Psychiatric Association Annual Review*, Vol 6. Edited by Hales RE, Frances AJ. Washington, DC, American Psychiatric Press, 1987, pp. 491–509. Used with permission.

Organic brain disorders are strongly associated with agitation and aggression. Common etiologies of neurologically induced agitation and aggression are summarized in Table 10–7, and medications associated with agitation and aggression are reviewed in Table 10–8. Clinical features that alert the consultation-liaison psychiatrist to the potential presence of neurologically induced agitation or aggression are summarized in Table 10–9.

TABLE 10–7. Common etiologies of neurologically induced agitation and aggression

Alzheimer's disease
Brain tumors
Chronic neurological disorders (e.g., Huntington's disease, Wilson's disease, Parkinson's disease, multiple sclerosis, systemic lupus erythematosus)
Delirium (e.g., hypoxia, electrolyte imbalance, anesthesia and surgery, uremia)
Epilepsy (ictal, postictal, and interictal)
Infectious diseases (e.g., encephalitis, meningitis, acquired immunodeficiency syndrome)
Medications and drugs (see Table 10–8)
Metabolic disorders (e.g., hyperthyroidism or hypothyroidism, hypoglycemia, vitamin deficiencies, porphyria)
Stroke and other cerebrovascular disease
Traumatic brain injury

Source. Adapted from Yudofsky SC, Silver JM, Hales RE: "Pharmacologic Management of Aggression in the Elderly." *Journal of Clinical Psychiatry* 51 (suppl):22–28, 1990. Copyright 1990, Physicians Postgraduate Press. Used with permission.

TABLE 10–8. Drugs associated with agitation and aggression

Type of drug	Clinical effect or symptom
Alcohol	Intoxication and withdrawal
Analgesics	Delirium
Amphetamines	Intoxication or paranoia
Antianxiety agents	Disinhibition
Anticholinergic drugs	Delirium
Antidepressants	Delirium
Antipsychotics	Delirium and akathisia
Cocaine	Intoxication or paranoia
Hypnotics	Disinhibition
Steroids	Mania or delirium

Source. Adapted from Yudofsky SC, Silver JM, Hales RE: "Pharmacologic Management of Aggression in the Elderly." *Journal of Clinical Psychiatry* 51 (suppl):22–28, 1990. Copyright 1990, Physicians Postgraduate Press. Used with permission.

TABLE 10–9. Characteristic features of neurologically induced agitation and aggression

Reactive	Triggered by modest stimuli
Nonreflective	Usually does not involve premeditation
Nonpurposeful	Is associated with no obvious short- or long-term aims or goals
Explosive	Buildup is *not* gradual
Periodic	Brief outbursts of rage and aggression punctuated by long periods of relative calm
Ego-dystonic	After outbursts, patients are upset or embarrassed

Source. Adapted from Yudofsky SC, Silver JM, Hales RE: "Pharmacologic Management of Aggression in the Elderly." *Journal of Clinical Psychiatry* 51 (suppl):22–28, 1990. Copyright 1990, Physicians Postgraduate Press. Used with permission.

In soliciting a history of agitation or aggression, it is critical to interview family members, teachers, friends, and co-workers because patients with aggressive disorders—as opposed to their families—tend to minimize the presence and importance of the disorder (Silver and Yudofsky 1994a). In addition, to develop a treatment plan, the clinician must learn from the patient and observers the context in which aggression occurs. Essential information includes the mental status of the patient before the agitated or aggressive event, the nature of precipitants, the physical and social environment in which agitation or aggression occurs, ways in which the agitated or aggressive event is mitigated, and primary and secondary gains related to agitation or aggression. If agitation or aggression occurs in the context of a psychiatric disorder, the clinician should obtain a thorough psychiatric history for the individual and the family. For *all* patients with agitation or aggression, the consultation-liaison psychiatrist must conduct a thorough review of physical symptoms, obtain a detailed review of neurological signs and symptoms, and conduct a thorough physical examination. The neurological examination deserves emphasis; relevant laboratory tests should be ordered on the basis of information from the history and physical and neurological examinations. We find that neuropsychological batteries, such as the Halstead-Reitan or the Luria-Nebraska tests, are more useful than psychological tests like the Minnesota Multiphasic Personality Inventory (MMPI) or projective psychological tests for evaluating patients with aggressive symptoms or disorders.

Staff and clinician safety should remain the first priority in any assessment of an aggressive or agitated patient. The staff member or clinician performing the assessment should remain vigilant and assess the potentially violent patient with other staff or a security guard present.

TREATMENT

Treatment of aggressive symptoms and disorders is guided by the four D's (see Table 10–10). Almost without exception, treatment of patients with aggressive disorders requires a multifaceted approach that combines pharmacological treatments, behavioral treatments, psychodynamically informed psychotherapy, family treatment, and, as indicated, other specific approaches such as spiritual counseling, occupational therapy, and couples treatment. Although psychopharmacological management of agitation and aggression is the main focus of this chapter, other approaches have considerable efficacy.

Nonpharmacological Treatment

Agitation and aggression can be caused and influenced by a combination of environmental and biological factors. Because of the dangerous and unpredictable nature of agitation and aggression, caretakers, both in institutions and at home, have intense and sometimes injudicious reactions to agitation and aggression when they occur. Behavioral treatments have been shown to be highly effective in patients with neurologically induced agitation or aggression and may be useful when combined with pharmacotherapy. Behavioral strategies, including a token economy, aggression replacement strategies, and decelerative techniques, may reduce aggression and can be combined effectively with pharmacological treatment (Corrigan and Jakus 1994; Corrigan et al. 1993). A review of this subject is found elsewhere (Corrigan et al. 1993).

TABLE 10–10. Four D's in the treatment of aggressive symptoms and disorders

Determine the etiologies of the psychological and/or central nervous system dysfunction that contributes to the aggression.

Delineate the biopsychosocial context in which the aggressive events occur.

Document and rate the aggression with the Overt Aggression Scale.

Develop a multifaceted treatment plan.

Source. Adapted from Silver JM, Yudofsky SC: "The Overt Aggression Scale: Overview and Guiding Principles." *Journal of Neuropsychiatry and Clinical Neurosciences* 3 (suppl 1):S22–S29, 1991. Used with permission.

Deciding which strategy to use depends on the clinical setting as well as the clinical problems of the patient. Settings that have highly structured environments usually foster more appropriate social behavior. Several strategies attempt to teach the patient how to replace agitated or aggressive behavior with nonviolent behavior. For example, staff reinforce all behaviors of the patient except the agitated or aggressive ones. However, it is not feasible in most hospitals for staff to frequently reinforce nonaggressive behaviors. Another strategy is for staff to reinforce behaviors that are incompatible with the aggressive ones. For example, patients would be praised for sitting quietly and asking for something rather than pacing and yelling demands. Using soothing music, companion animals, and other calming influences can also be successful strategies for managing aggression (Fritz et al. 1995; Ragneskog and Kihlgren 1997).

It is important to identify previolent behaviors, such as yelling, swearing, or threatening, so that staff or families can intervene before the patient becomes aggressive. Patients can be taught alternative and more appropriate behaviors to replace or discharge agitation or aggression. In addition, positive behaviors, such as sitting quietly and talking pleasantly, should be actively praised and reinforced. Patients are told that aggressive behaviors are not acceptable, will be ignored by the staff (or family), and will lead to a reduction in positive reinforcers. Staff should be prepared for short-term exacerbation of agitation or aggressive behavior; improvement will occur over a longer time. Patients can occasionally be "talked down" from an agitated or aggressive state. More serious and dangerous violence necessitates more active measures to protect the safety of both staff and patient.

Interventions may be required to stop assaults. In the use of time-outs, the patient is removed from an overstimulating environment. It is best if the patient initiates this request. The judicious use of seclusion and the application of restraints may be necessary to protect the patient from hurting himself or herself or others. The clinician must be thoroughly aware of the state regulations that guide the use of these methods. The application of restraints must be used in a setting where the patient can be carefully and frequently observed, with appropriate monitoring of vital signs and physical status. Clinicians must remember that patients have intense reactions to these interventions, and they should always treat patients with appropriate respect and dignity. Patients may feel relieved that they are not allowed to hurt themselves or others. When these interventions are used, staff interaction with the patient should be minimal so that staff do not reinforce the aggressive behavior.

Pharmacological Treatment

In conceptualizing an approach to the pharmacological treatment of agitation and aggression, the consultation-liaison psychiatrist must separate the management of acute agitation or aggression (which often constitutes a medical emergency) from the pharmacological treatment of chronic agitation or aggression. Currently, no medication is approved by the Food and Drug Administration for the treatment of these behaviors. When medications are administered to treat agitation or aggression, frequently it is their sedating side effects and not their direct pharmacological actions that are being used. Although this may be appropriate in emergency or acute situations, prolonged use of sedation to treat chronic agitation or aggressive behaviors has disadvantages. For example, when neuroleptics are used to manage agitation or aggression, side effects including oversedation, hypotension, confusion, neuroleptic malignant syndrome, parkinsonism, akathisia, dystonia, and tardive dyskinesia may emerge. When benzodiazepines are used for prolonged periods to manage agitation or aggression, side effects such as oversedation, motor disturbances (including poor coordination), mood disturbances, memory impairment, confusion, dependency, overdoses, withdrawal syndromes, and paradoxical violence complicate treatment (Silver et al. 1997).

Acute Aggression and Agitation

Physicians commonly use the sedative side effects of neuroleptics and benzodiazepines for the management of acute aggressive behavior and agitation. These agents are not specific in their capacities to inhibit agitation or aggressive behaviors but rather "cover over" the respective behaviors and symptoms. Therefore, the clinician must establish time limitations when prescribing medications for their sedative properties.

Neuroleptics

Consultation-liaison psychiatrists often prescribe neuroleptic medications to treat acute and chronic agitation or aggression. These agents are appropriate and effective in the treatment of agitation or aggression that is a result of psychosis. For example, a physically aggressive patient who presents in the emergency room with acute, manic psychosis with irritability would benefit from treatment with a neuroleptic medication. It would also be appropriate to administer a neuroleptic medication to a patient with paranoid schizophrenia who uses physical force to protect himself or herself from nurses because the patient believes they are agents sent from another planet to kidnap him or her. However, it is unfortunate that neuroleptic medications are commonly used to treat patients with chronic agitation or aggression associated with organic brain disorders, especially schizophrenia. If the increased irritability and agitation associated with akathisia are mistaken for the underlying illness, a vicious cycle can emerge. One study demonstrated a marked increase in violent behavior when patients with schizophrenia were treated with haloperidol at dosages up to 60 mg/day. Much lower rates of violent behavior occurred during treatment with chlorpromazine at dosages up to 1,800 mg/day or clozapine at dosages up to 900 mg/day (Herrera et al. 1988). Thus, patients who are taking haloperidol appear to be at higher risk for akathisia than patients who are taking chlorpromazine or clozapine.

These complications and side effects can be avoided by establishing a treatment plan (before initiating treatment with neuroleptics) that includes 1) operationalized ratings of agitation or aggression with the OAS or OASS, 2) reduction of neuroleptic doses when symptoms remit, and 3) specified dates to taper the dose of and discontinue the neuroleptic. Unless agitated or aggressive behavior is clearly related to psychotic ideation that responds to treatment with neuroleptic agents, consultation-liaison psychiatrists should limit the use of neuroleptics to a maximum of 6 weeks. After this period, the psychiatrist should determine whether the agitation or aggression is chronic and alter the treatment plan accordingly.

The essence of managing acute episodes of agitation and aggression with neuroleptics is to increase the dose of the neuroleptic, often every 1–2 hours, to establish the lowest dosage that will produce the sedation necessary to control the agitated or aggressive behaviors. Despite the aforementioned disadvantages of haloperidol in the management of chronic agitation or aggression, this drug is often used because it can be administered in oral, intramuscular, and intravenous forms and has few cardiovascular side effects compared with other classes of neuroleptics. Administering the combination of haloperidol and lorazepam is a particularly effective and rapid way to produce sedation, and the combination may be used if high doses of haloperidol are undesirable (Bieniek et al. 1998). Guidelines for the use of haloperidol in the management of acute agitation or aggression are given in Table 10–11.

Benzodiazepines

Benzodiazepines are also used to manage acute agitation and aggression. Intramuscular lorazepam has advantages over other benzodiazepines as a medication in the emergency treatment of the violent patient (Bick and Hannah 1986). Like haloperidol, lorazepam has flexible routes of

TABLE 10–11. Use of haloperidol in the management of acute agitation or aggression

Initially administer 1 mg (po) or 0.5 mg (iv or im) qh.

Increase dose by 1 mg qh until control of agitation or aggression is achieved.

Maintain dosage of 2 mg (po) or 1 mg (iv or im) q8h.

When patient is not agitated or aggressive for 48 hours, decrease highest total daily dose at rate of 25% per day.

If agitation or aggression reemerges when drug dose is tapered, reassess etiology and consider changing to a more specific medication to manage chronic agitation or aggression.

Do not continue to treat patient with haloperidol for more than 6 weeks—except in cases of agitation or aggression secondary to psychosis.

Note. im = intramuscular; iv = intravenous; po = per os (oral); qh = every hour; q8h = every 8 hours.

Source. Adapted from Yudofsky SC, Silver JM, Hales RE: "Pharmacologic Management of Aggression in the Elderly." *Journal of Clinical Psychiatry* 51 (suppl):22–28, 1990. Copyright 1990, Physicians Postgraduate Press. Used with permission.

administration (intravenous, intramuscular, or oral). In addition, lorazepam has a relatively brief duration of action and elimination half-life compared with other benzodiazepines, such as diazepam or chlordiazepoxide, which oversedate the patient through the buildup of active metabolites. Guidelines for the use of lorazepam in the management of acute agitation and aggression are given in Table 10–12. In a randomized, double-blind study, Lenox et al. (1992) compared lorazepam with haloperidol in the treatment of manic agitation in 20 hospitalized patients with bipolar disorder who were also taking lithium. The investigators found no significant difference between the treatment groups in the degree of or time to response.

Other Medications

Other medications, such as paraldehyde, chloral hydrate, and diphenhydramine, are also used to sedate patients who exhibit acute aggressive behaviors; however, in general, benzodiazepines and neuroleptics are preferable because they are safe and convenient and psychiatrists and hospital staff are more familiar with their benefits and risks.

Individual case reports suggest certain pharmacological approaches for specific clinical conditions. For example, amantadine, a dopamine agonist, reportedly reduced aggressive behavior in patients recovering from traumatic brain injury (T. Gualtieri et al. 1989). Intensive care unit physicians occasionally administer succinylcholine to achieve a pharmacological paralysis in patients who are agitated after traumatic brain injury or surgical proce-

TABLE 10–12.   Use of lorazepam in the management of acute agitation or aggression

1. Initially administer 1–2 mg (po or im).
2. Repeat every hour until control of agitation or aggression is achieved.
3. If iv dose is given, push slowly! Do not exceed 2 mg (1 mL) per minute, to avoid respiratory depression and laryngospasm; repeat in 30 minutes if required.
4. When patient is no longer agitated or aggressive, maintain at maximum of 2 mg (po or im) q4h.
5. When patient is not agitated or aggressive for 48 hours, decrease highest total daily dose at rate of 10% per day.
6. If agitation or aggression reemerges when drug dose is tapered, reassess etiology and consider changing to a more specific medication to manage chronic agitation or aggression.
7. If lorazepam dose cannot be tapered without reemergence of agitation or aggression after 6 weeks, reevaluate and revise treatment plan to include a more specific medication to manage chronic agitation or aggression.

Note.   im = intramuscular; iv = intravenous; po = per os (oral); q4h = every 4 hours.
Source.   Adapted from Yudofsky SC, Silver JM, Hales RE: "Pharmacologic Management of Aggression in the Elderly." *Journal of Clinical Psychiatry* 51 (suppl):22–28, 1990. Copyright 1990, Physicians Postgraduate Press. Used with permission.

dures and who do not respond to less dramatic treatments. Clearly, such interventions are best limited to physicians who, by virtue of subspecialty focus, have broad experience and the requisite resources to manage aggression and agitation safely in patients while employing novel approaches.

Chronic Aggression and Agitation

When a patient's agitation or aggression persists beyond several weeks, clinicians should consider treating the agitation or aggression with medications that have more selective activity. When selecting a specific psychopharmacological agent, consultation-liaison psychiatrists must determine the underlying cause of the chronic agitation or aggression (e.g., mania or depression). An approach in the pharmacological treatment of chronic aggression is outlined in Table 10–13.

Neuroleptics

The use of antipsychotic medications should be restricted to the treatment of aggression that is directly associated with psychosis. The atypical neuroleptics may be especially useful, given the decreased risk of tardive dyskinesia associated with them. Risperidone, clozapine, and tiapride have all been reported to be effective in agitated elderly patients with dementia and in aggressive schizophrenic patients (Fava 1997; Goldberg and Goldberg 1997; Hector 1998; Herrmann et al. 1998; Roger et al. 1998; Stoppe et al. 1999). At regular intervals, the dose of the neuroleptic medication should be tapered to gauge the efficacy of the agent in treating the psychosis and the associated agitation or aggression.

Antianxiety Medications

In several reported cases, buspirone, a 5-HT$_{1A}$ (serotonin) partial agonist, was effective in the management of aggression and agitation associated with traumatic brain injury (C. T. Gualtieri 1991; Ratey et al. 1992a; Stanislav et al. 1994), dementia (Colenda 1988; Tiller et al. 1988), and developmental disabilities and autism (Pfeffer et al. 1997; Ratey et al. 1989; Realmuto et al. 1989). Because some patients become more agitated in the initial phases of treatment with buspirone, the consultation-liaison psychiatrist may need to begin treatment at low doses (i.e., 5 mg bid) and increase the dose by 5 mg every 3–5 days. Dosages ranging from 45 to 60 mg/day are sometimes required for effective treatment; a latency period of 3–6 weeks before therapeutic effects are observed is common.

Although no double-blind, controlled studies have examined the use of clonazepam in the management of chronic agitation or aggression, several case reports have indicated that it has benefits in the treatment of agitation in elderly patients (Freinhar and Alvarez 1986) and in a patient with schizophrenia and seizures (Keats and Mukherjee 1988).

Clonazepam is also used when agitation or aggression is associated with pronounced anxiety or when agitation or aggression is present with neurologically induced tics and disinhibited motor behavior. Treatment is initiated at doses of 0.5 mg bid, and total daily doses rarely exceed 6 mg.

Anticonvulsant Medications

The consultant-liaison psychiatrist should consider using anticonvulsant medications, particularly carbamazepine, to treat patients whose chronic agitation or aggression is associated with seizure disorders or whose chronic agitation or aggression is related to diffuse neuronal destruction (such as that which occurs with traumatic brain injury, middle cerebral artery stroke, and Alzheimer's disease). Several studies indicate that carbamazepine therapy is effective in reducing aggressive behavior associated with organic brain disorders (Mattes 1988), schizophrenia (Hakoloa and Laulumaa 1982; Luchins 1983), developmental disabilities (Folks et al. 1982), and dementia (Gleason and Schneider 1990; Leibovici and

TABLE 10–13.   Psychopharmacological treatment of chronic agitation and aggression

Agent	Indications	Special clinical considerations
Antipsychotics	Psychotic symptoms	Oversedation and multiple side effects
Benzodiazepines	Anxiety symptoms	Paradoxical rage
Buspirone	Persistent, underlying anxiety and/or depression	Delayed onset of action
Carbamazepine	Seizure disorder	Bone marrow suppression and hepatotoxicity
Valproate	Seizure disorder	Hepatotoxicity
Lithium	Manic excitement or bipolar disorder	Neurotoxicity and confusion
Propranolol (and other β-blockers)	Chronic or recurrent aggression	Latency of 4–6 weeks
Selective serotonin reuptake inhibitors (SSRIs)	Depression or mood lability with irritability	May need usual doses
Trazodone	Depression with insomnia	Oversedation, brief half-life
Nefazodone	Depression with agitation and insomnia	Twice-a-day dosing

Source.   Adapted from Yudofsky SC, Silver JM, Hales RE: "Pharmacologic Management of Aggression in the Elderly." *Journal of Clinical Psychiatry* 51 (suppl):22–28, 1990. Copyright 1990, Physicians Postgraduate Press. Used with permission.

Tariot 1988; Lemke 1995; Tariot et al. 1998). One non-randomized, placebo-controlled crossover study involving 25 patients with dementia showed that low dosages of carbamazepine (modal dosage [most commonly used dosage] of 300 mg/day) reduced agitated behavior in some patients (Tariot et al. 1994). Carbamazepine should be prescribed at the same dosages used to treat patients with bipolar disorder (with the aim of achieving the same blood levels as in those patients).

Several studies have found that valproate is effective in the treatment of agitation and aggression in patients with a wide variety of medical disorders. Most of these studies were published as case reports in which valproate's usefulness in reducing agitation and aggression in patients with dementias or other organic brain syndromes was described (Giakas et al. 1990; Guay 1995; Kahn et al. 1988; Kunik et al. 1998; Mattes 1992; Mellow et al. 1993). Lott et al. (1995) conducted a prospective, open-label trial involving 10 elderly nursing home patients with dementia and agitation. These patients were treated with valproate at dosages ranging from 375 to 750 mg/day. Eight of the patients had at least a 50% reduction in the frequency of agitation, and the intensity of the behavioral outbursts also diminished in many of these patients. Valproate was well tolerated by all patients in the study. Because of valproate's favorable side-effect profile (e.g., low incidence of ataxia, rashes, and behavioral changes and fewer drug interactions), valproate may be preferred by consultation psychiatrists over carbamazepine in the treatment of agitation and aggression.

Antimanic Medications

Several authors suggest that lithium is effective in the treatment of agitated or aggressive patients without bipo-

lar disorder, such as patients with mental retardation who exhibit self-directed aggression (Luchins and Dojka 1989) or aggression toward others (Dale 1980) and patients with traumatic brain injury (Haas and Cope 1985). In addition, children and adolescents (Vetro et al. 1985) and prison inmates (Sheard et al. 1976) with aggression reportedly respond to lithium.

Aggressive behavior may occur during manic episodes in patients with bipolar disorder, and agitation frequently occurs during manic and depressive episodes. Mood-stabilizing medications such as lithium and valproate (Wilcox 1994) treat these behaviors in such patients by treating the underlying illness. In general, the same dosage of lithium and blood level monitoring that are recommended for patients with bipolar disorder without agitation or aggression should be used. One caveat is that patients with brain injury have increased sensitivity to the neurotoxic effects of lithium (Hornstein and Seliger 1989) and therefore must be observed much more closely with neuropsychiatric evaluations and measurement of serum lithium levels.

Antidepressant Medications

Many antidepressants are suggested for the treatment of aggression, especially those agents that act either preferentially or specifically on the serotonergic system. Amitriptyline (Szlabowicz and Stewart 1990) and trazodone (Lebert et al. 1994; Pinner and Rich 1988) are reported to be useful in the treatment of agitation and aggression; however, most relatively recent reports focus on the use of selective serotonin reuptake inhibitors (SSRIs). Fluoxetine has been used successfully in patients whose aggression is associated with brain lesions (Bass and Beltis 1991; Coccaro et al. 1990). Other SSRIs, such as paroxetine and sertraline, also are effective (Silver and Yudofsky 1994b). Treatment should begin at relatively low doses (e.g., 10 mg of fluoxetine, 25 mg of sertraline, or 10 mg of paroxetine). If antiaggressive effects are not achieved over several weeks, the dosage should be increased gradually at 1- or 2-week intervals to relatively high ranges (80–100 mg of fluoxetine per day, 200–300 mg of sertraline per day, 60–80 mg of paroxetine per day). Another effective agent is the 5-HT$_2$ (serotonin) antagonist nefazodone, which reportedly is well tolerated by some patients with agitated depression. The usual starting dose is 50 mg bid; the dose can be increased weekly by 100 mg until a total daily dosage of 400–600 mg is reached.

β-Blockers

Since the first report of the use of β-adrenergic receptor antagonists to treat aggression in 1977, more than 25 articles have been published in both the neurological and psychiatric literature on the use of β-blockers for this purpose (Silver and Yudofsky 1994b; Yudofsky et al. 1987). The β-blockers studied using prospective, placebo-controlled designs include propranolol, a lipid-soluble, nonselective receptor antagonist (Brooke et al. 1992b; Greendyke et al. 1986; Mattes 1988; Shankle et al. 1995); nadolol, a water-soluble, nonselective receptor antagonist (Alpert et al. 1990; Brooke et al. 1992b; Ratey et al. 1992b); and pindolol, a lipid-soluble, nonselective antagonist with partial sympathomimetic activity (Greendyke and Kanter 1986). These adrenergic receptor antagonists are specific and effective agents for the treatment of aggression and agitation in patients with central nervous syndromes and are now accepted as first-line drugs for treatment of organically induced agitation and aggression.

Guidelines for the use of propranolol in patients with chronic aggression are given in Table 10–14. Key clinical points related to the use of propranolol are as follows: First, the peripheral effects of β-blockage (e.g., lowered blood pressure or bradycardia) are frequently maximized when the patient achieves a dosage of about 280 mg/day. Thereafter, increasing the dose of the β-blocker is not usually associated with cardiovascular side effects. Second, because of the long latency of 6–8 weeks before a therapeutic response is achieved, consultation-liaison psychiatrists should remind the family and other members of the treatment team that their support is an essential component of care. Third, although it is reported that depression is commonly associated with the use of β-blockers, controlled trials and clinical expe-

TABLE 10–14.   Clinical use of propranolol

1. Conduct a thorough medical evaluation.
2. Exclude patients with bronchial asthma, chronic obstructive pulmonary disease, insulin-dependent diabetes mellitus, congestive heart failure, persistent angina, significant peripheral vascular disease, or hyperthyroidism.
3. Avoid sudden discontinuation of propranolol (particularly in patients with hypertension).
4. Begin with a single test dose of 20 mg/day in patients who may be at risk for hypotension or bradycardia. Increase dose by 20 mg/day every 3 days.
5. For patients without cardiovascular or cardiopulmonary disorder, begin propranolol on a 20-mg tid schedule.
6. Increase the dose by 60 mg/day as often as every 3 days.
7. Increase the dose unless the pulse rate is reduced to below 50 beats per minute or systolic blood pressure is less than 90 mm Hg.
8. Do not administer medication if severe dizziness, ataxia, or wheezing occurs. Reduce or discontinue propranolol if such symptoms persist.
9. Increase the dose to 12 mg/kg or until aggressive behavior is under control.
10. Doses of more than 800 mg are not usually required to control aggressive behavior.
11. Maintain the patient on the highest dose that he or she can tolerate for 4–8 weeks before concluding that the patient is not responding to propranolol. Some patients respond rapidly.
12. Use concurrent medications with caution. Monitor plasma levels of all antipsychotic and anticonvulsant medications.

Source.   Adapted from Silver JM, Hales RE, Yudofsky SC: "Neuropsychiatric Aspects of Traumatic Brain Injury," in *The American Psychiatric Press Textbook of Neuropsychiatry*, 3rd Edition. Edited by Yudofsky SC, Hales RE. Washington, DC, American Psychiatric Press, 1997, pp. 521–560. Copyright 1997, American Psychiatric Press. Used with permission.

rience indicate that depression is a rare side effect of β-blocker use (Yudofsky 1992). Finally, because the use of propranolol is associated with a significant increase in plasma levels of thioridazine, which has an absolute dosage ceiling of 800 mg/day, the combination of these two medications should be avoided whenever possible (Silver et al. 1986).

Antiandrogen Medications

There is limited but interesting evidence that antiandrogen agents may be effective in treating some forms of aggression in men (Amadeo 1996). The use of these medications, which include medroxyprogesterone and leuprolide, must be considered largely experimental at this time.

CONCLUSION

Agitation and aggression occur commonly in the general hospital setting and have serious and far-reaching consequences for patients whom consultation-liaison psychiatrists evaluate. When assessing patients who exhibit agitation or aggression, consultation-liaison psychiatrists should obtain careful histories, perform thorough physical examinations, and request relevant laboratory tests to diagnose any medical condition that could underlie and/or aggravate these symptoms. Although pharmacological intervention is often highly effective in the treatment of agitation and aggression, medications are used in the context of a carefully crafted treatment plan involving a full range of biopsychosocial approaches. In pharmacological treatment of acute agitation and aggression, sedative side effects of neuroleptic drugs or benzodiazepines are often required. However, prolonged use of neuroleptics or benzodiazepines frequently leads to undesirable side effects; therefore, neuroleptics and benzodiazepines are avoided in the treatment of chronic agitation and aggression. A wide range of medications are helpful in the management of chronic agitation and aggression, including β-blockers, SSRIs, nefazodone, buspirone, and anticonvulsants. Determining the underlying etiology of the aggression guides the consultation-liaison psychiatrist in selecting the appropriate pharmacological agent.

REFERENCES

Alexander RW, Davis JN, Lefkowitz RJ: Direct identification and characterization of β-adrenergic receptors in rat brain. Nature 258:437–440, 1979

Alpert M, Allan ER, Citrome L, et al: A double-blind, placebo-controlled study of adjunctive nadolol in the management of violent psychiatric patients. Psychopharmacology Bulletin 28:367–371, 1990

Amadeo M: Antiandrogen treatment of aggressivity in men suffering from dementia. J Geriatr Psychiatry Neurol 9:142–145, 1996

American Psychiatric Association: Diagnostic and Statistical Manual of Mental Disorders, 4th Edition, Text Revision. Washington, DC, American Psychiatric Association, 2000

Bareggi SR, Porta M, Selenati A, et al: Homovanillic acid and 5-hydroxyindole-acetic acid in the CSF of patients after a severe head injury, I: lumbar CSF concentration in chronic brain post-traumatic syndromes. Eur Neurol 13:528–544, 1975

Bass JN, Beltis J: Therapeutic effect of fluoxetine on naltrexone-resistant self-injurious behavior in an adolescent with mental retardation. J Child Adolesc Psychopharmacol 1:331–340, 1991

Bick PA, Hannah AL: Intramuscular lorazepam to restrain violent patients (letter). Lancet 1:206, 1986

Bieniek SA, Ownby RL, Penalver A, et al: A double-blind study of lorazepam versus the combination of haloperidol and lorazepam in managing agitation. Pharmacotherapy 18:57–62, 1998

Brooke MM, Questad KA, Patterson DR, et al: Agitation and restlessness after closed head injury: a prospective study of 100 consecutive admissions. Arch Phys Med Rehabil 73:320–323, 1992a

Brooke MM, Patterson DR, Questad KA, et al: The treatment of agitation during initial hospitalization after traumatic brain injury. Arch Phys Med Rehabil 73:917–921, 1992b

Brown GL, Goodwin FK, Ballenger JC, et al: Aggression in humans correlates with cerebrospinal fluid amine metabolites. Psychiatry Res 1:131–139, 1979

Chandler JD, Chandler JE: The prevalence of neuropsychiatric disorders in a nursing home population. J Geriatr Psychiatry Neurol 1:71–76, 1988

Coccaro EF, Astill JL, Herbert JL, et al: Fluoxetine treatment of impulsive aggression in DSM-III-R personality disorder patients (letter). J Clin Psychopharmacol 10:373–375, 1990

Colenda CC: Buspirone in treatment of agitated demented patients (letter). Lancet 1:1169, 1988

Corrigan PW, Jakus MR: Behavioral treatment, in Neuropsychiatry of Traumatic Brain Injury. Edited by Silver JM, Yudofsky SC, Hales RE. Washington, DC, American Psychiatric Press, 1994, pp 733–769

Corrigan PW, Yudofsky SC, Silver JM: Pharmacological and behavioral treatments for aggressive psychiatric inpatients. Hospital and Community Psychiatry 44:125–133, 1993

Dale PG: Lithium therapy in aggressive mentally subnormal patients. Br J Psychiatry 137:469–474, 1980

Eichelman BS Jr: Effect of subcortical lesions on shock-induced aggression in the rat. Journal of Comparative and Physiologic Psychology 74:331–339, 1971

Eichelman B[S] Jr: Neurochemical and psychopharmacologic aspects of aggressive behavior, in Psychopharmacology: The Third Generation of Progress. Edited by Meltzer HY. New York, Raven, 1987, pp 697–704

Eichelman BS Jr, Thoa NB, Ng KY: Facilitated aggression in the rat following 6-hydroxydopamine administration. Physiol Behav 8:1–3, 1972

Elliott FA: The neurology of explosive rage. Practitioner 217:51–59, 1976

Elliott FA: Violence: the neurologic contribution: an overview. Arch Neurol 49:595–603, 1992

Fava M: Psychopharmacologic treatment of pathologic aggression. Psychiatr Clin North Am 20:427–451, 1997

Folks DG, King LD, Dowdy SB, et al: Carbamazepine treatment of selective affectively disordered inpatients. Am J Psychiatry 139:115–117, 1982

Freinhar JP, Alvarez WA: Clonazepam treatment of organic brain syndromes in three elderly patients. J Clin Psychiatry 47:525–526, 1986

Fritz CL, Farver TB, Kass PH, et al: Association with companion animals and the expression of noncognitive symptoms in Alzheimer's patients. J Nerv Ment Dis 183:459–463, 1995

Ghosh TB, Victor BS: Suicide, in The American Psychiatric Press Textbook of Psychiatry, 3rd Edition. Edited by Hales RE, Yudofsky SC, Talbott JA. Washington, DC, American Psychiatric Press, 1999, pp 1383–1404

Giakas WJ, Seibyl JP, Mazure CM: Valproate in the treatment of temper outbursts (letter). J Clin Psychiatry 51:525, 1990

Gleason RP, Schneider LS: Carbamazepine treatment of agitation in Alzheimer's outpatients refractory to neuroleptics. J Clin Psychiatry 51:115–118, 1990

Goldberg RJ, Goldberg J: Risperidone for dementia-related disturbed behavior in nursing home residents: a clinical experience. Int Psychogeriatr 9:65–68, 1997

Greendyke RM, Kanter DR: Therapeutic effects of pindolol on behavioral disturbances associated with organic brain disease: a double-blind study. J Clin Psychiatry 47:423–426, 1986

Greendyke RM, Kanter DR, Schuster DB, et al: Propranolol treatment of assaultive patients with organic brain disease: a double-blind crossover, placebo-controlled study. J Nerv Ment Dis 174:290–294, 1986

Gualtieri CT: Buspirone for the behavior problems of patients with organic brain disorders (letter). J Clin Psychopharmacol 11:280–281, 1991

Gualtieri T, Chandler M, Coons TB, et al: Amantadine: a new clinical profile for traumatic brain injury. Clin Neuropharmacol 12:258–270, 1989

Guay DR: The merging role of valproate in bipolar disorder and other psychiatric disorders. Pharmacotherapy 15:631–647, 1995

Haas JF, Cope N: Neuropharmacologic management of behavior sequelae in head injury: a case report. Arch Phys Med Rehabil 66:472–474, 1985

Hakoloa HP, Laulumaa VA: Carbamazepine in treatment of violent schizophrenics (letter). Lancet 1:1358, 1982

Hales RE: Psychiatric systems interface disorders (PSID), in DSM-IV Sourcebook, Vol 2. Washington, DC, American Psychiatric Press, 1996, pp 871–884

Hales RE, Yudofsky SC, Talbott JA (eds): The American Psychiatric Press Textbook of Psychiatry, 3rd Edition. Washington, DC, American Psychiatric Press, 1999

Hamill RW, Woolf PD, McDonald JV, et al: Catecholamines predict outcome in traumatic brain injury. Ann Neurol 21:438–443, 1987

Hector RI: The use of clozapine in the treatment of aggressive schizophrenia. Can J Psychiatry 43:466–472, 1998

Herrera JN, Sramek JJ, Costa JF, et al: High potency neuroleptics and violence in schizophrenics. J Nerv Ment Dis 176:558–561, 1988

Herrmann N, Rivard MF, Flynn M, et al: Risperidone for the treatment of behavioral disturbances in dementia: a case series. J Neuropsychiatry Clin Neurosci 10:22–31, 1998

Higley JD, Mehlman PT, Taum DM, et al: Cerebrospinal fluid monoamine and adrenal correlates of aggression in free-ranging rhesus monkeys. Arch Gen Psychiatry 49:436–441, 1992

Hornstein A, Seliger G: Cognitive side effects of lithium in closed head injury (letter). J Neuropsychiatry Clin Neurosci 1:446–447, 1989

Kahn D, Stevenson E, Douglas CJ: Effect of sodium valproate in three patients with organic brain syndromes. Am J Psychiatry 145:1010–1011, 1988

Kavoussi R, Armstead P, Coccaro E: The neurobiology of impulsive aggression. Psychiatr Clin North Am 20:395–403, 1997

Keats MM, Mukherjee S: Antiaggressive effect of adjunctive clonazepam in schizophrenia associated with seizure disorder. J Clin Psychiatry 49:117–118, 1988

Kopecky HJ, Kopecky CR, Yudofsky SC: Reliability and validity of the Overt Agitation Severity Scale in adult psychiatric inpatients. Psychiatr Q 69:301–323, 1998

Kruesi MJP, Hibbs ED, Zahn TP, et al: A 2-year prospective follow-up study of children and adolescents with disruptive behavior disorders: prediction by cerebrospinal fluid 5-hydroxyindoleacetic acid, homovanillic acid, and autonomic measures? Arch Gen Psychiatry 49:429–435, 1992

Kunik ME, Puryear L, Orengo CA, et al: The efficacy and tolerability of divalproex sodium in elderly demented patients with behavioral disturbances. Int J Geriatr Psychiatry 13:29–34, 1998

Leavitt ML, Yudofsky SC, Maroon JC, et al: Effect of intraventricular nadolol infusion on shock-induced aggression in 6-hydroxydopamine-treated rats. J Neuropsychiatry Clin Neurosci 1:167–172, 1989

Lebert F, Pasquier F, Petit H: Behavioral effects of trazodone in Alzheimer's disease. J Clin Psychiatry 55:536–538, 1994

Leibovici A, Tariot PN: Carbamazepine treatment of agitation associated with dementia. J Geriatr Psychiatry Neurol 1:110–112, 1988

Lemke MR: Effect of carbamazepine on agitation in Alzheimer's inpatients refractory to neuroleptics. J Clin Psychiatry 56:354–357, 1995

Lenox RH, Newhouse PA, Creelman WL, et al: Adjunctive treatment of manic agitation with lorazepam versus haloperidol: a double-blind study. J Clin Psychiatry 53:47–52, 1992

Linnoila VMI, Virkkunen M: Aggression, suicidality, and serotonin. J Clin Psychiatry 53 (suppl):46–51, 1992

Lion JR, Reid WH: Assaults With Psychiatric Facilities. New York, Grune & Stratton, 1983

Lott AD, McElroy SL, Keys MA: Valproate in the treatment of behavioral agitation in elderly patients with dementia. J Neuropsychiatry Clin Neurosci 7:314–319, 1995

Luchins DJ: Carbamazepine for the violent psychiatric patient (letter). Lancet 2:755, 1983

Luchins DJ, Dojka D: Lithium and propranolol in aggression and self-injurious behavior in the mentally retarded. Psychopharmacology Bulletin 25:372–375, 1989

Malmquist CP: Homicide: A Psychiatric Perspective. Washington, DC, American Psychiatric Press, 1996

Mattes JA: Carbamazepine vs propranolol for rage outbursts. Psychopharmacology Bulletin 24:179–182, 1988

Mattes JA: Valproic acid for nonaffective aggression in the mentally retarded. J Nerv Ment Dis 180:601–602, 1992

Mellow AM, Solano-Lopez C, Davis S: Sodium valproate in the treatment of behavioral disturbance in dementia. J Geriatr Psychiatry Neurol 6:205–209, 1993

Oddy M, Caughlan T, Tyerman A, et al: Social adjustment after closed head injury: a further follow-up seven years after injury. J Neurol Neurosurg Psychiatry 44:564–568, 1985

Ovsiew F, Yudofsky SC: Aggression: a neuropsychiatric perspective, in Rage, Power and Aggression. Edited by Glick RA, Roose SP. New Haven, CT, Yale University Press, 1993, pp 213–230

Pfeffer CR, Jiang H, Domeshek LJ: Buspirone treatment of psychiatrically hospitalized prepubertal children with symptoms of anxiety and moderately severe aggression. J Child Adolesc Psychopharmacol 7:145–155, 1997

Pinner E, Rich CL: Effects of trazodone on aggressive behavior in seven patients with organic mental disorders. Am J Psychiatry 145:1295–1296, 1988

Rabins PV, Mace NL, Lucas MJ: The impact of dementia on the family. JAMA 248:333–335, 1982

Ragneskog H, Kihlgren M: Music and other strategies to improve the care of agitated patients with dementia: interviews with experienced staff. Scandinvian Journal of Caring Sciences 11:176–182, 1997

Rao N, Jellinek HM, Woolson DC: Agitation in closed head injury: haloperidol effects on rehabilitation outcome. Arch Phys Med Rehabil 66:30–34, 1985

Ratey JJ, Sovner R, Mikkelsen E, et al: Buspirone therapy for maladaptive behavior and anxiety in developmentally disabled persons. J Clin Psychiatry 50:382–384, 1989

Ratey JJ, Leveroni CL, Miller AC, et al: Low-dose buspirone to treat agitation and maladaptive behavior in brain-injured patients: two case reports. J Clin Psychopharmacol 12:362–364, 1992a

Ratey JJ, Sorgi P, O'Driscoll GA, et al: Nadolol to treat aggression and psychiatric symptomatology in chronic psychiatric inpatients: a double-blind, placebo-controlled study. J Clin Psychiatry 53:41–46, 1992b

Realmuto FM, August GJ, Garfinkle BD: Clinical effect of buspirone in autistic children. J Clin Psychopharmacol 9:122–124, 1989

Reid HW, Bollinger MF, Edwards G: Assaults in hospitals. Bulletin of the American Academy of Psychiatry and Law 13:1–4, 1985

Reisberg B, Borenstein J, Salob SP, et al: Behavioral symptoms in Alzheimer's disease: phenomenology and treatment. J Clin Psychiatry 48 (suppl):9–15, 1987

Roger M, Gerard D, Leger JM: Value of tiapride for agitation in the elderly. Encephale 24:462–468, 1998

Shankle WR, Nielson KA, Cotman CW: Low-dose propranolol reduces aggression and agitation resembling that associated with orbitofrontal dysfunction in elderly demented patients. Alzheimer Dis Assoc Disord 9:233–237, 1995

Sheard MH, Marini JL, Bridges C, et al: The effect of lithium on impulsive aggressive behavior in man. Am J Psychiatry 133:1409–1413, 1976

Silver JM, Yudofsky SC: Aggressive behavior in patients with neuropsychiatric disorders: the scope of the problem. Psychiatric Annals 17:367–370, 1987a

Silver JM, Yudofsky SC: Documentation of aggression in the assessment of the violent patient. Psychiatric Annals 17:375–384, 1987b

Silver JM, Yudofsky SC: The Overt Aggression Scale: overview and guiding principles. J Neuropsychiatry Clin Neurosci 3 (suppl 1):S22–S29, 1991

Silver JM, Yudofsky SC: Aggressive disorders, in Neuropsychiatry of Traumatic Brain Injury. Edited by Silver JM, Yudofsky SC, Hales RE. Washington, DC, American Psychiatric Press, 1994a, pp 313–356

Silver JM, Yudofsky SC: Pharmacology, in Neuropsychiatry of Traumatic Brain Injury. Edited by Silver JM, Yudofsky SC, Hales RE. Washington DC, American Psychiatric Press, 1994b, pp 631–670

Silver JM, Yudofsky SC, Kogan M, et al: Elevation of thioridazine plasma levels by propranolol. Am J Psychiatry 143: 1290–1292, 1986

Silver JM, Hales RE, Yudofsky SC: Neuropsychiatric aspects of traumatic brain injury, in The American Psychiatric Press Textbook of Neuropsychiatry, 3rd Edition. Edited by Yudofsky SC, Hales RE. Washington, DC, American Psychiatric Press, 1997, pp 521–560

Stanislav SW, Fabre T, Crismon ML, et al: Buspirone's efficacy in organic-induced aggression. J Clin Psychopharmacol 14: 126–130, 1994

Stoppe G, Brandt CA, Staedt JH: Behavioral problems associated with dementia: the role of newer antipsychotics. Drugs Aging 14:41–54, 1999

Szlabowicz JW, Stewart JT: Amitriptyline treatment of agitation associated with anoxic encephalopathy. Arch Phys Med Rehabil 71:612–613, 1990

Tardiff K, Swelliam A: The occurrence of assaultive behavior among chronic psychiatric inpatients. Am J Psychiatry 139:212–215, 1982

Tariot PN, Erb R, Leibovici A, et al: Carbamazepine treatment of agitation in nursing home patients with dementia: a preliminary study. J Am Geriatr Soc 42:1160–1166, 1994

Tariot PN, Erb R, Podgorski CA, et al: Efficacy and tolerability of carbamazepine for agitation and aggression in dementia. Am J Psychiatry 155:54–61, 1998

Tiller JWG, Dakis JA, Shaw JM: Short-term buspirone treatment in disinhibition with dementia (letter). Lancet 2:510, 1988

Vetro A, Szentistvanyi L, Pallag L, et al: Therapeutic experience with lithium in childhood aggressivity. Neuropsychobiology 14:121–127, 1985

Victoroff J, Zarow C, Mack WJ, et al: Physical aggression is associated with preservation of substantia nigra pars compacta in Alzheimer disease. Arch Neurol 53:428–434, 1996

Wilcox J: Divalproex sodium in the treatment of aggressive behavior. Ann Clin Psychiatry 6:17–20, 1994

Wise MG, Tierney JG: Impulse control disorders not otherwise classified, in the American Psychiatric Press Textbook of Psychiatry, 3rd Edition. Edited by Hales RE, Yudofsky SC, Talbott JA. Washington, DC, American Psychiatric Press, 1999, pp 774–776

Yudofsky SC: β-Blockers and depression: the clinician's dilemma. JAMA 267:1826–1827, 1992

Yudofsky SC, Silver JM, Jackson M, et al: The Overt Aggression Scale: an operationalized rating scale for verbal and physical aggression. Am J Psychiatry 143:35–39, 1986

Yudofsky SC, Silver JM, Schneider SE: Pharmacologic treatment of aggression. Psychiatric Annals 17:397–407, 1987

Yudofsky SC, Silver J, Yudofsky B: Organic personality disorder, explosive type, in Treatments of Psychiatric Disorders: A Task Force Report of the American Psychiatric Association, Vol 2. Washington, DC, American Psychiatric Association, 1989, pp 839–852

Yudofsky SC, Silver JM, Hales RE: Pharmacologic management of aggression in the elderly. J Clin Psychiatry 51 (suppl):22–28, 1990

Yudofsky SC, Kopecky JH, Kumik M, et al: The Overt Agitation Severity Scale for the objective rating of agitation. J Neuropsychiatry Clin Neurosci 9:541–548, 1997

11

Legal and Ethical Issues

Robert I. Simon, M.D.

Consultation-liaison psychiatrists encounter several thorny medicolegal issues in their practice. The delivery of competent mental health services requires a knowledgeable psychiatrist who is comfortable with the legal requirements surrounding consultation-liaison duties. For example, a patient's competency plays a large role in the right to refuse treatment, in informed consent, and in end-of-life decisions about treatment or withholding treatment.

The consultation-liaison psychiatrist may be exposed to an increased risk of legal liability in the evaluation and treatment of violent patients. Appropriate risk assessment and intervention for suicidal patients or potentially violent patients will reduce significantly the likelihood of a successful malpractice claim (Simon 1992a). Legally informed consultation-liaison psychiatrists are in a much better position to provide good clinical care without being encumbered by unrealistic fears and defensive practices (Simon 1992a), which increases the likelihood of a successful clinical outcome.

ETHICAL ISSUES

Ethical issues arise daily for psychiatrists who are involved in consultations on patients who are medically ill. Medical decision making, informed consent, resuscitation, "brain death," organ transplantation, the withholding or withdrawing of life support, and the allocation of medical resources all give rise to complex ethical and legal problems (Luce 1990). Moreover, what is considered ethical in clinical practice today may become a legal requirement tomorrow.

During the first half of the twentieth century, the principle of patient autonomy was clearly recognized in the medical malpractice case *Schloendorff v. Society of New York Hospital* (1914). Justice Cardozo firmly enunciated the principle of patient self-determination by stating that "every human being of adult years and sound mind has a right to determine what shall be done with his own body, and a surgeon who performs an operation without his patient's consent commits an assault, for which he is liable in damages" (pp. 92–93).

Since the late 1950s and early 1960s, the medical profession has moved away from an authoritarian, physician-oriented stance toward more collaboration between physician and patient in health care decisions. This is reflected in contemporary ethical principles (American Psychiatric Association 1997). Thus, on ethical grounds, competent patients have the legal right to autonomy in determining their medical care. Quite apart from any legal obligation, unless otherwise indicated, most psychiatrists disclose pertinent medical information to their patients as a way to enhance the therapeutic alliance (Simon 1987, 1989).

The ethical principles of beneficence, nonmaleficence (no misconduct), and respect for the dignity and autonomy of the patient provide the moral-ethical foundation for the doctor-patient relationship. For example, the consultation-liaison psychiatrist or attending physician has a legal and ethical duty to obtain consent from substitute decision-makers when a patient cannot make an informed decision. The rights of all patients are the same—only how these rights are exercised is different (Parry and Beck 1990).

The ethics of social justice call for the fair allocation of medical resources in accord with medical need (Ruchs 1984). The ethical concerns about equitable health care distribution may seem to be a new development, but they are found in the Hippocratic oath and in the tradition of medicine and psychiatry (Dyer 1988). Thus, psychiatric patients are ethically entitled to have the same access to medical resources as are medical-surgical patients.

DEFINITIONS

- *Competency*—Having the mental capacity to understand the nature of an act.
- *Informed consent*—A competent person's voluntary agreement based on full disclosure of facts needed to make that decision.
- *Right to refuse treatment*—The right of every patient to determine what is or is not done to his or her body (also referred to as the right of self-determination).
- *Confidentiality and testimonial privilege*—Confidentiality refers to the ethical duty of the psychiatrist to not disclose information obtained in the course of evaluating or treating the patient without the patient's express or implied permission. The duty of confidentiality is protected by law.

  Testimonial privilege is established by state statute and is a patient's right. The physician cannot be questioned about confidential information in certain legal proceedings unless the patient consents.
- *Voluntary hospitalization*—Patient admissions that are classified as either pure (also called informal) or as conditional voluntary admissions. A pure or informal voluntary admission permits the patient to leave the hospital at any time. A conditional voluntary admission usually allows the psychiatrist to detain the patient for a specified period after the patient presents a written request for discharge.
- *Involuntary hospitalization*—Hospitalization of a mentally ill person who is a danger to self or others against his or her will for a legally established period of time.
- *Seclusion and restraint*—Treatment interventions that involve isolating the patient or physical immobilization.
- *Advance directives*—Health care decision instruments such as a health care proxy, durable power of attorney, or living will used by individuals who are competent as a method to make health care decisions and choose substitute health care decision-makers in the event of future incompetence.
- *Managed care*—A system of cost-controlled health care delivery that uses cost-containment measures, patient management review, and competitive marketplace techniques.
- *Risk management*—Measures to control or, it is

hoped, lessen the exposure to legal liability. Optimally, these measures do not interfere with good clinical care or unduly raise the cost of evaluation or treatment.

CONFIDENTIALITY AND TESTIMONIAL PRIVILEGE

As noted above, confidentiality refers to the right of a patient to have confidential communications withheld from outside parties without implied or expressed authorization. Testimonial privilege is a legally created rule of evidence that gives the patient the right to prevent the psychiatrist, to whom confidential information was given, from disclosing it in a judicial proceeding.

Breaching Confidentiality

Once the doctor-patient relationship is created, the clinician assumes an automatic duty to safeguard a patient's disclosures. This duty is not absolute, and in some circumstances, breaching confidentiality is both ethical and legal (see Table 11–1).

TABLE 11–1.   Common statutory exceptions to confidentiality between psychiatrist and patient

Child abuse
Competency proceedings
Court-ordered examination
Danger to self or others
Patient-litigant exception
Intent to commit a crime or harmful act
Civil commitment proceedings
Communication with other treatment providers

Psychiatrists do not appear to protect confidentiality as carefully when treating patients in the hospital as compared with outpatient treatment. This is partially because the attending physician initiated the consultation, not the patient. However, the reasons for this disparity go beyond the necessity of involving family and other medical and nonmedical mental health practitioners. Severely ill psychiatric and medical-surgical patients can induce sufficient anxiety to interfere with the professional judgment of the psychiatrist in maintaining confidentiality.

Unless extenuating circumstances arise, the psychiatrist should obtain the competent patient's permission before speaking to the patient's family or other third parties. When this is not possible, a note should be recorded that explains the reasons for not obtaining the patient's permission. Maintaining confidentiality in the hospital is a complex issue because various staff members need to have information in order to develop evaluation and treatment plans. Psychiatrists should not assume that they possess carte blanche authorization when speaking to hospital staff members about all matters revealed by the patient. Information should be provided that will enable the staff to function effectively on behalf of the patient. It is often unnecessary to disclose intimate details of the patient's mental life. As a rule, the staff spends more time with the patient than does the psychiatrist, allowing trust to develop between staff and patient. Under these circumstances, patients often choose to reveal more information about themselves.

Testimonial Privilege

As stated earlier in this chapter, testimonial privilege is the privilege to withhold information that applies only to the judicial setting. The patient, not the psychiatrist, holds the testimonial privilege that controls the release of confidential information. Privilege statutes represent the most common recognition by the state of the importance of protecting information provided by a patient to a psychotherapist. This recognition moves away from the essential purpose of the American system of justice (e.g., "truth finding") by insulating certain information from disclosure in court. This protection is justified on the basis that the special need for privacy in the doctor-patient relationship outweighs the unbridled quest for an accurate outcome in court.

Exceptions to Testimonial Privilege

There are specific exceptions to testimonial privilege. Although exceptions vary, the most common include

- Child abuse reporting
- Civil commitment proceedings
- Court-ordered evaluations
- Criminal proceedings
- Cases in which a patient's mental state is part of the litigation

This last exception, known as the *patient-litigant exception*, commonly occurs in will contests, worker's compensation cases, child custody disputes, personal injury actions, and malpractice actions in which the psychiatrist is sued by the patient.

Liability

An unauthorized or unwarranted breach of confidentiality can cause a patient considerable emotional harm. As a result, a physician typically can be held liable for such a breach based on at least four theories:

1. Malpractice (breach of confidentiality)
2. Breach of statutory duty
3. Invasion of privacy
4. Breach of (implied) contract

INFORMED CONSENT AND THE RIGHT TO REFUSE TREATMENT

The right to refuse treatment is intimately connected with the doctrine of informed consent. By withholding consent, patients express their right to refuse treatment except under certain circumstances. In rare situations, courts have authorized treatment against the wishes of a competent patient. Generally, these cases involve situations in which the life of a fetus is at risk, a patient is encumbered or responsible for the care of dependent children and can be restored to full health through the intervention in question (most often, blood transfusion), and a patient who has attempted suicide is otherwise considered to be healthy. The right to refuse treatment also reflects the exercise of basic constitutional rights. As Stone (1981) pointed out, the right to refuse psychiatric medication is not an isolated issue. Protection of individual autonomy includes not only the right to refuse emergency lifesaving treatment but also advance directives, the right to die, manifold problems involving the rights of children, participation in experimentation, and other issues.

Informed consent provides patients with a legal cause of action if they are not adequately informed about the nature and consequences of a particular medical treatment or procedure. The legal theory of informed consent is based on two distinct principles. First, every patient has the right to determine what is or is not done to his or her body (also referred to as the right of self-determination) (*Schloendorff v. Society of New York Hospital* 1914). The second principle emanates from the fiduciary nature of the doctor-patient relationship. Inherent in a physician's fiduciary duty is the responsibility to disclose honestly and in good faith all requisite facts about a patient's condition. The primary purpose of the doctrine of informed consent is to promote individual autonomy and, secondarily, to facilitate rational decision making (Appelbaum et al. 1987).

Informed consent has three essential ingredients:

1. *Competency:* clinicians provide the first level of screening to establish patient competency and to decide whether to accept a patient's treatment decision.
2. *Information:* the patient or a bona fide representative must be given adequate information (see Table 11–2).
3. *Voluntariness:* the patient must voluntarily consent to or refuse the proposed treatment or procedure.

TABLE 11–2. Informed consent: reasonable information to be disclosed

Although no consistently accepted set of information to be disclosed for any given medical or psychiatric situation exists, as a rule, five areas of information are generally provided:

1. **Diagnosis:**   description of the condition or problem
2. **Treatment:**   nature and purpose of proposed treatment
3. **Consequences:**   risks and benefits of the proposed treatment
4. **Alternatives:**   viable alternatives to the proposed treatment, including risks and benefits
5. **Prognosis:**   projected outcome with and without treatment

Source.   Adapted from Simon 1992b.

Exceptions and Liability

Table 11–3 shows the four basic exceptions to the requirement of obtaining informed consent.

When emergency treatment is necessary to save a life or prevent imminent serious harm, and it is impossible to obtain either the patient's consent or that of someone authorized to provide consent for the patient, the law will typically "presume" that consent is granted. Two qualifications are necessary to apply this exception. First, the emergency must be serious and imminent, and second, the patient's condition and not other circumstances (e.g., adverse environmental conditions) must determine that an emergency exists.

The second exception to informed consent exists when a patient lacks sufficient mental capacity to give consent or is legally incompetent. Someone who is incompetent is incapable of giving informed consent. Under these circumstances, consent is obtained from a substitute decision-maker.

The third exception, therapeutic privilege, is the most difficult to apply. Informed consent may not be required if a psychiatrist determines that a complete disclosure of possible risks and alternatives might have a deleterious effect on the patient's health and welfare. Juris-

TABLE 11–3. Basic exceptions to obtaining informed consent

Emergencies
Incompetency
Therapeutic privilege
Waiver

Source.   Reprinted from Simon RI: *Concise Guide to Psychiatry and Law for Clinicians.* Washington, DC, American Psychiatric Press, 1992b. Copyright 1992, American Psychiatric Press. Used with permission.

dictions vary in their application of this exception. When specific case law or statutes outlining the factors relevant to such a decision are absent, a doctor must substantiate a patient's inability to psychologically withstand being informed of the proposed treatment. Some courts have held that therapeutic privilege may be invoked only if informing the patient will worsen his or her condition or so frighten the patient that rational decision making is precluded (*Canterbury v. Spence* 1972; *Natanson v. Kline* 1960). Therapeutic privilege is not a means of circumventing the legal requirement for obtaining informed consent from the patient before initiating treatment.

Finally, a physician need not disclose risks of treatment when the patient has competently, knowingly, and voluntarily waived his or her right for information (e.g., when the patient does not want information on drug side effects).

Aside from these four exceptions, a physician who treats a patient without obtaining informed consent is subject to legal liability. In some jurisdictions, however, case law or statutes specify that informed consent is unnecessary if a reasonable person under the given circumstances would have consented to treatment. As a rule, treatment without any consent or against a patient's wishes may constitute a battery (intentional tort), whereas treatment commenced with inadequate consent is treated as an act of medical negligence.

Prescribing Medication for Unapproved Uses

Prescribing a Food and Drug Administration (FDA)–approved medication for an unapproved purpose does not violate federal law (Macbeth et al. 1994). In 1961, the FDA established regulations to provide a package insert for all prescription drugs. The package insert must contain adequate information about use, dosages, method of administration, frequency, duration, relevant risks, contraindications, side effects, and precautions in prescribing the drug. The FDA evaluates only the clinical indications that the drug company wants listed in the insert, thus not precluding other specific uses. Failure to describe a particular use may mean that the FDA has not been requested to review the data, usually because the pharmaceutical company does not believe a market exists for a particular use. The FDA abides by the principle that good medical practice requires that a physician prescribe medication according to the best information available. However, the physician who deviates from the package insert may have to explain such a departure should a lawsuit arise.

Psychiatrists should understand that treatment latitude is available in regard to the *Physicians' Desk Reference* (PDR; 2000) and the drug insert. FDA guidelines should not be considered as absolutely authoritative (Simon 1992a). A psychiatrist may prescribe a drug for a use that is not yet approved by the FDA. For example, no drug is currently approved by the FDA for the treatment of aggression (Yudofsky et al. 1995). However, a number of drugs, including neuroleptics, benzodiazepines, β-blockers, anticonvulsants, and lithium, are used effectively to treat aggressive episodes.

The decision to prescribe drugs for nonapproved uses is based on sound knowledge of the drugs backed by firm scientific rationale and established medical studies. The psychiatrist should have texts or journal articles available to substantiate that a nonapproved use is based on the accepted practice of psychiatry. For example, fluoxetine has been approved by the FDA for the treatment of depression and obsessive-compulsive disorder. Nevertheless, psychiatrists have found this medication effective in the treatment of bulimia, premature ejaculation, premenstrual syndrome, smoking cessation, and other conditions. Such off-labeling prescribing can be safe and effective, particularly when based on scientific studies reported in the psychiatric literature. The prescribing of non-FDA-approved drugs, however, poses significant legal and risk management issues that are discussed elsewhere (King 1998).

The FDA does not have the power to control psychiatrists or to dictate the practice of psychiatry, particularly with regard to prescribing drugs. The use of a drug after it is marketed is the responsibility of physicians and prescribed at their sole discretion. The PDR, official guidelines, or any other reference cannot serve as a substitute for the psychiatrist's sound clinical judgment, training, and experience.

The standard for obtaining informed consent is correspondingly heightened when a medication is prescribed for an unapproved use. The patient or guardian must be informed that the patient will be taking a drug that has not been approved by the FDA and should be warned of reasonably foreseeable risks. Although a consent form may provide added protection, the nature of the disclosure should be recorded in the patient's chart. Whether the disclosure is given orally or provided in a consent form, the chart notes should also contain an assessment indicating whether the information was understood by the patient, whether consent was freely given, and the rationale for using a medication for unapproved purposes. This procedure also should be followed when prescribing drugs at higher-than-recommended doses.

Consultation-liaison practice, however, presents unique clinical problems. Consultation-liaison psychiatrists are faced daily with patients with delirium and dementia who require psychotropic medications. No medications are FDA approved specifically for delirium or dementia. Yet neuroleptic drugs are used regularly and effectively. The seriously medically ill patient may be incompetent to provide informed consent. If the psychiatrist approaches the patient's family to obtain consent to give the patient intravenous haloperidol, for example, the recommendation may be quickly rejected: "My father is not crazy!" or "Don't experiment on my mother with psychiatric (or mind-altering) drugs!" Consent options in the treatment of patients who lack decision-making capacity are discussed in the following section.

Informed Consent in Biomedical and Behavioral Research

Research is not a major part of consultation-liaison psychiatry, except in a few large medical schools. Consultation-liaison psychiatry is a clinical specialty. As such, research usually consists of collecting data during routine clinical activities. The opportunities for clinical investigation are practically limitless. In consultation-liaison psychiatry, biomedical research is aimed at the psychiatric aspects of medical illness. Behavioral research is defined as scientific inquiry into factors motivating and determining human attitudes and behavior, without physically intruding on the subject (Reisner and Slobogin 1990).

Systematic human experimentation is guided by self-regulation, statutory and administrative regulations, scientific peer review, local institutional review boards (IRBs), and case law that defines the rights of research subjects (Reisner and Slobogin 1990). Regulatory guidelines promulgated by the U.S. Department of Health and Human Services currently exert the most significant influence on the conduct of research (President's Commission 1982).

Behavioral research is not innocuous and may expose subjects to the risk of compensable psychological harm.

Behavioral research that uses passive observation studies, surveys, and manipulation studies with and without overt deception may raise a number of litigation issues. Passive observation studies may lead to legal actions for invasion of privacy in cases in which the subject is able to be identified in a published study or the study exposes the subject to embarrassment, legal liability, or financial loss. The researcher conducting a survey has a legal duty to protect the subject's anonymity when sensitive personal issues are involved. For a detailed discussion of informed consent in psychiatric research, see Pinals and Appelbaum (2000).

PATIENT COMPETENCY IN HEALTH CARE DECISION MAKING

Consultation-liaison psychiatrists frequently are asked to assess patients' competency. Nearly every area of human endeavor is affected by the law and, as a fundamental condition, requires that the patient be mentally competent (Table 11–4). Essentially, competency is defined as "having sufficient capacity, ability...(or) possessing the requisite physical, mental, natural, or legal qualifications" (Black 1990, p. 284). This definition is deliberately vague and ambiguous because the term *competency* is a broad concept encompassing many different legal issues and contexts. As a result, its definition, requirements, and application can vary widely depending on the circumstances (e.g., making health care decisions, executing a will, or confessing to a crime).

In general, competency refers to some minimal mental, cognitive, or behavioral ability, trait, or capability required to perform a particular legally recognized act or to assume a legal role. The determination of incompetency requires a judicial decision. In this regard, it is clinically useful to distinguish the terms *incompetence* and *incapacity*. Incompetence refers to a court decision, whereas incapacity refers to a clinical determination (Mishkin 1989). Legally, only competent persons may give informed consent. An adult patient is considered legally competent unless adjudicated incompetent or temporarily incapacitated due to a medical condition. Incapacity does not prevent treatment. It merely means that the clinician must obtain substitute consent. Legal competence is very narrowly defined in terms of cognitive capacity. This definition derives largely from the laws governing transactions. Important clinical concepts such as incompetence due to an affective illness may not be recognized by the law unless the disorder significantly diminishes cognitive capacity. For example, a severely

TABLE 11–4. Some areas of law in which competency is an issue

Civil law
Act in public or professional capacity
Authorize disclosure of medical records
Consent to treatment
Contract
Guardianship—care for oneself and one's property
Make a will
Obtain a driver's license
Receive benefits
Retain private counsel
Sue or be sued
Testify in court
Vote

Criminal law
Assume responsibility for a criminal act
Be executed
Be sentenced
Consent to sexual intercourse
Entertain premeditation or "specific intent" of a crime
Make a confession
Make a plea
Provide testimony in court
Stand trial
Waive the insanity defense
Waive the right to counsel

Family law
Adopt
Divorce
Marry
Terminate parental relations with a child

Source. Adapted from Bisbing SB: *Competency and Capacity in Legal Medicine,* 2nd Edition. St. Louis, MO, Mosby Year Book, 1991.

depressed but cognitively intact patient may refuse antidepressant medication because of profound feelings of hopelessness, helplessness, and worthlessness. Manic patients emphasize risks of medications while downplaying benefits. Schizophrenic patients tend to be fearful that medication will cause them serious harm. They are often unable to make a balanced assessment that considers both risks and benefits of a proposed drug. One study that used three assessment instruments of competency for treatment decisions found that the schizophrenia and depression groups had poorer understanding of treatment disclosures, poorer reasoning in making decisions about treatment, and a greater likelihood of failing to appreciate their illness or the potential treatment benefits (Grisso and Appelbaum 1995a). Denial of illness often interferes with insight and the ability to appreciate the significance of information provided to the patient. In *In the Guardianship of John Roe* (1992), the Massachusetts Supreme Judicial Court recognized that denial of illness can render a patient incompetent to make treatment decisions.

Competency is not a scientifically determinable state; it is situation specific. The issue of competency arises in a number of legal contexts (Table 11–4). Although there are no hard and fast rules, germane to determining competency is the patient's ability to

- Understand the particular treatment choice being proposed
- Make a treatment choice
- Be able to verbally or nonverbally communicate that choice

The above standard, however, obtains only a simple consent from the patient rather than an informed consent because alternative treatment choices are not provided.

A review of case law and scholarly literature reveals four standards for determining mental incapacity in decision making (Appelbaum et al. 1987). In the order of levels of mental capacity required, these standards include

1. Communication of choice
2. Understanding of information provided
3. Appreciation of options available
4. Rational decision making

Psychiatrists are generally most comfortable with a rational decision-making standard in determining mental incapacity. Most courts, however, prefer the first two standards. A truly informed consent that considers the patient's autonomy, personal needs, and values occurs when rational decision making is applied by the patient to the risks and benefits of appropriate treatment options provided by the clinician. Grisso and Applebaum (1995a) found that the choice of standards determining competence affected the type and proportion of patients classified as impaired. When compound standards were used, the proportion of patients identified as impaired increased. They advise that clinicians should be aware of the applicable standards in their jurisdictions.

Because severely mentally disordered patients frequently deny their illnesses, they may communicate a choice and understand the information provided but lack the insight or ability to appreciate the information provided. Rational decision making is impaired as well. For example, as noted above, schizophrenic patients tend to fear harm from the treatment while ignoring the risk of medication side effects (Grisso and Applebaum 1995b).

A valid consent is either expressed (orally or in writing) or implied from the patient's actions. The issue of competency, whether in a civil or criminal context, is commonly raised in two situations: when the person is a minor or is mentally disabled and lacks the requisite cognitive capacity for health care decision making. In many situations, minors are not considered legally competent, and therefore, the consent of a parent or designated guardian is required. However, there are exceptions to this general rule, such as minors who are considered emancipated (Smith 1986) or mature (*Gulf S I R Co. v. Sullivan* 1928), or in some cases of medical need, such as abortion (*Planned Parenthood v. Danforth* 1976) or mental health counseling (*Jehovah's Witnesses v. King County Hospital* 1968).

Mentally disabled patients, including mentally impaired psychiatric patients and psychiatrically impaired medically ill patients, present a slightly different problem in evaluating competency. Lack of capacity or competency *cannot* be presumed from either treatment for mental illness (*Wilson v. Lehman* 1964) or institutionalization of such persons (*Rennie v. Klein* 1978). Mental disability or illness does *not* in itself render a person incompetent in all areas of functioning. Instead, the patient must be examined to determine whether specific functional incapacities render a person incapable of making a particular kind of decision or performing a particular type of task. The legal designation of "incompetent" is applied to an individual who fails one of the mental tests of capacity and is therefore considered by law to be not mentally capable of performing a particular act or assuming a particular role. Often, an authorized representative or guardian may provide substitute consent. The adjudication of incompetence by a court is subject or issue specific. In other words, the fact that a patient is adjudicated incompetent to execute a will does not automatically mean that patient is incompetent to do other things, such as consent to treatment, testify as a witness, marry, drive a car, or make a legally binding contract.

Generally, the law will recognize only those decisions or choices that are made by a competent individual. The law seeks to protect incompetent individuals from the harmful consequences of their acts. Persons older than 18 years (U.S. Department of Health and Human Services 1981) are presumed to be competent (*Meek v. City of Loveland* 1929). This presumption, however, is rebuttable by evidence of an individual's incapacity (*Scaria v. St. Paul Fire and Marine Ins Co* 1975). Evidence of impaired perception, short- and long-term memory, judgment, language comprehension, verbal fluency, and reality orientation are mental functions that a court will scrutinize regarding mental capacity and competency.

Medically ill patients who are found to lack the requisite functional mental capacity to make a treatment decision, except in cases of an emergency (*Frasier v. Department of Health and Human Resources* 1986), must have an authorized representative or guardian appointed to make health care decisions on their behalf (*Aponte v. United States* 1984). Table 11–5 lists several consent options available for patients who lack the mental capacity for health care decisions, depending on the jurisdiction. In most states, proxy consent for the evaluation and treatment of a medical condition is available for the patient lacking health care decision-making capacity. However, in many states, proxy consent for the evaluation and treatment of a psychiatric condition in the patient lacking health care decision-making capacity is specifically prohibited.

RIGHT TO DIE

Legal decisions addressing the issue of a patient's right to die fall into one of two categories: 1) patients who are incompetent (i.e., removal of life-support systems) (*In re Conroy* 1985; *In re Quinlan* 1976) or 2) patients who are competent.

Incompetent Patients

On the very difficult and personal question of patient autonomy, the U.S. Supreme Court ruled in *Cruzan v. Director, Missouri Department of Health* (1990) that the state of Missouri may refuse to remove a food and water tube surgically implanted in the stomach of Nancy Cruzan without clear and convincing evidence of her wishes. She was in a persistent vegetative state for 7 years. Without clear and convincing evidence of a patient's decision to have life-sustaining measures withheld in a particular circumstance, the state has the right to maintain that individual's life, even to the exclusion of the family's wishes.

The importance of the *Cruzan* decision for physicians treating severely or terminally impaired patients is that they must seek clear and competent instructions from the patient regarding foreseeable treatment decisions. For example, physicians treating patients with progressive degenerative brain diseases should attempt to obtain the patient's wishes regarding the use of life-sustaining measures while that patient can still competently articulate those wishes. This information is best provided in the form of a living will, durable power of attorney agreement, or health care proxy. However, any written document that clearly and convincingly sets forth the patient's wishes would serve the same purpose.

TABLE 11–5. Common consent options for patients who lack the mental capacity for health care decisions

Proxy consent of next of kin
Adjudication of incompetence; appointment of a guardian
Institutional administrators or committees
Treatment review panels
Substituted consent of the court
Advance directives (living will, durable power of attorney, health care proxy)
Statutory surrogates (spouse or court-appointed guardian)[a]

[a]Medical Statutory Surrogate Laws (when treatment wishes of the patient are unstated).
Source. Reprinted from Simon RI: *Clinical Psychiatry and the Law,* 2nd Edition. Washington, DC, American Psychiatric Press, 1992a. Copyright 1992, American Psychiatric Press. Used with permission.

Although physicians fear civil or criminal liability for stopping life-sustaining treatment, liability now may arise from overtreating critically or terminally ill patients (Weir and Gostin 1990). Legal liability may occur for providing unwanted treatment to a competent patient or treatment that is against the best interests of an incompetent patient.

Competent Patients

A small but growing body of cases has emerged involving competent patients who usually have excruciating pain and terminal diseases and seek to stop further medical treatment. The single most significant influence in the development of this body of law is the doctrine of informed consent. Beginning with the fundamental tenet that "no right is held more sacred…than the right of every individual to the possession and control of his own person" (*Schloendorff v. Society of New York Hospital* 1914, pp. 92–93; *Union Pacific Ry Co v. Botsford* 1891, pp. 250–251), courts have fashioned the present-day informed consent doctrine and applied it to right-to-die cases.

Notwithstanding these principles, the right to decline life-sustaining medical intervention, even for a competent person, is not absolute. As noted in *In re Conroy* (1985), four countervailing interests may limit the exercise of that right: 1) preservation of life, 2) prevention of suicide, 3) safeguarding the integrity of the medical profession, and 4) protection of innocent third parties. In each of these situations, and depending on the surrounding circumstances, the trend is to support a competent patient's right to have artificial life-support systems discontinued (*Bartling v. Superior Court* 1984; *Bouvia v. Superior Court* 1986; *In re Farrell* 1987; *In re Jobes* 1987; *In re Peter* 1987; *Tune v. Walter Reed Army Medical Hosp* 1985).

As a result of the *Cruzan* decision, courts will focus on primarily the reliability of the evidence presented to establish the patient's competence—specifically, the clarity and certainty with which a decision to withhold medical treatment was made. Assuming that a terminally ill patient chose to forego any further medical intervention *and* the patient was competent at the time of the decision, courts are unlikely to overrule or subvert the patient's right to privacy and autonomy.

Do-Not-Resuscitate Orders

Cardiopulmonary resuscitation (CPR) is a medical life-saving technology. Immediate initiation of CPR at the time of a cardiac arrest leaves no time to think about the consequences of reviving a patient. Usually, patients requiring CPR have not thought about or expressed a preference for or against its use.

The ethical principle of patient autonomy justifies the position that the patient or substitute decision-maker should make the decision about the use of CPR. However, some patients and families who are not offered CPR may feel helpless and abandoned. Psychiatrists must remain aware of this reaction and properly assist the patient and family. The competent patient's decision about do-not-resuscitate (DNR) orders should be followed. Malpractice liability for withholding unwanted and futile care is unlikely, whereas the psychiatrist is exposed to greater liability if care is provided against the patient's wishes (March and Staver 1991).

Schwartz (1987) noted that two key principles have emerged concerning DNR decisions:

1. DNR decisions are reached consensually by the attending physician and the patient or substitute decision-maker.
2. DNR orders, including date and time, are written on the doctor's order sheet, and the reasons for the DNR order are documented in the chart.

Hospital CPR policies make DNR decisions discretionary (Luce 1990). Psychiatrists should become familiar with the specific hospital policy whenever a DNR order is written. Medicolegal-ethical principles for CPR and emergency cardiac care are available (Council on Ethical and Judicial Affairs 1991).

PHYSICIAN-ASSISTED SUICIDE

With the increasing legal recognition of physician-assisted suicide, psychiatrists are likely to be called on to become gatekeepers as part of their consultation-liaison practice. Such a role would be a radical departure from the physician's code of ethics that prohibits participation by an ethical doctor in any intervention that hastens death. Previously, the Supreme Court ruled in *Cruzan* that terminally ill persons could refuse life-sustaining medical treatment. Courts and legislatures will determine whether hastening death is an unwarranted extension of the right to refuse treatment. Every proposal for physician-assisted suicide requires a psychiatric screening or consultation to determine the terminally ill person's competence to commit suicide. The presence of psychiatric disorders associated with suicide, particularly depression, will have to be ruled out as the driving factor behind physician-assisted suicide. Much controversy rages over the ethics of this gatekeeping function (American Medical Association 1994).

ADVANCE DIRECTIVES

Advance directives such as a living will, health care proxy, or a durable medical power of attorney are recommended in order to avoid ethical and legal complications associated with requests to withhold life-sustaining treatment measures (Simon 1992a; Solnick 1985). The Patient Self-Determination Act that became effective on December 1, 1991, requires all hospitals, nursing homes, hospices, managed care organizations, and home health care agencies to advise patients or family members of their right to accept or refuse medical care in the form of an advance directive (LaPuma et al. 1991). Advance directives provide a method for individuals, while they are competent, to choose alternative health care decision-makers in the event of future incompetency. A living will may be contained as a subsection of a durable power of attorney agreement. The ordinary power of attorney created for the management of business and financial matters, unlike advance directives, becomes null and void if the person creating it becomes incompetent.

Federal law does not specify the right to formulate advance directives; therefore, state law applies. State legislators have recognized that individuals may want to stipulate who should make important health care decisions if they become incapacitated and unable to act in their own behalf. All 50 states and the District of Columbia permit individuals to create a durable power of attorney (i.e., one that endures even if the competence of the creator does not) (*Cruzan v. Director, Missouri Department of Health* 1990). Several states and the District of Columbia do have durable power of attorney statutes that expressly authorize the appointment of proxies for making health care decisions (*Cruzan v. Director, Missouri Department of Health* 1990).

Generally, durable power of attorney is construed to empower an agent to make health care decisions. Such a document is much broader and more flexible than a living will, which covers just the period of a diagnosed terminal illness and specifies only that no "extraordinary treatments" be used to prolong the act of dying (Mishkin 1985). To clarify the uncertain status of the durable power of attorney for health care decisions, several states have passed health care proxy laws. The health care proxy is a legal instrument akin to the durable power of attorney but is specifically created for the delegation of health care decisions (see Appendix). Despite the growing use of advance directives, increasing evidence suggests that physician values rather than patient values are more decisive in end-of-life decisions (Orentlicher 1992).

In a durable power of attorney or health care proxy, general or specific directions are set forth about how future decisions are to be made in the event that one becomes unable to make these decisions. The determination of a patient's competence, however, is not specified in most durable power of attorney and health care proxy statutes. Because this is a medical or psychiatric question, an examination by two physicians to determine the patient's ability to understand the nature and consequences of the proposed treatment or procedure, ability to make a choice, and ability to communicate that choice usually is sufficient. This information, like all significant medical observations, should be clearly documented in the patient's chart.

Because advance directives are frequently absent, statutory surrogate laws exist in a number of states. These laws authorize certain persons, such as a spouse or court-appointed guardian, to make health care decisions when the patient has not stated his or her wishes in writing.

The application of advance directives to patients with psychiatric syndromes presents difficulties. A situation may arise in which a currently asymptomatic patient with an organic personality disorder and occasional bouts of severe affective instability draws up a durable power of attorney agreement or health care proxy directing that "If I become mentally unstable again, administer medications even if I strenuously object or resist." Gutheil (personal communication, September 1985) described this agreement as the "Ulysses Contract." In Greek mythology, Ulysses was bound to the mast of his ship so he could hear the beautiful, although lethal, sirens' song. All the other sailors covered their ears. When Ulysses heard the irresistibly fetching song of the sirens, he tried to struggle loose. When that failed, Ulysses demanded to be untied. Similarly, when mood

instability recurs, the patient with an organic personality disorder may strenuously object to treatment.

Because durable power of attorney agreements or health care proxies are easily revoked, the treating psychiatrist or institution has no choice but to honor the patient's refusal, even if there is reasonable evidence that the patient is incompetent. If this situation occurs, legal consultation should be considered. If the patient is grossly confused and is an immediate danger to self and others, the physician or hospital is on firmer ground, both medically and legally, to temporarily override the patient's treatment refusal. Otherwise, it is generally better to seek a court order for treatment than to risk legal entanglement with the patient by attempting to enforce the advance directive's original terms. Typically, unless there are compelling medical reasons to do otherwise, courts will generally honor the patient's original treatment directions.

GUARDIANSHIP

Historically, the state or sovereign possessed the power and authority to safeguard the estate of incompetent persons (Regan 1972). In modern times, guardianship is a method of substitute decision making for individuals who are judicially determined to be unable to act for themselves (Parry 1985). In some states, there are separate provisions for the appointment of a "guardian of one's person" (e.g., health care decision making) and for a "guardian of one's estate" (e.g., authority to make contracts to sell one's property) (Sales et al. 1982). The latter guardian is frequently referred to as a *conservator*, although this designation is not uniformly used throughout the United States. Two further distinctions—*general (plenary)* and *specific* guardianship—are made in some jurisdictions (Sales et al. 1982). As the name implies, the latter guardian is restricted to making decisions about a particular subject area. For instance, the specific guardian is authorized to make decisions about major or emergency medical procedures, and the disabled person retains the freedom to make decisions about all other medical matters. The general guardian, by contrast, has total control over the disabled individual's person, estate, or both (Sales et al. 1982).

Guardianship arrangements are increasingly used with patients who have dementia, particularly AIDS-related dementia and Alzheimer's disease (Overman and Stoudemire 1988). Under the Anglo-American system of law, an individual is presumed to be competent unless adjudicated incompetent. Thus, incompetence is a legal determination made by a court of law based on evidence from health care providers and others that the individual's functional mental capacity is significantly impaired. The Uniform Guardianship and Protective Proceeding Act (UGPPA) or the Uniform Probate Code (UPC) is used as a basis for laws governing competency in many states (Mishkin 1989). The Uniform Acts were drafted by legal scholars and practicing attorneys to achieve uniformity among states by enactment of model laws (Uniform Guardianship and Protective Proceeding Act §5–101).

General incompetency is defined by the UGPPA as meaning

> impaired by reason of mental illness, mental deficiency, physical illness or disability, advanced age, chronic use of drugs, chronic intoxication, or other cause (except minority) to the extent of lacking sufficient understanding or capacity to make or communicate reasonable decisions. (Uniformed Guardianship and Protective Proceeding Act [UGPPA] Section 1–101(7); see also Uniform Probate Code [UPC] Section 5–101.)

A significant number of patients with severe medical or psychiatric disorders meet the above definition. Generally, the appointment of a guardian is limited to situations in which the individual's decision-making capacity is so impaired that he or she is unable to care for personal safety or provide necessities such as food, shelter, clothing, and medical care (*In re Boyer* 1981). The standard of proof required for a judicial determination of incompetency is clear and convincing evidence. Although the law does not assign percentages to proof, clear and convincing evidence is in the range of 75% certainty (Simon 1992a).

States vary with regard to the extent of their reliance on psychiatric assessments. Nonmedical personnel such as social workers, psychologists, family members, friends, colleagues, and even the individual who is the subject of the proceeding may testify.

SUBSTITUTED JUDGMENT

Psychiatrists often find that the process required to obtain an adjudication of incompetence is unduly burdensome, is costly, and frequently interferes with the provision of quality treatment. Moreover, families may be reluctant to face the formal court proceedings necessary to declare their family member incompetent, particularly when sensitive family matters are disclosed. Common consent options for patients lacking health care decision-making capacity are listed in Table 11–5. It can be legally risky to decide that a patient is incompetent and to rely on the consent of a family member (Macbeth et al. 1994).

Clear advantages are associated with having the family serve as decision-makers (Perr 1984). First, use of responsible family members as surrogate decision-makers maintains the integrity of the family unit and relies on the sources who are most likely to know the patient's wishes. Second, it is more efficient and less costly. There are some disadvantages, however. Proxy decision making requires synthesizing the diverse values, beliefs, practices, and prior statements of the patient for a specific circumstance (Emanuel and Emanuel 1992). As one judge characterized the problem, any proxy decision made in the absence of specific directions is at best only an optimistic approximation (*In re Jobes* 1987). Ambivalent feelings, conflicts within the family and with the patient, and conflicting economic interests may make certain family members suspect as guardians (Gutheil and Appelbaum 1980). Some family members are more impaired than the patient for whom proxy consent is being sought. In addition, relatives may not be available or may not want to get involved.

The President's Commission for the Study of Ethical Problems in Medicine and Biomedical and Behavioral Research (1982) recommended that the relatives of incompetent patients be selected as proxy decision-makers for the following reasons:

1. The family is generally most concerned about the good of the patient.
2. The family is usually most knowledgeable about the patient's goals, preferences, and values.
3. The family deserves recognition as an important social unit to be treated, within limits, as a single decision-maker in matters that intimately affect its members.

Some states permit proxy decision making by statute, mainly through their informed consent statute (Solnick 1985). Some state statutes specify that another person (e.g., specific relatives) may authorize consent on behalf of the incompetent patient. As noted earlier in this chapter, a number of states permit proxy consent by next of kin only for patients with medical conditions. Proxy consent is not available in many states for individuals with psychiatric conditions (Simon 2001).

Unless proxy consent by a relative is provided by statute or by case law authority within the state, the consultation-liaison psychiatrist should not rely on the good faith consent by next of kin in treating a patient believed to be incompetent (Macbeth et al. 1994). The legally appropriate procedure is to seek judicial recognition of the family member as the substitute decision-maker.

Some patients recover competency within a few days. As soon as the patient recovers sufficient mental capacity, consent for further treatment should be obtained directly from the patient. For the patient who continues to lack mental capacity for health care decisions, an increasing number of states have statutes that permit involuntary treatment of incompetent mentally ill patients who refuse treatment, even if the patient does not meet current standards for involuntary civil commitment (Hassenfeld and Grumet 1984; Zito et al. 1984). As noted above, in most jurisdictions, a durable power of attorney or health care proxy permits the next of kin to consent (Solnick 1985).

VOLUNTARY HOSPITALIZATION

Although an expressed or implied contract may be lacking, it is well established legally that a doctor is not obligated to accept a patient who simply seeks medical or psychiatric treatment (*Salas v. Gamboa* 1988). In some situations, however, an implied contractual arrangement does exist, even between a physician and a patient who have had no contact. The most common situation is a hospital's emergency room, where it is expected that medical services will be provided to all who seek treatment. This principle may extend to include physicians and psychiatrists who are on call for patient admissions or who consult to the emergency room staff (*Dillon v. Silver* 1987). Once a patient is admitted to a hospital, whether through voluntary or involuntary admission, the hospital is responsible to provide reasonable care to that patient.

Depending on the circumstances surrounding the admission or potential admission, liability issues associated with patient admission may arise. The most common cause of legal action involves the psychiatrist's failure to comply with civil commitment requirements. This situation typically gives rise to a lawsuit based on the theories of false imprisonment (*Gonzalez v. New York* 1983), malicious prosecution, or assault (*St. Vincent's Medical Center v. Oakley* 1979).

The medical-surgical patient who is transferred to a psychiatric unit may want to leave. Because these patients were originally admitted for a medical or surgical problem, transfer to a psychiatric unit can be a bewildering, frightening experience. If the psychiatric unit contains disturbed, noisy, or threatening patients, the medical-surgical patient may become terrified and demand immediate release. Grounds for a lawsuit may exist when a voluntary patient seeks to leave a hospital and is then coerced to remain in the hospital by threat of civil commitment. A patient should not be told that he or she will be involuntarily hospitalized unless that is the psychiatrist's actual intention. For example, an appeals court

ordered a new trial for a patient who alleged false imprisonment by her psychiatrist. The court held that material issues of fact existed in the patient's apprehension of force or coercion used to keep her in a hospital by threat of involuntary hospitalization (*Marcus v. Liebman* 1978).

In addition, a lawsuit may result when actual commitment proceedings are initiated without appropriate evidence for such an action (*Plumadore v. State* 1980). Liability also may occur if a patient represents a foreseeable risk of danger to self or others and the hospital does not hospitalize such a patient (*Clark v. State* 1985).

To protect a patient's civil rights, he or she should be informed of the types of voluntary admission. Pure or informal voluntary admission permits the patient to leave the hospital at any time. Only moral suasion is available to encourage the patient to stay. Conditional or formal voluntary admissions contain provisions that may require the patient to stay for a period of time after giving written notice of intention to leave. The latter provision is used when the patient is judged to be a danger to self or others.

In reality, the distinction between voluntary and involuntary admissions is not always clear. Patients are often induced or pressured into accepting voluntary admissions. If voluntary admission were maintained as truly voluntary, involuntary admissions would likely increase. The situation is analogous to plea bargaining in criminal cases. The criminal justice system would have to accommodate an increased number of cases if plea bargaining were eliminated.

Until recently, relatively few cases addressed the issue of informed consent for voluntary admission. In *In re Certification of William R* (1958), the court expressed disapproval for the procedure that admits an individual to a mental institution who makes no "positive objection" and thereby "shunts seniles into involuntary confinement without awareness by them of their plight and without their active approval or judicial surveillance." In addition to voluntary admissions procedures, an increasing number of states permit nonjudicial hospitalization of nonprotesting persons. The District of Columbia statute provides a simple, nontraumatic admission process for those individuals who either do not recognize their need for hospitalization or are unwilling to seek admission but nevertheless sign a "no objection" statement when others initiate the admission process (DC CODE ANN §21–513 [1981 and 1984 Supp]).

In a U.S. Supreme Court case, *Zinermon v. Burch* (1990), a mentally ill patient who was unable to give informed consent was permitted to proceed with a civil rights action against state officials who committed him to a state hospital under voluntary commitment procedures. The court held that Florida must have procedures to screen all voluntary patients for competency and exclude incompetent persons from the voluntary admission process. For the few states that require competent consent to voluntary admission, screening procedures to exclude incompetent patients are needed. Although the Supreme Court did not directly address whether a voluntary patient must be competent to consent to admission, Appelbaum (1990, p. 1060) opined that "Zinermon will refocus attention on the often-neglected process of voluntary admission."

Voluntary patients may demand to leave the hospital against medical advice (AMA). If the patient is not a danger to self or others and is competent, the psychiatrist cannot do much more than try to deal with the discharge as a treatment issue. Regardless of whether the patient signs an AMA form, a notation should be made in the record detailing the recommendations made to the patient about the need for further hospitalization as well as the possible risks of premature discharge. Voluntary patients who are incompetent but are not dangerous or gravely disabled can be kept in the hospital against their will if they have been adjudicated incompetent and a guardian gives consent for continued hospitalization. This authority also exists for individuals vested with durable power of attorney for health care decisions. Under these circumstances, family or another responsible party should be involved at the time of a premature discharge.

INVOLUNTARY HOSPITALIZATION

The consultation-liaison psychiatrist must consider the clinical intervention of involuntary hospitalization for patients who are judged violent to themselves or others, who are refusing treatment, and for whom a less restrictive alternative is unavailable or not appropriate. The consultation-liaison psychiatrist should be able to perform competent suicide and violence risk assessments that direct appropriate clinical interventions such as involuntary hospitalization (Simon 1998a, 2001; Tardiff 1996). Three main substantive criteria serve as the foundation for all statutory commitment requirements. These criteria require that the individual is 1) mentally ill, 2) dangerous to self or others, and/or 3) unable to provide for basic needs. Generally, each state determines which criteria are required and defines each criterion. Because terms such as *mentally ill* are often loosely described, the proper definition relies on the clinician's judgment.

Certain states have enacted legislation that permits the involuntary hospitalization of not only individuals with mental illness but also three other distinct groups: 1) developmentally disabled people (mentally retarded), 2) substance-addicted people (alcohol, drugs), and 3) mentally disabled minors. Special commitment provisions may exist governing requirements for the admission and discharge of mentally disabled minors as well as numerous due process rights of these individuals (*Parham v. J.R.* 1979).

Involuntary hospitalization of patients usually arises when violent behavior threatens to erupt and when patients become unable to care for themselves. These patients frequently have mental disorders and conditions that readily meet the substantive criteria for involuntary hospitalization.

Clinicians must remember that they cannot legally commit patients. This process is solely under the court's jurisdiction. The psychiatrist merely initiates a medical certification that brings the patient before the court, which usually occurs after a brief evaluation in a hospital. Psychiatrists who use reasonable professional judgment and act in good faith when requesting involuntary hospitalization are granted immunity from liability in many states.

Commitment statutes do not mandate involuntary hospitalization (Appelbaum et al. 1987). The statutes are permissive and enable mental health professionals and others to seek involuntary hospitalization for persons who meet certain criteria. On the other hand, the duty to seek involuntary hospitalization is a standard-of-care issue. That is, patients who are mentally ill and pose an imminent, serious threat to themselves or others may require involuntary hospitalization as a primary psychiatric intervention.

SECLUSION AND RESTRAINT

The psychiatric-legal issues surrounding seclusion and restraint are complex. There are both indications for and contraindications to the use of seclusion and restraint (see Tables 11–6 and 11–7). However, what the general psychiatrist may believe are contraindications to the use of restraints often are viewed as indications by the consultation-liaison psychiatrist. The consultation-liaison psychiatrist frequently recommends restraint in confused, medically unstable patients. These patients often have delirium or dementia. If restraints are not used in such patients, they may pull out their endotracheal tubes, arterial lines, and, in some instances, intra-aortic balloon pumps. Moreover, confused, medically ill patients also climb over bed rails and fall onto the floor. Falls may result in fractures and subdural hematomas.

TABLE 11–6.   Indications for seclusion and restraint

To prevent clear, imminent harm to patient or others

To prevent significant disruption to treatment program or physical surroundings

To assist in treatment as part of ongoing behavior therapy

To decrease sensory overstimulation[a]

To respond to patient's voluntary reasonable request for intervention

[a]Seclusion only.

Source.   Reprinted from Simon RI: *Clinical Psychiatry and the Law,* 2nd Edition. Washington, DC, American Psychiatric Press, 1992a. Copyright 1992, American Psychiatric Press. Used with permission.

TABLE 11–7.   Contraindications to seclusion and restraint

Extremely unstable medical and psychiatric conditions[a,b]

Patients with delirium or dementia who are unable to tolerate decreased stimulation[a,b]

Overtly suicidal patients[a,b]

Patients with severe drug reactions or overdoses[b] or those who require close monitoring of drug dosages[a]

Punishment of the patient or convenience of staff

[a]Unless close supervision and direct observation are provided.

[b]May be indications for restraint in medically ill patients in the general hospital.

Source.   Adapted from Simon RI: *Clinical Psychiatry and the Law,* 2nd Edition. Washington, DC, American Psychiatric Press, 1992a. Copyright 1992, American Psychiatric Press. Used with permission.

Stringent legal regulation of seclusion and restraint has increased during the past decade, as have legal challenges on the use of seclusion and restraint in institutionalized mentally ill and mentally retarded patients. These lawsuits usually are part of a challenge to a wide range of alleged abuses within a hospital. Generally, courts hold that restraints and seclusion are appropriate only when a patient presents a risk of harm to self or others and a less restrictive alternative is not available. Additional considerations include the following:

- Restraint and seclusion must be implemented by a written order from an appropriate medical official. However, a physician on call at night can give a verbal order for restraint, as long as the patient is examined soon thereafter and an order is written.
- Orders must be confined to specific, time-limited periods.
- A patient's condition must be regularly reviewed and documented.
- Extension of the original order must be reviewed and reauthorized.

The use of restraint or seclusion for the purposes of rehabilitative training was recognized in the landmark case *Youngberg v. Romeo* (1982). Youngberg challenged the treatment practices at the Pennhurst State School and Hospital in Pennsylvania. The Supreme Court held that restraint was unacceptable except to ensure a patient's safety or in certain undefined circumstances "to provide needed training." In the *Youngberg* case, the Supreme Court recognized that the defendant was entitled to safety and freedom from bodily restraint. The Supreme Court added that these interests were neither absolute nor in conflict with the need to provide training and that decisions made by professionals to use restraint are presumed correct. Psychiatrists and other mental health professionals have praised this decision because the Supreme Court recognized that professionals rather than the courts are better able to determine the needs of patients.

Most states have enacted statutes to regulate the use of restraints, which specify the circumstances in which restraints are appropriate. Most often, those circumstances occur only when a risk of harm to self or danger to others is imminent. Statutory regulation of the use of seclusion is far less common. Only about one-half of the states have laws relating to seclusion. Most states with laws regarding seclusion and restraint require documentation of their use.

Some courts and state statutes outline due process procedures before a restraint or seclusion order is implemented. Typical due process considerations include some form of notice, a hearing, and the involvement of an impartial decision-maker. Notably, patient due process protections are only required in cases in which restraint and seclusion are used for disciplinary purposes. Restrictions on the use of these procedures may be eased in cases of emergency, unless language to the contrary exists.

The American Psychiatric Association Task Force on the Psychiatric Uses of Seclusion and Restraint established national guidelines for the proper use of seclusion and restraint (Tardiff 1984). The Joint Commission on Accreditation of Healthcare Organizations (1991) promulgates detailed guidelines for hospitals regarding seclusion and restraint requirements. States and the federal government now regulate and limit the use of restraint and seclusion. Professional opinion about the clinical use of physical restraints and seclusion varies considerably. Unless precluded by regulations or by statutes, the use of seclusion and restraint may be justified on both clinical and legal grounds (Simon 1992a). However, the Joint Commission on Accreditation of Healthcare Organizations, state, and federal regulatory policies have developed new regulations that further limit the use of restraints. The new regulations are a response to a number of deaths occurring during or shortly after the use of restraints.

COLLABORATIVE, CONSULTATIVE, AND SUPERVISORY RELATIONSHIPS WITH NONMEDICAL THERAPISTS

The American Psychiatric Association (1980) formulated guidelines for psychiatrists who work with nonmedical mental health therapists. As mental health care is delivered increasingly by nonmedical therapists, psychiatrists will practice more within the framework of an organized health delivery system. Thus, the capacity to provide mental health care is enhanced. The cross-fertilization of different mental health disciplines fosters professional growth of the team members. However, an obvious limit exists to nonmedical mental health professionals' ability to appropriately consult on medically ill patients (e.g., patients with delirium).

In a collaborative relationship, responsibility for the patient's care is shared according to the qualifications and limitations of each discipline (American Psychiatric Association 1980). The patient is informed of the separate responsibilities of each therapist. The responsibilities of each discipline do not diminish the other. Periodic evaluation of the patient's clinical condition and needs by the psychiatrist and the nonmedical therapist is necessary to determine whether the collaboration should continue. On termination of the collaborative relationship, the health care providers should inform the patient either separately or jointly.

So-called split treatment has become commonplace in the managed care era. The psychiatrist provides the medication backup for the nonmedical therapist who conducts psychotherapy with the patient. Serious problems can exist with this arrangement, particularly confusion over responsibility for the patient's care and communication between the treaters (Meyer and Simon 1999). Fragmentation of care may result in ineffective or harmful treatment of the patient.

When performing single consultations, the consultation-liaison psychiatrist ordinarily does not enter into a treatment relationship with the patient and does not assume responsibility for care. Because most consultation-liaison psychiatrists do follow-up care in hospitals, a doctor-patient treatment relationship may be construed by a court from the consultation-liaison psychiatrist's continuing relationship with the patient, regardless of whether

actual orders are written. However, when orders are written, courts will likely find a doctor-patient relationship.

The consultation-liaison psychiatrist is not the primary physician. The consultation-liaison psychiatrist has a relationship with the consulting physician, not the patient. The consulting physician is free to accept or reject the findings and recommendations of the consultation-liaison psychiatrist. Consultation-liaison psychiatrists are not likely to be found ultimately liable for adverse outcomes when their suggestions are not acted on. They may, nonetheless, be sued along with the consulting physician. Follow-up and discussion with the consulting physician are important to avoid miscommunications. The consultation-liaison psychiatrist relies on information provided by the physician. The risk of liability for the consultation-liaison psychiatrist will arise only if the consultative advice provided is negligently based on inadequate or limited information. When the consultation-liaison psychiatrist sees the patient directly, liability may be assessed for a negligent consultation.

The American Psychiatric Association (1980) "Guidelines for Psychiatrists in Consultative, Supervisory, or Collaborative Relationships With Nonmedical Therapists" is now more than two decades old. Despite significant changes during this time, the guidelines have not been revised. Today, the relationship between psychiatrists and nonmedical therapists is infinitely more complex (Kleinman 1991). Furthermore, an important caveat that accompanies the guidelines states "that they do not represent official policy but rather a 'living document' to be adapted to local custom and practice."

The practice of psychiatry has changed a great deal since the guidelines were adopted, so that certain guidelines may no longer be applicable. The guidelines are not particularly helpful in defining the psychiatrist's obligations in providing supervision to a nonmedical therapist. For example, the responsibilities of a supervisor differ from those of a psychiatrist who is directly treating the patient. Yet the guidelines suggest that a psychiatrist in a supervisory relationship "remains ethically and medically responsible for the patient's care" (American Psychiatric Association 1980, p. 1490). The meaning of this statement is unclear. Important distinctions that exist in the psychiatrist's responsibilities between supervisory and treatment roles are ignored. Moreover, with the advent of biological treatments, the guidelines do not help to define the scope of nonsupervisory responsibilities of psychiatrists who may provide medication backup for nonmedical professionals (Goldberg et al. 1991). The psychiatrist's liability in cases in which the nonmedical professional is found to have practiced outside of the scope of his or her practice will likely depend on the nature and extent of the psychiatrist's relationship with the nonmedical professional and the patient. Appelbaum (1991, p. 282) recommends that "all responsibilities should be clearly specified, preferably in a written agreement among the patient, the psychiatrist, and the nonmedical therapist."

Unless psychiatrists are fully prepared to assume medical responsibility for the patient, they should not undertake the supervision of nonmedical therapists. In the supervision of nonmedical therapists, the issue of medical assessment is extremely important. Psychiatrists must not supervise in name only and allow themselves to be used as a means to obtain insurance payment for nonmedical providers. If the psychiatrist enters a collaborative, consultative, or supervisory relationship in which his or her role is misrepresented or the care provided by the nonmedical therapist is inadequate or inappropriate, the treatment is unethical unless the purpose is to raise the quality of care. Psychiatrists should not continue in these roles unless they are assured that they are appropriately informed about the nature of the treatment and the clinical course of the patient. Otherwise, there is no guarantee that the patient is receiving competent treatment. The frequency of collaboration, consultation, and supervision must fulfill the psychiatrist's medical, ethical, and legal responsibilities to the patient.

MANAGED CARE

Health maintenance organizations (HMOs), independent practice associations (IPAs), and preferred provider organizations (PPOs) may create additional ethical and legal dilemmas for psychiatrists. Managed care systems interject cost and contractual pressures into treatment and dispositional decisions. Psychiatrists must not allow themselves to be put in the position of choosing between a patient's need for quality care and the economic and administrative requirements of the health plan. Psychiatrists who do consultation-liaison work may find that they are practicing with greater regularity in managed care settings.

In *Wickline v. California* (1986), the treating physician, Dr. Polonsky, requested an extended stay of 8 days for his patient following surgery for Leriche's syndrome (occlusion of the terminal aorta). The Medi-Cal reviewer granted 4 days. The patient experienced complications following the premature release, resulting in amputation of her leg. She sued Medi-Cal. The jury ruled in her favor, but a California appellate court decided that the treating physician was liable, not Medi-Cal. The physician was not a defendant in the case.

In his testimony, Dr. Polonsky stated that he believed "that Medi-Cal had the power to tell him, as a treating doctor, when a patient must be discharged from the hospital." The appellate court noted that third-party payers of health care services can be held liable when appeals on the behalf of the patients for medical care "are arbitrarily ignored or unreasonably disregarded or over-ridden." The court added that "the physician who complies without protest with the limitations imposed by a third party payor, when his medical judgment dictates otherwise, cannot avoid his ultimate responsibility for his patient's care. He cannot point to the health care payor as the liability scapegoat when the consequences of his own determinative medical decision go sour."

The obvious misunderstanding of the surgeon, expressed in *Wickline*, is probably shared by other physicians about their duty and the authority of the third-party payer. The *Wickline* case holds that the physician has the unquestionable responsibility for a patient's health care. Accordingly, when a physician's decision and the position of a third-party payer conflict, it is the physician's duty to protest any compromise in patient care that might be presented by a third-party payer. All channels should be pursued to ensure that the physician's medical judgment (e.g., continued hospitalization) is carried out (Simon 1998b). It is the physician's professional and legal duty to provide competent care to the patient. Managed care organizations generally limit or deny payment for services but not the actual services themselves (Simon 1997).

In a subsequent case, *Wilson v. Blue Cross of Southern California et al.* (1990), a California appeals court chose not to follow the specific language of the *Wickline* case. In the *Wilson* case, a patient with anorexia, drug dependency, and major depression was hospitalized at College Hospital in Los Angeles, California. The treating physician determined that the patient required 3–4 weeks of hospitalization. After approximately 1½ weeks, utilization review determined that further hospitalization was unnecessary. The patient's insurance company refused to pay for further inpatient treatment. The patient was discharged and committed suicide a few weeks later.

The Appellate Division of the California Court of Appeals heard that third-party payers are not immune from lawsuits in regard to utilization review activities. The court determined that the insurer may be subject to liability for harm caused to the patient by premature termination of hospitalization. Although the fact pattern of this case differs from that of the *Wickline* case, it is clear from the *Wilson* decision that a third-party payer may be held legally liable for a negligent decision to discharge the patient either separately or along with the patient's physician, depending on the facts of the case. Although *Wickline* and *Wilson* are California cases only, they offer insight and, perhaps, precedence concerning future reasoning by other courts who will be increasingly confronted by complex liability issues associated with utilization review decisions.

Before signing a contract, the psychiatrist must be aware of plan requirements that may interfere with the provision of good clinical care and with the traditional doctor-patient relationship. Some plan agreements state that medical records must be made available to other providers in the plan. Psychiatrists who see patients under managed health care plans must explain to these patients that the same confidentiality that exists for other patients does not exist for them. Patients also may know other providers in the plan, and they may not want to have psychiatric information disseminated. Some contracts clearly state that the psychiatrist must provide information to administrators that may lead to loss of medical services to the patient. Patients who act in self-destructive or violent ways while refusing to follow a treatment plan may be dropped from the plan. Patients should be informed of any confidentiality limitations before embarking on treatment.

Psychiatrists must realize that their responsibilities to patients are not necessarily limited by the contractual services covered by a managed health care plan. If the plan decides to limit services to the suicidal or dangerous patient, the psychiatrist's legal duty remains the same as if treating the patient independently. The psychiatrist must take all necessary steps to care for the patient adequately. Most managed health care plans reserve the right to review all hospitalizations and may refuse coverage, even if the patient is admitted as an emergency, if the plan believes that further treatment is not necessary. If the patient is harmed as a result and a suit is filed, the plaintiff's attorney can claim that, to save money, the physician did not provide necessary care. Courts will not accept the argument that a plan prevents the physician from providing accepted treatments or from referring the patient to appropriate specialists outside of the plan.

Sometimes, plan contracts will state that the physician must not communicate anything or take any action that may adversely affect the confidence of patients in the plan. This requirement does not, however, supersede the psychiatrist's duty to report child abuse or to warn endangered third parties. States are enacting laws to make "gag rules" illegal that limit information on treatment options or prohibit physicians from revealing certain restrictions or financial incentives to limit care (Simon 1998b).

The treatment prerogatives of the psychiatrist may be limited by the conditions of a plan. Thus, a limit may be placed on patients requiring long-term hospitalization. The temptation to cut corners in patient treatment can become a malpractice trap. The plan may specify which hospital must be used or require that referrals be made to other providers in the plan. Psychiatrists must not suspend their judgment in making competent dispositions and referrals because the psychiatrist may be held responsible for making a negligent choice. During periods when the psychiatrist is away, nonparticipating psychiatrists who cover must understand that they will have to accept the fees designated by the health care plan and abide by its review procedures.

Psychiatrists should determine whether the contract contains a hold harmless provision that will require indemnification of the plan for any liability arising out of the psychiatrist's practice. Many malpractice policies will not cover any liability assumed under an oral or a written agreement such as a contract provision. If the plan is sued because of care provided by the psychiatrist, he or she may be held personally liable for any resulting judgment, which malpractice insurance will not cover. It is obvious that the psychiatrist should consult an attorney before signing any contract with a health provider organization.

RISK MANAGEMENT

Psychiatric Malpractice

Psychiatric malpractice is medical malpractice. Malpractice is the delivery of substandard professional care that causes a compensable injury to a person (Simon and Sadoff 1992). Although this definition may seem relatively clear and simple, confusion may exist. For example, the essential issue is *not* the existence of substandard care per se but whether actual compensable liability exists. In order for a psychiatrist to be found liable to a patient for malpractice, the four fundamental elements listed in Table 11–8 must be established by a preponderance of the evidence (e.g., more likely than not). Unless all of these four elements are met, the physician is not liable, even if negligence occurred. A psychiatrist may be negligent but is still not liable. For example, if the patient had no real injuries because of the negligence or if he or she had an injury but it was not directly due to the psychiatrist's negligence, then a claim of malpractice would likely be defeated.

Litigation Trend

During the past 25 years, there has been an ever-increasing number of medical malpractice lawsuits. Hospitals,

TABLE 11–8.   Four D's of malpractice

Duty—a duty of care was owed by the physician
Deviation—the duty of care was breached
Damages—the patient experienced actual damages
Direct causation—the deviation was the direct cause of the
damages

which provide the facilities in which physicians and nurses practice, also face a variety of malpractice actions (Sykes 1988). Unfortunately, no reliable data are available that list the number of lawsuits filed against psychiatric facilities annually. Many cases are settled out of court or dismissed.

CONCLUSION

Myriad clinical-legal issues arise in the practice of consultation-liaison psychiatry. In particular, the consultation-liaison psychiatrist must understand legal issues surrounding the competency of patients to make health care decisions. Informed consent, substitute decision-making, advance directives, and guardianship are areas in which frequent clinical-legal dilemmas arise. Although the consultation-liaison psychiatrist does not need to be a lawyer, a thorough understanding of commonly encountered clinical-legal issues is essential for effective practice.

REFERENCES

American Medical Association: Physician-assisted suicide, in Code of Medical Ethics Reports, Vol V, No 2. Chicago, IL, American Medical Association, July 1994, pp 269–275

American Psychiatric Association: Official actions: guidelines for psychiatrists in consultative, supervisory, or collaborative relationships with nonmedical therapists. Am J Psychiatry 137:1489–1491, 1980

American Psychiatric Association: The Principles of Medical Ethics: With Annotations Especially Applicable to Psychiatry. Washington, DC, American Psychiatric Press, 1997

Appelbaum PS: Voluntary hospitalization and due process: the dilemma of Zinermon v Burch. Hospital and Community Psychiatry 41:1059–1060, 1990

Appelbaum PS: General guidelines for psychiatrists who prescribe medication for patients treated by nonmedical therapists. Hospital and Community Psychiatry 42:281–282, 1991

Appelbaum PS, Lidz CW, Meisel A: Informed Consent: Legal Theory and Clinical Practice. New York, Oxford University Press, 1987

Black HC: Black's Law Dictionary, 6th Edition. St. Paul, MN, West, 1990

Council on Ethical and Judicial Affairs, American Medical Association: Guidelines for the appropriate use of do-not-resuscitate orders. JAMA 265:1868–1871, 1991

Dyer AR: Ethics and Psychiatry: Toward Professional Definition. Washington, DC, American Psychiatric Press, 1988

Emanuel EJ, Emanuel LL: Proxy decision making for incompetent patients—an ethical and empirical analysis. JAMA 267:2067–2071, 1992

Goldberg RS, Riba M, Tasman A: Psychiatrists' attitudes toward prescribing medication for patients treated by nonmedical psychotherapists. Hospital and Community Psychiatry 42:276–280, 1991

Grisso T, Appelbaum PS: Comparison of standards for assessing patients: capacities to make treatment decisions. Am J Psychiatry 152:1033–1037, 1995a

Grisso T, Appelbaum PS: The MacArthur treatment competence study, III: abilities of patients to consent to psychiatric and medical treatments. Law Hum Behav 19:149–174, 1995b

Gutheil TG, Appelbaum PS: Substituted judgment and the physician's ethical dilemma: with special reference to the problem of the psychiatric patient. J Clin Psychiatry 41:303–305, 1980

Hassenfeld IN, Grumet B: A study of the right to refuse treatment. Bulletin of the American Academy of Psychiatry and the Law 12:65–74, 1984

Joint Commission on Accreditation of Healthcare Organizations: Consolidated Standards Manual. Chicago, IL, Joint Commission on Accreditation of Healthcare Organizations, 1991, SC. 2.1–SC. 2.10, pp 146–147

Kleinman CC: Psychiatrists' relationships with nonmedical professionals, in American Psychiatric Press Review of Clinical Psychiatry and the Law, Vol 2. Edited by Simon RI. Washington, DC, American Psychiatric Press, 1991, pp 241–257

LaPuma J, Orentlicher D, Moss RJ: Advance directives on admission: clinical implications and analysis of the Patient Self-Determination Act of 1990. JAMA 266:402–405, 1991

Luce JM: Ethical principles in critical care. JAMA 263:696–700, 1990

Macbeth JE, Wheeler AM, Sither JW, et al: Legal and Risk Management Issues in the Practice of Psychiatry. Washington, DC, Psychiatrists Purchasing Group, 1994

March FH, Staver A: Physician authority for unilateral DNR orders. J Leg Med 12:115–165, 1991

Meyer D, Simon RI: Split treatment: clarity between psychiatrists and psychotherapists. Psychiatric Annals 29:241–245, 327–333, 1999

Mishkin B: Decisions in Hospice. Arlington, VA, The National Hospice Organization, 1985

Mishkin B: Determining the capacity for making health care decisions, in Issues in Geriatric Psychiatry (Advances in Psychosomatic Medicine Series, Vol 19). Edited by Billig N, Rabins PV. Basel, Switzerland, Karger, 1989, pp 151–166

Orentlicher D: The illusion of patient choice in end-of-life decisions. JAMA 267:2101–2104, 1992

Overman W, Stoudemire A: Guidelines for legal and financial counseling of Alzheimer's disease patients and their families. Am J Psychiatry 145:1495–1500, 1988

Parry J: Incompetency, guardianship, and restoration, in The Mentally Disabled and the Law, 3rd Edition. Edited by Brakel SJ, Parry J, Weiner BA. Chicago, IL, American Bar Foundation, 1985, p 370

Parry JW, Beck JC: Revisiting the civil commitment/involuntary treatment stalemate using limited guardianship, substituted judgment and different due process considerations: a work in progress. Medical and Physical Disability Law Reporter 14:102–114, 1990

Perr IN: The clinical considerations of medication refusal. Legal Aspects of Psychiatric Practice 1:5–8, 1984

Physicians' Desk Reference, 54th Edition. Oradell, NJ, Medical Economics Company, 2000

Pinals DA, Appelbaum PS: The history and current status of competence and informed consent in psychiatric research. Isr J Psychiatry Relat Sci 37:82–94, 2000

President's Commission for the Study of Ethical Problems in Medicine and Biomedical and Behavioral Research: Making Health Care Decisions. A Report on the Ethical and Legal Implications of Informed Consent in the Patient-Practitioner Relationship, Vol I: Report. Washington, DC, Superintendent of Documents, October 1982

Regan M: Protective services for the elderly: commitment, guardianship, and alternatives. William and Mary Law Review 13:569–573, 1972

Reisner R, Slobogin C: Law and the Mental Health System, 2nd Edition. St. Paul, MN, West, 1990, pp 223–232

Ruchs VR: The "rationing" of medical care. N Engl J Med 311:1572–1573, 1984

Sales BD, Powell DM, Van Duizend R: Disabled Persons and the Law: Law, Society, and Policy Services, Vol 1. New York, Plenum, 1982, p 461

Schwartz HR: Do not resuscitate orders: the impact of guidelines on clinical practice, in Geriatric Psychiatry and the Law. Edited by Rosner R, Schwartz HR. New York, Plenum, 1987, pp 91–100

Simon RI: The psychiatrist as a fiduciary: avoiding the double agent role. Psychiatric Annals 17:622–626, 1987

Simon RI: Beyond the doctrine of informed consent—a clinician's perspective. The Journal for the Expert Witness, The Trial Attorney, The Trial Judge 4:23–25, 1989

Simon RI: Clinical Psychiatry and the Law, 2nd Edition. Washington, DC, American Psychiatric Press, 1992a

Simon RI: Concise Guide to Psychiatry and Law for Clinicians. Washington, DC, American Psychiatric Press, 1992b

Simon RI: Discharging sicker, potentially violent psychiatric inpatients in the managed care era: standard of care and risk management. Psychiatric Annals 27:726–733, 1997

Simon RI: Psychiatrists awake! suicide risk assessments are all about a good night's sleep. Psychiatric Annals 28:479–485, 1998a

Simon RI: Psychiatrists' duties in discharging sicker and potentially violent inpatients in the managed care era. Psychiatr Serv 49:62–67, 1998b

Simon RI: Concise Guide to Psychiatry and Law for Clinicians, 3rd Edition. Washington, DC, American Psychiatric Press, 2001

Simon RI, Sadoff RL: Malpractice law: an introduction, in Psychiatric Malpractice: Cases and Comments for Clinicians. Washington, DC, American Psychiatric Press, 1992, pp 23–55

Smith JT: Medical Malpractice: Psychiatric Care. Colorado Springs, CO, Shephards McGraw-Hill, 1986

Solnick PB: Proxy consent for incompetent nonterminally ill adult patients. J Leg Med 6:1–49, 1985

Stone AA: The right to refuse treatment. Arch Gen Psychiatry 38:358–362, 1981

Sykes AO: The boundaries of vicarious liability: an economic analysis of the scope of employment rule and related legal doctrine. Harvard Law Review 101(3):563–609, 1988

Tardiff K (ed): The Psychiatric Uses of Seclusion and Restraint. Washington, DC, American Psychiatric Press, 1984

Tardiff K: Assessment and Management of Violent Patients, 2nd Edition. Washington, DC, American Psychiatric Press, 1996

U.S. Dept of Health and Human Services: The Legal Status of Adolescents 1980. Rockville, MD, USDHHS, 1981, p 41

Weir RF, Gostin L: Decisions to abate life-sustaining treatment for nonautonomous patients: ethical standards and legal liability for physicians after Cruzan. JAMA 264:1846–1853, 1990

Yudofsky SC, Silver JM, Hales RE: Treatment of aggressive disorders, in The American Psychiatric Press Textbook of Psychopharmacology. Edited by Schatzberg AF, Nemeroff CB. Washington, DC, American Psychiatric Press, 1995, pp 735–751

Zito JM, Lentz SL, Routt WW, et al: The treatment review panel: a solution to treatment refusal? Bulletin of the American Academy of Psychiatry and the Law 12:349–358, 1984

LEGAL CITE REFERENCES

Aponte v United States, 582 FSupp 555, 566–69 (D PR 1984)

Bartling v Superior Court, 163 Cal App 3d 186, 209 Cal Rptr 220 (1984)

Bouvia v Superior Court, 179 Cal App 3d 1127, 225 Cal Rptr 297 (1986)

Canterbury v Spence, 464 F2d 772 (DC Cir), cert denied, Spence v Canterbury, 409 US 1064 (1972)

Clark v State, No. 62962 Albany Court of Claims (NY 1985)

Cruzan v Director, Missouri Department of Health, 110 S Ct 284 (1990)

Dillon v Silver, 134 AD 2d 159, 520 NYS 2d 751 (1987)

Frasier v Department of Health and Human Resources, 500 So2d 858, 864, La Ct App (1986)

Gonzalez v New York, 121 Misc 2d 410, 467 NYS 2d 538 (1983), rev'd on other grounds, 110 AD 2d 810 488 NYS 2d 231

Gulf S I R Co. v Sullivan, 155 Miss 1, 119 So 501 (1928)

In re Boyer, 636 P2d 1085, 1089, Utah (1981)

In re Certification of William R, 9 Misc 2d 1084, 172 NYS 2d 896, NY Sup Ct (1958)

In re Conroy, 98 NJ 321, 486 A2d 1209, 1222–23 (1985)

In re Farrell, 108 NJ 335, 529 A2d 404 (1987)

In re Jobes, 108 NJ 365, 529 A2d 434 (1987)

In re Peter, 108 NJ 365, 529 A2d 419 (1987)

In re Quinlan, 70 NJ 10, 355 A2d 647, cert denied, 429 US 922 (1976)

In the Guardianship of John Roe, 411 MA 666 (1992)

Jehovah's Witnesses v King County Hospital, 278 FSupp 488 (WD Wash 1967), affd, 390 US 598 (1968)

Marcus v Liebman, 59 Ill App 3d 337, 375 NE2d 486 (Ill App Ct 1978)

Meek v City of Loveland, 85 Colo 346, 276 P 30 (1929)

Natanson v Kline, 186 Kan 393, 350 P2d 1093 (1960)

Parham v J.R., 442 US 584 (1979)

Planned Parenthood v Danforth, 428 US 52, 74 (1976)

Plumadore v State, 75 AD 2d 691, 427 NYS 2d 90 (1980)

Rennie v Klein, 462 FSupp 1131 (D NJ 1978), remanded, 476 FSupp 1294 (D NJ 1979) aff'd in part, modified in part and remanded, 653 F2d 836, 3rd Cir (1980), vacated and remanded, 458 U.S. 1119 (1982), 720 F2d 266, 3rd Cir (1983)

Salas v Gamboa, 760 SW2d 838, Tex App (1988)

Scaria v St. Paul Fire and Marine Ins Co, 68 Wis2d 1, 227 NW2d 647 (1975)

Schloendorff v Society of New York Hospital, 211 NY 125, 105 NE 92 (1914), overruled, Bing v Thunig, 2 NY2d 656, 143 NE2d 3, 163 NYS2d 3 (1957)

St. Vincent's Medical Center v Oakley, 371 So2d 590, Fla App (1979)

Tune v Walter Reed Army Medical Hosp, 602 FSupp 1452, DDC (1985)

Union Pacific Ry Co v Botsford, 141 US 250, 251 (1891)

Wickline v California, 183 Cal App 3d 1175, 228 Cal Rptr 661 (Cal Ct. App 1986)

Wilson v Blue Cross of Southern California et al., 222 Cal App 3d 660 (1990)

Wilson v Lehman, 379 SW2d 478, 479, Ky (1964)

Youngberg v Romeo, 457 US 307 (1982), on remand, Romeo v Youngberg, 687 F2d 33, 3rd Cir (1982)

Zinermon v Burch, 110 S Ct 975 (1990)

CIVIL STATUTES

DC CODE ANN §21–513 (1981 and 1984 Supp)

Uniform Guardianship and Protective Proceeding Act (UGPPA) §5–101

Appendix

Health Care Proxy

(1) I, _____ hereby appoint _____
_____

(Name, home address, and telephone number)

as my health care agent to make any and all health care decisions for me, except to the extent that I state otherwise. This proxy shall take effect when and if I become unable to make my own health care decisions.

(2) Optional instructions: I direct my agent to make health care decisions in accord with my wishes and limitations as stated below, or as he or she otherwise knows. [Attach additional pages if necessary.]

_____

_____

[Unless your agent knows your wishes about artificial nutrition and hydration (feeding tubes), your agent will not be allowed to make decisions about artificial nutrition and hydration. See instructions below for samples of language you could use.]

(3) Name of substitute or fill-in agent if the person I appoint above is unable, unwilling, or unavailable to act as my health care agent.

_____

(Name, home address, and telephone number)

(4) Unless I revoke it, this proxy shall remain in effect indefinitely, or until the date or conditions stated below. This proxy shall expire [specific date or conditions, if desired]:

_____

(5) Signature _____
    Address _____
    Date _____

Statement by Witness (must be 18 or older)

I declare that the person who signed this document is personally known to me and appears to be of sound mind and acting of his or her own free will.

He or she signed (or asked another to sign for him or her) this document in my presence.

Witness 1 _____
Address _____

Witness 2 _____
Address _____

Source. Reprinted from the New York State Department of Health.

About the Health Care Proxy

This is an important legal form. Before signing this form, you should understand the following facts:

1. This form gives the person you choose as your agent the authority to make all health care decisions for you, except to the extent you say otherwise in this form. "Health care" means any treatment, service, or procedure to diagnose or treat your physical or mental condition.
2. Unless you say otherwise, your agent will be allowed to make all health care decisions for you, including decisions to remove or provide life-sustaining treatment.
3. Unless your agent knows your wishes about artificial nutrition and hydration (nourishment and water provided by a feeding tube), he or she will not be allowed to refuse or consent to those measures for you.
4. Your agent will start making decisions for you when doctors decide that you are not able to make health care decisions for yourself.

You may write on this form any information about treatment that you do not desire and/or those treatments that you want to make sure you receive. Your agent must follow your instructions (oral and written) when making decisions for you.

If you want to give your agent written instructions, do so right on the form. For example, you could say:

If I become terminally ill, I do/don't want to receive the following treatments:...

If I am in a coma or unconscious, with no hope of recovery, then I do/don't want...

If I have brain damage or a brain disease that makes me unable to recognize people or speak and there is no hope that my condition will improve, I do/don't want...

I have discussed with my agent my wishes about _____, and I want my agent to make all decisions about these measures.

Examples of medical treatments about which you may wish to give your agent special instructions are listed below. This is not a complete list of the treatments about which you may leave instructions.

- Artificial respiration
- Artificial nutrition and hydration (nourishment and water provided by feeding tube)
- Cardiopulmonary resuscitation (CPR)
- Antipsychotic medication
- Electroconvulsive therapy
- Antibiotics
- Psychosurgery
- Dialysis
- Transplantation
- Blood transfusions
- Abortion
- Sterilization

Talk about choosing an agent with your family and/or close friends. You should discuss this form with a doctor or another health care professional, such as a nurse or social worker, before you sign it to make sure that you understand the types of decisions that may be made for you. You may also wish to give your doctor a signed copy. **You do not need a lawyer to fill out this form.**

You can choose any adult (over 18), including a family member, or close friend, to be your agent. If you select a doctor as your agent, he or she may have to choose between acting as your agent or as your attending doctor; a physician cannot do both at the same time. Also, if you are a patient or resident of a hospital, nursing home, or mental hygiene facility, there are special restrictions about naming someone who works for that facility as your agent. You should ask staff at the facility to explain those restrictions.

You should tell the person you choose that he or she will be your health care agent. You should discuss your health care wishes and this form with your agent. Be sure to give him or her a signed copy. Your agent cannot be sued for health care decisions made in good faith.

Even after you have signed this form, you have the right to make health care decisions for yourself as long as you are able to do so, and treatment cannot be given to you or stopped if you object. You can cancel the control given to your agent by telling him or her or your health care provider orally or in writing.

FILLING OUT THE PROXY FORM

Item (1) Write your name and the name, home address, and telephone number of the person you are selecting as your agent.

Item (2) If you have special instructions for your agent, you should write them here. Also, if you wish to limit your agent's authority in any way, you should say so here. If you do not state any limitations, your agent will be allowed to make all health care decisions that you could have made, including the decision to consent to or refuse life-sustaining treatment.

Item (3) You may write the name, home address, and telephone number of an alternative agent.

Item (4) This form will remain valid indefinitely unless you set an expiration date or condition for its expiration. This section is optional and should be filled in only if you want the health care proxy to expire.

Item (5) You must date and sign the proxy. If you are unable to sign yourself, you may direct someone else to sign in your presence. Be sure to include your address.

Two witnesses at least 18 years of age must sign your proxy. The person who is appointed agent or alternate agent cannot sign as a witness.

Consultation-Liaison Psychiatry Research

James R. Rundell, M.D.

Thomas N. Wise, M.D.

Historically, consultation-liaison psychiatry developed as a clinical discipline, not a research discipline. Psychiatrists attracted to consultation-liaison work generally enjoy its clinical challenges and satisfactions more than its research opportunities; it is difficult to persuade many consultation-liaison psychiatrists to conduct research. However, consultation-liaison psychiatrists must study the accuracy of their diagnostic methods and the efficacy of their interventions (M. Fava and Rosenbaum 1992; Freeman and Tyrer 1989; Glantz 1992; Levenson 1997; Muskin et al. 1997; Wright et al. 1996). Decisions by patients, health care providers, and payers are now more often based on valid and reliable data and less often based on tradition and historical practice patterns.

Psychiatric research is difficult because it must rely on more subjective outcome measures than other medical disciplines do. Consultation-liaison psychiatry research is more difficult than most general psychiatry research because researchers must account for impacts of medical status on the variables under study. In this chapter, we summarize research methodologies important to consultation-liaison psychiatry research. For each methodology defined, we provide specific research examples. Finally, we discuss potential research biases and ethical considerations.

CONSULTATION-LIAISON PSYCHIATRY RESEARCH METHODOLOGIES

Consultation-liaison psychiatry research takes advantage of research paradigms used by all biomedical disciplines. These include basic science research, case studies, population descriptive studies, intervention studies, and cost-effectiveness studies. A glance at scientific journals with direct relevance to consultation-liaison psychiatry reveals that many articles do not fit neatly into one of the categories discussed in this chapter. For example, some studies use more than one paradigm (Bowman 1993). Review articles compare or meta-analyze similar types of studies (Wool and Barsky 1994). There are also editorials (Levenson 1997; Nemiah 1995), obituaries (G. Fava 1993), exhortations and calls to arms (Blinder 1995), position statements (American Psychiatric Association 1995), reports of exotic or idiosyncratic clinical observations (Stern and Glick 1993), and articles that defy methodological classification (Fishbain et al. 1993).

In the following discussion, we aim to improve readers' abilities to understand published original research. The goal of original consultation-liaison psychiatry research is to increase understanding of biopsychosocial processes that cause or influence psychiatric syndromes in medically ill patients, to increase knowledge of categories of illness and their natural histories in consultation-liaison populations, or to evaluate interventions prescribed or administered by consultation-liaison psychiatrists.

Other types of medical journal articles, such as literature reviews and editorials, are derivative of and dependent on original research methodologies. Categories of original research important to the continuing viability of consultation-liaison psychiatry are summarized and defined in Table 12–1.

TABLE 12–1.   Consultation-liaison psychiatry research methodologies

Basic science research

Technologies and methods from neuroscience, behavioral science, and social science are applied to structural, metabolic, physiological, behavioral, and social correlates of psychiatric syndromes that occur in patients who have medical, surgical, or neurological disorders and events.

Case studies

Clinical presentations or treatment outcomes are reported that confirm, expand, or contradict existing knowledge. The power and general interpretability of these reports are always severely limited, but these reports are important because they frequently create a basis and justification for a more powerful hypothesis-generating study. They are also valuable in analyzing rare or idiosyncratic events not amenable to study in large populations.

Cross-sectional population descriptive studies

A sufficient number of individuals in a population or events in a system are studied to confirm or refute a hypothesis about an event or problem of interest. These studies cannot identify cause-and-effect relationships, but they attempt to establish prevalence of events or phenomena and may inform further studies that can infer causality.

Longitudinal population descriptive studies

A population or system is studied over time to determine whether associations or cause-and-effect relationships exist among variables of interest. Longitudinal studies may be retrospective or prospective, depending on aims and hypotheses. There are two types of longitudinal studies:

1.   Case-control studies: subjects are defined on the basis of presence or absence of a disease or other defined variable. Subjects who do not have the variable of interest (control subjects) are otherwise matched to the index cases for variables that should be controlled for, such as demographics.

2.   Cohort studies: subjects are always defined on the basis of initial absence of the variable of interest to the natural history of a shared disease or process. Study groups differ in some aspect (e.g., setting of health care delivery or degree of social support) hypothesized to be important to ultimate natural outcome of the baseline condition.

Clinical intervention studies

Two or more indistinguishable groups, one receiving a treatment or intervention and the other(s) receiving placebo or other treatment, are compared to determine the effect of the treatment under investigation. Potential biases are minimized when there are no distinguishing characteristics among comparison groups, when differences that might occur solely by chance are accounted for, and when neither researchers nor patients know which group is receiving the active intervention.

Cost-effectiveness studies

Health care activities (e.g., consultation-liaison psychiatry assessments and treatments) are studied to determine their impact on direct and indirect measures of health care costs. Outcome measures include reimbursement rates, numbers of bed-days saved, cost savings, outpatient health care utilization, and medication requirements. Cause-and-effect attributions are difficult to establish because pure experimental conditions that adequately control for all other possible contributing variables are rare.

Basic Science Research

A number of increasingly sophisticated technologies and methods are available to neuroscientists, behavioral scientists, and social scientists who study biopsychosocial phenomena. Basic research by these scientists helps to define structural, metabolic, physiological, behavioral, and social correlates of psychiatric syndromes that occur in patients who have medical, surgical, or neurological disorders. These basic science findings, in turn, inform clinical researchers. Three types of basic science research are of particular interest to the consultation-liaison psychiatrist: neuroscience, neuroimaging, and behavioral science.

Neuroscience

Psychiatric syndromes can result when the structure or function of the central nervous system is disturbed. Many disorders diagnosed by consultation-liaison psychiatrists are associated with demonstrable anatomical or physiological abnormalities (Johnstone and Lambert 1989; Mega and Cummings 1994; Weinberger 1993). Without these windows into central nervous system structure and function, current clinical research possibilities would be quite limited.

Contributions of neuroscientists to consultation-liaison psychiatry research are summarized elsewhere in this volume. The contributions of neuropsychology to consultation-liaison psychiatry research and clinical practice are discussed in detail in Chapter 7. In Chapters 15 and 16, structural and metabolic neuroscience research findings are related to the clinical evaluation and management of patients with delirium and dementia, respectively. In Chapter 20, neuroscience research is related to anxiety syndromes, such as panic attacks and obsessive-compulsive disorder, seen by consultation-liaison psychiatrists. Relevant consultation-liaison psychiatry, neurological, neurosurgical, and basic neuroscience research findings are integrated in Chapter 30.

Neuroimaging

Since the late 1980s, neuroimaging has rapidly moved from basic science theory to clinical practice and research tool. This trend is likely to continue, providing valuable consultation-liaison psychiatry clinical evaluation tools and research outcome measures. The basic science of neuroimaging modalities is described in considerable detail in Chapter 5. Clinical suspicions about relationships between cerebral dysfunction and specific psychiatric syndromes can now be studied with functional imaging technologies. For example, studies of regional cerebral glucose metabolism using positron emission tomography demonstrate bilateral hypometabolism of orbital-inferior prefrontal cortex and anterior temporal cortex among patients with major depression (Mayberg 1994). Hypometabolism occurs regardless of whether the depressive syndrome is primary major depression or secondary depression due to general medical or substance-induced conditions.

Behavioral Science

An important basic science research perspective in consultation-liaison psychiatry and the related discipline behavioral medicine is motivated behaviors (see Chapter 46). This research model, which investigates organized activity patterns that reduce psychic tension, is based on classic and operant learning theory. Stress management programs, chronic pain programs, and other clinical management strategies to decrease maladaptive health behaviors such as smoking have been greatly informed by basic behavioral science research (Gallagher 1990; Schwartz and Weiss 1978). Treatment of many psychiatric disorders has also benefited from behavioral science research. These disorders include obsessive-compulsive disorder, simple phobia, eating disorders, sleep disorders, sexual disorders, and panic disorder (Watson et al. 1991)

Central to some behavioral research is the belief that emotion fosters disease end points through either psychoneuroendocrine or behavioral pathways. For example,

many studies demonstrate psychosocial and behavioral risk factors in the etiology of ischemic heart disease (see Chapter 46; Blumenthal and Kamarck 1987). The best known of these is the type A personality construct (see Chapters 26 and 46). Other research applications of psychoneuroendocrine and behavioral pathway theory include noncompliance, stress response, illness progression (e.g., acquired immunodeficiency syndrome [AIDS]), and substance use.

Case Studies

Although case studies are commonly relegated to the "letters to the editor" section of most medical journals, they form a vital link between clinical practice and medical research. Some experts are so exasperated with misuse and misinterpretation of statistically based studies that they advocate more reliance on the case study method (Bromley 1986; Newcombe 1987). At times, single-case studies contribute more valid and useful knowledge to the literature than do comparisons of means of large populations (DiMartini and Twillman 1994; Mark et al. 1993), as demonstrated by the following clinical and research abstracts.

> A 41-year-old man developed subacute neurotoxicity associated with interleukin-2 and tumor necrosis factor therapy for metastatic renal cell carcinoma. Cognitive deficits revealed on neuropsychological testing and frontal lobe perfusion deficits revealed on SPECT [single photon emission computed tomography] resolved after 1 month. Findings suggest possible neuroanatomic and physiologic substrates of cytokine neurotoxicity. (Meyers et al. 1994, p. 285)

> Electroconvulsive therapy (ECT) was used to treat a patient with a large left frontal craniotomy and remaining frontal meningioma. Treatment was successful and uneventful. ECT should be considered in the treatment of drug-resistant depressed patients with craniotomies and remaining tumor. (Starkstein and Migliorelli 1993, p. 428)

> The authors present a follow-up of a previously described patient with obsessive-compulsive disorder (OCD). Her condition continued to worsen, and she died 5 years after disease onset. Neuropathological findings were consistent with the diagnosis of Pick's disease. They revealed, in addition to the "knife-edge" frontotemporal atrophy, striking atrophy with extensive neuronal loss and gliosis involving the caudate nuclei and, to a lesser degree, the putamens and globus pallidus. Neuroimaging data had showed isolated atrophy of the caudate nuclei in the early stages of Pick's disease in this patient when OCD was the leading clinical manifestation. Relevant literature is reviewed, and the role of caudate nuclei atrophy in

the development of OCD is discussed. (Tonkonogy et al. 1994, p. 176)

Effective case reports in the medical literature describe unusual case presentations, uncommon adverse effects of treatment, treatment that occurs in unusual circumstances, and rare or exotic syndromes. These situations are extremely difficult to study in large samples because they are rare. Case studies must be done with the same care and attention as studies involving larger groups of patients. Several techniques that increase the value of single-case studies are summarized in Table 12–2.

Cross-Sectional Population Descriptive Studies

When a hypothesis requires study of a population or group to determine the prevalence of an event or phenomenon, cross-sectional descriptive studies are used. The aims of such studies do not generally include detecting etiologies or cause-and-effect attributions. Often, only a single measurement is made (Backett and Robinson 1989). Observations made as part of these epidemiologic studies contribute to descriptive analysis of the event or phenomenon in question. Cross-sectional population descriptive studies have the advantages of being relatively quick and economical but are limited in their abilities to identify causal associations (Fink et al. 1999). However, they frequently provide pilot or preliminary data to inform further studies in which hypotheses can be more specifically applied to causality relationships. For example, cross-sectional studies detect the frequency of psychiatric disorders in a medically ill population, as well as in whom and when they occur. These data are then used to design subsequent studies to investigate why the disorders occur and what may ultimately prevent them.

A researcher who wants to generalize his or her findings to an entire population must use a representative study sample. Generally, this is accomplished by drawing random or probability samples from the population of interest. These samples are based on preexisting knowledge of demographic or other important selection variables so that the study population is unbiased and representative. Sometimes a stratified sample that deliberately oversamples subgroups is used to achieve statistical power to answer study questions. For example, because a small minority of men have somatization disorder, a study to compare outcomes of men and women with the disorder may include a disproportionate number of men. Within each stratum of a stratified study population, however, the subjects must be randomly selected so that appropriate statistical inferences can be made.

TABLE 12–2. Techniques to increase the value of the single-case study

1. Obtain measurements of the patient's problems before, during, and after the event or treatment of interest.
2. Obtain measurements repeatedly until reasonable stability is achieved.
3. Obtain as many longitudinal measurements as possible.
4. Conduct the case study prospectively when possible.
5. Remove the event or treatment and then reinstate it, if possible, and continue measurements throughout (e.g., if a medication is believed to cause a certain adverse effect that abates when treatment with the medication is discontinued, rechallenge the patient with the medication to confirm the findings, then discontinue therapy again, repeating study measures throughout).
6. Strive to not overgeneralize findings.
7. Record and account for potentially confounding events that could affect findings.
8. Suggest hypotheses based on the observations that could be studied or that have clinical or treatment implications.
9. Use the scientific method of hypothesis testing whenever possible.
10. Incorporate laboratory, vital sign, psychological testing, neuropsychological testing, psychiatric rating scale, and imaging data when indicated.

Source. Engel 1990; Peck 1989.

A common mistake in cross-sectional epidemiologic studies is underestimating necessary sample size (Backett and Robinson 1989). If the sample is too small, researchers cannot answer one or more of the study's questions. For example, general population data suggest that if a study to determine the prevalence of obsessive-compulsive disorder in a family practice clinic includes only 100 patients, researchers will be unlikely to detect any cases at all.

Another important aspect of developing an epidemiologic study is to first define an event or case. For example, if a study of neuroleptic malignant syndrome has no clear, operationalized case definition, it will be impossible to estimate its prevalence accurately, no matter how large or representative the study population may be.

Cross-sectional studies also compare prevalences of phenomena or diagnoses in subgroups of the study population. For example, a study of depression among liver transplant recipients could examine differences between men and women, between alcoholic and nonalcoholic patients, or between categories of patients with different severities of underlying illness.

Cross-sectional population descriptive studies are indispensable for psychiatrists designing marketing strategies and mental health care delivery systems. epidemiologic studies are also important precursors to longitudinal descriptive, intervention, and cost-effectiveness research. In general psychiatry, one of the most important examples of a cross-sectional population descriptive study is the Epidemiologic Catchment Area Program of the National Institute of Mental Health (Regier and Burke 1985). This multisite study assessed psychiatric disorder prevalence, incidence, and service use in approximately 20,000 community and institutional residents. This study used random probability samples and standard diagnostic measures to provide prevalence rates. These data provide a basis for designing mental health care delivery systems and health care utilization research.

Consultation-liaison psychiatry researchers use cross-sectional population descriptive studies to establish psychiatric disorder prevalences in specific medical-surgical populations. For example, Popkin et al. (1988) found that the lifetime prevalence of psychiatric illness in patients with long-standing insulin-dependent diabetes mellitus was 25%. The prevalence of depression among patients with Parkinson's disease following diagnosis varies from 25% to 70%, depending on the specific study design and the definition of depression (Cummings 1992).

Cross-sectional descriptive studies sometimes study phenomena other than disorder or syndrome prevalence. Physician behaviors and practice patterns are the focus of many studies. Ormel et al. (1991) found that primary care physicians recognized definable psychiatric disorders in only 47% of 1,994 primary care patients. Wells et al. (1994) found that among depressed outpatients treated with antidepressant medications, 39% received inappropriately low doses. (Note: The latter study was a descriptive study, not a treatment study. Therefore, the outcome measure of interest was presence or absence of a predefined adequate medication dose, not patient clinical improvement.)

Longitudinal Population Descriptive Studies

Sometimes researchers study a population or system over time to determine whether associations or cause-and-effect relationships exist among variables of interest. Longitudinal study data collection may be retrospective or prospective, depending on the study's aims and hypotheses. There are two types of longitudinal studies: cohort studies and case-control studies. Cohort studies follow well-defined samples from a population over time to establish incidence rates and risk ratios (risk factor status). In contrast, case-control studies use already identified cases rather than potential cases for retrospective or prospective longitudinal descriptions of natural history and potential risk factors. Differences between case-control and cohort longitudinal population descriptive studies are summarized in Table 12–3.

Case-Control Studies

Case-control studies are conducted over a defined period to compare a group of individuals with a disorder or variable of interest (cases) with a group of individuals without the disorder or variable of interest (control subjects). Cases and control subjects are compared on one or more outcome variables to define the relative importance of causal or contributory factors. The following simple case-control study illustrates this methodology. Two groups of patients with human immunodeficiency virus (HIV) disease were studied—a group of patients who had attempted suicide over a 2-year period (cases) and a group of patients who had not (control subjects) (Rundell et al. 1992). The two groups were matched by sex, age, and ethnic group. Several outcome variables of interest were statistically more likely to occur in the group of patients who attempted suicide: adjustment disorder, alcohol use disorder, personality disorder, major depressive disorder, multiple psychosocial stressors, and poor social supports.

Case-control studies have an advantage over cohort studies. They are generally less time-consuming and less expensive, especially when done retrospectively. However, retrospective case-control studies are difficult unless all important information was well recorded in a standard, consistent way for cases and control subjects.

TABLE 12–3. Differences between case-control and cohort longitudinal population descriptive studies

Study characteristic	Case-control studies	Cohort studies
Case definition	Cases possess the variable of interest	Free from variable of interest at beginning of study
Comparison group	Free from variable of interest	Do not develop/are not exposed to variable of interest
Retrospective or prospective?	Either	Usually prospective
Time and expense	Moderate	Great
Ability to infer causality	Limited	Great

Source. Backett and Robinson 1989; Regier and Burke 1985; Tohen 1992.

It is important to carefully consider which variables to control for when defining a control group for a case-control study (Troster et al. 1994). A balance must be achieved between controlling for enough variables to accurately assess the outcomes of interest and "over-matching" to such a degree that important factors are obscured. Once a variable is controlled for in a study, it cannot then become an outcome variable. For example, controlling for sex in the HIV disease suicide attempt study just described eliminates gender influences as possible confounders of study findings but prohibits the researchers from assessing potentially important gender differences.

Two types of control groups are possible in case-control studies—group control subjects and paired control subjects. Group control subjects are selected so that the control group as a whole is similar to the study group with regard to the variables being controlled for. A paired control subject is matched one-to-one with a study group subject. The latter method results in more precise matching but may prove exceedingly difficult, particularly as the number of "case" control variables increases. An example of a case-control study in consultation-liaison psychiatry research is described in the following research report abstract.

Although the two disease concepts have very different histories, many previous studies have mixed conversion disorder and somatization disorder and none has made direct comparison between them. The authors applied DSM-III criteria to inpatient and outpatient medical records and attempted to follow 98 patients who met criteria for somatization disorder or conversion disorder. Five of these patients died 4 years later and, of those who survived, 70 (75.3%) were given follow-up interviews by a rater blind to baseline diagnosis. The 32 patients with a baseline diagnosis of conversion disorder were significantly less likely than the 38 patients with somatization disorder to be given the same diagnosis at follow-up. Six of the conversion disorder patients were given follow-up diagnoses of somatization disorder and, in four other cases, subsequent developments revealed medical explanations for the presenting complaint. Of the two baseline diagnoses, somatization disorder predicted substantially more impairment in a variety of domains. (Kent et al. 1995, p. 138)

Cohort Studies

The main difference between cohort studies and case-control studies is that cohort studies begin with a group of patients or subjects who share a disease or other variable. Sometimes the absence of disease is the shared characteristic. Researchers monitor the subjects over time for the appearance of one or more outcome variables. The researchers can then draw conclusions about the relative importance of initial differences or events that accrue during the study period. More than any other study design discussed thus far, cohort studies provide information about possible causal associations. Most cohort studies are prospective, although retrospective cohort studies are possible if standard data were somehow collected on all study subjects, often as a result of some other prospective research study. Because of the planning, care, and precision necessary to conduct a cohort study, they are relatively expensive and time-consuming.

At the beginning of a cohort study, all subjects must be free of the outcome variable(s) of interest. The index and control groups then self-select on the basis of appearance or nonappearance of the specified variable(s). Cohort studies are particularly valuable in identifying risk factors because some noncases become new cases. The following two abstracts illustrate the nature and potential contributions of cohort studies.

Forty recipients of bone marrow transplants were recruited prospectively and assessed pretransplant, at 1 month postdischarge, and at 6 months postdischarge between 1989 and 1990. Assessments included a psychiatric interview, a variety of standardized questionnaires (Hospital Anxiety and Depression Scale, Mental Attitude to Cancer Scale, Psychosocial Adjustment to Illness Scale), and a standardized diagnostic interview. The influence of factors such as depression and anxiety upon length of stay, survival, psychosocial adjustment, and negative prognostic attitudes were examined. In contrast to other studies, little influence was found for psychiatric illness on physical outcome variables, but they did affect psychosocial outcome. The implications of these findings are discussed. (Jenkins et al. 1994, p. 361)

Objective: To determine if the diagnosis of major depression in patients hospitalized following myocardial infarction (MI) would have an independent impact on cardiac mortality over the first 6 months after discharge. Design: Prospective evaluation of the impact of depression assessed using a modified version of the National Institute of Mental Health Diagnostic Interview Schedule for major depressive episode. Cox proportional hazards regression was used to evaluate the independent impact of depression after control for significant predictors in the data set. Setting: A large, university-affiliated hospital specializing in cardiac care, located in Montreal, Quebec. Patients: All consenting patients (N = 222) who met established criteria for MI between August 1991 and July 1992 and who survived to be discharged from the hospital. Patients were interviewed between 5 and 15 days following the MI and were followed up for

6 months. There were no age limits (range, 24 to 88 years; mean, 60 years). The sample was 78% male. Primary outcome measure: Survival status at 6 months. Results: By 6 months, 12 patients had died. All deaths were due to cardiac causes. Depression was a significant predictor of mortality (hazard ratio, 5.74; 95% confidence interval, 4.61 to 6.87; $P = .0006$). The impact of depression remained after control for left ventricular dysfunction (Killip class) and previous MI, the multivariate significant predictors of mortality in the data set (adjusted hazard ratio, 4.29; 95% confidence interval, 3.14 to 5.44; $P = .013$). Conclusion: Major depression in patients hospitalized following an MI is an independent risk factor for mortality at 6 months. Its impact is at least as equivalent to that of left ventricular dysfunction (Killip class) and history of previous MI. Additional study is needed to determine whether treatment of depression can influence post-MI survival and to assess possible underlying mechanisms. (Frasure-Smith et al. 1993, p. 1819)

In the second study, all study subjects shared the characteristic of having had a myocardial infarction. The outcome variable of interest was death. The index group became those patients with myocardial infarction who died. The control group became those patients who lived. Variables likely to obscure or confound study results, such as age and illness severity, were controlled for in order to approximate an independent risk assessment for the presence of major depression. The elegant design of this study has made it a standard and model for consultation-liaison psychiatry cohort studies.

Clinical Intervention Studies

In contrast to longitudinal descriptive research, clinical intervention studies expose two or more groups of subjects to experimentally introduced preventive or therapeutic measures. Epidemiologic methods used in case-control and cohort descriptive studies are applied to a research design in which the outcome variables are affected by an experimentally introduced event or treatment rather than by a natural history event. Studying clinical interventions is uniquely important to consultation-liaison psychiatry because general psychiatry intervention study results may not apply to medically ill populations (Eisenberg 1991; McKegney and Beckhardt 1982). For example, consultation-liaison patients often have psychiatric syndromes due to toxic or medical causes that cannot necessarily be managed with treatment methods based on results of studies involving patients with equivalent primary psychiatric disorders. In addition, medical-surgical populations are usually receiving simultaneous treatments for their medical conditions that must be accounted for in consultation-liaison intervention studies.

In interpreting clinical trial results, it is important to understand the difference between statistical significance and clinical significance (Biedel 1992). Studies that proclaim attainment of the highly prized low P value may or may not include clinically important findings. For example, a mean depression rating scale change or difference of two or three points may be quite significant statistically but not mean much clinically.

In the intervention study research model, the intervention need not be a specific treatment. Frequently, exposure to a mental health system or to an educational effort is the intervention being assessed. Outcome measures may apply to a system of care rather than to patients. The following abstract illustrates one such instance, in which the intervention was to use a depression rating scale score to alert primary care physicians when patients were depressed. The outcome measure was physician recognition of depression.

A randomized clinical trial was performed to assess whether the results of a depression screening instrument, when provided to physicians, could influence their recognition and treatment of depression in a primary care setting. The intervention consisted of randomly informing or not informing physicians of the depression status of 100 patients who screened positively for depression on both the Zung Self-Rating Depression Scale (SDS) and a DSM-III screen. For 12 months patients were followed to assess depression status, and medical records were audited to assess depression recognition and treatment. Results show that feedback to physicians of SDS scores of previously unrecognized depressed patients makes a significant difference in greater recognition (56.2% vs. 34.6%) and treatment (56.2% vs. 42.3%) of depression over the 12-month study period. This was especially true for patients with high somatic ($P < .05$) or low psychologic symptoms of depression ($P < .05$). These results suggest that routine use of a depression screening instrument can improve physician recognition of depression, with increased initiation of treatment. (Magruder-Habib et al. 1990, p. 239)

Cost-Effectiveness Studies

A type of study that is receiving increasing emphasis in consultation-liaison psychiatry is the cost-effectiveness study (Hall and Wise 1995; Hall et al. 1994; Strain et al. 1994). Funding for health care, including consultation-liaison psychiatry services (see Chapter 3), is undergoing ever-increasing scrutiny. Consultation-liaison psychiatrists are under growing pressure to demonstrate not only their field's clinical effectiveness but also its cost-effectiveness (Katon and Gonzales 1994; Mumford et al. 1984; Saravay and Strain 1994). Although associations exist between clinical efficacy and cost-effectiveness, the two domains are not synonymous. A treatment that is highly effective clinically is not necessarily cost-effective. For instance, adding behavior therapy to pharmacological treatment of obsessive-compulsive disorder may increase the mean response rate. However, whether it improves outcome enough to be cost-effective is a separate research question. Similarly, adding a full-time consultation-liaison psychiatrist to a renal transplantation team may significantly improve clinical outcomes, but given today's bottom-line mentality, a consultation-liaison psychiatrist may not be approved unless cost savings can also be demonstrated.

Cost-effectiveness studies are frequently descriptive and focus on how psychiatric illness affects health care utilization and costs (Knapp and Harris 1998; Riesenberg and Glass 1989; Saravay and Lavin 1994; Stewart et al. 1989; Wells et al. 1989). On the basis of findings of these descriptive studies, investigators often conclude that psychiatric treatment should be more available to medical-surgical patients. Such conclusions are usually unwarranted, however, because descriptive studies do not prove that psychiatric interventions alter baseline utilization and costs. Prospective studies of the effects of psychiatric interventions on health care utilization and costs are more compelling (Dewan 1999; Huyse et al. 1996; Strain et al. 1994). An example of a study focusing on cost-effectiveness is described in the following abstract.

Objective: Managed care organizations prefer putatively less expensive treatment, i.e., a psychopharmacologist plus a non-M.D. psychotherapist. In this study the cost of integrated care by a psychiatrist was compared with split care. Method: Using 1998 fee schedules of seven large managed care organizations (with 54.3% market share and 67.8 million lives) plus Medicare (37 million people), the author modeled clinical scenarios of psychotherapy alone, medication alone, and combined treatment provided by a psychiatrist or split with a psychologist or social worker. Results: Brief psychotherapy by a social worker was the least expensive treatment. When treatment required both psychotherapy and medication, combined treatment by a psychiatrist cost about the same or less than split treatment with a social worker psychotherapist; it was usually less expensive than split treatment with a psychologist psychotherapist. Conclusions: The integrated biopsychosocial model practiced by psychiatry is both theoretically and economically the preferred model when combined treatment is needed. (Dewan 1999, p. 324)

It is a widely held belief that consultation-liaison psychiatry services have a large impact on cost savings rather than on salary-producing reimbursements (Hall et al.

1994; Strain et al. 1994). Unfortunately, it is exceedingly difficult to conclusively establish a causal relationship between an isolated consultation-liaison psychiatry intervention and cost savings resulting from improved health care utilization. Unless the control group is almost identical to the intervention group across many domains—demographic characteristics, medical diagnosis, severity of illness, and concurrent medical treatments—results will be confounded. For example, if control subjects in a chronic obstructive pulmonary disease study receive more steroids than do patients in the psychiatric intervention group, any difference in hospitalization costs could be at least partly accounted for by the difference in steroid use. This might obscure any effect of the psychiatric intervention. Similarly, a younger or less severely ill control group would likely obscure benefits to the intervention group derived from the psychiatric intervention.

RESEARCH BIAS

Research important to consultation-liaison psychiatry is sometimes confounded by bias. To avoid flawed research conclusions, it is imperative that bias be minimized. Countless well-meaning studies prove to be of little or no value because of unanticipated sources of bias. The most common sources of bias that affect research are summarized in Table 12–4.

Consultation-liaison psychiatry research is subject to bias more than general psychiatry research. It is difficult in medical-surgical populations to draw a proper study sample, to find outcome measures proven to be reliable and valid in those populations, and to avoid confounding biases. For example, in a study of the efficacy of a particular antidepressant medication in depressed medically ill patients, investigators face unique challenges: 1) defining the mood syndrome, 2) standardizing an outcome measure in the study population, and 3) accounting for effects of severity and types of medical illnesses and their treatments.

Consultation-liaison psychiatry researchers must consider the potential research biases summarized in Table 12–4. Fortunately, there are ways to minimize bias, even with the complexities of consultation-liaison psychiatry research. Steps to minimize bias are summarized in Table 12–5.

As Table 12–5 suggests, a great deal of effort must be expended for a study to have minimized bias and produce meaningful results. One of the most difficult and frustrating tasks for medical researchers is assuring that statistical tests are used appropriately. In general, medical

TABLE 12–4. Potential biases in consultation-liaison psychiatry research

Selection bias

Referral filter bias	Enrollment of patients referred from primary to secondary to tertiary care has the effect of concentrating rare cases, multiple diagnoses, and untreatable cases, which makes study populations nonrepresentative.
Diagnostic access bias	Individuals differ in geographical, social, and economic access to care and research, which introduces unexpected demographic differences.
Prevalence-incidence bias	Patients may be studied at differing points during their illness courses, which underestimates or overestimates psychopathology in medically ill patients.
Diagnostic purity bias	"Pure" diagnostic groups exclude comorbidity; thus, they may become nonrepresentative.
Missing data bias	Clinical data are missing because they are not measured, are excluded because they were normal, or are measured but not recorded, which leads to systematic underestimation of psychopathology in medically ill patients.
Noncontemporaneous control bias	Index and control cases are studied at different times; thus, changes in disease definition, exposures, diseases, and experiences may render study groups noncomparable.
Nonresponse bias	Nonrespondents in a specified sample may exhibit exposures or outcomes that differ from those of respondents.
Volunteer bias	Volunteers in a specified sample may exhibit exposures or outcomes that differ from those of nonvolunteers.

Information bias

Unacceptability bias	Measures that hurt, embarrass, or invade privacy may be refused or evaded systematically by study subjects.
Recall bias	How questions are asked, and how often, may differ between case subjects and controls (e.g., experimental subjects undergo more intensive examination than control subjects).
Attention bias (Hawthorne effect)	Study subjects systematically alter their behavior when they know they are being observed, which biases study results in the direction of perceived advantages to subjects.
Instrument bias	Defects in the validity or reliability of measurement instruments may lead to systematic deviations from true values, which underestimates or overestimates psychopathology in medically ill patients.
Expectation bias	Observers may err in measuring and recording observations so that they concur with their own prior expectations.
Confounding bias	When the effects of two or more procedures or factors are mixed together, it is concluded incorrectly that one of the factors is causal (e.g., not controlling for medical severity when studying effects of psychiatric interventions).

Source. Adapted from Levenson JL, Colenda C, Larson DB, et al: "Methodology in Consultation-Liaison Research: A Classification of Biases." *Psychosomatics* 31:367–376, 1990. Copyright 1990, Academy of Psychosomatic Medicine. Used with permission.

TABLE 12–5. Steps to minimize bias in consultation-liaison psychiatry research

1. **Invest time up front**	Effective planning for proper research design saves time and effort later.
2. **Randomize subjects**	Bias is far more likely to occur in nonrandomized samples.
3. **Balance information given to subjects**	Reveal enough information to subjects and care providers to elicit their support but not enough to introduce attention bias.
4. **Minimize contact with subjects**	The investigator's knowledge may introduce expectation bias. Use non–investigator-trained researchers to collect data.
5. **Conduct a pilot study**	A pilot study can evaluate whether unintended or unanticipated biases exist.
6. **Avoid excess in attempts to minimize bias**	Trying too hard to eradicate one source of bias can introduce another. For example, constructing an overhomogeneous subject population can increase diagnostic purity bias. Rather than try to eliminate bias entirely, try to reduce it in a balanced manner that recognizes these interrelationships.
7. **Obtain statistical consultation**	It takes less time to ask for advice in the beginning than to try to explain flawed data after the fact.

Source. Adapted from Levenson JL, Colenda C, Larson DB, et al: "Methodology in Consultation-Liaison Research: A Classification of Biases." *Psychosomatics* 31:367–376, 1990. Copyright 1990, Academy of Psychosomatic Medicine. Used with permission.

education does not provide a comprehensive grounding in biostatistics. Medical researchers must either acquire this knowledge while conducting research or rely on others who possess such training. A comprehensive discussion of biostatistics is beyond the scope of this chapter. For an excellent introduction to research design, with particular attention to statistics, consultation-liaison psychiatry researchers can refer to M. Fava and Rosenbaum (1992), Freeman and Tyrer (1989), and Glantz (1992).

ETHICAL CONSIDERATIONS

Ethical considerations in consultation-liaison psychiatry research are usually self-evident and straightforward. Federal statutes require written informed consent from subjects before they are enrolled in any clinical trial or prospective descriptive study. Subjects must understand treatment options, know all possible benefits and risks, and have the right to withdraw at any time without jeopardizing future eligibility for clinical care. Maximum disclosure should be provided when potential conflicts of interest exist (e.g., when pharmaceutical companies fund pharmacological clinical trials). "Any study which produces results that are misleading or incorrect as a result of avoidable methodologic errors—statistical or otherwise— is unethical" (Glantz 1992, pp. 392–393). These errors can produce risk and inconvenience for subjects. In addition, avoidable methodological errors may adversely affect future related research work and patient treatment.

Consultation-liaison psychiatry research sometimes involves subjects who cannot provide informed consent. For example, delirium treatment research may involve subjects whom the consultation-liaison psychiatrist considers not competent to consent. In those cases, it is important to gain the informed consent of the designated substitute decision-maker, as prescribed by state law (see Chapter 11). Patients with severe mental illnesses who participate as human subjects in research vary in their abilities to understand all aspects of informed consent. This situation may require input from families, primary care physicians, and the patients' psychiatrists. The National Alliance for the Mentally Ill (1995) has adopted policies on standards for protection of individuals with severe mental illnesses who participate as human subjects in research.

CONCLUSION

All methods of research described in this chapter are important in consultation-liaison psychiatry. Basic science research provides technologies and knowledge substrates to guide clinicians and clinical researchers. Case studies raise questions that can be more closely examined in cross-sectional population descriptive studies. Risk factors and possible cause-and-effect relationships are detected with longitudinal case-control and cohort studies. These studies inform clinical intervention research. Clinical intervention trials provide consultation-liaison psychiatrists with new tools to improve patient outcomes. Cost-effectiveness studies document whether and how improved clinical outcomes translate into cost savings. The degree to which consultation-liaison psychiatry can continue to demonstrate clinical effectiveness and cost-effectiveness will determine the future vitality and viability of the discipline.

REFERENCES

American Psychiatric Association: APA Official Actions—Position Statement on Nicotine Dependence. Am J Psychiatry 152:481–482, 1995

Backett S, Robinson A: Epidemiological methods in psychiatry, in Research Methods in Psychiatry. Edited by Freeman C, Tyrer P. Oxford, UK, Alden Press, 1989, pp 143–162

Biedel DC: Determining clinical outcome, in Research Designs and Methods in Psychiatry. Edited by Fava M, Rosenbaum JF. New York, Elsevier, 1992, pp 195–211

Blinder M: Gender differences in income for psychiatrists (letter). Am J Psychiatry 152:480, 1995

Blumenthal JA, Kamarck T: Assessment of the type A behavior pattern, in Applications in Behavioral Medicine and Health Psychology: A Clinician's Source Book. Edited by Blumental JA, McKee DC. Sarasota, FL, Professional Resource Exchange, 1987, pp 3–39

Bowman ES: Etiology and clinical course of pseudoseizures: relationship to trauma, depression, and dissociation. Psychosomatics 34:333–342, 1993

Bromley D: The Case-Study Method in Psychology and Related Disciplines. Chichester, UK, Wiley, 1986

Cummings JL: Depression in Parkinson's disease: a review. Am J Psychiatry 149:443–454, 1992

Dewan M: Are psychiatrists cost-effective? An analysis of integrated versus split treatment. Am J Psychiatry 156:324–326, 1999

DiMartini A, Twillman R: Organ transplantation and paranoid schizophrenia. Psychosomatics 35:159–161, 1994

Eisenberg L: Treating depression and anxiety in primary care: closing the gap between knowledge and practice. N Engl J Med 326:1080–1083, 1991

Engel GL: On looking inward and being scientific. Psychother Psychosom 54:63–69, 1990

Fava GA: Obituary—Robert Kellner, M.D., Ph.D., 1922–1992. Psychosomatics 34:287–289, 1993

Fava M, Rosenbaum JF: Research designs and methods in psychiatry, in Techniques in the Behavioral and Neural Sciences, Vol 9. Edited by Huston JP. New York, Elsevier, 1992, pp 119–211

Fink P, Sorensen L, Engberg M, et al: Somatization in primary care. Psychosomatics 40:330–338, 1999

Fishbain DA, Trescott J, Cutler B, et al: Do some chronic pain patients with atypical facial pain overvalue and obsess about their pain? Psychosomatics 34:355–359, 1993

Frasure-Smith N, Lesperance F, Talajic M: Depression following myocardial infarction: impact on 6-month survival. JAMA 270:1819–1825, 1993

Freeman C, Tyrer P (eds): Research Methods in Psychiatry. Oxford, UK, Alden Press, 1989

Gallagher RM: Training issues at the interface between consultation-liaison psychiatry and behavioral medicine. Adv Psychosom Med 20:33–52, 1990

Glantz SA: Primer of Biostatistics, 3rd Edition. New York, McGraw-Hill, 1992

Hall RCW, Wise MG: The clinical and financial burden of mood disorders. Psychosomatics 36:S11–S18, 1995

Hall RCW, Rundell JR, Hirsch TW: Developing a financially viable consultation-liaison service. Psychosomatics 35:308–318, 1994

Huyse FJ, Herzog T, Malt UF, et al: The European Consultation-Liaison Workgroup (ECLW) Collaborative Study—General Outline. Gen Hosp Psychiatry 18:44–55, 1996

Jenkins PL, Lester H, Alexander J, et al: A prospective study of psychosocial morbidity in adult bone marrow transplant recipients. Psychosomatics 35:361–367, 1994

Johnstone E, Lambert MT: Research methods appropriate to biological psychiatry, in Research Methods in Psychiatry. Edited by Freeman C, Tyrer P. Oxford, UK, Alden Press, 1989, pp 46–66

Katon W, Gonzales J: A review of randomized trials of psychiatric consultation-liaison studies in primary care. Psychosomatics 35:268–278, 1994

Kent DA, Tomasson K, Coryell W: Course and outcome of conversion and somatization disorders: a four-year follow-up. Psychosomatics 36:138–144, 1995

Knapp PK, Harris ES: Consultation-liaison in child psychiatry: a review of the past 10 years, part II: research on treatment approaches and outcomes. J Am Acad Child Adolesc Psychiatry 37:139–146, 1998

Levenson JL: Consultation-liaison psychiatry research: more like a ground cover than a hedgerow (editorial). Psychosom Med 59:563–564, 1997

Levenson JL, Colenda C, Larson DB, et al: Methodology in consultation-liaison research: a classification of biases. Psychosomatics 31:367–376, 1990

Magruder-Habib K, Zung WW, Feussner JR: Improving physicians' recognition and treatment of depression in general medical care: results from a randomized clinical trial. Med Care 28:239–250, 1990

Mark BZ, Kunkel EJ, Fabi MB, et al: Pimozide is effective in delirium secondary to hypercalcemia when other neuroleptics fail. Psychosomatics 34:446–450, 1993

Mayberg HS: Frontal lobe dysfunction in secondary depression. J Neuropsychiatry Clin Neurosci 6:428–442, 1994

McKegney FP, Beckhardt RM: Evaluative research in consultation-liaison psychiatry: review of the literature: 1970–1981. Gen Hosp Psychiatry 4:197–218, 1982

Mega MS, Cummings JL: Frontal-subcortical circuits and neuropsychiatric disorders. J Neuropsychiatry Clin Neurosci 6:358–370, 1994

Meyers CA, Valentine AD, Wong FCL, et al: Reversible neurotoxicity of interleukin-2 and tumor necrosis factor: correlation of SPECT with neuropsychological testing. J Neuropsychiatry Clin Neurosci 6:285–288, 1994

Mumford E, Schlesinger HJ, Glass GV, et al: A new look at evidence about reduced cost of medical utilization following mental health treatment. Am J Psychiatry 141:1145–1158, 1984

Muskin PR, Kunkel ES, Worley LL, et al: The multisite field trial of the consultation-liaison psychiatry assessment instrument. Gen Hosp Psychiatry 19:16–23, 1997

National Alliance for the Mentally Ill: Policies on strengthened standards for protection of individuals with severe mental illnesses who participate as human subjects in research. Adopted by the National Alliance for the Mentally Ill Board of Directors, February 4, 1995

Nemiah JC: A few intrusive thoughts on posttraumatic stress disorder (editorial). Am J Psychiatry 152:501–503, 1995

Newcombe RG: Towards a reduction in publication bias. BMJ 295:656–659, 1987

Ormel J, Koeter MW, van den Brink W, et al: Recognition, management, and course of anxiety and depression in general practice. Arch Gen Psychiatry 48:700–706, 1991

Peck DF: Research with single (or few) patients, in Research Methods in Psychiatry. Edited by Freeman C, Tyrer P. Oxford, UK, Alden Press, 1989, pp 92–104

Popkin MK, Callies AL, Lentz RD, et al: Prevalence of major depression, simple phobia, and other psychiatric disorders in patients with long-standing type 1 diabetes mellitus. Arch Gen Psychiatry 45:64–68, 1988

Regier DA, Burke JK: Quantitative and experimental methods in psychiatry, in Comprehensive Textbook of Psychiatry/III, 3rd Edition. Edited by Kaplan HI, Sadock BJ. Baltimore, MD, Williams & Wilkins, 1985, pp 295–312

Riesenberg D, Glass RM: The Medical Outcomes Study (editorial). JAMA 262:943, 1989

Rundell JR, Kyle KM, Brown GR, et al: Risk factors for suicide attempts in a human immunodeficiency virus screening program. Psychosomatics 33:24–27, 1992

Saravay SM, Lavin M: Psychiatric comorbidity and length of stay in the general hospital: a critical review of outcome studies. Psychosomatics 35:233–252, 1994

Saravay SM, Strain JJ: APM Task Force on Funding Implications of Consultation-Liaison Outcome Studies. Special series introduction: a review of outcome studies. Psychosomatics 35:227–232, 1994

Schwartz GE, Weiss SM: Yale Conference on Behavioral Medicine: a proposed definition and statement of goals. J Behav Med 1:3–12, 1978

Starkstein SE, Migliorelli R: ECT in a patient with a frontal craniotomy and residual meningioma. J Neuropsychiatry Clin Neurosci 5:428–430, 1993

Stern TA, Glick RL: Significance of stuffed animals at the bedside and what they can reveal about patients. Psychosomatics 34:519–521, 1993

Stewart AL, Greenfield S, Hays RD, et al: Functional status and well-being of patients with chronic conditions: results from the Medical Outcomes Study. JAMA 262:907–913, 1989

Strain JJ, Hammer JS, Fulop G: APM task force on psychosocial interventions in the general hospital inpatient setting. A review of cost-offset studies. Psychosomatics 35:253–262, 1994

Tohen M: Bias and other methodological issues in followup (cohort) studies, in Research Designs and Methods in Psychiatry. Edited by Fava M, Rosenbaum JF. New York, Elsevier, 1992, pp 119–125

Tonkonogy JM, Smith TW, Barreira PJ: Obsessive-compulsive disorders in Pick's disease. J Neuropsychiatry Clin Neurosci 6:176–180, 1994

Troster AI, Moe KE, Vitiello MV, et al: Predicting long-term outcome in individuals at risk for Alzheimer's disease with the Dementia Rating Scale. J Neuropsychiatry Clin Neurosci 6:54–57, 1994

Watson HE, Kershaw PW, Davies JB: Alcohol problems among women in a general hospital ward. British Journal of Addiction 86:889–894, 1991

Weinberger DR: A connectionist approach to the prefrontal cortex. J Neuropsychiatry Clin Neurosci 5:241–253, 1993

Wells KB, Stewart A, Hays RD, et al: The functioning and well-being of depressed patients: results from the Medical Outcomes Study. JAMA 262:914–919, 1989

Wells KB, Katon W, Rogers B, et al: Use of minor tranquilizers and antidepressant medications by depressed outpatients: results from the Medical Outcomes Study. Am J Psychiatry 151:694–700, 1994

Wool CA, Barsky AJ: Do women somatize more than men? Gender differences in somatization. Psychosomatics 35:445–452, 1994

Wright M, Samuels A, Streimer J: Clinical practice issues in consultation-liaison psychiatry. Aust N Z J Psychiatry 30:238–245, 1996

International Perspectives on Consultation-Liaison Psychiatry

Chapter Editors:

Frits J. Huyse, M.D.

Thomas Herzog, M.D.

Ulrik F. Malt, M.D.

Contributors:

Ruben Cesarco, M.D.

Francis Creed, M.D.

Peter de Jonge, Ph.D.

Trevor Friedman, M.D.

Thomas Herzog, M.D.

Takashi Hosaka, M.D.

Frits J. Huyse, M.D.

Yasutaka Iwasaki, M.D.

Antonio Lobo, M.D.

Ulrik F. Malt, M.D.

Marco Rigatelli, M.D.

Graeme C. Smith, M.D.

Wolfgang Söllner, M.D.

Barbara Stein, Ph.D.

Fritz Stiefel, M.D.

James J. Strain, M.D.

Paulo R. Zimmermann, M.D.

Consultation-liaison work, by definition, is making connections among different perspectives—the perspectives of medicine, psychiatry, and the patient. In this chapter, we propose to inform the United States reader about the different approaches to consultation-liaison work used throughout the world.

In the late 1970s and early 1980s, the United States paradigm for consultation-liaison psychiatry dominated the international scene. An important reason for this direction was the National Institute of Mental Health (NIMH) educational grant programs that were dedicated to the integration of mental health care into general medical care (Eaton et al. 1977). During that period, United States consultation-liaison psychiatry began to define its conceptual models, its target populations, and its methods of delivering appropriate and cost-effective services. Psychiatrists from many different countries visited the United States to observe consultation-liaison programs. Some psychiatrists even received full psychiatric training and then returned to their native country to focus on consultation-liaison psychiatry.

During the 1980s, several published articles described consultation-liaison services in different cultures, emphasizing the comparability of types of patients and differences in development of consultation-liaison and health care systems. Apart from these articles, communication between consultation-liaison psychiatrists in the United States and consultation-liaison psychiatrists in other countries was haphazard. Only a few international journals provided a scientific forum for consultation-liaison psychiatry; these journals were mainly Anglo-American. To the non-American, consult rates of 5% or more reported in the literature indicated ample resources (Torem et al. 1979). It took some time for non-American consultation-liaison psychiatrists to understand that the consultation-liaison health service research was generated by a relatively small group and did not represent the actual state of the art of consultation-liaison service delivery in the United States. This finding was confirmed by Wallen et al. (1987), who reported much lower average consultation rates in nonacademic and academic general hospitals (0.2% and 0.8%, respectively). This is an example of how United States domination of international scientific communication distorted reality and also neglected developments in other nations. In short, the diversity of consultation-liaison work in the international community is not well known.

This chapter was written by an international collaborative consultation-liaison group. It is designed to overcome communication problems and perhaps help to overcome the barriers already mentioned.

We begin the chapter with a brief review of the complex relations among consultation-liaison psychiatry, psychosomatics, and behavioral medicine. These relations are important in some European countries, notably the German-speaking ones.[1]

Next, we discuss consultation-liaison developments in some pertinent areas outside the United States: the northern (hereafter in this chapter, "Nordic") European countries, the German-speaking countries, the United Kingdom, the Netherlands, the European Mediterranean countries, Australia, Japan, and Latin America.

Finally, we cite experiences from a European research network of consultation-liaison psychiatrists who have conducted collaborative studies to highlight some of consultation-liaison psychiatry's needs, goals, and opportunities: 1) the assessment of the extent of consultation-liaison service delivery (see the subsection "ECLW Collaborative Study" under the section "European Studies" in this chapter), 2) the assessment of the risk of being a complex patient (COMPRI; see the subsection "Risk Factor Study" under "European Studies"), 3) the assessment of integrated health risk and needs (INTERMED; see the subsection "INTERMED" under "European Studies"), and 4) a model for quality management.

RELATION OF CONSULTATION-LIAISON PSYCHIATRY TO PSYCHOSOMATICS AND BEHAVIORAL MEDICINE

By and large, general hospital psychiatry is the result of a relatively recent effort by dedicated psychiatrists. This phenomenon has long and complex historical roots, which help to explain the differentiated development of the consultation-liaison mental health service delivery practices in various countries. During the nineteenth century, an empirically based medicine developed that focused on an external biological cause of diseases or defects on a cellular level (Koch 1987). Similarly, psychiatry adopted a biological perspective in the major psychiatric disorders. These developments left the neurotic disorders and illnesses, which were characterized by somatic symptoms and no physical findings, outside the mainstream of medicine and psychiatry. At the turn of the century, these symptoms were explained by an emerging psychoanalytical theory. Cannon's research on the physiologic responses to emotions and Pavlov's research with conditioning further broadened the concept of psychosomatic medicine. Unfortunately, psychological problems and psychiatric disorders in medical and surgical patients are still neglected by mainstream medicine and psychiatry. The extent of this neglect varies among countries.

In this chapter, we present a general overview of differences and interrelations among consultation-liaison psychiatry, psychosomatics, and behavioral medicine. We decided, for educational reasons, to focus on the German paradigm—which also dominates consultation-liaison psychiatry in Austria and the German-speaking part of Switzerland—to better elucidate transcultural differences in mental health service delivery to medically ill patients. In Germany, since the 1920s, practitioners with a background of internal medicine and/or psychoanalysis have tried to fill the gap left by psychiatrists. An additional and probably less-known fact is that clinical-medical psychologists, usually with a background in learning theories, also have filled this vacuum since the 1970s and are having an increasing influence. All of these developments have a considerable effect on both theoretical and practical aspects of mental health care delivery in the general hospital.

On a practical level, these developments influence relations and the use of psychological interventions, regardless of whether the intervention is primarily focused on the patient, team, family, or a combination thereof. In addition, terms used by the practitioners have various meanings in different places and contexts. In the following sections, we simplify and distinguish between 1) traditions and concepts influencing the field, 2) institutional developments and the participation of different professions, and 3) trends.

---

[1] We use the term *consultation-liaison psychiatry* because it corresponds to American usage. However, we include all services and professions involved that vary depending on local structures and traditions (e.g., psychosomatics, psychologists).

Traditions and Concepts[2]

The development of psychosomatics dates back to the 1920s. From its inception, psychosomatics has had much to do with a critical outlook on medicine and society and has been influenced by the attempt to come to terms with the Nazi experience, as discussed elsewhere (Herzog et al. 1994). In contrast to the United States, psychosomatics has its roots in two traditions outside psychiatry: 1) internists striving toward more holistic care—a *psychosomatic approach* to their patients—and 2) psychoanalysts applying psychodynamic thinking to patients with physical complaints and physical illness. There is enough cross-fertilization between these two traditions to discuss them here as one entity.

The psychosomatic approach takes into consideration the interactions between biological, psychological, and social factors in *every* patient, independent of the specialist involved. This implies a systems perspective and requires knowledge of the biological, psychological, and social subsystems and their interaction. The psychosomatic approach was clearly described in the United States consultation-liaison literature by Miller (1973). The doctor-patient relationship became a special focus. Teaching and training the clinician to integrate psychosocial aspects into his or her everyday work was highly valued (Uexküll et al. 1997) and, particularly in Germany, widely practiced. Consequences of this approach for clinical medicine are

1. *A different view of body and physical illness:* Specifically, all illnesses and traumas are viewed as having a function and a place in a given life situation, within the context of often unconscious intra- and interindividual conflicts.
2. *A different view of the interaction between doctor and patient:* The doctor monitors his or her experiences and feelings in dealing with the patient. These feelings provide important diagnostic information about the patient's relation to the environment. Other relevant interactions are understood and used in a similar way.
3. *A different view of the clinic:* Relationships and interactions are used as both diagnostic and therapeutic tools to examine the structure and organization of the medical institution and its effect on patients, staff, and their interactions (i.e., a systems perspective) (Köhle et al. 1997).

Behavioral medicine (Miltner et al. 1986; Wahl and Hautzinger 1989) is largely adapted from United States research (Schwartz and Weiss 1978). There is also considerable overlap with health psychology and clinical psychology. Essentially, behavioral medicine uses and integrates experimentally derived concepts and techniques from the psychological and behavioral sciences into the diagnosis and treatment of medical disorders. Its multifactorial models attempt to integrate biomedical and sociopsychological approaches. Both traditions—psychosomatics and, increasingly, behavioral medicine—strongly influence the training of physicians in psychosocial aspects of medicine. This influence is independent of institutional affiliations and developments.

Institutions and Professions

Radical advocates of the psychosomatic approach oppose psychosomatics as a distinct specialty because of their integrative view. According to this view, every physician should fully integrate psychosocial aspects into clinical practice and only needs psychiatric help for the core mental illnesses. Nevertheless, in many places, particularly in Germany, psychosomatics is increasingly institutionalized. This first occurred in the universities and then gradually spread to general hospital departments and special hospitals (Herzog 1991a). However, especially in older established institutions, the clear trend is away from competition and fixation on the "horse-race paradigm" (i.e., which approach is "winning"). Instead, the focus is on pragmatic approaches that combine or integrate what fits best with the needs of a particular patient and the capacities of a given team. This parallels the developments in empirical psychotherapy research and the evaluation of different therapies and settings (Orlinsky et al. 1994).

The scientific and clinical input of psychologists has been very important; in several places, although it remains controversial, the tendency is to integrate psychologists as consultants and allow them official status analogous to psychiatrists.

Institutionalized psychosomatics, which may have roots in one of several traditions, deals with a whole range of nonpsychotic and nonorganic psychological disorders and places special emphasis on patients with some type of physical complaint and on issues of coping and compliance. Patients with functional, neurotic, and personality disorders make up the largest part of the clientele. Psy-

---

[2] For more detailed information, see Herzog 1991a, 1991b; Richter and Wirsching 1991; Uexküll 1992; Uexküll et al. 1997; Wirsching and Herzog 1991.

chotherapy is the main treatment and is provided in a variety of settings. Psychotherapy uses many theoretical frameworks, although psychodynamic and cognitive-behavioral approaches are the most popular. Psychotherapy is used in four basic problem areas:

1. *Etiopathogenesis:* when psychological and social factors cause or influence the course of physical illness or when complex behavior problems (e.g., specific risk behaviors), life stresses, or psychosocial and psychophysiological maladaptations are present.
2. *Coping:* when the patient (or his or her relatives) cannot cope with an acute threat, chronic impairment, mourning, and situations in the family or in professional life.
3. *Compliance:* when psychological forces influence a patient's compliance with medical recommendations (e.g., taking prescriptions, changing lifestyle, making use of early detection programs).
4. *Psychological aspects and sequelae of physical illness:* for detection of substance-induced or medically related mental disorders.

In Germany, this use contrasts with the role of traditional psychiatry in the general hospital, where psychiatrists see all types of patients but mainly focus on patients with delirium, dementia, substance abuse, and severe mood disorders (i.e., those disorders with a fairly clear-cut biological basis and potential biological treatments).

Trends

Great diversity in types of mental health service delivery exists on the institutional level. In Germany, specialization carries the danger of fragmentation and the opportunity of specialized care, whereas the major issue elsewhere in Europe is the integration or splitting away of psychology. On the scientific level, different approaches are tested for their merits, taking into account social value and cultural preferences. There is hope that psychosocial and biomedical insights and approaches will continue together in consultation-liaison psychiatry, an undertaking that almost certainly requires subspecialization.

In contrast to the German situation, consultation-liaison services in Europe usually are satellites of psychiatric departments. However, this type of organizational structure is sometimes regarded as draining resources away from psychiatric to general medical and surgical care, and vice versa (Huyse and Smith 1997). Fully integrated services with comprehensive early screening are rare. Among the few exceptions are Engel's (1977) model in Rochester, New York; some departments of

behavioral medicine; and some German psychosomatic departments. In summary, consultation-liaison services often maintain a precarious balance and are often relatively isolated.

On the level of scientific work in the United States and other countries, consultation-liaison psychiatry is often on the periphery. The psychosomatic movements in the 1950s tended to neglect the clinical epidemiology of mental disturbances in the general medical population, mental health service delivery research that focused on dual diagnosis, treatment and health care delivery systems in the borderland between psychiatry and medicine, and the development of standards of services and training. Since the 1990s, in response to this situation, the specialist consultation-liaison groups in the United States, Europe, Australia, and Japan developed a collaborative effort.

International Networking

In the beginning of the 1990s, the MICRO-CARES Consortium—started as an American group—became an internationally active group through Australian and Canadian participation. Currently, the MICRO-CARES software is available in several languages.

Building on the network developed during the European Consultation-Liaison Workgroup (ECLW) Collaborative Study (see the section "European Studies" in this chapter), a European Association for Consultation-Liaison Psychiatry and Psychosomatics (EACLPP) was formed in 1992.

In the 1990s, as a result of increased international activities and the formalization of the Academy of Psychosomatic Medicine as the American forum for consultation-liaison psychiatry, the Academy of Psychosomatic Medicine's annual conferences became an informal meeting point for non–United States consultation-liaison psychiatrists. in November 1998, after consultation with the board of the Academy of Psychosomatic Medicine, national associations, and interest groups for consultation-liaison psychiatry, the International Organization for Consultation-Liaison Psychiatry (http://www.med.monash.edu.au/psychmed/ioclp) was launched.

In 2000 the informal EACLPP was formalized. The EACLPP is designed to be the official representative for consultation-liaison topics for the European Union, in addition to being a European umbrella organization for consultation-liaison psychiatry. The EACLPP organizes annual conferences in the beginning of the fall. Membership and other information can be obtained through the Web site http://www.eaclpp.org.

STATUS AND DEVELOPMENTS OF CONSULTATION-LIAISON PSYCHIATRY IN EUROPE, AUSTRALIA, JAPAN, AND SOUTH AMERICA[3]

One decisive background feature is shared by virtually all care delivery systems, namely, the consensus that medical care must be promptly available to all, according to need and independent of socioeconomic status. This care is provided by compulsory, usually income-related health insurance (e.g., Germany, the Netherlands, Greece, France, Australia and New Zealand, Japan), tax-financed systems (e.g., Scandinavia, United Kingdom, Portugal, Spain), or some mixture of the two. The way in which resources are allocated to consultation-liaison psychiatry mainly is related to negotiations within the national, regional, or local system, such as the individual hospital. Depending on the system, resource allocation also involves the insurance system and/or government authorities. University hospitals usually have more opportunities to allocate resources according to intramural negotiations. Since the psychiatric reform movements of the 1970s, psychiatric care has generally greatly improved. This improvement has led to better integration of psychiatric services with general medical care, including appropriate funding. Only in Japan has psychiatric treatment in the general hospital faired badly; in some cases, treatment of organic mental disorder is not reimbursed. Some countries plan to introduce fee-for-service payment or diagnosis-related group reimbursement (e.g., Germany). In Europe, the early 1990s have been a time of tremendous political and social change with repercussions on the organization and financing of public services, including medical care.

In the following sections, we present condensed reports on the status of consultation-liaison psychiatry in different countries. In reading these reports, do not underestimate the enormous diversity, the wealth of experience gained from different traditions, and the variety of approaches (even within one country). Up to now, taking part in the English-language-dominated international discourse has not been a priority for non-Anglo-Saxon consultation-liaison practitioners. This is especially true in countries or cultural regions with highly developed scientific and clinical infrastructures and large

native-language audiences, such as Germany, Spain, and Japan. For these reasons, we have provided a list of references, which includes some relevant reference texts in non-English languages. Pertinent English-language publications from European authors also are available (Strain et al. 1996).

Nordic Countries[4]

Relevant Background

The Nordic countries of Europe include three Scandinavian countries—Denmark, Norway, and Sweden—as well as Finland and Iceland. For decades, these countries have had close political and cultural collaboration. In fact, Danish, Norwegian, and Swedish languages are considered three Scandinavian dialects; the Icelandic language is actually old Norwegian. For centuries, Finland, with a Swedish minority, has had close connections with Sweden. This association has also strengthened Finland's bonds to Scandinavia. The citizens of these five countries can move freely among the different countries without a passport, gain employment in one of the countries without obtaining permission, and even change residence without obtaining permission. The health care systems are also similar. Almost all hospitals are owned by the government, counties, or local communities. Hospitals and their staff salaries are financed through taxes. This system explains why hospital care is available for all citizens at a low cost compared with the income level. Availability of care is independent of the socioeconomic status of the patient. Despite these similarities and close bonds between the Nordic countries, the status and development of consultation-liaison psychiatry differ among the five countries.

Psychiatry and General Hospital Patients

In Finland and Norway, psychiatry is largely psychodynamically oriented, but it also has strong social psychiatry roots. Sweden, with a closer historical relation to German psychiatry, is more biologically oriented. Denmark and Iceland are in an intermediate position. These differences in clinical orientation largely explain how consultation-liaison psychiatry has developed and is organized in the Nordic countries.

The strong psychodynamic orientation in Finland and Norway is associated with a marked interest in psychological and psychiatric aspects of physically ill

---

[3] This selection of countries was determined by participation in the international network and by space limitations.
[4] This section is by Ulrik F. Malt, M.D.

patients compared with the other countries (Malt 1991, 1993; Tienari 1993a, 1993b). Finland has at least one full-time consultation-liaison psychiatrist in most general hospitals (Viinamäki et al. 1993). Norway has full-time consultation-liaison psychiatrists in major academic hospitals, as well as the only chairperson of consultation-liaison psychiatry and psychosomatics among the Nordic countries (Malt and Weisæth 1989). In Sweden, some major general hospital departments have psychiatrists assigned to a specific department (e.g., gastroenterology, neurosurgery, gynecology) (Sjogren 1992; Stalhammar et al. 1988; Starmark et al. 1988; Weinryb et al. 1992). Nevertheless, in Denmark, Iceland, Norway, and Sweden, most hospitals do not have a special consultation-liaison service but rely on consultations from departments of psychiatry within the general hospitals (Gudmundsson et al. 1991; Mayou et al. 1991).

Official Status of Consultation-Liaison Psychiatry and Training

In none of the Nordic countries is consultation-liaison psychiatry an official subspecialty. However, in Finland, Sweden, and Norway, the psychiatric associations have divisions for general hospital psychiatry (Finland), consultation-liaison psychiatry, and psychosomatic medicine (Norway). In Finland, the status and amount of work for consultation-liaison psychiatrists will likely increase because of rapid deinstitutionalization.

None of the Nordic countries require that psychiatrists receive consultation-liaison training, but training in psychiatric outpatient services is mandatory. Basic training in psychological treatment of mental disorders (psychotherapy) also is now required in the Nordic countries. Every second year, after official approval from the five Nordic psychiatric associations' collaboration committee, Nordic conferences on consultation-liaison psychiatry and psychosomatics are organized.

Types of Patients Seen and Specific Services

The overall psychiatric consultation rate within the Nordic countries is unknown. Data from the European Consultation-Liaison Workgroup (ECLW) for General Hospital Psychiatry and Psychosomatics Collaborative Study suggest that rates are no higher than 1% of medical patients, when consultation-liaison services are available. Although no country has developed specialized services for specific patient groups, some services may be available. For example, in a few hospitals, patients who attempt suicide are referred to a psychiatrist; however, most consultation is on an ad hoc basis, relying on the best judgment of the attending physician or the nurse.

Quite often, patients who attempt suicide are referred to a general family physician because primary care (financed through taxes) is well developed in the Nordic countries (Rutz et al. 1990).

Research

As a consequence of the theoretical orientation of the psychiatrists in Finland and Norway, research in consultation-liaison psychiatry focuses on psychological aspects of physical illness and adjustment to illness more than on psychopathology, per se. In Norway, for historical reasons, there is a specific interest in disasters and the management of accidental injury (Malt 1993; Malt and Weisæth 1989). In Finland, cardiac surgery has developed a specialty area of consultation-liaison psychiatry (Tienari 1993b). As a result of the ECLW Collaborative Study, the characteristics, comorbidity, and functional status of substance abuse patients—a substantial number of consults on the Finnish consultation-liaison services—have been reported (Alaja et al. 1997, 1998a, 1998b, 1999). On the basis of these data, factors predictive for transfer to a psychiatric hospital among all patients referred were psychiatric hospital care during the last 5 years (odds ratio [OR] = 3.7), schizophrenic psychosis (OR = 2.9), and attempted suicide (OR = 2.1) (Viinamäki et al. 1998). In Sweden, consultation-liaison-related research had focused on more biological aspects, with emphasis on somatoform disorders (von Knorring 1989); more recent publications include psychology-based works (Weinryb et al. 1992). Epidemiological research on the frequency and interrelation of hospitalizations in general hospitals of patients with prior psychiatric hospitalizations and on patients' somatization was conducted in Denmark (Fink 1992; Fink et al. 1993). Recently, Fink et al. (1999) reported short screening tools for hypochondriasis and for somatoform disorders in general.

Two inter-Nordic research projects also should be mentioned. The first is a study of all patients who were admitted to four general hospitals in Denmark, Finland, Norway, and Sweden after attempting suicide (Stiles et al. 1993). The second is an assessment of the psychiatric morbidity in primary public health care (Fink et al. 1995).

In the beginning of the 1990s an important step was taken toward the use of standardized research instruments within the Nordic countries (Bech et al. 1993). The rather homogeneous population, high educational levels, low migration rate, and high acceptance and development of population registers within the Nordic countries create optimal conditions to compare interventions and longitudinal follow-up studies (Allgulander and Fischer

1990; Fink et al. 1993). Thus far, the full potential for this type of research in consultation-liaison psychiatry has not been realized.

Future Development

Many options are available to consultation-liaison psychiatry in the Nordic countries. Consultation-liaison psychiatry could focus on psychopathology, which might lead to the development of parallel departments of rehabilitation psychology and medical psychology. The alternative is to expand consultation-liaison psychiatry toward a more holistic, psychobiological approach, in which medical and rehabilitation psychology is an integrated part of the medical service. The concept of a consultation-liaison psychiatry and psychosomatics service could also include neuropsychobiological aspects. There is no general agreement on this latter issue. In countries where consultation-liaison psychiatry is developed (e.g., Finland and Norway), this integrated approach is the best way to secure a holistic perspective. Within the holistic concept, organizing consultation-liaison psychiatry as an integrated part of primary care may have important benefits for patients (Rutz et al. 1990). Clinical psychologists would need to be more actively used within this model. Thus, in the Nordic countries, development points toward a concept of consultation-liaison psychology, psychiatry, and psychosomatics or, simply, *consultation-liaison psychobiology.*

In line with this psychobiological approach, psychometric assessments are used more frequently in clinical consultation-liaison work. These assessments measure personality, cognitive, and emotional variables during the course of physical illness or injury and treatment. These tests have been most extensively developed in the consultation-liaison department of the University of Oslo, where investigators administer a battery of tests. Several measures are sensitive to change in quality of life and mental symptoms following interventions (i.e., outcome measures). Instruments used include the General Health Questionnaire (GHQ-30), Hospital Anxiety Depression Questionnaire (HAD), Eysenck Personality Questionnaire (EPQ-N and L scales), an expanded version of the Giessener symptom distress checklist (GBB), Toronto Alexithymia Scale (TAS), and the Multi Dimensional Health Locus of Control Scale (HLCS). Optical reading equipment is used to score tests. When a patient is referred to the consultation-liaison service, the battery is performed, and results are given to the patient's nurse. This test battery provides data for follow-up studies,

improves the "scientific status" of consultation-liaison service; and has led to an increased demand from colleagues in other departments for collaborative research. Science-driven practice and quality assurance are critical to the future of consultation-liaison psychiatry. In conclusion, we foresee the development of consultation-liaison psychiatry in the Nordic countries moving away from a narrow psychopathology focus toward a broader, holistic, science-driven service.

German-Speaking Countries[5]

Relevant Background

Although the organization, administration, and financing of services differ across Germany, Austria, and the German cantons of Switzerland, the services share clinical and theoretical traditions. Social psychiatry, psychodynamic orientation, and pragmatic psychotherapeutic approaches are each well represented, in addition to the more traditional biological orientation. The special clinical and theoretical tradition in Germany has led to the creation of two medical disciplines within consultation-liaison psychiatry: 1) general psychiatry and psychotherapy and 2) psychotherapeutic medicine/psychosomatics. A sketch of the psychosomatic tradition and institutionalization was discussed earlier in this chapter. The unification of Germany left little of the East German system intact, in contrast to the systems developed in West Germany. Inpatient and outpatient diagnosis and treatment are strictly separate (except for emergencies and special cases). Available medical services include extensive inpatient and outpatient psychotherapy and psychosomatics (Herzog 1991a, 1991b). Because of similar history and traditions, in Austria there is also a split into two separate consultation-liaison services: psychiatric services and psychotherapeutic services (Söllner et al. 1997). In Switzerland, unlike Germany, there is no tendency to split into two separate medical specialties (i.e., psychiatry and psychosomatics).

Psychological Medicine in the General Hospital

General hospital–based consultation-liaison services are underdeveloped in the German-speaking countries. Of the approximately 1,800 general hospitals in West Germany, only 15% have in-hospital mental health services. Most are served haphazardly by outside psychiatrists. The existing in-hospital consultation-liaison services are provided, with some overlap, by psychiatry (95%) and

---

[5] This section is by Thomas Herzog, M.D., Wolfgang Söllner, M.D., Barbara Stein, Ph.D., and Fritz Stiefel, M.D.

psychosomatics (20%). Most general hospital psychiatrists have some competence in psychotherapy and psychosomatics, and the psychosomatic departments usually have fully trained psychiatrists on their consultation-liaison staff. Compared with psychiatric departments, psychosomatic departments allocate a much larger proportion of their resources to consultation-liaison psychiatry (Herzog and Hartmann 1990).

In Austria, the first general hospital psychiatric unit outside a university was opened in 1994. Since 1996, a new law on the practice of and quality standards in psychotherapy has been passed; and in addition, there has been discussion of the results of empirical research demonstrating the gap between needs and the availability of consultation-liaison services in general hospitals (DeVries et al. 1998; Söllner et al. 1998a). These occurrences have led to a significant change: in central general hospitals, a growing number of psychotherapeutic units have been installed, and in smaller general hospitals, psychotherapeutic consultants have been employed in addition to the preexisting psychiatric consultants (Söllner et al. 1998b).

In Switzerland, consultation-liaison psychiatry, with some very notable exceptions in the French-speaking part, is also underdeveloped (Zumbrunnen 1992).

Consult rates depend on the availability of in-hospital consultation-liaison services. In hospitals where the consultation-liaison service lacks a "psychosomatic" orientation, patients with certain psychiatric diagnoses (neurotic, stress-related, and adjustment disorders; behavioral syndromes associated with physiologic disturbances and physical factors) are seldom referred. Independent of personnel, psychosomatic practitioners spend significantly more time on a consultation than do psychiatrists, partly because they assess indications for outpatient psychotherapy and try to motivate patients toward psychotherapy and partly because of their approach to medications. For instance, in a medically ill patient who is depressed, psychiatric consultants prescribe medication up to 60% of the time, whereas psychosomaticists prescribe medications less than 5% of the time. This is one of many indications that theoretical orientation has a great influence on treatment (Herzog et al. 1994, 1995). Notwithstanding the difficulties in obtaining cooperation between mental health and medical services, many consultees recognize the differences between psychiatric and psychosomatic services and make referrals accordingly.

Official Status of Consultation-Liaison Psychiatry Psychosomatics and Training

No organization specifically represents consultation-liaison psychiatry. Within the German College of Psychosomatic Medicine (DKPM), the German Psychiatric Association (DGPPN), and, recently, the German Association of Psychologists (BdP), informal committees focus on consultation-liaison issues. The DKPM unites doctors and psychologists from all theoretical orientations, which is an important prerequisite for collaborative research. The newly developed European infrastructure has an important effect on the professional organization.

In Germany, psychiatric training requires only some experience in consultation-liaison; there is no further specification. Basic qualification in psychotherapy, either psychodynamic or cognitive-behavioral, became mandatory in 1992. Specialist and general training in psychosomatics received a boost when a new medical specialty called *psychotherapeutic medicine* was created in 1992; this specialty requires 5 years of full-time training that focuses on biopsychosocial interventions in a medical setting. The medical specialty psychotherapeutic medicine is different from psychosomatic primary care. Every private-practice physician must be competent in psychosomatic primary care (e.g., outpatient internal medicine care). The training in psychosomatic primary care usually is provided by psychosomatics or psychotherapeutic medicine departments.

In Austria, training in basic knowledge and skills in psychotherapy is mandatory in the education of psychiatrists. Psychotherapists working in consultation-liaison services have to complete a full 5-year psychotherapeutic training. However, no specific training in consultation-liaison psychiatry and psychotherapy is obligatory for both professions. Currently, basic data on the training of consultation-liaison psychiatrists and psychotherapists are assessed in order to develop specific training programs.

Up to 5% of nonpsychiatrists, especially general practitioners, gynecologists, and internists, acquire psychotherapy training for use in their practice. Recently, a qualification in psychosomatic primary care was introduced in outpatient medicine. Psychotherapy training focuses on psychological aspects of complaints and illness, specifically using the doctor-patient relationship for treatment. Many residents participate in these programs. Members of the psychosomatics department contribute a great deal of the seminars, courses, and supervision necessary to obtain these qualifications.

In Switzerland, psychotherapy training is an established part of the psychiatric curriculum. Recently, a certificate for psychosocial and psychosomatic medicine has been created in Switzerland; this certificate is based on an extensive curriculum for general practitioners and should allow them to gain competence in psychosocial interventions with the medically ill. This certificate has been approved by the Swiss Medical Association and will ultimately allow these practitioners to bill their psychosocial interventions adequately.

Consultation-liaison psychiatry is an optional part of psychiatric training in some locations; nonpsychiatric residents from internal medicine and general practice sometimes receive consultation-liaison training. In all three countries, psychiatrists, internists, and psychologists may choose a career in psychosomatic departments.

Research

Research in consultation-liaison psychiatry is strongly influenced by the psychosomatic approach that emphazises the interaction of body and mind in the development, course, and treatment of mental disorders; psychotherapy is the main approach to treatment. Departments of psychosomatics, medical psychology, clinical psychology, and, to a lesser extent, general psychiatry are focused mainly on the epidemiology, etiology, course, and psychopathology of psychosomatic diseases and disorders; adjustment to somatic illness; quality of life; illness behavior; and problems with compliance and coping. These studies take place mostly in cooperation with general medicine, oncology, surgery, neurology, dermatology, and rehabilitative medicine. Recently, psychotraumatology is of growing research interest. Applied research has concentrated on the development of psychosocial interventions, especially for patients with cancer; renal, cardiovascular, or gastroenterological diseases; pain; eating disorders; and other chronic diseases and transplant patients. Multicenter randomized clinical trials examine different psychological interventions in patients with chronic medical illnesses, such as Crohn's disease, migraine, and eating disorders, with particular emphasis on cost-effectiveness.

To address the insufficient ability of general hospital physicians to recognize patients' psychiatric comorbidity (Söllner et al. 2001) as well as their deficits in communication skills, education programs at the undergraduate, postgraduate, and specialist levels were developed and their effects on mental health care delivery in primary care and general hospitals were evaluated (Langewitz et al. 1998; Söllner et al. 2000).

Another focus is the implementation of education programs at the undergraduate, postgraduate, and specialist levels and the evaluation of their effect on mental health care delivery in primary care and general hospitals. Because of the enormous changes in organization and financing of health services, the evaluation of service delivery in inpatient and outpatient mental health care becomes ever more important.

Consultation-liaison health service research led to the development of integrated consultation-liaison databases and of instruments for routine psychometric assessment as well as to the implementation and evaluation of quality management programs. In addition, under a systemic perspective, the specific needs of patients, patients' families, and the different caring professions are the object of assessment and intervention studies.

Future Development

Competing clinical approaches and research traditions have the potential to contribute to improved consultation-liaison care delivery, provided the competitiveness is productive and not destructive. The creation of the medical speciality psychotherapeutic medicine also was a result of the recognition of deficits in mental health care for general hospital and primary care patients. Currently, there are strong moves toward the implementation of specialized psychosomatic units based at secondary referral general hospitals and the provision of consultation-liaison care for the neighboring hospitals. This also places increased emphasis on collaboration with primary care, mainly through training in "psychosomatic basic care."

One of the most exciting recent developments in consultation-liaison psychiatry in Switzerland is the introduction of communication skills training for oncological nurses and medical oncologists. This training, based on a manual elaborated by a national task force, basically consists of a videotaped interview of each participant, with an actor playing a cancer patient. The videos are analyzed during the 3-day training in small groups and serve as a base for role playing. After six sessions of individual supervision, the participant again interviews an actor playing a patient; the session is videotaped and analyzed in a follow-up session of half a day. These training courses are financially supported by the pharmaceutical industry and organized by the Swiss Cancer League. They have now become mandatory for specialization in medical oncology.

Practice guidelines for psychosomatic consultation-liaison services, based on extensive analyses of the research literature, will contribute to improved service delivery. Although clearly, the medical specialities "psychiatry and psychotherapy" and "psychotherapeutic medicine" have different clinical and research tasks, their relation to each other and to behavioral medicine and health psychology needs further investigation and improvement. From the viewpoint of care delivery and applied research, close cooperation is a neccessity. However, there is real danger that competition for power and diminishing resources will interfere with the neccesary collaboration. Cost-effectiveness must consider culture, circumstances, and values of all parties involved—the patient, family, consultee and consultant, and society (Herzog and Scheidt 1991).

United Kingdom[6]

Relevant Background

Two aspects of the comprehensive National Health Service are important in understanding consultation-liaison psychiatry in the United Kingdom. One aspect is the dominance of general (family) practice, which integrates physical and psychological care; the other is that psychiatric services vary from one district to another. As emphasis on community-based psychiatric services increases, resources for hospital-based consultation-liaison services are threatened. In the average district, the consultation-liaison service typically offers consultations to patients with self-poisoning, psychiatric emergencies, and psychotic disorders. Psychosomatic services exist at only a few major teaching centers (Mayou 1989; Mayou et al. 1990). At best, services include biological, cognitive-behavioral, psychodynamic, and psychosocial approaches. Psychoanalytic treatment is uncommon.

Consultation-Liaison Psychiatry in the General Hospital

Consultation-liaison psychiatrists usually are based in general hospital psychiatric units and are rarely located in the community mental health setting. In district hospitals, consultation-liaison services are largely provided by duty (junior) psychiatrists or general psychiatrists with other responsibilities. Often, consultants provide consultation-liaison services on an individual basis without an organized service or unit within the hospital. Psychiatric consult rates in the general hospital are generally less than 1% (Mayou 1988). However, one-quarter of new patients to the psychiatric service pass through the general hospital, via emergency and accident departments or as admissions following self-poisoning (Gater and Goldberg 1991). Most psychiatry outpatient clinics, whether located in the general hospital psychiatric units or a psychiatric hospital, treat patients with combined physical and psychological problems referred by physicians in general hospitals or general (family) practitioners. Except for Leeds General Infirmary and Leicestershire Health Authority Mental Health Service Unit, very few psychiatric-medical units exist. Psychogeriatricians and psychiatric specialists in substance abuse, both subspecialties in psychiatry, provide specific consulta-

tion-liaison services. In contrast to consultation-liaison psychiatry, psychogeriatric consultation-liaison is comparatively well organized, whereas consultation-liaison for substance abuse services is usually unsatisfactory.

Over the last decade, referrals to consultation-liaison services indicated a continued predominance of self-poisoning patients (Hawton and Catalan 1987), psychological reactions to physical disease, or physical symptoms with no organic basis (Brown and Cooper 1987; Creed et al. 1993; Sensky et al. 1985; Thomas 1983). Psychiatric management in patients who deliberately injure themselves is not mandatory at most United Kingdom medical services. Doctors in casualty departments assess these patients and decide whether psychiatric referral is necessary. When referred, patients are seen by nurses, social workers, psychologists, or general psychiatrists, all of whom are usually supervised by a consultation-liaison psychiatrist.

Hospitals with a consultation-liaison service may have several psychiatrists who, among other tasks, offer ward consultation service to particular medical or surgical specialties. In this way, "liaison" develops, but traditional consultation-liaison psychiatry is uncommon because of limited resources. Liaison sometimes occurs with primary care (Creed and Marks 1989). A few consultation-liaison psychiatrists admit patients requiring inpatient psychiatric care to their own general hospital psychiatric unit and sometimes observe them after discharge. Specific cognitive-behavioral treatment, psychotherapy, education, and training are occasionally undertaken by consultation-liaison nurses who work collaboratively with general nurses or psychologists.

Well-developed consultation-liaison services provide specialist intervention (e.g., in oncology, renal, plastic surgery, and burn units). These services usually have expertise in psychological reactions to physical disease. Specialized outpatient services usually see patients with somatization disorders (Creed et al. 1993). Many hospitals have specific teams to treat women with puerperal psychiatric disorders. Prettyman and Friedman (1991) found that 19% of the health districts have dedicated facilities for admitting mentally ill mothers and their babies; only 9 of 201 health districts had no facilities for joint admissions or plans to establish this service. In some districts with these services, obstetric liaison also has developed. The Royal College of Psychiatrists recommended that all districts have the ability to admit mothers and babies to a specialized unit and that a psychiatric

---

[6] This section is by Trevor Friedman, M.D., and Francis Creed, M.D. In the United Kingdom, consultation-liaison psychiatry is referred to as liaison psychiatry.

consultant with specific responsibility be available. Areas with established consultation-liaison services also receive referrals from general practitioners and often play a crucial role in coordinating treatment of these patients.

Official Status of Consultation-Liaison Psychiatry Psychosomatics and Training

As a distinct specialty, consultation-liaison psychiatry is a small but growing group within the United Kingdom. There are a small number (probably fewer than 10) of full-time consultation-liaison psychiatrists. The national professional organization for consultation-liaison psychiatry is the Liaison Group of the Royal College of Psychiatrists. This organization started in the early 1980s and now has about 800 members, most of whom are general psychiatrists. An internal survey in 1994 identified 60 consultants—in addition to the above-mentioned 10— who spend a considerable portion of their time in consultation-liaison activities. The group is particularly active in holding joint meetings with other medical specialists— diabetologists, neurologists, transplant groups, gastroenterologists, and the Royal College of Physicians (Creed et al. 1992). Collaboration with the latter group has led to a joint working committee in the two Royal Colleges (Psychiatry and Physicians) to improve the psychological care of patients in the general hospital (Royal College of Physicians and Royal College of Psychiatrists 1995a, 1995b). As consultation-liaison organized activities increase, pressure for a separate subspecialty of consultation-liaison psychiatry is growing (Benjamin et al. 1994).

During training, medical students receive lectures on psychiatric aspects of medicine and surgery. The lack of large numbers of consultation-liaison psychiatrists within the United Kingdom limits training opportunities in consultation-liaison psychiatry. The Royal College of Psychiatrists published training recommendations for liaison psychiatry that state the psychiatrist should spend 6 months training in the specialty before taking higher qualifications. After passing higher qualifications, 4 years of further training are needed before appointment as a specialist. Approximately 25 one-year training placements are available in consultation-liaison psychiatry. In 1993, a postgraduate course in consultation-liaison psychiatry was begun in Manchester. It lasted 4 days and included design and management of consultation-liaison services, audit projects, and research relevant to local authorities.

Research

In contrast to levels of consultation-liaison service delivery, the level of research activity has been high. Much research has been done on risk factors, outcome, and specific interventions for deliberate self-harm (Hawton and Catalan 1987). Descriptive studies (Mayou and Hawton 1986) led to intervention studies, including cognitive-behavioral interventions for illnesses such as chronic fatigue syndrome, somatization disorder, and irritable bowel syndrome (Chick et al. 1985; Creed et al. 1992; Guthrie et al. 1991; Klimes et al. 1990; Mayou et al. 1995; Wessely and Powell 1989). Other areas of research interest included mental illness associated with childbirth, puerperal psychosis, and postnatal depression (Prettyman and Friedman 1991). Substantial work also has been done to investigate psychological treatment of patients with cancer and other illnesses (Maguire and Faulkner 1988). Generally, numerous small research studies are ongoing across the whole spectrum of consultation-liaison psychiatry; many focus on the health service aspects of consultation-liaison psychiatry. These studies are often described in the *Bulletin of the Royal College*. The Cochrane Centre in Oxford is coordinating the systematic review of randomized controlled trials in all areas of medicine, including mental health (Adams and Gelder 1994).

Future Development

An advisory publication by the Department of Health (1993) stated, "There is also evidence that the costs of providing high quality Liaison Psychiatry services is more than matched by the savings made in the reduction in inappropriate investigations and in length of stay." This conclusion encourages further intervention studies to examine reduction in service utilization as an outcome. Funding changes mean that purchasers of health care must be convinced of the importance of consultation-liaison services. It is likely that some consultation-liaison psychiatry will be funded within the mental health budgets and some within the general medical budgets. This provides an opportunity and a challenge to make the case for a well-developed consultation-liaison service within a general hospital (Benjamin et al. 1994). In 1995, a joint working party of the Royal College of Physicians and the Royal College of Psychiatrists produced a joint report titled *The Psychological Care of Medical Patients*, including a guide for purchasers. It provides the arguments and the guidelines for consultation-liaison psychiatry service delivery in the general hospital. It is a most remarkable step forward in the development of consultation-liaison service delivery because it is a joint statement by both groups of medical professionals and, therefore, a very important recognition of the importance of the development of consultation-liaison service delivery. As such, it can be seen as a real paradigm for the international consultation-liaison field (Royal College of Physicians and Royal College of Psychiatrists 1995a, 1995b).

The Netherlands[7]

Relevant Background

Even though an active Dutch psychosomatic movement occurred in the 1950s and 1960s and strong links existed between Dutch psychoanalysts and the German psychoanalytic and psychosomatic movement, the development of consultation-liaison psychiatry was unaffected (Huyse and Hengeveld 1989). Before the 1970s, a few consultations were handled by psychiatrists who worked on general hospital psychiatry units.

In addition to available Anglo-American literature, an important resource for consultation-liaison psychiatry was the work of Querido (1959; Boenink and Huyse 1997). In 1953, he screened about 2,000 consecutive admissions to a general hospital and followed up 1,650 patients about 6 months later. He reported that psychosocial status was a more powerful predictor of long-term medical outcome than the admission medical status of the patient. Consequently, he made a plea for the assignment of psychologists, psychiatrists, and social workers to general medical wards because he believed that physicians were too preoccupied with biomedical aspects of patient care to take psychosocial factors into account.

De facto consultation-liaison psychiatry did not exist in the Netherlands until the mid-1970s, when an academic curriculum for consultation-liaison psychiatry was started. By the 1980s, all university departments of psychiatry had consultation-liaison services. In 1983, a work group for consultation-liaison psychiatry was started that focused on the systematic documentation of clinical work (Huyse and Hengeveld 1989). This resulted in an audit study of six consultation-liaison services in 1984 (Hengeveld et al. 1988). The pragmatic empirical approach taken as well as ongoing international exchange with American leaders in the field further fertilized research and the scientific status of consultation-liaison psychiatry in the Netherlands.

Annual meetings became a stimulating place to discuss audit, health care policy, training, research, clinical cases, and consensus issues, such as the treatment of patients with delirium or somatic disorders and those who attempted suicide. An updated biopsychosocial schema, drawing on work of Leigh et al. (1980), became an important tool for clinical case conferences during the Netherlands Consortium for Consultation-Liaison Psychiatry (NCCP) meetings and for training and supervision purposes (Huyse et al. 1988, 1989).

Consultation-Liaison Psychiatry in the General Hospital

The clinical aspects of Dutch consultation-liaison psychiatry are extensively described elsewhere (Hengeveld et al. 1984, 1988; Huyse and Hengeveld 1989). The ECLW Collaborative Study found that the seven consultation-liaison services who participated in this study belonged, with those in Spain, to the services with the highest consult rates (2.4%; mean for all 56 participating consultation-liaison services = 1.4%). About one-third of the referrals to the Dutch consultation-liaison services were for attempted suicide or substance abuse. The Dutch consultation-liaison services also tended to see an older population (45% older than 65 years, mean = 28% for study; 25% older than 75 years, mean = 12.5% for study). Since the beginning of the 1990s, the close collaboration of consultation-liaison nursing with consultation-liaison psychiatric services has steadily developed. Currently, models are in the process of implementation and evaluation, in which these nurses train nursing staff in admission risk screening and the preventive approach to frequent clinical psychological and behavior problems, such as confusion, substance abuse, suicidal behavior, regression, and the use of physical restraints. From an international perspective, Dutch euthanasia policy and the role of the consultation-liaison psychiatrists in this process are significant (Bannink et al. 2000; Huyse and van Tilburg 1993).

Official Status of Consultation-Liaison Psychiatry and Training

As a result of the collaborative efforts within the NCCP, the audit study of 1984 became the foundation for a document prepared at the request of the secretary of health care. This document established the content and structure of the consultation-liaison sector of general hospital psychiatry in the Netherlands (Huyse and Hengeveld 1989). The major points in this document were as follows:

1. The general hospital consultation-liaison department should provide primary psychiatric services in support of medical-surgical wards and the emergency room.
2. General hospital psychiatric wards and outpatient clinics should shift focus and develop facilities, such as psychiatric-medical unit facilities, for the treatment of patients with combined psychiatric and physical morbidity.

---

[7] This section is by Frits J. Huyse, M.D.

3. An outreach consultation function in family practice should be developed for patients with combined morbidity, including somatization.
4. The activities of consultation-liaison nurses should be increased. Their tasks are twofold: 1) case management in complex patients with behavioral disturbances and 2) development of guidelines and related training for nursing staff, to include topics such as confusion (observation and treatment), use of physical restraints, and the approach to suicidal patients.

These recommendations were included in a government blue paper for mental health care published in March 1993. As a result, the Department of Health Mental Health Section initiated a work group that included government officials, health care funders, and representatives from general hospitals. The work group's task was to formulate a long-term strategy for general hospital psychiatry and consultation-liaison psychiatry in health care to ensure a structural basis for the cure and care of patients with medical and psychiatric comorbidity.

In 1992, the need for a consultation-liaison psychiatric residency in the psychiatric curriculum was emphasized by the Consilium Psychiatricum, the board responsible for psychiatric certification. In 1994, the status of consultation-liaison residencies was reinforced again through a Task Force of the Dutch Psychiatric Association (Psychiatric Profile) that emphasized the medical character of psychiatric training, in contrast to its major focus on psychotherapy training since the 1960s. Currently, consultation-liaison psychiatrists at several universities have a prominent and increasing role in teaching medical students. Since 1990, several training programs for general practitioners have consultation-liaison psychiatric courses in their curriculum. Recently, programs for training the housestaff of general hospitals are gaining interest. These include topics such as difficult treatment decisions, end-of-life questions, confusion, somatization, suicidality, aggression, and intercollegial issues.

Research

Consultation-liaison research is gradually increasing. An early focus was the outcome of bone marrow transplantation (Broers et al. 1998). The focus on somatization research is now growing, including intervention studies in outpatient general medicine and neurology departments, as well as primary care practice (Koopmans et al. 1995; Meeuwesen et al. 1994; Speckens et al. 1995a, 1995b,

1996a, 1996b, 1996c; van Hemert et al. 1993a, 1993b, 1995). Two alcohol abuse screening studies in elderly medical patients reported lower prevalence rates than previously suspected—8% and 9%, respectively (Smals et al. 1994; Speckens et al. 1991). A study of delirium in cardio-surgery patients ($N = 300$) reported a 14% incidence of delirium in the total population (age range = 23–83 years) and a 21% incidence rate in the population older than 60 years. Age was the main risk factor for the occurrence of delirium (van der Mast 1999; van der Mast and Fekkes 2000; van der Mast et al. 1991, 1999). In geriatric patients (75 years and older) admitted to internal medical wards, a randomized clinical trial showed that an integrated psychogeriatric intervention had significant and clinically relevant effects on length of stay, levels of daily functioning, and readmission rates in the 6-month period after discharge (Slaets et al. 1997). Finally, building on the guidelines presented in the national blue paper, a national survey has been performed to assess the extent and quality of psychiatric and other psychosocial services in the general hospital.

Future Development

As described earlier, a series of developments were initiated by the section for general hospital psychiatry of the Dutch Psychiatric Association, the NCCP, the Association for General Hospital Psychiatric Unit Managers, the Association of Consultation-Liaison Nurses, and the Dutch Federation for General Hospital Psychiatry to ensure that general hospital psychiatry is represented in negotiations with health care policymakers. A main emphasis of this negotiation is the interface between psychiatry and medicine. Closer links with psychologists who work in general hospitals are expected to follow, as are increasing consultations from primary care physicians. In the framework of the European collaboration and as a result of the national developments, a series of multicenter health service delivery studies were initiated (see the section "European Studies" in this chapter)

Southern European and Mediterranean Countries[8]

Relevant Background

Southern European and Mediterranean countries are heterogeneous in many respects; this also applies to consultation-liaison psychiatry. These countries have no psychosomatic wards. Community-based psychiatric clinics, often regionalized and organized by national

---

[8] This section is by Antonio Lobo, M.D., and Marco Rigatelli, M.D.

health services, are the usual form of mental health service delivery. These clinics provide some consultation on medical wards, particularly in small hospitals that do not have a psychiatric department. In Greece, few general hospitals have a psychiatric unit, and many have no psychiatrists at all. Italy is unique; psychiatric consultations in general hospitals have become routine since reform Law 180 (1978), which eliminated acute psychiatric beds and prompted patients with psychosis to be admitted to medical wards (Cazzullo et al. 1984). Community-based mental health clinics also take consultations and occasionally have liaison activities with primary care physicians. In Portugal, the development of a liaison between community mental health services and primary care is a priority (Guimaraes Lopes 1989), but in Greece, psychiatric consultations requested by primary care physicians are performed by private-practice psychiatrists.

From a theoretical perspective, all conceptual approaches are found in southern European psychiatrists; most could be described as eclectic. The ECLW Collaborative Study showed the restricted availability of psychological consultation-liaison services in the participating hospitals of Italy and Portugal.

Consultation-Liaison Psychiatry in the General Hospital

Where they exist, most general hospital psychiatric departments offer consultation services and 24-hour emergency psychiatric services. Sometimes, consultation-liaison services are provided by community-based psychiatrists, especially in small hospitals where no psychiatric ward is available. This is the case in Italy, for example, and is particularly so in Portugal, where 80% of the community mental health centers provide consultation-liaison services to general hospitals. No specific consultation-liaison services exist in France, but psychiatric departments have established links with particular medical departments. In this way, liaison has developed in areas such as oncology, acquired immunodeficiency syndrome (AIDS), and intensive care units. A few medical units in France, Italy, and Spain have developed a special interest in psychosomatic problems. In these countries, similar to the German experience, medical outpatients are treated in some well-developed consultation-liaison psychosomatic units; however, these units are seldom involved in consultation-liaison activities with primary care centers. Consultation-liaison professionals are mainly psychiatrists. Only the most developed units include psychiatric nurses and/or social workers; some of these units also may have clinical psychologists.

It is now estimated that 70% of the university hospitals in Italy and 50% in Spain have specialized consultation-liaison psychiatric services. Other hospitals have more informal consultation-liaison activities. In certain locations, consultation-liaison units have arisen haphazardly in response to unique clinical and academic demands. A growing number of university hospitals in Italy, Portugal, and Spain have full-time consultation-liaison psychiatrists; many offer liaison activities (Cardoso et al. 1988; De Bertolini et al. 1999; Mayou et al. 1991; Soldatos and Sakkas 1987). The ECLW Collaborative Study found that for the Portuguese consultation-liaison participating services, almost all consults came from a liaison ward. Some other data from the ECLW Collaborative Study shed light on consult rates in these countries. In Italy, the ECLW Collaborative Study reported a mean consult rate of 1.06% (SD = 0.60) in the five participating hospitals, but a more recent survey showed a rate of 0.72%. The same ECLW Collaborative Study reported the following rates for the participating consultation-liaison services in Portugal (1.09%, SD = 0.58), Spain (2.89%, SD = 0.58), and Greece (1.65%, SD = 0.93). Because the consultation-liaison services participating in this European study were, in general, quite active and well staffed, it is estimated that, as was the case in Italy, the rates are lower when all national hospitals are considered. Furthermore, consult rates vary widely, as the standard deviations in this database suggest. In any case, the rate is rapidly increasing as new consultation-liaison services are created (Garcia-Camba et al. 1997).

Well-staffed consultation-liaison units serve patients with typical psychiatric diagnoses. For less-developed services, psychiatrists consult only when urgent behavior problems develop, such as agitation or suicide attempts. Problems associated with psychogeriatrics, AIDS, drug abuse, and alcoholism are frequent reasons for consultation. In France, where alcohol abuse is a significant problem, consulting psychiatrists are inevitably involved in the assessment and management of substance abuse. In Portugal, specialized services for alcohol and drug abuse are separate, but they are rarely located on a consultation-liaison service in general hospitals. Since passage of Law 180 in Italy, consultations from medical services frequently include patients with psychosis, including schizophrenia. On an empirical basis, no significant differences between Italian consultation-liaison services and other European consultation-liaison services have been found with respect to the proportion of patients with schizophrenia (about 4%) (ECLW Collaborative Study).

Interventions vary depending on the target population and staffing of consultation-liaison services. Urgent referrals for agitation, suicidal behavior, and/or crisis interventions are common. Only France has the policy that all patients who attempt suicide must be assessed by psychiatric emergency services. On well-staffed services, psychological interventions and follow-up services for patients are available, and in some cases, liaison activities are available (Bourgeois 1990; Cardoso et al. 1988; Rigatelli et al. 1989). In Portugal, some mental health centers have Balint groups. Balint groups are groups of general practitioners who—under the guidance of a psychiatrist—regularly meet to discuss and explore their personal emotional reactions to specific patients to enhance their psychological approach toward patients. This approach, which was developed and promoted by Michael Balint from the Tavistock Clinic in London, has been quite popular in several European countries (Balint 1972).

Official Status of Consultation-Liaison Psychiatry Psychosomatics and Training

National consultation-liaison associations exist in southern European countries. In Spain, the main organization is the consultation-liaison section of the Spanish Society of Psychosomatic Medicine. Italy has one consultation-liaison association, and Portugal has two associations, as well as a Psychosomatic Society. Every 1 or 2 years, national congresses and seminars are organized in Italy, Portugal, and Spain. Two international congresses were organized in Portugal. The national psychiatric societies in all these countries have ongoing initiatives related to consultation-liaison psychiatry. These countries have several consultation-liaison journals: *Psichiatria di Consultazione, Psichiatria nella Practica Medica*, and *Rivista de Medicina Psicosomatica* in Italy and *Cuadernos de Medicina Psicosomatica y Psiquiatria de Enlace* in Spain. The first issue of the new journal of the Portuguese Psychosomatic Society appeared in 1999. Furthermore, consultation-liaison articles appear in the national psychiatric journals.

Only Spain includes psychosomatic and consultation-liaison teaching in the medical school curriculum. In Italy, psychiatrists are chairs of several psychosomatic medicine departments. Special postdoctoral courses are taught in several countries. Psychiatric programs recommend training in consultation-liaison psychiatry. This training is compulsory in some programs in Italy and Portugal and, at a national level, in Spain. In Spain, residents from specialties such as family and community medicine, as well as several other medical disciplines, spend time on well-developed consultation-liaison services (Rigatelli et al. 2000).

Research

Over the last few years, consultation-liaison research activities have grown in southern European countries. Reports on the prevalence and characteristics of psychological morbidity in patients who used different services are available from most countries (Grassi et al. 2000; Lobo et al. 1996). Several studies described models of intervention (Invernizzi et al. 1997; Lobo 1996; Rigatelli et al. 1980). In Italy, several studies described the experience of consulting on hospitalized patients with psychosis (Cazzullo et al. 1984). In Portugal, studies examined how patients adapt to hemodialysis and intensive care units (Cardoso et al. 1988). An extensive series of epidemiological studies was completed in Spain (Lobo et al. 1988). These Spanish studies focused on cancer, hemodialysis, and endocrine disorder patients. Similarly, psychiatric disorders, such as depression, organic disorders, somatization, and psychosomatic conditions, were reported in a number of studies. In southern Europe, standardized instruments are commonly used in consultation-liaison research; however, a generally accepted battery is not established. In Spain, some consultation-liaison services are very interested in using standardized international instruments and developing new ones (Lobo et al. 1993). In Portugal, ongoing studies include the measurement of cost-effectiveness. In Italy and Spain, multicenter studies incorporated ECLW methodology (see "European Studies" section later in this chapter) to derive conclusions on organization and models of intervention (Gala et al. 1999; Garcia-Camba et al. 1997; Lobo et al. 1997; Rigatelli et al. 1998).

Future Development

The prospects for consultation-liaison psychiatry seem good, largely as a result of an increased degree of collaboration among European countries. Besides consultation, liaison activities are expected to increase gradually in coming years, particularly in university hospitals, as are stronger links among the different associations. Data from research are expected to guide the future organization of services.

Australia and New Zealand[9]

Relevant Background

Australia is a multicultural country. The paradigms within psychiatry reflect this diversity. In the 1970s, consultation-liaison psychiatry flourished at centers where psychiatrists

---

[9] This section is by Graeme C. Smith, M.D.

had received postgraduate training in North America. At centers dominated by psychiatrists trained in the United Kingdom, consultation-liaison psychiatry made slower progress (Smith et al. 1993a). In New Zealand, consultation-liaison psychiatry developed in a similar way. Consultation-liaison psychiatry now faces significant challenges in New Zealand because health care delivery was reorganized from a free, universal access system to one in which users pay part of the charges and in Australia because diagnosis-related groups were introduced. In both countries, consultation-liaison services have been disadvantaged because public mental health services are rationed according to the concept of "a serious mental illness" (Smith 1998).

Consultation-Liaison Psychiatry in the General Hospital

In Australia, consultation-liaison psychiatry services exist in all university-affiliated general teaching hospitals (Smith et al. 1994). The same is true for the nine university-affiliated hospitals in New Zealand. These inpatient consultation-liaison services usually also provide consultation to an accident and emergency department and some outpatient services. The referral rate of medical inpatients for psychiatric consultation is approximately 1%–2%, but the range is large, which reflects the fact that the nature and staffing of consultation-liaison services vary greatly. For example, the median number of effective full-time consultation-liaison psychiatrists per 300 beds in 1992 was 0.45, whereas the number of referrals per each effective full-time psychiatrist varied from 300 to 1,500 per annum, according to site (Smith et al. 1994). Not all sites have full-time consultation-liaison psychiatrists. Most of the consultation work is performed by part-time staff. Consultation-liaison psychiatrists also supervise psychiatry trainees. The median number of psychiatry trainees in 1992 was 0.72 per 300 general hospital beds; it is now less. There is no fellowship scheme in Australia or New Zealand, but one is being developed. Some trainees undertake additional consultation-liaison training during the final years of the 5-year training program. A survey of consultation-liaison psychiatrists indicated that a 100% increase in current staffing is needed for optimal service. The level of staffing also dictates the intensity of liaison activities performed by consultation-liaison psychiatry services. Only a few sites can provide liaison to major medical inpatient units; many sites have no liaison at all. About one-third of medical facilities have a consultation-liaison nursing service; most would like to have one. Psychologists usually are involved in consultation-liaison

activity, but the level of integration with departments of psychiatry varies. Although it is not mandated that the consultation-liaison service see all patients who have attempted suicide, such patients are almost always seen by a psychiatrist, often as a part of a multidisciplinary team.

Official Status of Consultation-Liaison Psychiatry Psychosomatics and Training

Another reason to develop better services is the compulsory 6-month placement of psychiatry trainees on a consultation-liaison psychiatry service. To coordinate this endeavor and to promote research, a section of consultation-liaison psychiatry was formed within the Royal Australian and New Zealand College of Psychiatrists. This work group also will address the issue of subspecialty status and qualifications. Although there are no other national consultation-liaison psychiatry organizations, special groups such as the Australian Society for Psychosomatic Obstetrics and Gynecology, the Australian Pain Society, and the Australian Society for Traumatic Stress Studies exist.

Research

Gastrointestinal disorders (Bennett et al. 1998), posttraumatic stress disorder (McFarlane 1989), breast cancer (Kissane et al. 1998), and chronic fatigue syndrome (Hickie et al. 1999) have a strong psychosomatic research tradition. Some researchers use the MICRO-CARES clinical database system (Clarke et al. 1995; Dunsis and Smith 1996; Kissane and Smith 1996; Rustomjee and Smith 1996; Smith et al. 1993b). International collaboration with the MICRO-CARES Consortium (Strain et al. 1998) and the ECLW has been stimulating. Australia's use of both the DSM and the ICD classification systems permits psychiatrists to maintain research links with both American and European collaborators. At present, a major research thrust is the development of a multidiagnostic instrument for consultation-liaison psychiatry (Clarke et al. 1998). It is anticipated that this nonhierarchical instrument will improve the collection of outcome and intervention data, particularly in primary care settings.

Japan[10]

Relevant Background

Although Japan has about 10,000 active psychiatrists, the financial support for clinical psychiatry is inadequate.

---

[10] This section is by Takashi Hosaka, M.D., and Yasutaka Iwasaki, M.D.

The health insurance system, which covers all general psychiatric treatments, does not reimburse some psychiatric treatment when delivered in the general hospital. As a result, not many psychiatrists work in general hospitals. Despite this, it is interesting that psychiatrists were working in general hospitals before the concept of consultation-liaison psychiatry was introduced during the fourth congress of the International College of Psychosomatic Medicine in Kyoto in 1977. Since then, there has been an increasing number of consultation-liaison-related presentations and symposia at the scientific meetings of the Japanese Society of Psychiatry and Neurology and the Japanese Society of Psychosomatic Medicine. In addition, several monographs on consultation-liaison issues were published (Hosaka 1998; Iwasaki et al. 1989; Kurosawa 1996). A critical event for consultation-liaison psychiatry was the formation of the Japanese Society of General Hospital Psychiatry (JSGHP) in 1988. In 1989, the JSGHP started publication of *The Japanese Journal of General Hospital Psychiatry*, which is the only academic journal of consultation-liaison psychiatry and general hospital psychiatry in Japan. The journal has Japanese articles, with English abstracts and English-language articles by Japanese and other authors, in addition to special sections with perspectives, case conferences, and reviews of foreign articles. The most prominent Japanese consultation-liaison papers were reviewed in the *Supplement of General Hospital Psychiatry* in 1991 (Strain et al. 1991).

Consultation-Liaison Psychiatry in the General Hospital

Only 21% of the general hospitals in Japan have psychiatric inpatient wards, and 52% have psychiatric outpatient departments (Kuroki et al. 1997). Psychiatric departments located in general hospitals treat all types of patients (i.e., outpatients, inpatients, emergency room patients, and consultation-liaison patients), but for the reasons mentioned in the previous paragraph, consultation-liaison services are still limited. This is reflected in the referral rates; in one study, only 1.3% of general medical patients were referred for psychiatric consultation during a 10-year period (Yamashita et al. 1992). The need for consultation-liaison services is extensive; medical staffs are aware of the problem of psychiatric comorbidity and realize that management is very difficult without psychiatric treatment (Kurosawa et al. 1992). For example, in one study, the prevalence of psychiatric disorders among patients visiting primary care was 30.6% (Sato and Takeichi 1993). Because of limited resources, it is difficult to develop specific services for patients with psychiatric

comorbidity, such as patients who are severely injured during a suicide attempt, geriatric patients, diabetic patients, and schizophrenic patients with physical illness. The treatment available for these patients depends on the hospital. Some critical care medical centers have consultation-liaison psychiatrists available for consultation with patients who attempt suicide or patients who have delirium, but other facilities have no psychiatrists. The development of psychiatric-medical units is still experimental (Nomura et al. 1996). Currently, there is particular interest in critical care medicine, intensive care units, rehabilitation centers, and AIDS (Fukunishi et al. 1997) and geriatric wards or hospitals; this interest is often reflected in liaison work. Young psychiatrists are very interested in general hospital psychiatry.

Official Status of Consultation-Liaison Psychiatry Psychosomatics and Training

The JSGHP, as of December 1998, had about 1,300 members and is growing (Kurosawa 1998). Medical students and psychiatric residents receive training in teaching hospitals. These hospitals have divisions of psychiatry, but they do not have psychiatric wards. Education in consultation-liaison psychiatry is mandatory for medical students. Specifically, third- and fourth-year medical students receive 2–4 hours per week, including lectures and participation in consultation-liaison work, during a mandatory rotation of several weeks for psychiatry. However, psychiatric residents usually do not take consultation-liaison rotations or consultation-liaison-related seminars during their training. Yet, during their 2-year psychiatric residency (2 years to pass the board, followed by 4 additional clinical years), they must see patients on nonpsychiatric wards with their supervisors.

Research

Before the JSGHP was founded, research was limited. Now, consultation-liaison psychiatrists are actively involved in many research projects: delirium, attempted suicide (Kishi et al. 1996), psychooncology (Hosaka 1996), depressive illness in medical-surgical patients, and doctor-patient relationships (Hosaka 1989; Kurosawa et al. 1992; Matushima et al. 1985). As a result of the rapid growth of the geriatric population, many physicians (not only psychiatrists) are concerned about delirium. Delirium research, thus far, is oriented toward etiology more than treatment, although a shift is occurring. Clinical studies on severely injured patients who attempt suicide have been done in critical care medical centers (Iwasaki et al. 1992). Ongoing research includes multisite clinical surveys, intervention studies, family studies, and prevention studies (Kurosawa and Iwasaki 1991). In the past few years, follow-up studies and health-service-oriented studies have begun. Psychooncological research has focused on clinical aspects, such as the emotional state of cancer patients, psychiatric treatments for cancer patients, euthanasia (Hosaka 1997), and coping. Multisite clinical studies were started in the 1990s by a collaborative study group.

Future Development

The JSGHP is now one of seven major psychiatric associations in Japan. Thus, consultation-liaison psychiatrists can contribute to the development of health policy in psychiatry. One of the first steps planned by JSGHP is the modification of current insurance systems to allow proper reimbursement of consultation-liaison services in the general hospital. These modifications would increase the number of general hospitals that have psychiatric divisions. This would also encourage general hospital psychiatrists to do research, which would firmly establish consultation-liaison psychiatry in general medical settings. Finally, Japanese consultation-liaison psychiatrists should join international collaborative studies because cross-cultural understanding of consultation-liaison psychiatry would make this field more fruitful (Berger et al. 1997).

Latin America[11]

Brazil

Relevant background. Brazil is the largest country in Latin America, covering about 8,500,000 square kilometers. It has a population of 161 million. Until 1960, Brazil's psychiatric practice was dominated by large mental hospitals. In the 1970s, the focus for psychiatrists shifted to ambulatory care, day hospitals, and psychiatric units in general hospitals with emergency and consultation-liaison services (Botega 1997). In the 1980s, the number of consultation-liaison services increased significantly; this culminated in the first Brazilian meeting of Psychiatric Consultation in São Paulo in 1989 and biannual meetings. Nogueira-Martins and Freck (Nogueira-Martins 1989) published the first consultation-liaison paper. In 1989, Botega presented the first doctoral thesis in the area of consultation-liaison (Botega 1989). Since then, the books *Psicossomática Hoje* (Mello Filho 1992), *Saude Mental no Hospital Geral* (Botega and Dalgalarrondo 1993), and *Servicos de Saude Mental no Hospital Geral* (Fortes 1995) were published (Botega 1997). A section for con-

sultation-liaison psychiatry in the Brazilian Association of Psychiatry was established in 1991; this was an important event for the development of consultation-liaison psychiatry. This section has become an important meeting place for psychiatrists working in this area and has resulted in a national network for consultation-liaison psychiatrists.

Consultation-liaison psychiatry in the general hospital. In a 1982 survey, only 16% of the 48 respondents (48 of 75 medical schools) had a general hospital psychiatry unit. In an evaluation of fellowship programs in 1992, 35% of the responding general hospitals had a psychiatric unit and 55% had consultation-liaison services. Most existing information comes from surveys in university hospitals and hospitals in the public health sector. The most recent information—among them a study performed by the National Department of Mental Health (Botega and Schechtman 1997)—indicates that most facilities have general hospital psychiatry units. Consequently, since the 1980s (comparable with other parts of the world), there has been a gradual shift from large-scale mental hospitals to general hospital psychiatry units. However, in 1996, Brazil had 69,237 psychiatric beds, of which only 1,765 (2.5%) were found in general hospitals.

Reimbursement of consultation-liaison services is still a problem that affects the entry of psychiatrists into this field. However, this might change. A recent federal law regulating the services provided by private health insurance agencies compelled them to offer psychiatric services. In medical schools, medical psychologists mainly perform the training in the psychological aspects of the medically ill. Their focus is primarily the doctor-patient relationship and the emotional aspects of patients with physical illness. Many postgraduate psychiatric courses with a consultation-liaison focus are available (Nogueira-Martins 1993).

Research. Consultation-liaison research is almost totally tied to university services or public health. The research focuses on issues such as secondary depression, nephrology, and ethics.

Future development. Much developmental work remains to be done by the Section of Consultation-Liaison Psychiatry of the Brazil Psychiatric Association on the financial possibilities under the recent law. It is expected that these will increase both the number and the quality of the professionals working in this area. It is hoped that this increase, in combination with postgraduate courses related to consultation-liaison research, will attract new

---

[11] This section is by Ruben Cesarco, M.D., and Paulo R. Zimmermann, M.D.

colleagues. With a Portuguese version of MICRO-CARES, current ties with Portuguese colleagues are strengthened, and collaboration is expected to increase.

Uruguay

In the 1960s, psychoanalysts started courses in medical psychology to try to integrate psychodynamic concepts into medical curricula. This initiative was interrupted by 14 years of dictatorship. Currently, psychiatric consultations are performed in general hospitals in an unsystematic way by non-consultation-liaison-trained psychiatrists. Only one consultation-liaison service is located in the Hospital Maciel in Montevideo. It was founded 15 years ago by an internist trained in the Rochester program started by George Engel. This service provides courses for hospital doctors in indications for referrals.

Colombia

In Colombia, the situation is comparable to that in Uruguay. Yet, in 1995, the Colombian Association of Psychiatry established a committee for consultation-liaison psychiatry to promote the development of this area. Recently, the Medical School at the University of Bogotá started a 2-year course focusing on consultation-liaison topics.

Mexico

In Mexico, the development of consultation-liaison psychiatry has flourished during the last decade, and the Mexican Psychiatric Association has a section for consultation-liaison psychiatry. Although consultation-liaison psychiatry is not recognized as a subspecialty, its knowledge base is an important part of the training of general psychiatrists. In 1997, a successful international conference was organized.

EUROPEAN STUDIES

In this section, we describe developments that have helped establish an international forum for consultation-liaison clinical practice and research. In Europe, collaboration was established for many reasons. A main factor was the need for further integration because European exchange was nonexistent. Another important factor was that many consultation-liaison practitioners recognized the need to document and to compare work 1) as a tool to audit clinical practice and a guide for further training, 2) to establish areas for future research, and 3) to provide data for negotiations with administration and other relevant groups.

ECLW Collaborative Study

A lack of standardized assessment led groups in the United States (MICRO-CARES Consortium), the Netherlands (NCCP), and elsewhere to seek ways to systematically document consultation-liaison activities (Hammer et al. 1987; Hengeveld et al. 1988; Huyse and Hengeveld 1989; Taintor et al. 1979). This work became a standard for research in clinical database management systems and structured tracking of consultation-liaison service delivery.

An important breakthrough was the formation of the informal ECLW by consultation-liaison practitioners from nine countries in 1987. The ECLW exchanged information about national developments, differences, similarities, and needs (Huyse and Smith 1997; Mayou et al. 1991). Participants agreed to assess the extent and quality of consultation-liaison service delivery with structured instruments. The ECLW developed a collaborative study that assessed existing European consultation-liaison services; this research was funded by the European Union. It provides a survey of how consultation-liaison and other psychosocial services operate around Europe. In 1991, 56 European consultation-liaison services, including 7 German psychosomatic consultation-liaison services (see section "Relation of Consultation-Liaison Psychiatry to Psychosomatics and Behavioral Medicine" earlier in this chapter) and 11 European countries, participated. The 226 participants were trained and tested in the use of instruments specifically designed for this study (Huyse et al. 1996; Lobo et al. 1996; Malt et al. 1996). In addition to the description of the caseload for 1 year ($N = 14,717$), information on the logistics and other specifications of the consultation-liaison services, their personnel, and their hospitals was collected. Several earlier reported findings were confirmed in this multicenter study: 1) a consult rate of 1.4%, 2) a long time span between admission and referral (average = about 10 days), and 3) a longer length of stay for the referred population; consultation-liaison referred patients stayed two to three times longer than the average length of stay. The median consult rate of 1.4% underscores the discrepancy between the rates of mental disorders in the medically ill and the psychiatric services delivered.

The study led to the conclusion that the core purpose of consultation-liaison in general hospitals is a quick, comprehensive, emergency psychiatric service. This was supported by the following facts: 1) the main reasons for referral were deliberate self-harm (17%), substance abuse (7.5%), and current psychiatric symptoms (40%); 2) 30% of the patients referred for reasons other than deliberate self-harm had to be seen on the same day; 3) a significant portion of patients were old and seriously ill; 4) more serious mental disorders, including mood and organic mental disorders, were prominent (18%); and 5) only 5% of the patients seen were referred by means of the liaison function.

Consultation-liaison has a comprehensive function because most interventions included integrated—biopsychosocial—service delivery on the ward, as well as discharge management. This was evidenced by communications with primary care at referral and at discharge in half of the patients, discharges to mental health facilities for 10% of the patients, and outpatient mental health referrals in 30% of the patients. Consequently, the study documented that the consultation-liaison service provides an important bridge between mental health care and primary or general health care (Huyse et al. 2001b).

A large variation among consultation-liaison services was found on all variables assessed. Consequently, the types of patients referred to the consultation-liaison services and the services delivered had very marked differences; significant differences among countries were seen as well. One notable difference concerned whether patients were referred for deliberate self-harm or substance abuse. German psychosomatic consultation-liaison services rarely saw these patients. For other consultation-liaison services, these patients were one-quarter to one-third of the patients referred. The remaining referred patients could be best described by the following characteristics: the severity of psychopathology—consultations from surgery—and the clarity of medical diagnosis—consultations from medicine and neurology services (Figure 13–1). About 50% of the patients seen by the psychosomatic consultation-liaison services were referred for the evaluation of unexplained physical complaints, in contrast to the 20% for the average psychiatric consultation-liaison services. The psychiatric consultation-liaison services were more often consulted on patients with ongoing psychiatric symptoms who tended to be more elderly and surgical patients who more often had organic psychiatric disorders.

On a national level, the German psychosomatic services appeared to have their own identity. The Spanish and Portuguese services, in contrast to the Dutch, Finnish, Italian, and most of the participating services from the United Kingdom, had proportionally more patients referred for substance abuse. Variation in referral patterns, as well as the rather low consult rate, supports the hypothesis that referral of patients with psychiatric disorders is relatively haphazard. In addition, the results provide a blueprint for the development of future consultation-liaison services, which can specify more clearly which patients might be referred for consultation, as well

as populations that might benefit from preventive interventions (de Jonge et al. 2001a; Huyse et al. 2000a).

Finally, the data from the ECLW Collaborative Study provide information on the organization of consultation-liaison services. Consultation-liaison services can be described by their size, the maturity of their staff, and whether they have a multidisciplinary team. Monodisciplinary consultation-liaison services are organized according to the classic medical-consultant model, and multidisciplinary teams are more typically found in the mental health field. In several countries, these teams include consultation-liaison nurses; the functions of these nurses vary. Yet, their main tasks are assessment of specific diagnostic groups, such as the evaluation of patients after deliberate self-harm and for substance abuse, as well as the care of more complex patients (e.g., elderly delirious patients). In addition, they teach the nursing staff to better deal with more complex patients, a liaison function. The hospitals in the ECLW Collaborative Study can be described by their size and the availability of psychosocial services; these dimensions are not necessarily related. Hospitals with limited psychosocial services tend to have "medical-model" monodisciplinary consult teams. In this study, all Italian and all but one Belgian, Greek, and Portuguese consultation-liaison services belonged to such hospitals. All German psychosomatic consultation-liaison services had either monodisciplinary or small multidisciplinary consultation-liaison services. Consequently, the study provides support for the reported nonsystematic development of consultation-liaison psychiatric services in general hospitals (Huyse et al. 2000b). The political effect of the study is already evident. In several countries, the study has affected the relation between the consultation-liaison field and government policymakers, as discussed in earlier sections of this chapter.

Risk Factor Study

The risk factor study focused on the development and implementation of effective screening methods by nonpsychiatrist physicians and nurses to identify patients in need of psychiatric referral and treatment (Huyse et al. 1993). The study resulted in a paradigm that facilitates integrated care for more complex patients based on 1) an admission case finder and 2) a method to assess care needs and plan adequate care (Huyse 1997). The case finder developed for inpatient internal medicine wards is called the COMplexity PRediction Instrument (COMPRI). The premise behind its development was that hospitals (i.e., doctors, nurses, managers) are more interested in enhancing efficiency of care in patients who have high complex care rather than, specifically, in

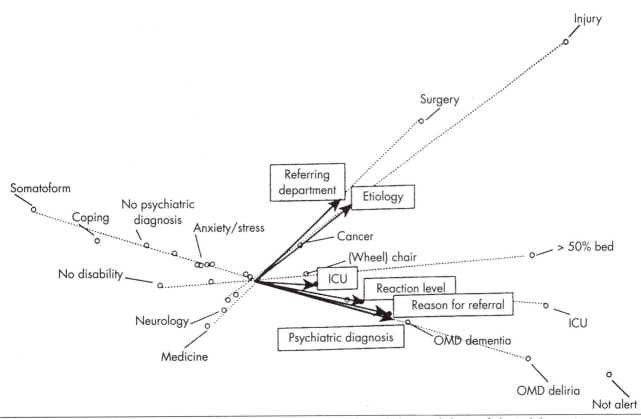

FIGURE 13–1. The status of the patient at referral: severity of psychopathology and clarity of physical diagnosis.

Source. Reprinted from Huyse FJ, Herzog T, Lobo A, et al: "European Consultation-Liaison Services and Their User Populations: the ECLW Collaborative Study." *Psychosomatics* 41:330–338, 2000a. Used with permission.

patients who might have or develop psychiatric disorders. The COMPRI was developed and tested in a cohort of 2,158 patients admitted to internal medicine wards in 11 European hospitals; it can be used at admission to predict complexity of care during hospitalization. Complexity of care is conceptualized as the (biomedical) reaction of the ward staff toward patients' problems and is operationally defined in terms of length of hospital stay, objective complexity (e.g., number of days with laboratory and diagnostic tests, number of nurse interventions beyond basic nursing care, number of consultants, and number of different types of medication), and perceived complexity by doctors and nurses at the time of discharge (de Jonge et al. 2001c; Huyse 1997). The COMPRI consists of 13 questions: 6 subjective predictions by doctors and nurses and 7 variables scored from the medical status and/or a patient interview (de Jonge et al. 2001b; Huyse et al. 2001a). All questions have a yes-or-no answer (Figure 13–2). The COMPRI explains about 20% of the variance in length of stay. The COMPRI can and will be used as a case finder for intervention studies, as an indicator for complexity of care; other indicators could be used to preselect populations on basis of service delivery characteristics.

INTERMED

INTERMED has been developed as a method to assess care needs and plan interdisciplinary care (Huyse et al. 1999, 2001c). INTERMED is an observer-rated instrument that classifies information from a structured medical history into four domains: biological, psychological, social, and health care (Table 13–1). It builds on the work of Engel (1977) on the biopsychosocial model of disease and allows documentation of the patient's biopsychosocial care needs and risks in a standardized way. In addition, the quantity and quality of the patient's relation to the health care system are scored. The four domains are assessed in the context of time (history, current state, and prognosis), resulting in 20 variables that are scored 0–3, depending on the vulnerabilities or needs in specific areas, based on a manual with clinical anchorpoints (Table 13–1). Domain scores are obtained by adding the five variables for each of the domains (range 0–15); the total score is the sum score of the domain scores (range 0–60). The INTERMED interview can be used with inpatients and outpatients and takes about 20 minutes, including the scoring.

The scoring leads to an indication for care coordination; an overview of the risks and needs of the patient,

Predictions Made by the Doctor		
Do you expect this patient to have a hospital stay of 2 weeks or more?	Yes	No
Do you think the organization of care during hospital stay will be complex?	Yes	No
Do you expect that this patient's mental health will be disturbed during this hospital stay?	Yes	No
Predictions Made by the Nurse		
Do you expect this patient to have a hospital stay of 2 weeks or more?	Yes	No
Do you think the organization of care during hospital stay will be complex?	Yes	No
Do you think this patient will be limited in activities of daily living after discharge?	Yes	No
Additional Questions		
Is this an unplanned admission?	Yes	No
Is the patient retired?	Yes	No
Is the patient known to have a currently active malignancy?	Yes	No
Did the patient		
have walking difficulties during the last 3 months?	Yes	No
have a negative health perception during the last week?	Yes	No
have more than 6 doctor visits during the last three months?	Yes	No
take more than three different kinds of medications the day prior to admission?	Yes	No

FIGURE 13–2. Complexity Prediction Instrument (COMPRI).

Source. Reprinted from Huyse FJ, de Jonge P, Slaets JPJ, et al: "COMPRI: An Instrument to Detect Patients With Complex Care Needs: Results From a European Study." *Psychosomatics* 42(3):222–228, 2001a. Used with permission.

which supports the communication between different professionals involved with the patient; and a case vignette, including a treatment plan. A 2-day training that has been developed ensures reliable scoring of INTERMED by doctors, nurses, and psychologists. A scoring manual has become available through a Web site (http://www.vumc.nl/intermed), and a computer program for scoring has been developed.

In the development of INTERMED, much attention has been directed to its psychometric quality in terms of reliability and validity (Fischer et al. 2000; Huyse et al. 1999; Stiefel et al. 1999a,1999b). Reliability has been studied in terms of 1) interrater agreement, since one of the main goals of INTERMED was to improve communication between health care professionals, 2) internal consistency, since a single concept of case complexity was

hypothesized to underlie the variables included in INTERMED, and 3) temporal stability or test-retest reliability, since it has been designed to support decision making on (long-term) health care policy for patients with specific health care risks.

A first interrater reliability study (Huyse et al. 1999) suggested some improvements, which have led to a final version that has been used in several studies. A recent study of the interrater reliability of this final version in a heterogeneous sample of patients with somatic illnesses resulted in a kappa of 0.85, indicating very good agreement between two independent raters—a psychologist and a clinical nurse specialist—who blindly rated patients on the basis of a joint interview. In order to study whether INTERMED measures a common underlying concept, case complexity, the inter-item reliability of INTERMED was assessed. Inter-item reliability coefficients (Cronbach's α) ranging from 0.78 to 0.94 were found in samples of patients (total $N = 829$) with several somatic illnesses and varying psychiatric comorbidities: low back pain patients (Stiefel et al. 1999a, 1999b); diabetic patients (Fischer et al. 2000); rheumatoid arthritis patients (Koch et al. 2001); internal medical inpatients (de Jonge et al. 2000); end-stage renal disease patients; and patients referred to a psychiatric consultation-liaison service (de Jonge et al. 2001d). The findings indicated that case complexity as measured with INTERMED is a unidimensional construct. Case complexity is influenced by biological, psychological, and social factors, as well as the patient's relationship with the health care system, and none of these domains can be excluded when an integral assessment of patient care needs is conducted. Test-retest reliability has been studied in a sample of outpatients with multiple sclerosis (MS), which resulted in a correlation coefficient of 0.75 of two measurements separated by the period of a year.

Studies aimed at the validity of INTERMED can be described as cross-sectional studies and longitudinal studies. Cross-sectional studies have demonstrated its validity in several patient samples, such as low back pain patients (correlations with physical, psychological, and social limitations) (Stiefel at al. 1999a), diabetic patients (compliance with treatment, as measured with HbA1c) (Fischer et al. 2000), rheumatoid arthritis patients (patient-rated severity of illness) (Koch et al. 2001), and MS patients (disability). Longitudinal studies have demonstrated the potential use of INTERMED to detect patients for whom interdisciplinary care such as case management is indicated—for example, low back pain patients (negative outcome of standard treatment) (Stiefel et al. 1999a) and medical inpatients (LOS, quality of life) and end-stage renal disease patients (quality of life after a year).

TABLE 13–1. INTERMED domains and variables

Domains	History	Current state	Prognoses
Biological	Chronicity	Severity of illness	Complications and life threat
	Diagnostic uncertainty	Clarity of diagnostic profile	
Psychological	Restrictions in coping	Treatment resistance	Mental health threat
	Premorbid level of psychiatric dysfunctioning	Severity of psychiatric symptoms	
Social	Family disruption	Residential instability	Social vulnerability
	Impairment of social support	Impairment of social integration	
Health care	Intensity of prior treatment	Organizational complexity at admission or referral	Care needs
	Prior treatment experience	Appropriateness of admission or referral	

Source. Reprinted from Huyse FJ, Lyons JS, Stiefel FC, et al: "'INTERMED': A Method to Assess Health Service Needs, I: Development and Reliability." *General Hospital Psychiatry* 21:39–48, 1999. Used with permission.

At the time of this writing, intervention studies are being conducted to assess the added effectiveness of early detection and treatment of patients with complex care needs in several patient populations, such as medical inpatients, diabetic patients, and patients with rheumatoid arthritis, in which a clinical nurse specialist uses INTERMED to plan interdisciplinary care, supervised by a consultation-liaison psychiatrist.

Quality Management Study

A collaborative study funded by the European Community (BIOMED1) and the Robert Bosch Stiftung (1994–1999) focused on the development and evaluation of programs for continuous quality improvement and standards for consultation-liaison mental health service delivery in the general hospital. After an intensive training in quality management, participating consultation-liaison services implemented local quality audits after defining goals of service delivery and objectives for quality improvement. Performance indicators were measured through a standardized instrument. Most areas selected for improvement were related to communications within the consultation-liaison service, the hospital at large, and communication between the consultation-liaison services and postdischarge providers. Solutions varied and included changing the referral procedure, standardizing consultation-liaison reports, and assessing consultees' needs. The study showed that quality management is feasible and can lead to substantial improvements of consultation-liaison care delivery if consultants have competence in quality management, access to instruments, and support from both quality experts and the relevant hierarchies. The instrumentation developed during the project is available in seven European languages and proved adaptable to local needs.

CONCLUSION

Consultation-liaison psychiatry outside the United States is developing rapidly. International consultation-liaison psychiatry is becoming organized, with particular areas of interest in reimbursement, training, subspecialty status, research, and the enhancement of clinical care. The ECLW and its European Community–funded health service delivery studies, through standardized instruments and methods, are crucial in the assessment of the current status and future development of consultation-liaison psychiatry in Europe. These studies have increased communication among consultation-liaison practitioners (such as psychiatrists, psychosomaticists, internists, psychologists) at an international and a professional level. Enhanced communications provide a broader forum for discussions and a mechanism to expand clinical knowledge beyond the published literature. The evolution of the United States health care service delivery system under the Clinton administration could serve as a stimulus for closer collaboration with non–United States systems (Malt 1986, 1991).

With regard to professional development, one might limit the scope of consultation-liaison psychiatry to the treatment of well-defined psychiatric disorders in medically ill or physically injured patients. However, such a narrow approach is not compatible with the reality of consultation-liaison work. Consultation-liaison psychiatrists are often faced with problems such as disturbed behavior, lack of compliance with treatment, and physical symptoms not explainable by biological findings. Disturbed behavior or lack of compliance may result from a concurrent psychiatric disorder but also may reflect family tension, conflicts with the staff, or even conflicts within the hospital (Smith 1998). Therefore, the consultation-liaison psychiatrist must sometimes adopt a family or systems perspective in addition to an individual perspective. Furthermore, modern theories of learning and behavior also can alter the course of medical disorders and symptom complaints (Blomhoff and Malt 1993). The course of the illness, or the injury, may be further complicated by the patient's response to the illness and the behavior of relatives, friends, or the health care system itself.

Different models in consultation-liaison work have far-reaching consequences for the conceptualization, organization, and training of consultation-liaison psychiatry. If consultation-liaison psychiatry is to exist in the future, it must broaden its focus to meet the needs of the patients, their relatives, and the health care system. This calls for a comprehensive approach in which psychology and medicine become an integral part of consultation-liaison psychiatry. Considering the complexity of these issues and the development toward psychology-based interventions for physical disorders, it is not likely—and not desirable—that consultation-liaison work be handled by a psychiatrist alone. Therefore, two options are available for the future development of mental health service delivery in the general medical sector: to unite or to split.

To unite is to acknowledge the complexity of the relation between physical and mental function. Instead of having separate services for different parts of mental function, united services are needed that incorporate consultation-liaison psychiatry and medical psychology into one service. Furthermore, to maintain a longitudinal perspective on the patient and illness rehabilitation, consultation-liaison nursing—including case management—health psychology, and social work must be integrated into consultation-liaison services as well. This integration will provide a mental health care sector for the general medical system (Hammer et al. 1987; Herzog and Scheidt 1991).

To split implies separate services for the different aspects of mental health care; it is a poor alternative. This solution is also expensive because the consultee must involve several services to comprehensively assess, treat, and rehabilitate the patient. This model does ensure that each specialty has its own service; the consultation-liaison service is directed by a psychiatrist, the department of medical psychology is directed by a psychologist, and so on.

Major innovations in consultation-liaison psychiatry will not occur where services are split. Innovations are the product of collaboration and cross-fertilization among all these health care professionals and systems. In the future, consultation-liaison psychiatry might be replaced by consultation-liaison sociopsychobiology. In such a field, the psychiatrist is important as one of several highly educated team members. In contrast to medicine,

consultation-liaison sociopsychobiology would focus on the "whole" patient, his or her family, and the health care system as a clinical and scientific arena.

REFERENCES

General; European Studies

de Jonge P, Huyse FJ, Ruinemans GMF, et al: The timing of psychiatric consultation: the impact of social vulnerability and level of psychiatric dysfunction. Psychosomatics 41(6):505–511, 2000

de Jonge P, Huyse FJ, Herzog T, et al: Referral pattern of neurological patients to psychiatric consultation-liaison services in 33 European hospitals. Gen Hosp Psychiatry 23:152–157, 2001a

de Jonge P, Huyse FJ, Herzog T, et al: Risk factors for complex care needs in general medical inpatients: results from a European study. Psychosomatics 42(3):213–221, 2001b

de Jonge P, Huyse FJ, Slaets JPJ, et al: Care complexity in the general hospital: results from a European study. Psychosomatics 42(3): 204–212, 2001c

de Jonge P, Huyse FJ, Stiefel FC, et al: INTERMED: a clinical instrument for biopsychosocial assessment. Psychosomatics 42(2):106–109, 2001d

Eaton JS, Daniels RS, Pardes H: Psychiatric education: state of the art, 1976. Am J Psychiatry 134 (suppl):2–6, 1977

Engel GL: The need for a new medical model: a challenge for biomedicine. Science 196:129–136, 1977

Fink P, Jensen J, Poulsen CS: A study of hospital admissions over time, using longitudinal latent structure analyses. Scand J Soc Med 3:211–219, 1993

Fischer CJ, Stiefel FC, de Jonge P: Case complexity and clinical outcome in diabetes mellitus: a prospective study using the INTERMED. Diabetes and Metabolism 26(4):295–302, 2000

Hammer JS, Strain JJ, Lyons JS: Consortium-based consultation/liaison research. Int J Psychiatry Med 17:237–248, 1987

Hengeveld MW, Huyse FJ, van der Mast RC, et al: A proposal for standardization of psychiatric consultation-liaison data. Gen Hosp Psychiatry 10:410–422, 1988

Herzog T: Psychosomatic liaison services, in The European Handbook of Psychiatry and Mental Health. Edited by Seva A. Barcelona, Spain, Editorial Anthropos, 1991a, pp 1447–1455

Herzog T: Inpatient treatment with patients with severe psychosomatic and neurotic disorders. British Journal of Psychotherapy 8:189–198, 1991b

Herzog T, Creed F, Huyse FJ, et al: Psychosomatic medicine in the general hospital, in Psychiatry in Europe: Directions and Developments. Edited by Katona C, Montgomery S, Sensky T. London, England, Gaskell Press, 1994, pp 143–151

Herzog T, Huyse FJ, Malt UF, et al: Quality assurance in C-L psychiatry and psychosomatics: development and implementation of a European quality assurance system, in Biomedical and Health Research. The BIOMED1 Programme (Grant BMH1-CT94-1706). Edited by Baert EA. Amsterdam, the Netherlands, IOS Press Ohmsha, 1995, pp 525–526

Huyse FJ: From consultation to complexity of care prediction and health service needs assessment. J Psychosom Res 43:233–240, 1997

Huyse FJ, Smith GC: From C-L dream to C-L reality: the need for a systematic approach to the development of C-L mental health service delivery. Psychiatric Bulletin 21:529–531, 1997

Huyse FJ, Herzog T, Malt UF, et al: A screening instrument for the detection of psychosocial risk factors in patients admitted to general hospital wards. Biomedical and Health Research Programme (1990–1994), BMH1-CT93-1180, Commission of the European Communities, Brussels, Belgium, 1993b

Huyse FJ, Herzog T, Malt UF, et al: The European Consultation-Liaison Workgroup (ECLW) Collaborative Study, I: general outline. Gen Hosp Psychiatry 18:44–55, 1996

Huyse FJ, Lyons JS, Stiefel FC, et al: "INTERMED": a method to assess health service needs, I: development and reliability. Gen Hosp Psychiatry 21:39–48, 1999

Huyse FJ, Herzog T, Lobo A, et al: European consultation-liaison services and their user populations: the ECLW Collaborative Study. Psychosomatics 41:330–338, 2000a

Huyse FJ, Herzog T, Lobo A, et al: European consultation-liaison psychiatric services: the ECLW Collaborative Study. Acta Psychiatr Scand 101:360–366, 2000b

Huyse FJ, de Jonge de P, Slaets JPJ, et al: COMPRI: an instrument to detect patients with complex care needs: results from a European study. Psychosomatics 42:222–228, 2001a

Huyse FJ, Herzog T, Lobo A, et al: Consultation-liaison psychiatric service delivery: results from a European study. Gen Hosp Psychiatry 23:152–157, 2001b

Huyse FJ, Lyons JS, Stiefel FC, et al: Operationalizing the biopsychosocial model: the INTERMED. Psychosomatics 42(1):5–13, 2001c

Koch N, Stiefel FC, de Jonge P, et al: Identification of complex patients with rheumatoid arthritis and increased health care utilization. Arthritis Care and Research 45(3):216–221, 2001

Lobo A, Huyse FJ, Herzog T, et al: The European Consultation-Liaison Workgroup (ECLW) Collaborative Study, II: patient registration form (PRF) instrument, training and reliability. J Psychosom Res 40:143–156, 1996

Malt UF: Philosophy of science and DSM-III. Acta Psychiatr Scand 73 (suppl 328):10–17, 1986

Malt UF, Huyse FJ, Herzog T, et al: The European Consultation-Liaison Workgroup (ECLW) Collaborative Study, III: training and reliability of ICD-10 psychiatric diagnoses in the general hospital setting—an investigation of 220 consultants from 14 European countries. J Psychosom Res 41:451–464, 1996

Mayou R, Huyse FJ, and the European Consultation-Liaison Workgroup: Consultation-liaison psychiatry in Western Europe. Gen Hosp Psychiatry 13:188–208, 1991

Miller WB: Psychiatric consultation, part I: a general system approach. Psychiatry Med 4:135–145, 1973

Miltner W, Birbauer N, Gerber WD (eds): Verhaltens-medizin [Behavioral Medicine]. Berlin, Germany, Springer-Verlag, 1986

Orlinsky D, Grawe K, Parks B: Process and outcome in psychotherapy, in Handbook of Psychotherapy and Behavior Change. Edited by Bergin AE, Garfield SL. New York, Wiley, 1994, pp 270–376

Richter HE, Wirsching M (eds): Neues Denken in der Psychosomatik [New Thinking in Psychosomatics]. Frankfurt, Germany, Fischer Taschenbuch Verlag, 1991

Schwartz GE, Weiss SM: Yale Conference on Behavioral Medicine: a proposed definition and statement of goals. J Behav Med 1:3–12, 1978

Stiefel FC, de Jonge P, Huyse FJ, et al: "INTERMED": an assessment and classification system for case complexity: results in patients with low back pain. Spine 24:378–385, 1999a

Stiefel FC, de Jonge P, Huyse FJ, et al: "INTERMED": a method to assess health service needs, II: results on its validity and clinical use. Gen Hosp Psychiatry 21:49–56, 1999b

Strain JJ, Hammer JS, Himelein C, et al: Consultation-liaison psychiatry database (1996 update). Gen Hosp Psychiatry 18:293–384, 1996

Taintor Z, Spikes J, Gise LH, et al: Recording psychiatric consultations: a preliminary report. Gen Hosp Psychiatry 2:139–149, 1979

Torem M, Saravay SM, Steinberg H: Psychiatric liaison: benefits of an "active" approach. Psychosomatics 20:598–607, 1979

Uexküll T (ed): Integrierte Psychosomatische Medizin in Praxis und Klinik [Integrated Psychosomatic Medicine in Practice]. Stuttgart, Germany, Schattauer, 1992

Wahl R, Hautzinger M (eds): Verhaltensmedizin: Konzepte, Anwendungsgebiete, Perspektiven [Behavioral Medicine: Concepts, Applications, Perspectives]. Köln, Germany, Deutscher Ärzteverlag, 1989

Wallen J, Pincus HA, Goldman HH, et al: Psychiatric consultations in short-term general hospitals. Arch Gen Psychiatry 44:163–168, 1987

Wirsching M, Herzog T: Towards a new psychosomatics. Psychiatria Fennica 22:103–111, 1991

BY AREA

Nordic Countries

Alaja R, Seppa K, Sillanaukee P, et al: Psychiatric referrals associated with substance use disorders: prevalence and gender differences: European Consultation-Liaison Workgroup. Alcohol Clin Exp Res 21:620–626, 1997

Alaja R, Seppä K, Sillanaukee P, et al: Physical and mental co-morbidity of substance use disorders in psychiatric consultations. Alcohol Clin Exp Res 22:1820–1824, 1998a

Alaja R, Tienari P, Seppä K, et al: Patterns of comorbidity in psychiatric consultations: relation to functioning (GAF) among general hospital psychiatric referrals. Acta Psychiatr Scand 97:1–6, 1998b

Alaja R, Seppä K, Leppävuori A, et al: Pattern of comorbidity in relation to functioning (GAF) among general hospital psychiatric referrals. Acta Psychiatr Scand 99:135–140, 1999

Allgulander C, Fischer LD: Clinical predictors of completed suicide and repeated self-poisoning patients. Eur Arch Psychiatry Neurol Sci 239:270–276, 1990

Bech P, Malt UF, Dencker SJ, et al: Scales for Assessment of Diagnosis and Severity of Mental Disorders. Acta Psychiatr Scand 87 (suppl 372):1–87, 1993

Blomhoff S, Malt UF: Psychiatric perspectives on psychogenic seizures and their treatment, in Pseudo-Epileptic Seizures. Edited by Gram L, Johannessen SI, Osterman PO, et al. London, England, Wrightson Biomedical Publishing, 1993, pp 99–108

Fink P: The use of hospitalizations by persistent somatizing patients. J Psychosom Res 22:173–180, 1992

Fink P, Jensen J, Borgquist L, et al: Psychiatric morbidity in primary public health care: a Nordic multicentre investigation, part I: method and prevalence of psychiatric morbidity. Acta Psychiatr Scand 92:409–418, 1995

Fink P, Ewald H, Jensen J, et al: Screening for somatisation and hypochondriasis in primary care and neurological inpatients: a seven-item scale for hypochondriasis and somatization. J Psychosom Res 46:261–273, 1999

Gudmundsson OO, Karlsson L, Pétursson H: Psychiatric consultations in a general hospital. Nordic Journal of Psychiatry 45:445–450, 1991

Malt UF: Somatization: an old disorder in new bottles? Psychiatria Fennica 22:79–91, 1991

Malt UF: Traumatic effects of accidents, in Individual and Community Responses to Trauma and Disaster: The Structure of Human Chaos. Edited by Ursano RJ, McCaughey BG, Fullerton CS. Cambridge, MA, Cambridge University Press, 1993, pp 103–135

Malt UF, Weisæth L: Disaster psychiatry and traumatic stress studies in Norway: history, current status and future. Acta Psychiatr Scand 80 (suppl 355):7–12, 1989

Mayou R, Huyse F, and the European Consultation-Liaison Workgroup: Consultation-liaison psychiatry in Western Europe. Gen Hosp Psychiatry 13:188–208, 1991

Rutz W, von Knorring L, Walinder J, et al: Effect of an educational program for general practitioners on Gotland on the pattern of prescription of psychotropic drugs. Acta Psychiatr Scand 82:399–403, 1990

Sjogren B: Future use and development of prenatal diagnosis: consumers' attitudes.Prenat Diagn 12:1–8, 1992

Stalhammar D, Starmark JE, Holmgren E: Assessment of responsiveness in acute cerebral disorder: a multicenter study on the RLS85. Acta Neurochir (Wien) 90:73–80, 1988

Starmark JE, Stalhammar D, Holmgren E, et al: A comparison of the Glasgow Coma Scale and the Reaction Level Scale (RLS85). J Neurosurg 69:699–706, 1988

Stiles TC, Bille-Brahe U, Bjerke T, et al: WHO (Nordic) multicentre study on parasuicide. Nordic Journal of Psychiatry 47:281–286, 1993

Tienari P: Adjustment disorder in cardiac surgery, in Cerebral Damage Before and After Cardiac Surgery. Edited by Willner A. Dordrecht, The Netherlands, Kluwer, 1993a, pp 239–248

Tienari P: Somatic illness and family interaction. Nordic Journal of Psychiatry 47:273–279, 1993b

Viinamäki H, Niskanen L, Haatainen J, et al: Determinants of psychiatric hospital care in a general hospital. Nordic Journal of Psychiatry 47:95–99, 1993

Viinamäki H, Tienari P, Niskanen L, et al: Factors predictive of referral to psychiatric hospital among general hospital psychiatric consultations. Acta Psychiatr Scand 97:47–54, 1998

von Knorring L: The pathogenesis of chronic pain syndromes. Nordic Journal of Psychiatry 43 (suppl 20):35–42, 1989

Weinryb RM, Gustavsson JP, Åsberg M, et al: The concept of alexithymia: an empirical study using psychodynamic ratings and self-reports. Acta Psychiatr Scand 85:153–162, 1992

German-Speaking Countries

DeVries A, Söllner W, Steixner E, et al: Subjektiv erlebte Belastung und Bedarf an psychosozialer Unterstützung bei Tumorpatienten in strahlentherapeutischer Behandlung (Psychological distress and need for psychosocial support of cancer patients undergoing radiotherapy). Strahlenther Onkol 174:408–414, 1998

Herzog T, Hartmann A: Psychiatrische, Psychosomatische und Medizinpsychologische Konsiliar–und Liaisontätigkeit in der Bundesrepublik Deutschland: Ergebnisse einer Umfrage [Current status of consultation-liaison psychiatry and psychosomatics in West-Germany: a survey]. Nervenarzt 61:281–293, 1990

Herzog T, Scheidt CE: Consultation/liaison psychiatry and psychosomatics in Germany—separate or united? Nordic Journal of Psychiatry 45:423–431, 1991

Herzog T, Stein B, European Consultation Liaison Workgroup (ECLW): Psychotherapeutisch-psychosomatische Konsiliar/liaisondienste: Entwicklungen, empirische Befunde, Perspektiven für Praxis und Forschung [Psychotherapeutic-psychosomatic CL services: developments, empirical findings, perspectives for clinical practice and research]. Psychologie in der Medizin 5:10–17, 1994

Koch U: Entwicklung der Forschung im Fach Medizinische Psychologie in den Letzten 10 Jahren [Research in medical psychology—trends of the last 10 years]. Psychother Psychosom Med Psychol 37:284–288, 1987

Köhle K, Joraschky P, Reisinger E: Integration of psychosomatic medicine in various clinical disciplines (institutionalization), in Psychosomatic Medicine. Edited by von Uexküll T, Adler RH, Herrmann JM, et al. München Wien, Austria, Urban & Schwarzenberg, 1997, pp 310–335

Langewitz WA, Eich P, Kiss A, et al: Improving communication skills: a randomized controlled behaviorally oriented intervention study for residents in internal medicine. Psychosom Med 60:268–276, 1998

Söllner W, Kantner-Rumplmair W, Lampe A, et al: Liaison-Psychotherapie im Allgemeinkrankenhaus: Aufgaben und Probleme bei der Etablierung psychotherapeutischer Dienste [Implementation of liaison psychotherapy in the general hospital: tasks and problems]. Psychotherapie Forum 5:92–101, 1997

Söllner W, Zingg-Schir M, Rumpold G, et al: Need for supportive counselling: the professionals' versus the patients' perspective: a survey in a representative sample of 236 melanoma patients. Psychother Psychosom 67:94–104, 1998a

Söllner W, Leithner K, Springer-Kremser M, et al: Psychotherapeutische und klinisch-psychologische Konsiliar-/Liaisondienste an Allgemeinen Krankenhäusern in Österreich [Psychotherapeutic and psychological consultation-liaison services in Austrian general hospitals]. Psychologie in der Medizin 9(3):19–33, 1998b

Söllner W, Crombach G, Harrer M, et al: Effekte psychosomatischer Fortbildung für Ärzte: Selbsteinschätzung durch die Teilnehmer der Fortbildungskurse in Psychosozialer und Psychosomatischer Medizin in Tirol [Training physicians in psychosomatic medicine: results of a self-evaluation of the participants of a two-year training course in Tyrol]. Psychologische Medizin 11(3):51–56, 2000

Söllner W, DeVries A, Steixner E, et al: How successful are oncologists in identifying patient distress, perceived social support, and need for psychosocial counselling? Br J Cancer 84:179–185, 2001

Uexküll T, Adler RH, Herrmann JM, et al: Psychosomatic Medicine. München Wien, Austria, Urban & Schwarzenberg, 1997

Zumbrunnen R: Psychiatrie de Liaison [Liaison Psychiatry]. Paris, Milan, Barcelona, Bonn, Masson, 1992

United Kingdom

Adams C, Gelder M: The case for establishing a register of randomized controlled trials of mental health care. Br J Psychiatry 164:433–436, 1994

Benjamin S, House A, Jenkins P (eds): Liaison Psychiatry: Defining Needs and Planning Services. London, England, Gaskell Press, Royal College of Psychiatrists, 1994

Brown A, Cooper AF: The impact of a liaison psychiatry service on patterns of referral in a general hospital. Br J Psychiatry 150:83–87, 1987

Chick J, Lloyd G, Crombie E: Counseling problem drinkers on medical wards: a controlled study. BMJ 290:965–967, 1985

Creed F, Marks B: Liaison psychiatry in general practice: a comparison of the liaison-attachment scheme and shifted outpatient clinic models. J R Coll Gen Pract 39:514–517, 1989

Creed F, Mayou R, Hopkins A: Medical Symptoms Not Explained by Organic Disease. London, England, Royal Colleges of Physicians and Psychiatrists, 1992

Creed F, Guthrie EA, Black D, et al: Referrals within a general hospital—comparison to those from a general practitioner. Br J Psychiatry 162:204–211, 1993

Department of Health: The Health of the Nation: Key Area Handbook Mental Illness. London, England, HMSO, January 1993

Gater R, Goldberg D: Pathways to psychiatric care in south Manchester. Br J Psychiatry 259:90–96, 1991

Guthrie E, Creed FH, Dawson D, et al: A controlled trial of psychological treatment for the irritable bowel syndrome. Gastroenterology 100:450–457, 1991

Hawton KE, Catalan JP: Attempted Suicide: A Practical Guide to Its Nature and Management, 2nd Edition. Oxford, England, Oxford Medical Publications, Oxford University Press, 1987

Klimes I, Mayou R, Pearce MJ: Psychological treatment for atypical non-cardiac chest pain: a controlled study. Psychol Med 20:605–611, 1990

Maguire P, Faulkner A: Improve the counselling skills of doctors and nurses in cancer care. BMJ 297:847–849, 1988

Mayou R: Consultation Liaison Psychiatry: An International Perspective. Kalamazoo, MI, Upjohn International, 1988

Mayou R: The history of general hospital psychiatry. Br J Psychiatry 155:764–777, 1989

Mayou R, Hawton KE: Psychiatric disorder in the general hospital. Br J Psychiatry 149:172–190, 1986

Mayou R, Anderson H, Feinmann L, et al: The present state of consultation and liaison psychiatry. Bulletin of the British Journal of Psychiatry 14:321–325, 1990

Mayou R, Bass C, Sharp M (eds): Treatment of Functional Somatic Symptoms. Oxford, England, Oxford University Press, 1995

Prettyman RJ, Friedman T: Care of women with puerperal psychiatric disorders in England and Wales. BMJ 302:1245–1246, 1991

Royal College of Physicians and the Royal College of Psychiatrists (RCP and RC Psych): The psychological care of medical patients: recognition of need and service provision: report of a working party. London, England, Royal College of Physicians and Royal College of Psychiatrists, 1995a

Royal College of Physicians and the Royal College of Psychiatrists (RCP and RC Psych): The psychological care of medical patients: a guide for purchasers: report of a working party. London, England, Royal College of Physicians and Royal College of Psychiatrists, 1995b

Sensky T, Greer S, Cundy T, et al: Referrals to psychiatrists in a general hospital—comparison of two methods of liaison psychiatry. J R Soc Med 78:463–468, 1985

Thomas CJ: Referrals to a British liaison psychiatry service. Health Trends 15:61–64, 1983

Wessely S, Powell R: Fatigue syndromes: a comparison of chronic 'post viral' fatigue with neuromuscular and affective disorders. J Neurol Neurosurg Psychiatry 52:940–948, 1989

United Kingdom, Selected Readings

Bass C: Somatization: Physical Symptoms of Psychological Illness. Oxford, England, Blackwell Scientific, 1990

Creed F: Life events and appendectomy. Lancet 1:1381–1385, 1981

Creed F, Guthrie E: Psychological treatment for the irritable bowel syndrome. Gut 28:1307–1318, 1989

Creed F, Graig T, Farmer R: Functional abdominal pain, psychiatric illness and life events. Gut 29:235–242, 1988

Hawton K, Fagg J: Suicide and other causes of death following attempted suicide. Br J Psychiatry 152:359–366, 1988

Hotopf MH, Wessely S: Viruses, neurosis and fatigue. J Psychosom Res 38:499–514, 1994

House A, Dennis M, Warlow C, et al: Mood disorders in the first year after stroke: a CT scan study of the importance of lesion location. Brain 113:1113–1129, 1990

Lloyd GG: Liaison psychiatry from a British perspective. Gen Hosp Psychiatry 2:46–51, 1980

Mayou R: Invited review: the psychiatric and social consequences of coronary artery bypass graft surgery. J Psychosom Res 258:1611–1614, 1986

Strathdee G: Primary care–psychiatry interaction: a British perspective. Gen Hosp Psychiatry 9:102–110, 1987

Wieck A, Kumar R, Hirst AD, et al: Increased sensitivity of dopamine receptors and recurrence of affective psychosis after childbirth. BMJ 303:613–616, 1991

The Netherlands

Bannink M, Van Gool AR, van der Heide A, et al: Psychiatric consultation and quality of decision making in euthanasia. Lancet 356:2067–2068, 2000

Boenink AD, Huyse FJ: Arie Querido (1901–1983), a Dutch psychiatrist: the lasting impact of his work for nowadays C-L psychiatry. J Psychosom Res 43:551–557, 1997

Broers S, Hengeveld MW, Kaptein AA, et al: Are pretransplant psychological variables related to survival after bone marrow transplantation? A prospective study of 123 patients. J Psychosom Res 45:341–351, 1998

Hengeveld MW, Rooijmans HGM, Vecht van den Bergh R: Psychiatric consultations in a Dutch university hospital: a report on 1814 referrals, compared with a literature review. Gen Hosp Psychiatry 6:271–279, 1984

Hengeveld MW, Huyse FJ, van der Mast RC, et al: A proposal for standardization of consultation-liaison data. Gen Hosp Psychiatry 10:410–422, 1988

Huyse FJ, Hengeveld MW: Development of consultation-liaison psychiatry in the Netherlands: its social psychiatric heritage. Gen Hosp Psychiatry 11:9–15, 1989

Huyse FJ, van Tilburg W: Euthanasia policy in the Netherlands: the role of consultation liaison psychiatrists. Hospital and Community Psychiatry 44:733–739, 1993

Huyse FJ, Hengeveld MW, Strain JJ, et al: Interventions in consultation-liaison psychiatry: the development of a schema and checklist for operationalized interventions. Gen Hosp Psychiatry 10:88–101, 1988

Koopmans GT, Meeuwesen L, Huyse FJ, et al: Effects of psychiatric consultations on medical consumption in medical outpatients with abdominal pain. Psychosomatics 36:387–399, 1995

Leigh H, Feinstein AR, Reiser MF: The patient evaluation grid: a systematic approach to comprehensive care. Gen Hosp Psychiatry 2:3–9, 1980

Meeuwesen L, Huyse FJ, Meiland FJM, et al: Psychiatric consultations in medical outpatients with abdominal pain: a randomized clinical trial. Int J Psychiatry Med 24:339–356, 1994

Querido A: Forecast and follow-up: an investigation into the clinical, social, and mental factors determining the results of hospital treatment. British Journal of Preventive and Social Medicine 13:33–49, 1959

Slaets JP, Kaufmann HP, Duivenvoorden HJ, et al: A randomized trial of geriatric liaison intervention in elderly medical inpatients. Psychosom Med 59:585–591, 1997

Smals GLM, Mast van der RC, Speckens AEM, et al: Alcohol abuse among general hospital in-patients according to the Münich Alcoholism Test (MALT). Gen Hosp Psychiatry 16:125–130, 1994

Speckens AEM, Heeren TJ, Rooymans HG: Alcohol abuse among elderly patients in a general hospital as identified by the Münich Alcoholism Test. Acta Psychiatr Scand 83:460–462, 1991

Speckens AEM, van Hemert AM, Bolk JH, et al: The acceptability of psychological treatment in patients with medically unexplained physical symptoms. J Psychosom Res 39:855–863, 1995a

Speckens AEM, van Hemert AM, Spinhoven PH, et al: Cognitive behavioral therapy for medically unexplained physical symptoms: a randomized controlled trial. BMJ 311:1328–1332, 1995b

Speckens AEM, Spinhoven PH, Sloekers PPA, et al: A validation study of the Whitely Index, the Illness Attitude Scales, and the Somatosensory Amplification Scale in general medical and general practice patients. J Psychosom Res 40:95–104, 1996a

Speckens AEM, van Hemert AM, Bolk JH, et al: Unexplained physical symptoms: outcome, utilization of medical care and associated factors. Psychol Med 26:745–752, 1996b

Speckens AEM, van Hemert AM, Spinhoven PH, et al: The diagnostic and prognostic significance of the Whitely Index, the Illness Attitude Scales and the Somatosensory Amplification Scale. Psychol Med 26:1085–1090, 1996c

van der Mast RC: Pathophysiology of delirium. J Geriatr Psychiatry Neurol 11:138–145, 1999

van der Mast RC, Fekkes D: Serotonin and amino acids: partners in delirium pathophysiology? Semin Clin Neuropsychiatry 5:125–131, 2000 van der Mast RC, Fekkes D, Moleman P, et al: Is post-operative delirium related to reduced plasma tryptophan? Lancet 338:851–852, 1991

van der Mast RC, van den Broek WW, Fekkes D, et al: Incidence of and preoperative predictors for delirium after cardiac surgery. J Psychosom Res 46:479–483, 1999

van Hemert AM, Hawton KE, Bolk JH, et al: Key symptoms in the detection of affective disorders in medical patients. J Psychosom Res 37:397–404, 1993a

van Hemert AM, Hengeveld MW, Bolk JH, et al: Psychiatric disorders in relation to medical illness among patients of a general medical out-patient clinic. Psychol Med 23:167–174, 1993b

van Hemert AM, Den Heijer M, Vorstenbosch M, et al: Detecting psychiatric disorders in medical practice using the General Health Questionnaire: why do cut-off scores vary? Psychol Med 25:165–170, 1995

Southern European and Mediterranean Countries

Balint M: Psychotherapy in general medicine and Balint groups. Psychiatry in Medicine 3:277–430, 1972

Bourgeois M: Situations médicales particulières [Specific medical situations], in Précis de Psychiatrie Clinique de l'Adulte [Comprehensive Textbook of Adult Psychiatry]. Edited by Deniker P, Lempérière TH, Guyotat J. Paris, France, Masson, 1990, pp 392–401

Cardoso G, Barbosa A, Franca de Sousa J: Psiquiatria de ligacao num hospital geral: novas perspectivas [Liaison psychiatry in the general hospital: new perspectives]. Acta Med Port 4/5/6:296–303, 1988

Cazzullo CL, Comazzi A, Guaraldi GP, et al: General hospital psychiatry in Italy: on the hospitalization of psychiatric patients and consultation-liaison psychiatry after Law 180/1978. Gen Hosp Psychiatry 6:261–265, 1984

De Bertolini C, Rigatelli M, Rizzardo R, et al: Psichiatria di consultazione e collegamento [Consultation-liaison psychiatry], in Trattato Italiano di Psichiatria [Italian Textbook of Psychiatry], 2nd Edition, Vol 3. Edited by Pancheri P, Cassano GB. Milan, Italy, Editions Masson, 1999, pp 3841–3871

Gala C, Rigatelli M, De Bertolini C, et al: A multicenter investigation of consultation-liaison psychiatry in Italy. Gen Hosp Psychiatry 21:310–317, 1999

Garcia-Camba E, Crespo MD, Lobo A, et al: Resultados del estudio del European Consultation Liaison Workgroup en Espana, sobre efectividad de los servicios de Psiquiatria de Interconsulta y Enlace: datos preliminares [The ECLW Collaborative Study: preliminary Spanish data]. Archivos de Neurobiologia 2 (suppl):23–33, 1997

Grassi I, Gritti P, Rigatelli M, et al: Psychosocial problems secondary to cancer: an Italian multicentre survey of consultation-liaison psychiatry in oncology. Eur J Cancer 36:579–585, 2000

Guimaraes Lopes R: Bases programaticas da promaçao de Saude Mental [Bases of mental health development]. O Medico 40:120, 147–152, 1989

Invernizzi G, Gala C, Bressi C: La Psichiatria di Consultazione Nell' Ospedale Generale [Consultation-Liaison Psychiatry in the General Hospital]. Rome, Italy, CIC Ed Internazionali, 1997

Lobo A: Elucidating mental disorder in liaison psychiatry: the Johns Hopkins "Perspectives." J Psychosom Res 41:7–11, 1996

Lobo A, Perez-Echeverria MJ, Artal J, et al: Psychiatric morbidity among medical out-patients in Spain: a case for new methods of classification. J Psychosom Res 32:355–364, 1988

Lobo A, Perez-Echeverria MJ, Campos R, et al: A new interview for the multiaxial assessment of psychiatric morbidity in medical patients (SPPI). Psychol Med 23:505–510, 1993

Lobo A, García-Campayo J, Campos R, et al: Somatization in primary care in Spain, I: estimates of prevalences and clinical characteristics. Br J Psychiatry 168:344–348, 1996

Lobo A, Huyse FJ, Herzog TH, et al: Los nuevos estudios Europeos y nacionales sobre servicios de psicosomática y psiquiatría "de enlace" en el hospital general, I: desarrollo y estudio de la efectividad de un programa de formación de postgrado en "gestión de calidad," II: desarrollo y validación de un instrumento de temprana detección de pacientes con problemas psicosociales con potencial de complicar el curso de la enfermedad médica [The new European consultation-liaison work group studies, I: the development of a quality management program, II: the development of an instrument for psychosocial risk screening at admission]. Archivos de Neurobiología 2 (suppl):35–56, 1997

Rigatelli M, Curci P, De Bernardinis M : Some experiences of consultation-liaison psychiatry in a university hospital. Psychother Psychosom 33:1–6, 1980

Rigatelli M, Marcon M, Morriti AR: A clinical consultation-liaison experience in a rehabilitation service: selected papers from the 10th World Congress of the International College of Psychosomatic Medicine. Psychother Psychosom 52:36–40, 1989

Rigatelli M, Galeazzi GM, Barbieri C, et al: Studio Europeo sulla qualità in psichiatria di consultazione [European study on quality in consultation-liaison psychiatry]. Rivista Sperimentale di Freniatria 4:261–266, 1998

Rigatelli M, Ferrari S, Uguzzoni U, et al: Teaching and training in the psychiatric-psychosomatic consultation liaison setting. Psychother Psychosom 69:219–226, 2000

Soldatos U, Sakkas P: Psychiatry in the general hospital. Archives of Greek Medicine 4:107–109, 1987

Australia and New Zealand

Bennett EJ, Tennant CC, Piesse C, et al: Level of chronic life stress predicts clinical outcome in irritable bowel syndrome. Gut 43:256–261, 1998

Clarke DM, Smith GC: Consultation-liaison psychiatry in general medical units. Aust N Z J Psychiatry 29:424–432, 1995

Clarke DM, Smith GC, Herrman HE, et al: Monash Interview for Liaison Psychiatry (MILP): development, reliability and procedural validity. Psychosomatics 39:318–328, 1998

Dunsis A, Smith GC: Consultation-liaison psychiatry in an obstetric service. Aust N Z J Psychiatry 30:63–73, 1996

Hickie I, Bennett B, Lloyd A, et al: Complex genetic and environmental relationships between psychological distress, fatigue and immune functioning: a twin study. Psychol Med 29:269–277, 1999

Kissane DW, Smith GC: Consultation-liaison psychiatry in an Australian oncology unit. Aust N Z J Psychiatry 30:397–404, 1996

Kissane DW, Bloch S, Ikin J, et al: Psychological morbidity and quality of life in Australian women with early stage breast cancer: a cross-sectional survey. Med J Aust 169:192–196, 1998

McFarlane AC: The aetiology of post-traumatic morbidity: predisposing, precipitating and perpetuating factors. Br J Psychiatry 154:221–228, 1989

Rustomjee S, Smith GC: Consultation-liaison psychiatry to renal medicine: work with inpatient unit. Aust N Z J Psychiatry 30:229–237, 1996

Smith GC: From consultation-liaison psychiatry to psychosocial advocacy. Aust N Z J Psychiatry 32:753–761, 1998

Smith GC, Clarke DM, Herrman HE: Consultation-liaison psychiatry in Australia. Gen Hosp Psychiatry 15:121–125, 1993a

Smith GC, Clarke DM, Hermann HE: Establishing a consultation-liaison psychiatry clinical database in an Australian general hospital. Gen Hosp Psychiatry 15:243–253, 1993b

Smith GC, Ellis PM, Carr VJ, et al: Staffing and funding of consultation-liaison psychiatry services in Australia and New Zealand. Aust N Z J Psychiatry 28:398–404, 1994

Strain JJ, Smith GC, Hammer JS, et al: Adjustment disorder: a mulitisite study of its utilization and interventions in the consultation-liaison psychiatry setting. Gen Hosp Psychiatry 20:139–149, 1998

Japan

Berger D, Fukunishi I, Hosaka T, et al: A comparison of Japanese and American psychiatrists' attitudes toward patients wishing to die in the general hospital. Psychother Psychosom 66:319–328, 1997

Fukunishi I, Hosaka T, Negishi M, et al: Avoidance coping behaviors and low social support are related to depressive symptoms in HIV-positive patients in Japan. Psychosomatics 38:113–118, 1997

Hosaka T: Physician's attitudes toward psychiatric consultation. Shinshin-Igaku 29:351–358, 1989

Hosaka T: A pilot study of a structured psychiatric intervention for Japanese women with breast cancer. Psychooncology 5:59–64, 1996

Hosaka T: A cultural perspective on euthanasia. Tokai J Exp Clin Med 22:279–282, 1997

Hosaka T: Psychiatry for Non-Psychiatric Physicians. Tokyo, Japan, Life Science, 1998

Iwasaki T, Kurosawa H, Hosaka T: The Future Theme of Consultation Liaison Psychiatry. Tokyo, Japan, Tokaidaigaku-Shuppannkai, 1989

Iwasaki Y, Kurosawa H, Watanabe N: The delirium in a critical care medical center: incidence, demographic characteristics, outcome, length of stay. Japanese Journal of General Hospital Psychiatry 4:39–45, 1992

Kishi Y, Robinson RG, Kosier JT: Suicidal plans in patients with stroke: comparison between acute-onset and delayed-onset suicidal plans. Int Psychogeriatr 8:623–634, 1996

Kuroki N, Katsuragawa S, Kobori S, et al: Adequate arrangement in general hospital psychiatry and clinical training designated hospital psychiatry. Japanese Journal of General Hospital Psychiatry 9:104–118, 1997

Kurosawa H (ed): Consultation-Liaison Psychiatry. Tokyo, Japan, Seiwa-shoten, 1996

Kurosawa H: A decade of the Japanese Society of General Hospital Psychiatry. Presidential address at the 11th annual meeting of the Japanese Society of General Hospital Psychiatry, Tokyo, Japan, December 1998

Kurosawa H, Iwasaki Y: Suicide attempters in critical care medical center: the conclusion of 12 centers. Japanese Journal of Acute Medicine 15:651–653, 1991

Kurosawa H, Iwasaki Y, Watanabe N, et al: What's in the term 'ICU syndrome'? The relationship between ICU, postoperative and other mental disorders. Clinical Intensive Care 3:122–126, 1992

Matushima E, Moriya H, Sakurada H, et al: The clinical study of the effect of intravenous haloperidol to circulation. ICU and CCU 10:141–146, 1985

Nomura S, Shigemura J, Nakamura M, et al: Evaluation of the first medical psychiatry unit in Japan. Psychiatry Clin Neurosci 50:305–308, 1996

Sato T, Takeichi M: Lifetime prevalence of specific psychiatric disorders in a general medicine clinic. Gen Hospital Psychiatry 15:224–233, 1993

Strain JJ, Hammer J, Lewin C, et al: C-L database—1991 update. Gen Hosp Psychiatry 13 (suppl):S10–S11, 1991

Yamashita N, Morimoto N, Monji A, et al: A study of psychiatric consultation-liaison service with the passage of time in a university hospital. Japanese Journal of General Psychiatry 4:141–150, 1992

Latin American Countries

Botega NJ: A assistencia em Saude Mental nos Hospitais Gerais: a atual situacao no Brazil [Dealing with the mentally ill in the general hospital]. Cadernos do IPUB 6:1–7, 1989

Botega NJ, Dalgalarrondo P: Saude Mental no Hospital Geral: Espaco para o Psiquico [Mental Health in the General Hospital: A Space for the Psychic]. São Paulo, Brazil, Editoria Hucitec, 1993

Botega NJ, Schechtman A: Censo nacional de Unidades de Psiquiatria em Hospitais Gerais, I: situacao e tendencias [National survey of psychiatry in the general hospital: situation and tendencies]. Revista ABP-APAL 19(3):79–86, 1997

Fortes SL, Pereira MEC, Botega NJ: Ambulatorio de saude mental, in Servicos de Saude Mental no Hospital Geral [Mental health ambulatory, in Mental Health Services in the General Hospital]. Edited by Botega NJ. Campinas, Brazil, Papirus Campinas, 1995

Mello Filho J: Psicossomatica Hoy [Psychosomatics Today]. Artes Medicas, 1992

Nogueira-Martins LA: Consultoria psiquiatrica e psicologica no hospital geral: a experiencia do Hospital Sao Paullo. Revista ABP-APAL 11(4):160–164, 1989

Nogueira-Martins LA: Ensino e formacao em interconsulta [Teaching and formation in consultation]. Revista ABP-APAL 15(2):68–74, 1993

Conclusion

Blomhoff S, Malt UF: Psychiatric perspectives on psychogenic seizures and their treatment, in Pseudo-Epileptic Seizures. Edited by Gram L, Johannessen SI, Osterman PO, et al. London, England, Wrightson Biomedical Publishing, 1993, pp 99–108

Hammer JS, Strain JJ, Lyons JS: Consortium-based consultation/liaison research. Int J Psychiatry Med 17:237–248, 1987

Malt UF: Philosophy of science and DSM-III. Acta Psychiatr Scand 73 (suppl 328):10–17, 1986

Malt UF: Somatization: an old disorder in new bottles? Psychiatria Fennica 22:79–91, 1991

Smith GC: From consultation-liaison psychiatry to psychosocial advocacy. Aust N Z J Psychiatry 32:753–761, 1998

Psychiatric Disorders in General Hospital Patients

Epidemiology of Psychiatric Disorders in Medically Ill Patients

William R. Yates, M.D.

Knowledge of the epidemiology of psychiatric disorders in medically ill patients provides guidance for many important public health issues. Without a thorough understanding of epidemiology, it is impossible to answer many important questions, including the following: What psychiatric illnesses have the greatest impacts on medically ill populations? How can psychiatric comorbidity be prevented in medically ill patients? Why should consultation-liaison psychiatry services be available in general hospitals? What curriculum structure should be used for teaching psychiatry residents and consultation-liaison psychiatry fellows? In this chapter, I address the important epidemiologic issues for consultation-liaison psychiatry by focusing on the key components of epidemiology: methodology, prevalence, risk factors, and course and outcome.

EPIDEMIOLOGIC METHODOLOGY AND CONSULTATION-LIAISON PSYCHIATRY

Diagnosis in patients with combined medical and psychiatric illnesses and studies of prevalence, risk factors, and outcome among these patients present several methodological challenges. These challenges are summarized in Table 14–1.

One key issue is the interpretation of psychiatric symptoms in medically ill patients. Many medical illnesses, or their treatments, induce common psychiatric symptoms such as fatigue, sleep disturbance, and impair-

TABLE 14–1. Methodological issues in the epidemiology of psychiatric illness in patients with comorbid medical illnesses

Diagnosis
  Medically induced psychiatric signs and symptoms
  Medication-induced psychiatric symptoms
  Substance-induced psychiatric symptoms
  Patient expectation of a medical explanation for psychiatric illness
  Effects of medical illness on cognitive function
  Effects of medication or substance on cognitive function

Prevalence studies
  Community samples vs. clinical samples
  Referral bias
  Diagnostic bias (single-illness studies vs. multiple-illness studies)
  General consultation services and liaison services

Studies of risk factors
  Role of medical illness as stressor (fear of pain, death, disfigurement, adverse economic consequences, or disability and loss of independence)

Course and outcome studies
  Separation of medical and psychiatric effects (disability, morbidity, and mortality)

ment of appetite and sexual function. Clinicians and epidemiologists face a challenge when establishing psychiatric diagnoses in situations in which the source of psychiatric symptoms is unclear. Medications used to treat medical illnesses often have adverse psychiatric effects. Medically ill patients are more likely to drink heavily and use illicit drugs. These substances can also induce psychiatric symptoms.

Another factor that increases the difficulty of psychiatric diagnosis is patient expectation of a medical explanation for all symptoms experienced. Patients often interpret psychiatric symptoms as results of medical illness. They seek help from medical physicians and expect a medical explanation. They may minimize psychological factors because of this expectation or because they are in denial about a socially unacceptable psychiatric cause.

Often clinicians are asked to perform psychiatric assessments of medically ill patients who have cognitive impairment due to their medical illnesses. For example, a clinician might be asked to assess a patient with cognitive impairment but not be aware of important alcohol abuse history that led to acute liver failure, which in turn led to the cognitive impairment.

Prevalence studies important for consultation-liaison psychiatry involve community and clinical populations. In community studies, the risk of referral bias or Berkson's bias related to studying a hospital sample is reduced or eliminated. However, results of clinical sample studies may have more practical application for consultation-liaison psychiatrists, who work directly with clinical populations. Clinical prevalence studies are often limited by referral bias—the referring physician must note the presence of a psychiatric illness to request a psychiatric consultation. Prevalence estimates will be artificially low when referring physicians fail to search for and identify psychiatric comorbidity.

Many prevalence studies involving populations served by consultation-liaison psychiatrists focus on a single psychiatric illness rather than on multiple psychiatric conditions. Single-diagnosis studies fail to take into account the comorbidity and complexity of psychiatric disorders in medically ill populations.

The prevalence of psychiatric disorders among medically ill patients can vary widely depending on the clinical sample studied. Series of inpatients referred for consultation can differ from outpatient series. Studies involving general hospital samples differ from those involving samples obtained from a focused liaison service (e.g., a liaison service for human immunodeficiency virus [HIV]/acquired immunodeficiency syndrome [AIDS]). A study of consultations in an obstetrics service will reflect the general population sex differences in psychiatric diagnosis.

When studying the risk factors for psychiatric illness in medically ill patients, clinicians and researchers need to address the role of medical illness as a stressor. Patients with acute or chronic illness fear many of the actual and presumed consequences of the illness, including pain, death, disfigurement, economic strain, and loss of function in work and social spheres. These fears may induce psychiatric disorders, particularly in those vulnerable to psychiatric disorder.

Course and outcome studies involving populations served by consultation-liaison psychiatrists present several additional challenges. Psychiatric and medical factors must be evaluated as factors contributing to disability. Psychiatric factors appear to play a significant role in functional outcome among those with medical illness. Major depression in patients with coronary artery disease increases deficits in activities of daily living (Steffens et al. 1999). Depression in persons with arthritis increases disability and the number of days of restricted activity (Vali and Walkup 1998). Disability related to a medical condition may also contribute to psychological stress (Ormel et al. 1997). Separating medical and psychiatric factors and weighing their relative importance can be difficult. It is important to measure outcomes and costs of depression and other psychiatric disorders in a variety of domains (Booth et al. 1997).

Epidemiology forms the basis for the understanding of clinical disorders in both medicine and psychiatry. In this chapter, I focus on the issues involved in the diagnosis and treatment of illness in patients with both medical and psychiatric disorders. The term *secondary illness* is used in this chapter to indicate an illness occurring after a primary illness. There may or may not be a pathophysiologic relationship between a primary disorder and a secondary disorder.

MODELS OF MEDICAL-PSYCHIATRIC COMORBIDITY

In medically ill patients, psychiatric illnesses occur at rates higher than expected by chance. The high rates of comorbidity can be explained by several models of relationship between the two illness types (Figure 14–1).

Medical illnesses can result in a variety of psychiatric disorders, including mood, anxiety, psychotic, cognitive, sleep, and sexual disorders (Model 1). One example of this pathway to comorbidity is the development of depression after stroke. There is strong evidence of a pathophysiologic relationship between stroke and depression, particularly when stroke involves those localized brain structures thought to modulate mood. Another example of a Model 1 relationship is depression associated with Huntington's disease. Some investigators have postulated a common etiological mechanism for autoimmune disorders and depression (Cohen et al. 1998).

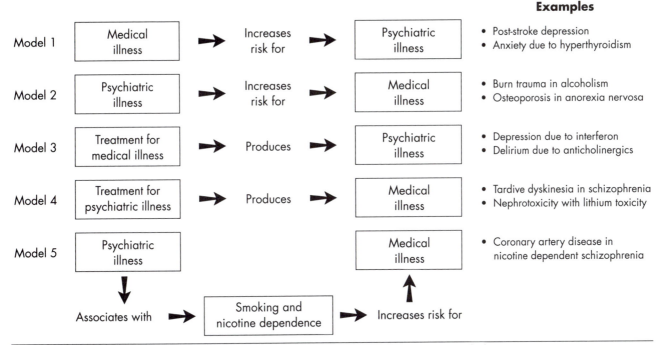

FIGURE 14–1.   Models of association to explain high rates of medical-psychiatric comorbidity.
Source.   Reprinted from Yates WR: "Epidemiology of Psychiatric Disorders in the Medically Ill," in *Psychiatric Treatment of the Medically Ill.* Edited by Robinson RG, Yates WR. New York, Marcel Dekker, 1999, pp. 41–64. Used with permission.

In a second model that explains a portion of the increased risk of comorbidity, psychiatric illnesses are designated that increase the risk of developing certain medical illnesses (Model 2). An example of this is alcohol dependence leading to alcoholic cirrhosis. Alcohol consumption is of course required for the development of alcoholic cirrhosis. The majority of patients with alcoholic cirrhosis meet criteria for alcohol abuse or dependence. Another example is the medical morbidity associated with suicide attempts. Affective disorder, personality disorder, and other psychiatric illnesses increase the risk of suicide attempts and suicide, and a significant number of admissions to medical intensive care units are for management of intentional overdose and self-inflicted trauma. Also noted in Figure 14–1 are the relationships between burn trauma and alcoholism and between osteoporosis and anorexia nervosa.

Medical treatments for medical illnesses can produce significant psychiatric symptomatology and psychiatric disorders (Model 3). In this instance, the psychiatric comorbidity occurs as a result of the adverse effect of treatment for the medical illness. Examples of this mechanism are the development of depression with treatment with interferon for hepatitis C and the development of delirium in a geriatric patient given an anticholinergic medication for the purposes of sedation. Often one cannot predict that a medication used to treat a medical disorder will have an adverse psychiatric effect. Certain

drugs and drug classes present higher risk. Nevertheless, when medical and psychiatric illnesses occur simultaneously, a medication-induced psychiatric syndrome should be considered.

Another mechanism for comorbidity is the development of medical complications related to the treatment for psychiatric illness (Model 4). Although the use of psychotropic drugs is usually safe, the risk of significant medical morbidity due to adverse effects and toxicity is present. An example of this mechanism is the development of tardive dyskinesia in association with long-term antipsychotic therapy for schizophrenia. In this example, the psychiatric illness requires a treatment that increases the risk of a medical disorder. Another example is renal complications linked to lithium therapy. Lithium can produce significant polyuria and even renal insufficiency.

A final mechanism that might explain some of the increased risk of medical-psychiatric comorbidity is the possibility of a link between psychiatric illnesses and behaviors or habits that increase the risk of medical illness (Model 5). One behavioral problem that is increased in psychiatric disorders is smoking and nicotine dependence. The medical complications associated with smoking are well documented. Breslau (1995) conducted an epidemiologic survey of the psychiatric correlates of nicotine dependence in a sample of more than 1,000 young adults in Michigan. DSM-III-R (American Psychiatric Association 1987) diagnoses including nicotine dependence were made using the Diagnostic Interview Schedule. The lifetime prevalence of nicotine dependence was 20%. Individuals with nicotine dependence were three times more likely than those without nicotine dependence to have a major depressive disorder. Additionally, nicotine dependence was associated with an odds ratio of 2.6 for any anxiety disorder, an odds ratio of 4.0 for drug abuse or dependence, and an odds ratio of 2.6 for alcohol abuse or dependence. Smoking and nicotine dependence appear to be associated with a variety of personality traits and disorders (Jorm et al. 1999; Yates et al. 1998). Adolescent depression and anxiety are associated with increased rates of smoking later in life (Patton et al. 1998).

The reason for increased rates of psychiatric disorders among persons with nicotine dependence is unclear. Gilbert and Gilbert (1995) proposed several mediators of the genetic risk of smoking, namely personality, psychopathology, and individual nicotine response. Nicotine dependence appears to be linked to neurotic traits (e.g., depression, anxiety, and anger), social alienation, and low achievement or socioeconomic status. Nicotine may be used by those with psychopathology to self-medicate for psychiatric symptoms. High rates of nicotine dependence among patients with psychiatric disorders increase the risk of smoking-related medical illness.

Studies of the prevalence of psychiatric illnesses in medically ill patients provide the basis for understanding medical-psychiatric comorbidity. In the next sections, I focus on general population and clinical studies of medical-psychiatric comorbidity.

PREVALENCE

General Population Studies

Few studies of psychiatric comorbidity in the general population have been completed. In the National Institute of Mental Health's Epidemiologic Catchment Area (ECA) study (Robins et al. 1984), a multicenter, population-based study, investigators focused on patients with DSM-III (American Psychiatric Association 1980) disorders and used a structured interview (the Diagnostic Interview Schedule). The prevalence of psychiatric disorders among subjects with general medical conditions was compared with that among subjects without general medical conditions (Wells et al. 1988). The eight medical disorder categories were arthritis, cancer, lung disease, neurological disorder, heart disease, physical handicap, hypertension, and diabetes.

Thirty-four percent of the approximately 2,500 persons in the study reported having one of the eight medi-

cal disorders. Twenty-one percent endorsed current treatment for their medical disorders. The most common medical conditions were arthritis (14.8% of the study sample) and hypertension (10.4%). The least common medical conditions were cancer (1.3%) and neurological disorder (1.3%). The presence of a medical condition was associated with significantly increased lifetime rates of any psychiatric disorder, mood disorders, substance use or dependence disorders, and anxiety disorders. Lifetime rates of mood disorders, anxiety disorders, substance abuse or dependence, and any psychiatric disorder were increased by 54%, 47%, 34%, and 28%, respectively. Rates of psychiatric disorders, particularly anxiety disorders, were also increased in the medically ill population during the 6 months before the interview. Recent anxiety disorders occurred in 11.9% of the patients with chronic medical illness and in 6.0% of the population without chronic medical illness. This represents a 98% increase for the group with chronic medical illness.

Wells et al. (1988) also focused on specific medical conditions. They found that all of the chronic medical conditions except hypertension and diabetes were associated with increased rates of psychiatric disorders. Rates of any recent psychiatric disorder were highest for heart disease (46%), arthritis (43%), physical handicap (40%), chronic handicap (32%), and neurological disorder (32%). In contrast, the rate of any psychiatric disorder among subjects with none of the general medical conditions was 18%. The authors of the study concluded that the rates of psychiatric disorders are increased in a variety of general medical conditions. They emphasized that investigators must pay attention to anxiety disorders when studying the epidemiology of psychiatric conditions in medically ill populations.

One weakness of the ECA study of medical and psychiatric conditions is the lack of information about the timing and sequencing of these two types of conditions. It is impossible to determine the mechanism for the development of the two types of conditions. Did the medical condition cause the increase in the rate of the associated psychiatric disorder? Did the psychiatric disorder lead to an increased risk of the medical disorder? Did treatment for either disorder lead to the other? More general population studies of the relationship between medical and psychiatric conditions are necessary, with attention paid to sequencing, timing, and causality.

Clinical Population Studies

Multiple Psychiatric Disorders

A study of DSM-IV (American Psychiatric Association 1994) psychiatric illness demonstrated the heterogeneity of psychiatric disorders in medical inpatients (Silverstone 1996). Three hundred thirteen consecutive medical patients admitted for treatment of medical illness participated in a study of DSM-IV diagnosis. Rates of psychiatric illnesses in the 7 days after admission were compared with rates of psychiatric illnesses before admission. Twenty-seven percent of the patients met criteria for DSM-IV diagnoses. The most frequent diagnoses were adjustment disorder (14%), anxiety disorder (6%), alcohol abuse or dependence (5%), and major depressive disorder (5%). In most of the cases of depression, the illness was present before admission. When medical staff and nursing staff were asked to identify patients with psychiatric illness, nurses recognized 61% of the cases and medical staff recognized 41%.

Barrett et al. (1988) conducted a well-designed two-stage study of the prevalence of psychiatric disorders in a primary care practice. The population sampled included adult patients of physicians in an internal medicine group practice. More than 1,000 patients were screened, and those with high screening scores were assessed with a direct psychiatric interview. The prevalence for all psychiatric disorder diagnoses was 26.5%. The majority of psychiatric disorders were depressive disorders or anxiety disorders.

Mood Disorders

After the onset of many medical illnesses, it is common for depression to occur (see Chapter 17). Depression secondary to medical illness appears to have some distinct clinical features. Winokur et al. (1988) summarized the differences between depression secondary to medical illness and primary major depression (major depression without medical illness). Depression secondary to medical illness is more likely to begin at a later age, respond to electroconvulsive therapy, and present with impaired cognition. It is less likely to be associated with a family history of alcoholism or depression and is less likely to result in suicide (Winokur 1990). Depression in medically ill patients may be preventable with the use of cognitive-behavioral interventions (Cuijpers 1998).

Many prevalence studies of depression in patients with particular medical illnesses have been completed. Although the methodologies of such studies often differ, findings appear to indicate that depression is common in a variety of disorders. In several studies involving patients with coronary artery disease, the rate of major depression was estimated to be 16%–19% (Carney et al. 1987; Forrester et al. 1992; Frasure-Smith et al. 1993; Schleifer et al. 1989). The rate of depression in patients with congestive heart failure appears to be higher (i.e., approximately

37% [Koenig 1998]). In patients with cancer, the estimated rate is in the 25%–38% range (Kathol et al. 1990; Massie and Holland 1990). The highest estimated rates of secondary depression in medically ill individuals occur in patients with neurological disorders such as Parkinson's disease (Sano et al. 1989), epilepsy (Mendez et al. 1986), and Huntington's disease (Folstein et al. 1983). These rates range from 40% to 55%. Haskett (1985) noted one of the highest rates of depression in a series of patients with Cushing's syndrome (67%). Depression in patients with Cushing's disease appears to be related to older age, female sex, and higher urinary cortisol levels (Sonino et al. 1998). Depression seems to be more common in patients with end-stage renal disease than in those with other medical conditions (Kimmel et al. 1998).

Katon and Schulberg (1992) summarized the findings of the studies of depression in primary care populations. The rate of major depression in the community has been estimated to be between 2% and 4%. In primary care studies involving ambulatory patients, the rate has been estimated to be between 5% and 10%. Among medical inpatients, the rate appears to be even higher, in the range of 10%–14%. The authors reported that two to three times as many primary care patients exhibit depressive symptoms but do not meet criteria for major depressive disorder. These findings indicate that there is a high rate of major depression and depression symptoms in primary care populations.

Geriatric populations tend to have the highest rates of medical disorders and also appear to have significant medical-psychiatric comorbidity (Kominski et al. 2001). Lish et al. (1995) examined a series of geriatric and nongeriatric patients attending a general medical clinic of a Veterans Administration hospital. Geriatric patients had high rates of a variety of psychiatric disorders, including mood disorders (primarily depression), anxiety disorders, substance use disorders, and somatoform disorders. The authors concluded that screening for depression alone in geriatric populations identifies only approximately one-half of all geriatric patients with psychiatric disorders. Depressive symptoms in geriatric patients contribute to self-ratings of poor health (Mulsant et al. 1997) and to increased numbers of hospital days (Koenig and Kuchibhatla 1998). The 1-year death rate for depressed elderly medical inpatients has been estimated to be 53% (Cole and Bellavance 1997). Medical illness is estimated to be a motivating factor in 50% of suicides among those older than 50 years and in 70% of suicides among those older than 70 years (Hendin 1999). Physicians need to expand their screening and assessment methods to include substance abuse, anxiety disorders, somatoform disorders, and cognitive disorders in geriatric medical populations.

Studies of Specific Psychiatric Conditions

Anxiety Disorders

Sherbourne et al. (1996) examined the prevalence of anxiety disorders in a series of family practice patients. Nearly 2,500 adult patients with hypertension, diabetes, heart disease, or depression were administered a structured interview for panic disorder, phobia, and generalized anxiety disorder. Depending on the type of presenting problem, 14%–66% of patients had one concurrent anxiety disorder. Anxiety disorder was more common among depressed patients than among patients with a primary medical illness.

Anxiety disorders including panic disorder have been increasingly recognized as important components of psychiatric illness in medically ill populations. Gerdes et al. (1995) examined the prevalence of panic disorder in a series of patients referred for psychiatric consultation during 1980, 1985, and 1990. Over that decade, medical physicians referred an increasing number of patients for evaluation of anxiety symptoms (10.6% of consultation requests in 1980 and 14.9% of consultation requests in 1990). The rate of consultation requests for panic disorder increased from 2.5% to 5.1% during the same period. Referring physicians identified panic attacks as a key feature in panic disorder at a much higher rate in 1990 than in 1980. Only 5% of patients with panic disorder in 1980 had panic attacks identified in the consultation request. The rate of identification of panic attacks in all patients with panic disorder was 59% in 1990. The development of DSM-III and DSM-III-R along with increased psychiatric training for medical physicians probably contributed to the increase in the rate of identification of panic disorder.

Trauma and medical illness may precipitate posttraumatic stress disorder. Rates of this disorder were four times greater than rates at baseline in a series of burn-injured patients (Tedstone and Tarrier 1997).

Primary care populations appear to have significant rates of mixed anxiety and depression. Pure major depression or pure anxiety disorder may be the exception rather than the rule for the majority of primary care patients with psychiatric disorders. Stein et al. (1995) studied a series of patients in a primary care outpatient setting. Seventy-eight (9.8%) of 798 patients screened demonstrated evidence of an anxiety disorder or a depressive disorder. Of those with a mood or anxiety disorder, only 20% had a depressive disorder alone and only 25% had an anxiety disorder alone. The majority (55%) had evidence of both an anxiety disorder and a mood disorder or significant anxiety in the context of depression that met criteria for mixed affective disorder given by the *International Statistical Classification of Diseases and Related Health Problems,* 10th Revision (ICD-10; World Health Organization 1992). This study confirms the need to consider the contribution of anxiety disorder to the clinical presentation of psychiatric illness among medically ill patients.

Although anxiety disorders can produce physical symptoms that mimic medical illness, it is possible that some anxiety disorders are more common in patients with certain medical conditions. A study of the prevalence of medical illness in patients with anxiety disorder demonstrated a link between panic disorder and peptic ulcer disease, angina, and thyroid conditions (Rogers et al. 1994). Studies of panic disorder have found no increased rate of serious medical illness but have found increased rates of use of medical services, impairment, and hypochondriasis (Barsky et al. 1999; Furer et al. 1997). Somatic complaints in patients with panic disorder or other psychiatric illnesses must be examined carefully to rule out significant medical illness.

Substance Use Disorders

Alcohol abuse and dependence contribute directly to significant morbidity and mortality in the United States and throughout the world. In the United States, an estimated 200,000 deaths per year are alcohol related (U.S. Department of Health and Human Services 1990). Approximately 25,000 of these deaths are due to alcohol-related motor vehicle accidents. Adolescents and young adults appear to be most vulnerable to the behavioral complications of drinking. Behavioral complications of drinking common in adolescents include alcohol-related trauma, alcohol-related legal problems, and high-risk sexual behaviors while intoxicated. Medical complications such as cirrhosis tend to occur after a long career of heavy drinking.

An estimated 25% of general hospital inpatients and 20% of medical outpatients have alcohol-related disorders (Cleary et al. 1988; Franklin and Frances 1996; Moore et al. 1989). Seppa and Makela (1993) studied the prevalence of heavy drinking in a series of inpatients at a university hospital in Finland. Heavy drinking was defined as drinking more than 280 g (by men) or more than 140 g (by women) of alcohol per week. Twenty-seven percent of men and 11% of women admitted to the hospital met criteria for heavy drinking. Physicians identified only 43% of men and 26% of women with alcohol problems. Psychiatrists and neurologists had the highest rates of correctly identifying alcohol problems, whereas internal medicine specialists had lower rates.

This study confirms that alcoholism goes unrecognized by physicians in a significant percentage of medical patients. Several factors may contribute to this underrecognition. Patients may be reluctant to discuss their drinking and drinking problems. Physicians may not ask about their patients' drinking or may not collect information from family members that might lead to a diagnosis of alcoholism.

Alcoholism contributes to a significant number of medical illnesses in various body systems. The extent of alcohol's contribution to specific medical conditions is designated the *alcohol-attributable fraction*. The alcohol-attributable fractions for a variety of medical conditions and events are listed in Table 14–2.

Drugs other than alcohol also contribute to medical disorders. Cocaine use has been linked to a variety of medical disorders, including necrosis of the nasal septum, seizures, myocardial infarction, cardiac arrhythmias, and significant weight loss (with long-term use). Intravenous use of cocaine and other drugs increases the risk of complications related to self-injection, namely endocarditis, septicemia, HIV infection, hepatitis B and C, pulmonary embolus, and local cellulitis and vasculitis.

Amphetamine use appears to be on the increase in the United States (Anglin et al. 2000). In one study it was found that 15.6% of patients referred for psychiatric consultation in a general hospital had used amphetamines (Baberg et al. 1996). Amphetamine use was documented by urine drug screens and verbal reports. Patients who used amphetamines had high rates of suicide attempts with medical morbidity and were more likely to be referred for psychiatric consultation from departments of infectious disease, obstetrics and gynecology, and trauma surgery.

The use of alcohol or drugs in pregnancy increases the risk of fetal and neonatal disorders. Heavy alcohol consumption during pregnancy increases the risk of premature labor and delivery and low birth weight. Cocaine use during pregnancy results in an increased risk of abruptio placentae and behavioral abnormalities in the infant (Chasnoff et al. 1985)

TABLE 14–2. Alcohol-attributable fractions for medical disorders [and events]

Alcoholic cirrhosis	1.00
Esophageal cancer	0.80
Homicide	0.46
Fire deaths	0.45
Motor vehicle accidents	0.42
Suicide	0.28
Stroke	0.07

Source. Reprinted from Yates WR: "Epidemiology of Psychiatric Disorders in the Medically Ill," in *Psychiatric Treatment of the Medically Ill.* Edited by Robinson RG, Yates WR. New York, Marcel Dekker, 1999, pp. 41–64. Used with permission.

Personality Disorders

Personality disorders in medically ill populations have been the subject of relatively few studies. One reason may be that the development of reliable and valid instruments for diagnosing personality disorders trailed the development of Axis I diagnoses. Also, personality disorders often are incorrectly assumed to be less prevalent and less important than the major Axis I psychiatric disorders. Several community studies of the prevalence of personality disorder have been completed (Reich et al. 1989a; Samuels et al. 1994). These studies estimated the community prevalence of personality disorder to be between 5% and 12%.

Some studies have found significant correlations between personality psychopathology and use of medical services (Polatin et al. 1993; Reich et al. 1989b). Cluster B personality scores among women correlated highly with the number of outpatient visits to a primary care physician. These studies point to the need for further exploration of how personality affects somatic symptoms and medical care utilization.

The few studies involving clinical populations suggest that personality disorder is common in patients with certain medical disorders, particularly chronic pain disorders and substance abuse problems. Polatin et al. (1993) interviewed 200 patients with chronic low-back pain who were entering a rehabilitation program. Fifty-one percent of these patients met criteria for at least one personality disorder. Personality disorders, anxiety disorders, and substance use disorders in this study tended to emerge before the onset of back pain, whereas depression occurred both before and after the onset of back pain. Personality disorders develop early in life and tend to be chronic, potentially influencing a variety of medical conditions.

Personality disorders are associated with a variety of chronic medical conditions and a variety of presenting complaints. A high percentage of a series of patients with chronic insomnia demonstrated personality disorder characterized by internalization of stress with an anxious-depressed reaction style (Schramm et al. 1995).

Somatoform Disorders

Kirmayer and Robbins (1991) surveyed 685 patients attending two family practice clinics. Using the Diagnostic Interview Schedule, these investigators described three measures of somatization: high levels of functional somatic distress; hypochondriasis, defined as high levels of worry about illness in the absence of serious medical illness; and somatic presentations alone in patients with current major depression or anxiety. One percent of subjects met criteria for somatization disorder, 16.6%

met abridged criteria for subsyndromal somatization disorder (these patients had significant functional somatic symptoms but did not meet criteria for somatization disorder), and 7.7% of patients exhibited hypochondriacal worry. A purely somatic presentation in patients with major depression or anxiety disorder occurred in 8% of the sample. This survey underscores the variety of manifestations of somatic distress in primary care and the high prevalence in common clinical outpatient settings.

General practice attendees in England have also had high rates of somatization disorder and other somatic presentations of psychiatric disorders. Using the General Health Questionnaire, Weich et al. (1993) surveyed a series of consecutive general practice patients. Pure somatization was considered present when somatic symptoms were judged in a medical consultation to be attributable to a psychiatric disorder unrecognized by the patient. Twenty-five percent of patients were identified as somatic presenters. Four percent of attenders met criteria for pure somatization. The majority of the remainder of somatic presenters were considered to probably have psychiatric disorders. Somatic presentation of psychiatric disorders resulted in lower rates of accurate psychiatric diagnosis compared with psychiatric presentation. This survey documents the tendency of somatic presentation to confuse physicians about the presence of psychiatric morbidity.

Other Psychiatric Disorders

Sleep disorders and complaints of chronic insomnia commonly present with comorbid psychiatric disorders. In a large series of more than 2,500 general practice attenders, patients with complaints of chronic insomnia were interviewed for the presence of psychiatric disorders including personality disorder (Schramm et al. 1995). One hundred five patients reported chronic insomnia, and 66 of these patients met DSM-III-R criteria for chronic insomnia. Of the patients meeting these criteria, 50% had at least one Axis I or II disorder. Mood disorders and substance use disorders ranked highest in terms of prevalence in this group. Insomnia in geriatric populations may be related to psychiatric or medical disorders or to treatment with medication (Jensen et al. 1998).

Another study of insomnia found increased rates among patients with certain medical conditions (congestive heart failure, obstructive airway disease, back pain, hip impairment, and prostate problems) as well as among patients with depression (Katz and McHorney 1998). Impaired sleep due to a medical illness may induce affective syndromes in those vulnerable to mood disorders.

Studies in Specific Medical Populations

Seizure Disorders

Seizure disorders have been noted to be associated with psychiatric symptoms and psychiatric disorders for many years. In one study, 97 consecutive patients admitted for neurodiagnostic imaging because of seizures underwent psychiatric evaluation (Blumer et al. 1995). Sixty-five percent of the patients were in need of psychiatric treatment. Mood disorders ranked first in prevalence (34%), followed by conversion disorder, pseudoseizure type (22%), and other psychiatric diagnoses (9%).

Traumatic Brain Injury

A well-designed survey examined the prevalence of psychiatric comorbidity in 50 outpatients with traumatic brain injury (Fann et al. 1995). Thirteen subjects (26%) demonstrated current major depression, and an additional 28% reported posttraumatic depression that had resolved. Generalized anxiety was noted in 24% of the sample, and 8% reported current substance abuse. Comorbid depression or anxiety was associated with significantly higher self-ratings of injury severity and cognitive impairment. These self-reports were not validated by objective measures of illness severity and cognitive function. This effect has been noted in patients with other medical illnesses. Medically ill patients with psychiatric illnesses tend to overestimate the severity of their medical illnesses.

Stroke

Stroke provides a model for understanding psychiatric disorders produced by lesions in various brain sites. Several psychiatric disorders occur at high rates after stroke. The focus of the most extensive work has been on depression after stroke (Robinson and Starkstein 1990). Depression complicates recovery from stroke in up to 50% of stroke patients. Depression may occur immediately after stroke or develop in the year after the event. The risk of depression after stroke appears to be related to lesion location. Stroke involving the left frontal region of the brain produces depression more frequently than does stroke in other brain sites. In addition to depression, stroke can also, in rare circumstances, induce mania (Starkstein et al. 1989). Generalized anxiety disorder also appears to occur in some patients after stroke (Starkstein and Robinson 1992).

Respiratory Disease

Psychiatric illnesses, particularly anxiety disorder and panic disorder, frequently complicate chronic respiratory diseases such as asthma and chronic obstructive pulmonary disease. Some patients with panic disorder seek evaluation for the purpose of determining whether their respiratory symptoms, which are related to their panic disorder, are caused by pulmonary problems. In a study of a series of patients referred for pulmonary testing, 41% reported panic attacks and 17% met screening criteria for panic disorder (Pollack et al. 1996).

Among patients with chronic obstructive pulmonary disease, the prevalence of panic disorder has been estimated to be 8%–24%, a rate range that is 10 times higher than the prevalence ranges for panic disorder determined in community studies of panic disorder (Karajgi et al. 1990; Yellowlees et al. 1985, 1988). Similarly high rates of panic disorder have been described for patients with asthma (Shavitt et al. 1992). Dyspnea is a common symptom of anxiety disorders, and the association between pulmonary disease and subjective complaints regarding breathing may be part of the reason for higher rates of anxiety disorders among patients with pulmonary disease (Klein 1993).

Cancer

A multicenter study of the prevalence of psychiatric disorders among cancer patients confirmed clinicians' impressions of high rates of psychiatric disorders in this population (Derogatis et al. 1983). Forty-seven percent of a series of patients with various types of cancer met criteria for psychiatric disorders when assessed with a structured psychiatric interview. The psychiatric disorder most commonly identified was adjustment disorder (in 32% of patients); the disorders with the next highest prevalences were major depression (6%), organic mental disorder (4%), personality disorder (3%), and anxiety disorder (2%). Estimated rates of depression have been higher in other clinical samples of cancer patients. It appears that pancreatic cancer is particularly likely to be complicated by depression (Holland et al. 1986). One hypothesis put forward to explain this association is that pancreatic cancers produce an antibody or autoantibody that crosses the blood-brain barrier and interferes with serotonin synaptic functioning (Lesko et al. 1993).

Gastrointestinal Disease

Psychiatric disorders occur in the context of a variety of gastrointestinal conditions at rates higher than expected by chance. The rate of psychiatric comorbidity among patients with irritable bowel syndrome appears to be particularly high. Walker et al. (1992) performed a survey of ECA study data on gastrointestinal complaints, depression, and anxiety. Medically unexplained gastrointestinal

symptoms were noted in 6%–25% of the general population. Rates of major depression, panic disorder, and agoraphobia were three times higher among subjects with one medically unexplained gastrointestinal complaint than among subjects without such complaints, and these rates were four to five times higher among patients with two or more medically unexplained gastrointestinal complaints.

Diabetes and Other Endocrine Disorders

For many patients, insulin-dependent diabetes mellitus is a serious, lifelong, progressive, and disabling condition. Like patients with other chronic diseases, patients with diabetes are reminded daily of their illness, being required to give themselves insulin injections and measure their blood glucose levels. Gavard et al. (1993) reviewed studies of the prevalence of depression in clinical populations with diabetes and found the prevalence range for depression among patients with diabetes to be 8.5%–27.3%, more than three times the prevalence range in the general population. The rate of death by suicide also appears to be increased among diabetic patients. Kyvik et al. (1994) studied a cohort of Danish men with diabetes who had been born between 1949 and 1964. The rate of completed suicide was 60% higher in this group than in the general population.

Thyroid disease appears to be associated with a variety of psychiatric disorders, including panic disorder, simple phobia, obsessive-compulsive disorder, major depression, bipolar disorder, and cyclothymia (Placidi et al. 1998).

Studies of Series of Patients Referred for Psychiatric Consultation

Wallen et al. (1987) reviewed 19 studies of the epidemiology of psychiatric consultation. Subjects were hospitalized medical patients in the United States, Canada, and Great Britain. Series ranged in size from 230 to more than 29,000 patients. The percentage of admitted patients referred for psychiatric consultation ranged from 0.6%–10.3%, the average being approximately 3%. In most studies of series of patients referred for psychiatric consultation, the most frequently encountered psychiatric diagnosis is depression. However, hysteria was the most common psychiatric diagnosis in a study of a series of pediatric patients referred for psychiatric consultation (Monnelly et al. (1993).

Wallen et al. (1987) reported the results of a study of consultation in general hospitals using a sample of 263,000 medical admissions. This sample came from a national data set in the United States. The rate of psychiatric consultation in this large series was 0.9%. Medical and psychiatric diagnoses were obtained from discharge abstracts and had been coded using the *Hospital Adaptation of the International Classification of Diseases (ICDA)* (Commission on Professional and Hospital Activities 1983).

The principal medical diagnoses associated with the highest rates of psychiatric consultation were accidents, poisoning, and violence; endocrine, nutritional, and metabolic diseases; and symptoms of ill-defined conditions. The principal medical diagnoses associated with the lowest rates of psychiatric illness were genitourinary system diseases, neoplasms, and respiratory diseases. The most frequently occurring psychiatric disorders in this series were neurosis, psychosis, alcoholism, and organic brain syndrome. Patients with somatoform disorders probably made up a significant percentage of the group of patients with neurosis.

MICRO-CARES Database Studies

The MICRO-CARES database studies are important epidemiologic studies in consultation-liaison psychiatry. The MICRO-CARES database was developed by James Strain, M.D., and colleagues at the Mount Sinai School of Medicine and represents an important advancement in the field of consultation-liaison psychiatry. In the MICRO-CARES database system, a structured interview with a standardized set of variables is used to collect information, using optical scanning technology or pen-based entry (Hammer et al. 1993b, 1995). The database is also linked to a literature database for consultation-liaison psychiatry and a checklist for operationalized interventions (Hammer et al. 1993a; Huyse et al. 1988). The MICRO-CARES database has been used to collect data in several sites, most notably Australia (Smith et al. 1993a, 1993b).

Several studies using the MICRO-CARES database system in specific populations have been published (Table 14–3). These studies examined psychiatric consultations regarding patients referred from a variety of settings, including general medical inpatient units (Clarke and Smith 1995; Smith et al. 2000; Strain et al. 1998) and specialty units such as oncology, obstetrics, renal, and HIV/AIDS units (Dunsis and Smith 1996; Judd et al. 1997; Kissane and Smith 1996; Rustomjee and Smith 1996). Mood disorders ranked first in the majority of the MICRO-CARES database studies of prevalence of psychiatric disorders. Organic mental disorders also ranked high in several studies. Two diagnostic categories, adjustment disorder and V code diagnoses, were a significant component in several samples (Strain et al. 1998). The MICRO-CARES database study was one of the first to

underscore the importance of adjustment disorder and V code diagnoses in samples in consultation-liaison studies. Findings of more MICRO-CARES database studies will likely be published in the future.

University of Iowa Series of Patients Referred for Psychiatric Consultation

For a better understanding of the epidemiology of psychiatric illness in the medical setting, data were reviewed from a series of patients referred for psychiatric consultation at the University of Iowa Hospitals and Clinics (Yates 1999). This consultation-liaison service sees patients referred from medical and surgical physicians and performs approximately 1,200 new consultations per year. About two-thirds of these consultations occur in the medical or surgical inpatient setting, and about one-third are performed in the outpatient setting.

A database for July 1, 1993, through June 30, 1995, provided information on psychiatric diagnosis rates for approximately 2,400 patients referred for consultation. This academic consultation-liaison service includes family practice and psychiatry residents. Each patient referred for consultation is seen by a psychiatrist with expertise in diagnosis in the consultation setting. Diagnoses are made using DSM-III-R or DSM-IV criteria. When multiple psychiatric diagnoses are present, the diagnosis that is most predominant or most related to the consultation request is coded.

Reviewed for the purposes of analysis were 200 consultations in the internal medicine setting and 200 consultations in neurology units, 200 in surgery units, and 66 in obstetrics and gynecology units. With the exception of obstetrics and gynecology, all consultations were selected randomly, with half of the subjects referred for consultation being female patients and half being male patients. Additionally, the series of patients was stratified by referral site, with half of each group seen as inpatients and half of each group seen as outpatients.

The distribution of the major psychiatric diagnostic categories, by referral source and site of consultation, is shown in Table 14–4.

Mood disorders ranked first on the prevalence list for all specialties and in the inpatient and outpatient settings. Mood disorders made up about one-third of all consultation diagnoses. This finding is consistent with the findings of the MICRO-CARES database studies. Some variability in prevalences of other disorders existed. Seven diagnostic categories—substance use disorders, adjustment disorders, personality disorders, anxiety disorders, cognitive disorders, somatoform disorders, and psychotic disorders—ranked closely together, with prevalences of

TABLE 14–3. Psychiatric illness prevalences determined in MICRO-CARES database studies

				Prevalence rate for specific diagnostic groups (%)					
Study	Prevalence period	No. of patients	Sample source	Mood disorders	Organic mental disorders	Adjustment disorders	Somatoform disorders	Personality disorders	Other
Clarke and Smith 1994	12 months	165	Medical IP units	55	35	19	16	15	
Kissane and Smith 1996	3 years	271	Oncology IP units	23	10	16			V code diagnoses: 24
Rustomjee and Smith 1996	3 years	299	Renal IP units						V code diagnoses: 35
Dunsis and Smith 1996	3 years	90	Obstetrics units	17		13		19	Schizophrenia: 15
Judd et al. 1997	2 years	292	AIDS IP units	36	18				Substance use disorders: 23
Strain et al. 1998		1,039	Medical IP units			12			V code diagnoses only: 6.4

Note. IP = inpatient.

TABLE 14–4. Distribution of psychiatric consultation diagnoses, by referring specialty and site of contact

	Internal medicine		Neurology		Surgery		Obstetrics and gynecology	
Disorder category	IP	OP	IP	OP	IP	OP	IP	OP
Mood disorders	31	41	38	46	25	25	10	15
Personality disorders	7	3	5	17	7	14	3	6
Substance use disorders	12	9	5	8	13	11	1	2
Adjustment disorders	8	13	6	3	10	10	5	4
Cognitive disorders	15	2	13	1	23	1	0	0
Anxiety disorders	6	14	5	10	4	13	1	2
Somatoform disorders	9	6	12	7	2	6	3	0
Psychotic disorders	8	6	5	1	11	6	5	2
No disorder	2	5	4	3	4	9	4	0
Other psychiatric disorders	2	1	7	4	1	5	1	2
Total	100	100	100	100	100	100	33	33

Note. IP = inpatient; OP = outpatient.
Source. Adapted from Yates WR: "Epidemiology of Psychiatric Disorders in the Medically Ill," in *Psychiatric Treatment of the Medically Ill.* Edited by Robinson RG, Yates WR. New York, Marcel Dekker, 1999, pp. 41–64. Used with permission.

5%–10%. Prevalences of most disorders were similar in the inpatient and outpatient settings (Figure 14–2). However, cognitive disorders, including dementia and delirium, occurred more commonly in inpatients than outpatients. The outpatient group included more patients with personality disorder and anxiety disorder diagnoses.

Distribution of psychiatric diagnosis varied somewhat by referring specialty group. Inpatients referred from surgery units had the highest rates of cognitive dis-

orders. Inpatients referred from neurology units had the highest rates of somatoform disorders. Substance abuse diagnoses were made in all groups, with rates slightly lower among obstetrics and gynecology patients.

The distribution of the psychiatric disorders, by referring service and sex, is shown in Table 14–5.

Mood disorders were common across both sexes, and the rates did not reflect the higher rates of mood disorders among women in the general population. However,

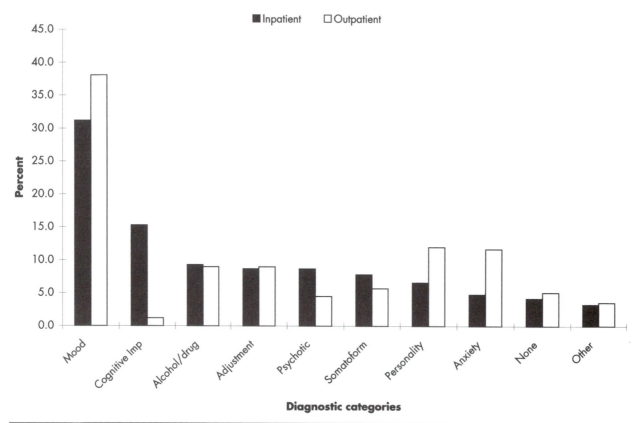

FIGURE 14–2.   Distribution of diagnosis in a University of Iowa series of patients referred for psychiatric consultation, by patient type.

TABLE 14–5.   Distribution of psychiatric consultation diagnoses, by referring specialty and sex

Disorder category	Internal medicine		Neurology		Surgery		Obstetrics and gynecology
	Female	Male	Female	Male	Female	Male	Female
Mood disorders	30	42	43	41	28	22	25
Anxiety disorders	16	4	8	7	9	8	9
Somatoform disorders	11	4	15	4	3	5	9
Adjustment	9	12	6	3	13	7	3
Cognitive disorders	9	8	9	5	13	11	0
Personality disorders	5	5	5	17	10	11	3
Substance use disorders	4	17	4	9	8	16	7
No disorder	6	1	5	2	8	5	3
Psychotic disorders	8	6	1	5	6	11	4
Other psychiatric disorders	2	1	4	7	2	4	3
Total	100	100	100	100	100	100	66

Source.   Adapted from Yates WR: "Epidemiology of Psychiatric Disorders in the Medically Ill," in *Psychiatric Treatment of the Medically Ill.* Edited by Robinson RG, Yates WR. New York, Marcel Dekker, 1999, pp. 41–64. Used with permission.

substance abuse diagnoses were more common among men in the series, as is the case in the general population (Figure 14–3). Anxiety disorders, adjustment disorders, and somatoform disorders were diagnosed at higher rates among women in the series.

The University of Iowa study provides a view of the spectrum of psychiatric illnesses in the medically ill population. Although the distribution of psychiatric disorders may vary by referring source, eight groups of disorders make up the majority of all diagnoses. In this

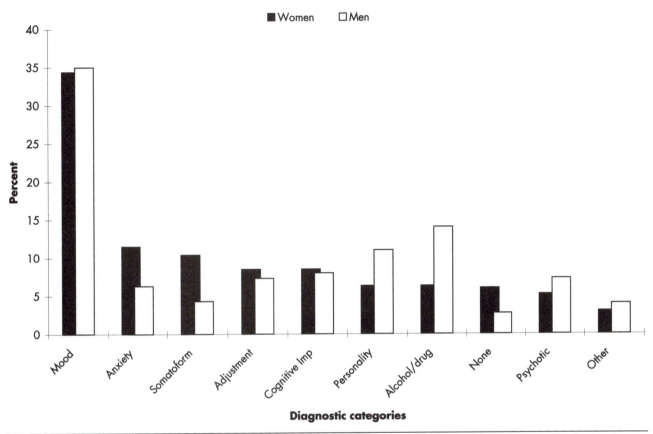

FIGURE 14–3.　Distribution of diagnosis in a University of Iowa series of patients referred for psychiatric consultation, by sex.

series, these eight groups made up more than 90% of the consultation diagnoses and formed the core group of psychiatric disorders in the medically ill population. In the next section, I address some of the risk factors for psychiatric illness in medical populations.

RISK FACTORS

Costello et al. (1988) conducted one of the few studies of risk factors for psychiatric disorders in pediatric primary care populations. Children ages 7–11 years were administered the Diagnostic Interview Schedule for Children, and 22% met criteria for at least one psychiatric diagnosis. Oppositional defiant disorder and conduct disorder were associated with male sex. Additionally, the risk of oppositional defiant disorder was increased in lower socioeconomic classes, among children who had repeated a grade, and among children without a father in the home. A parent reporting significant stress for his or her child was more likely to have a child with a behavior, anxiety, or mood disorder.

There has been limited study of the risk factors for psychiatric comorbidity among medical patients in general adult medical populations. However, risk factors for delirium have been studied and include severe medical illness, older age, premorbid dementia, male sex, and higher numbers of medications (Elie et al. 1998). In general, psychiatric illness appears more common in patients with more severe medical illness and patients with medical illness that results in significant impairment of daily functioning.

COURSE AND OUTCOME

Depression

Wells et al. (1993) studied the course of comorbid depression in patients with hypertension, diabetes, or myocardial infarction. More than 600 depressed patients from general medical practices were administered the Diagnostic Interview Schedule by telephone 1–2 years after an index interview. High rates of persistence of depressive symptoms occurred in both patients with medical comorbidity and those without. A history of myocardial infarction appeared to predict a more severe chronic course of depression. Myocardial infarction comorbidity in patients with depression predicted more episodes of depression, more symptoms during follow-up, and worse symptoms at the time of the follow-up interview. Comorbid hypertension and diabetes did not predict poorer outcome with regard to depression.

Recent studies continue to support the role of depression as important in the outcome of myocardial infarction (Lane et al. 2001; Penninx et al. 2001; Strik et al. 2001).

Patients hospitalized for depression have extended lengths of stay when concurrent medical illness is present. In a study by Schubert et al. (1995), depressed patients with physical illness were hospitalized nearly twice as long as depressed patients without physical illness (20.1 vs. 10.5 days). The investigators suggested that several mechanisms might explain the increased length of stay, including a tendency for depression to mask physical illness and a tendency to neglect physical symptoms when symptoms of a mood disorder are present.

Winokur et al. (1988) compared the clinical presentation and outcome of depression secondary to medical illness with those of depression secondary to psychiatric illness in a series of more than 400 patients. Patients with depression secondary to medical illness were older at the time of disease onset and had higher rates of cognitive impairment. However, the prognosis for depression secondary to medical illness appeared to be better. A higher percentage of patients with depression secondary to medical illness were improved at the time of discharge. Additionally, fewer patients in the medically ill group relapsed during the follow-up period, and in fewer cases was suicide the cause of death in this group.

Depression secondary to medical illness can be divided into two categories. In one category, the medical illness is a direct contributor to pathophysiologic changes in the brain that can induce depression. An example of secondary depression of this type is depression after stroke in the central nervous system sites thought to be important in the control and modulation of mood. Another category of secondary depression includes depression that does not seem to be due to a direct contribution to pathophysiologic changes in the brain. Examples of this type of secondary depression are depression in a patient with diabetes or depression in a patient with coronary artery disease. The clinical presentation and outcome of these two types of secondary depression may differ.

Yates et al. (1991) contrasted the clinical presentation and outcome of these two groups of secondary depression. Subjects in their study were identified from a series of patients referred for psychiatric consultation at a university hospital. Fifty subjects were identified with what was thought to be an "organic" depression due to a direct physiologic effect on the brain. The most common medical illnesses in this group were depression after stroke, seizure disorder, and corticosteroid use. The second group of 50 depressed subjects had medical illnesses *not* thought to have a direct pathophysiologic effect on the brain. The most common medical illnesses in this group were diabetes mellitus, hypertension, and coronary artery disease. Groups were matched by age and sex and compared on a variety of clinical and outcome measures.

The types of DSM-III-R symptoms did not differ between the two groups. Patients with organic depression had more severe Axis IV stress and received greater numbers of medications for their illnesses. They were also more likely to be having their initial episode of a mood disorder and to show evidence of cognitive impairment on cognitive tests. Despite similar exposure to adequate antidepressant treatment, fewer subjects in the group with organic secondary depression recovered during the year of follow-up. This study lends support to the concept of a poorer outcome and a poorer response to treatment in patients with secondary depressions thought to have an organic cause. The authors suggested that these differences add validity to the consideration of two types of secondary depression in medically ill populations.

Other studies support the idea that depression complicated by comorbid medical illness has a poorer prognosis than does depression without medical illness. Several studies examined the longitudinal course of depression among primary care patients (Mayou et al. 1988; Parker et al. 1986). Initial severity of depression predicts the outcome of depression: the most severe depression at the time of an index interview tends to have the poorest prognosis. Chronic medical illness appears to predict a poorer psychiatric outcome than do acute medical conditions. Chronic medical illness may produce a long-term psychological burden that prohibits complete recovery from depression. Further studies of the treatment of depression in patients with chronic medical illness are needed to determine whether this poor prognosis can be improved.

Anxiety Disorders

Up to 30% of patients develop generalized anxiety disorder after stroke. Generalized anxiety disorder can occur early or late in the course of recovery. Astrom (1996) found that early development of the disorder predicted poor functional outcome among patients with stroke. Only 23% of patients with early generalized anxiety disorder after stroke recovered by 1 year. Generalized anxiety disorder developing at any time was associated with dependence in daily activities and reduced social functioning.

Personality Disorders

Personality disorders in primary care settings can contribute to increases in medical morbidity, use of medical and psychiatric services, and psychotropic drug use. Seivewright et al. (1991) studied 357 primary care patients with psychiatric illness identified with a structured interview. Personality disorder predicted morbidity, psychiatric service use, and psychotropic drug use in this medical setting. Compared with their urban counterparts, rural primary care patients with personality disorder made more visits to their primary care physicians because of their medical illnesses. This study emphasizes the need for more study of the role of personality disorder in primary care settings.

Substance Use Disorders

The use of alcohol or drugs appears to complicate the course of many medical disorders. Alcohol plays a key role in the etiology of many medical conditions including hypertension, heart disease, peptic ulcer disease, alcoholic liver disease, pancreatitis, and cancer.

Jackson et al. (1995) studied the effect of current alcohol consumption on a series of family practice outpatients with hypertension, diabetes, heart disease, and/or major depression. Alcohol consumption predicted increased outpatient use of medical services in this primary care group.

In another study of alcohol use disorder in primary care, Sherbourne et al. (1993) examined 2,296 patients from a family practice. Subjects had diabetes, hypertension, heart disease, or depressive disorder. Both medical disorders and depression were associated with high rates of lifetime alcohol use disorder (14%–19%). Depressed patients with current alcohol problems were more likely to report a need for help with their drinking problem. Many patients in this primary care setting reported an unmet need for care for alcohol or drug problems. This study highlights the necessity for both accurate assessment of and treatment protocols for alcohol and drug abuse problems in primary care settings.

Medical Illnesses

Psychiatric disorders appear to influence the outcome of medical complaints and medical disorders. Clark et al. (1995) examined factors that predicted the persistence of fatigue in a series of patients followed for 30 months.

Seventy-eight patients who reported fatigue for 6 months or more were reevaluated 2.5 years after an index psychiatric examination. Persistence of fatigue symptoms was associated with DSM-III-R dysthymia at the time of the index interview. Other factors associated with symptom persistence included the following: presence of more than eight medically unexplained symptoms not associated with chronic fatigue syndrome, duration of symptoms of more than 1.5 years at the time of the index evaluation, less than 16 years of formal education, and age greater than 38 years. This well-designed study emphasizes the negative effects that comorbid psychiatric illness can have on medical outcome.

Several studies involving patients with insulin-dependent diabetes suggest that psychiatric factors contribute to poor compliance and adverse diabetic outcomes. Orlandini et al. (1995) studied a series of 77 patients with diabetes, using a structured self-report DSM-III-R personality inventory. Increased dramatic-dependent personality scores predicted high glycosylated hemoglobin levels (i.e., poor diabetic control).

ECONOMIC EFFECTS OF PSYCHIATRIC ILLNESS IN PRIMARY CARE

Psychiatric comorbidity can have significant effects on length of hospital stay among medical inpatients. Saravay and Lavin (1994) reviewed the studies of the effect of psychiatric comorbidity on length of hospital stay. More than 26 studies had been completed at the time of the review. The majority of studies in the United States found a significantly increased length of stay among patients in general hospitals. Psychiatric disorders associated with prolonged hospital stay included major depression, dementia, delirium, and personality disorder. Psychiatric morbidity may double the length of stay for trauma patients (Posel and Moss 1998). Well-designed research could lead to a better understanding of the mechanisms behind increased length of stay and provide strategies for accurate psychiatric assessment and prevention of long hospital stays.

Ormel et al. (1994) published results of a World Health Organization study of psychiatric disorders and disability in general practice populations. More than 25,000 patients from 14 countries were administered the General Health Questionnaire followed by the Composite International Diagnostic Interview. Psychopathology was a significant contributor to disability in this medical population, even when investigators controlled for effects of medical illness on disability. Disability was most significant in patients with major depression, panic disorder, generalized anxiety, or neurasthenia. A Canadian study confirmed the effect of depression on disability in long-term medical populations (Patten 1999). These studies underscore the impact of psychiatric factors on disability in medical populations throughout the world.

SUMMARY

Psychiatric morbidity occurs more commonly in persons with medical illness than in persons without medical illness. Comorbidity may develop when a primary psychiatric illness increases the risk of medical complications and when a primary medical illness increases the risk of a psychiatric illness. Treatment for medical and psychiatric illnesses can induce comorbidity. Psychiatric illnesses are associated with behavioral problems such as smoking and nicotine dependence that increase rates of medical complications.

Clinical population studies of medical-psychiatric comorbidity are more common than general population studies. However, clinical population studies are subject to various biases. For example, if psychiatric comorbidity increases the likelihood of seeking medical attention, clinical population studies would overestimate the extent of comorbidity. The ECA study provided evidence of true increased rates of medical-psychiatric comorbidity, in excess of what is expected by chance.

Clinical population studies of medical and psychiatric patients do support the concept of increased psychiatric comorbidity for a variety of medical conditions. Medical disorders that are chronic, disabling, and associated with significant pain appear to increase the rates of psychiatric comorbidity the most. Chronic pain of 6 months' duration is associated with a fourfold increase in depression and anxiety (Gureje et al. 1998). The rate of psychiatric disorders in patients with chronic daily headache approaches 90% (Verri et al. 1998).

In studies of patients referred for psychiatric consultation, mood disorders such as major depression and dysthymia ranked highest among all psychiatric conditions. The vast majority of psychiatric disorders in medical patients fall into seven categories: mood disorders, personality disorders, adjustment disorders, substance use disorders, anxiety disorders, somatoform disorders, and psychotic disorders. Studies of psychiatric patients have also documented a high rate of medical comorbidity.

Medical-psychiatric comorbidity predicts important aspects about clinical outcome and use of health services. Medical disorders accompanied by serious psychiatric illness are frequently associated with poorer outcomes, including increased mortality. In hospitalized medical patients, increased mortality may even be linked to higher numbers of depressive symptoms (Covinsky et al. 1999). High depression scores appear to increase hospital mortality in a variety of medical conditions (Roach et al. 1998). Self-reported depressive symptoms or substance abuse is estimated to increase yearly health care costs by $1,766 (Druss and Rosenheck 1999). Medical-psychiatric comorbidity increases the length and cost of hospitalization and the use of ambulatory medical services.

The epidemiology of psychiatric illness in medically ill populations underscores the need for further studies of the mechanisms of comorbidity and further studies of the treatment of psychiatric illness in specific medical populations. Such studies will address an important public health issue, help reduce morbidity and mortality, and provide strategies for the prevention of comorbid illness.

REFERENCES

American Psychiatric Association: Diagnostic and Statistical Manual of Mental Disorders, 3rd Edition. Washington, DC, American Psychiatric Association, 1980

American Psychiatric Association: Diagnostic and Statistical Manual of Mental Disorders, 3rd Edition, Revised. Washington, DC, American Psychiatric Association, 1987

American Psychiatric Association: Diagnostic and Statistical Manual of Mental Disorders, 4th Edition. Washington, DC, American Psychiatric Association, 1994

Anglin MD, Burke C, Perrochet B, et al: History of the methamphetamine problem. J Psychoactive Drugs 32:137–141, 2000

Astrom M: Generalized anxiety disorder in stroke patients: a 3-year longitudinal study. Stroke 27:270–275, 1996

Baberg HT, Nelesen RA, Dimsdale JE: Amphetamine use: return of an old scourge in a consultation psychiatry setting. Am J Psychiatry 153:789–793, 1996

Barrett JE, Barrett JA, Oxman TE, et al: The prevalence of psychiatric disorders in a primary care practice. Arch Gen Psychiatry 45:1100–1106, 1988

Barsky AJ, Delamater BA, Orav JE: Panic disorder patients and their medical care. Psychosomatics 40:50–56, 1999

Blumer D, Montouris G, Hermann B: Psychiatric morbidity in seizure patients on a neurodiagnostic monitoring unit. J Neuropsychiatry Clin Neurosci 7:445–456, 1995

Booth BM, Zhang M, Rost KM, et al: Measuring outcomes and costs for major depression. Psychopharmacol Bull 33:653–658, 1997

Breslau N: Psychiatric comorbidity of smoking and nicotine dependence. Behav Genet 25:95–101, 1995

Carney RM, Rich MW, Tevelde A, et al: Major depressive disorder in coronary artery disease. Am J Cardiol 60:1273–1275, 1987

Chasnoff IJ, Burns WJ, Scholl SH: Cocaine use in pregnancy. N Engl J Med 313:666–669, 1985

Clark MR, Katon W, Russo J, et al: Chronic fatigue: risk factors for symptom persistence in a 2½-year follow-up study. Am J Med 98:187–195, 1995

Clarke DM, Smith GC: Consultation-liaison psychiatry in general medical units. Aust N Z J Psychiatry 29:424–432, 1995

Cleary PD, Miller M, Bush BT, et al: Prevalence and recognition of alcohol abuse in a primary care population. Am J Med 85:466–471, 1988

Cohen P, Pine DS, Must A, et al: Prospective associations between somatic illness and mental illness from childhood to adulthood. Am J Epidemiol 147:232–239, 1998

Cole MG, Bellavance F: Depression in elderly medical patients: a meta-analysis of outcomes. CMAJ 157:1055–1060, 1997

Commission on Professional and Hospital Activities: Hospital Adaptation of ICDA, 2nd Edition. Ann Arbor, MI, Commission on Professional and Hospital Activities, 1983

Costello EJ, Costello AJ, Edelbrock C, et al: Psychiatric disorders in pediatric primary care: prevalence and risk factors. Arch Gen Psychiatry 45:1107–1116, 1988

Covinsky KE, Kahana E, Chin MH, et al: Depressive symptoms and 3-year mortality in older hospitalized medical patients. Ann Intern Med 130:563–569, 1999

Cuijpers P: Prevention of depression in chronic general medical disorders: a pilot study. Psychol Rep 82:735–738, 1998

Derogatis LR, Morrow GR, Fetting J, et al: The prevalence of psychiatric disorders among cancer patients. JAMA 249:751–757, 1983

Druss BG, Rosenheck RA: Patterns of health care costs associated with depression and substance abuse in a national sample. Psychiatr Serv 50:214–218, 1999

Dunsis A, Smith GC: Consultation-liaison psychiatry in an obstetric service. Aust N Z J Psychiatry 30:63–73, 1996

Elie M, Cole MG, Primeau FJ, et al: Delirium risk factors in elderly hospitalized patients. J Gen Intern Med 13:204–212, 1998

Fann JR, Katon WJ, Uomoto JM, et al: Psychiatric disorders and functional disability in outpatients with traumatic brain injuries. Am J Psychiatry 152:1493–1499, 1995

Folstein SE, Abbott MH, Chase GA, et al: The association of affective disorder with Huntington's disease in a case series and in families. Psychol Med 13:537–542, 1983

Forrester AW, Lipsey JR, Teitelbaum ML, et al: Depression following myocardial infarction. Int J Psychiatry Med 22:33–46, 1992

Franklin JE Jr, Frances RJ: Substance-related disorders, in The American Psychiatric Press Textbook of Consultation-Liaison Psychiatry. Edited by Rundell JR, Wise MG. Washington, DC, American Psychiatric Press, 1996, pp 426–465

Frasure-Smith N, Lesperance F, Talajic M: Depression following myocardial infarction impact on 6-month survival. JAMA 270:1819–1825, 1993

Furer P, Walker JR, Chartier MJ, et al: Hypochondriacal concerns and somatization in panic disorder. Depress Anxiety 6:78–85, 1997

Gavard JA, Lustman PJ, Clouse RE: Prevalence of depression in adults with diabetes: an epidemiological evaluation. Diabetes Care 16:1167–1178, 1993

Gerdes T, Yates WR, Clancy G: Increasing identification and referral of panic disorder over the last decade. Psychosomatics 36:480–486, 1995

Gilbert DG, Gilbert BO: Personality, psychopathology, and nicotine response as mediators of the genetics of smoking. Behav Genet 25:133–147, 1995

Gureje O, Von Korff M, Simon GE, et al: Persistent pain and well-being: a World Health Organization Study in Primary Care. JAMA 280:147–151, 1998

Hammer JS, Strain JJ, Lewin C, et al: The continuing evolution and update of a literature database for consultation-liaison psychiatry: MICRO-CARES Literature Search system 1993. Gen Hosp Psychiatry 15 (6 suppl):1S–73S, 1993a

Hammer JS, Strain JJ, Lyerly M: An optical scan/statistical package for clinical data management in C-L psychiatry. Gen Hosp Psychiatry 15:95–101, 1993b

Hammer JS, Strain JJ, Friedberg A, et al: Operationalizing a bedside pen entry notebook clinical database system in consultation-liaison psychiatry. Gen Hosp Psychiatry 17:165–172, 1995

Haskett RF: Diagnostic categorization of psychiatric disturbance in Cushing's syndrome. Am J Psychiatry 142:911–916, 1985

Hendin H: Suicide, assisted suicide, and medical illness. J Clin Psychiatry 60 (suppl 2):46–50, 1999

Holland JC, Korzun AH, Tross S, et al: Comparative psychological disturbance in patients with pancreatic and gastric cancer. Am J Psychiatry 143:982–986, 1986

Huyse FJ, Strain JJ, Hengeveld MW, et al: Interventions in consultation-liaison psychiatry: the development of a schema and a checklist for operationalized interventions. Gen Hosp Psychiatry 10:88–101, 1988

Jackson CA, Manning WG Jr, Wells KB: Impact of prior and current alcohol use on use of services by patients with depression and chronic medical illnesses. Health Serv Res 30:687–705, 1995

Jensen E, Dehlin O, Hagberg B, et al: Insomnia in an 80-year old population: relationship to medical, psychological and social factors. J Sleep Res 7:183–189, 1998

Jorm AF, Rodgers B, Jacomb PA, et al: Smoking and mental health: results from a community survey. Med J Aust 170:74–77, 1999

Judd FK, Cockram A, Mijeh A, et al: Liaison psychiatry in an HIV/AIDS unit. Aust N Z J Psychiatry 31:391–397, 1997

Karajgi B, Rifkin A, Doddi S, et al: The prevalence of anxiety disorders in patients with chronic obstructive pulmonary disease. Am J Psychiatry 147:200–201, 1990

Kathol RG, Mulgi A, Williams J, et al: Diagnosis of major depression in cancer patients according to four sets of criteria. Am J Psychiatry 147:1021–1024, 1990

Katon W, Schulberg H: Epidemiology of depression in primary care. Gen Hosp Psychiatry 14:237–247, 1992

Katz DA, McHorney CA: Clinical correlates of insomnia in patients with chronic illness. Arch Intern Med 158:1099–1107, 1998

Kimmel PL, Thamer M, Richard CM, et al: Psychiatric illness in patients with end-stage renal disease. Am J Med 105:214–221, 1998

Kirmayer LJ, Robbins JM: Three forms of somatization in primary care: prevalence, co-occurrence, and sociodemographic characteristics. J Nerv Ment Dis 179:647–655, 1991

Kissane DW, Smith GC: Consultation-liaison psychiatry in an Australian oncology unit. Aust N Z J Psychiatry 30:397–404, 1996

Klein DF: False suffocation alarms, spontaneous panics, and related conditions: an integrative hypothesis. Arch Gen Psychiatry 50:306–317, 1993

Koenig HG: Depression in hospitalized older patients with congestive heart failure. Gen Hosp Psychiatry 20:29–43, 1998

Koenig HG, Kuchibhatla M: Use of health services by hospitalized medically ill depressed elderly patients. Am J Psychiatry 155:871–877, 1998

Kominski G. Andersen R, Bastani R, et al: UPBEAT: the impact of a psychogeriatric intervention in VA medical centers. Unified Psychogeriatric Biopsychosocial Evaluation and Treatment. Med Care 39:500–512, 2001

Kyvik KO, Stenager EN, Green A, et al: Suicides in men with IDDM. Diabetes Care 17:210–212, 1994

Lane D, Carroll D, Ring C, et al: Mortality and quality of life 12 months after myocardial infarction: effects of depression and anxiety. Psychosom Med 63:221–230, 2001

Lesko LM, Massie MJ, Holland J: Oncology, in Psychiatric Care of the Medical Patient. Edited by Stoudemire A, Fogel B. New York, Oxford University Press, 1993, pp 565–590

Lish JD, Zimmerman M, Farber NJ, et al: Psychiatric screening in geriatric primary care: should it be for depression alone? J Geriatr Psychiatry Neurol 8:141–153, 1995

Massie MJ, Holland JC: Depression and the cancer patient. J Clin Psychiatry 51 (suppl 7):12–17, 1990

Mayou R, Hawton K, Feldman E: What happens to medical patients with psychiatric disorder? J Psychosom Res 32:541–549, 1988

Mendez MF, Cummings JL, Benson F: Depression in epilepsy: significance and phenomenology. Arch Neurol 43:766–770, 1986

Monnelly EP, Ianzito BM, Stewart MA: Psychiatric consultations in a children's hospital. Am J Psychiatry 130:789–792, 1993

Moore RD, Bone LR, Geller G, et al: Prevalence, detection and treatment of alcoholism in hospitalized patients. JAMA 261:403–407, 1989

Mulsant BH, Ganguli M, Seaberg MC: The relationship between self-rated health and depressive symptoms in an epidemiological sample of community-dwelling older adults. J Am Geriatr Soc 45:954–958, 1997

Orlandini A, Pastore MR, Fossati A, et al: Effects of personality on metabolic control in IDDM patients. Diabetes Care 18:206–209, 1995

Ormel J, VonKorff M, Ustun TB, et al: Common mental disorders and disability across cultures: results from the WHO Collaborative Study on Psychological Problems in General Health Care. JAMA 272:1741–1748, 1994

Ormel J, Kempen GI, Penninx BW, et al: Chronic medical conditions and mental health in older people: disability and psychosocial resources mediate specific mental health effects. Psychol Med 27:1065–1077, 1997

Parker G, Holmes S, Manicavasagar V: Depression in general practice attenders: "caseness," natural history and predictors of outcome. J Affect Disord 10:27–35, 1986

Patten SB: Long-term medical conditions and major depression in the Canadian community. Can J Psychiatry 44:151–157, 1999

Patton GC, Carlin JB, Coffey C, et al: Depression, anxiety, and smoking initiation: a prospective study over 3 years. Am J Public Health 88:1518–1522, 1998

Penninx BW, Beekman AT, Honig A, et al: Depression and cardiac mortality: results from a community-based longitudinal study. Arch Gen Psychiatry 58:221–227, 2001

Placidi GP, Boldrini M, Patronelli A, et al: Prevalence of psychiatric disorders in thyroid disease patients. Neuropsychobiology 38:222–225, 1998

Polatin PB, Kinney RK, Gatchel RJ, et al: Psychiatric illness and chronic low-back pain: the mind and the spine—which goes first? Spine 18:66–71, 1993

Pollack MH, Kradin R, Otto MW, et al: Prevalence of panic in patients referred for pulmonary function testing at a major medical center. Am J Psychiatry 153:110–113, 1996

Posel C, Moss J: Psychiatric morbidity in a series of patients referred from a trauma service. Gen Hosp Psychiatry 20:198–201, 1998

Reich J, Yates W, Nduaguba M: Prevalence of DSM-III personality disorders in the community. Soc Psychiatry Psychiatr Epidemiol 24:12–16, 1989a

Reich J, Boerstler H, Yates W, et al: Utilization of medical resources in persons with DSM-III personality disorders in a community sample. Int J Psychiatry Med 19:1–9, 1989b

Roach MJ, Connors AF, Dawson NV, et al: Depressed mood and survival in seriously ill hospitalized adults. The SUPPORT Investigators. Arch Intern Med 158:397–404, 1998

Robins LN, Helzer JE, Weissman MM, et al: Lifetime prevalence of specific psychiatric disorders in three sites. Arch Gen Psychiatry 41:949–958, 1984

Robinson RG, Starkstein SE: Current research in affective disorders following strokes. J Neuropsychiatry Clin Neurosci 2:1–14, 1990

Rogers MP, White K, Warshaw MG, et al: Prevalence of medical illness in patients with anxiety disorders. Int J Psychiatry Med 24:83–96, 1994

Rustomjee S, Smith GC: Consultation-liaison psychiatry to renal medicine: work with an inpatient unit. Aust N Z J Psychiatry 30:229–237, 1996

Samuels JF, Nestadt G, Romanoski AJ, et al: DSM-III personality disorders in the community. Am J Psychiatry 151:1055–1062, 1994

Sano M, Stern Y, Williams J, et al: Coexisting dementia and depression in Parkinson's disease. Arch Neurol 46:1284–1286, 1989

Saravay SM, Lavin M: Psychiatric comorbidity and length of stay in the general hospital: a critical review of outcome studies. Psychosomatics 35:233–252, 1994

Schleifer SJ, Macari-Hinson MM, Coyle DA, et al: The nature and course of depression following myocardial infarction. Arch Intern Med 149:1785–1789, 1989

Schramm E, Hohagen F, Kappler C, et al: Mental comorbidity of chronic insomnia in general practice attenders using DSM-III-R. Acta Psychiatr Scand 91:10–17, 1995

Schubert DS, Yokley J, Sloan D, et al: Impact of the interaction of depression and physical illness on a psychiatric unit's length of stay. Gen Hosp Psychiatry 17:326–334, 1995

Seivewright H, Tyrer P, Casey P, et al: A three-year follow-up of psychiatric morbidity in urban and rural primary care. Psychol Med 21:495–503, 1991

Seppa K, Makela R: Heavy drinking in hospital patients. Addiction 88:1377–1382, 1993

Shavitt RG, Gentil V, Mandetta R: The association of panic/agoraphobia and asthma: contributing factors and clinical implications. Gen Hosp Psychiatry 14:420–423, 1992

Sherbourne CD, Hays RD, Wells KB, et al: Prevalence of comorbid alcohol disorder and consumption in medically ill and depressed patients. Arch Fam Med 2:1142–1150, 1993

Sherbourne CD, Jackson CA, Meredith LS, et al: Prevalence of comorbid anxiety disorders in primary care outpatients. Arch Fam Med 5:27–34, 1996

Silverstone PH: Prevalence of psychiatric disorders in medical inpatients. J Nerv Ment Dis 184:43–51, 1996

Smith GC, Clarke DM, Herrman HE: Consultation-liaison psychiatry in Australia. Gen Hosp Psychiatry 15:121–124, 1993a

Smith GC, Clarke DM, Herrman HE: Establishing a consultation-liaison psychiatry clinical database in an Australian general hospital. Gen Hosp Psychiatry 15:243–253, 1993b

Smith GC, Strain JJ, Hammer JS, et al: Organic mental disorders in the consultation-liaison psychiatry setting: a multisite study. Psychosomatics 38:363–373, 1997

Smith GC, Clarke DM, Handrinos D, et al: Consultation-liaison psychiatrists' management of somatoform disorders. Psychosomatics 41:481–489, 2000

Sonino N, Fava GA, Raffi AR, et al: Clinical correlates of depression in Cushing's disease. Psychopathology 31:302–306, 1998

Starkstein SE, Robinson RG: Neuropsychiatric aspects of cerebral vascular disorders, in The American Psychiatric Press Textbook of Neuropsychiatry, 2nd Edition. Edited by Yudofsky SC, Hales RE. Washington, DC, American Psychiatric Press, 1992, pp 449–472

Starkstein SE, Robinson RG, Honig MA, et al: Mood changes after right-hemisphere lesions. Br J Psychiatry 155:79–85, 1989

Steffens DC, O'Connor CM, Jiang WJ, et al: The effect of major depression on functional status in patients with coronary artery disease. J Am Geriatr Soc 47:319–322, 1999

Stein MB, Kirk P, Prabhu V, et al: Mixed anxiety-depression in a primary-care clinic. J Affect Disord 34:79–84, 1995

Strain JJ, Smith GC, Hammer JS, et al: Adjustment disorder: a multisite study of its utilization and interventions in the consultation-liaison psychiatry setting. Gen Hosp Psychiatry 20:139–149, 1998

Strik JJ, Honig A, Maes M: Depression and myocardial infarction: relationship between heart and mind. Prog Neuropsychopharmacol Biol Psychiatry 25:879–892, 2001

Tedstone JE, Tarrier N: An investigation of the prevalence of psychological morbidity in burn-injured patients. Burns 23:550–554, 1997

U.S. Department of Health and Human Services: Seventh Special Report to the United States Congress on Alcohol and Health. Rockville, MD, National Institute on Alcohol Abuse and Alcoholism, 1990

Vali FM, Walkup J: Combined medical and psychological symptoms: impact on disability and health care utilization of patients with arthritis. Med Care 36:1073–1084, 1998

Verri AP, Proietti Cecchini A, Galli C, et al: Psychiatric comorbidity in chronic daily headache. Cephalalgia 18 (suppl 21):45–49, 1998

Walker EA, Katon KJ, Jemelka RP, et al: Comorbidity of gastrointestinal complaints, depression, and anxiety in the Epidemiologic Catchment Area (ECA) study. Am J Med 92:26S–30S, 1992

Wallen J, Pincus HA, Goldman HH, et al: Psychiatric consultations in short-term general hospitals. Arch Gen Psychiatry 44:163–168, 1987

Weich S, Lewis G, Donmall R, et al: Somatic presentation of psychiatric morbidity in general practice. Br J Gen Pract 45:143–147, 1993

Wells KB, Golding JM, Burnam MA: Psychiatric disorder in a sample of the general population with and without chronic medical conditions. Am J Psychiatry 145:976–981, 1988

Wells KB, Rogers W, Burnam MA, et al: Course of depression in patients with hypertension, myocardial infarction, or insulin-dependent diabetes. Am J Psychiatry 150:632–638, 1993

Winokur G: The concept of a secondary depression and its relationship to comorbidity. Psychiatr Clin North Am 123:567–583, 1990

Winokur G, Black DW, Nasrallah A: Depressions secondary to other psychiatric disorders and medical illnesses. Am J Psychiatry 145:233–237, 1988

World Health Organization: International Statistical Classification of Diseases and Related Health Problems, 10th Revision. Geneva, World Health Organization, 1992

Yates WR: Epidemiology of psychiatric disorders in the medically ill, in Psychiatric Treatment of the Medically Ill. Edited by Robinson RG, Yates WR. New York, Marcel Dekker, 1999, pp 41–64

Yates WR, Wesner RB, Thompson R: Organic mood disorder: a valid psychiatry consultation diagnosis? J Affect Disord 22:37–42, 1991

Yates WR, Cadoret R, Troughton E: Axis II comorbidity in nicotine dependence. Medicine + Psychiatry 1:30–35, 1998

Yellowlees PM, Alpers JH, Bowden JJ, et al: Psychiatric morbidity in patients with chronic airflow obstruction. Med J Aust 146:305–307, 1985

Yellowlees PM, Haynes S, Potts N, et al: Psychiatric morbidity in patients with chronic life-threatening asthma: initial report of a controlled study. Med J Aust 149:246–249, 1988

15

Delirium (Confusional States)

Michael G. Wise, M.D.

Donald M. Hilty, M.D.

Gabrielle M. Cerda, M.D.

Paula T. Trzepacz, M.D.

Delirium occurs in at least 10% of patients on medical and surgical wards, a figure derived from both referral and consecutive samples. Its prevalence is even higher in certain populations—30% among post–coronary artery bypass graft surgery patients (Smith and Dimsdale 1989) and 50% among post–hip surgery patients (Gustafson et al. 1988). The prevalence increases with advanced age and among individuals with existing or progressive brain disease (e.g., dementia of the Alzheimer's type) (Kolbeinsson and Jonsson 1993; Lipowski 1990). Therefore, as life expectancy increases—individuals older than 80 years (the "old old") are the fastest-growing age group in the population—the prevalence of delirium will also increase. The mortality associated with this psychiatric disorder is sobering: "Delirium is a common disorder in the hospitalized elderly and is a sign of impending death in 25% of cases" (Folstein et al. 1991, p. 169). Only dementia, when followed for several years, is associated with a higher mortality rate (Francis and Kapoor 1992; Roth 1955). In addition to an increased risk of mortality, patients with delirium have longer hospital stays (Francis et al. 1990; Franco et al. 2001; Marcantonio et al. 1994), face future cognitive decline (Francis and Kapoor 1992), use more hospital resources (Kane et al. 1993), have major postsurgical complications more frequently (Marcantonio et al. 1994), experience poor functional recovery (Cole and Primeau 1993; Inouye et al. 1998; Marcantonio et al. 1994; Murray et al. 1993), and are at increased risk for nursing home placement (Inouye et al. 1998; O'Keefe and Lavan 1997). Although delirium is commonly diagnosed by consultation psychiatrists and underdiagnosed by nonpsychiatric physicians, its phenomenology remains underresearched, and its treatment is largely empirically based. This is especially true of delirium in children.

A wide variety of physiologic and central nervous system (CNS) insults produce delirium, which helps to explain its high prevalence and extensive differential diagnosis. The latter is daunting to some physicians who are reluctant to investigate the multiple possible etiologies of an acute alteration in mental status. Diagnosis is further complicated because delirium may present as a hypoactive state (decreased arousal), as a hyperactive state (increased arousal), or as a mixed state with fluctuations between hypoactive and hyperactive forms (mixed variant). Accurate diagnosis must precede the etiological assessment and treatment. Without proper diagnosis and treatment, the prognosis for the patient with delirium is poor.

DEFINITION AND DIAGNOSTIC CRITERIA

DSM-IV-TR (American Psychiatric Association 2000) diagnostic criteria for delirium are listed in Table 15–1. The core symptom of delirium is impairment of consciousness with reduced ability to focus, sustain, or shift attention. Other DSM-IV-TR criteria include an acute change in cognition (onset usually over hours to days) that is not better accounted for by dementia, and a fluc-

---

TABLE 15–1. DSM-IV-TR criteria for delirium

A. Disturbance of consciousness (i.e., reduced clarity of awareness of the environment) with reduced ability to focus, sustain, or shift attention.

B. A change in cognition (such as memory deficit, disorientation, language disturbance) or the development of a perceptual disturbance that is not better accounted for by a preexisting, established, or evolving dementia.

C. The disturbance develops over a short period of time (usually hours to days) and tends to fluctuate during the course of the day.

D. There is evidence from the history, physical examination, or laboratory findings that the disturbance is caused by the direct physiological consequences of a general medical condition.

Coding note: If delirium is superimposed on a preexisting vascular dementia, indicate the delirium by coding 290.41 vascular dementia, with delirium.

Coding note: Include the name of the general medical condition on Axis I, e.g., 293.0 delirium due to hepatic encephalopathy; also code the general medical condition on Axis III (see Appendix G for codes).

---

tuating mental status during the day. When delirium is present, a specific diagnosis is made based on etiology. If an etiology is determined, the diagnosis is delirium due to a general medical condition (e.g., delirium due to hepatic encephalopathy or delirium due to hypoglycemia), substance-induced delirium (including medication side effects), or delirium due to multiple etiologies. If the clinician is unable to determine a specific etiology, a diagnosis of delirium not otherwise specified is made.

DSM-IV-TR states that various levels of psychomotor activity are associated with delirium, including hypoactive, hyperactive, and mixed behavioral states. Three lines of evidence support this subtyping:

1. The finding of equivalent degrees of cognitive impairment in hypoactive and hyperactive delirium (Ross et al. 1991)
2. The finding of diffuse electroencephalographic slowing for both hypoactive and hyperactive variants (Trzepacz 1994a), with the exception of delirium tremens
3. The finding of comparable responsiveness of subtypes to neuroleptic medication (Platt et al. 1994)

However, some neurologists do not classify delirium on the basis of its motoric presentation. They divide acute brain failure into two subtypes—an acute confusional state and an acute agitated delirium (R. D. Adams and Victor 1989; Mesulam 1985; Mori and Yamadori 1987). Delirium tremens, an example of hyperactive delirium, is the conceptual model used for delirium, even though it is the only type of hyperactive delirium that has associated electroencephalographic fast-wave activity and increased cerebral blood flow on single photon emission computed tomography (SPECT) scans (Trzepacz

1994a). These findings make delirium tremens an inappropriate model to use for other types of delirium. In patients who are acutely confused, incoherent, and disoriented but who do not have autonomic instability and hallucinations, some neurologists make the diagnosis of "acute confusional states" rather than delirium. This unfortunate disparity in the concept of delirium has historical roots, which were discussed by Lipowski (1980, 1990) and Berrios (1981). This disparity in terminology is especially notable in the limited literature on delirium in children.

EPIDEMIOLOGY AND RISK FACTORS

Within the last few years, systematic research into the prevalence and incidence of and risk factors for delirium has provided valuable insight into this disorder. The incidence of delirium depends on intraindividual factors and the specific etiologies involved. Engel (1967) estimated that 10%–15% of patients on acute medical and surgical wards have delirium. Lipowski (1990) suggested that this amount is an underestimate because the number of elderly people in the general medical population has increased. Listed in Table 15–2 are the ranges of prevalence for delirium in certain populations. The prevalence of the disorder across many studies ranges from 10% to 80% (American Psychiatric Association 1999). Cross-sectional studies of patients in emergency rooms have indicated a prevalence of delirium of between 10% and 14% (Lewis et al. 1995; Naughton et al. 1995). Of these patients, only 17% are recognized (i.e., have notations in their records) by emergency physicians as delirious (Lewis et al. 1995).

TABLE 15–2.   Prevalence of delirium in certain populations

Population	Prevalence (%)
Hospitalized medically ill patients	10–30
Hospitalized elderly patients	10–40
Cancer patients	25
Patients with acquired immunodeficiency syndrome	30–40
Postoperative patients	10–51
Terminally ill patients	Up to 80
Patients with coexistent structural brain disease	Up to 81

Patients who are at increased risk for delirium include the elderly (who often also have dementia and medical morbidity), patients with CNS disorders (e.g., stroke, Parkinson's disease, and human immunodeficiency virus [HIV] infection), postsurgical patients (e.g., postcardiotomy, posttransplantation, and post–hip surgery patients), burn patients, and drug-dependent patients who are experiencing withdrawal. Advancing age increases the risk; the group with the highest risk is usually patients age 60 years and older (Lipowski 1980, 1990). If children are excluded, the incidence of delirium increases with the age of the patient population studied. Sir Martin Roth (1955), while studying the natural history of mental disorders in older psychiatric patients, reported acute confusional states in 7.5% of patients ages 60–69 years, 9% of patients ages 70–79 years, and 12% of patients older than 80 years. More recent studies by Inouye et al. (1993) and Francis et al. (1990) using DSM-III-R criteria found that 25% and 23%, respectively, of patients older than 70 years had delirium during hospitalization. Increasing age is also associated with an increasing prevalence of dementia, which is an independent risk factor for delirium.

The aging brain has less "cerebral reserve" and flexibility in the face of external perturbations, including changes in vasculature, decreased cholinergic activity, and increased monoamine oxidase activity; all of these may increase an individual's vulnerability to delirium. Even with a relatively minor physiologic stress such as a urinary tract infection, elderly patients are more likely than younger adults to develop delirium. Preexisting brain damage, whether preoperative CNS neurological abnormalities (Koponen and Riekkinen 1993; Marcantonio et al. 1994) or dementia (Kolbeinsson and Jonsson 1993), also lowers the patient's threshold for developing delirium. Koponen and Riekkinen (1993) found that 81% of patients with delirium in their study had "coexistent structural brain disease" (p. 103). For many elderly individuals who live in the community, the first sign of

dementia is a delirious presentation to the emergency room (Rahkonen et al. 2000).

Brain damage related to HIV infection similarly increases the risk of delirium. Symptomatic HIV-1–seropositive individuals typically have significant cognitive deficits (Maj et al. 1994) that are consistent with a subcortical dementia. Perry (1990) reported that 90% of patients with advanced acquired immunodeficiency syndrome (AIDS) have organic mental disorders. In another study, delirium was the most frequent neuropsychiatric complication of AIDS (Fernandez et al. 1989).

In drug-dependent patients, discontinuation or rapid tapering of drugs, particularly alcohol and sedative-hypnotics, is a common cause of delirium and is often unsuspected in hospitalized patients. (For a more detailed discussion of substance-induced delirium, please see Chapter 21.)

Low serum albumin levels predispose patients to delirium, largely because of a reduction in drug-carrying capacity for protein-bound drugs, whose free serum levels then increase to cause toxicity, despite total serum levels in the normal therapeutic range (Trzepacz and Francis 1990). Malnutrition, chronic disease, aging, nephrotic syndrome, and hepatic insufficiency are common causes of low serum albumin levels.

DSM-IV-TR states that "children may be particularly susceptible to delirium compared with adults (other than the elderly), especially when it is related to febrile illnesses and certain medications (e.g., anticholinergics)" (p. 138); however, delirium in children is vastly understudied. Prugh et al. (1980) described the only systematic, controlled study of delirium in children using electroencephalograms (EEGs), cognitive tests, and neurological and psychiatric examinations. They found the same constellation of symptoms as that which has been described for adult delirium. In Kornfeld and colleagues' (1965) sample of 119 unselected patients who had open heart surgery, none of the 20 children developed delirium, whereas 30% of the adults did. However, children do experience delirium, as evidenced by reports of "encephalopathy," "confusion," or "posttraumatic amnesia" associated with, for example, AIDS; cancer chemotherapy; closed-head injury; emergence from anesthesia; organ failure; hypoxia due to status asthmaticus, near drowning, asphyxiation, or foreign body ingestion; CNS viral infections; fever; sepsis; seizures; alcohol dependence and withdrawal; anorexia nervosa; and inhalation of vapors from substances such as Wite-Out.

Although sleep deprivation and sensory deprivation may contribute to the severity of delirium, these conditions are not sufficient to cause delirium independently (Francis 1993). Sleep-wake abnormalities are a frequent component of delirium, which suggests brain stem and/or diencephalic dysfunction. Harrell and Othmer (1987) found that sleep disturbance developed after the onset of cognitive impairment (as determined by the Mini-Mental State Exam), which suggests that the disturbance was a symptom, rather than the cause, of delirium.

No personality or premorbid psychological variables, such as depression or anxiety, have been found to be associated with delirium or to predict its behavioral presentation (Dubin et al. 1979; Lipowski 1980). This suggests that the occurrence of delirium and its symptoms is more likely reflective of underlying neuropathophysiologic changes that produce a constellation of characteristic symptoms. Whether subtypes of delirium exist with differing symptom profiles based on particular biochemical categories of underlying neuropathophysiologic perturbations has not yet been clarified (Trzepacz 1994a).

CLINICAL FEATURES

Prodrome

Some patients manifest subclinical symptoms such as restlessness, anxiety, irritability, distractibility, or sleep disruption immediately before the onset of an overt delirium. In children, developmental issues, particularly regressive behavior, may contribute to the clinical and subclinical manifestations of delirium (Prugh et al. 1980). Review of the patient's hospital medical chart, particularly the nursing notes, may reveal prodromal features, although prospective studies to define a threshold for delirium have not been conducted.

Temporal Course

Two features of the temporal course of delirium are characteristic and assist in differential diagnosis: 1) abrupt or acute onset of symptoms and 2) fluctuation in symptom severity during an episode. The acute onset is sometimes more difficult to ascertain in the setting of preexisting dementia, but a stepwise decline or alteration in behavior can be elucidated retrospectively, even in nursing home patients. Waxing and waning of symptoms occurs often, with relatively lucid intervals fluctuating with more severe symptoms; careful examination usually reveals continued cognitive impairment even during lucid periods. Dementias do not characteristically fluctuate during a 24-hour period; an exception is Lewy body dementia, which can be difficult to distinguish from delirium.

Nocturnal agitation, also known as *sundowning*, occurs in patients with Alzheimer's disease, Parkinson's disease, or other disorders (Lipowski 1980, 1989). There are several differences between delirium and sundowning (Bliwise 1994). Patients with sundowning have agitation that is caused by or strongly associated with darkness, and they do not experience fluctuation throughout the 24-hour period or the diurnal variation that patients with delirium experience. Indeed, sundowning has been induced in patients with dementia by bringing these patients into a dark room during the daytime (D. E. Cameron 1941). Systematic observations of nursing home patients revealed that sleep is less likely between 3:00 and 7:00 P.M. (adjustments were made for potential disruption by dinner) (Bliwise et al. 1993). Vocalizations and physically aggressive behaviors are more likely to occur between 4:30 and 11:00 P.M. than earlier in the day (Cohen-Mansfield et al. 1992), and wandering is most likely between 7:00 and 10:00 P.M. (Martino-Saltzman et al. 1991). Other factors that could affect agitation include staff-induced awakening, the patient-to-staff ratio, shift changes, use of medication, the number and severity of medical conditions, and the physical environment. Circadian rhythmicity probably plays a part in sundowning; therefore, more information on the utility of exposure to bright light, administration of melatonin, and other interventions is needed.

Diffuse Cognitive Impairment

Attentional Deficits

Patients with delirium have difficulty sustaining attention and are usually distractible or unable to focus. The attentional deficits in delirium have not been well studied but may reflect a combination of prefrontal, parietal, and subcortical dysfunctions (Trzepacz 1994a). Poor performance on the Trail Making Test reflects poor concentration, visuomotor impairment, and difficulty switching mental sets (Trzepacz et al. 1988a; Weissenborn et al. 1998).

Memory Impairment

Both short- and long-term memory are impaired in patients with delirium. When impaired registration is present, memory difficulties may be secondary to attention deficits. Long-term declarative memory is often impaired, although procedural memory is rarely evaluated in general hospital settings. After recovering from delirium, some patients are amnestic for the entire episode; others have islands of memory for certain experiences. These experiences are generally remembered negatively; therefore, patients must be reassured that delirium is transient and occurs commonly in medically ill patients.

Disorientation

Disorientation to time and place is common in patients with delirium, with some fluctuation during relatively lucid intervals. Disorientation to person occurs often for doctors and nurses, less often for immediate family members, and rarely for the patient himself or herself. It is not unusual for a patient with delirium to believe that he or she is in a familiar place (e.g., a room at home) instead of in the hospital.

Visuoconstructional Impairment

Visuoconstructional impairment occurs often in patients with delirium. This finding lends support to the concept of diffuse cognitive deficits in delirium, because posterior cortical regions are important for spatial relations. Patients may be unable to copy simple geometric designs or to draw more complex figures such as a clock face (see Figure 15–1). Clock face drawing requires input from the nondominant parietal cortex for overall spatial proportions and relations, from the dominant parietal cortex for details such as numbers or hands, and from the prefrontal cortex for understanding the concept of time (e.g., placing the minute hand correctly even though only hours are numbered). Instructions and scoring of clock face drawing are described elsewhere (Trzepacz and Baker 1993).

Prefrontal Executive Functions

Many higher-level cognitive functions are subserved by the prefrontal cortices, especially the dorsolateral region. These functions are impaired in delirium (Trzepacz 1994b) and include switching of mental sets, abstraction, sequential thinking, verbal fluency, temporal memory, and judgment. Patients with delirium experience perseveration, concrete thinking, distractibility, and impaired performance on the Trail Making Test.

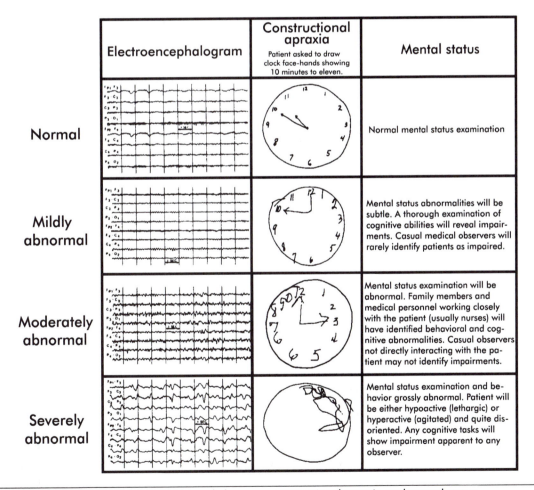

FIGURE 15–1. Comparison of electroencephalogram, constructional apraxia, and mental status.

Source. Reprinted from Wise MG, Brandt GT: "Neuropsychiatric Aspects of Delirium," in *The American Psychiatric Press Textbook of Neuropsychiatry*, 3rd Edition. Edited by Yudofsky SC, Hales RE. Washington, DC, American Psychiatric Press, 1997, p. 454. Copyright 1997, American Psychiatric Press. Used with permission.

Thought and Language Disturbances

Patients with delirium often have disorganized thought patterns. The disorganization can range from tangentiality and circumstantiality to loose associations. When thought disturbance is at its most severe level of disorganization, speech may resemble a fluent aphasia.

Language impairments range from mild dysarthria or mumbling to dysphasia or muteness. Word-finding difficulty, dysnomia with paraphasias, and reduced comprehension are common. Dysnomia and dysgraphia are not specific to delirium; however, the content of the writing may demonstrate some impairment, which may indeed be more specific to delirium (Patten and Lamarre 1989).

Perceptual Disturbances

Patients with delirium often experience misperceptions, usually illusions or hallucinations, and infrequently experience metamorphopsias or delusional misidentifications. Illusions and hallucinations can be auditory or visual, but the latter are more common and therefore raise the suspicion of organicity whenever they occur. Tactile, gustatory, and olfactory hallucinations are less common.

Hallucinations can be simple visual hallucinations or complex hallucinations. Delirium tremens is classically associated with often vivid visual hallucinations and misperceptions.

Psychomotor Disturbances

Many patients with delirium have changes in psychomotor behavior—either hypoactive or hyperactive, or some combination. Hypoactive patients appear apathetic, somnolent, and quietly confused and usually receive a misdiagnosis of "depression" by nonpsychiatric physicians and nurses. Koponen and Riekkinen (1993) found that those patients with the "silent," or hypoactive, form of delirium had the most severe cognitive impairment compared with patients with hyperactive or mixed forms. However, Ross et al. (1991) found comparable cognitive impairment, and Camus et al. (2000) found comparable outcome, in patients with hypoactive and those with hyperactive subtypes. In hyperactive delirium, the patient is agitated and hypervigilant and exhibits psychomotor hyperactivity. In one study of elderly patients with delirium, the disorder was classified as hyperactive in 15%, hypoactive in 19%, mixed in 52%, and neither in 14% (Liptzin and Levkoff 1992). In another study, Kobayashi et al. (1992) found that delirium was hyperactive in 78% of patients, hypoactive in 7%, and mixed in 15%. (Alcoholic patients were excluded in this study).

Disturbance of the Sleep-Wake Cycle

Sleep-wake disturbance is common in patients with delirium and ranges from insomnia to total disintegration of the sleep-wake cycle throughout a 24-hour period, with multiple periods of napping or drowsiness during the day and night. Reduction in external cues during the night may increase disorientation or paranoia, which may cause agitation. Restoration of the normal diurnal sleep cycle is an important goal in treatment.

Delusions

Delusions are generally of a paranoid type and are not as well systematized as those that occur in patients with schizophrenia, nor are they mood congruent, unlike typical delusions experienced by patients with depression or mania. Delusions occur in about one-fifth of patients with delirium. Persecutory ideas can lead to violent behavior and inadvertent harm to medical staff.

Affective Lability

Patients with delirium may exhibit rapid fluctuations in their emotional state (e.g., from fear to incongruent crying to irritability) consistent with affective lability characteristic of organicity. Emotional responses seen in patients with delirium include anxiety, panic, fear, anger, rage, sadness, apathy, and—rarely, except in steroid-induced delirium—euphoria. Medical and nursing staff often focus on the emotional or behavioral disturbance and do not recognize the underlying delirium. This leads to inappropriate consultation for "depression" (Nicholas and Lindsey 1995) or a "character problem." Prospective studies indicate that 23%–42% of patients referred by a staff-level physician to a consultation-liaison service for depression are subsequently given a diagnosis of delirium by the psychiatrist (Farrell and Ganzini 1995; Valan and Hilty 1996).

Neurological Abnormalities

Physical Examination

Neurological abnormalities that occur in delirium are indicative of the underlying etiology because no focal motor or sensory signs are specific to the syndrome. Motor findings include tremor, myoclonus, asterixis, and reflex or muscle tone changes. The tremor associated with delirium, particularly the toxic-metabolic tremor, is generally absent at rest but apparent during movement (action or intention tremors). Tremor types differ according to underlying conditions (e.g., delirium tremens or lithium toxicity), and the type of tremor may be a clue to the etiology of the delirium. Myoclonus and asterixis (liver flap) occur in toxic and metabolic conditions, especially uremia and hepatic insufficiency. Symmetric reflex and muscle tone changes can also occur—for example, in myxedema, carbon monoxide poisoning, neuroleptic malignant syndrome, and alcohol or sedative-hypnotic withdrawal. Nystagmus and ataxia accompany some drug intoxications. Cranial nerve palsies affecting extraocular movements occur in patients with Wernicke's encephalopathy and reverse promptly with thiamine administration. Lithium intoxication is associated with cerebellar signs.

Sensory abnormalities are difficult to detect during delirium. For example, delirium due to nondominant parietal-lobe infarction is accompanied by an inferior quadrantanopia that cannot be detected during acute confusion.

Electroencephalographic Abnormalities

Engel and Romano (1959), in their classic article entitled "Delirium, a Syndrome of Cerebral Insufficiency," proposed that the basic etiology of delirium was a derangement in metabolism manifested clinically by diffuse disturbances in cognitive functions and physiologically by generalized slowing of the electroencephalographic background rhythm. Pro and Wells (1977) reported that electroencephalographic changes virtually always accompany delirium. Hepatic encephalopathy is classically associated with severe slowing including triphasic delta waves. The electroencephalographic slowing illustrated in Figure 15–1 is representative of delirium with toxic-metabolic etiologies. Less typically, the electroencephalographic pattern in delirium is characterized by excess low-voltage beta waves, as seen most typically in delirium tremens (Kennard et al. 1945). This suggests that low-voltage fast activity is associated with hyperactive, agitated, heightened arousal (Pro and Wells 1977). However, fast activity is not associated with any hyperactive delirium other than delirium tremens. For example, patients with delirium caused by anticholinergic toxicity or posttraumatic brain injury exhibit electroencephalographic slowing (Trzepacz 1994a).

Unfortunately, an individual's normal dominant posterior rhythm could be slowed but still be in the alpha range and therefore be read as "normal." For example, a patient's normal background characteristic alpha rhythm is 13 Hz; when it slows to 9 Hz, it is technically still in the normal alpha range. Comparison with a prior baseline EEG or with a repeat EEG after the delirium clears is the only way to document the abnormality. Electroencephalographic slowing may also be out of phase temporally with the time course of severity of clinical symptoms (Andreasen et al. 1977).

DIAGNOSIS

The diagnosis of delirium requires recognition of the clinical features of the syndrome, as discussed in the previous section of this chapter, and a thorough evaluation of the patient's mental and physical status. In addition to conducting a routine bedside mental status examination, the examiner should test a broad range of cognitive functions to determine whether the patient meets the diagnostic criterion of diffuse impairment. Cognitive functions tested should include attention and concentration, short- and long-term memory, visuoconstructional ability (see Figure 15–1), abstraction, and language, such as writing and confrontational naming.

The gold standard for diagnosis is a clinical evaluation using DSM criteria, and the most useful diagnostic laboratory measure is the EEG. In addition to cognitive tests (e.g., Mini-Mental State Exam; Folstein et al. 1975), which document some symptoms of delirium but cannot alone distinguish delirium from dementia, several instruments measure a broader range of symptoms of delirium and can be used for screening purposes or to quantitate symptom severity. The Delirium Rating Scale (DRS; Trzepacz et al. 1988b) and the Confusion Assessment Method (CAM; Inouye et al. 1990) are two useful tests. The CAM is an algorithm of four cardinal symptoms of delirium that is used in high-risk settings by nonpsychiatric clinicians. It can be supplemented by more intensive interviews to diagnose delirium. The DRS, which requires psychiatric training to administer, rates the severity of a broad range of delirium symptoms using explicit descriptions for each item; it distinguishes delirium from other psychiatric disorders. The DRS is the most widely used delirium assessment instrument and is available in six languages (English, French, Spanish, Dutch, Japanese, and Italian). It will soon be translated into Mandarin Chinese (Trzepacz 1994b). In elderly patients, sensitivity and specificity improve when a cut point of 8 is used instead of the usual 10 (Rockwood et al. 1996).

DIFFERENTIAL DIAGNOSIS

Because the differential diagnosis of delirium is extensive, a reluctance to search carefully for etiologies sometimes exists. Confusional states, particularly in critically ill and elderly patients, often have multiple causes (Trzepacz et al. 1985). Francis et al. (1990) found that 56% of elderly patients with delirium had a single definite or probable etiology, and the remaining 44% had an average of 2.8 etiologies each. When no apparent etiology exists at the time of consultation, one often becomes apparent within a few days. Not uncommonly, unrecognized medication use or substance abuse is the cause of an intoxication or withdrawal delirium.

Laboratory and radiological evaluation of patients with delirium may be basic or may involve additional tests (see Table 15–3). The basic battery is ordered for virtually every patient with delirium. Additional tests are ordered depending on the specifics of a particular case. When information about the patient's mental and physical status is combined with the basic laboratory battery, the specific etiology (or etiologies) is often apparent. If not, the clinician should review the case and consider ordering further diagnostic studies. Computed tomography or magnetic resonance imaging of the brain and cerebrospinal fluid examination are of higher priority in immunosuppressed patients, such as patients who have undergone organ transplantation and patients with AIDS.

Terms such as *ICU* (intensive care unit) *psychosis* are inappropriately used to explain delirium. Such terms imply that no attempt at specific diagnosis is necessary because the environment is to blame. Koponen et al. (1989) found clear organic etiologies in 87% of patients with delirium. They also found that the few patients who became confused because of psychological and environmental events actually had severe dementia.

Organizing the large number of potential causes of delirium into a usable differential diagnosis might be enhanced by using the following two-tiered differential diagnostic system.

Emergent Items (WHHHHIMP)

The first level of this diagnostic system is the "emergent diagnoses" (mnemonic WHHHHIMP), which the physician must make early in the course of a delirium because failure to do so can result in irreversible injury to the patient. We describe each letter of this mnemonic here:

TABLE 15–3.   Assessment of the patient with delirium

Physical status

    History

    Physical and neurological examination

    Review of vital signs and anesthesia record if patient is postoperative

    Review of medical records

    Careful review of medications and correlation with behavioral changes

Mental status

    Interview

    Cognitive tests (e.g., clock face drawing, Trail Parts A and B)

Basic laboratory tests—*consider in every patient with delirium*

    Blood chemistries (electrolyte levels; glucose, calcium, albumin, blood urea nitrogen, creatinine, aspartate aminotransferase [AST], bilirubin, alkaline phosphatase, magnesium, and phosphate levels)

    Venereal Disease Research Laboratory (VDRL) test

    Complete blood count

    Measurement of serum drug levels (e.g., digoxin, theophylline, phenobarbital, cyclosporine)

    Arterial blood gas or oxygen saturation measurement

    Urinalysis and collection for culture and sensitivity

    Urine drug screen

    Electrocardiography

    Chest radiography

Additional laboratory tests—*order as indicated by clinical condition*

    Electroencephalography

    Lumbar puncture

    Brain computed tomography or magnetic resonance imaging

    Additional chemistries (e.g., heavy metal screen, B_{12} and folate levels, urinary porphyrin levels)

    Lupus erythematosus (LE) Prep, antinuclear antibody test, human immunodeficiency virus test

W—Wernicke's encephalopathy or Withdrawal: Patients with Wernicke's encephalopathy typically have the triad of confusion, ataxia, and ophthalmoplegia (usually lateral gaze paralysis). If Wernicke's encephalopathy is not immediately treated with parenteral thiamine, the patient develops a permanent amnestic disorder called Korsakoff's psychosis, which is termed *alcohol-induced persisting amnestic disorder* in DSM-IV-TR. Wernicke's encephalopathy may coexist with ethanol withdrawal syndromes. A history of alcohol-related arrests, alcoholic blackouts, medical complications associated with alcohol abuse, liver function abnormalities, and increased red blood cell mean corpuscular volume increase suspicion of ethanol-related syndromes. Hyperreflexia and increased sympathetic tone (e.g., tachycardia, tremor, sweating, or hyperarousal) occur in this hyperadrenergic withdrawal state. Sedative-hypnotic drugs are associated with delirium during withdrawal more than are other classes of drugs.

H—Hypoxemia, Hypertensive encephalopathy, Hypoglycemia, and Hypoperfusion: Arterial blood gas levels or oxygen saturation and current and past vital signs should be checked to establish whether hypoxemia or hypertensive encephalopathy is present. Patients with hypoglycemic-induced delirium usually have insulin-dependent diabetes mellitus, except for those who engage in factitious use of hypoglycemic agents. Hypoperfusion or hypoxemia of the brain can have many causes, such as decreased cardiac output, cardiac arrhythmias, pulmonary failure, carbon monoxide poisoning, and severe anemia.

I—Intracranial bleeding or Infection: Subarachnoid or intraparenchymal hemorrhage or subdural hematoma can present as delirium. If the patient had a brief period of unconsciousness, with or without headache, and now has delirium, or if the patient had or now has focal neurological signs, intracranial bleeding should be suspected. Brain scanning and immediate neurological or neurosurgical evaluation are needed. Infectious processes (e.g., increased white blood cell count or fever) that cause delirium via systemic or CNS etiologies should be investigated. These infections are viral, tubercular, bacterial, fungal, or protozoal and may be systemic or the result of seeding by an abscess.

M—Meningitis or Encephalitis: These are typically acute febrile illnesses (vital signs should be checked to determine whether there is fever) and usually have either nonspecific localizing neurological signs (e.g., meningismus with stiff neck) or more focal neurological signs. Oncological, tubercular, and viral causes should also be considered. Vasculitis, as in connective tissue diseases, can cause delirium.

P—Poisons or Medications: Probably the most common cause of delirium is use of certain exogenous substances—prescribed and over-the-counter medications or illicit substances and toxins. A less common cause is pesticide or solvent poisoning. In the emergency room, a toxicology screen should be ordered. Drug-drug interactions are a common cause of delirium. The importance of obtaining a thorough medication history, including calling the family, caregivers, or pharmacist, cannot be overemphasized. Drugs with anticholinergic activity, including meperidine and fentanyl, are especially likely to cause delirium (Tollefson et al. 1991; Tune et al. 1993). Nurses' medication lists most clearly document doses and times of administration.

Critical Items (I WATCH DEATH)

Many of the insults that can cause delirium are listed in Table 15–4 (mnemonic I WATCH DEATH). Delirium indicates acute brain failure. The same medical forces that are marshaled in the case of failure of any other vital organ, when such failure is associated with morbidity and mortality, should be brought together in the case of delirium.

TABLE 15–4. Differential diagnosis for delirium using the mnemonic I WATCH DEATH

Infection	Encephalitis, meningitis, syphilis, HIV, sepsis
Withdrawal	Alcohol, barbiturates, sedative-hypnotics
Acute metabolic	Acidosis, alkalosis, electrolyte disturbance, hepatic failure, renal failure
Trauma	Closed-head injury, heatstroke, postoperative, severe burns
CNS pathology	Abscess, hemorrhage, hydrocephalus, subdural hematoma, infection, seizures, stroke, tumors, metastases, vasculitis
Hypoxia	Anemia, carbon monoxide poisoning, hypotension, pulmonary or cardiac failure
Deficiencies	Vitamin B_{12}, folate, niacin, thiamine
Endocrinopathies	Hyper- or hypoadrenocorticism, hyper- or hypoglycemia, myxedema, hyperparathyroidism
Acute vascular	Hypertensive encephalopathy, stroke, arrhythmia, shock
Toxins or drugs	Medications, illicit drugs, pesticides, solvents
Heavy metals	Lead, manganese, mercury

Note. CNS = central nervous system; HIV = human immunodeficiency virus.

PREVENTION

Despite data on a variety of potential risk factors for delirium, little research into its prevention has been conducted until recently. Preoperative psychiatric interviews may reduce postoperative psychosis by 50% (Kornfeld et al. 1974; Layne and Yudofsky 1971). In a factor analysis of 28 risk factors from 44 studies, Smith and Dimsdale (1989) found that only preoperative psychiatric intervention decreased the occurrence of postcardiotomy delirium. Recently, potentially preventable problems and practices that lead to delirium were described, including dehydration, immobility, use of physical restraints, use of indwelling bladder catheters, sleep deprivation, and use of certain psychoactive medications (Inouye 2000; Inouye and Charpentier 1996; Inouye et al. 1999a). Medication-induced delirium is common because of inappropriate use and overuse of sedative-hypnotic, narcotic, anticholinergic, and other psychoactive medications; specifically, the use of more than two psychoactive medications, or the addition of three total medications to an existing regimen, increases the risk of delirium (Inouye and Charpentier 1996). Finally, despite the acuteness, number, and complexity of health problems experienced by patients older than 65 years, physicians spend less time with these patients than with younger patients (Keeler et al. 1982; Radecki et al. 1988).

In a recent randomized, controlled trial involving a multicomponent intervention, the number and duration of episodes of delirium in hospitalized older patients were reduced (Inouye et al. 1999b). The intervention consisted of standardized protocols for the management of six risk factors for delirium: cognitive impairment, sleep deprivation, immobility, visual impairment, hearing impairment, and dehydration. Delirium developed in 9.9% of the intervention group compared with 15.0% of the control group. The rate of adherence to the intervention was 87%.

TREATMENT AND MANAGEMENT

The treatment of patients with delirium has two separate and important aspects. The first is critical and bears directly on the survival of the patient: identify and reverse, when possible, the reason(s) for the delirium (discussed earlier in this chapter). The second aspect of treatment is to reduce psychiatric symptoms of delirium with medications and environmental manipulations regardless of whether psychosis or agitation is present (see Table 15–5).

TABLE 15–5. Medical management for delirium

Medical care

Monitor vital signs, fluid input and output, and oxygenation

Discontinue nonessential medications

Avoid addition of multiple medications at one time

Identify sources of pain (information might not be volunteered)

Avoid interruption of sleep whenever possible

Perform regular laboratory evaluations as indicated

Prevent and manage disruptive behaviors

Place patient in a room near the nursing station

If dangerous behaviors occur, consider a sitter

Keep bed in low position and use side rails only if patient insists on getting out of bed

Use restraints only if necessary (for emergencies or if treatment with medication fails)

Avoid placement of patient in a room with another delirious patient

Avoid placement of patient in a room cluttered with equipment or furniture

Use of medications

Use haloperidol for agitation; give intravenously whenever possible, to avoid side effects and to avoid antagonizing patient

Avoid use of benzodiazepines as sole agents, except in alcohol or sedative-hypnotic withdrawal delirium

Avoid use of narcotics unless there is significant pain

Avoid use of anticholinergic medications

Use low doses and increase slowly, except in emergencies

Facilitate reality

Encourage presence of family members

Provide familiar clues (e.g., clock, calendar)

Provide adequate day and night lighting (e.g., use a nightlight)

Minimize transfers (e.g., perform procedures in room whenever possible)

Maximize staff continuity

Reduce excessive environmental stimuli

Orient patient to staff, surroundings, and situations repetitively, particularly before procedures

Make available sensory aids (e.g., hearing aids, glasses)

Encourage use of personal belongings

Reassure patient

Because of the high mortality and morbidity associated with delirium, proper medical management is important (see Table 15–5). The patient should be placed in a room near the nursing station so that he or she can be observed for medical deterioration and dangerous behaviors, such as attempting to crawl over bed rails or pull out an intravenous line. If necessary, a sitter should be employed. Vital signs and fluid input and output should be monitored and good oxygenation ensured. All nonessential medications should be discontinued. If an etiology for the confusional state is not immediately identified, further laboratory, radiological, and physical examinations are recommended.

Agitation is a particularly disruptive delirium symptom in the general hospital, although not necessarily more worthy of treatment than other delirium symptoms. The impact of cognitive impairment on care, the comparability of cognitive deficits in both hypoactive and hyperactive variants of delirium (Ross et al. 1991), and a possibly graver prognosis for the hypoactive type support the need to treat delirium even in the absence of agitation or psychosis. Platt et al. (1994) showed that haloperidol therapy and chlorpromazine therapy were effective treatments for delirium symptoms even before underlying medical causes were corrected, with similar efficacy for hypoactive and hyperactive variants.

A task force of more than 40 individuals reviewed the literature in order to develop practice parameters for intravenous sedation in adult patients in the intensive care setting (Shapiro et al. 1995). Recommendations presented in individual publications in the literature were divided into three levels by a consensus process, with consideration being given to the methodology of the research, which ranged from randomized, prospective, controlled investigations to non–peer-reviewed published opinions (e.g., textbook statements or official organizational publications). The levels were as follows: Level 1—recommendation convincingly justifiable on the basis of scientific evidence alone; Level 2—recommendation reasonably justifiable on the basis of available scientific evidence and strongly supported by expert critical care opinion; and Level 3—adequate scientific evidence lacking but recommendation widely supported by available data and expert critical care opinion. Recommendations included administration of haloperidol for delirium (Level 1), lorazepam for anxiety (Level 2), and midazolam or propofol for short-term sedation (less than 24 hours) (Level 2).

Haloperidol is the drug of first choice to treat a patient with delirium (Lipowski 1980, 1990) because it is a potent antipsychotic with virtually no anticholinergic or hypotensive properties, does not suppress respirations, has minimal cardiotoxicity, and can be given parenterally. Use of intravenous haloperidol in megadoses (e.g., 1,200 mg in a 24-hour period) in seriously ill patients resulted in no harmful side effects (Levenson 1995; Sanders and Cassem 1993; Sos and Cassem 1980; Tesar et al. 1985). Intravenous haloperidol can be given as a bolus injection or by continuous infusion drip. Continuous intravenous infusion of haloperidol is occasionally required to control severe refractory agitation and confusion (Fernandez et al. 1988; Riker et al. 1994). (Note: haloperidol is not approved for intravenous use by the Food and Drug Administration.) Although extrapyramidal side effects are more likely with higher- than with lower-potency antipsychotic drugs, the actual occurrence rate in medically ill patients, particularly with intravenous administration, is strikingly low. When extrapyramidal symptoms after oral versus intravenous haloperidol were measured in a blind fashion, intravenous administration of haloperidol was found to be associated with fewer severe extrapyramidal symptoms (Menza et al. 1987). However, patients with HIV dementia and Lewy body dementia are more sensitive to extrapyramidal side effects from haloperidol that is used to treat delirium. In small numbers of vulnerable patients with a history of alcohol abuse or cardiomyopathy, intravenous haloperidol caused lengthening of the Q-T interval and torsades de pointes (Hunt and Stern 1995; Metzger and Friedman 1993). However, in a study of 1,100 consecutive intensive care unit patients, intravenous haloperidol was implicated in the development of torsades de pointes in only 4 patients (Wilt et al. 1993). A recent review of records of 18 patients with arrhythmia associated with haloperidol administration led to the suggestion that a pretreatment check of the Q-Tc interval and serum magnesium and potassium concentrations be performed (Lawrence and Nasraway 1997). If the baseline Q-Tc interval is 440 msec or longer and the patient has electrolyte disturbances or is receiving other drugs that may prolong the Q-Tc interval, caution is recommended.

Droperidol is used by anesthesiologists as a preanesthetic agent and by other physicians to control nausea and vomiting. Like haloperidol, it is a butyrophenone, and it has comparable antidopaminergic potency but seems to have lower antipsychotic activity. The Food and Drug Administration approved droperidol for intravenous use. The drug is more sedating, has a faster onset of action, has a shorter half-life, and has significantly greater α_1-adrenergic activity, thereby inducing hypotension, compared with haloperidol. Droperidol has been given as a continuous intravenous infusion for severe delirium without complications (Frye et al. 1995). In a double-blind study comparing (intramuscular) haloperidol with droperidol in actively agitated emergency room patients (not necessarily with delirium), droperidol offered somewhat quicker relief (Resnick and Burton 1984).

Other medications have been used for delirium, with varying levels of success. Antipsychotic medications that are less potent, such as chlorpromazine and thioridazine, are more likely to cause hypotension and anticholinergic and quinidine-like side effects and are not available in parenteral form. Used in low doses (e.g., 10–100 mg), chlorpromazine appears efficacious and well tolerated (Breitbart et al. 1996), but it is not routinely recommended for delirium. Although risperidone and olanzapine are not available in parenteral formulation, open trials have found that they are clinically useful in treating delirium and may have fewer side effects than traditional antipsychotic medication (Sipahimalani and Masand 1997, 1998). Other medications reportedly beneficial are a combination of buspirone and carbamazepine in cases of agitation secondary to traumatic brain injury (Pourcher et al. 1994), ondansetron in postcardiotomy delirium (Bayindir et al. 2000), and propofol in cases of benzodiazepine-refractory delirium tremens (McCowan 2000).

Regardless of the route of administration, the usual initial dose of haloperidol for younger adult patients is 0.5–1 mg for mild, 2–5 mg for moderate, and 5–10 mg for severe confusion or agitation. The initial dose for frail or elderly patients is 0.5 mg for mild, 1 mg for moderate, and 2 mg for severe confusion or agitation. The dose is repeated at regular intervals, but not before 30 minutes, until the patient is calmer. Often only twice-a-day or three-times-a-day dosing is needed in patients whose level of agitation does not mandate more emergent care. After the confusion has cleared, haloperidol is continued and tapered over several days, depending on the severity of the episode. Abrupt discontinuation of medication immediately after improvement may, within 24 hours, be followed by recurrence of the delirium. A larger bedtime dose or the addition of lorazepam can be used in patients whose sleep-wake cycle has not normalized with haloperidol therapy alone.

The use of benzodiazepines in patients with delirium is most appropriate in sedative-hypnotic or ethanol withdrawal delirium. In other cases, the sedation and mild cognitive impairment associated with benzodiazepine therapy may further compromise the patient's sensorium or disinhibit his or her behaviors. Therefore, with the exceptions of certain drug withdrawal states, benzodiazepines are not recommended as sole agents in the treatment of patients with delirium. Benzodiazepines have been used successfully as adjuncts to high-potency neuroleptics such as haloperidol in a subset of patients with severe delirium (F. Adams 1984; Garza-Trevino et al. 1989). Small doses of intravenous lorazepam, particularly in patients who have not responded to treatment with haloperidol alone, help to decrease agitation. A fluctuation in symptom severity is inherent in delirium; thus, one assessment will evoke management and medical recommendations that are time-limited in efficacy, and follow-up monitoring and dose adjustments are recommended.

Environmental interventions are sometimes helpful but are not a primary treatment for delirium (Ribby and Cox 1996). Nurses and family members can frequently reorient patients to date and surroundings. It may help to place a clock, a calendar, and familiar objects in the room. Adequate light in the room during the night may decrease frightening illusions or hasten reorientation during awakenings. A private room for the patient with delirium is not recommended unless adequate supervision is provided. Rooms with windows assist in orientation because they allow diurnal cues (Wilson 1972). Returning sensory aids such as eyeglasses or hearing aids to patients who normally use them may improve the quality of sensory input and help patients better understand their surroundings.

A common error on medical and surgical wards is to place more than one patient with delirium in the same room, sometimes to save money by using one sitter for two patients. Reorientation is more difficult, and confused patients may confirm each other's distortions of reality.

Psychological support during and after a delirium episode is important. The presence of a calm family member can reassure the paranoid, agitated patient. In lieu of a family member, close supervision by reassuring nursing staff is essential. After the delirium has cleared, the patient should be helped to understand the bizarre experience (MacKenzie and Popkin 1980) and reassured about its transience and frequent occurrence among hospitalized medically ill patients, to prevent the belief that he or she is "going crazy." Family education also helps.

COURSE (PROGNOSIS)

The course of delirium ranges from less than 1 week to 2 months, with a typical course of 10–12 days (American Psychiatric Association 1999). The outcome possibilities are full recovery; progression to stupor, coma, or death; seizures; chronic brain syndromes; and associated injuries (e.g., fracture or subdural hematomas from falls). The majority of patients who experience delirium may have a full recovery (Lipowski 1990), but only 4%–40% of patients have a full recovery by the time of hospital discharge, and the rate of recovery at the time of discharge is closer to 15% among elderly patients (American Psychiatric Association 1999; Levkoff et al. 1992). Persistent cognitive deficits are common, particularly in patients with AIDS, with only 27% having full recovery of cognition (American Psychiatric Association 1999; Rockwood 1993). Cognitive deficits may also be due to previously unrecognized dementia that was heralded by the delirium. Seizures can accompany delirium but are more likely to occur with drug withdrawal, particularly alcohol withdrawal, and burn encephalopathy (Antoon et al. 1972).

Morbidity

Delirium in patients who undergo orthopedic surgery is a harbinger of poor recovery and long-term outcome. Rogers et al. (1989) reported that patients who were cognitively healthy when tested preoperatively but who developed postoperative delirium showed no improvement in level of physical function 6 months postoperatively. Gustafson et al. (1988) found that delirium was the best predictor of outcome in patients who had femoral neck fractures. These investigators found that 37 of 111 patients had preoperative delirium and another 31 developed delirium postoperatively. The group with delirium but not dementia had longer hospital stays (21.7 days vs. 13.5 days for patients without delirium) and were more likely to require walking aids, be bedridden, require rehabilitation, or die. The group with delirium spent four times as much time in recuperation before discharge. In addition, Fernandez et al. (1989) found that only 37% of patients with AIDS who developed delirium had complete recovery of cognitive function.

Some behaviors in patients with delirium, such as striking caregivers, can interfere with ongoing medical care. These patients may pull out intravenous lines, urinary catheters, nasogastric tubes, arterial lines, nasopharyngeal tubes, and intra-aortic balloon pumps. Inouye et al. (1989) reported that the risk of complications, such as decubiti and aspiration pneumonia, was more than six times greater among patients with delirium. Data on morbidity in children are not available.

Mortality

Most psychiatrists, and physicians in general, are unaware of the mortality associated with delirium. Of 77 patients who received a DSM-III diagnosis of delirium from a consultation psychiatrist, 19 (25%) died within 6 months (Trzepacz et al. 1985). Three months after diagnosis, the mortality rate for delirium is 14 times higher than the mortality rate for affective disorders (Weddington 1982). The risk of dying in the hospital is 5.5 times greater for a patient with a diagnosis of delirium during a hospital stay than for a patient with a diagnosis of dementia (Rabins and Folstein 1982). Furthermore, an elderly patient who develops delirium in the hospital has a 22% (Rabins and Folstein 1982) to 76% (Flint and Richards 1956) chance of dying during that hospitalization. D. J. Cameron et al. (1987) reported that 13 (65%) of 20

patients with delirium died during hospitalization. Patients who survive hospitalization have a very high death rate during the months immediately after discharge. Patients with a diagnosis of delirium who were followed up for several months showed a mortality rate equal to that of patients with dementia who were followed up for several years (Roth 1955; Varsamis et al. 1972). Data on mortality in children are not available.

SUMMARY

Delirium is a ubiquitous, underrecognized clinical syndrome that accompanies potentially life-threatening medical conditions. Delirium is especially common in patients who are elderly, have impaired cognition or structural brain disorders, are seriously burned, have HIV-related illness, or are dependent on sedative-hypnotics or alcohol. Because these patients often exhibit bizarre behavior during delirium, psychiatric consultation is appropriate. Psychiatrists must be able to diagnose delirium correctly on the basis of specific signs and symptoms, organize a prioritized differential diagnosis, assist the primary physician in identifying the probable cause(s) of the delirium, and recommend and monitor treatment for symptoms. Correct management and treatment of delirium is lifesaving and can reduce hospital costs by shortening hospital stays (Thomas et al. 1988). Although the literature states that delirium is common in children, no epidemiologic studies support this statement. Early signs of delirium in children may be mistaken for "normal" regression. With the exception of such early signs, delirium in children generally manifests as it does in adults.

REFERENCES

Adams F: Neuropsychiatric evaluation and treatment of delirium in the critically ill cancer patient. The Cancer Bulletin 36:156–160, 1984

Adams RD, Victor M: Principles of Neurology. New York, McGraw-Hill, 1989

American Psychiatric Association: Practice Guideline for the Treatment of Patients With Delirium. Washington, DC, American Psychiatric Association, 1999

American Psychiatric Association: Diagnostic and Statistical Manual of Mental Disorders, 4th Edition, Text Revision. Washington, DC, American Psychiatric Association, 2000

Andreasen NJC, Hartford CE, Knott JR, et al: EEG changes associated with burn delirium. Diseases of the Nervous System 38:27–31, 1977

Antoon AY, Volpe JJ, Crawford JD: Burn encephalopathy in children. Pediatrics 50:609–616, 1972

Bayindir O, Akpinar B, Can E, et al: The use of 5-HT3-receptor antagonist ondansetron for the treatment of postcardiotomy delirium. J Cardiothorac Vasc Anesth 14:288292, 2000

Berrios GE: Delirium and confusion in the 19th century: a conceptual history. Br J Psychiatry 139:439–449, 1981

Bliwise DL: What is sundowning? J Am Geriatr Soc 42:1009–1011, 1994

Bliwise DL, Carroll JS, Lee KA, et al: Sleep and "sundowning" in nursing home patients with dementia. Psychiatry Res 48:277–292, 1993

Breitbart W, Marotta R, Platt MM, et al: A double-blind trial of haloperidol, chlorpromazine, and lorazepam in the treatment of delirium in hospitalized AIDS patients. Am J Psychiatry 153:231–237, 1996

Cameron DE: Studies in senile nocturnal delirium. Psychiatr Q 5:47–53, 1941

Cameron DJ, Thomas RI, Mulvihill M, et al: Delirium: a test of the Diagnostic and Statistical Manual III criteria on medical inpatients. J Am Geriatr Soc 35:1007–1010, 1987

Camus V, Gonthier R, Dubos G, et al: Etiologic and outcome profiles in hypoactive and hyperactive subtypes of delirium. J Geriatr Psychiatry Neurol 13:3842, 2000

Cohen-Mansfield J, Marx MS, Werner P, et al: Temporal patterns of agitated nursing home residents. Int Psychogeriatr 4:197–206, 1992

Cole MG, Primeau FJ: Prognosis of delirium in elderly hospital patients. CMAJ 149:41–46, 1993

Dubin WR, Field NL, Gastfriend DR: Postcardiotomy delirium: a critical review. J Thorac Cardiovasc Surg 77:586–594, 1979

Engel GL: Delirium, in Comprehensive Textbook of Psychiatry. Edited by Freedman AM, Kaplan HS. Baltimore, MD, Williams & Wilkins, 1967, pp 711–716

Engel GL, Romano J: Delirium, a syndrome of cerebral insufficiency. Journal of Chronic Disease 9:260–277, 1959

Farrell KR, Ganzini L: Misdiagnosing delirium as depression in medically ill elderly patients. Arch Intern Med 155:2459–2464, 1995

Fernandez F, Holmes V, Adams F, et al: Treatment of severe, refractory agitation with a haloperidol drip. J Clin Psychiatry 49:239–241, 1988

Fernandez F, Levy J, Mansell P: Management of delirium in terminally ill AIDS patients. Int J Psychiatry Med 19:165–172, 1989

Flint FJ, Richards SM: Organic basis of confusional states in the elderly. BMJ 2:1537–1539, 1956

Folstein MF, Folstein SE, McHugh PR: "Mini-mental state": a practical method for grading the cognitive state of patients for the clinician. J Psychiatr Res 12:189–198, 1975

Folstein MF, Bassett SS, Romanoski AJ, et al: The epidemiology of delirium in the community: the eastern Baltimore mental health survey, in International Psychogeriatrics. Edited by Miller NE, Lipowski ZJ, Lebowitz BD. New York, Springer, 1991, pp 169–176

Francis J: Sensory and environmental factors in delirium. Paper presented at a conference sponsored by the Minneapolis Veterans Affairs Medical Center, Minneapolis, MN, September 1993

Francis J, Kapoor WN: Prognosis after hospital discharge of older medical patients with delirium. J Am Geriatr Soc 40:601–606, 1992

Francis J, Martin D, Kapoor W: A prospective study of delirium in hospitalized elderly. JAMA 263:1097–1101, 1990

Franco K, Litaker D, Locala J, et al: The cost of delirium in the surgical patient. Psychosomatics 42:68–73, 2001

Frye MA, Coudreaut MF, Hakeman SM, et al: Continuous droperidol drip infusion for management of agitated delirium in an ICU. Psychosomatics 36:301–305, 1995

Garza-Trevino E, Hollister L, Overall J, et al: Efficacy of combinations of intramuscular antipsychotics and sedative-hypnotics for control of psychotic agitation. Am J Psychiatry 146:1598–1601, 1989

Gustafson Y, Berggren D, Brannstrom B, et al: Acute confusional states in elderly patients treated for femoral neck fracture. J Am Geriatr Soc 36:525–530, 1988

Harrell R, Othmer E: Postcardiotomy confusion and sleep loss. J Clin Psychiatry 48:445–446, 1987

Hunt N, Stern TA: The association between intravenous haloperidol and torsades de pointes. Psychosomatics 36:541–549, 1995

Inouye SK: Prevention of delirium in hospitalized older patients: risk factors and targeted intervention strategies. Ann Med 32:257–263, 2000

Inouye SK, Charpentier PA: Precipitating factors for delirium in hospitalized elderly persons. JAMA 275:852–857, 1996

Inouye SK, Horwitz RI, Tinetti ME, et al: Acute confusional states in the hospitalized elderly: incidence, factors, and complications (abstract). Clinical Research 37:524A, 1989

Inouye SK, van Dyck CH, Alessi CA, et al: Clarifying confusion: the confusion assessment method. A new method for detection of delirium. Ann Intern Med 113:941–948, 1990

Inouye SK, Viscolo CM, Horwitz RI, et al: A predictive model for delirium in hospitalized elderly medical patients based on admission characteristics. Ann Intern Med 119:474–481, 1993

Inouye SK, Rushing J, Foreman M, et al: Does delirium contribute to poor hospital outcomes? A three-site epidemiologic study. J Gen Intern Med 13:234–242, 1998

Inouye SK, Schlesinger MJ, Lydon TJ: Delirium: a symptom of how hospital care is failing older persons and a window to improve quality of hospital care. Am J Med 106:565–573, 1999a

Inouye SK, Bogardus ST, Charpentier PA, et al: A multicomponent intervention to prevent delirium in hospitalized older patients. N Engl J Med 340:669–676, 1999b

Kane FJ, Remmell R, Moody S: Recognizing and treating delirium in patients admitted to general hospitals. South Med J 86:985–988, 1993

Keeler EB, Solomon DH, Beck JC, et al: Effect of patient age on duration of medical encounters with physicians. Med Care 20:1101–1108, 1982

Kennard MA, Bueding E, Wortis WB: Some biochemical and electroencephalographic changes in delirium tremens. Quarterly Journal of Studies on Alcohol 6:4–14, 1945

Kobayashi K, Takeuchi O, Suzuki M, et al: Retrospective study on delirium type. Japanese Journal of Psychiatry and Neurology 46:911–917, 1992

Kolbeinsson H, Jonsson A: Delirium and dementia in acute medical admissions of elderly patients in Iceland. Acta Psychiatr Scand 87:123–127, 1993

Koponen HJ, Riekkinen PJ: A prospective study of delirium in elderly patients admitted to a psychiatric hospital. Psychol Med 3:103–109, 1993

Koponen H[J], Stenback U, Mattila E, et al: Delirium among elderly persons admitted to a psychiatric hospital: clinical course during the acute stage and one-year follow-up. Acta Psychiatr Scand 79:579–585, 1989

Kornfeld DS, Zimberg S, Malm JR: Psychiatric complications of open-heart surgery. N Engl J Med 273:287–292, 1965

Kornfeld DS, Heller SS, Frank KA, et al: Personality and psychological factors in postcardiotomy delirium. Arch Gen Psychiatry 31:249–253, 1974

Lawrence K, Nasraway S: Conduction disturbances associated with administration of butyrophenone antipsychotics in the critically ill: a review of the literature. Pharmacotherapy 17:531–537, 1997

Layne OL, Yudofsky SC: Postoperative psychosis in cardiotomy patients: the role of organic and psychiatric factors. N Engl J Med 284:518–520, 1971

Levenson JL: High-dose intravenous haloperidol for agitated delirium following lung transplantation. Psychosomatics 36:66–68, 1995

Levkoff SE, Evans DA, Liptzin B, et al: Delirium: the occurrence and persistence of symptoms among elderly hospitalized patients. Arch Intern Med 152:334–340, 1992

Lewis LM, Miller DK, Morley JE, et al: Unrecognized delirium in ED geriatric patients. Am J Emerg Med 13:142–145, 1995

Lipowski ZJ: Delirium: Acute Brain Failure in Man. Springfield, IL, Charles C Thomas, 1980

Lipowski ZJ: Delirium in the elderly patient. N Engl J Med 320:378–382, 1989

Lipowski ZJ: Delirium: Acute Confusional States. New York, Oxford University Press, 1990

Liptzin B, Levkoff SE: An empirical study of delirium subtypes. Br J Psychiatry 161:843–845, 1992

MacKenzie TB, Popkin MK: Stress response syndrome occurring after delirium. Am J Psychiatry 137:1433–1435, 1980

Maj M, Satz P, Janssen R, et al: WHO Neuropsychiatric AIDS study, cross-sectional phase II. Neuropsychological and neurological findings. Arch Gen Psychiatry 51:51–61, 1994

Marcantonio ER, Goldman L, Mangione CM, et al: A clinical prediction rule for delirium after elective noncardiac surgery. JAMA 271:134–139, 1994

Martino-Saltzman D, Blasch BB, Morris RD, et al: Travel behavior of nursing home residents perceived as wanderers and nonwanderers. Gerontologist 31:666–672, 1991

McCowan C: Refractory delirium tremens treated with propofol: a case series. Crit Care Med 28:1781–1784, 2000

Menza M, Murray G, Holmes V, et al: Decreased extrapyramidal symptoms with intravenous haloperidol. J Clin Psychiatry 48:278–280, 1987

Mesulam M-M: Patterns in behavioral neuroanatomy: association areas, the limbic system, and hemispheric specialization, in Principles of Behavioral Neurology. Edited by Mesulam M-M. Philadelphia, PA, FA Davis, 1985, pp 1–70

Metzger E, Friedman R: Prolongation of the corrected QT and torsades de pointes cardiac arrhythmia associated with intravenous haloperidol in the medically ill. J Clin Psychopharmacol 13:128–132, 1993

Mori E, Yamadori A: Acute confusional state and acute agitated delirium. Arch Neurol 44:1139–1143, 1987

Murray AM, Levkoff SE, Wetle TT, et al: Acute delirium and functional decline in the hospitalized elderly patient. Journal of Gerontology 48:M181–M186, 1993

Naughton BJ, Moran MB, Kadah H, et al: Delirium and other cognitive impairment in older adults in an emergency department. Ann Emerg Med 25:751–755, 1995

Nicholas LM, Lindsey BA: Delirium presenting with symptoms of depression. Psychosomatics 36:471–479, 1995

O'Keefe S, Lavan J: The prognostic significance of delirium in older hospital patients. J Am Geriatr Soc 45:174–178, 1997

Patten S, Lamarre C: Dysgraphia (letter). Can J Psychiatry 34:746, 1989

Perry S: Organic mental disorders caused by HIV: update on early diagnosis and treatment. Am J Psychiatry 147:696–710, 1990

Platt MM, Breitbart W, Smith M, et al: Efficacy of neuroleptics for hypoactive delirium (letter). J Neuropsychiatry Clin Neurosci 6:66–67, 1994

Pourcher E, Filteau MJ, Bouchard RH, et al: Efficacy of the combination of buspirone and carbamazepine in early posttraumatic delirium (letter). Am J Psychiatry 151:150–151, 1994

Pro JD, Wells CE: The use of the electroencephalogram in the diagnosis of delirium. Diseases of the Nervous System 38:804–808, 1977

Prugh DG, Wagonfeld S, Metcalf D, et al: A clinical study of delirium in children and adolescents. Psychosom Med 42 (suppl):177–197, 1980

Rabins PV, Folstein MF: Delirium and dementia: diagnostic criteria and fatality rates. Br J Psychiatry 140:149–153, 1982

Radecki SE, Kane SL, Solomon DH, et al: Do physicians spend less time with older patients? J Am Geriatr Soc 36:713–718, 1988

Rahkonen T, Luukkainen-Markkula R, Paanila S, et al: Delirium episode as a sign of undetected dementia among community dwelling elderly subjects: a 2 year follow up study. J Neurol Neurosurg Psychiatry 69:519–521, 2000

Resnick M, Burton B: Droperidol vs. haloperidol in the initial management of acutely agitated patients. J Clin Psychiatry 45:298–299, 1984

Ribby KJ, Cox KR: Development, implementation, and evaluation of a confusion protocol. Clinical Nurse Specialist 10:241–247, 1996

Riker RR, Fraser GL, Cox PM: Continuous infusion of haloperidol controls agitation in critically ill patients. Crit Care Med 22:433–440, 1994

Rockwood K: The occurrence and duration of symptoms in elderly patients with delirium. Journal of Gerontology 48:M162–M166, 1993

Rockwood K, Goodman J, Flynn M, et al: Cross-validation of the Delirium Rating Scale in older patients. J Am Geriatr Soc 44:839–842, 1996

Rogers M, Liang M, Daltroy L: Delirium after elective orthopedic surgery: risk factors and natural history. Int J Psychiatry Med 19:109–121, 1989

Ross CA, Peyser CE, Shapiro I, et al: Delirium: phenomenologic and etiologic subtypes. Int Psychogeriatr 3:135–147, 1991

Roth M: The natural history of mental disorder in old age. Journal of Mental Science 101:281–301, 1955

Sanders KM, Cassem EH: Psychiatric complications in the critically ill cardiac patient. Tex Heart Inst J 20:180–187, 1993

Shapiro BA, Warren J, Egol AB, et al: Practice parameters for intravenous analgesia and sedation for adult patients in the intensive care unit: an executive summary. Society of Critical Care Medicine. Crit Care Med 23:1596–1600, 1995

Sipahimalani A, Masand PS: Use of risperidone in delirium: case reports. Ann Clin Psychiatry 9:105–107, 1997

Sipahimalani A, Masand PS: Olanzapine in the treatment of delirium. Psychosomatics 39:422–430, 1998

Smith L, Dimsdale J: Postcardiotomy delirium: conclusions after 25 years? Am J Psychiatry 146:452–458, 1989

Sos J, Cassem NH: Managing postoperative agitation. Drug Therapy 10:103–106, 1980

Tesar GE, Murray GB, Cassem NH: Use of high-dose intravenous haloperidol in the treatment of agitated cardiac patients. J Clin Psychopharmacol 5:344–347, 1985

Thomas RI, Cameron DJ, Fahs MC: A prospective study of delirium and prolonged length of hospital stay. Arch Gen Psychiatry 45:937–940, 1988

Tollefson GD, Montague-Clouse J, Lancaster SP: The relationship of serum anticholinergic activity to mental status performance in an elderly nursing home population. J Neuropsychiatry Clin Neurosci 3:314–319, 1991

Trzepacz PT: Neuropathogenesis of delirium: a need to focus our research. Psychosomatics 35:375–391, 1994a

Trzepacz PT: A review of delirium assessment instruments. Gen Hosp Psychiatry 16:397–405, 1994b

Trzepacz PT, Baker RW: The Psychiatric Mental Status Examination. New York, Oxford University Press, 1993

Trzepacz PT, Francis J: Low serum albumin and risk of delirium (letter). Am J Psychiatry 147:675, 1990

Trzepacz PT, Teague GB, Lipowski ZJ: Delirium and other organic mental disorders in a general hospital. Gen Hosp Psychiatry 7:101–106, 1985

Trzepacz PT, Brenner R, Coffman G, et al: Delirium in liver transplantation candidates: discriminant analysis of multiple test variables. Biol Psychiatry 24:3–14, 1988a

Trzepacz PT, Baker RW, Greenhouse J: A symptom rating scale for delirium. Psychiatry Res 23:89–97, 1988b

Tune L, Carr S, Cooper T, et al: Association of anticholinergic activity of prescribed medications with postoperative delirium. J Neuropsychiatry Clin Neurosci 5:208–210, 1993

Valan MN, Hilty DM: Incidence of delirium in patients referred for evaluation of depression. Psychosomatics 37:190–191, 1996

Varsamis J, Zuchowski T, Maini KK: Survival rates and causes of death in geriatric psychiatric patients: a six-year follow-up study. Canadian Psychiatric Association Journal 17:17–21, 1972

Weddington WW: The mortality of delirium: an under-appreciated problem? Psychosomatics 23:1232–1235, 1982

Weissenborn K, Ruckert N, Hecker H, et al: The number connection tests A and B: interindividual variability and use for the assessment of early hepatic encephalopathy. J Hepatol 28:646–653, 1998

Wilson LM: Intensive care delirium. Arch Intern Med 130:225–226, 1972

Wilt JL, Minnema AM, Johnson RF, et al: Torsades de pointes associated with the use of intravenous haloperidol. Ann Intern Med 119:391–394, 1993

16

Dementia

Kevin F. Gray, M.D.

Jeffrey L. Cummings, M.D.

Changes in mental status and behavior are among the most frequently encountered phenomena in a general medical hospital setting, especially in elderly or postoperative patients (Lipowski 1990). Dementia is therefore frequently part of the differential diagnosis considered by consultation-liaison psychiatrists. The emergence of delirium in a hospitalized patient may be the first indication of a previously undiagnosed dementing illness. The detection of dementia by the psychiatric consultant becomes critical when considering treatment, prognosis, placement, rehabilitation, or even the patient's ability to comply with a medication regimen.

DEFINITIONS

Dementia

Dementia is a syndrome of acquired persistent impairment in intellectual function. Multiple spheres of mental activity, including memory and at least one other domain—language, visuospatial skills, emotion or personality, and executive function—must be compromised for a diagnosis of dementia to be considered (Cummings et al. 1980). The notion of acquired impairment removes congenital retardation from the realm of dementia; persistent impairment distinguishes dementia from delirium; and impairment in multiple spheres separates dementia from unitary disorders such as amnesia and aphasia. Although some dementias are chronic, irreversible, and progressive conditions, the term *dementia* does not automatically imply irreversibility. Of all the patients initially presenting for evaluation, 10%–30% have at least partially reversible dementia syndromes (Rabins 1983); however, since patients are increasingly evaluated in out-patient settings, and with the use of stricter diagnostic methods, truly reversible dementia is seen in less than 1% of cases (Weytingh et al. 1995). The principal causes of dementia are listed in Table 16–1.

Dementia reflects the effect of pathological processes on the brain and is not the result of normal aging. Age-related cognitive and memory decline is distinct from dementia (Bamford and Caine 1988; Crook et al. 1986). Psychomotor slowing, diminished performance on tests of executive functions, and reduced cognitive flexibility are the changes associated with normal aging (Van Gorp and Mahler 1990). The "normal elderly" are a heterogeneous group in whom intrinsic age-related processes may be complicated by the effects of illness and medications. Studies on optimally healthy elderly show only slowed information processing and some signs of inefficiency in generating problem-solving strategies (Boone et al. 1990). Naming, attention, and predominantly verbal neuropsychological tasks are all unaffected by age.

Cortical Dementia

Cortical dementias are disorders producing dysfunction of the cerebral cortex, as characterized by the "A's": amnesia, aphasia, apraxia, and agnosia. Alzheimer's disease is the classic example of a cortical dementia; dementia with cortical Lewy bodies, and the focal cortical atrophy syndromes, including frontotemporal dementias such as Pick's disease, are also included in this category (Black 1996). The "cortical" designation is a clinical concept that emphasizes the predominance of cortical dysfunction in these disorders despite coexisting pathology in subcortical regions (Cummings and Benson 1984).

TABLE 16–1. Etiological classification of the principal dementia syndromes

Degenerative disorders
  Cortical
    Alzheimer's disease
    Dementia with Lewy bodies
    Pick's disease
    Frontotemporal dementia
    Primary progressive aphasia
    Posterior cortical atrophy
  Subcortical
    Parkinson's disease
    Huntington's disease
    Progressive supranuclear palsy
    Spinocerebellar degenerations
    Idiopathic basal ganglia calcification
    Striatonigral degeneration
    Wilson's disease
    Thalamic dementia
    Corticobasal degeneration
    Multiple system atrophy

Vascular dementias
  Multiple large vessel occlusions
  Strategic infarct dementia
  Lacunar state (multiple subcortical infarctions)
  Binswanger's disease (white matter ischemic injury)
  Mixed cortical and subcortical infarctions
  CADASIL syndrome (cerebral autosomal dominant arteriopathy with subortical infarcts and leukoencephalopathy)

Myelinoclastic disorders
  Demyelinating
    Multiple sclerosis
    Marchiafava-Bignami disease
  Dysmyelinating
    Metachromatic leukodystrophy
    Adrenoleukodystrophy
    Cerebrotendinous xanthomatosis

Traumatic conditions
  Posttraumatic encephalopathy
  Subdural hematoma
  Dementia pugilistica

Neoplastic dementias
  Meningioma (particularly subfrontal)
  Glioma
  Metastatic deposits
  Meningeal carcinomatosis

Hydrocephalic dementias
  Communicating
    Normal-pressure hydrocephalus
  Noncommunicating
    Aqueductal stenosis
    Intraventricular neoplasm
    Intraventricular cyst
    Basilar meningitis

Inflammatory conditions
  Systemic lupus erythematosus
  Antiphospholipid antibody syndrome
  Temporal arteritis
  Sarcoidosis
  Granulomatous arteritis

Infection-related dementias
  Syphilis
  Chronic meningitis
  Postencephalitic dementia syndrome
  Whipple's disease
  Acquired immunodeficiency syndrome (AIDS)
  Creutzfeldt-Jakob disease
  Subacute sclerosing panencephalitis
  Progressive multifocal leukoencephalopathy

Toxic conditions
  Alcohol-related syndromes
  Polydrug abuse
  Iatrogenic dementias
    Anticholinergic agents
    Antihypertensive drugs
    Psychotropic agents
    Anticonvulsant agents
    Miscellaneous agents
  Metals
  Industrial solvents

Metabolic disorders
  Cardiopulmonary failure
  Uremia
  Hepatic encephalopathy
  Endocrine disorders
    Thyroid
    Adrenal
    Parathyroid
  Anemia and hematological conditions
  Deficiency states (vitamin B_{12})
  Porphyria

Psychiatric disorders
  Depression
  Mania
  Schizophrenia
  Conversion disorder
  Malingering

Source. Adapted from Cummings 1987.

Subcortical Dementia

Subcortical dementias reflect pathological processes primarily involving the white and deep gray matter structures, including basal ganglia, thalamus, and frontal lobe projections of these subcortical structures. The clinical findings in subcortical dementia reflect the disruption of fundamental cerebral functions such as arousal, attention, motivation, and rate of information processing. This disruption results in psychomotor retardation, defective recall, poor abstraction and strategy formation, and mood and personality alterations such as apathy and depression. The dementias due to human immunodeficiency virus (HIV) infection, Huntington's disease, and Parkinson's disease are all examples of subcortical dementias (Mandell and Albert 1990). Table 16–2 illustrates the features that distinguish cortical and subcortical dementias.

Mixed Dementia

Mixed dementia includes disease processes that produce a mixed clinical syndrome with both cortical and subcortical features. The most common entity in this category is vascular dementia, the syndrome of multiple strokes producing cognitive dysfunction. Vascular disease not only affects several brain regions but also can coexist with other pathological processes. Vascular dementia tends to affect subcortical gray matter structures and white matter tracts preferentially, producing a subcortical dementia; when cortical and subcortical structures are affected, mixed dementia results. Alzheimer's disease can occur in conjunction with Parkinson's disease and other Lewy body syndromes, or in elderly patients with stroke. Neoplastic, traumatic, infectious, and toxic-metabolic processes also may involve both cortical and subcortical structures (Cummings 1990).

Dementia Associated With Psychiatric Disorders: "Pseudodementia"

The term *pseudodementia* refers to cognitive deficits caused by clinical depression and other psychiatric disorders and is characterized by a reversible syndrome of cognitive impairment indistinguishable from primary dementia (Caine 1981; Wells 1979). However, because there is nothing "pseudo" about the cognitive impairment seen in patients with depression, the term *dementia syndrome of depression* (DSD) is preferable (M.F. Folstein and McHugh 1978). Sometimes the term *pseudodementia* is applied to any patient manifesting cognitive impairment secondary to psychiatric disturbance. In this context, mania, schizophrenia, hysterical conversion reactions, Ganser's "syndrome of approximate answers," and malingering all may be included (Lishman 1988).

EPIDEMIOLOGY

Dementia is a major public health challenge, not only for clinicians but also for society as a whole. Estimates suggest that up to 4 million Americans have severe dementia, and an additional 1–5 million patients have mild to moderate dementia. The number of people with dementia is expected to increase to 9 million by 2030.

Incidence/Prevalence

The most commonly occurring dementia is Alzheimer's disease, which accounts for approximately 70% of the elderly patients evaluated for progressive cognitive decline. Perhaps another 15%–20% have a combination of Alzheimer's disease and vascular pathology at autopsy (Tomlinson et al. 1970); more recent findings suggest that the presence of cerebrovascular disease plays an important role in determining the presentation and severity of the clinical symptoms of Alzheimer's disease (Snowdon et al. 1997). The risk of developing dementia of the Alzheimer's type increases dramatically with age. Numerous studies show that roughly 7% of the population ages 65 and over have Alzheimer's disease and that both prevalence and incidence rates double roughly every 5 years after age 65 (McDowell 2001).

Vascular dementia is the second most common cause of dementia. It occurs in 17%–29% of the patients with dementia; an additional 10%–23% of patients have vascular dementia mixed with Alzheimer's disease. Thus, the frequency of vascular dementia syndromes reported in the literature ranges from 10% to 52%—figures that arguably underestimate or overestimate the true prevalence (Brust 1988; O'Brien 1988). Finally, lack of uniformity in implementing diagnostic criteria makes it difficult to draw firm conclusions about the prevalence of vascular dementia (Rocca and Kokmen 1999).

Together, Alzheimer's disease and vascular dementia account for 70%–90% of the patients with dementia, whereas all the other syndromes listed in Table 16–1 account for the remaining 10%–30%. This latter group invites the special attention of the consultant because it contains the potentially reversible causes of dementia such as metabolic, structural, or psychiatric conditions (Rabins 1983). The consultant also must be mindful that the prevalence, severity, and likely etiology of dementia are all variable, depending on whether a patient resides at home, in an institution, in a hospital, or in a nursing home.

Other causes of dementia likely to be encountered by the consultant deserve mention. Dementia with Lewy bodies is now being recognized with increasing frequency and indeed may prove to be the second most common cause of dementia in elderly patients, accounting for 15%–20% of late-onset dementias (Campbell et al. 2001; McKeith et al. 1994, 1996). The frontotemporal dementias, which are more common than previously recognized, may account for up to 25% of all presenile dementia cases

TABLE 16–2. Distinguishing features of cortical and subcortical dementias

Characteristic	Subcortical	Cortical
Language	No aphasia	Aphasia early
Memory	Recall impaired; recognition is better preserved than recall	Amnesia: recall and recognition impaired
Visuospatial skills	Impaired	Impaired
Calculation	Preserved until late	Involved early
Frontal systems	Disproportionately affected	Impaired to the same degree as other abilities
Cognitive processing speed	Slowed early	Response time normal until late in disease course
Personality	Apathetic, inert	Unconcerned or disinhibited
Mood	Depressed	Euthymic
Speech	Dysarthric	Normal articulation[a]
Posture	Bowed or extended	Normal, upright[a]
Coordination	Impaired	Normal[a]
Gait	Abnormal	Normal[a]
Motor speed	Slowed	Normal[a]
Movement disorders	Common (chorea, tremor, tics, rigidity)	Absent[a]

[a]Motor system involvement occurs late in the course of the cortical dementias.
Source. Adapted from Cummings 1990.

(Chow et al. 1999). Dementia occurs in roughly two-thirds of elderly alcoholics, nearly half of whom have alcohol dementia in the absence of other brain disease (Kasahara et al. 1996). Significant neuropsychological deficits occur in at least 60% of the patients with Parkinson's disease (Mahler and Cummings 1990). A recent population survey found that the incidence of dementia among patients with Parkinson's disease was sixfold greater than the incidence in subjects without the disease (Aarsland et al. 2001). HIV disease is now a global epidemic, and an estimated 1.5–2 million Americans are infected with HIV-1 (American Academy of Neurology AIDS Task Force 1991). A substantial number of these patients have HIV-related dementia or secondary opportunistic brain infections with dementia (see Chapter 36 in this volume). Head trauma results in 400,000 to 500,000 patients being hospitalized in the United States each year and is an important cause of cognitive impairment among younger individuals (Kraus and Sorenson 1994).

Dementia in Medically Ill Patients

A large-scale study of 2,000 consecutive patients ages 55 years and older admitted to a university hospital medical service found that the occurrence of moderate to severe dementia was 9.1% for all age groups taken as a whole. This figure ranged from 0.8% in patients of ages 55–64 years to 31.2% in patients ages 85 years and older. Nearly 75% of these inpatients with dementia had vascular dementia, probably due to the high morbidity from cardiovascular disease in older age groups. Both mean hospitalization time and daily nursing care needs were significantly increased in the patients with dementia (Erkinjuntti et al. 1986).

Predisposition/Risk Factors

An age-associated risk for the development of Alzheimer's disease is compelling, but whether this risk ultimately plateaus, continues to increase, or finally declines in the oldest old is unknown. A family history for dementia is also convincingly associated with Alzheimer's disease; individuals with dementia are three to four times more likely to have an affected relative than are control subjects (Mendez et al. 1992). Down's syndrome and low level of education as well as head trauma with loss of consciousness appear to be associated with an increased risk for the development of Alzheimer's disease (Cummings 1995b; Van Duijn et al. 1992). It has been shown that inheritance of the apolipoprotein E4 allele, a gene involved in cholesterol metabolism, also is a risk factor for Alzheimer's disease (Corder et al. 1993; Saunders et al. 2000). The risk for cerebrovascular disease also increases with age. Vascular dementia is most commonly encountered in patients who are older than 60 years; men are affected more often than women. Typically, vascular dementia is associated with stroke risk factors: age, hypertension, heart disease, cigarette smoking, diabetes mellitus, excessive alcohol consumption (more than three drinks per day), and hyperlipidemia. Nephropathy, atrial fibrillation, previous mental decline, and stroke severity also appear to contribute to dementia risk; often, several of these risk factors are present in the patient with vascular dementia (Barba et al. 2000; Meyer et al. 1988). The percentage of alcoholics with dementia increases with age, comorbid hypertension, myocardiopathy, and hepatic injury (Kasahara et al. 1996).

Familial Associations

Researchers have explored the association between Alzheimer's disease and a family history of dementia and have identified possible genetic loci for familial Alzheimer's disease on chromosomes 21, 19, 14, and 1 (Levy-Lahad et al. 1995; Schellenberg et al. 1992; Whatley and Anderton 1990). Alzheimer's disease–causing mutations have been discovered on chromosomes 21, 14, and 1. Apolipoprotein genotype is coded on chromosome 19, and there is emerging evidence for a late-onset Alzheimer's disease susceptibility gene located on chromosome 12 (Pericak-Vance et al. 1997). Huntington's disease is inherited as an autosomal dominant trait with complete penetrance, so that half the offspring of Huntington's disease patients are affected; the mutation responsible for Huntington's disease is an elongated and unstable trinucleotide (CAG) repeat on the short arm of chromosome 4 (Haskins and Harrison 2000). Wilson's disease is inherited as an autosomal recessive trait (Dening and Berrios 1989); the defective gene is localized on chromosome 13 (Brewer 2000). Significant advances in the genetics of other dementias include the identification of tau gene mutations on chromosome 17 in some familial cases of frontotemporal dementia (Rosen et al. 2000); although most cases of Parkinson's disease appear to be sporadic, a number of important genetic loci have been identified (Lev and Melamed 2001). There are also familial associations for disorders that produce dementia, such as alcoholism and major depression, as well as cerebrovascular risk factors, including diabetes, hyperlipidemia, and heart disease.

CLINICAL FEATURES

Cortical Dementia

Alzheimer's Disease

According to DSM-IV-TR (American Psychiatric Association 2000), the clinical diagnosis of Alzheimer's disease requires the gradual, progressive development of multiple cognitive deficits, including both memory impairment and nonmemory cognitive disturbances. The diagnostic criteria for dementia of the Alzheimer's type are shown in Table 16–3.

The memory impairment found in Alzheimer's disease is manifested by disorientation for time and place

and failure to remember three unrelated words for 3 minutes, even with cues (Petersen et al. 1994). Recall usually is not helped by clues. The typical language disturbance is a fluent aphasia with anomia; speech has an empty quality and lacks specific content words. Naming and comprehension are progressively impaired, whereas the ability to repeat is relatively preserved; paraphasic errors are common (Cummings and Benson 1986). The gradual development of an isolated, progressive aphasia may be the precursor of a more generalized dementia syndrome in some patients (Green et al. 1990). Agnosia and apraxia in Alzheimer's disease are difficult to distinguish clinically from disabilities related to aphasia, amnesia, and visuospatial impairment. Patients retain the ability to recognize objects and to use them appropriately at a time when they can no longer name them accurately (Rapcsak et al. 1989). Disturbances in executive cognitive functions include abnormalities of planning, organizing, sequencing, and abstracting. Clinically, these executive functions help to orchestrate and to maintain goal-directed behavior. Apathy, distractibility, purposeless stereotypy, overreliance on environmental cues, agitation, and a tendency to perseverate all may arise from disturbed executive cognitive systems (Royall et al. 1992). Alzheimer's disease is relentlessly progressive, advancing through mild, moderate, and severe stages. The principal clinical findings in each stage of dementia of the Alzheimer's type are summarized in Table 16–4.

Increasingly, clinical and research attention is being focused on the critical stage of cognitive impairment that exists between normal aging and very early Alzheimer's disease, so-called mild cognitive impairment (MCI). MCI refers to individuals with memory impairment who are otherwise functioning well and do not meet clinical criteria for dementia. Patients with MCI should be recognized and monitored for cognitive and functional decline, since they have a high rate of progression to dementia or Alzheimer's disease—between 6% and 25% per year (Petersen et al. 2001).

Frontotemporal Dementia

Pick's disease, frontotemporal dementia with nonspecific histological changes, and frontotemporal dementia with motor neuron disease are the principal neurodegenerative conditions now diagnosed clinically as frontotemporal dementia. These frontotemporal dementia syndromes are indistinguishable clinically and present with marked personality changes that may precede the development of overt cognitive decline by at least 2 years. Disinhibition and irritability are common, as are wandering, impulsivity, and poor judgment. Social withdrawal, loss

---

TABLE 16–3.   DSM-IV-TR diagnostic criteria for dementia of the Alzheimer's type

A. The development of multiple cognitive deficits manifested by both

   (1) memory impairment (impaired ability to learn new information or to recall previously learned information)
   (2) one (or more) of the following cognitive disturbances:

      (a) aphasia (language disturbance)
      (b) apraxia (impaired ability to carry out motor activities despite intact motor function)
      (c) agnosia (failure to recognize or identify objects despite intact sensory function)
      (d) disturbance in executive functioning (i.e., planning, organizing, sequencing, abstracting)

B. The cognitive deficits in Criteria A1 and A2 each cause significant impairment in social or occupational functioning and represent a significant decline from a previous level of functioning.
C. The course is characterized by gradual onset and continuing cognitive decline.
D. The cognitive deficits in Criteria A1 and A2 are not due to any of the following:

   (1) other central nervous system conditions that cause progressive deficits in memory and cognition (e.g., cerebrovascular disease, Parkinson's disease, Huntington's disease, subdural hematoma, normal-pressure hydrocephalus, brain tumor)

   (2) systemic conditions that are known to cause dementia (e.g., hypothyroidism, vitamin B_{12} or folic acid deficiency, niacin deficiency, hypercalcemia, neurosyphilis, HIV infection)

   (3) substance-induced conditions

E. The deficits do not occur exclusively during the course of a delirium.
F. The disturbance is not better accounted for by another Axis I disorder (e.g., Major Depressive Disorder, Schizophrenia).

Code based on presence or absence of a clinically significant behavioral disturbance:

   294.10   Without behavioral disturbance: if the cognitive disturbance is not accompanied by any clinically significant behavioral disturbance.
   294.11   With behavioral disturbance: if the cognitive disturbance is accompanied by a clinically significant behavioral disturbance (e.g., wandering, agitation).

Specify subtype:

   With early onset: if onset is at age 65 years or below
   With late onset: if onset is after age 65 years
   Coding note: Also code 331.0 Alzheimer's disease on Axis III. Indicate other prominent clinical features related to the Alzheimer's disease on Axis I (e.g., 293.83 mood disorder due to Alzheimer's disease, with depressive features, and 310.1 personality change due to Alzheimer's disease, aggressive type).

---

of drive, and even major depression may be the first symptoms in some patients. Features of the Klüver-Bucy syndrome, such as hyperorality, hypersexuality, compulsory exploration of the environment, and visual agnosia, are not uncommon. Disproportionate impairment of frontal/executive skills is present on neuropsychological testing. Aphasia is present in some patients. The clinical presentation plus the relatively late onset of memory and visuospatial disturbances in frontotemporal dementia help to distinguish frontotemporal dementia from Alzheimer's disease (Baldwin and Forstl 1993; Neary et al. 1998).

Increasingly, the use of clinical inventories, along with ever more sophisticated neuropsychological testing, is enhancing the accurate diagnosis of the frontotemporal dementias; further refinements include recognition of left, right, and temporal lobe variants (Edwards-Lee et al. 1997; Kertesz et al. 2000; Razani et al. 2001).

Subcortical Dementia

Huntington's Disease

The clinical triad of dementia, chorea, and a "positive" family history should suggest the diagnosis of Huntington's disease to the consultant. Huntington's disease is a typical subcortical dementia, with diminished cognitive speed, a memory retrieval deficit (characterized by poor spontaneous recall but preserved recognition memory), poor executive functions, and motor symptoms. The absence of aphasia and other cortical features further distinguishes Huntington's disease from Alzheimer's disease (Savage 1997). Personality changes such as irritability or apathy are common and may antedate the onset of chorea (Cummings 1995a). Depression is common in Huntington's disease, and the risk of suicide is increased; mania and a syndrome with persecutory delusions resembling schizophrenia are seen as well (Rosenblatt and Leroi 2000).

TABLE 16–4. Principal clinical findings in each stage of dementia of the Alzheimer's type

Stage I (duration of disease 1–3 years)

Memory—new learning defective, remote recall mildly impaired

Visuospatial skills—topographic disorientation, poor complex constructions

Language—poor word list generation, anomia

Personality—indifference, occasional irritability

Psychiatric features—sadness or delusions in some patients

Motor system—normal

EEG—normal

CT/MRI—normal

PET/SPECT—bilateral posterior parietal hypometabolism/ hypoperfusion

Stage II (duration of disease 2–10 years)

Memory—recent and remote recall more severely impaired

Visuospatial skills—poor constructions, spatial disorientation

Language—fluent aphasia

Calculation—acalculia

Praxis—ideomotor apraxia

Personality—indifference or irritability

Psychiatric features—delusions in some patients

Motor system—restlessness, pacing

EEG—slowing of background rhythm

CT/MRI—normal and ventricular dilatation and sulcal enlargement

PET/SPECT—bilateral parietal and frontal hypometabolism/ hypoperfusion

Stage III (duration of disease 8–12 years)

Intellectual functions—severely deteriorated

Motor system—limb rigidity and flexion posture

Sphincter control—urinary and fecal incontinence

EEG—diffusely slow

CT/MRI—ventricular dilatation and sulcal enlargement

PET/SPECT—bilateral parietal and frontal hypometabolism/ hypoperfusion

Note. CT = computed tomography; EEG = electroencephalogram; MRI = magnetic resonance imaging; PET = positron-emission tomography; SPECT = single photon emission computed tomography.
Source. Adapted from Cummings JL, Benson DF: *Dementia: A Clinical Approach.* Boston, MA, Butterworth-Heinemann, 1992, pp. 217–265. Used with permission.

Wilson's Disease

Wilson's disease is a recessively inherited defect in the copper-carrying serum protein ceruloplasmin. Although Wilson's disease is an uncommon cause of dementia, the consultant must be aware of this diagnosis because its progression can be halted by treatment with chelating agents. Wilson's disease usually begins during adolescence or early adulthood. Dementia in Wilson's disease is variable but tends to be mild; additional neurological findings include dysarthria, dystonia, rigidity, cerebellar abnormalities, tremor, and gait and postural disturbances (Starosta-Rubinstein et al. 1987). Psychiatric symptoms of Wilson's disease include personality and behavioral changes such as irritability, aggression, disinhibition, and recklessness. Depressive features are common, whereas psychosis is infrequently seen. Almost invariably, the severity of psychiatric symptoms is associated with severity of neurological symptoms, especially dystonic and bulbar manifestations (Dening and Berrios 1989).

Parkinson's Disease

Assessment of dementia in Parkinson's disease is complex because the effects of aging, depression (in perhaps half of all Parkinson's disease patients), and chronic disability must be considered in addition to the profound motor deficits. Although Parkinson's disease dementia generally is classified as a subcortical dementia, the presentation and course of cognitive decline in Parkinson's disease are highly variable, and cortical-type deficits may occur. Coexistent Alzheimer's disease pathology can produce dementia in Parkinson's disease, whereas dementia with Lewy bodies itself can produce a spectrum of "cortical" dementia findings resembling Alzheimer's disease in patients with Parkinson's disease features (Forstl et al. 1993; Gibb et al. 1989; McKeith et al. 1996). The emerging clinical picture of dementia with Lewy bodies is one of delirium-like fluctuating cognitive impairment, with periods of both episodic confusion and lucid intervals; unlike in delirium, no physical cause can be found to account for the fluctuating cognitive state, which can persist for days or weeks. Psychotic features are common and include visual and/or auditory hallucinations, accompanied by paranoid delusions. Parkinsonism is common—either mild spontaneous extrapyramidal features or exaggerated sensitivity to standard doses of neuroleptic medications. Falling and unexplained losses of consciousness are seen significantly more often than in Alzheimer's disease, as is the early onset of urinary incontinence (Del Ser et al. 2001). Prominent depressive symptoms occur in perhaps 40% of the patients with dementia with Lewy bodies. The illness progresses, often rapidly, to an end stage of severe dementia (Byrne et al. 1991; Del Ser et al. 2000; McKeith et al. 1992b).

Progressive Supranuclear Palsy

Progressive supranuclear palsy (PSP) is a progressive extrapyramidal syndrome usually beginning in the sixth decade of life. PSP is characterized by supranuclear gaze paresis, pseudobulbar palsy, axial rigidity, and a dementia with subcortical features (Albert et al. 1974; Steele et al. 1964). In addition to the loss of volitional down gaze, the most common presenting symptoms are postural instability and falling, gait abnormalities, depression, dysarthria, and memory disturbances (Maher and Lees 1986). The profound rigidity and bradykinesia that develop during the course of PSP may impart a superficial resemblance to Parkinson's disease; however, the abnormal eye findings, absence of tremor, spastic dysarthria, and erect posture are more indicative of PSP, especially when coupled with a minimal response to L-dopa (Litvan et al. 1996, 1997).

Limbic Encephalopathy

Limbic encephalopathy is a relatively rare, nonmetastatic complication of carcinoma. This dramatic paraneoplastic syndrome usually is associated with small cell lung cancer and is characterized by cognitive, affective, and behavioral changes. Central nervous system (CNS) pathological changes include extensive neuronal loss, perivascular infiltration, astrocytosis, and glial nodules. The earliest and most prominent feature is the sudden onset of memory loss that is often severe. Limbic encephalopathy should be considered in any patient who presents with a pure amnestic syndrome. Other common symptoms include spells of confusion or disorientation, seizures, depression, bizarre behaviors, hallucinations, paranoia, and anxiety.

These symptoms may precede the diagnosis of cancer by as many as 6 years; therefore, it is important for the consultant to recognize limbic encephalopathy because it may be the first sign of a malignancy that is still at an early, possibly curable stage (Camara and Chelune 1987).

Mixed Dementia

Vascular Dementia

Although ischemia, hemorrhage, and anoxia can all cause vascular dementia, this disorder is most often associated with ischemic vascular disease. There is considerable heterogeneity in both the pathological and the clinical expression of vascular dementia. The accumulation of cerebral infarctions can produce the progressive cognitive impairment termed *multi-infarct dementia*. Chronic ischemia without frank infarction can impair cognition, focal infarcts in critical areas subserving multiple cognitive functions can produce the syndrome of strategic infarct dementia, and ischemic injury can coexist with other dementias such as Alzheimer's disease (Chui et al. 1992; Roman et al. 1993; Tatemichi et al. 1995). DSM-IV-TR diagnostic criteria for vascular dementia are listed in Table 16–5.

TABLE 16–5.   DSM-IV-TR diagnostic criteria for vascular dementia

A. The development of multiple cognitive deficits manifested by both

   (1) memory impairment (impaired ability to learn new information or to recall previously learned information)
   (2) one (or more) of the following cognitive disturbances:

      (a) aphasia (language disturbance)
      (b) apraxia (impaired ability to carry out motor activities despite intact motor function)
      (c) agnosia (failure to recognize or identify objects despite intact sensory function)
      (d) disturbance in executive functioning (i.e., planning, organizing, sequencing, abstracting)

B. The cognitive deficits in Criteria A1 and A2 each cause significant impairment in social or occupational functioning and represent a significant decline from a previous level of functioning.
C. Focal neurological signs and symptoms (e.g., exaggeration of deep tendon reflexes, extensor plantar response, pseudobulbar palsy, gait abnormalities, weakness of an extremity) or laboratory evidence indicative of cerebrovascular disease (e.g., multiple infarctions involving cortex and underlying white matter) that are judged to be etiologically related to the disturbance.
D. The deficits do not occur exclusively during the course of a delirium.

   Code based on predominant features:

      290.41 With delirium: if delirium is superimposed on the dementia
      290.42 With delusions: if delusions are the predominant feature
      290.43 With depressed mood: if depressed mood (including presentations that meet full symptom criteria for a major depressive episode) is the predominant feature. A separate diagnosis of mood disorder due to a general medical condition is not given.
      290.40 Uncomplicated: if none of the above predominates in the current clinical presentation

   Specify if:

      With behavioral disturbance
      Coding note: Also code cerebrovascular condition on Axis III.

Vascular dementia is characterized by an abrupt onset, a stepwise progression, pseudobulbar palsy, a history of hypertension, a history of strokes, focal neurological symptoms, and focal neurological signs on examination. These features together constitute an ischemia score (Table 16–6) that is valuable in differentiating vascular dementia from Alzheimer's disease (Hachinski et al. 1975; Knopman et al. 2001; Rosen et al. 1980). The ischemia score does not differentiate vascular dementia from vascular dementia plus Alzheimer's disease (Erkinjuntti et al. 1988). The presence of infarctions and white matter ischemia can be identified by magnetic resonance imaging (MRI) and is required in some diagnostic schema for a diagnosis of vascular dementia (Roman et al. 1993).

The clinical presentation of vascular dementia depends on the mechanism of cerebral injury. Deep hemispheric infarction, ischemia causing a lacunar state, or Binswanger's disease will produce a subcortical dementia associated with pseudobulbar palsy, spasticity, and weakness (Fisher 1989). Superficial cortical infarctions will produce a cortical dementia associated with hemimotor and hemisensory dysfunction. Dominant hemisphere insults produce aphasia, acalculia, apraxia, and verbal amnesia, whereas nondominant hemisphere damage causes aprosodia; disturbances in recognition of face, voice, and place; nonverbal amnesia; visuospatial deficits; and left hemineglect. Mixed cortical and subcortical syndromes are not uncommon (Cummings 1987). The mechanical aspects of speech are more abnormal in vascular dementia, whereas linguistic changes are more profound in Alzheimer's disease. The presence of an articulatory deficit and abnormal speech melody supports the diagnosis of vascular dementia; patients with vascular dementia have more information content in spontaneous speech and are less anomic than patients with Alzheimer's disease (Powell et al. 1988). Psychotic features are common in vascular dementia, although neither the nature and prevalence of delusions nor the occurrence of hallucinations distinguishes vascular dementia from Alzheimer's disease (Cummings et al. 1987). Depression is common following stroke and occurs most often with left cortical and subcortical lesions. The severity of depression is correlated with proximity of the lesion to the left frontal pole. A history of stroke or preexisting cortical atrophy may be an important risk factor for the subsequent development of poststroke depression (Robinson 1997).

Trauma

Serious head trauma can cause dementia. Amnesia and personality alterations are the most common neurobe-

TABLE 16–6. Hachinski Ischemia Score

Abrupt onset	2
Stepwise progression	1
Somatic complaints	1
Emotional incontinence	1
History of hypertension	1
History of strokes	2
Focal neurological symptoms	2
Focal neurological signs	2
Alzheimer's disease scores 4 or less	
Vascular dementia scores 7 or more	

Source.   Adapted from Hachinski et al. 1975.

havioral deficits following traumatic brain injury (TBI). Posttraumatic amnesia includes a variable period of unconsciousness caused by the injury, a period of retrograde amnesia for information acquired from a few minutes to a few years before the injury, and a period of anterograde amnesia lasting from hours to months after recovery from unconsciousness (Levin et al. 1982). Recovery is not always complete, and a degree of permanent anterograde memory disturbance may persist (Levin 1989). Aphasia can occur in up to 30% of TBI patients (Jennett and Teasdale 1981). Personality changes, attentional disturbances, and other cognitive impairments suggestive of frontal lobe damage are common (Mattson and Levin 1990). TBI increases the risk for developing secondary psychiatric syndromes, including depression, mania, and psychosis (McAllister 1992). Posttraumatic seizures further complicate recovery in 2%–5% of the patients with TBI (Slagle 1990). Subjective symptoms such as headache, dizziness, easy fatigability, and disordered sleep persist in some patients for several months, even after mild head trauma; this *postconcussional syndrome* is a complex blend of physiologic and psychological factors that results in significant chronic disability for a small proportion of patients (Lishman 1988).

Three other important dementia syndromes are associated with head trauma. The chronic, repeated head trauma experienced by boxers can lead to dementia pugilistica, a syndrome characterized by ataxia and dysarthria that progresses to dementia with parkinsonian-type extrapyramidal features (Jordan 1987). A potentially reversible cause of dementia following head trauma is subdural hematoma, a condition that may manifest as dementia, delirium, or psychosis (Black 1984). A history of head trauma may be minimal or entirely absent, especially in elderly patients. Although a head computed tomography (CT) scan may be diagnostic, MRI is the technique of choice for demonstrating these lesions (Traynelis 1991). Finally, an uncommon but potentially treatable dementia associated with head trauma is normal-pressure hydrocephalus (NPH), a condition that also may occur following subarachnoid hemorrhage or intracranial infection or may have no known precipitant. NPH produces a triad of clinical symptoms: 1) a gait disturbance, often described as "magnetic," that appears early; 2) a subcortical dementia; and 3) urinary incontinence that may not appear until late in the course (Benson 1985). This triad is not specific to NPH, and vascular dementia is a more commonly associated with these features.

Dementias Associated With Infectious Diseases

Infection with HIV-1 produces a dementing illness initially termed the *AIDS (acquired immunodeficiency syndrome) dementia complex* (Navia et al. 1986) and more recently designated *HIV-1-associated cognitive/motor complex* (American Academy of Neurology AIDS Task Force 1991). Two clinical categories are recognized: 1) a more severe form known as *HIV-1-associated dementia complex* and 2) a less severe form termed *HIV-1-associated minor cognitive/motor disorder*, in which only the most demanding activities of daily living are impaired despite the presence of demonstrable cognitive, motor, or behavioral abnormalities. HIV-1-associated dementia is the most frequent neurological complication of HIV infection; in some patients, it may be the earliest or only clinical manifestation of HIV-1 infection.

Neuropsychological deficits include impaired attention and concentration, psychomotor slowing, slowed complex reaction time, memory disturbance, and personality or mood alterations such as apathy and irritability (Faulstich 1987). This combination of cognitive impairment, motor dysfunction, and behavioral change is typical of a subcortical type of dementia. However, recent analysis suggests that there may be two relatively distinct subtypes of HIV-1-seropositive individuals with dementia: 1) a "subcortical, depressed" group, with depressed mood, psychomotor slowing, and forgetfulness; and 2) a "cortical" group, with verbal and visuospatial deficits, some psychomotor slowing, and euthymic mood. Thus, HIV dementia may be heterogeneous in its clinical presentation (Van Gorp et al. 1993).

Primary HIV-1-associated dementia complex is now the most common dementia associated with infectious diseases, but several other clinically important conditions deserve mention. Creutzfeldt-Jakob disease is an uncommon prion-related dementia characterized by extremely rapid progressive deterioration and death, usually within 1 year. Patients show intellectual devastation, myoclonic jerks, muscle rigidity, and ataxia (Brown et al. 1986; Prusiner 1998).

Progressive multifocal leukoencephalopathy (PML) is a subacute viral disorder that occurs in adults with chronic systemic illness. AIDS, chronic lymphocytic leukemia, Hodgkin's disease, lymphosarcoma, chronic myelocytic leukemia, sarcoidosis, and tuberculosis are the conditions most commonly associated with PML (Richardson 1974; von Einsiedel et al. 1993). The lesions of PML are distributed randomly in the nervous system, which results in highly variable clinical manifestations. PML usually progresses to death in 2–4 months, with dementia, blindness, and impaired motility present in the advanced stages.

Chronic meningitis caused by fungal, parasitic, or chronic bacterial infections can present as dementia. Slow, progressive compromise of intellectual function, with fluctuations in arousal, apathy, lethargy, disorientation, and poor memory, is typical; cranial nerve abnormalities are common, and focal signs may be present. The consultant must consider this diagnosis when evaluating immunocompromised or debilitated patients (Luby 1992).

Acute herpes simplex encephalitis preferentially damages the medial, temporal, and orbitofrontal regions of the cortex, and neurological sequelae are often seen among survivors of the acute illness. Although amnesia is the most common residual deficit, aphasia or other cognitive deficits can occur. Recovery of intellect is variable, and dementia can be a long-term consequence of the disease (Skoldenberg 1991).

Syphilitic infection of the CNS ultimately can manifest as dementia in a variety of ways. All forms of neurosyphilis begin as a meningitis that usually is asymptomatic but if left untreated may evolve into meningovascular syphilis or general paresis. Meningovascular syphilis usually occurs 6–7 years after the original infection and always should be considered in a young person who has one or more cerebrovascular accidents. General paresis usually becomes evident 15–20 years after infection, beginning with the insidious onset of a memory defect, inattention, and indifference; facial quivering, hand tremor, and myoclonus may be present. As the deterioration continues, intellectual function decays completely, and cortical deficits become apparent; perhaps two-thirds of these patients become psychotic, with expansive-grandiose or depressive-hypochondriacal delusions. The final progression of symptoms includes pupillary abnormalities, tremor of the tongue, dysarthria, muscular hypotonia, and seizures, and the disease culminates in a bedridden state (Adams and Victor 1993).

Toxic-Metabolic Dementias

Because toxic-metabolic dementias are common in the hospital setting, and many are potentially treatable or reversible to some extent, this category is especially important for the consultant. Whereas acute, overwhelming toxic-metabolic states present as delirium, more chronic, insidious toxic-metabolic conditions produce a slowly progressive dementia that has subcortical features (Cummings and Benson 1992). The principal toxic-metabolic conditions associated with dementia are listed in Table 16–7.

These dementias are diagnosed with DSM-IV-TR diagnostic criteria for substance-induced persisting dementia or dementia due to a general medical condition (American Psychiatric Association 2000). The DSM-IV-TR criteria for substance-induced persisting dementia are listed in Table 16–8. Although cognitive disturbances in toxic-metabolic dementias vary with the specific etiology of the dementia, these patients generally show impaired attention and concentration, forgetfulness, and disturbed executive functioning. Chronic intoxication from ingestion of medications is the most common cause of reversible dementia.

A frequent cause of toxic-metabolic dementia is alcoholism, a diagnosis that is often unrecognized in elderly patients (Beresford et al. 1988). Traditionally, Wernicke-Korsakoff syndrome is considered to be an isolated amnesia rather than a true dementia. It is produced by dietary thiamine deficiency. The acute phase of Wernicke-Korsakoff syndrome—Wernicke's encephalopathy—is characterized by ophthalmoplegia, ataxia, and confusion. Only 25% of the patients who eventually develop the chronic amnesia of Wernicke-Korsakoff syndrome have a prior clinical diagnosis of Wernicke's encephalopathy (Blansjaar et al. 1992a). Korsakoff's syndrome is the chronic amnestic phase of Wernicke-Korsakoff syndrome and is characterized by a severe disability in learning new material and by a retrograde amnesia with relative sparing of remote memories. Confabulation is common in the early phases of Korsakoff's syndrome, and variable degrees of apathy, loss of insight, and diminished initiative frequently accompany the amnesia (Bowden 1990; Butterworth 1995; Victor 1993). Further refinement of the Wernicke-Korsakoff syndrome diagnosis is needed because the clinical and cognitive manifestations are highly variable. Wernicke-Korsakoff syndrome appears to be clinically underdiagnosed because Wernicke-Korsakoff syndrome pathology is found in perhaps 10%–15% of all alcoholic patients at autopsy. With abstinence, a significant proportion of patients with Wernicke-Korsakoff syndrome show improvement in cognitive deficits, usually within the first year.

Alcoholic dementia not a part of Wernicke-Korsakoff syndrome occurs as well. Marchiafava-Bignami degeneration of the corpus callosum and anterior commissure, pellagrous encephalopathy, and acquired hepatocerebral degeneration are all distinct cerebral diseases associated with chronic alcoholism. In each of these syndromes, as in Wernicke-Korsakoff syndrome, the etiological role of alcohol is a secondary one. Currently, no clear evidence suggests that any persistent dementia is attributable to the direct toxic effects of alcohol on the brain; this is because of the lack of any distinctive, well-defined pathology for a primary alcoholic dementia (Victor 1994). Alcoholic dementia may be more common in women and typically occurs during the sixth or seventh decade of life. These patients describe failing intellect for about a year, with a drinking history of more than 10 years. Impairment on memory, visuoperceptual, and frontal/executive tests is seen on mental status examination (MSE), along with variable mood changes. Electroencephalogram (EEG) findings may be abnormal. Abstinence or dramatically reduced drinking may produce a favorable outcome. Medical illnesses, including organ failure syndrome (renal, cardiac, pulmonary) and endocrinopathies (especially thyroid dysfunction), are the most common metabolic causes of dementia.

Neoplastic Dementias

In addition to the paraneoplastic syndromes noted previously, brain tumors can present clinically as dementia. As many as 1%–2% of the patients given a psychiatric diagnosis may have undiagnosed CNS tumors (Keschner et al. 1938; Selecki 1965). Tumors may cause a variety of behavioral changes, but no mental syndromes are strictly characteristic of tumors located in specific areas of the brain. Psychiatric symptom formation is influenced greatly by the extent of tumor involvement, the rapidity of tumor growth, and the propensity of a given tumor to cause increased intracranial pressure; tumor location plays a less important role. Nevertheless, psychiatric disturbances are more commonly associated with frontal- and temporal-lobe tumors than with tumors of the parietal or occipital lobes. When elaborating a differential diagnosis in the patient with dementia, the consultant must keep in mind that frontal lobe tumors may produce executive cognitive dysfunction as well as apathetic and akinetic syndromes, whereas temporal lobe tumors may affect memory and language functions (Price et al. 1992).

Dementia Associated With Psychiatric Disorders: "Pseudodementia"

Depression

Depression often is encountered among patients evaluated for impaired cognition. In one large series, 27% of the patients referred to a dementia clinic met criteria for

TABLE 16–7.   Toxic-metabolic conditions associated with dementia

Conditions associated with anoxia	**Porphyria**
Anoxic anoxia	**Drugs**
Pulmonary insufficiency	Psychotropic agents
Stagnant anoxia	Anticholinergic compounds
Cardiac disease	Antihypertensive agents
Hyperviscosity states	Anticonvulsants
Anemic anoxia	Antineoplastic therapies
Postanoxia dementia	Antibiotics
Chronic renal failure	Polydrug abuse
Uremic encephalopathy	Histamine H_2 receptor antagonists
Dialysis dementia	Cardiac medications (digoxin, β-blockers)
Hepatic diseases	Corticosteroids
Portosystemic encephalopathy	Nonsteroidal anti-inflammatory agents
Acquired hepatocerebral degeneration	**Alcohol**
Pancreatic disorders	**Metals**
Insulinoma and recurrent hypoglycemia	Lead
Pancreatic encephalopathy	Mercury
Electrolyte abnormalities	Manganese
Hyponatremia	Arsenic
Hypernatremia	Nickel
Cerebral effects of systemic malignancies	Cadmium
Metabolic changes	Thallium
Structural abnormalities	Aluminum
Mass lesions	Gold
Hydrocephalus	Tin
Central nervous system infections	Bismuth
Remote effects: limbic encephalitis	**Industrial agents and pollutants**
Vitamin deficiency states	Perchloroethylene
Thiamine (B_1)	Toluene
Cyanocobalamin (B_{12})	Carbon tetrachloride
Folate	Methyl chloride
Niacin	Acrylamide
Endocrinopathies	Trichloroethane
Thyroid disturbances	Trichloroethylene
Parathyroid abnormalities	Carbon disulfide
Adrenal diseases	Organophosphate insecticides
Panhypopituitarism	Organochlorine pesticides
	Ethylene oxide
	Formaldehyde
	Hydrogen sulfide
	Jet fuels
	Carbon monoxide

Source.   Adapted from Cummings and Benson 1992.

a depressive disorder (Reding et al. 1985). Several potential relations exist between depression and dementia: 1) depression can occur in response to the onset of cognitive impairment; 2) depression and dementia can be produced by the same underlying condition, as in stroke or Parkinson's disease; 3) clinical symptoms of dementing illnesses overlap with those of depression and can lead to the misdiagnosis of either; and 4) dementia is a syndrome that can be caused by depression (i.e., dementia syndrome of depression [DSD]). Currently, DSD can only be established with certitude retrospectively because the patient recovers intellectual function after successful antidepressant therapy (Cummings 1989).

Several salient clinical features are associated with DSD: 1) the elapsed time between onset and seeking medical help is shorter than is typical for degenerative dementias; 2) many patients have a history of primary mood disorder; 3) a high frequency of current depressed

TABLE 16–8. DSM-IV-TR diagnostic criteria for substance-induced persisting dementia

A. The development of multiple cognitive deficits manifested by both

(1) memory impairment (impaired ability to learn new information or to recall previously learned information)

(2) one (or more) of the following cognitive disturbances:

(a) aphasia (language disturbance)

(b) apraxia (impaired ability to carry out motor activities despite intact motor function)

(c) agnosia (failure to recognize or identify objects despite intact sensory function)

(d) disturbance in executive functioning (i.e., planning, organizing, sequencing, abstracting)

B. The cognitive deficits in Criteria A1 and A2 each cause significant impairment in social or occupational functioning and represent a significant decline from a previous level of functioning.

C. The deficits do not occur exclusively during the course of a delirium and persist beyond the usual duration of Substance Intoxication or Withdrawal.

D. There is evidence from the history, physical examination, or laboratory findings that the deficits are etiologically related to the persisting effects of substance use (e.g., a drug of abuse, a medication).

Code [Specific substance]–induced persisting dementia:

(291.2 alcohol; 292.82 inhalant; 292.82 sedative, hypnotic, or anxiolytic; 292.82 other [or unknown] substance)

mood and delusions is present; and 4) severe early-morning awakening is common (Emery and Oxman 1992). Neuropsychological features distinguishing DSD from Alzheimer's disease include differential memory and language impairments. Unlike the patient with Alzheimer's disease, the patient with DSD retains self-awareness, has memory performance improved by prompting and organization of material, and lacks aphasia. Patients with Alzheimer's disease manifest characteristic "empty" speech, often with paraphasic errors not typically seen in patients with DSD (Cummings 1989; O'Brien et al. 2001). The consultant should keep in mind that nearly half of all patients with an initial diagnosis of DSD will develop irreversible dementia within 3 years; recommendations for thorough evaluation and close follow-up of the patient with DSD are essential (Alexopoulos et al. 1993).

Conversion Disorder

Conversion ("hysterical") dementia is a rare syndrome. Marked disparity between the ability to answer questions on mental status testing and abilities shown in casual or unstructured situations should suggest this diagnosis to the consultant. Caution must be exercised because despite the presence of apparent primary gain, secondary gain, or bizarre symptoms, between 50% and 70% of patients given a diagnosis of conversion disorder eventually manifest a related physical disorder (McEvoy and Wells 1979; Merskey and Buhrich 1975; B. L. Miller et al. 1986).

Ganser's syndrome, or the "syndrome of approximate answers," is sometimes considered to be a variant of hysterical dementia, even though the syndrome has been described in a wide variety of neurological and toxic-metabolic conditions and in psychotic states. Unusual "nearly correct" answers suggesting an awareness of the correct response is the hallmark of this condition (Sigal et al. 1992; Whitlock 1967).

Acute Psychosis

During the acute psychotic phase, both mania and schizophrenia may be mistaken for primary dementia syndromes, especially in elderly patients. Patients with mania can have memory impairment, aggressive outbursts, hypersexuality, and disinhibited behavior. Patients with these "typical" symptoms of dementia may present with little history available, which makes it difficult to diagnose a primary mood disorder (Casey and Fitzgerald 1988; Fortin 1990). Schizophrenia can produce acute disturbances of language, thought, memory, and movement, as well as a chronic neuropsychological impairment that is not well characterized. The mild to moderate cognitive dysfunction seen in most older patients with schizophrenia differs from the more severe, progressive deterioration seen in patients with Alzheimer's disease (Bienfeld and Hartford 1982; Granholm and Jeste 1994; Purohit et al. 1993).

Malingering

Entirely conscious simulation of dementia is rare, and careful observation usually reveals much that is inconsistent with genuine cognitive impairment. Isolated symptoms, such as loss of speech or memory, are produced more commonly than a full dementia syndrome. An underlying disorder always should be sought; the absence of obvious disease, an accompanying motive, and evidence of awareness on the part of the patient serve to alert the consultant to the diagnosis of malingering (Lishman 1998).

PATHOPHYSIOLOGY

Alzheimer's Disease

On gross inspection, the brain in Alzheimer's disease is characterized by cortical atrophy, with widened sulci and ventricular enlargement. Microscopic examination identifies neuronal loss, neurofibrillary tangles, neuritic plaques, granulovacuolar degeneration, and amyloid angiopathy. Within the cortex, the most severe pathological changes occur in the medial temporal lobe, including the hippocampus, amygdala, entorhinal cortex, and parahippocampal gyrus. Areas of association cortex in the parietotemporal and frontal lobes are involved to an intermediate degree (Pearson and Powell 1989). Tangles are located within neurons and are composed of paired helical filaments that contain abnormally phosphorylated microtubule-associated tau proteins. Plaques are located extracellularly and consist of a core of amyloid peptide and aluminosilicates surrounded by dystrophic nerve processes, terminals, and organelles (Dickson 2001a). Granulovacuolar degeneration consists of intracytoplasmic vacuoles, particularly in neurons of the hippocampus. Amyloid angiopathy is present in nearly all cases of Alzheimer's disease; this cerebrovascular amyloid is identical to that found in neuritic plaques (Mirra et al. 1993; Vinters et al. 1988). Findings indicate that the amyloid β-peptide of Alzheimer's disease is produced by normal cell metabolism rather than via pathological processes, implicating chronically enhanced production and/or decreased clearance mechanisms in the formation of neuritic plaques and vascular deposits (Haass et al. 1992). Virtually all of these neuropathological changes are found in the brains of individuals without dementia; the location and abundance of these lesions determine the postmortem histological diagnosis of Alzheimer's disease (Cummings et al. 1998; Khachaturian 1985; Vinters 1991).

Frontotemporal Dementia

Perhaps 20% of the frontotemporal dementias are Pick's disease, diagnosed by the presence of distinctive intraneuronal Pick bodies and ballooned Pick cells on microscopic examination; the remaining 80% are designated as frontotemporal dementias of the non-Alzheimer's type or dementia lacking distinctive histological features (Brun 1987). Mutations on chromosome 17 are responsible for approximately 20% of familial frontotemporal dementia and 3% of sporadic frontotemporal dementia (Dickson 2001b; Foster et al. 1997; Houlden et al. 1999).

Huntington's Disease

Pathologically, in Huntington's disease, atrophy of the caudate nucleus and loss of the γ-aminobutyric acid (GABA)–ergic interneurons with an inhibitory function in movement mechanisms from the striatum occur. Subcortical dopaminergic and cholinergic systems are dynamically balanced so that dopamine agonists increase chorea, whereas cholinergic and GABAergic compounds diminish spontaneous movements (Perry et al. 1973). Huntington's disease is caused by an increased CAG repeat number in a gene coding for a protein with unknown function, called huntingtin; it is likely that the Huntington's disease mutation confers a deleterious gain of function on the protein. The exact process whereby the abnormal gene on chromosome 4 ultimately produces the characteristic Huntington's disease neuropathology remains to be elucidated (Ho et al. 2001).

Wilson's Disease

The primary biochemical defect in Wilson's disease is a disorder of copper metabolism resulting from the absence or dysfunction of a copper-transporting P-type ATPase encoded on chromosome 13. This ATPase is expressed in hepatocytes where it transports copper into the secretory pathway for incorporation into ceruloplasmin and excretion into the bile. When the ability of the liver to handle copper and excrete it into the bile is impaired, unbound copper accumulates in the CNS, liver, cornea, and kidneys, where levels reach toxic proportions (Loudianos and Gitlin 2000; Starosta-Rubinstein et al. 1987).

Parkinson's Disease

Parkinson's disease is an idiopathic disorder characterized by progressive loss of dopaminergic neurons in the substantia nigra and other pigmented brain stem nuclei. Parkinson's disease represents an example of a long-latency neurological disease because tremor, rigidity, and bradykinesia emerge only when a 70%–80% reduction in dopamine occurs. The pathological hallmark of Parkinson's disease is the presence of Lewy bodies in the cytoplasm of the remaining nigral neurons, where they are considered to represent a marker for neuronal cell degeneration (Gibb 1989).

Progressive Supranuclear Palsy

In PSP, neurofibrillary tangles, granulovacuolar degeneration, cell loss, and gliosis are found in the subthalamic nucleus, red nucleus, substantia nigra, and dentate nucleus, but the cortex is unaffected (Steele et al. 1964). Both the nigrostriatal dopaminergic and the cholinergic systems are impaired (Ruberg et al. 1985). Recent insights into PSP pathogenesis implicate mitochondrial dysfunction as well as tau protein abnormalities (Albers and Augood 2001).

HIV-Associated Dementia

The severity of clinical deterioration generally correlates with the severity of brain pathology, and levels of plasma HIV RNA and CD4 lymphocyte counts appear to be predictive of HIV-associated dementia. Some degree of cerebral atrophy is present in almost all HIV-infected patients with dementia. Histological examination demonstrates diffuse pallor of the centrum semiovale with a mononuclear inflammatory response in the white matter and the deep gray nuclei (Navia 1990; Wesselingh and Thompson 2001).

Vascular Dementia

Several dimensions of cerebral injury relevant to vascular dementia are recognized, including the location of cerebral injury, the volume of cerebral tissue involved, the number of cerebral insults, and the co-occurrence of vascular dementia and Alzheimer's disease (Tatemichi 1990). Subcortical lacunar infarctions are found in approximately 70% of the patients with vascular dementia. This so-called lacunar state is produced by multiple small infarctions involving the basal ganglia, thalamus, and internal capsule and is the most frequent cause of vascular dementia. Vascular dementia also may result from the cumulative effects of watershed or border zone infarctions that are caused by critical reductions in cerebral perfusion in association with severe extracranial atherosclerosis; this pathology is seen in up to 40% of the patients with vascular dementia (Meyer et al. 1988). A diagnosis of Binswanger's disease is made on the basis of extensive ischemic white matter damage in the subcortical periventricular regions of the centrum semiovale. These periventricular areas are susceptible to damage produced by occlusion or hypoperfusion of the blood vessels supplying the deep white matter (Tatemichi 1990). Vascular dementia also may result from the cumulative effects of multiple cerebral emboli; these embolic infarcts are found in approximately 20% of the patients with vas-

cular dementia and represent the third most frequent cause of vascular dementia. Embolic infarcts usually are larger than lacunae and have a bilateral hemispheric distribution. An identifiable cardiac source for emboli is found in one-fourth of these patients. Combinations of two or more different types of strokes are common and occur in nearly one-third of the patients with vascular dementia (Meyer et al. 1988). Additional causes of vascular dementia to consider include 1) the hypercoagulable state associated with the antiphospholipid antibody syndrome, especially in young stroke patients or in older stroke patients with few vascular risk factors (Gorman and Cummings 1993), and 2) cerebral autosomal dominant arteriopathy with subcortical infarcts and leukoencephalopathy (CADASIL), an inherited arterial disease of the brain recently mapped to chromosome 19. CADASIL typically becomes evident in early or middle adulthood with migraine or an ischemic event, and it later manifests itself through recurrent subcortical ischemic strokes leading to a stepwise decline and dementia (Desmond et al. 1999).

Both the total volume of cerebral injury, with infarct size reaching a critical threshold that exceeds the brain's compensatory capacities, and the total number of infarctions, with additive and/or multiplicative effects, have considerable face validity as mechanisms of vascular dementia. Although study findings confirm that total infarction area correlates with poststroke dementia, the location of cerebral infarction (especially involvement of the posterior cortical region of the dominant hemisphere) rather than the total volume of infarcted brain appears to be more critically correlated with the development of vascular dementia (Liu et al. 1992; Meyer et al. 1988).

Trauma

Rapid acceleration or deceleration of the brain produces stretching and twisting of neuronal axons. The resulting spectrum of diffuse axonal injury ranges from brief interruption of physiologic function without obvious anatomic disruption to frank axonal tearing (Graham et al. 1987). Cortical contusions and intracerebral hemorrhage contribute to the dementia in some cases.

Creutzfeldt-Jakob Disease

Creutzfeldt-Jakob disease is caused by a transmissible infectious agent—the *prion*. Prions are proteinaceous particles containing no nucleic acid that reproduce by recruiting normal cellular prion protein and stimulating its conversion to the disease-causing isoform; the normal and prion polypeptide chains are identical in composition, but they differ critically in their three-dimensional, folded conformations (Prusiner 2001). Most cases of Creutzfeldt-Jakob disease arise sporadically, without any infectious source identified, although in Great Britain a number of patients have contracted a new variant form of Creutzfeldt-Jakob disease, apparently from prion-tainted beef products (Brown et al. 2001). Direct transmission of Creutzfeldt-Jakob disease had formerly occurred only iatrogenically, as from contaminated neurosurgical instruments or tissue (Hsiao and Prusiner 1990). Microscopic neuropathology includes neuronal loss, astrocytic proliferation, and spongiform change in the cells of the cortex, striatum, and thalamus (Masters and Richardson 1978).

Toxic-Metabolic Dementias

Anoxia causes a breakdown of energy-dependent membrane functions, with loss of ionic homeostasis and neuronal death (Espinoza and Parer 1991). Hippocampal neurons appear to be most vulnerable to anoxic injury (Zola-Morgan et al. 1986).

Alcoholic Dementia

At autopsy, the brains of chronic alcohol abusers show cortical atrophy and nerve fiber disintegration with dissolution of myelin sheaths (Lishman 1981). Wernicke-Korsakoff syndrome is caused by thiamine deficiency associated with prolonged, heavy ingestion of alcohol. The characteristic pathology of Wernicke-Korsakoff syndrome involves punctate lesions of the gray nuclei in the periventricular regions surrounding the third and fourth ventricles and the Sylvian aqueduct (Victor et al. 1989).

Chronic Drug Intoxications

Benzodiazepines are among the most widely prescribed medications in the world. Despite having valuable sedative, hypnotic, and anxiolytic properties, benzodiazepines negatively affect memory in two distinct ways: 1) anterograde amnesia after benzodiazepine administration and 2) impairment of memory consolidation and subsequent memory retrieval (American Psychiatric Association Task Force 1990). Benzodiazepines impair memory consolidation and delayed recall without affecting memory acquisition or short-term memory (Angus and Romney 1984). This memory impairment is not associated with sedation or psychomotor impairment (Roache and Griffiths 1985). Benzodiazepines have no effect on the retrieval of information learned before the drug is taken (Petersen and Ghoneim 1980). High-potency, short-half-life benzodiazepines are more likely to impair memory, even after a single dose (Scharf et al. 1987). Memory impairment depends on the dose and the route of benzodiazepine administration, with higher doses and intravenous administration causing the greatest impairment. Duration of benzodiazepine treatment is also a significant factor; this is especially true in elderly patients, who may experience an insidious, gradual decrease in memory function, even at a constant benzodiazepine dose (American Psychiatric Association Task Force 1990).

Endocrine-Related Dementias

Repeated or severe episodes of hypoglycemia can produce permanent amnesia; therefore, patients with poorly controlled type I diabetes mellitus are at risk for this complication (Sachon et al. 1992). Hypoglycemia has its greatest effect on hippocampal neurons and thus affects cognitive processes much more than motor or sensory processes (Blackman et al. 1990; Chalmers et al. 1991). In addition to the neurotoxic effects of hypoglycemia, poorly controlled diabetes makes elderly patients vulnerable to the osmotic effects of hyperglycemic episodes; acute fluid shifts can produce a subclinical delirium that can worsen cognition and may take weeks to fully resolve.

Although psychosis ("myxedema madness") is more common, hypothyroidism can produce a subcortical dementia, with psychomotor slowing, poor attention, memory impairment, and impaired abstraction (Hall 1983; Mintzer 1992).

Pernicious Anemia

In the elderly, atrophy of the gastric mucosa with loss of intrinsic factor secretion predisposes to vitamin B_{12} deficiency and subsequent development of pernicious anemia. Pathological lesions found in the CNS consist of focal areas of myelin degeneration scattered throughout the cortical white matter, the optic tracts, and the cerebellar peduncles. It is speculated that dementia early in the course of B_{12} deficiency may be reversible, unlike chronic deficiency states with established myelinolysis (Martin et al. 1992; O'Neill and Barber 1993). The strongest association between dementia and low B_{12} levels may occur in young, but not older, subjects. Low serum B_{12} levels are common in the elderly but are unlikely to be associated with dementia in the absence of macrocytosis and anemia or a significant neurological disorder (Crystal et al. 1994).

Neoplastic Dementias

Approximately 80% of all brain tumors are primary brain tumors, and the remaining 20% are metastatic. The most common primary brain tumors are supratentorial and include astrocytomas, glioblastomas, meningiomas, and pituitary adenomas. Metastases occur most commonly from the lung or breast. Perhaps one-third of intracranial tumors occur in the posterior fossa, where acoustic neuromas and medulloblastomas are most often diagnosed (Lohr and Cadet 1987).

DIFFERENTIAL DIAGNOSIS

Clinical Examination

Mental Status Examination

Use of the mental status examination (MSE) for effective cognitive screening is the cornerstone of neuropsychiatric assessment and diagnosis. The MSE serves as a probe of brain function and may be conceptualized as a structure built on a solid foundation of intact attentional systems. The consultant first must confirm that attention is undiminished, then the other major cognitive domains are assessed in a logical sequence (Figure 16–1).

A patient with poor attention can be expected to show deficits in most cognitive domains. Attention is a complex and multifaceted ability that includes two primary components—*arousal* and *concentration* (directed attention). Arousal is mediated by the ascending reticular activating system and is recorded along a spectrum of alertness as hyperaroused, alert, lethargic (obtunded), stuporous, or comatose (Plum and Posner 1982). Arousal should be tested by inspection, and the forward digit span should be used (i.e., the patient's ability to hear and repeat correctly at least five random numbers presented in a steady monotone at the rate of one per second) (G.A. Miller 1956). It is not unusual for patients with mild to moderate dementia of the Alzheimer's type to repeat five digits correctly. Directed attention (or mental control) should be tested by having the patient spell "WORLD" backward (or, alternatively, reciting the days of the week or the months of the year in reverse order) after the patient first performs the task forward correctly (M.F. Folstein et al. 1975). Failure of performance on these directed attention tasks usually indicates dysfunction in the frontal lobes or frontal-subcortical systems.

For screening purposes, the three chief language domains are fluency, comprehension, and repetition. The consultant can use these three basic elements to distinguish among the major aphasia syndromes (Figure 16–2). Comprehension becomes especially important in clinical settings and is tested along a spectrum of difficulty, first by pointing (1, 2, 3-step commands), then by pointing by description (e.g., "Point to the exit from this room." or

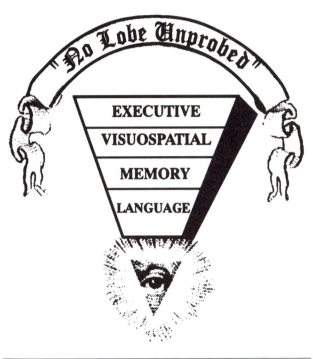

FIGURE 16–1. Mental status examination.

"Point to a source of illumination."), then by asking yes-or-no questions (e.g., "Are the lights on in this room?" or "Do you put on your socks before your shoes?"), and finally by asking passive questions (e.g., "A lion and tiger were fighting; the lion was killed by the tiger. Which animal is dead?") or possessive questions (e.g., "Is my brother's sister a man or a woman?"). Language testing probes the integrity of left-hemispheric functions. Naming deficits are anatomically nonspecific, but they may be diagnostically helpful in more extensive MSE testing (Benson 1979).

Recent memory is tested by stating three to five words and then asking the patient to recall them in 5–10 minutes. This task may be structured along a spectrum of difficulty (depending on the patient's expected level of performance) by giving more words with a longer time interval before recall is tested. Failure to encode and store the words may be distinguished from failure to recall learned material by providing recall cues; the clinician should give categorical prompts (e.g., "One of the words was a color."), then three choices to determine whether the patient has retrieval problems or a true amnesia. The patient with dementia of the Alzheimer's type is not reliably aided by cues on memory testing (Petersen et al. 1994). The consultant must be aware of temporal gradients when screening memory ability. Patients commonly can discuss remote life events or other "overlearned" material yet forget more recent information. Memory testing establishes the integrity of medial temporal structures.

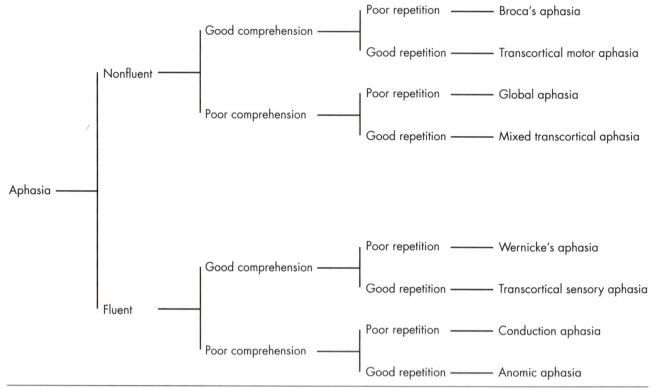

FIGURE 16–2. Systematic approach to differential diagnosis and localization of common aphasia syndromes.

Source. Reprinted from Cummings JL: *Clinical Neuropsychiatry.* Boston, MA, Allyn & Bacon, 1985, pp. 17–35. Copyright 1985, Allyn & Bacon. Used with permission.

Constructional tasks are useful clinical tools because they provide information about right-hemispheric and visuospatial function. Drawing a three-dimensional cube is a good screening item, as is clock drawing (Esteban-Santillan et al. 1998). The patient is told to draw the face of a clock and then to put hands on the clock to indicate a time of "10 minutes past 11." In addition to the constructional aspects of this task, the presence of tremor or hemispatial neglect can be detected; executive cognitive functioning can be observed as well. A patient with executive impairment may be "stimulus bound" and may put a hand on the 10 rather than the 2. Often, one can demonstrate poor strategy in the placement of the numbers or perseveration in the drawing itself (Figure 16–3). All drawing tasks are exquisitely sensitive to delirium from any source.

The frontal/executive cognitive domain includes planning, anticipation, sequencing, abstraction, and goal-directed activity. *Patients may be substantially impaired clinically by subtle dysfunction in this domain.* The consultant should remain alert for the patient who appears to be intact but who requires constant prompting, cuing, and supervision because frontal-system dysfunction may be the culprit. The consultant should look for problems with directed attention tasks, poor performance on clock

drawing, and problems with "motor programming" tasks. Two such tasks are 1) reciprocal programs (e.g., "When I raise one finger, you raise two fingers, and when I raise two fingers, you raise one finger, etc."—impaired patients will tend to imitate the examiner: echopraxia) and 2) serial hand sequences (e.g., the patient watches the examiner cycle repeatedly through a "fist-cut-slap" hand sequence [see Figure 16–4], then attempts to perform the task—impaired patients cannot continue performing the sequence despite instructions to continue; patients with executive dysfunction will fail even when cuing themselves verbally).

Neurological Examination

The extent of the neurological examination will vary, but important elements to include in a dementia workup are cranial nerve testing; observation of gait, posture, and motor speed; testing of muscle strength and tone; inspecting for tremor or other abnormal movements such as dyskinesias or myoclonus; testing of muscle stretch reflexes and extensor plantar responses; and noting pathological signs such as the grasp, snout, jaw jerk, or glabellar reflexes. Sensory examination also should be included when warranted by clinical information (Knopman et al. 2001; Paulson 1977; Thomas 1994).

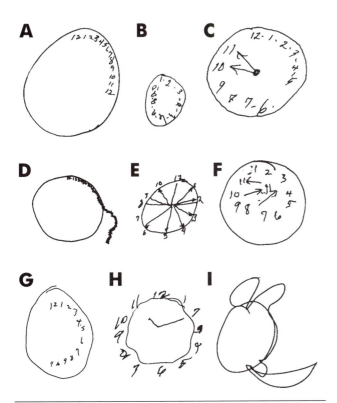

FIGURE 16–3. Clock drawing on command yields important clinical information.

Clocks A and B are from patients with dementia and prominent frontal/executive deficits and show poor planning and organization; clock C is from a patient with early-stage dementia and shows subtle problems with planning as well as "stimulus-bound" error in placing the hands to indicate the time 11:10; clocks D and E are two examples of perseverative errors seen in patients with executive dysfunction; clock F is from a patient with early dementia of the Alzheimer's type and shows obvious disorganization; clock G is from a patient with vascular dementia and left hemi-neglect who drew the circle "automatically" but was unable to use the left regions of the clock despite multiple trials; clock H is from a patient after a cerebellar stroke that left him cognitively intact but with a prominent action tremor; clock I is from a patient with frontal lobe degeneration and dramatic personality changes, including marked disinhibition and impulsivity. This patient began "teaching" the examiner how to draw various animals rather than completing his clock drawing.

Source. Clocks courtesy of Kevin Gray, M.D. Clock D first appeared in Sultzer DL: "Mental Status Examination," in *The American Psychiatric Press Textbook of Geriatric Neuropsychiatry*. Edited by Coffey CE, Cummings JL. Washington, DC, American Psychiatric Press, 1994, pp. 112–127. Used with permission.

Longitudinal History

Clinical history is invaluable to the consultant who must evaluate the patient with dementia; the history should be obtained or corroborated through reliable caregivers. The consultant must inquire about features of onset (gradual vs. sudden) and pattern of progression (relentless vs. "stepwise"). The consultant must understand the typical features of an illness such as Alzheimer's disease in order to address potentially reversible supervening processes and to avoid the therapeutic nihilism that sometimes accompanies the dementias. Although the onset of dementia is recorded as "early" (age 65 or younger) or "late," the distinction between Alzheimer's disease (presenile onset) and "senile dementia" is no longer made because the pathology of the two disorders is not qualitatively different (Amaducci et al. 1986). In the past, the diagnosis of Alzheimer's disease was one of exclusion; however, the refinement of diagnostic criteria has enabled clinicians to use specific clinical features to identify the disease (McKhann et al. 1984). The use of modern criteria yields a diagnostic accuracy rate approaching 85% when compared with postmortem studies (Joachim et al. 1988).

Reversible Etiologies

Of the dementia syndromes listed in Table 16–1, many are reversible to some degree (Barry and Moskowitz 1988). When rare or complicated dementia syndromes are encountered, a systematic approach to diagnosis is essential; additional neuroimaging studies, specific enzymatic or immunological assays, or biopsy of brain or extraneural tissues may be required for diagnosis (Reichman and Cummings 1990).

Laboratory Data

The laboratory evaluation in dementia is used to detect possibly reversible causes of cognitive compromise or to identify common conditions that may be amplifying intellectual deficits. Laboratory assessment is particularly valuable in consultation-liaison psychiatry because a disproportionate number of patients with dementia will have adverse cognitive consequences of systemic medical illnesses or drug effects. A battery of tests commonly used to assess patients with dementia is shown in Table 16–9 (Cummings and Benson 1992). If specific clinical evidence for the cause of the dementia is found (e.g., evidence of hypothyroidism), then the appropriate tests are ordered. If no compelling evidence suggests a specific cause of dementia, then the screening battery is used. The consultant should recommend lumbar puncture as part of the dementia workup in cases of suspected metastatic cancer, CNS infection or vasculitis, hydrocephalus, immunosuppression, and positive syphilis serology. Lumbar puncture should also be considered for patients with early onset, unusually rapid progression, or atypical features (Corey-Bloom et al. 1995).

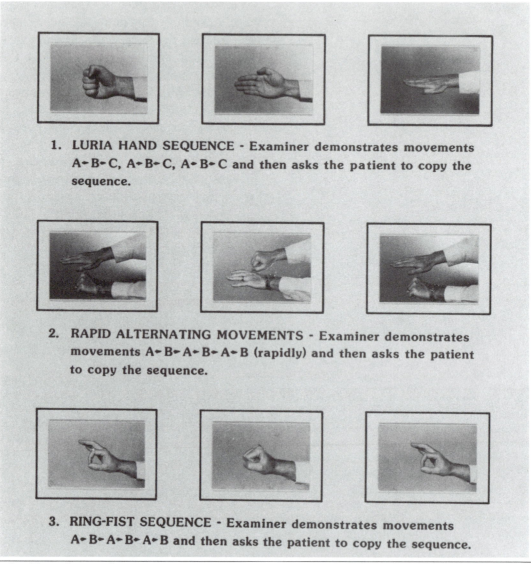

1. **LURIA HAND SEQUENCE** - Examiner demonstrates movements A→B→C, A→B→C, A→B→C and then asks the patient to copy the sequence.

2. **RAPID ALTERNATING MOVEMENTS** - Examiner demonstrates movements A→B→A→B→A→B (rapidly) and then asks the patient to copy the sequence.

3. **RING-FIST SEQUENCE** - Examiner demonstrates movements A→B→A→B→A→B and then asks the patient to copy the sequence.

FIGURE 16–4. Tests of motor fluency.

Source. Reprinted from Wise MG: "Delirium," in *The American Psychiatric Press Textbook of Neuropsychiatry.* Edited by Hales RE, Yudofsky SC. Washington, DC, American Psychiatric Press, 1987, pp. 89–105. Used with permission.

Additional Diagnostic Studies

Imaging

Because no laboratory test is yet available for Alzheimer's disease, diagnosis is aided by the use of neuroimaging techniques. Atrophy is present on CT and MRI in most patients with Alzheimer's disease, but age-related brain atrophy may be of similar magnitude. In addition, some patients with dementia will have normal CT scan results, whereas some control subjects without dementia will have atrophic changes similar to those associated with dementia (DeCarli et al. 1990). Patients with Alzheimer's disease usually have significantly larger ventricles than do age-matched control subjects. In general, correlations between ventricular enlargement and cognitive function are stronger than those between cortical atrophy and cognition (Burns 1990; Giacometti et al. 1994).

Neuroimaging plays an especially important role in diagnosing vascular dementia. CT detects actual infarctions in fewer than half of the patients with clinical evidence of vascular dementia (Radue et al. 1978). Nonetheless, areas of decreased lucency in the white matter—"leuko-araiosis"—are seen on CT in most patients with vascular dementia. Enlargement of the lateral and third ventricles correlates significantly with severity of cognitive impairment in vascular dementia (Aharon-Peretz et al. 1988). MRI is the most sensitive structural imaging technique for diagnosing vascular dementia (Kertesz et al. 1987). T2-weighted MRI images are best for the

TABLE 16–9. Laboratory tests in the assessment of dementia

Screening battery
    Complete blood count
    Erythrocyte sedimentation rate
    Blood glucose
    Blood urea nitrogen (BUN)
    Electrolytes
    Serum calcium
    Thyroid-stimulating hormone
    Vitamin B_{12}

If unexplained fever or urinary symptoms present
    Urinalysis
    Urine culture and sensitivity

If unexplained fever or pulmonary symptoms present
    Chest X ray

If cardiovascular symptoms present or evidence of vascular dementia
    Electrocardiogram (ECG)

If risk factors for HIV encephalopathy present
    Serum HIV test

If drug intoxication suspected
    Serum drug level

Tests selected on the basis of specific symptoms or history
    Blood gases
    Heavy metals
    Fluorescent treponemal antibody absorption (FTA-ABS)
    Disease-specific tests (e.g., serum copper and ceruloplasmin for Wilson's disease)
    Lumbar puncture (usually after computed tomography or magnetic resonance imaging) if evidence of infection, demyelinating disease, inflammatory disease, or neoplasm

Note. HIV = human immunodeficiency virus.

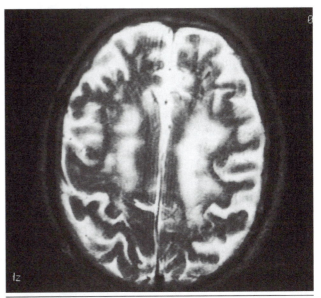

FIGURE 16–5. T2-weighted magnetic resonance image (MRI) of a patient with vascular dementia. Extensive areas of ischemic injury are visible as regions of increased signal intensity.

detection of hyperintensities in the white matter (Figure 16–5) that reflect ischemic changes and dysmyelination (Gupta et al. 1988; Kertesz et al. 1988). The magnitude of white matter changes in vascular dementia exceeds that seen in Alzheimer's disease or normal aging, although these white matter changes are not specific to vascular dementia and may occur to some extent in patients with Alzheimer's disease as well as in healthy elderly control subjects (Erkinjuntti et al. 1987; Hunt et al. 1989; Pantoni and Garcia 1995).

Imaging is also variably helpful in evaluating other forms of dementia. Frontal atrophy on CT or MRI usually is apparent late in the course of frontotemporal dementia (B.L. Miller et al. 1991). CT or MRI can show gross atrophy of the caudate nucleus in Huntington's disease (Gray and Cummings 1994). MRI studies have not detected any specific pattern of abnormalities in patients with dementia and Parkinson's disease (Huber et al. 1989); however, functional imaging techniques in Parkinson's disease may aid in identifying concomitant Alzheimer's disease (Pizzolato et al. 1988). MRI is becoming the primary diagnostic instrument in NPH and demonstrates enlarged ventricles, increased signal adjacent to the ventricles, and evidence of cerebrospinal fluid (CSF) flow disturbances within the ventricular system (Kunz et al. 1989).

In HIV-1 dementia, structural imaging studies using CT or MRI show atrophy and evidence for demyelination of subcortical white matter. Positron-emission tomography (PET) studies indicate relative hypermetabolism of the thalamus and basal ganglia in the early and middle stages of HIV infection. As the dementia worsens, the temporal lobes become metabolically hypoactive (Van Gorp et al. 1992).

CT imaging in abstinent chronic alcohol abusers shows lateral ventricular enlargement with widening of the cortical sulci; this atrophy does not correlate with intellectual impairment and may improve in some patients with abstinence (Carlen et al. 1978). To date, MRI studies are unable to consistently distinguish patients with Wernicke-Korsakoff syndrome from patients who chronically abuse alcohol but do not have cognitive impairment (Blansjaar et al. 1992b; Jernigan et al. 1991).

Structural imaging studies in patients with DSD show diminished brain density and increased ventricular-to-brain ratio values more similar to those of patients with Alzheimer's disease than to those of age-matched control subjects (Pearlson et al. 1989). The prognostic significance of these findings is unclear. Functional imaging studies with PET in patients with depression show asymmetric frontal hypometabolism, which is greater on the left, that resolves with successful therapy (Martinot et al. 1990). This hypofrontality and other metabolic alterations seen in DSD are distinct from the biparietal hypometabolism of Alzheimer's disease and may prove helpful in distinguishing these disorders in elderly patients (Dolan et al. 1992). Application of newer techniques such as polysomnographic sleep studies may eventually prove useful in this regard because diminished rapid eye movement (REM) sleep latency is a common feature of depression (Buysse et al. 1992).

The EEG in patients with Creutzfeldt-Jakob disease frequently shows a characteristic intermittent periodic burst pattern (Brown et al. 1986). Neuroimaging is non-diagnostic, although functional imaging techniques may be useful for directing brain biopsy (Holthoff et al. 1990; Jibiki et al. 1994). An immunoassay for the detection of the 14-3-3 protein in the CSF of patients is emerging as potentially useful for confirming the diagnosis of Creutzfeldt-Jakob disease (Burkhard et al. 2001).

Although the yield of potentially treatable conditions found with routine CT or MRI is low, the consultant should always recommend imaging in patients with impaired cognition for less than 3 months; rapid onset of impairment over 48 hours or less; head trauma during the week before the decline in mental state; a clinical history of stroke, seizures, or malignant tumor; urinary or fecal incontinence; and neurological abnormalities such as headache, visual field deficit, papilledema, abnormal gait, postural instability, or any focal findings on neurological examination (Alexander et al. 1995; Dietch 1983).

Dementia Rating Scales

Several brief standardized screens are reviewed in the literature. The Mini-Mental State Exam (MMSE) and the Orientation-Memory-Concentration test (commonly called the Short Blessed test) are two good examples (M.F. Folstein et al. 1975; Katzman et al. 1983). Despite a lack of sensitivity and specificity, the MMSE is the current "standard" used in most scientific reports. Newer tests such as the Executive Interview (EXIT), the CLOX, and the Frontal Assessment Battery are emerging to improve screening of subtle executive deficits (Dubois et al. 2000; Royall et al. 1992, 1998). The Clinical Dementia Rating (CDR) scale is emerging as the preferred scale for staging of dementia and is increasingly used to record meaningful responses to therapeutic interventions

(Hughes et al. 1982). The Neuropsychiatric Inventory (NPI) allows for comprehensive assessment of noncognitive psychopathology in patients with dementia (Cummings et al. 1994), and performance-based instruments like the Texas Functional Living Scale may improve the reliable measurement of functional abilities in patients with Alzheimer's disease (Cullum et al. 2001). Newer brief cognitive assessment instruments useful for screening patients for dementia include the Time and Change Test (Froehlich et al. 1998), the 7-minute screen (Solomon et al. 1998), and the modified WORLD test (Leopold and Borson 1997). Clinical personnel may use these screens to document deficits, to establish baselines, and to chart decline over time. These screens and all the previously mentioned tests must be interpreted in the light of educational and cultural factors (Tombaugh and McIntyre 1992). They are never a substitute for a full clinical MSE for patients seen by consultation-liaison psychiatrists.

Neuropsychological Testing

Neuropsychological testing can be a useful adjunct to mental status testing of patients with known or suspected intellectual impairment (Zec 1993). It does not replace a thorough MSE and should be used to amplify the results of clinical testing or to clarify questions that have arisen. Neuropsychological testing is particularly valuable as a means of 1) distinguishing between mild dementia and normal aging in elderly individuals, 2) differentiating mild dementia from the effects of low educational level or limited natural cognitive capacities, 3) providing detailed quantitative information that may help to differentiate among types of dementias, and 4) establishing a baseline description of cognitive function that may be followed over time to determine whether the patient is undergoing progressive decline. A comprehensive neuropsychological assessment should document the intelligence of the individual (Verbal IQ, Performance IQ, Full-Scale IQ, and IQ subscale test scores), language function, memory abilities, visuospatial skills, executive function, and psychomotor speed. The report should be quantitative and should include the raw data and their interpretation. Neuropsychological testing is excellent for distinguishing between dementia and normal aging; it cannot by itself establish the specific etiology of the dementia (i.e., differentiate among causes of dementia). Neuropsychological test performance can be affected by anxiety, depression, delirium, low educational level, or sociocultural influences, and interpretation must take these factors into account (Levin 1994).

CLINICAL COURSE AND PROGNOSIS

Alzheimer's disease usually begins after age 50, with an insidious and gradually progressive decline in mental abilities. The patient and family members often are unaware of the evolving cognitive impairment, and the onset of the illness is identified only in retrospect. Memory difficulties are manifest by forgetting tasks, repeating questions, or losing the thread of a telephone conversation or a television program. The patient may complain about memory problems very early in the course of the disease, but insight is rapidly lost. In fact, the patient's lack of insight in the face of gross cognitive impairments is characteristic of Alzheimer's disease. Typically, the patient's daily responsibilities increasingly are assumed by colleagues and family members, who do not yet recognize the presence of a progressive disease and may think only that the patient is "slipping" with age. Other common early findings include bungled finances or getting lost while driving. Alcohol may produce an exaggerated emotional response, whereas a family vacation or trip to visit relatives often will reveal problems with orientation and memory. Intercurrent illness that requires hospitalization or anesthesia may provoke episodes of sundowning or delirium (Bliwise 1994).

Deterioration progresses over months and years. Tasks performed easily in the past, such as grocery shopping, preparing meals, and selecting appropriate clothing to wear, become impossible for the patient with Alzheimer's disease to perform independently. Personal hygiene and grooming are neglected, with the patient no longer able to shave, bathe, or use the toilet properly. Delusional beliefs often develop (Burns et al. 1990; Mega et al. 1996). Patients commonly are convinced that others are trying to steal from them or harm them, that their spouse is unfaithful, that family members are not who they claim to be (Capgras' syndrome), that their house is not really their home, or that family members are plotting to abandon them. Hallucinatory experiences may arise, with the patient hearing or talking to people who are not there. Patients may cling to family members, often not letting the spouse or primary caregiver out of their sight ("shadowing"). The patient often will pace around the house without apparent purpose ("touring"); engage in repetitive, stereotyped activities such as opening and closing drawers; or wander from the house and get lost in formerly familiar surroundings.

The patient's responses become increasingly erratic and exaggerated, and well-intentioned attempts by family members or caregivers to insist or "force" the patient to perform tasks such as bathing or getting into a car may precipitate "catastrophic reactions." These reactions are abrupt, possibly even violent, outbursts of verbal and/or physical aggression. This overreaction may be misinterpreted by caregivers as stubbornness, criticism, or ingratitude. However, because these episodes are not premeditated, they may cease almost as abruptly as they arise, which may confuse and frustrate caregivers (Mace and Rabins 1991).

Eventually, patients become unable to recognize close family members, and they may even misidentify their own reflection in a mirror. Primitive reflexes, such as the grasp, snout, and suck emerge, and new-onset seizures may appear (Romanelli et al. 1990). In the final stage of the illness, the patient becomes incontinent of urine and feces, loses all intelligible vocabulary, and is unable to walk or to sit up (Reisberg 1988). Death from pneumonia or another infectious process frequently occurs after a period of total confinement to bed.

Studies of patients with Alzheimer's disease consistently show an annual rate of decline on mental status testing approximately equivalent to three points per year on the MMSE. This occurs independently of the patient's age, sex, education, or residence in a nursing home (Katzman et al. 1988). Although individual patients vary in their rate of decline, dramatic deviations from this rate warrant investigation. Currently, dementia of the Alzheimer's type is the fourth leading cause of death among the elderly.

Less is known about the course of other cortical degenerative dementias, but preliminary evidence suggests that they generally follow a course similar to that of Alzheimer's disease. Patients with dementia with Lewy bodies and frontotemporal dementia usually survive about 10 years from the time of diagnosis.

Parkinson's disease symptoms respond to treatment with dopaminergic agents, and these drugs have improved overall survival in patients with the disease. Patients with Parkinson's disease survived an average 9–10 years after diagnosis in the pre-L-dopa era and now survive for 13–14 years (Martilla 1992). Treatment with penicillamine before irreversible hepatic or neurological injury has occurred will allow a normal life span in many individuals with Wilson's disease (Patten 1993). This outcome contrasts with 8- to 12-year survival typical of patients with Wilson's disease before the advent of efficacious treatment. Specific interventions for other degenerative subcortical dementias have not emerged, and patients with these illnesses experience gradual decline in intellectual and motor function. Huntington's disease symptoms typically begin at about age 35–40; the disease course tends to last about 15 years (Rosenblatt and Leroi 2000). Patients with other movement disorders such as the spinocerebellar degenerations, PSP, and striatonigral degeneration typically survive 6–10 years from the time of diagnosis (Cummings and Benson 1992).

Vascular dementia has a poor prognosis. Patients generally succumb to cardiovascular events (myocardial infarction, congestive heart failure) rather than their brain disease, but it is not unusual for them to sustain additional strokes before death. Mean survival in patients with vascular dementia is 5–7 years (Nielsen et al. 1991).

Infectious dementias have disease-specific prognoses. Patients with CNS syphilis or chronic meningitis that is detected early and properly treated may have a complete reversal of intellectual changes. However, several of the infectious dementias have no curative treatment, and patients will eventually succumb to their disease. The course of HIV encephalopathy is highly variable; some patients survive for several years after the onset of cognitive deficits, whereas others survive only 2–9 months after the onset of the dementia. Ninety percent of the patients with Creutzfeldt-Jakob disease die within 1 year of the onset of symptoms, and 50% die within 6 months (Brown et al. 1986).

TREATMENT AND MANAGEMENT

Medical Therapy

Treatment and management of dementia aim to control the underlying disease and to manage the associated cognitive and behavioral manifestations. No current interventions halt the underlying disease process of degenerative disorders, but many manifestations of dementing processes can be effectively treated. Halting the progression of cognitive deterioration and optimizing the function of remaining cognitive capacity are the goals of treatment in vascular dementia. Medical and surgical treatments are focused on management of associated risk factors and disease-specific interventions for associated medical conditions (Skoog 1994). Individual patients may benefit from speech therapy or physical therapy. Use of daily aspirin therapy (325 mg/day) to inhibit platelet aggregation is recommended (Meyer et al. 1989). Although the benefit of aspirin in vascular dementia has been questioned (Hébert et al. 2000), ticlopidine or clopidogrel may ameliorate progressive ischemic injury in patients who cannot tolerate or do not respond to aspirin (Flores-Runk and Raasch 1993).

Surgical shunting of CSF produces improvement in 40%–50% of the patients with NPH; dementia is the least likely of the NPH triad to improve with shunting, whereas gait disturbance has the best outcome. Although no absolute guidelines define accurately those patients who are most responsive to surgery, as a rule, patients with good surgical prognosis present with the full clinical triad, with a short duration of symptoms, and have a known cause of their NPH (Clarfield 1989; Friedland 1989; Vanneste 1994).

Given the insidious course of Wernicke-Korsakoff syndrome and the high prevalence rate of undiagnosed Wernicke-Korsakoff syndrome, all alcohol-dependent patients should be given thiamine (Ambrose et al. 2001; Blansjaar and van Dijk 1992). The physician must always be alert to the possibility of any supervening illness (e.g., infection, electrolyte disturbance) that might cause sudden changes in behavior or mental status (Small 1988).

Pharmacotherapy

Therapy for Alzheimer's disease is divided into two main categories: control of behavioral manifestations of the illness and attempts to restore cognitive function. Behavioral disturbances, such as agitation, wandering, suspiciousness, hallucinations, and hostility, that arise during the course of dementia may be treated with low-dose neuroleptic medications or atypical antipsychotics (Katz et al. 1999; Madhusoodanan et al. 2000; Schneider et al. 1990; Street et al. 2000). Initial treatment with low doses of a high-potency agent (haloperidol 0.5–2 mg/day) or an atypical antipsychotic (risperidone 1–2 mg/day; olanzapine 5–15 mg/day; quetiapine 25–100 mg/day) is usually recommended. If troublesome extrapyramidal side effects emerge, dose reduction or changing to an atypical agent is preferable to the use of anticholinergic drugs (Carlyle et al. 1993). These drugs must be scheduled properly to produce the desired effects (e.g., improved sleep, diminished agitation during bathing and dressing). Whenever possible, clinicians should avoid the use of medications on an "as-needed" basis; consultants should help caregivers to recognize times when problems regularly arise so that they can administer medication to the patient in anticipation of agitation. This helps to minimize the total amount of medication required. The cautious, adjunctive use of low doses of short-acting benzodiazepines such as lorazepam or oxazepam also may prove beneficial. Clonazepam (0.5 mg) can be used to maintain sleep in patients with frequent awakening or nocturnal wandering; trazodone (50–250 mg) is useful for agitation and for patients with difficulty falling asleep (Sultzer et al. 1997). Other medications reported to help modify agitated behavior include buspirone, carbamazepine, valproate, fluoxetine, estrogen, leuprolide, medroxyprogesterone, and gabapentin (Hawkins et al. 2000; Kunik et al.

1994; Kyomen et al. 1991; Mazure et al. 1992; Rich and Ovsiew 1994; Schneider and Sobin 1991; Sobin et al. 1989; Tiller et al. 1988; Weiner et al. 1992). Novel antipsychotics and nonpharmacological therapies are particularly important alternatives to neuroleptic treatment in patients with dementia with Lewy bodies who are excessively sensitive to the effects of neuroleptics; approximately half of the patients experience severe adverse side effects (McKeith et al. 1992a). Creative use of medications can often achieve control of an individual patient's specific target symptoms. Control of unwanted behavioral symptoms is a key to helping patients with dementia remain with their families (Zubenko et al. 1992).

Nonsedating antidepressants and psychostimulants are useful for treating the dysphoric mood symptoms, irritability, and labile affect commonly seen in patients with vascular dementia, Parkinson's disease, HIV/AIDS, or other CNS disease (Cummings 1994; Holmes et al. 1989; Panzer and Mellow 1992). Use of antidepressant or electroconvulsive therapy for DSD should be initiated on the basis of intrapsychic depressive symptoms and characteristic sleep disturbance rather than for the mere complaint or presence of cognitive impairment (Emery and Oxman 1992). Evidence of confusion while taking low doses of tricyclic antidepressants may identify patients with DSD at high risk for development of primary dementia (Reding et al. 1985). However, the availability of newer antidepressant agents (with more favorable side-effect profiles) should prompt a medication trial in cognitively impaired patients whenever the relative contribution of depression to the overall clinical picture is uncertain (Jones and Reifler 1994).

Attempts to find an effective treatment for Alzheimer's disease have largely focused on augmentation of cerebral cholinergic neurotransmission (Davis and Mohs 1982). Various cholinomimetic strategies have been tried, including acetylcholine precursors, cholinergic agonists, and cholinesterase inhibitors; however, the therapeutic potential of these agents is limited by potentially toxic side effects and poor penetration across the blood-brain barrier.

Donepezil, a cholinesterase inhibitor that is administered once daily, is initiated at 5 mg/day and increased to 10 mg after 1 month if no significant side effects occur. The most common adverse effects are nausea, vomiting, and diarrhea; hepatotoxicity is not a concern, and no serum monitoring of liver enzymes is required (Rogers et al. 1996, 1998). Rivastigmine and galantamine are newer reversible cholinesterase inhibitors administered twice daily with meals. The doses are increased every 4 weeks until the maximum dose is reached (12 mg/day for rivastigmine; 24 mg /day for galantamine) or side effects

occur (Corey-Bloom et al. 1998; Raskind et al. 2000; Rosler et al. 1999; Tariot et al. 2000). These agents produce modest but significant improvements in cognition, behavior, and function in most patients with Alzheimer's disease and are showing promise as effective treatments in Lewy body disease and other dementias (McKeith et al. 2000).

Vitamin E (2,000 IU/day) has been shown in one study to delay the time to specific end points in the course of Alzheimer's disease (death, institutionalization, severe dementia, loss of activities of daily living) (Sano et al. 1997). Vitamin E is an antioxidant and may act by ameliorating amyloid-related oxidative neuronal injury. Current clinical practice guidelines recommend that the use of cholinesterase inhibitors and vitamin E should be considered in every case of Alzheimer's disease (Doody et al. 2001). Low doses of a nonsteroidal anti-inflammatory drug and possibly even aspirin may offer some protection against dementia of the Alzheimer's type (Broe et al. 2000).

Many neurotransmitter deficits are present in Alzheimer's disease, including norepinephrine and serotonin; thus, the utility of single neurotransmitter replacement therapy appears limited. Future strategies for cognitive restoration likely will target multiple neurotransmitter systems with drug combinations as well as precursors and pro-drugs (Schneider et al. 1993; Whitehouse and Geldmacher 1994). To date, clinical trials of other agents, including psychostimulants, cerebral vasodilators, and nootropics such as piracetam and ergoloid mesylates (hydergine), do not show consistent beneficial effects. Early and more accurate identification of patients with incipient Alzheimer's disease will allow therapeutic intervention before the degenerative processes are advanced beyond the brain's reserve capacity (Stern and Davis 1991). Antiamyloid and neuroprotector therapy, aimed at retarding neuronal degeneration, and preventive therapy to eliminate neuronal degeneration entirely, will be the ultimate treatment strategies for the future (Cutler and Sramek 2001; Growdon 1992).

Ward Management

The consultant must pay attention to the patient's environment; too much or too little stimulation may result in withdrawal or agitation. Patients with dementia do best in familiar and constant surroundings with regular daily routines. Clocks, calendars, night-lights, checklists, and diaries all aid in orientation and memory during the early phase of the illness. Appropriately balancing the use of psychosocial and pharmacological interventions in the patient with dementia requires using a frame of reference that includes information about where, when, and with whom troublesome behaviors arise. The consultant also must consider how often medications or medical conditions cause problems; how dangerous medications or medical conditions are to patients, caregivers, or others; and which medications or medical conditions are associated with problems and must keep in mind that the patient with dementia has the ability to communicate, learn, and comprehend (Weiner and Gray 1994). Caregivers must learn the patient's (and their own) limitations. Caregivers should be encouraged to simplify tasks and to avoid rushing the patient or forcing the patient to do things beyond his or her ability (Mace and Rabins 1991; Small 1989).

Family Therapy/Support

The consultant's most crucial allies in working with patients who have dementia are family members because they provide most of the care for these progressively dependent individuals. Consultation-liaison psychiatrists also must facilitate the care of the caregivers (Scott et al. 1986). Family members of patients with dementia frequently become depressed, experience enormous burden in the course of providing care, and need referral to psychological, social, and legal services (Overman and Stoudemire 1988). They may be sufficiently depressed or anxious to require pharmacotherapy and psychiatric care, but more frequently, support groups or family therapy to help families respond with mutual support is indicated. Referral to the Alzheimer Association provides a critical link between families and support services. Social service referrals help to inform the family about community resources such as home health services, day care, respite care, and nursing home care. Advice from an attorney is helpful for establishing wills, establishing trusts, and dealing with other estate management issues. Families also should be encouraged to provide advance directives regarding the care of hospitalized patients with dementia and should be counseled about the importance of autopsy (Raia 1994).

REFERENCES

Aarsland D, Andersen K, Larsen JP, et al: Risk of dementia in Parkinson's disease: a community-based, prospective study Neurology 56(6):730–736, 2001

Adams RD, Victor M: Principles of Neurology, 5th Edition. New York, McGraw-Hill, 1993

Aharon-Peretz J, Cummings JL, Hill MA: Vascular dementia and dementia of the Alzheimer type. Arch Neurol 45:719–721, 1988

Albers DS, Augood SJ: New insights into progressive supranuclear palsy. Trends Neurosci 24:347–353, 2001

Albert ML, Feldman RG, Willis AL: The "subcortical dementia" of progressive supranuclear palsy. J Neurol Neurosurg Psychiatry 37:121–130, 1974

Alexander EM, Wagner EH, Buchner DM, et al: Do surgical brain lesions present as isolated dementia? A population-based study. J Am Geriatr Soc 43:138–143, 1995

Alexopoulos GS, Meyers BS, Young RC, et al: The course of geriatric depression with "reversible dementia": a controlled study. Am J Psychiatry 150:1693–1699, 1993

Amaducci LA, Rocca WA, Schoenberg BS: Origin of the distinction between Alzheimer's disease and senile dementia: how history can clarify nosology. Neurology 36:1497–1499, 1986

Ambrose ML, Bowden SC, Whelan G: Thiamin treatment and working memory function of alcohol-dependent people: preliminary findings. A

American Academy of Neurology AIDS Task Force: Nomenclature and research case definitions for neurologic manifestations of human immunodeficiency virus–type 1 (HIV-1) infection. Neurology 41:778–785, 1991

American Psychiatric Association: Diagnostic and Statistical Manual of Mental Disorders, 4th Edition, Text Revision. Washington, DC, American Psychiatric Association, 2000

American Psychiatric Association Task Force: Benzodiazepine Dependence, Toxicity, and Abuse. Washington, DC, American Psychiatric Press, 1990, pp 42–44

Angus WR, Romney DM: The effect of diazepam on patient's memory. J Clin Psychopharmacol 4:203–206, 1984

Baldwin B, Forstl H: "Pick's disease"—101 years on—still there, but in need of reform. Br J Psychiatry 163:100–104, 1993

Barba R, Martinez-Espinosa S, Rodriguez-Garcia E, et al: Post-stroke dementia: clinical features and risk factors. Stroke 31:1494–1501, 2000

Bamford KA, Caine ED: Does "benign senescent forgetfulness" exist? Clin Geriatr Med 4:897–916, 1988

Barry PP, Moskowitz MA: The diagnosis of reversible dementia in the elderly: a critical review. Arch Intern Med 148:1914–1918, 1988

Benson DF: Aphasia, Alexia, and Agraphia. New York, Churchill Livingstone, 1979

Benson DF: Hydrocephalic dementia, in Handbook of Clinical Neurology, Vol 46: Neurobehavioral Disorders. Edited by Vinken PJ, Bruyn GW, Klawans HL. New York, Elsevier, 1985, pp 323–333

Beresford TP, Blow FC, Brower KJ, et al: Alcoholism and aging in the general hospital. Psychosomatics 29:61–72, 1988

Bienfeld D, Hartford JT: Pseudodementia in an elderly woman with schizophrenia. Am J Psychiatry 139:114–115, 1982

Black DW: Mental changes resulting from subdural haematoma. Br J Psychiatry 145:200–203, 1984

Black SE: Focal cortical atrophy syndromes. Brain Cogn 31:188–229, 1996

Blackman JD, Towle VL, Lewis GF, et al: Hypoglycemic thresholds for cognitive dysfunction in humans. Diabetes 39:828–835, 1990

Blansjaar BA, van Dijk JG: Korsakoff minus Wernicke syndrome. Alcohol Alcohol 27:435–437, 1992

Blansjaar BA, Takens H, Zwinderman AH: The course of alcohol amnestic disorder: a three-year follow-up study of clinical signs and social disabilities. Acta Psychiatr Scand 86:240–246, 1992a

Blansjaar BA, Vielvoye GJ, van Dijk JG, et al: Similar brain lesions in alcoholics and Korsakoff patients: MRI, psychometric and clinical findings. Clin Neurol Neurosurg 94:197–203, 1992b

Bliwise DL: What is sundowning? J Am Geriatr Soc 42:1009–1011, 1994

Boone KB, Miller BL, Lesser IM, et al: Performance on frontal lobe tests in healthy, older individuals. Dev Neuropsychol 6:215–223, 1990

Bowden SC: Separating cognitive impairment in neurologically asymptomatic alcoholism from Wernicke-Korsakoff syndrome: is the neuropsychological distinction justified? Psychol Bull 107:355–366, 1990

Brewer GJ: Recognition, diagnosis, and management of Wilson's disease. Proc Soc Exp Biol Med 223:39–46, 2000

Broe GA, Grayson DA, Creasey HM, et al: Anti-inflammatory drugs protect against Alzheimer disease at low doses. Arch Neurol 57(11):1586–{1591, 2000

Brown P, Cathala F, Castaigne P, et al: Creutzfeldt-Jakob disease: clinical analysis of a consecutive series of 230 neuropathologically verified cases. Ann Neurol 20:597–602, 1986

Brown P, Will RG, Bradley R, et al: Bovine spongiform encephalopathy and variant Creutzfeldt-Jakob disease: background, evolution, and current concerns. Emerg Infect Dis 7:6–16, 2001

Brun A: Frontal lobe degeneration of non-Alzheimer type, I: neuropathology. Archives of Gerontology and Geriatrics 6:193–208, 1987

Brust JCM: Vascular dementia is overdiagnosed. Arch Neurol 45:799–801, 1988

Burkhard PR, Sanchez JC, Landis T, et al: CSF detection of the 14-3-3 protein in unselected patients with dementia. Neurology 56:1528–1533, 2001

Burns A: Cranial computerized tomography in dementia of the Alzheimer's type. Br J Psychiatry 157 (suppl 9):10–15, 1990

Burns A, Jacoby R, Levy R: Psychiatric phenomena in Alzheimer's disease, I: disorders of thought content; II: disorders of perception. Br J Psychiatry 157:72–81, 1990

Butterworth RF: Pathophysiology of alcoholic brain damage: synergistic effects of ethanol, thiamine deficiency and alcoholic liver disease. Metab Brain Dis 10:1–8, 1995

Buysse DJ, Reynolds CF III, Hoch CC, et al: Rapid eye movement sleep deprivation in elderly patients with concurrent symptoms of depression and dementia. J Neuropsychiatry Clin Neurosci 4:249–256, 1992

Byrne EJ, Lennox GG, Godwin-Austen RB, et al: Dementia associated with cortical Lewy bodies: proposed clinical diagnostic criteria. Dementia 2:283–284, 1991

Caine ED: Pseudodementia: current concepts and future directions. Arch Gen Psychiatry 38:1359–1364, 1981

Camara EG, Chelune GJ: Paraneoplastic limbic encephalopathy. Brain Behav Immun 1:349–355, 1987

Campbell S, Stephens S, Ballard C: Dementia with Lewy bodies: clinical features and treatment. Drugs Aging 18:397–407, 2001

Carlen PL, Wortzman G, Holgate RC, et al: Reversible cerebral atrophy in recently abstinent chronic alcoholics measured by computed tomography scans. Science 200:1076–1078, 1978

Carlyle W, Ancill RJ, Sheldon L: Aggression in the demented patient: a double-blind study of loxapine versus haloperidol. Int Clin Psychopharmacol 8:103–108, 1993

Casey DA, Fitzgerald BA: Mania and pseudodementia. J Clin Psychiatry 49:73–74, 1988

Chalmers J, Risk MT, Kean DM, et al: Severe amnesia after hypoglycemia: clinical, psychometric, and magnetic resonance imaging correlations. Diabetes Care 14:922–925, 1991

Chow TW, Miller BL, Hayashi VN, et al: Inheritance of frontotemporal dementia. Arch Neurol 56:817–822, 1999

Chui HC, Victoroff JI, Margolin D, et al: Criteria for the diagnosis of ischemic vascular dementia proposed by the state of California Alzheimer's Disease Diagnostic and Treatment Centers. Neurology 42:473–480, 1992

Clarfield AM: Normal-pressure hydrocephalus: saga or swamp? JAMA 262:2592–2593, 1989

Corder EH, Saunders AM, Strittmatter WJ, et al: Gene dose of apolipoprotein E type 4 allele and the risk of Alzheimer's disease in late onset families. Science 261:921–923, 1993

Corey-Bloom J, Thal LJ, Galasko D, et al: Diagnosis and evaluation of dementia. Neurology 45:211–218, 1995

Corey-Bloom J, Anand R, Veach J, for the ENA 713 B352 Study Group: A randomized trial evaluating the efficacy and safety of ENA 713 (rivastigmine tartrate), a new acetylcholinesterase inhibitor, in patients with mild to moderately severe Alzheimer's disease. International Journal of Geriatric Psychopharmacology 1:55–65, 1998

Crook T, Bartus RT, Ferris SH, et al: Age-associated memory impairment: proposed diagnostic criteria and measures of clinical change—report of a National Institute of Mental Health work group. Developmental Neuropsychol 2:261–276, 1986

Crystal HA, Ortof E, Frishman WH, et al: Serum vitamin B12 levels and incidence of dementia in a healthy elderly population: a report from the Bronx Longitudinal Aging Study. J Am Geriatr Soc 42:933–936, 1994

Cullum CM, Saine K, Chan LD, et al: Performance-based instrument to assess functional capacity in dementia: the Texas Functional Living Scale. Neuropsychiatry Neuropsychol Behav Neurol 14:103–108, 2001

Cummings JL: Dementia syndromes: neurobehavioral and neuropsychiatric features. J Clin Psychiatry 48 (no 5, suppl):3–8, 1987

Cummings JL: Dementia and depression: an evolving enigma. J Neuropsychiatry Clin Neurosci 1:236–242, 1989

Cummings JL: Introduction, in Subcortical Dementia. New York, Oxford University Press, 1990, pp 1–16

Cummings JL: Depression in neurologic diseases. Psychiatric Annals 24:525–531, 1994

Cummings JL: Behavioral and psychiatric symptoms associated with Huntington's disease. Adv Neurol 65:179–186, 1995a

Cummings JL: Dementia: the failing brain. Lancet 345:1481–1484, 1995b

Cummings JL, Benson DF: Subcortical dementia: review of an emerging concept. Arch Neurol 41:874–879, 1984

Cummings JL, Benson DF: Dementia of the Alzheimer's type: an inventory of diagnostic clinical features. J Am Geriatr Soc 34:12–19, 1986

Cummings JL, Benson DF: Dementia: A Clinical Approach. Boston, MA, Butterworth-Heinemann, 1992

Cummings JL, Benson DF, LoVerme S Jr: Reversible dementia. JAMA 243:2434–2439, 1980

Cummings JL, Miller B, Hill MA, et al: Neuropsychiatric aspects of multi-infarct dementia and dementia of the Alzheimer's type. Arch Neurol 44:389–393, 1987

Cummings JL, Mega M, Gray KF, et al: The neuropsychiatric inventory: comprehensive assessment of psychopathology in dementia. Neurology 44:2308–2314, 1994

Cummings JL, Vinters HV, Cole GM, et al: Alzheimer's disease: etiologies, pathophysiology, cognitive reserve, and treatment opportunities. Neurology 51:S2–S17, 1998

Cutler NR, Sramek JJ: Review of the next generation of Alzheimer's disease therapeutics: challenges for drug development. Prog Neuropsychopharmacol Biol Psychiatry 25:27–57, 2001

Davis KL, Mohs RC: Enhancement of memory processes in Alzheimer's disease with multiple-dose intravenous physostigmine. Am J Psychiatry 139:1421–1424, 1982

DeCarli C, Kaye JA, Horowitz B, et al: Critical analysis of the use of computer-assisted transverse axial tomography to study human brain in aging and dementia of the Alzheimer's type. Neurology 40:872–883, 1990

Del Ser T, McKeith I, Anand R, et al: Dementia with Lewy bodies: findings from an international multicentre study. Int J Geriatr Psychiatry 15:1034–1045, 2000

Del Ser T, Hachinski V, Merskey H, et al: Clinical and pathologic features of two groups of patients with dementia with Lewy bodies: effect of coexisting Alzheimer-type lesion load. Alzheimer Dis Assoc Disord 15:31–44, 2001

Dening DC, Berrios GE: Wilson's disease: psychiatric symptoms in 195 cases. Arch Gen Psychiatry 46:1126–1134, 1989

Desmond DW, Moroney JT, Lynch T, et al: The natural history of CADASIL: a pooled analysis of previously published cases. Stroke 30:1230–1233, 1999

Dickson DW: Neuropathology of Alzheimer's disease and other dementias. Clin Geriatr Med 17:209–228, 2001a

Dickson DW: Neuropathology of Pick's disease. Neurology 56:S16–S20, 2001b

Dietch JT: Computerized tomographic scanning in cases of dementia. West J Med 138:835–837, 1983

Dolan RJ, Bench CJ, Brown RG, et al: Regional cerebral blood flow abnormalities in depressed patients with cognitive impairment. J Neurol Neurosurg Psychiatry 55:768–773, 1992

Doody RS, Stevens JC, Beck C, et al: Practice parameter: Management of dementia (an evidence-based review): Report of the Quality Standards Subcommittee of the American Academy of Neurology. Neurology 56:1154–1166, 2001

Dubois B, Slachevsky A, Litvan I, et al: The FAB: a Frontal Assessment Battery at bedside. Neurology 55:1621–1626, 2000

Edwards-Lee T, Miller BL, Benson DF, et al: The temporal variant of frontotemporal dementia. Brain 120:1027–1040, 1997

Emery VO, Oxman TE: Update on the dementia spectrum of depression. Am J Psychiatry 149:305–317, 1992

Erkinjuntti T, Wikstrom J, Palo J, et al: Dementia among medical inpatients: evaluation of 2000 consecutive admissions. Arch Intern Med 146:1923–1926, 1986

Erkinjuntti T, Ketonen L, Sulkava R, et al: Do white matter changes on MRI and CT differentiate vascular dementia from Alzheimer's disease? J Neurol Neurosurg Psychiatry 50:37–42, 1987

Erkinjuntti T, Haltia M, Palo J, et al: Accuracy of the clinical diagnosis of vascular dementia: a prospective clinical and post-mortem neuropathological study. J Neurol Neurosurg Psychiatry 51:1037–1044, 1988

Espinoza MT, Parer JT: Mechanisms of asphyxial brain damage and possible pharmacologic interventions in the fetus. Am J Obstet Gynecol 164:1582–1591, 1991

Esteban-Santillan C, Praditsuwan R, Ueda H, et al: Clock drawing test in very mild Alzheimer's disease. J Am Geriatr Soc 46:1266–1269, 1998

Evans DA, Funkenstein HH, Albert MS, et al: Prevalence of Alzheimer's disease in a community population of older persons. JAMA 262:2551–2556, 1989

Faulstich ME: Psychiatric aspects of AIDS. Am J Psychiatry 144:551–556, 1987

Fisher CM: Binswanger's encephalopathy: a review. J Neurol 236:65–79, 1989

Flores-Runk P, Raasch RH: Ticlopidine and antiplatelet therapy. Ann Pharmacother 27:1090–1098, 1993

Folstein MF, McHugh PR: Dementia syndrome of depression, in Alzheimer's Disease: Senile Dementia and Related Disorders. Edited by Katzman R, Terry RD, Bick KL. New York, Raven, 1978, pp 87–93

Folstein MF, Folstein SE, McHugh PR: Mini-Mental State: a practical method for grading the cognitive state of patients for the clinician. J Psychiatr Res 12:189–198, 1975

Forstl H, Burns A, Luthert P, et al: The Lewy-body variant of Alzheimer's disease: clinical and pathological findings. Br J Psychiatry 162:385–392, 1993

Fortin L: Manic disorder in the aged: a review of the literature. Can J Psychiatry 35:679–683, 1990

Foster NL, Wilhemsen K, Sima AAF, et al: Frontotemporal dementia and parkinsonism linked to chromosome 17: a consensus conference. Ann Neurol 41:706–715, 1997

Friedland RP: "Normal"-pressure hydrocephalus and the saga of the treatable dementias. JAMA 262:2577–2581, 1989

Froehlich TE, Robison JT, Inouye SK: Screening for dementia in the outpatient setting: the time and change test. J Am Geriatr Soc 46:1506–1511, 1998

Giacometti AR, Davis PC, Alazraki NP, et al: Anatomic and physiologic imaging of Alzheimer's disease. Clin Geriatr Med 10:277–298, 1994

Gibb WRG: Dementia and Parkinson's disease. Br J Psychiatry 154:596–614, 1989

Gibb WRG, Luthert PJ, Janota I, et al: Cortical Lewy body dementia: clinical features and classification. J Neurol Neurosurg Psychiatry 52:185–192, 1989

Gorman DG, Cummings JL: Neurobehavioral presentations of the antiphospholipid antibody syndrome. J Neuropsychiatry Clin Neurosci 5:37–42, 1993

Graham DI, Adams JH, Gennarelli TA: Pathology of brain damage in head injury, in Head Injury, 2nd Edition. Edited by Cooper PR. Baltimore, MD, Williams & Wilkins, 1987, pp 72–88

Granholm E, Jeste DV: Cognitive impairment in schizophrenia. Psychiatric Annals 24:484–490, 1994

Gray KF, Cummings JL: Neuroimaging in dementia, in Localization and Neuroimaging in Neuropsychology. Edited by Kertesz A. San Diego, CA, Academic Press, 1994, pp 621–651

Green J, Morris JC, Sandson J, et al: Progressive aphasia: a precursor of global dementia? Neurology 40:423–429, 1990

Growdon JH: Treatment for Alzheimer's disease? N Engl J Med 327:1306–1308, 1992

Gupta SR, Naheedy MH, Young JC, et al: Periventricular white matter changes and dementia: clinical, neuropsychological, radiological and pathological correlation. Arch Neurol 45:637–641, 1988

Haass CH, Schlossmacher MG, Hung AY, et al: Amyloid beta-peptide is produced by cultured cells during normal metabolism. Nature 359:322–325, 1992

Hachinski VC, Iliff LD, Zilhka E, et al: Cerebral blood flow in dementia. Arch Neurol 32:632–637, 1975

Hall RC: Psychiatric effects of thyroid hormone disturbance. Psychosomatics 24:7–11, 1983

Haskins BA, Harrison MB: Huntington's disease. Current Treatment Options in Neurology 2:243–262, 2000

Hawkins JW, Tinklenberg JR, Sheikh JI, et al: A retrospective chart review of gabapentin for the treatment of aggressive and agitated behavior in patients with dementias. Am J Geriatr Psychiatry 8:221–225, 2000

Hébert R, Lindsay J, Verreault R, et al: Vascular dementia: incidence and risk factors in the Canadian study of health and aging. Stroke 31(7):1487–1493, 2000

Ho LW, Carmichael J, Swartz J, et al: The molecular biology of Huntington's disease. Psychol Med 31:3–14, 2001

Holmes VF, Fernandez F, Levy JK: Psychostimulant response in AIDS-related complex patients. J Clin Psychiatry 50:5–8, 1989

Holthoff VA, Sandmann J, Pawlik G, et al: Positron emission tomography in Creutzfeldt-Jakob disease. Arch Neurol 47:1035–1038, 1990

Houlden H, Baker M, Adamson J, et al: Frequency of tau mutations in three series of non-Alzheimer's degenerative dementia. Ann Neurol 46:243–248, 1999

Hsiao K, Prusiner SB: Inherited human prion diseases. Neurology 40:1820–1827, 1990

Huber SJ, Shuttleworth EC, Christy JA, et al: Magnetic resonance imaging in dementia of Parkinson's disease. J Neurol Neurosurg Psychiatry 52:1221–1227, 1989

Hughes CP, Berg L, Danziger WL, et al: A new clinical scale for the staging of dementia. Br J Psychiatry 140:566–572, 1982

Hunt AL, Orrison WW, Yeo RA, et al: Clinical significance of MRI white matter lesions in the elderly. Neurology 39:1470–1474, 1989

Jennett B, Teasdale G: Management of Head Injuries. Philadelphia, PA, FA Davis, 1981, pp 271–288

Jernigan TL, Schafer K, Butters N, et al: Magnetic resonance imaging of Korsakoff patients. Neuropsychopharmacology 4:175–186, 1991

Jibiki I, Fukushima T, Kobayashi K, et al: Utility of 1231-IMP SPECT brain scans for the early detection of site-specific abnormalities in Creutzfeldt-Jakob disease (Heidenhain type): a case study. Neuropyschobiology 29:117–119, 1994

Joachim CL, Morris JH, Selkoe DJ: Clinically diagnosed Alzheimer's disease: autopsy results in 150 cases. Ann Neurol 24:50–56, 1988

Jones BN, Reifler BV: Depression coexisting with dementia: evaluation and treatment. Med Clin North Am 78:823–840, 1994

Jordan BD: Neurologic aspects of boxing. Arch Neurol 44:453–459, 1987

Kasahara H, Karasawa A, Ariyasu T, et al: Alcohol dementia and alcohol delirium in aged alcoholics. Psychiatry Clin Neurosci 50:115–123, 1996

Katz IR, Jeste DV, Mintzer JE, et al: Comparison of risperidone and placebo for psychosis and behavioral disturbances associated with dementia: a randomized double-blind trial. J Clin Psychiatry 60:107–115, 1999

Katzman R, Brown T, Fuld P, et al: Validation of a short orientation-memory-concentration test of cognitive impairment. Am J Psychiatry 140:734–739, 1983

Katzman R, Brown T, Thal LJ, et al: Comparison of rate of annual change of mental status score in four independent studies of patients with Alzheimer's disease. Ann Neurol 24:384–389, 1988

Kertesz A, Black SE, Nicholson L, et al: The sensitivity and specificity of MRI in stroke. Neurology 37:1580–1585, 1987

Kertesz A, Black SE, Tokar G, et al: Periventricular and subcortical hyperintensities on magnetic resonance imaging. Arch Neurol 45:404–408, 1988

Kertesz A, Nadkarni N, Davidson W, et al: The Frontal Behavioral Inventory in the differential diagnosis of frontotemporal dementia. J Int Neuropsychol Soc 6:460–468, 2000

Keschner M, Bender MB, Strauss I: Mental symptoms associated with brain tumor: a study of 530 verified cases. JAMA 110:714–718, 1938

Khachaturian ZS: Diagnosis of Alzheimer's disease. Arch Neurol 42:1097–1105, 1985

Knopman DS, DeKosky ST, Cummings JL, et al: Practice parameter: diagnosis of dementia (an evidence-based review): Report of the Quality Standards Subcommittee of the American Academy of Neurology. Neurology 56:1143–1153, 2001

Kraus JF, Sorenson SB: Epidemiology, in Neuropsychiatry of Traumatic Brain Injury. Edited by Silver JM, Yudofsky SC, Hales RE. Washington, DC, American Psychiatric Press, 1994, pp 3–41

Kunik ME, Yudofsky SC, Silver JM, et al: Pharmacologic approach to management of agitation associated with dementia. J Clin Psychiatry 55 (suppl):13–17, 1994

Kyomen HH, Nobel KW, Wei JY: The use of estrogen to decrease aggressive physical behavior in elderly men with dementia. J Am Geriatr Soc 39:1110–1112, 1991

Kunz U, Heintz P, Ehrenheim C, et al: MRI as the primary diagnostic instrument in normal pressure hydrocephalus? Psychiatry Res 29:287–288, 1989

Leopold NA, Borson AJ: An alphabetical 'WORLD'. A new version of an old test. Neurology 49:1521–1524, 1997

Lev N, Melamed E: Heredity in Parkinson's disease: new findings. Isr Med Assoc J 3:435–438, 2001

Levin HS: Memory deficit after closed-head injury. J Clin Exp Neuropsychol 12:129–153, 1989

Levin HS: A guide to clinical neuropsychological testing. Arch Neurol 51:854–859, 1994

Levin HS, Benton AL, Gassman RG: Neurobehavioral Consequences of Closed Head Injury. New York, Oxford University Press, 1982, pp 73–122

Levy-Lahad E, Wijsman EM, Nemens E, et al: A familial Alzheimer's disease locus on chromosome 1. Science 269:970–973, 1995

Lipowski ZJ: Delirium: Acute Confusional States. New York, Oxford University Press, 1990, pp 47–53

Lishman WA: Cerebral disorder in alcoholism: syndromes of impairment. Brain 104:1–20, 1981

Lishman WA: Physiogenesis and psychogenesis in the "postconcussional syndrome." Br J Psychiatry 153:460–469, 1988

Lishman WA: Organic Psychiatry. Oxford, England, Blackwell Science, 1998, pp 479–490

Litvan I, Agid Y, Calne D, et al: Clinical research criteria for the diagnosis of progressive supranuclear palsy (Steele-Richardson-Olszewski syndrome): report of the NINDS-SPSP international workshop. Neurology 47:1–9, 1996

Litvan I, Campbell G, Mangone CA, et al: Which clinical features differentiate progressive supranuclear palsy (Steele-Richardson-Olszewski syndrome) from related disorders? a clinicopathological study. Brain 120:65–74, 1997

Liu CK, Miller BL, Cummings JL, et al: A quantitative MRI study of vascular dementia. Neurology 42:138–143, 1992

Lohr JB, Cadet JL: Neuropsychiatric aspects of brain tumors, in The American Psychiatric Press Textbook of Neuropsychiatry. Edited by Hales RE, Yudofsky SC. Washington, DC, American Psychiatric Press, 1987, pp 351–364

Loudianos G, Gitlin JD: Wilson's disease. SeminLiver Dis 20:353–364, 2000

Luby JP: Infections of the central nervous system. Am J Med Sci 304:379–391, 1992

Mace NL, Rabins PV: The 36-Hour Day. Baltimore, MD, Johns Hopkins University Press, 1991, pp 116–143

Madhusoodanan S, Brenner R, Alcantra A: Clinical experience with quetiapine in elderly patients with psychotic disorders. J Geriatr Psychiatry Neurol 13:28–32, 2000

Maher ER, Lees AJ: The clinical features and natural history of the Steele-Richardson-Olszewski syndrome (progressive supranuclear palsy). Neurology 36:1005–1008, 1986

Mahler ME, Cummings JL: Alzheimer disease and the dementia of Parkinson disease: comparative investigations. Alzheimer Dis Assoc Disord 4(3):133–149, 1990

Mandell AM, Albert ML: History of subcortical dementia, in Subcortical Dementia. Edited by Cummings JL. New York, Oxford University Press, 1990, pp 17–30

Martilla RJ: Epidemiology, in Handbook of Parkinson's Disease, 2nd Edition. Edited by Koller WC. New York, Marcel Dekker, 1992, pp 35–57

Martin DC, Francis J, Protetch J, et al: Time dependency of cognitive recovery with cobalamin replacement: report of a pilot study. J Am Geriatr Soc 40:168–172, 1992

Martinot J-L, Hardy P, Feline A, et al: Left prefrontal glucose hypometabolism in the depressed state: a confirmation. Am J Psychiatry 147:1313–1317, 1990

Masters CL, Richardson EP Jr: Subacute spongiform encephalopathy (Creutzfeldt-Jakob disease)—the nature and progression of spongiform change. Brain 101:333–344, 1978

Mattson AJ, Levin HS: Frontal lobe dysfunction following closed head injury: a review of the literature. J Nerv Ment Dis 178:282–291, 1990

Mazure CM, Druss BG, Cellar JS: Valproate treatment of older psychotic patients with organic mental syndromes and behavioral dyscontrol. J Am Geriatr Soc 40:914–916, 1992

McAllister TW: Neuropsychiatric sequelae of head injuries. Psychiatr Clin North Am 15:395–413, 1992

McDowell I: Alzheimer's disease: insights from epidemiology. Aging (Milano) 13:143–162, 2001

McEvoy JP, Wells CE: Case studies in neuropsychiatry, II: conversion pseudodementia. J Clin Psychiatry 40:447–449, 1979

McKeith I, Fairburn A, Perry R, et al: Neuroleptic sensitivity in patients with senile dementia of Lewy body type. BMJ 305:673–678, 1992a

McKeith IG, Perry RH, Fairbairn AF, et al: Operational criteria for senile dementia of Lewy body type (SDLT). Psychol Med 22:911–922, 1992b

McKeith IG, Fairbairn AF, Perry RH, et al: The clinical diagnosis and misdiagnosis of senile dementia of Lewy body type (SDLT). Br J Psychiatry 165:324–332, 1994

McKeith IG, Galasko D, Kosaka K, et al: Consensus guidelines for the clinical and pathologic diagnosis of dementia with Lewy bodies (DLB): report of the Consortium on DLB International Workshop. Neurology 47:1113–1124, 1996

McKeith I, Del Ser T, Spano P, et al: Efficacy of rivastigmine in dementia with Lewy bodies: a randomised, double-blind, placebo-controlled international study. Lancet 356:2031–2036, 2000

McKhann G, Drachman D, Folstein M, et al: Clinical diagnosis of Alzheimer's disease: report of the NINCDS-ADRDA Work Group under the auspices of Department of Health and Human Services Task Force on Alzheimer's Disease. Neurology 34:939–944, 1984

Mega MS, Cummings JL, Fiorello T, et al: The spectrum of behavioral changes in Alzheimer's disease. Neurology 46:130–135, 1996

Mendez MF, Underwood KL, Zander BA, et al: Risk factors in Alzheimer's disease. Neurology 42:770–775, 1992

Merskey H, Buhrich NA: Hysteria and organic brain disease. Br J Med Psychol 48:359–366, 1975

Meyer JS, McClintic KL, Rogers RL, et al: Aetiological considerations and risk factors for multi-infarct dementia. J Neurol Neurosurg Psychiatry 51:1489–1497, 1988

Meyer JS, Rogers RL, McClintic K, et al: Randomized clinical trial of daily aspirin therapy in multi-infarct dementia: a pilot study. J Am Geriatr Soc 37:549–555, 1989

Miller BL, Benson DF, Goldberg MA, et al: The misdiagnosis of hysteria. Am Fam Physician 34:157–1620, 1986

Miller BL, Cummings JL, Villanueva-Meyer J, et al: Frontal lobe degeneration: clinical, neuropsychological, and SPECT characteristics. Neurology 41:1374–1382, 1991

Miller GA: The magic number seven, plus or minus two: some limits on our capacity for processing information. Psychol Rev 63:81–97, 1956

Mintzer MJ: Hypothyroidism and hyperthyroidism in the elderly. J Fla Med Assoc 79:231–235, 1992

Mirra SS, Hart MN, Terry RD: Making the diagnosis of Alzheimer's disease: a primer for practicing pathologists. Arch Pathol Lab Med 117:132–144, 1993

Navia BA: The AIDS dementia complex, in Subcortical Dementia. Edited by Cummings JL. New York, Oxford University Press, 1990, pp 181–198

Navia BA, Jordan BD, Price RW: The AIDS dementia complex, I: clinical features. Ann Neurol 19:517–524, 1986

Neary D, Snowden JS, Gustafson L, et al: Frontotemporal lobar degeneration: a consensus on the clinical diagnostic criteria. Neurology 51:1546–1554, 1998

Nielsen H, Lolk A, Pederson I, et al: The accuracy of early diagnosis and predictors of death in Alzheimer's disease and vascular dementia—a follow-up study. Acta Psychiatr Scand 84:277–282, 1991

O'Brien MD: Vascular dementia is underdiagnosed. Arch Neurol 45:797–798, 1988

O'Brien J, Thomas A, Ballard C, et al: Cognitive impairment in depression is not associated with neuropathologic evidence of increased vascular or Alzheimer-type pathology. Biol Psychiatry 49:130–136, 2001

O'Neill D, Barber RD: Reversible dementia caused by vitamin B-12 deficiency (letter). J Am Geriatr Soc 41:192–193, 1993

Overman W Jr, Stoudemire A: Guidelines for legal and financial counseling of Alzheimer's disease patients and their families. Am J Psychiatry 145:1495–1500, 1988

Pantoni L, Garcia JH: The significance of cerebral white matter abnormalities 100 years after Binswanger's report: a review. Stroke 26:1293–1301, 1995

Panzer MJ, Mellow AM: Antidepressant treatment of pathologic laughing or crying in elderly stroke patients. J Geriatr Psychiatry Neurol 5:195–199, 1992

Patten BM: Wilson's disease, in Parkinson's Disease and Movement Disorders, 2nd Edition. Edited by Jankovic J, Tolosa E. Baltimore, MD, Williams & Wilkins, 1993, pp 217–233

Paulson GW: The neurological examination in dementia, in Dementia, 2nd Edition. Edited by Wells CE. Philadelphia, PA, FA Davis, 1977, pp 169–188

Pearlson GD, Rabins PV, Kim WS, et al: Structural brain CT changes and cognitive deficits in elderly depressives with and without reversible dementia ("pseudodementia"). Psychol Med 19:573–584, 1989

Pearson RCA, Powell TPS: The neuroanatomy of Alzheimer's disease. Rev Neurosci 2:101–122, 1989

Perry TL, Hansen S, Kloster M: Huntington's chorea: deficiency of gamma-aminobutyric acid in brain. N Engl J Med 288:337–342, 1973

Pericak-Vance MA, Bass MP, Yamaoka LH, et al: Complete genomic screen in late-onset familial Alzheimer disease: evidence for a new locus on chromosome 12. JAMA 278:1237–1241, 1997

Petersen RC, Ghoneim MM: Diazepam and human memory: influence on acquisition, retrieval, and state-dependent learning. Prog Neuropsychopharmacol Biol Psychiatry 4:81–89, 1980

Petersen RC, Smith GE, Ivnik RJ, et al: Memory function in very early Alzheimer's disease. Neurology 44:867–872, 1994

Petersen RC, Stevens JC, Ganguli M, et al: Practice parameter: early detection of dementia: mild cognitive impairment (an evidence-based review). Report of the Quality Standards Subcommittee of the American Academy of Neurology. Neurology 56:1133–1142, 2001

Pizzolato G, Borsato N, Saitta B, et al: [99mTc]-HM-PAO SPECT in Parkinson's disease. J Cereb Blood Flow Metab 8:S101–S108, 1988

Plum F, Posner JB: The Diagnosis of Stupor and Coma, 3rd Edition. Philadelphia, PA, FA Davis, 1982

Powell AL, Cummings JL, Hill MA, et al: Speech and language alterations in multi-infarct dementia. Neurology 38:717–719, 1988

Price TRP, Goetz KL, Lovell MR: Neuropsychiatric aspects of brain tumors, in The American Psychiatric Press Textbook of Neuropsychiatry, 2nd Edition. Edited by Yudofsky SC, Hales RE. Washington, DC, American Psychiatric Press, 1992, pp 473–497

Prusiner SB: The prion diseases. Brain Pathology 8:499–513, 1998

Prusiner SB: Shattuck Lecture: neurodegenerative diseases and prions. N Engl J Med 344:1516–1526, 2001

Purohit DP, Davidson M, Perl DP, et al: Severe cognitive impairment in elderly schizophrenic patients: a clinicopathological study. Biol Psychiatry 33:255–260, 1993

Rabins PV: Reversible dementia and the misdiagnosis of dementia: a review. Hospital and Community Psychiatry 34:830–835, 1983

Radue EW, duBoulay GH, Harrison MJG, et al: Comparison of angiographic and CT findings between patients with multi-infarct dementia and those with dementia due to primary neuronal degeneration. Neuroradiology 16:113–115, 1978

Raia PA: Helping patients and families to take control. Psychiatric Annals 24:192–196, 1994

Rapcsak SZ, Croswell SC, Rubens AB: Apraxia in Alzheimer's disease. Neurology 39:664–668, 1989

Raskind MA, Peskind ER, Wessel T, et al: Galantamine in AD: a 6-month randomized, placebo-controlled trial with a 6-month extension. The Galantamine USA–1 Study Group. Neurology 54:2261–2268, 2000

Razani J, Boone KB, Miller BL, et al: Neuropsychological performance of right- and left-frontotemporal dementia compared to Alzheimer's disease. J Int Neuropsychol Soc 7:468–480, 2001

Reding M, Haycox J, Blass J: Depression in patients referred to a dementia clinic: a three-year prospective study. Arch Neurol 42:894–896, 1985

Reichman WE, Cummings JL: Diagnosis of rare dementia syndromes: an algorithmic approach. J Geriatr Psychiatry Neurol 3:73–84, 1990

Reisberg B: Functional assessment staging (FAST). Psychopharmacology Bulletin 24:653–659, 1988

Rich S, Ovsiew F: Leuprolide acetate for exhibitionism in Huntington's disease. Mov Disord 9:353–357, 1994

Richardson EP Jr: Our evolving understanding of progressive multifocal leukoencephalopathy. Ann N Y Acad Sci 230:358–364, 1974

Roache JD, Griffiths RR: Comparison of triazolam and pentobarbital: performance impairment, subjective effects, and abuse liability. J Pharmacol Exp Ther 234:120–133, 1985

Robinson RG: Neuropsychiatric consequences of stroke. Annu Rev Med 48:217–229, 1997

Rocca WA, Kokmen E: Frequency and distribution of vascular dementia. Alzheimer Dis Assoc Disord 13(suppl 3):S9–S14, 1999

Rogers SL, Friedhoff LT, The Donepezil Study Group: The efficacy and safety of donepezil in patients with Alzheimer's disease: results of a US multicentre, randomized, double-blind, placebo-controlled trial. Dementia 7:293–303, 1996

Rogers SL, Farlow MR, Doody RS, et al: A 24-week, double-blind, placebo-controlled trial of donepezil in patients with Alzheimer's disease. Neurology 50:136–145, 1998

Roman GC, Tatemichi TK, Erkinjuntti T, et al: Vascular dementia: diagnostic criteria for research studies: report of the NINDS-AIREN international workshop. Neurology 43:250–260, 1993

Romanelli MF, Morris JC, Ashkin K, et al: Advanced Alzheimer's disease is a risk factor for late-onset seizures. Arch Neurol 47:847–850, 1990

Rosen WG, Terry RD, Fuld PA, et al: Pathological verification of ischemic score in differentiation of dementias. Ann Neurol 7:486–488, 1980

Rosen HJ, Lengenfelder J, Miller B: Frontotemporal dementia. Neurol Clin 18:979–992, 2000

Rosenblatt A, Leroi I: Neuropsychiatry of Huntington's disease and other basal ganglia disorders. Psychosomatics 41:24–30, 2000

Rosler M, Anand R, Cicin-Sain A, et al: Efficacy and safety of rivastigmine in patients with Alzheimer's disease: international randomized controlled trial. BMJ 318:633–640, 1999

Royall DR, Mahurin RK, Gray KF: Bedside assessment of executive cognitive impairment: the Executive Interview. J Am Geriatr Soc 40:1221–1226, 1992

Royall DR, Cordes JA, Polk M: CLOX: an executive clock drawing task. Journal of Neurology, Neurosurgery, and Psychiatry 64:588–594, 1998

Ruberg RM, Javoy-Agid F, Hirsh E, et al: Dopaminergic and cholinergic lesions in progressive supranuclear palsy. Ann Neurol 18:523–529, 1985

Sachon C, Grimaldi A, Digy JP, et al: Cognitive function, insulin-dependent diabetes and hypoglycaemia. J Intern Med 231:471–475, 1992

Sano M, Ernesto C, Thomas RG, et al: A controlled trial of selegiline, alpha-tocopherol, or both as treatment for Alzheimer's disease. N Engl J Med 336:1216–1222, 1997

Saunders AM, Trowers MK, Shimkets RA, et al: The role of apolipoprotein E in Alzheimer's disease: pharmacogenomic target selection. Biochim Biophys Acta 1502:85–94, 2000

Savage CR: Neuropsychology of subcortical dementias. Psychiatr Clin North Am 20:911–931, 1997

Scharf MB, Saskin P, Fletcher K: Benzodiazepine-induced amnesia: clinical laboratory findings. J Clin Psychiatry 5 (monograph):14–17, 1987

Schellenberg GD, Bird TD, Wijsman EM, et al: Genetic linkage evidence for a familial Alzheimer's disease locus on chromosome 14. Science 258:668–671, 1992

Schneider LS, Sobin PB: Non-neuroleptic medications in the management of agitation in Alzheimer's disease and other dementia: a selective review. Int J Geriatr Psychiatry 6:691–708, 1991

Schneider LS, Pollock VE, Lyness SA: A metaanalysis of controlled trials of neuroleptic treatment in dementia. J Am Geriatr Soc 38:553–563, 1990

Schneider LS, Olin JT, Pawluczyk S: A double-blind crossover pilot study of L-deprenyl (selegiline) combined with cholinesterase inhibitor in Alzheimer's disease. Am J Psychiatry 150:321–323, 1993

Scott JP, Roberto KA, Hutton JT: Families of Alzheimer's victims: family support to the caregivers. J Am Geriatr Soc 34:348–354, 1986

Selecki BR: Intracranial space-occupying lesions among patients admitted to mental hospitals. Med J Aust 1:383–390, 1965

Sigal M, Altmark D, Alfici S, et al: Ganser syndrome: a review of 15 cases. Compr Psychiatry 33:134–138, 1992

Skoldenberg B: Herpes simplex encephalitis. Scand J Infect Dis Suppl 80:40–46, 1991

Skoog I: Risk factors for vascular dementia: a review. Dementia 5:137–144, 1994

Slagle DA: Psychiatric disorders following closed head injury: an overview of biopsychosocial factors in their etiology and management. Int J Psychiatry Med 20:1–35, 1990

Small GW: Psychopharmacological treatment of elderly demented patients. J Clin Psychiatry 49 (suppl 5):8–13, 1988

Small GW: Dementia and amnestic syndromes, in Treatments of Psychiatric Disorders: A Task Force Report of the American Psychiatric Association. Washington, DC, American Psychiatric Association, 1989, pp 815–831

Snowdon DA, Greiner LH, Mortimer JA, et al: Brain infarction and the clinical expression of Alzheimer disease: the Nun Study. JAMA 277:813–817, 1997

Solomon PR, Hirschoff A, Kelly B, et al: A 7 minute neurocognitive screening battery highly sensitive to Alzheimer's disease. Arch Neurol 55:349–355, 1998

Sobin P, Schneider L, McDermott H: Fluoxetine in the treatment of agitated dementia (letter). Am J Psychiatry 146:1636, 1989

Starosta-Rubinstein S, Young AB, Kluin K, et al: Clinical assessment of 31 patients with Wilson's disease. Arch Neurol 44:365–370, 1987

Steele JC, Richardson JC, Olszewski J: Progressive supranuclear palsy: a heterogeneous degeneration involving the brain stem, basal ganglia, and cerebellum with vertical gaze and pseudobulbar palsy, nuchal dystonia and dementia. Arch Neurol 10:333–359, 1964

Stern RG, Davis KL: Treatment approaches in Alzheimer's disease: past, present, and future, in The Dementias: Diagnosis and Management. Edited by Weiner MF. Washington, DC, American Psychiatric Press, 1991, pp 227–248

Street JS, Clark WS, Gannon KS, et al: Olanzapine treatment of psychotic and behavioral symptoms in patients with Alzheimer disease in nursing care facilities: a double-blind, randomized, placebo-controlled trial. The HGEU Study Group. Arch Gen Psychiatry 57:968–976, 2000

Sultzer DL: Mental status examination, in The American Psychiatric Press Textbook of Geriatric Neuropsychiatry. Edited by Coffey CE, Cummings JL. Washington, DC, American Psychiatric Press, 1994, pp 112–127

Sultzer DL, Gray KF, Gunay I, et al: A double-blind comparison of trazodone and haloperidol for treatment of agitation in patients with dementia. Am J Geriatr Psychiatry 5:60–69, 1997

Tariot PN, Solomon PR, Morris JC, et al: A 5-month, randomized, placebo-controlled trial of galantamine in AD. The Galantamine USA-10 Study Group. Neurology 54:2269–2276, 2000

Tatemichi TK: How acute brain failure becomes chronic: a view of the mechanisms of dementia related to stroke. Neurology 40:1652–1659, 1990

Tatemichi TK, Desmond DW, Prohovnik I: Strategic infarcts in vascular dementia: a clinical and brain imaging experience. Arzneimittelforschung 45:371–385, 1995

Thomas RJ: Blinking and the release reflexes: are they clinically useful? J Am Geriatr Soc 42:609–613, 1994

Tiller JWG, Dakis JA, Shaw JM: Short-term buspirone treatment in disinhibition with dementia (letter). Lancet 2:510, 1988

Tombaugh TN, McIntyre NJ: The Mini-Mental Status Examination: a comprehensive review. J Am Geriatr Soc 40:922–935, 1992

Tomlinson BE, Blessed G, Roth M: Observations on the brains of demented old people. J Neurol Sci 11:205–242, 1970

Traynelis VC: Chronic subdural hematoma in the elderly. Clin Geriatr Med 7:583–598, 1991

Van Duijn CM, Tanja TA, Haaxma R, et al: Head trauma and the risk of Alzheimer's disease. Am J Epidemiol 135:775–782, 1992

Van Gorp WG, Mahler M: Subcortical features of normal aging, in Subcortical Dementia. Edited by Cummings JL. New York, Oxford University Press, 1990, pp 231–250

Van Gorp WG, Mandelkern MA, Gee M, et al: Cerebral metabolic dysfunction in AIDS: findings in a sample with and without dementia. J Neuropsychiatry Clin Neurosci 4:280–287, 1992

Van Gorp WG, Hinken C, Satz P, et al: Subtypes of HIV-related neuropsychological functioning: a cluster analysis approach. Neuropsychology 7:62–72, 1993

Vanneste JA: Three decades of normal pressure hydrocephalus: are we wiser now? J Neurol Neurosurg Psychiatry 57:1021–1025, 1994

Victor M: Persistent altered mentation due to ethanol. Neurol Clin 11:639–661, 1993

Victor M: Alcoholic dementia. Can J Neurol Sci 21:88–99, 1994

Victor M, Adams RD, Collins GH: The Wernicke-Korsakoff Syndrome and Related Neurologic Disorders Due to Alcoholism and Malnutrition, 2nd Edition. Philadelphia, PA, FA Davis, 1989

Vinters HV: Pathologic issues in the diagnosis of Alzheimer disease. Bulletin of Clinical Neurosciences 56:39–47, 1991

Vinters HV, Miller BL, Pardridge WM: Brain amyloid and Alzheimer disease. Ann Intern Med 109:41–54, 1988

von Einsiedel RW, Fife TD, Aksamit AJ, et al: Progressive multifocal leukoencephalopathy in AIDS: a clinicopathologic study and review of the literature. J Neurol 240:391–406, 1993

Weiner MF, Gray KF: Balancing psychosocial and psychopharmacologic measures in Alzheimer's disease. American Journal of Alzheimer's Care and Related Disorders and Research 9:6–12, 1994

Weiner MF, Denke M, Williams K, et al: Intramuscular medroxyprogesterone acetate for sexual aggression in elderly men. Lancet 339:1121–1122, 1992

Wells CE: Pseudodementia. Am J Psychiatry 136:895–900, 1979

Wesselingh SL, Thompson KA: Immunopathogenesis of HIV-associated dementia. Curr Opin Neurol 14:375–379, 2001

Weytingh MD, Bossuyt PM, van Crevel H: Reversible dementia: more than 10% or less than 1%? A quantitative review. J Neurology 242:466–471, 1995

Whatley SA, Anderton BH: The genetics of Alzheimer's disease. Int J Geriatr Psychiatry 5:145–159, 1990

Whitehouse PJ, Geldmacher DS: Pharmacotherapy for Alzheimer's disease. Clin Geriatr Med 10:339–350, 1994

Whitlock FA: The Ganser syndrome. Br J Psychiatry 113:19–29, 1967

Wise MG: Delirium, in The American Psychiatric Press Textbook of Neuropsychiatry. Edited by Hales RE, Yudofsky SC. Washington, DC, American Psychiatric Press, 1987, pp 89–105

Zec RF: Neuropsychological functioning in Alzheimer's disease, in Neuropsychology of Alzheimer's Disease and Other Dementias. Edited by Parks RW, Zec RF, Wilson RF. New York, Oxford University Press, 1993, pp 3–80

Zola-Morgan S, Squire LR, Amaral DG: Human amnesia and the medial temporal region: enduring memory impairment following a bilateral lesion limited to the CA1 field of the hippocampus. J Neurosci 6:2950–2967, 1986

Zubenko GS, Rosen JR, Sweet RA, et al: Impact of psychiatric hospitalization on behavioral complications of Alzheimer's disease. Am J Psychiatry 149:1484–1491, 1992

Depression

Alvin M. Rouchell, M.D.

Richard Pounds, M.D.

John G. Tierney, M.D.

Depression in medically ill patients is an important clinical entity (N.H. Cassem 1991; Sutor et al. 1998). Although major depressive disorder occurs in 3.7%–6.7% of the general population (Robins et al. 1984), the prevalence of major depressive disorder is 5%–10% among general medical inpatients (Silverstone et al. 1996) and 9%–16% among general medical outpatients (Katon 1987; Katon and Schulberg 1992).

UNDERDIAGNOSIS AND UNDERTREATMENT

Even though depression occurs commonly in medically ill patients, it is underdiagnosed and undertreated (Hirschfeld et al. 1997). In one study, only 34.9% of patients with major depressive disorder were identified and adequately treated by primary care physicians (Coyne et al. 1995). Several explanations are offered for this problem (Table 17–1). Primary care patients typically emphasize somatic complaints and deny mood or cognitive symptoms. In addition, some patients report mild or nonspecific symptoms of depression. Some primary care physicians focus on physical signs and symptoms (Katon 1987) and are reluctant to stigmatize the patient with a psychiatric diagnosis (Docherty 1997). Also, some physicians avoid the diagnosis of depression because of the potentially hazardous side effects of tricyclic antidepressants (TCAs) in medically compromised patients (Freedland et al. 1991). Furthermore, some physicians deliberately substitute alternative diagnoses for major depressive disorder in order to improve reimbursement (Rost et al. 1994). Unfortunately, the most common reason for underdiagnosis and undertreatment of depression in medical patients is the mistaken notion that if a depression is understandable, explainable, and reactive to environmental circumstances, it neither is pathological nor requires treatment (Rifkin 1992).

TABLE 17–1. Reasons for underdiagnosis and undertreatment of depression in medically ill patients

Emphasis on somatic rather than cognitive and mood complaints

Reluctance to stigmatize patient with psychiatric diagnosis

Mild or nonspecific symptoms of depression

Fear of antidepressant side effects

Mistaken notion that reactive depressions are not pathological (e.g., "She should be depressed; she has cancer")

Time limitations in primary care

Inadequate training in psychiatry among primary care physicians

Inaccurate coding for purposes of reimbursement improvement

MORBIDITY AND MORTALITY

Major or minor depression in a medically ill patient has a significant effect on the patient's morbidity and mortality. In one study involving patients with coronary artery disease (CAD), major depressive disorder was the best predictor of myocardial infarction, angioplasty, and death during the 12 months after cardiac catheterization (Carney et al. 1988). In addition, depressed patients with CAD were six times more likely than nondepressed patients to have episodes of ventricular tachycardia as shown by 24-hour Holter monitoring (Carney et al. 1993). In two other studies, major depressive disorder in patients following myocardial infarction was an independent risk factor for mortality at 6- and 18-month follow-up (Frasure-Smith et al. 1993, 1995). Possible pathophysiologic mechanisms for this increased mortality are exaggerated platelet reactivity and alterations in heart rate variability (Musselman et al. 1996, 1998; Nemeroff et al. 1998). Morris et al. (1993a) reported that patients with either major or minor depression after a stroke were 3.4 times more likely to die during a 10-year period than were poststroke patients without depression. Patients with poststroke depression and few social contacts and personality introversion were particularly vulnerable—more than 90% died (Morris et al. 1993b). Silverstone (1990) examined the effect of depressive mood on patients with acute, life-threatening medical illnesses (myocardial infarction, subarachnoid hemorrhage, pulmonary embolus, and upper gastrointestinal hemorrhage). He reported that 47% of these depressed patients either died or had further life-threatening complications, whereas only 10% of the nondepressed patients died or had further complications. Depressed mood is also associated with an increased risk of death in home dialysis patients. In addition to depressed mood, these high-risk patients typically exhibit preoccupation with somatic complaints, degradation of self, despondency, and pessimism (Burton et al. 1986). Besides higher mortality rates, depressed cancer patients experience a poorer quality of life, are less compliant with medical care, and have longer hospital stays (Newport and Nemeroff 1998).

The increased risk of morbidity and mortality in medically ill patients is probably mediated by changes in the neuroendocrine and immune systems (Miller et al. 1993). In vitro alterations in immunological functioning associated with depression include reduced lymphocyte response to mitogen stimulation, decreased killer cell activity, and diminished neutrophil activity (Maes et al. 1994; Schleifer et al. 1996; Weisse 1992). Furthermore, the degree of immunosuppression may correlate with depression severity (Kiecolt-Glaser and Glaser 1986). In addition to these biological factors, depression may adversely affect the course of a medical illness by reducing the patient's motivation and compliance with medical regimens (Carney et al. 1988).

ECONOMICS

Overutilization of medical resources occurs when depression complicates the inpatient or outpatient course of a

medical illness (Henk et al. 1996). Von Korff et al. (1992) estimated that high utilizers of medical resources, who made up 15% of their health maintenance organization (HMO) patient population, accounted for 64% of the total health care costs. Moreover, in this same HMO patient population, 23.5% of the high utilizers had current major depressive disorder, and 16.8% had dysthymic disorder (Katon et al. 1990). These depressed individuals not only overutilized medical services but also exhibited a poor perception of their physical health, a more distorted view of their disability, and more impairment of their vocational and social roles compared with patients without depression. Among patients in one family practice clinic, depressed high utilizers scheduled nearly twice as many visits, placed more telephone calls, and underwent more laboratory testing than did the remainder of the patients in the clinic population (Katon 1991). Successful treatment of depressed high utilizers significantly reduced the number of disability days as well as scores on disability scales at 1-year follow-up (Von Korff et al. 1992).

DEPRESSION AS THE INITIAL MANIFESTATION OF PHYSICAL ILLNESS

Depression may precede the other signs and symptoms of many medical conditions. In many cases of cancer of the pancreas, the symptoms of depression come before the physical findings (Passik and Breitbart 1996). Major depressive disorder is sometimes present in patients with Cushing's syndrome (Kelly 1996), Addison's disease, hyperthyroidism, or hypothyroidism even before the classic endocrine signs and symptoms are evident (G.A. Fava et al. 1987). In cases of Huntington's disease (HD), primary or secondary depression may appear decades before the neurological symptoms (S.E. Folstein et al. 1983).

PRESENTATIONS AND DEFINITIONS

Major Depressive Episode

Depression is common in medically ill patients as an affective experience (e.g., sadness), as a symptomatic complaint, or as a clinical syndrome (Rodin and Voshart 1986). Psychiatrists are interested primarily in identifying the clinical syndrome. According to Kathol et al. (1990a), psychiatrists must identify those depressed medical patients who are likely to benefit from a psychiatric intervention. DSM-IV-TR (American Psychiatric Association 2000) nomenclature goes beyond DSM-III-R (American Psychiatric Association 1987) in directly addressing the diagnosis of a primary major depressive episode in patients with medical illness. DSM-III-R excludes symptoms from the diagnosis of major depressive episode if they are "due to a physical condition." DSM-IV-TR excludes symptoms of depression if they are "due to direct physiological effects of a substance…or a general medical condition." For the diagnosis of a major depressive episode, DSM-IV-TR requires at least five of nine depressive symptoms during the same 2-week period; one of the symptoms must be either 1) depressed mood or 2) loss of interest or pleasure. The nine symptoms are listed in Table 17–2.

DSM-IV-TR exclusion criteria for a major depressive episode pose two problems for the consultation-liaison psychiatrist: 1) the criteria require a conclusion about etiological or causal relations between the general medical condition and the depressive syndrome, and 2) the criteria restrict the diagnosis of a major depressive episode in medically ill patients. These problems are a likely reason that many consultation-liaison psychiatrists use the primary versus secondary terminology when diagnosing depression in medically ill patients. Several authors have credited Munroe (1966) with the development of the concept of secondary depression (Black et al. 1987; E.H. Cassem 1990; Winokur 1990). In the Research Diagnostic Criteria (RDC), secondary depression is defined as "a depression occurring in a person who has a preexisting nonaffective psychiatric disorder or a life-threatening medical illness that precedes and parallels the symptoms of depression" (Feighner et al. 1972, p. 59). It is unfortunate for the consultation-liaison psychiatrist that the concept of secondary depression has been absent from DSM beginning with DSM-III (American Psychiatric Association 1980). Organic mood disorder (DSM-III-R), mood disorder due to a general medical condition (DSM-IV-TR), and substance-induced mood disorder (DSM-IV-TR) are the diagnoses most similar to secondary depression. However, these diagnoses are very general and require only that dysphoric mood or decreased interest or pleasure be present.

Fortunately, consultation-liaison psychiatrists have developed alternative clinical approaches to categorize depressive syndromes in medically ill patients. Cohen-Cole and Stoudemire (1987) described four approaches to the diagnosis of major depressive disorder in medically ill patients: 1) inclusive, 2) exclusive, 3) etiological, and 4) substitutive. The authors advocated the use of an inclusive approach in clinical practice (i.e., inclusion of

TABLE 17–2. Signs and symptoms of depression syndromes (summarized from DSM-IV-TR criteria for major depressive episode)

Depressed mood
Diminished interest or pleasure
Significant weight loss or gain
Insomnia or hypersomnia
Psychomotor agitation or retardation
Fatigue or loss of energy
Feelings of worthlessness or excessive or inappropriate guilt
Diminished ability to think or concentrate, or indecisiveness
Recurrent thoughts of death, recurrent suicidal ideation, suicide attempt, or specific plan for suicide

symptoms of depression regardless of whether they are due to a physical or a psychiatric process). This approach may lead to some false-positive diagnoses but is preferable to the alternative of denying treatment to medically ill patients with depression who might benefit. For research, Cohen-Cole and Stoudemire (1987) recommended the use of an exclusive approach to obtain a "pure culture" of depressed patients; the disadvantage is decreased sensitivity and the risk of false-negative diagnoses (i.e., exclusion of some truly depressed patients from treatment). For example, Buckberg et al. (1984) used an exclusive approach to diagnosis in their study involving cancer patients; they eliminated anorexia and fatigue from the list of depressive symptoms and required four of the remaining six symptoms for the diagnosis of a major depressive episode.

The etiological approach is that taken by DSM-III-R and DSM-IV-TR. A symptom meets the criteria for depression only if it is not "caused" by the primary illness (E.H. Cassem 1990). In other words, the diagnostician must infer causality. The reliability of this approach is likely to be low (Cohen-Cole and Stoudemire 1987). The etiological approach was used by Robinson et al. (1984) in their work with patients with poststroke depression. This work is further discussed later in this chapter, in the section entitled "CNS and Neurological Disorders."

In the substitutive approach, alternative diagnostic criteria are substituted for the diagnosis of depression in medically ill patients (Endicott 1984). For example, when symptoms of depression are concurrent with a physical condition, change in appetite or weight is replaced with tearfulness or depressed appearance, sleep disturbance with social withdrawal, indecisiveness with lack of reactivity to events, and loss of energy or fatigue with brooding pessimism. Kathol et al. (1990b) used Endicott's (1984) substitutive criteria in a study of major depressive disorder in cancer patients and detected similar prevalence rates for depression using either a substitutive or inclusive approach to diagnosis.

Clarification of these diagnostic issues is critical to the comparison of epidemiology, clinical features, etiology, treatment, course, and prognosis of depression between medically ill patients and the general medically healthy population. Unlike primary mood disorders, relatively little systematic research has been done on the syndrome of secondary depression. Research in this area is hampered by factors such as ill-defined diagnostic criteria, the absence of standardized assessment measures (scales) for medically ill populations, heterogeneity of populations, and limited use of control groups (Rodin and Voshart 1986). Summarized in Table 17–3 are epidemiologic data on point prevalence of major depressive disorder in specific medical conditions; marked differences in prevalence exist. These differences are partially due to varying research methodologies. Winokur (1990) reported marked differences between clinical features of depression secondary to life-threatening medical illness and those of primary major depressive disorder (Table 17–4).

Dysthymic Disorder and Minor Depression

The diagnosis of dysthymic disorder in medically ill patients is restricted by the same exclusion criteria that complicate the diagnosis of major depressive disorder in medical-surgical patients (i.e., the symptoms cannot be due to the direct effects of a substance or a general medical condition). Dysthymic disorder has its roots in the concept of neurotic depression (Akiskal et al. 1980); however, the terminology has evolved in DSM, and *dysthymia* currently denotes a chronic depressive illness of at least 2 years' duration (in adults; 1 year in children and adolescents) and of insufficient severity to meet the criteria for a major depressive episode. Two views of dysthymia are used in the medical setting: 1) dysthymia as a chronic mild or moderate characterological mood syndrome and 2) dysthymia as a form of minor depression or depression that almost satisfies the diagnostic criteria for major depressive disorder.

Akiskal et al. (1980) proposed that chronic depression could be subtyped into chronic unipolar depression and chronic characterological depression. Furthermore, they suggested dividing characterological depression into 1) "subaffective dysthymia," or chronic depression, which can begin at any point in life, and 2) character spectrum disorder, with a developmental origin implied. The authors reported that the epidemiology, clinical features, and response to treatment of these two subtypes are dif-

TABLE 17–3. Likelihood of developing major depression after diagnosis of specific medical conditions

Condition	Prevalence (%)	Reference
Hemodialysis	6.5	Hinrichsen et al. 1989
	6–34	O'Donnell and Chung 1997
Coronary artery disease	18	Carney et al. 1987
	19	Forrester et al. 1992
	18	Schleifer et al. 1989
	16	Frasure-Smith et al. 1993
	23	Gonzalez et al. 1996
Cancer	25–38	Kathol et al. 1990b
	20	Massie and Holland 1990
Chronic pain	32	Katon et al. 1985
	21	Sullivan et al. 1992
Neurological disorders		
Stroke	27	Robinson et al. 1990
Parkinson's disease	28.6	Mayeux et al. 1986
	51	Sano et al. 1989
Multiple sclerosis	6–57	Minden and Schiffer 1990
	37	Schiffer et al. 1983
Epilepsy	55	Mendez et al. 1986
Huntington's disease	41	S.E. Folstein et al. 1983
Dementia	11	Greenwald et al. 1989
Endocrine conditions		
Hyperthyroidism	31	Kathol et al. 1986
Hypothyroidism	56	Haggerty et al. 1993
Diabetes mellitus	8.5–27.3	Goodnick 1997
Cushing's syndrome	66.6	Haskett 1985
Cushing's disease	54	Sonino et al. 1998
HIV disease	30.3	Atkinson et al. 1988
Chronic fatigue	17.2	Cathebras et al. 1992
	46.4	Kreusi et al. 1989

Note. HIV = human immunodeficiency virus.

TABLE 17–4. Characteristics of depression secondary to medical illness compared with primary major depression

Older age at onset

More likely to respond to electroconvulsive therapy

More likely to be improved at discharge

More likely to show "organic" features in the mental status examination

More likely to have a much lower incidence of a family history of alcoholism and depression (19% of medically ill patients vs. 36% of psychiatrically ill patients)

Less likely to have suicidal thoughts and commit suicide (10% death by suicide in medically ill sample vs. 45% in psychiatrically ill group)

ferent. Patients with subaffective dysthymia are described as similar to those with primary affective illness. Patients with character spectrum disorder are described as having a mix of personality disorders (Table 17–5).

TABLE 17–5. Characteristics of subaffective dysthymia compared with those of character spectrum disorder

Patients with subaffective dysthymia
 Respond to tricyclics and lithium
 Have shortened rapid eye movement (REM) latency
 Are evenly distributed by sex
 Frequently have superimposed depressed episodes (i.e., "double-depression")

Patients with character spectrum disorder
 Respond poorly to treatment interventions (e.g., tricyclic and lithium therapy)
 Are more often women
 Have inconstant depressive features
 Frequently have complications of alcohol and substance abuse

TABLE 17–6. Medical conditions etiologically related to depression

Neurological disorders
 Stroke
 Parkinson's disease
 Multiple sclerosis
 Epilepsy
 Huntington's disease
 Dementia

Endocrine disorders
 Hyperthyroidism
 Hypothyroidism
 Cushing's syndrome
 Addison's disease
 Hyperparathyroidism

Cancer

Conditions due to use of medications or psychoactive substances (see Table 17–7)

TABLE 17–7. Medications and psychoactive substances associated with depression

Antihypertensive medications
 Resperpine
 Methyldopa
 β-Blockers (in predisposed individuals)

Contraceptives

Corticosteroids

Benzodiazepines

Histamine$_2$ receptor antagonists
 Cimetidine
 Ranitidine

Cancer chemotherapeutic agents
 Vincristine
 Vinblastine
 Procarbazine
 L-Asparaginase
 Amphotericin B
 Interferon

Psychoactive substances
 Alcohol
 Opiates
 Amphetamine or cocaine (withdrawal)
 Anabolic steroids

The RDC as outlined by Spitzer et al. (1978) contained criteria independent of etiology and based on a temporal distinction between primary and secondary depression. This group also proposed the category of minor depression, defined as "nonpsychotic episodes of illness in which the most prominent disturbance is a relatively sustained mood of depression without the full depressive syndrome, although some associated features must be present" (Spitzer et al. 1978, p. 778). E.H. Cassem (1990) advocated continued use of the term *minor depression*, with the recommendation that the duration requirement of 2 years be eliminated for medically ill patients. E.H. Cassem pointed to the work of Robinson and colleagues (Robinson and Price 1982; Robinson et al. 1983, 1985, 1987) with stroke patients and noted the utility of distinctions between major and minor depression, as well as differences in course and treatment response identified with this nomenclature.

Mood Disorder Due to a General Medical Condition and Substance-Induced Mood Disorder

Mood disorder due to a general medical condition and *substance-induced mood disorder* are DSM-IV-TR diagnostic terms for depression caused by certain medical illnesses and some medications and psychoactive substances. These two diagnoses replace the terms *organic affective disorder* from DSM-III and *organic mood disorder* from DSM-III-R. Listed in Tables 17–6 and 17–7 are the medical conditions, medications, and psychoactive substances that are recognized as being etiologically related to depression. Rundell and Wise (1989) found that in 3.5% of 775 consecutive psychiatric consultations, a diagnosis of DSM-III-R organic mood disorder was made; this figure represented one-third of all patients

with a diagnosis of depressive disorder. Of the 27 patients with organic mood disorder, 23 had medical conditions or trauma affecting the central nervous system (CNS). Of the remaining 4 patients, 2 had hypothyroidism, 1 was receiving propranolol, and 1 was taking corticosteroids. In a similar study, 70% of patients with DSM-III-R organic mood disorder had CNS lesions

(Yates et al. 1991). Factors that suggest an underlying medical cause of a depression are an atypical clinical picture, resistance to standard treatment modalities, unexplained personality changes, subtle cognitive findings on mental status examination (Goldman 1992), and a negative mental health or substance use treatment history (Rundell and Hall 1997).

An issue that almost always arises in the diagnosis of medically induced depression is causality. How is a medical condition determined to cause a depression? Hall et al. (1987) offered the following practical suggestion: a causal relation can be postulated if the clinician demonstrates the presence of a medical condition known to cause depression and if the symptoms improve as the medical condition is treated.

Adjustment Disorder With Depressed Mood

Illness and hospitalization are stressful events. Both experiences often trigger passivity and feelings of helplessness and loss. The patient initially attempts to cope with illness by mobilizing personality traits (Geringer and Stern 1986). Even so, psychological regression often occurs (see also Chapters 8 and 45). Regression calls forth less mature ego defense mechanisms, anger, excessive praise or undue criticism of the physician, and over-dependence (Corradi 1983). When these defenses fail, the patient can become depressed. This depressive reaction to illness and hospitalization frequently meets the criteria for adjustment disorder. Adjustment disorder with depressed mood is one of the most common diagnoses made by consultation-liaison psychiatrists in the general hospital setting (G.C. Smith et al. 1998; Wise and Rundell 1994). This diagnosis identifies individuals who may be good candidates for psychotherapy (see Chapter 45).

DIAGNOSIS

History of Present Illness

To properly evaluate depression in a medically ill patient, it is essential to obtain a thorough history of the present illness. The history confirms the presence of depressive symptoms and excludes other psychiatric disorders. Suicidal potential must be assessed. In addition, the clinician should identify psychosocial factors that contribute to the depression. Furthermore, the history and review of systems may provide the first clues to an underlying medical condition (Rodin and Voshart 1986). A complete list of drugs—prescribed, over-the-counter, and illicit—may help in identifying substances that exacerbate or cause depression (N.H. Cassem 1991). In medically ill patients, symptoms that indicate depressive disorders are a wish for death or suicidal thoughts, guilt, dysphoria, distractibility, and discouragement (Hinrichsen et al. 1989).

Neurovegetative symptoms of depression are often difficult to differentiate from the physical symptoms of medical conditions and the side effects from the treatment of those medical disorders (Silverstone 1996). At times, however, careful exploration of the vegetative symptoms may suggest a medical etiology, especially if the consultation-liaison psychiatrist is knowledgeable about these effects. Vegetative symptoms in the medically ill patient with depression are usually multiple and more severe than symptoms arising solely from the medical condition (Cameron 1990).

Mental Status Examination

When Winokur (1990) compared depressive syndromes that followed medical conditions with those that were preceded by other psychiatric disorders, he found that subtle cognitive changes were more common in the medically ill group. Minor changes in speech production, fluency, or word finding are often the only mental status findings indicative of DSM-III general medical or substance-related organic mood disorder (Dietch and Zetin 1983).

Past History

Past history is an important consideration in the differential diagnosis of the patient's current condition. Most patients with primary depression have a history of mood disorder (Wise and Rundell 1994). In contrast, only 20% of patients with a DSM-III-R organic mood disorder have a history of depression (Yates et al. 1991). It is obvious that if a patient has a history of a medical condition that is known to cause depression (e.g., hypothyroidism), that condition should be carefully considered as a cause of the current depression.

Family History

The family history in patients with secondary depression is often negative for mood disorders (Popkin et al. 1987). A family history of depression increases the likelihood that the patient's current difficulties are due to a primary depression (Cameron 1990).

Physical Examination

Among patients with depression, the physical examination, with emphasis on the neurological portion, is crucial for detecting medical conditions that are sometimes missed by the referring physician (Koranyi 1979).

Routine Laboratory Studies

A complete blood count, blood chemistries, thyroid function tests, and urinalysis with toxicology screen identify many toxic and medically induced depressions. In addition, some clinicians routinely obtain chest X rays, electrocardiograms, and cortisol levels. With newer, more accurate assaying techniques, measurement of thyroid-stimulating hormone (TSH) levels is usually sufficient for thyroid disorder screening (Goldman 1992). Arterial blood gas or oxygen saturation measurements are sometimes necessary to rule out respiratory causes of fatigue and weakness (Dietch and Zetin 1983). An electroencephalogram is needed when the history suggests a diagnosis of epilepsy or a hypoactive delirium misdiagnosed as depression. Toxicology screening and determination of blood levels are helpful in the diagnosis of drug abuse and medication-induced depression. Computed tomography and magnetic resonance imaging are sometimes necessary to evaluate depressed patients with CNS disorders.

Biological Markers

The utility of biological markers in clinical psychiatry is debatable. Hopes that a laboratory value or a physiologic response could be used to diagnose depression with reasonable specificity are not yet a reality. In spite of this, research on the dexamethasone suppression test (DST), the thyroid-releasing hormone stimulation test, rapid eye movement (REM) latency, and platelet imipramine binding continue. These tests and features are sometimes selectively used by the clinician to aid in diagnosis.

Clinical depression typically causes hypercortisolism. The DST measures cortisol levels. A 1-mg dose of dexamethasone is given at 11:00 P.M., and serum cortisol levels are measured at 4:00 P.M. and 11:00 P.M. the next day. This dose of dexamethasone usually suppresses cortisol levels. Nonsuppression, sometimes referred to as a positive DST, suggests an escape from the normal feedback on the hypothalamic-pituitary axis and is associated with depression. It is more often associated with endogenous than nonendogenous depression (Rush et al. 1996). Unfortunately, many medical conditions also result in nonsuppression, including alcoholism, dementia,

Parkinson's disease (PD), and even nonspecific stress (Rupprecht and Lesch 1989). The best use of the DST is in patients who already have a diagnosis of depression and exhibit DST nonsuppression; repeated DSTs can forecast clinical improvement and relapse.

The thyroid-releasing hormone (TRH) stimulation test involves administration of a test dose of TRH followed by determination of serum TSH levels at 30-minute intervals. A blunted TSH response to TRH, in the absence of thyroid abnormalities, has been associated with depression. TSH blunting is reported in 25%–75% of depressed patients; physical conditions can also cause blunting (Schildkraut et al. 1989).

^{3}HImipramine platelet binding is believed to be an indirect measure of neuronal serotonin uptake. Therefore, decreased platelet serotonin uptake may parallel a decrease in neuronal serotonin uptake and central serotonin turnover. Early studies involving depressed patients found decreased density of binding sites on platelets, but more recent studies indicate otherwise (Healy et al. 1990).

REM latency—the time between sleep onset and the first REM period—is usually accepted as a reliable marker of depression. Up to 60% of depressed patients have decreased REM latency. Unfortunately, shortened REM latency is not specific for depression and may also indicate nonspecific stress (Benson and Zarcone 1993).

SPECIFIC MEDICAL CONDITIONS AND DEPRESSION

Major depressive disorder is seen more commonly in patients with certain medical conditions (Table 17–3). Several possible relations exist between depression and medical illnesses. The depression can predate the medical condition and thus represent a contributing cause or an early manifestation of that illness. At other times, the depression may occur after the onset of the medical condition. In these cases, the depression can be a pathophysiologic result of the medical illness or a psychological reaction to the physical disorder. In some patients, depression and a medical illness coexist but are etiologically unrelated (Dietch and Zetin 1983; Rodin et al. 1991).

End-Stage Renal Disease and Dialysis

Depression is the most prevalent psychological problem in patients with end-stage renal disease treated with hemodialysis and is associated with increased mortality (Kimmel et al. 1993). Hinrichsen et al. (1989) used the

RDC (Spitzer et al. 1978) to evaluate 124 patients with end-stage renal disease and found a prevalence for current major depressive disorder of 6.5% and for minor depression of 17.7%. O'Donnell and Chung (1997) found that rates of major depressive disorder in patients with end-stage renal disease varied between 6% and 34%, depending on the diagnostic criteria used (see also "Renal Disease" section in Chapter 26). The presence of suicidal ideation, depressed mood, and discouragement helped to discriminate depressed from nondepressed dialysis patients. The importance of identifying depressed dialysis patients is indicated by a suicide rate that may be 100–400 times that in the general population (Burton et al. 1986). For the treatment of depressed patients with renal failure who are undergoing hemodialysis, fluoxetine has been shown to be efficacious and safe (Blumenfield et al. 1997).

Coronary Artery Disease

Depression in patients with coronary artery disease (CAD) is associated with poor psychosocial rehabilitation and increased mortality (see also "Heart Disease" section in Chapter 26, as well as discussion of the topic in Chapter 27). Gonzalez et al. (1996) administered structured psychiatric interviews to 99 inpatients with CAD and diagnosed major depressive episode, using DSM-IV (American Psychiatric Association 1994) criteria, in 23%. CAD patients with histories of depression were more likely to be female, to be severely depressed, to have feelings of hopelessness and failure, and to experience self-blame (Freedland et al. 1992). Forrester et al. (1992) obtained similar findings in 129 patients following myocardial infarction; 19% of these patients met DSM-III criteria for major depressive disorder. The depressed group was characterized by a history of depression, female sex, large infarcts, severe functional physical impairment, and poor social relationships. In another study, half of patients with catheterization-proven CAD and major depressive disorder either were still depressed or had relapsed 12 months later (Hance et al. 1996).

There is convincing evidence that in patients with CAD, depression not only is common but also is associated with increased morbidity and mortality (Dwight and Stoudemire 1997). Treatment of depression in these patients appears to be effective, improves the quality of life, and may increase longevity (Nemeroff et al 1998). Serotonergic antidepressants are the medications of choice because of the absence of cardiac effects, the favorable influence of these drugs on platelets and clotting, and the reduction of anger and aggression (Shapiro et al. 1997).

Cancer

The frequency of depressive disorders reported in cancer patients varies widely, depending on tumor type, patient population, and diagnostic criteria (see also Chapter 29). The diagnosis of depression in cancer patients is further complicated by the presence of physical symptoms of the cancer or its treatment that are difficult to distinguish from the vegetative symptoms of depression. In a review, McDaniel et al. (1995) documented the prevalence of depression among patients with pancreatic cancer (50%), patients with oropharyngeal cancer (22%–40%), and patients with breast cancer (13%–26%).

Massie and Holland (1990) diagnosed DSM-III-R major depressive disorder in 20% and adjustment disorder with depressed mood in 27% of 546 inpatient and outpatient psychiatric consultations provided to cancer patients. They indicated that risk factors for depressive disorders in cancer patients include a mood disorder history, alcoholism, advanced stages of cancer, poorly controlled pain, and concurrent medical illnesses or use of medications, such as chemotherapy agents, known to cause depression. Additional risk factors are social isolation, recent losses, pessimism, certain socioeconomic factors, and a history of a suicide attempt (McDaniel et al. 1997).

Chronic Pain

Pain is a frequent complaint in patients in medical settings and often occurs in patients with major depressive disorder or alcoholism (see also Chapter 43). Katon et al. (1985) diagnosed DSM-III major depressive disorder in 32.4% of 37 patients with chronic pain; 43.2% of all the chronic pain patients had a history of major depressive disorder, and 40.5% of the total were concurrently abusing alcohol. Twenty-four (64.9%) of the 37 patients with chronic pain had a previous diagnosis of either alcohol abuse or major depressive disorder or both before the onset of the chronic pain. The family history was also markedly positive among these patients with chronic pain: 59.5% had at least one first-degree relative with chronic pain, 29.5% had at least one first-degree relative with a mood disorder history, and 37.8% had at least one first-degree relative with an alcohol abuse history. In a review of the literature, Sullivan et al. (1992) concluded that cognitive-behavioral therapy and tricyclic antidepressant (TCA) therapy were effective treatments for both depression and pain in patients with chronic low back pain. Furthermore, among patients with chronic low back pain, the response rate to a combination of TCA therapy and cognitive-behavioral therapy was about the same as the response rate of depressed patients who did not have chronic pain. However, in a study involving 15 chronic pain patients with major depressive disorder, carbamazepine was found to be effective for both the depression and the pain (Kudoh et al. 1998).

CNS and Neurological Disorders

Stroke

Of the CNS disorders, depression subsequent to stroke is the most extensively studied (see also Chapter 30). Many of these data were gathered in the last two decades by Robinson and colleagues (Robinson and Price 1982; Robinson et al. 1983, 1984a, 1984b, 1985, 1987, 1990). Their work is an excellent model for depression research in the setting of medical illness. In a review of this work, Beckson and Cummings (1991, p. 6) observed that "the similarities in symptomatology, natural history, cognitive impairment, biological markers, and treatment response between post-stroke-depression and idiopathic depression imply that the neurobiology of mood changes after stroke may be highly relevant in understanding the pathophysiology of 'idiopathic' or 'functional' depressive disorders."

Robinson et al. (1983) applied modified DSM-III criteria to poststroke patients in light of the DSM-III restriction that the depression should not be due to an organic mental disorder. They also modified the DSM-III definition of dysthymia by eliminating the 2-year-duration criterion; this definition is consistent with the earlier RDC concept of minor depression (Robinson et al. 1983). The examiners used clinical judgment to decide whether symptoms satisfied criteria for depression, based on how the stroke contributed to the symptom (i.e., an etiological approach to diagnosis) (Cohen-Cole and Stoudemire 1987).

Estimates of depression prevalence among poststroke patients range from 30% to 50% (mean, 38%) (Robinson and Price 1982; Robinson et al. 1983, 1984a, 1987). At the time of initial in-hospital evaluation, 26% of the 103 patients examined met the examiner's criteria for major depressive disorder, whereas 20% had minor depression. At 6-month follow-up, 34% had symptoms of major depressive disorder and 26% had symptoms of minor depression; thus, 60% of the sample received a diagnosis of a depressive syndrome.

Over the years, the Robinson group reported differences in clinical features of poststroke depression based on neuroanatomical location of the stroke and the time of onset of the depressive syndrome. Early in the 1980s, they reported a higher frequency and severity of depression among patients with left- versus right-hemisphere lesions. They also reported that major depressive disorder was most frequent in patients with left anterior lesions (Robinson and Price 1982; Robinson et al. 1983, 1984a). However, the mechanism and neuroanatomical correlates of poststroke depression have proven more complicated than originally thought; other researchers have failed to replicate results or have even reported reverse findings (Gordon and Hibbard 1997). These conflicting results led Robinson (1997) to write that although studies show a relationship between lesion location and size and poststroke depression, more work is still needed to determine both the mechanism and anatomical substrates.

As with depression seen in other medical illnesses, clinicians frequently assume that poststroke depression is a "natural" reaction to physical impairment; for example, "He should be depressed; he can't talk and walk as well anymore." This logic is often used to justify withholding treatment. The work of the Robinson group implicates multiple etiologies for poststroke depression, with evidence heavily weighted toward an intrinsic biological contribution to depressive syndromes (M.F. Folstein et al. 1977; Robinson et al. 1985). Specifically, when a stroke injures catecholamine pathways and temporarily causes the brain's catecholamine system to reduce transmitter release drastically, depression is likely (Robinson et al. 1983, 1985).

Numerous studies, albeit limited ones, have shown that psychiatric treatment of patients with poststroke depression is beneficial. Three of these studies were double-blind, prospective trials. First, Lipsey et al. (1984) showed that nortriptyline was more effective than placebo. Second, Reding et al. (1986) showed that trazodone was more effective than placebo. Finally, G. Andersen et al. (1994) demonstrated the efficacy of citalopram compared with placebo in 66 poststroke patients. Studies also support the use of psychostimulants in poststroke depression; for example, Lingam et al. (1988) found that poststroke depression improved in patients who were given methylphenidate compared with patients who received placebo. Smaller, randomized or retrospective studies also suggest that psychostimulants are useful in this population (Johnson et al. 1992; Lazarus et al. 1992, 1994). Murray et al. (1986) conducted a retrospective chart review that demonstrated the efficacy of electroconvulsive therapy (ECT). Studies that demonstrate how psychiatric interventions alter the rehabilitation, course, and prognosis of patients after stroke remain to be done.

Studies of the course and prognosis of poststroke depression have revealed that 1) poststroke patients are at high risk for depression for 2 years after the stroke;

2) major depressive disorder, left untreated, has a natural course of about 1 year; and 3) minor depression, left untreated, has a chronic course of about 2 years (Lipsey et al. 1984; Robinson et al. 1984b, 1987). In a 10-year follow-up of stroke patients, Morris et al. (1993a) found that depression during acute phase poststroke recovery was associated with a more than threefold greater mortality during this 10-year period. This study highlighted the importance of psychiatric treatment to reduce morbidity and mortality after a stroke and the need for research into the relative efficacy of various interventions, including psychotherapy.

Dementia

Wragg and Jeste (1989) reviewed 30 studies of Alzheimer's disease and found that the frequency of depressed mood ranged from 0% to 87%, with a median of 41%. Later that same year, Greenwald et al. (1989) reviewed the literature and found that the estimated prevalence of depression as a complication of dementia ranged from 0% to 85%. As with other medical disorders, definitions are problematic, and estimates of prevalence vary widely as a consequence of problems with study design and diagnostic criteria for depression and dementia. For example, the prevalence of depression varies between dementia of the Alzheimer's type (DAT) and multi-infarct dementia (MID). In a study involving 30 patients with DAT and 15 patients with MID, Cummings et al. (1987) found that 0% of patients with DAT had major depressive disorder and 17% had depression symptoms, whereas 26% of patients with MID had major depressive disorder and 60% had depression symptoms. N. H. Cassem (1991, p. 244) pointed out that "MID so commonly includes depression as a symptom that Hachinski et al. (1975) included it as part of their ischemia scale."

The task of separating clinical features of dementia from features of depression is difficult; however, it is as important as distinguishing among subtypes of dementia. The task is complicated because depression can masquerade as dementia. Specifically, depression (i.e., pseudodementia or dementia of depression) is likely a reversible cognitive mental disorder (McAllister 1983). Alexopoulos et al. (1993) conducted a controlled study of geriatric depression and "reversible dementia." Their results suggest that depression with reversible cognitive impairment may be a prodrome of dementia rather than a distinct disorder. According to the authors, nearly 50% of elderly patients with reversible dementia and depression will develop irreversible dementia within 5 years. Hirono et al. (1998) prospectively examined 53 Alzheimer's disease patients for depression and found significant glucose

hypometabolism in the bilateral superior gyri and left anterior cingulate gyrus of the 19 depressed patients. This finding is consistent with the finding of frontal hypometabolism in depression associated with other neurological illnesses and may prove supportive of the findings of the Alexopoulos group (Alexopoulos et al. 1993).

Whether or not the depression syndrome associated with dementia is a distinct disorder, the biochemical underpinnings of depression in patients with DAT are similar to those of primary depression. Zubenko et al. (1990) compared depressed patients who had dementia with nondepressed patients who had dementia and reported a 10- to 20-fold reduction in the level of norepinephrine in the cortices of the depressed patients, as well as relative preservation of choline O-acetyltransferase activity in subcortical regions. According to Cummings et al. (1987), the marked decrease in cholinergic function found in DAT may have clinical and biological implications; the cholinergic deficit in patients with DAT may offer some protection from severe depression and may help to explain the relative increase in the occurrence of depression syndromes in patients with MID.

The same problems that complicate the diagnosis of depression and dementia hamper treatment studies. Nevertheless, Katz (1998) determined in a recent review that three of five placebo-controlled studies found significant drug-placebo differences. The author concluded that this finding supports the treatment of depression in patients with DAT and related disorders. Greenwald et al. (1989) concluded that although initial treatment failures and intolerance of side effects are common, syndromal depressions that complicate dementia are treatable. These investigators compared 10 patients with depression and dementia, 10 nondepressed patients with dementia, and 33 age-matched, depressed control subjects without dementia. All depressed patients were treated with conventional somatic antidepressant therapy (i.e., antidepressant medications or ECT). Seventy percent of the patients with depression and dementia responded to antidepressant treatment, and 73% of the depressed control group without dementia responded. Perhaps most compelling to date is the American Psychiatric Association's (1997) conclusion that antidepressant medication should be used to treat patients with severe or persistent depressed mood with or without the full complement of neurovegetative symptoms.

Parkinson's Disease

In the 1950s, Oleh Hornykiewicz reported the depletion of three biogenic amines (dopamine, norepinephrine, and serotonin) in the postmortem brains of patients with PD

(L. Cote and Crutcher 1991). This discovery, arguably, launched modern neurotransmitter hypotheses of depression and other brain disorders and may yet prove central to the understanding of the etiology of both PD and depression. In addition to the neurotransmitter hypotheses, depression is important to a discussion of PD because depression is probably the most commonly encountered mental change in patients with PD (Mayeux 1990).

Estimates of the prevalence of depression among patients with PD range from 25% to 70% (Cummings 1992); Cummings found that the average prevalence across nine studies was approximately 40%. Two 1990 studies also found that about half of the patients with depression met criteria for major depressive disorder and the other half met criteria for "minor depression" (Mayeux 1990; Starkstein et al. 1990).

Patients with PD who are at increased risk for depressive illness have a history of depression (Mayeux et al. 1981; Starkstein et al. 1990) and greater functional disability (Cummings 1992). The clinical features common to depressed patients with PD include shortened REM latency (Kostic et al. 1991), increased anxiety, sadness, loss of appetite, weight change, fatigue, sleep disturbance, and loss of self-esteem. However, self-punitive ideation does not appear to be common relative to other depressive disorders (Barbosa et al. 1997; Cummings 1992). Depression seems to be more common among patients with dopamine-responsive signs (i.e., gait changes, akinesia, and rigidity) (Cummings 1992). However, depression does not always correlate with the severity of motor symptoms, because depression may occur before the first motor symptoms appear (Barbosa et al. 1997).

Some clinicians attribute depression in patients with PD to an "understandable" reaction to the progressive physical impairment (Mindham 1970); others suggest an intrinsic or neurochemical etiology (Mayeux et al. 1984, 1986; Starkstein et al. 1990). Mayeux et al. (1986) examined 49 consecutive patients with PD and reported a significant inverse correlation between cerebrospinal fluid 5-hydroxyindoleacetic acid (5-HIAA) levels and depression. In their study, 5-HIAA levels were 50% lower in patients with PD than in patients without PD, and 5-HIAA levels were 20% lower in PD patients with depression than in PD patients without depression. In a similar investigation of the etiology of PD depression, Starkstein et al. (1990) studied 105 patients with PD. They reported a bimodal distribution of depression in this sample. One group manifested depression early in the course of PD, and the other group developed depression late in the course. The group with early depression had significantly more left-hemisphere pathology (i.e.,

right-sided symptoms) and received higher doses of L-dopa; the late-course depression group was more strongly associated with impairment in activities of daily living.

In addition to changes in concentrations of biogenic amines, Mayberg et al. (1990) demonstrated that metabolic activity in the caudate and orbito-inferior region of the frontal lobe was significantly lower in depressed PD patients relative to nondepressed PD patients and control subjects. Furthermore, the researchers noted that the metabolic pattern of depressed PD patients was distinct from that of PD patients with dementia. These findings implicate an important role for basal ganglia circuits of the inferior frontal lobe in the regulation of mood.

Four studies demonstrated the efficacy of psychopharmacological interventions in depressed patients with PD (Cummings 1992). Imipramine (Strang 1965) and desipramine (Laitinen 1969) decreased both depression and motor symptoms to below baseline levels. Bupropion reportedly reduced depression in less than one-half and motor symptoms in less than one-third of depressed patients with PD (Goetz et al. 1984). In a study of nortriptyline, features of depression decreased but PD symptoms remained unchanged (J. Andersen et al. 1980). According to the review by Cummings (1992), ECT relieved both mood and motor symptoms of PD in patients with depressive syndromes. However, reduction in motor symptoms is usually short-lived (Burke et al. 1988; Cummings 1992; Douyon et al. 1989; Faber and Trimble 1991).

Few studies have focused on the course and prognosis of depression in PD, but patients with PD may be divided into groups with and without depression (Cummings 1992). In one study involving 132 patients with PD who underwent a preliminary assessment and then a follow-up evaluation at approximately 14 months, the overall ratio of patients with depression (27%) to patients without depression (61%) remained constant (Brown et al. 1988). The individuals with depression varied; a core of 16% (21 patients) were depressed on both occasions. However, depression remitted in 11% (15) of the original patients, whereas an equal number had developed depression by the time of the follow-up evaluation.

Huntington's Disease

HD, a genetically transmitted autosomal dominant disorder (with 100% penetrance), was first described by George Huntington in 1872 (Whitehouse et al. 1992). HD is a rare disorder; consequently, estimates of the disorder's prevalence vary, and estimates of the occurrence of depression are even less precise. However, according to Cummings' (1995) review of the literature, the frequency of major depressive disorder in HD is approximately 30%. Thus, depression is the second most common psychiatric manifestation of HD (next to alterations of personality) and the most common mood disorder in the disease. The works cited by Cummings include a report on a series of 88 patients with HD, in which S.E. Folstein et al. (1983) noted a prevalence of 41% for "major affective disorder." Caine and Shoulson (1983) reported that 24 of 30 patients had substantial behavioral abnormalities and 11 of 30 met DSM-III criteria for dysthymic syndrome or major depressive syndrome. A retrospective study of suicide deaths among patients with HD revealed a suicide rate 2–23 times greater than that for age-matched groups without HD (Schoenfeld et al. 1984).

Along with the high frequency of depression in HD, Mayberg et al. (1992) demonstrated orbitofrontal–inferior prefrontal cortex hypometabolism of glucose that differentiated depressed HD patients from nondepressed HD patients and age-matched control subjects. The authors concluded that the metabolic pattern was similar to that in depression in PD and suggested that the pathways between paralimbic frontal cortex basal ganglia may be key to normal regulation of mood.

The duration of HD varies from 17 to 30 years (Martin and Gusella 1986), and to date there is no known treatment (S.E. Folstein 1989; Martin and Gusella 1986; Whitehouse et al. 1992). However, depressive syndromes associated with HD have been treated with some success. Caine and Shoulson (1983) reported that antidepressants were beneficial in terms of treating the somatic signs of depression but that the drugs did not alter the patient's dysphoric outlook. S.E. Folstein (1989) and S.E. Folstein et al. (1983) reported that TCAs and ECT were effective but called for formal trials of somatic therapies. Ford (1986) reported that treatment with monoamine oxidase inhibitors (MAOIs) was effective in three patients with HD and affective syndromes. Given the high rate of suicide among such patients, vigilance for depression is clearly indicated.

Epilepsy

Epilepsy is common and affects approximately 1% of the population (Cummings 1985). Among patients with epilepsy, depression is the most common and important psychiatric disorder (Blumer 1991; Mendez et al. 1986). Even though the literature contains descriptions of ictal and interictal behavioral changes, we have limited this discussion to interictal depressive syndromes.

Although the actual prevalence is unknown, Currie et al. (1971), who conducted a retrospective survey, reported depression in 11% of 666 patients with tempo-ral lobe epilepsy (TLE). In a study of suicide among patients with epilepsy, Matthews and Barabas (1981) noted a suicide rate of 5%, compared with 1.4% in the general population. Mendez et al. (1986) compared 175 outpatients who had epilepsy with control subjects without epilepsy and found that the patients who had epilepsy were hospitalized for depression four times more often than were patients who did not have epilepsy. These authors also compared clinical features between depressed patients with epilepsy and depressed control subjects without epilepsy (Table 17–8).

Some investigators reported an increased incidence of depression among patients with left-sided seizure foci versus patients with right-sided foci (Mendez et al. 1986; Robertson and Trimble 1983). Schmitz et al. (1997) reported a relation between depression scores and bilateral frontal hypoperfusion in a group of patients with left-sided seizure focus. The issue of left brain lesions and higher risks of depressive syndromes remains controversial but intriguing.

The course, prognosis, and treatment of epileptic depression are less well studied than those of other CNS disorders such as stroke. However, Blumer (1997, p. 3) concluded from his literature review and trials of mixed TCA and selective serotonin reuptake inhibitor (SSRI) treatment of depressed patients with epilepsy that "antidepressants are the psychotropic drugs of choice for the affective disorder of epilepsy and can be effective in combined forms (TCA and SSRI) for otherwise intractable patients."

Multiple Sclerosis

The prevalence rate of multiple sclerosis (MS) in the general population varies from 1 to 80 per 100,000, depending on the latitude (Adams and Victor 1993). The likelihood of developing clinical major depressive disorder after a diagnosis of MS is 27%–54% (Joffe et al. 1987; Minden and Schiffer 1990; Minden et al. 1987; Schiffer et al. 1983; Whitlock and Siskind 1980). In 1987, Minden et al. conducted a study involving 50 outpatients with MS and found that 54% of patients had had at least one major depressive episode since the onset of their illness. On the basis of data obtained using a structured clinical interview, Minden and colleagues (1987) characterized these depressions as typically moderate to severe and marked by anger, irritability, emotionality, worry, and discouragement (as opposed to self-criticism, withdrawal, and loss of interest). They also found that the most robust predictors of MS-related depressive episodes were a history of major depressive disorder and an acute exacerbation of MS treated with adrenocorticotropic hormone (ACTH) or prednisone.

TABLE 17–8. Clinical features of depressed patients with epilepsy versus depressed control subjects without epilepsy

Depressed patients with epilepsy

Had "endogenous" neurovegetative symptoms

Had significantly fewer "neurotic" symptoms (e.g., somatization, anxiety, brooding, self-pity)

Demonstrated atypical features (e.g., chronic dysthymia, irritability, emotionality)

Attempted suicide more often

The etiology of depression in patients with MS is unknown. However, several studies have added to the growing body of evidence that the brain injury associated with MS directly contributes to the prevalence of depression. For example, a meta-analysis conducted by Schubert and Foliart (1993) supported the conclusion that MS patient groups have higher rates of depression even when compared with other groups of chronically ill patients. Minden et al. (1987), whose report was among those studied in the meta-analysis, observed that the severity of depressive symptoms in MS was not associated with disability, type of disability, duration of illness, type of MS, clinical status, fatigability, sex, age, or socioeconomic status. Schiffer and Babigian (1984) performed a retrospective comparison of depression in MS, TLE, and amyotrophic lateral sclerosis (ALS) and reported that "the significantly increased rate of depression diagnoses among patients with MS can't be easily dismissed as reactive depression…when compared with much lower rates of depressive features in diseases with comparable disability such as TLE and ALS" (p. 1069). Similarly, higher rates of depression were reported among patients with CNS lesions when patients with "cerebral" MS were compared with patients with "noncerebral" MS and non-CNS disorders (Schiffer et al. 1983; Whitlock and Siskind 1980). In addition to increased rates of depression, Stenager et al. (1992) reported an increased risk of suicide, especially among young men in the first 5 years after the diagnosis of MS.

As with many CNS disorders, studies of treatment of MS and depression are limited. However, Schiffer and Wineman (1990) conducted a double-blind trial of desipramine in patients with MS and major depressive disorder. A significantly greater proportion of treated patients had improvement of depressive symptoms compared with untreated control subjects, independent of degree of disability. In summary, research suggests that

- Patients with MS have more depressive disturbances than does the general population (Minden et al. 1987).

- Patients with MS have more depressive syndromes than do patients with similarly disabling non-CNS lesions (Rabins et al. 1986).

- Patients with MS who have predominantly cerebral disease have increased rates of depression compared with patients with MS who have predominantly spinal disease (Schiffer et al. 1983).

HIV Disease

The challenge for the consultation-liaison psychiatrist is to differentiate depressive syndromes from other human immunodeficiency virus (HIV) syndromes, such as HIV encephalopathy (Cummings and Benson 1992), HIV-associated dementia, constitutional features of HIV-related infections (Price et al. 1988), and antiviral medication side effects (Searight and McLaren 1997) (see also Chapter 36).

According to Atkinson and Grant (1994), rates of current major depressive disorder in HIV-positive patients are comparable to those among individuals with other chronic medical illnesses (Atkinson et al. 1988; Perry et al. 1990; Williams et al. 1991). Perry and Tross (1984) conducted a retrospective review and noted that 17.3% of patients with acquired immunodeficiency syndrome (AIDS) met DSM-III criteria for major depressive disorder (Holmes et al. 1989). Dilley et al. (1985) reported that 7 of 13 AIDS patients who underwent consultation had adjustment disorder, 2 of 13 had major depressive disorder, and 1 of 13 had dysthymia.

Suicide rates are also higher among HIV-seropositive individuals than in the general population. During the early years of the AIDS epidemic, Marzuk and associates (1988) reported that men ages 20–59 years with a diagnosis of AIDS were approximately 36 times more likely to commit suicide than were age-matched men in the general population. In subsequent years, presumably because of improved care and reduced stigma, the suicide rate apparently decreased. T.R. Cote et al. (1992) surveyed death certificates and reported that the suicide rate was only 7.4 times higher among persons with AIDS than among demographically similar men in the general population.

As with other medical illnesses, it is difficult to differentiate depressive symptoms from other medical and psychiatric conditions in HIV-positive patients. According to Navia et al. (1986), the dementia syndrome characteristic of HIV infection is readily stereotyped and is dominated by features of subcortical dysfunction, such as

- Forgetfulness
- Poor concentration
- Loss of trains of thought

- Slowed thinking
- Social withdrawal

The consultation-liaison psychiatrist must decide whether to exclude these features or to consider them vegetative symptoms of depression.

AIDS patients with depressive syndromes have responded favorably to interpersonal therapy, TCAs, SSRIs, stimulants, and ECT (Fernandez et al. 1988; Markowitz et al. 1998; Rabkin and Harrison 1990; Rabkin et al. 1994a, 1994b; Schaerf et al. 1989). In general, as with many other medically ill patients, AIDS patients are especially sensitive to anticholinergic side effects, sedation, orthostatic hypotension, extrapyramidal side effects of neuroleptics, and decreased clearance of prescription medications.

Endocrine Disorders

Hyperthyroidism

Major depressive episodes are seen in as many as 31% of patients with hyperthyroidism (Kathol et al. 1986). Depressed patients with hyperthyroidism tend to be older, appear more ill, and lose more weight than nondepressed patients with hyperthyroidism. The severity of the hyperthyroidism correlates more closely with the number and severity of the anxiety symptoms than with the depressive symptoms (Kathol and Delahunt 1986). Depressed, thyrotoxic patients should be treated with care because antidepressant medications may exacerbate the symptomatology of hyperthyroidism (Folks 1984). Fortunately, major depressive disorder in these patients almost always responds favorably to antithyroid therapy alone (Kathol et al. 1986).

Hypothyroidism

Hypothyroidism is usually the result of ablation of the thyroid gland, autoimmune thyroiditis, or lithium therapy. Hypothyroidism may occur in as many as 10% of patients taking lithium and is much more likely to occur in women (Goldman 1992). The association between clinical hypothyroidism and depression is well known. Haggerty and colleagues (1993) found that 56% of patients with subclinical hypothyroidism had a lifetime history of major depressive disorder, compared with only 20% of control subjects. Subclinical hypothyroidism is an increased response of thyrotropin (TSH) to thyroid-releasing hormone (TRH) in the absence of clinical evidence of hypothyroidism. In addition to depression, subclinical hypothyroidism can also cause cognitive dysfunction and rapid cycling in patients with bipolar disor-

der (Haggerty et al. 1990). A corollary to the hypothesis that decreased levels of thyroid functioning cause depression is the concept that supplemental thyroid hormone favors recovery from depression. This is the rationale for augmentation of TCA therapy with thyroid hormone replacement in the treatment of drug-resistant depression (Joffe 1990).

In many patients with hypothyroidism, depression responds to thyroid hormone replacement alone, but the response may take a prolonged time. When that is the case, antidepressant therapy is indicated and efficacious (Goldman 1992; Joffe 1990).

Although the prevalence of depressive disorders is high among patients with thyroid disease, thyroid abnormalities are a rare finding in depressed inpatients and outpatients. Among 277 consecutive inpatients who met criteria for DSM-III-R major depressive disorder, there were two patients (0.4%) with laboratory findings consistent with hyperthyroidism and none with hypothyroidism (Ordas and Labbate 1995). Similarly, no cases of hyperthyroidism or hypothyroidism were detected in a group of 200 outpatients who met DSM-III-R criteria for major depressive disorder (M. Fava et al. 1995).

Hyperparathyroidism

In addition to "stones, bones, and abdominal groans" (St. Goar 1957, pp.112–113), depression occurs in about 30% of patients with primary hyperparathyroidism and is the most common neuropsychiatric clinical feature (Palmer 1983). The severity of the cognitive and depressive symptoms parallels increases in the serum calcium concentration. Because lithium can induce an increase in parathyroid hormone levels, some authors advocate that patients taking lithium be monitored for hypercalcemia (Goldman 1992). Depression in patients with hyperparathyroidism usually abates quickly after correction of the calcium level. Occasionally, an antidepressant is necessary (G. A. Fava et al. 1987).

The prevalence of major depressive disorder in hyperparathyroidism is high, as it is in thyroid disease, but the prevalence of increased calcium levels among patients with major depressive disorder is low (Widmer et al. 1997).

Diabetes Mellitus

The prevalence of major depressive disorder among patients with diabetes mellitus is about 8.5%–27.3% (Goodnick 1997). The level of depression correlates with the severity of the complications of the diabetes (Leedom et al. 1991) and the length of the illness (Palinkas et al. 1991). There is a weakly positive relation between level of depression and blood glucose levels. This effect could be explained by neuroendocrine changes or poor compliance with drug therapy, blood sugar monitoring, and exercise regimens (Eaton et al. 1992). Even though all antidepressants are efficacious in the treatment of major depressive disorder in diabetic patients, the clinician should be careful in prescribing these medications, because noradrenergic antidepressants increase glucose levels and serotonergic antidepressants decrease glucose levels (Goodnick 1997). A combination of cognitive-behavioral therapy and diabetes education is also effective (Lustman et al. 1998).

Cushing's Syndrome

Cushing's syndrome refers to hypercortisolism from any cause. *Cushing's disease* is the term used specifically for hypercortisolism due to ACTH-secreting tumors of the pituitary gland. Other causes of Cushing's syndrome are paraneoplastic, nonpituitary tumors that produce ACTH; adrenal adenomas; and corticosteroid therapy. Exogenous steroids, especially prednisone at dosages greater than 40 mg/day, are more commonly linked to manic syndromes, but Cushing's disease is highly associated with depression (Goldman 1992). Sonino and colleagues (1998) reported that 88 (54%) of 162 patients with Cushing's disease had major depressive disorder according to DSM-IV criteria. Patients with Cushing's syndrome and depression were more irritable and emotionally labile compared with patients who had primary mood disorders. Patients with Cushing's syndrome were less likely to have histories and family histories of mood disorders (Haskett 1985). Kelly and associates (1983) pointed out that depressive symptoms were greatly reduced 12 months after successful treatment of Cushing's syndrome.

Chronic Fatigue Syndrome

Fatigue is common in patients in primary care settings. Cathebras et al. (1992) studied 686 patients who visited a family practice clinic and noted that 13.6% complained of fatigue. In almost half of these fatigued patients, anxiety or depression had been diagnosed sometime during their lives. At the time of the complaint of fatigue, 17.2% fulfilled DSM-III criteria for major depressive disorder.

Chronic fatigue syndrome is a condition in which fatigability, fever, sore throat, tender lymph nodes, headaches, allergies, and unusual titers of the Epstein-Barr virus antibody are usually evident. Kreusi et al. (1989) reviewed the case histories of 28 patients who met the Centers for Disease Control criteria for chronic fatigue syndrome (i.e., who had had disabling fatigue and the aforementioned constitutional complaints for at least

6 months, in the absence of other immunological dysfunction or medical problems). The lifetime prevalence of major depressive disorder was 46.4% among these 28 patients with chronic fatigue. The physical symptoms of chronic fatigue preceded the psychiatric disorder in only 2 of 21 patients. Thus, the authors concluded that the psychiatric problems were more likely a cause of chronic fatigue syndrome, not only a psychological reaction to it. Determining whether cortisol levels are increased can help the clinician identify major depressive disorder in patients complaining of fatigue (Jorge and Goodnick 1997).

MEDICATIONS AND SUBSTANCES ASSOCIATED WITH DEPRESSION

Consultation-liaison psychiatrists must be cautious in implicating medications in the development of clinical depression. Although more than 100 medications are associated with depression, only a few have been clearly shown to cause depressive syndromes (Zelnik 1987) (Table 17–7). Many studies, especially the older ones, have serious methodological flaws. To substantiate depression as a true side effect of a medication or substance, the following guidelines are suggested for research studies:

- A positive correlation should exist between the degree of depression and changes in the dosage of the medication.
- An appropriate temporal relation is necessary between exposure to the medication and onset of the depression (Maricle et al. 1988).
- Rechallenge or reintroduction of the medication should again precipitate depression (Zelnik 1987).
- Formal psychiatric evaluations, rating scales, recognized diagnostic criteria, and adequate control groups are necessary.
- The clinician must consider other possible causes of the depression, such as the illness itself or a psychological reaction to the illness (Paykel et al. 1982).

Few studies meet standards necessary to establish cause-and-effect relations.

Antihypertensive Medications

Reserpine

Depressive syndromes occur in 20% of patients taking reserpine; an additional 7% have a psychotic depression (Goodwin et al. 1972). Patients with psychotic depression have severely depressed mood, psychomotor changes, and worsening of depressed mood in the morning (Hall et al. 1980). In reserpine-induced depression—unlike in primary depression—anxiety, lack of guilt, and lack of self-deprecation are typical (Beers and Passman 1990). The depression is dose related and is more prevalent at doses greater than 0.5 mg/day (Ganzini et al. 1993). The latency period between exposure to reserpine and onset of the depression is generally 4–6 months (Zelnik 1987). This period may be the length of time required for depletion of serotonin, norepinephrine, and dopamine from CNS presynaptic storage vesicles (Hall et al. 1980). A previous episode of depression is the most reliable predictor of reserpine-induced depression; more than 50% of patients who experience this adverse effect have had a previous depressive episode (Pascualy and Veith 1989). Hence, a hypertensive patient who is depressed, has had a previous depressive episode, or has a family history of depression should not receive reserpine. Rather, calcium-channel blockers or angiotensin converting enzyme (ACE) inhibitors are the drugs of choice (Rauch et al. 1991).

Methyldopa

Ten percent of patients taking methyldopa become mildly to moderately depressed, and 7% develop severe depression (Hall et al. 1980). In an extensive review of the literature, Paykel and colleagues (1982) identified 83 depressed patients among 2,320 taking methyldopa, a prevalence of only 3.6%. The onset of the depressive symptoms was fairly rapid; they occurred within a few days of starting treatment with the drug. The patients frequently manifested agitation, apprehension, weeping, and suicidal ideation; a history of depression was common. Once methyldopa therapy was stopped, the depressive symptoms resolved within a week in most patients. DeMuth and Ackerman (1983) found that methyldopa-induced depressive symptoms rarely met DSM-III criteria for major depressive disorder. Two mechanisms for depression are proposed: 1) depletion of serotonin and dopamine through inhibition of the enzyme dopamine decarboxylase (Beers and Passman 1990) and 2) formation of the false neurotransmitter methylnorepinephrine (Rauch et al. 1991). Like reserpine, methyldopa should not be prescribed for hypertensive patients who are depressed or have a history of depression (Beers and Passman 1990).

Propranolol and Other β-Blockers

Whether propranolol and the other β-blockers cause depression is controversial. Hall et al. (1980) indicated that some degree of depression occurred in 30%–50% of patients taking significant amounts of propranolol. Petrie and associates (1982) evaluated 34 patients taking propranolol in a medical clinic setting and determined that only 3 patients met DSM-III criteria for major depressive disorder. These investigators established that propranolol can cause nonspecific fatigue and lassitude and cautioned against diagnosing depression on the basis of these nonspecific symptoms. They also concluded that there was a dose-response relation between the severity of the depression and the dose of the β-blocker. In a literature review, Paykel et al. (1982) found 19 cases of depression among 1,773 patients taking propranolol. Schleifer et al. (1991) interviewed 190 patients 3–4 months after myocardial infarction; digitalis, and not β-blockers, predicted depression in this group. Recent studies have failed to demonstrate an association between β-blockers and depression (Gerstman et al. 1996; Reid et al. 1998).

Before the low prevalence of depression among individuals taking β-blockers was established through epidemiologic surveys (Prisant et al. 1991), case reports of patients taking β-blockers who met DSM-III criteria for major depressive disorder appeared in the literature (Petrie et al. 1982; Pollack et al. 1985). Zelnik (1987) reviewed these case reports and concluded that patients taking β-blockers who became depressed often had histories or family histories of depression. Furthermore, he noted that the latency period between initiation of therapy and onset of depressive symptoms was a few days to several months. The depressive symptoms typically cleared within a week after treatment with the medication was stopped.

Other Antihypertensives

Less than 2% of patients taking clonidine or guanethidine become depressed (Paykel et al. 1982). Calcium-channel blockers and ACE inhibitors are rarely associated with depression (Hallas 1996). On the contrary, ACE inhibitors may elevate mood, and caution is recommended with regard to use in patients with bipolar disorder (Rauch et al. 1991). Diuretics can cause weakness and apathy because of electrolyte changes. These symptoms are sometimes confused with depression (Beers and Passman 1990).

Contraceptives

Shortly after the introduction of oral contraceptives into clinical practice, depressive symptoms were reported as a frequent side effect; they occurred in 7%–34% of users (Herzberg and Coppen 1970). Depressive symptoms were associated with the high amounts of estrogen compared with the amounts of progesterone (Hall et al. 1980). Modern low-dose estrogen preparations usually do not cause mood changes that satisfy DSM-III-R criteria for major depressive disorder (Patten and Lamarre 1992).

Norplant is a long-acting subdermal implant system that is widely used for contraception. In a case report, Wagner (1996) described five women who developed major depressive disorder and a variety of anxiety disorders while using this system. The women had not previously had depression. The depressions resolved within 1–2 months after the implants were removed.

Steroids

Corticosteroid reactions are diverse; of patients with steroid-related psychiatric syndromes, 40% have depression, 28% have hypomania, 8% have mixed manic and depressive features, 14% have psychosis, and 10% have delirium (Lewis and Smith 1983). The overall prevalence of steroid side effects is 6% (Kershner and Wang-Cheng 1989). Risk factors for steroid reactions are female sex, high doses of steroids, systemic lupus erythematosus (Lewis and Smith 1983), and possibly premorbid personality disorder (Kershner and Wang-Cheng 1989). The most discriminating factor is dosage. Less than 2% of patients who receive less than 40 mg of prednisone per day develop psychiatric symptoms, compared with 4%–6% who receive 41–80 mg/day and 18.4% who receive more than 80 mg/day (Boston Collaborative Drug Surveillance Program 1972). Steroid reactions begin within the first week of treatment but may require 4–6 weeks to resolve after cessation of drug therapy (Hall et al. 1979). Administration of neuroleptic medication at low doses is the treatment of choice for the acute episode; lithium prophylaxis can be useful in patients requiring high doses of steroids (Kershner and Wang-Cheng 1989).

Benzodiazepines

Although all benzodiazepines have been implicated in depression, Hall and Joffe (1972) described a specific depressive syndrome in patients receiving more than 40 mg of diazepam per day. They identified marked apprehension, impaired concentration, feelings of worthlessness, and suicidal ideation. B.D. Smith and Salzman (1991) reviewed the relation between benzodiazepines and depression and concluded that 1) benzodiazepines are occasionally associated with depression and even suicide, 2) no one benzodiazepine is more likely to cause depression than any other, 3) higher doses of the medication are associated with greater risk of depression, and

4) decreasing the dose or stopping treatment with the benzodiazepine eliminates the depression in most cases. In contrast, Tiller and Schweitzer (1992) proposed that the benzodiazepines do not induce depression but rather unmask the depressive symptomatology in agitated patients with depression.

Cimetidine and Ranitidine

Although delirium is the most common psychiatric side effect of the histamine$_2$ receptor antagonists, case reports of depression have also been published (Pascualy and Veith 1989). Cimetidine-induced depression begins within 3 days to several weeks after administration of medication. The depression clears 1–14 days after treatment with the medication is stopped (Zelnik 1987). Stocky (1991) reported three cases and reviewed the literature and found that depressive symptoms occurred in 1%–5% of patients receiving ranitidine, the onset of depressive symptoms occurred in 4–8 weeks, and reduction in symptoms occurred 7–14 days after discontinuation of therapy.

Cancer Chemotherapy Medications

Depression is reportedly seen with a variety of chemotherapy medications: vincristine, vinblastine, procarbazine, L-asparaginase, amphotericin B, and interferon (see also Chapter 29). In addition, corticosteroids are commonly coprescribed (Massie and Holland 1990). Besides major depressive disorder, interferon can cause memory impairment, cognitive slowing, and disturbed executive functions (Valentine et al. 1998).

Psychoactive Substances

Depression is common among people who abuse drugs (Dackis and Gold 1992; see also Chapter 21). In particular, alcohol (K.M. Davidson and Ritson 1993), opiates (Rounsaville et al. 1982), amphetamine withdrawal (Kramer et al. 1967), cocaine withdrawal (Gawin and Kleber 1986), and anabolic steroids (Pope and Katz 1994) can cause a substance-induced mood disorder with depressive features (American Psychiatric Association 1994; see Table 17–7). In people who abuse drugs, major depressive disorder increases the risk of suicide, causes more marital discord, and reduces the likelihood of abstinence (Mueller et al. 1993).

Alcohol

Ingestion of alcohol in small amounts enhances mood; however, at higher amounts, alcohol causes dysphoric mood states (K.M. Davidson and Ritson 1993). According to various rating scales, more than half of alcoholic patients have symptoms of depression (Schuckit 1983b). Some alcoholic patients develop an alcohol-induced depression that is indistinguishable from DSM-III major depressive disorder (Dackis et al. 1986; Schuckit 1983b). Schuckit et al. (1997) studied 2,945 alcohol-dependent individuals and found that 26.4% reported at least one substance-induced major depressive episode by DSM-III-R criteria. When the researchers compared patients with primary alcoholism who had secondary depression and patients with primary alcoholism who did not have depression, they found that the depressed group had slightly more alcohol-related problems and that the occurrence of alcoholism in first-degree male relatives was slightly greater in the depressed group than in the nondepressed group. The depressed group more often used drugs in addition to alcohol (Schuckit 1983a). Furthermore, alcoholic individuals with major depressive disorder are more likely to act on suicidal ideation (Cornelius et al. 1996).

Most alcohol-induced depressions resolve between 2 days and 2 weeks after abstinence has begun (Schuckit 1983b). The focus of treatment is on sobriety (Dackis and Gold 1992). Antidepressants are usually not necessary unless the patient has a history of major depressive disorder occurring during a period of abstinence (Dackis and Gold 1992; K.M. Davidson and Ritson 1993).

Opiates

Opiate addicts have high rates of depression. In a study involving 716 opioid abusers, 15.8% met DSM-III-R criteria for major depressive disorder and 25.1% had antisocial personalities (Brooner et al. 1997). The depression is possibly due to alterations in endorphin, noradrenergic, and cortisol systems in the brain (Dackis and Gold 1992). Because opiate-induced depressions generally persist during abstinence, use of antidepressants is indicated, and these drugs are usually effective (Dackis and Gold 1992; Rounsaville et al. 1982).

Cocaine: Withdrawal

People who are addicted to cocaine typically binge until their supply of cocaine is exhausted. The resulting "crash" begins within hours of the start of abstinence, lasts for about 3 days, and is characterized by depressive symptoms, irritability, and anxiety (Satel et al. 1991). Gawin and Kleber (1986) evaluated 30 chronic cocaine abusers during withdrawal and determined that 13% fulfilled DSM-III criteria for major depressive disorder and 20% met DSM-III criteria for dysthymic disorder. The

depressive symptoms are likely caused by depletion of CNS dopamine and norepinephrine (Dackis and Gold 1992). However, Satel et al. (1991) measured levels of prolactin, growth hormone, and homovanillic acid in 22 cocaine-dependent patients (DSM-III-R criteria) during abstinence that began abruptly. They found a small but significant increase in prolactin levels but no change from baseline in levels of growth hormone or homovanillic acid. Symptoms of withdrawal are usually mild (Satel et al. 1991), and the emphasis in treatment is on abstinence (Dackis and Gold 1992). Even so, bromocriptine (Giannini et al. 1989), amantadine (Tennant and Sagherian 1987), and desipramine (Gawin and Kleber 1984) can attenuate the depressive symptoms and drug craving that occur in cocaine withdrawal.

Anabolic Steroids

Anabolic steroids are increasingly being used to enhance athletic performance. In a study involving 88 athletes who used anabolic-androgenic steroids, Pope and Katz (1994) noted more gynecomastia, decreased testicular length, higher ratios of cholesterol to high-density lipoprotein, and a strikingly high rate of major mood syndromes, compared with 68 athletes who did not use the steroids. Among the 88 users, 4 (5%) became manic, 9 (10%) developed hypomania, and 11 (13%) met DSM-III-R criteria for major depressive disorder while taking the drugs.

COURSE AND PROGNOSIS

When depression accompanies a medical illness, each disorder complicates the course of the other. Katon and Schulberg (1992) showed that initial depressive symptoms of greater severity and the existence of a comorbid medical condition were the best predictors of persistence of depression. Yates et al. (1991) demonstrated that depression due to medical conditions or substance abuse was particularly persistent. They found that significantly fewer patients with secondary mood disorders recovered after 4 years compared with a group of medically ill, depressed individuals. In another study, one-half of 309 enrollees in prepaid group practice plans who initially had depressive symptoms continued to report depressive symptoms after a year (Hankin and Locke 1982). This persistently depressed group had more cognitive deficits and more physical illness. Maricle et al. (1988) studied patients with drug-induced depressions. Although the sample sizes were small, at 2.5-year follow-up all patients no longer taking depression-causing medications were free of depression, whereas all those still taking the implicated medications remained depressed.

Conversely, depression is associated with higher morbidity and mortality in patients with CAD (Carney et al. 1988), myocardial infarction (Frasure-Smith et al. 1993), stroke (Morris et al. 1993a; Robinson et al. 1990), acute life-threatening illness (Silverstone 1990), renal failure (Burton et al. 1986), or cancer (Newport and Nemeroff 1998).

TREATMENT

Underlying Medical Conditions

Treatment of depression in medically ill patients is complex and requires an understanding of diagnostic nosology, medicine, psychiatry, pharmacology, and psychotherapy. Once the diagnosis of depression is established, the initial step in treatment is the identification of causative toxic or medical factors. All medical conditions should be treated. If the medical condition is chronic, the depression should be treated in a manner similar to that for primary depression. Clinicians should reduce doses of or discontinue administering medications thought to contribute to the depression. If the medical condition requires continued treatment, the offending medication should be replaced with another medication that has comparable pharmacological activity but does not cause depression (Cameron 1990; G.A. Fava et al. 1987).

Psychopharmacology

Research into the molecular biology of neurotransmitter receptor systems is progressing at an astounding pace. The number of receptor subtypes and agents selective for these specific receptors is similarly expanding. As these new agents join the list of established antidepressant drugs, the clinician gains more flexibility in the pharmacological treatment of depression (see also Chapter 42). Selecting the correct medication is particularly important in treating depression in medically ill patients. Proper selection depends on side-effect profile, concurrent conditions and medications, target symptoms, and previous treatment responses.

Tricyclic and Related Agents

Tricyclic and related agents include the tricyclic agents imipramine, amitriptyline, desipramine, nortriptyline, doxepin, clomipramine, and protriptyline. Trazodone and amoxapine are also included in this group. These agents are equally efficacious when given at therapeutically equivalent doses. They are more effective than the selective serotonin reuptake inhibitors (SSRIs) in melancholic and severe depression (Nobler and Roose 1998). The differences among these medications lie in the relative activity of each agent at the muscarinic, histamine, noradrenergic, and serotonergic receptors.

Each of these compounds, except trazodone, has significant anticholinergic activity; amitriptyline and clomipramine are particularly potent. Therapeutic doses of these agents are equivalent to several milligrams of atropine. Symptoms of anticholinergic action such as dry mouth, blurred vision, and constipation are often tolerated and may subside with time. More severe symptoms such as urinary retention, ileus, and anticholinergic delirium are particularly worrisome. Elderly patients and individuals taking other medications that have anticholinergic side effects are especially vulnerable to these complications (Bernstein 1995).

Orthostatic hypotension is another serious potential complication of treatment with tricyclic agents. Antidepressants can block the α_1-adrenergic receptors, an action that is partially responsible for orthostasis. The resulting increased risk of falls in medically ill patients, especially the elderly, is a significant problem. Although the secondary amine nortriptyline is not entirely free of orthostatic properties, use of this drug is less likely than use of other TCAs to result in orthostasis (Chutka 1990). The consultant must monitor supine and standing blood pressures at the initiation of treatment, because significant changes typically begin at low doses.

Sedation is another common side effect that results in complications and noncompliance. Amitriptyline, clomipramine, doxepin, and trazodone are highly sedating. This effect is often advantageous in the early stages of treatment because it decreases insomnia, but early-morning "hangover" at higher doses can significantly interfere with a patient's functioning. Sedation and appetite stimulation relate to the antidepressant's activity at the CNS histamine$_1$ receptor.

The other major problem is that tricyclic agents have a quinidine-like antiarrhythmic activity. This activity slows conduction and can prolong the QRS duration and the Q-T and P-R intervals. These effects are often evident at therapeutic levels and are of great concern in overdose. The use of tricyclic agents in patients with first-degree heart block or bundle branch block could result in a higher-degree heart block. Use of tricyclic agents should be avoided in patients with second- and third-degree heart block or bifascicular or trifascicular block (Chutka 1990). Patients with hereditary prolongation of Q-T intervals are also at risk (Moss and Robinson 1992); because 90% of these cases are familial, a thorough family history, with exploration of sudden death and syncope, is necessary. The ultimate evaluation of cardiac conduction is an electrocardiogram. The use of TCAs should be avoided when the corrected Q-T interval is greater than 440 msec. Given that the use of antiarrhythmics in post–myocardial infarction patients can increase mortality, treatment with tricyclics should be avoided in such patients.

Selective Serotonin Reuptake Inhibitors

The SSRIs are a class of agents with a unique side-effect profile. Overall, these agents are well tolerated by medically ill patients with major depressive disorder. The most common complaints are gastrointestinal upset, nervousness, sexual dysfunction, and insomnia. There is little clinical difference in the frequency of these side effects among the different SSRIs except for citalopram's decreased frequency of gastrointestinal effects (Dewan and Anand 1999). SSRIs do differ in terms of elimination half-life and the presence of active metabolites. For example, fluoxetine, which has an elimination half-life of 1–3 days, is converted to norfluoxetine, an SSRI with a half-life of 7–9 days. Therefore, steady-state plasma levels are not reached for 5–6 weeks; a similar amount of time is required to eliminate norfluoxetine from the patient's system after discontinuation. Sertraline, paroxetine, and citalopram do not have this liability (Nemeroff 1993).

A troublesome aspect of many SSRIs is their inhibition of the cytochrome P450 system, especially CYP2D6. Fluoxetine, paroxetine, sertraline, and citalopram each inhibit this system to some degree. This enzyme system metabolizes antiarrhythmics, antidepressants, neuroleptics, codeine, oxycodone, and hydroxycodone (Ottson et al. 1993). In addition, as many as 7% of Caucasians are deficient in this enzyme and are considered slow metabolizers (Ottson et al. 1993). When SSRIs are used in medically ill patients, drugs metabolized by the cytochrome P450 system can accumulate to toxic levels; therefore, concentrations must be monitored. Codeine, oxycodone, and hydroxycodone, which require biotransformation for full activity, are less effective (Ottson et al. 1993).

Other Antidepressants

Bupropion is a monocyclic phenylethylamine of the aminoketone type that is structurally similar to amphetamine (Weintraub and Evans 1989). Although the exact mechanism of action is unknown, the interaction of bupropion and its primary active metabolite, hydroxybupropion, with the noradrenergic system is likely involved.

Norepinephrine reuptake blockade and weak dopaminergic reuptake blockade are known effects (Asher et al. 1995). After initial concerns were raised about the incidence of seizures in bulimic patients (Horne et al. 1988), a subsequent study showed the actual risk to be 0.4% among depressed patients when the dosage was less than 450 mg/day (Johnston et al. 1991). This incidence is comparable to that seen among patients receiving 200–300 mg of a TCA per day (J. Davidson 1989). Nevertheless, patients who have a history of seizures or head trauma, have electroencephalographic findings suggestive of epilepsy, have anorexia or bulimia, or are taking medications—or have a neurological condition—known to lower the seizure threshold should not receive bupropion (Stoudemire 1995). The advantages of bupropion are the result of its benign side-effect profile. In 36 patients with serious cardiac disease, bupropion rarely caused orthostatic hypotension, did not have an adverse effect on left ventricular function, did not cause or worsen conduction abnormalities, and did not affect pulse rate (Roose et al. 1991). Two of the hypertensive patients, however, had modest increases in blood pressure. Unlike the SSRIs, bupropion is associated with a low incidence of sexual dysfunction (Walker et al. 1993) and may actually improve erectile function in diabetic male patients (Rowland et al. 1997). Additionally, bupropion is efficacious in patients with attention-deficit/hyperactivity disorder (Barrickman et al. 1995). The side effects of bupropion are excessive stimulation, insomnia, tremor, and perceptual abnormalities in susceptible individuals (Weintraub and Evans 1989).

Venlafaxine is a phenylamine antidepressant that inhibits the presynaptic reuptake of serotonin, norepinephrine, and, to a lesser extent, dopamine without significant effects on the postsynaptic cholinergic, histamine, or α-adrenergic receptors (Cunningham 1994). The more common side effects of venlafaxine, like those of the other newer antidepressants, generally are not serious; these side effects are nervousness, nausea, sweating, anorexia, dry mouth, and dizziness (Montgomery 1993). Up to one-third of patients experience significant nausea, and up to one-half of those individuals discontinue treatment as a result. Cisapride, a serotonin$_3$ (5-HT$_3$) antagonist, can be useful in treating this side effect (Russell 1996). Another significant potential side effect is a dose-related increase in diastolic blood pressure; 19% of patients receiving 200 mg or more of venlafaxine daily had sustained hypertension (Feighner 1994). Another meta-analysis, involving 3,744 patients, found that the incidence of increased supine diastolic blood pressure was clinically and statistically significant only at doses greater than 300 mg/day (Thase 1998). Venlafaxine is only 30% protein bound, allowing safer administration in patients taking highly protein-bound drugs such as warfarin and digoxin (Ereshefsky et al. 1995). The combination of venlafaxine with a monoamine oxidase inhibitor (MAOI), which can result in serotonin syndrome, should be avoided (Ereshefsky et al. 1995).

Nefazodone is a phenylpiperazine antidepressant structurally similar to trazodone. Nefazodone is a selective serotonin (5-HT$_{2A}$) postsynaptic receptor antagonist that also blocks the presynaptic reuptake of serotonin and norepinephrine (Ayd 1995). In vitro studies indicate that nefazodone is devoid of affinity for the muscarinic, cholinergic, H$_1$, and α$_1$-adrenergic receptors. Consequently, compared with TCAs, nefazodone less often causes dry mouth, constipation, urinary retention, exacerbation of glaucoma, excessive sedation, weight gain, or priapism (D.P. Taylor et al. 1995). Furthermore, nefazodone does not suppress REM sleep and improves overall sleep quality (Armitage et al. 1994). Its efficacy in hospitalized depressed patients was demonstrated in a placebo-controlled study (Feighner et al. 1998). The more common adverse effects seen with nefazodone therapy are mild sedation, dry mouth, nausea, headache, constipation, and dizziness (Ereshefsky et al. 1995). Because of nefazodone's inhibition of CYP3A4, plasma levels of coadministered alprazolam, triazolam, ketoconazole, terfenadine, and astemizole increase. In particular, the combination of nefazodone with either terfenadine or astemizole should be avoided, because of the risk of cardiotoxicity (Ayd 1995).

Mirtazapine is the first noradrenergic and specific serotonergic antidepressant available. It blocks both α$_1$ and α$_2$ autoreceptors, enhancing both noradrenergic and serotonergic transmission. Additionally, it blocks 5-HT$_2$ and 5-HT$_3$ receptors, which reduces the incidence of serotonin-related agitation, nausea, and sexual dysfunction. Its efficacy has been found to be comparable to that of amitriptyline (Fawcett and Barkin 1998) and is perhaps superior to that of fluoxetine (Wheatley et al. 1998). This possible superiority is probably similar to the superiority in efficacy of TCAs over SSRIs in patients with severe or melancholic depression (Nobler and Roose 1998). Increased appetite and weight gain, sedation, and agranulocytosis are the major liabilities of this agent.

Monoamine Oxidase Inhibitors

MAOIs were developed after antidepressant activity was observed during their use as antitubercular agents during the 1950s. Although MAOIs are the oldest of the antidepressants, they are poorly understood. Phenelzine, tranylcypromine, and isocarboxazid irreversibly inhibit both MAO A and MAO B. Deprenyl, used in PD, at low doses irreversibly inhibits MAO B; it is not currently recommended for the treatment of depression. MAOIs have no significant anticholinergic activity, have no effect on cardiac conduction, and tend to be activating depressants. Orthostasis and hypotension are the only cardiovascular side effects associated with MAOIs. These side effects are particularly problematic in elderly patients, who are sensitive to these effects and for whom the consequences of falls are so devastating (Chutka 1990).

An important concern in using MAOIs is the hypertensive crisis that results from exposure to tyramine in the diet. Tyramine-containing foods such as aged fermented products, organ meats, overripe fruit, and broad beans are especially problematic (Shelman et al. 1989). Another source of difficulty is the concomitant use of sympathomimetics, other psychotropic agents, or meperidine. The use of sympathomimetics with MAOIs can result in a hypertensive crisis; when TCAs, SSRIs, or meperidine are combined with MAOIs, serotonin syndrome can result, with symptoms similar to those of neuroleptic malignant syndrome (D.W. Nierenberg and Semprebon 1993). Despite these hazards, MAOIs are very effective in atypical depression and anxiety disorders, especially panic disorder.

Psychostimulants

The use of psychostimulants to treat primary depressive disorders is not well supported by the literature (Satel and Nelson 1989); however, their safety and efficacy in treating secondary mood disorder symptoms in medical settings are well documented (Lazarus et al. 1992; Masand and Tesar 1996). Psychostimulants are fast acting and safe in elderly and medically ill patients and are well tolerated by these groups as well. In a large review of records of medically hospitalized patients, Masand et al. (1991) found that 70% of patients were rated as markedly or moderately improved with psychostimulant therapy; only 10% of patients discontinued treatment because of side effects. Of 198 patients, only 6 developed any form of cardiovascular side effect. Insomnia and anorexia, two concerns often raised with regard to prescribing stimulants, were reported in 1 and 0 patients, respectively. No differences were found between methylphenidate and dextroamphetamine. The rapid remission of depressive symptoms, usually in 1–3 days, allows patients to participate in rehabilitation much sooner than if conventional antidepressant therapy had been used (Masand et al. 1991). Adding antidepressants to the regimen allows the stimulant to jump-start therapy while the conventional agent is taking effect.

Treatment-Resistant Depression

Treatment-resistant depression (TRD) is a frequently used term that can, unfortunately, mean inadequately treated depression or an overlooked secondary depression in medically ill patients. In this chapter, we consider TRD to be any depressive episode that does not respond to appropriate pharmacological treatment administered at adequate levels for a sufficient time. The reader is referred to a review by A. A. Nierenberg and Amsterdam (1990) for a discussion of criteria for TRD.

The clinician has several options when a patient does not respond adequately to an antidepressant. The most important therapeutic intervention is for the clinician to maximize the potential efficacy of the current medication. The patient should be encouraged to take the medicine. Measuring serum levels of the newer agents can be of limited utility. Typically, the dose should be increased until either a response occurs or the side effects become intolerable. The clinician can then change agents, consider ECT, or augment with mood stabilizers or thyroid hormone. A lack of responsiveness to one member of a class of antidepressants, particularly SSRIs, does not necessarily predict a lack of response to all members of that class. In a study by Thase et al. (1997), 63% of patients who failed to respond to sertraline responded to fluoxetine. On the other hand, if a patient exhibits a complete lack of response or experiences intolerable side effects, a shift to a different class of antidepressant may be warranted. A partial response makes augmentation more attractive. Failure of multiple drug therapies, depression that is life-threatening, or a psychotic depression suggests ECT as an option.

The two agents most commonly used for antidepressant augmentation are lithium (Nemeroff 1991; Stein and Bernadt 1993) and thyroid hormone (Nemeroff 1991). Typically, lithium and the other mood stabilizers are used at full therapeutic doses; lithium augmentation is reported to be successful in 44%–66% of patients with TRD (Stein and Bernadt 1993). Thyroid augmentation is probably less effective, but it is worth consideration in cases of high-normal thyroid-stimulating hormone (TSH) levels or other indications of poor thyroid function.

Electroconvulsive Therapy

The efficacy of ECT is well established (see also Chapter 44). ECT remains among the most effective treatments available for depression. Despite more than 60 years of experience, the curative mechanism of action of ECT is unknown (Lerer 1987). ECT is unfortunately considered

a second-line treatment for depression; however, it is considered a first-line therapy in several clinical situations commonly encountered in consultation-liaison settings (Table 17–9). Psychotic depressions frequently are poorly responsive to medications. In addition, a patient with psychosis is at risk for self-injury or injury of others. The rate of response to ECT is as high as 83% (Avery and Lubrano 1985), which is superior to the rate of response to antidepressant medications in patients with nonpsychotic depression. ECT also deserves early consideration in depressed patients with unrelenting intense suicidality. Similarly, the rapid response to ECT in a malnourished, anorexic medically ill patient is lifesaving and obviates the need for a more invasive stopgap intervention such as use of an enteral feeding tube.

TABLE 17–9. Indications for electroconvulsive therapy as a first-line treatment

Psychotic/delusional depression
Intense suicidal tendencies associated with depression
Severe malnutrition/dehydration associated with depression
Catatonia of most functional and some organic etiologies
Severe manic excitement
Failure to respond to antidepressant therapy
History of depression responsive to electroconvulsive therapy
Medical conditions in which exposure to antidepressant medication is problematic (e.g., severe coronary artery disease, pregnancy)

ECT is an effective, often life-saving treatment for some of the medical causes of catatonia, such as lethal catatonia (Rummans 1993). The "functional" catatonias—primarily caused by depression, mania, or schizophrenia—are exquisitely sensitive to ECT. Once an organic etiology for the catatonia is ruled out (usually by electroencephalography), ECT is the treatment of choice (M. Taylor 1990).

Treatment resistance, as defined earlier, is a frequent indication for ECT. Many studies of the efficacy of ECT have demonstrated efficacy in patients who failed to respond to pharmacotherapy. The response rate is good, but the 1-year relapse rate, even with maintenance antidepressant therapy after ECT, is as high as 50% (Sackeim et al. 1990). Most relapses occur within the first 2–4 months after ECT. Options to decrease the risk of relapse include maintenance ECT and lithium or carbamazepine augmentation and antidepressant therapy.

There are no absolute contraindications to ECT (American Psychiatric Association Task Force on ECT 1990). Some conditions increase the morbidity associated with ECT and require thoughtful review of the risks and benefits in individual patients. These conditions are divided into three groups that are not mutually exclusive: 1) conditions that cause increased intracranial pressure, 2) conditions that increase the risk of serious hemorrhage, and 3) conditions involving pathophysiologic change that causes hemodynamic compromise, such as acute myocardial infarction or malignant arrhythmia. The addition of β-blockers and antiarrhythmics before ECT reduces some of these risks.

Mortality associated with ECT is less than 0.05% and is essentially the risk of brief general anesthesia. Arrhythmias, myocardial infarction, and congestive heart failure are the most frequent causes of death (Selvin 1987).

Transcranial Magnetic Stimulation

Transcranial magnetic stimulation (TMS) is an evolving treatment option for depression. TMS has numerous neuropsychiatric effects that can be used for functional mapping when applied to different regions of the brain (Pascual-Leone et al. 1999). In TMS, a large wire coil is placed next to the scalp to generate the magnetic field. The lack of stigma, seizures, cognitive complaints, and other serious sequelae makes this an attractive alternative to ECT. Results of efficacy studies have been mixed, but a recent study involving 28 patients with TRD showed a response rate of 56% (Epstein et al. 1998). The role of this emerging treatment for depression in medically ill patients remains to be established.

Psychotherapy

Psychotherapy for depression in the medically ill patient requires a flexible, eclectic approach (see also Chapter 45). Because of the shortening of hospital stays and the emergent nature of the medical situation, therapy is focused and brief. This approach demands a rapid assessment of the presenting problem, exploration of the precipitating events, and a comprehensive psychosocial history (Liberzon et al. 1992). The typical goals of the brief therapy are to improve self-esteem, correct misunderstandings about the illness, help the patient accept limitations imposed by the illness and the hospital (Massie and Holland 1990), reduce isolation, assist the patient in coping with loss and disability, and facilitate the expression of fears and concerns (Haig 1992). Sutor and associates (1998) identified four components essential for effective psychotherapy in depressed medical patients: social support, emotional expression, cognitive restructuring, and training in coping skills.

Therapy with a cognitive-behavioral emphasis is showing promise in the treatment of the depressed med-

ical patient in the outpatient consultation-liaison setting. Larcombe and Wilson (1984), in a controlled study, demonstrated the effectiveness of cognitive-behavioral therapy in 22 patients with depression and multiple sclerosis compared with similar patients on a waiting list. Cognitive therapy is particularly useful in patients with false assumptions about their illness. Such patients may believe that the illness represents punishment or weakness, may have unrealistic or distorted fears and expectations, or may have exaggerated or inappropriate responses to loss (G.A. Fava et al. 1987).

Rodin (1984) reviewed the technical problems unique to conducting psychotherapy in an inpatient consultation-liaison setting. Therapy with medically ill patients is emotionally demanding on the therapist. The therapist is often too supportive too quickly. In addition, therapy is frequently interrupted by medical setbacks, tests, or medical procedures. The therapist must have an understanding of the medical situation and incorporate the limitations of the illness into a reasonable psychosocial treatment plan. Furthermore, therapy is conducted with little or no privacy. Finally, hospitalized patients and medically ill outpatients are often regressed, which makes even supportive psychotherapy more difficult.

In the case of cancer patients, group therapy promotes support, improves interpersonal relationships, decreases loneliness, and helps patients develop a sense of meaning in life (Haig 1992). Spiegel (1990) used psychoeducational group therapy to treat depressed women with metastatic breast cancer. He unexpectedly found that the patients in group therapy lived twice as long as the patients who received only routine oncological care. Also, a group of 68 distressed patients with malignant melanoma who participated in a 6-week structured psychiatric group had fewer metastases and a lower mortality rate 6 years afterward, compared with a control group who only underwent standard surgery (Fawzy et al. 1993). Similarly, in patients with hematological malignancies, the use of special educational and supportive programs significantly improved both adherence to treatment and survival (Richardson et al. 1990). Levine et al. (1991) used a psychoeducational approach to treat depressed HIV-positive patients. This approach helped the patients function better in employment and social situations, alleviated abandonment issues, and improved social support. Levine et al. (1991) concluded that homogeneous psychoeducational groups are a cost-effective way to treat depressed HIV-positive patients.

The family of the medically ill patient with depression is also often in turmoil and may need care. Family therapy can provide emotional support, relieve guilt, expedite communications between the patient and the family, prepare the family for change, decrease alienation from the patient, and prevent displacement of anger toward hospital staff (Haig 1992).

CONCLUSION

Although depression in medically ill patients is an all too common condition, it is underdiagnosed and under-treated. Failure to diagnose and treat the depression is associated with higher morbidity and mortality. Even though many studies have methodological shortcomings, it can be concluded that depression appears often in patients with medical conditions, especially when a direct chemical or structural insult to the CNS occurs. By better understanding the pathophysiology, clinical presentations, diagnosis, management, course, and prognosis of depression in medically ill patients, the consultation-liaison psychiatrist is better able to provide the treatment these patients require.

REFERENCES

Adams RD, Victor M: Principles of Neurology, 5th Edition. New York, McGraw-Hill, 1993, pp 776–798

Akiskal HS, Rosenthal TI, Haykal RF, et al: Characterological depression: clinical and sleep EEG findings separating sub-affective dysthymias from character spectrum disorders. Arch Gen Psychiatry 37:777–783, 1980

Alexopoulos GS, Meyers BS, Young RC, et al: The course of geriatric depression with "reversible dementia": a controlled study. Am J Psychiatry 150:1693–1699, 1993

American Psychiatric Association: Diagnostic and Statistical Manual of Mental Disorders, 3rd Edition. Washington, DC, American Psychiatric Association, 1980

American Psychiatric Association: Diagnostic and Statistical Manual of Mental Disorders, 3rd Edition, Revised. Washington, DC, American Psychiatric Association, 1987

American Psychiatric Association: Diagnostic and Statistical Manual of Mental Disorders, 4th Edition. Washington, DC, American Psychiatric Association, 1994

American Psychiatric Association: Practice guideline for the treatment of patients with Alzheimer's disease and other dementias of late life. Am J Psychiatry 154:1–39, 1997

American Psychiatric Association: Diagnostic and Statistical Manual of Mental Disorders, 4th Edition, Text Revision. Washington, DC, American Psychiatric Association, 2000

American Psychiatric Association Task Force on ECT: The practice of ECT: recommendations for treatment, training and privileging. Convulsive Therapy 7:85–120, 1990

Andersen G, Vestergaard K, Lauritzen L: Effective treatment of poststroke depression with the selective serotonin reuptake inhibitor citalopram. Stroke 25:1099–1104, 1994

Andersen J, Aabro E, Gulmann N, et al: Anti-depressive treatment in Parkinson's disease treated with L-dopa. Acta Neurol Scand 62:210–219, 1980

Armitage R, Rush AJ, Trivedi M, et al: The effects of nefazodone on sleep architecture in depression. Neuropsychopharmacology 10:123–127, 1994

Asher J, Cole J, Colin J, et al: Bupropion: a review of its mechanism of antidepressant activity. J Clin Psychiatry 56:395–401, 1995

Atkinson JH [Jr], Grant I: Natural history of neuropsychiatric manifestations of HIV disease. Psychiatr Clin North Am 17:17–33, 1994

Atkinson JH Jr, Grant I, Kennedy CJ, et al: Prevalence of psychiatric disorders among men infected with human immunodeficiency virus: a controlled study. Arch Gen Psychiatry 45:859–864, 1988

Avery D, Lubrano A: Depression treated with imipramine and ECT: the DeCarolis study reconsidered. Am J Psychiatry 142:430–436, 1985

Ayd FJ: Nefazodone: the latest FDA approved antidepressant. International Drug Therapy Newsletter 30:17–20, 1995

Barbosa ER, Limongi CJ, Cummings JL: Parkinson's disease. Psychiatr Clin North Am 20:769–790, 1997

Barrickman LL, Perry PJ, Allen AJ, et al: Bupropion versus methylphenidate in the treatment of attention-deficit hyperactivity disorder. J Am Acad Child Adolesc Psychiatry 34:649–657, 1995

Beckson M, Cummings JL: Neuropsychiatric aspects of stroke. Int J Psychiatry Med 21:1–15, 1991

Beers MH, Passman LJ: Antihypertensive medications and depression. Drugs 40:792–799, 1990

Benson KL, Zarcone VP: Rapid eye movement sleep eye movements in schizophrenia and depression. Arch Gen Psychiatry 50:474–482, 1993

Bernstein JG: Tricyclic, heterocyclic, and serotonin selective antidepressants, in Handbook of Drug Therapy in Psychiatry, 3rd Edition. St. Louis, MO, Mosby Year-Book, 1995, pp 112–152

Black DW, Winokur G, Nasrallah A: Treatment and outcome in secondary depression: a naturalistic study of 1087 patients. J Clin Psychiatry 48:438–441, 1987

Blumenfield M, Levy NB, Spinowitz B, et al: Fluoxetine in depressed patients on dialysis. Int J Psychiatry Med 27:71–80, 1997

Blumer D: Epilepsy and disorders of mood. Adv Neurol 55:185–195, 1991

Blumer D: Antidepressant and double antidepressant treatment for the affective disorder of epilepsy. J Clin Psychiatry 58:3–11, 1997

Boston Collaborative Drug Surveillance Program: Acute adverse reactions to prednisone in relation to dosage. Clin Pharmacol Ther 13:694–698, 1972

Brooner RK, King VL, Kidorf M, et al: Psychiatric and substance use comorbidity among treatment-seeking opioid abusers. Arch Gen Psychiatry 54:71–80, 1997

Brown RG, MacCarthy B, Gotham AM, et al: Depression and disability in Parkinson's disease: a follow-up study of 132 cases. Psychol Med 18:49–55, 1988

Buckberg J, Penman D, Holland JC: Depression in hospitalized cancer patients. Psychosom Med 46:199–212, 1984

Burke WJ, Peterson J, Rubin EH: Electroconvulsive therapy in the treatment of combined depression and Parkinson's disease. Psychosomatics 29:341–346, 1988

Burton HJ, Kline SA, Lindsay RM, et al: The relationship of depression to survival in chronic renal failure. Psychosom Med 48:261–269, 1986

Caine ED, Shoulson I: Psychiatric syndromes in Huntington's disease. Am J Psychiatry 140:728–733, 1983

Cameron OG: Guidelines for diagnosis and treatment of depression in patients with medical illness. J Clin Psychiatry 51 (suppl 7):49–54, 1990

Carney RM, Rich MW, Tevelde A, et al: Major depressive disorder in coronary artery disease. Am J Cardiol 60:1273–1275, 1987

Carney RM, Rich MW, Freedland KE, et al: Major depressive disorder predicts cardiac events in patients with coronary artery disease. Psychosom Med 50:627–633, 1988

Carney RM, Freedland KE, Rich MW, et al: Ventricular tachycardia and psychiatric depression in patients with coronary artery disease. Am J Med 95:23–28, 1993

Cassem EH: Depression and anxiety secondary to medical illness. Psychiatr Clin North Am 13:597–612, 1990

Cassem NH: Depression, in Massachusetts General Hospital Handbook of General Hospital Psychiatry, 3rd Edition. Edited by Cassem NH. St. Louis, MO, Mosby Year-Book, 1991, pp 237–268

Cathebras PJ, Robbins JM, Kirmayer LJ, et al: Fatigue in primary care: prevalence, psychiatric comorbidity, illness behavior and outcome. J Gen Intern Med 7:276–286, 1992

Chutka DS: Cardiovascular effects of the antidepressants: recognition and control. Geriatrics 45:55–67, 1990

Cohen-Cole SA, Stoudemire A: Major depression and physical illness: special considerations in diagnosis and biologic treatment. Psychiatr Clin North Am 10:1–17, 1987

Cornelius JR, Salloum IM, Day NL, et al: Patterns of suicidality and alcohol use in alcoholics with major depression. Alcohol Clin Exp Res 20:1451–1455, 1996

Corradi RB: Psychological regression with illness. Psychosomatics 24:353–355, 358–359, 362, 1983

Cote L, Crutcher MD: The basal ganglia, in Principles of Neural Science. Edited by Kandel ER, Schwartz JH, Jessell TM. New York, Elsevier, 1991, pp 654–655

Cote TR, Biggar RJ, Dannenberg AL: Risk of suicide among persons with AIDS. JAMA 268:2066–2068, 1992

Coyne JC, Schwenk TL, Fechner-Bates S: Nondetection of depression by primary care physicians reconsidered. Gen Hosp Psychiatry 17:3–12, 1995

Cummings JL: Ictal and interictal behavioral alterations, in Clinical Neuropsychiatry. Edited by Cummings JL. Boston, MA, Allyn & Bacon, 1985, pp 95–116

Cummings JL: Depression in Parkinson's disease: a review. Am J Psychiatry 149:443–454, 1992

Cummings JL: Behavioral and psychiatric symptoms associated with Huntington's disease, in Advances in Neurology. Edited by Weiner WJ, Lang AE. New York, Raven, 1995, pp 179–186

Cummings JL, Benson DF: HIV encephalopathy, Jakob-Creutzfeldt disease, and other infectious dementias, in Dementia: A Clinical Approach, 2nd Edition. Boston, MA, Butterworth-Heinemann, 1992, pp 177–188

Cummings JL, Miller B, Hill MA, et al: Neuropsychiatric aspects of multi-infarct dementia and dementia of the Alzheimer type. Arch Neurol 44:389–393, 1987

Cunningham LA: Depression in the medically ill: choosing an antidepressant. J Clin Psychiatry 55 (suppl A):90–100, 1994

Currie S, Heathfield KW, Henson RA, et al: Clinical course and prognosis of temporal lobe epilepsy: a survey of 666 patients. Brain 94:173–190, 1971

Dackis CA, Gold MS: Psychiatric hospitals for treatment of dual diagnosis, in Substance Abuse—A Comprehensive Textbook, 2nd Edition. Edited by Lowinson JH, Ruiz P, Millman RB, et al. Baltimore, MD, Williams & Wilkins, 1992, pp 479–485

Dackis CA, Pottash AL, Gold MS, et al: Evaluating depression in alcoholics. Psychiatry Res 17:105–109, 1986

Davidson J: Seizures and bupropion: a review. J Clin Psychiatry 50:256–261, 1989

Davidson KM, Ritson EB: The relationship between alcohol dependence and depression. Alcohol Alcohol 28:147–155, 1993

DeMuth GW, Ackerman SH: Alpha-methyldopa and depression: a clinical study and review of the literature. Am J Psychiatry 140:534–538, 1983

Dewan MJ, Anand VS: Evaluating the tolerability of the newer antidepressants. J Nerv Ment Dis 187:96–101, 1999

Dietch JT, Zetin M: Diagnosis of organic depressive disorders. Psychosomatics 24:971–979, 1983

Dilley JW, Ochitill HN, Perl M, et al: Findings in psychiatric consultations with patients with acquired immune deficiency syndrome. Am J Psychiatry 142:82–86, 1985

Docherty JP: Barriers to the diagnosis of depression in primary care. J Clin Psychiatry 58 (suppl 1):5–10, 1997

Douyon R, Serby M, Klutchko B, et al: ECT and Parkinson's disease revisited: a "naturalistic" study. Am J Psychiatry 146:1451–1455, 1989

Dwight MM, Stoudemire A: Effects of depressive disorders on coronary artery disease: a review. Harv Rev Psychiatry 5:115–122, 1997

Eaton WW, Mengel M, Mengel L, et al: Psychosocial and psychopathologic influences on management and control of insulin-dependent diabetes. Int J Psychiatry Med 22:105–117, 1992

Endicott J: Measurement of depression in patients with cancer. Cancer 53:2243–2248, 1984

Epstein C, Figiel G, McDonald W, et al: Rapid rate transcranial magnetic stimulation in young and middle-aged refractory depressed patients. Psychiatric Annals 28:36–39, 1998

Ereshefsky L, Benefield WH, Laird LK: Update on drug therapy for depression. Primary Psychiatry 2:28–36, 1995

Faber R, Trimble MR: Electroconvulsive therapy in Parkinson's disease and other movement disorders. Mov Disord 6: 293–303, 1991

Fava GA, Sonino N, Morphy MA: Major depression associated with endocrine disease. Psychiatric Developments 5:321–348, 1987

Fava M, Labbate LA, Abraham ME, et al: Hypothyroidism and hyperthyroidism in major depression revisited. J Clin Psychiatry 56:186–192, 1995

Fawcett J, Barkin RL: A meta-analysis of eight randomized, double-blind, controlled clinical trials of mirtazapine for the treatment of patients with major depression and symptoms of anxiety. J Clin Psychiatry 59:123–127, 1998

Fawzy FI, Fawzy NW, Hyun CS, et al: Malignant melanoma: effects of an early structured psychiatric intervention, coping, and affective state on recurrence and survival six years later. Arch Gen Psychiatry 50:681–689, 1993

Feighner JP: The role of venlafaxine in rational antidepressant therapy. J Clin Psychiatry 55 (suppl A):62–68, 1994

Feighner JP, Robins E, Guze SB, et al: Diagnostic criteria for use in psychiatric research. Arch Gen Psychiatry 26:57–63, 1972

Feighner JP, Targum S, Bennett M, et al: A double blind placebo-controlled trial of nefazodone in the treatment of patients hospitalized for major depression. J Clin Psychiatry 59:246–253, 1998

Fernandez F, Adams F, Levy JK, et al: Cognitive impairment due to AIDS-related complex and its response to psychostimulants. Psychosomatics 29:38–46, 1988

Folks DG: Organic affective disorder and underlying thyrotoxicosis. Psychosomatics 25:243–249, 1984

Folstein MF, Miaberger R, McHugh PR: Mood disorder as a specific complication of stroke. J Neurol Neurosurg Psychiatry 40:1018–1020, 1977

Folstein SE: Huntington's Disease: A Disorder of Families. Baltimore, MD, Johns Hopkins University Press, 1989

Folstein SE, Abbott MH, Chase GA, et al: The association of affective disorder with Huntington's disease in a case series and in families. Psychol Med 13:537–542, 1983

Ford MF: Treatment of depression in Huntington's disease with monoamine oxidase inhibitors. Br J Psychiatry 149:654–656, 1986

Forrester AW, Lipsey JR, Teitelbaum ML, et al: Depression following myocardial infarction. Int J Psychiatry Med 22:33–46, 1992

Frasure-Smith N, Lesperance F, Talajic M: Depression following myocardial infarction: impact on 6-month survival. JAMA 270:1819–1825, 1993

Frasure-Smith N, Lesperance F, Talajic M: Depression and 18-month prognosis after myocardial infarction. Circulation 91:999–1005, 1995

Freedland KE, Lustman PJ, Carney RM, et al: Underdiagnosis of depression in patients with coronary artery disease: the role of nonspecific symptoms. Int J Psychiatry Med 22: 221–229, 1991

Freedland KE, Carney RM, Lustman PJ, et al: Major depression in coronary artery disease: patients with vs. without a prior history of depression. Psychosom Med 54:416–421, 1992

Ganzini L, Walsh JR, Millar SM: Drug-induced depression in the aged. Drugs Aging 3:147–158, 1993

Gawin FH, Kleber HD: Cocaine abuse treatment: open pilot trial with desipramine and lithium carbonate. Arch Gen Psychiatry 41:903–909, 1984

Gawin FH, Kleber HD: Abstinence symptomatology and psychiatric diagnosis in cocaine abusers. Arch Gen Psychiatry 43:107–113, 1986

Geringer ES, Stern TA: Coping with medical illness: the impact of personality types. Psychosomatics 27:251–261, 1986

Gerstman BB, Jolson HM, Bauer M, et al: The incidence of depression in new users of beta-blockers and selected antihypertensives. J Clin Epidemiol 49:809–815, 1996

Giannini AJ, Folts DJ, Feather JN, et al: Bromocriptine and amantadine in cocaine detoxification. Psychiatry Res 29:11–16, 1989

Goetz GG, Tanner CM, Klawans HL: Bupropion in Parkinson's disease. Neurology 34:1092–1094, 1984

Goldman MB: Neuropsychiatric features of endocrine disorders, in The American Psychiatric Press Textbook of Neuropsychiatry, 2nd Edition. Edited by Yudofsky SC, Hales RE. Washington, DC, American Psychiatric Press, 1992, pp 519–540

Gonzalez MB, O'Connor CM, Krishnan KR, et al: Depression in patients with coronary artery disease. Depression 4:57–62, 1996

Goodnick PJ: Diabetes mellitus and depression: issues in theory and treatment. Psychiatric Annals 27:353–359, 1997

Goodwin FK, Ebert MH, Bunney WE: Mental effects of reserpine in man: a review, in Psychiatric Complications of Medical Drugs. Edited by Shader RI. New York, Raven, 1972, pp 73–101

Gordon WA, Hibbard MR: Poststroke depression: an examination of the literature. Arch Phys Med Rehabil 78:659–663, 1997

Greenwald BS, Kramer-Gunsberg E, Marin DB, et al: Dementia with coexistent major depression. Am J Psychiatry 146:1472–1478, 1989

Hachinski VC, Iliff LD, Zilhka E, et al: Cerebral blood flow in dementia. Arch Neurol 32:632–637, 1975

Haggerty JJ, Garbutt JC, Evans DL, et al: Subclinical hypothyroidism: a review of neuropsychiatric aspects. Int J Psychiatry Med 20:193–208, 1990

Haggerty JJ, Stern RA, Mason GA, et al: Subclinical hypothyroidism: a modifiable risk factor for depression? Am J Psychiatry 150:508–510, 1993

Haig RA: Management of depression in patients with advanced cancer. Med J Aust 156:499–503, 1992

Hall RC, Joffe JR: Aberrant response to diazepam: a new syndrome. Am J Psychiatry 129:114–118, 1972

Hall RC, Popkin MK, Stickney SK, et al: Presentation of steroid psychoses. J Nerv Ment Dis 167:229–236, 1979

Hall RC, Stickney SK, Gardner ER: Behavioral toxicity of nonpsychiatric drugs, in Psychiatric Presentations of Medical Illness: Somatopsychic Disorders. Edited by Hall RC. New York, Spectrum, 1980, pp 337–349

Hall RC, Beresford TP, Blow FC: Depression and medical illness: an overview, in Presentations of Depression: Depressive Symptoms in Medical and Other Psychiatric Disorders. Edited by Cameron OG. New York, Wiley, 1987, pp 401–414

Hallas J: Evidence of depression provoked by cardiovascular medication: a prescription sequence symmetry analysis. Epidemiology 7:478–484, 1996

Hance M, Carney RM, Freedland KE, et al: Depression in patients with coronary heart disease: a 12-month follow-up. Gen Hosp Psychiatry 18:61–65, 1996

Hankin JR, Locke BZ: The persistence of depressive symptomatology among prepaid group practice enrollees: an exploratory study. Am J Public Health 72:1000–1007, 1982

Haskett RF: Diagnostic categorization of psychiatric disturbance in Cushing's syndrome. Am J Psychiatry 142:911–916, 1985

Healy D, Theodorou AE, Whitehouse AM, et al: 3H-Imipramine binding to previously frozen platelet membranes from depressed patients, before and after treatment. Br J Psychiatry 157:208–215, 1990

Henk HJ, Katzelnick DJ, Kobak KA, et al: Medical costs attributed to depression among patients with a history of high medical expenses in a health maintenance organization. Arch Gen Psychiatry 53:899–904, 1996

Herzberg B, Coppen A: A change in psychological symptoms in women taking oral contraceptives. Br J Psychiatry 116:161–164, 1970

Hinrichsen GA, Lieberman JA, Pollack S, et al: Depression in hemodialysis patients. Psychosomatics 30:284–289, 1989

Hirono N, Mori E, Ishii K, et al: Frontal lobe hypometabolism and depression in Alzheimer's disease. Neurology 50:380–383, 1998

Hirschfeld RM, Keller MB, Panico S, et al: The national depressive and manic-depressive association consensus statement on the undertreatment of depression. JAMA 277:333–340, 1997

Holmes VF, Fernandez F, Levy JK: Psychostimulant response in AIDS-related complex patients. J Clin Psychiatry 50:5–8, 1989

Horne RL, Ferguson JM, Pope HG, et al: Treatment of bulimia with bupropion: a multi-center controlled trial. J Clin Psychiatry 49:262–266, 1988

Joffe RT: A perspective on the thyroid and depression. Can J Psychiatry 35:754–758, 1990

Joffe RT, Lippert GP, Gray TA, et al: Mood disorder and multiple sclerosis. Arch Neurol 44:376–378, 1987

Johnson ML, Roberts MD, Ross AR, et al: Methylphenidate in stroke patients with depression. Am J Phys Med Rehabil 71:239–241, 1992

Johnston JA, Lineberry CG, Ascher JA, et al: A 102-center prospective study of seizure in association with bupropion. J Clin Psychiatry 52:450–456, 1991

Jorge CM, Goodnick PJ: Chronic fatigue syndrome and depression: biological differentiation and treatment. Psychiatric Annals 27:365–371, 1997

Kathol RG, Delahunt JW: The relationship of anxiety and depression to symptoms of hyperthyroidism using operational criteria. Gen Hosp Psychiatry 8:23–28, 1986

Kathol RG, Turner R, Delahunt J: Depression and anxiety associated with hyperthyroidism: response to antithyroid therapy. Psychosomatics 27:501–505, 1986

Kathol RG, Noyes R, Williams J, et al: Diagnosing depression in patients with medical illness. Psychosomatics 31:434–440, 1990a

Kathol RG, Mulgi A, Williams J, et al: Diagnosis of major depression in cancer patients according to four sets of criteria. Am J Psychiatry 147:1021–1024, 1990b

Katon W[J]: The epidemiology of depression in medical care. Int J Psychiatry Med 17:93–112, 1987

Katon WJ: The development of a randomized trial of consultation-liaison psychiatry trial in distressed high utilizers of primary care. Psychiatr Med 9:577–591, 1991

Katon W[J], Schulberg H: Epidemiology of depression in primary care. Gen Hosp Psychiatry 14:237–247, 1992

Katon W[J], Egan K, Miller D: Chronic pain: lifetime psychiatric diagnoses and family history. Am J Psychiatry 142:1156–1160, 1985

Katon W[J], Von Korff M, Lin E, et al: Distressed high utilizers of medical care: DSM-III-R diagnoses and treatment needs. Gen Hosp Psychiatry 12:355–362, 1990

Katz IR: Diagnosis and treatment of depression in patients with Alzheimer's disease and other dementias. J Clin Psychiatry 59 (suppl 9):38–44, 1998

Kelly WF: Psychiatric aspects of Cushing's syndrome. QJM 89:543–551, 1996

Kelly WF, Checkley SA, Bender DA, et al: Cushing's syndrome and depression: a prospective study of 26 patients. Br J Psychiatry 142:16–19, 1983

Kershner P, Wang-Cheng R: Psychiatric side effects of steroid therapy. Psychosomatics 30:135–139, 1989

Kiecolt-Glaser JK, Glaser R: Psychological influences on immunity. Psychosomatics 27:621–624, 1986

Kimmel PL, Weihs K, Peterson RA: Survival in hemodialysis patients: the role of depression. J Am Soc Nephrol 4:12–27, 1993

Koranyi EK: Morbidity and rate of undiagnosed physical illnesses in a psychiatric clinic population. Arch Gen Psychiatry 36:414–419, 1979

Kostic VS, Susic V, Przedborski S, et al: Sleep EEG in depressed and nondepressed patients with Parkinson's disease. J Neuropsychiatry Clin Neurosci 3:176–179, 1991

Kramer JC, Fischman VS, Littlefield DC: Amphetamine abuse: pattern and effects of high doses taken intravenously. JAMA 201:305–309, 1967

Kreusi MJ, Dale J, Straus SE: Psychiatric diagnoses in patients who have chronic fatigue syndrome. J Clin Psychiatry 50:53–56, 1989

Kudoh A, Ishihara H, Matsuki A: Effect of carbamazepine on pain scores of unipolar depressed patients with chronic pain: a trial of off-on-off-on design. Clin J Pain 14:61–65, 1998

Laitinen L: Desipramine in treatment of Parkinson's disease: a placebo-controlled study. Acta Neurol Scand 45:109–113, 1969

Larcombe NA, Wilson PH: An evaluation of cognitive-behaviour therapy for depression in patients with multiple sclerosis. Br J Psychiatry 145:366–371, 1984

Lazarus LW, Winemiller DR, Lingam VR, et al: Efficacy and side effects of methylphenidate for poststroke depression. J Clin Psychiatry 53:447–449, 1992

Lazarus LW, Moberg PJ, Langsley PR, et al: Methylphenidate and nortriptyline in the treatment of poststroke depression: a retrospective comparison. Arch Phys Med Rehabil 75:403–406, 1994

Leedom L, Meehan WP, Procci W, et al: Symptoms of depression in patients with type II diabetes mellitus. Psychosomatics 32:280–286, 1991

Lerer B: Neurochemical and other neurobiological consequences of ECT: implications for the pathogenesis and treatment of affective disorders, in Psychopharmacology: The Third Generation of Progress. Edited by Meltzer HY. New York, Raven, 1987, pp 577–588

Levine SH, Bystritsky A, Baron D, et al: Group psychotherapy for HIV-seropositive patients with major depression. Am J Psychother 45:413–424, 1991

Lewis DA, Smith RE: Steroid-induced psychiatric syndromes: a report of 14 cases and a review of the literature. J Affect Disord 5:319–322, 1983

Liberzon I, Goldman RS, Hendrickson WJ: Very brief psychotherapy in the psychiatric consultation setting. Int J Psychiatry Med 22:65–75, 1992

Lingam VR, Lazarus LW, Groves L, et al: Methylphenidate in treating post-stroke depression. J Clin Psychiatry 49:151–153, 1988

Lipsey JR, Robinson RG, Pearlson GD, et al: Nortriptyline treatment of post-stroke depression: a double blind study. Lancet 84:297–300, 1984

Lustman PJ, Griffith LS, Freedland KE, et al: Cognitive behavior therapy for depression in type 2 diabetes mellitus: a randomized, controlled trial. Ann Intern Med 129:613–621, 1998

Maes M, Meltzer HY, Stevens W, et al: Natural killer cell activity in major depression: relation to circulating natural killer cells, cellular indices of the immune response, and depressive phenomenology. Prog Neuropsychopharmacol Biol Psychiatry 18:717–730, 1994

Maricle RA, Kinzie JD, Lewinsohn P: Medication associated depression: a two and one half year follow-up of a community sample. Int J Psychiatry Med 18:283–292, 1988

Markowitz JC, Kocsis JH, Fishman B, et al: Treatment of depressive symptoms in human immunodeficiency virus-positive patients. Arch Gen Psychiatry 55:452–457, 1998

Martin JB, Gusella JF: Huntington's disease. N Engl J Med 315:1267–1276, 1986

Marzuk PM, Tierney H, Tardiff K, et al: Increased risk of suicide in persons with AIDS. JAMA 259:1333–1337, 1988

Masand PS, Tesar GE: Use of stimulants in the medically ill. Psychiatr Clin North Am 19:515–547, 1996

Masand P[S], Pickett P, Murray GB: Psychostimulants for secondary depression in medical illness. Psychosomatics 32:203–208, 1991

Massie MJ, Holland JC: Depression and the cancer patient. J Clin Psychiatry 51 (suppl 7):12–17, 1990

Matthews WS, Barabas G: Suicide and epilepsy: a review of the literature. Psychosomatics 2:515–524, 1981

Mayberg HS, Starkstein SE, Sadzot B, et al: Selective hypometabolism in the inferior frontal lobe in depressed patients with Parkinson's disease. Ann Neurol 28:57–64, 1990

Mayberg HS, Starkstein SE, Peyser CE, et al: Paralimbic frontal lobe hypometabolism in depression associated with Huntington's disease. Neurology 42:1791–1797, 1992

Mayeux R: Depression in the patient with Parkinson's disease. J Clin Psychiatry 51 (suppl):20–23, 1990

Mayeux R, Stern Y, Rosen J, et al: Depression, intellectual impairment, and Parkinson disease. Neurology 31:645–650, 1981

Mayeux R, Stern Y, Cote C, et al: Altered serotonin metabolism in depressed patients with Parkinson's disease. Neurology 34:642–646, 1984

Mayeux R, Stern Y, Williams JB, et al: Clinical and biochemical features of depression in Parkinson's disease. Am J Psychiatry 143:756–759, 1986

McAllister TW: Overview: pseudodementia. Am J Psychiatry 140:528–533, 1983

McDaniel JS, Musselman DL, Porter MR, et al: Depression in patients with cancer: diagnosis, biology, and treatment. Arch Gen Psychiatry 52:89–99, 1995

McDaniel JS, Musselman DL, Nemeroff CB: Cancer and depression: theory and treatment. Psychiatric Annals 27:360–364, 1997

Mendez MF, Cummings JL, Benson DF: Depression in epilepsy: significance and phenomenology. Arch Neurol 43:766–770, 1986

Miller AH, Spencer RL, McEwen BS, et al: Depression, adrenal steroids, and the immune system. Ann Med 25:481–487, 1993

Minden SL, Schiffer RB: Affective disorders in multiple sclerosis. Arch Neurol 47:98–104, 1990

Minden SL, Orav J, Reich P: Depression in multiple sclerosis. Gen Hosp Psychiatry 9:426–434, 1987

Mindham RH: Psychiatric symptoms in parkinsonism. J Neurol Neurosurg Psychiatry 33:188–191, 1970

Montgomery SA: Venlafaxine: a new dimension in antidepressant pharmacotherapy. J Clin Psychiatry 54:119–126, 1993

Morris PL, Robinson RG, Andrzejewski P, et al: Association of depression with 10 year post-stroke mortality. Am J Psychiatry 150:124–129, 1993a

Morris PL, Robinson RG, Samuels J: Depression, introversion, and mortality following stroke. Aust N Z J Psychiatry 27:443–449, 1993b

Moss AJ, Robinson J: Clinical features of the idiopathic long QT syndrome. Circulation 85 (suppl):140–144, 1992

Mueller TI, Brown RA, Recupero PR: Depression and substance abuse. Rhode Island Medicine 76:409–413, 1993

Munroe A: Some familial and social factors in depressive illness. Br J Psychiatry 112:429–441, 1966

Murray GB, Shea VS, Conn DK: Electroconvulsive therapy for post-stroke depression. J Clin Psychiatry 47:258–260, 1986

Musselman DL, Tomer A, Manatunga AK, et al: Exaggerated platelet reactivity in major depression. Am J Psychiatry 153:1313–1317, 1996

Musselman DL, Evans DL, Nemeroff CB: The relationship of depression to cardiovascular disease: epidemiology, biology, and treatment. Arch Gen Psychiatry 55:580–592, 1998

Navia BA, Cho E-S, Petito CK, et al: The AIDS dementia complex, II: neuropathology. Ann Neurol 19:525–535, 1986

Nemeroff CB: Augmentation regimens for depression. J Clin Psychiatry 52 (suppl 5):21–27, 1991

Nemeroff CB: Paroxetine: an overview of the efficacy and safety of a new selective serotonin reuptake inhibitor in the treatment of depression. J Clin Psychopharmacol 13 (suppl 2):18–22, 1993

Nemeroff CB, Musselman DL, Evans DL: Depression and cardiac disease. Depress Anxiety 8 (suppl 1):71–79, 1998

Newport DJ, Nemeroff CB: Assessment and treatment of depression in the cancer patient. J Psychosom Res 45:215–237, 1998

Nierenberg AA, Amsterdam JD: Treatment resistant depression: definition and treatment approaches. J Clin Psychiatry 51 (suppl 6):39–47, 1990

Nierenberg DW, Semprebon M: The central nervous system serotonin syndrome. Clin Pharmacol Ther 53:84–88, 1993

Nobler M, Roose S: Differential response to antidepressants in melancholic and severe depression. Psychiatric Annals 28:84–88, 1998

O'Donnell K, Chung JY: The diagnosis of major depression in end-stage renal disease. Psychother Psychosom 66:38–43, 1997

Ordas DM, Labbate LA: Routine screening of thyroid function in patients hospitalized for major depression or dysthymia. Ann Clin Psychiatry 7:161–165, 1995

Ottson SV, Wu D, Joffe RT, et al: Inhibition by fluoxetine of cytochrome $P_{450}2D6$ activity. Clin Pharmacol Ther 53:401–409, 1993

Palinkas LA, Barrett-Connor E, Wingard DL: Type 2 diabetes and depressive symptoms in older adults: a population based study. Diabet Med 8:532–539, 1991

Palmer FJ: The clinical manifestations of primary hyperparathyroidism. Compr Ther 9:56–64, 1983

Pascual-Leone A, Tarazona F, Keenan J, et al: Transcranial magnetic stimulation and neuroplasticity. Neuropsychologia 37:207–217, 1999

Pascualy M, Veith RC: Depression as an adverse drug reaction, in Aging and Clinical Practice: Depression and Coexisting Disease. Edited by Robinson RG, Rabins PV. New York, Igaku-Shoin, 1989, pp 132–151

Passik SD, Breitbart WS: Depression in patients with pancreatic carcinoma. Cancer 78:615–626, 1996

Patten SB, Lamarre CJ: Can drug-induced depressions be identified by their clinical features? Can J Psychiatry 37:213–215, 1992

Paykel ES, Flemenger R, Watson JP: Psychiatric side effects of antihypertensive drugs other than reserpine. J Clin Psychopharmacol 2:14–39, 1982

Perry SW, Tross S: Psychiatric problems of AIDS inpatients in the New York Hospital: preliminary report. Public Health Rep 99:200–205, 1984

Perry S[W], Jacobsberg LB, Fishman B, et al: Psychiatric diagnosis before serological testing for the human immunodeficiency virus. Am J Psychiatry 147:89–93, 1990

Petrie WM, Maffucci RJ, Woosley RL: Propranolol and depression. Am J Psychiatry 139:92–93, 1982

Pollack MH, Rosenbaum JF, Cassem NH: Propranolol and depression revisited: three cases and a review. J Nerv Ment Dis 173:118–119, 1985

Pope HG, Katz DL: Psychiatric and medical effects of anabolic-androgenic steroid use: a controlled study of 160 athletes. Arch Gen Psychiatry 51:375–382, 1994

Popkin MK, Callies AL, Colon EA: A framework for the study of medical depression. Psychosomatics 28:27–33, 1987

Price RW, Brew B, Sidtis J, et al: The brain in AIDS: central nervous system HIV-1 infection and AIDS dementia complex. Science 239:586–592, 1988

Prisant LM, Spruill WJ, Fincham JE, et al: Depression associated with antihypertensive drugs. J Fam Pract 33:481–485, 1991

Rabins PV, Brooks BR, O'Donnell P, et al: Structural brain correlates of emotional disorder in multiple sclerosis. Brain 109:585–597, 1986

Rabkin JG, Harrison WM: Effect of imipramine on depression and immune status in a sample of men with HIV infection. Am J Psychiatry 147:495–497, 1990

Rabkin JG, Rabkin R, Wagner G: Effects of fluoxetine on mood and immune status in depressed patients with HIV illness. J Clin Psychiatry 55:92–97, 1994a

Rabkin JG, Wagner G, Rabkin R: Effects of sertraline on mood and immune status in patients with major depression and HIV illness: an open trial. J Clin Psychiatry 55:433–439, 1994b

Rauch SL, Stern TA, Zusman RM: Neuropsychiatric considerations in the treatment of hypertension. Int J Psychiatry Med 21:291–308, 1991

Reding MJ, Orto LA, Winter SW, et al: Antidepressant therapy after stroke—a double blind trial. Arch Neurol 43:763–765, 1986

Reid LD, McFarland BH, Johnson RE, et al: Beta-blockers and depression: the more the murkier? Ann Pharmacother 32: 699–708, 1998

Richardson JL, Shelton DR, Krailo M, et al: The effect of compliance with treatment on survival among patients with hematological malignancies. J Clin Oncol 8:356–364, 1990

Rifkin A: Depression in physically ill patients. Postgrad Med 92:147–154, 1992

Robertson MM, Trimble MR: Depressive illness in patients with epilepsy: a review. Epilepsia 24:190–196, 1983

Robins LN, Helzer JE, Weissman MM, et al: Lifetime prevalence of specific psychiatric disorders in three sites. Arch Gen Psychiatry 41:949–958, 1984

Robinson RG: Neuropsychiatric consequences of stroke. Annu Rev Med 48:217–229, 1997

Robinson RG, Price TR: Post-stroke depressive disorders: a follow-up study of 103 patients. Stroke 13:635–641, 1982

Robinson RG, Starr LB, Kubos KL, et al: A two-year longitudinal study of post-stroke mood disorders: findings during the initial evaluation. Stroke 14:736–741, 1983

Robinson RG, Kubos KL, Starr LB, et al: Mood disorders in stroke patients—importance of lesion location. Brain 107:81–93, 1984a

Robinson RG, Starr LB, Price TR: A two year longitudinal study of mood disorders following stroke: prevalence and duration at six months follow-up. Br J Psychiatry 144:256–262, 1984b

Robinson RG, Lipsey JR, Price TR: Diagnosis and clinical management of post-stroke depression. Psychosomatics 26: 769–778, 1985

Robinson RG, Bolduc P, Price TR: A two-year longitudinal study of post-stroke depression: diagnosis and outcome at one and two year follow-up. Stroke 18:837–843, 1987

Robinson RG, Morris PL, Federoff JP: Depression in cerebrovascular disease. J Clin Psychiatry 51 (suppl 7):26–31, 1990

Rodin G: Expressive psychotherapy in the medically ill: resistances and possibilities. Int J Psychiatry Med 14:99–108, 1984

Rodin G, Voshart K: Depression in the medically ill: an overview. Am J Psychiatry 143:696–705, 1986

Rodin G, Craven J, Littlefield C: Introduction, in Depression in the Medically Ill: An Integrated Approach. New York, Brunner/Mazel, 1991, p xi

Roose SP, Dalack GW, Glassman AH, et al: Cardiovascular effects of bupropion in depressed patients with heart disease. Am J Psychiatry 148:512–516, 1991

Rost K, Smith R, Matthews DB, et al: The deliberate misdiagnosis of major depression in primary care. Arch Fam Med 3:333–337, 1994

Rounsaville BJ, Weissman MM, Crits-Christoph K, et al: Diagnosis and symptoms of depression in opiate addicts. Arch Gen Psychiatry 39:151–156, 1982

Rowland DL, Myers L, Culver A, et al: Bupropion and sexual function: a placebo-controlled prospective study on diabetic men with erectile dysfunction. J Clin Psychopharmacol 17:350–357, 1997

Rummans TA: Medical indications for electroconvulsive therapy. Psychiatric Annals 23:27–32, 1993

Rundell JR, Hall RC: Past mental health or substance use treatment history and psychiatric differential diagnosis in consultation-liaison patients. Psychosomatics 38:262–268, 1997

Rundell JR, Wise MG: Causes of organic mood disorder. J Neuropsychiatry Clin Neurosci 1:398–400, 1989

Rupprecht R, Lesch KP: Psychoneuroendocrine research in depression, I: hormone levels of different neuroendocrine axes and the dexamethasone suppression test. Journal of Neural Transmission General Section 75:167–178, 1989

Rush A, Giles D, Schlesser M, et al: The dexamethasone suppression test in patients with mood disorders. J Clin Psychiatry 57:470–484, 1996

Russell J: Relatively low doses of cisapride in the treatment of nausea in patients treated with venlafaxine for treatment-refractory depression. J Clin Psychopharmacol 16:35–37, 1996

Sackeim HA, Prudic J, Devanand DP, et al: The impact of medication resistance and continuation medication on relapse following response to electroconvulsive therapy in major depression. J Clin Psychopharmacol 10:96–104, 1990

Sano M, Stern Y, Williams J, et al: Coexisting dementia and depression in Parkinson's disease. Arch Neurol 46:1284–1286, 1989

Satel SL, Nelson JC: Stimulants in the treatment of depression: a critical overview. J Clin Psychiatry 50:241–249, 1989

Satel SL, Price LH, Palumbo JM, et al: Clinical phenomenology and neurobiology of cocaine abstinence: a prospective inpatient study. Am J Psychiatry 148:1712–1716, 1991

Schaerf FW, Miller RR, Lipsey JR, et al: ECT for major depression in four patients infected with human immunodeficiency virus. Am J Psychiatry 146:782–784, 1989

Schiffer RB, Babigian HM: Behavioral disorders in multiple sclerosis, temporal lobe epilepsy, and amyotrophic lateral sclerosis. Arch Neurol 41:1067–1069, 1984

Schiffer RB, Wineman NM: Antidepressant pharmacotherapy of depression associated with multiple sclerosis. Am J Psychiatry 147:1493–1497, 1990

Schiffer RB, Caine ED, Bamford KA, et al: Depressive episodes in patients with multiple sclerosis. Am J Psychiatry 140: 1498–1500, 1983

Schildkraut JJ, Green AI, Mooney JJ: Mood disorders: biochemical aspects, in Comprehensive Textbook of Psychiatry/V, 5th Edition, Vol 1. Edited by Kaplan HI, Sadock BJ. Baltimore, MD, Williams & Wilkins, 1989, pp 868–879

Schleifer SJ, Macari-Hinson MM, Coyle DA, et al: The nature and course of depression following myocardial infarction. Arch Intern Med 149:1785–1789, 1989

Schleifer SJ, Slater WR, Macari-Hinson MM, et al: Digitalis and β-blocking agents: effects on depression following myocardial infarction. Am Heart J 121:1397–1402, 1991

Schleifer SJ, Keller SE, Bartlett JA, et al: Immunity in young adults with major depressive disorder. Am J Psychiatry 153:477–482, 1996

Schmitz EB, Moriarty, Costa DC, et al: Psychiatric profiles and patterns of cerebral blood flow in focal epilepsy: interactions between depression, obsessionality, and perfusion related to the laterality of the epilepsy. J Neurol Neurosurg Psychiatry 62:458–463, 1997

Schoenfeld M, Myers RH, Cupples LA, et al: Increased rate of suicide among patients with Huntington's disease. J Neurol Neurosurg Psychiatry 47:1283–1287, 1984

Schubert DS, Foliart RH: Increased depression in multiple sclerosis patients: a meta-analysis. Psychosomatics 34:124–130, 1993

Schuckit M[A]: Alcoholic patients with secondary depression. Am J Psychiatry 140:711–714, 1983a

Schuckit M[A]: Alcoholism and other psychiatric disorders. Hospital and Community Psychiatry 34:1022–1027, 1983b

Schuckit MA, Tipp JE, Bergman M, et al: Comparison of induced and independent major depressive disorders in 2,945 alcoholics. Am J Psychiatry 154:948–957, 1997

Searight HR, McLaren LA: Behavioral and psychiatric aspects of HIV infection. Am Fam Physician 55:1227–1237, 1997

Selvin BL: Electroconvulsive therapy—1987. Anesthesiology 67:367–385, 1987

Shapiro PA, Lidagoster L, Glassman AH: Depression and heart disease. Psychiatric Annals 27:347–352, 1997

Shelman KI, Walker SE, MacKenzie S, et al: Dietary restriction, tyramine, and the use of monoamine oxidase inhibitors. J Clin Psychopharmacol 9:397–402, 1989

Silverstone PH: Depression increases mortality and morbidity in acute life threatening medical illness. J Psychosom Res 34:651–657, 1990

Silverstone PH: Concise assessment for depression (CAD): a brief screening approach to depression in the medically ill. J Psychosom Res 41:161–170, 1996

Silverstone PH, Lemay T, Elliott J, et al: The prevalence of major depressive disorder and low self-esteem in medical inpatients. Can J Psychiatry 41:67–74, 1996

Smith BD, Salzman C: Do benzodiazepines cause depression? Hospital and Community Psychiatry 42:1101–1102, 1991

Smith GC, Clarke DM, Handrinos D, et al: Consultation-liaison psychiatrists management of depression. Psychosomatics 39:244–252, 1998

Sonino N, Fava GA, Raffi AR, et al: Clinical correlates of major depression in Cushing's disease. Psychopathology 31:302–306, 1998

Spiegel D: Can psychotherapy prolong cancer survival? Psychosomatics 31:361–366, 1990

Spitzer RL, Endicott J, Robins E: Research diagnostic criteria: rationale and reliability. Arch Gen Psychiatry 35:773–782, 1978

Starkstein SE, Preziosi TJ, Bolduc PL, et al: Depression in Parkinson's disease. J Nerv Ment Dis 178:27–31, 1990

Stein G, Bernadt M: Lithium augmentation therapy in tricyclic-resistant depression: a controlled trial using lithium in low and normal doses. Br J Psychiatry 162:634–640, 1993

Stenager EN, Stenager E, Koch-Henriksen N: Suicide and multiple sclerosis: an epidemiological investigation. J Neurol Neurosurg Psychiatry 55:542–545, 1992

St. Goar WT: Gastrointestinal symptoms as a clue to the diagnosis of primary hyperparathyroidism: a review of forty-five cases. Ann Intern Med 46:102–118, 1957

Stocky A: Ranitidine and depression. Aust N Z J Psychiatry 25:415–418, 1991

Stoudemire A: Expanding psychopharmacologic treatment options for the depressed medical patient. Psychosomatics 36:519–526, 1995

Strang RR: Imipramine in treatment of parkinsonism: a double-blind placebo study. BMJ 3:33–34, 1965

Sullivan MJ, Reesor K, Mikail S, et al: The treatment of depression in chronic low back pain: review and recommendations. Pain 50:5–13, 1992

Sutor B, Rummans TA, Jowsey SG, et al: Major depression in medically ill patients. Mayo Clin Proc 73:329–337, 1998

Taylor DP, Carter RB, Eison AS, et al: Pharmacology and neurochemistry of nefazodone, a novel antidepressant drug. J Clin Psychiatry 56 (suppl 6):3–11, 1995

Taylor M: Catatonia: a review of a behavioral neurologic syndrome. Neuropsychiatry Neuropsychol Behav Neurol 3:48–72, 1990

Tennant FS, Sagherian AA: Double-blind comparison of amantadine and bromocriptine mesylate for ambulatory withdrawal from cocaine dependence. Arch Intern Med 147:109–112, 1987

Thase ME: Effects of venlafaxine on blood pressure: a meta-analysis of original data from 3744 depressed patients. J Clin Psychiatry 59:502–508, 1998

Thase ME, Blomgren SL, Birkett MA, et al: Fluoxetine treatment of patients with major depressive disorder who failed initial treatment with sertraline. J Clin Psychiatry 58:16–21, 1997

Tiller JW, Schweitzer I: Benzodiazepines: depressants or antidepressants? Drugs 44:165–169, 1992

Valentine AD, Meyers CA, Kling MA, et al: Mood and cognitive effects of interferon-alpha therapy. Semin Oncol 25:39–47, 1998

Von Korff M, Ormel J, Katon W, et al: Disability and depression among high utilizers of health care: a longitudinal analysis. Arch Gen Psychiatry 49:91–100, 1992

Wagner KD: Major depression and anxiety disorders associated with Norplant. J Clin Psychiatry 57:152–157, 1996

Walker PW, Cole JQ, Gardiner EA, et al: Improvement in fluoxetine-associated sexual dysfunction in patients switched to bupropion. J Clin Psychiatry 54:459–465, 1993

Weintraub M, Evans P: Bupropion: a chemically and pharmacologically unique antidepressant. Hospital Formulary 24:254–259, 1989

Weisse CS: Depression and immunocompetence: a review of the literature. Psychol Bull 111:475–489, 1992

Wheatley DP, van Moffaert M, Timmerman L, et al: Mirtazapine: efficacy and tolerability in comparison with fluoxetine in patients with moderate to severe major depressive disorder. Mirtazapine-Fluoxetine Study Group. J Clin Psychiatry 59:306–312, 1998

Whitehouse PJ, Friedland RP, Strauss ME: Neuropsychiatric aspects of degenerative dementias associated with motor dysfunction, in The American Psychiatric Press Textbook of Neuropsychiatry, 2nd Edition. Edited by Yudofsky SC, Hales RE. Washington, DC, American Psychiatric Press, 1992, pp 585–604

Whitlock FA, Siskind MM: Depression as a major symptom of multiple sclerosis. J Neurol Neurosurg Psychiatry 43:861–865, 1980

Widmer J, Mouthon D, Raffin Y, et al: Weak association between blood sodium, potassium, and calcium and intensity of symptoms in major depressed patients. Neuropsychobiology 36:164–171, 1997

Williams JB, Rabkin JG, Remien RH, et al: Multidisciplinary baseline assessment of homosexual men with and without human immunodeficiency virus infection, II: standardized clinical assessment of current lifetime psychopathology. Arch Gen Psychiatry 48:124–130, 1991

Winokur G: The concept of a secondary depression and its relationship to comorbidity. Psychiatr Clin North Am 123:567–583, 1990

Wise MG, Rundell JR: Concise Guide to Consultation Psychiatry, 2nd Edition. Washington, DC, American Psychiatric Press, 1994, p 3

Wragg RE, Jeste D: Overview of depression and psychosis in Alzheimer's disease. Am J Psychiatry 146:577–587, 1989

Yates WR, Wesner RB, Thompson R: Organic mood disorder: a valid psychiatry consultation diagnosis? J Affect Disord 22:37–42, 1991

Zelnik T: Depressive effects of drugs, in Presentations of Depression: Depressive Symptoms in Medical and Other Psychiatric Disorders. Edited by Cameron OG. New York, Wiley, 1987, pp 355–399

Zubenko GS, Mossy J, Kopp U: Neurochemical correlates of major depression in primary dementia. Arch Neurol 47:209–214, 1990

18

Mania

J. Stephen McDaniel, M.D.

Sanjay M. Sharma, M.D.

Patients with primary and secondary mania are seen frequently by consultation-liaison psychiatrists, thus requiring a thorough understanding of medical and toxic etiologies of mood syndromes and associated treatment strategies. In this chapter, we address the diagnosis, epidemiology, pathophysiology, and treatment of secondary mania.

DEFINITIONS

In a *manic episode*, as defined by DSM-IV-TR (American Psychiatric Association 2000), the essential feature is a distinct period lasting at least 1 week during which the predominant mood is either elevated, expansive, or irritable. Associated symptoms are outlined in Table 18–1. *Hypomania* is an episode in which the disturbance is not severe enough to cause marked impairment in social or occupational functioning or to require hospitalization, and delusions are absent. Number of criteria is not a distinguishing characteristic of either a hypomanic or a manic episode.

Manic episodes are sometimes phases of primary bipolar disorder (manic-depressive illness) or secondary to a particular medical or toxic etiology (i.e., secondary mania). *Bipolar disorder* is a syndrome characterized by one or more manic episodes usually accompanied by one or more major depressive episodes. Some individuals have seasonal patterns of bipolar disorder, in which the onset is temporally related to a particular 60-day period. Some patients in their manic phase have considerable dysphoria or depressive symptoms—so-called mixed states, often accompanied by psychomotor pressure, psychosis, and irritable aggression (Cassidy et al. 1998). Moreover, for bipolar patients who show frequent cycling between manic and depressive episodes (e.g., four or

more episodes in a year), a modifier of "rapid cycling" is used for classification.

Cyclothymia is a chronic mood syndrome characterized by alternating hypomanic episodes and periods of depressed mood. Symptoms that occur during phases of this disorder are not of sufficient severity or duration to meet the criteria for a major depressive or a manic episode; therefore, they also do not meet criteria for bipolar disorder. Some researchers have suggested that cyclothymia is an early manifestation of bipolar disorder that predisposes patients to secondary mania or depression (Winokur and Clayton 1986).

Secondary mania is a diagnosis of importance to consultation-liaison psychiatrists. This condition resembles primary mania; however, it occurs secondary to specific identifiable medical or toxic factors. According to DSM-IV-TR, secondary mania is called "mood disorder due to a general medical condition, with manic features" (Table 18–2), when caused by a medical illness, or "substance-induced mood disorder, with manic features" (Table 18–3), when caused by substance intoxication or withdrawal (American Psychiatric Association 2000). Like primary mania, the essential feature of this syndrome is a prominent and persistent elevated or expansive mood. According to DSM-IV-TR, a secondary mania diagnosis is not made in the context of delirium or dementia; however, mild cognitive impairment is often observed.

EPIDEMIOLOGY

Weissman et al. (1988) examined the Epidemiologic Catchment Area (Eaton et al. 1981) data to calculate the lifetime prevalence for primary bipolar disorder. For this study, bipolar disorder was defined as having a history of

---

TABLE 18–1. DSM-IV-TR criteria for manic episode

A. A distinct period of abnormally and persistently elevated, expansive, or irritable mood, lasting at least 1 week (or any duration if hospitalization is necessary).

B. During the period of mood disturbance, three (or more) of the following symptoms have persisted (four if the mood is only irritable) and have been present to a significant degree:

  (1) inflated self-esteem or grandiosity
  (2) decreased need for sleep (e.g., feels rested after only 3 hours of sleep)
  (3) more talkative than usual or pressure to keep talking
  (4) flight of ideas or subjective experience that thoughts are racing
  (5) distractibility (i.e., attention too easily drawn to unimportant or irrelevant external stimuli)
  (6) increase in goal-directed activity (either socially, at work or school, or sexually) or psychomotor agitation
  (7) excessive involvement in pleasurable activities that have a high potential for painful consequences (e.g., engaging in unrestrained buying sprees, sexual indiscretions, or foolish business investments)

C. The symptoms do not meet criteria for a mixed episode.

D. The mood disturbance is sufficiently severe to cause marked impairment in occupational functioning or in usual social activities or relationships with others, or to necessitate hospitalization to prevent harm to self or others, or there are psychotic features.

E. The symptoms are not due to the direct physiological effects of a substance (e.g., a drug of abuse, a medication, or other treatment) or a general medical condition (e.g., hyperthyroidism).

  Note: Manic-like episodes that are clearly caused by somatic antidepressant treatment (e.g., medication, electroconvulsive therapy, light therapy) should not count toward a diagnosis of bipolar I disorder.

TABLE 18–2. DSM-IV-TR diagnostic criteria for mood disorder due to a general medical condition

---

A. A prominent and persistent disturbance in mood predominates in the clinical picture and is characterized by either (or both) of the following:

  (1) depressed mood or markedly diminished interest or pleasure in all, or almost all, activities
  (2) elevated, expansive, or irritable mood

B. There is evidence from the history, physical examination, or laboratory findings that the disturbance is the direct physiological consequence of a general medical condition.

C. The disturbance is not better accounted for by another mental disorder (e.g., adjustment disorder with depressed mood in response to the stress of having a general medical condition).

D. The disturbance does not occur exclusively during the course of a delirium.

E. The symptoms cause clinically significant distress or impairment in social, occupational, or other important areas of functioning.

  Specify type:

    With depressive features: if the predominant mood is depressed but the full criteria are not met for a major depressive episode
    With major depressive–like episode: if the full criteria are met (except Criterion D) for a major depressive episode
    With manic features: if the predominant mood is elevated, euphoric, or irritable
    With mixed features: if the symptoms of both mania and depression are present but neither predominates
    Coding note: Include the name of the general medical condition on Axis I, e.g., 293.83 mood disorder due to hypothyroidism, with depressive features; also code the general medical condition on Axis III (see Appendix G for codes).
    Coding note: If depressive symptoms occur as part of a preexisting vascular dementia, indicate the depressive symptoms by coding the appropriate subtype, i.e., 290.43 vascular dementia, with depressed mood.

---

any manic episode, which retrospectively could have included secondary mania or the mania of primary bipolar disorder. A lifetime prevalence of 1.2% was calculated, and a similar rate was documented in a subsequent international study (Weissman et al. 1996). A lifetime prevalence of 1.6% was calculated in the National Comorbidity Survey (Kessler et al. 1994).

Goodwin and Jamison (1990) found the annual risk of having a manic episode to be 0.24%–0.77% in the general United States population. Unfortunately, available data reflect findings in the general population; therefore, translating these numbers to include medically ill populations is difficult. No studies to date have examined the epidemiology of secondary manic states in a population-

---

TABLE 18–3. DSM-IV-TR diagnostic criteria for substance-induced mood disorder

A. A prominent and persistent disturbance in mood predominates in the clinical picture and is characterized by either (or both) of the following:

    (1) depressed mood or markedly diminished interest or pleasure in all, or almost all, activities

    (2) elevated, expansive, or irritable mood

B. There is evidence from the history, physical examination, or laboratory findings of either (1) or (2):

    (1) the symptoms in Criterion A developed during, or within a month of, substance intoxication or withdrawal

    (2) medication use is etiologically related to the disturbance

C. The disturbance is not better accounted for by a mood disorder that is not substance induced. Evidence that the symptoms are better accounted for by a mood disorder that is not substance induced might include the following: the symptoms precede the onset of the substance use (or medication use); the symptoms persist for a substantial period of time (e.g., about a month) after the cessation of acute withdrawal or severe intoxication or are substantially in excess of what would be expected given the type or amount of the substance used or the duration of use; or there is other evidence that suggests the existence of an independent non-substance-induced mood disorder (e.g., a history of recurrent major depressive episodes).

D. The disturbance does not occur exclusively during the course of a delirium.

E. The symptoms cause clinically significant distress or impairment in social, occupational, or other important areas of functioning.

    Note: This diagnosis should be made instead of a diagnosis of substance intoxication or substance withdrawal only when the mood symptoms are in excess of those usually associated with the intoxication or withdrawal syndrome and when the symptoms are sufficiently severe to warrant independent clinical attention.

Code [Specific substance]–induced mood disorder:

    (291.89 alcohol; 292.84 amphetamine [or amphetamine-like substance]; 292.84 cocaine; 292.84 hallucinogen; 292.84 inhalant; 292.84 opioid; 292.84 phencyclidine [or phencyclidine-like substance]; 292.84 sedative, hypnotic, or anxiolytic; 292.84 other [or unknown] substance)

Specify type:

    With depressive features: if the predominant mood is depressed
    With manic features: if the predominant mood is elevated, euphoric, or irritable
    With mixed features: if symptoms of both mania and depression are present and neither predominates

Specify if:

    With onset during intoxication: if the criteria are met for intoxication with the substance and the symptoms develop during the intoxication syndrome
    With onset during withdrawal: if criteria are met for withdrawal from the substance and the symptoms develop during, or shortly after, a withdrawal syndrome

---

based sample with a standardized diagnostic instrument. However, in their retrospective chart review of 755 patients evaluated an inpatient psychiatric consultation-liaison service in a general hospital over a 1-year period, Rundell and Wise (1989) found that 13 of 15 (87%) patients identified as having mania met diagnostic criteria for secondary mania.

Several associated features and risk factors have been identified for primary bipolar disorder. Understanding these factors can be helpful in differentiating primary and secondary mania. Patients with primary bipolar disorder have a mean age at onset of 30 years (Goodwin and Jamison 1990), and with increasing age, the interval between manic episodes tends to decrease and duration of episodes tends to increase (Krauthammer and Klerman 1978).

Women are at increased risk for recurrence during the postpartum period (L. S. Cohen et al. 1995). Initial bipolar manic episodes rarely occur after age 50 (Wise and Rundell 1994). A positive family history of mood disorder is associated with earlier age at onset of the initial manic episode among bipolar patients (Stone 1989), and earlier age at onset is associated with a higher lifetime number of manic episodes (Mendlewicz et al. 1972). Although early reports suggested differences in prevalence among ethnic and socioeconomic categories, current evidence argues against sociodemographic risk factors for developing bipolar disorder.

Although precise genetic mechanisms have eluded investigators, bipolar disorder occurs at much higher rates in first-degree biological relatives of bipolar patients than in the general population. Recent research suggests that chromosome 18 carries the genetic risk for bipolar disorder, and the tryptophan hydroxylase gene may be involved as well (Bellivier et al. 1998; Berrettini et al. 1997). Among primary bipolar patients, 52% can be expected to have a parent with a mood disorder history, 54% have two generations of affected family members, and 63% have parents or an extended family member with a mood disorder (Winokur and Clayton 1986). Large-scale national research collaborations funded through the National Institute of Mental Health are under way to study further the complex genetic mechanisms of bipolar disorder (Simpson and DePaulo 1998), which may have implications regarding individuals who are vulnerable to developing secondary mania.

CLINICAL FEATURES

Manic syndromes in medical-surgical patients may be exacerbations of underlying bipolar disorder or secondary mania of new onset. The essential clinical feature of a manic episode is a distinctly expansive, elevated, or irritable mood. This disturbance is sufficiently severe to cause impairment in occupational or social functioning or to require hospitalization to prevent harm to oneself or others. In addition, DSM-IV-TR lists seven other signs or symptoms (Table 18–1). Frequently, the manic person does not recognize that he or she is ill and resists treatment. When delusions or hallucinations are present, the content usually is consistent with the mania (mood-congruent).

Manic episodes often develop in stages, beginning with mild hypomania, progressing through moderate manic symptoms, including grandiose or paranoid delusions, to severe mania accompanied by profound psychosis. Manic episodes develop more abruptly than depressive episodes. The time frame to progression to a full manic syndrome varies from days to hours. Estimates of the average duration of untreated manic episodes in primary bipolar disorder range from 4 to 13 months (Goodwin and Jamison 1990). The median lifetime number of affective (depressive plus manic) episodes in a bipolar patient is 9 (Wise and Rundell 1994); bipolar manic episode duration is fairly stable across consecutive episodes, decreasing slightly if 10 or more episodes occur (Angst 1981). A sizable literature has examined the possible role of psychosocial or physical stress in precipitating episodes of bipolar disorder; however, it is now generally accepted that environmental conditions contribute more to the timing of an episode than to underlying vulnerability (Roy et al. 1985). Sleep reduction may be the common denominator in many of the environmental stresses that precipitate mania (Wehr et al. 1987).

The course and prognosis of secondary mania have not been well defined. As in primary bipolar mania, manic symptoms caused by medical illness or a medication can occur rapidly within hours or days; secondary mania is not generally believed to be a chronic illness, as is primary bipolar disorder. Once the etiology is determined and treated, secondary mania usually resolves. However, some secondary manic syndromes, such as those attributed to the human immunodeficiency virus (HIV) or structural brain insults, can become chronic because the underlying organic pathology cannot be eradicated. In determining a differential diagnosis, a history of bipolar disorder is believed to increase the risk for secondary mania. Toxic and metabolic exacerbations of underlying mood disorders occur frequently and can occur simultaneously with a primary mood disorder. Even a patient whose primary bipolar disorder is successfully managed with a mood stabilizer can develop secondary mania from medical or toxic etiologies (e.g., stroke, steroids).

PATHOPHYSIOLOGY

Interest in the neuropathology and anatomy of mania grew out of the observation that lesions of the central nervous system (CNS) are frequently accompanied by signs of abnormal cognitive, behavioral, or motor functioning. For example, structural CNS lesions are associated with secondary depression and mania. Studies that have examined the prevalence of secondary mania in patients with structural CNS lesions are outlined in Table 18–4. Lesions in the limbic-related areas of the nondominant hemisphere have been implicated in mania (Cummings and Mendez 1984; Robinson et al. 1988a) and usually occur in the orbitofrontal and basotemporal cortices, the head of the caudate, and the thalamus.

Lesions in the frontal, limbic, and temporal lobes are more frequently associated with mood disorders than are lesions in other brain regions. Left-sided lesions are often associated with increased relative risk for depression, and right-sided lesions are associated with risk for mania (Cummings 1986; Starkstein and Robinson 1989). However, the left-right differences may be reversed in regions closer to the posterior poles (Goodwin and Jamison 1990). Thus, in right-handed patients, depression risk is relatively increased by left frontotemporal or right parietooccipital lesions, whereas manic symptoms are more likely to follow right frontotemporal or left parietooccipital lesions.

TABLE 18–4. Prevalence studies of secondary mania and hypomania

Investigators	No. of patients	Lesion type/location	Comments
Feuchtwanger 1923	400	Gunshot wounds, frontal lobes, in 200 patients	Euphoria more common in frontal lobe injuries
Kolodny 1928	38	Tumor, temporal lobes	8 patients with "depressed euphoria"
Kleist 1931	300	Trauma, frontal lobes, in 105 patients	Euphoria more common with orbitofrontal damage
Minski 1933	58	Tumor, frontal and temporal lobes	7 "excited" patients (5 had frontal and 2 had temporal tumors)
Strauss and Keschner 1935	85	Tumor, frontal lobes	5 manic or hypomanic patients
Keschner et al. 1936	110	Tumor, temporal lobes	6 hypomanic patients; depression more common with left-sided tumors
Flor-Henry 1969	100	Psychomotor epilepsy, temporal lobes	Bipolar symptoms associated with right-sided lesions
Gainotti 1972	160	Different lesion types; left hemisphere in 80, right hemisphere in 80	Indifference; euphoria more frequent with right-sided lesions
Sackeim et al. 1982	19	Hemispherectomy; left hemispherectomy in 5, right hemispherectomy in 14	12 of 14 with right hemispherectomy showed euphoria
Shukla et al. 1987	20	Trauma, different regions	Manic episodes were irritable, not euphoric
Starkstein et al. 1988b	12	Different lesion types; left hemisphere in 1, right hemisphere in 7, bilateral in 4	All developed mania; damage to structures functionally connected to orbitofrontal cortex
Robinson et al. 1988b	17	Tumor or trauma, different regions	All developed mania associated with areas in right hemisphere connected to limbic system
Starkstein et al. 1989	93	Stroke, right hemisphere	19 developed "undue cheerfulness"
Starkstein et al. 1991	19	Vascular or neoplastic lesion or trauma, different regions	Patients with "unipolar mania" had higher frequency of cortical involvement (mainly right basotemporal and orbitofrontal cortices), whereas patients with "bipolar mania" had more subcortical lesions
Jorge et al. 1993	66	Trauma, different regions	6 developed mania; significant association between diagnosis of mania and lesions in temporal basal polar location; duration of mania was brief, lasting approximately 2 months

Source. Adapted from Goodwin FK, Jamison KR: *Manic-Depressive Illness.* New York, Oxford University Press, 1990, p. 505. Copyright 1990, Oxford University Press. Used with permission.

Because not every patient with right-hemisphere limbic lesions develops secondary mania, premorbid risk factors are believed to play a key role. Two such risk factors were identified through comparison studies—genetic predisposition and brain atrophy. In a study that compared patients with secondary mania, patients with secondary major depression, and patients with no mood disturbance, manic patients had a significantly higher frequency of mood disorders in their family than did patients in the other groups (Robinson et al. 1988a). In another study (Starkstein et al. 1987), patients with secondary mania were matched for size, location, and etiology of brain lesion with patients who had no mood disturbance. These groups also were compared with patients who had primary mania and control subjects. Patients with secondary mania had significantly more subcortical atrophy than did other study patients. Moreover, among patients who developed secondary mania, those with a family history of psychiatric disorders had significantly less atrophy than did those without such a family history,

which suggests that genetic predisposition to mood disorders and brain atrophy may be independent risk factors (Starkstein and Robinson 1992). Furthermore, in a chart review at one hospital's HIV clinic, Lyketsos et al. (1993) found that manic syndromes affected 8% of the patients with AIDS. Those manic patients without a family history or personal history of mood disorder presented later in the course of HIV infection and had a higher prevalence of comorbid dementia.

Neurochemical abnormalities in primary bipolar disorder involve ascending monoaminergic pathways that are also probably involved in secondary mania (Larson and Richelson 1988). These pathways, which pass through the midbrain, connect the limbic system, basal ganglia, and cerebral hemispheres. In a rat model of focal brain injury, Starkstein et al. (1988a) found that right, but not left, frontolateral cortical lesions produced locomotor hyperactivity and bilateral increases in dopaminergic turnover in the nucleus accumbens. These investigators have postulated that in the presence of risk factors for secondary mania (e.g., subcortical atrophy or family history of mood disorder), increases in biogenic amine turnover produced by right-hemisphere lesions may play a role in the development of secondary mania. This biogenic amine dysfunction also may be most pronounced in the basotemporal cortex, one of the cortical regions that has the highest concentration of serotonergic terminals (Starkstein and Robinson 1992).

Neurochemical theories of mania focus on an association between increases in the functional output of basotemporal cortex pathways resulting in excess catecholamines (norepinephrine or dopamine) or indoleamines (serotonin), whereas depression is associated with functional deficits of these neurotransmitters (Goodnick 1998). Pharmacological studies support these associations; antidepressants increase the activity of one or more of these neurotransmitters via reuptake inhibition or inhibition of amine degradation. Measurements of amine metabolites in body fluids before and after treatment of depression or mania also support this theoretical model. Associations, however, do not necessarily infer a direct cause-and-effect relation. Other pathways and neurotransmitters are almost certainly involved in the etiologies of mood syndromes. For example, deficiency of γ-aminobutyric acid (GABA), an inhibitory neurotransmitter, has been implicated in mania. Medications that reduce manic symptoms, such as lithium, carbamazepine, and valproate, all enhance GABAergic transmission.

Many investigators believe that sleep deprivation is the final common pathway in the pathophysiology of mania. Patients with primary bipolar disorder often shift from depression to mania after they miss a night of sleep. Total sleep deprivation and sleep deprivation in the second half of the night can induce temporary remissions in depressed patients as well (Gillin 1983). Goodwin and Jamison (1990) reported that sleep deprivation is probably an important precipitant in the manic states that occasionally accompany bereavement, postpartum states, and jet lag. Sleep architecture abnormalities are associated with depression; however, because patients may be uncooperative or sleep so little, sleep in mania is difficult to monitor polygraphically. Nonetheless, insomnia and decreased need for sleep are almost invariably present during mania. Sleep deprivation is a common characteristic of medical-surgical hospitalization, particularly in intensive care units, so documenting a recent sleep history may be an important tool for consultation-liaison psychiatrists.

In summary, data on the phenomenology of secondary mania suggest that several general principles hold true. Numerous studies of patients with brain damage have found that patients who develop secondary mania have a greater frequency of lesions in the right hemisphere than do patients with brain injury who become depressed or develop no mood disturbance at all. The right-hemisphere lesions associated with mania are in specific right-hemisphere structures that are connected to the limbic system. The right basotemporal cortex appears to be particularly important because direct lesions of this cortical region are associated frequently with secondary mania (Starkstein and Robinson 1992).

DIFFERENTIAL DIAGNOSIS

The presentation of secondary mania includes any of the symptoms found in primary bipolar mania. Clinical history, physical examination, and laboratory evaluations are important elements in differentiating primary and secondary mania. Because one-third of bipolar manic patients have either disorientation or memory blanks during a manic episode, the differential diagnosis of primary and secondary mania is often difficult (Winokur and Clayton 1986). The onset of mania in a patient older than 35 years without a personal or family history of mood disorder strongly suggests secondary mania, as does the onset of mania during a medical hospitalization or illness. Patients with primary bipolar disorder usually have their first manic episode between late adolescence and early adulthood, with a mean age at onset of 30 years (Goodwin and Jamison 1990). The distinction between the two is important because eradication of the etiology is the treatment of choice for secondary mania. However, manic symptoms are treatable, so intervention need not be delayed while completing the medical evaluation.

Psychiatric disorders other than bipolar disorder can have symptoms that mimic a manic episode. Stimulant abuse, delirium, schizophrenia, schizoaffective disorder, anxiety disorders, some personality disorders (borderline personality disorder and histrionic personality disorder), and adolescent conduct disorders should be considered before establishing a diagnosis of secondary mania (Strakowski et al. 1994).

Several medical conditions are temporally associated with manic and hypomanic syndromes. These conditions are outlined in Table 18–5. Unfortunately, many of these reported causes are from single case reports or small series of patients. Among the multiple potential etiologies reportedly associated with secondary mania, several have proven to be consistent and frequent causes. These frequent conditions, listed in Table 18–6, have been temporally associated with onset of mania in series of patients or in clinical studies (i.e., more than single case reports).

TABLE 18–5. Reported causes of secondary mania

Neurological conditions

Focal neurological lesions	*Nonfocal neurological lesions*
Tumors (gliomas, meningiomas, thalamic metastases)	Posttraumatic encephalopathy
Cerebrovascular lesions (temporal, right hemispheric), including stroke and head trauma	General paresis
	Neurosyphilis
Temporal lobe seizure	Multiple sclerosis
Thalamotomy	Viral meningoencephalitis
Right hemispherectomy	Cryptococcal meningoencephalitis
Huntington's disease	Pick's disease
Wilson's disease	Klinefelter's syndrome
Postencephalopathic parkinsonism	Kleine-Levin syndrome
Idiopathic calcification of basal ganglia	HIV encephalopathy
	Post-St. Louis type A encephalitis

Medications

Alcohol	*Hypericum* (St. John's wort)
Alprazolam[a]	Iproniazid
Amantadine	Isoniazid
Amphetamines	Levodopa
Anabolic steroids	Lorazepam
Baclofen	Methylphenidate
Bromide	Metoclopramide[a]
Buspirone	Metrizamide
Captopril	Phencyclidine
Carbamazepine	Procainamide
Cimetidine	Procarbazine
Clonidine withdrawal	Procyclidine
Cocaine	Propafenone
Corticosteroids/corticosteroid withdrawal	Sympathomimetic amines
Cyclobenzaprine	Thyroid preparations
Cyproheptadine	Tolmetin
Dextromethorphan	Triazolam[a]
Dronabinol	Yohimbine[a]
Fenfluramine/phentermine	Zidovudine
Hallucinogens	

Systemic conditions

Hyperthyroidism	Niacin deficiency
Hyperthyroidism with starvation diet	Vitamin B_{12} deficiency
Uremia	Carcinoid
Hemodialysis	Use of hyperbaric chamber
Cushing's syndrome	Postoperative excitement
Puerperal psychosis	Premenstrual psychosis
Infectious mononucleosis	

Other

Aspartame	L-Glutamine

[a]Mania occurred in patients with histories of mood disorders.
Source. Adapted from Cassem NH: "Depression," in *Massachusetts General Hospital Handbook of General Hospital Psychiatry*, 3rd Edition. Edited by Cassem NH. St. Louis, MO, Mosby Year Book, 1991, pp. 237–268; Goodwin FK, Jamison KR: *Manic-Depressive Illness*. New York, Oxford University Press, 1990, p. 505; Larson EW, Richelson E: "Organic Causes of Mania." *Mayo Clinic Proceedings* 63:906–912, 1988. Used with permission.

Few studies of relative risks of all these potential causes have been done. As mentioned earlier in this chapter, patients with family or personal histories of mood disorders are at higher risk for mania. Many medications, particularly those that modulate central monoaminergic metabolism, are reported to produce mania. Corticosteroid use has long been associated with secondary mania (Rundell and Wise 1989). Anabolic steroids, popular

TABLE 18–6.   Most frequent causes of secondary mania[a]

Medications
 Levodopa
 Decongestants containing phenylephrine
 Sympathomimetics/bronchodilators
 Corticosteroids
 Adrenocorticotropic hormone
 Antidepressants

Metabolic abnormalities
 Hyperthyroidism

Neurological disorders
 Temporal lobe seizures
 Multiple sclerosis
 Right-hemispheric strokes or injuries

Central nervous system tumors
 Gliomas
 Meningiomas
 Thalamic metastases

[a]These causes are temporally associated with mania in either a series of patients or clinical studies.
Source.   Adapted from Stoudemire GA: "Selected Organic Mental Disorders," in *The American Psychiatric Press Textbook of Neuropsychiatry.* Edited by Hales RE, Yudofsky SC. Washington, DC, American Psychiatric Press, 1987, pp. 125–140. Used with permission.

TABLE 18–7.   Evaluation of secondary mania

Medical-psychiatric history
 Current medical symptoms
 Recent infections
 Use of prescribed medications
 Use of drugs of abuse
 History of psychiatric disorders, especially mood disorders
 Family history of psychiatric disorders, especially mood disorders
 Vital signs

Physical examination, with attention to focal neurological deficits

Mental status examination, with emphasis on mood, psychotic symptoms, and cognition

Laboratory evaluation
 Blood glucose
 Electrolytes
 Renal/hepatic function tests
 Complete blood count
 Serum calcium
 Serum cortisol
 Serum thyroxine
 Vitamin B_{12}
 Folate
 Toxicology screen
 Blood alcohol
 Pregnancy test
 Levels of antimanic drug(s) if already prescribed

Electrocardiogram

Computed tomography and magnetic resonance imaging scans

Cerebrospinal fluid examination

Electroencephalogram

among some athletes, also have been shown to cause mania as well as other psychiatric symptoms, including irritability, aggressiveness, and grandiosity (Pope and Katz 1988; Uzych 1992). Alternative drugs, such as *hypericum* (St. John's wort), have antidepressant effects and may be associated with new-onset mania (Lieberman 1998).

Investigating causes of secondary manic states requires a thorough assessment (Table 18–7), which should begin with a careful medical and psychiatric history; chart review, with special attention to medications prescribed or surreptitiously taken; and physical examination. The neurological examination should investigate possible focal deficits, especially findings associated with nondominant hemispheric lesions, such as left-sided hemiparesis with hyperactive deep tendon reflexes and Babinski's sign, attention disturbance (left-sided neglect), anosognosia, and constructional dyspraxia. Other brain regions associated with manic symptoms include lesions of the anterior cerebral artery and associated frontal lobe dysfunction, as well as basal ganglia lesions that may yield signs of movement disorders, such as athetosis, chorea, parkinsonism, or hemiballismus. When the etiology of mania is a stroke, lateralized focal lesions are found in the right hemisphere involving regions of the basal ganglia, thalamus, or midbrain nuclei or limbic portions of the frontal or temporal lobes (Starkstein and Robinson 1992).

Associated symptoms include neurological deficits that reflect the size and location of the cerebrovascular compromise. Mental status examination should evaluate mood, psychosis, and cognitive impairment to distinguish between primary psychiatric diagnoses and secondary conditions such as delirium and dementia (see Chapters 15 and 16, this volume).

Diagnostic laboratory testing should include screening of glucose, electrolytes, renal and hepatic function tests, complete blood count with differential, serum calcium, and serum levels of vitamin B_{12} and folate. Toxicology screening should be done to detect cocaine, amphetamines, phencyclidine, other hallucinogens, alcohol, sedative-hypnotics, and prescription medications such as antidepressants and corticosteroids that may cause manic symptoms (Tables 18–5 and 18–6). Brain imaging (computed tomography or magnetic resonance imaging [MRI]) should be done if neurological conditions with structural CNS changes are suspected. An electroencephalogram (EEG) may differentiate the diagnosis of seizures or delirium. Many medical illnesses linked to secondary mania have cardiac manifestations, so an electrocardiogram (ECG) is indicated; it is a component of the pretreatment lithium evaluation as well. If a patient is taking lithium, carbamazepine, or valproate, the medication level should be checked.

TREATMENT AND MANAGEMENT

In all cases of secondary mania, the treatment focuses on elimination of the underlying medical etiology (surgery to remove tumors and hematomas, medications or procedures to correct metabolic and endocrinologic abnormalities, medications to treat infections, or removal of toxins or drugs to eradicate substance-induced mania) and the attenuation of symptoms whenever elimination is not possible. Even though removing remediable etiologies is the first line of treatment, pharmacological intervention usually is necessary to control manic symptoms. Antimanic drugs usually lead to rapid resolution of symptoms. Complications such as sleep deprivation, dehydration, weight loss, and fatigue may make patients more vulnerable to medication side effects and to underlying medical illness. Several medication options are available for treatment of secondary mania (see also Chapter 42 in this volume). Table 18–8 describes dosing strategies and serum levels for some of these antimanic agents. Pharmacological intervention is recommended for up to 6 months beyond symptom resolution to prevent relapse.

The most important considerations in selecting a treatment for manic symptoms are the nature and severity of symptoms and the side-effect profile of antimanic medications (American Psychiatric Association 1994).

Mild manic symptoms may respond well to lithium or valproate alone. Hudson and colleagues (1989) reported that restoring a normal sleep pattern often averts escalation to more severe manic symptoms; short-term adjunctive treatment with a bedtime dose of a benzodiazepine, such as clonazepam, may help to normalize sleep. For more severe symptoms, especially hyperactivity and psychotic features, an antipsychotic is indicated. Anticonvulsants may be particularly helpful for patients who are lithium intolerant or lithium nonresponders. Many clinicians consider anticonvulsants to be first-line treatment modalities, especially for secondary mania. A discussion of pharmacological guidelines for the treatment of secondary mania follows.

Lithium Carbonate

Lithium has had widespread use in the United States for more than three decades (Nemeroff 2000). The only placebo-controlled, parallel-group study of lithium for patients with acute primary mania (secondary mania patients were excluded) compared lithium with valproate and placebo and found marked improvement with lithium and valproate treatment (49% and 48%, respectively) compared with placebo (25%) (Bowden et al. 1994). Lithium is the most widely used antimanic agent and generally is the first line of treatment for primary mania and for some cases of secondary mania. For example, lithium is beneficial in the treatment of manic syndromes secondary to corticosteroids (Greenberg et al. 1994) and organic brain syndromes (M.R. Cohen and Niska 1980). In their literature review of lithium treatment for secondary mania, Price et al. (1992) recommended the use of lithium in patients who have brain tumors without seizures. Dosages of lithium should begin at 300 mg/day and be increased gradually over several weeks to serum levels of 0.8–1.2 mEq/L. If seizures are present, anticonvulsants are preferable.

TABLE 18–8. Antimania medications

Drug	Daily dosage (mg)	Half-life[a] (hours)	Serum level
Lithium	300–1,800	18–36	0.6–1.2 mEq/L
Carbamazepine	400–1,200	25–65[a]	8–12 µg/mL
Gabapentin	900–2,400	5–9	
Lamotrigine	100–200	15–70	
Valproate	1,000–1,500	6–16	50–120 mg/mL
Clonazepam	1.5–6.0	18–58	[b]

[a]With repeated doses, half-life declines because carbamazepine usually induces its own metabolism.
[b]Serum levels less meaningful than for carbamazepine, lithium, or valproate.
Source. Adapted from Wise MG, Rundell JR: *Consultation Psychiatry,* 2nd Edition. Washington, DC, American Psychiatric Press, 1993. Used with permission.

Patients who are given lithium should have the pretreatment evaluation outlined in Table 18–9. Although contraindications are rare, an assessment of organ systems most often adversely affected (kidney, cardiovascular system, and CNS) is necessary. This assessment is particularly important in medically ill populations. Lithium is titrated within a narrow therapeutic range (i.e., toxic effects occur at doses only moderately higher than therapeutic levels). Serum levels are carefully monitored and are usually drawn 12 hours after the last dose. The half-life of lithium is 18–36 hours; therefore, steady-state serum levels are usually achieved 5–8 days after a dosage change. Because the therapeutic benefits of lithium may take 10–14 days to appear, concomitant antipsychotic use usually is necessary for acute management of mania. The generally accepted therapeutic range of serum lithium concentrations is 0.6–1.2 mEq/L. Patients in an acute manic phase are best treated with dosages that achieve serum concentrations at the upper end of this therapeutic range. However, in severely ill medical patients, including those with cancer and HIV infection; in elderly patients; or in those with renal disease, careful monitoring and lower doses should be used when possible (Greenberg et al. 1994). Treating medically ill patients with lithium requires knowledge of potential drug-drug interactions; these interactions are outlined in Table 18–10.

The primary metabolic consideration in the use of lithium in medically ill patients is renal function (A. Stoudemire et al. 1993). Lithium is excreted by the kidney, and excretion rates are affected by age and creatinine clearance. Therefore, pretreatment renal function screening is absolutely necessary. Sodium depletion increases the reabsorbed fraction of both sodium and lithium ions up to 95%, thereby decreasing lithium clearance. Thiazide diuretics, which act primarily at the distal tubule, enhance proximal reabsorption of lithium because they deplete sodium. Loop diuretics such as furosemide appear to have less effect on lithium clearance. Potassium-sparing diuretics (e.g., spironolactone, triamterene) also may reduce lithium clearance. Other clinically significant medications known to interact with lithium are listed in Table 18–10. Patients taking thiazide diuretics usually need approximately half the amount of lithium to attain therapeutic levels, but there is considerable individual variation (A. Stoudemire et al. 1993). When coadministered with a diuretic agent, the lithium dose should be started low and increased slowly, and lithium levels should be monitored at least twice weekly. Thereafter, frequent monitoring should be resumed after any change in diuretic dosage or in diet.

Lithium is dialyzable and should be given to patients on renal dialysis *after* their dialysis treatments; the usual

TABLE 18–9. Pretreatment evaluation for lithium maintenance

Laboratory

Minimum recommendations
Blood urea nitrogen
Creatinine
T_4/free T_4
T_3 resin uptake
Thyroid-stimulating hormone
Urinalysis including protein and microscopic examination
Electrocardiogram

Additional tests recommended by some authorities
24-hour urine volume
Creatinine clearance, if any history or risk of renal disease
Urine osmolality
Complete blood count
Electrolytes
Blood pressure

Clinical

Medical history focusing on renal, thyroid, cardiac, and central nervous systems

Catalog of present and past drug use
Prescription drugs
Over-the-counter preparations
Illicit drugs
Caffeine, nicotine, alcohol

Baseline weight and history of recent weight change

Dietary habits, including estimate of salt intake

Exercise and recreation habits

Note. T_4 = thyroxine; T_3 = triiodothyronine.
Source. Adapted from Goodwin FK, Jamison KR: *Manic-Depressive Illness.* New York, Oxford University Press, 1990, p. 669. Copyright 1990, Oxford University Press. Used with permission.

dosage is 300–600 mg/day (A. Stoudemire et al. 1993). The dose is typically not given until after the next dialysis. Serum levels of lithium are tested several hours after dialysis because plasma levels may rise in the postdialysis period when equilibration between tissue stores occurs (W.M. Bennett et al. 1980). The dialyzability of lithium makes dialysis the treatment of choice in cases of life-threatening lithium toxicity.

In most patients treated with lithium, the kidneys lose some ability to concentrate urine. Occasionally, this leads to polyuria (nephrogenic diabetes insipidus) as a result of lithium's action on the loop of Henle and the distal tubule. This effect is dose related and, in rare cases, is irreversible. Once-a-day dosing may partially mitigate this problem. If the polyuria threatens lithium treatment and there are compelling clinical reasons to continue lithium instead of alternative agents, several options are

TABLE 18–10. Reported drug interactions with antimanic agents

Medication	Interactive effect
Lithium	
Thiazide diuretics	Raise lithium levels
Spironolactone	
Triamterene	
Enalapril	
Nonsteroidal antiinflammatory drugs (e.g., indomethacin, ibuprofen, phenylbutazone, piroxicam)	
Acetazolamide	Lower lithium levels
Theophylline	
Aminophylline	
Calcium channel blockers	May either raise or lower lithium levels; effects not clear; verapamil may cause bradycardia when used with lithium
Metronidazole	May increase lithium levels; may increase chances of nephrotoxicity
Tetracycline	Minor elevation of lithium level
Carbamazepine	
Erythromycin	May raise carbamazepine levels and precipitate heart block
Antiarrhythmics	May cause additional delay in cardiac conduction time
Diltiazem	May raise carbamazepine levels to toxic levels
Verapamil	
Danazol	
Valproate	Lower valproate levels when used with carbamazepine; valproate increases metabolites of carbamazepine
Valproate	
Carbamazepine	May lower valproate levels
Phenobarbital	
Aspirin	May raise total and free valproate levels, yielding toxicity
Benzodiazepines (clonazepam)	
Cimetidine	May raise serum levels of benzodiazepines metabolized predominantly by oxidation
Disulfiram	
Isoniazid	
Ethanol[a]	
Estrogens	Tend to lower benzodiazepine levels
Cigarettes	
Methylxanthine derivatives	
Rifampin	

[a]Acute alcohol ingestion may elevate benzodiazepine levels; however, chronic alcohol use typically lowers some benzodiazepines via enzyme induction.

Source. Adapted from Stoudemire A, Moran MG, Fogel BS: "Psychotropic Drug Use in the Medically Ill, Part II." *Psychosomatics* 32:34–46, 1991. Copyright 1991, Academy of Psychosomatic Medicine. Used with permission.

available. First, thiazide diuretics may be used with the previously noted precautions to enhance lithium reabsorption at the proximal tubule, thereby protecting the distal nephron from high lithium concentrations. The total lithium dose is reduced by as much as 50% if this strategy is used. Second, potassium-sparing diuretics such as amiloride may be used; the usual dosage is 10–20 mg/day (Kosten and Forrest 1986). In refractory cases, 50 mg/day of hydrochlorothiazide should be added. With or without adjunctive thiazide therapy, amiloride increases lithium levels, which may lead to lithium toxic-

ity if levels are not monitored. If amiloride is used alone, hyperkalemia is a risk; electrolytes should be checked frequently after starting the drug. If amiloride is used with hydrochlorothiazide, the lithium dosage should be reduced.

Adverse Effects

Although side effects of lithium are usually mild and transient, medically ill patients should be monitored closely for adverse effects. The most common side effects are tremor, nausea, vomiting, diarrhea, polyuria, and polydipsia. Hypothyroidism, rashes, nephrogenic diabetes insipidus, interstitial nephritis, and weight gain are less common. Nonspecific ST segment and T-wave changes are commonly seen on the ECG; actual conduction defects and arrhythmias are rare. However, Cassem (1991) recommends caution in elderly patients or patients with cardiac disease because lithium may have an inhibitory effect on impulse generation and transmission within the atrium. The most commonly reported adverse cardiac effects are sinus node dysfunction or first-degree atrioventricular block.

Many of lithium's side effects decrease with dosage reduction, but that is not always possible, especially in patients prone to relapse. β-Blockers (atenolol 50 mg/day) sometimes help to control lithium-induced tremor, and, as discussed above, diuretics may help control polyuria. The use of slow-release lithium formulations diminishes some side effects and the postdose variation in serum lithium concentrations while allowing simpler dosing schedules (twice a day vs. three times a day).

Lithium is labeled a teratogen and is to be avoided in the first trimester of pregnancy. Use of lithium during the first trimester has been linked to fetal cardiac anomalies, which can be detected as early as the eighteenth week. Lithium used in the second and third trimesters is generally benign; however, its use during pregnancy should be measured against the risks of adverse events (Gelenberg 1988; Llewellyn et al. 1998).

Lithium toxicity markedly affects the CNS and is a life-threatening emergency in consultation-liaison settings. Symptoms of lithium-induced CNS toxicity include ataxia, slurred speech, and nystagmus and can proceed to convulsions, coma, and death if lithium levels are greater than 2.5 mEq/L. The threshold for more serious side effects is lower in predisposed or medically ill patients. Clearly understanding the organ system effects of lithium and carefully monitoring serum levels should preclude toxicity; even in medically ill patients, the effects on the kidney are almost always reversible after discontinuing the drug.

Anticonvulsants

Anticonvulsants are widely used in the treatment of both primary bipolar disorder and secondary mania, including lithium-unresponsive mania (Prien and Gelenberg 1989). Sometimes these agents are used in combination with lithium. One anticonvulsant, valproate, has received U.S. Food and Drug Administration (FDA) approval for its use in acute manic states. Carbamazepine has been used for many years in bipolar illness, particularly in cases of refractory illness or mixed states. New anticonvulsants whose use in bipolar illness is supported by emerging data include gabapentin and lamotrigine. Each of these agents is discussed below. General dosage recommendations and therapeutic levels are outlined in Table 18–8. The therapeutic anticonvulsant levels listed in Table 18–8 are used for treating seizures; considerable variability in the appropriate levels for treating mania may exist. The clinician must monitor symptom response and side-effect profiles closely. For those anticonvulsants that are hepatically metabolized (e.g., valproate, carbamazepine, lamotrigine), a pretreatment liver function assessment is necessary.

Valproate

Valproate has been used as an anticonvulsant since the early 1960s. Both its anticonvulsant and its antimanic activity are believed to be related to its GABAergic effects (Bernstein 1991). Although clinical trials are lacking, many consider valproate a drug of first choice in the management of secondary mania (Evans et al. 1995; Janicak and Levy 1998). It may offer a particular clinical advantage when combined with lithium as maintenance polypharmacy for patients with bipolar I disorder (Solomon et al. 2000).

Recently, valproate has been administered in a more rapid manner for the specific management of acute manic states. Data from clinical trials suggest that the antimanic effects of divalproex (an enteric-coated formulation of valproate) may be accelerated by administering the drug via the oral loading strategy of 20 mg/kg/day (which produces serum valproate concentrations of approximately 80 mg/L after 1 day). One group of investigators found this treatment strategy to produce results comparable to those with haloperidol but with fewer side effects (McElroy et al. 1996). Trials of valproate loading have not included patients with secondary mania; therefore, the strategy should be used carefully in patients with comorbid medical illnesses.

Adverse effects.   When prescribing valproate to medically ill patients, the clinician must be alert to gastrointestinal side effects, hepatotoxicity, coagulation effects, and possible drug-drug interactions. The most troublesome side effect of valproate for most patients is nausea. Medically ill patients, particularly those predisposed to nausea, are at increased risk. Depakote (divalproex) is less likely to cause gastrointestinal upset than Depakene (valproate), and more frequent dosing, preferably after meals, is better tolerated than larger doses taken fewer times a day.

Although hepatic toxicity is a concern when prescribing valproate, it is relatively rare. Hepatic necrosis is a major risk for children younger than 2 years, but in adults, it is an uncommon complication that occurs in only 1 in 10,000 patients (Eadie et al. 1988). Other investigators report the incidence of hepatic necrosis to be as low as 1 in 50,000, with 95% of patients developing symptoms within the first 6 months of therapy (Scheffner et al. 1988). Therefore, periodic liver function tests should be done during the first 6 months of therapy. Aside from this rare hepatic complication, a more common and benign hepatic effect of valproate is an increase in serum ammonia levels resulting from valproate's inhibition of urea synthesis. Although serum ammonia elevation usually does not cause any difficulties in patients, it can be problematic for patients with preexisting liver disease, especially those prone to hepatic encephalopathy. Therefore, significant liver disease is a relative contraindication to valproate therapy. Valproate can adversely affect coagulation by increasing prothrombin time, decreasing fibrinogen levels, and reducing platelet counts.

In contrast to carbamazepine, which is an enzyme inducer, valproate inhibits liver enzymes that metabolize drugs. Therefore, valproate can prolong the half-life of drugs that are hepatically metabolized. For example, prolonged and elevated benzodiazepine levels can cause increased sedation and ataxia. Valproate also can increase the levels of other anticonvulsants. For example, valproate increases phenobarbital levels by inhibiting its metabolism (Redenbaugh et al. 1980) and raises the free fraction of phenytoin by displacing the drug from protein binding sites (Bruno et al. 1980). Valproate also increases the 10,11-epoxide metabolite of carbamazepine, which is not usually measured with routine testing (Pisani et al. 1986). Thus, carbamazepine toxicity is sometimes produced at "therapeutic" levels when given concomitantly with valproate. Valproate should be used cautiously in women of reproductive age because it is associated with neural tube defects when used during the first trimester of pregnancy.

Carbamazepine

Carbamazepine is structurally similar to tricyclic antidepressants. Although the precise mechanism of action of carbamazepine in affective illness is not clear, it blocks the reuptake of norepinephrine, inhibits stimulation-induced release of norepinephrine at synaptic sites, and appears to decrease GABA turnover (Post 1982). Carbamazepine is considered an alternative to valproate in the treatment of rapid cycling and mixed episodes of bipolar illness (Expert Consensus Guideline Series 1996). Carbamazepine has shown effectiveness in the treatment of acute mania in most trials; however, its side-effect profile has made it a less popular choice

than valproate, particularly among the elderly and medically ill.

Adverse effects. When prescribing carbamazepine to medically ill patients, its potential hematological toxicity, quinidine-like effects on cardiac conduction, antidiuretic actions, and enzyme induction that alters the effects of other drugs must be considered (Table 18–10). Particularly common problems in the consultation-liaison setting are carbamazepine's interaction with the calcium channel blockers diltiazem and verapamil—two agents that may elevate carbamazepine levels into the toxic range (A. Stoudemire et al. 1993).

Carbamazepine administration may result in two different hematological reactions. One is a predictable and usually transient decrease in both red blood cell and white blood cell (WBC) counts when treatment is initiated; the other is aplastic anemia—a rare side effect that can occur at any time after initiation of therapy. Leukopenia (defined as WBC count < 50) occurs in 7%–12% of treated patients (Sobotka et al. 1990), and it is seemingly unrelated to aplastic anemia. The latter occurs in approximately 1 in 575,000 treated patients per year (Seetharam and Pellock 1991). Patients who have preexisting anemia or neutropenia do not appear to be at greater risk for the life-threatening complications of aplastic anemia or agranulocytosis (A. Stoudemire et al. 1993). A hematological consultation should be obtained before initiating carbamazepine therapy in any patient with a baseline hemoglobin level below 12 g/dL or a WBC count below 4,000/mm³. Preexisting neutropenia is a relative but not an absolute contraindication to carbamazepine.

Hepatic side effects related to carbamazepine usually are limited to a benign, asymptomatic elevation of alanine aminotransferase or aspartate aminotransferase, usually less than twice the upper limit of normal values. This reaction occurs in fewer than 5% of patients; however, a rare, idiosyncratic, and life-threatening acute hepatic necrosis is reported to occur in fewer than 1 in 10,000 patients, usually within the first month of therapy (Jeavons 1983). Regular blood monitoring is suggested for patients with risk factors for liver disease or with abnormal baseline liver function. Carbamazepine use in patients with preexisting liver disease has two risks: 1) any hepatic reaction to carbamazepine adds to preexisting problems if the patient has low baseline liver function, so a mild reaction can become symptomatic, and 2) carbamazepine is metabolized more slowly because its primary metabolic route is the liver (A. Stoudemire et al. 1993). This leads to a risk of toxic serum levels, even with low doses. Therefore, significant liver disease is a relative contraindication to carbamazepine.

The quinidine-like effects of carbamazepine are related to its tricyclic structure; therefore, precautions similar to those for tricyclics are indicated (Levenson 1993). These effects have the potential to slow cardiac conduction and to suppress ventricular automaticity (Benassi et al. 1987); however, the QRS complex or Q-T interval at normal heart rates is not affected (Kenneback et al. 1991). Pretreatment ECGs are indicated before initiating carbamazepine therapy because of the possibility of potentiating baseline cardiac conduction abnormalities. Conditions warranting cardiology consultation include block greater than first-degree atrioventricular block, right bundle branch block, left anterior hemiblock, or Mobitz type I block (A. Stoudemire et al. 1993).

Carbamazepine has an antidiuretic action associated with both clinically significant hyponatremia and mild, asymptomatic hyponatremia. The effect is probably mediated via a direct action on the renal tubules. Risk factors that predispose a patient to hyponatremia include advanced age, diuretic use, and congestive heart failure. These patients should have weekly electrolyte determinations during the first month of therapy.

Because carbamazepine is a potent inducer of the cytochrome P450 system, it influences the metabolism of many drugs that rely on this system. Therefore, the blood levels of some drugs may decline if carbamazepine is added to a patient's medication regimen (see Table 18–10). Carbamazepine even induces its own metabolism, necessitating gradual increases in dosage over the first few weeks of treatment to maintain a steady blood level. This phenomenon is problematic for women taking oral contraceptives (which may have reduced effectiveness if taken concomitantly with carbamazepine). Patients and their gynecologists must be apprised of the potential for birth control failure unless a higher-dose formulation of birth control medication is prescribed. Furthermore, drug metabolites that are not usually clinically significant might be present in larger quantities as a result of carbamazepine induction of metabolic enzymes. Hydroxymetabolites of desipramine have been reported to cause ECG changes in a patient concurrently treated with carbamazepine and desipramine, despite a therapeutic desipramine level (Baldessarini et al. 1988). Like valproate, carbamazepine should be used cautiously in women of reproductive age because it has been associated with neural tube defects.

Newer Anticonvulsants

Gabapentin and lamotrigine are two of the most recent anticonvulsants under investigation for their efficacy in treating refractory bipolar disorder. Studies indicate that both agents have mood-stabilizing effects; gabapentin may be beneficial for treating mania, whereas lamotrigine may provide more benefits in treating bipolar depression (Calabrese et al. 1999; Sachs and Cosgrove 1998). Both anticonvulsants are marketed as adjunctive therapy for refractory partial seizures (Belanoff and Glick 1998). Three new anticonvulsant agents—felbamate, topiramate, and tiagabine—may have potential use in the treatment of bipolar illness (Morris 1998); however, limited clinical data are currently available describing these newest agents.

Gabapentin. The precise mechanism of action of gabapentin is not well understood, although it is hypothesized to work through inhibition of excitatory amino acid release (J. Bennett et al. 1997). Gabapentin has several favorable pharmacokinetic properties. For example, it is not necessary to monitor gabapentin plasma concentrations, and it is not bound to plasma proteins. Gabapentin is not metabolized in humans, and it is excreted virtually unchanged in urine. Plasma clearance is linearly related to renal creatinine clearance, so dosage should be adjusted based on renal function. Additionally, gabapentin does not induce the hepatic microsomal enzyme system and does not inhibit the metabolism of other anticonvulsants or drugs used concomitantly (McLean 1994).

Gabapentin is generally well tolerated; the most common adverse side effects noted in clinical trial data are somnolence, dizziness, and ataxia (Ramsay 1994). Side effects generally are transient, resolving within 2 weeks of onset during continued treatment. Because of its short half-life (5–9 hours), gabapentin is administered in three divided daily doses. Initiation of treatment at 300 mg on the first day, 600 mg in two divided daily doses on the second day, and 900 mg in three divided daily doses on the third day is recommended. Maintenance dosages often range from 900 to 2,400 mg/day and are determined by clinical response.

Because gabapentin is not metabolized in the liver and is not protein bound, it may be particularly useful in medically ill patients, those taking multiple medications, or patients with impaired hepatic metabolism in whom drug-drug interactions are common. Gabapentin has dose-limited absorption, thus reducing the risk of overdose, and possibly making this medication a safer choice for manic patients at risk for suicide.

Lamotrigine. Clinical reports involving more than 200 patients suggest that lamotrigine may have a broad spectrum of mood-stabilizing efficacy in bipolar disorder when given as adjunct treatment or as monotherapy (Calabrese et al. 1999; Post et al. 1998). One case report described the use of lamotrigine as prophylaxis against steroid-induced mania (Masand 1999). Lamotrigine is believed to act by stabilizing the presynaptic neuronal membrane through blockade of sodium channels, thereby preventing the release of the excitatory neurotransmitter glutamate (Gilman 1995). Plasma protein binding is approximately 55%. Lamotrigine is metabolized in a linear fashion with glucuronidation as the rate-limiting step. It may induce its own metabolism to some degree.

Lamotrigine is generally well tolerated; adverse effects are primarily dose related and associated with the CNS: dizziness, headache, diplopia, ataxia, and nausea. The most important side effect is an 11% rate of skin rash, with a risk of Stevens-Johnson syndrome (Gilman 1995). Most rashes are transient and resolve despite continued treatment. The incidence of rash is notably higher in patients concomitantly receiving valproate, which inhibits the metabolism of lamotrigine and reduces its clearance, thereby leading to higher serum concentrations. Therefore, if lamotrigine and valproate are coadministered, the lamotrigine dosage should be reduced. A slow dosage escalation schedule at the onset of therapy is likely to reduce the potential for the development of rashes.

Lamotrigine may be given either once or twice daily, depending on concomitant anticonvulsant drug treatment. A higher maintenance dose is required when coadministered with hepatic enzyme inducers such as carbamazepine, and a lower maintenance dose is required when coadministered with hepatic enzyme inhibitors such as valproate. When used in monotherapy, lamotrigine may be dosed at 50 mg/day at the onset of treatment and gradually increased by 50 mg/week to a maintenance dosage of 100–200 mg/day.

Because lamotrigine inhibits ischemia-induced release of glutamate, it reduces neuronal damage and has been associated with improved recovery after cerebral ischemia in animals (Shuaib et al. 1995). For this reason, Dubovsky and Buzan (1997) highlighted the possibility of lamotrigine being a treatment for mania secondary to stroke; however, no clinical data to support this consideration are currently available.

Benzodiazepines

Although a number of benzodiazepines have been used in the treatment of acute mania, only clonazepam has been critically studied. Lorazepam, in the dosage range of 1–4 mg, has been used as an adjunct to lithium in the treatment of acute mania in case reports but not in controlled trials. Clonazepam, initially marketed as an anticonvulsant, is a useful agent for the rapid, although perhaps non-

specific, control of acute manic symptoms; it is relatively safe and easy to use (no blood monitoring). Clonazepam is often used in the dosage range of 2–5 mg/day to restore sleep in patients with acute mania. This medication is used safely and effectively in combination with the other antimanic agents.

Adverse Effects

Like other benzodiazepines, clonazepam can potentiate CNS depression or disinhibition when used with other psychotropic agents. Tolerance can develop when clonazepam is used for maintenance therapy. In medically ill patients, clinicians must monitor for clonazepam's long half-life and hepatic metabolism, drug-drug interactions (Table 18–10), and effects on respiratory drive.

Clonazepam has a long half-life (18–58 hours) in healthy adults. Because it is metabolized in the liver, the half-life in elderly patients or in patients with impaired hepatic function or metabolic inhibition from other drugs is even longer. Therefore, the effects of drug accumulation such as ataxia, sedation, confusion, or stupor must be monitored closely in such patients. Clonazepam's discontinuation raises the potential for withdrawal symptoms. Clonazepam should be tapered as slowly as 0.25 mg every 2 weeks in patients who have had months or years of clonazepam therapy (A. Stoudemire et al. 1993). Like other benzodiazepines, clonazepam can decrease hypoxic respiratory drive; therefore, it is relatively contraindicated in patients with chronic obstructive pulmonary disease who are at risk for carbon dioxide retention. If used in such patients, clinicians must monitor blood oxygen levels to ensure that pulmonary function is not compromised.

Antipsychotics

Antipsychotic medications are frequently administered to manic patients, usually to control agitation before other antimanic medications take effect and to treat the psychotic symptoms that are common in manic patients. Psychosis and hyperactivity are dangerous in hospitalized patients, particularly in critical care settings. Medically ill patients are more vulnerable to many of the side effects of antipsychotics, including extrapyramidal side effects (EPS) and neuroleptic malignant syndrome, so medication dosage and duration of therapy should be closely monitored.

Typical Antipsychotics

Most of the evidence documenting the usefulness of antipsychotics in the treatment of mania comes from studies that have used older or typical antipsychotics. Whether to choose a typical antipsychotic of high potency (e.g., haloperidol, thiothixine) or low potency (e.g., chlorpromazine, thioridazine) depends on the clinical setting. High-potency antipsychotics infrequently cause hypotension and sedation; thus, rapid dose escalation is possible. Low-potency antipsychotics, on the other hand, are more sedating, actually an advantage in achieving early control in acute mania if patients are healthy enough to tolerate side effects. However, low-potency antipsychotics have a higher frequency of anticholinergic and α-blockade side effects, which are particularly troublesome in elderly and medically compromised patients. Clinicians should base the antipsychotic dose on the clinical situation. In some medically ill patients with secondary mania, lower doses are indicated.

Atypical Antipsychotics

Newer atypical antipsychotics (e.g., risperidone, olanzapine, clozapine, quetiapine) may offer advantages over typical antipsychotics in the treatment of secondary mania because of their more favorable side-effect profiles. Although clinical experience supports their use, minimal empirical data are currently available.

Risperidone is an atypical agent that has dopamine, serotonin, and α1 and α2 antagonistic activities with minimal anticholinergic effects. Potential side effects may include somnolence, orthostasis, fatigue, tachycardia, nausea, diarrhea, weight gain, sexual dysfunction, and rhinitis. At doses greater than 6 mg, risperidone may be associated with an increased risk of EPS. Risperidone, when used as adjunctive therapy (2–6 mg/day) with concomitant mood-stabilizing agents, was shown to be well tolerated and effective in the treatment of mania in 15 patients who had relapsed while receiving mood stabilizers; it also has been used in the treatment of affective symptoms associated with bipolar disorder in the absence of psychotic symptoms (Tohen and Gannon 1998; Tohen et al. 1996). In one report, risperidone was effective in the treatment of manic psychosis secondary to HIV infection (Singh and Catalan 1994). It should be noted also that risperidone may have inherent antidepressant properties because it has been implicated in the development or exacerbation of mania in case studies in patients with schizoaffective disorder and psychotic depression (Dwight et al. 1994; Koek and Kessler 1996).

Olanzapine has been approved by the U.S. Food and Drug Administration for the treatment of acute mania associated with bipolar I disorder, showing markedly superior efficacy over placebo (Tohen et al. 1999). Olanzapine is structurally and pharmacologically related to

clozapine. Olanzapine has greater affinity for serotonin receptor sites compared with dopamine receptor sites. Principle side effects of olanzapine include weight gain and sedation. Akathisia also may occur in a dose-dependent fashion. Olanzapine has been shown to be equivalent to haloperidol in the treatment of positive symptoms of schizophrenia and superior to haloperidol in the treatment of negative symptomatology. Few, if any, significant EPS have been noted with olanzapine, especially when compared with haloperidol. McElroy et al. (1998) reported the successful use of olanzapine (mean dosage = 14.1 mg/day) in 14 bipolar manic patients who had failed two previous treatments; similar findings have been documented for a cohort of patients with rapid-cycling bipolar disorder (Sanger et al. 1998).

Clozapine, an atypical agent used in antipsychotic-resistant schizophrenia, has been used to some extent in patients with bipolar illness and schizoaffective disorder. Limited data support its use in refractory bipolar manic patients, including patients who have had no response to lithium, valproate, or typical antipsychotics (Banov et al. 1994; McElroy et al. 1991)

Other Treatments

Medications

Several other medications are occasionally used to treat mania. Calcium channel blockers (e.g., verapamil, diltiazem) may be effective treatment for some patients with mania; however, one randomized controlled trial found that lithium was a more effective antimanic agent than verapamil for treating acute mania (Walton et al. 1996). Calcium channel blockers are generally reserved for patients who are refractory or intolerant to lithium or anticonvulsants (Currier and Goodnick 1998).

Electroconvulsive Therapy

Electroconvulsive therapy (ECT) is a valuable and rapid treatment alternative in managing acute mania. ECT is especially useful for severely manic patients with unremitting, frenzied physical activity. This behavior is especially dangerous in medically ill patients and is considered a medical emergency (Akiskal 1988). Other indications for ECT are acutely manic patients who are unresponsive to antimanic agents or who are at high risk for suicide, patients who need a rapid antimanic response, and pregnant women who do not want medications (Llewellyn et al. 1998). If ECT is used, lithium should not be administered; lithium can prolong neuromuscular blockade induced by succinylcholine (Blackwell and Schmidt 1984; Rudorfer and Linnoila 1986). Two studies—a randomized trial (Small et al. 1988) and a large retrospective study (Black et al. 1989)—found favorable comparisons between ECT and lithium in treating acute primary mania. In treating drug-refractory primary mania, Mukherjee et al. (1988) found that in more than 50% of their patients, mania remitted with ECT. However, consultation-liaison psychiatrists who use ECT to treat primary and secondary mania in medical-surgical populations must maintain a firm understanding of medical contraindications to ECT, such as space-occupying intracerebral lesions, a recent myocardial infarction, and a leaky or otherwise unstable aneurysm (Weiner and Coffey 1987).

Psychotherapy

In many cases of primary and secondary mania in the general hospital or medical-surgical clinic setting, supportive psychotherapy is a powerful adjunct to pharmacotherapy. Behavioral and psychological manifestations of mania produce profound changes in perception, attitudes, personality, mood, and cognition. Psychological interventions are of unique value to patients undergoing such devastating changes in the way they perceive themselves and are perceived by others. For example, empathic education targeted to patients with secondary mania can relieve fears of losing control or losing one's mind. Working psychotherapeutically with these individuals requires an awareness of common psychological reactions to stressful events, especially hospitalization-related events, such as fear, anger, denial, and ambivalence. Supportive psychotherapy also helps to develop a therapeutic alliance, an important tool in managing behavioral manifestations of mania. In addition, because manic patients frequently resist medications that will decrease euphoria, a strong alliance may help to enhance adherence. Clinicians may find it helpful to offer relief for symptoms that the patient finds bothersome and not to focus on symptoms the patient finds pleasurable. Supportive psychotherapy allows a forum in which consultation-liaison psychiatrists can educate patients about mania, its underlying etiologies, and potential treatment measures. The psychotherapeutic relationship also is a safe environment to examine concerns about how the manic symptoms have affected the patient's family and to address fears of recurrence. Family therapy in clinical and hospital settings can comfort the patient and family, particularly if they are attempting to cope with the stress of underlying medical illness (Miklowitz 1998).

Behavioral Management

When a hospitalized patient is medically stable, psychiatric hospitalization often is required to manage acute manic symptoms, particularly if those symptoms include psychosis or suicidality. Transferring the patient to an inpatient psychiatric or medical-psychiatric unit provides a more controlled environment for treatment.

In medically ill patients, physical restraints are generally not used unless other interventions have failed. In some instances, particularly for the extremely agitated or violent patient, physical restraints are necessary to maintain patient and staff safety. For the extremely agitated and psychotic patient, a sense of comfort is often achieved by the controlled environment that restraints provide. Similarly, for the manic patient whose level of physical hyperactivity is a threat to his or her physical safety or underlying medical condition, restraints are mandatory. (For a more detailed discussion of aspects of treating agitated patients, see Chapters 10 and 15 in this volume.)

Because patients with secondary mania are often hospitalized for medical reasons at the time of symptom onset, consultation-liaison psychiatrists are called on to help manage the patients' symptoms. In such instances, close patient monitoring is essential. Psychiatric units are sometimes asked to provide staff or sitters experienced in working with psychiatric patients. The consultation-liaison psychiatrist must make clear treatment recommendations and openly communicate these to the referring clinicians. A staff unit meeting is often necessary to educate the patient's treatment team about etiology, symptoms, treatment strategies, and prognosis. This will often improve patient care and decrease the potential for staff-patient conflicts. The ideal setting for treating patients with secondary mania is a medical-psychiatry unit (see Chapter 38 in this volume), where patients can receive specialized care delivered by a staff accustomed to handling both the medical and the psychiatric sequelae of psychiatric illness.

SUMMARY

Mania, particularly in the general hospital patient, is a serious condition necessitating accurate diagnosis and treatment. Consultation-liaison psychiatrists are in a unique position to care for such patients. Diagnostic evaluations must carefully assess the multiple possible etiologies. Treatment options include somatic therapies used alone or in combination. Supportive psychotherapy is a valuable tool, as is the treating clinician's liaison relationship with the staff of medical-surgical wards. For some manic patients in the general hospital setting, treatment is best rendered on inpatient psychiatric or medical-psychiatric units.

REFERENCES

Akiskal HS: The clinical management of affective disorders, in Psychiatry, Vol I. Edited by Michels R, Cavenar JO, Cooper AM, et al. Philadelphia, PA, JB Lippincott, 1988, pp 1–27

American Psychiatric Association: Practice guidelines for the treatment of patients with bipolar disorder. Am J Psychiatry 151 (suppl):1–36, 1994

American Psychiatric Association: Diagnostic and Statistical Manual of Mental Disorders, 4th Edition, Text Revision. Washington, DC, American Psychiatric Association, 2000

Angst J: Course of affective disorders, in Handbook of Biological Psychiatry. Edited by Van Praag HM, Lader MH, Rafaelsen OJ, et al. New York, Marcel Dekker, 1981, pp 225–242

Baldessarini RJ, Teicher MH, Cassidy JW, et al: Anticonvulsant cotreatment may increase toxic metabolites of antidepressants and other psychotropic drugs. J Clin Psychopharmacol 8:381–382, 1988

Banov MD, Zarate CA, Tohen M, et al: Clozapine therapy in refractory affective disorder: polarity predicts response to long-term follow-up. J Clin Psychiatry 55:295–300, 1994

Belanoff JK, Glick ID: New psychotropic drugs for Axis I disorders: recently arrived, in development, and never arrived, in The American Psychiatric Press Textbook of Psychopharmacology, 2nd Edition. Edited by Schatzberg AF, Nemeroff CB. Washington, DC, American Psychiatric Press, 1998, pp 1015–1027

Bellivier F, Leboyer M, Courtet P, et al: Association between the tryptophan hydroxylase gene and manic-depressive illness. Arch Gen Psychiatry 55:33–37, 1998

Benassi E, Bo GP, Cocito L, et al: Carbamazepine and cardiac conduction disturbances. Ann Neurol 22:280–281, 1987

Bennett J, Goldman W, Suppes T: Gabapentin for treatment of bipolar and schizoaffective disorders. J Clin Psychopharmacol 17:141–142, 1997

Bennett WM, Muther RS, Parker RA: Drug therapy in renal failure: dosing guidelines for adults, part II: sedatives, hypnotics, and tranquilizers; cardiovascular, antihypertensive, and diuretic agents; miscellaneous agents. Ann Intern Med 93:286–325, 1980

Bernstein JG: Psychotropic drug prescribing, in Massachusetts General Hospital Handbook of General Hospital Psychiatry, 3rd Edition. Edited by Cassem NH. St. Louis, MO, Mosby Year Book, 1991, pp 527–570

Berrettini WH, Ferraro TN, Goldin LR, et al: A linkage study of bipolar illness. Arch Gen Psychiatry 54:27–35, 1997

Black DW, Hulbert J, Nasrallah A: The effect of somatic treatment and comorbidity on immediate outcome in manic patients. Compr Psychiatry 30:74–79, 1989

Blackwell B, Schmidt GL: Drug interactions in psychopharmacology. Psychiatr Clin North Am 7:625–637, 1984

Bowden CL, Brugger AM, Swann AC, et al: Efficacy of divalproex vs lithium and placebo in the treatment of mania. JAMA 271:917–924, 1994

Bruno J, Gallo JM, Lee CS, et al: Interactions of valproic acid with phenytoin. Neurology 30:1233–1236, 1980

Calabrese JR, Bowden CL, Sachs GS, et al: A double-blind, placebo-controlled study of lamotrigine monotherapy in outpatients with bipolar I depression. J Clin Psychiatry 60:79–88, 1999

Cassem NH: Depression, in Massachusetts General Hospital Handbook of General Hospital Psychiatry, 3rd Edition. Edited by Cassem NH. St. Louis, MO, Mosby Year Book, 1991, pp 237–268

Cassidy F, Forest K, Murry E, et al: A factor analysis of the signs and symptoms of mania. Arch Gen Psychiatry 55:27–32, 1998

Cohen LS, Sichel DA, Robertson LM, et al. Postpartum prophylaxis for women with bipolar disorder. Am J Psychiatry 152:1641–1645, 1995

Cohen MR, Niska RW: Localized right cerebral hemisphere dysfunction and recurrent mania. Am J Psychiatry 137:847–848, 1980

Cummings JL: Organic psychoses: delusional disorders and secondary mania. Psychiatr Clin North Am 9:293–311, 1986

Cummings JL, Mendez MF: Secondary mania with focal cerebrovascular lesions. Am J Psychiatry 141:1084–1087, 1984

Currier MB, Goodnick PJ: Calcium antagonists and newer anticonvulsants, in Mania: Clinical and Research Perspectives. Edited by Goodnick PJ. Washington, DC, American Psychiatric Press, 1998, pp 337–363

Dubovsky SL, Buzan RD: Novel alternatives and supplements to lithium and anticonvulsants for bipolar affective disorder. J Clin Psychiatry 58:224–242, 1997

Dwight MM, Keck PE, Stanton SP, et al: Antidepressant activity and mania associated with risperidone treatment of schizoaffective disorder. Lancet 344:554–555, 1994

Eadie MJ, Hooper WD, Dickinson RG: Valproate-associated hepatotoxicity and its biochemical mechanisms. Medical Toxicology and Adverse Drug Experience 3:85–106, 1988

Eaton WW, Reigier DA, Locke BZ, et al: The Epidemiologic Catchment Area Program of the National Institute of Mental Health. Public Health Rep 96:319–325, 1981

Evans DL, Byerly MJ, Greer RA: Secondary mania: diagnosis and treatment. J Clin Psychiatry 56 (suppl 3):31–37, 1995

Expert Consensus Guideline Series: Treatment of bipolar disorder. J Clin Psychiatry 57 (suppl 12A):1–88, 1996

Feuchtwanger E: Die Funktionen des Stirnhirns [The functions of the frontal lobes]. Gesamtgebiete der Neurologie und Psychiatrie 38:1–194, 1923

Flor-Henry P: Psychosis and temporal lobe epilepsy: a controlled investigation. Epilepsia 10:363–395, 1969

Gainotti G: Emotional behavior and hemispheric side of the lesion. Cortex 8:41–55, 1972

Gelenberg AJ: Lithium efficacy and adverse effects. J Clin Psychiatry 49 (suppl 11):8–9, 1988

Gillin JC: The sleep therapies of depression. Prog Neuropsychopharmacol Biol Psychiatry 7:351–364, 1983

Gilman J: Lamotrigine: an antiepileptic agent for the treatment of partial seizures. Ann Pharmacother 29:144–151, 1995

Goodnick PJ: Serotonin, in Mania: Clinical and Research Perspectives. Edited by Goodnick PJ. Washington, DC, American Psychiatric Press, 1998, pp 103–117

Goodwin FK, Jamison KR: Manic-Depressive Illness. New York, Oxford University Press, 1990

Greenberg DB, Younger J, Kaufman SD: Management of lithium in patients with cancer. Psychosomatics 34:388–394, 1994

Hudson JI, Lipinski JF, Frankenburg FR, et al: Effects of lithium on sleep in mania. Biol Psychiatry 25:665–668, 1989

Janicak PG, Levy NA: Rational copharmacy for acute mania. Psychiatric Annals 28:204–212, 1998

Jeavons PM: Hepatotoxicity in antiepileptic drugs, in Chronic Toxicity of Antiepileptic Drugs. Edited by Oxley J, Janz D, Meinardi H. New York, Raven, 1983, pp 1–46

Jorge RE, Robinson RG, Starkstein SE, et al: Secondary mania following traumatic brain injury. Am J Psychiatry 150:916–921, 1993

Kenneback G, Bergfeldt L, Vallin H, et al: Electrophysiologic effects and clinical hazards of carbamazepine treatment for neurologic disorders in patients with abnormalities of the cardiac conduction system. Am Heart J 121:1421–1429, 1991

Keschner M, Bender MB, Strauss I: Mental symptoms in cases of tumours in the temporal lobe. Archives of Neurology and Psychiatry 35:572–596, 1936

Kessler RC, McGonagle KA, Zhao S, et al: Lifetime and 12-month prevalence of DSM-III-R psychiatric disorders in the United States: results from the National Comorbidity Study. Arch Gen Psychiatry 51:8–19, 1994

Kleist K: Gehirnpathologische und Lokalisatorische Ergebnisse: die Storungen der Ichleistungen und Ihre Localisation in Orbita, Innen- und Zwischenhirn [Outcomes of brain pathology and localization: disorders of ego performances and their localization in the orbits, inner, and middle brain]. Monatsschrift fur Psychiatrie und Neurologie 79:338–343, 1931

Koek RJ, Kessler CC: Possible induction of mania by risperidone. J Clin Psychiatry 57:174–175, 1996

Kolodny A: The symptomatology of tumour in the temporal lobe. Brain 52:385–417, 1928

Kosten TR, Forrest JN: Treatment of severe lithium-induced polyuria with amiloride. Am J Psychiatry 143:1563–1568, 1986

Krauthammer C, Klerman GL: Secondary mania: manic syndromes associated with antecedent physical illness or drugs. Arch Gen Psychiatry 35:1333–1339, 1978

Larson EW, Richelson E: Organic causes of mania. Mayo Clin Proc 63:906–912, 1988

Levenson JL: Cardiovascular disease, in Psychiatric Care of the Medical Patient. Edited by Stoudemire A, Fogel BS. New York, Oxford University Press, 1993, pp 539–564

Lieberman S: Nutriceutical review of St. John's wort (Hypericum perforatum) for the treatment of depression. Journal of Women's Health 7:172–177, 1998

Llewellyn A, Stowe ZN, Strader JR: The use of lithium and management of women with bipolar disorder during pregnancy and lactation. J Clin Psychiatry 59 (suppl 6):57–64, 1998

Lyketsos CG, Hanson AL, Fishman M, et al: Manic syndrome early and late in the course of HIV. Am J Psychiatry 150:326–327, 1993

Masand PS:Lamotrigine as prophylaxis against steroid-induced mania. J Clin Psychiatry 60:708–709, 1999

McElroy SL, Dessain ED, Pope HG, et al: Clozapine in the treatment of psychotic mood disorders, schizoaffective disorder, and schizophrenia. J Clin Psychiatry 52:411–414, 1991

McElroy SL, Keck PE, Stanton S, et al: A randomized comparison of divalproex oral loading versus haloperidol in the initial treatment of acute psychotic mania. J Clin Psychiatry 57:142–146, 1996

McElroy SL, Frye M, Denicoff K, et al: Olanzapine in treatment-resistant bipolar disorder. J Affect Disord 49:119–122, 1998

McLean M: Clinical pharmacokinetics of gabapentin. Neurology 44 (suppl 5):S17–S22, 1994

Mendlewicz J, Fieve RR, Rainer J, et al: Manic-depressive illness: a comparative study of patients with and without a family history. Br J Psychiatry 120:523–530, 1972

Miklowitz DJ: Psychosocial approaches to the course and treatment of bipolar disorder. CNS Spectrums 3:48–65, 1998

Minski L: Mental symptoms associated with 58 cases of cerebral tumors. Journal of Neurology and Psychiatry 13:330–343, 1933

Morris H: Pharmacokinetics of new anticonvulsants in psychiatry. Cleve Clin J Med 65 (suppl 1):SI15–SI20, 1998

Mukherjee S, Sackeim HA, Lee C: Unilateral ECT in the treatment of manic episodes. Convulsive Therapy 4:74–80, 1988

Nemeroff C: Introduction: fifty years of lithium use in the treatment of bipolar disorder. J Clin Psychiatry 61(suppl): 3–5, 2000

Pisani F, Fazio A, Oteri G, et al: Sodium valproate and valpromide: differential interactions with carbamazepine in epileptic patients. Epilepsia 27:548–552, 1986

Pope HG, Katz DL: Affective and psychotic symptoms associated with anabolic steroid use. Am J Psychiatry 145:487–490, 1988

Post RM: Use of the anticonvulsant carbamazepine in primary and secondary affective illness: clinical and theoretical implications. Psychol Med 12:701–704, 1982

Post RM, Frye MA, Leverich GS, et al. The role of complex combination therapy in the treatment of refractory bipolar illness. CNS Spectrums 3:66–86, 1998

Price TRP, Goetz KL, Lovell MR: Neuropsychiatric aspects of brain tumors, in The American Psychiatric Press Textbook of Neuropsychiatry, 2nd Edition. Edited by Yudofsky SC, Hales RE. Washington, DC, American Psychiatric Press, 1992, pp 473–497

Prien RF, Gelenberg AJ: Alternatives to lithium for preventive treatment of bipolar disorder. Am J Psychiatry 146:840–848, 1989

Ramsay R: Clinical efficacy and safety of gabapentin. Neurology 44 (suppl 5):S23–S30, 1994

Redenbaugh JE, Sato S, Penry JK, et al: Sodium valproate: pharmacokinetics and effectiveness in treating intractable seizures. Neurology 30:1–6, 1980

Robinson RG, Boston JD, Starkstein SE, et al: Comparison of mania with depression following brain injury: causal factors. Am J Psychiatry 145:172–178, 1988a

Robinson RG, Starkstein SE, Price TR: Post-stroke depression and lesion location. Stroke 19:125–126, 1988b

Roy A, Breier A, Doran AR, et al: Life events in depression. J Affect Disord 9:143–148, 1985

Rudorfer MV, Linnoila M: Electroconvulsive therapy, in Lithium Therapy Monographs, Vol I: Lithium Combination Treatment. Edited by Johnson FN. Basel, Switzerland, Karger, 1986, pp 164–178

Rundell JR, Wise MG: Causes of organic mood disorder. J Neuropsychiatry Clin Neurosci 1:398–400, 1989

Sachs G, Cosgrove V: Bipolar disorder: current treatments and new strategies. Cleve Clin J Med 65 (suppl 1):SI31–SI37, 1998

Sackeim HA, Greenberg MS, Weisman AL, et al: Hemispheric asymmetry in the expression of positive and negative emotions: neurologic evidence. Arch Neurol 39:210–217, 1982

Sanger TM, Tohen M, Tollefson GD, et al: Olanzapine versus placebo in rapid-cycling bipolar disorder. Schizophr Res 29:152, 1998

Scheffner D, Konig S, Rauterberg-Rutland I, et al: Fatal liver failure in 16 children with valproate therapy. Epilepsia 29:520–542, 1988

Seetharam MN, Pellock JM: Risk-benefit assessment of carbamazepine in children. Drug Saf 6:148–158, 1991

Shuaib A, Mahmood RH, Wishart T, et al: Neuroprotective effects of lamotrigine in global ischemia in gerbils: a histological, in vivo microdialysis and behavioral study. Brain Res 702:199–206, 1995

Shukla S, Cook BL, Mukherjee S, et al: Mania following head trauma. Am J Psychiatry 144:93–96, 1987

Simpson SG, DePaulo JR: Genetics, in Mania: Clinical and Research Perspectives. Edited by Goodnick PJ. Washington, DC, American Psychiatric Press, 1998, pp 81–102

Singh AN, Catalan J: Risperidone in HIV-related manic psychosis. Lancet 344:1029–1030, 1994

Small JG, Klapper MH, Kellams JJ, et al: Electroconvulsive treatment compared with lithium in the management of manic states. Arch Gen Psychiatry 45:727–732, 1988

Sobotka JL, Alexander B, Cook BL: A review of carbamazepine's hematologic reactions and monitoring recommendations. DICP 24:1214–1217, 1990

Solomon DA, Keitner GI, Ryan CE, et al: Lithium plus valproate as maintenance polypharmacy with bipolar disorder: a review. CNS Spectrums 5:19–28, 2000

Starkstein SE, Robinson RG: Affective disorders and cerebrovascular disease. Br J Psychiatry 154:170–172, 1989

Starkstein SE, Robinson RG: Neuropsychiatric aspects of cerebral vascular disorders, in The American Psychiatric Press Textbook of Neuropsychiatry. Edited by Yudofsky SC, Hales RE. Washington, DC, American Psychiatric Press, 1992, pp 449–472

Starkstein SE, Pearlson GD, Boston JD, et al: Mania after brain injury: a controlled study of causative factors. Arch Neurol 44:1069–1073, 1987

Starkstein SE, Moran TH, Bowersox JA, et al: Behavioral abnormalities induced by frontal cortical and nucleus accumbens lesions. Brain Res 473:74–80, 1988a

Starkstein SE, Boston JD, Robinson RGG: Mechanisms of mania after brain injury: 12 case reports and review of the literature. J Nerv Ment Dis 176:87–100, 1988b

Starkstein SE, Robinson RG, Honig MA, et al: Mood changes after right hemisphere lesions. Br J Psychiatry 155:79–85, 1989

Starkstein SE, Federoff P, Berthier ML, et al: Manic-depressive and pure manic states after brain lesions. Biol Psychiatry 29:149–158, 1991

Stone K: Mania in the elderly. Br J Psychiatry 155:220–224, 1989

Stoudemire A, Moran MG, Fogel BS: Psychotropic drug use in the medically ill, part II. Psychosomatics 32:34–46, 1991

Stoudemire A, Fogel BS, Gulley LR, et al: Psychopharmacology in the medical patient, in Psychiatric Care of the Medical Patient. Edited by Stoudemire A, Fogel B. New York, Oxford University Press, 1993, pp 155–206

Stoudemire GA: Selected organic mental disorders, in The American Psychiatric Press Textbook of Neuropsychiatry. Edited by Hales RE, Yudofsky SC. Washington, DC, American Psychiatric Press, 1987, pp 125–140

Strakowski SM, McElroy SL, Keck PW, et al: The co-occurrence of mania with medical and other psychiatric disorders. Int J Psychiatry Med 24:305–328, 1994

Strauss H, Keschner M: Mental symptoms in cases of tumor of the frontal lobe. Archives of Neurology and Psychiatry 33:986–1105, 1935

Tohen M, Gannon KS: Pharmacologic approaches for treatment-resistant mania. Psychiatric Annals 28:629–632, 1998

Tohen M, Zarate C, Centorrino F, et al: Risperidone in the treatment of mania. J Clin Psychiatry 57:249–253, 1996

Tohen M, Sanger TM, McElroy SL, et al: Olanzapine versus placebo in the treatment of acute mania. Am J Psychiatry 156:702–709, 1999

Uzych L: Anabolic steroids and psychiatric-related effects: a review. Can J Psychiatry 37:23–27, 1992

Walton SA, Berk M, Brook S: Superiority of lithium over verapamil in mania: a randomized, controlled, single-blind trial. J Clin Psychiatry 57:543–546, 1996

Wehr TA, Sack DA, Rosenthal NE: Sleep reduction as a final common pathway in the genesis of mania. Am J Psychiatry 144:201–204, 1987

Weiner RD, Coffey CE: Electroconvulsive therapy in the medically ill, in Principles of Medical Psychiatry. Edited by Stoudemire A, Fogel BS. Orlando, FL, Grune & Stratton, 1987, pp 113–134

Weissman MM, Leaf PJ, Tischler GL, et al: Affective disorders in five United States communities. Psychol Med 17:141–153, 1988

Weissman MM, Bland RC, Canino GJ, et al: Cross-national epidemiology of major depression and bipolar disorder. JAMA 276:293–299, 1996

Winokur G, Clayton P: The Medical Basis of Psychiatry. Philadelphia, PA, WB Saunders, 1986

Wise MG, Rundell JR: Concise Guide to Consultation Psychiatry, 2nd Edition. Washington, DC, American Psychiatric Press, 1994

19

Somatization and Somatoform Disorders

Susan E. Abbey, M.D., F.R.C.P.C.

Somatization is a poorly understood "blind spot" of medicine (Quill 1985, p. 3075), and somatoform disorders remain poorly understood. Recent critiques have raised important conceptual and clinical questions about the validity and utility of the concepts, particularly in the clinical setting. There have been calls to develop new paradigms that might lead to more effective management (Epstein et al. 1999; Sharpe and Carson 2001). These areas challenge the consultation-liaison psychiatrist, who often wades into emotionally charged clinical situations in which diagnosis is difficult and both the referring physician and the patient are frustrated and angry. The complex set of emotions that patients with somatoform disorder engender has resulted in disparaging names for these patients (e.g., "crocks") (Lipsitt 1970) and for the discipline (e.g., "psychoceramic medicine"). However, consultation-liaison psychiatrists can effectively work with these patients, produce substantial improvements in their quality of life and that of their families, and decrease direct and indirect costs of the disorder. The increasing awareness of somatization's high costs to the health care system has spurred an explosion of literature, including monographs (Bass 1990; Creed et al. 1992; Ford 1983; Kellner 1986, 1991; Kirmayer and Robbins 1991a; Mayou et al. 1995; Shapiro and Rosenfeld 1987; Smith 1991) and commentaries (Barsky 1998; Barsky and Borus 1999; Epstein et al. 1999; Folks and Houck 1993; Mayou 1993; Murphy 1989; Sharpe and Carson 2001), to guide consultation-liaison psychiatrists and primary care practitioners.

This chapter begins with a review of somatization as a process, followed by a review of DSM-IV-TR somatoform disorders (American Psychiatric Association 2000). Somatization can be conceptualized as a way of respond-

ing or living. It is a ubiquitous human phenomenon that, at times, becomes problematic and warrants clinical attention. Somatization is extremely common in medical settings and among the patients referred to consultation-liaison psychiatrists (Katon et al. 1984). Not all somatizing patients have a somatoform disorder. Many have another Axis I disorder (see Table 19–1) or transiently somatize in the context of significant life stress. Patients who meet DSM-IV-TR diagnostic criteria for somatoform disorders are less common but are an important component of the consultation-liaison psychiatrist's work. The medical training of the consultation-liaison psychiatrist facilitates the management of the most difficult cases—those patients who somatize or have a somatoform disorder and have a concurrent general medical condition.

SOMATIZATION AS A PROCESS

Definitions and Clinically Useful Theoretical Concepts

Somatization

Historically, *somatization* was defined by Steckel as a deep-seated neurosis that produced bodily symptoms (Lipowski 1988). More recently, somatization has been used as a descriptive term for patients who have a tendency to experience and communicate psychological and interpersonal distress in the form of somatic distress and medically unexplained symptoms for which they seek medical help (Katon et al. 1984; Kleinman 1986; Lipowski 1988). In essence, somatization is a culturally sanctioned idiom of psychosocial distress (Katon et al. 1984;

TABLE 19–1. DSM-IV-TR Axis I psychiatric disorders and other conditions that may be a focus of clinical attention associated with persistent physical symptoms

Mood disorders
    Major depressive episode
    Dysthymic disorder

Anxiety disorders
    Panic disorder
    Generalized anxiety disorder
    Obsessive-compulsive disorder
    Posttraumatic stress disorder

Psychotic disorders
    Schizophrenia
    Delusional disorder, somatic type

Somatoform disorders
    Somatization disorder
    Undifferentiated somatoform disorder
    Hypochondriasis
    Conversion disorder
    Body dysmorphic disorder
    Pain disorder
    Somatoform disorder not otherwise specified

Adjustment disorder
    All subtypes may have associated physical complaints

Substance-related disorders
    Alcohol dependence and abuse
    Opioid dependence and abuse
    Sedative-hypnotic dependence and abuse
    Polysubstance dependence and abuse

Factitious disorders
    Factitious disorder with predominantly physical signs and symptoms or with combined psychological and physical signs and symptoms

Malingering

Psychological factors affecting a medical condition

TABLE 19–2. Clinical implications of the components of somatization

Component	Potential intervention
Experiential	Techniques to decrease somatic sensations (e.g., biofeedback, pharmacotherapy for concomitant psychiatric disorder)
Cognitive	Reattribution of sensation from sinister to benign
	Distraction techniques
Behavioral	Operant techniques to reduce medication consumption
	Contract to "save" symptoms for regular visit with primary care physician rather than visiting emergency room

Somatization has a variety of patterns. A study of 685 family practice patients described three forms of somatization associated with different sociodemographic and illness behavior characteristics. Most patients met criteria for only one form of somatization (Kirmayer and Robbins 1991b). The three forms of somatization were

1. *Medically unexplained symptoms*—somatic symptoms not explained after appropriate assessment (There is some disagreement as to whether this represents a discrete category or is better understood in terms of a dimensional characteristic.)
2. *Hypochondriacal somatization*—bodily preoccupation and a tendency to worry about the possibility of or vulnerability to serious physical illness
3. *Somatic presentation of psychiatric disorder*—primary psychiatric disorders other than somatoform disorders in which somatic symptoms are the most prominent part of the clinical picture (e.g., major depressive disorder, panic disorder)

Medically Unexplained Symptoms

Medically unexplained symptoms, also known as functional somatic symptoms, are extremely common in patients in both community and clinic settings. In a study of 14 common symptoms in 1,000 patients in an ambulatory medical clinic, 74% were medically unexplained (Kroenke and Mangelsdorff 1989). A study of 100 patients admitted to a neurology ward reported that 14% had physical symptoms that could not be medically explained, and 26% had both medically explained and unexplained symptoms (Ewald et al. 1994). There has been a recent resurgence of interest in functional somatic symptoms and paradigms for better understanding and managing such symptoms (Barsky and Borus 1999; Epstein et al. 1999; Wessely et al. 1999).

Kleinman 1986). The term *somatothymia* has been proposed to describe the use of somatic language to communicate affective distress (Stoudemire 1991). Everyone somatizes at times, but its frequency, the intensity of the stressor eliciting somatization, and the symptoms experienced vary. Many people experience somatic symptoms in response to the loss of an important relationship (e.g., the death of a loved one, a broken love affair), with the sensation of a "broken heart." Experiencing headaches or stomachaches is common in many people who do not feel prepared for a task for which there is no acceptable excuse except illness.

Three components of somatization described by Lipowski (1988) can be targeted for intervention: 1) experiential, 2) cognitive, and 3) behavioral (Table 19–2).

Somatosensory Amplification

Symptoms are the result of bodily sensations and their subsequent cortical interpretation. *Somatosensory amplification*, which refers to the tendency to experience somatic sensations as intense, noxious, or disturbing (Barsky et al. 1988a), is composed of three elements: 1) hypervigilance to bodily sensations, 2) predisposition to select out and concentrate on weak or infrequent bodily sensations, and 3) reaction to sensations with cognitions and affect that intensify them and make them more alarming (Barsky et al. 1988a). It has both trait and state components.

Illness Behavior

The distinction between *illness* and *disease* (Eisenberg 1977) is useful for consultation-liaison psychiatrists. Illness has been described as the response of the individual and his or her family to symptoms. This contrasts with disease, which is defined by physicians and is associated with pathophysiologic processes and documentable lesions. Mismatches between illness and disease are common and are at the root of many management problems. Patients with a disease such as hypertension may not perceive themselves as ill and thus may be noncompliant with treatment. Patients with somatoform disorders view themselves as very ill despite not having a disease. In somatizing patients with some disease component, their subjective illness experience is assessed to be disproportionate to the degree of disease.

Illness behavior refers to "the manner in which individuals monitor their bodies, define and interpret their symptoms, take remedial action, and utilize sources of help as well as the more formal health care system. It also is concerned with how people monitor and respond to symptoms and symptom change over the course of an illness and how this affects behaviour, remedial actions taken, and response to treatment" (Mechanic 1986, p. 1). Illness behavior may be regarded as a syndrome, as a symptom, as a dimension, or as an explanation of behavior (Mayou 1989). Illness behavior is affected by a wide variety of social, psychiatric, and cultural factors (Eisenberg 1977; Kleinman 1986; Mayou 1989; Mechanic 1986) and can be used as a means of negotiating tensions in relationships (Mechanic 1986). As Mechanic (1986) noted, "illness is often used to achieve a variety of social and personal objectives having little to do with biological systems of the pathogenesis of disease" (p. 3).

Abnormal illness behavior is when a physician identifies an inappropriate or maladaptive mode of perceiving, evaluating or acting in relation to one's own health status, which persists despite the fact that a doctor (or other appropriate social agent) has offered an accurate and reasonably lucid explanation of the nature of the illness and the appropriate course of management to be followed, based on a thorough examination of all parameters of functioning, and taking into account the individual's age, educational and sociocultural background. (Pilowsky 1987, p. 89)

Abnormal illness behavior may be somatically or psychologically focused and may be either illness-affirming or illness-denying. The construct has been criticized as dangerous in that it places physicians in the position of defining "abnormal" and judging their own behavior as adequate when in fact they may be exhibiting "abnormal treatment behavior" (Pilowsky 1987).

The consultation-liaison psychiatrist is often called because of "abnormal illness behavior" and must determine whether such behavior is abnormal within the individual's social world. The consultation-liaison psychiatrist's explanation that a behavior is culturally appropriate may be more readily accepted when the patient is of an obviously different ethnic or racial group. Patients who appear to be part of the dominant culture but espouse complementary or alternative medicine may be particularly difficult for traditional health care providers to deal with. For example, an American-born, Caucasian senior business executive alarmed the surgical team by insisting that a small velvet bag be suspended from the bed directly above his head. This caused considerable consternation among the nursing staff and surgeons, and a consultation was requested for "new-onset psychosis." When the consultation-liaison psychiatrist asked what the bag was, the executive proudly described that it contained crystals, soil, and rocks from "healing places," which he had been collecting for 10 years as part of his involvement in "New Age healing." He was aware that it "must seem pretty strange to have a CEO into this stuff." This explanation relieved the team.

Psychological Factors Affecting a Medical Condition

The DSM-IV-TR diagnosis psychological factor affecting medical condition is used when psychological or behavioral factors adversely affect a general medical condition (American Psychiatric Association 2000). Such factors include Axis I and II disorders, psychological symptoms that do not meet diagnostic criteria, personality traits or coping styles, and maladaptive health behaviors. The adverse effect may occur by 1) influencing the development or exacerbation of the medical condition, 2) interfering with the treatment, 3) increasing health risk, and 4) causing stress-related psychophysiological changes. DSM-IV-TR diagnostic criteria are shown in Table 19–3.

TABLE 19–3. DSM-IV-TR diagnostic criteria for psychological factor affecting medical condition

A. A general medical condition (coded on Axis III) is present.

B. Psychological factors adversely affect the general medical condition in one of the following ways:

    (1) the factors have influenced the course of the general medical condition as shown by a close temporal association between the psychological factors and the development or exacerbation of, or delayed recovery from, the general medical condition

    (2) the factors interfere with the treatment of the general medical condition

    (3) the factors constitute additional health risks for the individual

    (4) stress-related physiological responses precipitate or exacerbate symptoms of the general medical condition

Choose name based on the nature of the psychological factors (if more than one factor is present, indicate the most prominent):

    Mental disorder affecting . . . *[indicate the general medical condition]* (e.g., an Axis I disorder such as major depressive disorder delaying recovery from a myocardial infarction)

    Psychological symptoms affecting . . . *[indicate the general medical condition]* (e.g., depressive symptoms delaying recovery from surgery; anxiety exacerbating asthma)

    Personality traits or coping style affecting . . . *[indicate the general medical condition]* (e.g., pathological denial of the need for surgery in a patient with cancer; hostile, pressured behavior contributing to cardiovascular disease)

    Maladaptive health behaviors affecting . . . *[indicate the general medical condition]* (e.g., overeating; lack of exercise; unsafe sex)

    Stress-related physiological response affecting . . . *[indicate the general medical condition]* (e.g., stress-related exacerbations of ulcer, hypertension, arrhythmia, or tension headache)

    Other or unspecified psychological factors affecting . . . *[indicate the general medical condition]* (e.g., interpersonal, cultural, or religious factors)

DSM-IV-TR emphasizes that psychological and behavioral factors play a potential role in almost every general medical condition and that this diagnosis should be used only when psychological or behavioral factors have a clinically significant impact (American Psychiatric Association 2000).

The Problem of Defining New Diagnoses at the Borderline of Psychiatry and Medicine

Consultation-liaison psychiatrists are asked to assess and manage disorders that exist at the interface of medicine and psychiatry and that are poorly understood, such as fibromyalgia, chronic fatigue syndrome, functional gastrointestinal disorders, noncardiac chest pain, chronic headache, dizziness, and chronic unexplained pelvic pain. Studies of tertiary care patients typically show increased current and lifetime prevalence of psychiatric disorders, increased nonspecific emotional distress, and increased psychosocial stressors. The most common Axis I diagnoses identified in these populations are mood and anxiety disorders and somatoform disorders. Multifactorial models for the etiology of these conditions have been proposed. All of the models include factors such as psychiatric disorder, psychosocial stressors or trauma, somatosensory amplification, and misattribution of symptoms. An example of a multifactorial model for noncardiac chest pain is shown in Figure 19–1 (Mayou 1992). In some patients, these diagnoses may represent an emotional disorder misdiagnosed as a medical condition (Stewart 1990a). Patients with medically unexplained symptoms may adopt diagnoses popularized by the media (e.g., multiple chemical sensitivity) and often show considerable pathoplasticity of these diagnoses over time (Stewart 1990b). It has recently been argued that these disorders share more similarities than differences (Barsky and Borus 1999; Sharpe and Carson 2001; Wessely et al. 1999).

Somatization as a Clinical Problem

Somatization is a ubiquitous phenomenon that in and of itself does not necessarily constitute a clinical problem. Kirmayer and Young (1998) note that "depending upon circumstances" somatization "can be seen as an index of disease or disorder, an indication of psychopathology, a symbolic condensation of intrapsychic conflict, a culturally coded expression of distress, a medium for expressing social discontent, and a mechanism through which patients attempt to reposition themselves within their local worlds" (p. 420). Somatization becomes clinically significant when it is associated with significant occupational and social dysfunction or excessive health care use. Persistent somatization should be distinguished from transient somatization, which may occur as part of an acute response to a variety of significant life stressors, including bereavement (Lipowski 1988). Persistent somatization becomes a way of life and is a burden to patients,

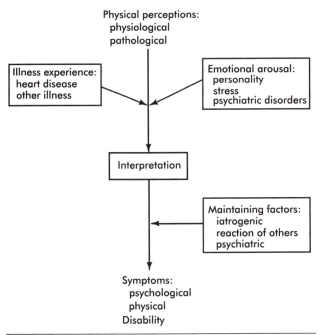

FIGURE 19–1. An etiological model for noncardiac atypical chest pain.

Source. Reprinted from Mayou R: "Patients' Fears of Illness: Chest Pain and Palpitations," in *Medical Symptoms Not Explained by Organic Disease.* Edited by Creed F, Mayou R, Hopkins A. London, England, The Royal College of Psychiatrists and The Royal College of Physicians of London, 1992, pp. 25–33. Used with permission.

families, the health care system, employers, and society at large.

The relation between acute and persistent forms of somatization is unclear. They may be part of a continuum or exist as discrete conditions. A longitudinal study of primary care "somatizers" (defined as patients with emotional disorder presenting with recent-onset physical symptoms) found that 16 of 44 patients went on to develop chronic somatoform disorders over 2-year follow-up. The physical symptoms of the somatizers were less likely to attenuate than those of control group patients, and changes in physical symptoms seemed to mirror changes in emotional arousal (Craig et al. 1993).

There is increasing concern about the economic burden of somatization (Barsky et al. 1986b; Shaw and Creed 1991). Somatization accounts for about 10% of total direct health care costs (Ford 1983) and has the potential to bankrupt the health care financing system (Cummings and van den Bos 1981). Patients with somatization disorder have higher average health carecosts than other patients: total charges 9 times greater, hospital charges 6 times greater, and physician services 14 times greater. In one study, somatizing patients spent an average of 7 days per month sick in bed compared

with the general population average of 0.48 days (Smith et al. 1986).

A variety of psychiatric disorders are associated with somatization, as noted in Table 19–1. Mood and anxiety disorders are the most common psychiatric disorders associated with somatization in primary care settings (Bridges and Goldberg 1985; Katon et al. 1984). Katon et al. (1984) studied a group of 261 primary care patients and documented somatization in the context of major depressive disorder in 38% of the sample, conversion disorder in 5%, psychogenic pain in 4%, and factitious disorder in 1.5%.

Relation Between Psychiatric Disorders and Somatization

Strong interrelations exist among somatization, psychiatric disorders, and health care utilization, with four models advanced to explain these relations (Simon 1991) (see Figure 19–2).

Somatization as a Masked Presentation of Psychiatric Illness

Physical symptom reporting and health care seeking may result from the physical symptoms that are an integral part of most psychiatric disorders. The somatizing patient focuses on these symptoms to the exclusion of the psychological symptoms and may in fact attribute psychological symptoms to the distress of having the physical symptoms (e.g., "Yes, doctor, I am sad, but you would be too if you couldn't sleep or eat and had no energy!"). Major depressive disorder and anxiety disorders are significantly underrecognized in patients presenting with somatic complaints. In a primary care study, physician recognition of major depressive disorder was 77% in patients with a psychosocial presentation and only 22% among patients with somatic symptoms (Kirmayer et al. 1993).

Somatization as an Amplifying Personal Perceptual Style

In this model, somatization is thought to result from an amplifying personal perceptual style, which is conceived of as a stable personality trait or a consequence of abnormal neuropsychological information processing (Barsky et al. 1988a). There is evidence of a lowered threshold for reporting physical symptoms in some of these patients (Barsky et al. 1988a; Pennebaker and Watson 1991).

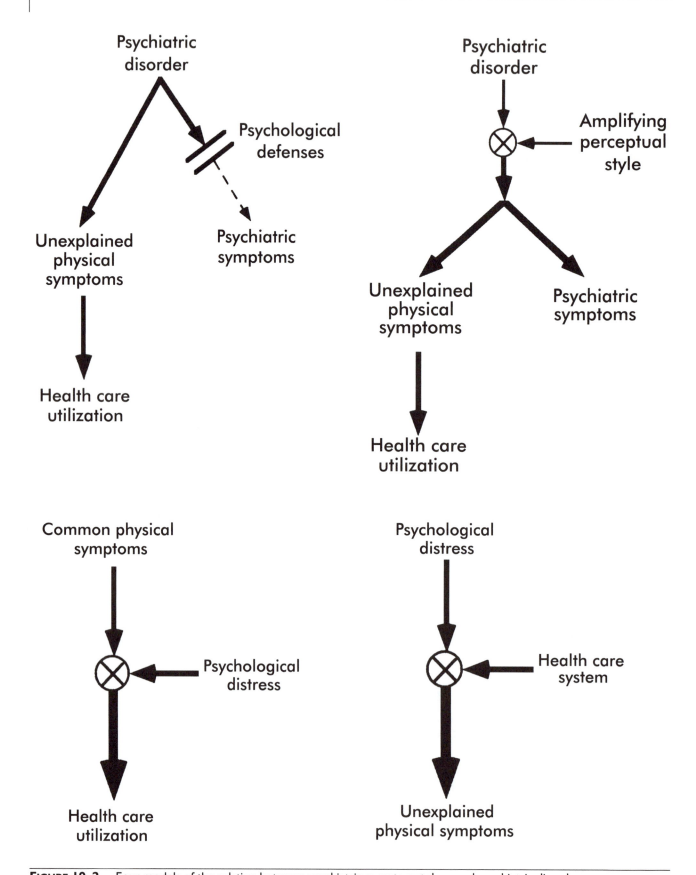

FIGURE 19–2. Four models of the relation between psychiatric symptomatology and psychiatric disorder.

Source. Reprinted from Simon GE: "Somatization and Psychiatric Disorder," in *Current Concepts of Somatization: Research and Clinical Perspectives.* Edited by Kirmayer LJ, Robbins JM. Washington, DC, American Psychiatric Press, 1991, pp. 37–62. Used with permission.

Somatization as a Tendency to Seek Care for Common Symptoms

This model posits that emotional distress prompts people to seek care for common symptoms for which they would not seek care in the absence of emotional distress. This model is supported by research in patients with irritable bowel syndrome. Medical help seeking in patients with irritable bowel syndrome is associated with higher levels of emotional distress despite levels of physical symptomatology similar to those in patients in the community with irritable bowel syndrome who do not seek medical care (Drossman et al. 1988).

Somatization as a Response to the Incentives of the Health Care System

This model proposes that somatic symptom reporting is caused by the health care system, which tends to reinforce illness behavior and symptom reporting and may produce "iatrogenic somatization" (Simon 1991).

Depression and Somatization

There has been considerable interest in the relation between somatization and depression (Katon et al. 1982, 1986; Simon et al. 1999; Smith 1992). Although somatic symptoms are noted to be common in major depressive disorder (Mathew et al. 1981), the mechanism by which they are produced is unclear and may be related to 1) psychophysiological concomitants of depression, 2) somatosensory amplification, and 3) a depressive attributional style in which symptoms are perceived as indicating poor health. Primary care patients with depression have higher health care utilization and more nonspecific complaints, vague complaints, and psychophysiological symptoms than do control patients (Katon et al. 1986). It is estimated that 50% or more of the patients presenting in primary care settings with major depressive disorder do so with predominantly somatic complaints rather than cognitive or affective symptoms of depression (Bridges and Goldberg 1985; Schurman et al. 1985; Simon et al. 1999). These somatic presentations of depression have been referred to as *masked depression* or *depressive equivalents*.

Smith (1992) evaluated the relation between depression and somatization by reviewing the literature from 1975 to 1990. He identified 14 studies addressing the relation between depression and somatization and 13 studies addressing the relation between depression and pain and concluded that 1) patients with somatization disorder have a high prevalence of depression (current prevalence ranging from 48% to 94%); 2) patients with major depressive disorder have substantial levels of somatization (63%–94%) and hypochondriacal symptoms (30%–80%); 3) depression can be treated successfully when it coexists with somatization disorder; 4) patients with chronic pain have a significant current prevalence of depressive disorders, but estimates range widely (8%–50%); 5) more than half of the patients with major depressive disorder complain of pain; and 6) pain is reduced with the treatment of depression (Smith 1992).

Anxiety and Somatization

Anxiety disorders are accompanied by prominent physical symptoms and are frequently mistaken for, or associated with, somatization in patients presenting in primary care and medical subspecialty settings (R. Goldberg et al. 1990; Sullivan et al. 1993). Somatization and hypochondriacal fears and beliefs are common among patients with panic disorder (Katon 1984), particularly those who also have agoraphobia and focus more on seeking an explanation for, rather than treatment of, their symptoms (Starcevic et al. 1992). Hypochondriacal fears and beliefs are reported to decrease with effective treatment of panic disorder (Noyes et al. 1986).

Substance Abuse and Somatization

Substance abuse occurs in a subset of patients with somatization disorder. In a sample of 25 patients with alcohol abuse or dependence, 33% of the men and 19% of the women met abridged criteria for somatization (Katon and Russo 1989). The relation between substance abuse and somatization appears to be associated with anxiety disorders in some patients (Katon 1984).

Posttraumatic Stress Disorder and Somatization

Individuals with posttraumatic stress disorder diagnoses appear to be at increased risk for somatization symptoms (Andreski et al. 1998). Medically unexplained somatic symptoms are more likely in cross-sectional comparisons with individuals without posttraumatic stress disorder, and prospectively, the incidence of new-onset medically unexplained somatic symptoms is greater than in control groups (Andreski et al. 1998).

Psychosis and Somatization

Patients with schizophrenia may present with medically unexplained symptoms typically described in a bizarre manner. They may occur in younger individuals in prodromal stages of psychotic decompensation.

Etiological Factors in Somatization and Somatoform Disorders

Pathophysiologic Mechanisms

Understanding and acknowledging physiologic mechanisms underlying somatization help both patient and physician avoid dualistic "mind versus body" (i.e., "imaginary" vs. "real") thinking and develop a therapeutic alliance. Table 19–4 summarizes some of the proposed pathophysiologic mechanisms of somatization.

Genetic Factors

Somatoform disorders have a genetic component (Torgersen 1986). An adoption study of Swedish women identified two clusters of somatizers with different genetic and environmental characteristics: 1) "high-frequency somatizers," who had a high frequency of psychiatric, abdominal, and back complaints and constituted 5% of the sample; and 2) "diversiform somatizers," who had less frequent disability but a greater diversity of complaints per occasion and accounted for 13% of the sample (Cloninger et al. 1984). High-frequency somatizers were more likely than diversiform somatizers to have biological mothers with increased rates of high-frequency somatization and biological fathers with increased rates of criminality (Bohman et al. 1984). Adoption studies with Swedish men suggested that the psychiatric processes associated with somatization in men and women may be qualitatively different (Cloninger et al. 1986). Further studies are needed.

TABLE 19–4.   Pathophysiologic mechanisms of somatization

Physiologic mechanisms
    Autonomic arousal
    Muscle tension
    Hyperventilation
    Vascular changes
    Cerebral information processing
    Physiologic effects of inactivity
    Sleep disturbance

Psychological mechanisms
    Perceptual factors
    Beliefs
    Mood
    Personality factors

Interpersonal mechanisms
    Reinforcing actions of relatives and friends
    Health care system
    Disability system

Source.   Adapted from Mayou 1993; Sharpe and Bass 1992.

Developmental and Social Learning and Attachment Behavior

Many cognitive appraisals patients make about somatic symptoms have their roots in early family experiences. For example, many patients with somatic symptoms report that their mothers were worried about health-related issues and had catastrophic interpretations for illness (e.g., every cough was likely to herald pneumonia). By the same token, physical symptoms are a major form of interpersonal communication in some families (Stuart and Noyes 1999). For example, a child receiving inattentive parenting may learn that complaining of physical symptoms leads to parental attention. Childhood exposure to parental chronic illness or illness behavior appears to increase the risk of somatization in later life (Bass and Murphy 1995; Craig et al. 1993). Anxious attachment behavior arising from early life experiences may be the basis for persistent care-seeking behavior that frustrates health care professionals and family members (Stuart and Noyes 1999).

Personality Characteristics

A variety of psychological traits or personality factors have been linked with somatization, although linkages have not been explored in detail, and it is unclear whether they are important in symptom production, influence help-seeking behavior, or result from dealing with chronic symptoms. Introspectiveness (i.e., the tendency to think about oneself) is associated with increased symptom reporting, greater physical and psychological distress, and more medical help seeking (Mechanic 1986). Negative affectivity is a construct based on negative mood, poor self-concept, and pessimism, which is associated with increased symptom reporting and greater worry about perceived symptoms (Pennebaker and Watson 1991). Several studies reported increased rates of personality disorder diagnoses (Stuart and Noyes 1999). Difficulties in relationships with medical caregivers often lead to psychiatric referral.

Psychodynamics

Bodily symptoms may represent metaphors through which a patient expresses emotional distress or psychic conflict (McDougall 1989). Self psychologists argue that bodily preoccupation develops in response to a fragmented sense of self and can be understood as an attempt to restore a sense of integration (Adler 1981). Rodin (1984) applied this paradigm, stating that somatization may arise from "a defective and fragile sense of self and from the relative inability to distinguish physical from psychological experiences" (p. 257). The theoretical construct of alexithymia refers to impairment in the ability to verbalize affect and elaborate fantasies (Taylor 1984). It has been implicated in some forms of somatization. Although repressed anger or aggression was thought by classical psychodynamic theorists to be important in somatization, Kellner et al. (1985) found no evidence that anger or hostility plays a specific etiological role in somatization and hypochondriasis.

Sexual and Physical Abuse

Both sexual and physical abuse have been linked with somatization. A potential association exists between sexual abuse and childhood and adult somatoform disorders (Morrison 1989), chronic pelvic pain syndromes (Toomey et al. 1993; Walker et al. 1988), functional gastrointestinal disorders (Drossman et al. 1990), and increased health care utilization (Drossman et al. 1990). Individuals who had been raped or molested before age 17 years were more likely to view common and benign symptoms as indicative of disease than were individuals who had not experienced childhood sexual or physical trauma (Barsky et al. 1993).

Physical abuse in both childhood and adulthood has been associated with somatization disorder (Walling et al. 1994), and childhood physical trauma has been associated with hypochondriasis (Barsky et al. 1994). Insight into the relation of abuse to somatization is helpful for many patients and may decrease health care use (Walling et al. 1994).

Particularly in gynecology and gastroenterology settings, patients should be specifically asked about sexual and physical abuse. The mechanism by which childhood sexual abuse and physical trauma are translated into somatization and adult somatoform disorders remains poorly understood. Sexual abuse effects "embodiment" (i.e., the experience of the self in and through the body) (Young 1992). Childhood sexual abuse typically occurs in a disturbed psychosocial milieu that may be characterized by other factors important in the development of adult somatoform syndromes (Drossman et al. 1990). However, higher rates of childhood sexual and physical trauma were found in patients with DSM-III-R (American Psychiatric Association 1987) hypochondriasis compared with control subjects, even when sociodemographic differences were controlled for (Barsky et al. 1994).

Sociocultural Factors

Although earlier writers argued that somatization was more common among non-Western cultures, more recent work suggests that somatization is ubiquitous, although prevalence and specific features vary across cultures (Kirmayer and Young 1998). The World Health Organization Cross-National Study of Mental Disorders in Primary Care found that all sites reported high rates of somatization (Gureje et al. 1997) and correlation of somatic symptoms and emotional distress (Simon et al. 1996), but rates of somatization disorder varied from 0% to 3.8% (Gureje et al. 1997). The stigmatization of psychiatric distress in Western culture is a powerful factor promoting somatization. "Organic" or physical illnesses are seen as more real and less blameworthy than psychiatric disorders, which are seen as under voluntary control and often are associated with connotations of malingering and weak moral fiber (Kirmayer and Robbins 1991a). Somatization may be the only form of communication permissible for the socially powerless (e.g., a headache that requires one to rest and remove oneself from the situation is more acceptable in many situations than openly expressing the view that the behavior of one's mate or employer is intolerable). Somatization may elicit caregiving.

Gender

The relation between gender and somatization is complex and poorly understood. Although traditionally, women have been thought to somatize more than men, the literature is problematic (Wool and Barsky 1994). A recent international study of somatization in primary care found few sex differences (Piccinelli and Simon 1997). A longitudinal study of primary care attendees found that somatizers were more likely to be men (Kirmayer and Robbins 1996), whereas data from the Epidemiologic Catchment Area study found that women report more unexplained symptoms overall (Liu et al. 1997).

Iatrogenesis

The health care insurance and disability systems foster somatization by providing reinforcement and a substrate on which this psychopathology may thrive (Ford 1983; Simon 1991). Insurance reimbursement patterns that cover physical but not psychiatric disorders foster somatization (Folks and Houck 1993; Ford 1992).

Diagnostic Process

Assessment for somatization or somatoform disorder is often difficult and requires additional interviewing skills (Creed and Guthrie 1993; Sharpe et al. 1992).

Collaborate With Referral Sources

Collaboration with the referral source is essential for a clear understanding of the reason for referral and of what the patient has been told about it. Consultation-liaison psychiatrists can provide guidance about how to explain the referral to the patient so as to make it more acceptable.

Review the Medical Records

Medical records should be reviewed before the consultation. Review helps the consultant to devise an approach to the patient. Familiarity with the history fosters an alliance. The type, number, and frequency of the patient's symptoms as well as comments about the patient's prior attitude toward symptoms and behavior should be documented (Creed and Guthrie 1993). The importance of a thorough chart review cannot be overestimated. The consultation-liaison psychiatrist may be the first person to thoroughly review the typically thick chart and thus may be in a better position than any other member of the medical team to reach a diagnosis of either a general medical condition or a psychiatric disorder.

Collaborate With Family and Friends

Collaboration with family and friends is almost always crucial to obtain an accurate assessment of the patient's history, current and past functional capacity, and current and past psychosocial stressors.

Build an Alliance With the Patient

The patient's ambivalence about seeing a psychiatrist must be addressed directly early in the examination. It is essential to know what the patient has been told about the consultation process. The specific approach to the examination will vary according to the patient. For very resistant patients, the initial interview is often dominated by gaining sufficient cooperation to allow a more detailed assessment to take place at a later time. The initial phase of the examination focuses on the history of physical symptoms. Allowing the patient to report a detailed history of his or her physical symptoms and concerns provides reassurance that the consultation-liaison psychiatrist is taking the symptoms seriously, which aids immeasurably in later phases of the assessment and treatment process. The psychiatrist's use of empathic comments such as "You have had a terrible time" or "The symptoms sound very difficult" help to build a working alliance with the patient and may lead the patient to volunteer information (Creed and Guthrie 1993). The question "How has this illness or symptom affected your life?" may go a long way toward answering the question "How has your life affected this illness?" Making interpretive or linking statements that bring together the patient's physical and emotional states may encourage

the patient to be more forthcoming with regard to emotional distress and may further the sense of engagement (Creed and Guthrie 1993). However, caution must be exercised because premature or maladroit interpretations can threaten the developing therapeutic alliance. An example of a comment that was found to be helpful by a patient with somatization disorder, pain disorder, and an extremely difficult early life was "You have had such a painful and difficult life; I wonder if some of this pain is being held in your body." This statement caused the patient to begin crying and to further reveal her history of early trauma. For skeptical patients, the consultation-liaison psychiatrist can emphasize his or her expertise in helping people develop the skills they need to minimize the effect of symptoms regardless of the "cause" of the symptoms (Fishman 1992).

Perform a Mental Status Examination

In addition to routine psychiatric observations, the mental status examination of the patient with somatic symptoms should include the components shown in Table 19–5. It is essential to evaluate the individual's ideas about the meaning, cause, implications, and significance of his or her symptoms and the individual's emotional response to his or her situation (Barsky 1998).

TABLE 19–5. Specific components of the mental status examination in the patient with somatic symptoms

Signs of abnormal illness behavior
Quality of the patient's descriptions of his or her symptoms
Thoughts, behaviors, and emotions associated with symptom occurrence
Range and depth of emotional response
Level of denial
Patient's explanations for his or her physical symptoms and the meaning of negative tests
Presence of abnormal hostility to physicians

Source.   Adapted from Creed and Guthrie 1993; Sharpe et al. 1992.

Complete a Physical Examination

A complete physical examination of the patient is a prerequisite for accurate diagnosis and treatment for several reasons. The consultation-liaison psychiatrist may be in the best position to diagnose a general medical condition because "something about the patient (personality, behavior, affect, odd cognition) has effectively distracted the primary physician and other consultants" (Cassem and Barsky 1991, p. 132). The physician who is managing a persistently somatizing patient must tolerate the patient's perpetual concern about symptoms with some degree of equanimity. Based on a medical education that emphasizes "missed diagnoses" and the current medicolegal climate, the physician must be confident that a thorough evaluation has been done. A contract should be established with the patient that further evaluations will be at the discretion of the physician and will occur only when the physician discovers a symptom complex that raises "red flags" or "bells and whistles."

The physical examination may help to establish a positive diagnosis of somatization disorder. For example, awareness of physical signs associated with stress (e.g., tender anterior chest wall, tender abdomen, spurious breathing, short breath-holding time) leads to a more confident diagnosis rather than a diagnosis of exclusion, which always has an implication of doubt associated with it (Sharpe and Bass 1992). A variety of physical signs may be useful, but some are controversial, in making a diagnosis of a somatoform disorder, including nonanatomical physical signs of low-back pain (Waddell et al. 1980), downward ocular deviation in simulated coma (Henry and Woodruff 1978), and Hoover's test in "paralysis" (Weintraub 1983). It is important to remember that physical findings reported to be suggestive of hysteria in patients also have been reported in patients with acute neurological illness (Gould et al. 1986; Jones and Barklage 1990). Somatization or a somatoform disorder should be diagnosed only if the examination also proves normal function of the system being tested (Newman 1993).

Use Psychometric Tests

The most commonly used psychometric instruments are listed in Table 19–6. The Minnesota Multiphasic Personality Inventories (MMPI, MMPI-2) are particularly useful in the assessment of patients who may be malingering and/or who have severe characterological problems. The Symptom Checklist—90 (SCL-90) has the advantage of being brief and readily scored in the office either by hand or by computer.

Clinical Management

The key to clinical management is to adopt caring rather than curing as a goal. Management is a much more realistic goal than treatment in this population (Bass and Benjamin 1993; Creed and Guthrie 1993; Epstein et al. 1999; Sharpe et al. 1992; Smith et al. 2000). Management must be tailored to the individual's somatic symptoms, thoughts and beliefs, behavior, and emotional state (Barsky 1998; Epstein et al. 1999). Three potential management approaches to the patient with somatization disorder have been described:

TABLE 19–6. Psychometric instruments useful in the clinical and research assessment of patients with unexplained medical symptoms

Measures of somatic amplification
  Somatosensory Amplification Scale (Barsky et al. 1988a)

Measures of preoccupation with health issues and illness
  Illness Behaviour Questionnaire (Pilowsky 1967)
  Illness Attitudes Scale (Kellner 1987)

Measures of somatic symptoms
  Symptom Checklist—90 somatization subscale (Derogatis et al. 1974)
  Pennebaker Inventory of Limbic Languidness (PILL) (Pennebaker 1982)
  Minnesota Multiphasic Personality Inventory (MMPI)—Version 1 (Hathaway and McKinley 1940) or 2 (Butcher et al. 1991)

Measures of increased sympathetic activity and heightened awareness of bodily functioning
  Modified Somatic Perception Questionnaire (MSPQ) (Main 1983)

Measures of pain
  McGill Pain Questionnaire (Melzack 1975)
  West Haven–Yale Multidimensional Pain Inventory (WHYMPI) (Kerns et al. 1985)

Depression rating scales
  Beck Depression Inventory (Beck et al. 1961)
  Hamilton Rating Scale for Depression (Hamilton 1960)

Anxiety rating scales
  State-Trait Anxiety Inventory (STAI) (Spielberger et al. 1970)
  Hamilton Anxiety Scale (Hamilton 1959)

Measures of personality attributes
  Minnesota Multiphasic Personality Inventory (MMPI)—Version 1 (Hathaway and McKinley 1940) or 2 (Butcher et al. 1991)
  Millon Clinical Multiaxial Inventory II (MCMI-II) (Millon 1987)

1. A *reattribution approach* emphasizes helping the patient to link his or her physical symptoms with psychological or stressful factors in his or her life. This is accomplished via a three-step process that links psychosocial stressors (e.g., marital strife) through physiologic mechanisms (e.g., increased muscle tension) to physical symptoms (e.g., headache) (D. Goldberg et al. 1989).

2. A *psychotherapeutic approach* concentrates on developing a close and trusting relationship with the patient (Guthrie et al. 1991).

3. A *directive approach* treats the patient as though he or she has a physical problem, and interventions are framed in a medical model (Benjamin 1989).

The three management approaches vary in their suitability for different patients. The reattribution approach is particularly useful in primary care settings, in medical or surgical inpatients with a fair degree of insight, and in psychiatric settings with patients who have less lengthy histories of somatization. The reattribution technique can be easily taught to primary care practitioners (Gask et al. 1989). The psychotherapeutic approach is most suitable for patients with persistent somatization who are willing to explore the effect of psychosocial factors on their symptoms. The directive approach is most useful for hostile patients who deny the importance of psychological or social factors in their symptomatology.

Principles of Management

The fundamental principles of management of patients with somatization and somatoform disorders are shown in Table 19–7 and are discussed in detail in the following sections.

TABLE 19–7.   Principles of management of somatization and somatoform disorders

---

Emphasize explanation
Arrange for regular follow-up
Treat mood or anxiety disorders
Minimize polypharmacy
Provide specific therapy when indicated
Change social dynamics
Resolve difficulties in the doctor-patient relationship
Recognize and control negative reactions and countertransference

---

Emphasize explanation of symptoms.   In order to engage in treatment, patients require a sense that their primary physician and consultation-liaison psychiatrist are taking them seriously, appreciate the magnitude of their distress, and have a rationale for the proposed management plan. Most somatizing patients hold explanatory models of their symptoms that are in conflict with their physicians' models (Salmon et al. 1999). The clinical challenge is to provide explanations that empower patients with tangible mechanisms, exculpation, and encouragement of self-management rather than explanations that reject or collude with the patient's model (Salmon et al. 1999). Reassurance, which is often thought of as helpful, may in fact be harmful for some patients. The appropriateness of reassurance must be evaluated for each patient (Warwick 1992). Confrontation generally is not a useful technique (Eisendrath 1989; Lazare 1981). According to Lazare (1981):

> Confrontation with the information that the symptom is psychological in origin is rarely helpful and gen-

erates an adversarial relationship. It is more useful to work somewhat obliquely by inquiring about the situation of the patient's life while listening for possible symbolic meanings of the symptoms, the unbearable affects against which the symptom defends, and the social communication inherent in the symptom. (p. 746)

It is important to emphasize to patients that the psychiatrist is not dismissing their symptoms as "all in their head" but rather sees the symptoms as "real" and "in their body" and wants to explore all opportunities for symptom control. The use of metaphors and analogies is often helpful. The metaphor of a radio is particularly useful—the channel playing is the symptom that is of concern (N.H. Cassem, personal communication, May 1983). The goal of the patient and physician is not to change the channel because investigations have not shown any role for "channel changers," such as surgery or specific medical techniques, but rather to gain greater control over the volume control knob (i.e., factors that exacerbate or relieve symptoms) and the sensitivity of the antenna (i.e., factors that amplify symptoms). Physiologic mechanisms underlying symptoms may be explained (see Table 19–4) (Sharpe and Bass 1992). Understanding the meaning of the symptom(s) to the patient and tailoring one's explanation in light of this meaning may improve the doctor-patient relationship (Epstein et al. 1999; Priel et al. 1991).

Ensure regular follow-up.   Regular follow-up is key to effective management, results in decreased health care utilization overall, and is less stressful for patients and physicians. The site of management depends on the availability of resources and the clinical characteristics of the patient. The best choice for most patients is management by their primary care practitioner in consultation with a consultation-liaison psychiatrist. The consultation-liaison psychiatrist may provide primary follow-up if significant comorbid Axis I or Axis II pathology is present or if the primary care physician cannot manage the symptoms.

Treat mood or anxiety disorders.   Mood or anxiety disorders have significant morbidity in their own right and interfere with participation in rehabilitation and psychotherapy. Their physiologic concomitants may fuel the somatization process or heighten somatic amplification.

Minimize polypharmacy.   Polypharmacy may produce iatrogenic complications. The classic stereotype of the patient with somatization disorder arriving with a shopping bag filled with pills is unfortunately all too common. Unnecessary medications should be tapered and withdrawn. This process may be long and complicated (i.e., months to several years), and it is important to take a staged approach with small, realistically achievable steps.

Provide specific therapy when indicated.   A variety of specific therapies have been recommended for the somatoform disorders, which are discussed later in this chapter. Physiotherapy or massage may be helpful in diminishing musculoskeletal pain for patients with somatoform disorders.

Change social dynamics that reinforce symptoms.   Many patients' lives come to revolve around their symptoms and use of the health care system. Regularly scheduled follow-up means that the patient no longer has to present a symptom as a "ticket of admission" to the physician's office. Important members of the patient's social support system may be persuaded to consistently reward nonillness-related behaviors. Social skills building, life skills training, assertiveness training, and physical reactivation programs may be indicated. Group therapy may be useful because it provides social support, increases interpersonal skills, and provides a nonthreatening environment in which to learn to experience and express emotions and desires more directly (Ford 1984).

Resolve difficulties in the doctor-patient relationship. Somatizing patients often have difficult relationships with their caregivers because of attention seeking, demands, and anger. These difficulties have multiple determinants, including attachment disorders (Stuart and Noyes 1999), differences in expectations and beliefs about the meaning and management of symptoms, and prior frustrating experiences with the health care system (Noyes et al. 1995).

Recognize and control negative reactions or countertransference.   Patients with somatization and somatoform disorders evoke powerful emotional responses in physicians, which may result in less than optimal clinical care (Hahn et al. 1994; Sharpe et al. 1994). The range of emotions experienced by physicians may include guilt for failing to "help" the patient, fear that the patient will make a complaint, and anger at the patient's entitlement. The physician may be dismissive of the patient or, alternatively, may collude with the patient in excessive investigations to exclude physical disease in "a suspension of professional judgment" (Bass and Murphy 1990). The decision to pursue further investigations may be an attempt at a conscious level to avoid a "painful, embarrassing and time-consuming confrontation" (Bass and Murphy 1990) or may be an unconscious solution to the conflicts and emotions that the patient evokes in the physician. The treating physician must identify something about the patient that is either likable or interesting that will help

to sustain his or her involvement—in the most difficult patients, it may simply be a sense of amazement at the degree of somatization. A physician caring for these patients must set clear limits as to his or her availability. If all else fails, the physician should transfer the care of the patient to a colleague, either temporarily or permanently.

SOMATOFORM DISORDERS

Somatoform disorders entered psychiatric nosology in 1980 with the publication of DSM-III (American Psychiatric Association 1980). The common feature shared by the somatoform diagnoses is "the presence of physical symptoms that suggest a general medical condition (hence, the term *somatoform*) and are not fully explained by a general medical condition, by the direct effects of a substance, or by another mental disorder (e.g., Panic Disorder)...the physical symptoms are not intentional (i.e., under voluntary control)" (American Psychiatric Association 2000, p. 485). DSM-IV-TR somatoform disorder diagnoses include somatization disorder, undifferentiated somatoform disorder, hypochondriasis, conversion disorder, body dysmorphic disorder (BDD), pain disorder, and somatoform disorder not otherwise specified (American Psychiatric Association 2000). The disorders are grouped together based on "clinical utility (i.e., the need to exclude occult general medical conditions or substance-induced etiologies for the bodily symptoms) rather than on assumptions regarding shared etiology" (American Psychiatric Association 2000, p. 485).

Relatively few patients seen on consultation-liaison services have primary diagnoses of somatoform disorders (Ford and Parker 1991). Conversion disorder is the most commonly diagnosed somatoform disorder in general hospital settings, and it is typically associated with other psychiatric or physical comorbidity (Ford and Parker 1991). Of 1,000 consecutive consultations in one general hospital, 5% received a conversion disorder diagnosis (Folks et al. 1984).

Clinicians frequently have problems with this diagnostic category. Most patients do not have "classical" presentations but have a mixed presentation of symptoms of a variety of somatoform disorders as well as somatization as a process. The question of intentionality or consciousness in symptom production is a vexing one, but it is an important basis for distinguishing these disorders from the factitious disorders and malingering (Ford 1992). Researchers have criticized the diagnostic category of somatoform disorders for six major reasons (Murphy 1990):

1. The division of patients on the basis of presenting symptoms is superficial.
2. The individual disorders are not qualitatively distinct but rather tend to merge with one another.
3. Many of the concepts embedded within the somatoform disorders such as hypochondriasis, medically unexplained symptoms, and medical help seeking are better described in dimensional rather than categorical terms.
4. The clinical descriptions of specific disorders are largely derived from tertiary care or psychiatric hospital samples and emphasize chronicity.
5. Making diagnoses gives the "spurious impression of understanding and leads to naive assumptions about disease entities" (p. 13).
6. The diagnostic criteria for somatization disorder are described as too restrictive for clinical use.

The separate existence of a discrete category of somatoform disorders reinforces the mind-body dualism of Western medicine and implies a separation of affective, anxiety, dissociative, and somatic symptoms (Kirmayer and Young 1998). Somatic symptoms and somatization cut across DSM-IV-TR.

In this chapter, I focus on adults. Recent reviews discuss child and adolescent somatization (Campo and Fritsch 1994; Garralda 1999) and somatoform disorders (Fritz et al. 1997).

Somatization Disorder

Definition

Somatization disorder has a lengthy history and is based on Briquet's syndrome. The psychiatric diagnostic criteria of Feighner et al. (1972) for Briquet's syndrome, which required 25 of 59 physical symptoms, an illness onset before age 30 years, and a pattern of recurrent physical complaints, were shown to have validity, reliability, and internal consistency. The long-term stability of the diagnosis was documented by the finding that 80%–90% of the patients continued to meet diagnostic criteria at 6- to 8-year follow-up (Guze et al. 1986). DSM-III criteria for somatization disorder were a modification of Feighner's criteria and required an onset of symptoms before age 30 and a total symptom count of 14 symptoms in women and 12 symptoms in men from a total list of 36 physical symptoms. DSM-III-R further modified the criteria by simplifying the requirement to 13 of 35 physical symptoms and specifically excluded symptoms occurring only during a panic attack (American Psychiatric Association 1987). DSM-IV further simplified the diagnostic

criteria for somatization disorder (Table 19–8), and they have been found to be concordant with prior criteria (Yutzy et al. 1995).

Epidemiology

The general population lifetime prevalence of somatization disorder is estimated at 0.1%–2.0% (Regier et al. 1988; Robins et al. 1984; Swartz et al. 1986). Because patients with somatization disorder seek out medical help, their prevalence in medical settings is higher than in the general population. It has been diagnosed in 1.4% of primary care patients (Simon and Gureje 1999), 5% of outpatient medical clinic patients (deGruy et al. 1987a), and 9% of one sample of 213 medical and surgical inpatients (deGruy et al. 1987b). Recent work has emphasized the instability of recall of somatic symptoms, with implications for diagnosing somatization disorder (Simon and Gureje 1999). The disorder is uncommon in men (Golding et al. 1991), with estimates of lifetime prevalence of 0.2%–2.0% in women and less than 0.2% in men (American Psychiatric Association 2000). Women and men with somatization disorder have similar clinical characteristics including comorbid psychopathology (Golding et al. 1991). Individuals with somatization disorder tend to be unmarried, nonwhite, from a rural area, and less educated than individuals without the diagnosis (Swartz et al. 1986). By definition, the syndrome must begin before age 30, but most often symptoms begin in the teens, often with menarche, or less commonly in the early 20s. The risk for depression, alcohol abuse, and antisocial personality disorder is increased in the first-degree relatives of individuals with somatization disorder (Golding et al. 1992).

Clinical Features

The classic patient with somatization disorder is a woman who began to experience medically unexplained symptoms in early adolescence and has shown a fluctuating, waxing and waning course over the years with a medical history that documents repeated unexplained physical complaints. Accompanying this chronic polysymptomatic pattern is the patient's subjective assessment of herself as "sickly." Numerous clinical descriptions emphasize the dramatic and vague presentations of these patients (Cassem and Barsky 1991), but others have noted that the patient with somatization disorder may present as odd or anxious (Rost et al. 1992).

Associated Features

Patients with somatization disorder have high rates of psychiatric comorbidity for both Axis I and Axis II diag-

TABLE 19–8. DSM-IV diagnostic criteria for somatization disorder

A. A history of many physical complaints beginning before age 30 years that occur over a period of several years and result in treatment being sought or significant impairment in social, occupational, or other important areas of functioning.

B. Each of the following criteria must have been met, with individual symptoms occurring at any time during the course of the disturbance:

   (1) *four pain symptoms:* a history of pain related to at least four different sites or functions (e.g., head, abdomen, back, joints, extremities, chest, rectum, during menstruation, during sexual intercourse, or during urination)

   (2) *two gastrointestinal symptoms:* a history of at least two gastrointestinal symptoms other than pain (e.g., nausea, bloating, vomiting other than during pregnancy, diarrhea, or intolerance of several different foods)

   (3) *one sexual symptom:* a history of at least one sexual or reproductive symptom other than pain (e.g., sexual indifference, erectile or ejaculatory dysfunction, irregular menses, excessive menstrual bleeding, vomiting throughout pregnancy)

   (4) *one pseudoneurological symptom:* a history of at least one symptom or deficit suggesting a neurological condition not limited to pain (conversion symptoms such as impaired coordination or balance, paralysis or localized weakness, difficulty swallowing or lump in throat, aphonia, urinary retention, hallucinations, loss of touch or pain sensation, double vision, blindness, deafness, seizures; dissociative symptoms such as amnesia; or loss of consciousness other than fainting)

C. Either (1) or (2):

   (1) after appropriate investigation, each of the symptoms in Criterion B cannot be fully explained by a known general medical condition or the direct effects of a substance (e.g., a drug of abuse, a medication)

   (2) when there is a related general medical condition, the physical complaints or resulting social or occupational impairment are in excess of what would be expected from the history, physical examination, or laboratory findings

D. The symptoms are not intentionally produced or feigned (as in factitious disorder or malingering).

Source. Reprinted from American Psychiatric Association: *Diagnostic and Statistical Manual of Mental Disorders*, 4th Edition. Washington, DC, American Psychiatric Association, 1994.

noses. As many as 75% of the patients with somatization disorder have comorbid Axis I diagnoses (Katon et al. 1991; Swartz et al. 1986), of which the most common comorbid diagnoses are major depressive disorder, dysthymia, panic disorder, simple phobia, and substance abuse. Because patients with somatization disorder have a low threshold for endorsing symptoms, in some cases comorbid diagnoses may reflect a response tendency rather than significant symptomatology. Personality disorders appear to be more common in patients with somatization disorder than in control subjects with mood and anxiety disorders (J. Stern et al. 1993). Studies have examined the prevalence of specific personality disorders. Antisocial personality disorder was diagnosed in 25% of the men and in 8.2% of the women in one study of patients with somatization disorder seen by a psychiatrist. These rates are significantly higher than general population rates of 0.5%–1.5% in women and 3.9%–5.9% in men (Smith et al. 1991). The association between personality disorder and somatization disorder has been suggested to result from a common biological substrate or social-environmental factors (Smith et al. 1991). A primary care study of 94 patients with somatization disorder found that 60% of the patients met criteria for one or more personality disorders, with the most frequent being: avoidant 26.7%, paranoid 21.3%, self-defeating

19.1%, obsessive-compulsive 17.1%, histrionic 12.8%, and antisocial 7.4% (Rost et al. 1992). Histrionic and antisocial personality disorders may have lower rates in primary care settings because these disorders are associated with more dramatic acting out, which would lead patients into the mental health care system. These findings are important in emphasizing that in primary care settings, patients with somatization disorder may present with anxious or odd characteristics rather than in a dramatic fashion (Rost et al. 1992). Patients with somatization disorder often have multiple social problems and chaotic lifestyles characterized by poor interpersonal relationships, disruptive or difficult behavior, and substance abuse (Cassem and Barsky 1991; Ford 1983) and show significant occupational and social impairment. Women with somatization disorder are more likely to have a history of sexual abuse than are women with primary mood disorders (Morrison 1989).

Clinical Course and Prognosis

"Somatization Disorder is a chronic but fluctuating disorder that rarely remits completely. A year seldom passes without the individual's seeking some medical attention prompted by unexplained somatic complaints" (American Psychiatric Association 2000, p. 488). Patients may have iatrogenic disease or injury secondary to unnecessary medical investigations, treatments (e.g., dependence on psychoactive substances that may have initially been unwittingly prescribed for symptom control), and surgical procedures.

Differential Diagnosis

The differential diagnosis of somatization disorder includes

- General medical disorders presenting with confusing or vague symptomatology or characterized by multiple symptoms in various organ systems (e.g., systemic lupus erythematosus, multiple sclerosis, acute intermittent porphyria, hyperparathyroidism). Factors suggesting a diagnosis of somatization disorder rather than a general medical condition include multiple organ system involvement, early onset and chronic course without development of physical signs or structural abnormalities, and absence of laboratory abnormalities (American Psychiatric Association 2000).
- Anxiety disorders—panic disorder is characterized by multiple somatic symptoms, but the symptoms are specifically limited to the panic attack. Generalized anxiety disorder may be characterized by multiple somatic symptoms but is accompanied by unrealistic worry, which is not limited to health concerns or symptoms.
- Depressive disorders—physical complaints may be prominent during depressed mood states but are limited to these episodes.
- Schizophrenia with multiple somatic delusions—the delusions are typically bizarre.
- Other somatoform disorders—by definition, somatization disorder includes symptoms compatible with other somatoform diagnoses. If the symptoms occur exclusively during the course of somatization disorder, then additional diagnoses are not made.
- Factitious disorder with predominantly physical symptoms—intentional symptom production occurs for the purpose of assuming the sick role and obtaining medical care.
- Malingering—intentional symptom production is motivated by external incentives.

Undifferentiated Somatoform Disorder

Definition

Undifferentiated somatoform disorder is a residual category for individuals who do not meet full criteria for somatization disorder or another somatoform disorder.

TABLE 19–9. DSM-IV-TR diagnostic criteria for undifferentiated somatoform disorder

A. One or more physical complaints (e.g., fatigue, loss of appetite, gastrointestinal or urinary complaints).

B. Either (1) or (2):

  (1) after appropriate investigation, the symptoms cannot be fully explained by a known general medical condition or the direct effects of a substance (e.g., a drug of abuse, a medication)

  (2) when there is a related general medical condition, the physical complaints or resulting social or occupational impairment is in excess of what would be expected from the history, physical examination, or laboratory findings

C. The symptoms cause clinically significant distress or impairment in social, occupational, or other important areas of functioning.

D. The duration of the disturbance is at least 6 months.

E. The disturbance is not better accounted for by another mental disorder (e.g., another somatoform disorder, sexual dysfunction, mood disorder, anxiety disorder, sleep disorder, or psychotic disorder).

F. The symptom is not intentionally produced or feigned (as in factitious disorder or malingering).

Epidemiology

No studies of undifferentiated somatoform disorder have been done, but studies of subsyndromal somatization disorder used a cutoff score of four DSM-III somatization symptoms for men and six symptoms for women to identify a group of patients with sociodemographic and clinical characteristics including increased medical utilization similar to patients meeting the full criteria for somatization disorder (Escobar et al. 1987, 1989). Further support for this concept has come from the study of distressed high utilizers of medical care, which documented significant increased health care utilization by patients endorsing functional somatic symptoms but falling below the DSM-III-R cutoff of 13 symptoms (Katon et al. 1991). It is probable that 4%–11% of the population have multiple, medically unexplained symptoms consistent with a subsyndromal form of somatization disorder (Escobar et al. 1987, 1989). Multisomatoform disorder, characterized by three or more medically unexplained, currently bothersome physical symptoms plus a greater than 2-year history of somatization, has been suggested to be more useful than undifferentiated somatoform disorder in primary care settings (Kroenke et al. 1997).

Clinical and Associated Features

DSM-IV-TR diagnostic criteria are listed in Table 19–9. Patients with undifferentiated somatoform disorder may have one symptom or multiple symptoms.

Clinical Course and Prognosis

The course of this disorder varies given that it is probably quite heterogeneous. DSM-IV-TR notes that the "course of individual unexplained physical complaints is unpredictable. The eventual diagnosis of a general medical condition or another mental disorder is frequent" (American Psychiatric Association 2000, p. 491).

Differential Diagnosis

The differential diagnosis of undifferentiated somatoform disorder includes

- Mood and anxiety disorders—medically unexplained symptoms commonly occur in these disorders.
- Factitious disorder with predominantly physical symptoms—intentional symptom production occurs for the purpose of assuming the sick role and obtaining medical care.
- Malingering—intentional symptom production is motivated by external incentives.

Hypochondriasis

Definition

Hypochondriasis is characterized by fears of having a disease or the belief that one has a serious disease based on the misinterpretation of bodily symptoms that persists despite medical reassurance (American Psychiatric Association 2000). DSM-IV-TR criteria for hypochondriasis are shown in Table 19–10. The validity of the construct in medical outpatients has been documented (Barsky et al. 1986b; Noyes et al. 1993). Secondary hypochondriasis (i.e., hypochondriasis developing in the context of another Axis I psychiatric disorder, a major life stress, or a medical disorder) has been described (Barsky et al. 1992), although it is not recognized in DSM-IV-TR.

Epidemiology

No large-scale epidemiologic studies of hypochondriasis have been done. Prevalence rates for primary and secondary forms of hypochondriasis of 3%–13% have been reported for study samples from medical and psychiatric settings (Kellner 1986). The prevalence in the general population is 1%–5% (American Psychiatric Association 2000). Data on the sex distribution of hypochondriasis

TABLE 19–10. DSM-IV-TR diagnostic criteria for hypochondriasis

A. Preoccupation with fears of having, or the idea that one has, a serious disease based on the person's misinterpretation of bodily symptoms.
B. The preoccupation persists despite appropriate medical evaluation and reassurance.
C. The belief in Criterion A is not of delusional intensity (as in delusional disorder, somatic type) and is not restricted to a circumscribed concern about appearance (as in body dysmorphic disorder).
D. The preoccupation causes clinically significant distress or impairment in social, occupational, or other important areas of functioning.
E. The duration of the disturbance is at least 6 months.
F. The preoccupation is not better accounted for by generalized anxiety disorder, obsessive-compulsive disorder, panic disorder, a major depressive episode, separation anxiety, or another somatoform disorder.

Specify if:

With poor insight: if, for most of the time during the current episode, the person does not recognize that the concern about having a serious illness is excessive or unreasonable

conflict, but the disorder occurs in both men and women (American Psychiatric Association 2000). The disorder can begin at any age, but the most common age at onset is in early adulthood (American Psychiatric Association 2000). Few demographic and clinical differences have been found between those individuals with primary hypochondriasis, which develops de novo, and those with secondary hypochondriasis (Barsky et al. 1992). The data on ethnic and cultural differences are equivocal (Barsky et al. 1986a; Kellner 1986), and these factors may be most important when an individual's concerns are reinforced by a traditional healer who disagrees with the medical reassurance provided. Hypochondriacal concerns are quite prevalent in medical inpatient wards (36% of the patients in one study) and are associated with emotional distress and learned social behavior (Mabe et al. 1988).

Clinical Features

The core feature of hypochondriasis is fear of disease or conviction that one has a disease despite normal physical examination results and investigations and physician reassurance. Bodily preoccupation (i.e., increased observation of and vigilance toward bodily sensations) is common. The preoccupation may be with a particular bodily function or experience (e.g., heartbeat); a trivial abnormal physical state (e.g., cough), which is taken as evidence of disease; a vague physical sensation; or a preoccupation with a particular disease (e.g., cancer). Patients with hypochondriasis believe that good health is a relatively symptom-free state and in comparison to control patients, they are more likely to consider symptoms to be indicative of disease (Barsky et al. 1993). The concern about the feared illness "often becomes a central feature of the individual's self-image, a topic of social discourse, and a response to life stresses" (American Psychiatric Association 2000, p. 504).

Associated Features

Patients with hypochondriasis have a high rate of psychiatric comorbidity (Barsky et al. 1992; Kellner 1986). In hypochondriacal patients from a general medical outpatient clinic, 88% had one or more concurrent Axis I diagnoses, the most common being generalized anxiety disorder (71.4%), dysthymia (45.2%), major depressive disorder (42.9%), somatization disorder (21.4%), and panic disorder (16.7%) (Barsky et al. 1992). Somatization disorder in this population was found to be phenomenologically distinct from hypochondriasis (Barsky et al. 1992). Personality disorders as assessed by questionnaire were three times more likely to be diagnosed in hypochondriacal patients compared with the control group (Barsky et al. 1992). High medical utilization is common, and the potential exists for iatrogenic damage from repeated investigations. Interpersonal relationships typically deteriorate because of the preoccupation with disease. Occupational functioning is often compromised with increased time taken off from work and decreased performance when the individual is at work because of the preoccupation with disease.

Clinical Course and Prognosis

Primary hypochondriasis appears to be a chronic condition, and thus, some have argued that it might be better understood in terms of a personality style or characteristic (Barsky and Klerman 1983; Barsky et al. 1992; P. Tyrer et al. 1990). Some forms of secondary hypochondriasis remit with resolution or treatment of the underlying condition (e.g., major life stressors, mood or anxiety disorders). A prospective 4- to 5-year study of hypochondriasis found that hypochondriacal patients had a considerable decline in symptoms and improvement in role functioning over 4–5 years, but two-thirds still met diagnostic criteria (Barsky et al. 1998).

Differential Diagnosis

The differential diagnosis of hypochondriasis includes

- General medical conditions—often the early stages of a variety of rheumatological, immunological, endocrine, and neurological diseases may be associated with subtle pathology that may not be detected by physical examination or laboratory investigation but may be noticeable in some way to patients. Hypochondriasis may coexist with medical pathology (Barsky et al. 1986a), but transient preoccupations related to medical illness do not constitute hypochondriasis (American Psychiatric Association 2000).
- Axis I disorders—a number of Axis I disorders may be characterized by a degree of hypochondriacal concern. These disorders include major depressive disorder, dysthymia, anxiety disorders (including panic disorder, generalized anxiety disorder, obsessive-compulsive disorder), and somatization disorder. Both diagnoses should be made only when the patient's health concerns are not better accounted for by the other disorder.
- Psychotic disorders, including major depressive disorder, with psychotic features; schizophrenia; and delusional disorder, somatic type, are characterized by the fixed quality of the delusional belief in contrast to the hypochondriacal patient, who is convinced of the veracity of his or her concerns but is able to consider the possibility that the feared disease is not present.

Conversion Disorder

Definition

Conversion symptoms have been described since antiquity (Mace 1992). DSM-IV-TR diagnostic criteria for conversion disorder (Table 19–11) are very similar to those of DSM-III-R, with the exception that DSM-IV-TR symptoms are limited to voluntary motor or sensory function that suggest a neurological or other general medical condition.

Controversies surrounding the diagnosis of conversion disorder include 1) whether it is in fact a disorder at all or rather a symptom because it has not been validated on the basis of longitudinal or family studies (Martin 1992); 2) where it should be placed in a given nosological system (i.e., should it be grouped with somatoform disorders as in DSM-IV-TR or with dissociative disorders as in ICD-10?) (Toone 1990); and 3) whether the need for the diagnostician to determine that the symptom is unconsciously produced leads to diagnostic heterogeneity—one clinician's con-

TABLE 19–11. DSM-IV-TR diagnostic criteria for conversion disorder

A. One or more symptoms or deficits affecting voluntary motor or sensory function that suggest a neurological or other general medical condition.

B. Psychological factors are judged to be associated with the symptom or deficit because the initiation or exacerbation of the symptom or deficit is preceded by conflicts or other stressors.

C. The symptom or deficit is not intentionally produced or feigned (as in factitious disorder or malingering).

D. The symptom or deficit cannot, after appropriate investigation, be fully explained by a general medical condition, or by the direct effects of a substance, or as a culturally sanctioned behavior or experience.

E. The symptom or deficit causes clinically significant distress or impairment in social, occupational, or other important areas of functioning or warrants medical evaluation.

F. The symptom or deficit is not limited to pain or sexual dysfunction, does not occur exclusively during the course of Somatization Disorder, and is not better accounted for by another mental disorder.

Specify type of symptom or deficit:

With motor symptom or deficit
With sensory symptom or deficit
With seizures or convulsions
With mixed presentation

version disorder is another clinician's factitious disorder or malingering.

Epidemiology

The prevalence of conversion disorder varies among studies, and the incidence in any given setting is likely influenced by several factors. Toone (1990) reviewed the studies and noted rates of 0.3% in the general population, 1%–3% in medical outpatient settings, and 1%–4.5% in inpatient neurological and medical settings. Much higher rates have been described in developing countries (Murphy 1990) and in isolated rural American settings (Ford 1983). Settings such as the military, in which substantial secondary gain may be involved, have increased rates of conversion symptomatology (Ford 1983). Women outnumber men with the disorder in a ratio varying from 2:1 to 10:1 (Murphy 1990). Men are more likely to present with conversion symptoms related to military service and industrial accidents (Folks and Houck 1993). Studies of associations between social class and urban versus rural distribution are equivocal (Murphy 1990).

Onset is typically in adolescence or early adulthood, but cases have been described in children (Shapiro and Rosenfeld 1987) as well as in later life. Early studies

argued for caution because significant numbers of patients given a conversion disorder diagnosis subsequently received a diagnosis of a medical condition that explained the symptom (Slater and Glithero 1965), although this has not been found in recent studies of medically unexplained motor symptoms. In the largest such study, 4.6% of a sample of 64 patients with medically unexplained motor symptoms subsequently developed a new organic neurological disorder that explained their previous symptoms (Crimlisk et al. 1998). This more recent finding may be partially explained by increasing caution on the part of clinicians in making a diagnosis of conversion disorder and by more sophisticated biomedical investigations, including neuroimaging.

Clinical Features

Conversion symptoms are neurological in nature and affect voluntary motor or sensory functioning. Common conversion symptoms include motor symptoms (e.g., paralysis, disturbances in coordination or balance, localized weakness, akinesia, dyskinesia, aphonia, urinary retention, and difficulty swallowing), sensory symptoms (e.g., blindness, double vision, anesthesia, paresthesia, deafness), and seizures or convulsions that may have voluntary motor or sensory components. Unilateral symptoms may be more likely to occur on the left side of the body, as is true for somatoform pain, hyperventilation, and hypochondriasis (Toone 1990). The neurophysiologic basis for the lateralization is unclear (Toone 1990), if it exists at all (Roelofs et al. 2000). The diagnosis of conversion is "predicated on two sets of negatives: (i) signs and symptoms of physical ill health which the physician refuses to accept, and (ii) inferences (by the physician) of psychological disturbance which the patient (usually) rebuts" (Toone 1990, p. 215). Psychological mechanisms were specifically implicated in prior diagnostic definitions, but the definition according to DSM-IV-TR only requires that psychological factors be associated with symptom onset or exacerbation. Earlier discussions of conversion focused on the etiological role of primary gain, which refers to "the effectiveness of the conversion symptom in providing a satisfactory symbolic expression for the repressed wishes" (Engel 1970, p. 660). For example, a conflict about aggression might be symbolically expressed through a paralyzed arm. Secondary gain refers to the benefits accruing from the sick role, which may include alterations in the interpersonal behavior of significant others which are deemed positive by the patient (e.g., increased attentiveness) and the permission to withdraw from disliked responsibilities. Secondary gain is intrinsic to the sick role and thus is present in many general medical conditions and psychiatric disorders. Secondary gain may occur in conversion disorder patients, but it is not consciously sought. This contrasts with malingering, in which symptoms are produced intentionally, motivated by external incentives, or factitious disorders, in which symptoms are produced intentionally from the unconscious motivation of assuming the sick role.

Associated Features

Little systematic study of comorbid Axis I diagnoses has been done. The literature on associated personality features suggests that "hysterical personality may be seen, but only in a minority of conversion cases; other forms of personality disorder of immature, dependent type are more usual" (Toone 1990, p. 229). Protracted conversion reactions may be associated with secondary physical changes (e.g., disuse atrophy).

Clinical Course and Prognosis

The course of conversion disorder is unknown, but individual episodes of conversion are usually of short duration with sudden onset and resolution, although recurrence of symptoms over time is common (American Psychiatric Association 2000; Murphy 1990). In some cases, conversion symptoms may last years. Factors reported to predispose to conversion disorder are antecedent physical disorders in the individual or a close contact, which provide a model for the symptoms occurring; and severe social stressors including bereavement, rape, incest, warfare, and other forms of psychosocial trauma (Toone 1990). The prognosis of conversion disorder depends on a number of factors, including 1) acuteness of onset, 2) presence of major stressors, 3) duration of symptoms before treatment, 4) symptom pattern, 5) personality, and 6) the sociocultural context within which the illness developed (Toone 1990). Good prognosis has been linked to acute and recent onset, traumatic or stressful life event at onset, good premorbid health, and absence of other major medical or psychiatric illnesses (Lazare 1981). Most patients show a rapid response to treatment, but some do not. Patients with pseudoseizures, tremor, and amnesia are particularly likely to have a poor outcome (Toone 1990). Recent neuroimaging studies are defining the neural networks involved and demonstrating differences between conversion and feigned symptoms (Ron 2001).

Differential Diagnosis

The differential diagnosis of conversion disorder includes

- General medical disorder—occult presentations of a variety of neurological, substance-induced, and general

medical conditions may be mistakenly diagnosed as conversion disorder. Conversion symptoms may occur in individuals with documented medical disorders (e.g., "pseudoseizures" in individuals with epilepsy).
- Other somatoform disorders—pain disorder is diagnosed if the conversion symptom is limited to pain. Conversion symptoms that occur exclusively during the course of somatization disorder do not warrant an additional diagnosis.
- Mood, anxiety, and psychotic disorders—conversion symptoms may occur in these other disorders, but a conversion disorder is not diagnosed if the symptoms are better accounted for by another mental disorder.
- Dissociative disorders—share with conversion disorder symptoms that suggest neurological dysfunction. If both conversion and dissociative symptoms occur, both disorders may be diagnosed if criteria are met for both diagnoses.
- Factitious disorder with predominantly physical symptoms—intentional symptom production occurs for the purpose of assuming the sick role and obtaining medical care.
- Malingering—intentional symptom production is motivated by external incentives.

Body Dysmorphic Disorder

Definition

The hallmark of BDD is the preoccupation with an imagined defect in appearance (if a slight physical anomaly is present, the individual's concern with it is judged to be markedly excessive) that is accompanied by significant distress or impairment in social or occupational functioning (American Psychiatric Association 2000). DSM-IV-TR diagnostic criteria are shown in Table 19–12. Although classified in DSM-IV-TR as a somatoform disorder, increasingly, it is seen as an obsessive-compulsive disorder spectrum disorder (Phillips 1998; Phillips and Hollander 1996).

TABLE 19–12. DSM-IV-TR diagnostic criteria for body dysmorphic disorder

A. Preoccupation with an imagined defect in appearance. If a slight physical anomaly is present, the person's concern is markedly excessive.

B. The preoccupation causes clinically significant distress or impairment in social, occupational, or other important areas of functioning.

C. The preoccupation is not better accounted for by another mental disorder (e.g., dissatisfaction with body shape and size in anorexia nervosa).

Epidemiology

The prevalence of BDD is unknown, although it is probably not rare (Phillips 1998). Structured interviewing is more likely to identify cases (Zimmerman and Mattia 1998) supporting the claim that it is an underrecognized disorder. The sex distribution of BDD varies across case series (Phillips 1998). Syndrome onset is typically in adolescence (Phillips 1998); although it may begin in childhood (Albertini and Phillips 1999). Many years may pass before diagnosis because of reluctance to reveal symptoms (American Psychiatric Association 2000).

Clinical Features

Most patients with BDD have concerns about more than one body part (Phillips 1998). The intensity of the preoccupation with the bodily "defect" has been described as "torturing" and "tormenting," dominating their lives and severely limiting social and occupational functioning. Many patients engage in "checking" behaviors, such as observing themselves in the mirror or measuring the body part of concern. Delusional BDD, classified as delusional disorder, somatic type, may reflect a difference in insight rather than a distinct syndrome (Phillips et al. 1994). Although BDD is remarkably similar in women and men, some differences suggest the influence of cultural norms on the content of BDD symptoms; for example, women are more likely to be preoccupied with their hips and weight and men with body build, genitals, and thinning hair (Phillips and Diaz 1997).

Associated Features

Phillips (1998) has reviewed data on comorbidity. Major depressive disorder is the most common comorbid disorder, with a current rate of about 60% and a lifetime rate of more than 80% (Phillips et al. 1994). Other disorders with lifetime rates of more than 30% include social phobia, substance use disorders, and obsessive-compulsive disorder. Studies of personality disorder in BDD have not been reported, but earlier studies of related disorders suggested that patients showed a wide range of abnormal personality traits. Psychosocial dysfunction is often profound, with social withdrawal and occupational functioning below capacity (Phillips 1998). In the study by Phillips et al. (1993), avoidance of usual social and occupational activities was reported by 97% of the patients with BDD, being housebound by 30%, and suicide attempts by 17%.

Clinical Course and Prognosis

No long-term prospective studies of clinical course have been done, but case series suggest that BDD is usually chronic, with few symptom-free intervals. The intensity of the symptoms may vary over time (American Psychiatric Association 2000). Patients with BDD often seek and obtain inappropriate medical and surgical treatment (Phillips et al. 1993).

Differential Diagnosis

The differential diagnosis of BDD includes

- Other Axis I disorders—concerns about bodily appearance or the belief that one has a bodily defect can occur in a variety of Axis I disorders, including mood disorders, schizophrenia, anorexia nervosa, and mental disorders due to a general medical condition. A diagnosis of BDD is not made when another Axis I disorder better accounts for the behavior.
- Bodily dissatisfaction that is "normal"—concerns about appearance are common within our society, and there is a divergence of opinion as to what constitutes "normal" appearance (Murphy 1990).
- Delusional disorder, somatic type—this additional diagnosis can be made when the preoccupation reaches delusional intensity. Distinguishing between BDD and delusional disorder, somatic type, may be difficult (Phillips et al. 1993).

Pain Disorder

Definition

Pain disorder in DSM-IV-TR is the latest incarnation of somatoform pain disorder (DSM-III-R) and psychogenic pain disorder (DSM-III). DSM-IV-TR diagnostic criteria are shown in Table 19–13. Psychological factors are judged to be important in the onset, severity, exacerbation, or maintenance of the pain, and some patients also will have a medical condition that is judged to be etiologically significant. DSM-IV criteria were designed to address criticisms of DSM-III-R diagnostic criteria (King and Strain 1992), which included the following:

- Lack of operationalization of criteria, leaving them open to clinician interpretation
- Requirement that a patient's pain exceed what would be expected from the physical findings, the determination of which can be problematic
- Requirement that evaluation uncover "no organic pathology or pathophysiologic mechanism...to account for the pain" (DSM-III-R, p. 266), which does not take into account that inadequate evaluation or the patient's failure to reach the threshold for

---

TABLE 19–13.   DSM-IV-TR diagnostic criteria for pain disorder

---

A. Pain in one or more anatomical sites is the predominant focus of the clinical presentation and is of sufficient severity to warrant clinical attention.

B. The pain causes clinically significant distress or impairment in social, occupational, or other important areas of functioning.

C. Psychological factors are judged to have an important role in the onset, severity, exacerbation, or maintenance of the pain.

D. The symptom or deficit is not intentionally produced or feigned (as in factitious disorder or malingering).

E. The pain is not better accounted for by a mood, anxiety, or psychotic disorder and does not meet criteria for dyspareunia.

Code as follows:

    307.80   **Pain disorder associated with psychological factors:**   psychological factors are judged to have the major role in the onset, severity, exacerbation, or maintenance of the pain. (If a general medical condition is present, it does not have a major role in the onset, severity, exacerbation, or maintenance of the pain.) This type of pain disorder is not diagnosed if criteria are also met for somatization disorder.

Specify if:

    Acute: duration of less than 6 months

    Chronic: duration of 6 months or longer

    307.89   **Pain disorder associated with both psychological factors and a general medical condition:**   both psychological factors and a general medical condition are judged to have important roles in the onset, severity, exacerbation, or maintenance of the pain. The associated general medical condition or anatomical site of the pain (see below) is coded on Axis III.

Specify if:

    Acute: duration of less than 6 months

    Chronic: duration of 6 months or longer

    Note: The following is not considered to be a mental disorder and is included here to facilitate differential diagnosis. **Pain disorder associated with a general medical condition:**   a general medical condition has a major role in the onset, severity, exacerbation, or maintenance of the pain. (If psychological factors are present, they are not judged to have a major role in the onset, severity, exacerbation, or maintenance of the pain.) The diagnostic code for the pain is selected based on the associated general medical condition if one has been established (see Appendix G) or on the anatomical location of the pain if the underlying general medical condition is not yet clearly established—for example, low back (724.2), sciatic (724.3), pelvic (625.9), headache (784.0), facial (784.0), chest (786.50), joint (719.40), bone (733.90), abdominal (789.0), breast (611.71), renal (788.0), ear (388.70), eye (379.91), throat (784.1), tooth (525.9), and urinary (788.0).

---

detection could result in the physical condition causing the pain not being detected

- Inapplicability of the diagnosis for patients who react dysfunctionally to lesion-associated pain
- Use of the term *somatoform*, which suggested that the pain was different from that caused by an identifiable etiology, although there is no support for this view and its perpetuation further stigmatizes patients
- Inclusion of the 6-month requirement associated with chronicity, which precluded more acute forms of pain in which psychological factors also may have played an important role

There is debate about whether the diagnosis should even be within the somatoform category or be listed as with other conditions that may be a focus of diagnosis and treatment (King and Strain 1992).

Epidemiology

Pain is the most common symptom in medical settings and is associated with both physical and mental illness

(Benjamin 1989). The prevalence of pain disorder is unknown. Somatoform pain disorder was described as probably common in general practice (American Psychiatric Association 1987), although the diagnosis was not commonly made in pain clinic patients (King and Strain 1992). The disorder may begin at any age. First-degree biological relatives of patients with chronic pain disorder may have increased rates of depressive disorders, alcohol dependence, and chronic pain compared with the general population (American Psychiatric Association 2000).

Clinical Features

Studies are awaited of the clinical features of patients who meet DSM-IV-TR criteria for pain disorder. Patients with chronic pain who were diagnosed previously as having psychogenic or somatoform pain disorder were described as having "the disease of the *D's*" (Brena 1983):

- **Disability**
- **Disuse** and degeneration of functional capacity secondary to pain behavior

- **D**rug misuse
- **D**octor shopping
- **D**ependency (emotional)
- **D**emoralization
- **D**epression
- **D**ramatic accounts of illness

Associated Features

Depression is diagnosed frequently in patients with chronic pain syndromes; estimates range widely between 8% and 80%, with most studies finding that at least half of their chronic pain sample is depressed (Smith 1992). Psychodynamic conflicts between a rigid ego ideal of activity, independence, and caregiving and unmet early dependency needs have been described as a pain-prone personality (Blumer 1982). In most cases, pain disorder is associated with significant occupational and/or social impairment and has persisted for months or years before the patient is referred to a mental health professional.

Clinical Course and Prognosis

Little is known about the course of DSM-IV-TR pain disorder. Iatrogenic complications are likely not uncommon and include dependence on narcotic analgesics and benzodiazepines and unnecessary surgical interventions. Few longitudinal studies of chronic pain patients have been done, and no studies of somatoform pain disorder have been done. Poor outcome has been associated with untreated pain of long duration, somatization, unemployment at the start of treatment, and receiving compensation (S. Tyrer 1992).

Differential Diagnosis

The differential diagnosis of pain disorder is discussed in greater detail elsewhere in this volume (see Chapter 43, this volume). It includes the following:

- Other somatoform disorders—pain complaints may be part of somatization disorder or conversion disorder and, in such a case, do not warrant separate diagnoses.
- Nonsomatoform Axis I disorders—pain complaints may occur in major depressive episode, anxiety disorders, adjustment disorder with physical complaints, and psychotic disorders. The additional diagnosis of pain disorder is made only when the pain is an independent focus of clinical attention, leads to significant distress or impairment, and seems excessive (American Psychiatric Association 2000).
- Factitious disorder with predominantly physical symptoms—intentional symptom production occurs for the purpose of assuming the sick role and obtaining medical care.

- Malingering—intentional symptom production is motivated by external incentives.

Somatoform Disorder Not Otherwise Specified

Somatoform disorder not otherwise specified is diagnosed in patients with somatoform symptoms that do not meet diagnostic criteria for any of the specific somatoform disorders. Examples of such symptoms include 1) pseudocyesis (classified in DSM-III-R as a conversion symptom), 2) nonpsychotic hypochondriacal symptoms lasting less than 6 months, and 3) unexplained somatic symptoms (e.g., fatigue, weakness) that are of less than 6 months' duration and are not due to another mental disorder. Because of heterogeneity of the category, little is known about its epidemiology, clinical course, or prognosis.

MANAGEMENT AND TREATMENT

The management of the somatoform disorders shares many features with the management of somatization outlined earlier in the chapter (see Table 19–7). It has traditionally focused on caring rather than curing, and limit setting (Adler 1981), although newer pharmacological and psychotherapeutic approaches offer the potential for substantial improvement in some patients. The consultation-liaison psychiatrist often develops a management plan that integrates multiple treatment modalities and different health care disciplines (Abbey and Lipowski 1987). In this section, issues specific to the management of somatoform disorders are summarized.

Therapeutic Role of Consultation With a Consultation-Liaison Psychiatrist

Psychiatric consultation has been shown to reduce health care expenditures in patients with somatization disorder without compromising patients' health status or satisfaction with health care. An intervention consisting of a psychiatric consultation and a letter to the referral source that described basic information about somatization disorder and outlined recommendations for management similar to those shown in Table 19–14 led to a decline of 53% in quarterly health charges, mostly accounted for by decreased hospitalization costs (Smith et al. 1986).

Approach to the Patient

In addition to the general comments made about the patient with somatic symptoms, specific approaches have

TABLE 19–14.   Writing a consultation report for patients with somatization disorder

Based on the study by Smith et al. (1986), the consultation report to the physician referring a patient for psychiatric assessment for multiple, medically unexplained symptoms should include the following:

1. A description of somatization disorder, including a description of its chronic relapsing course, the multiple symptoms associated with the diagnosis, its low morbidity and mortality, and the likelihood of periods when other psychiatric diagnoses may develop and be appropriate targets for treatment
2. Recommendations for regularly scheduled appointments, with frequency based on the patient's current frequency of visits and an explanation that this schedule is designed to remove the need to have symptoms present before visiting the doctor
3. Recommendations that symptoms not be taken at face value but that a physical examination be performed to assess for disease
4. Recommendations that further diagnostic procedures, hospitalizations, and surgery be avoided unless there are clear medical indications to do so
5. Recommendations that medications be kept to the minimum
6. Suggestions as to how the physician may communicate with the patient about his or her symptoms based on the consultant's understanding of the patient's psychology; such suggestions might include the recommendation that the patient not be told that the symptoms are "all in your head" but rather "the symptoms are in your body, but we have to pay attention to all of the factors that might be affecting them." The radio metaphor might be included if the patient found it helpful.

been described for patients with conversion disorder, including 1) explaining to the patient that his or her conversion symptoms are not caused by a serious disease, 2) refraining from confronting the patient, and 3) providing some form of "face-saving" mechanism for symptom resolution such as physical therapy or the suggestion that the patient will improve over a specified period. Eisendrath (1989, p. 386) observed that "When dealing with behavior with prominent unconscious motivation such as conversion reactions…the therapist provides no benefit by revealing understanding of the psychological processes too early in the treatment." Although many clinicians feel uncomfortable about the risks inherent in "legitimizing" the illness, this approach seems justified based on considerable anecdotal experience of good outcome with treatment and prolonged disability without it. The consultation-liaison psychiatrist often must help the referring physician and other health care professionals manage their emotional response to these patients whom they may view as deceiving them.

Pharmacotherapy for Somatoform Disorders

Pharmacotherapy for somatoform disorders is in its infancy. Treatments for hypochondriasis have included high-dose fluoxetine, which was reported to improve the conditions in 10 of 16 patients meeting DSM-III-R criteria who did not have marked depressive features (Fallon et al. 1993). Secondary hypochondriasis in patients with depression has been treated with amitriptyline (Kellner et al. 1986). A number of studies of BDD have reported success with serotonin reuptake blocking antidepressants (see review in Phillips 1998). Analgesics have a very limited role to play in somatoform pain disorder. The use of narcotic analgesics in nonmalignant chronic pain states is controversial. They are generally thought to be inappropriate (France et al. 1988), although there may be individual cases in which closely monitored use is associated with improved functioning. Psychotropic medications are frequently used in pain disorder (France and Krishnan 1988). Tricyclic antidepressants decrease pain in patients with chest pain and normal angiography (Cannon et al. 1994) and in women with chronic pelvic pain (Walker et al. 1991). The mechanisms of action are unclear and may include visceral analgesia (Cannon et al. 1994) and improvement in sleep, which results in a reduction in the level of pain or the distress associated with it.

Physical Reactivation and Physical Therapy

Physical reactivation via a gradually escalating program of exercise (e.g., walking, swimming) often improves the quality of life in patients with a variety of somatoform disorders. It may be difficult to engage patients in exercise, but once they become more active, they often find it pleasurable and report feelings of accomplishment, reduced stress, and greater confidence in their body. Physical therapy is invaluable for patients who have conversion disorder and may be the only treatment required (Delargy et al. 1986; Dvonch et al. 1991). One trial of an inpatient rehabilitation program for six patients with prolonged conversion paralysis (mean=3 years; range=1–6 years) returned all patients to walking (mean=41 days; range=10–70 days) and maintained their improvement on follow-up (mean=10 months; range=8–15 months) (Delargy et al. 1986).

Relaxation Therapies, Meditation, and Hypnotherapy

Various forms of relaxation therapies, biofeedback, meditation, and hypnotherapy have been used with somatoform disorder patients. Relaxation therapies modulate somatic sensations and may be used as part of a more comprehensive group treatment program for hypochondriasis (Barsky et al. 1988b). Relaxation therapy, biofeedback, meditation, and hypnotherapy all have been used in patients with somatoform pain (Andrasik 1986). These therapies may be used as either a primary form of treatment based on a psychophysiological model or an adjuvant to other forms of treatment. Hypnosis has been used diagnostically and therapeutically in patients with conversion disorder (see review by Van Dyck and Hoogduin 1989). It may be combined with intravenous sedation (Toone 1990). Although abreaction or catharsis under hypnosis or sedation has had dramatic anecdotal effects in individuals in whom the conversion was precipitated by extreme trauma, it is not helpful for most patients (Toone 1990). Behavioral stress management is helpful in hypochondriasis (Clark et al. 1998).

Behavioral Treatment

Learning theory models have been proposed for the treatment of several somatoform disorders (Wooley et al. 1978). Hypochondriasis has been treated with exposure and response prevention individually tailored to the patient's specific problem behaviors (Visser and Bouman 1992; Warwick and Marks 1988). Prevention of reassurance seeking was a key component of treatment because it is conceptualized as an anxiety-reducing ritual that is reinforced by the reassurance received (Warwick 1992). This program, which required a median of seven treatment sessions and 11 therapist hours, was associated with improvement that was maintained in half of the patients at follow-up (mean duration = 5 years; range = 1–8 years). Exposure therapy decreases hypochondriacal fears and beliefs in agoraphobic patients (Fava et al. 1988). Exposure plus response prevention for hypochondriasis was found to be as effective as cognitive therapy, and both treatments were superior to a waiting list control group (Visser and Bouman 2001). BDD has been successfully treated in some patients with behavioral techniques such as desensitization, live and fantasy exposure, and assertiveness training (Marks and Mishan 1988). Operant treatments of somatoform pain seek to remove positive reinforcers of pain (Roberts 1986) and are more effective than other forms of treatment at increasing physical activity and reducing medication consumption (Benjamin 1989).

Suggestion

The "suggestion of cure" has been described as possibly the most important factor in treatment of conversion disorder (Folks and Houck 1993). It is also reported to be helpful in patients with hypochondriasis (e.g., "If you remain relaxed and distract your thinking, you will worry less.") (Kellner 1986).

Cognitive Therapy

Cognitive therapy has been used in both individual and group formats for functional somatic symptoms and several somatoform disorders (see critical review of controlled trials by Kroenke and Swindle 2000). The use of cognitive therapy is predicated on cognitive models such as the one shown in Figure 19–3 for hypochondriasis. A cognitive model directs attention to factors that maintain preoccupation with worries about health, including attentional factors, avoidant behaviors, beliefs, and misinterpretation of symptoms, signs, and medical communications (Salkovskis 1989). Cognitive therapy programs for hypochondriasis have been described in considerable detail (Salkovskis 1989) and are based on a model of hypochondriasis as a disorder of perception and cognition in which somatic sensations are perceived as abnormally intense and attributed to serious medical disease. A 6-week program concentrates on modulating somatic sensations and altering cognitive appraisals by focusing on attention, relaxation, cognition, and symptom attribution; developing an understanding of the way in which the situational context may modulate symptom experience and attribution; and discussing how dysphoric affects and dependency conflicts can amplify somatic symptoms (Barsky et al. 1988b). The program has been successful in a clinical sample, and a controlled intervention trial has been advocated (Barsky et al. 1988b). Clark et al. (1998) demonstrated that cognitive therapy (up to 16 weekly 1-hour sessions and up to three booster sessions over the next 3 months) is an effective specific treatment for hypochondriasis. A group cognitive-behavioral program was effective for somatizing patients in primary care (Lidbeck 1997). Cognitive therapy may be helpful in BDD (see review in Phillips 1998). Cognitive therapy for somatoform pain is used to help the patient identify and replace inappropriate negative beliefs or attributions with more appropriate ideas or coping strategies (Benjamin 1989; Holzman et al. 1986) and produces greater reduction in pain complaints than do other forms of treatment (Benjamin 1989).

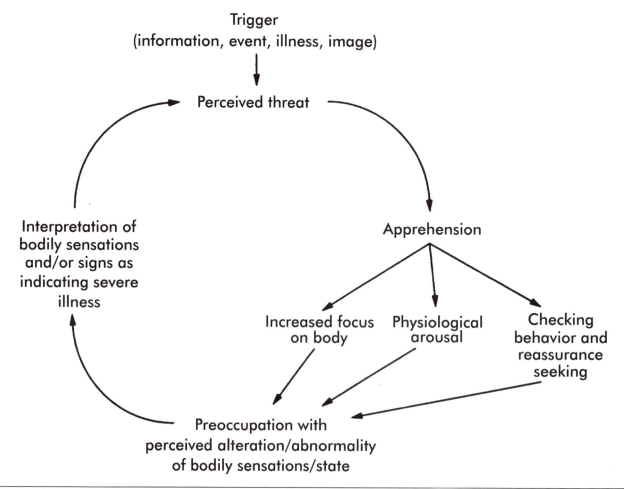

FIGURE 19–3. A cognitive model of hypochondriasis.

Source. Reprinted from Salkovskis PM: "Somatic Problems," in *Cognitive Behaviour Therapy for Psychiatric Problems.* Edited by Hawton K, Salkovskis PM, Kirk J, et al. Oxford, England, Oxford University Press, 1989, pp. 235–276. Used with permission.

Individual Psychotherapy

Individual psychotherapy plays a role in the management of some somatoform disorders. In general, psychoeducational and supportive techniques predominate, although insight-oriented therapy may be indicated in some patients. The psychotherapeutic treatment of hypochondriasis has been described (Kellner 1986). Psychotherapy plays a role in a relatively small proportion of patients with conversion disorder, but when indicated, it may have a very dramatic positive effect (Ford 1983). (Psychotherapy with chronic pain patients is discussed in Chapter 43.)

Group Psychotherapy

Group therapy may be particularly useful in the management of somatoform disorders. When social and affiliative needs are gratified via the group, patients' need to somatize to establish or maintain relationships may be reduced (Ford 1984). Confrontation by fellow group members about secondary gain is usually better tolerated than that by an individual therapist. Anger at physicians and family and dependency needs may be better tolerated in the group setting, which tends to diffuse intense affects. Group therapy also may be useful in increasing interpersonal skills and in enhancing more direct forms of communication regarding thoughts, feelings, and desires (Ford 1984). Helplessness has been identified as a central psychotherapeutic issue that can be effectively addressed in group therapy for patients with somatoform disorder (Levine et al. 1993). Various forms of group therapy have been reported for patients with somatoform disorder (see review by Levine et al. 1993) and for patients with somatoform pain (Benjamin 1989). Short-term group therapy appears to be effective in primary care somatization disorder patients (Kashner et al. 1995).

Marital and Family Therapy

Most families will benefit from information and psycho-educational approaches. More intensive forms of therapy are required when patients have significant marital or family pathology and when somatic symptoms are an important form of social communication within the family (Lazare 1981). It is important to identify the family's attitude and response because they may have a conscious or unconscious interest in maintaining a symptom in a patient (Toone 1990).

REFERENCES

Abbey SE, Lipowski ZJ: Comprehensive management of persistent somatization: an innovative inpatient program. Psychother Psychosom 48:110–115, 1987

Adler G: The physician and the hypochondriacal patient. N Engl J Med 304:1394–1396, 1981

Albertini RS, Phillips KA: Thirty-three cases of body dysmorphic disorder in children and adolescents. J Am Acad Child Adolesc Psychiatry 38:453–459, 1999

American Psychiatric Association: Diagnostic and Statistical Manual of Mental Disorders, 3rd Edition. Washington, DC, American Psychiatric Association, 1980

American Psychiatric Association: Diagnostic and Statistical Manual of Mental Disorders, 3rd Edition, Revised. Washington, DC, American Psychiatric Association, 1987

American Psychiatric Association: Diagnostic and Statistical Manual of Mental Disorders, 4th Edition. Washington, DC, American Psychiatric Association, 1994

American Psychiatric Association: Diagnostic and Statistical Manual of Mental Disorders, 4th Edition, Text Revision. Washington, DC, American Psychiatric Association, 2000

Andrasik F: Relaxation and biofeedback for chronic headaches, in Pain Management: A Handbook of Psychological Treatment Approaches. Edited by Holzman AD, Turk DC. New York, Pergamon, 1986, pp 213–239

Andreski P, Chilcoat H, Breslau N: Post-traumatic stress disorder and somatization symptoms: a prospective study. Psychiatry Res 79:131–138, 1998

Barsky AJ: A comprehensive approach to the chronically somatizing patient. J Psychosom Res 45:301–306, 1998

Barsky AJ, Borus JF: Functional somatic syndromes. Ann Intern Med 130:910–921, 1999

Barsky AJ, Klerman GL: Overview: hypochondriasis, bodily complaints, and somatic styles. Am J Psychiatry 140:273–283, 1983

Barsky AJ, Wyshak G, Klerman GL: Hypochondriasis: an evaluation of the DSM-III criteria in medical outpatients. Arch Gen Psychiatry 43:493–500, 1986a

Barsky AJ, Wyshak G, Klerman GL: Medical and psychiatric determinants of outpatient medical utilization. Med Care 24:548–560, 1986b

Barsky AJ, Goodson JD, Lane RS, et al: The amplification of somatic symptoms. Psychosom Med 50:510–519, 1988a

Barsky AJ, Geringer E, Wood CA: A cognitive-educational treatment for hypochondriasis. Gen Hosp Psychiatry 10:322–327, 1988b

Barsky AJ, Wyshak G, Klerman GL: Psychiatric co-morbidity in DSM-III-R hypochondriasis. Arch Gen Psychiatry 49:101–108, 1992

Barsky AJ, Coeytaux RR, Sarnie MK, et al: Hypochondriacal patients' beliefs about good health. Am J Psychiatry 150:1085–1089, 1993

Barsky AJ, Wool C, Barnett MC, et al: Histories of childhood trauma in adult hypochondriacal patients. Am J Psychiatry 151:397–401, 1994

Barsky AJ, Fama JM, Bailey ED, et al: A prospective 4- to 5-year study of DSM-III-R hypochondriasis. Arch Gen Psychiatry 55:737–744, 1998

Bass C (ed): Somatization: Physical Symptoms and Psychological Illness. Oxford, England, Blackwell Scientific, 1990

Bass C, Benjamin S: The management of chronic somatisation. Br J Psychiatry 162:472–480, 1993

Bass C, Murphy M: The chronic somatizer and the Government White Paper. J R Soc Med 83:203–205, 1990

Bass C, Murphy M: Somatoform and personality disorders; syndromal comorbidity and overlapping developmental pathways. J Psychosom Res 39:403–427, 1995

Beck AT, Ward CH, Mendelson M, et al: An inventory for measuring depression. Arch Gen Psychiatry 4:561–571, 1961

Benjamin S: Psychological treatment of chronic pain: a selective review. J Psychosom Res 33:121–131, 1989

Blumer D: Chronic pain as a psychobiologic phenomenon: the pain-prone disorder, in Psychiatric Aspects of Neurologic Disease, Vol II. Edited by Benson DF, Blumer D. New York, Grune & Stratton, 1982, pp 179–194

Bohman M, Cloninger R, von Knorring A-L, et al: An adoption study of somatoform disorders, III: cross-fostering analysis and genetic relationship to alcoholism and criminality. Arch Gen Psychiatry 41:872–878, 1984

Brena SF: The mystery of pain: is pain a sensation? in Management of Patients With Chronic Pain. Edited by Brena SF, Chapman SL. New York, Spectrum, 1983, pp 1–9

Bridges KW, Goldberg DP: Somatic presentation of DSM-III psychiatric disorders in primary care. J Psychosom Res 29:563–569, 1985

Butcher JN, Dahlstrom WG, Graham JR, et al: Minnesota Multiphasic Personality Inventory—2: Manual for Administration and Scoring. Minneapolis, MN, University of Minnesota Press, 1991

Campo JV, Fritsch SL: Somatization in children and adolescents. J Am Acad Child Adolesc Psychiatry 33:1223–1235, 1994

Cannon RO, Quyyumi AA, Mincemoyer R, et al: Imipramine in patients with chest pain despite normal coronary angiograms. N Engl J Med 330:1411–1417, 1994

Cassem NH, Barsky AJ: Functional somatic symptoms and somatoform disorders, in Massachusetts General Hospital Handbook of General Hospital Psychiatry, 3rd Edition. Edited by Cassem NH. Boston, MA, Mosby Year Book, 1991, pp 131–157

Clark DM, Salkovskis PM, Hackmann A, et al: Two psychological treatments for hypochondriasis: a randomised controlled trial. Br J Psychiatry 173:218–225, 1998

Cloninger CR, Sigvardsson S, von Knorring A-L, et al: An adoption study of somatoform disorders, II: identification of two discrete somatoform disorders. Arch Gen Psychiatry 41:863–871, 1984

Cloninger CR, Martin RL, Guze SB, et al: A prospective follow-up and family study of somatization in men and women. Am J Psychiatry 143:873–878, 1986

Craig TK, Boardman AP, Mills K, et al: The South London somatisation study, I: longitudinal course and the influence of early life experiences. Br J Psychiatry 163:579–588, 1993

Creed F, Guthrie E: Techniques for interviewing the somatising patient. Br J Psychiatry 162:467–471, 1993

Creed F, Mayou R, Hopkins A (eds): Medical Symptoms Not Explained by Organic Disease. London, The Royal College of Psychiatrists and The Royal College of Physicians of London, 1992

Crimlisk HL, Bhatia K, Cope H, et al: Slater revisited: 6 year follow up study of patients with medically unexplained motor symptoms. BMJ 316:582–586, 1998

Cummings NA, van den Bos GR: The twenty years Kaiser-Permanente experience with psychotherapy and medical utilization: implications for national health policy and national health insurance. Health Policy Quarterly 1:159–175, 1981

deGruy F, Columbia L, Dickinson P: Somatization disorder in a family practice. J Fam Pract 25:45–51, 1987a

DeGruy F, Crider J, Hashimi DK, et al: Somatization disorder in a university hospital. J Fam Pract 25:579–584, 1987b

Delargy MA, Peatfield RC, Burt AA: Successful rehabilitation in conversion paralysis. BMJ 292:1730–1731, 1986

Derogatis LR, Lipman RS, Rickels K, et al: The Hopkins Symptom Checklist (HSCL): a self-report symptom inventory. Behavioral Science 19:1–15, 1974

Drossman DA, McKee DC, Sandler RS, et al: Psychosocial factors in the irritable bowel syndrome. Gastroenterology 95:701–708, 1988

Drossman DA, Leserman J, Nachman G, et al: Sexual and physical abuse in women with functional or organic gastrointestinal disorders. Ann Intern Med 113:828–833, 1990

Dvonch VM, Bunch WH, Siegler AH: Conversion reactions in pediatric athletes. J Pediatr Orthop 11:770–772, 1991

Eisenberg L: Disease and illness: distinctions between professional and popular ideas of sickness. Cult Med Psychiatry 1:9–23, 1977

Eisendrath SJ: Factitious physical disorders: treatment without confrontation. Psychosomatics 30:383–387, 1989

Engel GL: Conversion symptoms, in Signs and Symptoms: Applied Pathologic Physiology and Clinical Interpretation, 5th Edition. Edited by MacBryde CM. Philadelphia, PA, JB Lippincott, 1970, pp 650–668

Epstein RM, Quill TE, McWhinney IR: Somatization reconsidered: incorporating the patient's experience of illness. Arch Intern Med 159:215–222, 1999

Escobar JI, Burnam MA, Karno M, et al: Somatization in the community. Arch Gen Psychiatry 44:713–718, 1987

Escobar JI, Manu P, Matthews D, et al: Medically unexplained physical symptoms, somatization disorder and abridged somatization: studies with the Diagnostic Interview Schedule. Psychiatric Developments 3:235–245, 1989

Ewald H, Rogne T, Ewald K, et al: Somatization in patients newly admitted to a neurological department. Acta Psychiatr Scand 89:174–179, 1994

Fallon BA, Liebowitz MR, Salman E, et al: Fluoxetine for hypochondriacal patients without major depressive disorder. J Clin Psychopharmacol 13:438–441, 1993

Fava GA, Kellner R, Zielezny M, et al: Hypochondriacal fears and beliefs in agoraphobia. J Affect Disord 14:239–244, 1988

Feighner JP, Robins E, Guze SB, et al: Diagnostic criteria for use in psychiatric research. Arch Gen Psychiatry 26:57–63, 1972

Fishman B: Therapy for an anxious patient who believes his symptoms are caused by a medical problem. Hospital and Community Psychiatry 43:583–585, 1992

Folks DG, Houck CA: Somatoform disorders, factitious disorders, and malingering, in Psychiatric Care of the Medical Patient. Edited by Stoudemire A, Fogel BS. New York, Oxford University Press, 1993, pp 267–287

Folks DG, Ford CV, Regan WM: Conversion symptoms in a general hospital. Psychosomatics 25:285–295, 1984

Ford CV: The Somatizing Disorders: Illness as a Way of Life. New York, Elsevier, 1983

Ford CV: Somatizing disorders, in Helping Patients and Their Families Cope With Medical Problems. Edited by Roback HB. Washington, DC, Jossey-Bass, 1984, pp 39–59

Ford CV: Illness as a lifestyle: the role of somatization in medical practice. Spine 17:S338–S343, 1992

Ford CV, Parker PE: Somatization in consultation-liaison psychiatry, in Current Concepts of Somatization: Research and Clinical Perspectives. Edited by Kirmayer LJ, Robbins JM. Washington, DC, American Psychiatric Press, 1991, pp 143–157

France RD, Krishnan KRR: Psychotropic drugs in chronic pain, in Chronic Pain. Edited by France RD, Krishnan KRR. Washington, DC, American Psychiatric Press, 1988, pp 322–374

France RD, Krishnan KRR, Manepalli AN: Analgesics in chronic pain, in Chronic Pain. Edited by France RD, Krishnan KRR. Washington, DC, American Psychiatric Press, 1988, pp 414–444

Fritz GK, Fritsch S, Hagino O: Somatoform disorders in children and adolescents: a review of the past 10 years. J Am Acad Child Adolesc Psychiatry 36:1329–1338, 1997

Garralda ME: Assessment and management of somatisation in childhood and adolescence: a practical perspective. J Child Psychol Psychiatry 40:1159–1167, 1999

Gask L, Goldberg D, Porter R, et al: The treatment of somatization: evaluation of a teaching package with general practice trainees. J Psychosom Res 33:697–703, 1989

Goldberg D, Gask L, O'Dowd T: The treatment of somatization: teaching techniques of reattribution. J Psychosom Res 33:689–695, 1989

Goldberg R, Morris P, Christian F, et al: Panic disorder in cardiac outpatients. Psychosomatics 31:168–173, 1990

Golding JM, Smith GR Jr, Kashner TM: Does somatization disorder occur in men? Clinical characteristics of women and men with multiple unexplained somatic symptoms. Arch Gen Psychiatry 48:231–235, 1991

Golding JM, Rost K, Kashner TM, et al: Family psychiatric history of patients with somatization disorder. Psychiatr Med 10:33–47, 1992

Gould R, Miller BL, Goldberg M, et al: The validity of hysterical signs and symptoms. J Nerv Ment Dis 174:593–597, 1986

Gureje O, Simon GE, Ustun TB, et al: Somatization in cross-cultural perspective: a World Health Organization study in primary care. Am J Psychiatry 154:989–995, 1997

Guthrie EA, Creed F, Dawson D, et al: A controlled trial of psychological treatment for the irritable bowel syndrome. Gastroenterology 100:450–457, 1991

Guze SB, Cloninger CR, Martin RL, et al: A follow-up and family study of Briquet's syndrome. Br J Psychiatry 149:17–23, 1986

Hahn SR, Thompson KS, Wills TA, et al: The difficult doctor-patient relationship: somatization, personality and psychopathology. J Clin Epidemiol 47:647–657, 1994

Hamilton M: The assessment of anxiety states by rating. Br J Med Psychol 32:50–55, 1959

Hamilton M: A rating scale for depression. J Neurol Neurosurg Psychiatry 23:56–62, 1960

Hathaway SR, McKinley JC: A multiphasic personality schedule (Minnesota), 1: construction of the schedule. J Psychol 10:249–254, 1940

Henry JA, Woodruff GHA: A diagnostic sign in states of apparent unconsciousness. Lancet 2:920–921, 1978

Holzman AD, Turk DC, Kerns RD: The cognitive-behavioral approach to the management of chronic pain, in Pain Management: A Handbook of Psychological Treatment Approaches. Edited by Holzman AD, Turk DC. New York, Pergamon, 1986, pp 31–50

Jones JB, Barklage NE: Conversion disorder: camouflage for brain lesions in two cases. Arch Intern Med 150:1343–1345, 1990

Kashner TM, Rost K, Cohen B, et al: Enhancing the health of somatization disorder patients: effectiveness of short-term group therapy. Psychosomatics 36:462–470, 1995

Katon W: Panic disorder and somatization: review of 55 cases. Am J Med 77:101–106, 1984

Katon W, Russo J: Somatic symptoms and depression. J Fam Pract 29:65–69, 1989

Katon W, Kleinman A, Rosen G: Depression and somatization: a review: part I. Am J Med 72:127–135, 1982

Katon W, Ries RK, Kleinman A: The prevalence of somatization in primary care. Compr Psychiatry 25:208–215, 1984

Katon W, Berg AO, Robins AJ, et al: Depression—medical utilization and somatization. West J Med 144:564–568, 1986

Katon W, Lin E, Von Korff M, et al: Somatization: a spectrum of severity. Am J Psychiatry 148:34–40, 1991

Kellner R: Somatization and Hypochondriasis. New York, Praeger, 1986

Kellner R: Psychological measurements in somatization and abnormal illness behavior. Adv Psychosom Med 17:101–118, 1987

Kellner R: Psychosomatic Syndromes and Somatic Symptoms. Washington, DC, American Psychiatric Press, 1991

Kellner R, Slocumb J, Wiggins RG, et al: Hostility, somatic symptoms and hypochondriacal fears and beliefs. J Nerv Ment Dis 173:554–560, 1985

Kellner R, Fava GA, Lisansky J, et al: Hypochondriacal fears and beliefs in DSM-III melancholia: changes with amitriptyline. J Affect Disord 10:21–26, 1986

Kerns RD, Turk DC, Rudy TE: The West Haven–Yale Multidimensional Pain Inventory (WHYMPI). Pain 23:345–356, 1985

King SA, Strain JJ: Revising the category of somatoform pain disorder. Hospital and Community Psychiatry 43:217–219, 1992

Kirmayer LJ, Robbins JM (eds): Current Concepts of Somatization: Research and Clinical Perspectives. Washington, DC, American Psychiatric Press, 1991a

Kirmayer LJ, Robbins JM: Three forms of somatization in primary care: prevalence, co-occurrence, and sociodemographic characteristics. J Nerv Ment Dis 179:647–655, 1991b

Kirmayer LJ, Robbins JM: Patients who somatize in primary care: a longitudinal study of cognitive and social characteristics. Psychol Med 26:937–951, 1996

Kirmayer LJ, Young A: Culture and somatization: clinical, epidemiological and ethnographic perspectives. Psychosom Med 60:420–430, 1998

Kirmayer LJ, Robbins JM, Dworkind M, et al: Somatization and the recognition of depression and anxiety in primary care. Am J Psychiatry 150:734–741, 1993

Kleinman A: Social Origins of Distress and Disease: Depression, Neurasthenia, and Pain in Modern China. New Haven, CT, Yale University Press, 1986

Kroenke K, Mangelsdorff D: Common symptoms in ambulatory care: incidence, evaluation, therapy and outcome. Am J Med 86:262–266, 1989

Kroenke K, Swindle R: Cognitive-behavioral therapy for somatization and symptom syndromes: a critical review of controlled clinical trials. Psychother Psychosom 69:205–215, 2000

Kroenke K, Spitzer RL, deGruy FV, et al: Multisomatoform disorder: an alternative to undifferentiated somatoform disorder for the somatizing patient in primary care. Arch Gen Psychiatry 54:352–358, 1997

Lazare A: Current concepts in psychiatry: conversion symptoms. N Engl J Med 305:745–748, 1981

Levine JB, Irving KK, Brooks JD, et al: Group therapy and the somatoform patient: an integration. Psychotherapy 30:625–634, 1993

Lidbeck J: Group therapy for somatization disorders in general practice: effectiveness of a short cognitive-behavioural treatment model. Acta Psychiatr Scand 96:14–24, 1997

Lipowski ZJ: Somatization: the concept and its clinical application. Am J Psychiatry 145:1358–1368, 1988

Lipsitt DR: Medical and psychological characteristics of "crocks." Psychiatr Med 1:15–25, 1970

Liu G, Clark MR, Eaton WW: Structural factor analyses for medically unexplained somatic symptoms of somatization disorder in the Epidemiologic Catchment Area study. Psychol Med 27:617–626, 1997

Mabe PA, Hobson DP, Jones R, et al: Hypochondriacal traits in medical inpatients. Gen Hosp Psychiatry 10:236–244, 1988

Mace CJ: Hysterical conversion, I: a history. Br J Psychiatry 161:369–377, 1992

Main CJ: The Modified Somatic Perception Questionnaire (MSPQ). J Psychosom Res 27:503–514, 1983

Marks I, Mishan J: Dysmorphophobic avoidance with disturbed bodily perception: a pilot study of exposure therapy. Br J Psychiatry 152:674–678, 1988

Martin RL: Diagnostic issues for conversion disorder. Hospital and Community Psychiatry 43:771–773, 1992

Mathew RJ, Weinman ML, Mirabi M: Physical symptoms of depression. Br J Psychiatry 139:293–296, 1981

Mayou R: Illness behavior and psychiatry. Gen Hosp Psychiatry 11:307–312, 1989

Mayou R: Patients' fears of illness: chest pain and palpitations, in Medical Symptoms Not Explained by Organic Disease. Edited by Creed F, Mayou R, Hopkins A. London, The Royal College of Psychiatrists and The Royal College of Physicians of London, 1992, pp 25–33

Mayou R: Somatization. Psychother Psychosom 59:69–83, 1993

Mayou RA, Bass C, Sharpe M: Treatment of Functional Somatic Symptoms. Oxford, England: Oxford University Press, 1995

McDougall J: Theaters of the Body: A Psychoanalytic Approach to Psychosomatic Illness. New York, WW Norton, 1989

Mechanic D: The concept of illness behaviour: culture, situation and personal predisposition. Psychol Med 16:1–7, 1986

Melzack R: The McGill Pain Questionnaire: major properties and scoring methods. Pain 1:277–299, 1975

Millon T: Millon Clinical Multiaxial Inventory II: Manual for the MCMI-II. Minneapolis, MN, National Computer Systems, 1987

Morrison J: Childhood sexual histories of women with somatization disorder. Am J Psychiatry 146:239–241, 1989

Murphy M: Somatisation: embodying the problem. BMJ 298:1331–1332, 1989

Murphy MR: Classification of the somatoform disorders, in Somatization: Physical Symptoms and Psychological Illness. Edited by Bass C. Oxford, England, Blackwell Scientific, 1990, pp 10–39

Newman NJ: Neuro-ophthalmology and psychiatry. Gen Hosp Psychiatry 15:102–114, 1993

Noyes R, Reich J, Clancy J, et al: Reduction in hypochondriasis with treatment of panic disorder. Br J Psychiatry 149:631–635, 1986

Noyes R, Kathol RG, Fisher MM, et al: The validity of DSM-III-R hypochondriasis. Arch Gen Psychiatry 50:961–970, 1993

Noyes R, Holt CS, Kathol RG: Somatization: diagnosis and management. Arch Fam Med 4:790–795, 1995

Pennebaker JW: The Psychology of Physical Symptoms. New York, Springer-Verlag, 1982

Pennebaker JW, Watson D: The psychology of somatic symptoms, in Current Concepts of Somatization: Research and Clinical Perspectives. Edited by Kirmayer LJ, Robbins JM. Washington, DC, American Psychiatric Press, 1991, pp 21–36

Phillips KA: Body dysmorphic disorder: clinical aspects and treatment strategies. Bull Menninger Clin 62 (4, suppl A):A33–A48, 1998

Phillips KA, Diaz SF: Gender differences in body dysmorphic disorder. J Nerv Ment Dis 185:570–577, 1997

Phillips KA, Hollander E: Body dysmorphic disorder, in DSM-IV Sourcebook, Vol 2. Edited by Widiger RA, Frances AJ, Pincus R, et al. Washington, DC, American Psychiatric Association, 1996, pp 949–960

Phillips KA, McElroy SL, Keck PE, et al: Body dysmorphic disorder: 30 cases of imagined ugliness. Am J Psychiatry 150:302–308, 1993

Phillips KA, McElroy SL, Keck PE, et al: A comparison of delusional and nondelusional body dysmorphic disorder in 100 cases. Psychopharmacology Bulletin 30:179–186, 1994

Piccinelli M, Simon G: Gender and cross-cultural differences in somatic symptoms associated with emotional distress: an international study in primary care. Psychol Med 27:433–444, 1997

Pilowsky I: Dimensions of hypochondriasis. Br J Psychiatry 113:89–93, 1967

Pilowsky I: Abnormal illness behavior. Psychiatr Med 5:85–91, 1987

Priel B, Rabinowitz B, Pels RJ: A semiotic perspective on chronic pain: implications for the interaction between patient and physician. Br J Med Psychol 64:65–71, 1991

Quill TE: Somatization disorder: one of medicine's blind spots. JAMA 254:3075–3079, 1985

Regier DA, Boyd JH, Burke JD, et al: One-month prevalence of mental disorders in the United States based on five Epidemiologic Catchment Area sites. Arch Gen Psychiatry 45:977–986, 1988

Roberts AH: The operant approach to the management of pain and excess disability, in Pain Management: A Handbook of Psychological Treatment Approaches. Edited by Holzman AD, Turk DC. New York, Pergamon, 1986, pp 10–30

Robins LN, Helzer JE, Weissman MM, et al: Life-time prevalence of specific psychiatric disorders in three sites. Arch Gen Psychiatry 41:949–958, 1984

Rodin G: Somatization and the self: psychotherapeutic issues. Am J Psychother 38:257–263, 1984

Roelofs K, Naring GW, Moene FC, et al: The question of symptom lateralization in conversion disorder. J Psychosom Res 49:21–25, 2000

Ron M: Explaining the unexplained: understanding hysteria [editorial]. Brain 124:1065–1066, 2001

Rost KM, Akins RN, Brown FW, et al: The comorbidity of DSM-III-R personality disorders in somatization disorder. Gen Hosp Psychiatry 14:322–326, 1992

Salkovskis PM: Somatic problems, in Cognitive Behaviour Therapy for Psychiatric Problems. Edited by Hawton K, Salkovskis PM, Kirk J, et al. Oxford, England, Oxford University Press, 1989, pp 235–276

Salmon P, Peters S, Stanley I: Patients' perceptions of medical explanations for somatisation disorders: qualitative analysis. BMJ 318:372–376, 1999

Schurman RA, Kramer PD, Mitchell JB: The hidden mental health network: treatment of mental illness by non-psychiatrist physicians. Arch Gen Psychiatry 42:89–94, 1985

Shapiro EG, Rosenfeld AA: The Somatizing Child: Diagnosis and Treatment of Conversion and Somatoform Disorders. New York, Springer-Verlag, 1987

Sharpe M, Bass C: Pathophysiological mechanisms in somatization. International Review of Psychiatry 4:81–97, 1992

Sharpe M, Carson A: "Unexplained" somatic symptoms, functional syndromes, and somatization: do we need a paradigm shift? Ann Intern Med 134:926–930, 2001

Sharpe M, Peveler R, Mayou R: The psychological treatment of patients with functional somatic symptoms: a practical guide. J Psychosom Res 36:515–529, 1992

Sharpe M, Mayou R, Seagroatt V, et al: Why do doctors find some patients difficult to help? Quarterly Journal of Medicine 87:187–193, 1994

Shaw J, Creed F: The cost of somatization. J Psychosom Res 35:307–312, 1991

Simon G, Gater R, Kisely S, et al: Somatic symptoms of distress: an international primary care study. Psychosom Med 58:481–488, 1996

Simon GE: Somatization and psychiatric disorders, in Current Concepts of Somatization: Research and Clinical Perspectives. Edited by Kirmayer LJ, Robbins JM. Washington, DC, American Psychiatric Press, 1991, pp 37–62

Simon GE, Gureje O: Stability of somatization disorder and somatization symptoms among primary care patients. Arch Gen Psychiatry 56:90–95, 1999

Simon GE, Von Korff M, Piccinelli M, et al: An international study of the relation between somatic symptoms and depression. N Engl J Med 341:1329–1335, 1999

Slater E, Glithero E: A follow-up of patients diagnosed of suffering from "hysteria." J Psychosom Res 9:9–14, 1965

Smith GR: Somatization Disorder in Medical Settings. Washington, DC, American Psychiatric Press, 1991

Smith GR: The epidemiology and treatment of depression when it coexists with somatoform disorders, somatization, or pain. Gen Hosp Psychiatry 14:265–272, 1992

Smith GR, Monson RA, Ray DC: Psychiatric consultation in somatization disorder: a randomized controlled study. N Engl J Med 314:1407–1413, 1986

Smith GR, Golding JM, Kashner TM, et al: Antisocial personality disorder in primary care patients with somatization disorder. Compr Psychiatry 32:367–372, 1991

Smith GC, Clarke DM, Handrinos D, et al: Consultation-liaison psychiatrists' management of somatoform disorders. Psychosomatics 41:481–489, 2000

Spielberger CD, Gorsuch RL, Luchene RE: Manual for the State-Trait Anxiety Inventory. Palo Alto, CA, Consulting Psychologist Press, 1970

Starcevic V, Kellner R, Uhlenhuth EH, et al: Panic disorder and hypochondriacal fears and beliefs. J Affect Disord 24:73–85, 1992

Stern J, Murphy M, Bass C: Personality disorders in patients with somatisation disorder: a controlled study. Br J Psychiatry 163:785–789, 1993

Stewart DE: The changing faces of somatization. Psychosomatics 31:153–158, 1990a

Stewart DE: Emotional disorders misdiagnosed as physical illness: environmental hypersensitivity, candidiasis hypersensitivity, and chronic fatigue syndrome. International Journal of Mental Health 19:56–68, 1990b

Stoudemire A: Somatothymia: parts I and II. Psychosomatics 32:365–381, 1991

Stuart S, Noyes R: Attachment and interpersonal communication in somatization. Psychosomatics 40:34–43, 1999

Sullivan M, Clark MR, Katon WJ, et al: Psychiatric and otologic diagnoses in patients complaining of dizziness. Arch Intern Med 153:1479–1484, 1993

Swartz M, Blazer D, George L, et al: Somatization disorder in a community population. Am J Psychiatry 143:1403–1408, 1986

Taylor GJ: Alexithymia: concept, measurement and implications for treatment. Am J Psychiatry 141:725–732, 1984

Toomey TC, Hernandez JT, Gittelman DF, et al: Relationship of sexual and physical abuse to pain and psychological assessment variables in chronic pelvic pain patients. Pain 53:105–109, 1993

Toone BK: Disorders of hysterical conversion, in Somatization: Physical Symptoms and Psychological Illness. Edited by Bass C. Oxford, England, Blackwell Scientific, 1990, pp 207–234

Torgersen S: Genetics of somatoform disorders. Arch Gen Psychiatry 43:502–505, 1986

Tyrer P, Fowler-Dixon R, Ferguson B, et al: A plea for the diagnosis of hypochondriacal personality disorder. J Psychosom Res 34:637–642, 1990

Tyrer S: Psychiatric assessment of chronic pain. Br J Psychiatry 160:733–741, 1992

Van Dyck R, Hoogduin K: Hypnosis and conversion disorders. Am J Psychother 93:480–493, 1989

Visser S, Bouman TK: Cognitive-behavioural approaches in the treatment of hypochondriasis: six single case cross-over studies. Behav Res Ther 30:301–306, 1992

Visser S, Bouman TK: The treatment of hypochondriasis: exposure plus response prevention vs cognitive therapy. Behav Res Ther 39:423–442, 2001

Waddell G, McCulloch JA, Kummel E, et al: Nonorganic physical signs in low-back pain. Spine 5:117–125, 1980

Walker E, Katon W, Harrop-Griffiths J, et al: Relationship of chronic pelvic pain to psychiatric diagnoses and childhood sexual abuse. Am J Psychiatry 145:75–80, 1988

Walker EA, Roy-Byrne PP, Katon WJ, et al: An open trial of nortriptyline in women with chronic pelvic pain. Int J Psychiatry Med 21:245–252, 1991

Walling MK, O'Hara MW, Reiter RC, et al: Abuse history and chronic pain in women, II: a multivariate analysis of abuse and psychological morbidity. Obstet Gynecol 84:200–206, 1994

Warwick H: Provision of appropriate and effective reassurance. International Review of Psychiatry 4:76–80, 1992

Warwick HMC, Marks IM: Behavioural treatment of illness phobia and hypochondriasis: a pilot study of 17 cases. Br J Psychiatry 152:239–241, 1988

Weintraub MI: Hysterical Conversion Reactions: A Clinical Guide to Diagnosis and Treatment. Jamaica, NY, SP Medical & Scientific Books, 1983

Wessely S, Nimnuan C, Sharpe M: Functional somatic syndromes: one or many? Lancet 354:936–939, 1999

Wool CA, Barsky AJ: Do women somatize more than men? Gender differences in somatization. Psychosomatics 35:445–452, 1994

Wooley SC, Blackwell B, Winget C: A learning theory model of chronic illness behavior: theory, treatment and research. Psychosom Med 40:379–401, 1978

Young L: Sexual abuse and the problem of embodiment. Child Abuse Negl 16:89–100, 1992

Yutzy SH, Cloninger CR, Guze SB, et al: DSM-IV field trial: testing a new proposal for somatization disorder. Am J Psychiatry 152:97–101, 1995

Zimmerman M, Mattia JI: Body dysmorphic disorder in psychiatric outpatients: recognition, prevalence, comorbidity, demographic, and clinical correlates. Compr Psychiatry 39:265–270, 1998

20

Anxiety and Panic

Eduardo A. Colón, M.D.

Michael K. Popkin, M.D., F.A.P.M.

To the consultation-liaison psychiatrist, anxiety is a ubiquitous part of clinical presentations encountered on the medical-surgical inpatient units of the general hospital. Ironically, that very ubiquity has dampened, if not precluded, systematic study of the issue of anxiety within the general hospital. Surprisingly little research effort has been directed toward exploring or establishing the boundaries between the "primary" anxiety disorders encountered elsewhere in psychiatry and those disturbances of anxiety emerging within the medical-surgical setting. Are these entities identical or equivalent in phenomenological or pathophysiologic terms? Should anxiety and panic in the medical-surgical setting be conceptualized differently? Are they distinct discrete clinical entities?

In this chapter, we focus on anxiety and panic encountered by the consultation-liaison psychiatrist working in the hospital's medical-surgical wards. The psychiatric consultant must be able to discern 1) whether anxiety is of sufficient degree to exceed what constitutes a normative response to the challenges presented by medical illness and hospitalization, and 2) if such a threshold is crossed, to what etiological factor or factors it may be ascribed. The first task often rests with clinical judgments honed by years of consultation-liaison work. Objective parameters are tenuous here; the decision about what is pathological is frequently facilitated by the recognition that the patient is not coping effectively with the demands of hospitalization and that symptomatology is accelerating (or that the patient is visibly struggling and losing ground). The second task involves considering several clinical factors. Is the anxiety a reactive (psychological) response to medical illness as stressor? Is the anxiety a concomitant of a preexisting or established psychiatric

disorder that has been exacerbated or unmasked by the medical illness process? Is the anxiety derivative of the pathophysiology of the medical illness or a by-product (albeit untoward) of the treatment process?

Anxiety is a nonspecific symptom, and its presence (and/or persistence) obligates the psychiatric consultant to consider an extensive differential diagnosis (Table 20–1). The likelihood that anxiety in the medical-surgical patient involves more than one of the above-mentioned categories compounds the clinician's dilemma. Anxiety, like delirium, often has a multifactorial etiology. Even the patient with a well-established "organic" etiology is prone to additional symptomatology created by maladaptive or unsuccessful efforts at coping with the effect of the illness.

In short, anxiety and panic in the medical-surgical setting are often overlooked; it is an area beset with diagnostic, if not treatment, complexities. The consultant must attend to the possibility that both psychiatric and medical bases exist for anxiety and panic.

TABLE 20–1. Major differential diagnostic considerations for anxiety symptoms in the consultation-liaison setting

Acute stress disorder
Adjustment disorder with anxious or mixed features
Anxiety disorder due to a general medical condition
Generalized anxiety disorder
Obsessive-compulsive disorder
Panic disorder
Posttraumatic stress disorder
Specific phobias
Substance-induced anxiety disorder

DEFINITIONS AND CENTRAL ELEMENTS

Anxiety usually is defined as a state of fear or a subjective feeling of apprehension, dread, or foreboding. It is manifested by a wide array of physical signs and measures of autonomic activation. In terms of psychiatry, pathological anxiety (primary) is identical to fear except that its precipitant is an unknown intrapsychic conflict (e.g., the danger or threat is not external or "real").

Regardless of etiology, anxiety "can present with disruption of practically any bodily system" (Hall 1980, p. 147). Which specific somatic symptoms may emerge in a given individual is not readily anticipated or explained. We conceptualize anxiety partly in terms of an unduly labile or overactive autonomic nervous system. Given specific internal or external challenges, some individuals respond with a degree of autonomic activation that yields overt physical symptomatology (Table 20–2). Autonomic overactivation can take either an acute or a chronic form. In the former, alarm (fight or flight) features predominate; in the latter, heightened vigilance is the predominant element of the presentations. Panic attacks have been carefully investigated within the medical illness framework (National Institute of Mental Health 1989) and are known to be associated with specific medical conditions. Anxiety, of course, has both psychological and cognitive disturbances among its manifestations. These disturbances are less varied than the somatic concomitants but, again, are not readily foreseen. Some individuals are inclined to more psychological symptoms of anxiety; for others, the somatic symptoms may predominate. In some patients, both types of symptoms are prominent parts of the clinical picture.

Table 20–3 lists the diagnoses found in the anxiety disorders section of DSM-IV-TR (American Psychiatric Association 2000). Several of these diagnoses are the regular domain of the consultation psychiatrist; we review them in the following paragraphs in terms of their central elements.

Panic disorder is classified in DSM-IV-TR as either with or without agoraphobia. These disorders entail recurrent unexpected panic attacks followed by worry, concern, and behavior changes related to the attacks. The attacks are not due to a general medical condition or the direct effects of a substance. Table 20–4 presents DSM-IV-TR criteria for a panic attack.

A diagnosis of *posttraumatic stress disorder* (PTSD) requires that a trauma is "persistently reexperienced" and that there is avoidance of stimuli linked to the trauma, numbing, and persistent arousal.

TABLE 20–2.   Physical signs and symptoms of anxiety

Anorexia
"Butterflies" in stomach
Chest pain or tightness
Diaphoresis
Diarrhea
Dizziness
Dry mouth
Dyspnea
Faintness
Flushing
Hyperventilation
Light-headedness
Muscle tension
Nausea
Pallor
Palpitations
Paresthesias
Sexual dysfunction
Shortness of breath
Stomach pain
Tachycardia
Tremulousness
Urinary frequency
Vomiting

Source.   Adapted from Wise MG, Taylor SE: "Anxiety and Mood Disorders in Medically Ill Patients." *Journal of Clinical Psychiatry* 51 (suppl 1):27–32, 1990. Copyright 1990, Physicians Postgraduate Press. Used with permission.

TABLE 20–3.   DSM-IV-TR anxiety disorders

Panic disorder without agoraphobia
Panic disorder with agoraphobia
Posttraumatic stress disorder
Acute stress disorder
Generalized anxiety disorder
Anxiety disorder due to a general medical condition
Substance-induced anxiety disorder
Specific phobia
Agoraphobia without history of panic disorder
Social phobia
Obsessive-compulsive disorder
Anxiety disorder not otherwise specified

Acute stress disorder involves exposure to a traumatic event plus resultant dissociative symptoms, reexperiencing of the trauma, avoidance of associated stimuli, increased arousal, significant distress, or social or occupational impairment. Symptoms must last for more than 2 days but less than 4 weeks and emerge within a month of the trauma. As in PTSD, the condition is not substance induced or the result of a general medical condition.

TABLE 20–4. DSM-IV-TR criteria for panic attack

Note: A panic attack is not a codable disorder. Code the specific diagnosis in which the panic attack occurs (e.g., 300.21 panic disorder with agoraphobia).

A discrete period of intense fear or discomfort, in which four (or more) of the following symptoms developed abruptly and reached a peak within 10 minutes:

   (1) palpitations, pounding heart, or accelerated heart rate

   (2) sweating

   (3) trembling or shaking

   (4) sensations of shortness of breath or smothering

   (5) feeling of choking

   (6) chest pain or discomfort

   (7) nausea or abdominal distress

   (8) feeling dizzy, unsteady, lightheaded, or faint

   (9) derealization (feelings of unreality) or depersonalization (being detached from oneself)

 (10) fear of losing control or going crazy

 (11) fear of dying

 (12) paresthesias (numbness or tingling sensations)

 (13) chills or hot flushes

Generalized anxiety disorder is characterized by excessive anxiety plus "apprehensive expectation" about a number of events or activities. The worrying is difficult to control and commonly evokes restlessness, fatigue, irritability, muscle tension, and sleep dysfunction.

Anxiety disorder due to a general medical condition is the new title for what DSM-III-R (American Psychiatric Association 1987) identified as organic anxiety disorder and early drafts of DSM-IV (American Psychiatric Association 1994) labeled secondary anxiety disorder. This diagnosis incorporates generalized anxiety, panic attacks, and obsessions or compulsions thought to be etiologically related to general medical conditions.

Substance-induced anxiety disorder is reserved for instances in which a clinical constellation of generalized anxiety, panic attacks, or obsessive-compulsive symptoms is linked to substance intoxication or withdrawal. The symptoms must emerge within a month of substance intoxication or withdrawal and are not better accounted for by another anxiety disorder that is not substance induced.

Other anxiety disorders, particularly *specific phobias*, are frequently encountered by consultation-liaison psychiatrists. For example, patients who have claustrophobia often have difficulty completing a magnetic resonance imaging (MRI) scan. Other anxiety disorders that may be clinically important in some settings, particularly outpatient consultations, include agoraphobia without history of panic disorder, social phobia, obsessive-compulsive disorder, and anxiety disorder not otherwise specified.

EPIDEMIOLOGY: ISSUES OF COMORBIDITY AND CAUSALITY

Prevalence of Anxiety Disorders in the General and Medical-Surgical Populations

Data gleaned from the National Comorbidity Survey (NCS; Kessler et al. 1994) are instructive for consultation-liaison psychiatrists. The NCS was "the first survey to administer a structured psychiatric interview to a representative national sample in the United States" (Kessler et al. 1994, p. 8). It was designed to supersede the Epidemiologic Catchment Area (ECA) study of 1982 (Robins et al. 1984) as the main data source on the prevalence of psychiatric disorders and use of services for these disorders for the past decade. The NCS used a stratified, multistage area probability sample of persons aged 15–54 years and found that the prevalence of psychiatric disorders was greater than previously appreciated. Nearly one-half of the respondents reported at least one lifetime disorder, and almost 30% reported at least one 12-month disorder. "More than half of all lifetime disorders occurred in the 14% of the sample who had a history of three or more comorbid disorders" (Kessler et al. 1994, p. 98). Table 20–5 presents lifetime and 12-month prevalence rates of anxiety disorders by sex and in total reported in the NCS data set. Rates for simple and social phobias are among the highest ones for all psychiatric disorders. Women have higher prevalence rates of anxiety disorders than do men, and socioeconomic status is

TABLE 20–5. Lifetime and 12-month prevalence of UM-CIDI/DSM-III-R disorders[a]

| | Male | | | | Female | | | | Total | | | |
| | Lifetime | | 12 mo | | Lifetime | | 12 mo | | Lifetime | | 12 mo | |
Anxiety disorders	%	SE	%	SE	%	SE	%	SE	%	SE	%	SE
Panic disorder	2.0	0.3	1.3	0.3	5.0	1.4	3.2	0.4	3.5	0.3	2.3	0.3
Agoraphobia without panic disorder	3.5	0.4	1.7	0.3	7.0	0.6	3.8	0.4	5.3	0.4	2.8	0.3
Social phobia	11.1	0.8	6.6	0.4	15.5	1.0	9.1	0.7	13.3	0.7	7.9	0.4
Simple phobia	6.7	0.5	4.4	0.5	15.7	1.1	13.2	0.9	11.3	0.6	8.8	0.5
Generalized anxiety disorder	3.6	0.5	2.0	0.3	6.6	0.5	4.3	0.4	5.1	0.3	3.1	0.3
Any anxiety disorder	19.2	0.9	11.8	0.6	30.5	1.2	22.6	0.1	24.9	0.8	17.2	0.7

[a]UM-CIDI indicates University of Michigan Composite International Diagnostic Interview.
Source. Adapted from Kessler RC, McGonagle KA, Zhao S, et al: "Lifetime and 12-Month Prevalence of DSM-III-R Psychiatric Disorders in the United States: Results From the National Comorbidity Survey." *Archives of General Psychiatry* 51:8–19, 1994. Used with permission.

linked to the likelihood of anxiety disorder. The lifetime prevalence of any anxiety disorder in the respondents was 24.9%; 17.2% had an anxiety disorder in the preceding 12 months.

A range of studies in the ambulatory or outpatient setting have addressed the prevalence and nature of psychiatric conditions, including anxiety disorders, in primary care populations. These studies suggest that one-quarter to one-third of such patients have a formal psychiatric disorder that is often unrecognized by the primary care physician. Notable efforts in this regard include work by Hoeper et al. (1979), Bridges and Goldberg (1985), Schulberg et al. (1985), and Barrett et al. (1988). Helzer et al. (1987) reported that the prevalence rate of a history of PTSD was 1% in the total (general) population, about 3.5% in civilians who were exposed to physical attack and in Vietnam War veterans who were not wounded, and 20% in veterans who were wounded in the Vietnam War. Lecrubier and Ustun (1998) reported survey data from primary care settings in 14 countries; they noted an average prevalence rate of 24% for anxiety and/or depression, accompanied by significant disability.

Although the consultation setting has not had the benefit of epidemiologic efforts on the scale of the ECA or NCS, over the years various consultation-liaison investigators have attempted to gauge the extent of anxiety in the general hospital inpatient areas. For example, Schwab et al. (1966) determined that 20% of a consecutive series of admissions to a medical unit of a teaching hospital had some degree of anxiety. Perhaps the studies that have called the most attention to the issue of anxiety in the medical setting are those of Hackett et al. (1968) and Cassem and Hackett (1971), which explored psychiatric presentations in the coronary care unit (CCU) of Massachusetts General Hospital. In a 1971 report, Cassem and Hackett detailed a "hypothetical schedule of the onset of

emotional and behavioral reactions" in the CCU patient with a myocardial infarction (p. 12). They characterized a trajectory of anxiety peaking within 48 hours and then diminishing, giving way to depressive symptoms. Almost half of the psychiatric consultations in their series were prompted by anxiety, which centered on the threat of death and responses to the symptoms of cardiac failure and dysfunction. The Boston studies are landmarks not only in their descriptions of psychiatric symptoms in the CCU but also in terms of the investigators' therapeutic strategies.

Subsequently, several investigators have estimated or reported the prevalence of anxiety disorders or anxiety symptoms among medical-surgical inpatients and outpatients. More recent estimates have ranged between 10% and 70% as a function of patient sample (Ballenger 1991, 1998; Zaubler and Katon 1998). Sherbourne et al. (1996) found that 14%–66% of a sample of primary care patients had at least one concurrent anxiety disorder. Meredith et al. (1997) observed that general medical patients with comorbid anxiety disorders were more likely to receive treatment for anxiety compared with those presenting with anxiety without accompanying medical illness. Using ECA data, Wells and colleagues (1988) found that patients with a chronic medical condition had a significantly higher adjusted lifetime prevalence of anxiety disorders than those without such a medical condition (P<0.01). Eighteen percent of the group with a chronic medical condition (n=841) had a lifetime prevalence of an anxiety disorder compared with 12% of those without a chronic medical condition (n=1,711). They also observed that "more than eleven percent of the persons with chronic medical conditions had a recent anxiety disorder" (Wells et al. 1988, p. 979). Subsequently, Wells's group also studied the prevalence of eight chronic medical conditions in a sample of adults with anxiety disorder relative to the prevalence rates in adults without anxiety. In the second study, the authors noted that "the only psychiatric disorders uniquely associated with current active chronic medical conditions were anxiety disorders, suggesting that the association between anxiety disorders and chronic medical conditions develops *more quickly* than associations between medical conditions and other psychiatric disorders" (Wells et al. 1988, p. 980). Wells et al. (1989) suggested that persons with primary anxiety disorders merit careful evaluation for diseases such as diabetes and heart disease.

Patients with anxiety disorders have been reported to be more likely to develop upper respiratory infections, chronic obstructive lung disease, and migraines (Zaubler and Katon 1998). They also appear to have impaired immunological functioning, which normalizes with clinical improvement of the anxiety (LaVia et al. 1996).

The prevalence rates of anxiety or symptoms of anxiety per se in medically ill patients do not distinguish between those instances in which the medical illness physiologically caused the psychiatric symptoms and those in which the anxiety is a reactive response or in which the anxiety antedates the physical disorder. As Wells et al. (1989) noted with regard to chronic medical conditions and psychiatric illness, "This finding alone does not provide information concerning the *nature* of these relationships, i.e., *which is primary* or whether or not they occur *contemporaneously*" (p. 1445).

Schuckit (1983) reported that 10%–40% of medical patients with anxiety had medical or toxic etiologies for their psychiatric symptoms. Hall (1980) identified a hierarchy of medical conditions that induce anxiety. He stated that neurological and endocrine disorders accounted for most of the "medical causes" of anxiety; other contributors were chronic infections (12%), rheumatic-collagen-vascular disorders (12%), and circulatory disorders (12%).

Studies of the prevalence of adjustment disorder in the medical setting have been limited. In theory, such disturbances would encompass the psychological issues cited above; by definition, an adjustment disorder is a maladaptive response to an identifiable stressor. The stressors in question are the medical illness, the hospitalization, and its treatment. In a study of 1,072 consultations (Popkin et al. 1984), adjustment disorder was the fourth most frequent DSM-III (American Psychiatric Association 1980) diagnosis, exceeded by organic mental disorder, affective disorder, and personality disorder. In a collaborative three-site study (Derogatis et al. 1983), the prevalence of adjustment disorder in a random sample of newly hospitalized cancer patients was reported to be 32%. Earlier studies (reviewed by Popkin et al. 1990)

have shown that between 9% and 21% of medical-surgical patients referred for psychiatric consultation received a diagnosis of adjustment disorder. In DSM-III and DSM-III-R, adjustment disorder included eight subtypes, among them adjustment disorder with anxious features and adjustment disorder with mixed features. We reviewed a series of 121 medical-surgical inpatients given a diagnosis of adjustment disorder by psychiatric consultants and found that medical illness was the primary stressor in 69% (Popkin et al. 1990). These patients were largely free of preceding psychiatric problems and had protracted hospitalizations for advanced illnesses, particularly malignancy and diabetes. Two-thirds of these patients had prompt resolution of their psychiatric symptoms. Short courses of psychotropic drugs were frequently used in this population. We concluded that

> in the medically ill hospitalized patient, this disruption of autonomic and emotional regulation may relate to any number of factors, including the uncertainty surrounding the physical illness, its treatment and its course; issues of dependency, regression and infantilization associated with hospitalizations; and physiological concomitants of the illness and its treatment. "Maladaptive" responses may resolve with clarification, improvement of the medical status, closure of the hospitalization or a process of accommodation (with or without psychotropic medication). (Popkin et al. 1990, pp. 412–413)

Frequencies of Medical and Toxic Etiologies of Anxiety Disorders

As several writers have emphasized, the roster of medical disorders that can directly or indirectly produce anxiety is extensive (Table 20–6). In their recent review, Hall and Hall (1999) noted the range of endocrine disorders that have been associated with anxiety; they focused on anxiety disorders in patients with diabetes mellitus and in patients with thyroid hormone disturbances. Lustman et al. (1986) used the Diagnostic Interview Schedule (DIS; Robins et al. 1981) and reported lifetime prevalence rates of 26.5% for phobic disorders and 41% for generalized anxiety disorder in type 1 and 2 diabetic patients. Popkin et al. (1993) found a lifetime prevalence rate of 28% for generalized anxiety disorders in 140 candidates for pancreas transplantation. Peyrot and Rubin (1997) observed anxiety disorders in 49.2% of a sample of 634 diabetic outpatients; the probability of an anxiety disorder was linked to those with higher "risk profiles." Okada et al. (1995) found that suppressing anxiety with a psychotropic medication reduced patients' glycosylated hemoglobin levels.

TABLE 20–6.   Medical conditions presenting with anxiety

Adrenal dysfunction/Cushing's disease

Angina

Brucellosis

Carcinoid syndrome

Cerebral arteriosclerosis

Collagen-vascular disease

Coronary insufficiency

Diabetes mellitus

Drug effects: stimulants—caffeine, cocaine, amphetamines

Drug withdrawal: antianxiety agents, caffeine, alcohol, sedatives, opiates

Hyperparathyroidism, pseudohyperparathyroidism

Hypoglycemia, hyperinsulinemia

Pancreatic tumor

Pheochromocytoma

Psychomotor epilepsy, complex partial seizures

Pulmonary emboli

Thyroid disease: hyperthyroidism, hypothyroidism, thyroiditis

Source.   Adapted from Popkin 1993.

With regard to thyroid disturbances, Rogers et al. (1994) found that patients in a longitudinal anxiety disorders research program had increased rates of thyroid disease, angina, and peptic ulcer disease compared with patients without panic disorder and comorbid major depression. In this study, 9% of the women had thyroid disease, far exceeding the rate in the general population. Hall and Hall (1999) observed that anxiety disorders are present in 30%–40% of patients with hypothyroidism and 60%–75% of patients with hyperthyroidism. Anxiety disorders in hypothyroid states often may be related to the rapidity of change of thyroid hormone levels compared with the absolute level encountered; anxiety usually resolves within days to months following initiation of treatment to restore a euthyroid state. Patients with hyperthyroidism can be differentiated from those with primary anxiety states in several ways. In patients with thyroid dysfunction, sleeping pulse will remain accelerated, sedated pulse will exceed 80, palms will be warm and dry (not cold and clammy), and fatigue will be accompanied by a desire to be active (Popkin and Mackenzie 1980). Generalized anxiety disorder is three to four times more likely among hyperthyroid patients than in the general population (Kathol and Dalahunt 1986).

Another group of disorders likely to give physiologic rise to anxiety are neurological diseases; these include encephalitis, multiple sclerosis, Wilson's disease, Huntington's disease, poliomyelitis, myasthenia gravis, porphyria, cerebral syphilis, combined systems disease, and tumors of the central nervous system (CNS). Wise and Rundell (1999) noted that "anxiety disorders occur in patients with neurologic disorders far more frequently than individuals without neurologic conditions" (p. 98). Richard et al. (1996) reported that anxiety disorders, particularly generalized anxiety disorder, panic disorder, and social phobia, occur in up to 40% of the patients with Parkinson's disease. This study confirmed observations by M.B. Stein et al. (1990), who found that 38% of an unselected sample of patients with idiopathic Parkinson's disease had a DSM-III-R anxiety disorder diagnosis. Those with anxiety disorders were no more severely disabled than the others and were not differentiated by duration or intensity of L-dopa treatment. The authors noted, "It remains to be seen…whether the rate of anxiety disorders is genuinely higher in PD [Parkinson's disease] than in other chronic medical conditions" (p. 220). Swedo et al. (1989) suggested that basal ganglia dysfunction was instrumental in the genesis of obsessive-compulsive symptoms in patients with Sydenham's chorea. Autoantibodies may thus have a part in the evolution of anxiety disorders.

With respect to stroke and anxiety, Astrom (1996) reported the prevalence of generalized anxiety disorder to be 28% in acute poststroke patients. At 3 months, the rate was 31%; at 1 year, it was 24%; and at 3 years, it was 19%. Astrom concluded that generalized anxiety disorder is common, is long lasting, and tends to interfere with recovery from stroke. Merikangas and Stevens (1997) reported an association between anxiety disorder and migraine headaches. Marazziti et al. (1993) found that of the patients presenting with migraines, 27% met criteria for panic, 25% met criteria for generalized anxiety disorder, 10% met criteria for obsessive-compulsive disorder, and 5% met criteria for social phobia. Riether (1999) reviewed the increasing evidence linking specific lesion location on MRI to psychiatric presentations (including anxiety) in patients with multiple sclerosis.

The prevalence of anxiety disorders among cancer patients varies widely in the literature (Kerrihard et al. 1999). Most authors, however, estimate the current prevalence of any anxiety disorder in a cancer patient sample to be within a range of 15%–28%. Kerrihard et al. (1999) used the Hospital Anxiety/Depression Scale and noted that five studies identified between 9% and 19% of cancer patients as having anxiety disorders. Large collaborative oncology data sets suggest that 47% of the patients had a clinically apparent psychiatric disorder and two-thirds of these had "reactive anxiety." Whether anxiety disorders are more common in patients with cancer than in those with other medical illnesses is unclear (Kerrihard et al. 1999).

In patients with human immunodeficiency virus (HIV) and acquired immunodeficiency syndrome

(AIDS), the prevalence of anxiety disorders has been reported to range from 0% to 39% (Kerrihard et al. 1999). Atkinson et al. (1988) found that 36% of the patients with AIDS and AIDS-related complex qualified for an anxiety disorder diagnosis compared with only 17.6% of the asymptomatic seropositive subjects and 9% of the seronegative homosexual subjects. Other data regarding the relation of anxiety to stage of HIV infection have conflicted with these early findings; some authors reported significant anxiety among patients with HIV disease that appeared to be independent of disease stage (Perdices et al. 1992). Anxiety has been associated with treatment and specific interventional procedures (Kerrihard et al. 1999).

Recent literature also has noted the prominent comorbidity of respiratory disease and anxiety disorders (Smoller et al. 1999). Respiratory disease appears to be a risk factor for the development of panic disorder (Carr 1998). A recent study of 150 consecutive anxiety patients found that respiratory disease predated the development of an anxiety disorder in 43% of those with panic disorder as compared with only 16% of those with other anxiety disorders (Verburg et al. 1995).

The prevalence of panic disorder in patients with asthma is 3 to 10 times greater than that in the general population (Shavitt et al. 1992; Van Peski-Osterbaan et al. 1996; Yellowlees et al. 1988). Thirteen percent of the patients with asthma met criteria for agoraphobia (Shavitt et al. 1992). Children with asthma are twice as likely as are children without asthma to meet criteria for an anxiety disorder (Bussing et al. 1996). Of particular import, "anxiety disorders adversely affect the course of asthma" (Smoller et al. 1999 p. 85).

With respect to chronic obstructive pulmonary disease (COPD), the prevalence of anxiety has usually been observed to range between 10% and 40%, although some observers reported rates approaching 90%. Yellowlees et al. (1987) studied 50 COPD patients and found that one-third had an anxiety disorder and one-fourth met criteria for panic disorder. Anxiety symptoms also have been linked to decreased quality of life and more problematic dyspnea in COPD (Howell 1990; Prigatano et al. 1984). Sleep apnea has been associated with nocturnal panic attacks in middle-aged men (Edlund et al. 1991). Some 30% of the patients on mechanical ventilators report panic (or agony), triggered by intratracheal suctioning, asynchrony between spontaneous and mechanical ventilation, and the inability to communicate (Smoller et al. 1999).

Increasingly, the careful delineation of anxiety disorders in patients with Axis III conditions suggests that these presentations encompass more than merely reactive response to medical illness as stressor. Many involve intrinsic pathophysiologic processes that are part of the Axis III conditions. In addition, evidence is increasing that anxiety disorders may be independent risk factors in the progression of the Axis III illnesses.

It has long been recognized that anxiety symptoms and syndromes may be caused by medications and/or substances of abuse. These are often encountered in the consultation-liaison setting, although accurate frequency data are not available. The list of such causes includes aspirin intolerance, drug intoxication, caffeinism, and withdrawal from CNS depressant drugs. Many medications are capable of engendering anxiety (Table 20–7). Ray et al. (1989) underscored the hazards associated with medications directed to modulate anxiety. In a Canadian study, they reported that the risk of hip fracture was nearly doubled in elderly current long-term users of benzodiazepines.

Levenson et al. (1992) studied the relation between psychopathology and resource use in general medical inpatients and identified 22% of a sample of 1,020 inpatients as very anxious (based on the revised Symptom Checklist—90 [SCL-90-R]; Derogatis 1983). Seventy percent of the patients with anxiety had significant depression scores as well. Similarly, 60% of those with elevated depression scores had an anxiety score above the designated cutoff. They found that depression and anxiety frequently occurred together. Their data showed that patients with high levels of psychopathology had longer stays and higher costs during the index hospitalization. This finding, which was not a function of difference in severity of medical illness, applied to the anxious patients as a subcategory.

BIOLOGY OF ANXIETY

Neurotransmitters

The understanding of neurotransmitter systems, including their function and role in anxiety and other psychiatric disorders, has increased dramatically, prompted by the development of a variety of experimental methods and techniques for their study in animal models and human subjects (Coupland et al. 1992). Attention has focused particularly on noradrenergic, serotonergic, and γ-aminobutyric acid (GABA) systems, with more recent interest in a variety of peptides. Panic disorder stands out as the anxiety disorder most extensively studied. Unfortunately, very little attention has been directed toward the study of the neurobiology of anxiety disorders in medically ill patients.

TABLE 20–7.   Medications associated with anxiety

Anesthetics/analgesics
Antidepressants (tricyclics, SSRIs, bupropion)
Antihistamines
Antihypertensives
Antimicrobials
Bronchodilators
Caffeine preparations
Calcium-blocking agents
Cholinergic-blocking agents
Digitalis
Estrogen
Ethosuximide
Heavy metals and toxins
Hydralazine
Insulin
Levodopa
Muscle relaxants
Neuroleptics
Nonsteroidal anti-inflammatories
Procaine
Procarbazine
Sedatives
Steroids
Sympathomimetics
Theophylline
Thyroid preparations

Note.   SSRIs = selective serotonin reuptake inhibitors.

Interest in stress and its physiologic concomitants led to early attention to the role of administered catecholamines and their physiologic effect, although the results were at times contradictory (Kopin 1980). The role of noradrenergic systems has been the focus of many panic disorder studies (Gorman et al. 1987). Locus coeruleus stimulation in animals generates behavioral responses consistent with clinical anxiety (Redmond et al. 1976a, 1976b). Locus coeruleus ablation, conversely, decreases fearful responses (Redmond et al. 1976a, 1976b). Drugs that increase noradrenergic function in humans increase anxiety symptoms. Yohimbine, an α_2-receptor antagonist, increases anxiety in patients with panic disorder and results in plasma 3-methoxy-4-hydroxyphenylglycol (MHPG) elevations (Breier 1991; Charney et al. 1984). These studies all suggest an association between anxiety and noradrenergic systems. However, the interpretability of animal physiology studies and human pharmacological induction models of panic and anxiety has limitations (Gorman et al. 1987).

Pharmacological provocation of panic attacks has generated valuable information about phenomenology, physiology, pathophysiology, medication response, and

panic prevention. Sodium lactate has become the most widely studied and accepted agent for panic induction (Pitts and McClure 1967). Other induction methods include carbon dioxide (CO_2), caffeine, and cholinomimetic agents (Gorman et al. 1987). Papp et al. (1993) studied respiratory changes in panic disorder and proposed a unifying biochemical hypothesis. These authors underscored the presence of an unstable autonomic system, with a hypersensitive respiratory control system and hypersensitive CO_2 chemoreceptors.

Chlordiazepoxide's introduction as a treatment for anxiety in the 1960s ushered in the development of various benzodiazepine compounds, which have played a central role in managing anxiety disorders. The recognition of the role of GABA in the pharmacological effect of benzodiazepines, as well as the identification of receptors for benzodiazepines and GABA, led to a surge of information about the molecular effects of these compounds (Hommer et al. 1987; Zorumski and Isenberg 1991).

GABA is a major inhibitory CNS neurotransmitter that is used by up to 40% of neurons (Zorumski and Isenberg 1991). Benzodiazepine receptors are linked to GABA receptors, and their interactions result in alterations in neuronal inhibition (Figure 20–1). Activation of benzodiazepine receptors results in increased affinity of GABA to its receptors, resulting in augmentation of chloride flow into the neuron through open chloride channels. This process causes electrochemical hyperpolarization of the neuron and, ultimately, neuronal inhibition. Multiple subunits of the GABA receptor and subtypes of benzodiazepine receptors have been identified. The identification of compounds with different selectivity for the various receptor subtypes will lead to the understanding of the receptors' diverse roles and interactions (Salzman et al. 1993). In addition, studies in animals and humans, using functional imaging techniques, are beginning to demonstrate the presence of alterations in GABA receptor function in anxiety disorders (Tilhonen et al. 1997). The use of antagonists and inverse agonists sheds light on the clinical effect of alterations in this receptor system.

Antagonists that block the actions of benzodiazepines, such as flumazenil, a diazepam-binding inhibitor, and benzodiazepine inverse agonists, such as β-carboline derivatives, cause anxiety in animals and humans (Coupland et al. 1992; Zorumski and Isenberg 1991). It has been hypothesized that patients with panic disorder experience alterations in benzodiazepine receptor sensitivity, with their set point shifted toward an inverse agonist position (Coupland et al. 1992). Reduced sensitivity to the effects of diazepam on saccadic eye movements and norepinephrine appearance rate has been shown in

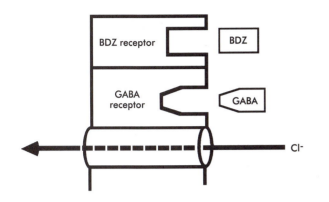

FIGURE 20–1. Schematic representation of benzodiazepine (BDZ)–γ-aminobutyric acid (GABA) complex.

patients with panic disorder but not in those with generalized anxiety disorder. Several compounds have been proposed as modulators or ligands of benzodiazepine receptors, with studies pursuing clarification of the effect of stress on their concentration (Marazziti et al. 1990). Hypotheses regarding the possible alterations in the GABA–benzodiazepine receptor complex were summarized by Salzman et al. (1993) and Malizia et al. (1995). These include abnormalities in benzodiazepine receptor activity, dysregulation of linkage between the subunits of the GABA-benzodiazepine complex, abnormal ligands, alteration in endogenous agonists, and changes in sensitivity to endogenous ligands.

The successful treatment of anxiety disorder with agents affecting serotonin function suggests that serotonin function plays an important role in anxiety disorders (Power and Cowen 1992). Hypersensitivity to serotonin, excess activity of the serotonin type 2 (5-HT$_2$) receptor, and functional serotonin deficiency all have been proposed. Serotonin is postulated to play a crucial role in regulating brain mechanisms that modulate responses to stressors in panic, generalized anxiety, and depression (Deakin 1998). Animal and human studies verify the effect of manipulation of serotonin function in these conditions. The effects of buspirone, an azaspirodecanedione compound, and related compounds support this hypothesis, in the light of their lack of direct effect on GABA systems. Behavioral, electrophysiological, and biochemical studies suggest that buspirone acts as an agonist at presynaptic 5-HT$_{1A}$ receptors (Tunnicliff 1991).

Ongoing interest in the neurophysiology of anxiety states has led to the study of other systems, such as cholecystokinin, corticotropin-releasing hormone (CRH), somatostatin, and neuropeptide Y. CNS application of cholecystokinin in animals leads to neuronal excitation. Peripheral administration can induce panic attacks in humans, with increased sensitivity shown in patients with panic disorder (Bradwejn et al. 1991). Gold et al. (1988) proposed a role for the CRH system in panic disorder by describing this system's role in the physiologic response to stress. Evidence supportive of CRH involvement includes the presence of a blunted adrenocorticotropic hormone (ACTH) response to CRH, as well as the suppression of CRH by alprazolam. These investigators proposed a "reverberatory positive feedback loop" between CRH and the locus coeruleus–norepinephrine system. These data, however, are contradicted by other findings, such as the absence of significant pituitary-adrenal activation during panic (Gold et al. 1988). However, animal data suggest that elevated corticosterone levels during development have effects on the expression of fear, whereas CRH and corticosterone have each been shown to play a significant role in determining behavioral responses to fearful stimuli (Rosen and Schulkin 1998). CRH effects may be modulated by the actions of neuropeptide Y (Helig et al. 1994). Abelson et al. (1990) suggested a modulating role for somatostatin; they demonstrated suppression of panic with a somatostatin analogue.

Anatomic Substrate

As noted in the previous section, pharmacological challenge studies, as well as electrical lesions and stimulation studies, have suggested a significant role for the locus coeruleus in modulating anxiety and panic disorder. Redmond (1987, p. 973) described the potential role of this nucleus as an "alarm system that filters and discriminates potentially noxious from irrelevant stimuli" and identifies various points at which aberrations in the locus coeruleus may produce pathological anxiety. The results of pharmacological interventions and electrical stimulation studies in humans are consistent with this concept (Charney and Deutch 1996). This nucleus has close interconnections with many other systems, which highlights the need to more completely understand the integrated role of multiple systems in brain function.

It has long been postulated that the limbic system plays a central role in emotional responses. Multiple interconnections between the amygdala, the hippocampus, and other limbic structures facilitate the processing of exteroceptive and interoceptive stimuli (Charney and Deutch 1996). Projections from the amygdala and hypothalamus modulate autonomic and endocrine responses involved in the regulation of anxiety (Reiman 1988). Amygdala stimulation in humans induces anxiety and fear (Chapman et al. 1954). Amygdala stimulation in animals also is associated with significant behavioral changes

(Kopchia et al. 1992). Interestingly, the amygdala contains a large number of benzodiazepine receptors. However, although lesions of the central nucleus of the amygdala in animals resulted in anxiolytic effects, the effects of chlordiazepoxide, phenobarbital, and carbamazepine on anxiety do not appear to depend on the integrity of this structure (Kopchia et al. 1992).

The study of human brain function with imaging techniques such as positron-emission tomography (PET) provides the opportunity for correlational studies of structure and function. CNS imaging technology will likely greatly enhance the understanding of anxiety disorders (Reiman 1997; Reiman et al. 1989). Functional imaging studies have detected abnormalities in metabolic rates in areas such as the hippocampus, parahippocampal area, and inferior prefrontal cortex in patients with panic disorder (Bisaga et al. 1998; Nordahl et al. 1998). These studies also found relations between cerebral benzodiazepine receptor binding and generalized anxiety and panic disorder (Tilhonen et al. 1997).

The frontal lobes also have been implicated in the genesis and modulation of anxiety. An apparent reduction in cerebral metabolic rate of glucose in the orbitomedial region occurs in patients who undergo capsulotomy for severe anxiety disorders (Mindus et al. 1986), which suggests that the frontal lobe system has a role in the modulation of anxiety. It is hoped that studies of volunteers without anxiety, as well as ongoing studies in pathological states, will help to elucidate the anatomic/functional substrate for anxiety (Mindus et al. 1986). Ultimately, an integrated model of anxiety and anxiety disorders (Charney and Deutch 1996; Rosen and Schulkin 1998; Stein and Bouwer 1997) may allow for a better understanding of the complexities of anxiety states in the medically ill: the role of genetic, developmental, and premorbid factors; the physiologic and emotional effect of chronic stressors; the effect of medications; and anatomic and physiologic changes secondary to medical illness.

CLINICAL CONSIDERATIONS

Anxiety Disorder Due to a General Medical Condition

"Focus on anxiety secondary to medical illness as a specific nosologic category is far more recent than its counterpart, secondary depression" (Cassem 1990, p. 607). The consultation-liaison psychiatrist who encounters significant anxiety in the medical patient must entertain the possibility that the anxiety is mediated by the medical illness. However, the requisite steps to address such a pros-

pect are not delineated in DSM-IV-TR. DSM-IV renamed what had formerly been called organic anxiety disorder. Whether a diagnosis of "anxiety due to a general medical condition" is made more readily or with more validity remains to be shown. For the most part, the clinician is left to gauge or determine whether clinical anxiety is "an integral part" of the medical illness's pathophysiology. If it is possible to redress the medical condition and note the cessation of the anxious symptomatology, then the psychiatric diagnosis is secure (if post hoc). For example, restoring the patient to a euthyroid or eucalcemic state will occasionally stop the anxiety; in this case, the diagnosis seems secure in retrospect. Should another variation in thyroid or calcium level again evoke anxiety, it would be difficult to argue that the relation was not causal. However, in many instances, such clarity is not forthcoming. Yet the clinician is remiss if he or she conceptualizes anxiety in the medical-surgical setting in terms of psychological response or psychogenic issues without first touching the "organic" base.

DSM-IV-TR permits identification of specific anxiety constellations (generalized anxiety disorder, phobias, panic disorder, or obsessive-compulsive disorder) under the "general medical" rubric. DSM-III-R confined itself to "anxiety" as the prominent or predominant feature of an organic presentation without further specifying the nature of the symptoms. Hall (1980) suggested that secondary anxiety can be differentiated from primary anxiety by 1) onset before age 18 or after age 35 years in patients with no personal or familial psychiatric histories, 2) characteristic fluctuations in severity and duration, 3) duration of less than 2 years, 4) absence of other psychiatric symptoms (e.g., phobias, conversion disorder), and 5) absence of a recent major psychosocial stressor. Starkman et al. (1990) found that anxiety was a qualitatively different experience for a patient with pheochromocytoma and that these symptoms did not correlate with peripheral norepinephrine or epinephrine levels. Studies of DSM-III-R organic anxiety disorder are almost exclusively case reports (Popkin and Tucker 1992). Although investigators and pharmaceutical companies have shown growing interest in anxiety associated with irritable bowel syndrome, COPD, cardiac disease, and asthma, the approach has not been directed to anxiety physiologically induced by a medical disease.

A clinical note of caution is in order. Many clinicians are inclined to rely heavily on a temporal relation to establish an organic-etiological relation. Although temporal relation is an instructive parameter, it may be misleading and subject to errors of recall. It is also apparent that psychiatric symptomatology may antedate the clinical recognition of the physical illness—that is, anxiety and depression may be the first presenting features of a medical illness. Likewise, it is by no means clear that correction or treatment of the medical illness will result in the elimination of the psychiatric symptoms. The symptoms may develop a life of their own.

The advent of DSM-IV has not to date prompted the hoped-for further study of anxiety disorders due to general medical conditions. Data are particularly needed regarding course of the conditions and the distribution of patients by subtypes (e.g., generalized anxiety disorder, panic disorder).

Panic Disorder

Panic has probably received the most attention of the anxiety disorders emerging in association with medical illness (Venkatesh et al. 1981; Wooley 1983, 1987). The most convincing report involved a group of patients ($n = 35$) with idiopathic cardiomyopathies awaiting cardiac transplantation (Kahn et al. 1987). Eighty-three percent of the group met criteria for at least probable panic disorder. In several other medical conditions, panic disorder was diagnosed at rates of 10%–25% (Cassem 1990). These rates far exceed those found in the general population. Rates of panic disorder have been estimated to be between 33% and 43% among patients with chest pain whose cardiac catheterizations indicated normal coronary arteries (Bass and Wade 1984; Beitman et al. 1987; Carter et al. 1992; Cormier et al. 1988; Katon 1984; Mukerji et al. 1987; Roll and Theorell 1987). In turn, this raises an interesting question about etiology of the panic. Is there something in the autonomic or CNS substrate of diverse conditions such as Parkinson's disease, epilepsy, COPD, and cirrhosis that has a common thread? PET may shed light on this issue in the future. In terms of phenomenology, few current data indicate whether panic emerging in the medical patient differs from that seen in the primary psychiatric setting. In addition, no data are available about factors such as course and onset in the medical setting. Note that sleep deprivation may worsen anxiety in patients with panic disorder (Uhde and Nemiah 1989). Therefore, admission to the general hospital may pose a special challenge to patients with established primary panic disorder.

Generalized Anxiety Disorder

Generalized anxiety disorder has traditionally been underdiagnosed by consultation-liaison psychiatrists. The diagnostic criteria for the disorder were modestly revised in DSM-IV, which has increased use of the category. Brawman-Mintzer and Lydiard (1997) suggested that patients at risk for generalized anxiety disorder may have deficits in the hypothalamic-pituitary-adrenal axis and its regulatory mechanisms in response to stress.

Generalized anxiety disorder that is encountered in consultation-liaison psychiatry is an established condition that is often intensified or unmasked in the general hospital setting. A full range of somatic and psychosensory complaints are common accompaniments. Motor tension is typical of generalized anxiety disorder and may include trembling and twitching. In addition, autonomic hyperactivity, vigilance, and scanning are part of the overall clinical picture. Age at onset usually is during the 20s or 30s. Few studies about either the natural history or the course of this condition have been done; however, there is some indication that symptomatology abates or is reduced with aging, particularly if the individual has achieved personal success (Uhde and Nemiah 1989). Studies of generalized anxiety disorder in the consultation setting are lacking and needed. Trzepacz et al. (1988) reported a very high prevalence of generalized anxiety disorder in a series of patients with untreated Graves' disease. We reported a lifetime prevalence of 32% and a 6-month prevalence of 17% for generalized anxiety disorder in a series of patients with type I diabetes mellitus seen as candidates for pancreas transplantation (Popkin et al. 1988).

Posttraumatic Stress Disorder and Acute Stress Disorder

Consultation-liaison psychiatrists occasionally encounter acute stress disorder, PTSD, or their variants. Clinicians usually have little difficulty in recognizing the constellation that is still best grasped in terms of Horowitz's model of information overload and its processing. In his seminal work on stress response, Horowitz (1976) conceptualized stress as a situation in which the individual is suddenly confronted (or assaulted) with information that is affectively overwhelming or extremely powerful. In the hospital setting, this might encompass, for example, being told that one requires radical surgery (e.g., an amputation), that one has a terminal illness or a malignancy, or that a new round of chemotherapy is needed. In short, any number of instances that threaten one's physical integrity and sense of stability would produce stress.

Like other powerful insults, such information is likely to initially elicit a period of disbelief and/or outcry. This is generally followed by "numbing" and brief immobilization. For example, after the loss of a loved one, for moments or even hours after the news is initially conveyed, as well as the ensuing day or days, activities seem remote and mechanical, and emotionality is constricted. Horowitz (1976) described how, after this initial period, the individual experiences a protracted period of oscillation. In this phase of stress response, the affectively charged information alternately is repressed from consciousness and then (in pendular fashion) swings back intrusively, unsolicited, into consciousness. This intrusive process may involve flashbacks or vivid imagery.

Horowitz recommended that the clinician or therapist facilitate information processing in a safe, structured fashion. He or she must preclude the "pendulum" from becoming fixed at either repression or persistent awareness. In the former, denial holds court, and no information processing or grief work can be done; in the latter, the painful affects are too pervasive and threaten to force decompensation. Horowitz urged that treatment or therapy consist of tolerable doses of awareness in which the overwhelming affect is slowly processed or gradually incorporated. Ultimately, cognitive restructuring occurs; the new information is integrated. Its accompanying affect is addressed. In the model, the pendulum of processing then comes to rest—dead center. Although DSM-IV-TR criteria are more detailed, the essence of both PTSD and the newer category, acute stress disorder, revolves around these constructs. The psychiatric consultant will see variants of both disorders on medical-surgical units. Some will involve war experiences; some will involve sexual abuse or assault; more will involve the challenges posed by the patient's medical illness, trauma, hospitalizations, and treatment.

Phobias

Phobias are characterized by persistent avoidance behavior "secondary to irrational fears of a specific object, activity, or situation" (Uhde and Nemiah 1989, p. 973). Intellectually, the individual usually recognizes that such fears are unreasonable, but he or she cannot dispel or surmount them. DSM-IV-TR identifies three groupings for phobias: 1) agoraphobia without history of panic disorder, 2) specific phobia (with five categories or types), and 3) social phobia.

Agoraphobia is the fear of being in places or situations from which escape might be difficult (or embarrassing) or in which help might not be available should incapacitating symptoms arise. DSM-IV-TR criteria for agoraphobia without history of panic disorder have been expanded; of particular interest to consultation-liaison psychiatry is the addition of a criterion that states, "If an associated general medical condition is present, the fear described in Criterion A is clearly in excess of that usually associated with the condition" (p. 443). An exclusion

criterion also has been added; it states that "the disturbance is not due to the direct physiological effects of a substance (e.g., a drug of abuse, a medication) or a general medical condition" (p. 443).

In the consultation-liaison setting, specific phobias are undoubtedly common, but they rarely seem to prompt or necessitate psychiatric consultations. Specific and social phobias tend to be shrouded by the patient and are unlikely to be identified by the primary physician unless the degree of impairment is pronounced or interferes with clinical care—for example, when a claustrophobic patient cannot tolerate an MRI procedure or when phobias involve blood, injection, or injury. These fears are especially likely to be revealed during a medical-surgical hospitalization and also may trigger concern regarding a diagnosis of factitious disorder with predominantly physical signs and symptoms. In the rigors of hospitalization, phobic disorders often take a back seat; these conditions are frequently ignored. Primary physician and psychiatric consultant alike may neglect to ask the crucial questions to establish the presence of these problems.

Obsessive-Compulsive Disorder

Obsessive-compulsive disorder centers on recurrent obsessions or compulsions that cause marked distress, are time-consuming, or significantly interfere with functioning or relationships. Obsessions are "recurrent and persistent thoughts, impulses, or images that are experienced…as intrusive and inappropriate and that cause marked anxiety or distress. The thoughts, impulses, or images are not simply excessive worries about real-life problems" (American Psychiatric Association 2000, p. 462). The individual seeks to ignore or to suppress thoughts or impulses but recognizes that they are a product of his or her own mind. Compulsions are "repetitive behaviors (e.g., hand washing, ordering, checking) or mental acts (e.g., praying, counting, repeating words silently) that the person feels driven to perform in response to an obsession, or according to rules that must be applied rigidly. The behaviors or mental acts are aimed at preventing or reducing distress or preventing some dreaded event or situation" (American Psychiatric Association 2000, p. 462).

In short, these behaviors are ego-dystonic phenomena; the individual recognizes obsessions as foreign to his or her personality and compulsions as unreasonable. DSM-IV-TR allows the clinician to specify a "poor insight" type, which signals the individual's failure to recognize his or her obsessions and compulsions as unreasonable or excessive. In addition, DSM-IV-TR (p. 463) requires that "if another Axis I disorder is present, the content of the obsessions or compulsions is not restricted to it." It also adds the standard exclusion criterion—not due to the direct effects of a substance or a general medical condition. This last step is an acknowledgment that a range of biological and physiologic factors can evoke these symptoms that have long been viewed from a predominantly psychodynamic perspective.

Before concluding the clinical considerations section, it is important to underscore the need for further careful studies of anxiety disorders in the general hospital setting. Some data suggest that these presentations may not be identical in phenomenology or pathophysiology to disturbances of anxiety seen in primary psychiatric populations. It behooves us to keep open the possibility that these anxiety disorders may (with their comorbidity) merit separate and distinct categorization in the future—even beyond anxiety disorder due to a general medical condition.

ASSESSMENT AND DIFFERENTIAL DIAGNOSIS

Assessing anxiety in medically ill patients requires a comprehensive evaluation with particular focus on medical, psychological, and environmental contributors to the patient's presentation. The hospital environment itself fosters various degrees of anxiety (Table 20–8). At first glance, anxiety symptoms may appear to be "understandable" in this context. This should not, however, lead the clinician to neglect the exploration of other possible contributors or to minimize the importance of interventions for the patient with anxiety. Even "understandable" anxiety is distressing and can complicate the course and management of medical conditions.

DSM-IV-TR provides guidelines for diagnoses in the differential diagnosis of anxiety. However, the acute onset of anxiety may preclude diagnoses that have duration criteria, such as panic disorder, major depression, and generalized anxiety disorder. In addition, the etiological roles of toxic and medical contributors are not always clear, as required in the diagnosis of anxiety disorder due to a general medical condition. From the clinical standpoint, assessing the effect of anxiety on the patient's condition and clinical course becomes a crucial factor in defining potential interventions. Anxiety is often the presenting symptom of a mood disorder, an impending or fully developed delirium, or a substance-induced mental disorder. In addition, anxiety symptoms in the medical setting may represent the recurrence or exacerbation of a preexisting psychiatric condition.

TABLE 20–8. Hospital environment factors associated with anxiety

Financial burden
Intrusive medical procedures
Isolation
Loss of autonomy
Loss of privacy
Physical discomfort, pain
Possibility of death
Uncertainty regarding cause, prognosis

The patient's psychiatric history provides information and clues about biological vulnerability and whether the current symptoms are the result of a preexisting condition. Family history may likewise help the clinician to broaden or further define the diagnostic possibilities. Significant anxiety in a patient with no personal or family psychiatric history should heighten suspicion that toxic or medical factors might be contributing to the presenting symptoms. Similarly, a positive psychiatric history should not blind the examiner to other possible medical etiologies and contributing factors.

As discussed earlier in this chapter, a variety of medical disorders, toxic substances, and medications may cause or exacerbate anxiety (Tables 20–6 and 20–7). In addition to acute toxicity from drugs such as cocaine and amphetamines, over-the-counter preparations for the treatment of cold symptoms, weight suppression, or sleep induction may generate significant anxiety or agitation (Abramowicz 1984; Aronson and Craig 1986; R.J. Goldberg 1987). Patients withdrawing from alcohol, opiates, benzodiazepines, and barbiturates usually present with marked anxiety, delirium, or seizures. Patients frequently underreport their actual use of any of these agents or may be unable to provide this information because their medical condition is too severe. Benzodiazepines may be discontinued inadvertently or may be regarded by attending physicians as not essential, which leads to the emergence of withdrawal syndromes. Clinicians must thoroughly review the patient's medications and substance use history to be able to assess acute anxiety in the medical setting. Families or friends can be of great assistance in this regard. They should be asked to bring in all of the patient's medications, prescribed or otherwise.

The presence of a toxic or metabolic cause for a patient's anxiety provides the opportunity for specific therapeutic interventions. An essential aspect of treatment is to explore the patient's beliefs, fears, and overall psychological response. The experience of cognitive dysfunction in delirium, for example, presents an overwhelming psychological threat to some patients, which may be ameliorated by anticipating its likelihood, symptoms, and course (Popkin 1993). Clinicians should provide ongoing reassurance, information, and assistance in coping. Patients may experience significant anxiety after the delirium resolves, as they attempt to integrate their recollections, discomfort, or anxiety due to the sense of lost time and as they try to integrate and understand experiences that have been particularly threatening or confusing (Mackenzie and Popkin 1980).

A variety of potential stressors in the medical setting play a significant role in patients' sense of fear and anxiety. A number of central themes may appear (Derogatis and Wise 1989a; R.J. Goldberg 1987), including a sense of alienation and separation anxiety, loss of physical control, physical damage or loss of vitality, threats to narcissistic integrity, and the threat of death. Often, patients' lack of understanding of their situation, or their personal interpretation of their conditions, will generate undue fear and apprehension. Understanding the patients' fears and expectations may pave the way for direct interventions and help clinicians to understand patients' anxiety or hostility toward care providers.

As part of the assessment of a patient's anxiety, the psychiatric consultant must attempt to understand the patient's typical repertoire of coping strategies. This will guide the psychiatrist's interventions to help the patient use previously helpful and adaptive strategies or to encourage the development of new strategies.

Corroborative history is essential in the consultation setting because access to an acutely ill patient is limited by time constraints, reduced endurance, pain, or sedation. In addition, patients may attempt to present themselves in the most favorable light, minimizing or denying relevant psychiatric history. Contacting a spouse, close relative, or friend will almost always provide important information and will establish a personal contact who may be important as the patient's course progresses. Access to these sources, however, may be constrained by the need for confidentiality.

Diagnostic tests in the assessment of patients with anxiety include laboratory examination, electrocardiogram (ECG), brain imaging studies (computed tomography, MRI), analysis of cerebrospinal fluid, psychiatric rating scales, and sometimes electroencephalogram (EEG). Laboratory examination should be based on suspected metabolic and electrolyte disturbances, including sodium, calcium, magnesium, phosphorus, thyroid function tests, liver function tests, albumin, creatinine, and blood urea nitrogen (BUN). Monitoring of the ECG and cardiac status is essential in patients presenting with chest pain, shortness of breath, and anxiety, especially in patients at high risk for cardiac illness. Brain imaging studies will help to exclude CNS structural lesions and to establish the presence of hydrocephalus, atrophy, or demyelination. Examination of cerebrospinal fluid is essential in suspected CNS infection, subarachnoid hemorrhage, or the diagnosis of demyelinating or inflammatory processes. The EEG may be helpful when seizure activity is suspected or to establish generalized cerebral dysfunction in delirium.

Several instruments have been developed to assist in the evaluation and monitoring of anxiety symptoms (Derogatis and Wise 1989b; Kellner and Uhlenhuth 1991). These instruments include self-rating and clinician rating scales (Table 20–9).

Among self-rating instruments, those commonly used include the State-Trait Anxiety Inventory (STAI; Spielberger et al. 1970), the SCL-90-R (Derogatis 1983), the Beck Anxiety Inventory (Beck et al. 1988), and the General Health Questionnaire (GHQ; D.P. Goldberg and Hillier 1979). Clinician-based rating scales include the Hamilton Anxiety Scale (HAS; Hamilton 1959) and the Anxiety Status Inventory (ASI; Zung 1971). These instruments help to quantify and monitor the course of anxiety but vary in their length and degree of emphasis on somatic or psychological symptoms. Although many of these scales are used in medical and surgical settings, there is no gold standard. This leads to difficulties in comparing studies in this area. Direct observation by the examiner and nursing staff and reports from family, friends, or significant others usually are more helpful in the overall assessment and monitoring of clinical course than are rating scale scores alone.

TREATMENT AND MANAGEMENT

Recognition of medical or toxic causes of anxiety should lead to attempts to correct the underlying etiology or to remove any offending agents. For example, managing anxiety secondary to hyperthyroidism must target the underlying pathophysiology, with palliative treatment until the primary process resolves. Adequate management of the anxiety that commonly accompanies acute angina and myocardial infarction may result in reduced morbidity. Even after resolution of the acute medical process, patients may continue to experience anticipatory anxiety or become hypervigilant about changes in somatic function and may require ongoing treatment and monitoring.

Pharmacological interventions include the possible use of a variety of agents. The clinical uses of and indications for some of these agents are summarized below. (For a

TABLE 20–9. Commonly used anxiety rating scales

Self-rating
State-Trait Anxiety Inventory (STAI)
Symptom Checklist–90—Revised (SCL-90-R)
Beck's Anxiety Inventory (BAI)
Self-Rating Anxiety Scale (SRAS)
General Health Questionnaire (GHQ)

Clinician rating
Hamilton Anxiety Scale (HAS)
Anxiety Status Inventory (ASI)

TABLE 20–10. Benzodiazepine characteristics

Drug	Dose equivalent (mg)	Active metabolites	Half-life (hours)
Triazolam	0.25	–	1.5–5
Midazolam		+	2–5
Oxazepam	15.0	–	5–15
Temazepam	15.0	–	9–12
Alprazolam	0.5	+	12–15
Halazepam	20.0	+	12–15
Lorazepam	1.0	–	10–20
Estazolam	0.33	+	10–24
Chlordiazepoxide	10.0	+	5–30
Clonazepam	0.5	–	18–50
Diazepam	5.0	+	20–70
Clorazepate[a]	7.5	+	30–100
Prazepam[a]	10.0	+	30–100
Flurazepam[a]	15.0	+	30–120

[a]Metabolites are active agents.
Source. Adapted from Wise MG, Taylor SE: "Anxiety and Mood Disorders in Medically Ill Patients." *Journal of Clinical Psychiatry* 51 (suppl 1):27–32, 1990. Copyright 1990, Physicians Postgraduate Press. Used with permission.

more detailed review of psychopharmacology in the consultation-liaison setting, please see Chapter 42 in this volume.)

Benzodiazepines, Hypnotics, and Barbiturates

Among the agents most commonly used to treat acute anxiety in the medical setting are the benzodiazepines (Sheehan et al. 1993) (Table 20–10). Their rapid onset of action, ease of administration, and effectiveness make these agents practical and useful in the medical setting. They can alleviate anxiety associated with procedures, assist with sleep, and provide relief in the short-term management of acute stressors. High-potency agents such as alprazolam, clonazepam, and lorazepam also are effective in the management of panic disorder symptoms (Gorman 1997).

Agents with longer half-lives can be administered less frequently and may be easier to taper after prolonged use. These agents take longer to reach steady state and are metabolized to active products. They are more likely to accumulate in patients with impaired hepatic function and in patients taking multiple other medications that undergo hepatic metabolism. Agents with shorter elimination half-lives reach steady state much more rapidly and can be eliminated in a shorter time; thus, they are reasonable options for the short-term management of anxiety (R.J. Goldberg 1987; Rickels and Schweizer 1987; Salzman et al. 1993). Lorazepam and oxazepam have no active metabolites, whereas alprazolam has active metabolites of little apparent clinical significance (Rickels and Schweizer 1987). These compounds are therefore best suited for patients who have liver impairment, who are taking multiple medications, or in whom careful titration of sedative effects is required.

Midazolam has a very rapid onset and a short duration of sedative action, with profound amnestic potential (Khanderia and Pandit 1987). Therefore, it is used for anesthesia and for acute sedation during procedures such as endoscopy. It is only available in parenteral form. Because of the potential for acute reversal of sedation when the drug is discontinued, midazolam is sometimes used for the management of acute agitation in the intensive care unit. However, this use can often lead to prolonged administration, tolerance, dose escalation, withdrawal syndromes, and worsening of confusion (Finley and Nolan 1989). Midazolam is also very expensive when administered around the clock.

Among these agents, only midazolam and lorazepam are reliably absorbed when administered intramuscularly (R.J. Goldberg 1987; Greenblat et al. 1982). Temazepam, triazolam, quazepam, and flurazepam are sedative-hypnotic benzodiazepines. Use of these agents over a prolonged period can lead to disturbed sleep patterns and rebound insomnia when discontinued. Hypnotic agents with a shorter duration of action and without active metabolites would be less likely to cause daytime sedation but may be more likely to cause memory problems. The appropriate use of hypnotics, particularly regarding the potential for CNS impairment, is the subject of considerable controversy and systematic review (Dement 1992; Jonas et al. 1992; Rothschild 1992).

Benzodiazepine use can cause oversedation and other direct effects on CNS function, such as confusion, ataxia, decreased coordination, decreased swallowing, and diminished respiratory drive, which are all significant problems for medically ill patients (R.J. Goldberg 1987).

Physiologically, benzodiazepines reduce the ventilatory response to hypoxia (Lakshminarawan et al. 1976). Patients with moderate to severe lung disease are at risk for CO_2 retention with longer-acting benzodiazepines, even at relatively low doses (Thompson and Thompson 1987). Intermediate-acting benzodiazepines without active metabolites (oxazepam and lorazepam) may be less likely than other benzodiazepines to cause hypoxia (Denaut et al. 1975). The potential for inducing cognitive changes, including amnesia, is particularly problematic when agents with a shorter duration of action are used intravenously (Healy et al. 1983; Wolkowitz et al. 1987). Monitoring patients for potential side effects, particularly CNS impairment, especially in debilitated and elderly patients, is essential (Maletta et al. 1991). Abrupt discontinuation of benzodiazepines, especially when used for prolonged periods, may result in rebound anxiety and withdrawal syndromes, including irritability, increased anxiety, confusion, and seizures (Petursson and Lader 1981).

Caution is mandatory when administering benzodiazepines to patients with respiratory impairment because of the potential for decreased ventilatory drive. This risk is of particular concern in patients with significant CO_2 retention, although low doses may be helpful in other patients with lung disease (Mitchells-Heggs et al. 1980). Anxiety may cause difficulties in weaning patients from ventilatory support, but oversedation will hinder weaning and should be avoided.

Although barbiturates have long been used for their antianxiety effects, they do not offer an advantage in treating anxiety disorders. Their potential for cognitive impairment, abuse, respiratory depression, and severe withdrawal make barbiturates undesirable in the treatment of anxiety.

Antidepressants

Serotonin reuptake inhibitors and the newer antidepressants have emerged as primary interventions for the treatment of various anxiety disorders, including panic disorder (Gorman 1997), generalized anxiety disorder (Lydiard 1998), obsessive-compulsive disorder (Leonard 1997), and social phobia (Davidson 1998). In the medically ill, use of low starting doses with subsequent titration to therapeutic doses seems prudent to minimize potential side effects such as nausea, diarrhea, headaches, jitteriness, or initial worsening of anxiety symptoms (Rickels and Schweizer 1987, 1990). The potential for drug-drug interactions needs to be highlighted in this population (Greenblat et al. 1998). The choice of an antidepressant agent should therefore reflect an assessment of other medications taken by the patient, as well as the medication's side-effect profile.

Unfortunately, data regarding the use of these agents in specific medical conditions are still somewhat limited, although their clinical use is widespread and some systematic data are emerging. For example, selective serotonin reuptake inhibitors appear to be relatively safe in patients with cardiac illness, based on small series of patients treated with fluoxetine, paroxetine, and sertraline (Glassman 1998), although the outcome of larger trials of sertraline following myocardial infarction is still pending. Recent data suggest decreased dyspnea in patients with COPD treated with a selective serotonin reuptake inhibitor (Smoller et al., in press). Clinical judgment, however, continues to guide the use of these agents in the medically ill population, based on the efficacy of these agents in general psychiatric populations.

The use of tricyclic or heterocyclic antidepressants in the medically ill requires particular attention to potential problems such as delirium, anticholinergic side effects (Popkin et al. 1985), conduction delays, cardiac arrhythmias, and orthostatic hypotension (Glassman 1998). Although concerns about decreased efficacy and heightened potential for side effects persist, these agents can be helpful adjuncts in the management of chronic pain (Egbunike and Chaffee 1990) or as alternatives when selective serotonin reuptake inhibitors are not tolerated.

Although the risk of seizures from bupropion appears lower than initially feared (Johnston et al. 1991), caution is still warranted in patients with bulimia, head injuries, or other seizure risks.

Antipsychotic Medications

The routine use of antipsychotic medications for the treatment of anxiety is not advocated in the light of the propensity of typical antipsychotics to produce extrapyramidal symptoms, tardive dyskinesia, and neuroleptic malignant syndrome (Silver and Simpson 1988). These agents, however, can be used judiciously in specific situations.

Antipsychotics are the pharmacological treatment of choice for agitation and anxiety in delirium; higher-potency agents such as haloperidol minimize the potential for anticholinergic side effects and hypotension. The combination of haloperidol with benzodiazepines such as lorazepam provides additional sedation, decreases agitation, and lowers the likelihood of extrapyramidal symptoms (Menza et al. 1988; Silver and Simpson 1988).

In addition, antipsychotics are particularly useful in treating anxiety and other psychiatric disorders resulting from high-dose steroid therapy (Hall et al. 1979). Clinical experience indicates that patients with HIV infection may be more susceptible to side effects from typical antipsychotics; therefore, low doses should be used initially (Edelstein and Knight 1987).

Newer antipsychotics such as risperidone, olanzapine, and quetiapine may provide an alternative in the medically ill because these drugs have a lower incidence of extrapyramidal side effects and greater sedative properties (Verma et al. 1998; Zarate et al. 1997). However, when administering these agents, hypotension, oversedation, and anticholinergic side effects need to be considered as potential complications. To date, the absence of parenteral forms of these agents limits their use in patients unable to take medications orally. Clinical use of the newer antipsychotics for the management of anxiety in patients with severe symptoms, or when benzodiazepines are contraindicated, appears to be increasing. However, controlled trials establishing their safety and effectiveness in this population are currently lacking.

β-Blockers

Because of their direct blockade of catecholaminergic effects, β-blockers are sometimes used to mitigate the peripheral manifestations of anxiety. They are particularly helpful in the treatment of conditions accompanied by increased adrenergic stimulation, such as hyperthyroidism. The effect of these agents in anxiety disorders, particularly panic disorder, however, is disappointing at best (Rickels and Schweizer 1987). Further research into the potential use of β-blockers in the medical setting is necessary.

Nonbenzodiazepine Anxiolytics

The potential use of nonbenzodiazepine anxiolytics, such as buspirone, presents some theoretical advantages in the management of anxiety in the medical patient. Buspirone is quite attractive because of its apparent lack of abuse potential, sedative effects, and psychomotor dysfunction (Wheatley 1988). Buspirone's usefulness, however, is limited by the delay in onset of therapeutic response; demonstrable effects require 2 or more weeks. The most common side effects of buspirone include gastrointestinal distress, headaches, dizziness, and nervousness (Newton et al. 1986). Some studies have suggested that ventilatory drive might increase with buspirone administration (Garner and Eldridge 1989). Therefore, this agent may be useful in anxious patients with lung disease or who require ventilatory support (Craven and Sutherland 1991; Mendelson et al. 1991). Unfortunately, buspirone is not particularly helpful in the treatment of panic disor-

der, although it can reduce anxiety and agitation in patients with dementia (Sakauye et al. 1993).

Psychotherapy

Along with elucidating the nature, severity, and possible etiology of the patient's anxiety, the psychiatric consultant must assess the potential role of psychotherapeutic interventions in the patient's care and management (see also Chapter 45 in this volume). Supportive psychotherapy can help patients cope with the emergence of acute stressors during the hospitalization. Faced with fear and physical discomfort, the anxious patient may benefit from attempts to bolster his or her coping strategies. The effects of this complex environment require the consultation psychiatrist to assume a flexible approach, adjusting goals and interventions to the patient's changing needs. The consultation psychiatrist's tasks may include ensuring ongoing communication between the patient and care providers; providing or facilitating ongoing education about the patient's condition or treatment; and clarifying the patient's perceptions, fears, and needs. Although loosely defined, and often undervalued, supportive psychotherapy plays a central role in the management of anxiety in the hospitalized patient and has been described as essential to the clinical practice of consultation-liaison psychiatry (Popkin 1993).

Brief psychodynamic psychotherapy can help a patient develop insight into the personal meaning or importance of specific events or situations. Psychodynamic psychotherapy can be accomplished, or at least begun, with attentive patients during hospitalization. Patients who can ambulate can be brought to the consultation-liaison psychiatrist's office for their psychotherapy appointment. Psychotherapy begun in the hospital can be continued in the outpatient consultation-liaison clinic after discharge. Observing interaction patterns between patients and care providers (including the consultant) provides information that can help to clarify maladaptive strategies and patterns. These clarifications may become the focus of acute psychotherapeutic intervention. The need for active involvement and intervention by the psychiatric consultant must be underscored, with attention focused on issues related to the patient's immediate needs and overwhelming fears. Resistance generally should not be interpreted directly in hospitalized patients. Hospitalization tends to induce regression; anxious regressed patients need to have their current level of psychological defensive functioning supported.

Behavioral psychotherapy provides an opportunity for acute anxiety reduction, enhancement of the patient's sense of mastery, and clarification of measurable goals.

Behavioral interventions commonly used in consultation-liaison psychiatry include relaxation techniques, systematic desensitization, biofeedback, meditation, hypnosis, and establishment of graded goals with simple reinforcement schedules.

Recent attention has focused on the potential efficacy of cognitive-behavioral therapy in the treatment of anxiety disorders (Sokol et al. 1989; Welkowitz et al. 1991). Although several different approaches are encompassed under this heading, all approaches assume that cognitions play a central role in the patient's affect. Cognitive-behavioral psychotherapy involves active exploration, clarification, and testing of the patient's perceptions and beliefs (Turk et al. 1983).

In addition, during symptomatic management and direct involvement with the anxious patient, the consultant becomes the link to the medical team caring for the patient. In a busy medical service, the escalating anxiety manifested by the patient can be perceived as based on unreasonable demands or uncooperativeness with care and may lead to further isolation of the patient, avoidance of the patient, or decreased intensity of care. The psychiatric assessment of the anxious patient can provide a framework that will lead to a better understanding of the patient's behavior and symptoms, resulting in the development of specific treatment plans. Specific management suggestions can be instituted by the nurses to manage the patient's discomfort, demands, and fears. Designation of primary nurses; provision of schedules; and ongoing notification of test results, planned procedures, or delays in anticipated procedures are simple interventions that may be overlooked in the context of the patient's acute medical needs. The consultant can assist nursing staff in providing structure and setting limits and in facilitating the provision of adequate medical care; offering reassurance and predictable care also may help to allay some of the patient's anxiety. In addition, medical and nursing personnel may find it helpful to discuss with the psychiatric consultant their own difficulties in managing the symptoms or behavior of particular patients, which helps to circumvent the direct escalation of difficulties that may affect the physician/nurse-patient relationship.

Attention to the nature and quality of the anxious patient's social support network, reliance on support from specific persons, or conflicts generated by the presence or involvement of specific family members or friends will help to optimize the patient's resources and facilitate the patient's symptom management on a medical ward. The concept of social support encompasses a broad spectrum of characteristics, such as type of support, quantity, quality, and perceived need (Rowland 1989). The effect of social support on emotional well-being and health outcomes has received significant empiric and clinical support (Rowland 1989; Wortman 1984). Clarifying the patient's perception of the level and quality of social support available, as well as the perceived need for support, can lead to direct attempts to bolster the patient's environment or to minimize stimulation or visits when patients feel overwhelmed by existing conflicts with members of this network. Lewis and Beavers (1977, p. 402) identified the family as "the most neglected component of the treatment system." The family's presence and involvement can be a source of support and reassurance but can also heighten the patient's or the caregivers' anxiety. Attention to family members' perceptions of the patient's condition and needs, as well as their own level of anxiety and how this is communicated to the patient, may result in a significant decrease in anxiety or minimized difficulties in management.

REFERENCES

Abelson LM, Nesse RM, Vinik A: Treatment of panic-like attacks with a long-acting analogue of somatostatin. J Clin Psychopharmacol 10:128–132, 1990

Abramowicz M: Drugs that cause psychiatric symptoms. Med Lett Drugs Ther 26:75–78, 1984

American Psychiatric Association: Diagnostic and Statistical Manual of Mental Disorders, 3rd Edition. Washington, DC, American Psychiatric Association, 1980

American Psychiatric Association: Diagnostic and Statistical Manual of Mental Disorders, 3rd Edition, Revised. Washington, DC, American Psychiatric Association, 1987

American Psychiatric Association: Diagnostic and Statistical Manual of Mental Disorders, 4th Edition. Washington, DC, American Psychiatric Association, 1994

American Psychiatric Association: Diagnostic and Statistical Manual of Mental Disorders, 4th Edition, Text Revision. Washington, DC, American Psychiatric Association, 2000

Aronson TA, Craig TJ: Cocaine precipitation of panic disorder. Am J Psychiatry 143:643–645, 1986

Astrom M: Generalized anxiety disorder in stroke patients: a 3 year longitudinal study. Stroke 27:270–275, 1996

Atkinson JH, Grant I, Kennedy CJ, et al: Prevalence of psychiatric disorders among men infected with human immunodeficiency virus. Arch Gen Psychiatry 45:859–864, 1988

Ballenger JC: Long-term pharmacologic treatment of panic disorder. J Clin Psychiatry 52 (suppl):18–23, 1991

Ballenger JC: Treatment of panic disorder in the general medical setting. J Psychosom Res 44:5–15, 1998

Barrett JE, Barrett JA, Oxman TE, et al: The prevalence of psychiatric disorders in a primary care practice. Arch Gen Psychiatry 45:1100–1106, 1988

Bass C, Wade C: Chest pain with normal coronary arteries: a comparative study of psychiatric and social morbidity. Psychol Med 14:51–61, 1984

Beck AT, Brown G, Epstein, N, et al: An inventory for measuring clinical anxiety: psychometric properties. J Consult Clin Psychiatry 56:893–897, 1988

Beitman BD, Lamberti JW, Mukerji V, et al: Panic disorder in patients with angiographically normal coronary arteries: a pilot study. Psychosomatics 28:480–484, 1987

Bisaga A, Katz J, Antonini A, et al: Cerebral glucose metabolism in women with panic disorders. Am J Psychiatry 155:1178–1183, 1998

Bradwejn J, Koszycki D, Shriqui C: Enhanced sensitivity to cholecystokinin tetrapeptide in panic disorder: clinical and behavioral findings. Arch Gen Psychiatry 48:603–610, 1991

Brawman-Mintzer O, Lydiard RB: Biological basis of generalized anxiety disorder. J Clin Psychiatry 58 (suppl 3):16–26, 1997

Breier A: Panic disorder: clinical features, neurobiology, and pharmacotherapy. New York State Journal of Medicine 91:43S–47S, 1991

Bridges KW, Goldberg DP: Somatic presentation of DSM-III psychiatric disorders in primary care. J Psychosom Res 29:563–569, 1985

Bussing R, Burket R, Kelleher E: Prevalence of anxiety disorders in a clinic-based sample of pediatric asthma patients. Psychosomatics 37:108–115, 1996

Carr R: Panic disorder and asthma: causes, effects and research implications. J Psychosom Res 44:43–52, 1998

Carter C, Maddock R, Amsterdam E, et al: Panic disorder and chest pain in the coronary care unit. Psychosomatics 33:302–309, 1992

Cassem NH: Depression and anxiety secondary to medical illness. Psychiatr Clin North Am 13:597–612, 1990

Cassem NH, Hackett TP: Psychiatric consultation in a CCU. Ann Intern Med 75:9–14, 1971

Chapman WP, Scroeder HR, Geyer G, et al: Physiological evidence concerning the importance of the amygdaloid nuclear region in the integration of circulating function and emotion in man. Science 120:949–950, 1954

Charney DS, Deutch A: A functional neuroanatomy of anxiety and fear: implications for the pathophysiology and treatment of anxiety disorders. Crit Rev Neurobiol 10:419–446, 1996

Charney DS, Heninger GR, Breier A: Noradrenergic function in panic anxiety. Arch Gen Psychiatry 41:751–763, 1984

Cormier LE, Katon W, Russo J, et al: Chest pain with negative cardiac diagnostic studies: relationship to psychiatric illness. J Nerv Ment Dis 176:351–358, 1988

Coupland N, Glue P, Nutt D: Challenge tests: assessment of the noradrenergic and GABA systems in depression and anxiety disorders. Mol Aspects Med 13:221–247, 1992

Craven J, Sutherland A: Buspirone for anxiety disorders in patients with severe lung disease (letter). Lancet 338:249, 1991

Davidson J: Pharmacotherapy of social anxiety disorder. J Clin Psychiatry 59:47–51, 1998

Deakin J: The role of serotonin in panic, anxiety and depression. International Clinical Pharmacology 13 (suppl 4):S1–S5, 1998

Dement WC: The proper use of sleeping pills in the primary care setting. J Clin Psychiatry 53 (suppl):50–60, 1992

Denaut M, Yernault J, DeCoster A: A double-blind comparison of the respiratory effects of parenteral lorazepam and diazepam in patients with COLD. Curr Med Res Opin 2:611–615, 1975

Derogatis LR: SCL-90-R Manual II. Towson, MD, Clinical Psychometric Research, 1983

Derogatis LR, Wise TN: Clinical assessment of anxiety and depression in the medical patient, in Anxiety and Depressive Disorders in the Medical Patient. Washington, DC, American Psychiatric Press, 1989a, pp 99–139

Derogatis LR, Wise TN: Screening and psychological assessment of anxiety and depression, in Anxiety and Depressive Disorders in the Medical Patient. Washington, DC, American Psychiatric Press, 1989b, pp 71–98

Derogatis LR, Morrow GR, Felting J, et al: The prevalence of psychiatric disorders among cancer patients. JAMA 249:751–757, 1983

Edelstein H, Knight RT: Severe parkinsonism in two AIDS patients taking prochlorperazine (letter). Lancet 2:341–342, 1987

Edlund MJ, McNamara E, Millman RP: Sleep apnea and panic attacks. Compr Psychiatry 32:130–132, 1991

Egbunike IG, Chaffee BJ: Antidepressants in the management of chronic pain syndromes. Pharmacotherapy 10:262–270, 1990

Finley PR, Nolan PE Jr: Precipitation of benzodiazepine withdrawal following sudden discontinuation of midazolam. DICP 23:151–152, 1989

Garner SJ, Eldridge FL: Buspirone, an anxiolytic drug that stimulates respiration. Am Rev Respir Dis 139:945–950, 1989

Glassman A: Cardiovascular effects of antidepressant drugs: updated. J Clin Psychiatry 59 (suppl 15):13–18, 1998

Gold PW, Pigott TA, Kling MA, et al: Basic and clinical studies with corticotropin-releasing hormone. Psychiatr Clin North Am 11:327–334, 1988

Goldberg DP, Hillier VF: A scaled version of the General Health Questionnaire. Psychol Med 9:139–145, 1979

Goldberg RJ: Anxiety in the medically ill, in Principles of Medical Psychiatry. Edited by Stoudemire A, Fogel BS. Orlando, FL, Grune & Stratton, 1987, pp 177–203

Gorman JM: The use of newer antidepressants for panic disorder. J Clin Psychiatry 58 (suppl 14):54–58, 1997

Gorman JM, Fyer MR, Liebowitz MR, et al: Pharmacologic provocation of panic attack, in Psychopharmacology: The Third Generation of Progress. Edited by Meltzer HY. New York, Raven, 1987, pp 985–993

Greenblat DJ, Divoll M, Harmatz JS, et al: Pharmacokinetic comparison of sublingual lorazepam with intravenous, intramuscular and oral lorazepam. J Pharm Sci 71:248–252, 1982

Greenblat D, von Moltke L, Harmatz J, et al: Drug interactions with newer antidepressants: role of human cytochromes p450. J Clin Psychiatry 59 (suppl 15):19–27, 1998

Hackett TP, Cassem NH, Wishnie HA: The coronary care unit: an appraisal of its psychological hazards. N Engl J Med 279:1365–1370, 1968

Hall RCW: Anxiety, in Psychiatric Presentations of Medical Illness. New York, Spectrum, 1980, pp 180–210

Hall RCW, Hall RCW: Anxiety and endocrine disease. Seminars in Clinical Neuropsychiatry 4(2):72–83, 1999

Hall RCW, Popkin MK, Stickney SK, et al: Presentation of the steroid psychoses. J Nerv Ment Dis 167:229–236, 1979

Hamilton M: The assessment of anxiety states by rating. Journal of Medical Psychology 32:50–55, 1959

Healy M, Pickens R, Meisch R, et al: Effects of clorazepate, diazepam, lorazepam and placebo on human memory. J Clin Psychiatry 44:436–439, 1983

Helig M, Koob G, Britton K: Corticotropin-releasing factor and neuropeptide Y: role in emotional integration. Trends Neurosci 17:80–85, 1994

Helzer JE, Robins LN, McEvoy MA: Post traumatic stress disorder in the general population. N Engl J Med 17:1630–1634, 1987

Hoeper EW, Nyczc GR, Cleary PD: Estimated prevalence of RDC mental disorder in primary care. International Journal of Mental Health 8:6–15, 1979

Hommer DW, Skolnick P, Paul SM: The benzodiazepine/GABA receptor complex and anxiety, in Psychopharmacology: The Third Generation of Progress. Edited by Meltzer HY. New York, Raven, 1987, pp 977–983

Horowitz M: Stress Response Syndrome. New York, Jason Aronson, 1976

Howell J: Behavioral breathlessness. Thorax 45:287–290, 1990

Johnston JA, Lineberry CG, Ascher JA, et al: A 102-center prospective study of seizure in association with bupropion. J Clin Psychiatry 52:450–456, 1991

Jonas JM, Coleman BS, Sheridan AQ, et al: Comparative clinical profile of triazolam versus other shorter-acting hypnotics. J Clin Psychiatry 33 (suppl):19–33, 1992

Kahn JP, Drusin RE, Klein DF: Idiopathic cardiomyopathy and panic disorder: clinical association in cardiac transplant candidates. Am J Psychiatry 144:1327–1330, 1987

Kathol RG, Delahunt JW: The relationship of anxiety and depression to symptoms of hyperthyroidism using operational criteria. Gen Hosp Psychiatry 8:23–28, 1986

Katon W: Panic disorder and somatization: review of 55 cases. Am J Med 77:101–106, 1984

Kellner R, Uhlenhuth EH: The rating and self-rating of anxiety. Br J Psychiatry 159 (suppl 12):15–22, 1991

Kerrihard T, Brietbart W, Dent R, et al: Anxiety in patients with cancer and human immunodeficiency virus. Seminars in Clinical Neuropsychiatry 4(2):114–132, 1999

Kessler RC, McGonagle K, Zhao S, et al: Lifetime and 12 month prevalence of DSM-III-R psychiatric disorders in the United States: results from the National Comorbidity Survey. Arch Gen Psychiatry 51:8–19, 1994

Khanderia U, Pandit SK: Use of midazolam hydrochloride in anesthesia. Clin Pharm 6:533–547, 1987

Kopchia KL, Altman HJ, Commissaris RL: Effects of lesions of the central nucleus of the amygdala on anxiety-like behaviors in the rat. Pharmacol Biochem Behav 43:452–461, 1992

Kopin IJ: Catecholamines, adrenal hormones, and stress, in Neuroendocrinology: The Interrelationships of the Body's Two Major Integrative Systems in Normal Physiology and in Clinical Disease. Edited by Krieger DT, Hughes JC. Sunderland, MA, Sinauer Associates, 1980, pp 159–166

Lakshminarawan S, Sahn S, Hudson L: Effects of diazepam on ventilatory responses. Clin Pharmacol Ther 20:173–183, 1976

LaVia MF, Munno I, Lydiard RB, et al: The influence of stress intrusion on immunodepression in generalized anxiety disorder patients and controls. Psychosom Med 58:138–142, 1996

Lecrubier Y, Ustun TB: Panic and depression: a world-wide primary care perspective. Int Clin Psychopharmacol 13 (suppl 14):S7–11, 1998

Leonard HL: New developments in the treatment of obsessive-compulsive disorder. J Clin Psychiatry 58 (suppl 14):39–45, 1997

Levenson JL, Hamer RM, Rossiter C: Psychopathology and pain in medical inpatients: predict resource use during hospitalization but not rehospitalization. J Psychosom Res 36:585–592, 1992

Lewis JM, Beavers WR: The family of the patient, in Psychiatric Medicine. Edited by Usdin G. New York, Brunner/Mazel, 1977, pp 401–424

Lustman PJ, Griffith LS, Clouse RE, et al: Psychiatric illness in diabetes mellitus: relationship to symptoms and glucose control. J Nerv Ment Dis 174:736–742, 1986

Lydiard R: The role of drug therapy in social phobia. J Clin Psychiatry 50:35–39, 1998

Mackenzie TB, Popkin MK: Stress response syndrome occurring after delirium. Am J Psychiatry 137:1433–1435, 1980

Maletta G, Mattox KM, Dysken M: Guidelines for prescribing psychoactive drugs in the elderly: part 1. Geriatrics 46:40–47, 1991

Malizia A, Coupland N, Nutt D: Benzodiazepine receptor function in anxiety disorders, in GABA-A Receptors and Anxiety: From Neurobiology to Treatment. Edited by Biggion G, Sanna E, Erra M, et al. New York, Raven, 1995, pp 115–133

Marazziti D, Michelini S, Giannaccini G, et al: Stress-related changes of benzodiazepine binding inhibitory activity (BBIA) in humans. Life Sci 46:1833–1836, 1990

Marazziti D, Toni C, Pedri S, et al: Headache, panic disorder and depression: comorbidity or a spectrum. Biol Psychiatry 34:465–470, 1993

Mendelson WB, Maczaj M, Holt J: Buspirone administration to sleep apnea patients. J Clin Psychopharmacol 11:71–72, 1991

Menza MA, Murray GB, Holmes VF, et al: Controlled study of extrapyramidal reactions in the management of delirious, medically ill patients: intravenous haloperidol versus intravenous haloperidol plus benzodiazepines. Heart Lung 17:238–241, 1988

Meredith LS, Sherbourne CD, Jackson CA, et al: Treatment typically provided for co-morbid anxiety disorder. Arch Fam Med 6:231–237, 1997

Merikangas KR, Stevens DE: Comorbidity of migraine and psychiatric disorders. Neurologic Clinics 15(1):115–123, 1997

Mindus P, Ericson K, Greitz T, et al: Regional cerebral glucose metabolism in anxiety disorders studied with positron emission tomography before and after psychosurgical intervention: a preliminary report. Acta Radiol Suppl 369: 444–448, 1986

Mitchells-Heggs P, Murphy K, Minty K, et al: Diazepam in the treatment of the dyspnea in the "pink-puffer" syndrome. Quarterly Journal of Medicine 49:9–20, 1980

Mukerji V, Beitman BD, Alpert MA, et al: Panic disorder: a frequent occurrence in patients with chest pain and normal coronary arteries. Angiology 38:236–240, 1987

National Institute of Mental Health: Panic disorder in the medical setting (DHHS Publ No ADM-89-1629). Edited by Katon W. Washington, DC, U.S. Government Printing Office, 1989

Newton RE, Marunycz JD, Alderdice MT, et al: Review of the side-effect profile of buspirone. Am J Med 80 (suppl 3B):17–21, 1986

Nordahl T, Stein M, Benkelfat C, et al: Regional cerebral metabolic asymmetries replicated in an independent group of patients with panic disorders. Biol Psychiatry 44:998–1006, 1998

Okada S, Ichiki K, Tankuchi S, et al: Improvement of stress reduces glycosylated hemoglobin levels in patients with Type 2 diabetes. J Int Med Res 23(2):119–122, 1995

Papp LA, Klein DF, Gorman JM: Carbon dioxide hypersensitivity, hyperventilation, and panic disorder. Am J Psychiatry 150:1149–1157, 1993

Perdices M, Dunbar N, Grungeit A, et al: Anxiety, depression and HIV related symptomatology across the spectrum of HIV disease. Aust N Z J Psychiatry 26:560–566, 1992

Petursson H, Lader MH: Withdrawal from long-term benzodiazepine treatment. BMJ 283:643–645, 1981

Peyrot M, Rubin RR: Levels and risks of depression and anxiety symptomatology among diabetic adults. Diabetes Care 20: 585–590, 1997

Pitts FN, McClure JN: Lactate metabolism in anxiety neurosis. N Engl J Med 227:1329–1336, 1967

Popkin MK: Consultation-liaison psychiatry, in Comprehensive Textbook of Psychiatry, 6th Edition. Edited by Kaplan HI, Sadock BJ. Baltimore, MD, Williams & Wilkins, 1993, pp 1592–1605

Popkin MK, Mackenzie TB: Psychiatric presentation of endocrine dysfunction, in Psychiatric Presentations of Medical Illness. Edited by Hall RCW. New York, Spectrum, 1980, pp 142–143

Popkin MK, Tucker G: Secondary and drug-induced mood, anxiety, psychotic, catatonic and personality disorders: a review of the literature. J Neuropsychiatry Clin Neurosci 4: 369–385, 1992

Popkin MK, Mackenzie TB, Callies AL: Psychiatric consultation to geriatric medically ill inpatients in a university hospital. Arch Gen Psychiatry 41:703–707, 1984

Popkin MK, Callies AL, Mackenzie TB: The outcome of antidepressant use in the medically ill. Arch Gen Psychiatry 42:1160–1163, 1985

Popkin MK, Callies A, Lentz RD, et al: Prevalence of major depression, simple phobia, and other psychiatric disorders in patients with longstanding type I diabetes mellitus. Arch Gen Psychiatry 45:64–68, 1988

Popkin MK, Callies AL, Colón EA, et al: Adjustment disorders in medically ill inpatients referred for consultation in a university hospital. Psychosomatics 31:410–414, 1990

Popkin MK, Callies AL, Colón EA, et al: Psychiatric diagnosis and the surgical outcome of pancreas transplantation in patients with type 1 diabetes mellitus. Psychosomatics 34:251–258, 1993

Power AC, Cowen PJ: Neuroendocrine challenge tests: assessment of 5-HT function in anxiety and depression. Mol Aspects Med 13:205–220, 1992

Prigatano GP, Wright EC, Levin D: The quality of life and its predictors in patients with mild hypoxemia and chronic obstructive pulmonary disease. Arch Intern Med 144:613–619, 1984

Ray WA, Griftin MR, Downey W: Benzodiazepines of long and short elimination half life and the risk of hip fracture. JAMA 262:3303–3307, 1989

Redmond DEJ: Studies of the nucleus coeruleus in monkeys and hypotheses for neuropsychopharmacology, in Psychopharmacology: The Third Generation of Progress. Edited by Meltzer HY. New York, Raven, 1987, pp 967–975

Redmond DEJ, Huang YH, Snyder DR, et al: Behavioral changes following lesions of the locus coeruleus in Macaca arctoides (abstract). Neuroscience Abstracts 1:472, 1976a

Redmond DEJ, Huang YH, Snyder DR, et al: Behavioral effects of stimulation of the locus coeruleus in the stumptail monkey (Macaca arctoides). Brain Res 116:502–510, 1976b

Reiman E: The quest to establish the neural substrates of anxiety. Psychiatr Clin North Am 11:295–307, 1988

Reiman E: The application of positron emission tomography to the study of normal and pathologic emotions. J Clin Psychiatry 58 (suppl 16):4–12, 1997

Reiman EM, Fusselman MJ, Fox PT, et al: Neuroanatomical correlates of lactate-induced anxiety attacks. Arch Gen Psychiatry 46:493–500, 1989

Richard IH, Schiffer RB, Kurlan R: Anxiety and Parkinson's disease. J Neuropsychiatry Clin Neurosci 8:383–392, 1996

Rickels K, Schweizer EE: Current pharmacotherapy of anxiety and panic, in Psychopharmacology: The Third Generation of Progress. Edited by Melzer HY. New York, Raven, 1987, pp 1193–1203

Rickels K, Schweizer E: Clinical overview of serotonin reuptake inhibitors. J Clin Psychiatry 51 (suppl B):9–12, 1990

Riether AM: Anxiety in patients with multiple sclerosis. Seminars in Clinical Neuropsychiatry 4(2):103–113, 1999

Robins LN, Helzer JE, Croughan J, et al: National Institute of Mental Health Diagnostic Interview Schedule: its history, characteristics, and validity. Arch Gen Psychiatry 38:381–389, 1981

Robins LN, Helzer JE, Weissman MM, et al: Lifetime prevalence of specific psychiatric disorders in 3 sites. Arch Gen Psychiatry 41:949–958, 1984

Rogers MP, White K, Warsaw WMG, et al: Prevalence of medical illness in patients with anxiety disorders. Int J Psychiatry Med 24:83–96, 1994

Roll M, Theorell T: Acute chest pain without obvious organic cause before age 40—personality and recent life events. J Psychosom Res 31:215–221, 1987

Rosen J, Schulkin J: From normal fear to pathological anxiety. Psychol Rev 105:325–350, 1998

Rothschild AJ: Disinhibition, amnestic reactions and other adverse reactions secondary to triazolam: a review of the literature. J Clin Psychol 53 (suppl):69–79, 1992

Rowland J: Interpersonal resources: social support, in Handbook of Psychooncology: Psychological Care of the Patient With Cancer. Edited by Holland JC, Rowland JH. New York, Oxford University Press, 1989, pp 58–71

Sakauye K, Camp C, Ford P: Effects of buspirone on agitation associated with dementia. Am J Geriatr Psychiatry 1:82–84, 1993

Salzman C, Miyawake EK, le Bars P, et al: Neurobiologic basis of anxiety and its treatment. Harv Rev Psychiatry 1:197–206, 1993

Schuckit M: Anxiety related to medical disease. J Clin Psychiatry 44:31–37, 1983

Schulberg HC, Saul M, McClelland M: Assessing depression in primary medical and psychiatric practices. Arch Gen Psychiatry 12:1164–1170, 1985

Schwab JJ, McGinness NH, Marder L, et al: Evaluation of anxiety in medical patients. Journal of Chronic Disease 19:1049–1057, 1966

Shavitt RG, Gentil V, Mandetta R: The association of panic/agoraphobia and asthma: contributing factors and clinical implications. Gen Hosp Psychiatry 14:420–423, 1992

Sheehan D, Raj A, Harnett-Sheehan K, et al: The relative efficacy of high-dose buspirone and alprazolam in the treatment of panic disorder: a double blind placebo-controlled study. Acta Psychiatr Scand 88:1–11, 1993

Sherbourne CD, Jackson CA, Meredith LS, et al: Prevalence of co-morbid anxiety disorders in primary care outpatients. Arch Fam Med 5:27–34, 1996

Silver PA, Simpson GM: Antipsychotic use in the medically ill. Psychother Psychosom 49:120–136, 1988

Smoller JW, Simon NM, Pollack MH, et al: Anxiety in patients with pulmonary disease: co-morbidity and treatment. Seminars in Clinical Neuropsychiatry 4(2):84–97, 1999

Sokol L, Beck AT, Greenberg RL, et al: Cognitive therapy of panic disorder: a nonpharmacological alternative. J Nerv Ment Dis 177:711–716, 1989

Spielberger CD, Gorsuch RL, Luchene RE: Manual for the State-Trait Anxiety Inventory. Palo Alto, CA, Consulting Psychologist Press, 1970

Starkman MN, Cameron OG, Nesse RM, et al: Peripheral catecholamine levels and the symptoms of anxiety: studies in patients with and without pheochromocytoma. Psychosom Med 52:129–142, 1990

Stein D, Bouwer C: A neuro-evolutionary approach to the anxiety disorders. J Anxiety Disord 11:409–429, 1997

Stein MB, Heuser IJ, Juncos JL, et al: Anxiety disorders in patients with Parkinson's disease. Am J Psychiatry 147:217–220, 1990

Swedo SE, Rappaport JL, Cheslow DL, et al: High prevalence of obsessive-compulsive symptoms in patients with Syndenham's chorea. Am J Psychiatry 146:246–249, 1989

Thompson W, Thompson T: Pulmonary disease, in Principles of Medical Psychiatry. Edited by Stoudemire A, Fogel B. Orlando, FL, Grune & Stratton, 1987, pp 553–570

Tilhonen J, Kuikka J, Rasanen R, et al: Cerebral benzodiazepine receptor binding and distribution in generalized anxiety disorder: a fractal analysis. Mol Psychiatry 2:463–471, 1997

Trepacz PT, McCue M, Klein I: A psychiatric and neuropsychological study of patients with untreated Graves' disease. Gen Hosp Psychiatry 10:39–55, 1988

Tunnicliff G: Molecular basis of buspirone's anxiolytic action. Pharmacol Toxicol 69:149–156, 1991

Turk DC, Meichenbaum D, Genest M: Pain and Behavioral Medicine. New York, Guilford, 1983

Uhde TW, Nemiah JC: Panic and generalized anxiety disorders, in Comprehensive Textbook of Psychiatry/V, 5th Edition. Edited by Kaplan HI, Sadock BJ. Baltimore, MD, Williams & Wilkins, 1989, pp 952–973

Van Peski-Osterbaan A, Spinhoven P, VanderDoes A, et al: Is there a specific relationship between asthma and panic disorder? Behav Res Ther 34:333–340, 1996

Venkatesh A, Pauls DL, Crowe R, et al: MVP in anxiety neurosis (panic disorder). Am Heart J 37:1361–1365, 1981

Verburg K, Griez E, Meijer J, et al: Respiratory disorders as a possible predisposing factor for panic disorder. J Affect Disord 33:129–134, 1995

Verma S, Davidoff D, Kambhampati K: Management of the agitated elderly patient in the nursing home: the role of the atypical antipsychotics. J Clin Psychiatry 59 (suppl 15):50–55, 1998

Welkowitz LA, Papp LA, Cloitre M, et al: Cognitive-behavior therapy for panic disorder delivered by psychopharmacologically oriented clinicians. J Nerv Ment Dis 179:472–476, 1991

Wells KB, Golding JM, Burnham MA: Psychiatric disorder in a sample of the population with and without chronic medical conditions. Am J Psychiatry 145:976–981, 1988

Wells KB, Golding JM, Burnam MA: Chronic medical conditions in a sample of the general population with anxiety, affective and substance use disorders. Am J Psychiatry 146:1440–1446, 1989

Wheatley D: Use of anti-anxiety drugs in the medically ill. Psychother Psychosom 49:63–80, 1988

Wise MG, Rundell JR: Anxiety and neurological disorders. Seminars in Clinical Neuropsychiatry 4(2):98–102, 1999

Wise MG, Taylor SE: Anxiety and mood disorders in medically ill patients. J Clin Psychiatry 51 (suppl 1):27–32, 1990

Wolkowitz OM, Weingartner H, Thompson K, et al: Diazepam-induced amnesia: a neuropharmacological model of "organic amnestic syndrome." Am J Psychiatry 144:25–29, 1987

Wooley CF: The mitral valve prolapse syndrome. Hosp Pract (Off Ed) 18:163–174, 1983

Wooley CF: From irritable heart to mitral valve prolapse: World War I—the US experience and the origin of neurocirculatory asthenia. Am J Cardiol 59:1183–1186, 1987

Wortman CB: Social support and the cancer patient: conceptual and methodologic issues. Cancer 53 (suppl 10):2339–2362, 1984

Yellowlees PM, Alpers JH, Bowden JJ, et al: Psychiatric morbidity in patients with chronic airflow obstruction. Med J Aust 146:305–307, 1987

Yellowlees PM, Haynes S, Potts N, et al: Psychiatric morbidity in patients with life threatening asthma: initial report of a controlled study. Med J Aust 149:246–249, 1988

Zarate C Jr, Baldessarini R, Siegel A, et al: Risperidone in the elderly: a pharmacoepidemiolgic study. J Clin Psychiatry 58:311–317, 1997

Zaubler TS, Katon W: Panic disorder in the general medical setting. J Psychosom Res 44:5–15, 1998

Zorumski CF, Isenberg KE: Insights into the structure and function of GABA-benzodiazepine receptors: ion channels and psychiatry. Am J Psychiatry 148:162–173, 1991

Zung WKW: A rating instrument for anxiety disorders. Psychosomatics 12:371–379, 1971

21

Substance-Related Disorders

John E. Franklin Jr., M.D.

Martin H. Leamon, M.D.

Richard J. Frances, M.D.

The extent of substance-related illnesses in the general hospital setting is mind-boggling. Alcohol and tobacco use alone contributes to a host of medical illnesses. Illegal drug use, particularly intravenous drug abuse, taxes the health care system. Increases in the National Institute on Drug Abuse budget are, in large part, due to growing recognition that certain illnesses, such as acquired immunodeficiency syndrome (AIDS) and tuberculosis, are associated with drug abuse. Emergency rooms have seen a steady increase in drug overdoses. In addition, the extent of current perinatal drug abuse has consequences far into the future.

Substance-related disorders in the general hospital present unique challenges to consultation-liaison psychiatrists. Because of the number of consultation problems, a thorough knowledge of substance abuse, especially signs and symptoms and acute management, is essential. Fortunately, consultation-liaison work with other caregivers and patients offers many opportunities for therapeutic interventions and education. Hospital staff are prone to misunderstand, neglect, and be biased toward substance-abusing patients. In addition, the span of issues faced by the consultation-liaison psychiatrist includes drug overdose; withdrawal regimens; initial diagnosis; engaging patients in a therapeutic process; evaluating pain medication; assessing patients for liver and kidney transplantation, patients with trauma and burns (who have a high frequency of drug dependency), and pregnant substance abusers; drug abuse problems in geriatric or adolescent patients; and referral or triage to substance abuse specialists.

Consultation-liaison psychiatrists are often members of a multidisciplinary team of professionals treating these patients. These professionals include nurses, social workers, other physicians, nutritionists, and administrators, who are often also involved in important aspects of the substance abuser's care. An integrated, multidisciplinary approach is needed for thorough medical evaluation and education, for nutritional assessment, for housing and family assessment, and to address complex legal issues that arise.

Alcohol and drug education plays an increasingly important part in medical school curricula. However, there is a lag in educational efforts in many residency programs. As of March 2001, there were 43 accredited addiction psychiatry fellowship programs, which add subspecialists to the many physicians who have already passed the American Society of Addiction Medicine certification examination. In addition, approximately 2,000 psychiatrists have taken the added qualification examination in addiction medicine given by the American Board of Psychiatry and Neurology. Some hospitals have specialized addiction consultation services (Fleming et al. 1995; M.G. Fuller and Jordan 1994). Other addiction specialists, such as certified drug and alcohol counselors (who are themselves often recovering substance abusers), often play an important role in the general hospital setting. They can conduct routine evaluations and make referrals to the local drug-treating community in a cost-effective manner. They also provide hope of recovery to patients newly diagnosed with substance abuse. It is also important to note that the American Psychiatric Association (1995a, 1995b) has published practice guidelines for the treatment of alcohol, cocaine, and opioid use disorders.

In this chapter, we provide an update on addiction medicine for the practicing consultation-liaison psychiatrist. We highlight issues that arise in consultations on general medical units. We discuss assessment of intoxication and withdrawal, complications, psychological and psychiatric factors, treatment resistance, recovery environment, and relapse potential. We pay particular attention to treatment recommendations and planning on general medical-surgical units.

DSM-IV-TR SUBSTANCE-RELATED DISORDERS

In DSM-IV-TR (American Psychiatric Association 2000), the broad diagnostic category of substance-related disorders includes disorders caused by substances taken by individuals to alter mood or behavior as well as disorders caused by unintentional use of a substance or medication side effects. For example, over-the-counter and prescription medications (e.g., steroids, antihistamines, and anticholinergics) that have psychoactive effects are classified using an *other (or unknown) substance–related category*. Substance-related disorders are divided into *substance use disorders*, which include abuse and dependence, and *substance-induced disorders*, which include intoxication, withdrawal, delirium, dementia, sexual dysfunction, and amnestic, psychotic, mood, anxiety, and sleep disorders.

DSM-IV-TR criteria for substance dependence are listed in Table 21–1. Because not all substances of dependence are associated with physiologic dependence (i.e., tolerance and withdrawal), the clinician must specify whether physiologic dependence is part of the substance dependence. Other specifiers include remission type (early or sustained, full or partial) and whether the patient is receiving agonist therapy (such as L-α-acetylmethadol [LAAM] for opiate dependence) or is in a controlled environment (such as the hospital [for a long time] or prison). Idiosyncratic alcohol intoxication was eliminated from DSM-IV (American Psychiatric Association 1994) because empirical data do not support the existence of this diagnosis. The diagnosis of substance abuse is a diagnosis of exclusion, to be used only when a patient does not meet, and has never met, criteria for substance dependence. This distinction can be confusing, because the term *substance abuse* is often used in a nondiagnostic sense to refer to a broad spectrum of substance use patterns.

Definitions

Withdrawal

Withdrawal symptoms are substance-specific constellations of symptoms that may occur after cessation or a decrease in use of alcohol or drugs in individuals who are physiologically dependent. Withdrawal can sometimes precipitate delirium, psychotic disorders, mood disorders, anxiety disorders, and sleep disorders. After acute withdrawal from alcohol, opiates, and stimulants, many milder physiologic and psychological disruptions can persist for weeks to months. Some authors have proposed the concept of a protracted withdrawal syndrome, but its existence as a substance-specific syndrome and its management remain controversial (Begleiter and Porjesz 1979; Geller 1994).

Tolerance

Tolerance is an acquired decrease in the effects of a substance caused either by lower blood or brain substance levels after ingestion or by increased cellular resistance. For example, Minion et al. (1989) reported on a series of patients in an emergency room whose average blood alcohol concentration (BAC) was 467 mg/dL—a level known to cause coma or death in an alcohol-naive individual; 88% of these patients were oriented to time, person, and place. Tolerance is influenced by innate, acquired, and learned factors (Kalant 1998).

GENERAL CONSULTATION PRINCIPLES

Consultation-liaison psychiatrists are called on to evaluate and treat patients with substance-related disorders in a variety of settings and for a variety of reasons. Examples include evaluating a patient with impotence in a urology clinic or managing acute alcohol withdrawal in patients on an oncology service, trauma service, or burn unit. The consultation-liaison psychiatrist must have an appropriate attitude and possess specific knowledge to work with patients who have substance use disorders (Table 21–2). At times, especially in critically ill patients, medical problems overshadow substance abuse issues.

In the general hospital, there are a number of barriers to detection and treatment of substance use disorders, so consultations can pose unique challenges. The consultant may encounter strong feelings on the part of the patient or members of the medical team, and the psychiatrist may enter a clinical situation in which considerable misunderstanding and animosity have developed between the patient and the physician. Nurses and physicians may over- or underestimate the impact of a patient's substance use or may be overly frustrated by rebuffs of attempts to engage an unmotivated patient. Patients may acknowledge their substance use but either not realize or deny its

---

TABLE 21–1. DSM-IV-TR criteria for substance dependence

A maladaptive pattern of substance use, leading to clinically significant impairment or distress, as manifested by three (or more) of the following, occurring at any time in the same 12-month period:

(1) tolerance, as defined by either of the following:

    (a) a need for markedly increased amounts of the substance to achieve intoxication or desired effect

    (b) markedly diminished effect with continued use of the same amount of the substance

(2) withdrawal, as manifested by either of the following:

    (a) the characteristic withdrawal syndrome for the substance (refer to Criteria A and B of the criteria sets for withdrawal from the specific substances)

    (b) the same (or a closely related) substance is taken to relieve or avoid withdrawal symptoms

(3) the substance is often taken in larger amounts or over a longer period than was intended

(4) there is a persistent desire or unsuccessful efforts to cut down or control substance use

(5) a great deal of time is spent in activities necessary to obtain the substance (e.g., visiting multiple doctors or driving long distances), use the substance (e.g., chain-smoking), or recover from its effects

(6) important social, occupational, or recreational activities are given up or reduced because of substance use

(7) the substance use is continued despite knowledge of having a persistent or recurrent physical or psychological problem that is likely to have been caused or exacerbated by the substance (e.g., current cocaine use despite recognition of cocaine-induced depression, or continued drinking despite recognition that an ulcer was made worse by alcohol consumption)

Specify if:

    With physiological dependence: evidence of tolerance or withdrawal (i.e., either Item 1 or 2 is present)

    Without physiological dependence: no evidence of tolerance or withdrawal (i.e., neither Item 1 nor 2 is present)

Course specifiers (see text for definitions):

    Early full remission
    Early partial remission
    Sustained full remission
    Sustained partial remission
    On agonist therapy
    In a controlled environment

TABLE 21–2. General consultant issues for patients with substance use disorders

---

Have a high suspicion for drug abuse.

Perform urine toxicology screens whenever possible, immediately after admission.

Know general principles of detoxification (i.e., know indications for inpatient versus outpatient and pharmacological versus observational detoxification).

Realize that tailored detoxification is often needed in medically ill patients.

When treating polysubstance dependence, be aware that sedative detoxification occurs first.

Use challenge tests or estimate conservatively if unsure of initial detoxification dose.

Know equivalent doses of sedatives and opiates.

Recognize drug-drug interactions.

Be able to differentiate major psychopathology, metabolic and neurological conditions, and withdrawal and intoxication.

---

relation to their medical and other psychosocial problems. Patients whose parents were active substance abusers often distrust authority figures (i.e., nurses and doctors) and rely on friends who also often abuse substances. Substance-abusing patients typically do not request psychiatric consultations and often are not told that a psychiatric consultation was requested. In general, the earlier the consultation, the better. While they are acutely sick, medically ill patients are often more open to treatment recommendations. Some patients are reluctant to fully disclose substance abuse or dependence because of potential legal problems (e.g., relating to motor vehicle accidents) or fear of job loss. This makes gathering factual information more difficult. Feelings of anger toward patients are usually uncomfortable for caregivers.

Acute Assessment

The elements of a basic substance abuse history are listed in Table 21–3. Important aspects of assessment include

TABLE 21–3. Elements of a basic substance use history

Chief complaint

History of present illness

Current medical signs and symptoms

Substance abuse review of symptoms for all psychoactive substances

Dates of first use, regular use, heaviest use, longest period of sobriety, pattern, amount, frequency, time of last use, route of administration, circumstances of use, reactions to use

Medical history, medications, human immunodeficiency virus (HIV) status, hepatitis B and C status

History of past substance abuse treatment, response to treatment

Family history, including substance abuse history

Psychiatric history

Legal history

Object-relations history

Personal history

Source. Adapted from Frances RJ, Franklin JE Jr: *Concise Guide to Treatment of Alcoholism and Addictions.* Washington, DC, American Psychiatric Press, 1989, p. 62. Used with permission.

identifying and resolving significant negative countertransference before treating substance abusers, ensuring brief but comprehensive triage, and establishing patient eligibility for follow-up care (this is an administration function, but a consultant must not make unrealistic recommendations). It is sometimes difficult during the initial consultation to differentiate the effects of substance intoxication, withdrawal, or chronic use from other psychiatric disorders.

Evaluation of the patient's family is essential because a family system that accommodates the patient's substance use may also reinforce it. Including the family in treatment increases the chances that the patient will remain abstinent.

Treatment

Proper implementation of treatment always involves the medical treatment staff and the patient. For both, treatment includes several stages: 1) educating the patient; 2) motivating the patient to accept the recommended treatment plan; 3) encouraging the staff to work collaboratively with the patient; 4) suggesting pharmacological treatments, when needed; 5) integrating substance abuse treatment into the overall treatment plan; and 6) facilitating transfers to appropriate treatment facilities when appropriate.

Detoxification alone does not constitute treatment of an addiction. Some patients with mild substance abuse may resolve drug- or alcohol-related problems without additional treatment (Sobell et al. 1996) or with brief intervention by the consultant or another physician (Barnes and Samet 1997). Substance dependence, however, is best viewed as a chronic medical illness (McLellan et al. 2000), and many substance-dependent patients will benefit from referral to specialized treatment. Failure to refer can reinforce in the patient's mind the denial of substance-related problems and enable continued addiction.

A consultation-liaison psychiatrist must be familiar with local substance abuse treatment resources. It is difficult to arrange proper aftercare during a short hospitalization or when financial resources are limited. Patients' insurance coverage of substance abuse treatment varies considerably. Patients with little or no coverage usually must wait until public treatment slots are available. While waiting, patients often relapse. This is especially true of patients who have poor psychosocial supports and problems with housing, employment, and income (Humphreys et al. 1996).

Recovery from addiction is a process in which patients must develop responsibility for their own addiction. Therefore, the role of the consultation-liaison psychiatrist is to empathically confront the patient about substance-related problems and to provide support, information, and access to resources but not to assume total responsibility for patient follow-up. Education and a motivational approach, rather than continuous confrontation, usually work best. The psychiatric consultant is typically not directly involved in a patient's aftercare, so a brief intervention model is needed. An early treatment goal is to have the patient accept that his or her substance use is causing problems and that some form of treatment is needed.

The most common referrals are to a specialized substance abuse treatment program or to a 12-step group such as Alcoholics Anonymous (AA). Most United States drug and alcohol treatment programs emphasize a combination of psychoeducation, participation in a 12-step program, and individual, group, and family counseling. Although resource availability is often a determining factor in follow-up treatment recommendations, guidelines like those developed by the American Society of Addiction Medicine (Mee-Lee et al. 1994) can be used in referring patients to different levels of care. Because most treatment programs require that patients themselves call for services, the role of the consultant is to provide resources and encourage patients to contact programs directly.

AA is a worldwide self-help group of recovering alcoholic individuals that was started in 1936 by Bill Wilson. The only requirement for membership is a desire to stop drinking. Meetings provide members with acceptance, understanding, forgiveness, confrontation, and a means for positive identification. AA uses a 12-step program: 12 tenets of recovery that members work through sequentially on their way to overcoming addiction. The steps include admitting powerlessness over alcohol, conducting a personal assessment, making amends, and eventually helping others. Members may contact one another outside meetings for sobriety support, and newer members team up with more experienced AA members, sponsors who guide them through the process. Although AA is not affiliated with any religion (25% of AA members identify themselves as atheists), the organization allows for spiritual reevaluation. Members frequently remain active in AA for many years, and AA involvement is generally associated with favorable outcome (Humphreys et al. 1996; Vaillant 1995). A prospective study of employed alcoholic patients found that treatment plus AA participation was more effective than AA involvement alone in helping such individuals attain and continue abstinence (Walsh et al. 1991). In some hospitals, AA members visit inpatients; many general hospitals host AA meetings.

Other organizations have been modeled on AA. Narcotics Anonymous (NA), founded in 1947, and Cocaine Anonymous (CA), founded in 1982, are two examples. Contacts for AA, NA, and CA can usually be found in local telephone directories or on the organizations' respective Web sites.

Patients with a substance-related disorder and another psychiatric disorder have better outcomes when both disorders are treated simultaneously (Mueser et al. 1997; Nunes and Quitlin 1997). Nevertheless, integrated long-term treatment programs for such patients can be difficult to find. Many psychiatric inpatient units, psychiatric halfway houses, outpatient clinics, and other mental health facilities in the community are unable or unwilling to treat psychiatric patients who have alcohol or drug problems. In many substance abuse treatment facilities, there is little if any contact with a psychiatric consultant, and treatment is provided by counselors who have minimal psychiatric training. Integrated programs combine rehabilitation, psychiatric evaluation, and the appropriate use of other treatment modalities, such as psychotherapy and pharmacotherapy. AA, NA, and CA officially support the use of psychotropic medications when necessary. Dual-diagnosis or "double-trouble" groups also use a 12-step approach.

Recommendations for patients after a suicide attempt and a recent history of alcohol or drug use or abuse range from discharge with outpatient mental health follow-up to inpatient psychiatric involuntary commitment (i.e., if there is a strong suicidal risk). When ambivalence exists about the correct disposition, a brief inpatient psychiatric stay for further evaluation is usually prudent.

Patients with concomitant chronic medical illnesses that limit participation in formal substance treatment programs pose special problems. Patients may encounter difficulties with transportation (e.g., physical limitations or unreliable transportation) or difficulty sustaining the concentration necessary to take full advantage of formal rehabilitation programs. These patients often feel estranged from the "world of the well." Devising aftercare programs tailored to patients' needs is often difficult. Patients are sometimes seen individually and attend meetings of AA or professional groups as tolerated. Frequently, the primary concern of patients and staff is the medical illness.

Additional difficulties emerge when patients have spinal cord injuries, blindness, deafness, or other physical disabilities. Some caregivers involved in the treatment of paraplegic patients experience excessive sympathy that causes them to ignore significant substance abuse problems. It is possible to successfully integrate paraplegic patients into standard treatment programs. Deaf patients often need specialized services, such as sign language interpreters, to utilize standard rehabilitation services. Some communities have AA groups for deaf or blind people. Patients with mental retardation pose special problems; they are taken advantage of on the streets, not identified as having alcoholism, or not given adequate attention in treatment programs. These patients often obtain more comprehensive care from services designed for mentally impaired people.

Patients in recovery from addiction who are abstinent often face the dilemma of whether to take mood-altering substances (e.g., narcotics for pain, anxiolytics for sedation) when hospitalized. Recovery teaches people to avoid all mood-altering substances because they can lead to relapse or a substitute addiction. If the hospitalization is elective, such as for ambulatory surgery, the issue can be discussed beforehand with drug treatment staff members or AA sponsors. When the issue is discussed up front and adequate support is provided, these patients do well. The clinician should encourage AA members and sponsors to visit the patient and should halt treatment with mood-altering medication as soon as possible.

Treatment Outcome

Long-term studies have consistently shown that treatment for substance dependence is undeniably beneficial and cost-efficient from a public health or societal cost perspective (McLellan et al. 1996). Predicting which individual patients are more apt to benefit from which type of treatment has been more problematic. Patients who are more compliant with and receive more treatment generally do better, as do patients who receive additional treatment directed at specific ancillary problems, such as housing, employment, or comorbid psychiatric illness (McLellan et al. 1997). Other potential predictors, such as severity of addiction, social status, number of previous treatment attempts, coping style, family history, or patient self-selection of treatment type, have not been shown to have consistent associations with treatment outcomes.

Relapse prevention is essential in treating substance dependence. The goals of relapse prevention are to address ambivalence, reduce drug or alcohol availability, minimize high-risk situations, develop coping strategies, be able to recognize conditioned cues to craving and decision patterns that lead to use, establish alternatives to drug or alcohol use, and avoid the attitude that all is lost with drug use "slips" (Carroll et al. 1991).

ALCOHOL USE DISORDERS

The addiction field has attempted to more clearly define alcohol use problems; accuracy is even more important when making a diagnosis in a consultation-liaison setting. Several alcohol-related hospitalizations can occur before a direct connection is made between a patient's alcohol use and medical problems. Alcoholic patients tend to experience many alcohol-related problems before seeking professional help or attending AA meetings (Bucholz and Homan 1992). Resistance to the term *alcoholism* frequently inhibits physicians from exploring the connections between abuse and biopsychosocial consequences. Psychiatrists participating in a hospital survey conducted by Moore et al. (1989) positively identified alcohol abuse two-thirds of the time, whereas physicians treating gynecology patients diagnosed the disorder only 10% of the time.

The official psychiatric nomenclature for alcohol abuse and dependence evolved from the view of alcoholism as a personality disorder (DSM-I; American Psychiatric Association 1952), to recognition of episodic, habitual abuse (DSM-II; American Psychiatric Association 1968), to the more recent definitions in DSM-III (American Psychiatric Association 1980), DSM-III-R (American Psychiatric Association 1987), DSM-IV (American Psychiatric Association 1994), and DSM-IV-TR (American Psychiatric Association 2000) that stress the psychosocial consequences, as well as physiologic withdrawal, as hallmarks of the disease process. The National Council

on Alcoholism and Drug Dependence and the American Society of Addiction Medicine define alcoholism as a disease process (Morse and Flavin 1992). (Note: *Disease* is defined as an involuntary disability.) The definition states that

> alcoholism is a primary, chronic disease with genetic, psychosocial, and environmental factors influencing its development and manifestations. The disease is often progressive and fatal. It is characterized by impaired control over drinking, preoccupation with alcohol, use of alcohol despite adverse consequences, and distortions in thinking, most notably denial. Each of these symptoms may be continuous or periodic. (Morse and Flavin 1992, p. 1013)

Epidemiology

The Epidemiologic Catchment Area (ECA) study found that the lifetime prevalence of alcohol abuse or dependence in the general population is 13.6% (Robins et al. 1984). Follow-up data from the same ECA population revealed a 1-year prevalence for alcohol disorders of 7.4%. Only 22% of these people ever used any mental health or addiction service; of these, about half were seen by specialty mental health or addiction professionals, and the other half were examined by general medical professionals (Regier et al. 1993). In other words, people who seek consultation for alcohol problems are as likely to see general physicians as they are to see mental health or drug abuse specialists.

Alcohol-related problems usually begin between ages 16 and 30 years. In addition, Regier et al. (1990) reported that 53% of those with an alcohol or drug abuse disorder also have a comorbid psychiatric disorder. Women are more likely than men to present for treatment in mental health or medical settings (Weisner and Schmidt 1992). Men are more likely than women to receive treatment in jails and drug treatment programs. Alcoholism among elderly individuals is increasing and is often difficult to diagnose because symptoms are often less dramatic.

A conservative estimate is that 25% of general hospital inpatients and 20% of medical outpatients have alcohol-related disorders (Cleary et al. 1988; Moore et al. 1989). Unfortunately, only about 20%–50% of the general hospital population's alcohol problems are diagnosed (Moore et al. 1989). Diagnosis in patients seen in general hospital settings is challenging. For example, a patient presents with liver failure or gastrointestinal problems after several years of "moderate" alcohol intake, but no psychosocial sequelae are reported. Detailed, repeated, or collateral history is necessary before the diagnosis of alcohol dependence becomes clear. The consultation-liaison psychiatrist must always maintain a high index of suspicion and vigilance for substance-related disorders.

Patients with alcoholism usually resist and avoid doctors because of denial, embarrassment, problems with authority figures, and poor self-care. Occasionally, the medical condition is the only apparent indication of alcohol abuse. Despite this, the patient must come to the same realization as other alcoholic persons: "I just can't drink anymore." Vaillant's (1995) seminal study highlights the fact that medical complications are sometimes the main reason for abstinence. For example, a patient with sickle-cell disease may go into crisis after moderate alcohol consumption, or a patient with epilepsy may have a seizure after moderate alcohol use.

Medical and Other Complications

Common alcohol-related medical conditions include gastritis, pneumonia, liver failure, subdural hematoma, ulcer, pancreatitis, cardiomyopathy, anemia, peripheral neuropathy, fetal alcohol syndrome, Korsakoff's psychosis, and alcoholic dementia. Liver disease is the ninth leading cause of death; alcoholism is a major cause of liver disease. Seventy-five percent of patients with chronic pancreatitis have alcoholism (Van Thiel et al. 1981). Alcohol use also contributes to increased rates of oral cavity, laryngeal, esophageal, and liver cancer (Cole and Rodu 2001).

The total spending for health care services due to alcohol problems and the medical consequences of alcohol consumption was estimated at $22.5 billion for 1995 (National Institute on Drug Abuse and National Institute on Alcohol Abuse and Alcoholism 2001). There is an association between alcohol use and violent crime, including assault, rape, child molestation, attempted murder, and murder. One study of 2,095 trauma victims found that 41% were drinking before their injury (Meyers et al. 1990). Unfortunately, these patients' alcohol problems are underrecognized and undertreated on trauma services and burn units (Bernstein et al. 1992). Orthopedic injuries in alcohol and drug users are more severe and require longer hospitalizations than orthopedic injuries in nonusers (Levy et al. 1996).

Alcoholism, which is strongly associated with suicide, increases suicide rates between 60 and 120 times compared with those in the nonalcoholic population, particularly in synergy with other predisposing factors such as unemployment, impulsivity, or aggression (Caces and Harford 1998; Mann et al. 1999). The lifetime risk of suicide among alcoholic patients is estimated to be 2.0%–3.4% (Murphy and Wetzel 1990). Alcoholic patients who attempt suicide may have more severe alcohol problems and greater comorbidity than those who do not attempt suicide (Murphy et al. 1992). The increased rate of alcohol use among suicide attempters emphasizes the importance of detection, especially because the consultation-liaison psychiatrist often determines whether a patient is discharged after a suicide attempt.

Predisposition and Risk Factors

Alcoholism probably results from a complex interaction among biological vulnerability, family, environment, and culture. Studies involving men and women found that genetic variables significantly influence prevalence, although the mechanism for genetic transmission is unknown (Johnson et al. 1998; Merikangas et al. 1998b). Hypothesized heritable factors include abnormalities in the serotonergic (Lappalainen et al. 1998), dopaminergic (Edenberg et al. 1998), or opioidergic (Wand et al. 1998) systems. Inherited variations in alcohol-metabolizing enzymes, such as those common in Asian populations, confer reduced risk of alcoholism (Schuckit 1999).

In a prospective study, Vaillant (1995) found no personality style to be predictive of alcoholism; however, alcoholism occurs more commonly when other psychiatric disorders, such as somatization disorder, are present. Alcoholic patients are at increased risk in their lifetimes for bipolar disorder, panic disorder, and social phobia but not for non-substance-induced major depressive disorder (Schuckit et al. 1997). In a study involving general hospital patients with borderline personality disorder, 67% had a substance abuse diagnosis (Dulit et al. 1990). Antisocial personality disorder is also associated with alcohol abuse and with poorer treatment outcomes (Kranzler et al. 1996). The interaction between alcohol abuse and anxiety symptoms and anxiety disorders continues to be debated, with different investigators reaching different conclusions (Kopelman 1995; Merikangas et al. 1998a). Alcohol use is also common in patients with schizophrenia, in whom such use may transiently decrease social anxiety, dysphoria, insomnia, and other nonpsychotic but unpleasant experiences; however, alcohol use may also help to explain a poor outcome (Drake et al. 1989; Noordsy et al. 1991).

Intoxication

The effects of alcohol intoxication range from mild inebriation to respiratory depression, coma, and, rarely, death. γ-Aminobutyric acid (GABA)-activated neurotransmission, N-methyl-D-aspartate (NMDA) receptors, and second-messenger systems all mediate physiologic effects (Nestler and Self 1997). Alcohol activates GABA chloride ion channels, inhibits NMDA-activated ion channels, and potentiates 5-HT$_3$-activated ion channels. GABA subunits may change structurally as tolerance and dependence develop. Alcohol may combine with endogenous and exogenous chemicals such as dopamine or cocaine to produce toxic metabolites (Cami et al. 1998).

The body metabolizes alcohol at the rate of 100 mg/kg/hour. Approximately 1.5 hours are required to metabolize one shot of whiskey. Among individuals who have not developed tolerance, BACs of 0.03 mg% can lead to euphoria, 0.05mg% can cause mild coordination problems, and 0.1 mg% usually causes ataxia. Anesthesia, coma, and death are associated with BACs greater than 0.4 mg% (Adams et al. 1997). In chronic heavy drinkers who have developed tolerance, high blood levels are reached with fewer of these effects. The first-pass metabolism of alcohol by gastric tissue is lower in women with alcoholism than in men with alcoholism. This phenomenon may explain the increased bioavailability of alcohol, higher rates of liver cirrhosis, and lower thresholds for intoxication among women (Frezza et al. 1990).

Uncomplicated Withdrawal

In individuals who have developed tolerance, alcohol withdrawal symptoms develop when a relative decrease in blood alcohol levels occurs; therefore, symptoms can occur while drinking continues. A coarse, fast-frequency generalized tremor appears that increases during motor activity or stress (e.g., when the hand or the tongue is extended). The tremor typically peaks 24–48 hours after the last drink and subsides after 5–7 days of abstinence. Patients also often show signs of autonomic hyperactivity, including increased blood pressure, heart rate greater than 100 beats/minute, sweating, malaise, nausea, vomiting, anxiety, and disturbed sleep.

Histories are usually difficult to obtain during medical emergencies. A patient who is not suspected of having alcohol dependence often suddenly develops withdrawal symptoms 3 days after surgery. It is sometimes difficult to distinguish withdrawal from other postsurgical complications. Medical conditions such as infections and hypertension or treatments such as propranolol or clonidine therapy often alter vital signs, confusing the clinical picture. In addition, patients frequently receive benzodiazepines for preoperative insomnia or anxiety. These as-needed doses may mask or delay autonomic symptoms of withdrawal but not eliminate the potential for serious delayed withdrawal complications. In addition, the patient is sometimes so seriously ill that the possibility of withdrawal is not considered. The Clinical Institute Withdrawal Assessment for Alcohol–Revised (CIWA-Ar)

is a valuable clinical scale that helps the clinician quantify withdrawal and follow symptoms over time (Sullivan et al. 1991) (see Figure 21–1). Biological studies have suggested the occurrence of hypothalamic-pituitary-adrenal axis dysfunction (Adinoff et al. 1991) and hyperexcitability of NMDA receptors (Tsai and Coyle 1998) during alcohol withdrawal; in addition, decreased regional brain metabolism has been measured by positron-emission tomography (Volkow et al. 1997).

Withdrawal Seizures

Withdrawal seizures typically occur 7–38 hours after last alcohol use, with peak frequency at approximately 24 hours (Adams et al. 1997). Ten percent of patients with chronic alcoholism experience multiple seizures (Espir and Rose 1987). Hypomagnesemia, respiratory alkalosis, hypoglycemia, increased intracellular sodium concentration, and upregulation of NMDA receptors all potentially contribute to alcohol withdrawal seizures. One-third of patients who have withdrawal seizures develops alcohol withdrawal delirium.

Withdrawal Delirium (Delirium Tremens)

Delirium tremens (DT) is characterized by confusion, disorientation, fluctuating or clouded consciousness, and perceptual disturbances. Typical signs and symptoms include delusions, vivid hallucinations, agitation, insomnia, mild fever, and marked autonomic arousal. Patients frequently report vivid visual hallucinations of insects or small animals or other perceptual distortions; these hallucinations are associated with feelings of terror and agitation. Symptoms of DT usually appear 2–3 days after cessation of heavy drinking, with peak intensity on the fourth to fifth day. Patients often show a repetitive pattern of DT each time they withdraw from alcohol (Turner et al. 1989). Withdrawal symptoms, which can wax and wane, usually subside after 3 days of adequate treatment. Untreated DT can last as long as 4–5 weeks. Compared with other alcoholic patients, those with a history of DT or withdrawal seizures report a greater maximum number of drinks per day, more lifetime withdrawal episodes, more sedative-hypnotic abuse, and a greater number of medical problems (Schuckit et al. 1995). DT occurs more frequently and is particularly dangerous in patients who have infections, subdural hematomas, trauma, liver disease, or metabolic disorder. Palmstierna (2001) reported that of 334 alcohol-dependent patients presenting with alcohol withdrawal, 6.9% developed delirium tremens despite benzodiazepine treatment. All of the patients developing delirium tremens

Patient _____ Date ____/____/____ Time __:__
                          Y   M   D   (24-hour clock, midnight = 00:00)

Pulse or heart rate, taken for 1 minute: _____ Blood pressure _____/_____

NAUSEA AND VOMITING—Ask "Do you feel sick to your stomach? Have you vomited?" Observation.
0 No nausea and no vomiting
1 Mild nausea with no vomiting
2
3
4 Intermittent nausea with dry heaves
5
6
7 Constant nausea, frequent dry heaves, and vomiting

TREMOR—Arms extended and fingers spread apart. Observation.
0 No tremor
1 Not visible but can be felt fingertip to fingertip
2
3
4 Moderate, with patient's arms extended
5
6
7 Severe, even with arms not extended

PAROXYSMAL SWEATS—Observation.
0 No tremor
1 Barely perceptible sweating, palms moist
2
3
4 Beads of sweat obvious on forehead
5
6
7 Drenching sweats

ANXIETY—Ask "Do you feel nervous?" Observation.
0 No anxiety, at ease
1 Mildly anxious
2
3
4 Moderately anxious, or guarded, so anxiety is inferred
5
6
7 Equivalent to acute panic states as seen in severe delirium or acute schizophrenic reactions

AGITATION—Observation.
0 Normal activity
1 Somewhat more than normal activity
2
3
4 Moderately fidgety and restless
5
6
7 Paces back and forth during most of the interview, or constantly thrashes about

TACTILE DISTURBANCES—Ask "Have you any itching, any pins and needles sensations, any burning, any numbness, or do you feel bugs crawling on or under your skin?" Observation.
0 None
1 Very mild itching, pins and needles, burning, or numbness
2 Mild itching, pins and needles, burning, or numbness
3 Moderate itching, pins and needles, burning, or numbness
4 Moderately severe hallucinations
5 Severe hallucinations
6 Extremely severe hallucinations
7 Continuous hallucinations

AUDITORY DISTURBANCES—Ask "Are you more aware of sounds around you? Are they harsh? Do they frighten you? Are you hearing anything that is disturbing to you? Are you hearing things you know are not there?" Observation.
0 Not present
1 Very mild harshness or ability to frighten
2 Mild harshness or ability to frighten
3 Moderate harshness or ability to frighten
4 Moderately severe hallucinations
5 Severe hallucinations
6 Extremely severe hallucinations
7 Continuous hallucinations

VISUAL DISTURBANCES—Ask "Does the light appear to be too bright? Is its color different? Does it hurt your eyes? Are you seeing anything that is disturbing to you? Are you seeing things you know are not there?" Observation.
0 Not present
1 Very mild sensitivity
2 Mild sensitivity
3 Moderate sensitivity
4 Moderately severe hallucinations
5 Severe hallucinations
6 Extremely severe hallucinations
7 Continuous hallucinations

FIGURE 21–1. Addiction Research Foundation Clinical Institute Withdrawal Assessment for Alcohol—Revised (CIWA-Ar).

HEADACHE, FULLNESS IN HEAD—Ask "Does your head feel different? Does it feel like there is a band around your head?" Do not rate for dizziness or light-headedness. Otherwise, rate severity.
0   Not present
1   Very mild
2   Mild
3   Moderate
4   Moderately severe
5   Severe
6   Very severe
7   Extremely severe

ORIENTATION AND CLOUDING OF SENSORIUM—Ask "What day is this? Where are you? Who am I?"
0   Oriented and can do serial additions
1   Cannot do serial additions or is uncertain about date
2   Disoriented for date by no more than 2 calendar days
3   Disoriented for date by more than 2 calendar days
4   Disoriented for place and/or person

Total CIWA-Ar score _____

Rater's initials _____

Maximum possible score 67

FIGURE 21–1.   Addiction Research Foundation Clinical Institute Withdrawal Assessment for Alcohol—Revised (CIWA-Ar) *(continued)*.

Source.   Reprinted from Sullivan JT, Swift RM, Lewis DC: "Benzodiazepine Requirements During Alcohol Withdrawal Syndrome: Clinical Implications of Using a Standardized Withdrawal Scale." *Journal of Clinical Psychopharmacology* 11:291–295, 1991.

had the following five risk factors: 1) current infectious disease, 2) heart rate >120 beats per minute on admission, 3) withdrawal symptoms despite a Breathalyzer alcohol concentration >1 gram per liter body fluid, 4) history of seizures, and 5) history of delirious episodes. In the hospital, physical restraints and 24-hour sitters are sometimes needed to protect the patient and to ensure that intravenous lines are maintained.

Alcohol-Induced Psychotic Disorder

Chronic alcohol hallucinosis, designated *alcohol-induced psychotic disorder* in DSM-IV-TR, is defined as vivid auditory hallucinations that last at least 1 week and occur shortly after the cessation or reduction of heavy alcohol ingestion. The hallucinosis presents with a clear sensorium and few autonomic signs or symptoms. The hallucinations sometimes include familiar noises or clear voices; the patient usually responds to these hallucinations with fear, anxiety, and agitation (Victor 1992). Diagnosis is based on a history of recent heavy alcohol use and the absence of schizophrenia or mania.

Alcohol-Induced Persisting Amnestic Disorder

Alcohol-induced persisting amnestic disorder (Wernicke-Korsakoff syndrome) begins with an abrupt onset of truncal ataxia, ophthalmoplegia, and delirium (Wernicke's encephalopathy). Brew (1986) recommended that the clinician not require all three signs; the presence of two suggests a form of the disorder. The etiology of the disorder is thiamine deficiency due to dietary, medical, or other factors. Thiamine deficiency may cause death or, more commonly, a persisting severe anterograde amnesia

(Korsakoff's psychosis) in which memory is not transferred from immediate to long-term memory storage. Approximately 80% of patients with Wernicke's encephalopathy who are treated and survive develop this persisting amnesia (Reuler et al. 1985). Postmortem examinations show lesions in the brain stem, diencephalon, and frontal lobes (Kopelman 1995).

Neurological Disease

Alcohol-induced dementia is another example of a neuropsychiatric disorder found in patients with chronic alcoholism. Because alcoholic patients have complicated medical histories and are often poor historians, the diagnosis is often presumptive. Other nervous system disorders associated with chronic alcoholism include polyneuropathies, hepatic encephalopathy, acute or chronic subdural hematoma, and cerebellar degeneration with truncal ataxia. Rare conditions such as central pontine myelinolysis, Marchiafava-Bignami disease, and nutritional amblyopia also occur.

Liver Disease

Alcohol has direct toxic effects on the liver (Lieber 1988). Alcohol dehydrogenase, a liver enzyme, metabolizes alcohol to toxic acetaldehyde. Aldehyde dehydrogenase completes the transformation of acetaldehyde to acetic acid; lactic acid, uric acid, and fat accumulation are by-products in this process. In addition, alcoholic hepatitis can cause cirrhosis or death. Inflammation and liver cell destruction kill 10%–30% of patients who develop cirrhosis. The only definitive way to diagnose alcohol-induced cirrhosis is by liver biopsy. Hepatitis C may accelerate liver damage caused by alcohol consumption.

Liver and Kidney Transplantation

Despite early bias against liver transplantations in alcoholic patients, approximately 30% of the 3,000 orthotopic liver transplantations in the United States each year are performed in patients with alcoholism. There is reliable evidence that properly screened alcoholic patients rarely return to drinking and also have rates of survival and a quality of life comparable to those of nonalcoholic patients (DiMartini et al. 1998; Lucey et al. 1997).

Consultation-liaison psychiatrists often participate in transplantation evaluation and selection (see also Chapter 28). The psychiatrist does not typically recommend or discourage a transplantation but rather assesses what treatments are needed before and after transplantation. The psychiatric evaluation should include consideration of history of drinking, insight into illness, family insight and support, willingness to consider treatment, social stability, and long-term sobriety predictors such as substitute activities and a sense of hope (Roggla et al. 1996; Tringali et al. 1996). The consultation-liaison psychiatrist must also know the pharmacokinetics and pharmacodynamics of medications administered to patients with liver dysfunction (Trzepacz et al. 1993a, 1993b). Hepatic metabolism is dependent on the amount of blood flow to the liver and the capacity of hepatic enzymes. Cirrhosis decreases the activity and levels of hepatic enzymes, including the cytochrome P450 system. Decreased albumin concentrations, common in alcoholic patients with liver disease, increase the bioavailability of most psychotropic drugs. In patients with impaired liver function, the doses of hepatically metabolized medications are usually decreased; blood levels should be monitored whenever possible.

Several specific psychotropic medication issues exist with regard to patients with liver impairment. Ascites reduce lithium levels because of expanded spaces for water-soluble medications. Nefazodone and fluvoxamine increase levels of cyclosporine because these drugs inhibit the cytochrome P450 3A4 enzyme. The psychiatric consultant must also be familiar with the neuropsychiatric side effects of cyclosporine, corticosteroids, OKT3, FK-506, interferon, antibiotics, and acyclovir (see Chapter 28).

Interaction Between Alcohol and Medications

The interaction between alcohol and medications can have a wide range of effects (i.e., from lethal overdoses to undermedication; Table 21–4). Alcohol is partly metabolized through the hepatic microsomal enzyme system that metabolizes other drugs. Acutely, alcohol can slow metabolism and increase blood levels of medications, such as oral anticoagulants, diazepam, and phenytoin, which compete for cytochrome P450 enzymes. Chronically, because of cytochrome P450 enzyme induction, alcohol can lead to increased metabolism and decreased blood levels of these medications. Chronic alcohol intake can also lead to acetaminophen toxicity as a result of accumulation of toxic metabolites (Table 21–5).

Conversely, some medications can influence alcohol's metabolism. For example, chlorpromazine, chloral hydrate, and cimetidine increase blood alcohol levels by inhibiting alcohol dehydrogenase. Alcohol enhances diazepam absorption, which decreases its safety margin and increases the possibility of overdose. In addition, alcohol increases the potency of other central nervous system (CNS) depressants, such as narcotics and antihistamines, and has unpredictable effects when used with CNS stimulants. Mild disulfiram-like reactions can occur with oral hypoglycemics (e.g., tolbutamide, chlorpropamide), griseofulvin, metronidazole, and quinacrine. Continued use of salicylates and alcohol can lead to gastrointestinal bleeding. Because some alcoholic beverages contain tyramine, monoamine oxidase inhibitors are best avoided in the treatment of active or recovering alcoholic patients.

Physical Examination and Laboratory Testing

Spider nevi, palmar erythema, cigarette burns between the index and middle fingers, poor dental care, jaundice, enlarged liver, abdominal pain, peripheral neuropathy, and muscle weakness are clinical signs of alcoholism. When alcoholic patients present as severely intoxicated, semicomatose, or comatose, head injuries such as subdural hematoma, metabolic conditions such as hypoglycemia, diabetic coma, or hepatic encephalopathy, and other disorders such as cardiac arrhythmia, myasthenia, or polydrug intoxication can be ruled out.

Serum γ-glutamyltransferase (SGGT) levels are increased in more than 50% of patients who have an alcohol problem and in 80% of alcoholic patients with liver dysfunction (Trell et al. 1984); aspartate aminotransferase (AST) levels are increased in 46% of patients with alcoholism. Decreased white blood cell counts and increased mean corpuscular volume and uric acid, triglyceride, alanine aminotransferase (ALT), and urea levels are also common in alcoholism. In patients with advanced cirrhosis, liver function is sometimes normal; however, prothrombin time is prolonged. One-third of patients with alcoholism have increased blood glucose levels. It is

TABLE 21–4.   Effects of medication interactions with alcohol

Medication	Effects
Disulfiram (Antabuse)	Flushing, diaphoresis, vomiting, confusion
Anticoagulants (oral)	Increased anticoagulation effect with acute alcohol intoxication, decreased effect after chronic alcohol use
Griseofulvin	Minor Antabuse reactions
Tranquilizers, narcotics, antihistamines	Increased central nervous system depression
Diazepam	Increased absorption of diazepam
Phenytoin	Increased anticonvulsant effect with acute intoxication; after chronic alcohol abuse, alcohol intoxication or withdrawal may lower seizure threshold
Salicylates	Gastrointestinal bleeding
Chlorpromazine	Increased levels of alcohol
Monoamine oxidase inhibitors	Adverse reactions to tyramine in some alcoholic beverages

Source. Adapted from Franklin JE Jr, Frances RJ: "Alcohol and Other Psychoactive Substance Use Disorders," in *The American Psychiatric Press Textbook of Psychiatry*, 3rd Edition. Edited by Hales RE, Yudofsky SC, Talbott JA. Washington, DC, American Psychiatric Press, 1999, p. 372. Used with permission.

TABLE 21–5.   Alcohol effects on cytochrome P450 enzymes

Acute users
Slows P450 metabolism; therefore, increases levels of medications dependent on system for metabolism

Chronic users
Increases P450 metabolism; therefore, decreases levels of medications dependent on P450 metabolism or increases toxic metabolites (e.g., increases acetaminophen toxic metabolites)

TABLE 21–6.   Laboratory findings associated with alcohol abuse

Alcohol present in blood

Positive Breathalyzer test results

Increased mean corpuscular volume

Increased aspartate aminotransferase (AST), alanine aminotransferase (ALT), and lactate dehydrogenase levels

Increased serum γ-glutamyltransferase (SGGT) levels (particularly sensitive)

Increased serum carbohydrate-deficient transferrin levels

Decreased albumin, vitamin B_{12}, and folic acid levels

Increased uric acid and amylase levels, evidence of bone marrow suppression

Prolonged prothrombin time (cirrhosis)

Source. Adapted from Frances RJ, Franklin JE Jr: *Concise Guide to Treatment of Alcoholism and Addictions.* Washington, DC, American Psychiatric Press, 1989, p. 74. Used with permission.

not uncommon for alcoholic patients with inadequate calorie intake to have decreased blood glucose levels and mild hypertension (Table 21–6).

The search for reliable markers of recent heavy alcohol use led to the finding that both the total amount of carbohydrate-deficient transferrin and the ratio of carbohydrate-deficient transferrin to total serum transferrin can help identify heavy alcohol use over time. Stowell et al. (1997) found the test to be approximately 80% sensitive and 90% specific in detecting chronic consumption of more than 60 g of alcohol daily in a population of male drinkers. Although results may be influenced by tobacco use, age, sex, and other factors (Stowell et al. 1997; Whitfield et al. 1998), the test may be a useful monitor for relapse in men and women, particularly when combined with measurement of SGGT concentrations (Allen et al. 1999, 2001; Anton et al. 1998).

Screening Tests

Two widely used brief screening tests to detect alcoholism are the self-administered Michigan Alcoholism Screening Test (MAST) (Figure 21–2) and the clinician-administered CAGE questionnaire (Table 21–7). The MAST is a 25-question form that is 90% sensitive; the CAGE is a 4-item test. The 5-question TWEAK and the 10-question AUDIT have been found to be more useful in women and ethnically diverse populations than the CAGE (Bradley et al. 1998; Steinbauer et al. 1998). The addiction severity index (ASI) is a treatment planning assessment tool that examines seven areas of patient functioning, including drug and alcohol abuse (McLellan et al. 1980). A review of the various screening instruments is available on-line through the Center for Substance Abuse Treatment, Treatment Improvement Protocol series (Center for Substance Abuse Treatment 2001).

Points			Yes	No
	0.	Do you enjoy a drink now and then?		
(2)	1.	Do you feel you are a normal drinker? (By normal we mean you drink less than or as much as most people.)	_____	_____
(2)	2.	Have you ever awakened in the morning after some drinking the night before and found that you could not remember part of the evening?	_____	_____
(1)	3.	Does your wife, husband, a parent, or other near relative ever worry or complain about your drinking?	_____	_____
(2)	4.	Can you stop drinking without a struggle after one or two drinks?	_____	_____
(1)	5.	Do you ever feel guilty about your drinking?	_____	_____
(2)	6.	Do friends and relatives think you are a normal drinker?	_____	_____
(0)	7.	Do you ever try to limit your drinking to certain times of the day or to certain places?	_____	_____
(2)	8.	Have you ever attended a meeting of Alcoholics Anonymous?	_____	_____
(1)	9.	Have you gotten into physical fights when drinking?	_____	_____
(2)	10.	Has your drinking ever created problems between you and your wife, husband, a parent, or other relative?	_____	_____
(2)	11.	Has your wife, husband, or other family members ever gone to anyone for help about your drinking?	_____	_____
(2)	12.	Have you ever lost friends because of your drinking?	_____	_____
(2)	13.	Have you ever gotten into trouble at work or school because you were drinking?	_____	_____
(2)	14.	Have you ever lost a job because of drinking?	_____	_____
(2)	15.	Have you ever neglected your obligations, your family, or your work for two or more days in a row because you were drinking?	_____	_____
(1)	16.	Do you drink before noon fairly often?	_____	_____
(2)	17.	Have you ever been told you have liver trouble?	_____	_____
		Cirrhosis?	_____	_____
(2)[a]	18.	After heavy drinking, have you ever had delirium tremens (DT) or severe shaking, or heard voices or seen things that really weren't there?	_____	_____
(5)	19.	Have you ever gone to anyone for help about your drinking?	_____	_____
(5)	20.	Have you ever been in a hospital because of your drinking?	_____	_____
(2)	21.	Have you ever been a patient in a psychiatric hospital or on a psychiatric ward of a general hospital where drinking was part of the problem that resulted in hospitalization?	_____	_____
(2)	22.	Have you ever been seen at a psychiatric or mental health clinic or gone to a doctor, social worker, or clergyperson for help with an emotional problem in which drinking played a part?	_____	_____
(2)[b]	23.	Have you ever been arrested for drunk driving, driving while intoxicated, or driving under the influence of alcoholic beverages? (If YES, how many times? _____)	_____	_____
(2)[b]	24.	Have you ever been arrested, or taken into custody, even for a few hours, because of other drunk behavior? (If YES, how many times? _____)	_____	_____

[a]5 points for delirium tremens
[b]2 points for *each* arrest

SCORING SYSTEM: In general, five points or more would place that subject in an "alcoholic" category. Four points would suggest alcoholism; three points or less would indicate the subject was not alcoholic. Programs using the above scoring system find it very sensitive at the five-point level, and it tends to find more people alcoholics than anticipated. However, it is a screening test and should be sensitive at its lower levels.

FIGURE 21–2.   Michigan Alcoholism Screening Test (MAST).

Source.   Adapted from Franklin JE Jr, Frances RJ: "Alcohol and Other Psychoactive Substance Use Disorders," in *The American Psychiatric Press Textbook of Psychiatry*, 3rd Edition. Edited by Hales RE, Yudofsky SC, Talbott JA. Washington, DC, American Psychiatric Press, 1999, p. 370. Used with permission.

TABLE 21–7. CAGE screen for diagnosis of alcoholism

Have you ever

C   Thought you should CUT back on your drinking?

A   Felt ANNOYED by people criticizing your drinking?

G   Felt GUILTY or bad about your drinking?

E   Had a morning EYE-OPENER to relieve hangover or nerves?

Note.   Two or three positive responses = high index of suspicion; four positive responses = pathognomonic.

Source.   Reprinted from Ewing JA: "Detecting Alcoholism: The CAGE Questionnaire." *Journal of the American Medical Association* 252:1905–1907, 1984. Copyright 1984, American Medical Association. Used with permission.

Acute Management and Treatment

Intoxication

The behavior associated with intoxication is managed by decreasing external stimuli, interrupting alcohol ingestion, and protecting individuals from harming themselves and others until the toxic effects of alcohol disappear. Consultation-liaison psychiatrists are rarely called to see an acutely intoxicated patient, unless he or she is in an emergency room. In cases of potentially fatal overdoses, hemodialysis is sometimes attempted; otherwise, careful observation is all that is needed.

Withdrawal

Usually, the choice of inpatient versus outpatient treatment for withdrawal depends on the severity of symptoms, the stage of withdrawal, medical and psychiatric complications, the presence of polysubstance abuse, patient cooperation, the ability to follow instructions, social support systems, patient history, and, increasingly, insurance or managed care reimbursement policies. Consultation requests often involve patients whose withdrawal symptoms have been only partially eliminated during detoxification or patients who are not yet beyond danger of serious medical complications. Rapid transfer or admission to a psychiatric or addictions unit is often the referring physician's goal; rapid discharge is usually the patient's goal. The managed care system often insists on the least expensive alternative. It is useful to acknowledge these conflicting goals.

In a study involving 487 hospitalized alcohol-dependent patients, Benzer (1990) found that only 10.6% had withdrawal symptoms severe enough to require medication. Regardless of the medications requested on the doctor's order sheet, the nurse's medication log is the only reliable source to determine which medications a patient has actually received. Full detoxification, a mod-

ified detoxification schedule, or as-needed medication is used depending on the severity of dependence, medical condition, detoxification history, vital signs, and mental status. In alcoholic patients with histories of withdrawal seizures or complicated withdrawals or with other serious medical conditions, full medical detoxification should proceed; as-needed medications alone should not be relied on in these patients (Table 21–8).

TABLE 21–8. General principles of medical alcohol detoxification

Prevent complications of withdrawal, and increase patient comfort.

Select a cross-tolerant medication that has a longer half-life during tapering.

Know that clonazepam is useful in hospital settings because of self-tapering (Note: effective for alprazolam detoxification).

Select an intermediate-half-life benzodiazepine, such as lorazepam, for patients who are very sick, have compromised liver function, or are elderly (i.e., for patients who do not use long-half-life benzodiazepines).

Note that if lorazepam is used to manage withdrawal, it must be tapered (i.e., it does not self-taper).

Give explicit instructions to medical staff regarding signs and symptoms of withdrawal and medication schedule.

Adjust medications based on signs and symptoms; allow some flexibility in protocol.

Avoid as-needed dosing alone when detoxification is clearly needed (e.g., in patients with chronic severe use or history of withdrawal complications).

Avoid clonidine and propranolol, which mask symptoms and signs of withdrawal.

Although nonpharmacological inpatient treatment is sometimes used in patients with uncomplicated withdrawal (Hayashida et al. 1989), pharmacological treatment of withdrawal symptoms relieves discomfort and prevents complications such as seizures and DT. Some evidence suggests that repeated withdrawal may hasten cognitive decline, possibly mediated by high levels of cortisol (Linnoila 1989), and lead to subsequent more severe withdrawals. Safe detoxification occurs when patients' autonomic signs and symptoms are adequately controlled. Sedation is a clinically useful indicator for adequate treatment in early withdrawal.

Benzodiazepines are recommended for the treatment and prevention of withdrawal symptoms (Mayo-Smith 1997). Benzodiazepines are safe, are easy to administer (orally, intramuscularly, or intravenously), have anticonvulsant properties, and are efficacious. Diazepam and chlordiazepoxide are commonly used. Benzodiazepines such as lorazepam or oxazepam should be used in patients with severe liver disease and elderly patients, because these drugs are metabolized via conjugation versus oxidation; otherwise, no clear differences in efficacy have been found among benzodiazepines. Lorazepam is better absorbed intramuscularly than are other benzodiazepines. The benzodiazepines with longer half-lives, such as chlordiazepoxide or diazepam, may require less frequent administration. There may be relevant cost differences among the medications.

Candidates for outpatient detoxification should have good social supports, be highly motivated, and be able to make daily clinic visits during the withdrawal period. For outpatient treatment of alcohol withdrawal, a long-acting benzodiazepine is given orally and tapered

(Table 21–9). For example, 50 mg of chlordiazepoxide may be prescribed orally four times a day for four doses, followed by 25 mg orally for eight doses. When possible, inpatient withdrawal should follow a symptom-triggered medication protocol, using a standardized withdrawal rating scale, such as the CIWA-Ar (Figure 21–1 and Table 21–9). Ward staff must be trained in using such scales, but withdrawal will generally be faster and require less medication with the use of the scales (Saitz et al. 1994). The patient is observed for signs of agitation, tremulousness, or increased vital signs. Environmental stimulation should be avoided, frequent orientation should be provided, and a nonjudgmental approach should be taken.

TABLE 21–9.   Pharmacological management of alcohol withdrawal

Monitoring

Monitor the patient every 4–8 hours using the Clinical Institute Withdrawal Assessment for Alcohol–Revised (CIWA-Ar) until the score has been below 8–10 for 24 hours; perform further assessments as needed.

Symptom-triggered medication regimens

Administer one of the following medications every hour when the CIWA-Ar score is ≥8–10:

  Chlordiazepoxide (50–100 mg po)

  Diazepam (10–20 mg po)

  Oxazepam (30–60 mg po)

  Lorazepam (2–4 mg po)

Other benzodiazepines or routes of administration may be used at equivalent substitutions.

Repeat the CIWA-Ar 1 hour after every dose, to assess the need for further medication.

Structured medication regimens

In certain patients (e.g., patients experiencing myocardial infarction), it may be desirable to prevent even mild to moderate withdrawal, and medication therefore might be ordered to be given on a predetermined schedule. One of the following regimens could be used in such circumstances:

  Chlordiazepoxide 50 mg po every 6 hours for four doses, then 25 mg every 6 hours for eight doses

  Diazepam 10 mg po every 6 hours for four doses, then 5 mg every 6 hours for eight doses

  Lorazepam 2 mg po every 6 hours for four doses, then 1 mg every 6 hours for eight doses

Other benzodiazepines or routes of administration may be used at equivalent substitutions.

Patients receiving medication on a predetermined schedule must be monitored closely, and additional medication must be provided if the scheduled doses prove inadequate to control symptoms.

Structured regimens are also more commonly used for withdrawal management in the outpatient setting.

Agitation

For the patient with increasing agitation or hallucinations that have not improved with oral benzodiazepines alone, one of the following medications may be used:

  Haloperidol (2–5 mg im) alone or in combination with lorazepam (2–4 mg)

  Intravenous diazepam, given slowly every 5 minutes until the patient is lightly sedated. Begin with 5 mg for two doses, increase to 10 mg for two doses, if needed, and then administer 20 mg every 5 minutes. (Given the risk of respiratory depression, the patient should be closely monitored, with equipment for respiratory support immediately available.)

Source.   Adapted from Mayo-Smith MF: "Management of Alcohol Intoxication and Withdrawal," in *Principles of Addiction Medicine*, 2nd Edition. Edited by Graham AW, Schultz TK. Chevy Chase, MD, American Society of Addiction Medicine, Inc., 1998, p. 437

Nutritional deficiencies of thiamine, vitamin B$_{12}$, and folic acid should be corrected with oral thiamine (100 mg/day), folic acid (1 mg/day orally for 5 days), daily multivitamins, and adequate nutrition. Clinicians should administer thiamine 100–200 mg intramuscularly or intravenously for 3 days in cases of very poor nutrition; thiamine should be given before glucose infusion, because glucose depletes thiamine stores. Patients with histories of alcohol withdrawal seizures should receive intramuscular magnesium sulfate, 1 g/2 mL (50% solution) four times a day for 2 days. When sweating, fever, or vomiting causes severe dehydration, attention to rehydration and electrolyte replacement is essential.

Patients with a history of epilepsy may require additional anticonvulsant medication. However, for uncomplicated withdrawal seizures, adding anticonvulsants to benzodiazepines is not always necessary (D'Onofrio et al. 1999). Diazepam, 10 mg iv, usually inhibits status epilepticus; however, the addition of phenytoin is occasionally necessary (Table 21–10).

Alcohol-Induced Psychotic Disorder

When patients develop alcohol hallucinosis during detoxification, a potent antipsychotic such as haloperidol, 2–5 mg orally twice a day, is typically needed to control agitation and hallucinations. The clinician should reassess the use of medications shortly after cessation of symptoms; continued administration of neuroleptics is seldom needed (Table 21–11).

TABLE 21–10.   Diagnosis and treatment of alcohol seizures

Diagnosis

Alcohol can lower seizure threshold

Withdrawal lowers seizure threshold ("rum fit")

Underlying trauma (e.g., subdural hematoma)

Combinations of above

Idiopathic seizure

Electroencephalography may identify seizure focus

Seizures often herald delirium tremens (Note: 50% develop delirium tremens)

10% of seizures present as status epilepticus (Note: 10% develop status epilepticus)

Treatment

Diazepam 10 mg iv, repeat as necessary

Phenytoin loading if necessary; phenytoin should not be continued for maintenance after an uncomplicated alcohol seizure

For high seizure risk, 1 mg magnesium sulfate im every 6 hours for 2 days or 2 mL iv in 50% solution

---

Wernicke's Encephalopathy and Persistent Amnesia

Wernicke's encephalopathy should be treated with parenteral thiamine, 100 mg every hour, with titration upward until ophthalmoplegia has resolved; this usually prevents progression. Ophthalmoplegia usually responds fairly quickly; truncal ataxia may persist. Thiamine is always given before glucose loading.

Long-Term Management

Disulfiram is an important treatment adjunct for many patients with alcoholism. It provides an added buffer between the impulse to drink and alcohol use. However, consultation-liaison psychiatrists rarely recommend starting disulfiram therapy in the general hospital patient. Contraindications to disulfiram use include severe liver disease, pregnancy, heart disease, and psychosis. Disulfiram also is associated with important drug-drug interactions (e.g., it increases levels of phenytoin and isoniazid). A well-controlled, double-blind study of disulfiram raised questions about its effectiveness (R. K. Fuller et al. 1986). However, it has utility in selected patients and needs to be given in higher doses in some patients.

Naltrexone has been shown to reduce the risk of relapse to heavy drinking in alcohol-dependent patients (Garbutt et al. 1999). The usual dosage is 50 mg orally once a day; in patients with polysubstance dependence, the dose may need to be increased (Oslin et al. 1999). Side effects include headache, nausea, and mild dysphoria and can be minimized by starting with a dosage of 25 mg and proceeding slowly. For obvious reasons, naltrexone cannot be used in patients receiving opiate analgesics. Medication compliance significantly affects efficacy. Kranzler et al. (1998) have performed preliminary investigations of an injectable, sustained-release form of naltrexone.

Calcium acetylhomotaurinate (acamprosate) is a GABA analogue that has effects on multiple neurotransmitter systems, particularly glutamatergic and GABA-ergic receptors (Wilde and Wagstaff 1997). In multiple European studies, it has been shown to be useful for improving treatment retention (which also may be an important aspect of naltrexone effectiveness), reducing the risk of relapse and increasing abstinence rates (Pelc et al. 1997; Sass et al. 1996; Whitworth et al. 1996). Available in several countries in Europe, the drug is currently undergoing clinical trials in the United States.

Treatment Outcome

Approximately one-third of patients with alcoholism stop drinking without formal treatment intervention,

TABLE 21–11. Alcohol-induced disorders

Disorder	Onset	Treatment
Alcohol intoxication	Depends on tolerance, amount ingested, and amount absorbed	Time; protective environment; hemodialysis can be attempted in potentially fatal overdoses
Alcohol withdrawal	Several hours after cessation or a significant decrease in usual amount consumed; peak symptoms 24–48 hours after last drink	Refer to Table 21–8
Alcohol seizures	6–48 hours after cessation of alcohol use	Diazepam 10 mg iv if seizures do not cease; phenytoin load if multiple seizures; prevent seizures by benzodiazepine detoxification
Alcohol withdrawal delirium (DT)	Gradual onset 2–3 days after cessation of alcohol use; peak intensity at 4–5 days; may fluctuate over several weeks	Benzodiazepine detoxification; low-dose antipsychotic (e.g., haloperidol 2–5 mg orally twice daily) for psychotic symptoms
Alcohol hallucinosis	Usually within 48 hours of last drink; may last several weeks	Low-dose antipsychotic (e.g., haloperidol 2–5 mg orally twice daily)
Wernicke's encephalopathy	Abrupt onset; ataxia may precede mental confusion	Thiamine 100 mg iv; should be given before glucose loading

Source. Adapted from Franklin JE Jr, Frances RJ: "Alcohol and Other Psychoactive Substance Use Disorders," in *The American Psychiatric Press Textbook of Psychiatry*, 3rd Edition. Edited by Hales RE, Yudofsky SC, Talbott JA. Washington, DC, American Psychiatric Press, 1999, p. 377. Used with permission.

one-third improve with treatment, and one-third never achieve sobriety. Patients who are simply handed lists of community-based substance abuse facilities rarely follow through with treatment. The challenge for the consultation-liaison psychiatrist is to fill the cracks in the medical system through which patients fall and to increase patients' motivation for treatment.

SEDATIVE-, HYPNOTIC-, AND ANXIOLYTIC-RELATED DISORDERS

Anxiety is a very common symptom or complaint among hospitalized and medically ill patients. Benzodiazepines are a mainstay in the management of acute anxiety in hospitalized patients. In addition, benzodiazepines are regularly ordered (prn) for sleep. Because sedative use is so frequent in hospitalized patients, the detection of sedative abuse can be quite difficult.

Abuse rarely starts as a result of treatment for acute anxiety or insomnia in a hospitalized patient. The risk of sedative abuse in chronically medically ill outpatients is far greater. There are three major classes of benzodiazepine abusers: polysubstance abusers, pure sedative abusers, and therapeutic users who have lost control. Individuals prone to polysubstance abuse tend to use sedatives for their calming effects (i.e., to come down after use of a stimulant such as cocaine) and for their ability to decrease dysphoric affects, including anxiety, or to potentiate euphoric effects of other drug classes (e.g.,

benzodiazepines are used in combination with methadone to boost euphoria).

Pure sedative abusers usually have significant underlying psychopathology, and relapse is common. In a long-term follow-up study involving subjects with primary sedative-hypnotic dependence, 46% continued to abuse drugs after in-hospital rehabilitation treatment (Allgulander et al. 1987). Any individual can develop dependence with low-dose use over several years or high-dose use over weeks to months (Dietch 1983). Patients with a history of substance abuse are at increased risk for benzodiazepine abuse. In addition, children of alcoholic individuals may respond differently to benzodiazepines than control subjects and may be more prone to benzodiazepine abuse (Ciraulo et al. 1996).

Medical and Other Complications

Other sedative-hypnotics can cause intoxication, withdrawal, withdrawal delirium, and amnestic disorder, as can alcohol. Because the half-life of most benzodiazepines is much longer than that of alcohol, withdrawal symptoms are delayed. For example, withdrawal symptoms occur 7–10 days after abrupt cessation of diazepam. Seizures may herald withdrawal and are a potential complication of high-dose, unexpected, or poorly managed benzodiazepine withdrawal. Severe withdrawal can produce anxiety and psychosis and may possibly result in death from cardiovascular collapse. Cognitive deficits are not uncommon with benzodiazepine abuse and may improve or may persist for months after detoxification

(Tonne et al. 1995). In one study involving more than 4,000 insured patients age 65 years or older, more than 9% had been treated with benzodiazepines in the preceding year, and benzodiazepine use was associated with impaired functional status, independent of age and other medical conditions (Ried et al. 1998).

The high-potency benzodiazepine flunitrazepam has been used illegally to incapacitate women for the purpose of sexual assault. The drug can induce anterograde amnesia. Consultation-liaison psychiatrists should suspect covert flunitrazepam intoxication in sexual assault victims who are amnestic for the assault (Anglin et al. 1997).

Prevention and Acute Management

Preventing habituation to sedative-hypnotic drugs is the best prevention of abuse and dependence. Limited prescriptions, single-source policies (i.e., obtaining all benzodiazepine prescriptions from one provider), and appropriate follow-up are necessary. Generally, benzodiazepines are used to treat specific symptoms, are used only for short periods, and are avoided in patients with alcoholism and those with a history of substance abuse. In people recovering from anxiety disorders, benzodiazepines should be tried only after behavioral and other pharmacological treatments fail. Buspirone therapy is often helpful in such individuals (Kranzler et al. 1994). If benzodiazepines are prescribed, a single provider should closely monitor the patient, and the dose should not escalate (Dupont and Saylor 1991). Chronic therapeutic users frequently experience withdrawal symptoms requiring treatment, in the absence of other symptoms of abuse or dependence (Romach et al. 1995).

Treatment of sedative-hypnotic withdrawal is similar to that of withdrawal from alcohol. Because of the high prevalence of polysubstance abuse, a detailed substance use history should be obtained to determine the likelihood of polysubstance withdrawal (Busto et al. 1996). A cross-tolerant sedative is given to prevent benzodiazepine withdrawal symptoms, and the daily dose is gradually decreased; long-acting barbiturates or benzodiazepines are recommended (Table 21–12). Because of potential medical complications during detoxification, especially among high-dose abusers, inpatient treatment is preferred. Clonazepam, a benzodiazepine with a moderately long half-life (23 ± 5 hours), has shown promise as an agent for treating alprazolam withdrawal. Alprazolam is particularly difficult to taper after long-term use or high-dose abuse. It binds very tightly to the benzodiazepine–GABA receptor complex; therefore, significant rebound anxiety or withdrawal symptoms can occur with small decreases in dose.

TABLE 21–12. Dose conversions for sedative-hypnotic drugs

Drug	Oral dose (mg)
Benzodiazepines	
Alprazolam (Xanax)	0.5
Chlordiazepoxide (Librium)	25
Clonazepam (Klonopin)	1–2
Clorazepate (Tranxene)	15
Diazepam (Valium)	10
Estazolam (ProSom)	2
Flurazepam (Dalmane)	15
Lorazepam (Ativan)	2
Oxazepam (Serax)	10
Quazepam (Doral)	15
Temazepam (Restoril)	15
Triazolam (Halcion)	0.25
Barbiturates	
Amobarbital (Amytal)	100
Butalbital (Fiorinal[a])	100
Pentobarbital (Nembutal)	50–100
Phenobarbital	30
Secobarbital (Seconal)	100
Others	
Carisoprodol (Soma)	700
Chloral hydrate (Noctec)	500
Ethchlorvynol (Placidyl)	300
Glutethimide (Doriden)	250
Meprobamate (Miltown)	400
Methaqualone (Quaalude)	300
Methyprylon (Noludar)	200

[a]Also contains caffeine.
Source. Adapted from Eickelberg SJ, Mayo-Smith MF: "Management of Sedative-Hypnotic Intoxication and Withdrawal," in *Principles of Addiction Medicine*, 2nd Edition. Edited by Graham AW, Schultz TK. Chevy Chase, MD; American Society of Addiction Medicine, Inc., 1998, p. 450.

For inpatient detoxification of high-dose benzodiazepine abusers, a pentobarbital or diazepam challenge test can help to determine an initial dose of medication (Table 21–13). The most important factor in minimizing complications during benzodiazepine withdrawal is to decrease the dose by approximately 10% per day; the terminal 10% should be tapered slowly to zero over a 3- to 4-day period (Table 21–14). Generally, detoxification is accomplished within a 10- to 14-day period, but in certain individuals, longer detoxification is required. This is particularly true when patients have been taking benzodiazepines for many years or when the drug resists tapering (e.g., alprazolam and lorazepam). In such cases, tapering may take weeks or months.

During withdrawal, additional doses of a benzodiazepine are given as needed for marked increases in vital

TABLE 21–13. Clinical response patterns to 200-mg test dose of oral pentobarbital: relation to tolerance

Patient's condition 1–2 hours after dose	Degree of tolerance	24-hour pentobarbital requirement (estimated amount [mg])
Asleep, but able to be aroused	None or minimal	None
Drowsy, slurred speech, coarse nystagmus; ataxia; marked intoxication	Definite	400–600
Comfortable; fine lateral nystagmus is only sign of intoxication	Marked	600–1,000
No signs of drug effects; no sign of intoxication	Extreme	1,000–1,200 or more

Source. Adapted from Franklin JE Jr, Frances RJ: "Alcohol and Other Psychoactive Substance Use Disorders," in *The American Psychiatric Press Textbook of Psychiatry*, 3rd Edition. Edited by Hales RE, Yudofsky SC, Talbott JA. Washington, DC, American Psychiatric Press, 1999, p. 387. Used with permission.

TABLE 21–14. Benzodiazepine detoxification

Estimate usual daily dose by history or pentobarbital challenge test.

Convert dose into equivalent daily dose of diazepam (see Table 21–12); administer that dose daily for 2 days.

Decrease diazepam dose 10% per day thereafter.

Add diazepam 5 mg orally every 6 hours if signs of increased withdrawal (increased pulse, increase in blood pressure, diaphoresis) are noted.

When diazepam dose approaches 10% of starting dose, reduce dose slowly over 3–4 days and then discontinue.

Source. Adapted from Franklin JE Jr, Frances RJ: "Alcohol and Other Psychoactive Substance Use Disorders," in *The American Psychiatric Press Textbook of Psychiatry*, 3rd Edition. Edited by Hales RE, Yudofsky SC, Talbott JA. Washington, DC, American Psychiatric Press, 1999, p. 387. Used with permission.

signs or agitation. Phenobarbital substitution is also useful for withdrawal from high-dose or long-acting benzodiazepines. The computed phenobarbital equivalence is given in four daily doses and then generally decreased by 30 mg each day. Because of phenobarbital's long half-life, the drug is associated with a mild withdrawal. For withdrawal from shorter half-life benzodiazepines, clonazepam usually allows for a smooth withdrawal. Certain personality traits, such as dependency and passivity, are associated with higher daily doses, more severe withdrawal symptoms, and treatment failure (Schweizer et al. 1998). Detoxification with shorter-acting benzodiazepines, such as oxazepam or lorazepam, is often used in elderly patients and patients with severe liver or pulmonary disease. Carbamazepine and propranolol are reportedly useful in discontinuing long-term benzodiazepine therapy and appear to be useful in treating prolonged withdrawal symptoms (Schweizer et al. 1991). Benzodiazepine antagonists, such as flumazenil, can reverse coma in some individuals with hepatic coma or benzodiazepine overdose (Basile et al. 1991).

OPIOID-RELATED DISORDERS

Opiate abuse presents in various ways in patients on a general medical unit (Table 21–15). Consultation requests include the follow-up of patients taking methadone, patients thought or known to be dependent on prescription or illicit opiates, patients who engage in drug-seeking behavior, patients who require behavioral management of personality problems that interfere with medical care, and patients who overdose. Opioid-dependent patients often provoke angry reactions from staff, such as discharging a patient too soon or underprescribing pain medications. A chronic pain patient who is tolerant to usual doses of pain medications and who experiences opiate withdrawal is sometimes labeled an addict. Tolerance and withdrawal alone are not sufficient for the DSM-IV-TR diagnoses of either substance abuse or dependence. For example, a cancer patient with painful bone metastases may require high doses of narcotics; this individual is not psychologically dependent, and the requirement is a time-limited issue.

Deaths related to heroin overdose are common and result from variations in purity of and the presence of certain contaminants in street drugs. Purer forms of Asian heroin have appeared on the streets in recent years. Purity of street heroin ranges from 16% to 90%, with an average of about 60%. Purer forms of heroin can be snorted. This alternative route of administration is attractive to some heroin-addicted people who fear contracting AIDS or hepatitis C; snorting has also contributed to heroin's surge in popularity. Polysubstance abuse is extremely common among people addicted to opiates. The combination of heroin and cocaine is one of the most frequently used combinations in "speedballing," and concomitant alcohol use is common. A subset of heroin abusers exists among working middle- and upper-class individuals. Synthetic opiates, such as fentanyl, are abused by individuals who have easy access, such as nurses, physicians, and, especially, anesthesiologists.

TABLE 21–15.   Clinical cues to possible opiate abuse or dependence in general hospital patients

History

Exaggerated pain complaints in relation to physical findings

Drug-seeking behavior

Recent multiple outpatient medical visits for pain complaints requiring a narcotic prescription

"Allergic" to every analgesic except meperidine

Physical examination

Pupillary constriction

Withdrawal signs: hyperthermia, hypertension, tachycardia, diaphoresis, nausea, pupillary dilation

Hyperpigmentation over veins, tourniquet areas, tattoos, abscesses

Jaundice

Laboratory findings

Positive toxicology screen results

Increased transaminase levels

Decreased globulin levels

Hospital course

Demanding, unruly, or agitated behavior

Threats to leave against medical advice

Contaminated needles and impure drugs can lead to endocarditis, septicemia, pulmonary emboli, pulmonary hypertension, skin infections, hepatitis, and HIV infection. Twenty-two percent of AIDS cases in males and 43% of cases in females occur in intravenous drug users (Centers for Disease Control and Prevention 1998a). Non–drug-using partners of intravenous drug users are at high risk for HIV infection. Seventy-nine percent of intravenous drug users are infected with the hepatitis C virus (Centers for Disease Control and Prevention 1998b).

Epidemiology

Estimates of opioid use derive from overdose reports, surveys, the prevalence of medical complications, reports of arrests, and data on admissions into treatment programs. The majority, approximately 1 million chronic opioid users, are not in treatment. Difficult-to-reach addicts are an intense focus for HIV and tuberculosis education programs and intervention. Most opiate-dependent individuals come into the hospital at some time, and they are sometimes seen by a consultation-liaison psychiatrist. Most are generally lost to follow-up.

Pathophysiology

There are several subtypes of opioid receptors (i.e., mu, delta, kappa, iota, and epsilon). (Note: the sigma recep-

tor is no longer considered an opioid receptor.) The mu receptor—the classic morphine receptor—has selective affinity for heroin, meperidine, hydromorphone, and methadone. The mu receptor is very sensitive to naloxone (an opioid antagonist) and mediates analgesia, euphoria, sedation, meiosis, and respiratory depression. The dozen or so current endogenous opioids interact with these five major receptors and their subtypes (Simon 1997). Certain individuals may be prone to opioid addiction because of a hypothesized hypoactivity of the endogenous opioid system.

Neuroadaptive changes at receptor sites, in the postreceptor signal transduction system, and in other neurotransmitter systems (particularly the NMDA system) are hypothesized to produce dependence and tolerance. Once neuroadaptation occurs, removal of the opioid from receptors produces withdrawal symptoms. Neuroadaptation appears to result from changes in opioid receptor functioning and from enhanced activity of the postreceptor signal transduction system, including cyclic adenosine monophosphate (cAMP), G proteins, adenylate cyclase, and other protein kinases (Simon 1997).

Opioid receptors are located in the locus coeruleus; chronic administration of opioids inhibits the firing rates of the locus coeruleus's norepinephrine system. In contrast, opioid withdrawal increases noradrenergic activity in the locus coeruleus, which results in withdrawal symptoms. The concentration of CNS 3-methoxy-4-hydroxyphenylglycol (MHPG), the metabolite of norepinephrine, increases after naltrexone-precipitated withdrawal. The level of MHPG correlates positively with signs and symptoms of withdrawal (Charney et al. 1984). The rationale for the use of clonidine for detoxification derives from these findings. In one study of 3,372 male twin pairs, genetic factors were calculated to account for 38% of the variance in heroin abuse (Tsuang et al. 1998). Future work may help to further identify individuals at risk for opioid abuse.

Comorbidity

Among people addicted to opiates, the prevalence of other psychiatric disorders is high. However, it is often difficult to separate the symptoms of chronic intoxication and withdrawal from preexisting Axis I and II pathology. Rounsaville et al. (1982) found that 80% of opiate-addicted patients had histories of psychiatric disorders, frequently mood disorders. During initial rehabilitation, symptoms of major depressive disorder are not as likely to remit as they are in alcoholic patients. Rounsaville and Kleber (1985) found that opiate-addicted people who sought treatment in community programs were more depressed than an untreated community sample and had poorer social functioning, increased nonspecific anxiety symptoms, and more drug-related legal problems. These factors probably facilitate crises that lead patients to treatment.

Intoxication and Withdrawal

Physical signs of intoxication include pupillary constriction (so-called pinpoint pupils), decreased gastrointestinal motility, marked sedation, slurred speech, and impairment in attention and memory. Daily use of opioids for days to weeks, depending on the dosage and potency of the drug, can produce rather intense but non–life-threatening withdrawal syndromes after cessation. The onset of opioid withdrawal depends on the half-life of the opioid and the chronicity of use. For example, symptoms begin approximately 10 hours after the last dose of short-acting opioids, such as morphine and heroin.

Mild opioid withdrawal presents as a flulike syndrome, with symptoms of anxiety, dysphoria, yawning, sweating, rhinorrhea, lacrimation, pupillary dilation, piloerection, mild hypertension, tachycardia, and disrupted sleep. Severe withdrawal symptoms include hot and cold flashes, deep muscle and joint pain, nausea, vomiting, diarrhea, abdominal pain, weight loss, fever, and gooseflesh. Subacute, protracted withdrawal symptoms can last for several weeks.

The clinician should suspect an opioid overdose in any patient who presents in a coma, especially when associated with respiratory depression, pupillary constriction, or the presence of needle marks. In any comatose patient who has overdosed on opioids, naloxone 0.4 mg is given immediately and the dose is repeated because of naloxone's short duration of action. The clinician must remember that excessive naloxone can precipitate severe withdrawal symptoms.

In pregnant women, methadone doses of more than 20 mg/day are associated with moderate to severe withdrawal in newborns (Ostrea and Welch 1991). However, total withdrawal in pregnant women already taking methadone is not recommended (Center for Substance Abuse Treatment 1993). The outcome of infants' withdrawal improves when mothers are supervised in methadone maintenance programs (Harris-Allen 1991) compared with when mothers are using opiates but are not in methadone maintenance programs.

Acute Management and Treatment

Two methods of treatment are available for actively using opioid-dependent individuals in a general hospital—

detoxification and agonist maintenance. Detoxification is often needed for patients who are using street drugs such as heroin or prescription drugs such as oxycodone, meperidine, or codeine. Agonist maintenance is rarely initiated in the general hospital; more often, the consulting psychiatrist is asked to advise on the continuation or modification of ongoing outpatient maintenance. When opioid dependence is questionable, the consultant can perform a naloxone challenge test by administering naloxone 0.4 mg intravenously. Abrupt onset or worsening of withdrawal symptoms (Table 21–16) strongly supports a diagnosis of opioid dependence. Unfortunately, consultation-liaison psychiatrists are too often called at the last minute, before a discharge against medical advice, in the case of patients who abuse opioids. Table 21–17, a list of equal doses of opioids, is provided for conversion purposes during withdrawal or maintenance.

TABLE 21–16.   Objective signs of opiate withdrawal

Pulse 10 beats/minute over baseline or >90 beats/minute if baseline unknown
Systolic blood pressure >10 mm Hg over baseline or >160/ 95 mm Hg in absence of known hypertension
Dilated pupils
Sweating, gooseflesh, rhinorrhea, or lacrimation

TABLE 21–17.   Opioid potency conversion

Drug	Equal dose (mg)	
	Intramuscular	Oral
Morphine	10	60
Hydromorphone (Dilaudid)	1.5	7.5
Methadone (Dolophine)	10	20
Oxycodone (Percocet)	15	30
Levorphanol (Levo-Dromoran)	2	4
Oxymorphone (Numorphan)	1	10 (PR)
Heroin	5	60
Meperidine (Demerol)	75	—
Codeine	130	200

Note.   PR = per rectum.
Source.   Adapted from data published in Foley 1985.

Agonist Maintenance

In 1965, Dole and Nyswander first postulated that methadone would diminish drug-seeking behavior, increase personal productivity, and decrease illicit activities because wide fluctuations in opioid blood levels would cease. One hundred fifteen thousand people are currently undergoing methadone maintenance. In "hard-core addicts" (i.e., opioid-addicted patients who have been using drugs two or more times per day for more than a year or who are continuously involved in drug street life), methadone continues to contribute to improved health, decreased crime, increased employment, and decreased risk of HIV infection (Office of National Drug Control Policy 2001).

Methadone is relatively long acting and has a half-life of 24–36 hours. The long half-life prevents extreme fluctuation in opioid blood levels. Methadone also blunts the euphoric response to heroin. Unlike heroin, which has a half-life of 8–12 hours, methadone is taken once daily—orally, intramuscularly (in divided doses), or intravenously (one-third of oral maintenance dose). Once-daily administration provides a structure for rehabilitation. The addicted person no longer needs illegal activities to support a costly habit. Common side effects of methadone are sedation, mild euphoria, constipation, and reduced sweating.

A frequent mistake made by medical staff is to base a methadone dosage solely on how a patient looks, how a patient says he or she feels, or vital signs. Hospitalized patients who were taking methadone should continue to receive methadone based on their preadmission dose, which should be verified with the methadone clinic, unless methadone is medically contraindicated. For opioid-dependent patients hospitalized on a general medical unit who were not taking methadone, 30–40 mg/day is a reasonable starting dosage, and that amount should initially be given in divided doses. Additional doses of 5 mg twice a day are added, based on signs of withdrawal. Patients must be observed closely for oversedation or undertreatment. An average maintenance dosage is 60–80 mg; 80–120 mg is occasionally needed.

Several medications, such as rifampin, phenobarbital, phenytoin, and carbamazepine, increase methadone metabolism. Methadone also increases plasma desipramine concentrations (Kosten et al. 1990). Methadone should not be combined with monoamine oxidase inhibitors. Methadone maintenance in patients with liver disease is possible until the end stages of the disease; the dose should be reduced to one-half or more.

L-α-Acetyl-methadol (LAAM) is another synthetic opiate agonist. The half-lives of the parent compound (2.6 days) and its two active metabolites (approximately 4 days) are longer than those of methadone. Patients are treated with 25–100 mg three times a week (compared with daily methadone), with the Friday dose usually somewhat higher. One hundred milligrams of twice-weekly LAAM is roughly equivalent to 80 mg of daily methadone. Inhibitors of cytochrome P450 3A4 may reduce the efficacy of LAAM (Moody et al. 1997), whereas inducers of hepatic enzymes may have variable effects on its efficacy. LAAM has also been associated with Q-T prolongation and serious arrhythmia (Roxane Laboratories 2001).

Buprenorphine is a long-acting, mu opioid receptor mixed agonist-antagonist with properties similar to either methadone or naltrexone, depending on the dose. It has shown promise in clinical trials for use in outpatient maintenance therapy for opiate dependence, with sublingual administration daily to thrice weekly, at an average dosage of 9 mg/day (Ling et al. 1998).

Detoxification From Methadone

Consultation-liaison psychiatrists very rarely detoxify patients who are taking methadone. Methadone detoxification is a viable option for patients who have good pretreatment functioning, have long-term success at a low dose of methadone, are less connected to a "street culture," or were addicted to opioids other than heroin. Detoxification from methadone is very slow, and withdrawal symptoms are protracted. Slow outpatient detoxification (i.e., decreasing by 10% per week until the daily dosage is 10–20 mg and then decreasing by 3% per week) reduces relapse rates. Clonidine can be substituted toward the end of methadone detoxification, when the methadone dose is 20 mg or less (see Table 21–18).

Detoxification From Heroin and Other Opiates

Agonist detoxification from heroin, morphine, meperidine, and weak opioids (e.g., codeine and oxycodone) is generally accomplished by giving sufficient methadone to reduce withdrawal symptoms (Table 21–16), and then decreasing the dose by 20% each day over a 5- to 7-day period (Table 21–18). Higher initial doses are typically needed for high-dose heroin users—that is, those whose habit costs more than $50 per day or who use a gram or more per day (the heroin amount is approximate because of the widely varying purity of the street drug). The clinician must monitor the signs and symptoms of withdrawal; 5 mg should be given every hour to titrate signs during peak withdrawal (Table 21–18). Whenever possible, the same volume of medication should be given each time so that the patient is blind to the amount given. Patients may need medications to help with diarrhea, muscle and stomach cramps, or insomnia (e.g., dicyclomine, ibuprofen, Kaopectate, temazepam).

In hospitalized patients who are dependent on prescribed opioids, detoxification can be accomplished by converting the daily dose to a codeine dose and then tapering the liquid codeine amount by 20% per day (Table 21–18). People who are dependent on synthetic narcotics, such as oxycodone or hydrocodone, can slowly

TABLE 21–18. Treatment of opiate withdrawal

Agonist treatment

Methadone 10 mg orally every 4 hours when two or more withdrawal signs are present (see Table 21–16); once baseline dose is established, taper by 5 mg/day until zero.

   OR

Methadone 20 mg orally twice a day; methadone 5 mg prn every 1–6 hours when breakthrough withdrawal signs are noted. Hold methadone if patient is sedated or when withdrawal signs abate. Taper total daily dosage by 5 mg/day.

   OR

(For prescription opiates) Taper drug itself over several weeks or convert usual daily dosage to equivalent codeine oral dose (see Table 21–17). Use liquid form of codeine and taper 20% per day over 5–7 days.

Clonidine treatment

Start with 0.1–0.2 mg every 4 hours to maximum total daily dosage of 1.2 mg. Maintain dose for a minimum of 2–4 days, and then taper by 0.2 mg/day.

Blood pressure is limiting factor; hold if blood pressure is <90/60 mm Hg or orthostatic changes are >10 mm Hg.

   OR

Use Catapres transdermal patch (0.1, 0.2, or 0.3 mg, depending on body weight and withdrawal severity). Apply Catapres-TTS to hairless area; supplement with clonidine 0.1 mg orally every 4 hours as needed for breakthrough withdrawal symptoms.

Clonidine-naltrexone treatment

On day 1, load with oral clonidine 0.2–0.4 mg and oxazepam 30–60 mg or other equivalent benzodiazepine. Two hours later, give naltrexone 12.5 mg. Continue clonidine and adjuvant medications as with clonidine protocol. On day 2, give naltrexone 25 mg, and on day 3, give naltrexone 50 mg, while continuing clonidine protocol, as above.

---

taper the medication over several weeks, or more rapidly as inpatients. Outpatient detoxification from prescribed opioid drugs is seldom successful unless the patient is involved in a well-structured outpatient program. In most United States jurisdictions, only physicians practicing in licensed drug treatment facilities may prescribe opiates to outpatients for the treatment of addiction.

Detoxification Using Clonidine

Clonidine helps to suppress opioid withdrawal symptoms because it suppresses locus coeruleus activity and reduces autonomic activity. Although clonidine is very useful in patients on drug treatment units, it is very rarely used alone to treat opioid withdrawal in patients on a general medical floor. Several studies confirmed the usefulness of clonidine for inpatient detoxification from methadone and heroin (Charney et al. 1981), but results are less impressive in outpatient populations (Kleber et al. 1985). Although clonidine suppresses autonomic signs of withdrawal, it is less effective in relieving subjective discomfort (Jasinski et al. 1985). Clonidine may be administered orally, transdermally (via the Catapres TTS-1, -2, or -3 patch), or in combination (see Table 21–18). The advantage of the patch is once-a-week application, which is usually adequate. The patch is more problematic in elderly patients because it may cause orthostasis; in addition, the patch may have adverse interactions with other drugs and may not work in cases of severe dependence. Sedation and hypotension (blood pressure <90/60 mm

Hg) are common side effects and limit the dose of clonidine. Although clonidine is widely used, it does not currently have a U.S. Food and Drug Administration (FDA)–approved indication for opioid detoxification. As with agonist detoxification, patients detoxified with clonidine may need adjunctive medications to reduce auxiliary withdrawal symptoms (see previous section).

Detoxification Using Clonidine and Naltrexone

A combination of clonidine and low-dose naltrexone can also be used for opiate detoxification (Table 21–18). In one study, detoxification with this combination was associated with a better completion rate than was detoxification with clonidine alone (O'Connor et al. 1995). Naltrexone may help "reset" the opioid receptors. The combination may shorten the withdrawal period to 3 or 4 days. The clonidine blocks the precipitated withdrawal caused by naltrexone. This combination has been used successfully in outpatients; however, higher doses of clonidine are often necessary (Stine and Kosten 1992).

Ultrarapid opiate detoxification has been investigated in several studies. This protocol involves abrupt antagonist-precipitated withdrawal during general anesthesia. The procedure is relatively quick, and subjective experience of withdrawal symptoms is minimized, but it carries the additional costs and risks associated with general anesthesia. Although ultrarapid opiate detoxification may be appropriate for selected patients, further research is needed (O'Connor and Kosten 1998).

Detoxification From Combinations of Opioids and Other Substances

Detoxification from multiple drugs is best achieved in an inpatient setting. First, sedative-hypnotic medications should be tapered while methadone therapy is started or maintained. The clinician must monitor the combined administration of methadone and benzodiazepines very carefully because both are CNS depressants. Once sedative-hypnotic medication is successfully tapered, methadone should be withdrawn in accordance with the guidelines in Table 21–18.

Opiate Addiction and Pain

Treatment dilemmas can arise when opiate-addicted patients develop acute or chronic pain syndromes. The general principles of evaluation and treatment of pain in opiate-dependent individuals are similar to those in non-opiate-dependent individuals who develop pain (e.g., after trauma). In all cases, pain management is directed at the primary disorder. The consultant must ensure that adequate pain medications are prescribed and that as-needed medication schedules are avoided. Opiate-dependent patients are more demanding and drug-seeking; expectations and behavioral limits must be established early. Medical staff must assume responsibility for adequate pain management—they must avoid excessive negotiations. Opioid-dependent patients may require up to double amounts of narcotics for acute pain control as a result of opioid tolerance. When opioids are used for analgesia, such as for postoperative pain, the opioids should be tapered at the same percentage rate in both non-opioid-dependent and opioid-dependent patients.

COCAINE-RELATED DISORDERS

DSM-IV-TR describes the following cocaine-related disorders: *cocaine use disorders* (cocaine dependence and cocaine abuse) and *cocaine-induced disorders* (cocaine intoxication, cocaine withdrawal, cocaine intoxication delirium, cocaine-induced sexual dysfunction, and cocaine-induced psychotic, mood, anxiety, and sleep disorders).

Epidemiology

An estimated 161,087 emergency department visits for cocaine use were documented in the 1997 Drug Abuse Warning Network (Office of Applied Studies 1997). Frequent reasons for psychiatric consultation in the medical setting are cocaine overdose, positive urine toxicology screen results, cocaine-induced depression, and cocaine-induced psychosis. According to the 1998 National Household Survey on Drug Abuse, 1.8 million individuals in the United States used cocaine during a 1-month period (Office of Applied Studies 1999). Crack cocaine is used by a small subset of that population (Smart 1991). Cocaine use remained stable or slightly decreased between 1992 and 1997, after a steep decrease beginning in 1985. Many cocaine users are polysubstance abusers (Community Epidemiology Work Group 1999).

Pharmacology

Cocaine hydrochloride is a white crystal powder derived from coca leaves and coca paste. It is usually diluted to 20% purity by mixing with other local anesthetics, such as lidocaine or procaine, or various sugars. Freebase cocaine is prepared from the hydrochloride salt by alkalinization and extraction with organic solvents. Crack or rock cocaine is a prepackaged freebase form of cocaine that is ready for smoking. "Freebasing" is smoking freebase cocaine; intense euphoria begins within seconds. Because freebased cocaine is absorbed directly from the lungs, it goes immediately to the brain, bypassing the liver. Euphoric effects depend on blood levels and on the slope to peak concentration. Most cocaine is hydrolyzed in the body to benzoylecgonine, which is detected in the urine up to 36 hours after use. High doses are detectable for up to 3 weeks. Rapid tolerance develops to cocaine's euphoric effects. Cocaine and alcohol may combine to make a toxic metabolite called cocaethylene, which is potentially quite cardiotoxic (Cami et al. 1998).

Pathophysiology

Cocaine blocks reuptake of neuronal dopamine, serotonin, and norepinephrine. With repeated cocaine use, tolerance develops rapidly as a result of decreased reuptake inhibition and release of catecholamines and altered receptor sensitivity. Hypotheses to explain the severe craving associated with cocaine dependence include cortical kindling (Halikas et al. 1991), altered opioid receptor binding (Zubieta et al. 1996), and altered dopaminergic or serotonergic function (Satel et al. 1995). Decreases in cortical blood flow may help explain the "high" feeling; neuropsychological deficits and cortical tissue loss, as measured by magnetic resonance imaging, are reported.

Intoxication

Intoxication is characterized by euphoria, hyperalertness, grandiosity, and impaired judgment. Individuals are more gregarious or withdrawn; may have increased anxiety, restlessness, and vigilance; and exhibit stereotypical behavior. Maladaptive behavior includes fighting, psychomotor agitation, and impaired social or occupational functioning.

Cocaine binges can last for a few hours to several days. Tolerance to the euphoric effects develops during the course of a binge. Physical signs of use include tachycardia, pupillary dilation, increased blood pressure, perspiration or chills, nausea or vomiting, and visual or tactile hallucinations. Paranoia occurs with high doses and chronic or binge use of cocaine; it is usually of brief duration. In one study, experienced cocaine users given intravenous cocaine became uniformly paranoid (Sherer et al. 1988). These symptoms usually remit, but heavy, prolonged use or preexisting psychopathology may result in persistent psychosis. Bizarre obsessive and ritualistic behaviors, such as skin picking, are also reported.

Withdrawal or Abstinence

Medically uncomplicated withdrawal occurs with cessation of or decrease in cocaine use after regular, high doses. Efforts to systematically study and correlate abstinence phenomena with neurobiological findings have led to the identification of three phases:

1. *Phase 1* ("the crash") consists of depression, suicidal ideation, insomnia, anxiety, irritability, and intense cocaine craving usually during the first day of withdrawal.
2. *Phase 2* lasts for a few days and consists of cocaine craving, irritability, anxiety, and decreased capacity to experience pleasure.
3. *Phase 3* consists of milder episodic craving stimulated by conditioned environmental factors (Gawin and Kleber 1986).

Suicidal ideation peaks during the crash period. Another study found that the greatest cocaine craving occurred during the 24 hours before admission and that the greatest mood distress occurred on the first day after admission, with mood states, craving, and insomnia improving gradually (Weddington et al. 1990).

Medical and Other Complications

Cocaine use is associated with acute and chronic medical ailments (e.g., chronic intranasal use leads to septal necrosis). Anesthetic properties of cocaine can lead to oral numbness and dental neglect; cocaine binges can cause malnutrition, severe weight loss, and dehydration. Intra-

venous cocaine use, because of contaminants, can result in endocarditis, septicemia, HIV infection, local vasculitis, hepatitis B and C, emphysema, pulmonary emboli, and granulomas. Freebase cocaine is associated with decreased pulmonary gas exchange; pulmonary dysfunction can persist (Itkomen et al. 1984). Cocaine intravenous injection sites are characterized by prominent ecchymosis, whereas opioid users frequently have needle scars.

In New York City, one of every five individuals who committed suicide during a 1-year period used cocaine immediately before his or her death (Marzuk et al. 1992). Congenital deficiency of pseudocholinesterase slows metabolism of cocaine, which can result in toxic levels, sudden delirium, and hypothermia. Cocaine can cause acute agitation, diaphoresis, tachycardia, metabolic and respiratory acidosis, cardiac dysrhythmia, grand mal seizures, and, ultimately, respiratory arrest. Myocardial infarctions, likely caused by tachycardia, coronary vasoconstriction, and increased platelet "stickiness," as well as subarachnoid hemorrhages and acute rhabdomyolysis are all reported with cocaine use (Lichtenfeld et al. 1986; Nadamanee et al. 1989; Roth et al. 1988). Deaths in even recreational, low-dose users are reported. Pregnant women who use cocaine are at increased risk for abruptio placentae. Fetal growth is often decreased, and infants often exhibit decreased interactive behaviors (Eyler et al. 1998a, 1998b).

Acute Management and Referral

Agitation and anxiety associated with cocaine intoxication are treated with diazepam, lorazepam, or propranolol (Jonsson et al. 1983). Haloperidol therapy is usually an effective treatment for cocaine psychosis. Withdrawal depression generally does not necessitate use of antidepressant medication. In her review, McCance (1997) noted that although more than 30 medications have undergone clinical trials, no medication has shown consistent efficacy in treating cocaine dependence or in reducing craving for the drug. Medications investigated include tricyclic antidepressants such as desipramine; anticonvulsants such as carbamazepine and phenytoin; selective serotonin reuptake inhibitors; dopaminergic agents such as L-dopa, bromocriptine, and haloperidol; and miscellaneous agents such as bupropion, naltrexone, methylphenidate, and tyrosine. Novel approaches involving peripherally active immunological and enzymatic agents are under investigation (Sparenborg et al. 1997). When another psychiatric disorder—such as major depressive disorder, bipolar disorder, or schizophrenia—is present, optimal treatment of that disorder is essential to rehabilitation of cocaine users.

Gawin and Kleber (1986) recommended a trial of outpatient nonpharmacological treatment, especially for those who are new to treatment and have passed the cocaine crash and intense craving period. Indications for inpatient treatment are chronic freebase or intravenous use, concurrent dependence on other drugs or alcohol, concurrent serious medical or psychiatric problems, severe impairment in psychosocial functioning, insufficient motivation for outpatient treatment, lack of family and other supports, and failure of outpatient treatment.

Treatment Outcome

Treatment outcome is affected by factors such as severity of psychosocial problems, family support, intensity of withdrawal, and degree of antisocial features more than by initial motivation for treatment. In a multicenter trial involving 487 randomly assigned patients, Crits-Christoph et al. (1999) compared four manual-guided psychotherapeutic treatments of cocaine dependence. Individual drug counseling combined with group drug counseling proved more effective in reducing cocaine use than did cognitive psychotherapy, supportive-expressive psychotherapy, or group drug counseling alone. In a study involving 1,605 cocaine-dependent patients undergoing long-term residential, short-term residential, or outpatient treatment, relapse rates were lowest among patients with the fewest psychosocial problems (Simpson et al. 1999). Among those with more problems, longer treatment was related to more positive outcome.

People who abuse cocaine must avoid alcohol and other mood-altering drugs, which disinhibit behavior and lead to relapse. This concept is difficult for a cocaine-dependent individual to accept, because he or she merely wants to quit cocaine use. Treatment of clearly defined attention-deficit/hyperactivity disorder (Levin et al. 1998) or affective disorders proceeds in concert with treatment of cocaine dependence.

AMPHETAMINE-RELATED DISORDERS

Amphetamines ("speed") have stimulant and reinforcing properties similar to those of cocaine. Amphetamines block reuptake of dopamine, serotonin, and norepinephrine and have profound effects on dopamine storage release. The signs and symptoms of amphetamine use include tachycardia, increased blood pressure, pupillary dilation, agitation, elation, loquacity, and hypervigilance. Amphetamine psychosis can resemble acute paranoid schizophrenia. Visual hallucinations are common. Binge episodes ("runs"), which are similar to those experienced with cocaine use, often alternate with symptoms of a severe crash. Polysubstance use is common.

CNS stimulants, such as dextroamphetamine and methylphenidate, are manufactured for the treatment of medical conditions, such as narcolepsy and attention-deficit/hyperactivity disorder. Because prescriptions of this drug class are tightly controlled, legal use has decreased. Adverse side effects include insomnia, irritability, confusion, and hostility. Amphetamine abuse can start during weight-loss treatment or attempts at energy enhancement.

Abuse of methamphetamine is primarily a problem in the western and southwestern United States but has been spreading into other parts of the country (Community Epidemiology Work Group 1999). Methamphetamine can be readily manufactured ("cooked") in small kitchen or bathroom "labs," and the process can result in explosions, fires, or exposure of household residents to toxic chemicals. Intravenous amphetamine abuse can present with the same complications seen with other illicit substances taken intravenously.

Acute Management

Treatment in individuals who abuse amphetamines is similar to that in cocaine users. However, the effects of amphetamine may last longer. The consultant may be asked to assist with management of psychosis, violence, or withdrawal depression and suicidality. In the case of an amphetamine overdose, acidifying the urine with vitamin C speeds elimination. Antipsychotic medications should be used to treat paranoid or delusional symptoms, which can continue for days to weeks after the drug is no longer present in the urine. Rehabilitation requires a comprehensive treatment approach, as described for other substances earlier in this chapter (for example, see the subsection entitled "Long-Term Management").

PHENCYCLIDINE-RELATED DISORDERS

Phencyclidine (PCP) is an anesthetic agent that first appeared as a street drug in the 1960s; PCP abuse peaked between 1978 and 1980. Current street samples sold as PCP vary greatly in purity. Smoking marijuana cigarettes laced with PCP is the most common form of administration. Ketamine, a related compound, has recently gained popularity.

PCP is a noncompetitive NMDA/glutamate receptor antagonist and has effects on serotonergic and dopaminergic systems as well (Jentsch and Roth 1999; Nabeshima et al. 1996). PCP induces several mental disorders, including intoxication, delirium, delusions, flashbacks, mood disorders, and anxiety.

Medical and Other Complications

Psychoactive effects of PCP generally begin within 5 minutes and plateau 30 minutes after use. Volatile emotionality is the predominant behavioral presentation. Affects range from intense euphoria to anxiety, and behavior can include stereotypical repetitive activities and bizarre aggression. Distorted perceptions, numbness, and confusion are also common. Associated physical signs include high blood pressure, muscle rigidity, ataxia, and, at higher doses, hypersalivation, hyperthermia, involuntary movements, and coma; high-dose PCP toxicity can simulate neuroleptic malignant syndrome. Rhabdomyolysis in overdoses can lead to acute renal failure. Dilated pupils and nystagmus, particularly vertical nystagmus, should alert the consultation-liaison psychiatrist to PCP use. Chronic psychotic episodes are reported after use, as are long-term neuropsychological deficits (Davis 1982; Deutsch et al. 1998).

Acute Management

Acute reactions generally require pharmacological intervention. Intravenous diazepam is the drug of first choice; antipsychotics are occasionally necessary. Because supportive treatment is also needed, management in a medical setting is preferred. After ingestion of PCP, the urine may test positive for 7 days; false-negative results can occur. PCP elimination is initially enhanced by ammonium chloride and subsequently by ascorbic acid or cranberry juice (Aronow et al. 1980).

HALLUCINOGEN-RELATED DISORDERS

Hallucinogenic drugs include lysergic acid diethylamide (LSD) and synthetic derivatives such as 3,4-methylenedioxyamphetamine (MDA) and 3,4-methylenedioxymethamphetamine (MDMA) (called "ecstasy"). Since 1979, psychedelic drugs have decreased in popularity, but a modest resurgence in use has occurred since the early 1990s, particularly among youth.

Ecstasy is promoted as a "mood drug" without the distracting perceptual changes of other hallucinogens

(Grinspoon and Bakalar 1986). Parkinsonian syndromes are reported to occur secondary to MDMA use, and neuropsychological deficits may persist; however, the actual relationship to drug use is hotly debated (Halpern and Pope 1999; Rickert et al. 1999). MDMA use has been associated with hyperthermia, seizures, cardiac arrhythmias, myocardial infarction, and hyponatremia, among other medical complications (Burgess et al. 2000; Qasim et al. 2001; Shannon 2000).

In animal studies, hallucinogens are not reinforcing. In humans, the pattern of psychedelic use is most often infrequent use. Abuse patterns of psychedelic drugs are consistent with DSM-IV-TR substance abuse and dependence.

Intoxication and Persisting Perception Disorder

An individual's response to LSD, mescaline, and related drugs varies greatly with the user's expectations and the circumstances of use (set and setting). Rather intense changes in perception of time, space, and body image often occur. Generally, reality testing and orientation are preserved. The mechanism of action proposed for perceptual changes is disrupted serotonin action in the raphe nucleus, producing a disinhibition of cerebral occipital and limbic structures (Jacobs 1987). Physical signs of intoxication include increased heart rate, dilation of pupils, and sweating. Individuals having "bad trips" can present with severe anxiety or paranoia. The chance of a bad trip is increased by emotional distress before use, reluctant use, or an aversive setting. Hallucinogen persisting perception disorder (flashbacks) is characterized by recurrent psychedelic experiences, usually visual, after cessation of hallucinogenic drug use. Common precipitating factors include a prior psychedelic experience, marijuana smoking, and emotional stress.

Management

Hallucinogen-intoxicated patients should be placed in a quiet setting with minimal stimuli. Spoken to in a soft, calm voice, the individual is then "talked down" from frightening experiences. Occasionally, diazepam is needed as an adjunct. Antipsychotics are rarely necessary. Pure hallucinogen users are rarely treated in rehabilitation centers. In studies involving small numbers of patients, clonidine, naltrexone, and sertraline have been used successfully to treat flashbacks (Lerner et al. 1998, 2000); risperidone reportedly worsens symptoms (Morehead 1997).

CANNABIS-RELATED DISORDERS

The main psychoactive constituent in marijuana is Δ^9-tetrahydrocannabinol (Δ^9-THC), one of 60 cannabinoids. Marijuana sold on the street contains from 5% to 17% Δ^9-THC (Drug Enforcement Administration 2001). Hashish is a resin from the cannabis plant that contains a higher percentage of Δ^9-THC than does marijuana. Δ^9-THC binds to cannabinoid receptors, located primarily in hippocampal and striatal regions; an endogenous ligand for these receptors, anadamide, has been identified (Ameri 1999). Several studies suggest that there is a genetic vulnerability to cannabis dependence (Merikangas et al. 1998b; Tsuang et al. 1998).

Laboratory Findings

Cannabinoids were detected in the urine of chronic abusers 21 days after cessation, because of slow release from fat stores; in most occasional users, urine drug screen results remain positive for 1–5 days (Schwartz and Hawks 1985). Blood sampling is used to measure levels of cannabinoids.

Intoxication

Peak intoxication after smoking cannabis generally occurs in 10–30 minutes. Intoxication usually lasts 2–4 hours, depending on the dose; however, behavioral and psychomotor impairment may continue several hours longer. Δ^9-THC and its metabolites, which are highly liquid soluble, tend to accumulate in fat cells; this phenomenon extends the half-life to approximately 50 hours. Personality, past experience with the drug, and setting can alter the experience dramatically, although higher doses of Δ^9-THC increase the chances of a toxic reaction. Users experience slowed time, increased appetite, increased thirst, and a keener sense of color, sound, pattern, texture, and taste. They also experience euphoria, heightened introspection, absorbing sensual experiences, feelings of relaxation and floating, and increased self-confidence. Psychosis, derealization, and aggression occur rarely. Conjunctivitis, a strong odor of cannabis, dilated pupils, tachycardia, dry mouth, and coughing are physical signs of recent use.

Withdrawal

In chronic high-dose users, reported withdrawal symptoms include anxiety, dysphoria, insomnia, anorexia, tremulousness, and sweating, but no stereotypical syndrome has been described (Haney et al. 1999; Wiesbeck et al. 1996).

Consultation Requests

Consultation requests involving marijuana abusers are often exploratory. Controversy surrounds the existence of a behavioral syndrome associated with chronic cannabis use. The behavioral syndrome is described as an "amotivational syndrome," characterized by passivity, decreased drive, diminished goal-directed activity, fatigue, and apathy. Research into this amotivational syndrome is plagued by methodological problems, including selection bias and lack of control subjects. Long-term marijuana users may have residual cognitive deficits (Fletcher et al. 1996; Reilly et al. 1998) and other comorbid psychiatric symptoms (Troisi et al. 1998). There is little evidence that cannabis causes chronic psychosis in asymptomatic individuals (Gruber and Pope 1994).

Δ^9-THC is used in some medical settings to control severe nausea and vomiting, mainly in association with AIDS, cancer chemotherapy, and bone marrow transplantation. Δ^9-THC is no longer an approved treatment for glaucoma; more effective treatments are available. Other medical use remains highly controversial (Joy et al. 1999).

Acute Management

Marijuana intoxication does not usually require professional attention. Support, reassurance, and reality testing by friends or family are sufficient. Anxiolytic agents are occasionally needed, and neuroleptics are used in rare cases of protracted paranoia. Patients with cardiovascular disease often cannot tolerate the increased heart rate and blood pressure that are caused by marijuana. Acute intake can cause bronchodilation. Cannabis smoke contains carcinogens similar to those found in tobacco, and chronic heavy marijuana use can predispose an individual to chronic obstructive lung disease, bronchial constriction, sinusitis, and pulmonary neoplasm.

Long-Term Management

Treatment in people who abuse marijuana follows the general principles established for other substances, with special attention paid to developmental issues in adolescent abusers. Monitored detoxification or inpatient intervention is rarely needed, except for severe abuse or behavioral problems (e.g., in teenage populations). Outpatient treatment consists of 12-step self-help programs, group and individual therapy, family therapy, and periodic urine testing to monitor abstinence. Adolescent drug programs typically focus on promoting age-appropriate behavior and communication skills.

NICOTINE-RELATED DISORDERS

Tobacco addiction is the most preventable health problem in the United States. Approximately 60 million Americans smoke tobacco; 400,000 deaths per year are attributed to nicotine, and $50 billion per year are spent on smoking-attributable, direct medical-care expenditures—7% of the country's total health care costs ("Medical-Care Expenditures Attributable to Cigarette Smoking" 1994). In the United States, approximately 30% of men and 26% of women smoke cigarettes; the percentage of young adults smoking cigarettes significantly increased between 1994 (35%) and 1998 (42%) (Office of Applied Studies 1999). Because most general hospitals are smoke-free, nicotine withdrawal should be considered in the differential diagnosis of any anxious or dysphoric patient.

Nicotine is a psychoactive substance with euphoric and positive reinforcement properties, similar to those of cocaine and opiates (Benowitz 1988; Henningfield 1984). Tolerance develops to nicotine, and significant withdrawal syndromes occur. Craving for tobacco, irritability, anxiety, difficulty concentrating, restlessness, decreased heart rate, increased eating with a weight gain of 5–10 lb, and sleep disturbance are associated with withdrawal. Subjects with higher nicotine tolerance have more withdrawal discomfort. Similarities in the temporal pattern of relapse are found among nicotine, alcohol, and opioid abusers.

Predisposition or Risk Factors and Comorbidity

Cigarette smokers generally begin smoking as teenagers; use is associated with peer tobacco use, parental tobacco use, and symptoms of anxiety, depression, or conduct disorder. A strong association exists between smoking and other drug abuse, especially alcohol abuse. However, alcoholic patients quit smoking at the same rate as nonalcoholic patients.

Carmelli and colleagues (1992), using the United States twin registry, found that monozygotic twins were more concordant in their smoking behavior (i.e., more concordant for smoking, never smoking, or quitting smoking) than were dizygotic twins; these results suggest moderate genetic influences on lifetime smoking practices. There is a well-established relationship between nicotine dependence and major depressive disorder. For example, Kendler et al. (1993) found a strong association between average lifetime daily cigarette smoking and lifetime prevalence of depression. It is possible that a person might be genetically predisposed to both conditions. Nic-

otine withdrawal is typically more severe in persons with histories of major depressive disorder or anxiety disorders. Patients with histories of major depressive disorder are prone to recurrence of their depression after smoking cessation (Covey et al. 1997) and should therefore be more closely monitored.

A well-established association exists between tobacco use and chronic obstructive lung disease, lung cancer, oral cancers, and hypertension. Mothers who smoke are more likely than mothers who do not smoke to deliver low-birth-weight infants (U.S. Department of Health and Human Services 1988). The success rate with every attempt to quit is 5%, and 50% of individuals eventually quit.

Effects

Tobacco use can produce a calming, euphoric effect in chronic users; this effect is more pronounced after a period of tobacco deprivation. Symptoms of acute nicotine poisoning include nausea, salivation, abdominal pain, vomiting and diarrhea, headaches, dizziness, and sweating; inability to concentrate, confusion, and tachycardia can also occur (Hughes and Hatsukami 1986). Nicotine increases the activity of several neurotransmitters.

Tobacco smoke also contains polycyclic hydrocarbons that alter hepatic metabolism of many drugs (Carrillo et al. 1996; Hughes 1993). Patients who resume smoking after prolonged stays in smoke-free hospitals may experience clinically significant alterations in therapeutic blood levels of prescribed medications.

Management

Behavioral, cognitive, educational, self-help, and pharmacological approaches are all used to treat nicotine dependence (American Psychiatric Association 1996). Cognitive-behavioral treatments may be particularly suitable for patients with histories of depression (Hall et al. 1998). However, the vast majority (95%) of individuals who stop smoking receive no formal intervention; research is needed to clarify how and why these individuals discontinued use. All of the following factors are associated with poor long-term outcome: environmental stress, poor social support, smoking by family members, lack of educational information, female sex, poor overall adjustment, low self-confidence, poor motivation, and high pretreatment levels of cotinine (a metabolite of nicotine) (Porjesz and Begleiter 1981). Fear of weight gain frequently delays quitting. Cognitive-behavioral strategies, pharmacological strategies, or exercise regimens are sometimes used to treat weight gain associated with cessation.

Nicotine Replacement Therapy

We recommend nicotine replacement therapy for medically ill hospitalized patients with heavy nicotine addiction, because 50% of these patients will experience significant withdrawal. Most general hospitals have antismoking rules, but it is unfortunate that few have adequate smoking cessation programs. The transdermal nicotine patch is a nonprescription medication that reduces withdrawal symptoms and improves abstinence rates (Finn and Wilcock 1997). Nicotine patches have been found to be safe in patients with coronary artery disease (Tzivoni et al. 1998). Use of the patch alone doubles the chance of quitting; use of the patch plus behavioral treatment doubles the rate of cessation compared with use of the patch alone (Fiore et al. 1994).

Nicotine gum, which also requires no prescription, maintains blood nicotine levels to minimize withdrawal symptoms (Fortmann and Killen 1995; Raw 1985). It is prescribed for use every 30 minutes or as needed. Patients must be thoroughly instructed in the proper chewing technique to release the nicotine. One-year postintervention effectiveness is between 25% and 40% in most intensive smoking cessation programs, which is approximately the same rate as that for other substance abuse treatment (Fiore et al. 1990).

Nicotine intranasal spray and a nicotine inhaler are also available in the United States as prescribed alternative methods for nicotine replacement (Hughes et al. 1999). The spray, and possibly the inhaler, may be combined with other therapies (Blondal et al. 1999).

Other Pharmacological Treatments

Bupropion, an atypical antidepressant, improves abstinence rates, independent of its antidepressant effect (Hayford et al. 1999). The sustained-release form is approved for use for smoking cessation. The identical form is marketed as an antidepressant under a different brand name, which may cause confusion. Jorenby et al. (1999) showed that combining bupropion with the transdermal patch further improves abstinence rates while reducing weight gain. Hall et al. (1998) showed that nortriptyline may also be a useful adjunct in smoking cessation.

INHALANT-RELATED DISORDERS

Inhalants are a diverse group of chemicals and include gasoline, airplane glue, aerosols (e.g., spray paints), lighter fluid, fingernail polish remover, typewriter correction fluid, a variety of cleaners, amyl and butyl nitrites, and nitrous oxide. Hydrocarbons are the active ingredients.

Inhalant use has been increasing among both male and female adolescents (Neumark et al. 1998). A high rate of abuse is also found among Native Americans (Reed and May 1984). Nitrous oxide abuse occurs predominantly among medical personnel such as dentists. Inhalants are inexpensive and easily obtained. Fumes of glues and paint products are usually inhaled from bags or rags.

Intoxication

Typical signs and symptoms of inhalant intoxication include grandiosity, a sense of invulnerability and immense strength, euphoria, slurred speech, and ataxia. Visual distortions and faulty space perception are also common. Inhalant intoxication is associated with aggressive, disruptive, and antisocial behavior. Among adolescents, inhalant abuse is associated with arrests, poor performance in school, increased family disruption, and other drug abuse (Santos de Barona and Simpson 1984).

Intoxication can last from a few minutes to as long as 2 hours. Impaired judgment, poor insight, violence, and psychosis are common sequelae (Cohen 1984). Paint stains around the face are an obvious indication of inhalant abuse. Central respiratory depression, cardiac arrhythmia, and accidents can cause death, and long-term damage to bone marrow, kidneys, liver, neuromusculature, and the brain has also been reported (Brouette and Anton 2001; Espeland 1995). The lifetime course of an inhalant abuser is not clear. Reports suggest that inhalants are primarily abused by youths; inhalant abusers are likely to move on to other substances in later life.

SUMMARY

Substance-related disorders are commonly found in medically ill patients. The consultation-liaison psychiatrist must know how to identify such patients quickly, treat withdrawal symptoms, and initiate appropriate referral for long-term treatment. In this chapter, we have provided the consultation-liaison psychiatrist with a practical clinical approach to substance-related disorders in medically ill patients.

REFERENCES

Adams RD, Victor M, Ropper AH: Principles of Neurology, 6th Edition. New York, McGraw-Hill, 1997

Adinoff B, Risher-Flowers D, De Jong J, et al: Disturbances of hypothalamic-pituitary-adrenal axis functioning during ethanol withdrawal in six men. Am J Psychiatry 148:1023–1025, 1991

Allen JP, Sillamaukee P, Anton R: Contribution of carbohydrate deficient transferrin to gamma glutamyl transpeptidase in evaluating progress of patients in treatment for alcoholism. Alcohol Clin Exp Res 23:115–120, 1999

Allen JP, Litten RZ, Fertig JB, et al: Carbohydrate-deficient transferrin: an aid to early recognition of alcohol relapse. Am J Addict 10 (suppl):24–28, 2001

Allgulander C, Ljungberg L, Fisher LD: Long-term prognosis in addiction on sedative and hypnotic drugs analyzed with the Cox regression model. Acta Psychiatr Scand 75:521–531, 1987

Ameri A: The effects of cannabinoids on the brain. Prog Neurobiol 58:315–348, 1999

American Psychiatric Association: Diagnostic and Statistical Manual: Mental Disorders. Washington, DC, American Psychiatric Association, 1952

American Psychiatric Association: Diagnostic and Statistical Manual of Mental Disorders, 2nd Edition. Washington, DC, American Psychiatric Association, 1968

American Psychiatric Association: Diagnostic and Statistical Manual of Mental Disorders, 3rd Edition. Washington, DC, American Psychiatric Association, 1980

American Psychiatric Association: Diagnostic and Statistical Manual of Mental Disorders, 3rd Edition, Revised. Washington, DC, American Psychiatric Association, 1987

American Psychiatric Association: Diagnostic and Statistical Manual of Mental Disorders, 4th Edition. Washington, DC, American Psychiatric Association, 1994

American Psychiatric Association: Practice guideline for psychiatric evaluation of adults. Am J Psychiatry 152:63–80, 1995a

American Psychiatric Association: Practice guideline for the treatment of patients with substance use disorders: alcohol, cocaine, opioids. Am J Psychiatry 152:1–59, 1995b

American Psychiatric Association: Practice guideline for the treatment of patients with nicotine dependence. Am J Psychiatry 153:1–31, 1996

American Psychiatric Association: Diagnostic and Statistical Manual of Mental Disorders, 4th Edition, Text Revision. Washington, DC, American Psychiatric Association, 2000

Anglin D, Spears KL, Hutson HR: Flunitrazepam and its involvement in date or acquaintance rape. Acad Emerg Med 4:323–326, 1997

Anton RF, Stout RL, Roberts JS, et al: The effect of drinking intensity and frequency on serum carbohydrate-deficient transferrin and gamma-glutamyl transferase levels in outpatient alcoholics. Alcohol Clin Exp Res 22:1456–1462, 1998

Aronow R, Miceli JN, Done AK: A therapeutic approach to the acutely overdosed PCP patient. J Psychoactive Drugs 12:259–267, 1980

Barnes HN, Samet JH: Brief interventions with substance-abusing patients. Med Clin North Am 81:867–879, 1997

Basile AS, Hughes RD, Harrison PM, et al: Elevated brain concentrations of 1,4-benzodiazepines in fulminant hepatic failure. N Engl J Med 325:473–478, 1991

Begleiter H, Porjesz B: Persistence of a subacute withdrawal syndrome following chronic ethanol intake. Drug Alcohol Depend 4:353–357, 1979

Benowitz NL: Drug therapy: pharmacologic aspects of cigarette smoking and nicotine addiction. N Engl J Med 319:1318–1330, 1988

Benzer D: Quantification of the alcohol withdrawal syndrome in 487 alcoholic patients. J Subst Abuse Treat 7:117–123, 1990

Bernstein L, Jacobsberg L, Ashman T, et al: Detection of alcoholism among burn patients. Hospital and Community Psychiatry 43:255–256, 1992

Blondal T, Gudmundsson LJ, Olafsdottir I, et al: Nicotine nasal spray with nicotine patch for smoking cessation: randomised trial with six year follow up. BMJ 318:285–288, 1999

Bradley KA, Boyd-Wickizer J, Powell SH, et al: Alcohol screening questionnaires in women: a critical review. JAMA 280:166–171, 1998

Brew BJ: Diagnosis of Wernicke's encephalopathy. Aust N Z J Med 16:676–678, 1986

Brouette T, Anton R: Clinical review of inhalants. Am J Addict 10:79–94, 2001

Bucholz KK, Homan SM: When do alcoholics first discuss drinking problems? J Stud Alcohol 53:582–589, 1992

Burgess C, O'Donohoe A, Gill M: Agony and ecstasy: a review of MDMA effects and toxicity. European Psychiatry 15:287–294, 2000

Busto UE, Romach MK, Sellers EM: Multiple drug use and psychiatric comorbidity in patients admitted to the hospital with severe benzodiazepine dependence. J Clin Psychopharmacol 16:51–57, 1996

Caces F, Harford T: Time series analysis of alcohol consumption and suicide mortality in the United States, 1934–1987. J Stud Alcohol 59:455–461, 1998

Cami J, Farre M, Gonzalez ML, et al: Cocaine metabolism in humans after use of alcohol: clinical and research implications. Recent Dev Alcohol 14:437–455, 1998

Carmelli D, Swan GE, Robinette D, et al: Genetic influence on smoking—a study of male twins. N Engl J Med 327:829–833, 1992

Carrillo JA, Dahl ML, Svensson JO, et al: Disposition of fluvoxamine in humans is determined by the polymorphic CYP2D6 and also by the CYP1A2 activity. Clin Pharmacol Ther 60:183–190, 1996

Carroll KM, Rounsaville BJ, Keller DS: Relapse prevention strategies for the treatment of cocaine abuse. Am J Drug Alcohol Abuse 17:249–265, 1991

Center for Substance Abuse Treatment: Treatment Improvement Protocol for Pregnant, Substance-Using Women. Rockville, MD, CSAT, 1993

Center for Substance Abuse Treatment: CSAT TIPs (Web page). Available at: http://www.treatment.org/Externals/tips.html. Accessed January 5, 2001

Centers for Disease Control and Prevention: U.S. HIV and AIDS cases reported through December 1998. HIV/AIDS Surveillance Report (Year-End Edition) 10(2):14, 1998a

Centers for Disease Control and Prevention: Recommendations for prevention and control of hepatitis C virus (HCV) infection and HCV-related chronic disease. MMWR Morb Mortal Wkly Rep 47:1–39, 1998b

Charney DS, Sternberg DE, Kleber HD, et al: The clinical use of clonidine in abrupt withdrawal from opiates. Arch Gen Psychiatry 38:1273–1277, 1981

Charney DS, Redmond E, Galloway MP: Naltrexone precipitated opiate withdrawal in methadone addicted human subjects: evidence for noradrenergic hyperactivity. Life Sci 35:1263–1272, 1984

Ciraulo DA, Sarid-Segal O, Knapp C, et al: Liability to alprazolam abuse in daughters of alcoholics. Am J Psychiatry 153:956–958, 1996

Cleary PD, Miller M, Bush BT, et al: Prevalence and recognition of alcohol abuse in a primary care population. Am J Med 85:466–471, 1988

Cohen S: The hallucinogens and inhalants. Psychiatr Clin North Am 4:681–688, 1984

Cole P, Rodu B: Analytic epidemiology: cancer causes, in Cancer: Principles and Practice of Oncology, 6th Edition. Edited by Devita VT, Hellman S, Rosenberg SA. Philadelphia, PA, Lippincott Williams & Wilkins, 2001, pp 241–252

Community Epidemiology Work Group: Epidemiologic trends in drug abuse: advance report, December 2000 (Web page). Available at: http://www.nida.nih.gov/CEWG/AdvancedRep/1200ADV/1200adv.html. Accessed July 3, 2001

Covey LS, Glassman AH, Stetner F: Major depressive disorder following smoking cessation. Am J Psychiatry 154:263–265, 1997

Crits-Christoph P, Siqueland L, Blaine J, et al: Psychosocial treatments for cocaine dependence: National Institute on Drug Abuse Collaborative Cocaine Treatment Study. Arch Gen Psychiatry 56:493–502, 1999

Davis BL: The PCP epidemic: a critical review. Int J Addict 17:1137–1155, 1982

Deutsch SI, Mastropaolo J, Rosse RB: Neurodevelopmental consequences of early exposure to phencyclidine and related drugs. Clin Neuropharmacol 21:320–332, 1998

Dietch J: The nature and extent of benzodiazepine abuse: an overview of recent literature. Hospital and Community Psychiatry 34:1139–1145, 1983

DiMartini A, Jain A, Irish W, et al: Outcome of liver transplantation in critically ill patients with alcoholic cirrhosis: survival according to medical variables and sobriety. Transplantation 66:298–302, 1998

Dole VP, Nyswander ME: A medical treatment of heroin addiction. JAMA 193:646–650, 1965

D'Onofrio G, Rathlev N, Ulrich A, et al: Lorazepam for the prevention of recurrent seizures related to alcohol. N Engl J Med 340:915–919, 1999

Drake RE, Osher FC, Wallach MA: Alcohol use and abuse in schizophrenia: a prospective community study. J Nerv Ment Dis 177:408–414, 1989

Drug Enforcement Administration: Cannabis, in Drugs of Abuse (Web page). Available at: http://www.usdoj.gov/dea/concern/abuse/chap6/marijuan.htm. Accessed January 5, 2001

Dulit RA, Fyer MR, Haas GL, et al: Substance use in borderline personality disorder. Am J Psychiatry 147:1002–1007, 1990

Dupont RL, Saylor KE: Sedatives/hypnotics and benzodiazepines, in Textbook of Addictive Disorders. Edited by Frances RJ, Miller SI. New York, Guilford, 1991, pp 69–102

Edenberg HJ, Foroud T, Koller DL, et al: A family-based analysis of the association of the dopamine D2 receptor (DRD2) with alcoholism. Alcohol Clin Exp Res 22:505–512, 1998

Espeland K: Identifying the manifestations of inhalant abuse. Nurse Pract 20:49–50, 53, 1995

Espir ML, Rose FC: Alcohol, seizures and epilepsy. J R Soc Med 9:542–543, 1987

Eyler FD, Behnke M, Conlon M, et al: Birth outcome from a prospective, matched study of prenatal crack/cocaine use, I: interactive and dose effects on health and growth. Pediatrics 101:229–237, 1998a

Eyler FD, Behnke M, Conlon M, et al: Birth outcome from a prospective, matched study of prenatal crack/cocaine use, II: interactive and dose effects on neurobehavioral assessment. Pediatrics 101:237–241, 1998b

Finn P, Wilcock K: Levo-alpha acetyl methadol (LAAM): its advantages and drawbacks. J Subst Abuse Treat 14:559–564, 1997

Fiore MC, Novotny TE, Pierce JP, et al: Methods used to quit smoking in the United States: do cessation programs help? JAMA 263:2760–2765, 1990

Fiore MC, Smith SS, Jorenby DE, et al: The effectiveness of the nicotine patch for smoking cessation: a meta-analysis. JAMA 271:1940–1947, 1994

Fleming MF, Wilk A, Kruger J, et al: Hospital-based alcohol and drug specialty consultation service: does it work? South Med J 88:275–282, 1995

Fletcher JM, Page JB, Francis DJ, et al: Cognitive correlates of long-term cannabis use in Costa Rican men. Arch Gen Psychiatry 53:1051–1057, 1996

Foley KM: The treatment of cancer pain. N Engl J Med 313:84–95, 1985

Fortmann SP, Killen JD: Nicotine gum and self-help behavioral treatment for smoking relapse prevention: results from a trial using population-based recruitment. J Consult Clin Psychol 63:460–468, 1995

Frezza M, Di Padova G, Pozzato G, et al: High blood alcohol levels in women: the role of decreased gastric alcohol dehydrogenase activity and first-pass metabolism. N Engl J Med 322:95–99, 1990

Fuller MG, Jordan ML: The substance abuse consultation team: addressing the problem of hospitalized substance abusers. Gen Hosp Psychiatry 16:73–77, 1994

Fuller RK, Branchey L, Brightwell DR, et al: Disulfiram treatment of alcoholism. JAMA 256:1449–1455, 1986

Garbutt JC, West SL, Carey TS, et al: Pharmacological treatment of alcohol dependence: a review of the evidence. JAMA 281:1318–1325, 1999

Gawin FH, Kleber HD: Abstinence symptomatology and psychiatric diagnosis in cocaine abusers. Arch Gen Psychiatry 43:107–113, 1986

Geller A: Management of protracted withdrawal, in Principles of Addiction Medicine. Edited by Miller NS. Chevy Chase, MD, American Society of Addiction Medicine, 1994, pp 1–6

Grinspoon L, Bakalar JB: Psychedelics and arylcyclohexylamines, in Psychiatry Update: The American Psychiatric Association Annual Review, Vol 5. Edited by Frances AJ, Hales RE. Washington, DC, American Psychiatric Press, 1986, pp 212–225

Gruber AJ, Pope HG Jr: Cannabis psychotic disorder: does it exist? Am J Addict 3:72–83, 1994

Halikas JA, Crosby RD, Carlson GA, et al: Cocaine reduction in unmotivated crack users using carbamazepine versus placebo in a short term, double-blind crossover design. Clin Pharmacol Ther 50:81–95, 1991

Hall SM, Reus VI, Munoz RF, et al: Nortriptyline and cognitive-behavioral therapy in the treatment of cigarette smoking. Arch Gen Psychiatry 55:683–690, 1998

Halpern JH, Pope HJ: Do hallucinogens cause residual neuropsychological toxicity? Drug Alcohol Depend 53:247–256, 1999

Haney M, Ward AS, Comer SD, et al: Abstinence symptoms following smoked marijuana in humans. Psychopharmacology (Berl) 141:395–404, 1999

Harris-Allen M: Detoxification considerations in the medical management of substance abuse in pregnancy. Bull N Y Acad Med 67:270–276, 1991

Hayashida M, Alterman AI, McLellan AT, et al: Comparative effectiveness and costs of inpatient and outpatient detoxification of patients with mild to moderate alcohol withdrawal syndrome. N Engl J Med 320:358–365, 1989

Hayford KE, Patten CA, Rummans TA, et al: Efficacy of bupropion for smoking cessation in smokers with a former history of major depression or alcoholism. Br J Psychiatry 174:173–178, 1999

Henningfield JE: Pharmacologic basis and treatment of cigarette smoking. J Clin Psychiatry 45:24–34, 1984

Hughes JR: Tobacco abstinence and psychiatric treatment. J Clin Psychiatry 54:110–114, 1993

Hughes JR, Hatsukami D: Signs and symptoms of tobacco withdrawal. Arch Gen Psychiatry 43:289–294, 1986

Hughes JR, Goldstein MG, Hurt RD, et al: Recent advances in the pharmacotherapy of smoking. JAMA 281:72–76, 1999

Humphreys K, Moos RH, Finney JW: Life domains, Alcoholics Anonymous, and role incumbency in the 3-year course of problem drinking. J Nerv Ment Dis 184:475–481, 1996

Itkomen J, Schnoll S, Glassroth J: Pulmonary dysfunction in freebase cocaine users. Arch Intern Med 144:2195–2197, 1984

Jacobs BL: How hallucinogenic drugs work. American Scientist 75:386–392, 1987

Jasinski DR, Johnson RE, Kocher TR: Clonidine in morphine withdrawal. Arch Gen Psychiatry 42:1063–1066, 1985

Jentsch JD, Roth RH: The neuropsychopharmacology of phencyclidine: from NMDA receptor hypofunction to the dopamine hypothesis of schizophrenia. Neuropsychopharmacology 20:201–225, 1999

Johnson FW, Gruenewald PJ, Treno AJ, et al: Drinking over the life course within gender and ethnic groups: a hyperparametric analysis. J Stud Alcohol 59:568–580, 1998

Jonsson S, O'Meara M, Young JB: Acute cocaine poisoning. Am J Med 75:1061–1064, 1983

Jorenby DE, Leischow SJ, Nides MA, et al: A controlled trial of sustained-release bupropion, a nicotine patch, or both for smoking cessation. N Engl J Med 340:685–691, 1999

Joy JE, Watson SJ, Benson J (eds): Marijuana and Medicine: Assessing the Science Base. Washington, DC, National Academy Press, 1999

Kalant H: Research on tolerance: what can we learn from history? Alcohol Clin Exp Res 22:67–76, 1998

Kendler KS, Neale MC, MacLean CJ, et al: Smoking and major depression: a causal analysis. Arch Gen Psychiatry 50:36–43, 1993

Kleber HD, Riordan CE, Rounsaville B, et al: Clonidine in outpatient detoxification from methadone maintenance. Arch Gen Psychiatry 42:391–394, 1985

Kopelman MD: The Korsakoff syndrome. Br J Psychiatry 166:154–173, 1995

Kosten TR, Gawin FH, Morgan C: Evidence for altered desipramine disposition in methadone-maintained patients treated for cocaine abuse. Am J Drug Alcohol Abuse 16:329–336, 1990

Kranzler HR, Burleson JA, Del Boca FK, et al: Buspirone treatment of anxious alcoholics: a placebo-controlled trial. Arch Gen Psychiatry 51:720–731, 1994

Kranzler HR, Del Boca FK, Rounsaville BJ: Comorbid psychiatric diagnosis predicts three-year outcomes in alcoholics: a posttreatment natural history study. J Stud Alcohol 57:619–626, 1996

Kranzler HR, Modesto-Lowe V, Nuwayser ES: Sustained-release naltrexone for alcoholism treatment: a preliminary study. Alcohol Clin Exp Res 22:1074–1079, 1998

Lappalainen J, Long JC, Eggert M, et al: Linkage of antisocial alcoholism to the serotonin 5-HT1B receptor gene in 2 populations. Arch Gen Psychiatry 55:989–994, 1998

Lerner AG, Finkel B, Oyffe I, et al: Clonidine treatment for hallucinogen persisting perception disorder (letter). Am J Psychiatry 155:1460, 1998

Lerner A, Gelkopf M, Oyffe I, et al: LSD-induced hallucinogen persisting perception disorder treatment with clonidine: an open pilot study. Int Clin Psychopharmacol 15:35–37, 2000

Levin FR, Evans SM, McDowell DM, et al: Methylphenidate treatment for cocaine abusers with adult attention-deficit/hyperactivity disorder: a pilot study. J Clin Psychiatry 59:300–305, 1998

Levy RS, Hebert CK, Munn BG, et al: Drug and alcohol use in orthopedic trauma patients: a prospective study. J Orthop Trauma 10:21–27, 1996

Lichtenfeld J, Rubin DB, Feldman RS: Subarachnoid hemorrhage precipitated by cocaine snorting. Arch Neurol 41:223–224, 1986

Lieber C: Biochemical and molecular basis of alcohol-induced injury to liver and other tissues. N Engl J Med 319:1639–1647, 1988

Ling W, Charuvastra C, Collins JF, et al: Buprenorphine maintenance treatment of opiate dependence: a multicenter, randomized clinical trial. Addiction 93:475–486, 1998

Linnoila M: Alcohol withdrawal syndrome and sympathetic nervous system function. Alcohol Health Res World 13:355–357, 1989

Lucey MR, Carr K, Beresford TP, et al: Alcohol use after liver transplantation in alcoholics: a clinical cohort follow-up study. Hepatology 25:1223–1227, 1997

Mann JJ, Waternaux C, Haas GL, et al: Toward a clinical model of suicidal behavior in psychiatric patients. Am J Psychiatry 156:181–189, 1999

Marzuk PM, Tardiff K, Leon AC: Prevalence of cocaine use among residents of New York City who committed suicide during a one-year period. Am J Psychiatry 3:371–375, 1992

Mayo-Smith MF: Pharmacological management of alcohol withdrawal: a meta-analysis and evidence-based practice guideline. American Society of Addiction Medicine Working Group on Pharmacological Management of Alcohol Withdrawal. JAMA 278:144–151, 1997

McCance EF: Overview of potential treatment medications for cocaine dependence, in Medications Development for the Treatment of Cocaine Dependence: Issues in Clinical Efficacy Trials. Edited by Tai B, Chiang N, Bridge P. Rockville, MD, National Institute on Drug Abuse, 1997, pp 36–72

McLellan AT, Luborsky L, Woody GE, et al: An improved diagnostic evaluation instrument for substance abuse patients: the Addiction Severity Index. J Nerv Ment Dis 168:26–33, 1980

McLellan AT, Woody GE, Metzger D, et al: Evaluating the effectiveness of addiction treatments: reasonable expectations, appropriate comparisons. Milbank Q 74:51–85, 1996

McLellan AT, Grissom GR, Zanis D, et al: Problem-service 'matching' in addiction treatment: a prospective study in 4 programs. Arch Gen Psychiatry 54:730–735, 1997

McLellan AT, Lewis DC, O'Brien CP, et al: Drug dependence, a chronic medical illness: implications for treatment, insurance, and outcomes evaluation. JAMA 284:1689–1695, 2000

Medical-care expenditures attributable to cigarette smoking—United States, 1993. MMWR Morb Mortal Wkly Rep 43:469–472, 1994

Mee-Lee D, Shulman G, Gartner L: ASAM Patient Placement Criteria for the Treatment of Psychoactive Substance-Related Disorders, 2nd Edition. Chevy Chase, MD, American Society of Addiction Medicine, 1994

Merikangas KR, Mehta RL, Molnar BE, et al: Comorbidity of substance use disorders with mood and anxiety disorders: results of the International Consortium in Psychiatric Epidemiology. Addict Behav 23:893–907, 1998a

Merikangas KR, Stolar M, Stevens DE, et al: Familial transmission of substance use disorders. Arch Gen Psychiatry 55:973–979, 1998b

Meyers HB, Zepeda SG, Murdock MA: Alcohol and trauma: an endemic syndrome. West J Med 153:149–153, 1990

Minion GE, Slovid CM, Boutiette L: Severe alcohol intoxication: a study of 204 consecutive patients. J Toxicol Clin Toxicol 27:375–384, 1989

Moody DE, Alburges ME, Parker RJ, et al: The involvement of cytochrome P450 3A4 in the N-demethylation of L-alpha-acetylmethadol (LAAM), norLAAM, and methadone. Drug Metab Dispos 25:1347–1353, 1997

Moore RD, Bone LR, Geller G, et al: Prevalence, detection and treatment of alcoholism in hospitalized patients. JAMA 261:403–407, 1989

Morehead DB: Exacerbation of hallucinogen-persisting perception disorder with risperidone (letter). J Clin Psychopharmacol 17:327–328, 1997

Morse R, Flavin D: The definition of alcoholism. JAMA 268:1012–1014, 1992

Mueser KT, Drake RE, Miles KM: The course and treatment of substance use disorders in persons with severe mental illness, in Treatment of Drug-Dependent Individuals With Comorbid Mental Disorders. Edited by Onken LS, Blaine JD, Genser S, et al. Rockville, MD, National Institutes of Health, 1997, pp 86–109

Murphy GE, Wetzel R: The lifetime risk of suicide in alcoholism. Arch Gen Psychiatry 47:383–392, 1990

Murphy GE, Wetzel RD, Robine E, et al: Multiple risk factors predict suicide in alcoholism. Arch Gen Psychiatry 49:459–463, 1992

Nabeshima T, Kitaichi K, Noda Y: Functional changes in neuronal systems induced by phencyclidine administration. Ann N Y Acad Sci 801:29–38, 1996

Nadamanee K, Gorelick DA, Josephson MA: Myocardial ischemia during cocaine withdrawal. Ann Intern Med 111:876–880, 1989

National Institute on Drug Abuse and National Institute on Alcohol Abuse and Alcoholism: The economic costs of alcohol and drug abuse in the United States—1992 (Web page). Available at: http://www.nida.nih.gov/EconomicCosts/Table7_6.html. Accessed January 5, 2001

Nestler EJ, Self DW: Neurobiologic aspects of ethanol and other chemical dependencies, in The American Psychiatric Press Textbook of Neuropsychiatry, 3rd Edition. Edited by Yudofsky SC, Hales RE. Washington, DC, American Psychiatric Press, 1997, pp 773–798

Neumark YD, Delva J, Anthony JC: The epidemiology of adolescent inhalant drug involvement. Arch Pediatr Adolesc Med 152:781–786, 1998

Noordsy DL, Drake RE, Teague GB, et al: Subjective experiences related to alcohol use among schizophrenics. J Nerv Ment Dis 179:410–414, 1991

Nunes EV, Quitlin FM: Treatment of depression in drug-dependent patients: effects on mood and drug use, in Treatment of Drug-Dependent Individuals With Comorbid Mental Disorders. Edited by Onken LS, Blaine JD, Genser S, et al. Rockville, MD, National Institutes of Health, 1997, pp 61–85

O'Connor PG, Kosten TR: Rapid and ultrarapid opioid detoxification techniques. JAMA 279:229–234, 1998

O'Connor PG, Waugh ME, Carroll KM, et al: Primary care-based ambulatory opioid detoxification: the results of a clinical trial. J Gen Intern Med 10:255–260, 1995

Office of Applied Studies: Year-End 1997 Emergency Department Data From the Drug Abuse Warning Network. Rockville, MD, SAMHSA, U.S. Department of Health and Human Services, 1997

Office of Applied Studies: Summary Findings From the 1998 National Household Survey on Drug Abuse. Rockville, MD, SAMHSA, 1999

Office of National Drug Control Policy: Consultation document on opioid agonist treatment (Web page). Available at: http://www.whitehousedrugpolicy.gov/scimed/methadone/contents.html. Accessed January 5, 2001

Oslin DW, Pettinati HM, Volpicelli JR, et al: The effects of naltrexone on alcohol and cocaine use in dually addicted patients. J Subst Abuse Treat 16:163–167, 1999

Ostrea EM Jr, Welch RA: Detection of prenatal drug exposure in the pregnant woman and her newborn infant. Clin Perinatol 18:629–645, 1991

Palmstierna T: A model for predicting alcohol withdrawal delirium. Psychiatr Serv 52:820–823, 2001

Pelc I, Verbanck P, Le Bon O, et al: Efficacy and safety of acamprosate in the treatment of detoxified alcohol-dependent patients: a 90-day placebo-controlled dose-finding study. Br J Psychiatry 171:73–77, 1997

Porjesz B, Begleiter H: Human evoked brain potentials and alcohol. Alcoholism 5:304–316, 1981

Qasim A, Townend J, Davies M: Ecstasy induced acute myocardial infarction. Heart 85:E10, 2001

Raw M: Does nicotine chewing gum really work? BMJ 290:1231–1232, 1985

Reed BT, May PA: Inhalant abuse and juvenile delinquency: a control study in Albuquerque, New Mexico. Int J Addict 19:789–803, 1984

Regier DA, Farmer ME, Rae DS, et al: Comorbidity of mental disorders with alcohol and other drug abuse: results from the Epidemiologic Catchment Area (ECA) study. JAMA 264:2511–2518, 1990

Regier DA, Narrow WE, Rae DS, et al: The de facto US Mental and Addictive Disorders Service System: Epidemiologic Catchment Area prospective 1-year prevalence rates of disorders and services. Arch Gen Psychiatry 50:85–94, 1993

Reilly D, Didcott P, Swift W, et al: Long-term cannabis use: characteristics of users in an Australian rural area. Addiction 93:837–846, 1998

Reuler JB, Girard DE, Cooney TG: Wernicke's encephalopathy. N Engl J Med 312:1035–1039, 1985

Rickert VI, Wiemann CM, Berenson AB: Prevalence, patterns, and correlates of voluntary flunitrazepam use. Pediatrics 103:E6, 1999

Ried LD, Johnson RE, Gettman DA: Benzodiazepine exposure and functional status in older people. J Am Geriatr Soc 46:71–76, 1998

Robins LN, Helzer JE, Weissman MM, et al: Lifetime prevalence of specific psychiatric disorders in three sites. Arch Gen Psychiatry 41:949–958, 1984

Roggla H, Roggla G, Muhlbacher F: Psychiatric prognostic factors in patients with alcohol-related end-stage liver disease before liver transplantation. Wien Klin Wochenschr 108:272–275, 1996

Romach M, Busto U, Somer G, et al: Clinical aspects of chronic use of alprazolam and lorazepam. Am J Psychiatry 152:1161–1167, 1995

Roth D, Alarcon FJ, Fernandez JA: Acute rhabdomyolysis associated with cocaine intoxication. N Engl J Med 319:673–677, 1988

Rounsaville BJ, Kleber HD: Untreated opiate addicts: how do they differ from those seeking treatment? Arch Gen Psychiatry 42:1072–1077, 1985

Rounsaville BJ, Weissman MM, Kleber H, et al: The heterogenicity of psychiatric diagnoses in treated opiate addicts. Arch Gen Psychiatry 39:161–166, 1982

Roxane Laboratories, Inc.: Orlaam (package insert). Columbus OH, Roxane Laboratories, Inc., 2001

Saitz R, Mayo-Smith MF, Roberts MS, et al: Individualized treatment for alcohol withdrawal: a randomized double-blind controlled trial. JAMA 272:519–523, 1994

Santos de Barona M, Simpson DD: Inhalant users in drug abuse prevention programs. Am J Drug Alcohol Abuse 10:503–518, 1984

Sass H, Soyka M, Mann K, et al: Relapse prevention by acamprosate: results from a placebo-controlled study on alcohol dependence. Arch Gen Psychiatry 53:673–680, 1996

Satel SL, Krystal JH, Delgado PL, et al: Tryptophan depletion and attenuation of cue-induced craving for cocaine. Am J Psychiatry 152:778–783, 1995

Schuckit MA: New findings in the genetics of alcoholism. JAMA 281:1875–1876, 1999

Schuckit MA, Tipp JE, Reich T, et al: The histories of withdrawal convulsions and delirium tremens in 1648 alcohol dependent subjects. Addiction 90:1335–1347, 1995

Schuckit MA, Tipp JE, Bucholz KK, et al: The life-time rates of three major mood disorders and four major anxiety disorders in alcoholics and controls. Addiction 92:1289–1304, 1997

Schwartz RH, Hawks RL: Laboratory detection of marijuana use. JAMA 254:788–792, 1985

Schweizer E, Rickels K, Case WG, et al: Carbamazepine treatment in patients discontinuing long-term benzodiazepine therapy: effects on withdrawal severity and outcome. Arch Gen Psychiatry 48:448–452, 1991

Schweizer E, Rickels K, De Martinis N, et al: The effect of personality on withdrawal severity and taper outcome in benzodiazepine dependent patients. Psychol Med 28:713–720, 1998

Shannon M: Methylenedioxymethamphetamine (MDMA, "ecstasy"). Pediatr Emerg Care 16:377–380, 2000

Sherer MA, Kumor KM, Cone EJ, et al: Suspiciousness induced by four-hour intravenous infusions of cocaine: preliminary findings. Arch Gen Psychiatry 45:673–677, 1988

Simon EJ: Opiates: neurobiology, in Substance Abuse: A Comprehensive Textbook. Edited by Lowinson JH, Ruiz P, Millman RB, et al. Baltimore, MD, Williams & Wilkins, 1997, pp 148–158

Simpson DD, Joe GW, Fletcher BW, et al: A national evaluation of treatment outcomes for cocaine dependence. Arch Gen Psychiatry 56:507–514, 1999

Smart RG: Crack cocaine use: review of prevalence and adverse effects. Am J Drug Alcohol Abuse 17:13–26, 1991

Sobell LC, Cunningham JA, Sobell MB: Recovery from alcohol problems with and without treatment: prevalence in two population surveys. Am J Public Health 86:966–972, 1996

Sparenborg S, Vocci F, Zukin S: Peripheral cocaine-blocking agents: new medications for cocaine dependence. Drug Alcohol Depend 48:149–151, 1997

Steinbauer JR, Cantor SB, Holzer CE 3rd, et al: Ethnic and sex bias in primary care screening tests for alcohol use disorders. Ann Intern Med 129:353–362, 1998

Stine SM, Kosten TR: Use of drug combinations in treatment of opioid withdrawal. J Clin Psychopharmacol 3:203–209, 1992

Stowell LI, Fawcett JP, Brooke M, et al: Comparison of two commercial test kits for quantification of serum carbohydrate-deficient transferrin. Alcohol Alcohol 32:507–516, 1997

Sullivan JT, Swift RM, Lewis DC: Benzodiazepine requirements during alcohol withdrawal syndrome: clinical implications of using a standardized withdrawal scale. J Clin Psychopharmacol 11:291–295, 1991

Tonne U, Hiltunen AJ, Vikander B, et al: Neuropsychological changes during steady-state drug use, withdrawal and abstinence in primary benzodiazepine-dependent patients. Acta Psychiatr Scand 91:299–304, 1995

Trell E, Kristenson H, Fex G: Alcohol-related problems in middle-aged men with elevated serum gamma-glutamyltransferase: a preventive medical investigation. J Stud Alcohol 45:302–309, 1984

Tringali RA, Trzepacz PT, DiMartini A, et al: Assessment and follow-up of alcohol-dependent liver transplantation patients: a clinical cohort. Gen Hosp Psychiatry 18:70S–77S, 1996

Troisi A, Pasini A, Saracco M, et al: Psychiatric symptoms in male cannabis users not using other illicit drugs. Addiction 93:487–492, 1998

Trzepacz PT, DiMartini A, Tringali R: Psychopharmacologic issues in organ transplantation, part 1: pharmacokinetics in organ failure and psychiatric aspects of immunosuppressants and anti-infectious agents. Psychosomatics 34:199–207, 1993a

Trzepacz PT, DiMartini A, Tringali RD: Psychopharmacologic issues in organ transplantation, part 2: psychopharmacologic medications. Psychosomatics 34:290–298, 1993b

Tsai G, Coyle JT: The role of glutamatergic neurotransmission in the pathophysiology of alcoholism. Annu Rev Med 49:173–184, 1998

Tsuang MT, Lyons MJ, Meyer JM, et al: Co-occurrence of abuse of different drugs in men: the role of drug-specific and shared vulnerabilities. Arch Gen Psychiatry 55:967–972, 1998

Turner RG, Lichstein PR, Peden JG, et al: Alcohol withdrawal syndromes: a review of pathophysiology, clinical presentations and treatment. J Gen Intern Med 4:432–444, 1989

Tzivoni D, Keren A, Meyler S, et al: Cardiovascular safety of transdermal nicotine patches in patients with coronary artery disease who try to quit smoking. Cardiovasc Drugs Ther 12:239–244, 1998

U.S. Department of Health and Human Services: The health consequences of smoking: nicotine addiction: a report of the Surgeon General (DHHS Publ No CDC-88-8406). Washington, DC, U.S. Department of Health and Human Services, 1988

Vaillant GE: The Natural History of Alcoholism Revisited. Cambridge, MA, Harvard University Press, 1995

Van Thiel DH, Lipsitz HD, Porter LE, et al: Gastrointestinal and hepatic manifestations of chronic alcoholism. Gastroenterology 81:594–615, 1981

Victor M: The effects of alcohol on the nervous system, in Medical Diagnosis and Treatment of Alcoholism. Edited by Mendelson JH, Mello NK. New York, McGraw Hill, 1992, pp 201–262

Volkow ND, Wang GJ, Overall JE, et al: Regional brain metabolic response to lorazepam in alcoholics during early and late alcohol detoxification. Alcohol Clin Exp Res 21:1278–1284, 1997

Walsh DC, Ringson RW, Merrigan DM, et al: A randomized trial of treatment options for alcohol abusing workers. N Engl J Med 325:775–782, 1991

Wand GS, Mangold D, El Deiry S, et al: Family history of alcoholism and hypothalamic opioidergic activity. Arch Gen Psychiatry 55:1114–1119, 1998

Weddington WW, Brown BS, Haertzen CA, et al: Changes in mood, craving, and sleep during short-term abstinence reported by male cocaine addicts: a controlled, residential study. Arch Gen Psychiatry 47:861–868, 1990

Weisner C, Schmidt L: General disparities in treatment for alcohol problems. JAMA 268:1872–1876, 1992

Whitfield JB, Fletcher LM, Murphy TL, et al: Smoking, obesity, and hypertension alter the dose-response curve and test sensitivity of carbohydrate-deficient transferrin as a marker of alcohol intake. Clin Chem 44:2480–2489, 1998

Whitworth AB, Fischer F, Lesch OM, et al: Comparison of acamprosate and placebo in long-term treatment of alcohol dependence. Lancet 347:1438–1442, 1996

Wiesbeck GA, Schuckit MA, Kalmijn JA, et al: An evaluation of the history of a marijuana withdrawal syndrome in a large population. Addiction 91:1469–1478, 1996

Wilde MI, Wagstaff AJ: Acamprosate: a review of its pharmacology and clinical potential in the management of alcohol dependence after detoxification. Drugs 53:1038–1053, 1997

Zubieta JK, Gorelick DA, Stauffer R, et al: Increased mu opioid receptor binding detected by PET in cocaine-dependent men is associated with cocaine craving. Nat Med 2:1225–1229, 1996

22

Sexual Disorders and Dysfunctions

George R. Brown, M.D.

Gregory Gass, M.D.

Kemuel Philbrick, M.D.

Physicians have tended to focus on sexual dysfunction rather than evaluating or restoring sexual health. Sexual health is defined by the World Health Organization (WHO) as "the integration of the somatic, emotional, intellectual, and social aspects in ways that are positively enriching and that will enhance personality, communication, and love" (Jensen 1992, p. 135). The consultation-liaison psychiatrist has regular contact with patients whose somatic dysfunction is the principal focus of their hospital admission (T. Wise 1983). The high incidence of anxiety, mood, and substance abuse disorders in general hospital patients (Wells et al. 1988) suggests that chronic medical illnesses may pose a particular challenge to the successful integration of the necessary elements of satisfactory sexual function. All phases of the human sexual response are subject to influence by a variety of medical and psychiatric conditions (Table 22–1). Whether sexual dysfunction occurs as a direct consequence of chronic illness (e.g., impotence from diabetic neuropathy), a reflection of psychological struggle arising from chronic illness (e.g., fear of exposure during a flare of psoriasis), a comorbid psychiatric illness (Rosen et al. 1999), or a combination of two or more factors (e.g., surrender of libido in response to the chronic experience of inadequacy caused by a medical disability), the consultation-liaison psychiatrist has the unique opportunity to address the interrelation of these various areas, do battle with the tendency to compartmentalize, and enhance the patient's overall quality of life (Nankervis 1989).

Fagan et al. (1990) suggested seven factors that may indicate a psychological source of sexual dysfunction in patients with discrete medical illnesses:

TABLE 22–1. Human sexual response cycle

Desire
  Fantasies about sexual activity and desire for sex
Excitement
  Subjective sense of sexual pleasure and associated physiologic changes
Orgasm
  Peaking (climax) of sexual pleasure, with release of sexual tension
Resolution
  Sense of general well-being and muscular relaxation after orgasm

Source. Adapted from American Psychiatric Association 1994.

1. History of sexual trauma or abnormal sexual development
2. Restrictive religious or moral sexual attitudes
3. Preexisting sexual dysfunction
4. Situational or partner-specific dysfunction
5. Evidence of morning or masturbatory full tumescence
6. Evidence of masturbatory arousal and orgasm in women
7. Sexual dysfunction following the onset of another psychiatric disorder

The patient's propensity for privacy may collude with the general physician's tendency to focus on the medical precipitants of the patient's admission. Consequently, sexual dysfunction could easily escape evaluation unless the consultation-liaison psychiatrist remains alert for the possibility that the manifest reason for a consultation may have underlying associations with sexual dysfunction. Attending physicians may avoid discussing sexual health because of time limitations, discomfort with the topic, or fear of having little to offer even if a problem is identified. Therefore, it is important for the consultation-liaison psychiatrist to raise the issue. It is generally true that if the physician does not ask about sexual health issues, the patient will not tell.

In the following sections, we discuss many specific biological intrusions on sexual function. Of note, DSM-IV-TR (American Psychiatric Association 2000) lists specific categories for "sexual dysfunction due to a general medical condition." These diagnoses are to be used when patients have clinically significant sexual dysfunctions judged to be etiologically related to a general medical condition.

Jensen (1992, p. 136) went beyond the purely biological axis and reported that "disease acceptance (global evaluation) has been shown to be significantly related to the presence of sexual dysfunction. Only fifteen percent of couples with good disease acceptance reported a sexual dysfunction in contrast to 57% of those with moderate or poor disease acceptance." T. Wise (1977, p. 62) proposed a useful shorthand for conceptualizing the psychosocial context of a particular dysfunction, suggesting that the consulting physician next "identify what aspect of sexuality is being utilized—the reproductive, the interpersonal, or autistic—and at what stage of the life cycle the individual is at present." This multidimensional formulation lays the foundation for constructive intervention.

In addition to the sexual consequences of common disease entities, we discuss some primary sexual and gender identity disorders that may be encountered in the hospital setting and the treatments that are available for these patients.

SEXUAL DYSFUNCTIONS IN PATIENTS WITH MEDICAL AND SURGICAL ILLNESSES

Heart Disease

Patients who have recently experienced either crescendo angina or a myocardial infarction and those who have been hospitalized for procedures such as percutaneous angioplasty or coronary artery bypass surgery are common sources of consultation requests. Most studies of patients with heart disease to address sexual functioning have focused on men; however, evidence suggests that the physiologic measures used may not be substantially different in women (Skinner 1979). Although study designs and specific conclusions vary, frequent conclusions include 1) markedly decreased sexual activity and increased perception of sexual dysfunction after a myocardial infarction are common (Nankervis 1989; Skinner 1979); 2) resuming sexual activity postinfarction with one's prior partner and in the usual setting does not increase morbidity (Silber 1987); 3) most impediments to a satisfying sexual life are psychological rather than physiologic (Skinner 1979); 4) those with low ejection fraction and advanced heart disease experience marked changes in libido and in ability to perform sexually (Jaarsma et al. 1996); and 5) concerns about the safety of sexual activity are rarely discussed with patients and their spouses before discharge from the hospital (Silber 1987).

Although sexual dysfunction generally does not precipitate a consultation request in the heart disease population, the consulting psychiatrist should remember the ubiquity of this concern among these patients and their partners (McLane et al. 1980). The consultation-liaison psychiatrist can encourage patients to raise the issue of sexual concerns with their nonpsychiatric physicians by showing an awareness of fundamental facts (see Table 22–2) and by attaching importance to their discussion. This models for the patient the appropriateness of a discussion with the primary physician. Similarly, active liaison psychiatry provides an opportunity to tactfully remind one's colleagues of the effect that a myocardial infarction can have on the patient's sense of self and wholeness and on the patient's expression of his or her sexuality (Hackett and Cassem 1973).

TABLE 22–2. Sexuality and heart disease

Sexual questions are common.

Typically, return to full premorbid level of sexual activity can be anticipated at about 2–3 months.

Sexual energy expenditure/oxygen consumption for the average middle-aged married couple approximates that of a brisk walk.

When clinical circumstances dictate caution, experimenting with different techniques and positions may enable the couple to achieve satisfactory expression less strenuously.

Certain cardiotropic medications have potential effects.

Prophylactic sublingual nitroglycerin may be useful.

Coital or postcoital infarction or sudden death with established partners in familiar settings is relatively rare.

Source. Adapted from Silber E: "The Treatment of Ischemic Heart Disease," in *Heart Disease*, 2nd Edition. Edited by Silber E. New York, Macmillan, 1987, pp. 1663–1665. Copyright 1987, McGraw-Hill. Used with permission.

An increasing number of patients have received heart transplants. As survival after heart transplant continues to improve (≥50% 5-year survival), attention to subsequent quality of life also has increased. Mulligan et al. (1991) reported that libido that was generally strong before surgery remained strong afterward; however, most of their 71 male respondents perceived that their partner's libido increased further postoperatively. Sixty percent of the respondents noted anorgasmia posttransplant (Mulligan et al. 1991). Pretransplant erectile disability and anorgasmia appeared to increase at 3 and 12 months posttransplant (Mulligan et al. 1991). Patients commonly experience sexual concerns posttransplant but rarely pursue their questions (Tabler and Frierson 1990). Questions tend to be fueled by one or more of a few very common concerns, even though they are often raised in the context of a specific dysfunction (Table 22–3).

Cancer

Breast, cervical, ovarian, endometrial, and vulvar cancer all threaten female sexual function, but the biopsychosocial basis for the dysfunction varies considerably according to etiology (body image, radiation sequelae, anatomic limitations such as vaginal fibrosis) and focus (loss of desire, need for adjunctive aids such as lubricants) (Schover et al. 1987). Although treatments that maximize breast preservation would intuitively seem to favor maintenance of sexual function, a woman's premorbid adjustment and function may be a more accurate determinant of subsequent function and satisfaction (Schover 1991). Newer approaches to combining tumor removal and breast reconstruction in the same operation may affect this issue. Problematic sequelae of pelvic radiation for cervical cancer can be delayed for several months after treatment but may result in considerably more sexual dysfunction than does surgical treatment (Schover et al. 1989). One study that compared women with breast cancer treated with chemotherapy with those whose cancer was treated by other means found that those who received chemotherapy were more likely to report vaginal dryness, decreased libido, dyspareunia, and difficulty achieving orgasm (Young-McCaughan 1996).

Sexual function in men with reproductive system cancer may be threatened by the disease itself (including a period before formal diagnosis), hormonal therapy, radiation, or surgical procedures. Erectile dysfunction may herald prostatic cancer, accompany hormonal or surgical treatments, or trail radiation by several months because of progressive vascular scarring. One study of nerve-sparing surgical techniques in patients with prostatic cancer resulted in a difference in postsurgical fre-

TABLE 22–3. Sexual concerns of heart transplant patients

Inability to integrate the new heart into their sense of self
Fear of placing undue stress on the new heart
Anxiety about the particular sexual practices of the donor
Shift in roles and responsibilities in important relationships
Self-perception of sexual attractiveness
Medication effects on sexual desire and sexual performance
Depression and its sexual sequelae

Source. Adapted from Tabler J, Frierson R: "Sexual Concerns After Heart Transplantation." *Journal of Heart and Lung Transplantation* 9:397–403, 1990. Copyright 1990, Mosby Year-Book, Inc. Used with permission.

quency of impotence of 85% versus 32% (Ofman and Auchincloss 1992). In contrast, 30% of the demographically distinct group of young men with testicular cancer stated that sexual performance difficulties were bothersome 1 year postdiagnosis but were less prominent than the concerns about retrograde ejaculation and infertility (Rieker et al. 1989). Infertility among men with testicular cancer has been treated with some success by electroejaculation (Ohl et al. 1991). The consultation-liaison psychiatrist may be called on to assist patients in their decision between treatments that may be more effective in arresting their cancer but lead to sometimes irreversible sexual dysfunction and less effective treatments with higher probabilities of salvaging erectile and orgasmic capacity (Singer et al. 1991).

Nongenital tumor sites such as the bladder, colon, rectum, and systemic lymphoma also can be associated with sexual dysfunction, either as a direct consequence of treatment (e.g., retroperitoneal lymph node dissection) or as a result of negative effects on a patient's self-esteem and sense of propriety. For example, ostomy patients may have a particularly difficult struggle with regaining comfortable sexual expression (Ofman and Auchincloss 1992). The consultation-liaison psychiatrist should ask cancer patients specifically about sexual issues and then obtain a thorough sexual history, including questions to the patient's partner when possible. The consultant should not make any assumptions about sexual orientation and should convey a sense of openness to the range of human sexual expression. A positive stance should be used, and an informed capacity for basic counseling, and further referral when indicated, is necessary (Auchincloss 1989).

Renal Failure

Multiple body systems have been implicated in sexual dysfunctions when experienced by patients with acute and chronic renal failure. In men with uremia, endocrine disturbances (characterized by decreased testosterone, increased estradiol, and excessive parathyroid hormone), autonomic disruption, vascular insufficiency, and zinc deficiency all have been implicated (Campese and Liu 1990). In addition to estimates of erectile dysfunction that range from 20% to 80%, men with renal failure commonly experience decreased sexual interest, testicular atrophy, and impaired spermatogenesis, which lead to infertility (Campese and Liu 1990). More than half of the women with uremia are amenorrheic before menopause, bearing witness to the sensitivity of the female hypothalamic-pituitary-ovarian axis. A similar proportion are reported to complain of decreased sexual interest and anorgasmia (Finkelstein and Steele 1978). Sexual dysfunction in both men and women may be further aggravated by any of several medications typically required by patients with renal failure. An almost universal sequela, anemia, may also drain desire and energy for sexual activity. In one series of case reports, erythropoietin was used beneficially in three patients who had partial erectile dysfunction; the benefit may have been attributable to increased blood viscosity promoted by the erythropoietin (Imagawa et al. 1990).

Although hemodialysis corrects many metabolic derangements seen in chronic renal failure, it appears to offer little improvement in sexual function (Procci and Martin 1985). Some researchers suggest that sexual dysfunction may actually increase after dialysis is begun (Dillard et al. 1989). Other concomitant treatment efforts (e.g., clomiphene citrate, zinc, testosterone, bromocriptine) have had mixed anecdotal success (Menchini-Fabris et al. 1990).

Successful kidney transplantation is associated with general improvement in sexual function. In one study (Schover et al. 1990) of 54 men and 36 women who had undergone a successful transplant during the prior 5 years, the frequency of major sexual dysfunction was decreased by 50% to about 25% of pretransplantation levels. Sexual desire increased significantly for both men and women; many men also reported substantial improvement in the ability to achieve an erection and experience orgasm. Women enjoyed less definitive improvement in the ability to experience orgasm. Although frequency of sexual activity in transplanted women doubled to once per week, this did not achieve statistical significance; overall sexual satisfaction levels remained constant pre- and posttransplant. The challenge to negotiating the hurdles of appropriate intimacy in young adult patients with renal failure may be reflected in the fact that patients with end-stage renal disease (ESRD) diagnosed before adulthood are significantly less likely to marry (i.e., 37% of the patients with

ESRD diagnosed before adulthood are less likely to marry compared with 7% of those with ESRD diagnosed after adulthood). Schover et al. (1990, p. 11) advised that "younger renal patients may need special support and counseling on how to form committed relationships." In this group of young patients, although 75% expressed a broad interest in information about sexuality and ESRD, only one-third had received such information (Schover et al. 1990).

Diabetes Mellitus

A high level of awareness that impotence (erectile dysfunction) is common in patients with diabetes mellitus is generally found. However, sexual dysfunction in diabetic patients may be considerably more pleomorphic than is commonly recognized. Fairburn et al. (1982a, 1982b) studied 27 impotent and 7 nonimpotent diabetic men. They noted a variety of sexual complaints in addition to erectile dysfunction, including a range of ejaculatory disturbances, loss of sexual interest, persistent morning erections in one-half, and spontaneous erections in one-third. In general, erectile dysfunction did not parallel other general indicators of diabetic progression. Thus, psychological factors may contribute significantly to the presence of erectile dysfunction (e.g., premorbid sexual difficulties and/or marital discord). On the other hand, Forsberg et al. (1989) studied 37 diabetic men with erectile difficulties and concluded that psychosocial factors were the *sole* cause in only 2 patients. Nevertheless, despite identification of neuropathic, hormonal, and vascular contributors in the other 35 patients, nearly two-thirds of the men had psychosocial factors "of importance"; half of these factors were believed to be "of great importance" in the diagnosis and/or treatment of their sexual dysfunction (Forsberg et al. 1989).

The unfortunate but common assumption that diabetic impotence is "wholly organic" was examined further by Lustman and Clouse (1990). They used a standardized interview to study 37 impotent diabetic men with established peripheral neuropathy and/or peripheral vascular disease. All 8 patients with neuropathy who met criteria for either current major depression or generalized anxiety disorder were impotent. Of the 20 patients with neuropathy but without either of the above psychiatric diagnoses, only 6 were impotent. Although the study was hampered by its retrospective design, further statistical analysis nonetheless confirmed that the apparent association of neuropathy with erectile dysfunction was actually dependent on the psychiatric status of the patient (Lustman and Clouse 1990). This observation strengthens the need for caution in assigning undue emphasis to time-honored evaluations such as nocturnal penile tumescence studies (Thase et al. 1988). In a placebo-controlled study of 268 men with erectile dysfunction and diabetes, Rendell et al. (1999) reported that 56% reported improved erections with sildenafil and 10% improved with placebo. This response rate, which is 20%–40% lower than that found in random population studies (Marks et al. 1999), and the above correlation of psychiatric diagnosis and erectile dysfunction underscore the necessity for using a comprehensive biopsychosocial approach to the evaluation and treatment of diabetic patients with sexual dysfunction (Sarica et al. 1994).

Diabetic women have not been so well studied. In one report, Forsberg et al. (1989) concluded that women with diabetes do not have a greater incidence of sexual dysfunction than do women in the general population. Webster (1994), however, noted that problems with libido, arousal, and orgasm are common in both men and women with diabetes.

HIV Disease/AIDS

Persons infected with the human immunodeficiency virus (HIV) are common on nearly all wards of many general hospitals regardless of whether they have been admitted specifically for care of the medical and surgical complications of this infection. Patients with earlier stages of infection (defined as having > 400 T cells/mm^3 and usually physically asymptomatic) may express sexual concerns that have become both quality-of-life and relationship issues for themselves and their partners. New onset of hypoactive sexual desire disorder (HSDD)—operationally defined for this population as at least a one-third decrease in baseline levels of sexual fantasies and/or desire for sexual activity of any type persistently present for at least 1 month and commencing at least 1 month after notification of HIV seroconversion (among other specific criteria; Brown et al. 1992)—is one of the most common psychiatric diagnoses in both men and women with early-stage HIV disease. For example, 21.7% of 442 men (Brown et al. 1992) and 31%–41% of 25 women (Brown and Rundell 1990, 1993) were noted to have disorders of sexual desire in a United States Air Force population. Impaired sexual desire also has been reported in men with HIV disease in Australia (32% of 232 men; Dunbar et al. 1991) and The Netherlands (23% of 65 men; Van Buuren et al. 1991). Rosser and colleagues (1997) reviewed the sexual issues of gay men living with HIV.

Among non–chemically dependent women with early HIV disease, marital problems and HSDD may be the only psychiatric problems with substantial clinical frequency (Brown and Rundell 1993). When HSDD is present in HIV-infected women, they usually describe it in a typical fashion 4–18 months after learning of their HIV seropositivity: gradual onset over a 2- to 6-month period, usually in the presence of a willing partner and in the absence of comorbid medical or psychiatric conditions (Brown et al. 1995). HIV-infected women with HSDD do not differ demographically from those without it and are no more likely to have additional psychiatric diagnoses (except possibly marital conflicts, often secondary to the wife's sexual dysfunction). Their sexual desire complaints usually are not a component of mood or anxiety disorders. Most patients who develop HSDD a year or more after notification of seropositivity are puzzled by the symptoms and frequently convey that these symptoms threaten previously established levels of intimacy in important relationships. This phenomenon, possibly caused by direct infection of the brain by HIV, has been noted in women from middle-class backgrounds free of poverty and drug abuse as well as in the inner-city populations of injection drug users who often face the challenges of poverty and instability in all areas of life (Goggin et al. 1998). Patients with late-stage HIV disease (acquired immunodeficiency syndrome [AIDS]) may be physically debilitated by the opportunistic infections, wasting, and fatigue that often bring them into the hospital (Tindall et al. 1994).

Sexual health is often overlooked in both the psychiatric and the medical care of HIV-infected patients. HIV-seropositive patients may be reluctant to discuss their sexual dysfunction, especially when the topic is not broached by their physician. Communication is further hampered when their primary care physician suggests that complete abstinence from interpersonal expressions of sexuality is the only acceptable "safe" alternative. Such absolutism serves only to jeopardize informed, collaborative sexual and reproductive behavior decision making (Minkoff and Moreno 1990). With the success of prenatal and postnatal antiretroviral treatments as first discovered in AIDS Clinical Trials Group-76 (ACTG-76), perinatal transmission in the United States has been reduced to about 7%–8%, making the decision to have children substantially safer than in earlier years of the epidemic. Negative or moralistic attitudes on the part of the consultant could also lead to dangerous sexual "acting out." The consulting psychiatrist can make a useful contribution by opening a dialogue on sexual issues and communicating the view that sexual health may incorporate responsible, "safer-sex" approaches that limit HIV transmission. For example, the potential benefits of masturbation and mutual masturbation with a partner should be emphasized. Major depression and dementia (Atkinson et al. 1988) also may complicate all stages of HIV infection, especially later stages. Sexual desire disorders and, less commonly, secondary erectile dysfunction may accompany these conditions.

The consultation-liaison psychiatrist caring for HIV/AIDS patients must be aware of the clear connection between increased high-transmission risk behaviors (e.g., unprotected intercourse with seronegative partners) and substance use. Volatile nitrites ("poppers") used at the point of orgasm to intensify the experience have been linked to higher-risk behaviors (Ostrow et al. 1991), as have alcohol and illicit drug use (Crosby et al. 1991).

MEDICATIONS AND SEXUAL FUNCTIONING

Many medications are associated with sexual dysfunctions in all phases of the human sexual response cycle. DSM-IV (American Psychiatric Association 1994) included a new diagnostic category that can be used to describe these disorders—substance-induced sexual dysfunction—as well as sexual side effects from nonprescribed substance use. Hospitalized patients are frequently taking several of the medications listed in Table 22–4 that may have sexual side effects or contribute to sexual dysfunction, but patients may be hesitant to discuss these problems.

In addition, some medications are reportedly associated with improved sexual response. One study reported prosexual side effects of the aminoketone antidepressant bupropion. Of 107 psychiatric outpatients, 77% reported improvements in at least one aspect of sexual response (Modell et al. 1997). However, the "true aphrodisiac" remains an elusive potion that does not reliably best placebo.

Sildenafil Citrate

Sildenafil citrate (Viagra) has revolutionized the treatment of erectile dysfunction in men with physiologic compromise, whether vascular or neurologically induced. The high levels of this disorder (39% of 40-year-olds, 67% of 70-year-olds; Feldman et al. 1994) contributed to this oral medication's resounding success in the marketplace, both licit and illicit.

Sildenafil is a selective inhibitor of cyclic guanosine monophosphate (cGMP)–specific phosphodiesterase type 5 (Ballard et al. 1998). Nitric oxide (NO) is a key component in erectile tissue functioning (both male and female) under the influence of sexual stimulation. Nitric oxide activates guanylate cyclase, resulting in higher levels of cGMP, which in turn produce smooth muscle relaxation in the corpora and a net increase of blood flow to the penis or clitoris. In the absence of sexual stimulation, sildenafil has no effect. Sildenafil has been shown to be more effective than placebo in restoring erectile function to men with radical prostatectomy (43% vs. 15%; Physicians' Desk Reference 1999), spinal cord injuries (83% vs. 12%), "psychogenic etiologies" (84% vs. 26%; Boolell et al. 1996), coronary artery disease, peripheral vascular disease, diabetes mellitus, and erectile dysfunction as a side effect from antidepressants, antipsychotics, and antihypertensives (Eid 2000; Goldstein et al. 1998). Doses range from 25 to 100 mg taken 30–90 minutes before sexual activity. Patients with renal and hepatic disease also can be given this generally safe agent. Pooled safety data from 18 studies involving more than 3,700 men showed a remarkable safety profile (Gregoire 1998). Typical side effects are minor and include headaches, flushing, nasal congestion, transient changes in color vision, and dyspepsia; only 2% of the men discontinued treatment because of side effects. Sildenafil is contraindicated in men who are taking any form of nitrates, including sublingual nitroglycerin (Kloner 1998). Through July 1998, after 3.6 million prescriptions, 69 deaths were reported, most of which were caused by potentiation of hypotensive effects of nitrates by sildenafil. This additive effect limits the usefulness of sildenafil in a large population of patients with unstable angina (Kloner and Jarow 1999; Morales et al. 1998).

Sildenafil also has been used in women with arousal difficulties, despite a lack of published controlled trials supporting this off-label use (Gregoire 1998). This is based on work indicating an analogous mechanism of clitoral cavernosum engorgement involving nitrogen oxide (Park et al. 1998). Anecdotally, many women with this type of sexual dysfunction appear to benefit from sildenafil, and controlled studies for this indication are nearing completion (Nurnberg et al. 1999).

One unanticipated side effect of sildenafil the prescribing psychiatrist should take into consideration is the effect of greatly increased sexual activity on the spouses of treated men. A sudden return of erectile functioning changes the dynamics of a relationship and may lead to unintended psychological and physical consequences (e.g., new onset of cystitis in female partners) ("Cystitis in Partners of Viagra Users" 1998; Wise 1999) or destabilization of a relationship that has accommodated long-term abstinence.

TABLE 22–4. Medications associated with sexual dysfunction

Medication	Reported adverse effect
Acetazolamide	Loss of libido; decreased potency
Acitretin	Decreased libido
Alcohol	Chronic abuse: decreased libido; impotence; premature or retarded ejaculation; dyspareunia (women)
Alprazolam	Inhibition of orgasm; delayed or no ejaculation; decreased libido
Amiloride	Impotence; decreased libido
Aminocaproic acid	Dry ejaculation
Amiodarone	Decreased libido
Amitriptyline	Loss of libido; impotence; no ejaculation
Amoxapine	Loss of libido; impotence; ejaculatory problems
Amphetamines	Chronic abuse: impotence; delayed or no ejaculation; no orgasm (women)
Amyl nitrite	Decreased libido; impotence
Anisotropine	Impotence
Atenolol	Impotence
Atorvastatin calcium	Decreased libido; impotence; abnormal ejaculation
Atropine	Impotence
Baclofen	Impotence; no ejaculation
Barbiturates	Decreased libido; impotence
Bendroflumethiazide	Impotence; ejaculatory and libido problems
Benztropine	Impotence
Bromocriptine	Painful clitoral tumescence; impotence
Bupropion	Decreased libido; impotence; priapism
Buserelin	Loss of libido; impotence
Buspirone	Priapism
Busulfan	Impotence
Butaperazine	Impotence; ejaculatory and libido problems
Cannabis	Increased libido
Captopril	Impotence; ejaculatory problems
Carbamazepine	Impotence
Carbidopa-levodopa	Priapism; increased libido
Carvedilol	Impotence
Cetirizine hydrochloride	Decreased libido
Chlorambucil	Impotence
Chlordiazepoxide	Decreased libido
Chlorothiazide	Impotence; ejaculatory and libido problems
Chlorpromazine	Decreased libido; impotence; no ejaculation; priapism
Chlorprothixene	Ejaculatory inhibition
Chlorthalidone	Decreased libido; impotence
Cimetidine	Decreased libido; impotence
Citalopram	Increased or decreased libido; clitoral priapism; delayed ejaculation; delayed or absent orgasm; erectile dysfunction
Clidinium	Impotence
Clofibrate	Decreased libido; impotence
Clomipramine	Decreased libido; impotence; retarded or no ejaculation or orgasm; orgasm precipitated by yawning; painful ejaculation
Clonidine	Impotence; delayed or retrograde ejaculation; decreased libido
Clozapine	Priapism; retrograde ejaculation
Cocaine	Priapism
Cyclophosphamide	Impotence
Cyproterone acetate	Decreased libido
Cytosine arabinoside	Impotence; decreased libido; dyspareunia
Danazol	Increased or decreased libido
Delavirdine mesylate	Decreased libido; impotence
Desipramine	Decreased libido; impotence; painful orgasm
Diazepam	Decreased libido; delayed ejaculation; retarded or no orgasm (women); erection problems
Dichlorphenamide	Decreased libido; impotence

TABLE 22–4.   Medications associated with sexual dysfunction *(continued)*

Medication	Reported adverse effect
Dicyclomine	Impotence
Diethylpropion	Impotence; delayed ejaculation; anorgasmia (women)
Digoxin	Decreased libido; impotence
Diphenhydramine	Impotence
Disopyramide	Impotence
Disulfiram	Impotence
Donepezil	Increased libido
Doxepin	Decreased libido; ejaculatory problems
Estrogens	Increased or decreased libido
Ethosuximide	Increased libido
Ethoxzolamide	Decreased libido
Etretinate	Erectile problems
Famotidine	Impotence
Fat emulsion	Priapism
Fenfluramine	Increased libido; loss of libido in women with large doses or long-term use; impotence
Fenofibrate	Decreased libido
Finasteride	Decreased libido; impotence; ejaculatory failure
Fluoxetine	Anorgasmia; delayed orgasm; spontaneous orgasm; ejaculatory problems; penile anesthesia; decreased libido
Fluphenazine	Decreased libido; erectile problems; ejaculatory inhibition; priapism
Fluvoxamine	Delayed ejaculation; inhibited orgasm; increased libido
Gemfibrozil	Impotence; loss of libido
Goserelin	Impotence; loss of libido and sexual fantasies
Glutethimide	Decreased libido
Glycopyrrolate	Impotence
Grepafloxacin hydrochloride	Impotence
Guanabenz	Impotence
Guanadrel	Decreased libido; delayed or retrograde ejaculation; delayed orgasm (women)
Guanethidine	Decreased libido; impotence; delayed, retrograde, or no ejaculation
Guanfacine	Impotence
Haloperidol	Impotence; painful ejaculation
Heroin	Increased or decreased libido; ejaculatory problems
Hexamethonium	Ejaculatory inhibition; impotence
Hexocyclium	Impotence
Homatropine methylbromide	Impotence
Hydralazine	Impotence; priapism
Hydrochlorothiazide	Impotence; ejaculatory and libido problems
Hydroxyzine	Impotence
Imipramine	Decreased libido; impotence; painful, delayed ejaculation; delayed orgasm (women)
Indapamide	Decreased libido; impotence
Indomethacin	Impotence; decreased libido
Interferon-α	Decreased libido; impotence
Isocarboxazid	Impotence; delayed ejaculation; no orgasm (women)
Ketoconazole	Impotence; decreased libido
Labetalol	Priapism; impotence; delayed or no ejaculation; decreased libido
Leuprolide	Impotence
Levodopa	Increased libido
Lithium	Decreased libido; impotence
Lorazepam	Loss of libido
LSD	Increased or decreased libido; erectile and ejaculatory problems
Maprotiline	Impotence; decreased libido
Mazindol	Impotence; spontaneous ejaculation; painful testes
MDA	Increased or decreased libido; erectile and ejaculatory problems
Mecamylamine	Impotence; decreased libido
Melphalan	Impotence

TABLE 22–4. Medications associated with sexual dysfunction *(continued)*

Medication	Reported adverse effect
Mepenzolate bromide	Impotence
Mesoridazine	No ejaculation; impotence; priapism
Methadone	Decreased libido; impotence; no orgasm; retarded ejaculation
Methaqualone	Impotence or inhibited ejaculation (men); decreased libido (women)
Methandrostenolone	Decreased libido
Methantheline bromide	Impotence
Methazolamide	Decreased libido; impotence
Methotrexate	Impotence; erectile problems
Methscopolamine	Impotence
Methyldopa	Decreased libido; impotence; delayed or no ejaculation; delayed or no orgasm (women)
Metoclopramide	Impotence; decreased libido
Metoprolol	Impotence
Metyrosine	Impotence; no ejaculation
Mexiletine	Impotence; decreased libido
Midazolam	Sexual fantasies (women)
Midodrine	Impotence
Mirtazapine	Increased libido; impotence
Molindone	Priapism
Morphine	Decreased libido; impotence
Nadolol	Decreased libido; impotence; ejaculatory problems
Nafarelin	Impotence; loss of libido
Nefazodone	Spontaneous ejaculation
Naltrexone	Delayed ejaculation; decreased potency
Naproxen	Impotence; no ejaculation
Naratriptan hydrochloride	Decreased libido; inflammation of breast, vagina, and fallopian tubes
Nifedipine	Priapism
Nilutamide	Decreased libido; testicular atrophy
Nisoldipine	Decreased libido; impotence
Nizatidine	Impotence
Norethandrolone	Decreased libido; impotence
Nortriptyline	Impotence; decreased libido
Olanzapine	Decreased libido; impotence; abnormal ejaculation
Omeprazole	Painful nocturnal erections
Oxybutynin	Impotence
Oxymetholone	Prepubertal males: phallic enlargement, increased frequency of erections; postpuberbertal males: inhibition of testicular function, testicular atrophy, oligospermia, impotence, chronic priapism; females: clitoral enlargement; both: increased or decreased libido
Oxyphencyclimine	Impotence
Papaverine	Priapism, especially with neurological disorders
Pargyline	No ejaculation; impotence
Paroxetine	Delayed ejaculation; inhibited orgasm
Pergolide	Hypersexuality; priapism; spontaneous ejaculation
Perphenazine	Decreased or no ejaculation
Phencyclidine	Increased or decreased libido; erectile and ejaculatory problems
Phenelzine	Impotence; retarded or no ejaculation; delayed or no orgasm; priapism
Phenmetrazine	Impotence; delayed ejaculation
Phenoxybenzamine	Dry ejaculation
Phentolamine	Impotence
Phenytoin	Decreased libido; impotence; priapism
Pimozide	Impotence; no ejaculation; decreased libido
Pindolol	Impotence
Pramipexole dihydrochloride	Decreased libido; impotence (in early Parkinson's disease)
Prazosin	Impotence; priapism
Primidone	Decreased libido; impotence
Probucol	Impotence

TABLE 22–4. Medications associated with sexual dysfunction *(continued)*

Medication	Reported adverse effect
Procarbazine	Decreased libido; impotence; dyspareunia
Progestins	Impotence
Propantheline bromide	Impotence
Propofol	Sexual disinhibition
Propranolol	Loss of libido; impotence
Protriptyline	Loss of libido; impotence; painful ejaculation
Quetiapine	Increased or decreased libido; impotence; abnormal ejaculation
Riluzole	Increased or decreased libido; impotence
Risperidone	Erectile dysfunction; delayed ejaculation; abnormal orgasm (dose-dependent)
Ritonavir	Decreased libido; impotence
Saquinavir mesylate	Decreased libido; impotence
Scopolamine	Impotence
Selegiline	Transient anorgasmia; decreased penile sensation
Sertindole	Abnormal or dry ejaculation (not retrograde)
Sertraline	Delayed ejaculation; inhibited orgasm
Sildenafil citrate	Abnormal ejaculation; genital edema; anorgasmia
Spironolactone	Decreased libido; impotence
Steroids	Increased or decreased libido
Sulfasalazine	Impotence
Tamoxifen	Priapism
Tamsulosin	Decreased libido, abnormal ejaculation
Terazosin	Impotence
Testosterone	Priapism
Thiabendazole	Impotence
Thiazide diuretics	Impotence
Thioridazine	Impotence; priapism; delayed, decreased, painful, retrograde, or no ejaculation; anorgasmia
Thiothixene	Spontaneous ejaculation; impotence; priapism
Tiagabine	Increased or decreased libido; impotence
Timolol	Decreased libido; impotence
Tolcapone	Increased or decreased libido; impotence
Trandolapril	Decreased libido; impotence
Tranylcypromine	Impotence; painful or retarded ejaculation
Trazodone	Priapism; clitoral priapism; increased libido; retrograde or no ejaculation; anorgasmia
Tridihexethyl chloride	Impotence
Trifluoperazine	Painful or spontaneous ejaculation
Trihexyphenidyl	Impotence
Trimethaphan	Impotence
Trimipramine	Decreased libido; impotence; anorgasmia
Triptorelin	Impotence; decreased libido; loss of sexual fantasies
Trovafloxacin mesylate	Decreased libido; impotence
Valsartan	Impotence
Venlafaxine	Decreased libido; impotence; abnormal ejaculation; delayed orgasm
Verapamil	Impotence
Vinblastine	Decreased libido; impotence; dyspareunia
Zolpidem	Decreased libido; impotence; anorgasmia

Note.   LSD = lysergic acid diethylamide; MDA = 3,4-methylenedioxyamphetamine.
Source.   Compiled from numerous sources, including Abramowicz 1992; Berk and Acton 1997; Buffum 1992; Herrod 1997; Jeffries et al. 1996; Kaplan and Sadock 1994; Michael and Herrod 1997; Michael and Ramana 1996; O'Farrell et al. 1997; Rosen 1999; Physicians' Desk Reference 1995, 1999; Segraves 1977, 1989; Steele 1989; Wilson 1991; Wilton et al. 1996; M.G. Wise and Rundell 1988.

Antidepressant-Induced Sexual Dysfunction

The selective serotonin reuptake inhibitors (SSRIs) as a class of antidepressants have become the first-line treatment and most widely prescribed medications for depression in patients with concurrent medical and surgical illnesses. Unlike tricyclic antidepressants, SSRIs are generally not associated with dangerous or debilitating side effects (e.g., anticholinergic effects, orthostasis, significant weight gain) or cardiac conduction disruptions. Roose et al. (1998a) clearly showed the substantial advantages of fluoxetine and paroxetine (Roose et al. 1998b) over tricyclic antidepressants in post–myocardial infarction patients, for example. However, SSRIs often are associated with one or more types of sexual dysfunction that can lead to noncompliance in some patients. Decreased sexual interest, diminished genital sensation, erectile dysfunction, decreased lubrication, and delayed or inhibited orgasm all have been reported (Rosen et al. 1999). The most common sexual dysfunction appears to be delayed ejaculation and orgasm in men and delayed or inhibited orgasm in women, reported in up to 50% of the patients who are specifically asked about their sexual functioning. Citalopram, introduced to the United States market in 1998, anecdotally has less sexual dysfunction liability than do other SSRIs; however, no data support this contention. In patients who already have compromised sexual functioning from concurrent medical illness, the SSRIs may add to their difficulties.

The etiology of dysfunction appears to be based on levels of drug in the periphery and is therefore related to dose and half-life. It has been found that ejaculatory delay in men is increased by paroxetine, sertraline, citalopram, and fluoxetine and that these agents could be used as treatments for premature ejaculation (Kara et al. 1996; Mendels 1995; Mendels et al. 1995; Waldinger et al. 1994, 1997). Venlafaxine, an agent with mixed serotonergic and noradrenergic effects, has a similar rate of sexual dysfunction as a side effect.

Antidepressants without appreciable sexual side effects and levels of efficacy similar to those of SSRIs include bupropion (immediate and sustained release), mirtazapine, and nefazodone. These antidepressants presumably operate through different mechanisms of action than SSRIs (and have different side-effect profiles) that do not include prominent serotonergic mechanisms. Bupropion has demonstrated benefits in reversing sexual dysfunction induced by SSRIs in controlled studies (Ashton and Rosen 1998; Coleman et al. 1999; Croft et al. 1999). These medications may be important considerations as first-line agents for depressed medically ill patients who express a desire to retain, or attain, "normal" sexual functioning. It behooves the consultation psychiatrist to therefore ask the patient about his or her sexual functioning before selecting months-long antidepressant treatment.

Some depressed medically ill patients have responded well to SSRIs in the past, and continuing this treatment despite sexual dysfunction may be appropriate. A variety of approaches may be effective in ameliorating this side effect (Rosen et al. 1999). Sequentially, first, the patient should be observed to determine whether the sexual dysfunction is part of his or her depression, associated with a comorbid psychiatric disturbance such as an adjustment disorder, or a definite medication side effect. Watchful waiting in the latter cases generally shows the tenacity of this side effect, unlike the other acute side effects of SSRI treatment. Second, the psychiatrist should consider lowering the dose, if possible, or changing the timing of the dose to be as distant as possible from anticipated sexual activity. In stable patients in remission from depressive symptoms who are taking short-half-life SSRIs (paroxetine, fluvoxamine, sertraline, citalopram), a "drug holiday" may be considered (Rothschild 1995, 2000). For example, patients may discontinue their medication on Fridays in anticipation of engaging in sexual relations on Saturday evening with a resumption of treatment on Sunday morning. It has been shown that central nervous system levels of short-half-life SSRIs remain high (therapeutic) well after the peripheral level has diminished to the point at which sexual dysfunction is normalized. Additional approaches include adding "antidotes" to SSRI treatment (e.g., amantadine [Balon 1996; Shrivistava et al. 1995], cyproheptadine, yohimbine, or bupropion). It is theorized that enhancing dopaminergic functioning can circumvent SSRI-induced sexual side effects. Following this hypothesis, bupropion 75–100 mg 1–2 hours before sexual activity has been suggested. Sildenafil also is being studied as an antidote for both men and women who have one or more types of SSRI-induced sexual dysfunction, with promising early reports.

SEXUAL DYSFUNCTIONS IN PATIENTS WITH NEUROLOGICAL DISORDERS

Disorders involving the central nervous system can have profound effects on sexuality, involving all phases of the sexual response cycle. Spinal cord injuries, multiple sclerosis (MS), cerebrovascular accidents, and dementias have all been studied in this regard.

Spinal Cord Injury

The central, peripheral, and autonomic nervous systems are all essential to sexual functioning. Injury to one or more components can disrupt an individual's patterns of function. When spinal cord injury occurs at the cervical or thoracic levels, ascending sensory and descending upper motor neuron tracts are compromised. The capacity for psychogenic erection or clitoral engorgement is compromised. However, the genital–spinal cord reflex allows genital arousal and orgasm to occur in response to mechanical stimulation (Higgins 1978). Unfortunately, the patient cannot feel genital sensations, and the reflexive erections usually are unpredictable and often insufficient to sustain intercourse. If the injury occurs at lumbar or sacral levels, the genital–spinal cord reflex is lost, and "reflexogenic" erections do not occur. However, if the injury has spared the autonomic nervous system, the capacity for psychogenic genital arousal is preserved; the loss of sensation will vary according to the lesion (Kaufman 1990; Stewart 1991).

The erectile disabilities and anorgasmia of patients with spinal cord injuries are compounded by the potential for bowel and bladder incontinence, the frequent necessity for urinary catheters, and the loss of accustomed mobility and protective benefits of normal sensation. Given this context, Stewart (1991) properly emphasized the value of discussing sexual possibilities with such patients "to affirm the reality of some retained sexual behavior and feelings after the injury, a reality the patient often doubts. This overture also presents the opportunity to share with the patient his sadness over what he has lost in both the sexual and nonsexual spheres of his life" (p. 484). A physical therapist with experience in the sexual problems of disabled persons can provide invaluable practical assistance.

Spinal cord injuries most often occur in active people younger than 40 years who are usually otherwise healthy. Premorbid sexual and reproductive functioning in most cases is normal. Although women with spinal cord injuries commonly report sexual dysfunctions in all phases of the sexual response cycle (including desire phase disorders, diminished lubrication/swelling, and anorgasmia), most of the available literature focuses on erectile dysfunction in paraplegic and quadriplegic men. Because the etiology of erectile dysfunction in these men is usually neurogenic, they are ideal candidates for a major treatment advance developed during the past decade: intracavernosal pharmacotherapy. These treatments are best accomplished in the form of home autoinjections for paraplegic men with adequate motivation and dexterity or as a partner-assisted erection program for quadriplegic men (Gerstenberg et al. 1992).

Pharmacological erection programs, described in detail elsewhere (Padma-Nathan and Kanellos 1992; Padma-Nathan et al. 1987), have proven to be effective for many patients in safely restoring adequate erectile function for intercourse. Originally, fixed combinations of phentolamine mesylate and papaverine hydrochloride were injected by 0.5-inch, 28-gauge needle into the lateral base of the penis at the level of the corpus cavernosum. A firm erection for an hour after treatment was the targeted outcome. Corporal scarring (3%) and extended priapism (variable rates) were the major side effects. Recent advances use a more "physiologic" combination of prostaglandin E_1 and phentolamine mesylate or a "trimixture" of papaverine, phentolamine, and alprostadil (prostaglandin E_1) (Chao and Clowers 1994). Test doses are increased until the optimal dose is achieved (erection of sufficient rigidity for intercourse for about 1 hour). The pharmacologically induced erection is often enhanced in both duration and rigidity by sexual stimulation, which then permits a decrease in medication dose. Although priapism remains a risk, the incidence of corporal scarring has been greatly reduced with the substitution of prostaglandin E_1. Average frequency of autoinjection or partner-assisted injection has been reported to be seven times per month, with partner and patient satisfaction ratings of more than 90% (Padma-Nathan and Kanellos 1992).

Sildenafil also may improve the quality of erections after spinal cord injury without the need for a complicated autoinjection regimen. Derry et al. (1998) studied a group of 27 patients who maintained at least a partial reflexogenic erectile response to penile vibratory stimulation after lesions from T6 to L5. After 28 days, 9 of 12 patients (75%) taking sildenafil and 1 of 14 patients (7%) taking placebo reported that treatment had improved their erections.

Other treatments available to patients with spinal cord injuries and erectile dysfunction include a variety of penile prostheses, topical applications of nitroglycerine (Meyhoff et al. 1992), and the negative-pressure, or vacuum erection, device (Witherington 1988). Vacuum devices produce negative pressure by using suction and causing mechanical entrapment of blood in the penis.

Multiple Sclerosis

MS generally affects individuals between ages 20 and 40 years, a time when base rates of sexual dysfunctions are otherwise relatively low. Because MS has a variable course and is associated with primary and secondary psychiatric disorders, psychiatrists are often involved in the care of hospitalized patients and outpatients with MS. Sexual dysfunction is rarely the initial symptom of MS but regularly appears during the course of illness. Deleterious effects on sexuality have been noted in 60%–91% of men and 52%–77% of women (Hulter and Lundberg 1995; Minderhoud et al. 1984). Even in cases of "mild MS" with minimal chronic neurological manifestations of the disease, the frequency of sexual dysfunction in both men and women may be high compared with that in the general population (43% of men, 52% of women; Minderhoud et al. 1984). Longitudinal studies of both male and female patients with MS indicate that the number of patients with at least one type of sexual dysfunction increases with time in both sexes (Stenager et al. 1996). Modern diagnostic techniques assist with the differential diagnosis of arousal phase disorders in MS patients. These include nocturnal penile tumescence and rigidity measurements, penile arterial pressure tests, venous out-flow studies, pudendal evoked potential, sacral (52–54) evoked response, and bulbocavernosus reflex testing.

Erectile dysfunction is the most common sexual complaint in men with MS; at least 90% of the erectile dysfunctions are diagnosed as neurogenic and fewer than 10% as "mainly psychogenic" (Kirkeby et al. 1988). In contrast, disorders in the orgasm phase (48%) and desire phase (58%) are most common in women. A minority of both men and women report that pelvic sensory defects (21% of men, 29% of women) and fatigue (26% of men, 29% of women) contribute to sexual dysfunction. In patients with MS, changes in sexual functioning are not highly correlated with overall ability to ambulate but are correlated with neurological symptoms that can be traced to the sacral segments and to the presence of vertigo and ataxia (Hulter and Lundberg 1995). It is interesting that few patients with MS report that the importance of sexual activity decreases after diagnosis, and only 5% endorse the view that chronic illness constitutes a "good reason" for reduced sexual interest and activity (Minderhoud et al. 1984). Dysfunction in the lumbosacral spine accounts for many of the sexual difficulties experienced by patients with MS. For example, patients with anal sphincter and bladder dysfunction are also likely to report sexual dysfunction (Schapiro and Langer 1994). For both men and women with MS, sexual dysfunction constitutes an important aspect of the disease that merits routine inquiry (Dupont 1996). As in most of the other conditions discussed in this chapter, sexual dysfunction in one sexual partner can jeopardize intimacy in spousal or other supportive relationships. A thorough review of sexual functioning in patients with MS can be found elsewhere (Dupont 1995).

Cerebrovascular Accident (Stroke)

Unlike MS and spinal cord injury, most patients who experience a cerebrovascular accident (CVA) are older than 50 years. Because American society tends to "asexualize" elderly and medically ill people, it is not surprising that studies of sexuality in elderly CVA patients are few. This lack of study is despite the fact that CVA is one of the commonest causes of long-term disability in patients in the United States. Sexual functioning post-CVA is generally characterized by reduced desire and decreased frequency of activity in both men and women. In a large study of sexual functioning in CVA patients, *all* phases of sexual response were impaired after CVA. Table 22–5 summarizes the changes noted by 113 CVA patients (78 men, 35 women) whose average age was about 68 years (Monga et al. 1986).

TABLE 22–5. Changes in sexual functioning after stroke

Phase	Pre-CVA (baseline) (%)	Post-CVA (%)
Normal desire, male	75	21
Normal desire, female	60	34
Normal erection	94	38
Normal lubrication	63	29
Normal orgasm, male	73	22
Normal orgasm, female	43	11
Anorgasmia, female	34	77
Premature ejaculation	13	43

Note. CVA = cerebrovascular accident.
Source. Adapted from Monga T, Lawson J, Inglis J: "Sexual Dysfunction in Stroke Patients." *Archives of Physical Medicine and Rehabilitation* 67:19–22, 1986. Copyright 1986, WB Saunders. Used with permission.

In women, right-hemisphere lesions appear to cause less sexual dysfunction than left-hemisphere CVA. The reverse may be true for men, in whom 75% with unilateral right-hemisphere CVA had sexual dysfunction compared with 29% of those with left-hemisphere CVA (Coslett and Heilman 1986). It has been hypothesized that "limbic activation" of the dominant hemisphere for sexual function is required for intact sexual functioning in men.

In addition to potential loss of independence or control over some body movements, CVA patients often experience the loss of their sexual life (Hawton 1984). Monga et al. (1986) noted that 95% of men and 76% of women in their late 60s were satisfied with their sexual lives before CVA, whereas only 26% of men and 37% of women remained satisfied post-CVA. The most common self-reported cause for both decreased satisfaction and increased dysfunction is fear of having another CVA that could be initiated by blood pressure elevations associated with sexual activity. Other reported causes include diminished self-esteem, anxiety about sexual performance, fear of partner rejection, and pharmacotherapy toxic to sexual functioning (e.g., antianxiety, hypotensive, antidepressant, and hypnotic medications). Therefore, unlike the clear neurogenic etiology for much of the sexual dysfunction experienced by patients with MS and spinal cord injury, those surviving one or more CVAs frequently have primary psychological concerns that account for their post-CVA problems. Although no guarantees can be offered, patients can be informed that the changes in heart rate, blood pressure, and oxygen uptake during most forms of conventional sexual activity with an established partner are similar to those experienced during light to moderate short-term exercise (Bohlen et al. 1984). Orgasm, lasting only seconds, is associated with the greatest increases in these physiologic parameters, which then quickly return to baseline values during the resolution phase of the sexual response cycle. To further decrease stroke risk, it has been suggested that couples engage in longer foreplay and minimize or eliminate the man-on-top coital position. Self-stimulation and partner stimulation to orgasm using noncoital techniques may further limit the risk of adverse circulatory events.

The consultation-liaison psychiatrist should also be aware that sexual morbidity after CVA may be largely unrelated to the CVA itself. Premorbid relationship problems, including sexual boredom, may be an important contributor, with the CVA presenting a convenient and socially acceptable reason to exempt oneself from a previously unsatisfactory sexual relationship. In these situations, it is often the spouse who seeks assistance for the identified patient's sexual dysfunction. In addition, loss of sexual desire is a common symptom of major depression syndromes, for which patients have a heightened risk following stroke (see Chapter 17, this volume).

Dementia

The emergence of disruptive sexual behavior in patients with dementing diseases causes significant distress for family members and hospital staff (Ehrenfeld et al. 1999). Nursing homes and chronic care settings consult psychiatrists to evaluate patients with compulsive public masturbation, frequent genital exposures, fondling of other patients and staff, or dangerous sexual behaviors (e.g., vaginal or rectal insertions of sharp objects, chair legs). Patients with the Klüver-Bucy syndrome, resulting from bilateral lesions of the temporal lobes, frequently act in inappropriate, hypersexual ways. Normal inhibitory controls appear to be impaired, with resultant primitive sexual displays. Problems related to hypersexuality may be the cause for hospital admission in patients with

Huntington's chorea. For example, a longitudinal study of patients with Huntington's chorea identified abnormal sexual behavior in 63% of the patients, including exhibitionism, sexual aggression, voyeurism, and hypersexuality (Dewhurst and Oliver 1970).

Sexual "acting out" in patients with Alzheimer's disease or multi-infarct dementia may frequently reflect disordered frontotemporal inhibitory mechanisms, causing a "release phenomenon" (Cooper 1987). Behavior is rarely predatory or dangerous but may involve inadvertent self-harm (e.g., during episodes of compulsive or aggressive masturbation). For example, we evaluated a patient with Alzheimer's disease who was hospitalized after public masturbation in a shopping mall. During the admission, the patient was found publicly masturbating while inserting the leg of his desk chair rectally.

Antiandrogen treatment may be effective in some men with dementia and sexual disorders. This treatment, described below, may decrease dangerous sexual behaviors. In one study, 300 mg of medroxyprogesterone acetate (MPA) administered intramuscularly each week suppressed dangerous and problematic sexual behaviors within 14 days in a series of four elderly patients with dementia ages 75–84 (Cooper 1987). After 1 year, MPA was discontinued, and three of the four patients' behavior remained under control for a 1-year, drug-free follow-up period, even though serum testosterone had returned to baseline normal levels within 4 weeks of discontinuation. Because of the obvious medicolegal issues associated with using pharmacological agents for behavioral "control" of patients with dementia, physicians are well advised to seek informed consent from guardians, next of kin, or the courts.

GENDER AND SEXUAL DISORDERS THAT MAY BE PRESENT IN MEDICAL-SURGICAL PATIENTS

Gender Identity Disorders

The consulting psychiatrist may be called on to assess patients admitted to surgical services after genital self-mutilation. Dramatic examples of autocastration and autopenectomy in men (Fisch 1987; Mellon et al. 1989) and autoamputation of the labia majora (T. Wise et al. 1989) or vulvar or vaginal lacerations (Standage et al. 1974) in women have appeared over the past 30 years. However, such cases are rare, albeit memorable, and are often associated with gender dysphoric symptoms with or without psychosis. Clinical considerations in the differential diagnosis of patients with gender dysphoria include conditions listed in Table 22–6 (Brown 2001).

TABLE 22–6. Differential diagnosis of gender dysphoria

Primary and secondary transsexualism

Transvestic fetishism with depression, regression, or substance abuse

Homophobic homosexuality (sexual identity disorder)

Schizophrenia with gender identity disturbance

Borderline personality disorder with severe gender identity issues

Body dysmorphic disorder

Gender identity disorder not otherwise specified

Ambiguous gender identity adaptation

Malingering/factitious disorder

Career female impersonators

Endocrine disorders, genetic or prenatal exposures

In hospitals where surgical procedures are performed as part of a comprehensive gender confirmation program, consultation may be requested in the pre- and perioperative periods. Standards of care for all mental health professionals involved in the evaluation and treatment of patients with gender identity disorder have been established and should be reviewed before providing consultation (Levine et al. 1998). Table 22–7 summarizes the common somatic treatments for patients with gender identity disorders. At the time a consultation is requested, patients may be at various stages of physical transition and are likely to be receiving one or more of the treatments listed (Brown 2001). Psychosis in the immediate postoperative period after castration, penectomy, and neovaginal construction is rarely seen but is a potential concern. Rejection by family members or loved ones contributes to depressive symptoms in some patients with gender identity disorders both before and after irreversible genital surgery. At times, antidepressant treatment has limited effectiveness, whereas cross-gender hormonal treatment, alone or in combination with antidepressants, can result in dramatic positive responses. Estrogens and androgens have substantial binding in the central nervous system and are clearly psychoactive agents that can affect mood.

Ideally, patients admitted to surgical or urological services for major genital surgery should already be receiving care from a mental health professional familiar with the case. Because patients often undergo these procedures at a considerable distance from their homes, local psychiatric consultation may be requested. Consultation-liaison psychiatrists who are not familiar with these patients should examine their potential negative countertransference reactions in advance (Lothstein 1977). Lothstein (1978) reported that countertransference anxiety in a male anesthesiologist nearly resulted in a lethal outcome for a male transsexual patient during

penectomy/orchiectomy. Bioethical issues surrounding the appropriateness of providing, or withholding, irreversible genital surgical procedures for gender dysphoric patients have been discussed elsewhere (Brown 1988; Lothstein 1982).

Other Sexual Disorders

Few of the sexual disorders and paraphilias listed in DSM-IV-TR are the primary reason for admission to general hospital wards. Most individuals with these disorders do not come to clinical attention in any setting. Those who are evaluated often submit under duress, either as court referrals or at family members' insistence. Paraphilias may be largely ego-syntonic and compatible with high levels of occupational functioning. Self-referral for treatment, however, does occur for some patients who experience their sexual fantasies and/or activities as highly disruptive and potentially destructive factors in their lives. In fact, paraphiliac patients may experience lethal levels of guilt and attempt suicide as self-punishment. Table 22–8 lists some of the sexual disorders that the consultation-liaison psychiatrist may encounter in the hospital or outpatient consultation-liaison setting. Comorbidity with other sexual disorders, mood disorders, substance use disorders, and attention-deficit disorders is common (Kafka and Prentky 1998) We discuss some of these disorders below.

Potentially harmful genital manipulation may be present as an active form of autoerotic behavior (a type of fetishistic interest) or as a masochistic instrumentation (i.e., a form of factitious disorder). T. Wise (1982) reported seven cases of urethral manipulation, including a woman with borderline personality disorder who would repeatedly insert injectable razor blades into her urethra and a 14-year-old boy who lodged a pencil in his bladder after urethral masturbation.

In contrast to active forms of urethral manipulation, T. Wise (1982) noted that individuals more frequently present with recurrent complaints of inability to void or persistent pain with urination. Such patients readily accept repeated cystoscopies and catheterizations and may report to several emergency rooms for these interventions. These "passive instrumenters" often show less obvious psychopathology (obsessional behavior, sadomasochistic fantasies, monosymptomatic hypochondriasis) than do "active instrumenters" (those with borderline personality disorder, schizophrenia, multiple paraphilias).

Psychiatric consultation in these cases usually is requested after medical and urological evaluations uncover no apparent physical causes for the complaints or when foreign objects are discovered in the bladder.

TABLE 22–7. Medical and surgical treatments for gender identity disorders (not all patients require all treatments)

Adult men with gender identity disorder	Adult women with gender identity disorder
Estrogen treatment (lifelong; reduced dose after orchiectomy)	Testosterone treatment (lifelong; reduced dose after oophorectomy)
Electrolysis (25–300 hours manually or 4–6 sessions with laser)	Facial cosmetic procedures
Laryngeal cartilage shaving	Hysterectomy
Vocal cord shortening or other voice alteration surgeries	Oophorectomy
Liposuction	Bilateral mastectomy
Rhinoplasty	Neophallus construction (multiple stages)
Jaw reconfiguration	Testicular implants
Other facial cosmetic procedures	Genitoplasty (maximizing clitoral prominence)
Orchiectomy	Chest wall contouring
Penectomy	
Neovaginal construction	
Augmentation mammoplasty	

TABLE 22–8. Other sexual disorders in the hospital setting

Hypoxyphilia (asphyxiophilia; autoerotic asphyxiophilia)
Sexual masochism
Paraphilia with suicidality (e.g., pedophilia)
Serendipitous finding of transvestic fetishism
Sexual disorder not otherwise specified
    Genital/rectal manipulations and injuries
    Substance-enhanced orgasm (e.g., volatile nitrites)
    Hypersexuality syndromes associated with central nervous system disease

Active inserters may initially deny self-instrumentation, but tactful and nonjudgmental questioning may yield a more complete clinical picture. Psychotherapy may be the treatment of choice and involves a dynamic understanding of "libidinal, structural and ego psychological constructs" (T. Wise 1982, p. 225). Although these behaviors appear to have fetishistic and sadomasochistic elements, analogies to factitious disorder (Munchausen syndrome) are clear, and engaging such patients in treatment may be difficult (see Chapter 25, this volume).

Hypoxyphilia, labeled in the literature as asphyxiophilia, autoerotic asphyxia, or eroticized repetitive hangings, involves the deliberate induction of cerebral anoxia during masturbation to heighten orgasmic intensity (Hucker and Stermac 1992). Practitioners of this potentially lethal sexual behavior rarely present for treatment, but near-fatal self-strangulation may be mistaken for a suicide attempt when encountered in the hospital setting (Johnstone and Huws 1997). However, evidence for suicidal intent was present in only 2 of 157 fatal cases of hypoxyphilia (Hazelwood et al. 1983). The literature provides few examples of specific treatment for hypoxyphilia and no long-term outcome studies (Hucker 1990). Treatment strategies for other paraphilias have been used with this disorder, including behavior therapy involving covert sensitization (Haydn-Smith et al. 1987) and antiandrogenic hormonal treatment (Hucker and Stermac 1992). Lithium carbonate also has been reported to be useful (Cesnick and Coleman 1989). Uva (1995) provides a review of this disorder as it presents in the United States.

PHARMACOLOGICAL TREATMENTS FOR PARAPHILIAS AND HYPERSEXUALITY

Antiandrogenic medications are used as an adjunctive treatment for some malignancies to limit tumor growth (e.g., prostate cancer) and as a primary treatment modality for moderate to severe sexual disorders and paraphilias (Bradford and Greenberg 1996). "Pure" antiandrogens, including flutamide and nilutamide, only block androgen's action at the target organs, which results in greatly elevated gonadotropin and circulating testosterone levels. These drugs are not adequate for the monotherapy of paraphilias. Other antiandrogens, including cyproterone acetate (CPA) and MPA, have progestogenic and antigonadotropic properties, which result in *both* inhibition of androgen biosynthesis and inhibition of androgen action in the periphery. In addition, CPA and MPA appear to block central androgen receptor sites that may be important in the generation of deviant sexual fantasies (Cooper 1986, 1987). Placebo-controlled trials support the use of antiandrogens for the treatment of moderate to severe paraphilias (Cooper 1981), and clinical use of antiandrogens in properly selected and informed patients with paraphilias can yield dramatic results (Neumann and Kalmas 1991).

MPA trials for the treatment of paraphilias began in 1966. Numerous reports documented the effectiveness of this medication in the intramuscular form, especially when combined with psychotherapy and relapse prevention programs. A typical treatment regimen for hypersexuality or a severe paraphilic disorder in a man would be 200 mg intramuscular MPA two or three times per week for 2 weeks, then 200 mg once or twice per week for 4 weeks, followed by 200 mg every 2 weeks. Thereafter, doses would range from 100 mg once per week to once per month, depending on clinical response. Testosterone levels should be reduced to the range observed in females. Most patients will require longer-term treatment because deviant fantasies or hypersexual desire patterns will reemerge as testosterone levels return to normal when treatment is discontinued. Long-term treatment with MPA is associated with weight gain, increases in systolic blood pressure, gallstone formation, infertility, and potential changes in glucose tolerance. For patients with intact cognition, the treatment of choice is multimodal therapy, including a variety of treatment modalities in addition to antiandrogen treatment (Gagne 1981). For example, referral to anonymous self-help groups (e.g., Sex and Love Addicts Anonymous) in conjunction with expressive psychotherapy groups may be helpful.

Leuprolide is a synthetic gonadotropin-releasing hormone analogue approved by the U.S. Food and Drug Administration (FDA) in 1985 for the treatment of prostatic cancer. It initially stimulates release of luteinizing hormone (LH) and follicle-stimulating hormone (FSH) and, therefore, testosterone, but further release of LH and FSH is blocked after 3–5 days (Allolio et al. 1985). Serum levels of testosterone then decrease to the castrate level. The most common side effect is hot flashes and an initial worsening of sexual symptoms because of the transient increase in testosterone. A depot preparation allows for once-monthly subcutaneous injections in most patients. Triptorelin and goserelin are long-acting gonadotropin-releasing hormone analogues that have shown substantial promise in centrally blocking the production of testosterone. Goserelin has been widely used in prostate cancer treatment (Brogden and Faulds 1995). Both agents are beginning to be used in patients with severe sexual disorders that respond to markedly lowering the circulating testosterone levels (Dickey 1992; Rosler and Witztum 1998). The initial month of treatment is associated with increased levels of testosterone prior to a rapid depletion of testicular stores.

In addition to antiandrogens and gonadotropin releasing hormone agents, orally administered estrogens (e.g., ethinyl estradiol 0.10 mg/day) have been used as monotherapy for some sexual disorders. Success rates have not been as good as with CPA or MPA, but more important is that the side-effect profile of estrogen is distinctly unfavorable compared with CPA or MPA. Specifically, estrogen treatment results in feminization (breast growth, decreased upper-body muscle mass, increased hip fat, changes in body hair), nausea, vomiting, and the potential for breast cancer in men. Use of hormonal agents is not without some controversy despite their efficacy in many cases. Cordier and colleagues (1996) reviewed some of these issues.

Because neuroleptic medications have nonspecific effects and unacceptable risks for acute and tardive dyskinesia, they are no longer recommended. Small, uncontrolled trials of fluoxetine for a variety of paraphiliac and nonparaphiliac "sexual addictions" have suggested that this medication may offer some promise in decreasing the compulsivity associated with these disorders. However, most patients who have responded have also met criteria for a mood disorder (Kafka and Prentky 1992). Additional studies are necessary before any definitive statements about the efficacy of SSRIs for sexual disorders, alone or in combination with hormonal treatments, can be made (Fedoroff 1995).

REFERENCES

Abramowicz M: Drugs that cause sexual dysfunction: an update. Med Lett Drugs Ther 34:73–78, 1992

Allolio B, Keffel D, Deuss U, et al: Treatment of sex behavior disorders with LH-RH superagonists. Dtsch Med Wochenschr 110:110–117, 1985

American Psychiatric Association: Diagnostic and Statistical Manual of Mental Disorders, 4th Edition. Washington, DC, American Psychiatric Association, 1994

American Psychiatric Association: Diagnostic and Statistical Manual of Mental Disorders, 4th Edition, Text Revision. Washington, DC, American Psychiatric Association, 2000

Ashton A, Rosen R: Bupropion as an antidote for serotonin reuptake inhibitor–induced sexual dysfunction. J Clin Psychiatry 59:112–115, 1998

Atkinson J, Grant I, Kennedy C, et al: Prevalence of psychiatric disorders among men infected with human immunodeficiency virus. Arch Gen Psychiatry 45:859–864, 1988

Auchincloss S: Sexual dysfunction in cancer patients: issues in evaluation and treatment, in Handbook of Psychooncology: Psychological Care of the Patient With Cancer. Edited by Holland JC, Rowland JH. New York, Oxford University Press, 1989, pp 383–413

Ballard S, Gingell C, Tang K, et al: Effects of sildenafil on the relaxation of human corpus cavernosum tissue in vitro and on the activities of cyclic nucleotide phosphodiesterase isoenzymes. J Urol 159:2164–2171, 1998

Balon R: Intermittent amantadine for fluoxetine-induced anorgasmia. J Sex Marital Ther 22:290–292, 1996

Berk M, Acton M: Citalopram-associated clitoral priapism: a case series. Int Clin Psychopharmacol 12:121–122, 1997

Bohlen J, Held J, Sanderson M, et al: Heart rate, rate pressure-product and oxygen uptake during four sexual activities. Arch Intern Med 144:1745–1748, 1984

Boolell M, Gepi-Atlee S, Gingell J, et al: Sildenafil, a novel effective oral therapy for male erectile dysfunction. Br J Urol 78:257–261, 1996

Bradford J, Greenberg D: Pharmacological treatment of deviant sexual behavior. Annual Review of Sex Research 7:283–303, 1996

Brogden R, Faulds D: Goserelin: a review of its pharmacodynamic and pharmacokinetic properties and therapeutic efficacy in prostate cancer. Drugs Aging 6:324–343, 1995

Brown G: Bioethical issues in the management of gender dysphoria. Jefferson Journal of Psychiatry 6:33–44, 1988

Brown G: Transvestism and gender identity disorder in adults, in Treatments of Psychiatric Disorders, 3rd Edition. Edited by Gabbard GO. Washington, DC, American Psychiatric Publishing, 2001, pp 2007–2067

Brown G, Rundell J: Prospective study of psychiatric morbidity in HIV-seropositive women without AIDS. Gen Hosp Psychiatry 12:30–35, 1990

Brown G, Rundell J: A prospective study of psychiatric aspects of early HIV disease in women. Gen Hosp Psychiatry 15:139–147, 1993

Brown G, Rundell J, McManis S, et al: Prevalence of psychiatric disorders in early stages of HIV infection. Psychosom Med 54:588–601, 1992

Brown G, Kendall S, Ledsky R: Sexual dysfunction in HIV-seropositive women without AIDS. Journal of Psychology and Human Sexuality 7:73–97, 1995

Buffum J: Prescription drugs and sexual function. Psychiatric Medicine 10:181–198, 1992

Campese V, Liu AS: Sexual dysfunction in uremia: endocrine and neurological alterations. Contrib Nephrol 77:1–14, 1990

Cesnick J, Coleman E: Use of lithium carbonate in the treatment of autoerotic asphyxia. Am J Psychother 43:277–286, 1989

Chao R, Clowers DE: Experience with intracavernosal trimixture for the management of neurogenic erectile dysfunction. Arch Phys Med Rehabil 75:276–278, 1994

Coleman C, Cunningham L, Foster V, et al: Sexual dysfunction associated with the treatment of depression: a placebo-controlled comparison of bupropion sustained release and sertraline treatment. Ann Clin Psychiatry 11:205–215, 1999

Cooper A: A placebo-controlled trial of the antiandrogen cyproterone acetate in deviant hypersexuality. Compr Psychiatry 22:458–465, 1981

Cooper A: Progestogens in the treatment of male sex offenders: a review. Can J Psychiatry 31:73–79, 1986

Cooper A: Medroxyprogesterone acetate (MPA) treatment of sexual acting out in men suffering from dementia. J Clin Psychiatry 48:368–370, 1987

Cordier B, Thibaut F, Kuhn J, et al: Hormonal treatments for disorders of sexual conduct. Bull Acad Natl Med 180:599–605, 1996

Coslett H, Heilman K: Male sexual function: impairment after right hemisphere stroke. Arch Neurol 43:1036–1039, 1986

Croft H, Settle E, Houser T, et al: A placebo-controlled comparison of the antidepressant efficacy and effects on sexual functioning of sustained-release bupropion and sertraline. J Clin Ther 21:643–658, 1999

Crosby M, Paul J, Midanik L, et al: A new method of measuring the association between alcohol use, drug use, and high-risk sex. Proceedings of the 7th International Conference on AIDS, 1991, MD 4044, p 401

Cystitis in partners of Viagra users. Health News 4:5, October 1, 1998

Derry F, Dinsmore W, Frazer M, et al: Efficacy and safety of oral sildenafil (Viagra) in men with erectile dysfunction caused by spinal cord injury. Neurology 51:1629–1633, 1998

Dewhurst K, Oliver J: Huntington's disease of young people. Eur Neurol 3:278–279, 1970

Dickey R: The management of a case of treatment resistant paraphilia with a long-acting LHRH agonist. Can J Psychiatry 37:567–569, 1992

Dillard F, Miller B, Sommer B, et al: Erectile dysfunction post-transplant. Transplant Proc 21:3961–3962, 1989

Dunbar N, Perdices M, Grunseit A, et al: The relationship between HIV symptomatology and affect. Proceedings of the 7th International Conference on AIDS, 1991, MD 4044, MB 2126, p 213

Dupont S: Multiple sclerosis and sexual functioning: a review. Clin Rehabil 9:135–141, 1995

Dupont S: Sexual function and ways of coping in patients with multiple sclerosis and their partners. J Sex Marital Ther 11:359–372, 1996

Ehrenfeld M, Bronner G, Tabak N, et al: Sexuality among institutionalized elderly patients with dementia. Nurs Ethics 6:144–149, 1999

Eid J: Sildenafil citrate: current clinical experience. Int J Impot Res 12(suppl 4):S62–S66, 2000

Fagan PJ, Wise T, Schmidt C: Sexual problems in spinal cord disease, in Current Therapy in Neurologic Disease—3. Edited by Johnson RT. Philadelphia, PA, BC Decker, 1990, pp 168–172

Fairburn C, Wu F, McCulloch D, et al: The clinical features of diabetic impotence: a preliminary study. Br J Psychiatry 140:447–452, 1982a

Fairburn C, Wu F, McCulloch D, et al: The effects of diabetes on male sexual function. Baillieres Clin Endocrinol Metab 11:749–757, 1982b

Fedoroff J: Antiandrogens vs. serotonergic medications in the treatment of sex offenders: a preliminary compliance study? Canadian Journal of Human Sexuality 4:111–122, 1995

Feldman H, Goldstein I, Hatzichristou D, et al: Impotence and its medical and psychosocial correlates: results of the Massachusetts Male Aging Study. J Urol 151:54–61, 1994

Finkelstein F, Steele T: Sexual dysfunction and chronic renal failure: a psychosocial study. Dialysis and Transplantation 7:877–878, 1978

Fisch R: Genital self-mutilation in males: psychodynamic anatomy of a psychosis. Am J Psychother 41:453–458, 1987

Forsberg L, Hojerback T, Olsson A, et al: Etiologic aspects of impotence diabetes. Scand J Urol Nephrol 23:173–175, 1989

Gagne P: Treatment of sex offenders with medroxyprogesterone acetate. Am J Psychiatry 138:644–646, 1981

Gerstenberg T, Metz P, Ottesen B, et al: Intracavernous self-injection with vasoactive intestinal polypeptide and phentolamine in the management of erectile failure. J Urol 147:1277–1279, 1992

Goggin K, Engelson E, Rabkin J, et al: The relationship of mood, endocrine, and sexual disorders in human immunodeficiency virus positive (HIV+) women: an exploratory study. Psychosom Med 60:11–16, 1998

Goldstein I, Lue T, Padma-Nathan H, et al: Oral sildenafil in the treatment of erectile dysfunction. N Engl J Med 338:1397–1404, 1998

Gregoire A: Viagra: on release. Evidence on the effectiveness of sildenafil is good. BMJ 317:759–760, 1998

Hackett T, Cassem N: Psychological adaptation to convalescence in myocardial infarction patients, in Exercise Testing and Exercise Training in Coronary Heart Disease. Edited by Naughton J, Hellerstein H, Mohler I. New York, Academic Press, 1973, pp 253–262

Hawton K: Sexual adjustment of men who have strokes. J Psychosom Res 28:243–249, 1984

Haydn-Smith P, Marks I, Buchaya A, et al: Behavioral treatment of life-threatening masochistic asphyxiation: a case study. Br J Psychiatry 150:518–519, 1987

Hazelwood R, Dietz P, Burgess A: Autoerotic Fatalities. Lexington, MA, Lexington Books, 1983, pp 110–115

Higgins G: Sexual response in spinal cord injured adults: a review. Arch Sex Behav 8:173–196, 1978

Hucker S: Sexual asphyxia, in Principles and Practice of Forensic Psychiatry. Edited by Bluglass R. London, England, Churchill-Livingstone, 1990, pp 717–721

Hucker S, Stermac L: The evaluation and treatment of sexual violence, necrophilia, and asphyxiophilia. Clinical Forensic Psychiatry 15:703–719, 1992

Hulter B, Lundberg P: Sexual function in women with advanced multiple sclerosis. J Neurol Neurosurg Psychiatry 59:83–86, 1995

Imagawa A, Kawanishi Y, Numata A: Is erythropoietin effective for impotence in dialysis patients? Nephron 54:95–96, 1990

Jaarsma T, Dracup K, Walden J, et al: Sexual function in patients with advanced heart failure. Heart Lung 25:262–270, 1996

Jeffries J, Vanderhaeghe L, Remington G, et al: Clozapine-associated retrograde ejaculation (letter). Can J Psychiatry 41:62–63, 1996

Jensen S: Sexuality and chronic illness: biopsychosocial approach. Semin Neurol 12:135–140, 1992

Johnstone J, Huws R: Autoerotic asphyxia: a case report. J Sex Marital Ther 23:326–332, 1997

Kafka M, Prentky R: Fluoxetine treatment of nonparaphiliac sexual addictions and paraphilias in men. J Clin Psychiatry 53:351–358, 1992

Kafka M, Prentky R: Attention-deficit/hyperactivity disorder in males with paraphilias and paraphilia-related disorders: a comorbidity study. J Clin Psychiatry 59:388–396, 1998

Kaplan H, Sadock B: Human sexuality, in Synopsis of Psychiatry, 7th Edition. Edited by Kaplan HI, Sadock BJ. Baltimore, MD, Williams & Wilkins, 1994, pp 653–681

Kara H, Aydin S, Yucel M, et al: The efficacy of fluoxetine in the treatment of premature ejaculation: a double-blind, placebo-controlled study. J Urol 156:1631–1632, 1996

Kaufman DM (ed): Neurologic aspects of sexual function, in Clinical Neurology for Psychiatrists, 3rd Edition. Philadelphia, PA, WB Saunders, 1990, pp 321–336

Kirkeby H, Poulsen E, Petersen T, et al: Erectile dysfunction in multiple sclerosis. Neurology 38:1366–1371, 1988

Kloner R: Viagra: what every physician should know. Ear Nose Throat J 77:783–786, 1998

Kloner R, Jarow J: Erectile dysfunction and sildenafil citrate and cardiologists. Am J Cardiol 83:576–582, 1999

Levine S, Brown G, Coleman E: The standards of care for gender identity disorders. International Journal of Transgenderism 2:2–20, 1998

Lothstein L: Countertransference reactions to gender dysphoric patients: implications for psychotherapy. Psychotherapy Theory, Research, and Practice 24:21–31, 1977

Lothstein L: The psychological management and treatment of hospitalized transsexuals. J Nerv Ment Dis 166:255–262, 1978

Lothstein L: Sex reassignment surgery: historical, bioethical, and theoretical issues. Am J Psychiatry 139:417–426, 1982

Lustman P, Clouse R: Relationship of psychiatric illness to impotence in men with diabetes. Diabetes Care 13:893–895, 1990

Marks L, Duda C, Dorey F, et al: Treatment of erectile dysfunction with sildenafil. Urology 53:19–24, 1999

McLane M, Krop H, Mehta J: Psychosexual adjustment and counseling after myocardial infarction. Ann Intern Med 92:514–519, 1980

Mellon C, Barlow C, Cook J, et al: Autocastration and autopenectomy in a patient with transsexualism and schizophrenia. Journal of Sex Research 26:125–130, 1989

Menchini-Fabris G, Turchi P, Giorgi P, et al: Diagnosis and treatment of sexual dysfunction in patients affected by chronic renal failure on hemodialysis. Contrib Nephrol 77:24–33, 1990

Mendels J: Sertraline for premature ejaculation. J Clin Psychiatry 56:591, 1995

Mendels J, Camera A, Sikes C: Sertraline treatment for premature ejaculation. J Clin Psychopharmacol 15:341–346, 1995

Meyhoff H, Rosenkilde P, Bodker A: Non-invasive management of impotence with transcutaneous nitroglycerin. Br J Urol 69:88–90, 1992

Michael A, Herrod J: Citalopram-induced decreased libido (letter). Br J Psychiatry 171:90, 1997

Michael A, Ramana R: Nefazodone-induced spontaneous ejaculation (letter). Br J Psychiatry 169:672–673, 1996

Minderhoud J, Leemhuis J, Kremer J, et al: Sexual disturbances arising from multiple sclerosis. Acta Neurol Scand 70:299–306, 1984

Minkoff H, Moreno J: Drug prophylaxis for human immunodeficiency virus–infected pregnant women: ethical considerations. Am J Obstet Gynecol 163:1111–1114, 1990

Modell JG, Katholi C, Modell JD, et al: Comparative sexual side effects of bupropion, fluoxetine, paroxetine, and sertraline. Clin Pharmacol Ther 61:476–487, 1997

Monga T, Lawson J, Inglis J: Sexual dysfunction in stroke patients. Arch Phys Med Rehabil 67:19–22, 1986

Morales A, Gingell C, Collins M, et al: Clinical safety of oral sildenafil citrate (Viagra) in the treatment of erectile dysfunction. Int J Impot Res 10:69–73, 1998

Mulligan T, Sheehan H, Hanrahan J: Sexual function after heart transplantation. J Heart Lung Transplant 10:125–128, 1991

Nankervis A: Sexual function in chronic disease. Med J Aust 151:548–549, 1989

Neumann F, Kalmas J: Cyproterone acetate in the treatment of sexual disorders: pharmacology base and clinical experience. Exp Clin Endocrinol 98:71–80, 1991

Nurnberg H, Hensley P, Lauriello J, et al: Sildenafil for women patients with antidepressant-induced sexual dysfunction. Psychiatr Serv 50:1076–1078, 1999

O'Farrell T, Choquette K, Cutter H, et al: Sexual satisfaction and dysfunction in marriages of male alcoholics: comparison with nonalcoholic maritally conflicted and nonconflicted couples. J Stud Alcohol 58:91–99, 1997

Ofman US, Auchincloss SS: Sexual dysfunction in cancer patients. Curr Opin Oncol 4:605–613, 1992

Ohl D, Denil J, Bennett C, et al: Electroejaculation following retroperitoneal lymphadenectomy. J Urol 145:980–983, 1991

Ostrow D, Beltran E, Chaniel J, et al: Predictors of volatile nitrite use among the Chicago MACS cohort of homosexual men. Proceedings of the 7th International Conference on AIDS, 1991, MD 4043, p 400

Padma-Nathan H, Kanellos A: The management of erectile dysfunction following spinal cord injury. Semin Urol 10:133–137, 1992

Padma-Nathan H, Payton T, Goldstein I: Intracavernosal pharmacotherapy: the pharmacologic erection program (PEP). World Journal of Urology 5:160–166, 1987

Park K, Moreland R, Goldstein I, et al: Sildenafil inhibits phosphodiesterase type 5 in human clitoral corpus cavernosum smooth muscle. Biochem Biophys Res Commun 249:612–617, 1998

Physicians' Desk Reference. Montvale, NJ, Medical Economics Company, 1995

Physicians' Desk Reference. Montvale, NJ, Medical Economics Company, 1999

Procci W, Martin DJ: Effect of maintenance hemodialysis on male sexual performance. J Nerv Ment Dis 173:366–372, 1985

Rendell M, Rajfer J, Wicker P, et al: Sildenafil for treatment of erectile dysfunction in men with diabetes: a randomized controlled trial. JAMA 281:421–426, 1999

Rieker R, Fitzgerald E, Kalish L, et al: Psychosocial factors, curative therapies, and behavioral outcomes: a comparison of testis cancer survivors and a control group of healthy men. Cancer 64:2399–2407, 1989

Roose S, Glassman A, Attia E, et al: Cardiovascular effects of fluoxetine in depressed patients with heart disease. Am J Psychiatry 155:660–665, 1998a

Roose S, Laghrissi-Thode F, Kennedy J, et al: Comparison of paroxetine and nortriptyline in depressed patients with ischemic heart disease. JAMA 279:287–291, 1998b

Rosen R, Lane R, Menza M: Effects of SSRIs on sexual function: a critical review. J Clin Psychopharmacol 19:67–85, 1999

Rosler A, Witztum E: Treatment of men with paraphilia with a long-acting analogue of gonadotropin-releasing hormone. N Engl J Med 338:416–422, 1998

Rosser B, Metz M, Bockting W, et al: Sexual difficulties, concerns, and satisfaction in homosexual men: an empirical study with implications for HIV prevention. J Sex Marital Ther 23:61–73, 1997

Rothschild A: Selective serotonin reuptake inhibitor–induced sexual dysfunction: efficacy of a drug holiday. Am J Psychiatry 152:1514–1516, 1995

Rothschild A: Sexual side effects of antidepressants. J Clin Psychiatry 61(suppl 11):28–36, 2000

Sarica K, Arikan N, Serel A, et al: Multidisciplinary evaluation of diabetic impotence. Eur Urol 26:314–318, 1994

Schapiro RT, Langer SL: Symptomatic therapy of multiple sclerosis. Curr Opin Neurol 7:229–233, 1994

Schover L: The impact of breast cancer on sexuality, body image, and intimate relationships. CA Cancer J Clin 41:112–120, 1991

Schover L, Evans R, von Eschenbach A: Sexual rehabilitation in a cancer center: diagnosis and outcome in 384 cases. Arch Sex Behav 16:445–461, 1987

Schover L, Fife M, Gershenson D: Sexual dysfunction and treatment for early stage cervical cancer. Cancer 63:204–212, 1989

Schover L, Novick A, Steinmuller D, et al: Sexuality, fertility and renal transplantation: a survey of survivors. J Sex Marital Ther 16:3–13, 1990

Segraves R: Pharmacologic agents causing sexual dysfunction. J Sex Marital Ther 3:177–186, 1977

Segraves R: Effects of psychotropic drugs on human erection and ejaculation. Arch Gen Psychiatry 46:275–284, 1989

Shrivastava R, Shrivastava S, Overweg N, et al: Amantadine in the treatment of sexual dysfunction associated with selective serotonin reuptake inhibitors. J Clin Psychopharmacol 15:83–84, 1995

Silber E (ed): The treatment of ischemic heart disease, in Heart Disease, 2nd Edition. New York, Macmillan, 1987, pp 1663–1665

Singer P, Tasch E, Stocking C, et al: Sex or survival: trade-offs between quality and quantity of life. J Clin Oncol 9:328–334, 1991

Skinner J: Sexual relations and the cardiac patient, in Heart Disease and Rehabilitation. Edited by Pollock ML, Schmidt DH. Boston, MA, Houghton Mifflin, 1979, pp 587–599

Standage K, Moore J, Cale M: Self-mutilation of the genitalia by a female schizophrenic. Canadian Psychiatric Association Journal 19:17–20, 1974

Steele D: Drugs causing sexual dysfunction and their alternatives: a reference tool. Urologic Nursing 9:10–12, 1989

Stenager E, Stenager EN, Jensen K: Sexual function in multiple sclerosis: a 5-year follow-up study. Ital J Neurol Sci 17:67–69, 1996

Stewart TD: The spinal cord–injured patient, in Handbook of General Hospital Psychiatry. Edited by Cassem NH. St. Louis, MO, Mosby Year-Book, 1991, pp 484–486

Tabler J, Frierson R: Sexual concerns after heart transplantation. J Heart Lung Transplant 9:397–403, 1990

Thase M, Reynolds C, Jennings J, et al: Nocturnal penile tumescence is diminished in depressed men. Biol Psychiatry 24:33–46, 1988

Tindall B, Forde S, Goldstein D, et al: Sexual dysfunction in advanced HIV disease. AIDS Care 6:105–107, 1994

Uva J: Review: autoerotic asphyxiation in the United States. J Forensic Sci 40:534–581, 1995

Van Buuren H, Lunter C, Groenhuijzen H: Prevalence of psychiatric complications among HIV-infected people in the Netherlands. Proceedings of the 1st International Conference on Biopsychosocial Aspects of HIV Infection, 1991, p 24

Waldinger M, Hengeveld M, Zwinderman A: Paroxetine treatment of premature ejaculation: a double-blind, randomized, placebo-controlled study. Am J Psychiatry 151:1377–1379, 1994

Waldinger M, Hengeveld M, Zwinderman A: Ejaculation-retarding properties of paroxetine in patients with primary premature ejaculation. Br J Urol 79:592–595, 1997

Webster L: Management of sexual problems in diabetic patients. Br J Hosp Med 51:465–468, 1994

Wells K, Golding J, Burnam M: Psychiatric disorder in a sample of the general population with and without chronic medical conditions. Am J Psychiatry 145:976–981, 1988

Wilson B: The effect of drugs on male sexual function and fertility. Nurse Pract 16:12–24, 1991

Wilton L, Pearce G, Edet E, et al: The safety of finasteride in benign prostatic hypertrophy: a non-interventional observational cohort study in 14,772 patients. Br J Urol 78:379–384, 1996

Wise MG, Rundell JR: Special consultation topics, in Concise Guide to Consultation Psychiatry. Washington, DC, American Psychiatric Press, 1988, pp 158–175

Wise T: Sexual difficulties with concurrent physical problems. Psychosomatics 18:56–64, 1977

Wise T: Urethral manipulation: an unusual paraphilia. J Sex Marital Ther 8:222–227, 1982

Wise T: Sexual dysfunction in the medically ill. Psychosomatics 24:797–805, 1983

Wise T: Psychosocial side effects of sildenafil therapy for erectile dysfunction. J Sex Marital Ther 25:145–150, 1999

Wise T, Dietrich A, Segall E: Female genital self-mutilation: case reports and literature review. J Sex Marital Ther 15:269–274, 1989

Witherington R: Suction device therapy in the management of erectile impotence. Urol Clin North Am 15:123–128, 1988

Young-McCaughan S: Sexual functioning in women with breast cancer after treatment with adjuvant therapy. Cancer Nurs 19:308–319, 1996

23

Eating Disorders

Richard C. W. Hall, M.D.

James R. Rundell, M.D.

Eating disorders are serious psychiatric disorders that are often encountered in a consultation-liaison setting. They are often unrecognized and produce multiple inexplicable symptoms, laboratory findings, and complications in patients admitted with other diagnoses. Such patients are admitted to the hospital with electrolyte imbalances, seizures, cardiac arrhythmias, unexplained gastrointestinal bleeding, or acute confusional states. The management of eating disorders is complicated and requires a familiarity with the pertinent medical literature. Although we do not discuss all management points in this chapter, essential aspects are covered. The reader is referred to the references marked with an asterisk at the end of this chapter for a more in-depth review of the management of eating disorders.

The commonly recognized eating disorders are anorexia nervosa, bulimia nervosa, pica, rumination disorder of infancy, and atypical eating disorders. Both anorexia nervosa and rumination disorder of infancy may have a severe, unremitting course and, without appropriate medical intervention, may progress to death. Simple obesity is not currently defined as an eating disorder. In this chapter, we focus on anorexia nervosa, bulimia nervosa and, to a lesser extent, pica.

DEFINITIONS

Anorexia nervosa is a disorder that is characterized by an intense fear of gaining weight that leads to faulty eating patterns, malnutrition, and excessive weight loss. It occurs predominantly in young women, usually beginning during the teens or early 20s. Diagnostic criteria for anorexia nervosa are listed in Table 23–1.

Bulimia nervosa is a disorder that usually begins in adolescence or early adult life. The disorder is characterized by recurrent episodes of rapid consumption of a large quantity of food in a short period (binge eating), often with the consumption of more than 1,000 kcal per episode. Patients report feeling out of control during the binge and often engage in either self-induced vomiting, the use of laxatives or diuretics, strict dieting, fasting, or vigorous exercise to prevent weight gain. Symptoms of anorexia and bulimia nervosa overlap; many patients have mixed presentations. Diagnostic criteria for bulimia nervosa are listed in Table 23–2.

Pica, "the eating of one or more nonnutritive substances on a persistent basis for a period of at least 1 month" (DSM-IV-TR [American Psychiatric Association 2000], p. 103), is a disorder that usually occurs in children and is often first seen between ages 12 and 24 months. It frequently remits early in childhood but on rare occasions persists into adolescence or adulthood. In psychiatrically ill patients, pica characteristically begins during adulthood. It has an increased incidence in children who have mental retardation, autism, or schizophrenia or who are neglected or poorly supervised. It may occur culturally in some groups of adults, particularly in the rural South (i.e., "clay eaters" of Georgia and "starch eaters" of Appalachia). Diagnostic criteria for pica are listed in Table 23–3.

ANOREXIA NERVOSA

Epidemiology

The incidence and prevalence of anorexia have remained relatively constant since the beginning of the twentieth

TABLE 23–1.   DSM-IV-TR criteria for anorexia nervosa

A. Refusal to maintain body weight at or above a minimally normal weight for age and height (e.g., weight loss leading to maintenance of body weight less than 85% of that expected; or failure to make expected weight gain during period of growth, leading to body weight less than 85% of that expected).

B. Intense fear of gaining weight or becoming fat, even though underweight.

C. Disturbance in the way in which one's body weight or shape is experienced, undue influence of body weight or shape on self-evaluation, or denial of the seriousness of the current low body weight.

D. In postmenarcheal females, amenorrhea, i.e., the absence of at least three consecutive menstrual cycles. (A woman is considered to have amenorrhea if her periods occur only following hormone, e.g., estrogen, administration.)

Specify type:

   Restricting Type: during the current episode of Anorexia Nervosa, the person has not regularly engaged in binge-eating or purging behavior (i.e., self-induced vomiting or the misuse of laxatives, diuretics, or enemas)

   Binge-Eating/Purging Type: during the current episode of Anorexia Nervosa, the person has regularly engaged in binge-eating or purging behavior (i.e., self-induced vomiting or the misuse of laxatives, diuretics, or enemas)

Source.   Adapted from American Psychiatric Association: *Diagnostic and Statistical Manual of Mental Disorders*, 4th Edition, Text Revision. Washington, DC, American Psychiatric Association, 2000. Used with permission.

TABLE 23–2.   DSM-IV-TR criteria for bulimia nervosa

A. Recurrent episodes of binge eating. An episode of binge eating is characterized by both of the following:

   (1) eating, in a discrete period of time (e.g., within any 2-hour period), an amount of food that is definitely larger than most people would eat during a similar period of time and under similar circumstances

   (2) a sense of lack of control over eating during the episode (e.g., a feeling that one cannot stop eating or control what or how much one is eating)

B. Recurrent inappropriate compensatory behavior in order to prevent weight gain, such as self-induced vomiting; misuse of laxatives, diuretics, enemas, or other medications; fasting; or excessive exercise.

C. The binge eating and inappropriate compensatory behaviors both occur, on average, at least twice a week for 3 months.

D. Self-evaluation is unduly influenced by body shape and weight.

E. The disturbance does not occur exclusively during episodes of Anorexia Nervosa.

Specify type:

   Purging Type: during the current episode of Bulimia Nervosa, the person has regularly engaged in self-induced vomiting or the misuse of laxatives, diuretics, or enemas

   Nonpurging Type: during the current episode of Bulimia Nervosa, the person has used other inappropriate compensatory behaviors, such as fasting or excessive exercise, but has not regularly engaged in self-induced vomiting or the misuse of laxatives, diuretics, or enemas

Source.   Adapted from American Psychiatric Association: *Diagnostic and Statistical Manual of Mental Disorders*, 4th Edition, Text Revision. Washington, DC, American Psychiatric Association, 2000. Used with permission.

TABLE 23–3.   DSM-IV-TR criteria for pica

A. Persistent eating of nonnutritive substances for a period of at least 1 month.

B. The eating of nonnutritive substances is inappropriate to the developmental level.

C. The eating behavior is not part of a culturally sanctioned practice.

D. If the eating behavior occurs exclusively during the course of another mental disorder (e.g., Mental Retardation, Pervasive Developmental Disorder, Schizophrenia), it is sufficiently severe to warrant independent clinical attention.

Source.   Adapted from American Psychiatric Association: *Diagnostic and Statistical Manual of Mental Disorders*, 4th Edition, Text Revision. Washington, DC, American Psychiatric Association, 2000. Used with permission.

century (Hall and Beresford 1989a). The reported lifetime prevalence of anorexia nervosa among women is 0.5% if the disease is narrowly defined and up to 3.7% if it is more broadly defined (Garfinkel et al. 1996; Walters and Kendler 1995). The disorder occurs most often in females between ages 13 and 18 years; cases are reported in patients as young as 5 years and as old as 60 years (Halmi et al. 1979; Palazzali 1978). In females between ages 12 and 18 years, the prevalence rate remains between 1 in 100 and 1 in 800.

Course

The onset of anorexia nervosa is often preceded by a period of dieting. Over time, the patient develops an intense fear of becoming obese, develops a disturbance of body image, experiences progressive and significant weight loss, and persistently refuses, in spite of encouragement, to maintain normal body weight.

The course of anorexia is episodic or unremitting until death. Although only a minority of anorexic patients fully recover, most patients who do not die improve symptomatically with time (Herzog et al. 1996). The most frequent pattern in patients who have anorexia for 3 years or more is a persistent, uncompromising maintenance of anorexic behavior. Anorexia that is treated early in adolescence is typified by a single episode with return to normal weight. Disordered anorexic thought processes, however, may persist for months to years after return to an acceptable weight.

Predisposing Factors

Predisposing factors include a history of sexual abuse (50% of these patients), difficulties negotiating psychosexual development, problems expressing aggression, and a recently stressful life situation such as a change of schools, a move, divorce, death of a parent, estrangement from parents, or loss of a boyfriend or girlfriend (Zerbe 1996). The personality profile suggests that patients with anorexia are often "the best and the brightest." These patients are characteristically model children who are perfectionistic, compulsive, careful, and "peacemakers." They are often self-sacrificing and rigidly incorporate parental values. They may harbor the feeling that they suffered some injustice—for example, that they modeled the family's values while siblings have not, yet the siblings are somehow better treated or more valued. Anorexic symptoms are a call for attention and help. The individual with anorexia is unable to meet his or her needs through any means other than self injury.

The patient often has a history of being mildly overweight, with chiding by important people to lose weight. The family is often body, diet, and fitness conscious. Anorexia is more commonly found in the mothers and sisters of anorexic patients (Strober et al. 1990). The first-degree biological relatives of anorexic patients are four times more likely to have major affective disorders

(unipolar or bipolar disorder) than are control subjects, and alcoholism is represented four to eight times more frequently in families with anorexic members than in control families.

Comorbid Psychiatric Conditions

Comorbid mood disorders have been reported in 50%–75% of anorexic and bulimic patients (Braun et al. 1994; Halmi et al. 1991; Herzog et al. 1992). As many as one-fourth of anorexic patients have a lifetime history of obsessive-compulsive disorder (Halmi et al. 1991), and obsessive-compulsive symptoms have been found in most anorexic patients at tertiary care treatment centers (Srinivasagam et al. 1995). It is estimated that 40%–75% of anorexic patients have comorbid personality disorders (Braun et al. 1994).

Outcome

Although the mortality from anorexia nervosa has diminished during the past 10 years, it is the highest among all psychiatric disorders. The death rate remains between 5% and 18%. Brotman et al. (1985) cautioned that as many as 22% of patients with persistent anorexia die as a result of the disorder. The mortality rate per decade has increased by 5%–6% among anorexic patients. The most frequent causes of death are cardiac arrhythmias with sudden cardiac death, seizures, gastrointestinal bleeding, renal failure, and secondary infection (Sullivan (1995).

Clinical Features

Severe weight loss associated with anorexia often necessitates hospitalization to prevent death by starvation. A variety of other behaviors place these patients at medical risk. The patients at greatest medical risk are those who have alternating episodes of anorexia and bulimia, the latter putting the greatest strain on the body's ability to maintain homeostasis. These patients often achieve their anorexic goals through total starvation, bizarre eating patterns (e.g., eating only lettuce), rumination of food (i.e., chewing, swallowing, and regurgitating food or chewing food and spitting it out), self-induced vomiting, or the use of diuretics, laxatives, emetics, enemas, and over-the-counter or prescription diet pills. In addition to restricting intake of food in general, these patients especially avoid foods that have a high fat content. They also often engage in excessive exercise; abuse diuretics, laxatives, and enemas; or induce vomiting. They commonly use stimulants such as caffeine, phenylpropanolamine, amphetamines, and cocaine to maintain energy and curb hunger.

Amenorrhea can occur before or after the onset of anorexia. Patients with anorexia, even when profoundly emaciated, report that they feel fat and often are preoccupied with particular parts of their bodies. They spend a considerable amount of time comparing themselves with others and often mirror gaze. Despite profound weight loss, patients with anorexia usually report a high energy level and pride themselves on their ability to function in spite of their progressive physical debilitation.

An important diagnostic feature is the absence of hunger. After a certain point in starvation, central peptides are released that diminish or obviate hunger. A second physiological plateau is reached when these patients enter the phase of terminal starvation, during which cachectin is released and interferes with the cells' ability to utilize energy.

Patients with anorexia deny the severity of their illness, and this denial and a stubborn resistance to therapy cause extreme difficulty during treatment. These patients often come to medical attention only after a crisis such as profound hypothermia; sudden, alarming, "marching" edema that begins in the legs and extends over the thighs to the lower back; profound cardiac disturbances; bradycardia; syncopal episodes associated with hypotension; confusional episodes; renal failure; or seizures.

Patients with anorexia can also have a variety of other psychiatric symptoms, including depression, obsessive-compulsive behavior (such as hand washing or hoarding food), and organic mental disorder with episodes of agitation, confusion, and disorientation. Organic mental disorder often responds to low doses of a phenothiazine such as perphenazine (2–6 mg/day). Zinc sulfate, 220 mg/day for 10 days, and oral thiamine, 100 mg/day, help to prevent this disorder. In contrast to bulimic patients, anorexic patients often show a marked loss of sexual interest and may have a history of delayed psychosexual development. They also have an increased frequency of urogenital abnormalities and Turner's syndrome.

BULIMIA NERVOSA

In the United States, bulimia nervosa is more likely to interfere with a young person's successful completion of college than any other medical or psychiatric disorder; it represents a major public health problem. Previously, bulimia was considered to be a relatively benign medical disorder; however, studies by Hall and Beresford (1990) and others demonstrated that it is a dangerous and often life-threatening disease.

Epidemiology

Estimates of the lifetime prevalence of bulimia among women range from 1.1% to 4.2%, depending on the narrowness of definition (Garfinkel et al. 1995). The prevalence of the disorder, particularly among college women, is increasing. The prevalence is estimated to be between 4% and 12% among college-age women and between 0.4% and 1% among college-age men (Casper et al. 1980; Hall and Beresford 1989b; Halmi et al. 1981; Heatherton et al. 1995; Herzog and Copeland 1985; Pyle et al. 1983).

Course

The disorder usually begins between early to mid-adolescence and early adult life and usually has a chronic intermittent course. Food binges may alternate with either periods of restrictive anorexia (which places the patient at greatest risk for medical complications) or periods of normal eating. Bulimic behavior usually begins as an attempt to control weight but rapidly progresses to a point at which it affects all aspects of the patient's life and is no longer voluntary (Hall and Beresford 1989b, 1990; Hall et al. 1989a; Mitchell et al. 1985; Striegel-Moore et al. 2001; Willard et al. 1990).

Predisposing Factors

Bulimic patients often have a family history of obesity. Major mood disorders occur two to four times more often in the first-degree biological relatives of bulimic patients than in the general population.

Bulimia often begins when important family members express concern about the patient's weight or appearance or after some disappointment, such as a disruption of interpersonal relationships. The patient may report a history of inappropriate sexual contact, rejection by a boyfriend or girlfriend, or that a significant other has commented he or she should "tone up and lose some weight."

Comorbid Psychiatric Conditions

Like patients with anorexia, bulimic patients have a high rate of comorbid mood disorders (50%–75%) (Braun et al. 1994; Halmi et al. 1991; Herzog et al. 1992). Obsessive-compulsive symptoms are common in patients with bulimia (Srinivasagam et al. 1995), and an estimated 40%–75% of bulimic patients also have personality disorders (Braun et al. 1994).

Clinical Features

Patients with bulimia are aware that their eating pattern is abnormal but are fearful of eating normally. They lose control of their eating behavior and begin to binge and purge. Bulimic patients often develop a significant lability of mood and profound alterations in mood state. At some time during their lives, 50%–70% of patients with bulimia experience a full-blown major depressive episode. Attention and concentration are diminished in patients with severe bulimia. This inability to concentrate is the most likely cause of their academic difficulties.

Approximately 80% of bulimic eating binges are planned; 20% occur as a reaction to emotional stress. The foods consumed during a binge are highly caloric, usually sweet or salty, and high in fat. The food is usually eaten rapidly. Once the binge begins, attempts by friends or relatives to stop it can cause disruptive behavior and/or violence. Patients stop bingeing when they experience abdominal pain, when they fall asleep, or after they induce vomiting.

Patients with bulimia often exercise excessively and abuse laxatives, diuretics, ipecac, and over-the-counter and illicit stimulants (e.g., phenylpropanolamine, amphetamines, or cocaine). Most bulimic patients are overweight at some time before the onset of bulimia. Most (60%–80%) are of normal weight or slightly overweight when first seen. Unlike patients with anorexia, bulimic patients maintain libido and desire interpersonal contact.

Hall and Beresford (1990), Mitchell et al. (1986), Willard et al. (1990), and others noted an increased medical risk in patients who routinely abuse laxatives. Hall et al. (1989a) demonstrated that, in a hospitalized population, 13% of patients with anorexia, 8% of patients with bulimia, and 25% of patients with restrictive anorexia alternating with bulimia chronically abused laxatives, compared with 8% of a control group of female patients with other psychiatric disorders. Profound physiological dependence on laxatives occurred in 3% of patients with anorexia, 1.2% of patients with bulimia, and 11% of patients with restrictive anorexia alternating with bulimia. Seventeen percent of outpatients with anorexia or bulimia were regular laxative users, compared with 7% of a general psychiatric control population. These findings are similar to those reported by Mitchell et al. (1986), who noted that laxative abusers were twice as likely to abuse diuretics, 2.5 times more likely to abuse diet pills, and 4 times more likely to experience serious medical complications than were non–laxative-abusing patients with anorexia or bulimia. The most significant medical findings in patients with eating disorders who abuse diuretics and laxatives are listed in Table 23–4.

PICA

Pica usually occurs very early in life and frequently remits between ages 4 and 6 years. However, it may persist into adolescence or even develop de novo during adolescence or adulthood.

Complications occur based on the substances ingested. For example, lead poisoning is common in children who ingest paint or plaster. Bezoars can cause intestinal obstruction. *Toxoplasma* and *Toxocara canis* infections can occur after ingestion of dirt. Clay eaters can develop a variety of both gastrointestinal malabsorption syndromes and helminthic infections. Individuals with psychosis reportedly have consumed substances such as glass, pins, cloth, string, feces, sand, and insects. Some patients with bulimia who want to injure themselves consume food that is likely to tear the esophagus on regurgitation (e.g., broken buttons or peanut shells); patients who thus injure themselves have a symptomatic form of pica (Hall et al. 1992).

The prevalence of pica is uncertain, but it is considered rare, particularly in adults. There is no known family pattern associated with the disorder. Mortality is rare.

TABLE 23–4. Significant medical findings in patients with eating disorders who abuse diuretics and laxatives

Anemia

Confusional states

Esophageal tears

Glucose intolerance

Granulocytic suppression

Hypocalcemia

Hypokalemia

Hyponatremia

Hypoproteinemia with or without massive edema and cardiovascular compromise

Hypotension

Localized or systemic infections

Lower gastrointestinal bleeding

Pancreatitis

Peptic ulcer

Persistent cardiac arrhythmias

Profound muscular weakness

Refractory hypokalemia associated with hypomagnesemia

Renal insufficiency

Rhabdomyolysis

MEDICAL COMPLICATIONS

Hospitalized Patients With Anorexia or Bulimia

Hall and Beresford (1990) carefully evaluated 276 anorexic and bulimic patients admitted to an eating disorders unit and compared them with 78 depressed control patients for the occurrence of medical disorders. Two hundred distinct medical diagnoses were made in the 276 patients studied. The diagnosis of previously unrecognized medical disorders in the patients with eating disorders was nearly twice that in patients in the control group (statistically significant at $P = .001$). Forty percent of the patients with bulimia had a severe medical complication that was dangerous to life or limb or, if left untreated, would likely have long-term medical sequelae. The results were highly significant because these patients were young and presented in large numbers to general hospitals. Almost 90% of the serious medical complications were previously unrecognized by the patient or his or her physician, even though the majority of these patients had ongoing medical care. Seventy percent of the patients with bulimia admitted to the hospital required some type of medical treatment.

On the basis of these study findings, Hall and Beresford (1990) stressed the importance of an effective laboratory evaluation for a newly hospitalized patient with a suspected eating disorder (Table 23–5).

Hypomagnesemia and hypokalemia are common problems; refractory hypokalemia is occasionally caused by persistent unrecognized hypomagnesemia (Boyd et al. 1983; Hall et al. 1988a, 1988b; Wong et al. 1983). Table 23–6 includes the medical complications found in patients during the study by Hall and Beresford (1990).

TABLE 23–5. Laboratory evaluation for a newly hospitalized patient with a suspected eating disorder

Complete blood count with differential
SMAC-21 or equivalent, including serum electrolyte levels; liver function studies; and blood urea nitrogen, creatinine, and serum calcium and magnesium levels
Thyroid function tests
Luteinizing hormone and follicle-stimulating hormone levels, in a patient with persistent amenorrhea at normal weight
Testosterone levels, in a male patient
Urinalysis
Electrocardiography
Urine toxicology
Pancreatic amylase levels (or amylase levels and, if elevated, lipase levels)

TABLE 23–6. Medical complications frequently encountered in hospitalized patients with anorexia or bulimia

Complication	Prevalence (%)
Persistent cardiac arrhythmia	33
Hypomagnesemia	25
Peptic ulcer disease	10–16
Severe anemia	5–10
Seizures	4
Esophageal tears	3
Pancreatitis (often associated with excessive thiazide diuretic abuse)	1
Renal insufficiency	1
Hypokalemia	30
Hyponatremia	20
Hypocalcemia	15
Leukopenia	35

The persistent hypokalemia can result in cardiac arrhythmias, profound muscular weakness, rhabdomyolysis, and glucose intolerance. Hypoproteinemia with massive "marching" edema is an ominous sign of impending cardiac decompensation and hypovolemic shock. This condition usually occurs in patients with severe anorexia who abuse laxatives and have profoundly low serum protein levels on admission.

Patients frequently have a moderate anemia with a hematocrit between 30 and 35. Severe anemia with a hematocrit below 25 occurs in 5%–10% of hospitalized patients; bone marrow biopsies show severely reduced or absent iron stores and low red blood cell folate levels. Routine replacement of iron, folate, vitamin B_{12}, and zinc is appropriate, as is routine replacement of thiamine (100 mg/day orally) to obviate starvation-induced mental changes.

Persistent cardiac arrhythmias occur in one-third of the hospitalized patients with anorexia and are often associated with substernal chest pain and a history of syncope. Profoundly ill patients with anorexia have difficulty maintaining body temperature and blood pressure; 60% of the severely ill patients with anorexia in the study by Hall and Beresford (1989a, 1990a) developed cardiac arrhythmias secondary to electrolyte disorders, particularly hypokalemia. Peptic ulcer occurs in patients hospitalized for eating disorders. Esophageal ulcerations and tears occur most frequently in patients with a history of alternating restrictive anorexia and bulimia. Cerebral cortical atrophy and ventricular dilatation occur in both anorexic and bulimic patients, particularly in patients with a history of restrictive anorexia alternating with bulimia (Nussbaum et al. 1980).

Profound hypomagnesemia is most likely to occur in patients with alternating anorexia and bulimia who abuse laxatives and diuretics (Hall et al. 1990a). Ten percent of patients with alternating anorexia and bulimia present with white blood cell counts below 3,500/mm^3. Severe leukopenia and granulocytopenia with total granulocyte counts that decrease to below 1,000/mm^3 are most frequent in these patients, who require double reverse isolation during refeeding. Less severe bone marrow suppression typically responds to refeeding within 1–2 weeks.

Patients With Anorexia

In 1698, Richard Morton (1920), in his first description of anorexia nervosa, commented that it was a disease with profound medical complications. *Consumption*, his original term for the condition, was considered a discrete entity of "will." Morton's description remains important to this date. The most frequent signs and symptoms encountered in patients with anorexia are listed in Table 23–7. Physical examination may evidence a variety of findings, such as cardiac arrhythmias, a mitral click or murmur (mitral valve prolapse), muscle wasting, tetany, scars over the dorsum of the hand (Russell's sign), calluses over the abdomen from digital pressure, and burns or scars from self-laceration.

The acute medical emergencies associated with eating disorders include arrhythmias, infections, persistent syncope, delirium, grand mal seizures, acute gastric rupture, toxic megacolon, esophageal tears with bleeding, development of Barrett's esophagus with bleeding, and acute upper or lower gastrointestinal bleeding. These patients often develop osteoporosis and may present with various pathological fractures, particularly of the small bones of the feet, as well as vertebral compression fractures (Brincat et al. 1983; Parsons et al. 1983; Rigotti et al. 1984). The clinician should thoroughly investigate complaints of bone or back pain. Mean bone density in these patients is diminished compared with control subjects. Rigotti et al. (1984) believed that osteopenia in these patients is caused by a combination of estrogen deficiency, dietary calcium deficiency, and excessive glucocorticoid secretion. The areas most vulnerable to osteoporosis are the lumbar spine and hip (Klibanski et al. 1995). Patients with anorexia whose symptoms are so severe that amenorrhea develops during adolescence are at greatest risk for osteoporosis because these patients fail to form bone at a critical phase of development (Treasure et al. 1996).

Polycystic ovaries occur commonly in patients with anorexia as a result of starvation (Rapaport 1985; Treasure et al. 1985). The menstrual pattern of anorexic

TABLE 23–7. Signs and symptoms frequently found in patients with anorexia

Most common

Progressive weight loss to the point of emaciation and organic mental impairment

Return to prepubescent levels of development, with regression of breasts and secondary sexual characteristics

Significant orthostatic hypotension

Inability to maintain body temperature, with lowered core temperature

Appearance of lanugo

Amenorrhea

Constipation

Acrocyanosis

Muscular weakness and wasting

Loss of subcutaneous fat throughout the body

Pericardial thinning

Bradycardia

Hypercarotenemia

Peripheral "marching" edema

Other

Petechiae

Ecchymoses

Tremor

Ataxia

Confusion

Auditory and/or visual hallucinations

Acute gastric dilatation with periumbilical and midepigastric tenderness or pain

Signs of "pigbel" (acute clostridial gastritis)

Associated with bulimia

Nausea

Spontaneous (i.e., nonvolitional) reflex vomiting of any food ingested

Persistent lancinating epigastric pain

Abdominal bloating and distension

Intractable constipation

Pyrosis

Flatulence

Belching or diarrhea alternating with constipation

patients is affected by both their degree of starvation and their level of physical activity. Litt and Glader (1986) demonstrated that athletic patients with anorexia have lower gonadotropin levels, have longer periods of amenorrhea before significant weight loss and after weight restoration, and require higher baseline weights to resume menses than do sedentary patients with anorexia. These findings are independent of the patient's malnutrition and suggest that increased physical activity worsens a patient's menstrual dysfunction. Studies have also found that bone density is better maintained in patients who continue to exercise (Hall and Beresford 1990).

Substance Use

Patients with anorexia or bulimia often poison themselves through consumption of stimulants or substances to induce purging. In addition, patients with eating disorders often consume large quantities of caffeine in diet sodas, coffee, and tea. The symptoms of caffeine toxicity include profound gastrointestinal upset, heartburn, tachycardia, arrhythmia, myoclonic twitching, and transient psychotic episodes. Patients have been reported to have consumed 3–10 g of caffeine a day and died (Shaul et al. 1984). The laboratory findings associated with acute caffeinism include hyperglycemia, hypokalemia, ketonuria, glycosuria, and transient leukocytosis. Central nervous system irritability and tonic posturing occur with caffeine concentrations of 1.5–1.7 mEq/dL, whereas severe persistent tachycardia and convulsions occur at levels of 4–4.6 mg/dL. At levels of severe caffeine intoxication (3–6 mg/dL), patients are likely to experience rigidity, posturing, convulsions, and fluctuating levels of coma; at somewhat lower levels, they may present with transient psychotic episodes characterized by tactile hallucinations, disorientation, paranoid delusions, confusion, and bizarre behavior.

Ipecac toxicity is also encountered in patients with anorexia or bulimia. Two toxic alkaloids of ipecac—emetine and cephaeline—accumulate because of slow excretion from the body. These substances can prolong the Q-T interval and produce atrial and ventricular arrhythmias. Both can produce sudden cardiac death by blocking calcium transport in the myocardium and thus causing a profound negative inotropic effect (Isner et al. 1985). Emetine becomes lethal when patients consume 10–25 mg/kg body weight. Signs and symptoms of emetine toxicity may not appear for days to weeks after a patient stops abusing ipecac; consequently, patients with a history of serious ipecac abuse should be monitored closely.

Laxative abuse is frequently associated with hypochloremic, metabolic acidosis and hypocalcemia, particularly in patients who abuse phosphate-containing laxatives (Oster et al. 1980). Laxative dependence represents a serious problem, and the sudden cessation of laxatives may result in impaction, adynamic ileus, or acute toxic megacolon. The phenothaline metabolites found in many laxatives may cause bone marrow suppression and persistent anemia.

Cardiac Abnormalities

Cardiac arrhythmias and grand mal seizures are frequent causes of death in patients with anorexia. Most cardiac arrhythmias are precipitated by the electrolyte abnormalities described earlier in this chapter. Fohlin (1977) dem-

onstrated that up to 87% of patients with anorexia nervosa develop cardiac abnormalities at some time during their disease (Pallosy and Oo 1977; Thurston and Marks 1974). Brotman and Stern (1983) recommend immediate medical hospitalization for patients with anorexia when 1) symptoms of dizziness, syncope, or chest pain develop; 2) arrhythmias occur in the setting of a dangerous medical condition such as an abnormal electrolyte level, coagulopathy, or infection; 3) arrhythmias develop in patients with anorexia who have been abusing laxatives or diuretics or are vomiting; or 4) more than 40% of premorbid body weight is lost and an electrolyte abnormality is present.

The high-protein liquid diets that many of these patients abuse can produce profound fatigue, dehydration, hair loss, orthostatic hypotension, arrhythmias, and myocarditis (Bistrian 1981). In addition, hypomagnesemia can induce coronary artery spasm leading to acute myocardial ischemia and chest pain. The clinician should remember that the triad of prolonged Q-T interval, arrhythmia, and hypomagnesemia can lead to sudden cardiac death in an anorexic patient (Chadda 1986).

Cardiac failure can occur during the refeeding phase of treatment; refeeding is a more dangerous time than the period of gradual starvation. During refeeding, the recovery of stroke volume lags behind the recovery of total heart volume, with end-systolic volume being increased disproportionately to stroke volume. The ejection fraction is diminished. If refeeding is too rapid, particularly in individuals who place stress on the heart by exercise, dyspnea followed by heart failure is common. Refeeding dyspnea usually begins between the second and fifth month of refeeding and is associated with elevated venous pressure. If refeeding is too zealous, myocardial reserve may not be adequate to keep up with increased myocardial demand. Thus, caution is essential with the use of intravenous fluids and hyperalimentation in severely starved anorexic patients (Hall and Beresford 1990). Because of the risks associated with refeeding, severely cachectic anorexic patients should be hospitalized on a unit that has cardiac monitoring and is capable of handling cardiac emergencies. Gradual refeeding of severely starved anorexic patients over a 2- to 4-month period, with an average weight gain of not more than 5 lb/week, is safest.

The electrocardiographic changes and coronary ischemia seen on admission in anorexic patients usually improve rapidly after hydration, renourishment, and the correction of electrolyte abnormalities (Hoffman and Hall 1990). The most frequent electrocardiographic abnormalities encountered include ST segment depression, inversion of T waves, low voltage, bradycardia, and the presence of U waves associated with hypokalemia and hypomagnesemia. The most dangerous findings encountered include superventricular arrhythmias with premature ventricular beats and ventricular tachycardia. Other frequently recorded abnormal cardiac rhythms include premature ventricular contractions (PVCs), coupled PVCs, premature atrial contractions (PACs), bigeminy, and atrial fibrillation. Patients with anorexia can have widening of the QRS interval with peaked T waves, prolongation of the P-R interval, and ST segment depression (Arik et al. 1985; Fonseca and Havard 1985; Kalager et al. 1978). Isner et al. (1985) and Hall et al. (1990a, 1990b) highlighted the fact that prolonged Q-T intervals are associated with, and may predict, sudden development of life-threatening arrhythmias in patients with anorexia. Bradycardia occurs in up to 87% of anorexic patients; a significant dimunition in myocardial mass (i.e., a decrease in left ventricular wall thickness and a reduction in cardiac chamber size) also occurs (Fohlin 1977; Thurston and Marks 1974). Hypotension, with blood pressure consistently below 90/60 mm Hg, is reported in as many as 85% of patients with anorexia (M.P. Warren and Vandewyle 1979); this may cause recurrent episodes of dizziness, near syncopal episodes, or frank syncope. Heart rates as low as 25 beats/minute occur in anorexic patients. It is surprising that individuals with sedentary lifestyles can adjust reasonably well to these low rates.

Several investigators believe that the bradycardia associated with anorexia is related to energy-conserving mechanisms that slow the metabolic rates in these patients. These changes are attributed to a diminution in circulating peripheral catecholamines and a change in the rate of conversion of thyroxine (T_4) to triiodothyronine (T_3). In patients who have anorexia, the peripheral conversion of T_4 to T_3 is inhibited, and T_3 levels are decreased to as much as 50% below normal values. In addition, total T_4 levels are often lower than expected but remain in the low end of the normal range. Free T_4 levels are normal. The resultant metabolic downregulation produces a variety of symptoms, including cold intolerance, drying of the skin, bradycardia, carotenemia, hypercholesterolemia, and constipation. This constellation of symptoms is called *euthyroid sick syndrome* (Croxson and Ibbertson 1977; Miyai et al. 1975; Moshang et al. 1975; Wartofsky and Burman 1982).

Renal Abnormalities

Renal abnormalities occur in up to 70% of patients who have chronic anorexia nervosa. Such patients present with increased levels of blood urea nitrogen, diminished glomerular filtration rates, diminished renal concentrating capability, pitting edema, renal calculi, hypokalemic nephropathy, diabetes insipidus–like states, and a variety of electrolyte abnormalities (Brotman et al. 1986; Mira et al. 1984; Schwartz and Relman 1967; Sheinin 1989; Silber and Kass 1984; S. E. Warren and Steinberg 1979).

Hypokalemic nephropathy with renal tubular vacuolization is a particularly ominous finding in patients with anorexia or bulimia who have abused diuretics and laxatives. Chronic renal failure often develops in these patients. Patients become profoundly dehydrated, with increased thirst, drying of the mucous membranes, diminished skin turgor, profound postural hypotension, and delirium. If untreated, the condition may progress to acute glomerular necrosis and death (Fleming et al. 1975; Grebb et al. 1984; Mars et al. 1982; Reyes and Leary 1984).

Electrolyte Abnormalities

Mitchell et al. (1983), in a study involving 168 patients with bulimia, anorexia, or atypical eating disorders, found that 49% of subjects had electrolyte abnormalities. They noticed increased bicarbonate (HCO_3) concentrations in 27%, hypochloremia in 24%, hyperchloremia in 5.4%, hypokalemia in 14%, and decreased HCO_3 concentrations in 8.3%. High phosphate levels are common in patients who vomit excessively. Laboratory values may be normal in patients with anorexia, despite the presence of significant malnutrition. For example, patients with low total potassium levels may have normal serum electrolyte levels and are still prone to arrhythmias (Powers et al. 1995).

Abnormal laboratory values in patients with bulimia or anorexia are almost always reversible when weight is restored (Kingston et al. 1996; Swayze et al. 1996). Hall et al. (1989a) defined the characteristic laboratory profile of patients who purge at least three times daily for a prolonged period (Table 23–8). This profile is useful as a laboratory indicator of ongoing vomiting.

TABLE 23–8. Common laboratory findings in patients who purge at least three times daily

Low white blood cell count (as low as 3,500/mm^3)
Moderate anemia with hematocrit in the range of 32–38
Diminished red blood cell mass
Macrocytic red blood cell indices
Atypical lymphocytes in the peripheral smear (2%–10%)
Hypochloremia
Hyperphosphatemia
Low total protein levels
Hypomagnesemia (25%)

Edema

Peripheral edema is seen in approximately 20% of patients with severe anorexia and is more likely to occur during the refeeding period than during starvation. Two forms of edema occur. In one form, levels of plasma proteins, including albumin, are normal; and in the second, a more serious type, levels of plasma proteins, particularly albumin, are profoundly decreased. In the first form, hyperaldosteronism and disturbances in glucose-to-insulin ratios cause the edema. In the second type, profound hypoproteinemia produces tissue edema, diminished plasma volume, cardiovascular collapse, renal insufficiency, and, ultimately, hypovolemic shock. The latter condition is life threatening, and immediate treatment with plasma or plasma volume expanders is essential (DeFronzo 1981; Gold et al. 1982; Mira et al. 1984).

Hematological Abnormalities

The hematological change most frequently accompanying severe anorexia (50% of cases) is pancytopenia; bone marrow biopsies show marrow hypoplasia (Bowers and Eckert 1978; Myers et al. 1981; Reiger et al. 1978).

Of hospitalized patients with anorexia, 40%–60% have white blood cell counts of approximately 3,500/mm^3. Diminished platelet counts occur in approximately 30% of patients with profound anorexia, but this thrombocytopenia is unlikely to produce significant bleeding; however, increased bruisability is common. Vitamin K–deficient coagulopathies may also occur and require immediate treatment.

Hematological changes are common in patients with bulimia and include leukopenia, relative lymphocytosis, and, in severe cases, particularly those associated with abuse of phenophthaline laxatives, a hypocellular bone marrow that is filled with large amounts of gelatinous mucopolysaccharide. In long-standing cases, fibrous changes may occur within the bone marrow spaces and reduce the patient's ability to repopulate the bone marrow cavities; this may result in chronic anemia. Other findings include a low erythrocyte sedimentation rate, a diminished level of plasma fibrinogen, and prolongation of prothrombin time as a result of vitamin K deficiency (Bowers and Eckert 1978; Reiger et al. 1978).

Endocrine Abnormalities

Patients with anorexia have many profound endocrine changes. The reader is referred elsewhere for a more detailed description of these changes (Danowski et al. 1972; Gerner and Gwirtsman 1981; Gwirtsman et al. 1983; Macaron et al. 1978; Neri et al. 1972; Russell 1969; Takahara et al. 1976; T. Walsh 1980).

In summary, the endocrine changes in patients with anorexia and anorexia alternating with bulimia include T_4 levels in the lower range of, or just below, clinical laboratory norms, as well as T_3 levels that are somewhat reduced. Elevated serum concentrations of 3,3',5'-triiodothyronine (reverse T_3) are often associated with diminished levels of serum T_3. Some clinical laboratory equipment does not detect reverse T_3 and may produce a false picture of hypothyroidism (euthyroid sick syndrome) (Wartofsky and Burman 1982). Administration of thyroid hormones to euthyroid starved patients is dangerous and should be avoided. If routine T_3 levels are low, the clinician should obtain T_3 levels by radioimmunoassay as well as thyroid-stimulating hormone levels before any thyroid replacement is begun.

Amenorrhea usually begins in patients who are more that 15% below median ideal body weight. Frisch and McArthur (1974) noted that body weight and age at menarche are directly related, with menarche requiring a mean weight of 48 kg regardless of patient height. In addition, they noted that menstruation ceases when body fat falls below 22% of total body weight. Other endocrine factors are also important in the cessation of menstruation in anorexic women, because almost 35% cease menstruating before they experience significant weight loss. In addition, many patients do not resume menses until they gain 8–10 lb over the weight at which menstruation ceased (Kay and Leigh 1954). Russell (1969, 1973) suggested that the primary disturbance of hypothalamic function that produces amenorrhea is caused by psychological factors that directly alter central neurochemistry, because the resumption of menses is often associated with profound psychological improvement. Halmi and Falk (1983) reported similar findings in their study of anorexic women 1 year after treatment. They noted that patients who are menstruating are significantly less likely to persist in their anorexic behaviors and attitudes than are amenorrheic patients.

Other common endocrine changes encountered in patients with anorexia include lowered levels of follicle-stimulating hormone, luteinizing hormone, and serum estrogen. Testosterone levels are lowered in male anorexic patients. All of these changes also occur with starvation. Nonsuppression on dexamethasone suppression tests occurs in anorexic and bulimic patients who do not meet DSM-IV-TR (American Psychiatric Association 2000) criteria for depression. Of patients with bulimia, 40%–70% have abnormal dexamethasone suppression test results. In both bulimia and anorexia, dexamethasone suppression test results revert to normal when the abnormal eating behavior ceases or the patient returns to median ideal body weight.

Growth hormone release is diminished in patients with anorexia following insulin-induced hypoglycemia and administration of L-dopa; these patients also secrete less growth hormone during rapid eye movement (REM) sleep. However, both patients with bulimia and patients with anorexia may show a paradoxical increase in growth hormone levels after administration of thyroid-releasing hormone (Macaron et al. 1978). Levels of prolactin, vasopressin, and 3-methoxy-4-hydroxyphenylglycol (MHPG) are diminished in patients with anorexia. These levels return to normal when patients reach median ideal body weight.

Patients With Bulimia

Many of the medical complications that occur in patients with bulimia are discussed in the previous section on anorexia. The most frequent serious medical complications of bulimia are electrolyte imbalances, profound dehydration, hypovolemic shock, cardiac arrhythmias, esophageal tears, gastric rupture, peptic ulcer, blood loss, anemia with syncope, seizures, and organic mental syndrome, particularly confusional states.

In addition, patients with bulimia are at risk for a variety of dental problems, such as erosion of tooth enamel, development of gum abscesses, and obstruction or inflammation of salivary ducts, which causes parotid inflammation and enlargement ("chipmunk cheeks"). They are also more likely to develop pyorrhea of the gums, ulcerations of the oral mucosa, and a loss of tongue papillae. Characteristically, tooth size is reduced and teeth are more sensitive because of thinning enamel. Patients often have sore throats, caused by the constant irritation from gastric acid, as well as a history of intermittent recurrent mid-periumbilical abdominal pain, esophageal irritation, crushing esophageal pain, and bouts of mild hematemesis. Mallory-Weiss tears of the esophagus are common, and Boerhaave's syndrome (esophageal rupture caused by vomiting) is reported (Russell 1979; Wilbur and Washburn 1978).

Parotid enlargement occurs in 10% of bulimic patients; 50% of these patients have elevated serum amylase levels. In patients who also report abdominal pain, measurement of serum lipase levels is useful to rule out pancreatitis. If lipase concentrations are elevated, the source of the elevated amylase is likely the pancreas. If lipase levels are within normal limits, the source is the parotid glands.

More than 60 cases of death as a result of acute gastric dilatation have occurred in bulimic patients. If gastric rupture occurs, the mortality rate exceeds 80%. The condition is more likely to occur in patients with a history of alternating anorexia and bulimia. As noted, bulimic patients are at risk for peptic ulcer (as many as 16% of patients). Other gastrointestinal disorders associated with bulimia include pancreatitis (secondary to dehydration and the use of thiazide diuretics), nutritional hepatitis, chronic cholecystitis, gastritis, irritable colon, rectal bleeding, adynamic ileus, toxic megacolon, nocturnal fecal soiling (secondary to laxative abuse), melena, ileitis, and superior mesenteric artery syndrome (Evans 1968; Gavish et al. 1987; Jennings and Klidjian 1974; Mitchell et al. 1982).

A variety of neurological and psychiatric symptoms are associated with severe bulimia. These include seizures; paresthesias; muscular weakness; changes in sensorium; delirium; dementia; headache; dizziness; gait disorders; tetany; unilateral pupillary dilation; facial weakness; auditory, visual, and tactile hallucinations; derealization; depersonalization; and depression (Rau and Green 1978; Remick et al. 1980).

TREATMENT

Anorexia

The treatment of patients with eating disorders is first directed toward stabilizing their medical conditions. Patients' conditions should be managed by a team experienced in the treatment of patients with eating disorders. It is important to try to establish and maintain a therapeutic alliance. Trust is difficult for anorexic patients, and countertransference frequently occurs (Zerbe 1993). The desire to rescue or abandon a patient should be avoided. The clinician should consult with other medical professionals, particularly internists and dentists, as required.

After initial medical stabilization, a complete blood count with differential and SMAC-21 are recommended, at least weekly during the acute stage of treatment, to monitor for surreptitious activity and abnormal physiological states. Treatment is directed toward medical management, nutritional rehabilitation, and psychoeducation, as well as family, individual, and group therapy. For patients with anorexia, an educational program taught by an experienced dietitian is crucial.

During the early stages of treatment, a weight gain of 2–5 lb/week is typically established. If the patient is unable to consume reasonable quantities of solid food, supplemental feedings with Ensure, Sustacal, or Glucerna are often helpful. My colleagues and I routinely have patients begin with 10 servings of Ensure daily (2,500 kcal), supplemented with 1,500 calories worth of solid food a day. If serum protein levels are low, Dalmark gelatin twice each day is added to the regimen. Patients are also given zinc sulfate 220 mg/day for 10 days, oral thiamine 100 mg/day, and a multivitamin with minerals. Vital signs are carefully monitored every 6 hours during the first 3–4 weeks of treatment. Patients are weighed daily in a gown. If the patient is unable to eat or if weight continues to decline, the patient is placed on strict one-to-one (i.e., a nurse is with the patient at all times) or bed rest.

Organic confusional states are treated with low doses of appropriate phenothiazines. In our experience, patients tolerate low-dose perphenazine (i.e., 2–4 mg at bedtime) quite well. The discharge goal weight is established on admission and is no less than 80% of the median ideal body weight; the goal is to reach median ideal body weight by the time of discharge, if possible, or within 1–3 months after discharge.

With nutritional rehabilitation and weight gain, other symptoms of eating disorders concurrently diminish, although they may not disappear. Distorted attitudes about weight and exercise are least likely to change; long-term, regular structured diets are important to prevent rapid relapse. Psychotherapy, discussed shortly, becomes crucial at this stage of treatment.

In this era of managed care, there is pressure to shorten inpatient treatment. The issue of whether management should consist of inpatient, partial hospital, or outpatient psychiatric treatment arises soon after diagnosis and medical stabilization. Outpatient management should be considered when weight is more than 80% of base weight, motivation for recovery is good, and a supportive social structure exists. Inpatient programs should be considered when weight is less than 75% of base weight, motivation for recovery is poor, there are clinically significant electrocardiographic or laboratory findings, and the patient does not have the social structure to help him or her eat and gain weight. Partial hospital treatment is appropriate for patients who do not meet all criteria for either outpatient or inpatient management. When outpatient treatment is possible, a more modest weight-gain goal of about 1 lb/week is set (Andolf et al. 1997).

Therapy is directed toward redefining interpersonal relationships; increasing self-esteem, providing specific coping tools; helping the patient cooperate with nutritional rehabilitation; redefining family interactions; and helping the patient become less fearful about normal body size and eating. Considerable effort is directed toward changing the anorexic patient's attitude and cognitions about his or her body size, food consumption, and weight. Most clinicians favor cognitive-behavioral therapies for maintaining healthy eating behaviors and either cognitive or interpersonal therapies for promoting more effective coping (Bowers 2001).

Other issues of psychotherapeutic importance are fear of separation, failure, autonomy, social and sexual development, and social isolation; the patient typically needs to develop better coping skills and assertiveness. The clinician must also carefully evaluate the factors that led to and perpetuated the eating disorder (Kennedy et al. 1995). The associated symptoms of mental rumination, obsessional thoughts and compulsive behaviors, substance and alcohol abuse, and depression also require specific intervention. If the patient has neurological symptoms, such as weakness or headache, the consultant should obtain a computed tomography scan or a magnetic resonance image. If the patient reports amenorrhea lasting 2 years or more or complains of bone or back pain, appropriate radiographs and a bone density scan should be ordered.

No proven pharmacological treatments are available for anorexia nervosa. Medications may be useful for adjunctive treatment or for managing comorbid psychiatric conditions such as major depressive disorder or obsessive-compulsive disorder.

The phenothiazines, particularly low-dose perphenazine or thioridazine, are helpful for treating the agitation and mental turmoil associated with starvation-induced organic mental syndromes. Patients should be monitored for hypotensive side effects. In addition, phenothiazines lower the seizure threshold and may produce dystonia and akathisia. Pimozide should be avoided because it may lengthen the Q-T interval and cause adverse cardiac effects. If major tranquilizers or antidepressants are given to patients with severe anorexia, the clinician should carefully monitor cardiac, hematopoietic, hepatic, and renal function.

Once weight gain is accomplished, patients who remain agitated, depressed, perplexed, or ruminative or have difficulty with decision making may respond well to antidepressant medications. Selective serotonin reuptake inhibitors (SSRIs) are currently favored because they lack significant cardiac or cardiovascular side effects and do not lower the seizure threshold. Patients with anorexia are particularly prone to adverse effects of medications; consideration should be given to beginning with low initial doses and limiting the use of medication to patients whose psychiatric symptoms persist after weight is restored.

Bulimia

Much of the treatment for anorexia also applies to patients with bulimia. Hospitalized patients usually have experienced significant medical consequences of bulimia; thus, medical stabilization is the most important issue. Once stabilized, either inpatient or outpatient treatment with careful monitoring and follow-up is necessary. Bulimic patients benefit from individual, group, and family therapy, as well as cognitive-behavioral restructuring techniques (Connors et al. 1984; Freeman et al. 1988; Lacey 1983; Lee and Rush 1986; Mitchell et al. 1990; Ordman and Kirschenbaum 1985; Yates and Sambraillo 1984). Although self-help groups are a useful adjunct, they do not substitute for psychotherapy. In addition, self-help groups that are based on 12-step models are counterproductive for many patients. Traditional group psychotherapy may be of significant benefit for many patients. A meta-analysis of 40 group-treatment studies suggested that moderate overall functional and symptomatic improvement occurred, and such improvement was typically maintained for 1 year (Oesterheld et al. 1987). Frequent visits early in treatment and integration of nutritional counseling into the group program predict better outcomes with group therapy (Fairburn et al. 1993; Laessle et al. 1987; Mitchell et al. 1993).

Cognitive-behavioral therapies are often used to help patients maintain healthy eating behaviors. Cognitive or interpersonal therapies also help improve coping skills. It is important to involve families, either in the patient's therapy or with more comprehensive family psychotherapy (Eisler et al. 1997). Some programs combine cognitive-behavioral approaches with features of addiction models such as 12-step principles (Johnson and Taylor 1996).

Outpatient therapy requires careful monitoring of physical and laboratory findings, regular appointments, and specific treatment goals (i.e., reduction and ultimately elimination of the binge-purge behavior). An eating diary often helps to identify triggers for bulimic behavior. An educational program to advise the patient of the seriousness of the disorder and the potential symptoms that may develop, with emphasis on the elimination of diuretic, laxative, and ipecac abuse, is crucial. Assistance with meal preparation and in controlling situations that produce binge-purge behavior is needed. Assertiveness and relaxation training are helpful. Underlying family conflicts usually respond well to family therapy. Patients need deconditioning to reduce fears of specific foods and assistance to master eating in moderation. Common issues in psychotherapy are a history of sexual abuse or assault, difficulty in dealing with interpersonal demands, a fear of confrontation, anger about emotional misuse by someone close to the patient, and competitiveness with other family members, as well as a fear of autonomy, loss of control, and failure.

The pharmacotherapy for bulimia is more effective than that for anorexia. Studies have shown that serotonin is an important transmitter in bulimic behavior (Kaye et al. 1984). It was suggested by Kaye et al. (1984) that serotonergic dysregulation is common in patients with bulimia. These investigators showed that cerebrospinal fluid levels of 5-hydroxyindoleacetic acid (5-HIAA), a serotonin metabolite, are lower in bulimic patients than in control subjects. Serotonin levels are also lower in patients with restrictive anorexia alternating with bulimia than in patients with pure restrictive anorexia (Blouin et al. 1988; Pope et al. 1985).

Randomized clinical trials have demonstrated that nondepressed as well as depressed patients with bulimia respond to antidepressant medications. In addition to their effects on depressive symptoms in bulimic patients, antidepressants are associated with reductions in binge eating and vomiting rates, in the range of 50%–75% (Fichter et al. 1991, 1996; Goldstein et al. 1995; Rothschild et al. 1994). Antidepressant classes and drugs with demonstrated efficacy in double-blind, placebo-controlled studies include tricyclics (Agras et al. 1987; B. T. Walsh et al. 1991), SSRIs (Goldstein et al. 1995; Hudson et al. 1998), monoamine oxidase inhibitors (Kennedy et al. 1988), bupropion (Horne et al. 1988), and trazodone (Pope et al. 1989). Bupropion is not recommended, because it has been associated with seizures in bulimic patients who purge. At least one antidepressant medication, fluvoxamine, has also been associated with decreased relapse rates (Fichter et al. 1996).

Outcome studies suggest that patients with bulimia do best when treated with a combination of individual, group, and family psychotherapy in addition to pharmacotherapy (Mitchell et al. 1990). At least two studies have demonstrated that a combination of cognitive-behavioral therapy and pharmacotherapy results in superior outcomes compared with either treatment alone. At the end of 2 years of intensive combined therapy, 40%–60% of patients achieve abstinence from purging behavior and an additional 10%–30% show marked improvement (Hall 1991). Among successfully treated patients, relapse rates are 30%–50% over 6 years (Hsu and Sobkiewicz 1989; Keel and Mitchell 1997, 1999).

REFERENCES[1]

Agras WS, Dorian B, Kirkley BG, et al: Imipramine in the treatment of bulimia: a double-blind controlled study. Int J Eat Disord 6:29–38, 1987

---

[1] An asterisk (*) indicates the references that were mentioned in the first paragraph of this chapter, which the reader can refer to for a more in-depth review of the management of eating disorders.

American Psychiatric Association: Diagnostic and Statistical Manual of Mental Disorders, 4th Edition. Washington, DC, American Psychiatric Association, 1994

Andolf E, Theander S, Aspenberg P: Outpatient treatment of bulimia nervosa. Eur J Obstet Gynecol Reprod Biol 73:49–53, 1997

Arik TH, Dresser KB, Benchimol A: Cardiac complications of intensive dieting and eating disorders. Arizona Medicine 42:72–74, 1985

*Ben-Tovim DI, Walker K, Gilchrist P, et al: Outcome in patients with eating disorders: a 5-year study. Lancet 357:1254–1257, 2001

Bistrian BR: The medical treatment of obesity (editorial). Arch Intern Med 141:429–430, 1981

Blouin AG, Blouin HJ, Perez EL, et al: Treatment of bulimia with fenfluramine and desipramine. J Clin Psychopharmacol 8:261–269, 1988

Bowers WA: Basic principles for applying cognitive-behavioral therapy to anorexia nervosa. Psychiatr Clin North Am 24:293–303, x, 2001

Bowers T, Eckert E: Leukopenia in anorexia nervosa. Arch Intern Med 138:1520–1524, 1978

Boyd JC, Bruns DE, Wills MR: Frequency of hypomagnesemia in hypokalemic states. Clin Chem 29:178–179, 1983

Braun DL, Sunday SR, Halmi KA: Psychiatric comorbidity in patients with eating disorders. Psychol Med 24:859–867, 1994

Brincat M, Parsons V, Studd J: Anorexia nervosa (letter). British Medical Journal (Clinical Research Edition) 287:1306, 1983

Brotman AW, Stern TA: Case report of cardiovascular abnormalities in anorexia nervosa. Am J Psychiatry 140:1227–1228, 1983

*Brotman AW, Rigotti NA, Herzog DB: Medical complications of eating disorders. Compr Psychiatry 26:258–272, 1985

*Brotman AW, Stern TA, Brotman DL: Renal disease and dysfunction in two patients with anorexia nervosa. J Clin Psychiatry 47:433–436, 1986

*Casper RC, Eckert ED, Halmi KA, et al: Bulimia: its incidence and clinical importance in patients with anorexia nervosa. Arch Gen Psychiatry 37:1030–1053, 1980

*Castillo-Duran C, Heresi G, Fisberg M, et al: Controlled trial of zinc supplementation during recovery from malnutrition: effects on growth and immune function. Am J Clin Nutr 45:602–608, 1987

Chadda KD: Clinical hypomagnesemia, coronary spasm and cardiac arrhythmia. Magnesium 5:47–52, 1986

Connors ME, Johnson CL, Stuckey MK: Treatment of bulimia with brief psycho-educational group therapy. Am J Psychiatry 141:1512–1516, 1984

*Cooper PJ, Fairburn CG: Cognitive behavior therapy for anorexia nervosa: some preliminary findings. J Psychosom Res 28:493–499, 1984

*Crisp AH: A treatment regimen for anorexia nervosa. Br J Psychiatry 112:505–510, 1965

Croxson MS, Ibbertson HK: Low serum triiodothyronine (T3) and hypothyroidism in anorexia nervosa. J Clin Endocrinol Metab 44:167–174, 1977

Danowski TS, Livstone E, Gonzales AR, et al: Fractional and partial hypopituitarism in anorexia nervosa. Hormones 3:105–118, 1972

DeFronzo RA: The effect of insulin on renal sodium metabolism. Diabetologia 21:165–171, 1981

*Eckert ED, Mitchell JE: An overview of the treatment of anorexia nervosa, in Clinical Diagnosis and Management of Eating Disorders. Edited by Hall RCW. Longwood, FL, Ryandic Publishing, 1990, pp 293–315

Eisler I, Dare C, Russell GF, et al: Family and individual therapy in anorexia nervosa: a 5-year follow-up. Arch Gen Psychiatry 54:1025–1030, 1997

*Esca SA, Brenner W, Mach K, et al: Kwashiorkor-like zinc deficiency syndrome in anorexia nervosa. Acta Derm Venereol 59:361–364, 1979

Evans DS: Acute dilatation and spontaneous rupture of the stomach. Br J Surg 55:940–942, 1968

Fairburn CG, Marcus MD, Wilson GT: Cognitive-behavioral therapy for binge eating and bulimia nervosa: a comprehensive treatment manual, in Binge Eating: Nature, Assessment and Treatment. Edited by Fairburn CG, Wilson GT. New York, Guilford, 1993, pp 361–404

Fichter MM, Leibl K, Rief W, et al: Fluoxetine versus placebo: a double-blind study with bulimic inpatients undergoing intensive psychotherapy. Pharmacopsychiatry 24:1–7, 1991

Fichter MM, Kruger R, Rief W, et al: Fluvoxamine in prevention of relapse in bulimia nervosa: effects on eating-specific psychopathology. J Clin Psychopharmacol 16:9–18, 1996

*Fishman J, Boyar RM, Hellman L: Influence of body weight on estradiol metabolism in young women. J Clin Endocrinol Metab 41:989–991, 1979

Fleming BJ, Genuth SM, Gould AB, et al: Laxative-induced hypokalemia, sodium depletion and hyperreninemia: effects of potassium and sodium replacement on the renin-angiotensin-aldosterone system. Ann Intern Med 83:60–62, 1975

Fohlin L: Body composition, cardiovascular and renal function in adolescent patients with anorexia nervosa. Acta Paediatrica Scandinavica Supplement 268:3–20, 1977

Fonseca V, Havard CWH: Electrolyte disturbances and cardiac failure with hypomagnesaemia in anorexia nervosa. BMJ 291:1680–1682, 1985

Freeman CPL, Barry F, Dunkeld-Turnbull J, et al: Controlled trial psychotherapy for bulimia nervosa. BMJ 296:521–525, 1988

Frisch RE, McArthur JW: Menstrual cycles: fatness as a determinant of minimum weight for height necessary for their maintenance or onset. Science 185:949–951, 1974

Garfinkel PE, Lin E, Goering P, et al: Bulimia nervosa in a Canadian community sample: prevalence and comparison of subgroups. Am J Psychiatry 152:1052–1058, 1995

Garfinkel PE, Lin E, Goering P, et al: Should amenorrhea be necessary for the diagnosis of anorexia nervosa? Br J Psychiatry 168:500–506, 1996

*Garner DM, Rockert W, Davis R, et al: Comparison of cognitive-behavioral and supportive-expressive therapy for bulimia nervosa. Am J Psychiatry 150:37–46, 1993

*Gavish D, Eisenberg S, Berry EM, et al: Bulimia: an underlying behavioral disorder in hyperlipidemic pancreatitis: a prospective multidisciplinary approach. Arch Intern Med 147: 705–708, 1987

Gerner RH, Gwirtsman HE: Abnormalities of dexamethasone suppression test and urinary MHPG in anorexia nervosa. Am J Psychiatry 138:650–653, 1981

Gold TP, Kay EW, Robertson GL, et al: Abnormalities in plasma and CSF arginine vasopressin in patients with anorexia nervosa. N Engl J Med 308:1112–1123, 1982

Goldstein DJ, Wilson MG, Thompson VL, et al: Long-term fluoxetine treatment of bulimia nervosa. Br J Psychiatry 166: 660–666, 1995

*Gordon EF, Gordon RC, Passal DB: Zinc metabolism: basic, clinical, and behavioral aspects. J Pediatr 99:341–349, 1981

*Grebb JA, Wangling CD, Reus VI: Electrophysiologic abnormalities in patients with eating disorders. Compr Psychiatry 25:216–224, 1984

Gwirtsman HE, Roy-Byrne P, Yager J, et al: Neuroendocrine abnormalities in bulimia. Am J Psychiatry 140:559–563, 1983

*Hall A, Crisp AH: Brief psychotherapy in the treatment of anorexia nervosa: outcome at one year. Br J Psychiatry 151: 185–191, 1987

*Hall RCW: Management of eating disorders (audiotape). Audio-Digest Psychiatry 20(14), July 19, 1991

*Hall RCW, Beresford TP: Anorexia nervosa: diagnostic, prognostic and clinical features. Psychiatr Med 7:3–12, 1989a

*Hall RCW, Beresford TP: Bulimia nervosa: diagnostic criteria, clinical features and discrete clinical subsyndromes. Psychiatr Med 7:13–25, 1989b

*Hall RCW, Beresford TP: Medical Management of Eating Disorders. Edited by Hall RCW. Longwood, FL, Ryandic Publishing, 1990, pp 165–192

*Hall RCW, Hoffman RS, Beresford TP, et al: Hypomagnesemia in patients with eating disorders. Psychosomatics 29:264–272, 1988a

*Hall RCW, Hoffman RS, Beresford TP, et al: Refractory hypokalemia secondary to hypomagnesemia in eating disorder patients. Psychosomatics 29:435–438, 1988b

*Hall RCW, Hoffman RS, Beresford TP, et al: Physical illness encountered in patients with eating disorders. Psychosomatics 39:174–191, 1989a

*Hall RCW, Hoffman RS, Beresford TP, et al: Unrecognized physical illness in patients with eating disorders, in Recent Advances in Psychiatric Medicine. Edited by Hall RCW. Littleton, MA, PSG Publishing, 1989b, pp 68–80

*Hall RCW, Beresford TP, Hall AK: Hypomagnesemia in eating disorder patients: clinical signs and symptoms, in Clinical Diagnosis and Management of Eating Disorders. Edited by Hall RCW. Longwood, FL, Ryandic Publishing, 1990a, pp 193–203

*Hall RCW, Beresford TP, Popkin MK, et al: Mitral valve prolapse and anxiety disorders in patients with anorexia nervosa, in Clinical Diagnosis and Management of Eating Disorders. Edited by Hall RCW. Longwood, FL, Ryandic Publishing, 1990b, pp 217–233

*Hall RCW, Blakey RE, Hall AK: Bulimia nervosa: four uncommon sub-types. Psychosomatics 33:428–435, 1992

*Halmi KA, Falk JR: Behavior in dietary discriminators of menstrual function in anorexia, in Proceedings of the International Eating Disorders Meeting, 1983, reported in Halmi KA: Anorexia nervosa in bulimia (Psychosomatic Illness Review #6). Psychosomatics 24:111–129, 1983

*Halmi KA, Brodlan G, Loney J: Prognosis in anorexia nervosa. Ann Intern Med 78:907–909, 1973

*Halmi KA, Powers P, Cunningham S: Treatment of anorexia nervosa with behavior modification. Arch Gen Psychiatry 32:93–96, 1975

*Halmi KA, Casper RC, Eckert ED, et al: Unique features associated with age of onset of anorexia nervosa. Psychiatry Res 1:209–215, 1979

*Halmi KA, Falk JR, Schwartz E: Binge eating and vomiting: a survey of a college population. Psychol Med 11:697–706, 1981

*Halmi KA, Eckert E, Laud T, et al: Anorexia nervosa: treatment efficacy of cyproheptadine and amitriptyline. Arch Gen Psychiatry 43:177–181, 1986

*Halmi KA, Eckert E, Marchi P, et al: Comorbidity of psychiatric diagnoses in anorexia nervosa. Arch Gen Psychiatry 48: 712–718, 1991

Heatherton TF, Nichols P, Mahamedi F, et al: Body weight, dieting, and eating disorder symptoms among college students, 1982 to 1992. Am J Psychiatry 152:1623–1629, 1995

*Henkin RI, Pattern BM, Re PK, et al: A syndrome of acute zinc loss. Arch Neurol 32:745–751, 1975

*Herzog DB, Copeland PM: Eating disorders. N Engl J Med 313:295–303, 1985

*Herzog DB, Keller MB, Sacks NR, et al: Psychiatric comorbidity in treatment-seeking anorexics and bulimics. J Am Acad Child Adolesc Psychiatry 31:810–818, 1992

*Herzog DB, Nussbaum KM, Marmor AK: Comorbidity and outcome in eating disorders. Psychiatr Clin North Am 19:843–859, 1996

Hoffman RS, Hall RCW: Reversible EKG changes in anorexia nervosa, in Clinical Diagnosis and Management of Eating Disorders. Edited by Hall RCW. Longwood, FL, Ryandic Publishing, 1990, pp 211–216

Horne RL, Ferguson JM, Pope HG Jr, et al: Treatment of bulimia with bupropion: a multicenter controlled trial. J Clin Psychiatry 49:262–266, 1988

Hsu LK, Sobkiewicz TA: Bulimia nervosa: a four- to six-year follow-up study. Psychol Med 19:1035–1038, 1989

Hudson JI, McElroy SL, Raymond NC, et al: Fluvoxamine in the treatment of binge-eating disorder: a multicenter placebo-controlled, double-blind trial. Am J Psychiatry 155:1756–1762, 1998

*Humphries L, Vivian B, Stuart M, et al: Zinc deficiency and eating disorders. J Clin Psychiatry 50:456–459, 1989

Isner JM, Roberts WC, Heymsfield SB, et al: Anorexia nervosa and sudden death. Ann Intern Med 103:49–52, 1985

Jennings KP, Klidjian AN: Acute gastric dilatation in anorexia nervosa. BMJ 2:477–478, 1974

Johnson CL, Taylor C: Working with difficult-to-treat eating disorders using an integration of twelve-step and traditional psychotherapies. Psychiatr Clin North Am 19:829–841, 1996

Kalager T, Brubakk O, Bassoe HH: Cardiac performance in patients with anorexia nervosa. Cardiology 63:1–4, 1978

Kay DW, Leigh D: The natural history, treatment and prognosis of anorexia nervosa. Journal of Mental Science 100:411–431, 1954

*Kaye WH, Ebert MH, Gwirtsman HE, et al: Differences in brain serotonergic metabolism between non-bulimic and bulimic patients with anorexia nervosa. Am J Psychiatry 141:1598–1601, 1984

Keel PK, Mitchell JE: Outcome in bulimia nervosa. Am J Psychiatry 154:313–321, 1997

Keel PK, Mitchell JE: Long-term outcome of bulimia nervosa. Arch Gen Psychiatry 56:63–69, 1999

Kennedy SH, Piran N, Warsh JJ, et al: A trial of isocarboxazid in the treatment of bulimia nervosa. J Clin Psychopharmacol 8:391–396, 1988

Kennedy SH, Katz R, Rockert W, et al: Assessment of personality disorders in anorexia nervosa and bulimia nervosa: a comparison of self-report and structured interview methods. J Nerv Ment Dis 183:358–364, 1995

Kingston K, Szmukler G, Andrews D, et al: Neuropsychological and structural brain changes in anorexia nervosa before and after refeeding. Psychol Med 26:15–28, 1996

Klibanski A, Biller BM, Schoenfeld DA, et al: The effects of estrogen administration on trabecular bone loss in young women with anorexia nervosa. J Clin Endocrinol Metab 80:898–904, 1995

Lacey JH: Bulimia nervosa, binge eating and psychogenic vomiting: a controlled treatment study and long term outcome. BMJ 286:1609–1613, 1983

Laessle RG, Zoettle C, Pirke KM: Meta-analysis of treatment studies for bulimia. Int J Eat Disord 6:647–654, 1987

Lee NF, Rush AJ: Cognitive-behavioral group therapy for bulimia. Int J Eat Disord 5:599–615, 1986

*Leibowitz SF: Brain monoamines and peptides: role in the control of eating behavior. Federation Proceedings 45:1396–1403, 1986

Litt IF, Glader L: Anorexia nervosa, athletics and amenorrhea. J Pediatr 109:150–153, 1986

Macaron C, Wicker JF, Green OH, et al: Studies of growth hormone, thyrotropin and prolactin secretion in anorexia nervosa. Psychoneuroendocrinology 3:181–185, 1978

Mars DR, Anderson MH, Riggall FC: Anorexia nervosa: a disorder with severe acid-base derangements. South Med J 75:1038–1042, 1982

*Mills IH: Amitriptyline therapy in anorexia nervosa (letter). Lancet 2:687, 1976

*Mira M, Stewart PM, Abraham SF: Hypokalemia and renal impairment in patients with eating disorders. Med J Aust 140:290–293, 1984

*Mitchell JE: Psychobiology of bulimia nervosa (audiotape). Audio-Digest Psychiatry 21(22), November 23, 1992

*Mitchell JE, Pyle RL, Mine RA: Gastric dilatation as a complication of bulimia. Psychosomatics 23:96–97, 1982

*Mitchell JE, Pyle RL, Eckert ED, et al: Electrolyte and other physiological abnormalities in patients with bulimia. Psychol Med 13:273–278, 1983

*Mitchell JE, Hatsukami D, Eckert ED, et al: Characteristics of 275 patients with bulimia. Am J Psychiatry 142:482–485, 1985

*Mitchell JE, Boutacoff LI, Hatsukami D, et al: Laxative abuse as a variant of bulimia. J Nerv Ment Dis 174:174–176, 1986

*Mitchell JE, Hoberman H, Pyle RL: An overview of the treatment of bulimia nervosa, in Clinical Diagnosis and Management of Eating Disorders. Edited by Hall RCW. Longwood, FL, Ryandic Publishing, 1990, pp 317–332

Mitchell JE, Pyle RL, Pomeroy C, et al: Cognitive-behavioral group psychotherapy of bulimia nervosa: importance of logistical variables. Int J Eat Disord 14:277–287, 1993

Miyai K, Yamamoto T, Azukizawa M, et al: Serum thyroid hormone and thyrotropin in anorexia nervosa. J Clin Endocrinol Metab 40:334–338, 1975

*Morgan HG, Purgold J, Wolbourne J: Management and outcome in anorexia nervosa: a standardized prognosis study. Br J Psychiatry 143:282–286, 1983

Morton R: Theologia: or a Treatise on Consumption, 2nd Edition. London, Smith, 1920

Moshang T Jr, Parks JS, Baker L, et al: Low serum triiodothyronine in patients with anorexia nervosa. J Clin Endocrinol Metab 40:470–473, 1975

Myers TJ, Perkerson MD, Witter BA, et al: Hematologic findings: anorexia nervosa. Conn Med 45:14–17, 1981

Neri V, Ambrosi B, Peck-Peccoz L, et al: Growth hormone regulation and hypothalamic-pituitary-adrenal function in anorexia nervosa. Nippon Naibunpi Gakkai Zasshi 25:143–151, 1972

*Nussbaum M, Shenker IR, Marc J, et al: Cerebral atrophy in anorexia nervosa. J Pediatr 5:867–869, 1980

Oesterheld JR, McKenna MS, Gould NB: Group psychotherapy of bulimia: a critical review. Int J Group Psychother 37:163–184, 1987

Ordman AM, Kirschenbaum DS: Cognitive-behavioral therapy for bulimia: an initial outcome study. J Consult Clin Psychol 53:305–313, 1985

Oster JR, Masterson BPJ, Rogers AI: Laxative abuse syndrome. Am J Gastroenterol 74:451–458, 1980

Palazzali MS: Self Starvation. New York, Jason Aronson, 1978

Pallosy B, Oo ME: ECG alterations in anorexia nervosa. Adv Cardiol 19:280–282, 1977

Parsons V, Szmukler G, Brown SJ, et al: Fracturing osteoporosis in young women with anorexia nervosa. Calcif Tissue Int 35 (suppl A):72, 1983

*Pillay M, Crisp AH: The impact of social skills training within an established inpatient treatment program for anorexia nervosa. Br J Psychiatry 139:533–539, 1981

*Pope HG Jr, Hudson JI, Jonas JM, et al: Antidepressant treatment of bulimia: a two-year follow-up study. J Clin Psychopharmacol 5:320–327, 1985

Pope HG Jr, Keck PE Jr, McElroy SL, et al: A placebo-controlled study of trazodone in bulimia nervosa. J Clin Psychopharmacol 9:254–259, 1989

Powers PS, Tyson IB, Stevens BA, et al: Total body potassium and serum potassium among eating disorder patients. Int J Eat Disord 18:269–276, 1995

*Pyle RL, Mitchell JE, Eckert ED: The incidence of bulimia in freshman college students. Int J Eat Disord 2:75–85, 1983

Rapaport MJ: Pellagra in a patient with anorexia nervosa. Arch Dermatol 121:255–257, 1985

Rau JH, Green RS: Soft neurological correlates of compulsive eaters. J Nerv Ment Dis 166:435–437, 1978

Reiger W, Brady JP, Weisberg E: Hematologic changes in anorexia nervosa. Am J Psychiatry 135:984–985, 1978

Remick RA, Jones NW, Campos PE: Postictal bulimia (letter). J Clin Psychiatry 41:256, 1980

Reyes AJ, Leary WP: Cardiovascular toxicity of diuretics related to magnesium depletion. Human Toxicology 3:351–371, 1984

Rigotti NA, Nussbaum SR, Herzog DB, et al: Osteoporosis in women with anorexia nervosa. N Engl J Med 311:1601–1606, 1984

Rothschild R, Quitkin HM, Quitkin FM, et al: A double-blind placebo-controlled comparison of phenelzine and imipramine in the treatment of bulimia in atypical depressives. Int J Eat Disord 15:1–9, 1994

*Russell GFM: Metabolism, endocrine and psychiatric aspects of anorexia nervosa. Scientific Basis Medicine 1:236–242, 1969

*Russell GFM: The management of anorexia nervosa, in Symposium/Anorexia Nervosa and Obesity: Royal Edinburgh, TA Constable Ltd., 1973, pp 44–60

*Russell GFM: Bulimia nervosa: an ominous variant of anorexia nervosa. Psychol Med 9:429–448, 1979

*Russell GFM, Szmukler GI, Dare C, et al: An evaluation of family therapy in anorexia nervosa and bulimia nervosa. Arch Gen Psychiatry 44:1047–1056, 1987

*Safai-Kutti S: Oral zinc supplementation in anorexia nervosa. Acta Psychiatr Scand Suppl 361:14–17, 1990

Schwartz WB, Relman AS: Effects of electrolyte disorders on renal structure and function. N Engl J Med 276:383–389, 452–458, 1967

Shaul PW, Farrell MK, Maloney MJ: Caffeine toxicity as a cause of acute psychosis in anorexia nervosa. J Pediatr 105:493–495, 1984

*Sheinin JC: Medical aspects of eating disorders. Adolescent Psychiatry 13:405–421, 1989

Silber TJ, Kass EJ: Anorexia nervosa and nephrolithiasis. Journal of Adolescent Health Care 5:50–52, 1984

Srinivasagam NM, Kaye WH, Plotnicov KH, et al: Persistent perfectionism, symmetry and exactness after long-term recovery from anorexia nervosa. Am J Psychiatry 152:1630–1634, 1995

*Steinhausen HC, Glanville K: Follow-up studies of anorexia nervosa: a review of research findings. Psychol Med 13:239–249, 1983

Striegel-Moore RH, Cachelin FM, Dohm FA, et al: Comparison of binge eating disorder and bulimia nervosa in a community sample. Int J Eat Disord 29:157–165, 2001

Strober M, Lampert C, Morrell W, et al: A controlled family study of anorexia nervosa: evidence of familial aggregation and lack of shared transmission with affective disorders. Int J Eat Disord 9:239–253, 1990

Sullivan PF: Mortality in anorexia nervosa. Am J Psychiatry 152:1073–1074, 1995

Swayze VW, Anderson A, Arndt S, et al: Reversibility of brain tissue loss in anorexia nervosa assessed with a computerized Talairach 3-D proportional grid. Psychol Med 26:381–390, 1996

Takahara J, Hosogi H, Yonuki S, et al: Hypothalamic pituitary adrenal function in patients with anorexia nervosa. Endocrinologica Japonica 23:451–456, 1976

*Theander S: Outcome and prognosis of anorexia nervosa and bulimia: some results of previous investigations, compared to those of a Swedish long term study. J Psychiatr Res 19:493–508, 1985

*Thurston J, Marks SP: Electrocardiographic abnormalities in patients with anorexia nervosa. British Heart Journal 36:719–723, 1974

Treasure JL, Kinj EA, Gordon PAL, et al: Cystic ovaries: a phase of anorexia nervosa. Lancet 2:1379–1382, 1985

*Treasure J[L], Schmidt U, Troop N, et al: Sequential treatment for bulimia nervosa incorporating a self-care manual. Br J Psychiatry 168:94–98, 1996

Walsh BT, Hadigan CM, Devlin MJ, et al: Long-term outcome of antidepressant treatment for bulimia nervosa. Am J Psychiatry 148:1206–1212, 1991

Walsh T: The endocrinology of anorexia nervosa. Psychiatr Clin North Am 3:299–309, 1980

Walters EE, Kendler KS: Anorexia nervosa and anorexic-like syndromes in a population-based female twin sample. Am J Psychiatry 152:64–71, 1995

Warren MP, Vandewyle RI: Clinical and metabolic features of anorexia nervosa. Am J Obstet Gynecol 117:415–418, 1979

Warren SE, Steinberg SM: Acid-base and electrolyte disturbances in anorexia nervosa. Am J Psychiatry 136:415–418, 1979

Wartofsky L, Burman KD: Alterations in thyroid function in patients with systemic illness: the "euthyroid sick syndrome." Endocr Rev 3:164–217, 1982

Wilbur TL, Washburn RN: Clinical features and treatment of functional or nervous vomiting. JAMA 110:477–480, 1978

*Willard SG, Winstead DK, Anding R, et al: Laxative abuse in eating disorders, in Clinical Diagnosis and Management of Eating Disorders. Edited by Hall RCW. Longwood, FL, Ryandic Publishing, 1990, pp 75–87

Wong ET, Rude RK, Singer FR, et al: A high prevalence of hypomagnesemia and hypermagnesemia in hospitalized patients. Am J Clin Pathol 79:348–352, 1983

Yates AJ, Sambraillo F: Bulimia nervosa: a descriptive and therapeutic study. Behav Res Ther 5:503–517, 1984

*Yen S: Neuroendocrine regulation of the menstrual cycle. Hospital Practice 14:83–97, 1979

*Zerbe KJ: The Body Betrayed: Women, Eating Disorders, and Treatment. Washington, DC, American Psychiatric Press, 1993

Zerbe KJ: Feminist psychodynamic psychotherapy of eating disorders: theoretic integration informing clinical practice. Psychiatr Clin North Am 19:811–827, 1996

24

Sleep Disorders

Jeffrey B. Weilburg, M.D.

John W. Winkelman, M.D., Ph.D.

The scientific study of sleep began in the 1930s, when it was first recognized that characteristic electroencephalogram (EEG) patterns appeared during sleep. Rapid eye movement (REM) sleep was discovered in 1953, and sleep apnea was described in 1965. Since then there has been an explosion of information about sleep and sleep disorders. In this chapter, we begin with a summary of the classification of sleep disorders and of sleep physiology; readers requiring comprehensive reviews may consult Kryger et al. (2000) or Thorpy (1990).

We follow this with a discussion of the sleep patterns characteristic of patients in intensive care units (ICUs) and in general medical and surgical settings. Next, we outline an approach to hospital patients with insomnia or hypersomnia. Finally, we present information about sleep changes that are associated with selected specific medical problems that the psychiatric consultant may encounter; additional information on this topic is available in the review by Regestein (1987).

CLASSIFICATION OF SLEEP DISORDERS

DSM-IV-TR (American Psychiatric Association 2000) contains a useful section on sleep disorders. An outline of DSM-IV-TR schema is provided in Table 24–1. In this chapter, we follow DSM-IV-TR classification whenever possible. The other current classification schema for sleep disorders is the International Classification of Sleep Disorders (ICSD; American Sleep Disorders Association 1990); an outline of this schema is shown in Table 24–2. The ICSD manual provides more detailed and comprehensive information than DSM-IV-TR, so it is also a valuable resource for consultation psychiatrists. DSM-IV-TR includes cross-references to the ICSD.

PHYSIOLOGY OF NORMAL SLEEP

Sleep is a dynamic process that is organized on the basis of EEG, electromyographic, and electrooculographic data into REM sleep and non-REM (NREM) sleep. NREM sleep is further divided into Stages I, II, III, and IV. NREM Stages III and IV are often considered together as delta (or slow-wave) sleep.

Sleep normally proceeds smoothly through NREM Stages I, II, and delta, returning to Stage II before entering the first REM period, typically 70–90 minutes after sleep onset. The rhythmic alternation of NREM and REM has a cycle length of about 90 minutes, and REM periods increase in length as the sleep period progresses. Delta sleep occurs mostly during the early part of the night and tapers off with successive cycles.

The circadian cycling of sleep and wakefulness directly affects the regulation of a wide variety of neuroendocrine functions (e.g., the secretion of cortisol, melatonin, and growth hormone). Sleep disruption may therefore secondarily affect endocrine status. Body temperature also follows a circadian rhythm in healthy adults, varying between 1.0°C and 1.2°C from its peak in the late afternoon to its nadir in the early morning. Abnormalities in temperature cycling may be correlated with some forms of insomnia, and disruption of sleep cycling may affect temperature cycling.

Age, premorbid sleep patterns, and general health status may affect sleep. For example, compared with younger individuals, elderly people generally sleep less efficiently and less deeply and have less delta sleep and more awakenings (Reynolds et al. 1985b). Daytime sleepiness tends to be more common in elderly persons, and it is more difficult for them to adjust to changes in the sleep-wake schedule. Some patients are normally short sleepers, sleeping

TABLE 24–1. DSM-IV-TR classification of sleep disorders

Primary sleep disorders

   Dyssomnias

307.42	Primary insomnia
307.44	Primary hypersomnia
347	Narcolepsy
780.59	Breathing-related sleep disorder
307.45	Circadian rhythm sleep disorder (formerly sleep-wake schedule disorder)
307.47	Dyssomnia NOS

   Parasomnias

307.47	Nightmare disorder (formerly dream anxiety disorder)
307.46	Sleep terror disorder
307.46	Sleepwalking disorder
307.47	Parasomnia NOS

Sleep disorders related to another mental disorder

307.42	Insomnia related to (Axis I or Axis II disorder)
307.44	Hypersomnia related to (Axis I or Axis II disorder)

Other sleep disorders

   Sleep disorder due to a general medical condition

780.52	Insomnia type
780.54	Hypersomnia type
780.59	Parasomnia type
780.59	Mixed type

   Substance-induced sleep disorder

xxx.xx	Insomnia type (refer to specific substances for codes)
xxx.xx	Hypersomnia type (refer to specific substances for codes)
xxx.xx	Parasomnia type (refer to specific substances for codes)
xxx.xx	Mixed type (refer to specific substances for codes)

(Modifiers: with onset during intoxication; with onset during withdrawal)

Note. NOS = not otherwise specified.

less than 7 hours each night without compromised daytime function. Significant weight loss—at times a consequence of chronic illness—has been associated with short, fragmented sleep. The consultant should consider these factors when evaluating the degree of sleep disruption in hospitalized patients. The consultant's goal in managing sleep disruption in such patients should be to restore sleep to a prehospitalization baseline, unless treatment of a sleep disorder itself is the reason for admission or a clinically significant sleep disorder has been identified in the workup.

SLEEP PATTERNS IN PATIENTS IN INTENSIVE CARE UNITS

Patients in ICUs tend to have several characteristic patterns in their sleep. These patterns appear in a similar fashion in patients with a variety of underlying medical and surgical problems and include decreased total sleep time (TST), disrupted day/night circadian cycles, and disrupted sleep architecture.

Decreased Total Sleep Time

Several investigators (Aurell and Elmquist 1985; Broughton and Baron 1978; Johns et al. 1974; Orr and Stahl 1977; Richards and Bairnsfather 1988) reported marked decreases in the TST of patients in ICUs. A mean TST of 2 hours was noted during the first 48 hours after noncardiac surgery (Aurell and Elmquist 1985). Decreased nighttime sleep was found in patients after open-heart surgery, valve replacement, and pneumonectomy (Johns et al. 1974; Orr and Stahl 1977). Investigators found that patients in ICUs typically appear to be sleeping, lying quietly with their eyes closed, but the EEG demonstrates a pattern consistent with drowsiness or Stage I sleep interrupted frequently by brief arousals (Broughton and Baron 1978).

Disrupted Day/Night Circadian Cycles

Many patients in the ICU have periods of sleep that are brief and distributed fairly evenly throughout the 24-hour day rather than consolidated at night (Broughton

TABLE 24–2.   International Classification of Sleep Disorders outline

I. **Dyssomnias**
   A. **Intrinsic sleep disorders**
      1. Psychophysiological insomnia
      2. Sleep state misperception
      3. Idiopathic insomnia
      4. Narcolepsy
      5. Recurrent hypersomnia
      6. Idiopathic hypersomnia
      7. Posttraumatic hypersomnia
      8. Obstructive sleep apnea syndrome
      9. Central sleep apnea syndrome
      10. Central alveolar hypoventilation syndrome
      11. Periodic limb movement disorder
      12. Restless legs syndrome
      13. Intrinsic sleep disorder NOS
   B. **Extrinsic sleep disorders**
      1. Inadequate sleep hygiene
      2. Environmental sleep disorder
      3. Altitude insomnia
      4. Adjustment sleep disorder
      5. Insufficient sleep syndrome
      6. Limit-setting sleep disorder
      7. Sleep-onset association disorder
      8. Food allergy insomnia
      9. Nocturnal eating (drinking) syndrome
      10. Hypnotic-dependent sleep disorder
      11. Stimulant-dependent sleep disorder
      12. Alcohol-dependent sleep disorder
      13. Toxin-induced sleep disorder
      14. Extrinsic sleep disorder NOS
   C. **Circadian rhythm sleep disorders**
      1. Time zone change (jet lag) syndrome
      2. Shift work sleep disorder
      3. Irregular sleep-wake pattern
      4. Delayed sleep phase syndrome
      5. Advanced sleep phase syndrome
      6. Non-24-hour sleep-wake disorder
      7. Circadian rhythm sleep disorder NOS
II. **Parasomnias**
   A. **Arousal disorders**
      1. Confusing arousals
      2. Sleepwalking
      3. Sleep terrors
   B. **Sleep-wake transition disorders**
      1. Rhythmic movement disorder
      2. Sleep starts
      3. Sleep talking
      4. Nocturnal leg cramps

   C. **Parasomnias usually associated with REM sleep**
      1. Nightmares
      2. Sleep paralysis
      3. Impaired sleep-related penile erections
      4. Sleep-related painful erections
      5. REM sleep-related sinus arrest
      6. REM sleep behavior disorder
   D. **Other parasomnias**
      1. Sleep bruxism
      2. Sleep enuresis
      3. Sleep-related abnormal swallowing syndrome
      4. Nocturnal paroxysmal dystonia
      5. Sudden unexplained nocturnal death syndrome
      6. Primary snoring
      7. Infant sleep apnea
      8. Congenital central hypoventilation syndrome
      9. Sudden infant death syndrome
      10. Benign neonatal sleep myoclonus
      11. Other parasomnia NOS
III. **Medical-psychiatric sleep disorders**
   A. **Associated with mental disorders**
      1. Psychoses
      2. Mood disorders
      3. Anxiety disorders
      4. Panic disorder
      5. Alcoholism
   B. **Associated with neurological disorders**
      1. Cerebral degenerative disorders
      2. Dementia
      3. Parkinsonism
      4. Fatal familial insomnia
      5. Sleep-related epilepsy
      6. Electrical status epilepticus of sleep
      7. Sleep-related headaches
   C. **Associated with other medical disorders**
      1. Sleeping sickness
      2. Nocturnal cardiac ischemia
      3. Chronic obstructive pulmonary disease
      4. Sleep-related asthma
      5. Sleep-related gastroesophageal reflux
      6. Peptic ulcer disease
      7. Fibrositis syndrome
IV. **Proposed sleep disorders**
      1. Short sleeper
      2. Long sleeper
      3. Subwakefulness syndrome
      4. Fragmentary myoclonus
      5. Sleep hyperhidrosis
      6. Menstrual-associated sleep disorder
      7. Pregnancy-associated sleep disorder
      8. Terrifying hypnagogic hallucinations
      9. Sleep-related neurogenic tachypnea
      10. Sleep-related laryngospasm
      11. Sleep choking syndrome

Note.   NOS = not otherwise specified; REM = rapid eye movement.
Source.   Abstracted from American Sleep Disorders Association: *International Classification of Sleep Disorders: ICSD Diagnostic and Coding Manual.* Rochester, MN, American Sleep Disorders Association, 1990. Used with permission.

and Baron 1978; Dlin et al. 1971; Dohno et al. 1977, 1979; Ellis and Dudley 1978; Johns et al. 1974; Karacan and Williams 1969; Karacan et al. 1974; Kavey and Altshuler 1979; Maggini et al. 1976/1977; Richards and Bairnsfather 1988). This pattern was common to patients in ICUs despite different surgical procedures, medications, and related complications (Aurell and Elmquist 1985; Broughton and Baron 1978; Dlin et al. 1971; Dohno et al. 1977, 1979; Ellis and Dudley 1978; Johns et al. 1974; Karacan et al. 1974; Kavey and Altshuler 1979; Maggini et al. 1976/1977). The clinical and physiologic consequences of the sleep disruption remain poorly understood, but it has been shown that the normal pattern of melatonin secretion may be lost in ICU patients with disrupted sleep (Shilo et al. 1999).

Disrupted Sleep Architecture

Patients in ICUs tend to have frequent awakenings and to spend very little time in REM and delta sleep (Broughton and Baron 1978; Dlin et al. 1971; Dohno et al. 1977, 1979; Ellis and Dudley 1978; Johns et al. 1974; Karacan et al. 1974; Kavey and Altschuler 1979; Maggini 1976/1977; Richards and Bairnsfather 1988). REM and delta sleep deteriorate regardless of differences in medications, type of illness, or procedures employed and may occur even when patients achieve several hours of uninterrupted sleep.

The severity of the degree of disruption of the sleep architecture tends to vary directly with the severity of the illness (Dohno et al. 1979). Furthermore, sleep disruption tends to resolve over a time course that varies with the severity of the initial insult. Compared with other hospital nights, REM sleep was maximally decreased on the nights immediately following a myocardial infarction (MI) (Johns et al. 1974). The sleep of less severely ill patients returns to baseline by the time of hospital discharge, whereas patients who are more severely ill usually have decreased REM and delta sleep persisting at 2–4 weeks after they have been discharged to home (Orr and Stahl 1977). Similarly, statistically significant improvement in TST, sleep architecture, and amount of REM sleep tends to appear on each successive night post-MI (Broughton and Baron 1978). When a patient remains in the ICU, sleep tends to improve over 4–7 days if the overall condition improves (Johns et al. 1974). However, if delirium or complications supervene, sleep often remains disrupted for prolonged periods.

Environmental factors can affect the quality and quantity of an individual's sleep (Gelling 1999). Noise can interfere with falling asleep and can produce arousals. Noise-induced arousal thresholds are lowest in light sleep

and when the noise has significance to the sleeper (e.g., a monitor alarm will be significant to a patient who has a cardiac monitor) (Dlin et al. 1971; Johns and Doré 1978; Jones et al. 1979). The high decibel level of noise in ICU settings probably does have a negative effect on sleep, and efforts to minimize unnecessary noise may improve sleep (Aaron et al. 1996; Kahn et al. 1998). Indwelling venous and arterial catheters may disrupt sleep if they produce pain or other discomfort; however, the mere presence of these devices appears to have minimal effects on sleep architecture (Jarrett et al. 1984; Johns and Doré 1978). Anxiety, emotional stress, and nursing routine may add to the disrupted sleep seen in patients in ICUs (Freedman et al. 1999; Yinnon et al. 1992). Attempts to minimize stress and interference by nursing routines may, however, improve patients' self-reported comfort (Simpson et al. 1996). Disruption of sleep similar to that seen in patients in ICUs may be induced by fever alone in some hospitalized patients who are not in ICUs. Small (0.2°C) increases in core temperature do by themselves fragment sleep in healthy subjects, but the effect of core temperature changes on ICU patients is unknown (A. Fletcher et al. 1999). The sleep changes seen in patients in ICUs occur even in those who are afebrile (Karacan and Wolff 1968).

However, most authors conclude that some endogenous derangement of sleep-wake regulating systems in the central nervous system (CNS) is the basis for sleep disruption in patients in ICUs (Aurell and Elmquist 1985; Broughton and Baron 1978; Dohno et al. 1979). The specific factors producing this derangement are poorly understood, but no specific disease process or drug can be found to account for the disturbances described earlier.

Therefore, when patients register complaints about disturbed sleep, the psychiatric consultant may verify that basic patient comfort has been reasonably attended to and that the nursing routine is adjusted to minimize unnecessary intrusion. However, the consultant should focus attention on identifying the specific physiologic and emotional factors underlying a patient's sleep complaints, as outlined below.

Clinical Consequences of Sleep Changes

The clinical consequences, if any, of the sleep changes seen in patients in ICUs are not clear. Early studies suggested that delirium or psychosis might be produced by sleep deprivation. Sleep deprivation was thus advanced as a cause of "ICU psychosis." Subsequent work indicates that healthy subjects who undergo prolonged sleep deprivation have brief periods when sleep intrudes into waking (microsleeps), during which time unusual or confused behavior may occur. Sleep deprivation also can produce mood lability, irritability, and cognitive changes, such as slow reaction time. More recent work (Pilcher and Huffcutt 1996) confirmed this by showing that sleep deprivation produced changes mostly in mood, cognition, and motor performance. Sleep deprivation itself does not appear to produce psychosis or delirium (L.C. Johnson 1982; Pasnau et al. 1968; Pilcher and Huffcutt 1996; Williams et al. 1967). In ICU patients, Johns and colleagues (1974) found that the severity of sleep deprivation did not distinguish patients who became delirious from those who did not. Indeed, Harrell and Othmer (1987) found that sleep loss results from postcardiotomy confusion, not vice versa. Furthermore, REM rebound appears to play no etiological role in ICU delirium (Johns et al. 1974; Orr and Stahl 1977). It is critical for the psychiatric consultant to recognize that psychosis and delirium are not a direct result of sleep disruption found in patients in ICUs. Patients with psychosis or delirium should have these problems addressed directly. Sleep will improve as the delirium or psychosis resolves (Cassem 1984; Tesar and Stern 1986). Both midazolam and propofol can improve nocturnal sleep (thereby correcting the loss of normal diurnal pattern) in some ICU patients, but improved sleep did not correlate with reduction in anxiety or depression (Treggiari-Venzi et al. 1996). (For a further discussion of delirium, please refer to Chapter 15, this volume.)

Patients occasionally will be admitted to an ICU for problems directly related to a primary sleep disorder. For example, serious injuries may occur during episodes of REM sleep behavior disorder, night terrors, or sleepwalking (Schenck and Mahowald 1991). REM sleep behavior disorder is a relatively uncommon condition that typically appears in older men; it may be elicited or worsened by stress, toxic or metabolic problems (including alcohol withdrawal), or CNS disease (e.g., Alzheimer's, Parkinson's) (Schenck et al. 1996). During an episode of REM sleep behavior disorder, patients may ambulate—sometimes in an agitated fashion—while they are in REM sleep. (For more information on this disorder, refer to the ICSD manual.) Pulmonary hypertension, right heart failure, and nocturnal cardiac arrest may occur secondary to severe sleep apnea. Although ICU post-MI patients with obstructive sleep apnea have no different outcomes (mortality, complications) than do those without obstructive sleep apnea (Marin et al. 1998), sleep disorders should be factored into a complete differential diagnosis, especially when more common causes have been ruled out.

SLEEP IN PATIENTS IN MEDICAL AND SURGICAL INPATIENT UNITS

The disturbances of sleep found in patients on the medical and surgical floors—for example, in studies involving patients in private and semiprivate rooms (Aurell and Elmquist 1985; Broughton and Baron 1978; Dohno et al. 1977; Johns et al. 1974; Kavey and Altshuler 1979; Orr and Stahl 1977)—are similar to those observed in ICU patients but are not as severe and tend to more readily resolve as patients' conditions improve. Indeed, most studies reported that, in many patients, sleep spontaneously returns to baseline despite continued hospitalization. Therefore, the consultant should not assume that a patient's presence on the medical or surgical ward is enough in itself to produce disrupted sleep. Likewise, the consultant should not assume that a patient's report of "not sleeping well" is in itself an indication of true sleep disruption or that disturbed sleep is the proximate cause of daytime distress. The consultant should first ascertain whether psychiatric problems (such as anxiety, depression, adjustment disorders, or delirium) or general medical and surgical management problems (such as pain or the side effects of medications) are the source of the discomfort. Taking the time to ask specific questions about psychiatric and medical issues as well as about sleep is critical, because most studies show that simply asking patients and staff general questions about sleep is insufficient. Indeed, according to Kavey and Altschuler (1979, pp. 686–687), "a hospitalized patient's summary statement of the quality of the night's sleep correlates poorly with the electrophysiological data," so "while asking how a patient slept is perhaps politic, it is unlikely to elicit a meaningful answer unless followed by a more detailed inquiry." Patients and nursing staff may make helpful observations regarding sleep-related respiration, movement, and behavior. Family members and bed partners may reveal details about the patient's sleep characteristics before hospitalization.

Transient insomnia (i.e., of a duration less than 1 week) is probably both common and underdiagnosed in medical and surgical patients. Berlin and colleagues (1984) diagnosed transient insomnia in 71% of 100 consecutive patients referred for psychiatric consultation in a general hospital. Hypersomnia was diagnosed in 6%, parasomnias (nightmares, enuresis) in 2%, and chronic persistent insomnia in 1%. Notably, no mention of sleep disturbance was found in the medical records of 54% of the patients who were found to have sleep disorders by the consulting psychiatrist.

In patients on surgical units, uncomplicated herniorrhaphy produced significant but transient changes in the sleep of otherwise healthy males (Kavey and Altshuler 1979). On the preoperative night, slight reductions in TST, REM sleep time, and delta sleep (with more time awake) were noted, which the investigators believed were caused by situational anxiety. On the afternoon after surgery, naps composed of Stage II sleep predominated. On the first 2 postoperative nights, REM and delta sleep were significantly decreased and in some cases were almost absent, and the patients alternated between brief periods of being awake and periods of light sleep (much like patients in ICUs). Some patients showed mild REM rebound on the fourth postoperative night. No delta rebound was observed. In all patients, sleep gradually returned to normal during the hospital stay. As in studies of patients in ICUs, no clear or significant differences were found between the patients who received general anesthesia and those who received local anesthetics. The use of meperidine correlated with the patients' subjective perception of improved sleep (probably mediated by meperidine's capacity to decrease pain and discomfort and to produce amnesia) but did not correlate with objectively improved sleep.

Hypnotic agents are often routinely prescribed for general hospital patients, but the rational basis for this practice has not been established. A retrospective randomly selected chart review conducted in 1982 on 23 medical and 20 surgical patients in a general hospital showed that prescriptions for hypnotics to be administered as needed were written for 46% of those on the medical service but were actually used by only 31% (Perry and Wu 1984). Among those on the medical service who used the hypnotics, the rate of use declined with increasing length of hospital stay. In contrast, orders were written for as-needed hypnotics for 96% of the surgical patients; 88% of those on the surgical service actually used a hypnotic at least once, and the frequency of hypnotic use increased with increasing length of hospital stay. However, no clear correlation was found between the writing of an as-needed prescription for hypnotics and the presence of sleep disturbance, perceived quality of sleep, primary diagnosis, or actual use of hypnotics. Another study showed that hypnotics were prescribed for 40% of the medical-surgical patients in a Veterans Administration (VA) hospital, but only 22% of the patients actually took the drugs (Lunberg et al. 1977). On a randomly selected weekday in 1981, 38% of the patients in a large teaching hospital took hypnotics, yet justification for and utility of prescribing hypnotics for these patients were undocumented (Salzman 1981).

More recently, a chart review of 856 elderly patients found that even when controlling for illness severity and comorbidities, hospital length of stay and cost of admission were increased when hypnotic use exceeded recommended doses and duration (Yuen et al. 1997). Some evidence indicates that nurses giving a back rub, providing a warm drink, and playing a relaxation tape for elderly hospitalized patients may be as effective as giving a hypnotic drug (McDowell et al. 1998). When hypnotics were rapidly withdrawn from a group of 120 terminal cancer patients, no change in sleep occurred, indicating that hypnotics may be overused in this group of patients (Bruera et al. 1996). However, a study of 357 adults given either zolpidem 10 mg, triazolam 0.25 mg, or placebo found that patients who received either hypnotic had no more adverse effects at night or the next morning than did those who received placebo but had longer and higher-quality sleep. More work is needed to determine whether to use the newer hypnotics routinely before surgery; it is probably reasonable to use them if the patient has or anticipates trouble with sleep (Morgan et al. 1997).

APPROACH TO THE PATIENT COMPLAINING OF INSOMNIA

Insomnia is generally defined as a complaint of trouble falling asleep or staying asleep or of nonrestorative sleep, with these sleep abnormalities being associated with daytime distress such as anergy, malaise, cognitive slowness, and irritability. Mild transient sleep disturbance secondary to anxiety or physical discomfort is very common in hospitalized patients. If the sleep disruption is self-limited and is not associated with daytime compromise, there is no need to make a diagnosis of insomnia or to treat with hypnotics. More severe or persistent sleep disruption that can be linked with daytime distress may be regarded as a clinical problem worth pursuing. In such cases, insomnia might be identified as a primary clinical problem.

Several subtypes of insomnia are found in hospitalized patients. The most common is mild, transient insomnia, which, in most cases, occurs secondary to adjustment disorder in patients in whom the medical illness or the hospitalization and the related psychosocial disruption are the stressors.

Insomnia secondary to anxiety or mood disorder is, in our experience, also seen commonly in hospitalized patients. Patients with preexisting anxiety disorders, including panic disorder, generalized anxiety disorder, and posttraumatic stress disorder (PTSD), often experience an exacerbation of their conditions during hospitalization, and complaints of insomnia among these patients are frequent. The stress of hospitalization may induce preexisting subclinical anxiety disorders to reach threshold. Nocturnal panic attacks may be initially reported as insomnia, so a careful history of nocturnal events and experiences is important.

Both major depression and dysthymia are common in hospitalized patients, and both frequently produce difficulty falling asleep, difficulty staying asleep, or early-morning waking. The degree of insomnia tends to be correlated with the severity of the depression. If complaints of daytime fatigue and malaise are also present, the patient may complain of insomnia rather than of depression. Because treatment decisions follow from the diagnosis, the consultant should be alert to the possibility that insomnia may be the presenting symptom of depression in the hospitalized patient.

Patients with narcissistic or obsessional disorders, especially when subjected to the stress of illness and hospitalization, may become angry, frustrated, or agitated if they are unable to sleep. Such patients focus on sleep and ruminate about being deprived of the rest they believe they need and deserve. This then begins a cycle in which they may become further stimulated and have even more difficulty achieving sleep. Angry complaints, manipulative behavior, and conflicts with the clinical staff may revolve around sleep. Such cases underscore the importance of carefully evaluating and managing Axis II issues in all patients who have complaints of insomnia.

Psychoses of any type may produce trouble falling and staying asleep, both before and during the episode of illness. Before ascribing insomnia to a patient's preexisting psychosis, however, it is important to rule out sleep disruption caused by toxic and medical factors such as delirium due to medication or direct adverse drug effects (e.g., neuroleptic-induced akathisia).

DSM-IV-TR specifies that the insomnia must be present for at least 4 weeks to justify a diagnosis of insomnia secondary to a mental disorder. However, for clinical purposes, it is probably reasonable to use this diagnosis in hospitalized patients who have insomnia for less than 4 weeks but who otherwise meet the criteria for this diagnosis.

The next most common insomnia subtype found in hospitalized patients is classified in DSM-IV-TR as sleep disorder due to a general medical condition, insomnia type. The specific nature of the medical disorder should be noted—for example, sleep disorder due to asthma, insomnia type. For this diagnosis to be made, the sleep disturbance and/or the related daytime distress must be significant in itself and sufficient to warrant being addressed as a new and distinct clinical problem, and the insomnia must be judged to be produced directly by the specific medical disorder. Evidence supporting the existence of a direct connection between the insomnia and the medical disorder may be the onset of sleep problems coincident with the onset or exacerbation of the medical disorder or a known association between the specific medical disorder and insomnia (as discussed in the following section, "Insomnia Caused by Specific Medical Disorders"). DSM-IV-TR does not include duration criteria for the insomnias produced by medical disorders, so these diagnoses may be made formally even when the insomnia is transient, as long as the problem is severe enough to require independent identification. Insomnias secondary to psychiatric problems (including adjustment disorders in which the medical disorder is the stressor), delirium, primary sleep disorders (e.g., primary or idiopathic insomnia), sleep-related breathing disorders, or narcolepsy (discussed later in this chapter in the section "Narcolepsy") are not included in this category.

In many cases, it may be difficult to determine whether a medical disorder or the medications used in treatment are causing the insomnia. For example, both Parkinson's disease and L-dopa can produce insomnia. If it appears that the insomnia is more a function of the drug than of the medical problem, a diagnosis of substance-induced sleep disorder, insomnia type, may be made instead. Patients who have been dependent on alcohol, caffeine, nicotine, or stimulants may experience withdrawal in the hospital and may experience insomnia as a withdrawal symptom. Patients with chronic alcoholism may have significantly disturbed sleep even after months of abstinence. Such patients also may be given a diagnosis of substance abuse–related insomnia. A careful history, with an interview of those who know the patient, may be required to make this diagnosis.

Patients who learn to associate sleep with frustration or dysphoria may develop conditioned, or psychophysiological, insomnia. Such patients may have only anxious or depressive traits rather than formal Axis II or adjustment disorders, but when stressed by illness or hospitalization, they may have significant insomnia. A careful history will reveal long-standing intermittent insomnia, which is sometimes better when the patient is in a novel environment such as a hotel. For practical purposes, the consultant may manage such patients in a manner similar to how patients with anxiety disorders are managed (see section "Treatment of Insomnia" later in this chapter). Some patients who complain of insomnia have "sleep state misperception," or lack of correlation between the complaints and the abnormalities of sleep documented by objective measures (such as polysomnography). Like psychophysiological insomnia, this type of insomnia complaint usually is long-standing and is unlikely to arise for the first time during hospitalization. Patients in whom this type of insomnia is suspected also may be managed in the hospital like those with anxiety-related insomnias and may be referred to a sleep clinic for further workup after discharge. The clinician should consider the possibility that medication-induced periodic leg movements of sleep (PLMS) is the cause of the insomnia. Table 24–3 lists medications that can cause insomnia. In our experience, medication-induced insomnia is much more commonly seen among outpatients than among hospitalized patients.

Delirium may be a subtle and transient problem in some patients. Nocturnal agitation with resultant insomnia may be the initial, and in some cases the major, presenting feature of delirium. The consultant should always have a high index of suspicion for delirium as a cause of insomnia in hospitalized medically ill patients. When disrupted sleep is reported by staff or insomnia is described by patients with CNS illness or compromise (e.g., anoxia or poor cerebral perfusion) or by patients following surgery or other procedures, delirium should be formally ruled out before other causes are cited to explain the insomnia. As noted above, sleep disturbance in seriously ill and ICU-confined patients is often related to delirium. Clues to the presence of nocturnal delirium include reports from patients or staff of agitation or vivid, often unpleasant dreams. Nurses may be instructed to perform careful mental status examinations at night, which can assist in proper diagnosis.

Most patients with sleep apnea complain of excessive daytime sleepiness, but some also complain of insomnia. Because sleep apnea is both potentially fatal if misdiagnosed or mismanaged and potentially correctable if discovered, and because sleep apnea may be present yet underrecognized in elderly patients or in those with pulmonary, cardiac, neurological, or other illness, the consultant should always consider it in the differential diagnosis of insomnia (see section "Sleep Apnea" later in this chapter for further discussion).

INSOMNIA CAUSED BY SPECIFIC MEDICAL DISORDERS

It is quite common for nonspecific symptoms such as pain, fever, cough, dysuria, or pruritus to induce mild, transient sleep disturbance. Patients with these symptoms may complain of insomnia, even if they do not meet

TABLE 24–3.   Insomnia secondary to drugs or medications: substance-induced sleep disorder, insomnia type

Alcohol (withdrawal, long-term abuse)

Antiasthmatics, decongestants (β_2-agonists, pseudoephedrine, phenylephrine)

Antidepressants: phenelzine, tranylcypromine, protriptyline, desipramine, imipramine, amoxapine, fluoxetine and other selective serotonin reuptake inhibitors (by direct stimulant properties and, in some, by induction of PLMS), tricyclic withdrawal

Antihypertensives, methyldopa, diuretics, reserpine, clonidine (nightmares, PLMS)

Cimetidine

Heavy metal toxicity: arsenic, mercury, lead, copper

L-Dopa, baclofen, methysergide

Neuroleptics: phenothiazines, butyrophenones (can induce PLMS)

Sedative-hypnotics (rebound insomnia following withdrawal after long-term abuse): barbiturates, benzodiazepines, narcotics

Stimulants: amphetamines; methylphenidate; pemoline; cocaine; caffeine and stimulant xanthines in coffee, tea, cola, chocolate

Tetracycline (nightmares)

Thyroxine, steroids, birth control pills

Tobacco (direct stimulation, withdrawal, conditioned awakening to smoke)

Note.   PLMS = periodic leg movements of sleep.

diagnostic criteria. From a practical point of view, the sleep disturbance resolves when the underlying offending symptom is brought under control. In such cases, the consultant can assist by helping the primary medical team to optimize the management of the disorder producing the sleep disturbance and by identifying improved sleep as a medical treatment goal. Some medical disorders are specifically associated with insomnia; these include cardiac disease, pulmonary disease, gastrointestinal disease, neurological disease, musculoskeletal disease, endocrine disease, and cancer. These disorders are summarized in Table 24–4.

Cardiac Disease

Patients with congestive heart failure (CHF) who develop orthopnea, paroxysmal nocturnal dyspnea, or Cheyne-Stokes respiration often complain of insomnia secondary to fragmented and nonrestorative sleep (Hanly et al. 1989). Diuretic-induced nocturia or cerebral hypoperfusion following overdiuresis also may produce insomnia (Pasnau et al. 1968; Williams 1988). Many patients with angina have insomnia resulting from nocturnal angina attacks, some of which may occur during

TABLE 24–4.   Causes of insomnia in hospitalized patients

Insomnia secondary to another mental disorder
  Adjustment disorder
  Mood disorders (including dysthymia)
  Anxiety disorder
  Personality disorder
  Psychotic disorder
Sleep disorder due to a general medical condition,
insomnia type
  Nonspecific symptoms: pain of any source, cough, pruritus,
    dyspnea, fever
  Cardiovascular disease
    Angina
    Congestive heart failure
    Myocardial infarction
    Postcardiotomy delirium
    Intra-aortic balloon pump delirium
  Pulmonary disease
    Chronic obstructive pulmonary disease (COPD)
    Asthma
    Cystic fibrosis
    Hypoventilation secondary to polio, scoliosis, or other
      (alveolar hypoventilation)
    Restrictive lung disease
  Gastrointestinal disease
    Duodenal ulcer
    Hiatal hernia and reflux syndromes
    Hepatic failure
  Neurological disease
    Migraine and cluster headache
    Epilepsy (partial, generalized)
    Parkinson's disease
    Alzheimer's disease and related dementias
    Stroke
    Tumors (thalamus, hypothalamus, brain stem, third
      ventricle)
    Delirium tremens and withdrawal states
    Head injury (open, closed)
    Meningoencephalitides (viral, bacterial, fungal)
	Sleep disorder due to a general medical condition,
	insomnia type *(continued)*
	  Musculoskeletal disease
	    Fibromyalgia
	    Arthritis (including degenerative, rheumatoid,
	      autoimmune types)
	  Renal disease
	    Uremia
	    Post–renal transplantation
	    Nephrolithiasis
	    Urinary tract infection (polyuria)
	  Endocrine disease and changes
	    Hyperthyroidism, hypothyroidism
	    Exogenous steroid use; endogenous hyperadrenalism,
	      hypoadrenalism
	    Diabetic peripheral neuropathy (and related restless
	      legs syndrome)
	  Pregnancy
	Insomnia secondary to delirium
	Substance abuse sleep disorder, insomnia type
	Primary sleep disorder
	  Sleep apnea
	  Narcolepsy
	  Periodic movements during sleep (nocturnal myoclonus,
	    restless legs)
	  Circadian rhythm disruption (phase shift)

dreams (Cassano et al. 1981; King et al. 1973; Murao et al. 1972; Nowlin et al. 1965). The sleep changes in patients post-MI and after cardiac surgery, which may produce the complaint of insomnia, have been reviewed earlier in this chapter. Preliminary evidence suggests that some patients who are treated with benzodiazepines post-MI may develop short but repetitive episodes of central apnea, so caution is advised in such cases.

Pulmonary Disease

Patients with chronic obstructive pulmonary disease (COPD) often have frequent arousals and decreased sleep efficiency (Declerk et al. 1982; Flenley 1989).

Those with comorbid obesity, heart disease, or depression may have severe insomnia. The role of nasal oxygen in treating the insomnia in such patients is controversial because some studies indicate benefit, whereas other studies do not. Preliminary studies suggest that it is safe to treat insomnia in patients with mild to moderate COPD with triazolam 0.25 mg at bedtime or zolpidem 10 mg at bedtime.

Insomnia is common in patients with asthma, 60%–70% of whom are awakened often by nocturnal asthma attacks (Clark 1985). Diurnal variation of airway flow rates (nadirs occur at 4:00 P.M. and 4:00 A.M.) (Clark 1985) is very common in patients with asthma and may be partly responsible for sleep fragmentation and frequent nocturnal awakenings (Montplaisir et al. 1982). The xanthines, β-adrenergic agents, and systemic steroids that are used to treat asthma and COPD can themselves frequently induce insomnia.

Patients with interstitial lung disease or cystic fibrosis may have sleep fragmentation, but this tends to be less severe than the sleep fragmentation that occurs in patients with COPD (Rosenblatt et al. 1973). Finally, snoring may indicate the presence of sleep apnea and may itself be associated with insomnia and nocturnal cardiopulmonary dysfunction in certain individuals (Koskenvuo et al. 1985). Benzodiazepines must be used cautiously in treating patients without apnea who snore heavily; in such patients, these drugs may induce serious obstructive sleep apnea.

Gastrointestinal Disease

Peptic ulcer disease, hiatal hernia, gastroesophageal reflux, or colitis may produce insomnia, often related to nocturnal pain (Orr 1989). Patients with hepatic failure often have insomnia; the insomnia worsens as the hepatic failure progresses. Even mild hepatic encephalopathy may produce insomnia, so supporting full compliance with protein restrictions may be clinically useful. Benzodiazepines such as lorazepam and oxazepam that do not require metabolism by the hepatic microsymal system are the preferred agents in treating insomnia in patients with hepatic failure or in the elderly with hepatic compromise.

Neurological Disease

Patients with Parkinson's disease who have nocturnal discomfort secondary to restricted movement in bed often develop insomnia. The drugs used to treat Parkinson's disease, such as L-dopa-containing compounds and bromocriptine, also produce insomnia (Nausieda et al. 1982). Degenerative disorders such as Huntington's disease—or any disorders that produce myoclonus or chorea—produce insomnia (Aldrich et al. 1989; Nausieda et al. 1982). Patients with Alzheimer's disease frequently have insomnia related to day/night sleep pattern shifts in the early phases of the disease and to delirium and agitation in the later phases (Masson et al. 1987). In our experience, the nocturnal agitation of patients with dementia, which is often called insomnia, is a frequent reason for requests for psychiatric consultation. Insomnia frequently accompanies migraine and cluster variety headaches, because headaches that occur during sleep—sometimes during REM sleep—interrupt sleep (Dexter 1986). Depending on the location of the lesion, some patients with stroke have frequent and prolonged nocturnal awakenings (Koerner et al. 1986). Although most patients

with encephalitis or head injuries have excessive daytime sleepiness, some develop disruption of their normal circadian rhythm generators and may have prolonged nocturnal wakefulness (Regestein 1987). Patients with epilepsy, partial or generalized, often have trouble both falling asleep and staying asleep (Montplaisir et al. 1985; Sterman et al. 1982).

Musculoskeletal Disease

Patients with fibromyalgia syndrome frequently complain of insomnia (Moldofsky 1989). Such patients may have sleep interruption from muscle and joint pain and may show the intrusion of alpha EEG activity into delta sleep (called alpha-delta sleep), which can interfere with the restorative quality of their sleep. Patients with arthritis of various types and with related rheumatic or connective tissue disease tend to have a relatively high prevalence of insomnia and sleep-related complaints (Hench 1996). Both rheumatoid arthritis and fibromyalgia are also associated with restless legs syndrome (RLS) (Salih et al. 1994; Yunus and Aldag 1996).

Endocrine Disease

Hyperthyroidism, not surprisingly, often causes insomnia, but in some cases, insomnia may appear in patients with hypothyroidism as well (Johns et al. 1975). Diabetes may cause insomnia when nocturia or nocturnal hypoglycemia is present. Peripheral and autonomic neuropathies may induce PLMS and paresthesias and may thereby exacerbate sleep fragmentation and multiple awakenings (Mouret 1975).

Cancer

Insomnia appears to be a common complaint of patients with a wide variety of malignancies; the mechanisms remain obscure (Derogatis et al. 1979; Silberfarb et al. 1993).

TREATMENT OF INSOMNIA

For patients with insomnia secondary to medical or psychiatric disorders, optimized treatment of the underlying disorder is the first step. Behavioral management techniques, such as progressive muscle relaxation, hypnosis, or guided imagery, along with attention to the rules of sleep hygiene may help some patients who have insomnia secondary to psychiatric disorders, particularly adjustment and anxiety disorders (Turner and Ascher 1979).

More elaborate behavioral techniques, such as sleep restriction therapy, are sometimes used in the outpatient setting. Caffeine appears to increase insomnia in hospitalized patients (Victor et al. 1981), so simply removing coffee, tea, and cola beverages from the diets of patients complaining of insomnia may be of practical utility. Similarly, nicotine interferes with nocturnal sleep, so prohibition of smoking also may be helpful for some patients (Cummings et al. 1985). Patients with anxiety disorders may be sensitive to the stimulant side effects of antidepressants used to treat mood or anxiety disorders and, as a result, may experience insomnia during the early phase of treatment. Trazodone 25–100 mg, the anticonvulsant gabapentin 200–600 mg, or a benzodiazepine may be added to moderate the insomnia-producing effects of potentially stimulating antidepressants such as fluoxetine (Nierenberg et al. 1994). Cyproheptadine may be helpful in some patients who have nightmares (Harsh 1986). (Please refer to Chapters 20 and 42 in this volume for a more extensive discussion of psychopharmacological management of anxiety disorders.)

Benzodiazepine hypnotics have been and remain a mainstay of drug treatment for insomnia secondary to psychiatric and medical disorders in hospitalized patients. Benzodiazepines may be used when insomnia symptoms persist despite treatment of the primary cause of insomnia, such as pain, depression, or CHF. Because they may induce significant nocturnal respiratory compromise, benzodiazepines should be used with caution when patients have significant COPD, obesity- or cardiac-related hypoventilation, or CHF (Guilleminault 1990). As noted above, triazolam and zolpidem may be less likely than other benzodiazepines to cause respiratory compromise in patients with mild to moderate COPD and insomnia. Benzodiazepines can impair ventilation in patients with sleep apnea and thus should be used with caution in such patients. Elderly patients are particularly sensitive to the cognitive compromise produced by benzodiazepines, and falls can result from impaired cognition or motor coordination. Therefore, in elderly patients, benzodiazepines should be used cautiously and in reduced dosages.

Most of the drugs classified as benzodiazepines are metabolized by the liver, so coadministration of medications that inhibit the cytochrome oxidation system (such as cimetidine, estrogen, disulfiram, isoniazid, erythromycin, and fluoxetine) may result in excessive daytime sedation secondary to reduced benzodiazepine clearance.

Benzodiazepines should be used at the lowest effective dose and only while the insomnia complaint remains acute. It has yet to be established whether the newer nonbenzodiazepine hypnotics—zaleplon and zolpidem—offer clear advantages over older agents for hospitalized patients with medical and surgical problems (Salazar-Gruesco et al. 1988). In general, drugs with a short half-life (such as zaleplon, triazolam, and zolpidem) are the agents of choice to help those who have trouble falling asleep, whereas drugs with a longer duration of action (such as estazolam, temazepam, and lorazepam) are useful for those who have sleep interruption. Withdrawal problems (rebound anxiety or insomnia) may occur when short-acting benzodiazepines such as triazolam or alprazolam are used to treat daytime anxiety. In our experience, patients with insomnia secondary to anxiety disorders may be particularly sensitive to withdrawal and rebound phenomena. Longer-acting benzodiazepines such as clonazepam may improve both daytime anxiety and insomnia for such patients (see Table 24–5).

Chloral hydrate, paraldehyde, and barbiturates should be used rarely, if at all, because these drugs have a greater tendency to depress respiration and are generally less effective than benzodiazepines. Clinical lore suggests that sedating antihistamines such as diphenhydramine and hydroxyzine may be useful in some patients, but their efficacy for the treatment of insomnia is not well established, and the possibility of their causing antihistamine-induced delirium in some patients makes these agents of questionable value (Nicholson et al. 1985; Rickels et al. 1983).

Neuroleptics should be used in hospitalized patients to control insomnia secondary to psychosis, psychotic depression, and acute mania. Neuroleptics also may be extremely helpful in controlling disturbed sleep secondary to delirium in elderly individuals and in ICU patients. This use is especially important if concomitant agitation and irritability pose a risk to a patient who is already compromised by medical illness or whose postsurgical status requires compliance with restrictions posed by drains, intravenous drug administration, and dressings. Neuroleptics also may be used to control mania secondary to steroids or other medications. Low to moderate doses of benzodiazepines such as lorazepam may be used adjunctively with neuroleptics to induce sleep and to manage nocturnal delirium or agitation.

In depressed patients with insomnia, sedating antidepressants (e.g., doxepin or trazodone) may be given along with benzodiazepines on the initial nights, if needed. Antidepressants may induce or worsen preexisting sleep-related movement disorders and thus may precipitate or worsen insomnia in some patients. Likewise, some antidepressants such as fluoxetine, imipramine, desipramine, protriptyline, and the monoamine oxidase inhibitors (MAOIs) may be stimulating and may produce insomnia (see Table 24–3). Lithium may disrupt sleep continuity if polyuria supervenes.

TABLE 24–5. Sedative-hypnotics

	Clonazepam	Estazolam	Flurazepam	Lorazepam	Quazepam	Temazepam	Triazolam	Zolpidem	Diphenhydramine	Hydroxyzine	Zaleplon
Onset of action	Intermediate	Intermediate	Rapid–intermediate	Intermediate	Rapid–intermediate	Slow–intermediate	Rapid	Rapid	Intermediate	Rapid	Rapid
Duration of action	Long	Intermediate	Long	Intermediate	Long	Intermediate	Short	Short	Intermediate	Intermediate	Ultrashort
Half-life (hours) (includes metabolites)	15–50	10–24	24–150	10–20	35–150	8–20	1.5–6	2.4–3	3.5–9.5	6–24	1
Excretion/metabolism	Oxidation/hydroxylation	Oxidation/hydroxylation	Oxidation/hydroxylation	Conjugation	Oxidation/hydroxylation	Conjugation	Oxidation/hydroxylation	Oxidation/hydroxylation	Oxidation/hydroxylation	Oxidation/hydroxylation	Oxidation/glucuronidation
Dose (adult) (mg)	0.5–1.0	1–2	15–30	1	15	15	0.125–0.5	10	50	25	10
Dose (elderly) (mg)	0.25–0.5	0.5	15	0.25–0.5	7.5	15	0.125	5	25	25	5

APPROACH TO THE PATIENT COMPLAINING OF EXCESSIVE DAYTIME SOMNOLENCE

Evaluating a patient who complains of excessive daytime somnolence (EDS) requires a careful history and, occasionally, objective measures of sleepiness. Multiple etiologies of EDS exist (Table 24–6), and the most common is inadequate TST; however, EDS that is caused by a primary sleep disorder is the result of an inability to obtain restorative sleep and therefore will not be relieved simply by the patient's achieving more sleep.

As with insomnia, the approach to the management of the patient with EDS begins with clarification of the nature of the complaint. EDS is characterized by falling asleep inappropriately during the day. Many patients fail to report the extent of their somnolence because of inattention, cognitive decline, and memory disturbance. On the other hand, fatigue, lethargy, depression, delirium, boredom, obtundation, and abulia are often described by patients as "sleepiness"; however, these patients may not have inappropriate episodes of sleep during the day. The sleepiness associated with psychiatric disorders is likely to be related to impaired attention, energy, or motivation. Other conditions, such as depression, can lead to sleeping excessive lengths of time or to spending excessive time awake in bed, but objective measures do not support the conclusion that the patient has EDS. These patients, if kept to a "normal" sleep schedule, will not have inappropriate levels of daytime somnolence (Nofzinger et al. 1991).

The hospital setting is a poor environment in which to assess EDS because hospitalized patients frequently sleep during the day for a variety of reasons that are no cause for concern. Patients generally lie in bed for prolonged periods, have little to intellectually or socially stimulate them, are often taking numerous medications, and have reduced social and physical circadian cues. Thus, daytime sleepiness is usually attributed to the hospital setting rather than to EDS; this contributes to the underdiagnosis of primary sleep disorders among hospitalized inpatients. Outpatient situations that help identify inappropriate daytime sleepiness include falling asleep while driving, watching a movie, or engaging in other sedentary activities. Additional sources of information are helpful. For example, interviews with family members or housemates can help define the extent and duration of sleep problems. Bed partners can describe snoring or abnormal behaviors during sleep. A history of job loss, injury, or motor vehicle accidents may reflect dysfunctions associated with EDS.

TABLE 24–6. Causes of excessive daytime somnolence

Sleep apnea syndromes (43%)
Narcolepsy (25%)
Idiopathic central nervous system hypersomnia (9%)
Periodic leg movements of sleep/restless legs syndrome (4%)
Depression (3%)
Substance use, including alcohol (2%)
Insufficient sleep syndrome (2%)

All others, less than 1%:
Medications
Posttrauma
Postviral (e.g., chronic fatigue syndrome)
Multiple sclerosis
Metabolic
    Hyponatremia
    Hypercalcemia
Endocrine
    Hypothyroidism
    Hyperglycemia

Note. Numbers in parentheses represent approximate percentage of patients with excessive daytime somnolence presenting to sleep disorders centers.
Source. Adapted from Coleman et al. 1982.

In addition to a careful history, objective measures are sometimes indicated. The gold standard for EDS evaluation is the Multiple Sleep Latency Test (MSLT), which determines latency to EEG-defined sleep averaged over five naps during the day (Carskadon 1986). Mean sleep latencies of less than 5 minutes are pathological. Once the presence of EDS is clearly established—on the basis of the history and, if necessary, evaluation with the MSLT—the differential diagnosis of the underlying cause of EDS can be considered (see Table 24–6).

SLEEP APNEA

Sleep apnea is classified in DSM-IV-TR under the category sleep-related breathing disorders. In 1965, Gastaut first associated sleep apnea with specific polysomnographic abnormalities in patients with obesity-hypoventilation syndrome (Pickwickian syndrome). The first successful treatment for this condition, tracheostomy, was performed in 1968. By the mid-1970s, the focus shifted away from Pickwickian syndrome to obese patients with normal daytime respiration. Obstructive sleep apnea is the result of obstruction at any point in the upper airway. Increased resistance at any one point (e.g., from nasal polyps) generates greater intrathoracic pressures and results in a higher likelihood of subsequent airway collapse. In these patients, upper airway obstruction during sleep produces hypoxia, repetitive arousals, poorly restorative sleep, and daytime somnolence. Continuous positive airway pressure (CPAP) was first developed in 1981 but was not widely used as the treatment of choice for sleep apnea until 1986. More recently, this treatment has been extended to include patients without apneas who snore and those who neither snore nor have apneas but have repetitive arousals due to increased airway resistance (Guilleminault et al. 1992).

Sleep-disordered breathing is identified by means of polysomnographic evaluation in a sleep laboratory in which the EEG, electrooculogram, electromyogram, respiratory effort, oxygen saturation, and airflow from the nares and mouth are recorded. Two types of apnea are recognized, although they commonly coexist in the same patient: 1) obstructive, in which airflow is compromised despite respiratory effort; and 2) central, in which little, if any, respiratory effort is made. Whereas hypopnea is a minimum of a one-third reduction in airflow, apnea is defined as a complete elimination of airflow, lasting for a minimum of 10 seconds, that causes a reduction in oxyhemoglobin saturation. These episodes are usually followed by a brief arousal. Sleep apnea is defined as more than five apnea or hypopnea episodes per hour of sleep. The severity of sleep apnea is determined by the respiratory index (number of hypopnea or apnea episodes per hour), the extent of the oxygen desaturation (oxygen nadir and number of desaturations below 85%), the sleep fragmentation caused by respiratory events, and any associated cardiac arrhythmia.

The reported prevalence of sleep apnea varies depending on the population studied, the cutoff respiratory index used to define sleep-disordered breathing, and whether daytime sleepiness is included as a diagnostic criterion. When both apneas/hypopneas and EDS are included (obstructive sleep apnea syndrome), the prevalence ranges from 1% to 4% of adults. Among hospitalized patients, the prevalence of sleep apnea increases as a result of the strong association between sleep apnea and medical illnesses (Hung et al. 1990; Partinen and Palomaki 1985).

Symptoms of sleep apnea are due to sleep fragmentation and cardiopulmonary stress associated with obstructed respiration (see Table 24–7). Reduced airflow produces oxyhemoglobin desaturation, and obstruction in the upper airway leads to compensatory increases in respiratory effort. Repetitive brief arousals produce daytime somnolence. Hypoxia and high intrathoracic pressures lead to increases in pulmonary artery pressure, which have been shown to produce right heart failure, systemic hypertension, and stroke, although the confounding variable of obesity limits conclusions of such

TABLE 24–7. Signs and symptoms of obstructive sleep apnea syndrome

Central nervous system
  Excessive daytime somnolence
  Nocturnal restlessness
  Depression
  Cognitive deterioration
  Morning headache
  Loss of sexual drive

Respiratory
  Snoring
  Dry mouth/sore throat

Cardiac
  Hypertension
  Right heart failure
  Arrhythmias

Gastrointestinal
  Gastroesophageal reflux

Autonomic nervous system
  Nocturnal diaphoresis

Renal
  Nocturia and nocturnal enuresis

Hematological
  Polycythemia

studies (Partinen and Palomaki 1985; Wright et al. 1997). Studies have indicated that one-quarter to one-third of the patients with a diagnosis of moderate to severe apnea do not survive beyond 8–10 years (He et al. 1988; Partinen and Guilleminault 1990). Finally, the severity of apnea and subsequent hypoxemia during the early morning might explain currently available population studies suggesting higher mortality rates (Mitler et al. 1987).

The pathophysiology of central sleep apnea differs from that of the obstructive form. Rather than an obstruction in the upper airway, the abnormality in central sleep apnea is in the central drive for respiration. Central sleep apnea usually produces less oxyhemoglobin desaturation and does not produce the high intrathoracic pressures of obstructive apnea. Most patients with pure central sleep apnea describe insomnia and not EDS (Roehrs et al. 1985). Cardiovascular, CNS, or pulmonary pathology are the most common underlying causes of central sleep apnea (Guilleminault and Robinson 1996).

Treatment of sleep apnea is multifaceted. The first step is an investigation of the potential underlying medical and anatomic etiologies (see Table 24–8). Minimum evaluation includes direct or endoscopic evaluation of the upper airway. If the patient is overweight, a referral to a nutritionist is essential. Patients should eliminate noctur-

TABLE 24–8. Risk factors for obstructive sleep apnea

General
Obesity
Increasing age
Male gender
Postmenopausal status (women)
Nocturnal alcohol or sedative-hypnotic use

Reduction in upper airway patency
Hypertrophic tonsils or adenoids
Nasal septum deviation
Nasal polyps
Neoplasms
Storage diseases (e.g., amyloidosis)
Craniofacial abnormalities (e.g., Pierre Robin syndrome,
    Treacher Collins syndrome)
Retrognathia
Micrognathia
Macroglossia (e.g., Down syndrome)

Metabolic abnormalities
Hypothyroidism
Acromegaly
Prader-Willi syndrome

Neurological disorders
Parkinson's disease
Syringomyelia
Shy-Drager syndrome
Mitochondrial encephalomyopathy

nal alcohol or sedatives because these reduce activity of the upper airway musculature and extend the duration of apneas.

The mainstay of treatment for both obstructive and central sleep apnea is nasal CPAP. Positive pressure is delivered via a plastic mask over the nose; the pressure is adjusted in the sleep laboratory to eliminate sleep-related obstructive events, including snoring. By mechanisms that are not clear, nasal CPAP "splints" the upper airway and prevents frequent arousals and episodic oxyhemoglobin desaturation. In addition to providing restorative sleep and producing near-normal levels of wakefulness (Issa and Sullivan 1986), CPAP prevents the long-term morbidity and mortality that is associated with untreated sleep apnea (He et al. 1988) and can even reverse associated advanced left ventricular dysfunction (Malone et al. 1991).

Resection of nasal polyps or hypertrophied adenoids and tonsils can reduce obstructive events and may enhance CPAP compliance. More aggressive surgical management—that is, uvulopalatopharyngoplasty—is reserved for CPAP treatment failures because of unpredictable efficacy of such procedures (the chance of a successful outcome is 50% in the hands of even a highly skilled surgeon).

It is unclear whether obstructive sleep apnea is associated with emergent or worsening psychiatric illness. Certainly, neurocognitive abnormalities, such as problems in attention, vigilance, and executive functions, are frequently observed. However, aside from anecdotal reports, depression is the only psychiatric disorder that has been investigated; studies are conflicting, with some suggesting a causal role, whereas others have not (Day et al. 1999).

NARCOLEPSY

Narcolepsy is a disorder characterized by both excessive daytime sleepiness and the associated REM symptoms of cataplexy, sleep paralysis, and hypnagogic hallucinations. The prevalence is approximately 0.05% in the general population. Onset occurs most commonly in the second decade of life, and a physical or psychological stressor is identified in about 50% of cases. About 1%–2% of patients have a first-degree family member with narcolepsy.

The REM-related symptoms of narcolepsy distinguish it from other disorders of daytime sleepiness. Cataplexy describes a sudden loss of motor tone, most commonly in the knees but possibly also in the arms, face, jaw, or any other voluntary muscles. These attacks are often elicited by emotion, can last from seconds to minutes, and can evolve into a sleep attack. Sleep paralysis is the presence of total muscular paralysis at sleep onset or awakening. When REM-related dreaming similarly intrudes into wakefulness, patients with narcolepsy describe vivid visual and auditory phenomena, known as hypnagogic or hypnopompic hallucinations.

There is no cure for narcolepsy, so treatment is directed toward relief of daytime sleepiness and REM-related phenomena. Dextroamphetamine (up to 60 mg/day) and methylphenidate (up to 60 mg/day) restore alertness to an average of 70% of normal (Mitler and Hajdukovic 1991). Both medications are available in sustained-release formulations; these are usually administered in twice-daily doses of 30 mg each. Modafinil (up to 400 mg/day) is a novel once-a-day alerting medication, which does not appear to interact with adrenergic systems and may be associated with fewer side effects (Fry 1998) than are sympathomimetic stimulants. The goal of treatment is to maximize alertness and minimize central (irritability, racing thoughts, insomnia) and peripheral (tremulousness, tachycardia, anorexia) side effects. Prophylactic naps, when feasible, can reduce the total daily dose of stimulants required. Because of their potent REM suppression effects, antidepressants are the treatment of choice for patients with cataplexy, sleep paralysis, and hypnagogic hallucinations. Tricyclic antidepressants, MAOIs, and serotonergic uptake inhibitors are all effective, although the greatest clinical experience has been amassed with protriptyline and clomipramine. Adjunctive use of a short- to intermediate-acting benzodiazepine may consolidate nocturnal sleep and permit lower doses of both stimulants and antidepressants.

RESTLESS LEGS SYNDROME AND PERIODIC LEG MOVEMENTS OF SLEEP

RLS is a movement disorder characterized by both sensory and motor components. Patients commonly describe an achy or "crawling" paresthesia, usually in the legs. Movement of the affected limb partially relieves such sensations and thus leads to the appearance and complaint of restlessness. Frequently, the sensory and motor aspects of the disorder are worse at night when immobility is necessary, so the presenting complaint of this movement disorder is sleep disturbance.

Many patients with RLS also manifest the associated movement disorder, PLMS, in which involuntary movements of the affected limbs occur episodically during sleep, approximately every 20–40 seconds. Such movements are brief (0.5–5.0 seconds) and are most common in the dorsiflexors of the foot and flexors of the lower leg. However, the movements can be quite disruptive of sleep continuity, producing nocturnal arousals or actual awakenings.

RLS occurs in association with several medical problems, such as renal failure, diabetes, chronic anemia, and peripheral nerve injuries. It may appear during otherwise uncomplicated pregnancy, with aging, or as an apparently idiopathic problem in its own right. RLS and PLMS also may be induced by various medications, including neuroleptics, antidepressants, lithium, and diuretics, and by narcotic withdrawal. The symptoms of RLS or PLMS do not appear to vary across the spectrum of etiologies, so RLS and PLMS are best considered as syndromes rather than as primary illnesses.

Treatment of the underlying causes of RLS and PLMS (removal of offending medications, correction of electrolyte disturbance or anemia) can at times eliminate the disturbance, but generally, only symptomatic relief is possible (Hanly and Zuberi 1992; Montplaisir et al. 1992). The primary therapeutic agents are benzodiazepines, dopamine agonists, and narcotics. Arousals from PLMS have been successfully reduced by clonazepam, temazepam, and triazolam in hypnotic doses. The

dopaminergic agents (L-dopa, pergolide, pramipexole) attenuate RLS and decrease the number of PLMS events during sleep. Narcotics (codeine, oxycodone) have shown effectiveness in both RLS and PLMS, although their dependence potentially limits their use to treatment-resistant cases (Silber 1997).

SLEEP IN PATIENTS WITH SELECTED MEDICAL CONDITIONS AND DISORDERS

Characteristic changes in the clinical and polysomnographic features of sleep are associated with some medical illnesses. Insomnia-related changes are reviewed in the section "Insomnia Caused by Specific Medical Disorders" earlier in this chapter. Other changes are outlined below. This information may assist consultants in explaining—and in some cases managing—sleep-related changes in patients with certain medical disorders.

Cardiac Disease

Dysrhythmias

Patients with ventricular arrhythmias may have a decreased rate of arrhythmias during sleep, but some—especially those with sleep apnea, alveolar hypoventilation, or COPD—can develop significant worsening of arrhythmias during either REM or NREM sleep (Bond et al. 1973; Lown et al. 1973; Nevins 1972; Smith et al. 1972). Ventricular tachycardia or fibrillation during frightening REM-related dreams has been reported (Guilleminault et al. 1984b; Reich et al. 1981). Ventricular tachycardia probably related to the sudden death of a nearby patient, highlighting the influence of psychological and environmental factors on sleep-related arrhythmias, has been reported (Lester et al. 1969). Atrial arrhythmias may worsen during sleep (Bond et al. 1973; Lown et al. 1973), although more recent work fails to find an association between sleep, sleep stage, and paroxysmal atrial tachycardia (Coccagna et al. 1997).

Conduction system abnormalities, especially in patients with comorbid nocturnal hypoxia, can worsen during sleep (Miller 1982). A case of cardiac pacemaker threshold increasing during sleep, resulting in pacemaker failure, has been reported (Somerdike et al. 1971). Benzodiazepines may precipitate or worsen hypoxia, so consultants should use these drugs with caution in patients with conduction system abnormalities.

Patients with sleep apnea can develop bradycardia at the beginning of an apneic spell, which may progress to asystole in severe cases. Dramatic increases in heart rate can occur as respiration resumes. Arrhythmias (ventricular or supraventricular) can appear during these times; such arrhythmias may be worsened by concomitant hypoxia and acidosis and may be fatal (Guilleminault et al. 1984a; Miller 1982).

Coronary Artery Disease

Cardiac ischemia frequently occurs during sleep in patients with coronary artery disease (CAD). The ischemia may produce angina pain, which awakens the patient, or the episode may be silent (e.g., signified only by ST segment depression on cardiac monitoring) (Figueras et al. 1979; King et al. 1973; Maggini et al. 1976/1977; Murao et al. 1972; Nowlin et al. 1965; Quuyumi et al. 1984; Stern and Tzivvoni 1973). Patients with sleep apnea, obesity, or daytime hypoxemia are particularly at risk for nocturnal angina (E.C. Fletcher et al. 1985; Koskenvuo et al. 1985). Furthermore, sleep apnea has a high incidence in males and females with CAD (Peker et al. 1999)

There is a relation between nocturnal angina and REM sleep in some patients (Broughton and Baron 1978; Cassano et al. 1981; Murao et al. 1972; Nowlin et al. 1965). Variant (spasm) angina can occur during REM sleep, sometimes in association with frightening dreams (King et al. 1973). The physiologic triggers of nocturnal angina attacks are not completely understood but may involve autonomic instability, increased myocardial oxygen demands during REM sleep, decreased heart rate and blood pressure during NREM sleep, as well as circadian, neural, and neurohumoral factors (Hemenway 1980).

Heart Failure

Cheyne-Stokes respiration is found in approximately 40% of the patients with significant CHF. It produces nocturnal apnea and daytime sedation and is associated with increased mortality. Nocturnal oxygen by nasal cannula, and CPAP, may be helpful (Quaranta et al. 1997).

Chronic Obstructive Pulmonary Disease

Patients with COPD have frequent arousals during sleep, decreased sleep efficiency, and significant sleep-related oxygen desaturations (especially during REM sleep) of uncertain etiology (Flenley 1989; Klink and Quan 1987; Perez-Padilla et al. 1985). The role of nasal oxygen as a treatment for these sleep-related desaturations is controversial. Benzodiazepines or other sedatives can precipitate clinically significant sleep apnea in patients with COPD and must be used with caution (Cohn et al. 1992;

Guilleminault 1990). Whether neuroleptics induce respiratory compromise in patients with COPD has not, to our knowledge, been studied, but no evidence of such compromise has been noted in our experience with neuroleptics in patients in ICUs.

Endocrine Disease

Hyperthyroidism typically increases and hypothyroidism decreases delta sleep, but the clinical significance of these effects is uncertain. Goiter, diabetes, and use of exogenous androgen can predispose to sleep apnea (Guilleminault et al. 1981; Johnson et al. 1984; Millman 1985; Regestein 1993; Young et al. 1986).

Pregnancy

Sleep changes, probably related to hormonal alterations, may occur in some women during pregnancy (Errante 1985). Increased sleep time and daytime sleepiness appear in the first trimester; after this time, sleep patterns normalize, and then in the third trimester, a shift toward decreased TST occurs. Stage IV sleep may decrease as term approaches, but this sleep change resolves postpartum. REM sleep also may decline before term and resolve in the first 2 weeks postpartum.

Neurological Disease

Epilepsy

In *generalized epilepsy*, convulsive seizures appear equally distributed during waking and sleep in most patients with epilepsy. Convulsive seizures occur exclusively during sleep in about 8% of patients (morpheic epilepsy) (Fisch and Pedley 1987). Patients with only nocturnal seizures may have normal daytime EEG findings. Nocturnal generalized seizures tend to occur during NREM sleep. Interictal discharges tend to increase during NREM sleep and decrease during REM sleep. Some patients have interictal discharges during early NREM cycles, whereas others have more frequent discharges as the night progresses. REM is sometimes decreased or abolished on nights when nocturnal seizures occur. Clinically, a wide range of changes—from significant sleep disruption to minimal change—has been reported in patients with generalized seizures (Sterman et al. 1982).

The 3-Hz synchronous bilateral and slow-wave discharges that are associated with absence seizures often worsen with drowsiness and with the onset of sleep. In patients with generalized epilepsy, interictal discharges also tend to appear during sleep onset and early NREM but not during REM sleep.

Most patients with *partial epilepsy* have daytime seizures exclusively, with exclusively nocturnal seizures occurring in 11% of this population (Baldy-Moulinier 1982). Rolandic epilepsy, or the benign focal epilepsy of childhood, is particularly likely to present with nocturnal seizures exclusively. REM may facilitate or inhibit partial seizures with a temporal lobe focus. Likewise, interictal discharges in partial epilepsy are often revealed during sleep onset and NREM sleep but may be either increased or decreased by REM sleep (Baldy-Moulinier 1982; Billiard et al. 1987).

Patients with partial epilepsy appear to have lighter, unstable sleep; a higher frequency of complaints of EDS; and subjectively unsatisfying sleep compared with subjects without epilepsy or patients with generalized epilepsy. The frequency and severity of partial seizures often increase after sleep deprivation (Shouse 1988). Frequent brief awakenings—some associated with spike and wave discharges—and disruption of sleep architecture appear in patients who have a temporolimbic seizure focus (Baldy-Moulinier 1982). Decreased delta sleep is sometimes seen in patients with a frontal seizure focus; anticonvulsant medications have minimal beneficial effects on sleep in such patients (Harding et al. 1985; Ruiz-Primo et al. 1985).

Headache

Vascular headaches often appear during sleep, either at night or during an afternoon nap. An association between REM and the onset of some migrainous headaches has been reported. Both cluster headache and chronic paroxysmal hemicrania also often have REM-related onset. Patients with vascular and mixed vascular/tension headaches often complain of insomnia and sometimes show frequent awakening, abnormal sleep architecture, and overall decreases in REM sleep (Dexter 1986). Patients with vascular headaches have an incidence of somnambulism, enuresis, and night terrors higher than that found in the general population (Pradalier et al. 1987). Many patients with sleep apnea complain of morning headache. There may be an association between cluster headache and sleep apnea, especially if apneic episodes occur during REM sleep (Kudrow et al. 1984).

Stroke

Strokes often begin during nocturnal sleep, and there is a high incidence of stroke among patients with snoring and sleep apnea. Strokes that affect medullary and pontine areas may produce sleep apnea or aggravate preexisting mild apnea. Sleep apnea is often present in patients following stroke or transient ischemic attacks, but the exact basis for the correlation is uncertain. Treating sleep apnea may, however, improve outcome in stroke patients (Bassetti and Aldrich 1999). Strokes in a variety of locations can produce alterations in the sleep-wake cycle, decreased sleep efficiency, decreased time, and drowsiness and, in rare cases, can induce narcolepsy (Aldrich and Naylor 1989; Kapen et al. 1990).

Trauma

Sleep apnea, Kleine-Levin syndrome, secondary narcolepsy, and EDS have been reported to appear following head injuries, but such cases are unusual (Guilleminault et al. 1983; Maccario et al. 1987; Rosomoff 1986; Will et al. 1988).

Degenerative Diseases

Degenerative CNS diseases such as Huntington's disease, progressive supranuclear palsy, spinocerebellar degeneration, olivopontocerebellar degeneration, and torsion dystonia often produce insomnia, EDS, circadian cycle disturbances, and parasomnias (Chokroverty 1996; Katayama et al. 1985; Lavigne et al. 1991). Abnormal activity in the extremities and respiratory muscles produces sleep fragmentation and sleep apnea, particularly with spinocerebellar and olivopontocerebellar degeneration (Salazar-Gruesco et al. 1988). Alterations in neurotransmitter balance and cell loss in sleep centers may produce disturbances of sleep.

Patients with Tourette's disorder may experience nocturnal tics, insomnia, and parasomnias, which remit or worsen as a function of the severity of the syndrome itself (Erenberg 1985). These problems tend to become less common as patients enter adulthood.

Senile dementia of the Alzheimer's type, multi-infarct dementia, alcoholic dementia, Pick's disease and other frontal degenerative processes, Creutzfeldt-Jakob disease, and obstructive hydrocephalus can all produce sleep problems secondary to nocturnal delirium (sundowning). The likelihood of sundowning increases as the dementing illness worsens or comorbid medical problems supervene (Evans 1987).

Sleep apnea exacerbates cognitive decline. There may be a direct correlation between apnea and dementia among women, beyond the increased incidence of both disorders that are present at baseline with advancing age (Bliwise 1993; Reynolds et al. 1985a).

Patients with dementia typically have fragmented nocturnal sleep. They are awake more during the night and nap frequently during the day. This disruption of the normal circadian sleep-wake cycle, and a decrease in total delta sleep, tends to worsen with the progression of the dementia (Prinz et al. 1982).

Parkinson's disease and related conditions (Shy-Drager syndrome, striatonigral degeneration, Parkinson's–amyotrophic lateral sclerosis–dementia complex) frequently produce insomnia characterized by frequent nocturnal awakenings and excessive daytime napping (Mouret 1975; Stocchi et al. 1998). Disordered breathing secondary to interference with the operation of the muscles of respiration may add to sleep fragmentation. Sudden death secondary to glottic failure may occur in multiple system atrophy (Sadaoka et al. 1996). Sleep disruption also may occur because of the inability to move normally in bed, painful leg cramps, nightmares, and PLMS. Dementia, which occurs in approximately one-third of the patients with Parkinson's disease, may further complicate matters. One of the most common sources of sleep disturbance among patients with Parkinson's disease and related conditions is the antiparkinsonian medications themselves. L-Dopa and bromocriptine can induce parasomnias (somnambulism, pavor nocturnus), PLMS, nightmares, visual hallucinations, dystonias, and choreiform movements.

Parkinsonian-related sleep changes tend to worsen as the disease progresses and as the duration of treatment lengthens. Careful timing of L-dopa compound administrations (earlier in the day), use of multiple classes of drugs (selegiline, amantadine, anticholinergic agents) concomitantly, and careful, short-term use of benzodiazepine hypnotics with short or intermediate duration of action may be helpful (Nausieda et al. 1982; Stocchi et al. 1998).

Other Neurological Conditions

Sleep apnea can occur during postpolio syndrome, years after the disease itself has resolved (Cosgrove et al. 1987; Hsu and Staats 1998). In a similar fashion, apnea and Kleine-Levin syndrome have been reported as late complications of encephalitis (Merriam 1986). Narcoleptic sleep attacks and cataplexy have been reported in some patients with multiple sclerosis (Poirier et al. 1987). Lesions involving brain stem respiratory centers may, in rare instances, produce "sleep-related neurogenic tachypnea" (a proposed diagnosis in the ICSD), which is characterized by an increase in respiratory rate during sleep of at least 20% over the rate in the waking state. Sleep fragmentation with a complaint of EDS may appear with this condition.

Other Diseases and Conditions

Gastroesophageal reflux is a very common problem and causes awakenings during sleep (Lavigne et al. 1991). *Peptic ulcer disease* also can produce pain-related awakenings during sleep (Orr 1989). There is a circadian rhythm to gastric acid secretion, with a maximum reached between 9:00 P.M. and midnight. Gastric acid secretion may be increased as a function of *rebound from antacid use*, and *sedatives* may inhibit esophageal acid clearance, so the alteration in the timing of administration of these agents may improve sleep in some patients.

Patients with *fibromyalgia* or *fibrositis syndrome* typically complain of fatigue and nonrestorative sleep. The unusual polysomnographic pattern of alpha activity appearing during Stages III and IV sleep, called *alpha-delta sleep*, has been associated with fibromyalgia and may be directly related to the nonrestorative quality of sleep (Goldenberg 1987; Moldofsky 1989). Patients with *osteoarthritis* often complain of insomnia, with frequent awakenings and a sense of not being refreshed on awakening, secondary to pain and muscle stiffness.

Obstructive sleep apnea from tonsillar enlargement is a potential complication of *amyloidosis* (Carbone et al. 1985). Patients with *uremic renal failure* may have decreased amounts of delta sleep and a relatively high incidence of RLS, producing complaints of insomnia or EDS (Winkelman et al. 1996). The incidence of sleep apnea also appears to be significantly increased in patients with renal failure (Kimmel et al. 1989). Large volume peritoneal dialysis may worsen sleep apnea, whereas renal transplantation may cure it (Kraus and Hamburger 1997).

SUMMARY

Psychiatric consultants should perform a formal assessment of sleep and related issues on each patient they see. A high index of suspicion for delirium as the cause of nocturnal agitation and related sleep complaints should be maintained, especially for patients in ICUs, elderly individuals, and patients taking multiple medications. An attempt to discover a particular etiology for a sleep or related problem—be it medical, drug related, or psychiatric—should be made, and treatment should be focused as specifically as possible on this etiology. Sedative-hypnotics should not be prescribed until this attempt is made and factors such as sleep-related respiratory status have been considered.

REFERENCES

Aaron JN, Carlisle CC, Carskadon M, et al: Environmental noise as a cause of sleep disruption in an intermediate respiratory care unit. Sleep 19:707–710, 1996

Aldrich MS, Naylor MW: Narcolepsy associated with lesions of the diencephalon. Neurology 18:1505–1508, 1989

Aldrich M, Eisler A, Lee M, et al: Effects of continuous, positive airway pressure on phasic events of sleep in patients with obstructive sleep apnea. Sleep 12:413–419, 1989

American Psychiatric Association: Diagnostic and Statistical Manual of Mental Disorders, 4th Edition, Text Revision. Washington, DC, American Psychiatric Association, 2000

American Sleep Disorders Association: International Classification of Sleep Disorders: ICSD Diagnostic and Coding Manual. Rochester, MN, American Sleep Disorders Association, 1990

Aurell J, Elmquist D: Sleep in the surgical intensive care unit: continuous polygraphic recording of sleep in nine patients receiving postoperative care. BMJ 2290:1029–1032, 1985

Baldy-Moulinier M: Temporal lobe epilepsy and sleep organization, in Sleep and Epilepsy. Edited by Sterman MB, Shouse MN, Passouant P. New York, Academic Press, 1982, pp 347–359

Bassetti C, Aldrich MS: Sleep apnea in acute cerebrovascular diseases: final report on 128 patients. Sleep 22:217–223, 1999

Berlin RM, Litovitz GL, Diaz MA, et al: Sleep disorders on a psychiatric consultation service. Am J Psychiatry 141:582–584, 1984

Billiard M, Besset A, Zachariev Z, et al: Relation of seizures and seizure discharge to sleep stages, in Advances in Epileptology. Edited by Wolf P, Dam M, Janz F, et al. New York, Raven, 1987, pp 665–670

Bliwise DL: Sleep in normal aging and dementia. Sleep 16:40–81, 1993

Bond WC, Bohs C, Ebey J, et al: Rhythmic heart rate variability related to stages of sleep. Conditional Reflex 8:98–107, 1973

Broughton R, Baron R: Sleep patterns in the intensive care unit and on the ward after acute myocardial infarction. Electroencephalography and Clinical Neurophysiology 45:348–360, 1978

Bruera E, Fainsinger RL, Schoeller T, et al: Rapid discontinuation of hypnotics in terminal cancer patients: a prospective study. Ann Oncol 7:855–856, 1996

Carbone JE, Barker D, Stauffer JL, et al: Sleep apnea in amyloidosis. Chest 87:401–403, 1985

Carskadon MA: Guidelines for the Multiple Sleep Latency Test (MSLT): a standard measure of sleepiness. Sleep 9:519–524, 1986

Cassano GB, Maggini C, Guazzelli M, et al: Nocturnal angina and sleep. Prog Neuropsychopharmacol Biol Psychiatry 5:99–104, 1981

Cassem NH: Critical care psychiatry, in Textbook of Critical Care. Edited by Shoemaker WC, Thompson WL, Holbrook PR. Philadelphia, PA, WB Saunders, 1984, pp 981–989

Chokroverty S: Sleep and degenerative neurologic disorders. Neurol Clin 14:807–826, 1996

Clark TJH: The circadian rhythm of asthma. British Journal of Diseases of the Chest 125:18–22, 1985

Coccagna G, Capucci A, Bauleo S, et al: Paroxysmal atrial fibrillation in sleep. Sleep 20:396–398, 1997

Cohn MA, Morris DD, Juan D, et al: Effects of estazolam and flurazepam on cardiopulmonary function in patients with chronic obstructive pulmonary disease. Drug Saf 7:152–158, 1992

Coleman RM, Roffwarg HD, Kennedy SJ, et al: Sleep-wake disorders based on a polysomnographic diagnosis: a national cooperative study. JAMA 247:997–1003, 1982

Cosgrove JL, Alexander MA, Kitts EL, et al: Late effects of poliomyelitis. Arch Phys Med Rehabil 68:4–7, 1987

Cummings KM, Giovino GJ, Jaen CR, et al: Reports of smoking withdrawal symptoms over a 21 day period of abstinence. Addict Behav 10:373–381, 1985

Day R, Gerhardstein R, Lumley A, et al: The behavioral morbidity of obstructive sleep apnea. Prog Cardiovasc Dis 41:341–354, 1999

Declerk AC, Wauguier A, Sijben-Kiggen R, et al: A normative study of sleep in different forms of epilepsy, in Sleep and Epilepsy. Edited by Sterman MB, Shouse MN, Passouant P. New York, Academic Press, 1982, pp 329–337

Derogatis LR, Feldstein M, Morrow G, et al: A survey of psychotropic drug prescriptions in an oncology population. Cancer 44:1919–1929, 1979

Dexter J: The relationship between disorders of arousal from sleep and migraine (abstract). Headache 26:322, 1986

Dlin BM, Rosen H, Dickstein K, et al: The problems of sleep and rest in the intensive care unit. Psychosomatics 2:155–163, 1971

Dohno S, Lynch JJ, Paskewitz DA, et al: Sleep-waking changes in cardiac arrhythmia in a coronary care patient. Psychosom Med 39:39–43, 1977

Dohno S, Paskewitz D, Lynch JJ, et al: Some aspects of sleep disturbance in coronary patients. Percept Mot Skills 18:199–205, 1979

Ellis BW, Dudley HAF: Some aspects of sleep research in surgical stress. J Psychosom Res 20:303–308, 1978

Erenberg G: Sleep disorders in Giles de la Tourette's syndrome (letter). Neurology 35:1397, 1985

Errante J: Sleep deprivation or post partum blues? Topics in Clinical Nursing 6(4):9–18, 1985

Evans K: Sundown syndrome in institutionalized elderly. J Am Geriatr Soc 35:101–108, 1987

Figueras J, Singh BN, Ganz W, et al: Mechanisms of rest and nocturnal angina: observations during continuous hemodynamic and electrocardiographic monitoring. Circulation 59:955–968, 1979

Fisch BJ, Pedley TA: Generalized tonic-clonic epilepsies, in Epilepsy: Electro-Clinical Syndromes. Edited by Luders H, Lesser RP. New York, Springer-Verlag, 1987, pp 151–185

Flenley C: Chronic obstructive pulmonary disease, in Principles and Practice of Sleep Medicine. Edited by Kryger M, Roth T, Dement WC. Philadelphia, PA, WB Saunders, 1989, pp 601–610

Fletcher A, van den Heuvel C, Dawson D: Sleeping with an electric blanket: effects on core temperature, sleep and melatonin in young adults. Sleep 22:313–318, 1999

Fletcher EC, DeBehnke RD, Lovoi MS, et al: Undiagnosed sleep apnea in patients with essential hypertension. Ann Intern Med 103:190–195, 1985

Freedman NS, Kotzer N, Schwab RJ: Patient perception of sleep quality and etiology of sleep disruption in the intensive care unit. Am J Respir Crit Care Med 159:1155–1162, 1999

Fry JM: Treatment modalities for narcolepsy. Neurology 50 (2 suppl 1):S43–S48, 1998

Gelling L: Causes of ICU psychosis: the environmental factors. Nursing in Critical Care 4:22–26, 1999

Goldenberg DL: Fibromyalgia syndrome. JAMA 257:2782–2787, 1987

Guilleminault C: Benzodiazepines, breathing, and sleep. Am J Med 88 (suppl 3A):25–28, 1990

Guilleminault C, Robinson A: Central sleep apnea. Neurol Clin 14:611–628, 1996

Guilleminault C, Briskin JG, Greenfield MS, et al: The impact of autonomic nervous system dysfunction on breathing during sleep. Sleep 4:263–278, 1981

Guilleminault C, Faull KF, Miles L, et al: Posttraumatic excessive daytime sleepiness: a review of 20 patients. Neurology 33:1584–1589, 1983

Guilleminault C, Connolly S, Winkle R, et al: Cyclical variation of the heart rate in sleep apnea syndrome. Lancet 2:126–131, 1984a

Guilleminault C, Pool P, Motta J, et al: Sinus arrest during REM sleep in young adults. N Engl J Med 311:1006–1010, 1984b

Guilleminault C, Stoohs R, Clerk A, et al: From obstructive sleep apnea syndrome to upper airway resistance syndrome: consistency of daytime sleepiness. Sleep 15:S13–S16, 1992

Hanly P, Zuberi N: Periodic leg movements during sleep before and after heart transplantation. Sleep 15:489–492, 1992

Hanly PJ, Millar TW, Steljes DG, et al: The effect of oxygen on respiration and sleep in patients with congestive heart failure. Ann Intern Med 111:777–782, 1989

Harding GFA, Alfon CA, Powell G, et al: The effect of sodium valproate on sleep, reaction times and visual evoked potential in normal subjects. Epilepsia 26:597–601, 1985

Harrell RG, Othmer E: Postcardiotomy confusion and sleep loss. J Clin Psychiatry 48:445–446, 1987

Harsh HH: Cyproheptadine for recurrent nightmares. Am J Psychiatry 143:1491–1492, 1986

He J, Kryger MH, Zorick FJ, et al: Mortality and apnea index in obstructive sleep apnea. Chest 94:9–14, 1988

Hemenway JA: Sleep and the cardiac patient. Heart Lung 9:453–463, 1980

Hench PK: Sleep and the rheumatic diseases. Bull Rheum Dis 45(8):1–6, 1996

Hsu AA, Staats BA: "Postpolio" sequelae and sleep-related disordered breathing. Mayo Clin Proc 73:216–224, 1998

Hung J, Whitford EG, Parsons RW, et al: Association of sleep apnea with myocardial infarction in man. Lancet 336:261–264, 1990

Issa GH, Sullivan CE: The immediate effects of nasal continuous positive airway pressure treatment on sleep patterns in patients with obstructive sleep apnea syndrome. Electroencephalography and Clinical Neurophysiology 63:10–17, 1986

Jarrett DG, Greenhouse JB, Thompson SB, et al: Effect of nocturnal intravenous cannulation on sleep EEG measures. Biol Psychiatry 19:1537–1550, 1984

Johns MW, Doré C: Sleep at home and in the sleep laboratory. Ergonomics 21:325–330, 1978

Johns MW, Large AA, Masterson JP, et al: Sleep and delirium after open heart surgery. Br J Surg 61:377–381, 1974

Johns MW, Masterson JP, Paddle-Ledinek JE, et al: Variations in thyroid function and sleep in healthy young men. Clinical Science and Molecular Medicine 49:629–632, 1975

Johnson LC: Sleep deprivation and performance, in Biological Rhythms, Sleep and Performance. Edited by Webb WB. New York, Wiley, 1982, pp 111–142

Johnson MW, Anch AM, Remmers JE, et al: Induction of the obstructive sleep apnea syndrome in a woman by exogenous androgen administration. American Review of Respiratory Diseases 128:1023–1025, 1984

Jones J, Hoggart B, Withey J, et al: What the patients say: a study of reactions to an intensive care unit. Intensive Care Med 5:89–92, 1979

Kahn DM, Cook TE, Carlisle CC, et al: Identification and modification of environmental noise in an ICU setting. Chest 114:535–540, 1998

Kapen S, Maas C, Nichols C, et al: Obstructive sleep apnea is a major risk factor for stroke. Neurology 40 (suppl 1):136, 1990

Karacan I, Williams RL: Sleep characteristics of patients with angina pectoris. Psychosomatics 10:280–284, 1969

Karacan I, Wolff SM: The effects of fever on sleep and dream patterns. Psychosomatics 9:331–339, 1968

Karacan I, Green JR, Gore JM, et al: Sleep in post-myocardial infarction patients, in Contemporary Problems in Cardiology: Stress and the Heart. Edited by Eliot RS. New York, Futura Publishers, 1974, pp 163–195

Katayama S, Yokoyana S, Hiramo Y, et al: TRH and Sleep Abnormalities in Spinocerebellar Degeneration. Amsterdam, The Netherlands, Elsevier, 1985, pp 227–230

Kavey NB, Altshuler KZ: Sleep in herniorrhaphy patients. Am J Surg 138:682–687, 1979

Kimmel PW, Miller G, Mendelson WB, et al: Clinical studies: sleep apnea syndrome in chronic renal disease. Am J Med 86:308–314, 1989

King M, Zir L, Kaltman AJ, et al: All-night polygraphic studies of nocturnal angina pectoris. Am J Med Sci 265:419–422, 1973

Klink M, Quan SF: Prevalence of reported sleep disturbances in a general adult population and their relationship to obstructive airway diseases. Chest 91:540–546, 1987

Koerner E, Flooh E, Reinhart B, et al: Sleep alternatives in ischaemic stroke. Eur Neurol 25 (suppl 2):104–110, 1986

Koskenvuo M, Kaprio J, Partinen M, et al: Snoring as a risk factor for hypertension and angina pectoris. Lancet 1:893–896, 1985

Kraus MA, Hamburger RJ: Sleep apnea in renal failure. Adv Perit Dial 13:88–92, 1997

Kryger MH, Roth T, Dement W: Principles and Practice of Sleep Medicine, 3rd Edition. Philadelphia, PA, WB Saunders, 2000

Kudrow L, McGinty DJ, Phillips ER, et al: Sleep apnea in cluster headache. Cephalalgia 4:33–38, 1984

Lavigne GJ, Velley-Miguel AM, Montplaisir J, et al: Muscle pain, dyskinesia, and sleep. Can J Physiol Pharmacol 69:678–682, 1991

Lester BK, Block R, Gunn CG, et al: The relationship of cardiac arrhythmias to the phases of sleep (abstract). Clinical Research 17:456, 1969

Lown B, Tykoscinski M, Garfein A, et al: Sleep and ventricular premature beats. Circulation 48:691–701, 1973

Lunberg P, Roth T, Kramer M, et al: A hospital survey of prescription vs administration of hypnotics used (abstract). Sleep Research 6:75, 1977

Maccario M, Ruggles KH, Merinether JA, et al: Post-traumatic narcolepsy. Mil Med 152:370–371, 1987

Maggini C, Guazzelli M, Castrogiovanni P, et al: Psychological and physiopathological study on coronary patients. Psychother Psychosom 27:210–216, 1976/1977

Malone S, Liu PP, Holloway R, et al: Obstructive sleep apnea in patients with dilated cardiomyopathy: effects of continuous positive airway pressure. Lancet 338:1480–1484, 1991

Marin JM, Carrizo SJ, Kogan I: Obstructive sleep apnea and acute myocardial infarction: clinical implications of the association. Sleep 21:809–815, 1998

Masson C, Mear JY, Masson M, et al: Symptomatic hypersomniac ictus of a posterior thalamic hemorrhage. Presse Med 16:79–80, 1987

McDowell JA, Mion LC, Lydon TJ, et al: A nonpharmacologic sleep protocol for hospitalized older patients. J Am Geriatr Soc 46:700–705, 1998

Merriam AE: Kleine-Levin syndrome following acute viral encephalitis. Biol Psychiatry 21:1301–1304, 1986

Miller WP: Cardiac arrhythmias and conduction disturbances in the sleep apnea syndrome. Am J Med 73:317–321, 1982

Millman RP: Sleep apnea in hemodialysis patients: the lack of testosterone effect. Nephron 40:401–410, 1985

Mitler M, Hajdukovic R: Relative efficacy of drugs for the treatment of sleepiness in narcolepsy. Sleep 14:218–220, 1991

Mitler MM, Hajdukovic RM, Shafor R, et al: When people die: cause of death versus time of death. Am J Med 82:266–274, 1987

Moldofsky H: Nonrestorative sleep and symptoms after a febrile illness in patients with fibrositis and chronic fatigue syndromes. J Rheumatol 16 (suppl 19):150–153, 1989

Montplaisir J, Walsh J, Malo JL, et al: Nocturnal asthma: features of attacks, sleep and breathing patterns. American Review of Respiratory Diseases 125:18–22, 1982

Montplaisir J, Laveriere M, Saint-Hilaire JM, et al: Sleep and epilepsy, in Long-Term Monitoring and Computer Analysis of the EEG Epilepsy. Edited by Gotman J, Ives JR, Gloor P. Amsterdam, The Netherlands, Elsevier, 1985, pp 215–239

Montplaisir J, Lapierre O, Warnes H, et al: The treatment of the restless leg syndrome with or without period leg movements in sleep. Sleep 15:391–395, 1992

Morgan PJ, Chapados R, Chung FF, et al: Evaluation of zolpidem, triazolam, and placebo as hypnotic drugs the night before surgery. J Clin Anesth 9:97–102, 1997

Mouret J: Difference in sleep in patients with Parkinson's disease. Electroencephalography and Clinical Neurophysiology 38:563–567, 1975

Murao S, Harumi K, Katayama S, et al: All-night polygraphic studies of nocturnal angina pectoris. Jpn Heart J 13:295–306, 1972

Nausieda P, Weiner W, Kaplan LR, et al: Sleep disruption in the course of chronic levodopa therapy: an early feature of the levodopa-induced psychosis. Clin Neuropharmacol 5:183–194, 1982

Nevins DB: First and second degree AV heart block with rapid eye movement sleep. Ann Intern Med 76:981–983, 1972

Nicholson AN, Pascoe PA, Stone BM, et al: Histaminergic systems and sleep. Neuropharmacology 24:245–250, 1985

Nierenberg A, Adler L, Peselow E, et al: Trazodone for antidepressant-associated insomnia. Am J Psychiatry 151:1069–1072, 1994

Nofzinger E, Thase M, Reynolds CF, et al: Hypersomnia in bipolar depression: a comparison with narcolepsy using the multiple sleep latency test. Am J Psychiatry 148:1177–1181, 1991

Nowlin J, Troyer W, Collins WS, et al: The association of nocturnal angina pectoris with dreaming. Ann Intern Med 631:1040–1046, 1965

Orr WC: Gastrointestinal disorders, in Principles and Practice of Sleep Medicine. Edited by Kryger MH, Roth T, Dement WC. Philadelphia, PA, WB Saunders, 1989, pp 622–629

Orr WC, Stahl ML: Sleep disturbance after open heart surgery. Am J Cardiol 39:196–201, 1977

Partinen M, Guilleminault C: Daytime sleepiness and vascular morbidity at seven-year follow up in obstructive sleep apnea patients. Chest 97:27–32, 1990

Partinen M, Palomaki H: Snoring and cerebral infarction. Lancet 2:1325–1326, 1985

Pasnau RO, Naitoh R, Stier S, et al: The psychological effects of 205 hours of sleep deprivation. Arch Gen Psychiatry 18:496–505, 1968

Peker Y, Kriaczi H, Hedner J, et al: An independent association between obstructive sleep apnea and coronary artery disease. Eur Respir J 14:179–184, 1999

Perez-Padilla R, West P, Lertzman M, et al: Breathing during sleep in patients with interstitial lung disease. American Review of Respiratory Diseases 132:224–229, 1985

Perry SW, Wu A: Rationale for the use of hypnotic agents in a general hospital. Ann Intern Med 100:441–446, 1984

Pilcher JJ, Huffcutt AI: Effects of sleep deprivation on performance: a meta-analysis. Sleep 19:318–326, 1996

Poirier G, Montplaisir J, Dumont M, et al: Clinical and sleep laboratory study of narcoleptic symptoms in multiple sclerosis. Neurology 37:693–695, 1987

Pradalier A, Giroud M, Dry J, et al: Somnambulism, migraine and propranolol. Headache 27:143–145, 1987

Prinz PN, Vitaliano P, Vitiello MV, et al: Sleep EEG and mental function changes in senile dementia of the Alzheimer's type. Neurobiol Aging 3:361–370, 1982

Quaranta AJ, D'Alonzo GE, Krachman SL: Cheyne-Stokes respiration during sleep in congestive heart failure. Chest 111:467–473, 1997

Quuyumi A, Mockus LJ, Wright CA, et al: Mechanisms of nocturnal angina pectoris: importance of increased myocardial oxygen demand in patients with severe coronary artery disease. Lancet 1:1207–1209, 1984

Regestein QR: Relationship between psychological factors and cardiac rhythm and electrical disturbances. Compr Psychiatry 16:137–148, 1987

Regestein QR: Sleep disorders in medicine, in Psychiatric Care of the Medically Ill Patient. Edited by Stoudemire A, Fogel BS. New York, Oxford University Press, 1993, pp 485–515

Reich P, DeSilva RA, Lown B, et al: Acute psychological disturbances preceding life threatening ventricular arrhythmias. JAMA 246:233–235, 1981

Reynolds CF, Kupfer DJ, Taska LS, et al: EEG sleep in elderly depressed, demented and healthy subjects. Biol Psychiatry 20:431–442, 1985a

Reynolds CF, Kupfer DJ, Taska LS, et al: Sleep of healthy seniors: a revisit. Sleep 8:20–29, 1985b

Richards KC, Bairnsfather L: A description of night sleep patterns in the critical care unit. Heart Lung 17:35–42, 1988

Rickels K, Morris RJ, Newman H, et al: Diphenhydramine in insomniac family practice patients: a double-blind study. J Clin Pharmacol 23:235–242, 1983

Roehrs T, Conway W, Wittig R, et al: Sleep complaints in patients with sleep-related respiratory disturbances. American Review of Respiratory Diseases 132:520–523, 1985

Rosenblatt G, Hartmann E, Zwilling GR, et al: Cardiac irritability during sleep and dreaming. J Psychosom Res 17:129–134, 1973

Rosomoff HL: Occult respiratory and autonomic dysfunction in craniovertebral anomalies and upper cervical spinal disease. Spine 11:345–347, 1986

Ruiz-Primo ME, Coria S, Torres O, et al: Prevalence of subjective sleep disorders in poorly controlled chronic epileptics (abstract). Sleep Research 14:243, 1985

Sadaoka T, Kakitsuba N, Fujiwara Y, et al: Sleep-related breathing disorders in patients with multiple system atrophy and vocal cord palsy. Sleep 19:479–484, 1996

Salazar-Gruesco EF, Rosenberg RS, Roos RP, et al: Sleep apnea in olivopontocerebellar degeneration: treatment with trazodone. Ann Neurol 123:399–401, 1988

Salih AM, Gray RE, Mills KR, et al: A clinical, serological and neurophysiological study of restless legs syndrome in rheumatoid arthritis. British Journal of Rheumatology 33:60–63, 1994

Salzman C: Psychotropic drug use and polypharmacy in a general hospital. Gen Hosp Psychiatry 3:1–9, 1981

Schenck CH, Mahowald MW: Injurious sleep behavior disorders (parasomnias) affecting patients on intensive care units. Intensive Care Med 17:219–224, 1991

Schenck CH, Bundlie SR, Mahowald MW: Delayed emergence of a parkinsonian disorder in 38% of 29 older men initially diagnosed with idiopathic rapid eye movement sleep behaviour disorder. Neurology 46:388–393, 1996

Shilo L, Dagan Y, Smorjik Y, et al: Patients in the intensive care unit suffer from severe lack of sleep associated with loss of normal melatonin secretion pattern. Am J Med Sci 317:278–281, 1999

Shouse MN: Sleep deprivation increases susceptibility to kindling and penicillin seizure events during all waking and sleep states in cats. Sleep 11:162–171, 1988

Silber MH: Restless legs syndrome. Mayo Clin Proc 72:261–264, 1997

Silberfarb P, Hauri PJ, Oxman TE, et al: Assessment of sleep in patients with lung cancer and breast cancer. J Clin Oncol 11:997–1004, 1993

Simpson T, Lee ER, Cameron C: Patients' perceptions of environmental factors that disturb sleep after cardiac surgery. Am J Crit Care 5:173–181, 1996

Smith R, Johnson L, Rothfeld D, et al: Sleep and cardiac arrhythmias. Arch Intern Med 130:751–753, 1972

Somerdike J, Ostermiller W, Camarata SJ, et al: Sleeping threshold change causing failure of artificial cardiac pacing (letter). JAMA 215:980, 1971

Sterman MB, Shouse MN, Passouant P (eds): Sleep and Epilepsy. New York, Academic Press, 1982

Stern S, Tzivvoni D: Dynamic changes in the ST-T segment during sleep in ischemic heart disease. Am J Cardiol 32:17–20, 1973

Stocchi F, Barbato L, Nordera G, et al: Sleep disorders in Parkinson's disease. J Neurol 245 (suppl 1):S15–S18, 1998

Tesar GA, Stern TA: Evaluation and treatment of agitation in the intensive care unit. J Intensive Care Med 1:137–148, 1986

Thorpy MJ: Handbook of Sleep Disorders. New York, Marcel Dekker, 1990

Treggiari-Venzi M, Borgeat A, Fuchs-Buder T, et al: Overnight sedation with midazolam or propofol in the ICU: effects on sleep quality, anxiety and depression. Journal of Intensive Care Medicine 22:1186–1190, 1996

Turner RM, Ascher M: Controlled comparison of progressive relaxation, stimulus control and paradoxical intention therapies for insomnia. J Consult Clin Psychol 47:500–508, 1979

Victor BS, Lubetsky M, Greden JF, et al: Somatic manifestations of caffeinism. J Clin Psychiatry 42:185–188, 1981

Will RG, Young JPR, Thomas DJ, et al: Kleine-Levin syndrome: report of two cases with onset of symptoms precipitated by head trauma. Br J Psychiatry 152:410–412, 1988

Williams RL: Sleep disturbances in various medical and surgical conditions, in Sleep Disorders: Diagnosis and Treatment, 2nd Edition. Edited by Williams RL, Karacan I, Moore CA. New York, Wiley, 1988, pp 265–292

Williams R, Agnew H, Webb WB: Effects of prolonged stage four and 1-REM sleep deprivation: EEG, task performance, and psychologic responses (Report No SAM-TR-67–59). United States Air Force School of Aerospace Medicine, Brooks Air Force Base, Texas, 1967

Winkelman JW, Chertow GM, Lazarus JM: Restless legs syndrome in end-stage renal disease. Am J Kidney Dis 28:372–378, 1996

Wright J, Johns R, Watt I, et al: Health effects of obstructive sleep apnoea and the effectiveness of continuous positive airways pressure: a systematic review of the research evidence. BMJ 314:851–860, 1997

Yinnon AM, Ilan Y, Tadmor B, et al: Quality of sleep in the medical department. British Journal of Clinical Practice 46:88–91, 1992

Young R, Waldron J, Baer S, et al: Obstructive sleep apnea in association with retrosternal goitre and acromegaly. J Laryngol Otol 100:861–863, 1986

Yuen EJ, Zisselman MH, Louis DZ, et al: Sedative-hypnotic use by the elderly: effects on hospital length of stay and costs. Journal of Mental Health Administration 24:90–97, 1997

Yunus MB, Aldag JC: Restless legs syndrome and leg cramps in fibromyalgia syndrome: a controlled study. BMJ 312:1339, 1996

25

Factitious Disorders and Malingering

Charles V. Ford, M.D.

Marc D. Feldman, M.D.

Self-induced, simulated, exaggerated, or totally fabricated illnesses have most likely existed throughout human history. Such "disease forgery" was well documented by the Roman physician Galen in the second century A.D. (Adams 1846). The manifestations and motivations of both factitious disorder and malingering were catalogued in Hector Gavin's 1838 book on medical deception.

Today, factitious disorders are among the Axis I diagnoses in DSM-IV-TR (American Psychiatric Association 2000), whereas malingering is assigned a V code. However, these two entities differ only in whether there are clear-cut external benefits accruing from the symptom production (malingering) or whether the symptoms are produced or feigned for the sole purpose of assuming the sick role (factitious disorders). When perceived incentives are used as a diagnostic criterion, imprecision in diagnosis is bound to arise; indeed, behavior is often motivated by a variety of conscious and unconscious objectives, and a person may feign illness in order to achieve different goals at different times (Eisendrath 1996) (see Figure 25–1). Although the medical literature contains numerous bizarre examples of simulated illness, these cases merely represent one end on a continuum of illness portrayals. On the other end are normal illness behaviors that are somewhat common, such as the use of physical symptoms to avoid undesired social obligations (e.g., a "tummyache" to avoid going to school).

There has been an increasing recognition and interest referable to factitious disorders. By early 1999, almost 1,300 journal articles had been published in which factitious illness was the predominant topic, and more recently, several books have been devoted to these disorders (e.g., Adshead and Brooke 1999; Artingstall 1998; Feldman and Eisendrath 1996; Feldman and Ford 1994; Schreier and Libow 1993).

The inventive capabilities of some persons to use deceptive means to seek attention and nurturance seem almost endless. Two additional syndromes that are related to factitious disorders are those of factitial (fictitious) allegations of sexual abuse and the use of the Internet and e-mail to create fictional identities and diseases. Several cases of factitial sexual abuse, stalking, and harassment have been reported (Feldman et al. 1994; Feldman-Schorrig 1996; Gibbon 1998), the primary object of which appears to be the pursuit of concern and care. Feldman (2000) reported four situations in which persons used Internet support groups to create fictional diseases to gain attention and sympathy. Discovery of the fraud proved deleterious to group members with genuine disease. Yet another syndrome that appears closely related to factitious disorder by proxy is that of the "angels of death": nurses who create emergency situations in their patients (Yorker 1996). Reuber et al. (2000) reported on a man who, claiming to be a physician, made numerous telephone calls to physicians and emergency rooms requesting advice on handling medical situations and/or alerting them to an imminent admission to their services. The man was known to have simulated status epilepticus.

Hardie and Reed (1998) noted the overlap in characteristics of persons with pseudologia fantastica, factitious disorders, and impostureship. Their proposal to use the term *deception syndrome* to describe many of the syndromes described above has some merit.

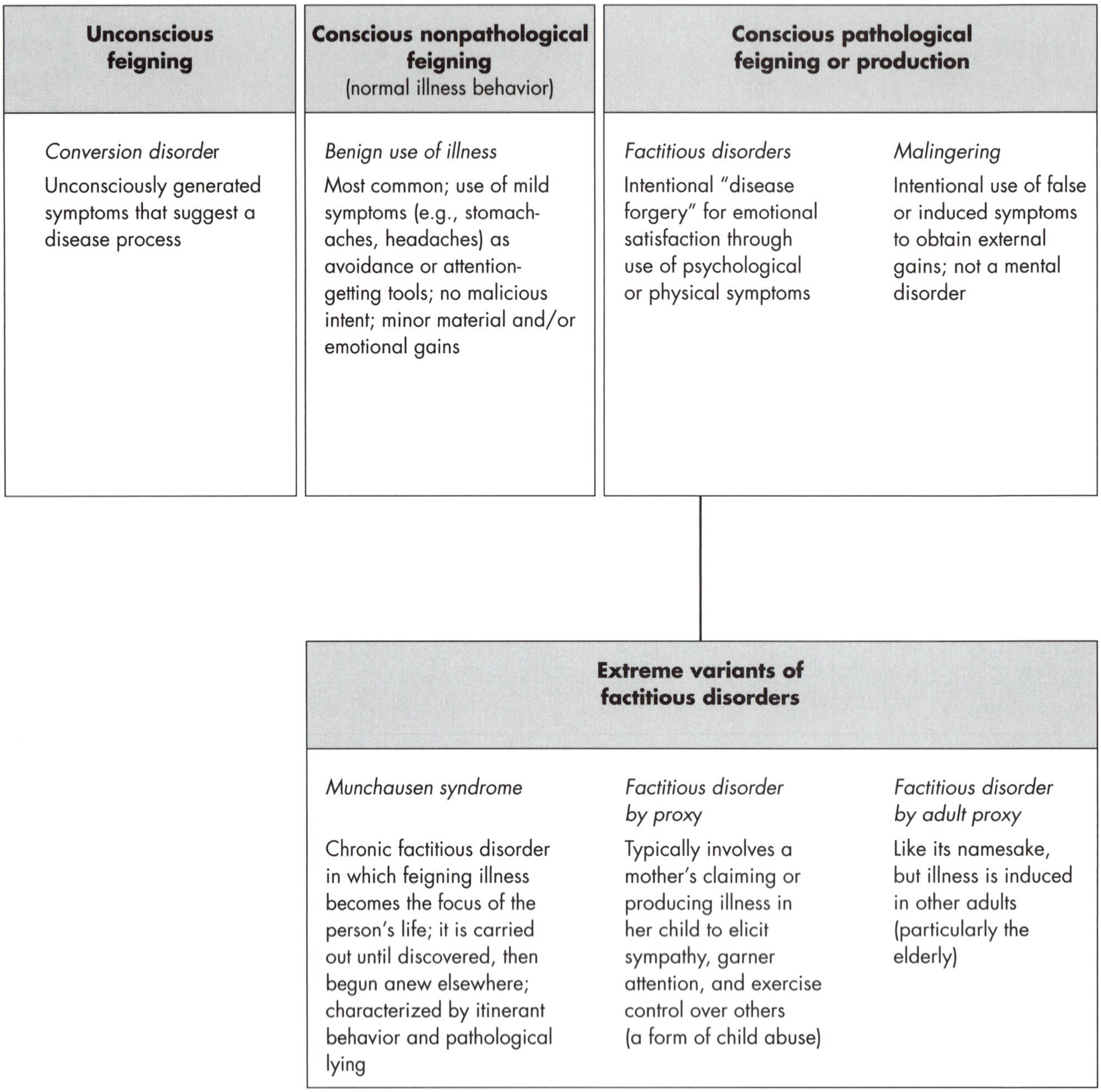

Unconscious feigning	**Conscious nonpathological feigning** (normal illness behavior)	**Conscious pathological feigning or production**	
Conversion disorder Unconsciously generated symptoms that suggest a disease process	*Benign use of illness* Most common; use of mild symptoms (e.g., stomach-aches, headaches) as avoidance or attention-getting tools; no malicious intent; minor material and/or emotional gains	*Factitious disorders* Intentional "disease forgery" for emotional satisfaction through use of psychological or physical symptoms	*Malingering* Intentional use of false or induced symptoms to obtain external gains; not a mental disorder

Extreme variants of factitious disorders		
Munchausen syndrome Chronic factitious disorder in which feigning illness becomes the focus of the person's life; it is carried out until discovered, then begun anew elsewhere; characterized by itinerant behavior and pathological lying	*Factitious disorder by proxy* Typically involves a mother's claiming or producing illness in her child to elicit sympathy, garner attention, and exercise control over others (a form of child abuse)	*Factitious disorder by adult proxy* Like its namesake, but illness is induced in other adults (particularly the elderly)

FIGURE 25–1. Simulation of disease.

Although the headings in this chapter are traditional diagnoses, the reader is advised that crisp delineations exist much more frequently in textbooks than in real-life clinical situations.

FACTITIOUS DISORDERS

Patients who have factitious disorders intentionally feign, exaggerate, aggravate, or self-induce diseases or symptoms. These patients are conscious of their behaviors, although their underlying motivations may be unconscious. By convention, a diagnosis of factitious disorder does not apply to individuals who readily acknowledge that they have produced their own medical signs and symptoms (e.g., patients who self-mutilate).

Inherent in factitious disorders is an unsettling paradox: the patient presents to a physician ostensibly for thorough medical care but simultaneously conceals the cause of the malady, making definitive care impossible. In chronic factitious disorder, or Munchausen syndrome, dramatic illness—typically associated with gratuitous lying and traveling or wanderlust—allows the patient to achieve the goal of multiple hospitalizations. More recent recognition of factitious disorder by proxy (or Munchausen syndrome by proxy), in which signs and symptoms are created in another person, has resulted in frightening insights about children whose recurrent illnesses had previously seemed inexplicable. It has also provided glimpses into the multigenerational web of abnormal illness behaviors that exists in many families.

Epidemiology

Because willful deception is inherent in factitious disorders, traditional epidemiologic techniques are unlikely to provide accurate data. Information about incidence, prevalence, and demographic features must therefore be inferred from single-case studies, a few reported series, and referral patterns. For example, Sutherland and Rodin (1990) noted that 10 of 1,288 inpatients (or 0.8%) at a large teaching hospital in Toronto, Ontario, who were referred consecutively for psychiatric consultation had a diagnosis of factitious disorder. A similar percentage (0.6%) was reported for a German university hospital psychiatric consultation service (Kapfhammer et al. 1998). At the National Institute of Allergy and Infectious Diseases, Aduan et al. (1979) diagnosed factitious disorders in 9.3% of the patients referred for evaluation of fever of unknown origin, and such higher prevalence statistics have been reported consistently in highly specialized treatment settings. A different mechanism for estimating frequency was used by Gault and colleagues (1988), who analyzed material submitted by patients as "kidney stones." Of these, 3.5% of the stones were obviously nonphysiologic and artifactual. Even when false stones that might have been presented innocently were eliminated, 2.6% remained as representing probable attempts to deceive physicians.

It is clear that the subtype of factitious disorder patients with Munchausen syndrome is relatively small (Kapfhammer et al. 1998). However, estimates of incidence are unreliable because the terms *factitious disorder* and *Munchausen syndrome* are used imprecisely, if not interchangeably, in much of the literature (Fink and Jensen 1989).

Factitious disorder by proxy is estimated currently to account for fewer than 1,000 of the more than 2.5 million cases of child abuse reported each year in the United States, but recognition of these cases is increasing worldwide, and approximately 100 published case reports have come from non-English-speaking and developing countries. For example, Rahilly (1991), who described infants brought to an Australian clinic because

of apparently life-threatening episodes, asserted that 1.5% of these cases represented possible factitious disorder by proxy. McClure et al. (1996) computed an annual incidence of Munchausen syndrome by proxy in the United Kingdom of at least 0.5 of 100,000 for children younger than 16 years and at least 2.8 of 100,000 for children younger than 1 year. Meadow (1999) carefully reviewed cases of sudden infant death and found that many deaths attributed to sudden infant death syndrome fit the phenomenological pattern of Munchausen syndrome by proxy. This suggests that cases of Munchausen syndrome by proxy often are misdiagnosed as spontaneous illness.

The two general phenomenological patterns of factitious disorder reflect different demographic characteristics. Factitious disorder patients with Munchausen syndrome tend to be middle-aged men who are usually unmarried and estranged from their families. The remaining patients with factitious disorders usually are women, aged 20–40 years, who work in medical occupations such as nursing or medical technology (Carney and Brown 1983; Ford 1983). Patients with factitious disorder by proxy are the mothers in almost all reported cases, although fathers or other caregivers (e.g., grandmothers, baby-sitters) are sometimes reported (Meadow 1998). The victim is generally a preverbal child, but some victims are older; in one infamous case, three adults were victimized by the same man (Sigal et al. 1991).

Child and adolescent illness falsification without the parents' knowledge may also occur. Libow (2000), in her review of the literature, identified 42 such cases, the majority of which involved females.

Clinical Features

Factitious Disorder With Predominantly Physical Symptoms

The range of physical symptoms and signs simulated or induced by factitious disorder patients challenges the imagination. Essentially, every known disease has been fabricated, including esoteric maladies unfamiliar to most physicians. Symptoms may be so bizarre as to include complaints such as "green sweat" (MacSween and Millard 2000). These ruses are reported in a variety of both general and subspecialty medical journals. In recent years, reflecting the times, sophisticated enactments of acquired immunodeficiency syndrome (AIDS) and systemic lupus erythematosus (Tlacuilo-Parra et al. 2000; Zuger and O'Dowd 1992). A partial list of diseases simulated by factitious disorder patients is provided in Table 25–1.

TABLE 25–1. Some signs, symptoms, and diseases simulated in or caused by factitious behavior

More common	Less common
Autoimmune diseases	Acquired immunodeficiency syndrome (AIDS)
Bleeding (e.g., hematuria)	Anaplastic anemia
Cancer	Cushing's disease
Chronic diarrhea	Diabetes mellitus
Dizziness or syncope	Gangrene
Epilepsy	Goodpasture's syndrome
Fever of unknown origin	Hemiplegia
Hypoglycemia	Hypersomnia
Impaired wound healing	Hypertension
Infection	Hyperthyroidism
Intestinal bleeding	Hypotension
Iron-deficiency anemia	Myocardial infarction
Kidney stones	Pheochromocytoma
Rashes	Pupillary dysfunction
Seizures	Reflex sympathetic dystrophy
	Septic arthritis
	Thrombocytopenia
	Torsion dystonia
	Uterine bleeding
	Ventricular tachycardia

Modern interest in factitious disorders was stimulated by Asher's (1951) whimsical article describing and naming Munchausen syndrome. Despite the misnomer—Baron von Munchausen (1720–1791) was really an honorable man and a war hero—and despite frequent criticism of the term, the Munchausen eponym persists when references are made to cases of chronic factitious disorder. Other features that are typically encountered in patients with Munchausen syndrome are included in Table 25–2.

TABLE 25–2. Characteristic features of Munchausen syndrome

Simulation or production of signs and symptoms that are plausible but unusual or dramatic

Pseudologia fantastica, which is engaging (but pathological) lying (e.g., the patient may falsely present himself or herself as a college president)

Peregrination, or widespread travel associated with numerous hospitalizations (more than 500 admissions have been reported for a single patient) (Von Maur et al. 1973)

Patients with Munchausen syndrome frequently present to the emergency room of large teaching hospitals during the evening hours or on the weekend, presumably because insurance offices are closed and more inexperienced members of the house staff are on duty. Dramatic signs and symptoms, such as gross bleeding, incapacitating chest pain, or apparent seizures or coma, may divert attention from other patients. Alternatively, the patient may provide a history typical of an unusual and intriguing disease, such as porphyria or Mediterranean fever. After admission to the hospital, the patient becomes widely known, sometimes offering claims such as being a former major league baseball player, an awardee of a Congressional Medal of Honor, or a foreign dignitary. Despite their reputed prominence, however, these patients infrequently receive visitors, and the physicians rarely receive telephone calls from concerned family members or friends. The patient is usually surprisingly willing to undergo invasive tests and procedures. Ultimately, inconsistencies in the personal history or medical findings create suspicions among the staff. When caregivers become more confrontational, the patient responds with irritation, renewed physical complaints, or disruptive behavior. The patient may belligerently demand discharge against medical advice, threaten to file a lawsuit, or simply disappear. The red-faced clinicians on the treatment team then console themselves by writing a case report for publication.

Although patients with classic Munchausen syndrome as described by Asher (1951) do exist, the more common form of factitious disorders is not so dramatic. With the more common form, the features of peregrination and pseudologia fantastica are typically less pronounced or absent. Whereas referrals for consultation to major diagnostic centers are common, the individual primarily seeks medical care within one community for symptoms that do not remit with usual treatments. Among the symptoms and signs frequently reported within this group of patients are hypoglycemic episodes (Freyberger et al. 1994; Grunberger et al. 1988), recurrent infections or abscesses (Freyberger et al. 1994; P. Reich and Gottfried 1983), blood dyscrasias (Freyberger et al. 1994), simulated renal colic (J.D. Reich and Hanno 1997), neurological syndromes (Bauer and Boegner 1996), and obstetrics and gynecology syndromes (Edi-Osagie et al. 1998).

These patients, usually single women, tend to have medical insurance and are often readmitted to the same hospitals; there, they become well known to the staff, regard themselves as "special" patients, and are commonly at the center of ward conflicts and emotional controversies among staff members. Some treatment team members have difficulty accepting the factitious nature of the symptoms even when presented with incontrovertible evidence. Family members may be involved but are often either overly enmeshed or peculiarly distant. Borderline personality traits are characteristic of these patients and may be evident on psychological testing. Although the patient may describe fantasized relationships, evidence of the capacity for intimacy and mature sexual relationships is almost always lacking. One discovers, with time, that although pseudologia fantastica is absent, more subtle prevarication is present, and the information presented is a rich mélange of fact and fantasy.

Factitious Disorder With Predominantly Psychological Symptoms

The bulk of the published cases of factitious disorder involve physical symptoms alone. Factitious psychological symptoms are most often seen by clinicians in conjunction with physical complaints (authentic or fabricated). As a result, psychiatrists are more likely to encounter patients with factitious psychological symptoms on medical-surgical wards or in the emergency room than to see such patients on psychiatric units.

Although reports of factitious disorder with psychological symptoms alone are infrequent, the traits that are typically manifested in such cases resemble those seen in Munchausen syndrome. Those traits include itinerancy, aggressiveness, a lack of intimate or sustained relationships, and falsification of background information (Popli et al. 1992).

As is common among patients with factitious disorder with physical symptoms, patients with this variant of factitious disorder may creatively fabricate a wide range of symptoms. The features most commonly reported—including depression and suicidal thinking—are frequently tied to claims of bereavement (Phillips et al. 1983; Snowden et al. 1978). The patient purports that his or her emotional distress is the result of the death of someone close, such as a parent or child. The distress appears genuine, is often accompanied by copious tears, and elicits sympathy from medical personnel. Later, the staff members discover that the mourned person is still very much alive or that the circumstances of the death were much less dramatic than the patient claims.

Case reports describe feigned multiple personality disorder (dissociative identity disorder), substance dependence, dissociative and conversion reactions, memory loss, and posttraumatic stress disorder. Multiple feigned psychological syndromes may occur in the same patient (Parker 1993). Some researchers urge great cau-

tion in diagnosing factitious disorder with predominantly psychological symptoms, especially factitious psychosis; some patients with these symptoms eventually manifest clear-cut psychotic disorders, such as schizophrenia (Nicholson and Roberts 1994; Rogers et al. 1989).

Patients with factitious disorder with predominantly psychological symptoms may have Ganser's syndrome, which is characterized by the provision of approximate answers, or *vorbeireden*, to questions (e.g., the examiner asks, "What is the color of snow?" and the patient answers "Green"). Amnesia, disorientation, and perceptual disturbance are generally present as well. This syndrome was originally described by Sigbert Ganser (1965) as a form of malingering used by prisoners; however, it has been described in other settings, including general hospital units (Dalfen and Anthony 2000; Weiner and Braiman 1955). Ganser's syndrome was described in one patient who also had clear-cut factitious physical and psychological symptoms (Parker 1993). The etiology has been questioned; in addition to malingering, it has been proposed to stem from hysteria (dissociation) or organic brain disease (Sigal et al. 1992).

Factitious Disorder With Combined Physical and Psychological Symptoms

When the patient presents with both physical and psychological factitious symptoms and neither predominates, the appropriate diagnosis is factitious disorder with combined physical and psychological symptoms. The aforementioned case reported by Parker (1993) included pseudodementia (Ganser's syndrome), feigned bereavement, factitious rape, and pseudoseizures.

Factitious Disorder Not Otherwise Specified

Meadow (1977) coined the term *Munchausen syndrome by proxy* (introduced as "factitious disorder by proxy" in DSM-IV [American Psychiatric Association 1994]) to refer to a form of child abuse in which an individual surreptitiously produces signs of disease in a child and then seeks medical care for that child. Associated with this invidious behavior are the risks associated with not only the original ailment but also the resultant procedures and medication trials. Meadow's description of this syndrome is reaffirmed by case reports from around the world, including from non-Western cultures (Bappal et al. 2001).

Typically, a child is admitted to the hospital with symptoms such as seizures, bleeding, diarrhea, or respiratory/apneic difficulties. The mother, who often has a history of some medical training, characteristically assists the nurses and readily consents to any invasive diagnostic procedures proposed for the child. Discovery of her role in the production of the child's symptoms may occur accidentally, such as finding her smothering the child with a pillow or introducing a toxic substance into the child's mouth or intravenous tubing. Suspicions also may arise if symptoms or episodes of illness arise only when the mother is alone with the child, if another child in the family has had unexplained illnesses, or if the child's medical problems do not respond to appropriate treatment.

Adults who perpetuate factitious disorder by proxy may seem superficially quite normal, and in fact, evaluation of them has not always resulted in a psychiatric diagnosis (Meadow 1985). Others meet criteria for a somatoform disorder or personality disorder or have previously produced factitious disease in themselves (Bools et al. 1994). Of ominous note is the fact that 9% of these children die if they are not taken out of the home (Rosenberg 1987). In addition, severe psychological morbidity, such as hyperactivity, symptoms of posttraumatic stress disorder, and personal adoption of Munchausen syndrome behavior, is reported in children and adults who have been subjected to factitious disorder by proxy (Bools et al. 1993; Libow 1995; McGuire and Feldman 1989).

Etiology

Most authors have emphasized psychodynamic factors as initiating and perpetuating factitious behavior. Some of the proposed psychodynamic explanations for factitious disorders are shown in Table 25–3.

Some recent explanations for Munchausen syndrome emphasize the possible role of underlying brain dysfunction. Approximately 20%–25% of the patients with Munchausen syndrome have some suggestion of brain dysfunction (Ford 1996b; King and Ford 1988). There are often findings on brain imaging (Babe et al. 1992; Fenelon et al. 1991) or neuropsychological testing. Pankratz and Lezak (1987) found that about one-third of their series of patients with Munchausen syndrome had deficits in conceptual organization and judgment. These authors postulated an interaction between impaired information processing and psychodynamic factors.

Differential Diagnosis and Diagnosis

The diagnosis of factitious disorders is generally established by one of four routes (Table 25–4). The consultation-liaison psychiatrist is usually asked for help either when suspicions are raised or after the diagnosis of factitious disorder is already established. When the diagnosis

TABLE 25–3.   Psychodynamic explanations for factitious disorders

Longing for nurturance and the use of illness to place demands on others to provide care

Reaction to loss; an attempt to deal with feelings of abandonment and helplessness

Use of deceit to create a feeling of power and superiority ("duping delight")

Use of deceit as a form of angry "acting out" toward physicians, who may also be serving as transference objects

Source.   Babe et al. 1992; Cramer et al. 1971; Feldman and Escalona 1991; Ford 1983.

is not yet confirmed, the psychiatric consultant may assist the medical team by providing ethical and legal guidelines for further investigations (see subsection "Ethical and Legal Issues" below). The consultants also should evaluate the patient for characteristics such as pseudologia fantastica and a concurrent personality disorder.

To develop a sound management plan, determination of both physical and psychiatric comorbidity in patients with factitious disorder is essential. Patients with factitious disorder may also have legitimate physical findings, the presence of which mislead their physicians. For example, a patient may learn that he or she has congenital nystagmus. When he or she presents at an emergency room complaining of a recent "head injury," admission to the hospital is a virtual certainty (Ford 1982). Another patient with genuine diabetes may manipulate hypoglycemic agents to create symptoms (Grunberger et al. 1988). Comorbid psychiatric findings that patients are likely to have include personality disorders, especially the borderline, histrionic, and antisocial subtypes (Carney and Brown 1983; Ford 1983).

TABLE 25–4.   Four methods to establish the diagnosis of factitious disorder

1. The patient is fortuitously discovered while engaging in factitious illness behavior (e.g., self-injecting air to create subcutaneous emphysema) (Karnik et al. 1990).
2. Incriminating paraphernalia, such as syringes and medications, are noted among the patient's belongings.
3. Laboratory findings suggest a factitious etiology (e.g., inappropriately high insulin levels and low C-peptide levels in a hypoglycemic individual surreptitiously injecting insulin) (Horwitz 1989).
4. The diagnosis is made by exclusion because there is no known disease that could explain the findings, which are also consistent with the known features of factitious disorder.

Management

Ethical and Legal Issues

Patients with factitious disorders often are approached with little attention to their personal rights. This cavalier attitude developed, in part, from a belief by health care practitioners that the patients falsified their histories and physical examinations so there is little danger of a malpractice suit. Thus, a patient suspected of having factitious disorder might be sent to have X rays so that his or her room can simultaneously be searched for medical paraphernalia. In one situation, to prove a patient's surreptitious insulin use, a vial of insulin found during a search was spiked with a radioactive compound and the patient was monitored for radioactivity (Berkowitz et al. 1971). Recent changes in medical practice in the United States have emphasized patients' rights and informed consent. As a result, it is now apparent that many practices, such as clandestine searches of personal articles, are not ethically or legally acceptable (Feldman and Ford 1994; Ford 1996a). An individual suspected of factitious behavior must be accorded the same rights as other patients; among these rights are 1) personal privacy, including that of one's belongings; 2) confidentiality; and 3) informed consent, which mandates that caregivers provide information about the nature of proposed diagnostic procedures, including those aimed solely at detecting factitious behavior.

Patients with factitious disorder can and do sue (Eisendrath and Feder 1996; *Ford v. United States of America* 1987; Lipsitt 1986). Because many of these patients have borderline personality dynamics, idealization of the physician may be followed by devaluation and vindictive behaviors such as malpractice suits (Feldman and Ford 1994). Thus, when a patient is suspected of factitious disorder, it is prudent to take the steps outlined in Table 25–5.

TABLE 25–5. Steps to take when factitious disorders are suspected

1. Involve the hospital administration from the start.
2. Seek legal advice from the hospital's risk management department and/or the physician's own attorney.
3. Consult with the hospital ethics committee early on.
4. Maintain confidentiality to the extent specified by law. The "blacklists" of Munchausen patients advocated by some authors (Mohammed et al. 1985) are not legally acceptable in the United States (Kass 1985).

When evaluating a patient suspected of factitious disorder, it is generally best to communicate one's concerns to the patient early in the diagnostic process. Physicians must keep in mind that they are healers and not amateur sleuths. A nonconfrontational, nonadversarial approach is unlikely to offend patients who are not engaging in any deception; however, patients with factitious disorder may choose to seek care elsewhere. If so, this decision limits the physician's role in maintenance of the ruse and may help set the stage for an effective therapeutic intervention later on.

An important legal issue for psychiatrists is whether patients with factitious disorder are subject to commitment for involuntary psychiatric hospitalization (Feldman and Ford 1994; Ford 1996a). Their behavior is indeed self-destructive, but the thresholds for commitment vary by jurisdiction. Few cases exist in the United States in which a patient was committed solely on the basis of a factitious disorder. Regardless, the outpatient commitment of one patient in Oregon, which resulted in lower medical costs and less iatrogenic morbidity to the patient, suggests that this method may hold promise in controlling illness behavior (McFarland et al. 1983).

Factitious disorder by proxy presents a unique medicolegal challenge because it is a form of child abuse. In cases of possible factitious disorder by proxy, physicians in the United States must, by law, share their suspicions with the proper civil authorities. It must also be kept in mind that the child is at risk and helpless to protect himself or herself; therefore, more aggressive investigative approaches are justified (Samuels et al. 1992). For example, one may consider hidden video surveillance of a hospitalized child (Southall et al. 1997). Hall and colleagues (2000) reported that a diagnosis of Munchausen syndrome by proxy was made in 23 of 41 patients monitored by covert video surveillance. In 4 patients, surveillance was instrumental in establishing the innocence of the parents. Hall et al. (2000) concluded that covert video surveillance is required to make a definitive and timely diagnosis in most cases and that without this diagnostic tool, many cases will go undetected, placing children at risk. It must be kept in mind that such procedures raise legal and ethical issues in regard to invasion of privacy (Anonymous 2000) and that it is essential to have in place a plan for intervention if illness-producing behavior is detected.

Confrontation

Recognition is the first step in treating any disorder. The second step might be a consultation-liaison psychiatrist's discussion of factitious illness with the team. In some situations, the psychiatrist may gently confront the patient directly, with a redefinition of the nature of distress as a psychological problem for which help will be provided. In these situations, a period of brief inpatient psychiatric treatment may facilitate a therapeutic alliance and subsequent outpatient psychotherapy. In other situations, a direct confrontation may be regarded as unwise, and more indirect ways of communicating the patient's behavior may allow the patient a face-saving mechanism to discontinue his or her disease-simulating behavior. Comorbid psychiatric diagnoses, such as major depression, should be vigorously treated with the appropriate modalities (Earle and Folks 1986). A similar approach is taken with factitious disorder by proxy perpetrators, although the denial in these cases is typically tenacious and is often buttressed by spouses or other physicians; for this reason, steps to protect the child must be in place before any degree of confrontation. The child generally must be removed from the home regardless of whether the perpetrator acknowledges the abusive behavior.

Techniques proposed for the psychotherapy of factitious disorders have ranged from vigorous, persistent confrontation (Stone 1977) to a supportive approach incorporating face-saving measures (Eisendrath and Feder 1996). The latter approach is in wider favor among clinicians because of the emotional fragility of these patients. As therapy proceeds, the factitious disorder patient may engage in new episodes of factitious illness behavior or may make suicidal gestures. These responses are more likely to occur with confrontation of prevarications or with perceived rejections, such as the therapist's vacations. In view of these patients' severe underlying personality disorders, therapeutic gains are customarily very modest. Ideally, the therapist's consistency in providing support reduces the patient's need for acting-out behaviors. The primary care physician's regularly scheduled examinations of the patient serve the same purpose.

Prognosis

Factitious disorders are *not* benign conditions. They are associated with considerable morbidity and even mortality (Grunberger et al. 1988; Meadow 1999; Nichols et al. 1990; Sutherland and Rodin 1990). Relatively few patients accept referral for psychiatric treatment, and of these, even fewer are "cured" of their factitious behavior (Grunberger et al. 1988; Sutherland and Rodin 1990). At present, we can do little more than echo Abram and Hollender's (1974) observation that, when confronted, some patients deny their behavior but stop it, some acknowledge it and enter psychiatric treatment, but most transfer their medical care elsewhere and continue their factitious illness behaviors. Some Munchausen patients who have

discontinued their deceptions have done so as a result of gradual life change or establishment of social support rather than psychiatric treatment per se.

MALINGERING

By definition, individuals with malingering are motivated by specific, recognizable external incentives to produce or simulate physical or psychological illness (American Psychiatric Association 2000; Gorman 1982). Examples of these incentives are deferment from military service, avoidance of hazardous work assignments, receipt of financial rewards such as disability payments, escape from incarceration (e.g., not guilty by reason of insanity), or procurement of controlled substances. As we explore the psychological aspects of malingering, we must also keep in mind the admonition of Szasz (1956) that malingering is not a psychiatric diagnosis but an accusation.

Epidemiology

Malingering occurs in settings where external, often tangible gains are accrued by illness. Among these settings are prisons, the military, courtrooms hearing personal or industrial injury disputes, and the offices of physicians who are performing disability evaluations. Flicken (1956) estimated that approximately 5% of the patients who were conscripted for military service attempted to avoid it by feigning or manufacturing symptoms.

Mayou (1995), who conducted a prospective study in the United Kingdom on the outcome of persons involved in motor vehicle accidents, found that malingering to gain compensation was remarkably uncommon. He suggested that high rates found in some tertiary care centers represent atypical samples. On the other hand, Kay and Morris-Jones (1998) found clear-cut surveillance videotape evidence that at least 20% of the medicolegal litigants in a pain clinic were overtly malingering their symptoms. Financial incentives do make a difference in symptoms and disability. Binder and Rohling (1996), in their meta-analysis of 2,353 subjects, found more abnormality and disability in patients with mild closed-head injury who had financial incentives than in those who did not have such an incentive.

Clinical Features

Malingered symptoms fall into four major categories (Table 25–6). The deliberate embellishment of previous or concurrent illness is probably the form of malingering most frequently encountered by consultation-liaison psy-

TABLE 25–6. Categories of malingered symptoms

Production or simulation of an illness (e.g., the use of thyroxine to mimic hyperthyroidism)

Exacerbation of a previous illness (e.g., deliberate infection of a surgical wound)

Exaggeration of symptoms of a previous or concurrent illness (e.g., embellished complaints of pain)

Falsification of laboratory samples or medical reports

chiatrists. The symptoms reported are usually difficult to quantify objectively. They include pain (particularly back pain), dizziness, weakness, seizures or "spells," and features of posttraumatic stress disorder (Sparr and Pankratz 1983). Patients may intensify their complaints when they are asked directly about their symptoms or when they think that they are being observed. When distracted by television or visitors, however, they become visibly more relaxed and are able to engage in physical activities incompatible with their symptom reports.

Etiology

The diagnosis of malingering is established by the presence of specific gain, but there is often considerable difficulty in distinguishing malingering from conversion or factitious disorder. Even consciously motivated malingerers may have unconscious motives as well. "Pseudomalingering" arises when the patient uses an external incentive as a rationalization for malingering symptoms, shielding himself or herself from awareness of unconscious determinants (Ford 1983; Schneck 1962). For example, a genuinely psychotic person may believe he or she is feigning psychosis to escape punishment for a crime.

Bellamy (1997) proposed that "most exaggerated illness behavior in compensation situations takes place because of a combination of suggestion, somatization and rationalization" (p. 94). Other factors influencing exaggeration include a victim status with a distorted sense of justice and an adversarial legal system that challenges the claimant to prove his or her disability. Lees-Haley (1997), who analyzed the Minnesota Multiphasic Personality Inventory—2 (MMPI-2; Hathaway and McKinley 1989) findings of a large number of personal injury plaintiffs, interpreted these profiles in a manner consistent with Bellamy's observations.

Diagnosis and Differential Diagnosis

The "mission impossible" often requested of the consulting psychiatrist is to determine whether a patient is malingering. The clinician should consider malingering when symptom complaints and objective data are incongruent. Suspicions also may be raised, at times unfairly, when the patient is engaged in litigation or is seeking disability funding. To convincingly suggest malingering in these situations, the consultation-liaison psychiatrist must verify an external motivation and show that there is limited or no objective evidence for the patient's symptoms. It must be kept in mind, however, that malingering is basically a legal rather than medical determination, and the psychiatric consultant is advised to report findings and a differential diagnosis but to be cautious in making accusations of motivations.

The differential diagnosis of malingering includes somatoform disorders (conversion disorder, hypochondriasis, somatization disorder, pain disorder, body dysmorphic disorder) and factitious disorders. These clinical syndromes have indistinct boundaries, so a person may meet the criteria for different disorders at different times (Ford 1992; Jonas and Pope 1985; Nadelson 1985).

Furthermore, Cameron (1947) stated that conversion disorder and malingering are on a continuum, representing opposite poles of purely unconscious and purely conscious motivation. It is difficult for the diagnostician to know the patient's location on the continuum at any moment. Relevant factors include evidence of past somatization, as well as the coexistence of anxiety, mood, substance, or personality disorders that may contribute to symptom presentations. Patients with unconsciously determined somatoform disorders (e.g., conversion) usually are consistent in their symptom presentation, irrespective of their audience; as noted, malingerers may show markedly different behaviors when they believe that they are being observed.

Evidence obtained by attorneys and insurance companies is often not readily available to the psychiatric consultant who is not, and cannot be, a detective. In "high stakes" litigation, it is not uncommon for private detectives to videotape an individual's activities outside the hospital. A jury may be powerfully influenced by photographs of a man taking a beautiful swing on the golf links but who is unable to raise his arms above his shoulders in the doctor's office.

Psychological testing is often helpful in identifying malingering patients. The MMPI-2 is a useful test for patients who distort their presentations (Lees-Haley and Fox 1990; McCaffrey and Bellamy-Campbell 1989; Wetzler and Marlowe 1990). This test and others have diagnostic value in those who exaggerate physical and/or psychological symptoms (Cliffe 1992; Perconte and Goreczny 1990; Rawling 1992). Screening instruments with face validity, such as the Beck Depression Inventory and the Symptom Checklist—90, are easily distorted by patients who embellish their symptoms (Lees-Haley 1989a, 1989b) and have very limited value in the determination of malingering.

It cannot be overemphasized that no single evaluation technique will unequivocally identify malingerers. This is particularly true when the examiner makes a subjective assessment of a feature such as sincerity of effort (Lechner et al. 1998; Main and Waddell 1998). Rather, patients must be evaluated from a complete physical and psychosocial perspective that includes various possibilities such as pseudomalingering (Ford 1983).

Management

Malingering is basically a legal rather than a medical issue. With this fact in mind, the primary physician and consultation-liaison psychiatrist must be circumspect in their approach to the patient. Every note must be written with the understanding that it will likely become a courtroom exhibit. Malingering is often listed among the diagnostic possibilities but is rarely proved conclusively in medical settings.

The patient who is suspected of malingering should not be confronted with a direct accusation. Instead, subtle communication indicates that the physician is "onto the game" (Kramer et al. 1979). One technique is to mention, almost in passing, that diagnostic tests indicate no "organic" basis for the symptoms. The malingerer may feel freer to discard the symptoms if the physician suggests that patients with similar problems usually recover after a certain procedure is performed or a particular length of time has passed. Such suggestions are often followed by perceptible improvement, if not recovery. Still, some patients—particularly those seeking drugs—will leave treatment and seek medical care elsewhere. Others, in an effort to prove the existence of their disease, may vastly intensify their symptoms. In doing so, they may create such caricatures of the illness that the effort to malinger becomes obvious to all.

Prognosis

No information is available about the long-term outcome of persons who malinger. One can presume that when a person is successful in the deception, his or her behavior is reinforced and is more likely to recur. Also, the morality of some cases of malingering is debatable. For instance, during periods when the draft is in force, malingering to avoid service in the United States military is illegal and has been viewed as immoral by most Americans. Would malingering to avoid conscription in a coun-

try like Nazi Germany be viewed in the same way? From this perspective, particular examples of malingering are viewed as adaptational mechanisms rather than as indications of pathology (Rogers 1990).

SUMMARY AND CONCLUSION

Requests for psychiatric consultation on patients with suspected factitious disorders or malingering are relatively infrequent. However, when the consultation-liaison psychiatrist becomes involved with one of these cases, a disproportionate amount of time is typically invested. Issues of diagnosis, legal and ethical considerations, and the need to provide liaison services for members of the medical care staff may make one of these patients the primary focus of one's clinical activities for several days. Nevertheless, they are fascinating patients who show the extreme end of the continuum of abnormal illness behavior. They are rarely forgotten.

REFERENCES

Abram HS, Hollender MH: Factitious blood disease. South Med J 67:691–696, 1974

Adams F: The Seven Books of Paulus Aegineta, Vol II. London, England, Sydenham Society, 1846

Adshead G, Brooke D (eds): Munchausen's Syndrome by Proxy: Current Issues in Assessment, Treatment and Research. London, England, Imperial College Press, 1999

Aduan RP, Fauci AS, Dale DC, et al: Factitious fever and self-induced infection: a report of 32 cases and a review of the literature. Ann Intern Med 90:230–242, 1979

American Psychiatric Association: Diagnostic and Statistical Manual of Mental Disorders, 4th Edition. Washington, DC, American Psychiatric Association, 1994

American Psychiatric Association: Diagnostic and Statistical Manual of Mental Disorders, 4th Edition, Text Revision. Washington, DC, American Psychiatric Association, 2000

Anonymous: Using hidden cameras to monitor suspected parental abuse: a security requirement or an invasion of privacy? Hospital Security and Safety Management 21:5–8, 2000

Artingstall K: Practical Aspects of Munchausen by Proxy and Munchausen Syndrome Investigation. Boca Raton, FL, CRC Press, 1998

Asher R: Munchausen's syndrome. Lancet 1:339–341, 1951

Babe KS Jr, Peterson AM, Loosen PT, et al: The pathogenesis of Munchausen syndrome: a review and case report. Gen Hosp Psychiatry 14:273–276, 1992

Bappal B, George M, Nair R, et al: Factitious hypoglycemia: a tale from the Arab world. Pediatrics 107:180–181, 2001

Bauer M, Boegner F: Neurological syndromes in factitious disorder. J Nerv Ment Dis 184:281–288, 1996

Bellamy R: Compensation neurosis: financial reward for illness as nocebo. Clin Orthop 336:94–106, 1997

Berkowitz S, Parrish JE, Field JB: Factitious hypoglycemia: why not diagnose before laparotomy. Am J Med 51:669–674, 1971

Binder LM, Rohling ML: Money matters: a meta-analytic review of the effects of financial incentives on recovery after closed-head injury. Am J Psychiatry 153:7–10, 1996

Bools CN, Neale BA, Meadow SR: Follow up of victims of fabricated illness (Munchausen syndrome by proxy). Arch Dis Child 69:625–630, 1993

Bools C, Neale B, Meadow R: Munchausen syndrome by proxy: a study of psychopathology. Child Abuse Negl 18:773–788, 1994

Cameron NA: The Psychology of Behavior Disorders. Boston, MA, Houghton Mifflin, 1947

Carney MWP, Brown JP: Clinical features and motives among 42 artifactual illness patients. Br J Med Psychol 56:57–66, 1983

Cliffe MJ: Symptom-validity testing of feigned sensory or memory deficits: a further elaboration for subjects who understand the rationale. Br J Clin Psychol 31:207–209, 1992

Cramer B, Gershberg MR, Stern M: Munchausen syndrome: its relationship to malingering, hysteria and the doctor-patient relationship. Arch Gen Psychiatry 24:573–578, 1971

Dalfen AK, Anthony F: Head injury, dissociation and the Ganser syndrome. Brain Inj 14:1101-1105, 2000

Earle JR Jr, Folks DG: Factitious disorder and coexisting depression: a report of a successful psychiatric consultation and case management. Gen Hosp Psychiatry 8:448–450, 1986

Edi-Osagie ECO, Hopkins RE, Edi-Osagie NE: Munchausen's syndrome in obstetrics and gynecology: a review. Obstet Gynecol Surv 53:45–49, 1998

Eisendrath SJ: When Munchausen becomes malingering: factitious disorders that penetrate the legal system. Bull Am Acad Psychiatry Law 24:471–481, 1996

Eisendrath SJ, Feder A: The management of factitious disorders, in The Spectrum of Factitious Disorders. Edited by Feldman MD, Eisendrath SJ. Washington, DC, American Psychiatric Press, 1996, pp 195–213

Feldman MD: Munchausen by Internet: detecting factitious illness and crisis on the Internet. South Med J 93:669–672, 2000

Feldman MD, Eisendrath SJ (eds): The Spectrum of Factitious Disorders. Washington, DC, American Psychiatric Press, 1996

Feldman MD, Escalona R: The longing for nurturance: a case of factitious cancer. Psychosomatics 32:226–228, 1991

Feldman MD, Ford CV: Patients or Pretender: Inside the Strange World of Factitious Disorders. New York, Wiley, 1994

Feldman MD, Ford CV, Stone T: Deceiving others/deceiving oneself: four cases of factitious rape. South Med J 87:736–738, 1994

Feldman-Schorrig S: Factitious sexual harassment. Bull Am Acad Psychiatry Law 24:387–482, 1996

Fenelon G, Mahieux F, Roullet E, et al: Munchausen's syndrome and abnormalities on magnetic resonance imaging of the brain. BMJ 302:996–997, 1991

Fink P, Jensen J: Clinical characteristics of the Munchausen syndrome: a review and 3 new case histories. Psychother Psychosom 52:164–171, 1989

Flicken DJ: Malingering: a symptom. J Nerv Ment Dis 123:23–31, 1956

Ford CV: Munchausen syndrome, in Extraordinary Disorders of Human Behavior. Edited by Friedmann CTH, Fagnet RA. New York, Plenum, 1982, pp 15–27

Ford CV: The Somatizing Disorders: Illness as a Way of Life. New York, Elsevier, 1983

Ford CV: Illness as a lifestyle: the role of somatization in medical practice. Spine 17:S338–S343, 1992

Ford CV: Ethical and legal issues in factitious disorders: an overview, in The Spectrum of Factitious Disorders. Edited by Feldman MD, Eisendrath SJ. Washington, DC, American Psychiatric Press, 1996a, pp 51–66

Ford CV: Lies! Lies!! Lies!!! The Psychology of Deceit. Washington, DC, American Psychiatric Press, 1996b

Ford v United States of America, Civil Action No. 84-1013, U.S. Dist. (Penn), 1987

Freyberger H, Nordmeyer JP, Freyberger HJ, et al: Patients suffering from factitious disorders in the clinico-psychosomatic consultation liaison service: psychodynamic processes, psychotherapeutic initial care and clinico-interdisciplinary cooperation. Psychother Psychosom 62:108–122, 1994

Ganser SJM: A peculiar hysterical state. British Journal of Criminology 5:120–126, 1965

Gault MH, Campbell NR, Aksu AE: Spurious stones. Nephron 48:274–279, 1988

Gavin H: On the Feigned and Factitious Diseases of Solders and Seamen. Edinburgh, Scotland, University Press, 1838

Gibbon KL: Munchausen's syndrome presenting as an acute sexual assault. Med Sci Law 38:202–205, 1998

Gorman WF: Defining malingering. J Forensic Sci 27:401–407, 1982

Grunberger G, Weiner SL, Silverman R, et al: Factitious hypoglycemia due to surreptitious administration of insulin: diagnosis, treatment and long term follow-up. Ann Intern Med 108:252–257, 1988

Hall DE, Eubanks L, Meyyazhagan LS, et al: Evaluation of covert video surveillance in the diagnosis of Munchausen syndrome by proxy: lessons from 41 cases. Pediatrics 105:1305–1312, 2000

Hardie TJ, Reed A: Pseudologia fantastica, factitious disorder and impostership: a deception syndrome. Med Sci Law 38:198–201, 1998

Hathaway SR, McKinley JC: Minnesota Multiphasic Personality Inventory—2. Minneapolis, MN, University of Minnesota, 1989

Horwitz DL: Factitious and artifactual hypoglycemia. Endocrinol Metab Clin North Am 18:203–210, 1989

Jonas JM, Pope HG: The dissimulating disorders: a single diagnostic entity? Compr Psychiatry 26:58–62, 1985

Kapfhammer HP, Rothenhauster HB, Dietrich E, et al: Artifactual disorders—between deception and self mutilation: experiences in consultation psychiatry at a university clinic (in German with English abstract). Nervenarzt 69:401–409, 1998

Karnik AM, Farah S, Khadadah M, et al: A unique case of Munchausen's syndrome. Br J Clin Pract 44:699–701, 1990

Kass FC: Identification of persons with Munchausen's syndrome: ethical problems. Gen Hosp Psychiatry 7:195–200, 1985

Kay NR, Morris-Jones H: Pain clinic management of medico-legal litigants. Injury 29:305–308, 1998

King BH, Ford CV: Pseudologia fantastica. Acta Psychiatr Scand 77:1–6, 1988

Kramer KK, La Piana FG, Appleton B: Ocular malingering and hysteria: diagnosis and management. Surv Ophthalmol 24:89–96, 1979

Lechner DE, Bradbury SF, Bradley LA: Detecting sincerity of effort: a summary of methods and approaches. Phys Ther 78:867–888, 1998

Lees-Haley PR: Malingering emotional distress on the SCL-90-R: toxic exposure and cancerphobia. Psychol Rep 65:1203–1208, 1989a

Lees-Haley PR: Malingering traumatic mental disorder on the Beck Depression Inventory: cancerphobia and toxic exposure. Psychol Rep 65:623–626, 1989b

Lees-Haley PR: MMPI-2 base rates for 492 personal injury plaintiffs: implications and challenges for forensic assessment. J Clin Psychol 53:745–755, 1997

Lees-Haley PR, Fox DD: MMPI subtle-obvious scales and malingering: clinical vs simulated scores. Psychol Rep 66:907–911, 1990

Libow JA: Munchausen by proxy victims in adulthood: a first look. Child Abuse Negl 19:1131–1142, 1995

Libow JA: Child and adolescent illness falsification. Pediatrics 105:336–342, 2000

Lipsitt DR: The factitious patient who sues (letter). Am J Psychiatry 143:1482, 1986

MacSween RM, Millard LG: A green man. Arch Dermatol 136:115, 118, 2000

Main CJ, Waddell G: Behavioral responses to examination: a reappraisal of the interpretation of "non-organic" signs. Spine 23:2367–2371, 1998

Mayou R: Medico-legal aspects of road traffic accidents. J Psychosom Res 39:789–798, 1995

McCaffrey RJ, Bellamy-Campbell R: Psychometric detection of fabricated symptoms of combat-related post-traumatic stress disorder: a systematic replication. J Clin Psychol 45:76–79, 1989

McClure RF, Davis PM, Meadow SR, et al: Epidemiology of Munchausen syndrome by proxy, non-accidental poisoning and non-accidental suffocation. Arch Dis Child 75:57–61, 1996

McFarland BH, Resnick M, Bloom JD: Ensuring continuity of care for a Munchausen patient through a public guardian. Hospital and Community Psychiatry 34:65–67, 1983

McGuire TL, Feldman KW: Psychologic morbidity of children subjected to Munchausen syndrome by proxy. Pediatrics 83:289–292, 1989

Meadow R: Munchausen syndrome by proxy: the hinterland of child abuse. Lancet 2:343–345, 1977

Meadow R: Management of Munchausen syndrome by proxy. Arch Dis Child 60:385–393, 1985

Meadow R: Munchausen syndrome by proxy perpetrated by men. Arch Dis Child 78:210–216, 1998

Meadow R: Unnatural sudden infant death. Arch Dis Child 80:7–14, 1999

Mohammed R, Goy JA, Walpole BG, et al: Munchausen's syndrome: a study of the casualty "black books" of Melbourne. Med J Aust 143:561–563, 1985

Nadelson T: False patients/real patients: a spectrum of disease presentation. Psychother Psychosom 44:175–184, 1985

Nichols GR II, Davis GJ, Corey TS: In the shadow of the Baron: sudden death due to Munchausen syndrome. Am J Emerg Med 8:216–219, 1990

Nicholson SD, Roberts GA: Patients who (need to) tell stories. Br J Hosp Med 51:546–549, 1994

Pankratz L, Lezak MD: Cerebral dysfunction in the Munchausen syndrome. Hillside Journal of Clinical Psychiatry 9:195–206, 1987

Parker PE: A case report of Munchausen syndrome with mixed psychological features. Psychosomatics 34:360–364, 1993

Perconte ST, Goreczny AJ: Failure to detect fabricated post-traumatic stress disorder with the use of the MMPI in a clinical population. Am J Psychiatry 147:1057–1060, 1990

Phillips MR, Ward NG, Ries RK: Factitious mourning: painless patienthood. Am J Psychiatry 140:420–425, 1983

Popli AP, Masand PS, Dewan MJ: Factitious disorders with psychological symptoms. J Clin Psychiatry 53:315–318, 1992

Rahilly PM: The pneumographic and medical investigation of infants suffering apparent life threatening episodes. J Paediatr Child Health 27:349–353, 1991

Rawling PJ: The Simulation Index: a reliability study. Brain Inj 6:381–383, 1992

Reich JD, Hanno PM: Factitious renal colic. Urology 50:858–862, 1997

Reich P, Gottfried LA: Factitious disorders in a training hospital. Ann Intern Med 99:240–247, 1983

Reuber M, Zeidler M, Chataway J, et al: Munchausen syndrome by phone (letter). Lancet 356:1358, 2000

Rogers R: Development of a new classificatory model of malingering. Bull Am Acad Psychiatry Law 18:323–333, 1990

Rogers R, Bagby RM, Rector N: Diagnostic legitimacy of factitious disorder with psychological symptoms. Am J Psychiatry 146:1312–1314, 1989

Rosenberg DA: Web of deceit: a literature review of Munchausen syndrome by proxy. Child Abuse Negl 11:547–563, 1987

Samuels MP, McClaughlin W, Jacobson RR, et al: Fourteen cases of imposed upper airway obstruction. Arch Dis Child 67:162–170, 1992

Schneck JM: Pseudo-malingering. Diseases of the Nervous System 23:396–398, 1962

Schreier HA, Libow JA: Hurting for Love: Munchausen by Proxy Syndrome. New York, Guilford, 1993

Sigal M, Altmark D, Gelkopf M: Munchausen syndrome by adult proxy revisited. Isr J Psychiatry Relat Sci 28:33–36, 1991

Sigal M, Altmark D, Alfici S, et al: Ganser syndrome: a review of 15 cases. Compr Psychiatry 33:134–138, 1992

Snowden J, Solomons R, Druce H: Feigned bereavement: twelve cases. Br J Psychiatry 133:15–19, 1978

Southall DP, Plunkett MC, Banks MW, et al: Covert video recordings of life-threatening child abuse: lessons for child protection. Pediatrics 199:735–760, 1997

Sparr L, Pankratz LD: Factitious posttraumatic stress disorder. Am J Psychiatry 140:1016–1019, 1983

Stone MH: Factitious illness: psychological findings and treatment recommendations. Bull Menninger Clin 41:239–254, 1977

Sutherland AJ, Rodin GM: Factitious disorders in a general hospital setting: clinical features and a review of the literature. Psychosomatics 31:392–399, 1990

Szasz TS: Malingering: "diagnosis" or social condemnation? Arch Neurol Psychiatry 76:432–443, 1956

Tlacuilo-Parra JA, Guevara-Gutierrez E, Garcia-De La Torre I: Factitious disorders mimicking systemic lupus erythematosus. Clin Exp Rheumatol 18:89–93, 2000

Von Maur K, Wasson KR, DeFord JW, et al: Munchausen's syndrome: a thirty year history of peregrination par excellence. South Med J 66:629–632, 1973

Weiner H, Braiman A: The Ganser syndrome. Am J Psychiatry 111:767–773, 1955

Wetzler S, Marlowe D: "Faking bad" on the MMPI, MMPI-2 and Million-II. Psychol Rep 67:1117–1118, 1990

Yorker BC: Hospital epidemics of factitious disorder by proxy, in The Spectrum of Factitious Disorders. Edited by Feldman MD, Eisendrath SJ. Washington, DC, American Psychiatric Press, 1996, pp 157–174

Zuger A, O'Dowd MA: The Baron has AIDS: a case of factitious human immunodeficiency virus infection and review. Clin Infect Dis 14:211–216, 1992

Clinical Consultation-Liaison Settings

Internal Medicine and Medical Subspecialties

Chapter Editor: Donna B. Greenberg, M.D.

onsultation-liaison psychiatrists must include psychiatric possibilities in the differential diagnosis of medical patients' complaints and must remain vigilant to both somatic presentations of mood disorders and medical causes of abnormal mood and delirium. The physician will draw on a psychological understanding of the patient and on behavioral techniques to maximize strengths and minimize weaknesses in mature management of chronic illness. In this chapter, we discuss psychiatric aspects of heart, lung, gastrointestinal, and renal disease. We then review psychiatric symptoms associated with endocrine disorders, systemic lupus erythematosus, cobalamin deficiency, and the differential diagnosis of chronic fatigue.

Heart Disease

Peter Halperin, M.D.

Consultation-liaison psychiatry offers a uniquely rich opportunity to treat at the mind-body interface, but in no medical specialty is this more true than in consultation to cardiology. Cardiac disease has a reciprocal relation with emotional distress, psychosocial state, and psychiatric pathology. The imminent threat of sudden death or illness commonly causes anxiety and dysphoria and often causes depression. The reverse is also true. Psychiatric pathology—ranging from major depressive disorder, panic disorder, and acute anxiety to more chronic problems such as poor social supports, low income, and hostility—is associated with cardiac abnormalities. Furthermore, the same symptoms can signal either primary psychiatric or primary cardiological conditions. A panic attack may present as chest discomfort, and cardiac ischemia can mimic acute anxiety. Consultation-liaison psychiatrists can make important contributions to the comprehensive care of patients with cardiac disease.

To provide effective consultations for such patients, the psychiatrist must be well grounded in heart disease and its treatment but also must be keenly aware of the interrelation between psychosocial state and cardiac pathophysiology, a subject reviewed by Henry and Stephens (1977) and more recently by Folkow (1987) and Rozanski et al. (1999). After briefly summarizing the relation between the stress response and cardiac pathophysiology, I will examine these interfaces in more detail.

Mammals have evolved the fight-or-flight response—a powerful set of physiologic reflexes that prepares the body for intense physical activity in anticipation of a chal-

lenging event. Through changes in norepinephrine, epinephrine, and corticosteroid levels, challenging stimuli increase heart rate, increase myocardial contractility, increase blood pressure, and regulate arterial tone so that blood goes preferentially to exercising skeletal muscle. Lipids and triglycerides are released from storage sites into the bloodstream to be used as a source of energy for the impending exercise. Norepinephrine also reduces the threshold for platelet aggregation, thus making clotting more likely, an advantage in situations in which physical injury might occur.

These responses are all helpful in the environments in which they evolved; however, the actions of norepinephrine, epinephrine, and cortisol have counterparts that relate to cardiovascular disease. For instance, a physiologic increase in heart rate can lead to pathological arrhythmias in vulnerable individuals, arterial tone changes can produce coronary artery spasm, positive inotropic effects cause intermittent hypertension and can contribute to sustained hypertension, increased lipid release can contribute to hyperlipidemias and other dyslipidemias (Pauletto et al. 1991), and a decreased threshold for platelet aggregation can be a factor in coronary artery thrombosis and myocardial infarction (MI) (S.O. Levine et al. 1985; Markovitz and Matthews 1991; Rozanski et al. 1999).

In modern human society, the triggers for this stress response are a myriad of mostly psychological stressors. The response that was designed to prepare people for physical activity and physical danger now usually occurs in arenas in which people are sedentary. Furthermore, the number of stressful events of psychological origin is far greater than the number of physical threats that have occurred throughout human evolution. Likewise, the opportunity for relaxation responses seems to decrease steadily as civilization progresses. This change, along with a more sedentary lifestyle and unhealthy dietary habits, coincided with a steady increase in the incidence of cardiac disease throughout most of the twentieth century. I will examine more fully the roles that these and other factors play in cardiac morbidity and mortality.

CARDIAC PATHOLOGY AND THE NERVOUS SYSTEM

Ventricular Arrhythmias and Sudden Cardiac Death

Arrhythmias are perhaps the most extensively studied, best understood area of psychophysiological cardiac disease. Mostly through the work of Lown and his group, it is well documented that sympathetic nervous system discharge lowers the threshold for ventricular arrhythmias, especially in hearts with prior ischemic damage (Lown et al. 1977, 1980). Adrenergic stimulation, which normally increases rate and rhythm, can trigger ectopic sites in the myocardium to override normal conductive pathways, producing sustained and often deadly arrhythmias.

Animal studies have demonstrated that intense emotional arousal predisposes to ventricular arrhythmias. In one paradigm, a dog with a previous experimentally induced myocardial infarct was tethered while it watched another dog eat its food. The tethered dog had ventricular arrhythmias that could be suppressed by β-adrenergic blockade (Lown et al. 1973; Matta et al. 1976). Although one can only conjecture, a good guess is that the dog experienced anger and helplessness, two emotional states that are often implicated as triggers for stress-induced cardiac pathology in humans.

Both the brain and the peripheral sympathetic nervous system are implicated as causes of stress-induced arrhythmias. In animal models, direct electrode stimulation of limbic structures, the hypothalamus, anterior temporal lobe, insula, and cingulate gyrus, as well as the frontal, orbital, motor, and premotor cortical areas, produces ventricular arrhythmias. Pretreatment with β-adrenergic blockers and physical ablation of peripheral sympathetic structures such as the stellate ganglion prevent the arrhythmias caused by cortical stimulation as well as arrhythmias caused by psychological stressors in animal models. However, other neurochemical mediators

of these arrhythmias are also suspect, because β-adrenergic blocking agents have not been sufficient to prevent such arrhythmias in humans.

Because major depressive disorder is associated with cardiac morbidity, the interactions among the serotonin system, depression, and the heart hold great interest. In animal models, pharmacological maneuvers to increase central nervous system (CNS) serotonin levels raise the threshold for induction of ventricular arrhythmias (Blatt et al. 1979; Rabinowitz and Lown 1978). Increased CNS serotonin concentrations are also associated with decreased sympathetic neural activity (Antonaccio and Robson 1973). The use of newer selective serotonin reuptake inhibitors (SSRIs) may have a specific role, clearly worthy of research, in the care of depressed (and perhaps even nondepressed) patients with ventricular arrhythmias.

Public speaking, recall of emotionally charged events, automobile driving, and other common stressors can produce ventricular arrhythmias in susceptible patients (Lown et al. 1980; Sigler 1967; Taggart et al. 1969, 1973). In one series of such patients, the Lown group (DeSilva and Lown 1978; Lown and DeSilva 1978) demonstrated that stressors—from mental arithmetic to the more potent interview involving discussion of illness and death—were much more reliable inducers of arrhythmias than were physical maneuvers such as carotid sinus massage, posture changes on a tilt table, the Valsalva maneuver, hyperventilation, breath holding, and dive reflex activation. It is no surprise, then, that aspects of hospital life such as an interview during walk rounds have been important triggers for arrhythmia and even sudden death in patients with cardiac disease (Jarvinen 1955).

In patients with cardiac pathology, even minor psychological stress can induce arrhythmias. An acute emotional trigger, often provoking anger, is the immediate precipitant for arrhythmias in patients with a relatively chronic state of helplessness, an underlying sense of entrapment without possible escape (Lown 1979; Reich et al. 1979). Lown and Graboys (1977) suggested a role for psychiatric treatment by showing that psychological management of particular triggers could reduce the frequency of life-threatening arrhythmias. Furthermore, patients who have had a cardiac arrest are at risk for depression and posttreatment cognitive deficits (Roine et al. 1993).

Stress and Hypertension

Given the effects of norepinephrine and epinephrine on the myocardium and on peripheral vascular resistance, it is not surprising that psychosocial factors correlate with transient and sustained increases in blood pressure. In one well-known animal model, mice were subjected to social manipulations that simulated modern urban society: forced crowding, exposure to threat by cats, development in isolation, and then exposure to established mouse societies. These stressors caused sustained hypertension (Henry et al. 1967). Human studies suggest that stable, safer, and rural societies have fewer hypertensive individuals than do urban societies with a higher crime rate and unstable social structures (Harburg et al. 1973; Henry and Cassel 1969; Stamler et al. 1967).

Genetic factors may add to the power of stress on the vascular system (Doyle and Fraser 1961). Some hypertensive patients, for instance, have a more prolonged vasoconstrictive response to psychological stress than normotensive patients (Brod 1970; Brod et al. 1959). Similar responses in normotensive offspring of hypertensive parents suggest genetic transmission of vulnerability in stress responsiveness (Ditto and Miller 1989). Hypertensive patients also have greater heart rate and blood pressure responses than do normotensive patients to psychological stress such as mental arithmetic and to experimental situations designed to cause anger or fear (Baumann et al. 1973; Nestel 1969; Schachter 1957). Behavioral studies involving hypertensive patients show the most consistent correlations between hypertension and expressed or internalized anger or hostility, especially in challenging situations that produce active, hostile coping responses (Esler et al. 1977; Light et al. 1985; Manuck et al. 1987).

Direct Effect on Myocardium-Myofibrillar Degeneration

Myocardial necrosis, caused by exogenously administered or stress-induced catecholamines, has been found at autopsy in people who were literally scared to death by psychological trauma (Raab 1966). This lesion, which is thought to be much more prevalent in humans than is diagnosed (Reichenbach and Bendit 1970), greatly increases the risk of ventricular arrhythmias and sudden death (Cebelin and Hirsch 1980). In animal models, white rats that were frustrated by interference with their ability to reach food, and gray rats that were frightened by tape recordings of noisy cat-rat fights, developed identical areas of ventricular necrosis that were not secondary to poor coronary blood flow (Raab 1966). Catecholamine-induced peroxidation of myocardial lipid membranes blocks the calcium-channel pump, causing "stone heart" calcification and necrosis in small and large areas of myocardium. Antioxidants, sympatholytic agents, and

calcium-channel blockers reduce these lesions in animal models (Meerson 1983).

Stress-Induced Ischemia

The mental stress of ordinary life is the most common precipitant of myocardial ischemia in patients with coronary artery disease (CAD) (Rozanski et al. 1988). In studies using ambulatory electrocardiograms (ECGs), investigators examined the incidence of ischemia in daily life (as defined by ST depression) in patients with angina; they found that angina is more likely to occur when patients are mentally rather than physically stressed and that most ischemic episodes are painlessly silent (Deanfield et al. 1983). Further work with positron emission tomography analysis of coronary blood flow also demonstrated mental stress–induced ischemia in patients with CAD (Deanfield et al. 1984).

Stress and the Pathogenesis of Coronary Artery Disease

Since the earliest descriptions of CAD, physicians have speculated that psychosocial factors play an important role in its pathogenesis. Near the beginning of the last century, William Osler (1910) stated that all cases of premature angina in physicians under age 50 were due to worry accompanied by an "incessant treadmill of practice" (p. 939). Osler often wrote about the connection between CAD and things such as overwork and failure to relax. When Osler developed angina, he made radical lifestyle changes, moving away from workaholism and toward increased tranquility in his life. Knowledge about psychosocial factors and CAD comes largely from animal studies.

Animal studies. Social and environmental manipulations have been linked to atherogenesis in studies involving subjects ranging from mice to primates (Bassett and Cairncross 1975; Henry et al. 1967, 1971; Kaplan et al. 1982, 1983; Manuck et al. 1983; Nerem et al. 1980). In general, arteriosclerosis in animals is associated with paradigms that increase aggression, decrease affiliation, disturb stable hierarchical relationships, increase fear, and cause subordinate, "given up" behavior (Schneiderman 1987). Sympathoadrenal activity is the proposed mechanism, with some studies specifically demonstrating increased production of catecholamines and associated hypertension in mice (Henry et al. 1971; Stephens 1967). In one animal study, monkeys that were moved repeatedly from one stable social monkey society to another had a higher rate of severe aggression and severe submission (as opposed to affiliate behaviors) and more CAD than did control monkeys (Kaplan et al. 1983). Taken as a whole, the data from animal studies make clear a powerful connection between arteriosclerosis, psychosocial stress, and behavior—specifically, heightened aggression, fear, and depression—all known to be associated with increased sympathetic nervous system activity.

Type A behavior. Early attempts to relate personality characteristics to coronary disease reflected the psychoanalytic and psychosomatic models prevailing in academic psychiatry at the time. In the 1940s, Dunbar (1943) described a typical patient with heart disease compulsively working long hours without taking vacations, without delegating responsibility, without taking care of his or her health, and without acknowledging a tendency to depression. The tendency to experience internal anger while controlling its expression was another cornerstone in the psychoanalytic understanding of patients with CAD. Given the animal research cited earlier, one might expect that anger and other states of increased sympathoadrenal drive would increase the risk of coronary disease.

Sympathetic arousal and anger are evident in Friedman and Rosenman's (1974) type A behavior pattern hypothesis, which came to dominate this line of research from the 1960s through the 1980s. The type A pattern was defined by these authors as "an action-emotion complex" characterized by expression of two underlying traits: hostility and "time urgency" or "hurry sickness." The cardiologists who developed this concept were not bound by prevalent psychodynamic or psychiatric paradigms but wanted to describe objectively the physical signs and symptoms of type A behavior, much as one would codify palpation and auscultation of the heart. They developed diagnostic indicators of type A behavior, elicited by a structured, videotaped, clinical interview in which signs such as facial expression, posture, speech prosody, stereotypical display of anger or anxiety, and the number of interruptions of the interviewer weigh more heavily in the scoring than does the content of the patient's answers to direct questioning about type A characteristics.

The type A concept has become an important anchor for research. The Western Collaborative Group Study found that over an 8-year period, type A men developed CAD between 1.7 and 4.1 times more frequently than type B men when other risk factors were controlled for (Rosenman et al. 1975). The data from the Framingham study supported the significance of type A behavior in men (Friedman et al. 1986). There were no comparable studies involving women. Type A scores were also related to physiologic variables that were relevant to coronary

disease (M. Fava et al. 1987). Compared with type B subjects, type A subjects exhibited an exaggerated sympathomimetic response to laboratory challenges and stressors such as harassment during competition and work- or goal-related tasks, including exercise (DeQuattro et al. 1985; Friedman et al. 1975; Glass et al. 1980; Seraganian et al. 1985; Simpson et al. 1974; Williams et al. 1982). That β-adrenergic blockade lowers both type A behavior scores and cardiovascular responsivity also suggests the existence of a type A–sympathoadrenal connection (Krantz et al. 1982). Associations between type A behavior and changes in adrenocorticotropic hormone (ACTH), cortisol, testosterone, growth hormone, and insulin secretion have been demonstrated less consistently (M. Fava et al. 1987). Two studies of global type A scores did not demonstrate a correlation with severity of angiographic findings (Dimsdale et al. 1979; Sherwitz et al. 1983). However, hostility and anger measures alone have been correlated with severity of CAD as shown by angiography (Dembroski et al. 1985; MacDougall et al. 1985). The Multiple Risk Factor Intervention Trial did not demonstrate a connection between type A behavior and subsequent CAD (Shekelle et al. 1985). Furthermore, an investigation involving the Western Collaborative Group Study cohort 20 years after that study did not show a continued worsened prognosis for those originally designated as type A (Miller et al. 1991; Ragland and Brand 1988). Findings of more recent prospective studies have also seriously challenged the hypothesized type A link to CAD, although none of these studies used the structured videotaped diagnostic interview, considered a more accurate measure of type A behavior than questionnaires. It might be wise to assume that chronic increases in sympathetic outflow, whether caused by anger, impatience, affective disorders, or situational reactivity, are likely to increase cardiac risk, and it may be time to de-emphasize the term *type A behavior* in clinical practice.

Perhaps the most important study to emerge from the type A literature was an extensive treatment study, the Recurrent Coronary Prevention Project (RCPP), which demonstrated that group psychotherapy that reduced type A behavior and other behavioral risks substantially decreased the incidence of recurrent MI and cardiac death in patients with a previous MI (Friedman et al. 1986). Patients who had a history of MI ($n = 862$) were randomized to group therapy directed at lessening type A behavior over a 3-year period ($n = 592$) or to cardiac counseling without psychotherapy ($n = 270$). A comparison group of 151 patients who refused either treatment was also followed. Over 4.5 years, the recurrent infarct rate in the therapy group was 12.9%, compared with 21.2% in the control group ($P < .005$) and

28.2% in the comparison group. After the first year, the therapy group had a significant reduction in cardiac deaths compared with the control group.

In addition to type A behavior, other important psychosocial factors that were addressed in treatment in the RCPP may have contributed to the beneficial outcome. First, denial of symptoms and delay in seeking medical attention were major foci of the therapy (J.J. Gill and M. Friedman, personal communication, May 1994). In the first year, patients tended to change their behavior toward increased acceptance of the meaning of symptoms, better communication with cardiologists, and less delay from pain onset to reaching the emergency room. In addition to decreased global type A scores and hostility, time urgency, and impatience, the researchers also documented significant decreases in depression, significant increases in self-efficacy, and marginal increases in social support (Mendes de Leon et al. 1991). Given the mounting evidence that depression increases cardiac risk, the reduction in depression among treated subjects in the RCPP may be critical to the measured outcomes. Another psychological treatment program, aimed at lowering stress rather than reducing type A behavior, resulted in reduced recurrent MI and cardiac death rates by almost 50% up to 7 years later (Frasure-Smith and Prince 1989). The outcomes of both of these treatment studies are significant; in fact, no medical or surgical intervention has achieved such a reduction in MI recurrence or cardiac death. Unfortunately, application of such psychotherapy programs to patients with cardiac disease is rare (Nunes et al. 1987).

Social support. The benefit of group psychotherapy may also be related to the benefit of social support. In a classic article, Ruberman and colleagues (1984) demonstrated that patients with MI who were more socially isolated and who had higher life stress and less education had more than four times the risk of death than their counterparts who had low levels of stress and were isolated. More recent studies have demonstrated that social isolation (living alone) is associated with greater risk of a recurrent cardiac event (Case et al. 1992) and that patients with cardiac disease who have fewer social and economic resources have significantly poorer outcomes (Williams et al. 1992).

Denial. Of all the psychological and emotional conditions that affect cardiac disease, perhaps none is more clinically important than denial. Patients ignore cardiac symptoms or attribute them to a more benign problem, such as heartburn, despite intellectual awareness of the symptoms of MI. Studies have disclosed a median delay

of 2.9–5.1 hours between the onset of symptoms and arrival at the emergency room (Hackett and Cassem 1969; Moss and Goldstein 1970; Simon et al. 1972). This issue is critical because 55%–80% of deaths from MI occur within 4 hours of the onset of symptoms (Wallace and Yu 1975). Techniques such as thrombolytic therapy are available in most emergency rooms and can minimize damage from an evolving infarct. The most likely explanation for patients not attributing their symptoms to their hearts is fear of an MI. Unconscious mechanisms of denial, displacement, and rationalization reduce anxiety by preventing conscious awareness of the danger (Hackett and Rosenbaum 1984).

However, denial may not always be detrimental to patients with cardiac disease. Hackett and co-workers (1968) demonstrated that once a patient is in the coronary care unit in the postinfarct stage, denial of the degree of danger is associated with a better in-hospital clinical course. Given the greatly heightened risk of ischemia and arrhythmias in the immediate postinfarct period, the lower anxiety resulting from denial presumably decreases risk by decreasing catecholamine release. However, in the day-to-day life of a patient with cardiac disease, denial can have a devastating effect on the acute response to symptoms and can prevent compliance with medical care in the long run (Shaw 1985). Psychotherapeutic and educational treatment instituted after the acute stages of recovery to reduce cardiac patients' denial can be lifesaving.

Depression. Depression has been associated with cardiac disease as a risk factor since at least 1937, when Malzberg compared the mortality among patients with involutional melancholia with the mortality of the general population of the state of New York, controlling for age and sex. Overall, he found that cardiac disease accounted for 40% of the total deaths among the depressed patients and that this rate of cardiac death was eight times higher than that in the general population. Cardiac patients have a high prevalence of major depressive disorder, which modern studies using Research Diagnostic Criteria or DSM-III (American Psychiatric Association 1980) criteria place at about 18% (Carney et al. 1988; Schleifer et al. 1989). Milder depressive syndromes not meeting the criteria for major depressive disorder occur at least this frequently in cardiac patients (Hance et al. 1996; Schleifer et al. 1989) and are associated with recurrent carciac events (Horsten et al. 2000). Although still generally considered an "understandable" reaction to cardiac events by most physicians, increasing numbers of modern studies are showing depression to be a significant risk factor for cardiac illness. Carney et al. (1988) determined that depression was an independent risk factor for coronary events—stronger than sex, hypertension, ventricular arrhythmias, or diabetes.

Avery and Winokur (1976) examined mortality among depressed patients who were adequately treated with medication or electroconvulsive therapy (ECT) and among inadequately treated depressed patients. They found that the rate of MI was significantly higher in the inadequately treated group over a 3-year observation period. Ahern et al. (1990) found that depression in patients with a history of MI was associated with a significantly increased risk of death or cardiac arrest. In a more recent study involving 222 hospitalized patients with MI, Lesperance and Frasure-Smith (1993) found that patients with severe depression were five times more likely to die within 6 months after discharge than were their nondepressed counterparts. Other studies have shown a significant prospective relationship between major depressive disorder and cardiac illness (Abramson et al. 2001; Anda et al. 1993; Aromaa et al. 1994; Barefoot and Schroll 1996; Everson et al. 1996; D.E. Ford 1998; Frasure-Smith et al. 1995; Lesperance et al. 2000; Vogt et al. 1995; L.A. Pratt et al. 1996; Wassertheil-Smoller et al. 1996). Taken as a whole, these studies implicate not only major depressive disorder but also minor depression as risk factors for coronary disease, and there may be a continuous risk varying with the severity of depression (Penninx et al. 2001).

Depression may increase cardiac risk indirectly: a depressed patient may be more likely to engage in risky behaviors such as smoking and may not comply with medical regimens including exercise, dietary changes, and drug therapy (Blumenthal et al. 1982; Glassman et al. 1990; Zigelstein et al. 1998). It is also likely that depression has a pathophysiologic effect; stress response mechanisms in depressed patients result in increased sympathetic and adrenocortical outflows. In patients with depression, the incidence of hypercortisolemia is greater (Carroll et al. 1976; Nemeroff et al. 1984). Peripheral catecholamine activity is increased as well (Esler et al. 1982; Veith et al. 1994). This increased sympathoadrenal activity may predispose patients to hypercholesterolemia, hypertension, and hypertriglyceridemia, all of which are atherogenic, and increased platelet reactivity. Depressed patients have in fact been shown to have increased platelet reactivity, an especially important focus of recent studies (Laghrissi-Thode et al. 1997; Musselman et al. 1996).

Panic disorder. Panic disorder, characterized by heightened sympathetic nervous system discharge and sensitivity and also perhaps by locus coeruleus dysregulation, has been associated with cardiac risk (Coryell et al. 1982) and cardiac disease (Goldberg et al. 1990). Panic disorder and myocardial ischemia can produce the same symptoms. Catecholamine-induced spasm of the coronary arterioles or microvascular angina in patients with panic disorder can be overlooked during cardiac catheterization (Cannon 1988). In one study, Chignon et al. (1993) examined the rate of panic disorder in a group of patients who were referred for ambulatory ECGs to identify CAD. The prevalence rate of panic disorder was approximately 15% among 200 consecutively referred patients. Panic was just as prevalent among those with electrocardiographic changes. The psychiatric consultant, who may be asked whether chest pains are "real," should treat the panic disorder but should not rule out coronary disease prematurely. Coronary disease and panic disorder may occur together, and the risk of overlooking coronary disease must always be considered.

Psychological factors affecting medical condition. Another Axis I diagnosis, psychological factors affecting medical condition, is common and by definition relevant to the risk profile of cardiac patients, given the proven risk of stressful life events, isolation, anger, and increased global type A scores. Psychotherapy and other behavioral treatments for stress reduction, anger, and type A behavior have been shown to be beneficial for cardiac patients (Blumenthal et al. 1997).

TREATMENT OF PATIENTS WITH CARDIAC DISEASE

Psychological Treatment

The psychiatric consultant can diagnose and often begin to treat patients in the hospital while laying the groundwork for outpatient treatment. Frasure-Smith (1991) showed that a modest treatment protocol to evaluate and reduce stress in patients after MI significantly decreased morbidity and mortality over the subsequent 5 years. Thus, in-hospital identification of psychiatric morbidity can significantly improve both the psychiatric and cardiac prognoses of patients with heart disease.

The patient who will undergo coronary artery bypass graft surgery may also benefit from the skills of the consultation-liaison psychiatrist, both preoperatively and postoperatively. Blacher (1987) wrote about the uniquely intense fears that patients have about heart surgery; patients invariably do not discuss these fears unless they are carefully invited to do so. The possible positive effect of routine psychological support on morbidity and length of stay for patients awaiting this operation is an important area for research and clinical work.

Two studies support the notion that psychotherapeutic and educational approaches improve the condition of hospitalized patients who have had an MI. Gruen (1975) examined the effect of individual supportive psychotherapy on such patients and found decreases in length of total hospitalization, time in intensive care, occurrence of congestive heart failure (CHF), and self-reported anxiety, as well as a faster return to normal activities 4 months after discharge. Oldenburg and co-workers (1985) compared therapy and education with routine care for hospitalized patients after MI and found that the treated group had fewer symptoms of CAD and better psychological measures after 1 year. Consultation-liaison psychiatrists can thus help to reduce health care costs as well as morbidity.

The psychiatric consultant should also be well versed in relaxation training (see Chapter 46). Simple meditation and muscle relaxation exercises can be quickly taught at the bedside. Patients who perform such exercises not only reduce sympathetic discharge directly but also gain a sense of autonomy and control in the passive environment of the hospital bed. In one study, patients who received in-hospital stress management and relaxation training after their MI improved at 6 months in both vocational and psychological status (Langosch et al. 1982). Other studies point toward an amelioration of ventricular arrhythmias among patients who practice meditation (Benson et al. 1975). The Lown group (Lown et al. 1980) reported the case of one patient whose ventricular tachycardia terminated during meditation. Taken together, these nonpharmacological, easily administered, completely safe, and inexpensive treatments, which are vastly underutilized in current routine inpatient and outpatient cardiac care, define a valuable role for the consultation-liaison psychiatrist.

A cardiac rehabilitation team can contribute to behavioral treatment. Patients benefit from witnessing or participating in monitored exercise. Rehabilitation programs also represent a unique opportunity to bring psychosocial treatment, such as group psychotherapy, into the regimen of behavioral treatment (exercise, dietary changes, smoking cessation). Informing inpatients about available outpatient treatments is a useful component of the psychiatric consultation. (For further discussion, see Chapters 45 and 46.)

Somatic Treatment

Depression

Determining when to begin somatic treatment of depression in patients with cardiac disease has always been difficult, but the decision is all the more important given the evidence suggesting that depression is a risk factor for CAD. In current practice, depression is both underdiagnosed and undertreated in cardiac patients, as in medical patients in general. Under investigation in a multicenter study ("Sad Heart") is whether the use of sertraline in depressed cardiac patients improves clinical cardiac outcomes, but preliminary evidence reported earlier in this chapter suggests that treating depression lowers cardiac risk. The possibility that untreated depression may expose depressed cardiac patients to increased cardiac risk must be considered in decision making about treating such patients. In practice, the diagnosis of major depressive disorder in patients with cardiac disease is more difficult because of the substantial overlap in the symptoms of the two illnesses (Freedland et al. 1992). It would seem wise to err on the side of diagnosis and treatment of depression. The neurovegetative symptoms of depression should not be discounted as being caused by cardiac illness in patients who demonstrate other emotional and behavioral symptoms of depression.

Selective serotonin reuptake inhibitors. The SSRIs, including fluoxetine, sertraline, and paroxetine, hold promise as being relatively safe for use in patients with cardiac disease. Notably, the SSRIs are devoid of α-adrenergic activity and, except for paroxetine, anticholinergic activity. In a recent study, paroxetine was compared with nortriptyline in depressed cardiac patients (Roose et al. 1998). The drugs achieved similar reductions in depression, but nortriptyline had significantly more cardiovascular side effects, including a sustained 11% increase in heart rate and a reduction in heart rate variability, leading to a significantly increased rate of discontinuation of treatment compared with paroxetine. On the ECGs of nondepressed patients, fluoxetine was noted to produce a small decrease in resting heart rate, with no change in conduction, P-R and Q-T intervals, or QRS duration (Fisch 1985; Upward et al. 1988). Likewise, in a large sample of depressed patients, sertraline had essentially no electrocardiographic effect (Upward et al. 1988). However, bradycardia was reported in two patients (Ellison et al. 1990), and atrial fibrillation was reported in one patient with heart disease who was treated with fluoxetine (Buff et al. 1991).

SSRIs are much safer for the heart in overdose situations than are other classes of antidepressants. Trials are under way to determine whether sertraline improves cardiac outcome in depressed cardiac patients and to determine whether paroxetine improves the platelet dysfunction seen in depression. Additionally, there is some evidence that fluoxetine is useful in decreasing anger associated with depression (M. Fava et al. 1993a). Given the relation between serotonin, anger, and cardiovascular risk, SSRIs may be indicated in depressed and nondepressed patients with cardiac disease who display high levels of anger and hostility. M. Fava et al. (1993b) demonstrated that clomipramine reduced anger attacks in two patients without cardiac disease in whom depression or panic disorder was not diagnosed.

Because they can displace other protein-bound drugs and may inhibit cytochrome P450 enzymes, SSRIs can cause increased blood levels of various cardiac drugs, including digoxin and warfarin. Owing to the narrow therapeutic windows of those drugs, serum levels in patients taking digoxin and prothrombin times in patients taking warfarin should be closely monitored when SSRIs are added. Levels of antiarrhythmics, metoprolol, and other β-adrenergic antagonists and calcium-channel blockers may be higher than expected because of inhibition of liver enzymes (Gram 1994). Newer drugs such as nefazodone and mixed serotonergic-adrenergic agents such as venlafaxine and mirtazapine have not been well studied in cardiac patients.

Tricyclic antidepressants.   In clinical practice, tricyclic antidepressant side effects result in discontinuation by 14%–60% of patients with cardiac disease (Roose et al. 1991a). Roose and Dalack (1992) detailed the major concerns in such patients.

- *Orthostatic hypotension:* Orthostatic blood pressure measurements should be obtained before and after treatment in any patient with cardiac disease who is given a tricyclic antidepressant. Falling is a serious side effect in elderly patients, who are more prone to hip fracture. Nortriptyline is the least likely among the tricyclic agents to cause orthostasis due to α-adrenergic blockade, but amitriptyline is one of the most likely, and that drug is often the one prescribed by nonpsychiatric physicians. Pretreatment changes in orthostatic blood pressure predict both posttreatment hypotension and, ironically, a positive antidepressant response to tricyclic agents (Jarvik et al. 1983; Schneider et al. 1986). Not everyone with postural signs feels dizzy on rising, and the dizziness may improve even when the standing blood pressure does not. Patients with CHF are especially vulnerable to such drug-induced postural changes in blood pressure (Roose et al. 1986, 1987).
- *Anticholinergic side effects:* Because tachycardia—typically 5 beats/minute over baseline—increases cardiac work and demand, the tricyclic antidepressants with the least anticholinergic activity (such as nortriptyline and desipramine) should be used.

- *Conduction system effects:* At therapeutic levels, tricyclic antidepressants prolong conduction in the HV portion of the His bundle. In patients with partial bundle-branch block, tricyclic drug–induced slowing of HV time can cause complete heart block.

   Tricyclic antidepressants, as type I antiarrhythmics, suppress premature ventricular contractions to therapeutic advantage; however, they may also be proarrhythmic, especially when used with another type I antiarrhythmic. When the drugs are given at toxic doses, the incidence of arrhythmias is high: 6%–16%. All tricyclic antidepressants appear to prolong atrial and ventricular depolarization, leading to predictably increased P-R, QRS, and Q-T intervals. A Q-Tc interval greater than 440 msec is associated with increased risk of sudden death (Schwartz and Wolf 1978). In patients with cardiac disease, a baseline ECG should be obtained, and additional ECGs should be obtained when therapeutic levels have been reached, and then at least yearly, to evaluate P-R, QRS, and Q-Tc durations and monitor for bundle branch block or complete atrioventricular block (Bigger et al. 1977, 1978; Burckhardt et al. 1987; Burrows et al. 1976, 1977; Giardina et al. 1979, 1981; Kantor et al. 1975, 1978; Luchins 1983; Raskind et al. 1982; Sigg et al. 1963; Thase and Perel 1982; Veith et al. 1982a).
- *Myocardial contractility:* Several studies have demonstrated that tricyclic antidepressants do not adversely affect left ventricular function, even in patients with low ejection fraction (Giardina et al. 1981; Veith et al. 1982b), so this is not a concern in patients with CHF.

Bupropion.   Thirty-six cardiac patients given bupropion had a low rate of orthostatic hypotension, few significant conduction disturbances, and no exacerbation of ventricular arrhythmias (Roose et al. 1991b); however, bupropion did cause a mild increase in supine blood pressure. Hypertension worsened in two of five patients who could not tolerate the drug.

Trazodone.   The main risk of trazodone to those with cardiac disease is related to α-adrenergic blockade and postural hypotension (Himmelhoch et al. 1984). Ventricular irritability has rarely been reported (Vitullo et al. 1990).

Monoamine oxidase inhibitors.   An important advantage of monoamine oxidase inhibitors (MAOIs) is the essential absence of anticholinergic side effects. The most notorious disadvantage is the possibility of diet-induced hypertensive crisis when foods containing large amounts of tyramine are consumed. Although this complication is rare and patients often cheat on their diets, a hypertensive crisis could precipitate a stroke or MI. A much more common problem is orthostatic hypotension (Robinson et al. 1982). Other cardiac effects include shortened P-R and Q-Tc intervals, a lower heart rate, and lower blood pressure (McGrath et al. 1987; Robinson et al. 1982). Atrial flutter and fibrillation were reported in one patient receiving tranylcypromine (Gorelick et al. 1981). When phenelzine was added to β-blockers, it caused marked bradycardia (Reggev and Vollhardt 1989). MAOIs should be considered for very reliable patients or for those who have not responded adequately to other agents.

Psychostimulants.   Cardiac side effects from the psychostimulants methylphenidate and dextroamphetamine are relatively rare, and these agents are probably underused in patients with cardiac disease (Ballard et al. 1976; Katon and Raskind 1980; Kaufman et al. 1982; Woods et al. 1986). Reported side effects, including hypertension, tachycardia, and arrhythmias, are rare in medically ill elderly patients. Psychostimulants have the advantages of little sedation, rapid onset of action (often within days), and relief of mood-related anorexia. Patients who do not tolerate tricyclic antidepressants have been shown to tolerate psychostimulants. In profoundly depressed hospitalized patients with cardiac disease in whom depression will affect medical recovery, psychostimulants can be rapidly effective; however, blood pressure and heart rate should be monitored.

Mood stabilizers.   Lithium carbonate is generally considered safe for treating bipolar disorder in patients with cardiac disease, but its use requires careful monitoring. At therapeutic levels, conduction abnormalities have been noted even in patients without cardiac disease, especially elderly individuals (Jaffe 1977; Mitchell and MacKenzie 1982; Roose et al. 1979a, 1979b; Tangedahl and Gau 1972; Wellens et al. 1975; J. Wilson et al. 1976). The most common abnormalities are sinus node dysfunction, atrioventricular block, and (rarely at therapeutic levels) ventricular ectopy. Benign T-wave flattening or inversion is also common. Any patients taking lithium who have cardiac disease or who are older than age 65 should have baseline ECGs and follow-up ECGs (every 6–12 months) to rule out conduction disturbances. Given these issues, either carbamazepine or valproic acid may have advantages over lithium, but they have not been adequately studied in cardiac patients.

Electroconvulsive therapy.   ECT has been seen as a safe alternative to drug therapy in severely depressed patients with cardiac disease, despite the absence of prospective studies. Zielinski and colleagues (1993) compared the cardiac complication rate of ECT among 40 depressed patients with and 40 patients without serious cardiac disease. Fifty-five percent of patients with cardiac disease had a cardiac complication, compared with 7.5% of subjects without heart disease. Minor transitory arrhythmias or ST–T-wave changes during or immediately after treatment that resolved within minutes accounted for all complications in the subjects without heart disease and for 66% of complications in the patients with cardiac disease. One-fifth of patients with cardiac disease ($n = 8$) developed major complications or persistent electrocardiographic changes lasting hours to days, accompanied by chest pain, asystole, or arrhythmia. No deaths occurred. Preexisting ischemic heart disease predicted ischemic events, and preexisting arrhythmias predicted arrhythmias. Only 2 of the 40 patients with cardiac disease actually discontinued ECT because of side effects. In summary, ECT with appropriate monitoring is relatively safe, even in patients with severe cardiac disease. ECT is an appropriate choice for patients with cardiac disease who cannot tolerate medications, who have psychotic depression, or who risk life-threatening complications if the depression should persist. (See Chapter 44 for further discussion of ECT.)

Delirium

Neuroleptic medications, particularly intravenous haloperidol and droperidol, are commonly used to treat cardiac patients with agitated delirium. These problems often occur in intensive care settings in patients with cardiac instability. (For further information on delirium, see Chapter 14; for more information about intensive care settings, see Chapter 34.)

The risk of hypotension is related to the degree of α-adrenergic blockade of the tranquilizer. Haloperidol has less of a hypotensive effect than does droperidol. At very high intravenous doses of haloperidol, torsades de pointes is a risk; the Q-T interval should be monitored carefully (Kriwisky et al. 1990).

Anxiety

Benzodiazepines.   Hospitalized patients with heart disease, especially those who are just recovering from an MI—and, even more, those who are too unstable to be discharged and who await surgical or other invasive procedures—often have acute anxiety. Severe anxiety can have lethal complications in patients with ventricular arrhythmia or in patients who are awaiting electrophysiological testing, surgery, or intra-abdominal defibrillator placement. Because of the risk of sympathetic arousal, benzodiazepine therapy has become an almost routine component of anxiety management in coronary care units and cardiac surgical units (Jefferson 1989). Benzodiazepines reduce not only anxiety but also, as has been shown in animal studies, stress-induced catecholamine levels and platelet activation (Baer and Cagen 1987; Vogel et al. 1984). These drugs have negligible cardiovascular effects but can contribute to respiratory depression, oversedation, and delirium. Recognition of patient dependence on benzodiazepines before hospitalization is also important. Withdrawal symptoms of generalized arousal or seizures are certainly undesirable when a patient's cardiac status is compromised.

Buspirone. Buspirone appears to be a benign agent, lacking anticholinergic or α-adrenergic effects. It is less likely to cause respiratory depression and is therefore safer to use than diazepam in patients with respiratory illness (Rapoport et al. 1991). Buspirone may also be preferable for patients with cardiac disease who are on respirators, but its onset of action is slow. Benzodiazepines or haloperidol may be started simultaneously with buspirone and then tapered after several weeks when buspirone begins to have an effect.

Selective serotonin reuptake inhibitors. SSRI treatment has become a front-line therapy for anxiety disorders of all types, including panic disorder. Their safety profiles in cardiac patients make them especially suitable in such patients.

Lung Disease

Donna B. Greenberg, M.D.

Richard L. Kradin, M.D.

Intuitively and clinically, physicians judge anxiety and grief by sighs; panic by rapid, shallow breathing; surprise by gasps; enthusiasm by full voice; and calm by easy breathing. Dyspnea connotes both physical fatigue and effort. Indeed, a patient's emotion is judged by the way he or she breathes, but the clues to such emotion may be obscured by the wheezes, pursed lips, and dyspnea that characterize chronic lung disease.

The chemistry of inefficient respiration affects mood. Chronic hypoxia compromises cognitive function and mood, at times leading to delirium and mood lability (Heaton et al. 1983; Prigatano et al. 1983). Changes in partial pressure of carbon dioxide (pCO_2) and acid-base balance have profound effects on cerebral blood flow and neuronal function. Acute increases in pCO_2 compromise consciousness and mental facility. Chronic hypercapnia leads to headache and dull, unmotivated, unproductive states (Burns and Howell 1969; Neff and Petty 1972). Hypocapnia also decreases ability to rehearse or recall (Posner 1972).

Hypoxia, strenuous exercise, sudden and unexpected thoracoabdominal trauma, or intense fear can cause dyspnea—the apperception of breathlessness. Severe dyspnea can occur even when patients have normal levels of gas exchange, if expiration becomes an energy-dependent process requiring mechanical work—for instance, in chronic bronchitis or asthma, when bronchospasm and secretions increase airway resistance, or in emphysema, when the connective tissue that supports the airways is lost. Dyspnea occurs invariably when the mechanical work of breathing increases, presumably mediated by increased firing of sensory neural elements in the lung and chest wall (Killian and Campbell 1983). Increased pulmonary arterial pressures and diminished fitness also contribute.

The patient's assessment of the severity of dyspnea affects his or her quality of life and functional status (Moody et al. 1990). The perception of severity correlates with mood, the tendency to hyperventilate, catastrophic cognition, fear of dyspnea, and the intrapsychic meaning of the symptom (Carr et al. 1992; Demers et al. 1990; Kellner et al. 1987, 1992; D.F. Klein 1993; Morgan et al. 1983; Porzelius et al. 1992; Yellowlees et al. 1987).

Not only does emotion affect breathing, but breathing also affects emotion (Bass and Gardner 1985). Because the breath, unlike the heartbeat or gastrointestinal motility, is easily perceived and easily altered by voluntary control, that ability can be used to advantage. Awareness of the breath is fundamental to virtually all meditation practices in the Judeo-Christian, Islamic, Hindu, and Buddhist traditions. Indeed, the "full awareness of breathing," as described in detail in the Anapanasati Sutra of the Buddhist Pali canon (Conze 1959), is one of the direct paths leading to nirvanic release and enlightenment.

The traditions of yoga, respiratory physical therapy, systematic desensitization, and behavioral treatments of agoraphobia all use awareness of breathing to augment a sense of control, reduce physiologic arousal, and reduce anticipatory anxiety. Yoga uses apnea at the end of full expiration and inspiration to calm, whereas behavior therapy uses rapid inhalation followed by slow exhalation to reduce anticipatory anxiety (Bass and Gardner 1985).

NEUROPHYSIOLOGY OF VENTILATION

Both the conscious and unconscious will, the cortex and the limbic system, affect the rhythmic respiratory centers of the medulla and pons. Breathing is automatic on the one hand and responsive to emotion and volition on the other. Centers controlling the rhythm of breathing are linked to the pontine reticular activating formation, so that arousal increases ventilation, and ventilation varies with the normal sleep cycle.

The psychologically important neurotransmitters cross-talk with the neurotransmitters of ventilation. Axons of the medullary respiratory centers project to the locus coeruleus (C.A. Ross et al. 1983). The majority of serotonergic 5-HT_{1B} receptors are located in the nuclei that regulate breathing (Peroutka 1988).

The lung itself is innervated largely by cholinergic fibers that course with the vagus nerve. Sympathetic adrenergic nerves are less plentiful in the lung but can be identified in the airways in the vicinity of the pulmonary vessels (Laitinen and Laitinen 1991).

Neurotransmitters modulate the activity of respiratory control centers. Cholinergic neurons are the primary excitatory neurons for the effector motor pacemakers of breathing (Burton et al. 1989). γ-Aminobutyric acid (GABA)ergic neurons inhibit firing of the pacemaker center (Hedner et al. 1984). β-Adrenergic neurotransmitters augment the output of cholinergic neurons (Katz and Black 1986). Finally, nonadrenergic, noncholinergic neuropeptides, including the tachykinins, can modulate, albeit more slowly, output from ventilatory neurons (Lindefors et al. 1986). In addition, endocrine hormones, including thyroxine and progesterone (Fadel et al. 1979), may directly increase the firing of respiratory center neurons.

RESPIRATION IN CLINICAL PSYCHIATRIC SYNDROMES

Respiration in Clinical Depression

Patients with clinical depression often display blunted ventilatory responses to inhaled CO_2. Depressed and grieving patients manifest lower respiratory rates, lower resting end tidal volumes, and increased pCO_2 (Damas-Mora et al. 1976, 1982). The lung and blood levels of CO_2 are normally tightly regulated by the minute ventilation, the product of the rate and volume of air exchanged each minute. Patients who experience depression or grief do not increase the minute ventilation appropriately when they breathe a mixture of gas with high pCO_2 or low partial oxygen pressure (pO_2) (Jellinek et al. 1985; Shershow et al. 1973, 1976). Patients with depression who experience sleep disturbance are more vulnerable to CO_2 retention, so patients who have both depression and lung disease are at increased risk for complications of respiratory depression (White et al. 1983).

Respiration in Anxiety Disorders

Increased respiratory rate and changes in tidal volume are key aspects of Selye's (1956) fight-or-flight response. Anxious patients have faster respiratory rates, smaller tidal volumes, and shorter breath-holding times than do control subjects (Tobin et al. 1983).

Anxious patients complain of an inability to get enough air and feelings of suffocation or oppression (Christie 1935). They breathe rapidly, sigh frequently, and only rarely develop tetany during an episode. Anxiety-driven hyperventilation can lead to diminished cerebral blood flow, light-headedness, and feelings of depersonalization. Gasping, sighing, and air hunger are clues to the presence of panic attacks. Phobic symptoms, which are often associated with panic attacks, are another clue to the presence of anxiety disorder in patients with pulmonary disease.

Patients with anxiety or panic disorder are often hypocapnic (van den Hout et al. 1992), and once a patient is hypocapnic, the respiratory alkalosis can be maintained without visible overbreathing (Saltzman et al. 1963). Sighing—that is, periodic alterations of the breath toward total lung capacity—can abrogate the normal tendency to alveolar collapse when an individual breathes at low lung volumes, but sighing can also maintain hypocapnia in a person who chronically hyperventilates. Patients with panic disorder sigh more often (Wilhelm et al. 2001). However, it is not clear that hypocapnia itself produces panic (Griez et al. 1988). Patients with panic disorder have intrinsic tidal volume irregularity (Abelson et al. 2001).

D.F. Klein (1993) suggested that the primary abnormality in patients with panic disorder is an enhanced central chemosensitivity to increased pCO_2. M.E. Cohen and White (1951) showed that breathing up to 4% CO_2 induced anxiety attacks in patients with anxiety neurosis.

In other studies, CO_2-induced panic closely resembled naturally occurring episodes but differed qualitatively from the dysphoria experienced by control subjects who breathed increased levels of CO_2 (Woods et al. 1988). The kinetics of response to breathing CO_2 also differed between groups, with panic disorder patients displaying maximal responses to increased pCO_2 sooner than control subjects, suggesting increased chemosensitivity to this agent. Sodium lactate is a potent panic-causing agent that secondarily increases pCO_2 by inducing a rapid metabolic alkalosis and decreased ventilation (Hollander et al. 1987). Panic induced by CO_2 could be blocked by tricyclic antidepressants, alprazolam, and clonazepam (Woods et al. 1990), all effective antipanic agents.

Although most panic research has focused on the central dysregulation of breathing in response to CO_2, we have hypothesized that this dysregulation may reflect a primary or acquired instability in both central and peripheral cholinergic pathways. Indeed, preliminary results from our laboratory suggest that a subset of patients with panic disorder also show abnormally increased bronchial motor responses to the inhaled cholinergic agent methacholine (R. L. Kradin, unpublished data, December 1994).

The patient with panic disorder who has CO_2 sensitivity may interpret the interoceptive sensation of dysphoria and breathlessness as catastrophic, foreshadowing suffocation; to alleviate symptoms, this cognition can be reinterpreted through behavioral and cognitive interventions (D.F. Klein 1993).

PSYCHIATRIC ASPECTS OF RESPIRATORY SYNDROMES

Chronic Obstructive Pulmonary Disease

In patients with chronic obstructive pulmonary disease (COPD), chronic hypoxia can compromise thinking and mood, producing delirium, mood lability, and restrictions in daily activities. These deficits were documented in a six-center trial involving more than 200 patients, in which continuous versus nocturnal supplemental oxygen administration was compared in subjects with a pO_2 of less than 55 mm Hg or incipient right heart failure. Patients with COPD have impaired abstracting ability and complex perceptual motor integration. These are impaired more than motor speed, strength, or gross coordination. Continuous oxygen treatment improves quality of life, neuropsychiatric function, and longevity more than nocturnal-only treatment. No change in mood has been documented (Grant et al. 1982, 1987; Heaton et al.

1983; Nocturnal Oxygen Therapy Trial Group 1980; Prigatano et al. 1983; Series and Cormier 1990).

However, the benefits of supplemental oxygen have a psychological cost. Supplemental oxygen use is a social embarrassment. Some patients believe that home oxygen marks the beginning of terminal illness, and they may withdraw socially. Others become psychologically dependent on the oxygen supply (Marchionno et al. 1985). Patients may limit their emotional expressiveness in order not to exceed lung capacity. Dyspnea implies helplessness. Sexual dysfunction, inhibited sexual excitement, premature ejaculation, and avoidance of intimacy have all been noted in patients with chronic lung disease (Thompson 1982). The dyspnea of diminished exercise tolerance may also compound the shortness of breath reported by patients with both COPD and associated anxiety and depression.

Borson and McDonald (1989) suggested that clues to the diagnosis of major depressive disorder in patients with COPD include the perception of activity as effortful, pervasive pessimism, diurnal mood variation with morning worsening, and early morning awakening. The prevalence of depression in individuals with COPD is 12%–15%, and panic symptoms are often linked to depression (Light et al. 1985). In an autopsy-documented community study of suicide in men older than 65 years, Horton-Deutsch and colleagues (1992) found that 14 of 73 patients had a chief complaint of dyspnea and undiagnosed major depressive disorder. Characterologically, these 14 men seemed to have avoided doing tasks unless they could do them with their usual vigor.

The prevalence of panic symptoms may be high. A history of panic attacks has been reported in 38% of patients with COPD (Porzelius et al. 1992; Yellowlees et al. 1987). Although the presence of underlying lung disease tends to disqualify this group from a diagnosis of primary panic disorder according to DSM-IV-TR (American Psychiatric Association 2000) criteria, it is likely that the experience of panic is similar in this population, particularly with respect to the catastrophic interpretation of interoceptive cues. Because a significant subset of patients with COPD are predisposed to CO_2 retention, the possibility that CO_2 sensitivity generates panic cannot be excluded. Furthermore, common and possibly genetically determined elements may link the tendency to smoke and predisposition to panic disorder (Pohl et al. 1992).

We have noted that GABAergic agents suppress the respiratory pacemaker. To treat panic, benzodiazepines are used conservatively for fear of respiratory depression, but the benefits for relief of panic, anticipatory anxiety, and phobia must be weighed against the risk of CO_2

retention in any individual patient. Newer SSRIs may be useful therapeutically in this setting. To diminish fear and agitation without risking respiratory suppression, neuroleptic medications can also be beneficial in low doses. When respiratory drive is marginal, any sedative must be used cautiously.

Protriptyline, a stimulating tricyclic antidepressant, improves diurnal and nocturnal hypoxemia at a dose of 20 mg in a small percentage of patients with COPD. This effect appears to be unrelated to pulmonary mechanics but may correlate with decreased rapid eye movement (REM) sleep (Series and Cormier 1990). Protriptyline has also been shown to be beneficial in patients with sleep apnea; however, the effect on mood has not been clarified.

Borson and McDonald (1989) reported preliminary data from a trial of nortriptyline in patients with COPD and major depressive disorder. There was a notable risk of hypotension, especially when other antihypertensive medications were used concomitantly.

Because of recent emphasis on treatment of inflammation in both chronic lung disease and asthma, patients with respiratory compromise commonly receive high-dose steroids. Because the psychiatric side effects of steroids are dose related, agitation and mania may be underestimated in the acute setting, and the subsequent labile or depressed states may contribute to morbidity. Steroid side effects may respond acutely to low-dose neuroleptics.

Smoking and Smoking Cessation

For historical and practical reasons, cigarette smoking was largely unaddressed by members of the psychiatric community, despite considerable evidence that nicotine is addictive. It has been argued that Freud's compulsive cigar smoking disposed psychotherapists to excuse the smoking habit in their patients. In addition, the extraordinarily high prevalence of cigarette smoking among hospitalized patients with chronic psychosis and substance-related disorders has been tacitly accepted (Goff et al. 1992).

Although cigarette smoke contains hundreds of bioactive substances, nicotine appears to be the major component with central and peripheral neuroactivity. Nicotine, which increases heart rate and blood pressure, acts as an acute stimulus for breathing (Stolerman and Shoaib 1991). Nicotine increases dopamine release in the prefrontal cortex and nucleus accumbens (Mifsud et al. 1989). Other addictive agents such as opiates, amphetamines, and cocaine also release dopamine (DiChiara and Imperato 1988).

Several large studies have found that cigarette smoking is associated with a history of major depressive disorder and with other negative states (Anda et al. 1990; Glassman et al. 1990; Kendler et al. 1993). In a review of this subject, Glassman (1993) made a convincing argument that depressive illness is highly correlated with having ever smoked, with addictive smoking, and with substantial difficulty with smoking cessation. On the basis of these highly significant correlations, it has been suggested that smokers may share a genetic vulnerability toward both behaviors, because little evidence suggests that smoking alone can predispose an individual to depression. Alcoholism (Covey et al. 1993), generalized anxiety disorder, and panic disorder all show an increased association with cigarette smoking (Carvajal et al. 1989; Glassman 1993). Most anxious smokers report that cigarette smoking allays anxiety, although experimental models do not support this observation (Frederick et al. 1988).

Even when the variables of anxiety and alcoholism are controlled for, the association between smoking and depression remains. Glassman (1993) pointed out that although depression was not listed as a criterion for nicotine withdrawal in DSM-III-R (American Psychiatric Association 1987), 75% of heavy cigarette smokers who attempt to quit will experience depressive symptoms. In some patients with severe psychiatric disease in remission, attempts at smoking cessation have led to severe exacerbation of symptoms (Glassman et al. 2001), which remitted with a return to smoking (Glassman 1993).

The effects of nicotine on adrenergic, serotonergic, and dopaminergic pathways modulate dysphoric symptoms. Nicotine-induced firing of dopaminergic neurons that project to prefrontal areas may also antagonize the negative symptoms in patients with schizophrenia and could help to explain the inordinately high prevalence of cigarette smoking in this population (Tung et al. 1990). Sustained-release bupropion (Hurt 1997), nortriptyline (Prochazka 1998), nicotine gum, nicotine inhaler, nicotine nasal spray, and nicotine patch have been effective in treatment programs for tobacco dependence. a U.S. Publisc Health Service consensus report underscored the dose-response relationship betwen intensity of counseling and effectiveness for three types of counseling: practical counseling and social support in and out of treatment (Tobacco Use and Dependence Clinical Practice Guideline Panel 2000). (For more information on behavioral methods for smoking cessation, see Chapter 46.)

Asthma

Asthma is one of the classic psychosomatic diseases. French and Alexander (1939–1941) hypothesized a specific central conflict: the strong, unconscious dependency wish toward the mother associated with the fear of separation. Asthma was seen as a struggle to have the last word. Emotional arousal (anxiety, fear, and anger) and suggestion can cause changes in airway tone. These changes have the greatest effect when they work synergistically with environmental or physical triggers. Airway reactivity to emotion may be mediated by the vagus nerve (Isenberg et al. 1992). Suggestion and emotion may preferentially affect the larger, upper airways (Lehrer et al. 1986), which are innervated by cholinergic neurons.

The challenge for patients with asthma is to lead a full life despite the tendency to wheeze. Boner and colleagues (1992) found that patients make judgments about their condition, assessments that correlate with objective markers of increased mortality risk and increased severity. Attack severity is associated with major depressive disorder, panic attacks, the number of emergency room visits, and self-assessment of risk of death. Psychoeducation, relaxation, biofeedback, and family therapy have each had a role in the care of asthma patients (Ewer and Stewart 1986; Lehrer et al. 1992). Appropriate management of prophylactic and as-needed medications is a critical aspect of education. The side effects of antiasthmatic drugs are jitteriness, palpitations, and insomnia. Those who become phobic about dyspnea may overuse bronchodilator inhalers. Table 26–1 summarizes adverse effects of pulmonary medications that have psychiatric implications.

Weiss (1994) described a sensible behavioral management program. He used a problem checklist to assess asthma medications, early signs of wheezing, triggers of an attack, individual behavior and behavior of other people during an attack, and the effects of asthma on social development, school, and the family (Creer 1979). A patient diary of attacks is an added resource. Weiss looks for core psychological issues that may prevent the patient from attending to early warning signals or from taking medication appropriately (e.g., fear of appearing inadequate, fear of rejection, and drive to excel athletically, such that there is a premium on keeping vulnerability secret). Weiss's advice to his patients is to know the facts and fallacies about asthma, the emotional and physical factors that precipitate and aggravate an attack, the early warning signs and what to do about them, and how to relax and breathe abdominally.

Factitious Asthma

Occasionally, asthma may be a feature of factitious illness. The distinguishing clinical and physiologic features

TABLE 26–1. Side effects of common pulmonary medications

Adrenergic bronchodilators

Mild tremor, palpitations, transient adrenergic rush with inhaler use

Danger of compulsive overuse, associated with risk of death from asthma

Corticosteroids

Dose- and duration-related insomnia, irritability, lability, maniform psychosis, depression

Brief treatment for exacerbation of pulmonary condition seems to be associated with few complications

Cycloserine

Irritability, excitement, drowsiness, nightmares, insomnia, depression, delirium

Ipratropium bromide

Systemic side effects uncommon

Isoniazid

Schizophreniform psychosis, delirium, euphoria, agitation, paranoia, auditory and visual hallucinations

Commonly given with vitamin B_6 or nicotinamide to prevent the neurological sequelae of vitamin B_6 deficiency

Rifampin

Concomitant use of nortriptyline may increase rifampin level

Theophylline

Jitteriness, difficulty falling asleep, trouble concentrating until tolerance develops

At toxic levels, nausea, vomiting, headache, diarrhea, irritability, then seizures, arrhythmia, and death

A study comparing cromolyn and theophylline in children with asthma suggested that theophylline was associated with cognitive impairment and depression (Furukawa et al. 1988)

were documented in three cases reported by Downing et al. (1982). These patients, all of whom had a history of psychiatric illness, had respiratory distress with wheezing and an apparent response to conventional therapy; however, features inconsistent with asthma included the absence of a significantly elevated alveolar-arterial oxygen tension difference, lack of hyperinflation on chest X ray, and normal small airway function immediately after attack. Self-induced wheezing was loudest at the neck, with transmission to the chest wall; in one patient, the sound was related to holding the vocal cords in apposition. There was no bronchial reactivity to methacholine inhalation. Intentional malingering is probably not as common a reason as panic attacks for repeated hospital visits.

Pulmonary Embolus

The differential diagnosis of sudden anxiety or a panic attack includes pulmonary embolus. A panic attack in a postoperative setting or in a patient known to have phlebitis should lead to measurement of blood gases and consideration of this often-overlooked diagnosis. Seizure, syncope, and dyspnea occur commonly in patients with pulmonary embolus.

Sleep Apnea

During normal sleep, oxygenation decreases and pCO_2 increases. In Stage IV sleep, breathing is regular (Fishman 1972; Hedgel and Cherniack 1988). During REM and Stage I and II non-REM sleep, irregular breathing and apnea—obstructive or central or both—occur. Daytime sleepiness, morning headache, restless sleep, snoring, and thrashing in bed should raise the suspicion of sleep apnea in those who complain of depression or memory loss, especially obese men. Medroxyprogesterone, a respiratory stimulant, has helped some patients with obstructive sleep apnea, especially those with CO_2 retention. Protriptyline helps about 50% of patients with mild to moderately severe disease, in part by stimulating upper airway inspiratory muscle activity or by decreasing REM sleep. Continuous positive airway pressure at night is another option. (For further information on the management of sleep apnea, see Chapter 24.)

Respiratory Dyskinesia

In patients with dyskinesia from neuroleptics or other drugs, the choreiform movement disorder of the chest may produce grunting, gasping breathing, and the respiratory alkalosis of hyperventilation (Godlee et al. 1989). As in other movement disorders, the signs are absent during sleep and are augmented as sympathetic tone increases. Usually, choreiform movements are also noted in the tongue, hands, or toes, bolstering the diagnosis (Jann and Bitar 1982). Respiratory dystonia may predispose a patient to aspiration. Patients with COPD have a higher prevalence of movement disorder (Campbell et al. 1983); the basal ganglia are perhaps more vulnerable in the setting of hypoxia (W.J. Weiner et al. 1978).

Gastrointestinal Disorders

Kevin W. Olden, M.D., F.A.C.G.

R. Bruce Lydiard, M.D., Ph.D.

The diagnosis of symptomatic gastrointestinal (GI) disorders without structural abnormalities has traditionally lacked precision. Some terms, such as *chronic gastritis*, *mucous colitis*, and *spastic colon*, widely used by clinicians to describe these disorders, have implied a physiologic explanation such as inflammation when no such explanation existed. Diagnostic criteria have varied widely among researchers. More than 25 functional GI disorders have been described. Since 1988, international working groups have been formulating diagnostic criteria for the major functional bowel disorders (Drossman et al. 2000), allowing a common nomenclature for the first time. These efforts, by providing a common language for clinical trials, hold promise for the development of more effective therapeutic modalities.

EPIDEMIOLOGY

Functional GI disorders are extremely common. A total of 69% of respondents to a survey of householders in the United States reported experiencing symptoms, in the 3 months before participation in the survey, that met the criteria for at least 1 of 25 distinct GI disorders (Drossman et al. 1993). Symptoms consistent with functional disorders of the large bowel were reported by 44% of the sample, of the esophagus by 42%, of the gastroduodenal region by 26%, and of the anorectal area by 26%.

In North America, the GI disorders that are more common in women than in men are globus, functional dysphagia, irritable bowel syndrome (IBS), constipation, abdominal pain, and functional biliary pain. Men, however, more commonly experience aerophagia and postprandial bloating (Drossman et al. 1993).

CONCOMITANT PSYCHIATRIC PATHOLOGY

Many investigators have contributed to the understanding of how the brain and gut interact (Heitkempe et al. 2001; Mertz et al. 2000; Naliboff et al. 2001; Rossel et al. 1999; Schmulson et al. 2000; Tougas 2000; Van Ginkel et al. 2001). The relation between GI complaints and psychiatric pathology is complex. Patients with concomitant GI complaints and psychiatric pathology are more likely to have learned illness behavior, to report more chronic medical problems, to avoid work or school as a result of medical complaints, and to have families in which illness behavior was rewarded and amplified (Levy et al. 2000). Patients with functional GI disorders tend to have a higher number of physician visits if they have concomitant psychiatric disorders (Herschbach et al. 1999). A significantly higher rate of physical or sexual abuse in childhood or adulthood has been found among patients with functional GI disorders. These patients have also had more lifetime surgeries and were more likely to develop chronic or recurrent abdominal pain with multiple somatic complaints (Drossman et al. 1990b). A substantial body of literature documents a high prevalence of psychiatric disorders among patients with functional bowel disorders compared with the general population (Bennett 1991; Fullwood and Drossman 1995; Irwin et al. 1996; Kaplan et al. 1996; Lydiard 1997; Lumley et al. 1997; Olden 1998; Olden and Drossman 2000; Slepoy et al. 1999; Talley et al. 1997; Whitehead 1996).

However, patients who seek medical care differ significantly from those who meet the diagnostic criteria for functional bowel disorders but who do not seek treatment. Only about half of the respondents to a community survey of individuals with bowel disturbances actually visited a doctor for their GI symptoms (Drossman et al. 1982). In one study, those who did not seek care for symptoms of diarrhea-predominant IBS did not differ psychologically from patients with lactose intolerance and a similar pattern of chronic diarrhea. However, by comparison, patients who presented to a university gastroenterology clinic with symptoms diagnosed as IBS tended to be significantly more psychologically distressed (Whitehead et al. 1988).

The psychological and psychosocial factors that lead patients to seek health care are critical to understanding these patients (Drossman et al. 1988; Talley et al. 1997; Whitehead and Schuster 1985). Consultation for bowel symptoms is often sought when symptoms are amplified by depression, anxiety, pain, and recent negative life events.

GLOBUS SENSATION

Globus is defined as a fullness, lump, or tickle in the throat at the level of the cricopharyngeal cartilage that is present for at least 3 months. It is not related to swallowing (i.e., symptoms occur between meals). There is no true dysphagia—that is, the patient has no difficulty swallowing solids or liquids. Any lifetime history of globus is common in healthy control subjects (46% in one study), and it occurs more commonly in women than in men (Thompson 1982). A complaint of globus accounts for 1%–3% of otolaryngology consultations (Freeland et al. 1974). Although globus has been classically associated with emotional distress, many patients with globus demonstrate anatomic pathology (Smit et al. 2000). The differential diagnosis includes achalasia (an esophageal dysmotility disorder); diffuse esophageal spasm; anatomic lesions of the tonsils, pharynx, or esophagus; cervical spondylolisthesis; gastroesophageal reflux disease; hypothyroidism; and neuromuscular dysfunction of cranial nerve IX, X, or XII (Greenberg et al. 1988; Janssen et al. 2000).

Although globus has classically been called *hystericus*, it occurs with anatomic findings, grief, conversion disorder, panic attacks, and depression (Greenberg et al. 1988; Kim et al. 196). In psychometric studies, patients with globus have nonspecific levels of "neuroticism"—for example, increased scores on depression and hypochondriasis scales (Deary et al. 1995; Thompson 1982).

Globus has a strong tendency to abate on its own. Biofeedback and behavior therapy have been used with reasonable success (Lichstein 1986), but no large-scale controlled trials have demonstrated the effectiveness of these interventions. antidepressants may also be of use (Cybulska 1997).

The responsible consultation-liaison psychiatrist should first confirm that no infection or neurological factor is responsible for the patient's complaint. This is best done by reviewing the case with the referring clinician. A mental status examination and a focused psychosocial history to identify any acute life stressors should follow. Particular attention should be paid to the diagnosis of anxiety and mood disorders. Most patients respond to a brief course of supportive psychotherapy. Anxiolytics and/or antidepressants should be considered for patients with diagnosed anxiety or mood disorder.

ESOPHAGEAL DYSFUNCTION

Five patterns of esophageal dysmotility have been described: achalasia, hypertensive lower esophageal sphincter, diffuse esophageal spasm, nutcracker esophagus, and nonspecific esophageal motility disorders. Of these, the last three are most often associated with psychiatric comorbidity. The diagnosis of esophageal dysmotility can be made only by esophageal motility testing—that is, by passing a pressure-sensitive motility catheter through the nose into the esophagus. Changes in pressure generated by esophageal peristaltic waves are measured by pressure receptors on the catheter, using constant water perfusion or electronic transducers. The use of tiny profusion catheters in combination with computer recorders has eliminated much of the technical difficulty of previous methods of motility testing, making the procedure much more comfortable for patients (Kahrilas et al. 1994).

The majority of patients with documented esophageal motility disorders have an Axis I psychiatric diagnosis. Clouse and Lustman (1983) found a prevalence of 84%, compared with 31% of a group of control subjects. Patients with esophageal motility disorders were likely to have major depressive disorder (52%), generalized anxiety disorder (36%), somatization disorder (20%), substance abuse disorders (20%), panic disorder (4%), or social phobia (4%). A subsequent study did not demonstrate an association between esophageal motility disorders and acute stress but confirmed the association between motility disorders and long-standing major psychiatric problems (Clouse and Lustman 1989).

Esophageal dysmotility is a common cause of noncardiac chest pain. Panic disorder is also frequently seen in patients with chest pain and angiographically normal coronary arteries. It is likely that both esophageal dysmotility and panic attacks contribute to the complaints of chest pain in many of these patients. Ringel and Drossman (1999) showed that psychiatric treatment could reduce chest pain complaints in these patients.

Clouse et al. (1987) treated 29 patients who had documented esophageal motility disorders with trazodone 100–150 mg/day for 6 weeks. Although esophageal motility tracings did not change, the treated patients, compared with those who received placebo, reported significant improvement in psychological well-being and a significant decrease in esophageal symptoms at 6 weeks.

Because calcium-channel blockers are potent smooth muscle relaxants, it was expected that use of these drugs would result in a decrease in abnormal esophageal motility patterns and, in turn, a decrease in GI complaints. In a study of nifedipine 10–30 mg tid compared with placebo, the esophageal motility tracings improved in the treated group, but the patients' psychological distress and esophageal complaints did not (Richter et al. 1987). This study, along with that of Clouse et al. (1987), would suggest that therapy targeted at the patient's emotional distress is much more efficacious in resolving symptoms than therapy targeted at the specific motility disorder.

Behavioral treatments using biofeedback and relaxation (Fang and Bjorkman 2001) hold theoretical promise for these disorders of the upper GI tract. However, further investigation in the form of large-scale, controlled trials is required to test this theory.

IRRITABLE BOWEL SYNDROME

IBS is a common and sometimes debilitating disorder that affects 8%–17% of the general population (Connell et al. 1965; Drossman et al. 1982; Thompson and Heaton 1980). It is second only to the common cold as a cause for absenteeism from work. IBS commonly occurs in early adulthood and affects women approximately twice as often as men (Fielding 1977; Hislop 1971). The diagnostic criteria for IBS have been refined (Drossman 1999) and are listed in Table 26–2. Psychiatric disorders in patients with IBS are shown in Table 26–3.

TABLE 26–2. Rome II diagnostic criteria for irritable bowel syndrome

At least 12 weeks, which need not be consecutive, in the preceding 12 months, of abdominal discomfort or pain that has two of three features:

1. Relieved with defecation; and/or
2. Onset associated with a change in frequency of stool; and/or
3. Onset associated with a change in form (appearance) of stool.

Source. Adapted from Thompson WG, Longstreth GF, Drossman DA, et al: "Functional Bowel Disorders and Functional Abdominal Pain," in *Rome II: The Functional Gastrointestinal Disorders.* McLean, Virginia, Degnon Associates, 2000, p. 360.

Most clinicians prefer using nonpharmacological modalities to treat patients with mild forms of IBS. These include education, dietary discretion, stress management techniques, and use of bulk-fiber products. In general, physicians request psychiatric consultation for patients whose conditions are refractory to such treatments.

Drossman and Thompson (1992) suggested that in the case of a patient with IBS, the clinician should 1) schedule regular appointments with the patient to indicate that the treating clinician is committed to the patient for the long term, 2) let the patient know that IBS is often a chronic condition that requires long-term management, 3) make a positive diagnosis of IBS to reassure the patient that he or she does not have a more serious illness such as cancer, and 4) identify reasonable treatment goals, such as better functioning, rather than complete relief from all symptoms. Psychotherapy may be indicated for some patients who have severe psychosocial stressors.

Psychiatric Morbidity in Patients With Irritable Bowel Syndrome

Treatment-seeking patients with IBS have high rates of psychiatric disorders. Earlier studies may have underestimated the prevalence of anxiety disorders because of the diagnostic hierarchies used before DSM-III-R, in which mood disorders, if present, were preferentially diagnosed. Lydiard et al. (1993) evaluated psychiatric disorders in treatment-resistant patients with IBS who were referred to a university-based gastroenterology practice. They found that 94% of the patients had a lifetime history of a major psychiatric illness (see Table 26–3). More than 80% were currently psychiatrically ill, primarily with anxiety and mood disorders. Many patients were unaware of their psychiatric diagnoses. Of the 27% of the IBS patients in the study who had panic disorder, nearly

TABLE 26–3. Psychiatric disorders among patients with irritable bowel syndrome

	Lifetime		Current	
DSM-III-R diagnosis (*n* = 35)	*n*	%	*n*	%
Panic disorder	11	31	9	26
Panic disorder with agoraphobia[a]	7	20	6	17
Limited-symptom panic attacks	5	14	5	14
Limited-symptom panic attacks with agoraphobia[a]	3	9	3	9
Generalized anxiety disorder	12	34	9	26
Social phobia	10	29	9	26
Major depression	16	46	8	23
Dysthymic disorder	5	14	3	9
Bipolar disorder	2	6	2	6
Cyclothymic disorder	3	9	3	9
Somatization disorder	9	26	6	17
Hypochondriasis	2	6	2	6
Obsessive-compulsive disorder	3	9	2	6
Any DSM-III-R diagnosis	33	94	32	91
Current anxiety disorder[b]			23	66
Current mood disorder[c]			12	34

[a]Subgroup of patients with panic disorder and not an additional group.
[b]Number of patients with any anxiety disorder (panic disorder with or without agoraphobia, limited-symptom panic attacks, generalized anxiety disorder, social phobia, or obsessive-compulsive disorder; several patients had more than one anxiety disorder diagnosis).
[c]Number of patients with any mood disorder (major depression, dysthymic disorder, bipolar disorder, or cyclothymic disorder; several patients had more than one mood disorder diagnosis).
Source. Adapted from Lydiard et al. 1993.

all had agoraphobia based on fear of loss of bowel control. Obsessive-compulsive disorder (OCD) has also been associated with IBS (Olden 1994); in that study, 42% of patients with OCD met diagnostic criteria for IBS, compared with 29% of control subjects who did not have OCD.

Patients with IBS who are referred for psychiatric consultation are more likely to have a psychiatric diagnosis than patients with IBS who are treated in primary care centers or who do not seek help (Drossman 1987). Those with significant anxiety or mood symptoms achieve only partial relief with first-line treatments. Several studies have shown the benefit of psychopharmacological medications, particularly antidepressants, for patients with IBS, but these studies were seriously flawed (Jailwala et al. 2000). The specific benefits have varied. Little attention was paid to psychiatric diagnoses. Even so, the few data available suggest that pharmacological treatment of the psychiatric disorder in patients with IBS leads to reduction in both GI and psychiatric symptoms (Jackson et al. 2000; Olden 2001).

Patients With Irritable Bowel Syndrome and Generalized Anxiety Disorder or Panic Disorder

Many patients with IBS exhibit symptoms of generalized anxiety without panic attacks. For these patients, agents

such as buspirone may be helpful, beginning at dosages of 5 mg tid, with dosages increased to 30–60 mg/day as tolerated. To date, no controlled trials of the use of buspirone have been done in this patient population, but clinical experience suggests that such therapy may be helpful. Antidepressants, which have also been shown to be effective in patients with generalized anxiety disorder, may be a useful alternative. Finally, in anxious patients (with either panic disorder or generalized anxiety disorder) who have IBS but not substance abuse disorder, antidepressants and benzodiazepines can relieve both anxiety and GI symptoms (Jackson et al. 2000).

Patients With Irritable Bowel Syndrome and Mood Disorders

Many treatment-seeking patients with IBS appear to exhibit major depressive disorder and dysthymic disorder with significant frequency. For patients with IBS who have depression and predominant diarrhea, imipramine or desipramine is used, starting at dosages of 10 mg/day, with dose increases as tolerated. These patients are often quite emotionally stimulated by antidepressants, so clinicians should explain in advance that stimulation may occur, and treatment should be initiated at very low doses. Sometimes, prescribed dosages must exceed 200 mg/day, but often patients will respond to lower doses. For patients with IBS who are sensitive to anticholinergic effects, especially those with constipation-predominant IBS, agents such as trazodone or fluoxetine (initiated at a low dose in the morning, with an increase over several days or weeks to 20 mg/day), sertraline (beginning at 12.5–25 mg in the morning, with an increase to 50–100 mg), or paroxetine (10 mg/day to start, with an increase to 20–40 mg over several days or weeks) may be reasonable alternatives. The strategy for all patients is to begin with low doses and increase as tolerated until the desired antipanic or antidepressant effect is achieved.

Patients With Irritable Bowel Syndrome and No Psychiatric Disorders

Patients with IBS who have no significant psychopathology may benefit from treatment with psychopharmacological agents. Clouse (1994) reported that of patients with treatment-refractory IBS who were referred to a university-based gastroenterology practice, of whom nearly half had no psychiatric disorder, more than 90% benefited from the addition of low-dose antidepressants or antianxiety agents. In this study, 92% of patients improved, 56% experienced complete remission of IBS symptoms, and 44% experienced remission after the first medication trial.

INFLAMMATORY BOWEL DISEASE

Patients with inflammatory bowel disease (IBD), Crohn's disease, or ulcerative colitis can develop marked abnormalities in fluid and electrolyte balance as a result of their diarrhea. Chronic hematochezia and malabsorption of nutrients can lead to significant anemia. In addition, these patients are at risk for poor absorption of calcium, phosphorus, folic acid, and cobalamin (Ginsberg and Albert 1989; Gitnick 1990). Patients with IBD also tend to have significant psychological impairment and disturbed social functioning (Drossman 1989).

The "specificity" theory proposed by Franz Alexander and co-workers of the Chicago psychoanalytic school was incorrect in assuming that IBD represents the somatic manifestation of an "organic neurosis" (Kollar et al. 1964). In a review of 138 studies exploring the relation between psychiatric problems and IBD, North et al. (1990) found that only 34 used control groups. Many studies also lacked precise diagnostic criteria for IBD and did not take disease severity into account. Rates of diagnosable psychiatric disorders are not significantly increased among patients with IBD compared with patients who have other chronic medical illnesses. Also, no relation has been found between severity of IBD and the presence or absence of a psychiatric diagnosis (Helzer et al. 1984). Investigators did find a suggestion of increased "obsessional thinking" in patients with ulcerative colitis. In addition, patients with ulcerative colitis who had undergone colectomy were more likely to have a diagnosable psychiatric disorder. However, North and colleagues (1990) did find in one study that patients with previously stable IBD were most likely to develop depressive symptoms as measured by the Beck Depression Inventory when they experienced an exacerbation of their IBD.

In the case of patients with IBD, psychiatric consultation involves more than establishing the presence or absence of a diagnosable psychiatric disorder. It includes assessing the patient's quality of life: his or her ability to perform activities of daily living, to achieve sexual satisfaction, and to ambulate freely. Screening for discrete psychiatric diagnoses should be done in addition to assessment of disease severity and functional limitations (Casati et al. 2000; Olden 1998; Walker et al. 1996). The clinician can give the best treatment recommendations if he or she uses this multimodal approach. A psychiatric consultant must work with all members of the multidisciplinary team—including ostomy nurses, surgeons, and gastroenterologists—to formulate treatment strategies. In addition to undergoing psychotherapy and psychopharmacological intervention, patients can seek help from patient advocacy groups such as the Crohn's & Colitis Foundation of America. The support that patients receive can greatly enhance their ability to cope. The goal is to maximize the patient's quality of life rather than merely reduce physical symptoms.

Renal Disease

Lewis M. Cohen, M.D.

Just a few short years ago, kidney failure meant death. One could no more conceive of an existence without functioning kidneys than consider life without a functioning heart. Renal transplantation and the various types of dialysis have transformed the fate of people with end-stage renal disease (ESRD) and have made it possible for consultation-liaison psychiatrists to attend to the psychiatric aspects of their new lives (Levy and Cohen 2000).

RENAL TRANSPLANTATION

Each year in the United States, approximately 20,000 transplantations of all kinds of organs are performed, and close to a million individuals are alive in the world as a result of artificial or natural substitution therapy (Bonomini 1991). Kidney transplantation is now an acknowledged successful treatment for ESRD (Kiley et al. 1993), with people who receive cadaveric grafts having a 1-year survival rate of 91%–96% (Sipes 1987). Whereas 70 years ago the Catholic Church was opposed to organ donation (Pope Pius XI 1930), Pope John Paul II (1980) declared spontaneous donation to be "an act of supreme charity." As long as financial profit is not a part of the transaction, living organ donation is now permitted or even encouraged by most major religions, including Islam, Buddhism, and Protestantism. Unfortunately, only 15% of Americans who need organ transplants to survive will receive them in any given year. The limiting factor is the availability of organs.

Many individuals have survived more than 20 years with a kidney transplant, and long-term reports are now appearing in the literature. For example, Gorlen et al. (1993), in Norway, examined the quality of life of 33 patients who had received kidney transplants an average of 15.6 years previously. Almost the entire sample reported a good quality of life, and three-quarters (76%) were fully rehabilitated and engaged in full-time work. Renal transplantations are now the standard of comparison for research on transplantation of other organs, such as allogeneic bone marrow transplantation (Andrykowski et al. 1990).

Renal transplantation is also offered to minors. Reynolds and co-workers (1991), in Manchester, England, examined the psychological aspects of transplantation in 29 children and adolescents. They compared children who underwent renal transplantation with those receiving hemodialysis and contrasted the data with those from a group of physically well classmates. Parents' and children's perceptions were evaluated. The improvement in physical health after transplantation was paralleled by improvement in the children's behavior and emotional state.

Although the conclusions of Reynolds and colleagues (1991) are encouraging, the team acknowledged that other studies have pointed to the difficulties of transplantation in children, including issues relating to appearance, such as short stature, hirsutism, and body image (S.D. Klein et al. 1984; Korsch et al. 1978). In the long-term outcome study by Henning et al. (1988), 25% of the children required physician intervention for emotional or psychological problems in early adulthood. As a result, pediatric transplantation programs need to provide psychosocial assistance and support for children and their families.

Psychiatric Participation in the Transplantation Team

Psychiatrists and social workers are currently members of most transplantation teams and provide screening and support of potential kidney transplant recipients and donors (Fricchione 1989). Psychiatric screening is still in a formative state, but transplantation is contraindicated in some obvious situations (Garcia et al. 1991)—for instance, when patients cannot intellectually or emotionally grasp the risks or the responsibilities that come with transplantation, or when they have irreversible psychoses or dementias. There is general agreement that patients with acute major psychiatric disorders, such as depression or delirium, need psychiatric treatment before transplantation.

In many programs, transplantation is not offered to patients who are actively abusing substances, although they do receive dialysis. There is some controversy about offering transplantation to patients infected with the human immunodeficiency virus (HIV), although these patients are legally entitled to dialysis treatment. Federal lawsuits have been directed at dialysis programs that discriminate against HIV-positive patients. Data from alcoholic patients who have received liver transplants should assist clinicians with many of these decisions in the future.

Nonadherence

The concern that people will not adhere to the necessary diet, medication regimen, or schedule of appointments has repeatedly been emphasized in the literature. Noncompliance is reported to be the third major cause, after simple graft rejection and systemic infection, of renal allograft failure (Didlake et al. 1988). Surman (1989) cited a 2%–5% incidence of allograft loss from noncompliance and listed risk factors including age less than 30 years, substance abuse history, and untreated major depressive disorder (Surman 1991). Rodriguez et al. (1991), in Puerto Rico, reported that the best predictor of noncompliance after transplantation is a history of noncompliance during dialysis. All of the patients in their "compliant" group had been scrupulously compliant when they were treated with dialysis, whereas 10 of 12 "noncompliant" patients had been less than conscientious.

Kiley et al. (1993) distinguished three subgroups of noncompliance: 1) noncompliance with medication,

2) noncompliance with diet, and 3) overall noncompliance. It is most troublesome that these authors believed that 75% of the 105 subjects in the study sample fit into a noncompliant category. The word *compliance* is itself paternalistic, suggesting that the patient is a naughty child and the staff are knowledgeable parents. Some medical writers use the word *adherence* (Christensen et al. 1990), which is almost as problematic, or speak of people "self-regulating" medications and diet, which is perhaps a little better.

The central dynamic for every patient who has been treated for kidney failure, whether by transplantation or by dialysis, is the conflict between independence and dependence (Abrams 1978). The noncompliant patient rebels and opposes the pull toward dependence. The key to this dilemma is for staff to acknowledge the conflict and to empower the patient along with his or her family (Christensen et al. 1992). Cognitive and behavioral approaches are often useful for managing these treatment issues (Hegel et al. 1992). (For further discussion regarding the issues involved in organ transplantation, see Chapter 28.)

PSYCHOLOGICAL ASPECTS OF DIALYSIS

When dialysis first became available, most attention was focused on the degree to which treatment might prolong life. Concerns have now shifted, and more effort is being devoted to improving quality of life. After the extension of Medicare coverage to practically all patients with ESRD, the population of patients undergoing dialysis grew 10-fold and now includes individuals with progressive and deteriorating disorders and a growing number of elderly individuals (Blagg et al. 1989). There are currently about 300,000 individuals with ESRD who are maintained with chronic dialysis, at an annual cost of approximately $45,00 per patient. The total estimated direct medical payments by public and private sources are more than $13 billion (NIH 2000; Pastan and Vaily 1998). These staggering numbers, combined with a consistently high mortality and morbidity that have not appeared to respond appreciably to improvements in dialysis technology, have prompted physicians, legislators, and medical-policy makers to question the value of dialysis ("Morbidity and Mortality of Dialysis" 1993).

The Agency for Healthcare Research and Quality (formerly the Agency for Health Care Policy and Research) has sponsored numerous research projects that go beyond the standard outcomes of mortality and morbidity to evaluate quality of life and patient satisfaction

(Kassirir 1993). Several questionnaires and research measures have been developed specifically for patients with ESRD (Laupacis et al. 1992), and a body of knowledge is accumulating about the different dialysis treatments (Wolcott 1991).

Sexual Function

Levy's (1973) important studies in the early 1970s were conducted when relatively few American patients were maintained with hemodialysis. Not many machines were available, the government did not fund dialysis, and patients were rigorously screened and selected by committees before they were allowed to begin treatment. Levy decided to study how these carefully chosen individuals had adapted to life with hemodialysis. He found that many were dysphoric. This result was due in part to the very high proportion of patients with kidney disease who also have sexual dysfunction.

Another psychiatric pioneer, Harry Abrams, conducted a study with colleagues at that same time and found that 75% of a sample of men with ESRD reported reduced potency (Abrams et al. 1975). Reduced potency was operationally defined as a decrease in the frequency of sexual intercourse by at least 50%. A more recent questionnaire study again underscored the problems of sexual dysfunction and infertility and demonstrated partial improvement after transplantation (Schover et al. 1990). Further amelioration of problems with potency may follow administration of testosterone or reduction of the corticosteroid or antihypertensive dose (Dubovsky and Penn 1980). Insertion of a penile prosthesis has also become an option (Gulledge et al. 1983). However, sexual problems continue to be largely ignored in most dialysis programs. (For further discussion of sexual disorders and dysfunctions, see Chapter 22.)

Quality of Life

The majority of psychosocial studies of ESRD have led investigators to conclude that the quality of life is best for patients with successful transplantations (Bentdal et al. 1991; Piehlmeier et al. 1991; Simmons et al. 1984), similarly good for home peritoneal dialysis patients (Bremer et al. 1989), and considerably worse for patients who receive hemodialysis (Barrett et al. 1990; Evans et al. 1985). Evans and colleagues (1985), who conducted one of the most rigorous studies, found that ESRD treatments were associated with numerous losses according to objective quality-of-life measures, such as active employment, yet, surprisingly, subjective quality-of-life measures were near normal (Hart and Evans 1987).

Clinicians should not believe that transplantation is a panacea. In an interesting methodological twist on the aforementioned studies, an Israeli team carefully matched 31 male nondiabetic patients with successful renal transplantations to 31 similar men who were receiving hospital-based hemodialysis (Sayag et al. 1990). Unlike in previous studies, the subjects in this study were paired according to age, religion, education, and time on dialysis or transplantation. When these demographic variables were accounted for, the psychological adjustment of patients in the two groups was remarkably similar. Sexual function was slightly improved after renal transplantation, but the vocational rehabilitation and psychological adjustment could not be distinguished.

Individuals who stay with hemodialysis may be more isolated and more receptive to the psychological and social benefits of structured dialysis programs. This was the conclusion drawn by Callender et al. (1989), who compared two groups of patients who had been offered transplantation; one group had accepted, the other refused and were on dialysis. The members of the group that refused transplantation were older, less educated, and more likely to be female than were those who had agreed to undergo the surgery.

Researchers involved in three prospective studies concluded that compared with a dialysis-treated population, people who receive kidney transplants experience improved physical and emotional outcomes (Parfrey et al. 1989; Russell et al. 1992; Simmons et al. 1981). A psychiatric history is a useful predictor of psychiatric symptomatology after transplantation (Sensky 1989).

Diminished quality of life and depression are particularly pronounced in people with failed transplantations who are now receiving dialysis (Bremer et al. 1989). This subgroup of dialysis patients must cope with the added disappointment of staff and family. Often they struggle with guilt over the "sacrificed" or "wasted" kidney.

Evaluation continues for patients receiving high-flux hemodialysis and recombinant human erythropoietin (Churchill et al. 1992). Erythropoietin not only helps patients to avoid the adverse effects of repeated transfusions but also appears to improve energy levels, psychological well-being, and sexual function (Evans et al. 1990). Both objective and subjective measures improve in patients who receive erythropoietin (McMahon and Dawborn 1992).

Ethical Issues and Discontinuation of Dialysis

The initial shortage of dialysis machines and the resulting need to screen patients made it necessary for hospitals to form dialysis selection committees. These committees included both medical staff and community representatives, such as members of the clergy. Many consultation-liaison psychiatrists play active roles in today's medical ethics committees based on this earlier model.

Nephrologists are sensitive to the reality that patients who are maintained with dialysis remain terminally ill. Statistics demonstrate that the life expectancy of a 65-year-old individual who requires treatment with dialysis is 3.5 years, or about one-fifth the life expectancy of a 65-year-old person who does not have ESRD (Nissenson 1993).

In 1999, 58% of the newly diagnosed chronic ESRD patients in New England are 65 or older, and 17% are 80 or older. As the population increasingly includes patients with diabetes and dementia, as well as geriatric patients, nephrologists have begun to accept that dialysis is a type of life-support treatment that may be electively discontinued (Chazan 1990; Epstein 1979; Galla 2000; Neumann 1992).

Although in some dialysis programs, discontinuing treatment is opposed (Fisher et al. 1986), 90% of surveyed nephrologists consider treatment cessation to be an option (Singer 1992). Kjellstrand and associates (Kjellstrand and Dossetor 1992; Neu and Kjellstrand 1986) reported that dialysis termination was the second leading cause of mortality in their sample, occurring in 23% of patient deaths. Data from the ESRD Network of New England indicate that approximately 20% of the patient population dies each year, and about one in four deaths are preceded by a decision to discontinue dialysis (ESRD Network of New England 1990). It would be ethically and emotionally comforting for staff and families if patients expressed their wishes relating to terminal care, but research—including our own—suggests that this expectation is probably unrealistic.

The large majority of people with ESRD do not articulate terminal care wishes, do not speak directly to their families about death, do not discuss this subject with medical staff, and do not complete the legal options available to them (L.M. Cohen et al. 1991; Holley et al. 1993; Husebye et al. 1987; Reilly 1990). Denial is a powerful coping mechanism for individuals with ESRD, and it is the rare patient who considers discontinuation of dialysis or seriously contemplates death (L.M. Cohen et al. 1993). People who receive dialysis are preoccupied not with death but with the ordinary activities of life (Norton 1969).

In our prospective study involving 19 patients and families who decided to terminate dialysis, none of the patients who were able to participate in making the decision were suicidal or irrational or had major psychiatric disorders. This was also the finding in our subsequent multicenter study at eight dialysis facilities in Canada and the United States (L. M. Cohen et al. 2000a, 2000b, 2000c). Patients had decided that progressive physical deterioration left them unable to enjoy life further and that dialysis was prolonging suffering rather than prolonging life (McKegney and Lange 1971).

Neuropsychiatric Syndromes

Chronic renal failure causes diffuse abnormalities in central nervous system (CNS) function. Most of the time, these abnormalities are subtle and subclinical, with comparatively mild abnormalities in concentration, problem solving, and calculation ability. Advanced uremia causes impaired mentation, lethargy, asterixis, multifocal myoclonus, and other neurobehavioral disturbances. Although these profound abnormalities may be reversible with the initiation of dialysis, subtle deficits remain in even well-dialyzed patients (Osberg et al. 1982). Adequacy of dialysis has an effect on these subtle abnormalities in the individual patient. As a whole, better-dialyzed patients have fewer electroencephalographic (EEG) abnormalities and improved concentration and sleep function (Teschan et al. 1983).

A deterioration in total intelligence as measured by the Wechsler Adult Intelligence Scale—Revised (Wechsler 1981) has also been found in patients with chronic renal failure who are undergoing dialysis. This decline is partly due to slowness in performing tests. Verbal skills are maintained at the original levels, but performance IQ scores deteriorate. Memory function, particularly working memory, is more severely affected. Many patients complain of problems in concentration, which increase demonstrably during the intervals between dialysis treatments (West 1978). Teschan et al. (1977) believed that the adequacy of dialysis treatments may be monitored by repeat neuropsychological measurements.

The differential diagnosis of neuropsychiatric syndromes in the patient with chronic renal failure includes hypercalcemia, hypophosphatemia, hypoglycemia, hyperglycemia, hyponatremia, hypernatremia, drug intoxication, hypertensive encephalopathy, cerebrovascular disease, subdural hematomas, meningitis, encephalitis, and normal-pressure hydrocephalus. In a susceptible person, HIV encephalopathy should also be considered. Some authors have suggested that hyperparathyroidism may be an important factor in the mental status changes of patients with chronic renal failure and that treatment of hyperparathyroidism may have a beneficial effect on mental symptoms (Massry 1984).

Dialysis dementia is a specific syndrome that was first reported in the early 1970s and is characterized by progressive encephalopathy, stuttering, dysarthria, dysphasia, impaired memory, depression, paranoia, myoclonic jerking, and seizures. In the course of approximately 1 year, the syndrome may progress to global dementia and death. A triphasic EEG abnormality is seen in this condition. This syndrome was found to correlate with high concentrations of aluminum in the brain tissue of patients and was clearly associated with outbreaks in dialysis units in which the water supply was contaminated with excess aluminum concentrations. Because water treatment in the United States now removes aluminum from dialysate water, the incidence of dialysis dementia has markedly diminished.

The pathophysiology of uremic encephalopathy is not known. Nonspecific EEG changes, such as diffuse slowing, occur commonly in uremia, can improve with dialysis treatment, and can be reversed entirely with successful renal transplantation. Structural changes in the CNS have not been noted in patients with uremic encephalopathy. Oxygen utilization in the brain is reduced in patients with uremia (Scheinberg 1954). These changes may be caused by uremic toxins, although the exact toxins are unknown. Urea itself is not believed to be a uremic toxin.

Psychotropic Medications

Antidepressants. Clinicians have always been alert to the possibility of depression in this patient population, and antidepressants have been used extensively. Unfortunately, patients maintained with dialysis seemed by anecdote to be more sensitive to the side effects associated with these medications (Levy and Cohen 2000; Stoudemire et al. 1990). The reason is unclear but may be related to an increase in concentrations of the hydroxylated tricyclic metabolites (Dawling et al. 1982). Anecdotal evidence also suggests that patients are better able to tolerate the serotonin reuptake inhibitors, as well as medications such as bupropion. A pharmacokinetic study involving depressed patients with severe renal dysfunction maintained with hemodialysis showed that plasma fluoxetine concentrations were unaffected at the normal adult dose (Bergstrom et al. 1993). As discussed in Chapter 44, electroconvulsive therapy (ECT) has a role to play in the treatment of these medically ill patients (R.D. Weiner and Coffey 1987).

Anxiety agents. It is probably best to avoid benzodiazepines that have pharmacologically active metabolites, such as diazepam (Levy 1985). Most clinicians rely on lorazepam, clonazepam, oxazepam, and temazepam. Doses are usually in a range of one-half to two-thirds of those used in patients with normal renal function (Levy 1985).

Antipsychotics. Neuroleptics have been used extensively, but cautiously, in patients who have renal failure or are receiving dialysis. One would imagine that patients are at greater risk for neuroleptic malignant syndrome because of the marked fluid shifts and dehydration associated with treatment (Stoudemire et al. 1991). Likewise, medications such as clozapine lower the seizure threshold (W.H. Wilson and Claussen 1994) and should warrant concern in a patient population in which dementias, other organic brain syndromes, and marked transient electrolyte shifts are often seen. Nevertheless, anecdotal evidence again suggests that these medications are commonly given, often at somewhat lower starting doses than usual, and that the high-potency agents, in particular, appear to be well tolerated (Levy 1985).

Mood stabilizers. Lithium poses an interesting challenge for the practitioner because the kidney is the primary route of excretion for this monovalent medication. Stoudemire et al. (1991) pointed out that patients maintained on dialysis do not eliminate lithium and therefore do not require daily lithium supplementation between treatments. The protocol requires determining an appropriate dose (usually 300–600 mg), which is administered after the dialysis. Serum lithium levels are checked 2–3 hours later. Some of the alternatives to lithium, such as valproate or verapamil, may also prove to be of value for these patients.

CONCLUSION

The vast majority of individuals who develop kidney failure have never had psychiatric disorders. Medical staff and psychiatrists are equally guilty of viewing patients through a pathological lens. Most patients in dialysis programs are psychologically healthy people who are suddenly faced with incredible new stresses and demands. Life becomes a repetitive and prolonged experience of having the blood removed from one's body and circulated through a machine. Life for the patient undergoing hemodialysis includes perhaps 17 different daily medications, enormous pharmaceutical and medical bills, intermittent pain and fatigue, uncertainty about the future, a long wait for a transplant, a rigid diet, dependency on others for basic care, and exposure to peers whose conditions deteriorate or who die.

It is a pleasure and a challenge for psychiatrists to work with patients who have ESRD and with the staff who care for them. Dialysis staff members are knowledgeable about their patients in a way that is increasingly uncommon in other fields of medicine. The medical technology associated with transplantation is very sophisticated, and the clinical management decisions, such as discontinuing treatment, are extremely complex. Nephrologists and their staffs and eager for assistance in the management of the psychosocial aspects of the ESRD patient population. There are currently several thousand dialysis and transplantation facilities in the United States that could become the settings for psychiatric consultations. We sincerely hope that psychiatry will take advantage of this stimulating opportunity.

Endocrine Disorders

Roger G. Kathol, M.D., C.P.E.

Patients with endocrine disorders often have psychiatric symptoms. Depression and anxiety are the most common psychiatric presentations of endocrine disorders. Mania occasionally occurs, either in association with specific endocrine diseases, such as Cushing's disease, or when patients are treated for other diseases such as hypothyroidism (Josephson and MacKenzie 1980). Dementia can also be found in a subpopulation of patients with endocrine disease. However, dementia related to these hormonal causes accounts for less than 1% of patients with dementia in case series (Clarfield 1988). Finally, psychosis and delirium can occur in patients with severe endocrinopathies, as in patients with other forms of serious medical illness. With the improved ability to identify endocrine disorders through physical examination and laboratory testing, fewer patients than in the past demonstrate delirium or psychosis primarily caused by their endocrine abnormality. Endocrine diseases are identified earlier in the course of the disorder than was previously possible.

It is important to recognize which endocrine disorders are associated with high frequencies of specific kinds of psychiatric syndromes (see Table 26–4), because these might cause or contribute to the symptoms of a patient who is first seen in psychiatric consultation. The differential diagnoses should always include questions pertinent to these endocrine disorders and, when appropriate, a physical examination to document the presence or absence of signs of the disorder in question. When the symptoms and/or signs suggest that an endocrine abnormality might be present, or when the patient presents with a psychiatric syndrome with aspects atypical for the primary psychiatric disorder (e.g., outside the age at risk, unusual symptoms, limited family history, nonresponse to usual treatment), further investigation with laboratory tests is warranted. Endocrine tests in the absence of signs or symptoms of a specific endocrine disease, including thyroid disease (Bauer et al. 1991), are generally not indicated. The psychiatrist must therefore perform at least focal physical examinations for endocrine signs when endocrine disorders are seriously considered in the differential diagnosis.

Difficulties can arise if appropriate psychiatric questions are not asked in interviews of patients with specific endocrine disorders. This is particularly true for patients with Cushing's disease, in whom mood disorder is a frequent serious complication and suicide a significant risk. Likewise, it is important to ask individuals with diabetes about anxiety and depression, because depressed patients with diabetes tend to have persistent depression, along with impairment in personal, social, and economic functioning and worse glucose control as demonstrated by increased hemoglobin A_1 levels (Lustman et al. 1986). Psychiatric questions should also be asked of patients with myxedema, because cognitive impairment occurs relatively frequently. Depending on the degree and the duration of the hypothyroid state, impairment may require adjustment of daily responsibilities. Finally, symptoms of mania should be reviewed in patients treated for newly diagnosed hypothyroidism. Behavior

TABLE 26–4.   Prevalence of psychiatric disorders among patients with endocrine disease, from studies with prospective systematic evaluations

Endocrine disorder	Anxiety disorder	Major depression	Cognitive impairment	Substance abuse	Psychosis/ delirium	Any disorder
Diabetes mellitus	0%–45%[a,b,c]	7%–33%[a,b,c]	0%[c]	1%–14%[a,b,c]	0%–1%[a,b,c]	33%–71%[a,b,c]
Hypothyroidism	20%–33%[d]	33%–43%[d]	29%[e]	—	5%[e]	—
Hyperthyroidism	53%–69%[f,g]	30%–70%[f,g]	0%[f]	0%–8%[f]	0%[f,g]	53%–100%[f,g]
Hyperparathyroidism	12%[h]	11%–43%[h,i,j]	3%–39%[h,i,j]	—	3%–9%[h,j]	23%–67%[h,j]
Cushing's syndrome	18%[k]	35%–86%[k,l,m,n]	—	3%–6%[k,m]	0%[k,l,m]	80%[k,m]
Addison's disease	—	48%[o]	—	—	4%[o]	—
Pheochromocytoma	12%*–29%†[p]	12%*–18%†[p]	—	—	—	—
Acromegaly	—	2.5%[q]	—	—	—	—

*Definite. †Probable plus definite.

Source.   [a]Popkin et al. 1988; [b]Wilkinson et al. 1988; [c]Lustman et al. 1986; [d]Jain 1972; [e]Nickel and Frame 1958; [f]Trzepacz et al. 1988; [g]Kathol and Delahunt 1986; [h]Joborn et al. 1986; [i]Brown et al. 1987; [j]Petersen 1968; [k]Hudson et al. 1987; [l]S.I. Cohen 1980; [m]Haskett 1985; [n]Jeffcoate et al. 1979; [o]Cleghorn 1951; [p]Starkman et al. 1985; [q]Abed et al. 1987.

control may be required, but because manic symptoms usually resolve spontaneously, pharmacotherapy is not necessary.

DIABETES MELLITUS

The most frequent psychiatric conditions associated with diabetes mellitus include anxiety and depression (Table 26–4). Because diabetes is controlled with treatment but not cured, patients experiencing persistent psychiatric symptoms who receive psychiatric intervention may have less disease morbidity (Table 26–5). Eating disorders affect young women with insulin-dependent diabetes, and intentional omission of insulin may lead to more diabetic complications (Rydall et al. 1997). At present, the most appropriate forms of intervention include syndrome-specific medication and cognitive-behavioral psychotherapy.

HYPOTHYROIDISM

Although depression and anxiety are seen with great frequency in patients with hypothyroidism, the greatest concern is the cognitive deficits that can occur as a result of the changes in metabolic activity in the central nervous system (CNS). For this reason, cognition should be assessed and lifestyle adjustments made until adequate treatment has been administered. Later assessment is important; follow-up studies of dementia suggest that treatment of hypothyroidism does not necessarily reverse memory deficits (Clarfield 1988).

In most patients who have either depression or anxiety with hypothyroid state, correction of the thyroid deficiency with thyroxine replacement therapy will reverse psychiatric symptoms. If, however, these symptoms do not improve after adequate replacement therapy for 1 month to 6 weeks, the clinician should consider alternative forms of direct psychiatric intervention (Table 26–5). Certainly, if a patient has life-threatening or highly debilitating symptoms of depression or anxiety, a short course of psychotropic medications could be tried during the wait for the effects of hormone replacement therapy to occur.

HYPERTHYROIDISM

As in patients with hypothyroidism, depression and anxiety are common in patients with hyperthyroidism. In most situations, it is not difficult to identify hyperthyroid patients, given the signs and symptoms of that disease. In more than 90% of people with symptoms of depression and anxiety associated with hyperthyroidism who do not have a preexisting psychiatric condition, these symptoms will resolve during the course of treatment for the hyperthyroidism alone (Kathol and Delahunt 1986). For this reason, no other psychiatric intervention is required until an adequate trial of antithyroid medication, radioactive iodine, or thyroid surgery has been completed. As might be expected, symptoms of anxiety will disappear in direct relation with the reduction in thyroid hormone levels. Depressive symptoms are not as linearly related to thyroxine levels.

TABLE 26–5. Important clinical factors among patients with endocrine disorders and psychiatric symptoms

Endocrine disease	Effect of psychiatric disorder on illness	Effect of treatment of endocrine disorder on psychiatric symptoms	When to treat psychiatric symptoms with psychiatric medications	Comments
Diabetes mellitus	Increased hemoglobin A_1 levels[a] Increased rate of diabetic complications	Depression persists[b]	Early after identification	Stressful situation does not affect glucose control[c]
Hypothyroidism	May lead to misdiagnosis Need to do physical examination and obtain medical history	Anxiety and depression resolve[d] Cognitive function stabilizes, but problems persist[e] Short period of mania may occur	If symptoms are life-threatening or persist > 1 month after thyroid replacement therapy	Psychiatric symptoms less severe now than before thyroid replacement therapy; take this into account when reading old literature Thyroid laboratory tests unnecessary unless signs of thyroid disease are present on examination, the patient is an elderly woman,[g] or presentation is atypical If mania occurs during treatment, continue replacement therapy; mania will typically subside
Hyperthyroidism	May lead to misdiagnosis Need to do physical exam and obtain medical history	Anxiety and depression resolve[h]	If symptoms are life-threatening or persist > 1 month after thyrotoxicosis is treated	Same as for hypothyroidism Anxiety symptoms correlate with free T_4 level
Hyperparathyroidism	Psychiatric symptoms may be first sign of hypercalcemia	Depression, but not cognitive problems,[i] resolves	If symptoms are life-threatening or persist > 1 month after calcium level has normalized	Calcium level should be determined in patients with newly diagnosed major depression, atypical presentations, or other symptoms of hypercalcemia Calcium level correlates with degree of psychiatric symptoms[j]
Pheochromocytoma	May lead to misdiagnosis if thorough history is not obtained and criteria for anxiety disorders are not used	Symptoms usually resolve with treatment	If symptoms are disabling or life-threatening	Anxiety disorder less common than originally suspected[k]
Cushing's syndrome	Mood symptoms may be severe, with increased suicide risk[l] May lead to misdiagnosis, particularly because HPA axis abnormalities also occur in primary depression Physical examination is necessary	Delayed (1–3 months), but eventual resolution[m,n]	If symptoms are disabling or life-threatening If symptoms persist after > 2 months of glucocorticoid control	Resolution of HPA axis abnormalities with depression treatment and blunted ACTH response after CRF- or insulin-induced hypoglycemia differentiate primary depression from Cushing's syndrome in patients without physical signs[n] Family history of mood disorder less likely than among primary mood disorder patients

Note. ACTH = adrenocorticotropic hormone; CRF = corticotropin-releasing factor; HPA = hypothalamic-pituitary-adrenal; T_4 = thyroxine.
Source. [a]Lustman et al. 1986; [b]Lustman et al. 1988; [c]Kemmer et al. 1986; [d]Jain 1972; [e]Haggerty et al. 1993; [f]Josephson and MacKenzie 1980; [g]Bauer et al. 1991; [h]Kathol and Delahunt 1986; [i]Brown et al. 1987; [j]Petersen 1968; [k]Starkman et al. 1985; [l]Haskett 1985; [m]Kelly et al. 1983; [n]Jeffcoate et al. 1979; [o]Hudson et al. 1987.

HYPERPARATHYROIDISM

Studies using criteria-based diagnoses of psychiatric illnesses in patients with hyperparathyroidism have not been performed. Data from patients who were interviewed prospectively but not systematically with structured instruments provide a general idea of the kinds of symptoms that might occur (see Table 26–4). From this incomplete literature, the impression is that mood symptoms are commonly seen in patients with this disorder. The several case series suggest that the severity of symptoms intensifies as the level of hypercalcemia increases. Delirium, psychosis, and cognitive impairment are more commonly seen in patients who have calcium levels greater than 15 or 16 mg/dL. Depressive symptoms but not cognitive symptoms tend to resolve with treatment (Brown et al. 1987). Cognitive symptoms may improve; however, some symptoms may remain. For this reason, identification of patients with hyperparathyroidism, which may cause psychiatric symptoms, is very important. Patients with atypical presentations of depression or changes in mental capabilities without a definite etiology should have serum calcium levels determined, because no other signs or symptoms of hypercalcemia may be present.

CUSHING'S SYNDROME

One of the best-substantiated associations between psychiatric symptoms and a physical disorder may be that between mood disorder and Cushing's syndrome. Most studies indicate that 50%–80% of patients with Cushing's syndrome also experience mild to severe depressive symptoms (see Table 26–4). It is also well documented that the depressive symptoms are moderate to severe in up to 50% of such patients. Many of these individuals exhibit psychotic features, unusual in depression associated with medical illness. For this reason, it is critical that clinicians assess mood in individuals with Cushing's syndrome as part of the medical evaluation.

In patients who demonstrate depression, it may be necessary to treat the depression while awaiting resolution of both the physical and psychiatric manifestations of Cushing's syndrome through surgery and/or medical therapy directed at the cause of hypercortisolemia. Such intervention may include medications or electroconvulsive therapy (ECT) in more severely ill patients. For less severely ill patients, supportive counseling or cognitive-behavioral therapy through the course of treatment for Cushing's syndrome may be sufficient. Ultimately, in all patients who have a mood syndrome related to Cushing's syndrome, the depression will resolve with control of the cortisol excess alone. Therefore, patients in whom the hypercortisolism has been controlled for several months can stop taking psychotropic medication with little likelihood of recurrence, unless there is a preexisting disorder.

Some patients with Cushing's syndrome have relatively few physiologic signs despite hypercortisolemia documented by increased urinary free cortisol levels or dexamethasone nonsuppression. Therefore, it is difficult to distinguish patients with Cushing's syndrome from those with hypothalamic-pituitary-adrenal axis hyperactivity related to primary depression. To differentiate these two conditions, the clinician should treat the patient's depressive symptoms and then, as the depression resolves, determine whether hypercortisolemia persists. If it does, this is suggestive evidence that Cushing's syndrome could be the cause of the patient's depression. Alternatively, the patient could be subjected to a corticotropin-releasing factor (CRF) infusion test. Patients with Cushing's syndrome have an augmented ACTH response to CRF infusion, whereas patients with primary depression have a blunted response.

ADDISON'S DISEASE

Few studies of psychiatric symptoms in patients with Addison's disease have been conducted since the mid-1950s. For this reason, it is impossible to determine whether psychiatric symptomatology is present with increased frequency in these patients or whether what was documented as psychiatric symptomatology was merely the apathy, fatigue, and lethargy associated with the underlying endocrine state.

PHEOCHROMOCYTOMA

Pheochromocytoma is typified by excess catecholamine production. It has long been assumed that because catecholamines are involved in the stress response, patients with pheochromocytomas are likely to have symptoms compatible with anxiety or panic disorder. However, Starkman et al. (1985) documented that few patients present with symptoms that meet the criteria for either generalized anxiety disorder or panic disorder (see Table 26–4). For this reason, when a thorough medical history is taken and a physical examination is performed in patients with pheochromocytoma, it is unlikely that these patients will appear to have anxiety disorder. Although no studies have been conducted, the anxiety symptoms that are present in patients with pheochromocytoma are likely to resolve with removal of the tumor causing the excess catecholamine production.

ACROMEGALY

Information about psychiatric aspects of acromegaly has largely been in the form of case reports and data from case series. Although the usefulness of the results of the investigation by Abed et al. (1987) is limited because of the methods used, the principal finding in that study involving 51 patients with acromegaly was that depression is no more commonly identified in this population than in the general population. This finding suggests that there is no increase in psychiatric morbidity in patients with acromegaly, in contrast to what was suggested by prior reports.

CONCLUSION

Several endocrine diseases are associated with a high frequency of psychiatric symptoms or syndromes. In most instances, these symptoms or syndromes resolve with adequate treatment of the endocrine disorder. However, in several endocrine disorders, psychiatric intervention may also be necessary. Two important facets of the assessment of patients with psychiatric symptoms are the physical examination and the medical history; these provide the most readily available data that will indicate whether further investigation into a potential endocrine etiology should be contemplated. In addition, patients who have an endocrine disorder should be questioned about commonly associated psychiatric symptoms. If psychiatric manifestations are recognized, the patient can be informed about the course of symptoms with treatment of the endocrine disorder and the likelihood of his or her requiring psychiatric care.

Systemic Lupus Erythematosus

Donna B. Greenberg, M.D.

Patients with systemic lupus erythematosus (SLE) can present with the neuropsychiatric complications of SLE itself, the complications of steroid treatment, or psychiatric syndromes associated with any chronic illness. The features of neuropsychiatric systemic lupus erythematosus (NPSLE) are delirium, psychosis, major depressive disorder, progressive cognitive dysfunction, seizures of all types, strokes, transverse myelitis, peripheral neuropathy, headache, and chorea. More rarely, aseptic meningitis, pseudotumor cerebri, autonomic neuropathy, or Guillain-Barré syndrome occurs (Boumpas et al. 1995). The American College of Rheumatology recently standardized the nomenclature, using DSM-IV (American Psychiatric Association 1994) criteria for psychiatric syndromes, so that NPSLE can be better studied (American College of Rheumatology Nomenclature and Case Definitions 1999). A case of NPSLE would be defined by one neuropsychiatric syndrome and three or more non-NPSLE criteria for SLE. The antiphospholipid antibody status of the patient should be reported, because the antiphospholipid antibody is associated with a high rate of recurrent thromboses. Antiribosomal P has been associated with NPSLE in some but not all studies. Cerebrospinal fluid (CSF) findings included increased cell counts and/or increased protein levels in only one-third of patients.

The pathology of NPSLE includes multifocal cerebral cortical microinfarctions from microvascular injury, vascular occlusion from vasculopathy, thrombosis, antibody-mediated neuronal injury, and, more rarely, vasculitis. Some autoantibodies may enter the central nervous system (CNS) through the injured vessels, which normally support the blood-brain barrier, or they may be produced locally within the nervous system (Bluestein 1987). The neuroimaging findings may correlate with the pathological findings but are often not specific.

Mood syndromes may be the most common psychiatric presentation of patients with lupus (Baker 1973; Grigor et al. 1978), but mood change is not always due to lupus involvement in the brain. Patients with SLE are often treated with steroids, which raises the risk of steroid-related mood syndromes and psychosis. Metabolic derangement—for instance, resulting from kidney impairment—may increase the likelihood of seizures and delirium. Convulsive seizures and complex partial seizures have their own psychiatric consequences (see Chapter 30 for further discussion). Patients with thrombosis are anticoagulated. Glucocorticoid treatment is the mainstay of treatment for active lupus; sometimes cyclophosphamide therapy or plasmapheresis is used. In practice, treatment options for CNS lupus include increasing doses of steroid medications; adding anticonvulsants, neuroleptics, and antidepressants, for psychiatric syndromes; and, for severe depression, administering electroconvulsive therapy (ECT) (Allen and Pitts 1978; Douglas and Schwartz 1982; Guze 1967).

Cobalamin (B$_{12}$) Deficiency

Donna B. Greenberg, M.D.

Cobalamin deficiency causes memory disturbance, paranoid depression, and dementia. Unsuspected cobalamin deficiency may contribute to treatment resistance in depressed patients (Herrera et al. 1991).

The minimal daily requirement of cobalamin is small, so deficiency is unlikely to occur in patients with normal absorption unless they are on a strict vegetarian diet. Deficiency occurs in patients with pernicious anemia (autoimmune loss of intrinsic factor and atrophic gastritis) and in patients with complete gastrectomy or bowel repairs that allow bacterial overgrowth in blind intestinal loops. Malabsorption from atrophic gastritis or ileal disease is an additional predisposing condition, which may be associated with *H. pylori* infection or the use of proton pump inhibitors or histamine$_2$ antagonists. Vitamin B$_{12}$ deficiency is also frequent among patients with acquired immunodeficiency syndrome (Mantero-Atienza et al. 1991). Even when opportunistic GI pathogens are absent, malabsorption may be due to HIV-induced mononuclear infiltration of the gut (Harriman et al. 1989).

Although cobalamin deficiency is associated with megaloblastic anemia, neuropsychiatric deficits from this vitamin deficiency do occur even when megaloblasts and anemia are absent (Stabler et al. 1990). Patients with vitamin B$_{12}$ levels between 100 and 200 pg/mL, not just patients with levels less than 100 pg/mL, may have cobalamin-reversible neurological deficits.

The sooner the treatment, the better. The ability to correct cerebral damage due to vitamin B$_{12}$ deficiency depends on how long the condition has been present. Reversal of longstanding dementia due to cobalamin deficiency may be difficult, but a clinician's alertness to clues may make this dementia preventable in some patients. Other than increased mean corpuscular volume, the clues to vitamin B$_{12}$ deficiency may be peripheral neurological deficits: symmetrical and progressive lower limb vibratory loss, paresthesias, and a deficit in postural sensation that produces a weak, unsteady, and awkward gait.

Cobalamin is a coenzyme in only two biochemical reactions: 1) the oxidation of odd-number carbon fatty acids (the conversion of methylmalonyl-CoA to succinate CoA) and 2) the methyl group transfer of methyltetrahydrofolate to homocysteine, which impairs conversion of homocysteine to methionine. The first defect causes defective DNA synthesis in red blood cells; the second impairs fatty acid synthesis and allows accumulation of defective fatty acids such that abnormal myelin is produced. Subacute combined degeneration of the spinal cord's posterior and lateral columns leads to vibratory loss and impaired postural sensation. Under the microscope, the pathology is diffuse, spongy degeneration of white matter near small vessels.

Treatment requires replacement of vitamin B$_{12}$, with frequent intramuscular injections over the first month and then monthly vitamin B$_{12}$ injections for maintenance. Studies have suggested that an oral regimen of 1 mg of B$_{12}$ orally each day may be sufficient maintenance for many patients (Hitchcock and Toendle 1991; Lederle 1991).

Fatigue

Donna B. Greenberg, M.D.

Fatigue is one of the most common complaints heard in the doctor's office ("National Ambulatory Medical Care Survey" 1978). The physician's task is to find serious explanations from the history, physical examination findings, and results of common blood tests. Three syndromes—fibromyalgia, chronic fatigue syndrome (CFS), and postviral fatigue syndrome—are contemporary diagnoses given to patients who continue to complain of fatigue without evidence of another specific medical diagnosis. In patients with any of these three syndromes, psychiatric diagnoses—particularly anxiety and mood disorders—occur more often than in the general population.

Chronic fatigue is a prominent feature of mood disorders. Anxiety and tension, per se, sap energy, and low energy state is associated with depressive syndromes (Thayer 1989).

One takes for granted energetic arousal and, after activity, calm tiredness. Those who come to the doctor to complain of fatigue are reporting some change in their usual physical endurance. The word *tired* has many meanings, with dimensions of tension, avoidance, or effort.

High-tension fatigue is a feature of anxiety and mood disorder. Criteria for depression have long included loss of energy and the feeling of being slowed down. A sensation of increased physical and mental effort also occurs in depressive syndromes (Borg 1982; Lewis and Haller 1991). Severe tension and the inability to relax were defined by multifactorial analysis to be features of anxiety (Roth et al. 1972). Fatigability, poor persistence, and marked reaction to minor physical complaints (e.g., heaviness in arms and legs) were seen as characterological features of anxious somatization (Prusoff and Klerman 1974). In panic disorder, fatigue occurs after a panic attack (e.g., "The attack took the wind out of my sails. I couldn't do anything. I thought I was going to die"). Patients with panic disorder talk in terms of tiredness as avoidance behavior increases and as the tendency for depression increases (Greenberg et al. 1991). Even the frenetic, disorganized, dysphoric, and anxious features of hypomania can be perceived as exhausting. In patients who are accustomed to mild hypomania, the change from chronic hypomania to euthymia may be perceived as fatigue.

Fatigue without tension can occur as a result of many medical conditions and as a response to drugs (Table 26–6). Laboratory examinations that are suggested when the medical diagnosis is still unclear are shown in Table 26–7. Magnetic resonance imaging of the brain may also be done to exclude multiple sclerosis (Dawson and Sabin 1993).

FIBROMYALGIA

Fibromyalgia is a syndrome of generalized muscle pain in which sleep dysfunction and fatigue are prominent but no sign of collagen vascular disease can be documented by rheumatologists. Nonrestorative sleep, associated with

TABLE 26–6. Causes of fatigue

Active cancer
Acute viral infection
Addison's disease
Drugs (e.g., antihistamines, sedatives, narcotics, alcohol, sympathetic antagonists, lithium)
Heart disease
Hypothyroidism
Infection
Lung disease
Myopathy
Neurological injury
Rheumatological disease

TABLE 26–7. Suggested laboratory examinations in cases of fatigue

Complete blood count
Blood chemistries (electrolyte, calcium, phosphorus, total protein, creatine kinase levels)
Serum protein electrophoresis
Liver function tests
Measurement of sedimentation rate
Antinuclear antibody test
Test for rheumatoid factor
Measurement of thyroid-stimulating hormone level
Venereal Disease Research Laboratory test for syphilis
Serological tests (human immunodeficiency virus, Epstein-Barr virus, cytomegalovirus, toxoplasmosis, Lyme disease)

EEG findings of persistent alpha waves during rapid-eye-movement (REM) and non-REM sleep, has been thought to be a key feature (Moldofsky and Lue 1980). Fatigue occurs in 81% of patients with fibromyalgia, sleep disturbance occurs in 75%, and anxiety occurs in 45%–55% (Wolfe et al. 1990). Fibromyalgia is a disease marked by relapses, but prospective studies are lacking. Two treatments have shown benefit in controlled studies: amitriptyline 25 mg, with and without naproxen (Carette et al. 1986; Goldenberg et al. 1986); and cyclobenzaprine plus another tricyclic (Bennett et al. 1988). In a more recent double-blind, placebo-controlled study involving 208 patients who met 1990 criteria, the benefit of amitriptyline 50 mg or cyclobenzaprine 30 mg was not sustained over 6 months compared with placebo (Carette et al. 1994).

Major depressive disorder (Goldenberg 1989; Hudson et al. 1985) and irritable bowel syndrome (IBS) (Veale et al. 1991; Yunus et al. 1989) are common in patients with fibromyalgia. Hudson and Pope (1990) suggested that fibromyalgia is a syndrome in an affective spectrum of syndromes that are responsive to antidepressants and that occur in patients with a family history of mood disorder.

The American College of Rheumatology defined fibromyalgia as a condition of generalized pain and specific tender points but eliminated fatigue as a criterion because this symptom is so common in patients with comparison diagnoses such as rheumatoid arthritis (Wolfe et al. 1990). The criteria for fibromyalgia include a history of widespread pain—left and right, above and below the waist, and in the axial-cervical spine, chest, or low back. Pain must be noted in 11 of 18 tender point sites on digital palpation—the examiner must use a force of 4 kg, acknowledged to be painful by the patient (Figure 26–1). Although the elimination of fatigue as a criterion places the focus on the muscle condition, patients who appear in rheumatology offices by referral will have high rates of fatigue complaints and psychiatric comorbidity.

CHRONIC FATIGUE SYNDROME

Researchers have continued to search for the causes of persistent fatigue. In the mid-1980s, EBV, the cause of mononucleosis and a known cause of prolonged fatigue with acute illness, was a suspect. However, studies did not support the hypothesis that chronic or recrudescent EBV infection accounted for chronic fatigue symptoms. The syndrome was renamed *chronic fatigue syndrome*. The working criteria were defined by consensus in 1988 (Holmes et al. 1988) and 1994 (Fukada et al. 1994) (Figure 26–2). The British delineated a postinfection fatigue syndrome, a specific CFS subtype lasting 6 months after an identified infectious illness (Sharpe et al. 1991). The CFS diagnostic criteria are largely symptoms. Signs of fever, pharyngitis, or lymphadenopathy are often absent. Neuropsychiatric symptoms in the list could just as easily be symptoms of a comorbid psychiatric diagnosis, although patients with bipolar disorder, substance abuse, or schizophrenia are meant to be excluded from consideration.

Patients with CFS often meet criteria for psychiatric illness: major depressive disorder (35%–75%), panic disorder (5%), dysthymia (5%), and somatization disorder (10%–15%) (Abbey and Garfinkel 1990). Because of myalgia and arthralgia, CFS criteria may overlap with fibromyalgia, allergic rhinitis, or fatigue after infection.

CFS is extremely heterogeneous. Katon and Russo (1992) pointed out that patients with a large number of medically unexplained physical symptoms, including patients who meet CFS criteria, have a high prevalence

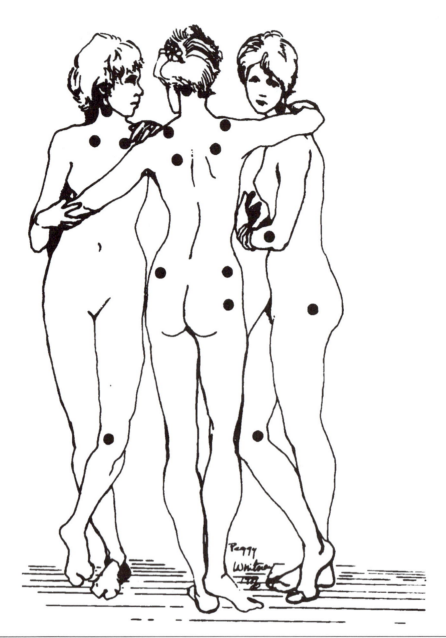

FIGURE 26–1.   Trigger points in fibromyalgia.

Tenderness must be noted at 11 of 18 sites.

Source.   Reprinted from Wolfe F, Smythe HA, Yunus MB, et al: "The American College of Rheumatology 1990 Criteria for the Classification of Fibromyalgia: Report of the Multicenter Criteria Committee." *Arthritis and Rheumatism* 33:160–172, 1990. Used with permission.

of lifetime psychiatric diagnoses, the tendency to amplify symptoms, and greater-than-expected degrees of disability.

Demitrack and colleagues (1991) found that one group of patients identified as having CFS had mild central adrenal insufficiency compared with control subjects. This insufficiency could be caused by subnormal levels of corticotropin-releasing hormone (CRH). In the Demitrack study, ACTH response to CRH stimulation was blunted. Adrenal function was more sensitive to exogenous ACTH among CFS patients than among control subjects, but the maximal response in the CFS group

was less. Because many of these patients had a lifetime history of mood disorder, depression-related blunting of endocrine function during and between depressive episodes may have accounted for this finding (Geracioti et al. 1992).

Treatment of chronic fatigue syndrome has many dimensions but no specific or exotic treatments. Pharmacological treatment for allergies, sleep, arthralgias, and depresson can be helpful. Occult diagnoses of substance abuse, primary sleep disorder, or depression with hypomania (bipolar II disorder) should be considered. The

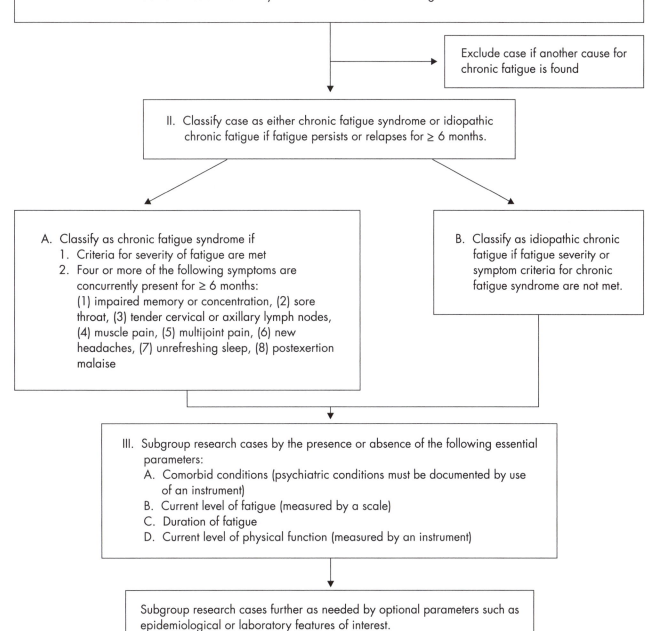

I. Clinically evaluate cases of prolonged or chronic fatigue by
   A. History and physical examination
   B. Mental status examination (abnormalities require appropriate psychiatric, psychological, or neurological examination)
   C. Tests (abnormal results that strongly suggest an exclusionary condition must be resolved)
      1. Screening laboratory tests: CBC, ESR, ALT, total protein, albumin, globulin, alkaline phosphatase, Ca, PO_4, glucose, BUN, electrolytes, creatinine, TSH, and UA
      2. Additional tests as clinically indicated to exclude other diagnoses

Exclude case if another cause for chronic fatigue is found

II. Classify case as either chronic fatigue syndrome or idiopathic chronic fatigue if fatigue persists or relapses for ≥ 6 months.

A. Classify as chronic fatigue syndrome if
   1. Criteria for severity of fatigue are met
   2. Four or more of the following symptoms are concurrently present for ≥ 6 months:
      (1) impaired memory or concentration, (2) sore throat, (3) tender cervical or axillary lymph nodes, (4) muscle pain, (5) multijoint pain, (6) new headaches, (7) unrefreshing sleep, (8) postexertion malaise

B. Classify as idiopathic chronic fatigue if fatigue severity or symptom criteria for chronic fatigue syndrome are not met.

III. Subgroup research cases by the presence or absence of the following essential parameters:
   A. Comorbid conditions (psychiatric conditions must be documented by use of an instrument)
   B. Current level of fatigue (measured by a scale)
   C. Duration of fatigue
   D. Current level of physical function (measured by an instrument)

Subgroup research cases further as needed by optional parameters such as epidemiological or laboratory features of interest.

FIGURE 26–2.　Evaluation and classification of unexplained chronic fatigue.

ALT = alanine aminotransferase; BUN = blood urea nitrogen; CBC = complete blood count; ESR = erythrocyte sedimentation rate; PO_4 = phosphorus; TSH = thyroid-stimulating hormone; UA = urinalysis.

Source.　Adapted from Fukada K, Straus SE, Hickie I, et al: "The Chronic Fatigue Syndrome: A Comprehensive Approach to Its Definition and Study." *Annals of Internal Medicine* 121:953–959, 1994.

treatment, like that for somatoform pain disorder, requires attention to emotional attributions and functional necessity, cognitive retraining, and graded increases in aerobic function. The benefits of cognitive-behavioral treatment have been documented in a randomized, controlled study (Deale et al. 1997; Wessely 1996). These patients often feel belittled if their physical symptoms are presumed to be psychological. Acknowledging the validity of their suffering is critical.

The new criteria exclude patients with major depressive disorder with psychotic or melancholic features, bipolar affective disorder, schizophrenia, dementia, anorexia nervosa, or bulimia nervosa. Substance abuse in the last 2 years excludes patients, but anxiety disorder or nonmelancholic depression does not (Fukada et al. 1994).

Factors most important in predicting persistent illness at 2.5 years are more than eight unexplained medical symptoms, a lifetime history of dysthymia, more than 1.5 years' duration of the syndrome, less education, and older age. No initial physical examination findings or negative immunological or viral measures predicted persistent symptoms (Clark et al. 1995).

POSTINFECTION SYNDROMES POTENTIALLY ASSOCIATED WITH CHRONIC FATIGUE SYNDROME

Postviral Syndrome

Certainly, acute viral malaise is a low-energy state associated with sleepiness and increased cytokine levels, but no single virus has been implicated in CFS. Patients with chronic fatigue, like much of the population, have serologies confirming exposure to a variety of viruses. The causes of clusters of CFS have also varied (P.H. Levine et al. 1992). The mechanism of fatigue appears to be central rather than peripheral (i.e., not merely neuromuscular impairment).

On the premise that viruses could be reactivated or persist when the immune system is stressed, scientists have looked for evidence of immune deficiency among patients with CFS. No measure of immune deficiency was consistent enough to be considered a constant feature of the syndrome (Arnason 1991; Herberman 1991; Holmes 1991); also, formal studies of memory and concentration have not verified specific cognitive deficits in attention or effortful processes (Barofsky and Legro 1991; Grafman et al. 1991). In a prospective study involving British patients who visited general practitioners because of viral syndromes, psychiatric morbidity,

belief in vulnerability to viruses, and attributional style were associated with postviral fatigue 6 months later. The need for certification of illness, less definite diagnosis by the physician, and a tendency to somatize were the most powerful predictors (Cope et al. 1994).

A prospective study involving 1,200 primary care patients yielded evidence that episodes of common infections were related to the onset of chronic fatigue. The strongest indicators of postinfectious fatigue were psychological distress and fatigue before infection (Wessely et al. 1995).

Epstein-Barr Virus Infection (Acute Mononucleosis)

The fatigue of acute mononucleosis may occur as a 3-week prodrome of malaise before exudative pharyngitis, lymphadenopathy, hepatosplenomegaly, hepatitis, or encephalitis develops; heterophile antibody test results are positive only after several weeks. Atypical lymphocytes may be noted. The best indicator of acute infection is the presence of antibodies to viral capsid antigen immunoglobulin (Ig) M, which persists for 4–8 weeks. Most patients return to work in 3 weeks, but some remain tired for months. Depression and anxiety syndromes have often been reported during the recovery phase. Recrudescent disease, with very high antibody titers, is associated with interstitial pneumonitis in immunocompromised hosts.

Chronic fatigue is not explained by persistence of acute mononucleosis. Because the virus is secreted intermittently in healthy people with a history of exposure (and because 90% of people have evidence of exposure by age 20), evidence of the virus in body fluids is not meaningful. High levels of antiviral capsid antigen, restricted early antigen titers, and anti-EBV nuclear antigen titers persist in a subset of patients, findings that are unrelated to symptoms.

Cytomegalovirus Infection

CMV infection mimics mononucleosis, but heterophile test results are negative, and sore throat and lymphadenopathy are less prominent. Hepatosplenomegaly, atypical lymphocytes, pneumonia, cough, and petechial rash also occur. Except among immunocompromised patients, encephalitis is not common, especially compared with its frequency in patients with acute mononucleosis. CMV is spread by sexual activity and transfusion. The diagnosis depends on detection of CMV antigens in urine, blood, and the respiratory tract (Drew 1988).

Human Herpesvirus-6 Infection

Human herpesvirus-6 (HHV-6) is the virus that causes rubeola in infants and nonspecific viral symptoms in children (Agut 1993). The role of the virus later in life is unclear. Like EBV, it is ubiquitous and remains in the body for the patient's entire life. It is found in lung biopsy specimens from immunosuppressed patients with pneumonitis. A primary illness like mononucleosis has been described with HHV-6 DNA in T cells, serum, peripheral blood mononuclear cells, and skin biopsy specimens. It is not yet clear whether HHV-6 is more than a passenger virus in these settings (Gerson 1993).

Lyme Disease

Lyme disease is caused by a spirochete, *Borrelia burgdorferi*, and, like neurosyphilis, has late neurotoxic features. The diagnosis of Lyme disease is clinical and relies on classical physical signs. Knowledge of a tick bite gives a clue to the diagnosis. An early sign of the disease is the appearance of erythema migrans, a red papule expanding concentrically and sometimes clearing in the center. A portion of patients with erythema migrans have early disseminated disease. Over a period of 6 months after infection, 15%–20% of patients develop lymphocytic meningitis, radicular pains, and cranial and peripheral neuropathies. Somnolence, emotionality, memory deficits, and depression are common. Other patients have facial palsy, meningitis, radiculoneuritis, chorea, cerebellar ataxia, seizures, dementia, hemiplegia, transverse myelitis, encephalomyelitis, or leukoencephalitis. Examination of cerebrospinal fluid (CSF) obtained by lumbar puncture reveals lymphocytic pleocytosis, IgG and IgM, and Lyme antibodies; 80% of patients with Lyme disease also have arthritis or arthralgias. An asymmetric sensory and motor peripheral neuropathy is also seen.

Late disease is characterized by knee, hip, or shoulder arthritis, which gradually improves. Encephalomyelitis can be a late consequence of untreated disease, appearing as late as 7 years after diagnosis and characterized by cognitive impairment, seizures, dementia, hemiplegia, dysphasia, hemianopsia, paresis, cranial nerve palsies, and radiculoneuropathy. CSF examination reveals lymphocytosis, excess protein, IgG, and specific Lyme antibody. Magnetic resonance imaging studies show infarct patterns, white matter disease, and hydrocephalus. Late neurological disease is treated with intravenous antibiotics, but patients respond slowly to therapy.

For a diagnosis of Lyme disease, a positive enzyme-linked immunosorbent assay (ELISA) result must be confirmed by Western blot technique. In the United States, Western blotting should be interpreted according to the standardized criteria of the Centers for Disease Control (Steer 2001). ELISA antibody screening may not yield postiive results in the first 6 weeks after infection, but most patients have an active IgG response after 1 month. A positive test does not differentiate active disease from old disease. After treatment, neither IgM nor IgG antibody titers are evidence of recent infection, since antibodies may persist after treatment. Test results are meaningful only if the patient presents with clinical signs likely to be due to Lyme disease in a community where exposure is likely. In a patient with vague symptoms, only a negative result would be meaningful. Although fatigue is common in late Lyme disease, isolated fatigue attributed to Lyme disease is probably rare (Reik 1993).

Fear of Lyme disease is common, and because no Lyme disease test is perfect, proving that the patient's symptoms are not due to Lyme disease is a problem (Shapiro 2001; Steere 2001). The American College of Rheumatology and the Infectious Diseases Society of America presented a joint statement arguing against treatment with intravenous antibiotics for nonspecific chronic fatigue, myalgia, and no clinical sign other than positive serological findings (Luft et al. 1994). A recent study confirmed that prolonged antibiotic treatment offers no benefit for those who formerly had Lyme disease and still have persistent symptoms (Klempner et al. 2001).

Acute Hepatitis

The malaise that appears as a prodrome of acute viral hepatitis may not be recognized until testing reveals increased liver enzyme levels. The diagnosis of acute hepatitis A depends on the presence of anti–hepatitis A virus IgM antibodies. Hepatitis B infection is indicated by the presence of hepatitis B surface antigen, which documents viral replication. High titers are noted in the sera of patients with active disease; low titers are found in patients with persistent disease. Anti–hepatitis B core antibody in the absence of hepatitis B surface antigen indicates acute infection (Lemon 1988).

Toxoplasmosis

Lymphadenopathy, fever, malaise, muscle discomfort, maculopapular rash, myocarditis, myositis, and brain, liver, and skin involvement characterize toxoplasmosis. Tests for the presence of toxoplasma IgM, which documents infection, may not yield positive results for 1 month.

Neurosyphilis

Ataxia, lightning pains, headache, dizziness, hearing loss, and seizures are presentations of neurosyphilis (R.L. Ross et al. 1990; Rundell and Wise 1985). The VDRL test is specific but not sensitive, with a false-negative rate of 5%–39%. Performance of a fluorescent treponemal antibody (FTA) absorption test on CSF is necessary if neurosyphilis is truly suspected. Primary or secondary infection progresses to neurosyphilis in 6% of untreated patients; neurosyphilis is asymptomatic in 31%. Dementia, with poor judgment or speech, memory, or behavior abnormalities, may be due to syphilis. Depression occurs in 27% of patients, and mania is noted in 3.3%–18%. A characteristic finding is Argyll Robertson pupils—pupils that react normally to convergence but do not react to light. Paralysis of cranial nerves III and VIII are common. Syphilis may have a more malignant course in HIV-positive patients (Johns et al. 1987).

Conclusion

Axis III, the medical axis of DSM, is the focus of this chapter. The consultation-liaison psychiatrist is in the best position to combine medical knowledge with knowledge of Axis I (psychiatric syndromes) and Axis II (personality traits and disorders) conditions to diagnose and treat conditions in medically ill patients with respect and technical understanding.

REFERENCES

Abbey SE, Garfinkel PE: Chronic fatigue syndrome and the psychiatrist. Can J Psychiatry 35:625–633, 1990

Abed RT, Clark J, Elbadawy HF, et al: Psychiatric morbidity in acromegaly. Acta Psychiatr Scand 75:635–639, 1987

Abrams HS: Repetitive dialysis, in Massachusetts General Hospital Handbook of General Hospital Psychiatry. Edited by Hackett TP, Cassem NH. St. Louis, MO, CV Mosby, 1978, pp 342–364

Abrams HS, Hester LR, Sheridan WF, et al: Sexual functioning in patients with chronic renal failure. J Nerv Ment Dis 160:220–226, 1975

Abramson J, Berger A, Krumholz HM, et al: Depression and risk of heart failure among older persons with isolated systolic hypertension. Arch Intern Med 161:1725–1730, 2001

Agut H: Puzzles concerning the pathogenicity of human herpesvirus 6. N Engl J Med 329:203–204, 1993

Ahern DK, Gorkin L, Anderson JL, et al: Biobehavioral variables and mortality or cardiac arrest in the Cardiac Arrhythmia Pilot Study (CAPS). Am J Cardiol 66:59–62, 1990

Allen RE, Pitts FN: ECT for depressed patients with lupus erythematosus. Am J Psychiatry 135:367–368, 1978

American College of Rheumatology nomenclature and case definitions for neuropsychiatric lupus syndromes. Arthritis Rheum 42:599–608, 1999

American Psychiatric Association: Diagnostic and Statistical Manual of Mental Disorders, 3rd Edition. Washington, DC, American Psychiatric Association, 1980

American Psychiatric Association: Diagnostic and Statistical Manual of Mental Disorders, 3rd Edition, Revised. Washington, DC, American Psychiatric Association, 1987

American Psychiatric Association: Diagnostic and Statistical Manual of Mental Disorders, 4th Edition. Washington, DC, American Psychiatric Association, 1994

American Psychiatric Association: Diagnostic and Statistical Manual of Mental Disorders, 4th Edition, Text Revision. Washington, DC, American Psychiatric Association, 2000

Anda RF, Williamson DF, Escobedo LG, et al: Depression and the dynamics of smoking: a national perspective. JAMA 264:1541–1545, 1990

Anda R[F], Williamson D[F], Jones D, et al: Depressed affect, hopelessness, and the risk of ischemic heart disease in a cohort of U.S. adults. Epidemiology 4:285–294, 1993

Andrykowski MA, Altmaier EM, Barnett RL, et al: The quality of life in adult survivors of allogeneic bone marrow transplantation. Transplantation 50:399–406, 1990

Antonaccio MJ, Robson RD: Centrally mediated cardiovascular effects of 5-hydroxy-tryptophan in anesthetized dogs. J Pharm Pharmacol 25:495–497, 1973

Arnason BGW: Nervous system-immune system communication. Rev Infect Dis 13 (suppl 1):S134–S137, 1991

Aromaa A, Raitasalo R, Reunanen A, et al: Depression and cardiovascular diseases. Acta Psychiatr Scand Suppl 377:77–82, 1994

Avery D, Winokur G: Mortality in depressed patients treated with electroconvulsive therapy and antidepressants. Arch Gen Psychiatry 33:1029–1037, 1976

Baer PG, Cagen LM: Platelet activating factor vasoconstriction of dog kidney: inhibition by alprazolam. Hypertension 9:253–260, 1987

Baker M: Psychopathology in SLE: psychiatric observations. Semin Arthritis Rheum 3:95–110, 1973

Ballard JE, Boileau RA, Sleator EK, et al: Cardiovascular responses of hyperactive children to methylphenidate. JAMA 236:2870–2874, 1976

Barefoot J, Schroll M: Symptoms of depression, acute myocardial infarction, and total mortality in a community sample. Circulation 93:1976–1980, 1996

Barofsky I, Legro MW: Definition and measurement of fatigue. Rev Infect Dis 12 (suppl 1):S94–S97, 1991

Barrett BJ, Vavasour HM, Major A, et al: Clinical and psychological correlates of somatic symptoms in patients on dialysis. Nephron 55:10–15, 1990

Bass C, Gardner W: Emotional influences on breathing and breathlessness. J Psychosom Res 29:599–609, 1985

Bassett JR, Cairncross KD: Morphological changes induced in rats following prolonged exposure to stress. Pharmacol Biochem Behav 3:411–424, 1975

Bauer MS, Halpern L, Schriger D: Screening Ambulatory Depressives for Causative Medical Illnesses: The Example of Thyroid Function Screening. A Report for the Agency for Health Care Policy and Research. Washington, DC, Agency for Health Care Policy and Research, 1991, pp 1–24

Baumann R, Ziprian H, Godicke W, et al: The influence of acute psychic stress situations on biochemical and vegetative parameters of essential hypertension at an early state of the disease. Psychother Psychosom 22:131–135, 1973

Bennett: Functional gastrointestinal disorders: psychological, social, and somatic features. Gut 42:414–420, 1991

Bennett RM, Gatter RA, Campbell SM, et al: A comparison of cyclobenzaprine and placebo in the management of fibrositis: a double blind controlled study. Arthritis Rheum 31:1535–1542, 1988

Benson H, Alexander S, Feldman CL: Decreased premature ventricular contractions through the use of the relaxation response in patients with stable ischemic heart disease. Lancet 2:380–382, 1975

Bentdal OH, Fauchald P, Brekke IB, et al: Rehabilitation and quality of life in diabetic patients after successful pancreas-kidney transplantation. Diabetologia 34 (suppl 1):S158–S159, 1991

Bergstrom RF, Beasley CM Jr, Levy NB, et al: The effects of renal and hepatic disease on the pharmacokinetics, renal tolerance, and risk-benefit profile of fluoxetine. Int Clin Psychopharmacol 8:261–266, 1993

Bigger JT, Giardina E-GV, Perel JM, et al: Cardiac antiarrhythmic effect of imipramine hydrochloride. N Engl J Med 296:206–208, 1977

Bigger JT, Kantor SJ, Glassman AH, et al: Cardiovascular effects of tricyclic antidepressant drugs, in Psychopharmacology: A Generation of Progress. Edited by Lipton MA. New York, Raven, 1978, pp 1033–1046

Blacher RS (ed): The Psychological Experience of Surgery. New York, Wiley, 1987

Blagg CR, Bovbjerg RR, FitzSimmons SC: Here are (almost all) the data: the evolution of the US Renal Data System. Am J Kidney Dis 14:347–353, 1989

Blatt CM, Rabinowitz SH, Lown B: Central serotonergic agents raise the repetitive extrasystole threshold of the vulnerable period of the canine ventricular myocardium. Circ Res 44:723–730, 1979

Bluestein HG: Neuropsychiatric manifestations of systemic lupus erythematosus. N Engl J Med 317:309–310, 1987

Blumenthal JA, Levenson RM: Behavioral approaches to secondary prevention of coronary heart disease. Circulation 1(pt 2):I130–I137, 1987

Blumenthal JA, Williams RS, Wallace AG, et al: Physiological and psychological variables predict compliance to prescribed exercise therapy in patients recovering from myocardial infarction. Psychosom Med 44:519–527, 1982

Blumenthal JA, Jiang W, Babyak MA, et al: Stress management and exercise training in cardiac patients with myopdcardial ischemia: effects on prognosis and evaluation of mechanisms. Arch Intern Med 157:2213–2223, 1997

Boner AL, DeStefano G, Piacentini GL, et al: Perception of bronchoconstriction in chronic asthma. J Asthma 29:323–330, 1992

Bonomini V: Ethical aspects of living donation. Transplant Proc 23:2497–2499, 1991

Borg GAV: Psychophysical bases of perceived exertion. Med Sci Sports Exerc 14:377–381, 1982

Borson S, McDonald GJ: Depression and chronic obstructive pulmonary disease, in Depression and Coexisting Disease. Edited by Robinson RG, Rabins PV. New York, Igaku-Shoin, 1989, pp 40–60

Boumpas DT, Austin HA 3rd, Fessler BJ, et al: Systemic lupus erythematosus: emerging concepts, part 1: renal, neuropsychiatric, cardiovascular, pulmonary, and hematologic disease. Ann Intern Med 122:940–950, 1995

Bremer BA, McCauley CR, Wrona RM, et al: Quality of life in end-stage renal disease: a reexamination. Am J Kidney Dis 13:202–209, 1989

Brod J: Hemodynamics and emotional stress. Bibliotheca Psychiatrica 144:13–16, 1970

Brod J, Fencl V, Jirka J: Circulatory changes underlying blood pressure elevation during acute emotional stress (mental arithmetic) in normotensive and hypertensive subjects. Clinical Science 18:269–278, 1959

Brown GG, Preisman RC, Kleerekoper M: Neurobehavioral symptoms in mild primary hyperparathyroidism: related to hypercalcemia but not improved by parathyroidectomy. Henry Ford Hosp Med J 35:211–215, 1987

Buff DD, Brenner R, Kirtane SS, et al: Dysrhythmia associated with fluoxetine treatment in an elderly patient with cardiac disease. J Clin Psychiatry 52:174–176, 1991

Burckhardt D, Raedler E, Muller V, et al: Cardiovascular effects of tricyclic and tetracyclic antidepressants. JAMA 239:213–216, 1987

Burns BH, Howell JBL: Disproportionately severe breathlessness in chronic bronchitis. Quarterly Journal of Medicine 38:277–294, 1969

Burrows GD, Vohra J, Hunt D, et al: Cardiac effects of different tricyclic antidepressant drugs. Br J Psychiatry 129:335–341, 1976

Burrows GD, Vohra J, Dumovic P, et al: Tricyclic antidepressant drugs in cardiac conduction. Progress in Neuropharmacology 1:329–334, 1977

Burton MD, Johnson DC, Kazemi H: CSF acidosis augments ventilation through cholinergic mechanisms. J Appl Physiol 66:2562–2572, 1989

Callender CO, Jennings PS, Bayton JA, et al: Psychologic factors related to dialysis in kidney transplant decisions. Transplant Proc 21:1976–1978, 1989

Campbell RJ, Fann WE, Thornby JI: Abnormal involuntary movements and chronic obstructive pulmonary disease. J Clin Psychopharmacol 3:179–182, 1983

Cannon RO: Causes of chest pain in patients with normal coronary angiograms: the eye of the beholder. Am J Cardiol 62:306–308, 1988

Carette S, McCain GA, Bell DA, et al: Evaluation of amitriptyline in primary fibrositis: a double-blind, placebo-controlled study. Arthritis Rheum 29:655–659, 1986

Carette S, Bell MJ, Reynolds J, et al: Comparison of amitriptyline, cyclobenzaprine, and placebo in the treatment of fibromyalgia: a randomized double-blind clinical trial. Arthritis Rheum 37:32–40, 1994

Carney RM, Rich MW, Freedland KE, et al: Major depressive disorder predicts cardiac events in patients with coronary artery disease. Psychosom Med 50:627–633, 1988

Carr RE, Lehrer PM, Hochron SM: Panic symptoms in asthma and panic disorder: a preliminary test of the dyspnea-fear theory. Behav Res Ther 30:251–261, 1992

Carroll BJ, Curtis GC, Davies BM, et al: Urinary free cortisol excretion in depression. Psychol Med 6:43–50, 1976

Carvajal C, Passig C, San Martin E, et al: Prevalence of cigarette smoking in psychiatric patients [in Spanish]. Acta Psiquiatr Psicol Am Lat 35:145–151, 1989

Casati J, Toner BB, De Rooy EC, et al: Concerns of patients with inflammatory bowel disease: a review of emerging themes. Dig Dis Sci 45:26–31, 2000

Case RB, Moss AJ, Case N, et al: Living alone after myocardial infarction: impact on prognosis. JAMA 267:515–519, 1992

Cebelin M, Hirsch CS: Human stress cardiomyopathy. Hum Pathol 11:123–132, 1980

Chazan JA: Elective withdrawal from dialysis: an important cause of death among patients with chronic renal failure. Dialysis and Transplantation 19:530–538, 1990

Chignon JM, Lepine JP, Ades J: Panic disorder in cardiac outpatients. Am J Psychiatry 150:780–785, 1993

Christensen AJ, Smith TW, Turner CW, et al: Type of hemodialysis and preference for behavioral involvement: interactive effects on adherence in end-stage renal disease. Health Psychol 9:225–236, 1990

Christensen AJ, Smith TW, Turner CW, et al: Family support, physical impairment, and adherence in hemodialysis: an investigation of main and buffering effects. J Behav Med 15:313–325, 1992

Christie RV: Some types of respiration in the neuroses. Quarterly Journal of Medicine 16:427–434, 1935

Churchill DN, Bird DR, Taylor DW, et al: Effect of high-flux hemodialysis on quality of life and neuropsychological function in chronic hemodialysis patients. Am J Nephrol 12:412–418, 1992

Clarfield AM: The reversible dementias: do they reverse? Ann Intern Med 109:476–486, 1988

Clark MR, Katon W, Russo J, et al: Chronic fatigue: risk factors for symptom persistence in a 2 1/2-year follow-up study. Am J Med 98:187–195, 1995

Cleghorn RA: Adrenal cortical insufficiency: psychological and neurological observations. Can Med Assoc J 65:449–454, 1951

Clouse RE: Spastic disorders of the esophagus. Gastroenterology 5:112–127, 1997

Clouse RE, Lustman PJ: Psychiatric illness and contraction abnormalities of the esophagus. N Engl J Med 309:1337–1342, 1983

Clouse RE, Lustman PJ: Value of recent psychological symptoms in identifying patients with esophageal contraction abnormalities. Psychosom Med 51:570–576, 1989

Clouse RE, Lustman PJ, Eckert TC, et al: Low-dose trazodone for symptomatic patients with esophageal contraction abnormalities: a double-blind, placebo-controlled trial. Gastroenterology 92:1027–1036, 1987

Clouse RE, Lustman P, Geisman RA, et al: Antidepressant therapy in 138 patients with irritable bowel syndrome: a five-year clinical experience. Aliment Pharmacol Ther 8:409–416, 1994

Cohen LM, Woods A, McCue J: The challenge of advance directives and ESRD. Dialysis and Transplantation 20:593–594, 1991

Cohen LM, Steinberg MD, Hails KC, et al: The psychiatric evaluation of death-hastening requests: lessons from dialysis discontinuation. Psychosomatics 41(3):195–203 (commentary: pp 193–194), 2000a

Cohen LM, Germain M, Poppel DM, et al: Dying well after discontinuing the life-support treatment of dialysis. Arch Intern Med 160:2513–2518, 2000b

Cohen LM, Germain M, Poppel DM, et al: Dialysis discontinuation and palliative care. Am J Kidney Dis 36(1):140–144, 2000c

Cohen ME, White PD: Life situations, emotions and neurocirculatory asthenia. Research Publications—Association for Research in Nervous and Mental Disease 12:335–357, 1951

Cohen SI: Cushing's syndrome: a psychiatric study of 29 patients. Br J Psychiatry 136:120–124, 1980

Connell AM, Hilton C, Irvine G, et al: Variation of bowel habits in two population samples. BMJ 5470:1095–1099, 1965

Conze E: Meditation in Buddhist Scriptures. New York, Penguin Books, 1959

Cope H, David A, Pelosi A, et al: Predictors of chronic postviral fatigue. Lancet 344:864–868, 1994

Coryell W, Noyes R, Clancy J: Excess mortality in panic disorder: a comparison with primary unipolar depression. Arch Gen Psychiatry 39:701–703, 1982

Covey LS, Glassman AH, Stetner F, et al: Effect of history of alcoholism or major depression on smoking cessation. Am J Psychiatry 150:1546–1547, 1993

Creed F, Craig T, Farmer R: Functional abdominal pain, psychiatric illness, and life events. Gut 29:235–242, 1988

Creer TL: Asthma Therapy: A Behavioral Health Care System for Respiratory Disorders. New York, Springer, 1979

Cybulska EM: Globus hystericus: a somatic symptom of depression? the role of electroconvulsive therapy and antidepressants. Psychosom Med 59:67–69, 1997

Dammen T, Ekeberg O, Arnesen H, et al: Personality profiles in patients referred for chest pain: investigation with emphasis on panic disorder patients. Psychosomatics 41:269–276, 2000

Deary IJ, Wilson JA, Kelly SW: Globus pharyngis, personality, and psychological distress in the general population. Psychosomatics 36:570–577, 1995

Dammen T, Ekeberg O, Arnesen H, et al: Personality profiles in patients referred for chest pain: investigation with emphasis on panic disorder patients. Psychosomatics 41:269–276, 2000

Damas-Mora J, Grant R, Kenyon P, et al: Respiratory ventilation and carbon dioxide levels in syndromes of depression. Br J Psychiatry 129:457–464, 1976

Damas-Mora J, Suster L, Jenne A: Diminished hypercapnic drive in endogenous or severe depression. J Psychosom Res 26:237–245, 1982

Dawling S, Lynn K, Rosser R, et al: Nortriptyline metabolism in chronic renal failure: metabolite elimination. Clin Pharmacol Ther 32:322–329, 1982

Dawson DM, Sabin TD: Summary and perspective, in Chronic Fatigue Syndrome. Edited by Dawson DM, Sabin TD. Boston, MA, Little, Brown, 1993, pp 195–211

Deale A, Chalder T, Marks I, et al: Cognitive behavior therapy for chronic fatigue syndrome: a randomized controlled trial. Am J Psychiatry 154:408–414, 1997

Deanfield JE, Maseri A, Selwyn AP, et al: Myocardial ischemia during daily life in patients with stable angina: its relation to symptoms and heart rate changes. Lancet 2:753–758, 1983

Deanfield JE, Kensett M, Wilson RA, et al: Silent myocardial ischemia due to mental stress. Lancet 2:1001–1004, 1984

Deary IJ, Wilson JA, Kelly SW: Globus pharyngis, personality, and psychological distress in the general population. Psychosomatics 36:570–577, 1995

Dembroski TM, MacDougall JM, Williams RB, et al: Components of Type A, hostility, and anger-in: relationship to angiographic findings. Psychosom Med 47:219–233, 1985

Demers RY, Fischetti LR, Neale AV: Incongruence between self-reported symptoms and objective evidence of respiratory disease among construction workers. Soc Sci Med 30:805–810, 1990

Demitrack MA, Dale JK, Straus SE, et al: Evidence for impaired activation of the hypothalamic-pituitary-adrenal axis in patients with chronic fatigue syndrome. J Clin Endocrinol Metab 73:1224–1234, 1991

DeQuattro V, Loo R, Foti A: Sympathoadrenal responses to stress: the linking of type A behavior pattern to ischemic heart disease. Clinical and Experimental Hypertension. Part A, Theory and Practice 7:469–481, 1985

DeSilva RA, Lown B: Ventricular premature beats, stress and sudden death. Psychosomatics 19:639–659, 1978

DiChiara G, Imperato A: Drugs abused by humans preferentially increase synaptic dopamine concentrations in the mesolimbic system of freely moving rats. Proc Natl Acad Sci U S A 85:5274–5278, 1988

Didlake RH, Dreyfus K, Kerman RH, et al: Patient noncompliance: a major cause of late graft failure in cyclosporine-treated renal transplants. Transplant Proc 20:63–69, 1988

Dimsdale JE, Hackett TP, Hutter AM, et al: Type A behavior and angiographic findings. J Psychosom Res 23:273–276, 1979

Ditto B, Miller SB: Forearm blood flow responses of offspring of hypertensives to an extended stress task. Hypertension 13:181–187, 1989

Douglas CJ, Schwartz HI: ECT for depression caused by lupus cerebritis: a case report. Am J Psychiatry 139:1631–1632, 1982

Downing ET, Braman SS, Fox MJ, et al: Factitious asthma. JAMA 248:2878–2881, 1982

Doyle AE, Fraser JRE: Essential hypertension and inheritance of vascular reactivity. Lancet 2:509–511, 1961

Drew WL: Diagnosis of cytomegalovirus infection. Rev Infect Dis 10 (suppl 3):S468–S476, 1988

Drossman DA: Psychosocial treatment of the refractory patient with irritable bowel syndrome. J Clin Gastroenterol 9:253–255, 1987

Drossman DA: Irritable bowel syndrome. Am Fam Physician 39:159–164, 1989

Drossman DA: The functional gastrointestinal disorders and the Rome II process. Gut 45(suppl 2):1–5, 1999

Drossman DA, Thompson WG: The irritable bowel syndrome: review and a graduated multicomponent treatment approach. Ann Intern Med 116:1009–1016, 1992

Drossman DA, Sandler RS, McKee DC, et al: Bowel patterns among subjects not seeking health care. Gastroenterology 83:529–534, 1982

Drossman DA, McKee DC, Sandler RS, et al: Psychosocial factors in the irritable bowel syndrome: a multivariate study of patients and nonpatients with irritable bowel syndrome. Gastroenterology 95:701–708, 1988

Drossman DA, Thompson WG, Talley NJ, et al: Identification of subgroups of functional gastrointestinal disorders. Gastroenterology International 3:159–172, 1990a

Drossman DA, Leserman J, Nachman G, et al: Sexual and physical abuse in women with functional or organic gastrointestinal disorders. Ann Intern Med 113:828–833, 1990b

Drossman DA, Li Z, Andruzzi E, et al: U.S. householder survey of functional gastrointestinal disorders: prevalence, sociodemography, and health impact. Dig Dis Sci 38:1569–1580, 1993

Dubovsky SL, Penn I: Psychiatric considerations in renal transplant surgery. Psychosomatics 21:481–491, 1980

Dunbar F: Psychosomatic Diagnosis. New York, Paul B Hoeber, 1943

Ellison JM, Milofsky JE, Ely E: Fluoxetine-induced bradycardia and syncope in two patients. J Clin Psychiatry 51:385–386, 1990

Epstein FH: Responsibility of the physician in the preservation of life. Arch Intern Med 139:919–920, 1979

Esler M[D], Julius S, Zweifler A, et al: Mild high-renin essential hypertension: neurogenic human hypertension? N Engl J Med 296:405–411, 1977

Esler M[D], Turbott J, Schwarz R, et al: The peripheral kinetics of norepinephrine in depressive illness. Arch Gen Psychiatry 39:295–300, 1982

ESRD Network of New England: Paper presented at the annual meeting of the Medical Review Board, Boston, MA, September 25, 1990

ESRD Network of New England: End Stage Renal Disease 1999 Annual Report. Health Care Financing Administration, 2000, p 84

Evans RW, Manninen DL, Garrison LP, et al: The quality of life in patients with end-stage renal disease. N Engl J Med 312:553–559, 1985

Evans RW, Rader B, Manninen DL: The quality of life of hemodialysis recipients treated with recombinant human erythropoietin. Cooperative Multicenter EPO Clinical Trial Group. JAMA 263:825–830, 1990

Everson SA, Goldberg DE, Kaplan GA, et al: Hopelessness and risk of mortality and incidence of myocardial infarction and cancer. Psychosom Med 58:113–121, 1996

Ewer TC, Stewart DE: Improvement in bronchial hyper-responsiveness in patients with moderate asthma after treatment with a hypnotic technique: a randomised controlled trial. BMJ 293:1129–1132, 1986

Fadel HE, Northrop G, Misenhimer HR, et al: Normal pregnancy: a model of sustained respiratory alkalosis. J Perinat Med 7:195–201, 1979

Fang J, Bjorkman J: A critical approach to noncardiac chest pain: pathophysiology, diagnosis and treatment. Am J Gastroenterol 96:958–968, 2001

Fava M, Littman AB, Halperin PH: Neuroendocrine correlates of the type A pattern: a review and new hypothesis. Int J Psychiatry Med 17:41–48, 1987

Fava M, Rosenbaum JF, Pava JA, et al: Anger attacks in unipolar depression, part 1: clinical correlates and response to fluoxetine treatment. Am J Psychiatry 150:1158–1163, 1993a

Fava M, Anderson K, Rosenbaum JF: Are thymoleptic-responsive "anger attacks" a discrete clinical syndrome? Psychosomatics 34:350–355, 1993b

Fisch C: Effects of fluoxetine on the electrocardiogram. J Clin Psychiatry 46:42–44, 1985

Fisher SH, Curry E, Batuman V: Stopping long-term dialysis (letter). N Engl J Med 314:1449, 1986

Fishman R: REM sleep inhibition. Exp Neurol 36:166–172, 1972

Folkow B: Psychosocial and central nervous influences in primary hypertension. Circulation 76:110–119, 1987

Ford DE, Mead LA, Chang PP, et al: Depression is a risk factor for coronary artery disease in men: the precursors study. Arch Intern Med 158:1422–1426, 1998

Frasure-Smith N: In-hospital symptoms of psychological stress as predictors of long-term outcome after acute myocardial infarction in men. Am J Cardiol 67:121–127, 1991

Frasure-Smith N, Prince R: Long-term follow-up of the ischemic Heart Disease Life Stress Monitoring Program. Psychosom Med 51:485–513, 1989

Frasure-Smith N, Lesperance F, Talajic M: Depression and 18-month prognosis after myocardial infarction. Circulation 91:999–1005, 1995

Frederick T, Frerichs RR, Clark VA: Personal health habits and symptoms of depression at the community level. Prev Med 17:173–182, 1988

Freedland KE, Lustman PJ, Carney RM, et al: Underdiagnosis of depression in patients with coronary artery disease: the role of nonspecific symptoms. Int J Psychiatry Med 22:221–229, 1992

French TM, Alexander F: Psychogenic factors in bronchial asthma. Psychosomatic Medicine Monographs 4:1–96, 1939–1941

Fricchione GL: Psychiatric aspects of renal transplantation. Aust N Z J Psychiatry 23:407–417, 1989

Friedman M, Rosenman RH: Type A Behavior and Your Heart. New York, Knopf, 1974

Friedman M, Byers SO, Diamant RH, et al: Plasma catecholamine response of coronary-prone subjects (type A) to a specific challenge. Metabolism 24:205–210, 1975

Friedman M, Thoresen CE, Gill JJ, et al: Alteration of type A behavior and its effect on cardiac recurrences in post myocardial infarction patients: summary results of the Recurrent Coronary Prevention Project. Am Heart J 112:653–665, 1986

Fukuda K, Straus SE, Hickie I, et al: The chronic fatigue syndrome: a comprehensive approach to its definition and study. Ann Intern Med 121:953–959, 1994

Fullwood A, Drossman DA: The relationship of psychiatric illness with gastrointestinal disease. Annu Rev Med 46:483–496, 1995

Furukawa CT, DuHamel TR, Weimer L, et al: Cognitive and behavioral findings in children taking theophylline. J Allergy Clin Immunol 81:83–88, 1988

Galla J: Clinical practice guideline on shared Decision-Making in the appropriate initiation and withdrawal from dialysis. J Am Soc Nephrol 11:1340–1342, 2000

Garcia LL, Agueru AE, Cavalli N, et al: Kidney transplantation: absolute and relative psychologic contraindications. Transplant Proc 23:1344–1345, 1991

Geracioti TD, Loosen PT, Gold PW, et al: Cortisol, thyroid hormone, and mood in atypical depression: a longitudinal case study. Biol Psychiatry 31:515–519, 1992

Gerson S: Puzzles concerning the pathogenicity of human herpesvirus 6. N Engl J Med 329:203–205, 1993

Giardina E-GV, Bigger JT, Glassman AH, et al: The electrocardiographic and antiarrhythmic effects of imipramine hydrochloride at therapeutic plasma concentrations. Circulation 60:1045–1052, 1979

Giardina E-GV, Bigger JT, Johnson LL: The effect of imipramine and nortriptyline on ventricular premature depolarizations and left ventricular function. Circulation 64 (suppl IV):316–320, 1981

Ginsberg AL, Albert MB: Treatment of patient with severe steroid-dependent Crohn's disease with nonelemental formula diet: identification of possible etiologic dietary factor. Dig Dis Sci 34:1624–1628, 1989

Gitnick G: Etiology of inflammatory bowel diseases: where have we been? Where are we going? Scand J Gastroenterol Suppl 175:93–96, 1990

Glass DC, Krakoff LR, Contrada R, et al: Effect of harassment and competition upon the cardiovascular and plasma catecholamine responses in type A and type B individuals. Psychophysiology 17:453–463, 1980

Glassman AH: Cigarette smoking: implications for psychiatric illness. Am J Psychiatry 150:546–553, 1993

Glassman AH, Helzer JE, Covey LS, et al: Smoking, smoking cessation, and major depression. JAMA 264:1546–1549, 1990

Glassman AH, Covey LS, Stetner F, et al: Smoking cessation and the course of major depression: a follow-up study. Lancet 357:1929–1932 (comment, 1900–1901), 2001

Godlee FN, Brooks DJ, Impallomeni M: Dyskinesia in the elderly presenting as respiratory disorder. Postgrad Med J 65:830–831, 1989

Goff DC, Henderson DC, Amico E: Cigarette smoking in schizophrenia: relationship to psychopathology and medication side effects. Am J Psychiatry 149:1189–1194, 1992

Goldberg R, Morris P, Christian F, et al: Panic disorder in cardiac outpatients. Psychosomatics 31:168–173, 1990

Goldenberg DL: Psychiatric and psychologic aspects of fibromyalgia syndrome. Rheum Dis Clin North Am 15:105–114, 1989

Goldenberg DL, Felson DT, Dinerman H: A randomized controlled trial of amitriptyline and naproxen in the treatment of patients with fibromyalgia. Arthritis Rheum 29:1371–1377, 1986

Gorelick DA, Marder SR, Sack D, et al: Atrial flutter/fibrillation associated with tranylcypromine treatment. J Clin Psychopharmacol 1:402–404, 1981

Gorlen T, Ekeberg O, Abdelnoor M, et al: Quality of life after kidney transplantation: a 10–20 years follow-up. Scand J Urol Nephrol 27:89–92, 1993

Grafman J, Johnson R Jr, Scheffers M: Cognitive and mood-state changes in patients with chronic fatigue syndrome. Rev Infect Dis 13 (suppl 1):S45–S52, 1991

Gram L: Fluoxetine. N Engl J Med 331:1354–1361, 1994

Grant I, Heaton RK, McSweeny AJ, et al: Neuropsychologic findings in hypoxemic chronic obstructive pulmonary disease. Arch Intern Med 142:1470–1476, 1982

Grant I, Prigatano GP, Heaton RK, et al: Progressive neuropsychologic impairment and hypoxemia. Arch Gen Psychiatry 44:999–1006, 1987

Greenberg DB, Stern TA, Weilberg JB: The fear of choking: three successfully treated cases. Psychosomatics 29:126–129, 1988

Greenberg DB, Eisenthal S, Tesar GE, et al: Linking panic disorder and depression: the fatigue dimension. Ann Clin Psychiatry 3:205–208, 1991

Griez E, Zandbergen J, Lousberg H, et al: Effects of low pulmonary CO_2 on panic anxiety. Compr Psychiatry 29:490–497, 1988

Grigor R, Edmonds J, Lewkonia R, et al: Systemic lupus erythematosus: a prospective analysis. Ann Rheum Dis 37:121–128, 1978

Gruen W: Effects of brief psychotherapy during the hospitalization period on the recovery process in heart attacks. J Consult Clin Psychol 43:223–232, 1975

Gulledge AD, Buszta C, Montague D: Psychological aspects of renal transplantation. Urol Clin North Am 10:327–335, 1983

Guze SB: The occurrence of psychiatric illness in systemic lupus erythematosus. Am J Psychiatry 123:1562–1570, 1967

Hackett TP, Cassem NH: Factors contributing to delay in responding to the signs and symptoms of acute myocardial infarction. Am J Cardiol 24:651–658, 1969

Hackett TP, Rosenbaum JF: Emotion, psychiatric disorders, and the heart, in Heart Disease. Edited by Braunwald E. Philadelphia, PA, WB Saunders, 1984, pp 1826–1844

Hackett TP, Cassem NH, Wishnie HA: The coronary care unit: an appraisal of its psychological hazards. N Engl J Med 279:1365–1370, 1968

Haggerty JJ, Stern RA, Mason GA, et al: Subclinical hypothyroidism: a modifiable risk factor for depression? Am J Psychiatry 150:508–510, 1993

Hance M, Carney RM, Freedland KE: Depression in patients with coronary heart disease: a 12-month follow-up. Gen Hosp Psychiatry 18:61–65, 1996

Harburg E, Erfurt JC, Hauenstein LS, et al: Socio-ecological stress, suppressed hostility, skin color, and Black-White male blood pressure: Detroit. Psychosom Med 35:276–296, 1973

Harriman GR, Smith PD, Horne MK, et al: Vitamin B12 malabsorption in patients with acquired immunodeficiency syndrome. Arch Intern Med 149:2039–2041, 1989

Hart LG, Evans RW: The functional status of ESRD patients as measured by the Sickness Impact Profile. Journal of Chronic Disease 40 (suppl 1):S117–S130, 1987

Haskett RF: Diagnostic categorization of psychiatric disturbance in Cushing's syndrome. Am J Psychiatry 142:911–916, 1985

Heaton RK, Grant I, McSweeny AJ, et al: Psychologic effects of continuous and nocturnal oxygen therapy in hypoxemic chronic obstructive pulmonary disease. Arch Intern Med 143:1941–1947, 1983

Hedgel DW, Cherniack NS: Sleeping and breathing, in Update: Pulmonary Diseases and Disorders. Edited by Fishman AP. New York, McGraw-Hill, 1988, pp 249–261

Hedner J, Hedner T, Wessberg P, et al: An analysis of the mechanism by which gamma-aminobutyric acid depresses ventilation in the rat. J Appl Physiol 56:849–856, 1984

Hegel MT, Ayllon T, Thiel G, et al: Improving adherence to fluid restrictions in male hemodialysis patients: a comparison of cognitive and behavioral approaches. Health Psychol 11:324–330, 1992

Heitkemper MM, Jarrett M, Cain KC, et al: Autonomic nervous system function in women with irritable bowel syndrome. Dig Dis Sci 46:1276–1284, 2001

Helzer JE, Chammas S, Norland CC, et al: A study of the association between Crohn's disease and psychiatric illness. Gastroenterology 86:324–330, 1984

Henning P, Tomlinson L, Rigden SPA, et al: Long term outcome of treatment of end-stage renal failure. Arch Dis Child 63:35–40, 1988

Henry JP, Cassel JC: Psychological factors in essential hypertension: recent epidemiological and animal experimental evidence. Am J Epidemiol 90:171–200, 1969

Henry JP, Stephens PM: Stress, Health, and the Social Environment: A Sociobiological Approach to Medicine. New York, Springer-Verlag New York, 1977

Henry JP, Meehan JP, Stephens PM: The use of psychosocial stimuli to induce prolonged systolic hypertension in mice. Psychosom Med 29:408–432, 1967

Henry JP, Ely DL, Stephens PM, et al: The role of psychosocial factors in the development of arteriosclerosis in CBA mice. Atherosclerosis 14:203–218, 1971

Herberman RB: Sources of confounding in immunologic data. Rev Infect Dis 13 (suppl 1):S84–S86, 1991

Herrera LA, Trundle D, Federico JJ, et al: Prevalence of biologic markers and biochemical abnormalities in depressed patients. Ann Clin Psychiatry 3:55–59, 1991

Herschbach P, Henrich G, Von Rad M: Psychological factors in functional gastrointestinal disorders: characteristics of the disorder or the illness behavior? Psychosom Med 61:148–153, 1999

Himmelhoch JM, Schechtman K, Auchenbach R: The role of trazodone in the treatment of depressed cardiac patients. Psychopathology 17 (suppl 2):51–63, 1984

Hitchcock JN, Toendle GJ: Oral cobalamin for treatment of pernicious anemia. JAMA 265:96–97, 1991

Hollander E, Liebowitz MRT, Gorman JM, et al: Cortisol and sodium lactate-induced panic. Arch Gen Psychiatry 21:23–52, 1987

Holley JL, Nespor S, Rault R: Chronic in-center hemodialysis patients' attitudes, knowledge, and behavior towards advance directives. J Am Soc Nephrol 3:1405–1408, 1993

Holmes GP: Defining the chronic fatigue syndrome. Rev Infect Dis 13 (suppl 1):S53–S55, 1991

Holmes GP, Kaplan JE, Gantz NM, et al: Chronic fatigue syndrome: a working case definition. Ann Intern Med 108:387–389, 1988

Horsten M, Mittleman MA, Wamala SP, et al: Depressive symptoms and lack of social integration in relation to prognosis of CHD in middle-aged women. (The Stockholm Female Coronary Risk Study.) Eur Heart J 21:1072–1080, 2000

Horton-Deutsch SL, Clark DC, Farran CL: Chronic dyspnea and suicide in elderly men. Hospital and Community Psychiatry 43:1198–1203, 1992

Hotopf M, Mayou R, Wadsworth M, et al: Psychosocial and developmental antecedents of chest pain in young adults. Psychosom Med 61:861–867, 1999

Hudson JI, Pope HG: Affective spectrum disorder: does antidepressant response identify a family of disorders with a common pathophysiology? Am J Psychiatry 147:552–564, 1990

Hudson JI, Hudson MS, Pliner LF, et al: Fibromyalgia and major affective disorders: a controlled phenomenology and family history study. Am J Psychiatry 142:441–446, 1985

Hudson JI, Hudson MS, Griffing GT, et al: Phenomenology and family history of affective disorder in Cushing's disease. Am J Psychiatry 144:951–953, 1987

Hunt RH: Eradication of Helicobacter pylori infection. Am J Med 100(5A):42S–51S, 1996

Hurt RD, Sachs DPL, Glover ED, et al: A comparison of sustained-release bupropion and placebo for smoking cessation. N Engl J Med 337:1195–1202

Husebye DG, Westlie L, Styrvoky TJ, et al: Psychological, social, and somatic prognostic indicators in old patients undergoing long-term dialysis. Arch Intern Med 147:1921–1924, 1987

Irwin C, Falsetti S, Lydiard RB, et al: Comorbidity of posttraumatic stress disorder and irritable bowel syndrome. J Clin Psychiatry 57:576–578, 1996

Isenberg SA, Lehrer PM, Hochron S: The effects of suggestion and emotional arousal on pulmonary function in asthma: a review of a hypothesis regarding vagal mediation. Psychosom Med 54:192–216, 1992

Jackson JL, O'Malley PG, Tomkins G, et al: Treatment of functional gastrointestinal disorders with antidepressant medications: a meta-analysis. Am J Med 108:65–72, 2000

Jaffe CM: First-degree atrioventricular block during lithium carbonate treatment. Am J Psychiatry 134:88–89, 1977

Jailwala J, Imperiale TF, Kroenke K: Pharmacologic treatment of the irritable bowel syndrome: a systematic review of randomized, controlled trials. Ann Intern Med 133:136–147, 2000

Jain VK: A psychiatric study of hypothyroidism. Psychiatr Clin (Basel) 5:121–130, 1972

Jann MW, Bitar AH: Respiratory dyskinesia. Psychosomatics 23:764–765, 1982

Janssen M, Baggen MGA, Veen HF, et al: Dysphagia lusoria: clinical aspects, manometric findings, diagnosis and therapy. Am J Gastroenterol 95:1411–1416, 2000

Jarvik LF, Read SL, Mintz J, et al: Pretreatment orthostatic hypotension in geriatric depression: predictor of response to imipramine and doxepin. J Clin Psychopharmacol 3:368–372, 1983

Jarvinen KAJ: Can ward rounds be a danger to patients with myocardial infarction? BMJ 2:318–320, 1955

Jeffcoate WJ, Silverstone JT, Edwards CRW, et al: Psychiatric manifestations of Cushing's syndrome: response to lowering of plasma cortisol. Quarterly Journal of Medicine 191:465–472, 1979

Jefferson JW: Cardiovascular effects and toxicity of anxiolytics and antidepressants. J Clin Psychiatry 50:368–378, 1989

Jellinek MS, Goldenheim PD, Jenicke MA: The impact of grief on ventilatory control. Am J Psychiatry 142:121–123, 1985

Joborn C, Hetta J, Palmer M, et al: Psychiatric symptomatology in patients with primary hyperparathyroidism. Ups J Med Sci 91:77–87, 1986

Johns DR, Teirney M, Felsenstein D: Alteration in the natural history of neurosyphilis by concurrent infection with the human immunodeficiency virus. N Engl J Med 316:1569–1572, 1987

Josephson AM, MacKenzie TB: Thyroid-induced mania in hypothyroid patients. Br J Psychiatry 137:222–238, 1980

Kahrilas PJ, Clouse RE, Hogan WJ: American Gastroenterological Association technical review on the clinical use of esophageal manometry. Gastroenterology 107:1865–1884, 1994

Kantor SJ, Bigger JT, Glassman AH, et al: Imipramine-induced heart block. JAMA 231:1364–1366, 1975

Kantor SJ, Glassman AH, Bigger JT, et al: The cardiac effect of therapeutic plasma concentrations of imipramine. Am J Psychiatry 135:534–538, 1978

Kaplan DS, Masand PS, Gupta S. The relationship of irritable bowel syndrome (IBS) and panic disorder. Ann Clin Psychiatry 8(2):81–88, 1996

Kaplan JR, Manuck SB, Clarkson TB, et al: Social status, environment and atherosclerosis in cynomolgus monkeys. Arteriosclerosis 2:359–368, 1982

Kaplan JR, Manuck SB, Clarkson TB, et al: Social stress and atherosclerosis in normocholesterolemic monkeys. Science 220:733–735, 1983

Kassirir JP: The quality of care and the quality of measuring it. N Engl J Med 329:1263–1265, 1993

Kathol RG, Delahunt JW: The relationship of anxiety and depression to symptoms of hyperthyroidism using operational criteria. Gen Hosp Psychiatry 8:23–28, 1986

Katon W, Raskind M: Treatment of depression in the medically ill elderly with methylphenidate. Am J Psychiatry 30:106–108, 1980

Katon W, Russo JS: Chronic fatigue syndrome criteria. Arch Intern Med 152:1604–1609, 1992

Katz DM, Black IB: Expression and regulation of catecholaminergic traits in primary sensory neurons: relationship to target innervation in vivo. J Neurosci 6:983–989, 1986

Kaufman MW, Murray GB, Cassem NH: Use of psychostimulants in medically ill depressed patients. Psychosomatics 23:817–819, 1982

Kellner R, Samet JM, Pathak D: Hypochondriacal concerns and somatic symptoms in patients with chronic airflow obstruction. J Psychosom Res 31:575–582, 1987

Kellner R, Samet J, Pathak D: Dyspnea, anxiety, and depression in chronic respiratory impairment. Gen Hosp Psychiatry 14:20–28, 1992

Kelly WF, Checkley SA, Bender DA: Cushing's syndrome and depression—a prospective study of 26 patients. Br J Psychiatry 142:16–19, 1983

Kemmer FW, Bisping R, Steingruber HJ, et al: Psychological stress and metabolic control in patients with type I diabetes mellitus. N Engl J Med 314:1078–1084, 1986

Kendler KS, Neale MC, MacLean CL, et al: Smoking and major depression: a causal analysis. Arch Gen Psychiatry 50:36–43, 1993

Kiley DC, Lam CS, Pollak R: A study of treatment compliance following kidney transplantation. Transplantation 55:51–56, 1993

Killian KJ, Campbell EJM: Dyspnea and exercise. Annu Rev Physiol 45:465–479, 1983

Kim CH, Hsu JJ, Wiliams DE, et al: A prospective psychological evaluation of patients with dysphagia of various etiologies. Dysphagia 11:34–40, 1996

Kjellstrand CM, Dossetor JB: Ethical Problems in Dialysis and Transplantation. Dordrecht, The Netherlands, Kluwer Academic, 1992

Klein DF: False suffocation alarms, spontaneous panics, and related conditions. Arch Gen Psychiatry 50:306–317, 1993

Klein KB: Controlled treatment trials in irritable bowel syndrome: a critique. Gastroenterology 95:233–241, 1988

Klein SD, Simmons RG, Anderson CR: Chronic kidney disease and transplantation in childhood and adolescence, in Chronic Illness and Disabilities in Childhood and Adolescence. Edited by Blum RW. New York, Grune & Stratton, 1984, pp 429–557

Klempner MS, Hu LT, Evans J, et al: Two controlled trials of antibiotic treatment in patients with persistent symptoms and a history of Lyme disease. N Engl J Med 345:85–92, 2001

Kollar EJ, Fullerton DT, DiCenso R, et al: Stress specificity in ulcerative colitis. Compr Psychiatry 5(2):101–112, 1964

Korsch BM, Fine RN, Negrete VF: Non-compliance in children with renal transplants. Pediatrics 61:872–876, 1978

Krantz DS, Durel LA, David JE, et al: Propranolol medication among coronary patients: relationship to type A behavior and cardiovascular response. Journal of Human Stress 8:4–12, 1982

Kriwisky M, Perry GY, Tarchitsky D, et al: Haloperidol-induced torsades de pointes. Chest 98:482–484, 1990

Laghrissi-Thode F, Wagner WR, Pollock BG, et al: Elevated platelet factor 4 and beta-thromboglobulin plasma levels in depressed patients with ischemic heart disease. Biol Psychiatry 42:290–295, 1997

Laitinen LA, Laitinen A: Neural system, in The Lung: Scientific Foundations. Edited by Crystal RG, West JB. New York, Raven, 1991, pp 759–767

Langosch W, Seer P, Brodner G, et al: Behavior therapy with coronary heart disease patients: results of a comparative study. J Psychosom Res 26:475–484, 1982

Laupacis A, Muirhead N, Keown P, et al: A disease-specific questionnaire for assessing quality of life in patients on hemodialysis. Nephron 60:302–306, 1992

Lederle FA: Oral cobalamin for pernicious anemia. Medicine's best kept secret? JAMA 265:94–95, 1991

Lehrer PM, Hochron SM, McCann B, et al: Relaxation decreases large airway but not small airway asthma. J Psychosom Res 30:13–25, 1986

Lehrer PM, Sargunaraj D, Hochron S: Psychological approaches to the treatment of asthma. J Consult Clin Psychol 60:639–643, 1992

Lemon SM: What is the role of testing for IgM antibody to core antigen of hepatitis B virus? (editorial) Mayo Clin Proc 63:201–204, 1988

Lesperance F, Frasure-Smith N: Depression and death post-myocardial infarction (NR457), in New Research Program and Abstracts, American Psychiatric Association, 146th Annual Meeting, San Francisco, CA, May 22–27, 1993. Washington, DC, American Psychiatric Association, 1993, p 175

Lesperance F, Frasure-Smith N, Juneau M, et al: Depression and 1-year prognosis in unstable angina. Arch Intern Med 160:1354–1360, 2000

Levy NB, Cohen LM: End-stage renal disease and its treatment: dialysis and transplantation, in Psychiatric Care of the Medical Patient, 2nd Edition. Edited by Stoudemire A, Fogel BS, Greenberg D. London, Oxford University Press, 2000, pp 791–800

Levy RL, Whitehead WE, Von Korff MR, et al: Intergenerational transmission of gastrointestinal illness behavior. Am J Gastroenterol 95(2):451–456, 2000

Levine PH, Jacobson S, Pocinki AG, et al: Clinical, epidemiologic, and virologic studies in four clusters of the chronic fatigue syndrome. Arch Intern Med 152:1611–1616, 1992

Levine SO, Towell BL, Suarez AM, et al: Platelet aggregation and secretion associated with emotional stress. Circulation 71:1129–1134, 1985

Levy NB: Sexual adjustment to maintenance hemodialysis and renal transplantation: national survey by questionnaire: preliminary report. Transactions of the American Society of Artificial Internal Organs 19:138–143, 1973

Levy NB: Use of psychotropics in patients with kidney failure. Psychosomatics 26:699–709, 1985

Lewis SF, Haller RG: Physiologic measurement of exercise and fatigue with special reference to chronic fatigue syndrome. Rev Infect Dis 13 (suppl 1):S98–S108, 1991

Lichstein KL, Eakin TL, Dunn ME: Combined psychological and medical treatment of oropharyngeal dysphagia. Clinical Biofeedback and Health: An International Journal 9:9–14, 1986

Light RW, Merrill EJ, Despars JA, et al: Prevalence of depression and anxiety in patients with COPD: relationship to functional capacity. Chest 87:35–38, 1985

Lindefors N, Yamamoto Y, Pantaleo R, et al: In vivo release of substance P in the nucleus tractus solitarii increases during hypoxia. Neurosci Lett 69:94–97, 1986

Lown B: Sudden cardiac death: the major challenge confronting contemporary cardiology. Am J Cardiol 43:313–328, 1979

Lown B, DeSilva RA: Roles of psychologic stress and autonomic nervous system changes in provocation of ventricular premature complexes. Am J Cardiol 41:979–985, 1978

Lown B, Graboys TB: Management of patients with malignant ventricular arrhythmias. Am J Cardiol 39:910–918, 1977

Lown B, Verrier RL, Corbalan R: Psychologic stress and the threshold for repetitive ventricular response. Science 132:834–836, 1973

Lown B, Verrier RL, Rabinowitz SH: Neural and psychologic mechanisms and the problem of sudden cardiac death. Am J Cardiol 39:890–902, 1977

Lown B, DeSilva RA, Reich P, et al: Psychophysiologic factors in sudden cardiac death. Am J Psychiatry 137:1325–1335, 1980

Luchins DJ: Review of clinical and animal studies comparing the cardiovascular effects of doxepin and other tricyclic antidepressants. Am J Psychiatry 140:1006–1009, 1983

Luft BJ, Gardner P, Lightfoot RW, et al: Empiric antibiotic treatment of patients who are seropositive for Lyme disease but lack classic features (abstract). Clin Infect Dis 18:112, 1994

Lumley MA, Torosian T, Ketterer MW, et al: Psychological factors related to noncardiac chest pain during treadmill exercise. Psychosomatics 38:230–238, 1997

Lustman PJ, Griffith LS, Clouse RE, et al: Psychiatric illness in diabetes mellitus: relationship to symptoms and glucose control. J Nerv Ment Dis 174:736–742, 1986

Lustman PJ, Griffith LS, Clouse RE: Depression in adults with diabetes. Diabetes Care 11:605–612, 1988

Lydiard RB: Anxiety and the irritable bowel syndrome: psychiatric, medical or both? J Clin Psychiatry 58(suppl 3):51–58, 1997

Lydiard RB, Fossey MD, Ballenger JC: Irritable bowel syndrome in patients with panic disorder (letter). Am J Psychiatry 148:1614, 1991

Lydiard RB, Fossey MD, Marsh W, et al: Prevalence of psychiatric disorders in patients with irritable bowel syndrome. Psychosomatics 34:229–234, 1993

MacDougall JM, Dembroski TM, Dimsdale JE, et al: Components of type A, hostility, and anger-in: further relationships to angiographic findings. Health Psychol 4:137–145, 1985

Malzberg B: Mortality among patients with involutional melancholia. Am J Psychiatry 93:1231–1238, 1937

Manning AP, Thompson WG, Heaton KW, et al: Towards positive diagnosis of the irritable bowel. BMJ 2:653–654, 1978

Mantero-Atienza E, Baum MK, Morgan R, et al: Vitamin B12 in early human immunodeficiency virus-1 infection. Arch Intern Med 151:1019–1020, 1991

Manuck SB, Kaplan JR, Clarkson TB: Behaviorally induced heart rate reactivity and atherosclerosis in cynomolgus monkeys. Psychosom Med 345:95–108, 1983

Manuck SB, Morrison RL, Bellack AS, et al: Behavioral factors in hypertension: cardiovascular responsivity, anger, and social competence, in Anger and Hostility in Cardiovascular and Behavioral Disorders. Edited by Chesney MA, Rosenman RH. New York, Hemisphere/McGraw-Hill, 1987, pp 149–172

Marchionno PM, Kirilloff LH, Openbrier DR, et al: Effects of continuous oxygen therapy on body image and lifestyle in patients with COPD (abstract). Am Rev Respir Dis 13 (part 2):A163, 1985

Markovitz JH, Matthews KA: Platelets and coronary heart disease: potential psychophysiologic mechanisms. Psychosom Med 53:643–668, 1991

Massry SG: Neurotoxicity of parathyroid hormone and uremia (abstract). Kidney Int 28:S5, 1984

Matta RJ, Lawler JE, Lown B: Ventricular electrical instability in the conscious dog: effects of psychologic stress and beta-adrenergic blockade. Am J Cardiol 34:594–598, 1976

McGrath PJ, Blood DK, Stewart JW, et al: A comparative study of the electrocardiographic effects of phenelzine, tricyclic antidepressants, mianserin, and placebo. J Clin Psychopharmacol 7:335–339, 1987

McKegney FP, Lange P: The decision to no longer live on chronic hemodialysis. Am J Psychiatry 128:47–53, 1971

McMahon LP, Dawborn JK: Subjective quality of life assessment in hemodialysis patients at different levels of hemoglobin following use of recombinant human erythropoietin. Am J Nephrol 12:162–169, 1992

Meerson FZ: Pathogenesis and prophylaxis of cardiac lesions in stress, in Advances in Neurocardiology, Vol 4. Edited by Chazov EI, Sachs P. New York, Plenum, 1983, pp 123–134

Mendes de Leon CF, Powell LH, Kaplan BH: Change in coronary-prone behaviors in the Recurrent Coronary Prevention Project. Psychosom Med 53:407–419, 1991

Mertz H, Morgan V, Tanner G, et al: Regional cerebral activation in irritable bowel syndrome and control subjects with painful and nonpainful rectal distention. Gastroenterology 118:842–848, 2000

Meyers S, Walfish JS, Sachar DB, et al: Quality of life after surgery for Crohn's disease: a psychosocial survey. Gastroenterology 78:1–6, 1980

Mifsud JC, Hernandez L, Hoebel BG: Nicotine infused into the nucleus accumbens increases synaptic dopamine as measured by in vivo microdialysis. Brain Res 478:365–367, 1989

Miller TQ, Turner CW, Tindale RS, et al: Reasons for the trend toward null findings in research on type A behavior. Psychol Bull 110:469–485, 1991

Mitchell JE, MacKenzie TB: Cardiac effects of lithium in man: a review. J Clin Psychiatry 43:47–51, 1982

Moldofsky H, Lue FA: The relationship of alpha and delta EEG frequencies to pain and mood in "fibrositis" patients treated with chlorpromazine and L-tryptophan. Electroencephalogr Clin Neurophysiol 50:71–80, 1980

Moody L, McCormick K, Williams A: Disease and symptom severity, functional status, and quality of life. J Behav Med 13:297–306, 1990

Morbidity and Mortality of Dialysis. NIH Consensus Development Conference, Rockville, MD, November 1–3, 1993

Morgan AD, Peck DF, Buchanan D, et al: Psychological factors contributing to disproportionate disability in chronic bronchitis. J Psychosom Res 27:259–263, 1983

Moser G, Vacariugranser GV, Schneider C, et al: High incidence of esophageal motor disorders in consecutive patients with globus sensation. Gastroenterology 101:1512–1521, 1991

Moss AJ, Goldstein S: The pre-hospital phase of acute myocardial infarction. Circulation 41:737–742, 1970

Musselman DL, Tomer A, Manatunga AK, et al: Exaggerated platelet reactivity in major depression. Am J Psychiatry 153:1313–1317, 1996

Naliboff BD, Derbyshire SWG, Munakata J, et al: Cerebral activation in patients with irritable bowel syndrome and control subjects during rectosigmoid stimulation. Psychosom Med 63:365–375, 2001

National Ambulatory Medical Care Survey: 1975 Summary. Hyattsville, MD, National Center for Health Statistics, 1978, pp 22–26

National Institutes of Health NIDDK/DKUHD: Excerpts from the United States Renal Date System 2000 Annual Data Report. Am J Kidney Dis 36(suppl 2):S1–S239, 2000

Neff TA, Petty TL: Tolerance and survival in severe chronic hypercapnia. Arch Intern Med 129:591–596, 1972

Nemeroff CB, Widerlow E, Bissette G, et al: Elevated concentrations of CSF corticotropin-releasing factor-like immunoreactivity in depressed patients. Science 226:1342–1344, 1984

Nerem RM, Levesque MJ, Cornhill JF: Social environment as a factor in diet-induced atherosclerosis. Science 208:1475–1476, 1980

Nestel PJ: Blood-pressure and catecholamine excretion after mental stress in labile hypertension. Lancet 1:692–694, 1969

Neu S, Kjellstrand CM: Stopping long-term dialysis: an empirical study of withdrawal of life-supporting treatment. N Engl J Med 314:14–20, 1986

Neumann ME: As dialysis becomes an extension of life, its use gains greater scrutiny (editorial). Nephrology News Issues 6:5, 1992

Nickel SN, Frame B: Neurologic manifestations of myxedema. Neurology 8:511–517, 1958

Nissenson AR: Dialysis therapy in the elderly patient. Kidney Int 43 (suppl 40):S51–S57, 1993

Nocturnal Oxygen Therapy Trial Group: Continuous or nocturnal oxygen therapy in hypoxemic chronic obstructive lung disease: a clinical trial. Ann Intern Med 93:391–398, 1980

North CS, Clouse RE, Spitznagel EL, et al: The relation of ulcerative colitis to psychiatric factors: a review of findings and methods. Am J Psychiatry 147:974–981, 1990

Norton CE: Attitudes toward living and dying in patients on chronic hemodialysis. Ann N Y Acad Sci 164:720–732, 1969

Noyes R Jr, Cook B, Garvey M, et al: Reduction of gastrointestinal symptoms with treatment for panic disorder. Psychosomatics 31:75–79, 1990

Nunes EV, Frank KA, Kornfield DS: Psychological treatment for the type A behavior pattern and for coronary heart disease: a meta-analysis of the literature. Psychosom Med 49:159–173, 1987

Olden KW: Brain-gut interactions. West J Med 160:55, 1994

Olden KW: Inflammatory bowel disease and psychiatry: from causality to comorbidity. Med Psychiatr 1:17–21, 1998

Olden KW: Antidepressants and functional gastrointestinal disorders. Practical Gastroenterology, April 2001, pp 16–23

Olden KW, Brotman AW: Irritable bowel/irritable mood: the mind/gut connection. Harv Rev Psychiatry 6:149–154, 1998

Olden KW, Drossman DA: Psychological and psychiatric aspects of gastrointestinal disease. Med Clin North Am 84(5): 1313–1327, 2000

Oldenburg B, Perkins RJ, Andrews G: Controlled trial of psychological intervention in myocardial infarction. J Consult Clin Psychol 53:852–859, 1985

Osberg JW, Mears GL, McKee DC, et al: Intellectual functioning in renal failure and chronic dialysis. Journal of Chronic Disease 35:445–447, 1982

Osler W: The Lumleian lectures on angina pectoris. Lancet 1:939–942, 1910

Osterberg E, Blomquist L, Kraukau I, et al: A population study on irritable bowel syndrome and mental health. Scand J Gastroenterol 35:264–268, 2000

Parfrey PS, Vavasour HM, Gault MH: A prospective study of health status in dialysis and transplant patients. Transplant Proc 20:1231–1232, 1989

Pastan S, Bailey J: Dialysis therapy. N Engl J Med 338:1428–1437, 1998

Penninx W, beekman AT, Honig A, et al: Depression and cardiac mortality: results from a community-based longitudinal study. Arch Gen Psychiatry 58:221–227, 2001

Peroutka SJ: 5-Hydroxytryptamine receptor subtypes. Annu Rev Neurosci 11:45–60, 1988

Petersen P: Psychiatric disorders in primary hyperparathyroidism. J Clin Endocrinol Metab 28:1491–1495, 1968

Piehlmeier W, Bullinger M, Nusser J, et al: Quality of life in type I (insulin-dependent) diabetic patients prior to and after pancreas and kidney transplantation in relation to organ function. Diabetologia 34 (suppl 1):S150–S157, 1991

Pohl RB, Yeragani VK, Balon R, et al: Smoking in panic disorder patients, in CME Syllabus and Scientific Proceedings in Summary Form. 145th Annual Meeting of the American Psychiatric Association, Washington, DC, May 2–7, 1992. Washington, DC, American Psychiatric Association, 1992, p 84

Pope John Paul II: Speech to blood and organ donors. Rome, Italy, October 15, 1980

Pope Pius XI: Litt Encycl "Casti Connubi." Atti della Accademia dei Fisiocritici in Siena 22:565, 1930

Popkin MK, Callies AL, Lentz RD, et al: Prevalence of major depression, simple phobia and other psychiatric disorders in patients with long-standing type I diabetes mellitus. Arch Gen Psychiatry 45:64–68, 1988

Porzelius J, Vest M, Nochomovitz M: Respiratory function, cognitions, and panic in chronic obstructive pulmonary patients. Behav Res Ther 30:75–77, 1992

Posner JB: Newer techniques of cerebral blood flow measurement. Stroke 3:227–237, 1972

Pratt LA, Ford DE, Crum RM, et al: Depression, psychotropic medication, and risk of myocardial infarction: prospective data from the Baltimore ECA follow-up. Circulation 94:3123–3129, 1996

Prigatano GP, Parsons O, Wright E, et al: Neuropsychological test performance in mildly hypoxemic patients with chronic obstructive pulmonary disease. J Consult Clin Psychol 51:108–116, 1983

Prochazka A, Weaver MJ, Keller RT, et al: A randomized trial of nortriptyline for smoking cessation. Arch Intern Med 158:2035–2039

Prusoff B, Klerman GL: Differentiating depressed from anxious neurotic outpatients. Arch Gen Psychiatry 30:302–309, 1974

Raab W: Emotional and sensory stress factors in myocardial pathology: neurogenic and hormonal mechanisms in pathogenesis, therapy, and prevention. Am Heart J 72:538–564, 1966

Rabinowitz SH, Lown B: Central neurochemical factors related to serotonin metabolism and cardiac ventricular vulnerability for repetitive electrical activity. Am J Cardiol 41:516–522, 1978

Ragland DR, Brand RJ: Type A behavior and mortality from coronary heart disease. N Engl J Med 318:65–69, 1988

Rapoport DM, Greenberg HE, Goldring RM: Differing effects of the anxiolytic agents buspirone and diazepam on control of breathing. Clin Pharmacol Ther 49:394–401, 1991

Raskind M, Veith RC, Barnes R, et al: Cardiovascular and antidepressant effects of imipramine in the treatment of secondary depression in patients with ischemic heart disease. Am J Psychiatry 139:1114–1117, 1982

Reggev A, Vollhardt BR: Bradycardia induced by an interaction between phenelzine and beta-blockers. Psychosomatics 30:106–108, 1989

Reich P, Murawski BJ, DeSilva RA, et al: Psychologic studies of patients with ventricular arrhythmias. Psychosom Med 41:74–79, 1979

Reichenbach D, Benditt EP: Myofibrillar degeneration, a common form of cardiac muscle injury. Ann N Y Acad Sci 156:164–176, 1970

Reik L: Lyme disease and fatigue, in Chronic Fatigue Syndrome. Edited by Dawson DM, Sabin TD. Boston, MA, Little, Brown, 1993, pp 161–177

Reilly GS: A questionnaire for dialysis patients on treatment cessation issues. Dialysis and Transplantation 19:533–545, 1990

Reynolds JM, Garralda ME, Postlethwaite RJ, et al: Changes in psychosocial adjustment after renal transplantation. Arch Dis Child 66:508–513, 1991

Richter JE, Dalton CB, Bradley LA, et al: Oral nifedipine in the treatment of noncardiac chest pain in patients with the nutcracker esophagus. Gastroenterology 93:21–28, 1987

Ringel Y, Drossman DA: Treatment of patients with functional esophageal symptoms: is there a role for a psychotherapeutic approach? J Clin Gastroenterol 28(3):189–193, 1999

Robinson DS, Nies A, Corcella J, et al: Cardiovascular effects of phenelzine and amitriptyline in depressed outpatients. J Clin Psychiatry 43:8–15, 1982

Rodriguez A, Diaz M, Colon A, et al: Psychosocial profile of noncompliant transplant patients. Transplant Proc 23:1807–1809, 1991

Roine RO, Kajaste S, Kaste M: Neuropsychological sequelae of cardiac arrest. JAMA 269:237–242, 1993

Rome II: The Functional Gastrointestinal Disorders. Edited by Drossman DA, Corazziari E, Talley NJ, et al. McLean, VA, Degnon Associates, 2000

Roose SP, Dalack GW: Treating the depressed patient with cardiovascular problems. J Clin Psychiatry 53 (suppl):25–31, 1992

Roose SP, Nurnberger JI, Dunner DL, et al: Cardiac sinus node dysfunction during lithium treatment. Am J Psychiatry 136:804–806, 1979a

Roose SP, Bone S, Haidorfer C, et al: Lithium treatment in older patients. Am J Psychiatry 136:843–844, 1979b

Roose SP, Glassman AH, Giardina E-GV, et al: Nortriptyline in depressed patients with left ventricular impairment. JAMA 256:3253–3257, 1986

Roose SP, Glassman AH, Giardina E-GV, et al: Tricyclic antidepressants in depressed patients with cardiac conduction disease. Arch Gen Psychiatry 44:273–275, 1987

Roose SP, Dalack GW, Glassman AH, et al: Cardiovascular effects of bupropion in depressed patients with heart disease. Am J Psychiatry 148:512–516, 1991a

Roose SP, Dalack GW, Woodring S: Death, depression, and heart disease. J Clin Psychiatry 52 (suppl):34–39, 1991b

Roose SP, Laghrissi-Thode F, Kennedy JS, et al: Comparison of paroxetine and nortriptyline in depressed patients with ischemic heart disease. JAMA 279:287–291, 1998

Rosenman RH, Brand RJ, Jenkins D, et al: Coronary heart disease in Western Collaborative Group Study: final follow-up experience of 8 1/2 years. JAMA 233:872–877, 1975

Ross CA, Ruggiero DA, Joh TH, et al: Adrenaline synthesizing neurons in the rostral ventrolateral medulla: a possible role in tonic vasomotor control. Brain Res 273:356–361, 1983

Ross RL, Smith R, Guggenheim FG: Neurosyphilis and organic mood syndrome: a forgotten diagnosis. Psychosomatics 31:448–450, 1990

Rossel P, Drewes AM, Petersen P, et al: Pain produced by electric stimulation of the rectum in patients with irritable bowel syndrome: further evidence of visceral hyperalgesia. Scand J Gastroenterol 10:1001–1006, 1999

Roth M, Gurney C, Garside RF, et al: Studies in the classification of affective disorders: the relationship between anxiety states and depressive illnesses, I. Br J Psychiatry 121:147–161, 1972

Rozanski A, Bairey CN, Krantz DS, et al: Mental stress and the induction of silent myocardial ischemia in patients with coronary artery disease. N Engl J Med 318:1005–1011, 1988

Rozanski A, Blumenthal JA, Kaplan J: Impact of psychological factors on the pathogenesis of cardiovascular disease and implications for therapy. Circulation 99:2192–2217, 1999

Ruberman W, Weinblatt AB, Goldberg JD, et al: Psychosocial influences on mortality after myocardial infarction. N Engl J Med 311:552–559, 1984

Rundell JR, Wise MG: Neurosyphilis: a psychiatric perspective. Psychosomatics 26:287–290, 1985

Russell JD, Beecroft ML, Ludlow D, et al: The quality of life in renal transplantation—a prospective study. Transplantation 54:656–660, 1992

Rydall AC, Rodin GM, Olmsted MP, et al: Disordered eating behavior and microvascular complications in young women with insulin-dependent diabetes mellitus. N Engl J Med 336:1849–1854, 1997

Saltzman HA, Heyman A, Sieker F: Correlation of clinical and physiologic manifestations with sustained hyperventilation. N Engl J Med 268:1431–1436, 1963

Sayag R, Kaplan De-Nour A, Shapira Z, et al: Comparison of psychosocial adjustment of male nondiabetic kidney transplant and hospital hemodialysis patients. Nephron 54:214–218, 1990

Schachter J: Pain, fear, and anger in hypertensives and normotensives. Psychosom Med 19:17–26, 1957

Scheinberg P: Effects of uremia on cerebral blood flow and metabolism. Neurology 4:101–115, 1954

Schleifer SJ, Macari-Hinson MM, Coyle DA, et al: The nature and course of depression following myocardial infarction. Arch Intern Med 149:1785–1789, 1989

Schmulson MW, Chang L, Naliboff BD, et al: Correlation of symptom criteria with perception thresholds during rectosigmoid distension in irritable bowel syndrome patients. Am J Gastroenterol 95:152–156, 2000

Schneider LS, Sloane RB, Stapes FR, et al: Pretreatment orthostatic hypotension as a predictor of response to nortriptyline in geriatric depression. J Clin Psychopharmacol 6:172–176, 1986

Schneiderman N: Psychophysiologic factors in atherogenesis and coronary artery disease. Circulation 76:41–47, 1987

Schover LR, Novick AC, Steinmuller DR, et al: Sexuality, fertility, and renal transplantation: a survey of survivors. J Sex Marital Ther 16:3–13, 1990

Schwartz PJ, Wolf S: QT interval prolongation as predictor of sudden death in patients with myocardial infarction. Circulation 57:1074–1077, 1978

Selye H: The Stress of Life. New York, McGraw-Hill, 1956

Sensky T: Psychiatric morbidity in renal transplantation. Psychother Psychosom 52:41–46, 1989

Seraganian P, Hanley JA, Hollander BJ, et al: Exaggerated psychophysiological reactivity: issues in quantification and reliability. J Psychosom Res 29:393–405, 1985

Series F, Cormier Y: Effects of protriptyline on diurnal and nocturnal oxygenation in patients with chronic obstructive pulmonary disease. Ann Intern Med 113:507–511, 1990

Shapiro ED: Doxycycline for tick bites: not for everyone. N Engl J Med 345:133–134, 2001

Sharpe MC, Archard LC, Banatvala JE, et al: A report—chronic fatigue syndrome: guidelines for research. J R Soc Med 84:118–121, 1991

Shaw R: The impact of denial and repressive style on information gain and rehabilitation outcomes in myocardial infarction patients. Psychosom Med 47:262–273, 1985

Shekelle RB, Hulley SB, Neaton J, et al: The MRFIT behavior pattern study, II: Type A behavior and incidence of coronary heart disease. Am J Epidemiol 122:559–579, 1985

Shershow JC, King A, Robinson S: Carbon dioxide sensitivity and personality. Psychosom Med 35:155–160, 1973

Shershow JC, Kanarek DJ, Kazemi H: Ventilatory response to carbon dioxide inhalation in depression. Psychosom Med 38:282–287, 1976

Sherwitz L, McKelvain R, Laman C, et al: Type A behavior, self-involvement and coronary atherosclerosis. Psychosom Med 45:47–57, 1983

Sigg EG, Osborne M, Porol B: Cardiovascular effects of imipramine. J Pharmacol Exp Ther 141:237–243, 1963

Sigler LH: Emotion and atherosclerotic heart disease, I: electrocardiovascular changes observed on the recall of past emotional disturbances. Br J Med Psychol 40:55–64, 1967

Simmons RG, Kamstra-Hennen L, Thompson CR: Psychosocial adjustment five to nine years posttransplant. Transplant Proc 13:40–43, 1981

Simmons RG, Anderson C, Kamstra L: Comparison of quality of life of patients on continuous ambulatory peritoneal dialysis, hemodialysis, and after transplantation. Am J Kidney Dis 4:253–255, 1984

Simon AB, Feinleib M, Thompson HK: Components of delay in the pre-hospital phase of acute myocardial infarction. Am J Cardiol 30:476–482, 1972

Simpson MT, Olewine DA, Jenkins CD, et al: Exercise-induced catecholamines and platelet aggregation in the coronary-prone behavior pattern. Psychosom Med 36:467–487, 1974

Singer PA: Nephrologists' experience with and attitudes towards decisions to forgo dialysis. J Am Soc Nephrol 2:1235–1240, 1992

Sipes DD: State, federal statutes guide organ donation procedures. Health Prog 68:46–50, 67, 1987

Slepoy VD, Pezzotto SM, Kraier L, et al: Irritable bowel syndrome: clinical and psychopathological correlations. Dig Dis Sci 44(5):1008–1012, 1999

Smit CF, Van Leeuwen AMJ, Mathus-Vliegen LMH, et al: Gastrophyaryngeal and gastroesophageal reflux in globus and hoarseness. Arch Otolaryngol Head Neck Surg 126:827–830, 2000

Stabler SP, Allen RH, Savage DG, et al: Clinical spectrum and diagnosis of cobalamin deficiency. Blood 76:871–881, 1990

Stamler J, Stamler R, Pullman T: The Epidemiology of Essential Hypertension. New York, Grune & Stratton, 1967

Starkman MN, Zelnik TC, Nesse RM, et al: Anxiety in patients with pheochromocytomas. Arch Intern Med 145:248–252, 1985

Steere AC: Lyme disease. N Engl J Med 345:115–125, 2001

Steere AC, Taylor E, McHugh GL, et al: The overdiagnosis of Lyme disease. JAMA 269:1812–1816, 1993

Stephens PM: The use of psychosocial stimuli to induce prolonged systolic hypertension in mice. Psychosom Med 29:408–432, 1967

Stolerman IP, Shoaib M: The neurobiology of tobacco addiction. Trends Pharmacol Sci 12:467–473, 1991

Stoudemire A, Moran MG, Fogel BS: Psychotropic drug use in the medically ill: part I. Psychosomatics 31:377–391, 1990

Stoudemire A, Moran MG, Fogel BS: Psychotropic drug use in the medically ill: part II. Psychosomatics 32:34–46, 1991

Surman OS: Psychiatric aspects of organ transplantation. Am J Psychiatry 146:972–982, 1989

Surman OS: Hemodialysis and renal transplantation, in Massachusetts General Hospital Handbook of General Hospital Psychiatry, 3rd Edition. Edited by Cassem NH. St. Louis, MO, CV Mosby, 1991, pp 401–430

Taggart P, Gibbons D, Somerville W: Some effects of motor car driving on the normal and abnormal heart. BMJ 4:130–134, 1969

Taggart P, Carruthers M, Somerville W: Electrocardiogram, plasma catecholamines and lipids, and their modification by oxyprenolol when speaking before an audience. Lancet 2:341–346, 1973

Talley NJ, Boyce PM, Jones M: Predictors of health care seeking for irritable bowel syndrome: a population based study. Gut 41:394–398, 1997

Tangedahl TN, Gau GT: Myocardial irritability associated with lithium carbonate therapy. N Engl J Med 287:867–868, 1972

Teschan PE, Ginn HE, Bourne JR, et al: Neurobehavioral probes for adequacy of dialysis. Transamerican Society of Artificial Internal Organs 23:556–559, 1977

Teschan PE, Bourne JR, Reed RB, et al: Electrophysiologic and neurobehavioral responses to therapy: the National Corroborative Dialysis Study. Kidney Int 23 (suppl 13):S58–S65, 1983

Thase ME, Perel JM: Antiarrhythmic effects of tricyclic antidepressants (letter). JAMA 248:429, 1982

Thayer RE: The Biopsychology of Mood and Arousal. New York, Oxford University Press, 1989

Thompson WG: Sexual problems in chronic respiratory disease: achieving and maintaining intimacy. Postgrad Med 79:41–44, 47, 50–52, 1982

Thompson WG, Longstreth GF, Drossman DA, et al: Functional bowel disorders and functional abdominal pain, in Rome II: The Functional Gastrointestinal Disorders. Edited by Drossman DA, Corazziari E, Talley NJ, et al. McLean, VA, Degnon Associates, 2000, pp 351–396

Tobacco Use and Dependence Clinical Practice Guideline Panel, Staff, and Consortium Representatives: A Clinical Practice Guideline for Treating Tobacco Use and Dependence. U.S. Public Health Service Report. JAMA 283:3244–3254, 2000

Tobin MJ, Chadha TS, Jenouri G, et al: Breathing patterns, 2: diseased subjects. Chest 84:286–294, 1983

Tougas G: The autonomic nervous system in functional bowel disorders. Gut 47(suppl IV):IV78–IV80, 2000

Trzepacz PT, McCue M, Klein I, et al: A psychiatric and neuropsychological study of patients with untreated Graves' disease. Gen Hosp Psychiatry 10:49–55, 1988

Tung CS, Grenhoff J, Svensson TH: Nicotine counteracts midbrain dopamine cell dysfunction induced by prefrontal cortex inactivation. Acta Physiol Scand 138:427–428, 1990

Upward JW, Edwards JG, Goldie A, et al: Comparative effects of fluoxetine and amitriptyline on cardiac function. Br J Clin Pharmacol 26:399–402, 1988

van den Hout MA, Hoekstra R, Arntz A, et al: Hyperventilation is not diagnostically specific to panic patients. Psychosom Med 53:182–191, 1992

Van Ginkel R, Voskuul WP, Benninga MA, et al: Alterations in rectal sensitivity and motility in childhood irritable bowel syndrome. Gastroenterology 120:31–38, 2001

Vanner SJ, Depew WT, Paterson WG, et al: Predictive value of the Rome criteria for diagnosing the irritable bowel syndrome. Am J Gastroenterol 94:2912–2917, 1999

Veale D, Kavanagh G, Fielding JF, et al: Primary fibromyalgia and the irritable bowel syndrome: different expressions of a common pathogenetic process. Br J Rheumatol 30:220–222, 1991

Veith RC, Raskind MA, Caldwell JH, et al: Cardiovascular effects of tricyclic antidepressants in depressed patients with chronic heart disease. N Engl J Med 306:954–959, 1982a

Veith RC, Bloom V, Bielski R, et al: ECG effects of comparable plasma concentrations of desipramine and amitriptyline. J Clin Psychopharmacol 2:394–398, 1982b

Veith RC, Lewis N, Linares OA, et al: Sympathetic nervous system activity in major depression: basal and desipramine-induced alterations in plasma norepinephrine kinetics. Arch Gen Psychiatry 51:411–422, 1994

Vitullo RN, Wharton JM, Allen NB, et al: Trazodone related exercise induced nonsustained ventricular tachycardia. Chest 98:247–248, 1990

Vogel WH, Miller J, DeTurck KH, et al: Effects of psychoactive drugs on plasma catecholamines during stress in rats. Neuropsychopharmacology 23:1105–1108, 1984

Vogt T, Pope C, Mullooly J, et al: Mental health status as a predictor of morbidity and mortality: a 15-year follow-up of members of a health maintenance organization. Am J Public Health 84:227–231, 1995

Walker EA, Gelfand MD, Gelfand AN, et al: The relationship of current psychiatric disorder to functional disability and distress in patients with inflammatory bowel disease. Gen Hosp Psychiatry 18(4):220–229, 1996

Wallace WA, Yu PA: Sudden death and the pre-hospital phase of acute myocardial infarction. Annu Rev Med 26:1–7, 1975

Wassertheil-Smoller S, Applegate WB, Berge K, et al: Change in depression as a precursor to cardiovascular events. SHEP Cooperative Research Group (Systolic Hypertension in the Elderly). Arch Intern Med 156:553–561, 1996

Wechsler D: Wechsler Adult Intelligence Scale—Revised. San Antonio, TX, Psychological Corporation, 1981

Weiner RD, Coffey CE: Electroconvulsive therapy in the medically ill, in Principles of Medical Psychiatry. Edited by Stoudemire A, Fogel BS. Orlando, FL, Grune & Stratton, 1987, pp 113–134

Weiner WJ, Goetz CG, Nausieda R, et al: Respiratory dyskinesias: extrapyramidal dysfunction and dyspnea. Ann Intern Med 88:327–331, 1978

Weiss JH: Behavioral management of asthma, in Behavioral Approaches to Breathing Disorders. Edited by Tenemon BH, Ley R. New York, Plenum, 1994, pp 205–219

Wellens HJ, Cats VM, Duren DR: Symptomatic sinus node abnormalities following lithium carbonate therapy. Am J Med 59:285–287, 1975

Wessely S: Chronic fatigue syndrome: a summary of a report of a joint committe of the Royal Colleges of Physicians, Psychiatrists & General Practitioners. J R Coll Physicians Lond 30:497–504, 1996

Wessely S, Chalder T, Hirsch S, et al: Postinfectious fatigue: prospective cohort study in primary care. Lancet 345:1333–1338, 1995

West TPJ: A comparison: pre dialysis, post dialysis cognitive abilities. Dialysis and Transplantation 7:809–821, 1978

White DP, Douglas NJ, Pickett CK, et al: Sleep deprivation and the control of ventilation. Am Rev Respir Dis 128:984–986, 1983

Whitehead WE: Psychosocial aspects of functional gastrointestinal disorders. Gastroenterol Clin North Am 25(l):21–34, 1996

Whitehead WE, Schuster MM: Gastrointestinal Disorders: Behavioral and Physiological Basis for Treatment. New York, Academic Press, 1985

Whitehead W[E], Bosmajian L, Zorderman AB, et al: Psychologic distress associated with irritable bowel syndrome: comparison of community and medical clinic samples. Gastroenterology 95:709–714, 1988

Wilkinson G, Borsey DQ, Leslie P, et al: Psychiatric morbidity and social problems in patients with insulin-dependent diabetes mellitus. Br J Psychiatry 153:38–43, 1988

Williams RB, Lane JD, Kuhn CM, et al: Type A behavior and elevated physiological and neuroendocrine responses to cognitive tasks. Science 218:483–485, 1982

Williams RB, Barefoot JC, Califf RM, et al: Prognostic importance of social and economic resources among medically treated patients with angiographically documented coronary artery disease. JAMA 267:520–524, 1992

Wilson J, Kraus E, Bailas M, et al: Reversible sinus node abnormalities due to lithium carbonate therapy. N Engl J Med 294:1223–1224, 1976

Wilson WH, Claussen AM: Seizures associated with clozapine treatment in a state hospital. J Clin Psychiatry 55:184–188, 1994

Wolcott DL: Psychiatric aspects of renal dialysis and organ transplantation. Psychiatr Med 9:623–640, 1991

Wolfe F, Smythe HA, Yunus MB, et al: The American College of Rheumatology 1990 Criteria for the Classification of Fibromyalgia: Report of the Multicenter Criteria Committee. Arthritis Rheum 33:160–172, 1990

Woods SW, Tesar GE, Murray GB, et al: Psychostimulant treatment of depressive disorders secondary to medical illness. J Clin Psychiatry 47:12–15, 1986

Woods SW, Charney DS, Goodman WK, et al: Carbon dioxide-induced anxiety: behavioral, physiologic, and biochemical effects of carbon dioxide in patients with panic disorders and healthy subjects. Arch Gen Psychiatry 45:43–52, 1988

Woods SW, Charney DS, Delgado PL, et al: The effect of long-term imipramine treatment on carbon dioxide-induced anxiety in panic disorder patients. J Clin Psychiatry 51:505–507, 1990

Yellowlees PM, Alpers JH, Bowden JJ, et al: Psychiatric morbidity in patients with chronic airflow obstruction. Med J Aust 146:305–307, 1987

Yunus MB, Masi AT, Aldag JC: A controlled study of primary fibromyalgia syndrome: clinical features and association with other functional syndromes. J Rheumatol Suppl 19:62–71, 1989

Zielinski RJ, Roose SP, Devanand DP, et al: Cardiovascular complications of ECT in depressed patients with cardiac disease. Am J Psychiatry 150:904–909, 1993

Zigelstein RC, Bush DE, Faurbach JA: Depression, adherence behavior, and coronary disease outcomes. Arch Intern Med 158:808–809, 1998

27

Surgery and Surgical Subspecialties

Charles L. Raison, M.D.

Robert O. Pasnau, M.D.

Fawzy I. Fawzy, M.D.

Christine E. Skotzko, M.D.

Thomas B. Strouse, M.D.

David K. Wellisch, Ph.D.

Alisa K. Hoffman, Ph.D.

In recent years, economic forces and changes in surgical technology have radically altered the hospital practice of general surgery. Examples include trends toward same-day admissions for planned surgical procedures, shortened hospitalization with management of complex medical regimens at home, and reliance on visiting nurses and home health care rather than hospital-based care. Technological advances, such as endoscopic procedures in lieu of open procedures, have shortened stays and reduced surgical morbidity (Phillips et al. 1993).

The effect of these changes on the patient's psychological experience of surgery is unknown. It is notable that these changes are occurring while the population grows older and is more likely to have medical diseases, two factors that independently predict a vulnerability to a number of postsurgical psychiatric disorders (Lipowski 1992; Schor et al. 1992; Zisselman 1993).

In his definitive chapter on the surgical patient, Surman (1987) discussed the varied psychological problems of the surgical patient. He noted the important role that surgeons play in a patient's life:

> Two aspects of surgery speak to the reality and the excess meaning of the experience: 1. Surgery repre-

sents a decisive approach to the relief of pain and suffering. 2. Surgery involves a transference relationship with the patient in a role of heightened dependency and expectation. (Surman 1987, p. 69)

The surgical patient typically experiences fear—fear of bodily injury and fear of death. Recognition and exploration of a patient's fears and anxieties are quite helpful. Strategies to reduce preoperative stress emphasize reassurance and education. The patient should feel comfortable speaking directly and honestly with the surgeon. Another anxiety-reduction measure is consultation with a psychiatrist who is familiar with the specific surgery and possible reactions. Preoperative preparation for a group of patients led by a psychiatrist, another physician, a nurse, or other informed staff is also helpful (Mumford et al. 1982). The importance of these types of interventions before surgery is underscored by research showing that poor preoperative psychological functioning predicts poor surgical outcome (Stengrevics et al. 1996).

Psychiatric complications that patients develop during the course of surgical treatment were termed *operative syndromes* by Hackett and Weisman (1960). These disorders frequently trouble the surgeon, impede the course of recovery, are sometimes as dangerous as the infectious or embolic complications of surgery, and make the nursing staff caring for these patients feel harassed (see Table 27–1). Operative syndromes range from acute psychotic episodes to problems of overdependence and addiction, from suicidal depression to disruptive ward behavior.

The tasks facing consultation-liaison psychiatrists in the management of surgical patients are multifaceted and often complex. Consultation-liaison team members are often called on to help patients with psychiatric problems that either interfere with the impending operation or hamper convalescence. This help can take the form of psychopharmacological interventions or of brief, focused psychotherapy or other behaviorally based strategies, such

as progressive relaxation. Often a multimodal approach is most beneficial. Consultation-liaison psychiatrists frequently serve as "delirium experts" in the hospital setting and play a key role in managing postoperative altered mental status. Although determination of patient competency to make medical decisions is a legal issue, psychiatrists are often asked to provide an expert opinion on whether patients have the ingredients of competency. Psychiatric management is articulated with surgical treatment in order to help the patient through an otherwise difficult hospital stay. Because the aims of the surgeon and the psychiatrist coincide, there should be no basic disagreement in patient management. However, without good communication and agreement about these goals, misunderstandings may occur.

TABLE 27–1.   General surgery categories: associated psychiatric symptoms and behavioral issues

Breast	**Small intestine/pancreas**
Body image issues	Eating disorders
Grief and loss	Alcoholism
Sexual adjustment	Secondary mood disorder
Living with cancer	**Irritable bowel syndrome**
Thyroid/parathyroid	Generalized anxiety disorders
Secondary psychiatric disorders such as	Panic disorder
Psychosis	Social phobia
Mood disorders	Mood disorders
Anxiety disorders	Eating disorders
Adrenal (pheochromocytoma,	**Colon/rectum**
hypoadrenalism/Cushing's syndrome)	Eating disorders
Secondary psychiatric disorders such as	Psychotic disorders
Generalized anxiety	Unconventional sexual practices
Panic	**Acute abdomen/trauma (accidental**
Depression	**injury, self-inflicted injury, assault)**
Morbid obesity	Depression
Body image issues	Psychosis
Mood disorders	Acute posttraumatic stress disorder
Impulse regulation problems	Group violence/gangs
Hopes for miracle	Antisocial behavior
Stomach/duodenum (gastritis, ulcer)	**Vascular access procedures, renal failure, organ**
Alcohol abuse/dependence	**transplantation, malignancies, HIV-positive status**
Cocaine abuse/dependence	Secondary psychiatric disorders
Anxiety disorders	Dementia/cognitive dysfunction
Esophagus/diaphragm (dysmotility,	Delirium
chemical/mechanical injury)	Depression
Eating disorders	Anxiety
"Functional globus"	
Alcohol abuse/dependence	
Anxiety	
Somatization	
Psychosis	

We have organized this chapter to provide some general principles of psychiatric consultation performed in surgical settings. Some of the special problems frequently encountered are detailed in the text and tables, although these problems are not exclusively limited to surgery. We have also included sections that detail the special issues involved in consultation to cardiothoracic surgery, orthopedic surgery, ophthalmology, burn units, cosmetic surgery, and head and neck surgery.

GENERAL PRINCIPLES

Preoperative Issues

Context of consultation. Because most planned surgical procedures involve same-day admissions, presurgical hospital-based psychiatric consultations are increasingly rare. One major exception to this is organ transplantation: psychiatrists are routinely involved in the prospective evaluation of candidates at most centers or when a complex medical course leads to the need for surgery during an extended hospitalization (Levenson and Olbrisch 1993). According to Jacobsen and Holland (1989), presurgical psychiatric consultation is most commonly requested in three major areas:

1. When patients experience preoperative panic or are refusing surgery
2. When questions arise about perioperative management of patients who are taking psychotropic drugs
3. When concern exists about a patient's capacity to give informed consent or refusal

Each of these areas is discussed here.

Preoperative anxiety and transient treatment refusal. Patients preparing to undergo surgery show higher levels of anxiety than the general population (Caumo et al. 2001; Jelicic and Bonke 1991). The psychodynamic origins of preoperative anxiety include a history of emotional trauma, expectations of loss versus gain as an outcome of surgery, and identification with others who have undergone similar procedures. Our understanding of such identification has been deepened by the studies by Wellisch and colleagues (1991, 1992) of the family experience of breast cancer. Additionally, an array of psychological stressors are inherent in the surgical situation and affect most patients; these stressors include basic threats to bodily and psychic integrity, fears of the unknown, loss of identity and control, and fear of pain and death (Johnston 1980).

Individual cognitive styles are also relevant to how patients make decisions about treatment. Some meta-analyses indicated that patients' cognitive and emotional processes in decision making are often governed by impulse, misperceived risk-benefit information, overemphasis of potential losses versus gains, and distorted memory of past experiences (Redelmeier et al. 1993; Wade 1990).

Preoperative panic or surgery refusal is estimated to occur in 5% of general surgery patients (Strain 1985). Less severe but still clinically significant anxiety is present in more than 30% of patients before surgery (Vingerhoets 1998). Frequently, these problems occur in patients with preexisting anxiety disorders or new-onset anxiety in the context of serious illness. Recent evidence suggests that the level of preoperative anxiety strongly predicts how anxious a patient will be postoperatively (Vingerhoets 1998), which suggests in turn that identification of presurgical anxiety not only aids in preoperative adjustment but also may identify patients uniquely at risk for postoperative psychological sequelae. Management of preoperative anxiety is directed at education, coordination of care, involvement of anesthesia personnel, and autonomy-enhancing behavioral techniques (such as self-guided relaxation exercises, effective pharmacological interventions, and efforts to introduce familiar persons into the medical setting). Psychoeducational interventions that permit rehearsal, desensitization, and orientation to the hospital environment are clearly associated with reduction in patient distress (Shipley et al. 1978). Self-help groups provide patients with preoperative and postoperative visitation and major communal support (Grosso-Haacker 1991).

Psychiatric illness in surgical patients. Personality disorders, mood disorders, anxiety disorders, cognitive impairment, and substance-related disorders warrant special attention because of the potential for significant related complications in the postoperative setting.

Examples of problems seen in patients with personality disorders include unrealistic expectations of surgery, struggles with staff over treatment decisions, noncompliance, and sign-outs against medical advice. These factors are particularly important in patients undergoing cosmetic surgery, as we describe later in this chapter. Patients with mood disorders may feel poorly understood, may experience significant psychological and physiologic distress at abrupt discontinuation of treatment with psychotropic agents, or may have significant avoidable iatrogenic morbidity caused by ill-informed treatment (such as mania induced by sleep deprivation or steroids) (Berlin 1984; Porter and Rosenthal 1993). Similarly, patients with anxiety disorder may develop panic attacks acutely when hospitalized or when drug therapy is discontinued. Panic attacks are frequently undertreated by nonpsychiatric physicians. The major risks for alcohol- and drug-dependent patients are unrecognized acute withdrawal symptoms and inadequate coping with hospitalization during enforced abstinence.

A subgroup of high-risk patients approach surgery with factitious symptoms (Baile et al. 1992b; Gattaz et al. 1990; J.Z. Sadler 1987; Schlesinger et al. 1989). The most malignant form of the desperate and complex psychological drive to undergo medical procedures is often referred to as Munchausen syndrome, a disorder that usually occurs with severe character pathology, mood disorder, and/or abuse history (American Psychiatric Association 1987, 1994). Such patients manage to undergo surgeries, acquire iatrogenic illnesses, and continue to manufacture symptoms in the hospital (Castor et al. 1990). (The etiology and management of this disorder are discussed thoroughly in Chapter 25.)

Psychotropic medications. Table 27–2 summarizes issues pertinent to psychotropic medications and surgical anesthesia. The clinical importance of these issues is highlighted by recent data showing that up to 50% of patients older than 21 years who present for elective surgery are taking one or more psychotropic medications ("Psychiatric Drug Use and Surgery" 1999). Reviews of the literature emphasize the need for open and careful discussion between patient, surgeon, anesthesiologist, and psychiatrist of the risks and benefits of presurgical continuation or cessation of treatment with psychotropic drugs (Sedgwick et al. 1990). The appreciable psychiatric risks of discontinuing psychotropic drug therapy in seriously ill patients are increasingly recognized. Recent guidelines suggest that most psychiatric patients should continue taking their psychotropic drugs until the time of surgery and should be carefully observed after surgery for medication interactions and emergent psychiatric symptoms. Abrupt discontinuation of maintenance psychotropic therapy can have adverse medical consequences, including malignant arrhythmias in vulnerable patients (Van Sweden 1988), withdrawal seizures (Shader and Greenblatt 1993), and a syndrome of cholinergic rebound (Dilsaver et al. 1983; Lawrence 1985).

In addition to specific drug-drug adverse reactions, many psychotropic medications have the potential for causing anesthetic complications through effects on the metabolism and elimination of anesthetic agents (Bovill 1997). Many psychotropics inhibit one or more cytochrome P450 enzymes in the liver. These enzymes are responsible for the metabolism of most pharmaceutical compounds, including many anesthetic agents. Coadministration of anesthetics and enzyme-inhibiting psychotropics can lead to enhanced anesthetic effect and possible toxicity. Agents known to significantly inhibit one or more P450 enzymes include the selective serotonin reuptake inhibitors fluoxetine, sertraline, paroxetine, and fluvoxamine and the atypical antidepressant nefazodone (Bohets et al. 2000; Caley and Silvia 2000). Antipsychotic agents, tricyclic antidepressants, and monoamine oxidase inhibitors are less potent enzyme inhibitors. The new antidepressants venlafaxine and mirtazapine appear not to possess clinically significant enzyme-inhibiting properties (Richelson 2001).

Certain medications have the ability to induce P450 enzymes in the liver, thereby increasing the metabolism of many anesthetic agents. Carbamazepine, which is commonly used in the treatment of bipolar disorder, is one such compound. Patients taking carbamazepine appear to be relatively resistant to a wide range of nondepolarizing neuromuscular blockers, such as pancuronium, vecuronium, and rocuronium (Spacek et al. 1999). Because carbamazepine increases hepatic metabolism, patients receiving carbamazepine therapy may require higher doses of some anesthetic agents.

Competency and informed consent. Few issues evoke more confusion among medical and surgical staff than a patient who refuses to undergo an apparently needed and reasonable procedure. In such a situation, a request for psychiatric consultation may represent the treating physician's wish to have the patient declared "incompetent," thus authorizing medical-surgical treatment over a patient's protests (Katz et al. 1995). Such a request often results from a widely held belief that psychiatrists determine competency. In fact, competency is a legal determination made by a judge. The psychiatrist can only authorize the civil commitment process, which permits time-limited involuntary detention for observation and emergency treatment of a defined psychiatric disorder. Despite the general misunderstanding of the legal authority of psychiatrists in a medical setting in which the capacity to consent to or refuse treatment is at issue, the psychiatric consultant's role is extremely important in assessing patients and in facilitating good outcomes for patients and their caregivers. An algorithm for decision making is outlined in Figure 27–1.

True emergencies in which treatment refusal or competency is an issue are resolved de facto by Good Samaritan standards (e.g., emergency room resuscitation), by patients becoming too ill to protest, or when authorized surrogates intervene (such as individuals with a durable power of attorney for health care). Psychiatric consulta-

TABLE 27-2. Psychotropic drugs and anesthesia

Category	Considerations	Recommendations
Antidepressants		
Tricyclic antidepressants (TCAs)	1. May interact with general and regional agents, leading to intraventricular conduction delays; may increase arrhythmias when used in conjunction with epinephrine 2. Chronic TCA administration can result in greater anesthetic requirements 3. TCAs may enhance anticholinergic properties of anticholinergic or inhalation agents, leading to toxicity 4. Abrupt discontinuation of TCA therapy can cause cholinergic rebound and withdrawal arrhythmias 5. TCAs lower seizure threshold and increase risk of perioperative seizures	1. Treat until time of surgery, as psychiatrically indicated 2. Presurgical anticholinergics may be unnecessary; glycopyrrolate, which does not cross blood-brain barrier, may be anticholinergic of choice 3. Consider avoiding use of enflurane, given increased seizure risk
Monoamine oxidase inhibitors (MAOIs)	1. Pressor effects of endogenous adrenergic discharge may be difficult to control 2. Exogenous pressors may cause hemodynamic lability during surgery 3. MAOIs potentiate action and duration of action of muscle blockers and opiates (not meperidine) 4. Surgical personnel may be unfamiliar with MAOI precautions (e.g., diet and avoidance of meperidine, serotonergic antidepressants, and dextromethorphan) 5. Abrupt withdrawal may cause delirium or psychosis	1. If feasible, discontinue therapy 7–14 days before surgery; may treat until time of surgery, if needed 2. Hypotension should be treated with direct (not indirect) vasopressors 3. Make extra effort to communicate with anesthesiologist 4. Medical chart should be *clearly labeled* regarding diet, no meperidine 5. Morphine and fentanyl appear to be safe at low doses (1/4–1/5 usual dose)
Selective serotonin reuptake inhibitors (SSRIs), bupropion, trazodone, nefazodone, venlafaxine, mirtazapine	1. Case report of serotonin syndrome in patient taking sertraline; treated with lidocaine, midazolam, and fentanyl 2. All newer antidepressants lower seizure threshold; no adverse anesthetic reactions yet reported 3. No adverse reactions yet reported for trazodone, nefazodone, venlafaxine, mirtazapine, or SSRIs other than sertraline; however, given sertraline case report, all SSRIs, as well as venlafaxine, may have potential to induce serotonin syndrome during anesthetic procedures	1. May be given until time of surgery, as psychiatrically indicated; resume as tolerated
Typical antipsychotic agents		
Butyrophenones	1. Haloperidol and droperidol are often used to potentiate fentanyl induction and are potent antiemetics 2. Malignant hyperthermia can be confused with neuroleptic malignant syndrome; patients with neuroleptic malignant syndrome tend to have normocapnia, and patients with malignant hyperthermia show increased end-tidal CO_2 pressure 3. All dopamine-blocking agents dysregulate thermoregulation 4. Vasopressor effect of exogenous dopamine may be blunted 5. Bolus injection of iv haloperidol or droperidol may increase risk of ventricular arrhythmia (torsades de pointes), especially in patients with preexisting heart disease 6. Lowers seizure threshold	1. No contraindication to maintenance use before surgery 2. Consider neuroleptic malignant syndrome and malignant hyperthermia in differential diagnosis of postoperative fevers and/or muscle rigidity; inquire about family history of atypical reactions to anesthetics 3. Treatments for neuroleptic malignant syndrome and malignant hyperthermia are similar 4. Patients receiving any class of neuroleptic may be subject to altered thermoregulation; extra intra- and postoperative warming blankets may be required

TABLE 27–2. Psychotropic drugs and anesthesia (continued)

Category	Considerations	Recommendations
Phenothiazines	1. Anticholinergic and α-adrenergic effects increase risk of delirium, hypotension (especially in combination with epinephrine), and falls; post spinal anesthesia urinary retention may be aggravated 2. May enhance tachycardia and arrhythmias associated with anticholinergic, sympathomimetic, or inhalant agents 3. Cholinergic rebound possible with abrupt discontinuation of therapy	1. No absolute contraindications to presurgical maintenance; a switch to high-potency agents is preferable before surgery 2. Observe for neuroleptic malignant syndrome, as with butyrophenone therapy 3. Consider avoiding use of enflurane, given increased seizure risk
Atypical antipsychotic agents		
Clozapine	1. Clozapine significantly lowers seizure thresholds, especially at dosages > 600 mg/day 2. Significant anticholinergic properties may lead to interactions described for phenothiazines 3. No unique interactions with anesthetic agents reported	1. Patients taking clozapine are generally psychiatrically refractory and clozapine therapy should probably be continued until time of surgery; weigh risk-benefit ratio of symptom recurrence without therapy
Risperidone, olanzapine, quetiapine	1. Less anticholinergic and less apt to cause seizures than clozapine 2. No reported interactions	1. No contraindication to maintenance use before surgery
Mood stabilizers		
Lithium	1. Lowers seizure threshold 2. Potentiates duration of action of muscle blockers 3. Serum levels and clinical toxicity depend on volume status and renal function; sodium overload due to perioperative administration of hypertonic saline may decrease lithium levels and increase risk of postoperative mania; nonsteroidal anti-inflammatory drugs, thiazide diuretics, and angiotensin-converting enzyme inhibitors can significantly increase lithium levels, leading to toxicity	1. Continue until time of surgery 2. If patient can take nothing by mouth, substitute parenteral benzodiazepines and/or neuroleptics to manage postsurgical mania 3. Encourage treatment team to frequently check volume and electrolyte status
Valproic acid, carbamazepine	1. Maintenance use associated with faster-than-normal recovery from effects of paralytic agents but also with greater need for higher doses of fentanyl during surgery 2. No known synergistic increase in risk of idiosyncratic hepatotoxic effects of inhalation anesthetics	1. Continue until time of surgery, as psychiatrically indicated
Anxiolytics		
Benzodiazepines	1. Chronic use and tolerance necessitate prophylaxis for withdrawal postoperatively 2. Many nonpsychiatrists are unfamiliar with dosing needs of patients with anxiety disorders 3. Alprazolam, in particular, has short half-life: may require larger doses of parenteral agents to substitute; may have limited cross-reactivity with other benzodiazepines	1. Continue until time of surgery, as psychiatrically indicated 2. For alprazolam-treated patients, presurgical transition to oral or parenteral agent is ideal 3. If brief period of NPO status is expected, alprazolam therapy can be continued (sublingual administration) 4. Give flumazenil for toxic sedation

Note. iv = intravenous; NPO = nil per os (nothing by mouth).

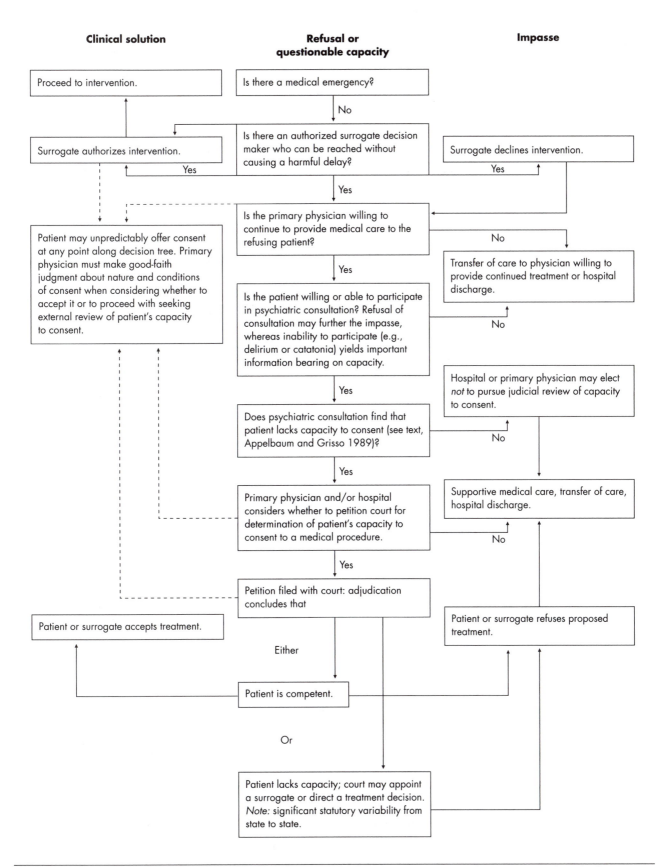

FIGURE 27–1. Decision tree for psychiatric consultation in a medical-surgical patient refusing proposed medical treatment or whose capacity to provide consent is questionable.

tion usually follows—for example, in cases in which resistance is expressed by the revived patient to the possibility of future needed interventions.

In other circumstances in which a duly authorized surrogate decision maker is absent, the capacity to provide informed consent or refusal is judicially determined. The psychiatrist must assess the entire situation, including the patient's current mental status and health beliefs. After assessment, the consultant is usually able to offer valuable observations about the nature of the impasse and can help to resolve it without legal recourse or without patient and primary physician dismissing each other. Preservation of the possibility of appropriate medical treatment is an important goal. When the surgeon and psychiatrist concur that it is appropriate to pursue judicial review of the patient's competency to consent to or to refuse a procedure or treatment, the psychiatrist must have already documented the findings of the patient's mental status examination focusing on the ingredients of capacity:

- The consistent ability to communicate a choice
- The capacity to demonstrate an understanding of relevant medical information, including risks and benefits
- The capacity to appreciate the current situation and its consequences
- The ability to manipulate information in a rational manner (Appelbaum and Grisso 1989; Hall and Ellman 1990)

A detailed description of how the patient demonstrates or fails to demonstrate these elements, with examples, should appear in the consultation report. A concise differential psychiatric diagnosis and the actual or expected results of psychiatric treatment, when relevant, are also critical. The psychiatrist's report is expert testimony that is commonly used in the judicial review. Sufficient detail and clarity in the consultation can obviate the need for a personal court appearance by the psychiatrist.

Rarely, the civil commitment process of the state is used to warrant neuropsychiatric evaluation, including circumscribed medical treatment, against a protesting patient's will. An example of this is a case of acute delirium, in which a high degree of medical concern exists that a life-threatening process requires rapid diagnosis and treatment (such as in an agitated patient with suspected bacterial meningitis who requires a diagnostic lumbar puncture and antibiotic treatment). (For further discussion of competency and informed consent, see Chapter 11.)

Although evaluating competency is usually viewed as an essentially nontherapeutic procedure, during which the clinician evaluates only the patient's current mental condition, Bostwick and Masterson (1998) recently demonstrated that psychiatrists may be able to play a more active role by actually restoring competency to patients with delirium. The authors reported on a series of delirious patients restored to competency through psychopharmacological intervention—use of the benzodiazepine-receptor antagonist flumazenil, in cases of hepatic coma; and administration of the high-potency neuroleptic haloperidol, in cases of delirium. Such active attempts to improve patients' mental status before judging competency seem a potentially invaluable and underused strategy, given that as many as 80% of patients for whom competency evaluations are requested have secondary psychiatric disorders (McKegney et al. 1992), many of which may respond to pharmacological intervention.

Psychiatric Morbidity in Postsurgical Patients

Psychiatric disorders secondary to medical treatment or substances of abuse.   Medical and substance-induced psychiatric disorders are commonly diagnosed postoperatively in surgical patients. Most frequent among these is delirium, with a prevalence in prospectively studied surgical patients ranging from 7% to 15% (Golinger 1989; Lipowski 1992; Schor et al. 1992; Seymour and Vaz 1989; Zisselman 1993). Withdrawal from alcohol or other substances is also commonly present and underdiagnosed (Reynaud et al. 2000). Immediate preoperative patient self-medication with alcohol was documented in approximately 11% of patients in a German series (Neukam et al. 1992). Nicotine withdrawal is also common (Fiore et al. 1992).

Other psychiatric disorders.   A variety of other problems, including disruptive ward behavior (acting-out), new-onset or recurrent depression, mania, anxiety symptoms, brief psychoses, intoxication with iatrogenic agents, acute posttraumatic stress disorder (PTSD), and others, can also occur (Porter and Rosenthal 1993; Strain 1985; Surman 1987; Vieta et al. 1993). Several studies convincingly demonstrated lengthened stays, increased costs, and excess morbidity among general hospital patients with undiagnosed or inadequately treated psychiatric disorders (Holmes and House 2000; Lyons et al. 1986; Thomas et al. 1988; Verboskey et al. 1993; Zatzick et al. 2000).

Treatment Considerations

Formal psychotherapy on the surgical service is often difficult to engage in because of noise, interruptions, the postoperative medical regimen, lack of recognition by the staff of the importance of psychological concerns, and other factors. Nonetheless, even brief, focused meetings are valuable and are sometimes of crucial importance in the postsurgical management of patients with borderline and other primitive personality disorders. Behavioral interventions such as treatment contracts, relaxation techniques, and guided imagery are also valuable. The principles of interpersonal therapy, with a focus on the management of critical relationships (medical staff, visiting family) and boundaries, are sometimes useful. The problem of psychiatric consultation with hospitalized surgical patients is addressed in more detail later in this chapter (see "Orthopedic Surgery"); an extended discussion of these issues is found in Chapter 45.

Psychopharmacological interventions in postoperative patients are complicated by factors such as orders to give nothing by mouth, absent or compromised gastrointestinal (GI) absorption, emerging medical problems (e.g., perioperative myocardial infarction or stroke), or drug interactions that may compromise previously effective treatments. Therefore, the psychiatrist must perform a complete assessment of the patient's postoperative physical and mental status before recommending psychopharmacological intervention and must then communicate recommendations in a clear and understandable way to surgical and nursing staff. This often requires education of colleagues about the nature, course, and contemporary strategies of treatment of psychiatric disorders. Compromised postoperative GI functioning often poses complicated therapeutic dilemmas. Although benzodiazepines and typical neuroleptics (e.g., haloperidol, chlorpromazine) can be administered parenterally, antidepressants, mood stabilizers, and atypical neuroleptics (clozapine, olanzapine, risperidone, quetiapine) are not routinely available in parenteral form in the United States. Patients are at significant risk for relapse if administration of these medications is discontinued perioperatively because of GI considerations. Bipolar patients are especially at risk for relapse into mania if treatment with mood stabilizers is rapidly discontinued: many bipolar patients relapse almost immediately if their mood stabilizers are withheld. Similarly, many data indicate that the risk of relapse among patients with unipolar depression is heightened significantly if drug therapy is discontinued for any extended period. Add to this an increased risk of developing depression in the perioperative period, and it becomes clear that the lack of readily available parenteral forms of many psychotropics is a significant clinical limitation.

The key guiding principles in managing patients with compromised GI function are 1) differentiating compromised absorption from situations in which nothing can be taken by mouth (NPO) and 2) estimating the length of time that a patient can take nothing orally. Treatment of patients who take mood stabilizers or atypical antipsychotics can be temporized during brief NPO periods with parenteral benzodiazepines or traditional neuroleptics such as haloperidol. The use of 1- to 2-day drug holidays to improve sexual functioning in patients taking selective serotonin reuptake inhibitors points to the fact that brief periods of abstinence from antidepressants do not appear to appreciably increase relapse risk. However, most antidepressants have been associated with withdrawal syndromes, and patients whose antidepressant therapy is suddenly terminated in the perioperative period are at risk for morbidity from this problem.

Several options are available for treating mood disorders in the face of prolonged periods of NPO status. Electroconvulsive therapy is probably the treatment of choice for these patients. In addition to having high efficacy rates, electroconvulsive therapy is an effective treatment for a wide range of mood syndromes, including melancholia, psychotic depression, mixed states, and mania. The tricyclic antidepressants imipramine, amitriptyline, and clomipramine are available in injectable form, although the use of these drugs in this form is limited in the United States. Studies of loading intravenous clomipramine suggest that not only is it effective for treating depression but it may actually decrease the time to therapeutic response (Pollock et al. 1989). We have used intramuscular imipramine to good effect in patients prescribed long-term bowel rest. We prefer imipramine because it has well-established therapeutic blood levels to help guide dosing schedules. Our experience conforms to published reports that parenteral tricyclics should be used at approximately half the oral dose (Thompson and DiMartini 1999). Recommendations are that patients should first be given a test dose of 0.5 mg/kg of body weight. If this is tolerated, patients should receive a dose of 2 mg/kg (Beliles and Stoudemire 1998). Blood levels should be assessed frequently, both to ensure that a therapeutic level has been attained and to decrease the risk of toxicity in a patient population vulnerable to volume and electrolyte disturbances.

Other options for pharmacological treatment of mood disorders in patients who can take nothing orally include the use of parenteral or sublingual psychostimulants, antidepressants, or mood stabilizers. Case reports suggest that each of these options may be effective, but controlled studies are lacking (Thompson and DiMartini 1999). A promising option for bipolar patients who require mood stabilization but can take nothing by mouth is the new intravenous form of valproic acid. Developed for seizure patients unable to take oral medications, intravenous valproic acid might be expected to be as effective as the oral form for the treatment of bipolar disorder, but studies confirming this have yet to be performed.

Patients with various malabsorption syndromes are at high risk for depressive and anxiety disorders (DiMartini et al. 1996). Pharmacological treatment of these patients is complicated by unpredictable absorption of oral medications and by volume and electrolyte disturbances that can increase the likelihood of untoward cardiac effects from psychotropics, especially from tricyclics (DiMartini 1997). Generally, these patients require higher oral doses of psychotropics to achieve therapeutic effect. Although associated with potential increased risk of cardiac morbidity in patients with short-gut syndromes, tricyclic antidepressants have the advantage of therapeutic blood levels that allow for a level of control of dose titration that is not possible with newer antidepressants. Similarly, at this time clozapine appears to be the only atypical antipsychotic with therapeutic blood levels that can guide treatment (>350 ng/dL). Accurate associations between clinical response and blood level have been established for valproic acid and lithium, suggesting that treatment with these agents might be preferable to carbamazepine therapy in patients with malabsorption syndromes. As with tricyclics, however, much care must be taken in administering lithium to patients with malabsorption syndrome, given the increased risk of toxicity in the presence of electrolyte and fluid imbalances.

Psychiatric consultants are sometimes asked to play a role in acute pain management, particularly when the patient is dissatisfied with previous pain management efforts, has an identified or suspected psychiatric history, is a suspected substance abuser, or is responding "atypically" to pain management (Agency for Health Care Policy and Research 1992). Because pain is a subjective somatosensory experience, staff doubtfulness about the patient's self-report carries the risk of significant undertreatment and unnecessary suffering. In such situations, the psychiatrist has multiple tasks: to form an alliance that helps restore the patient's credibility with the treatment team, to make an intelligible psychiatric diagnosis, to comment on the potential interplay between psychiatric factors and the patient's pain experience, and to help minimize acting-out by involved parties. Of value are rational pharmacotherapy (France and Krishnan 1988), relaxation techniques, appropriate education about the psychiatric diagnosis, autonomy-enhancing interventions such as patient-controlled analgesia (Chapman 1992; Gil et al. 1990; Voulgari et al. 1991), and assiduous attention to improvement of communication between the patient and the treatment team. These issues are particularly rel-

evant to the management of burn victims and patients hospitalized for head and neck surgery (both patient populations are discussed later in this chapter). (See Chapter 43 for a more extensive discussion of pain management.)

CARDIOTHORACIC SURGERY

The cardiothoracic surgery setting offers a particular challenge to the consultation-liaison psychiatrist. The patient who faces cardiovascular surgery usually has a life-threatening illness, and the surgery itself carries a risk of death or morbidity. Technology such as the intra-aortic balloon pump (IABP) permits medical support of patients through illnesses that were once fatal. These factors create a setting in which prompt, focused consultation can dramatically affect outcome and reduce costs (Lazarus and Hagens 1968; Mumford et al. 1982; Surman et al. 1974).

Conditions that bring individuals to cardiovascular surgeons are generally either congenital or acquired (Table 27–3). Among the acquired disorders, unhealthy behaviors such as noncompliance with medication regimens, smoking, excessive alcohol consumption, and intravenous drug use often cause profound cardiac damage that requires surgical treatment. Among patients with congenital heart disease, sophisticated pediatric cardiothoracic repair has resulted in improved longevity (Perloff 1991).

Thoracic surgery is confined predominantly to the chest wall, pleura, lungs, mediastinum, and, at some centers, the esophagus. Table 27–4 outlines some of the thoracic defects that prompt surgical procedures. There is a paucity of literature on psychiatric consultation with patients undergoing thoracic surgery, but because these patients share many issues with patients having cardiovascular surgery, these issues will be addressed together unless special attention is warranted concerning either population.

The consultation-liaison psychiatrist may be involved in the patient care system during one of three phases: the preoperative phase, the perioperative phase (12–72 hours after surgery), or the postoperative phase (more than 72 hours after surgery). Issues common in each phase are outlined below.

Preoperative Issues

Competency and compliance. Clinical issues differ somewhat depending on whether the patient is hospitalized. Consultation on competency to consent is usually

TABLE 27–3. Cardiovascular diseases by etiology

Acquired

Mitral stenosis/insufficiency
Aortic stenosis/insufficiency
Tricuspid stenosis/insufficiency
Trauma
Coronary artery disease
Left ventricular aneurysm
Pericarditis
Ventricular fibrillation
Heart block

Congenital

Atrial septal defect
Ventricular septal defect
Tetralogy of Fallot
Single ventricle
Bicuspid mitral valve
Eisenmenger's syndrome
Pulmonic stenosis
Aortic stenosis
Coarctation of the aorta
Transposition of the great vessels
Truncus arteriosus
Ebstein's anomaly
Double-outlet right ventricle

Source. Adapted from Spencer FC: "Congenital Heart Disease," in *Principles of Surgery*, 5th Edition. Edited by Schwartz SI, Shires GT, Spencer FC. New York, McGraw-Hill, 1989, pp. 771–842; Spencer FC, Culliford AT: "Acquired Heart Disease," in *Principles of Surgery*, 5th Edition. Edited by Schwartz SI, Shires GT, Spencer FC. New York, McGraw-Hill, 1989, pp. 843–908.

TABLE 27–4. Common diagnoses in patients undergoing thoracic surgery

Achalasia
Barrett's esophagus
Chest wall tumors
Congenital deformities: pectus excavatum and pectus carinatum
Emphysematous bullae
Esophageal rupture
Esophageal stricture/stenosis
Mediastinitis
Pleural effusions
Pneumothorax
Pulmonary infection
Shortened esophagus
Superior vena cava syndrome
Thoracic defects
Thoracic outlet syndrome
Trauma
Tumors: chest wall, trachea, esophagus, pleura, lung

Source. Adapted from King TC, Smith CR: "Chest Wall, Pleura, Lung and Mediastinum," in *Principles of Surgery*, 5th Edition. Edited by Schwartz SI, Shires GT, Spencer FC. New York, McGraw-Hill, 1989, pp. 627–770; Pairolero PC, Trastek VF, Payne WS: "Esophagus and Diaphragmatic Hernias," in *Principles of Surgery*, 5th Edition. Edited by Schwartz SI, Shires GT, Spencer FC. New York, McGraw-Hill, 1989, pp. 1103–1156.

related to preexisting psychiatric disorders or to secondary conditions such as delirium. (The factors that are relevant to competency are discussed in detail in Chapter 11.) Statutes and procedures vary from state to state. When faced with the possibility of the death of a very ill patient, physicians will often look to family members for consent. In dire circumstances in an unresponsive patient, in which immediate surgical intervention is required and/or in which death may be imminent, consent will often be presumed.

Another common consultation question, relative to both inpatients and outpatients, is whether a patient's future compliance with medication regimens can be predicted. Valve replacement and organ transplantation are areas in which concerns about patient compliance with treatment and medication regimens are especially important. (Compliance in the field of transplantation is addressed in more detail in Chapter 28.) Noncompliance may result in graft failure and death. If postoperative noncompliance is likely, the psychiatrist can communicate this to the surgeon so that the surgeon can place a

valvular prosthesis that does not require the patient to take anticoagulants postoperatively; this reduces such a patient's risk of future stroke or death. Similarly, individuals with a history of serious behavioral dyscontrol, such as head banging, frequent fights, or self-mutilation, are identified in order to eliminate the risk of serious hemorrhage during maintenance anticoagulation.

Preoperative anxiety. Contemplating impending cardiac surgery can cause significant anxiety for an individual or family. The general issue of preoperative anxiety has already been addressed in this chapter. The symbolic importance of the heart, and concerns when it is "broken," may foster additional discomfort. A small subpopulation of patients are at risk for anxiety-related silent ischemia; fortunately, preoperative anxiety does not appear to put the majority of individuals at risk for this phenomenon (Jolly et al. 1990).

The agitated patient. During the assessment of an agitated patient, it is important to ascertain whether a worsening medical condition is causing delirium or another disorder. Often, the underlying cardiothoracic process impairs circulation or oxygenation, putting other organs at risk for dysfunction and increasing the risk of delirium.

The psychiatric consultant must determine whether a psychiatric disorder, a central nervous system disorder, or personality traits are contributing to the clinical picture. Interventions include altering the treatment environment, eliminating toxic drugs from the treatment regimen, and maximizing patient comfort (Tesar and Stern 1986).

Tesar and Stern's review (1988) of literature on agitated patients in intensive care provides a practical protocol for assessment and treatment. Agitation is life-threatening in individuals with limited cardiac reserve; aggressive treatment is warranted (Tesar and Stern 1988). (A full discussion of delirium is found in Chapter 15.)

Another potential cause of agitation is antiemetic medication. Akathisia and other extrapyramidal side effects are often unrecognized adverse effects of antiemetics such as metoclopramide, prochlorperazine, and droperidol. Careful assessment of agitated patients will often reveal the relatively sudden onset of extreme physical discomfort and restlessness, often in the absence of a concomitant sense of cognitive anxiety and frequently in the context of no history of anxiety. Anticholinergic agents such as benztropine or β-blockers such as propranolol often provide rapid relief and bring about resolution of the agitation. Because these agents can have cardiac effects, they should be used only in close collaboration with the cardiothoracic team.

Inadequate pain control is an additional potential cause of agitation and is sometimes related to the patient's reluctance to inform the staff of increasing discomfort, problems in communication when a patient is receiving mechanical ventilation, or inadequate dosing. In general, physicians underestimate analgesic requirements and overestimate the duration of analgesic action. Pain is most effectively treated with regular rather than as-needed dosing of analgesics.

Fear of impending surgery or uncertainty regarding outcome must also be considered in the agitated patient. If discussion does not alleviate the patient's distress, benzodiazepines may be helpful. When panic is evident, a low dose of a high-potency neuroleptic is recommended.

Cardiac assist devices. Cardiac assist devices are generally used in individuals with cardiogenic shock, to support circulation to the body and prevent irreparable harm to other organ systems and the heart. These devices are used until a corrective procedure is performed or until the heart regains sufficient function. The types of assist devices include the IABP, left ventricular assist device, right ventricular assist device, extracorporeal membrane oxygenation, and total artificial heart. The nature of an assist device requires that patients lie quietly because interruption of blood flow or loosening of an attachment may result in extensive bleeding and death. For this reason, with the exception of the IABP, patients are kept heavily sedated and paralyzed. Numerous risks, including infection, bleeding, and embolization, are associated with use of any assist devices. Psychiatric consultation, other than to support family members, is generally limited. Nonetheless, these patients have high rates of psychiatric syndromes and will constitute an increasingly significant clinical concern in the years ahead. It is estimated that by 2010, as many as 70,000 patients per year will be candidates for ventricular support (Argenziano et al. 1997).

After the initial healing period, patients with total artificial hearts and certain ventricular assist devices are allowed to awaken and actually may become ambulatory (Hravnak and George 1989; Ruzevich et al. 1990). Psychiatric assessment and support are often helpful during this period. Delirium is common in this group, as are strokes and more subtle forms of neuropsychological and neurological impairment (Petrucci et al. 1999).

In assessing an agitated patient who has an IABP, it is necessary to ascertain whether the underlying difficulty is related to pain, to delirium, to frustration, or to other factors. Individuals may require intubation to maintain oxygenation, which makes assessment and communication even more difficult. Complaints of pain are quite common and are often attributed to position. Extension of the leg in which the device is inserted is imperative for adequate hemodynamic function. Prior back injuries and degenerative disk disease may be sources of extreme discomfort. The incidence of delirium is reportedly as high as 34% among individuals who have IABPs (Sanders et al. 1992). High-dose intravenous haloperidol is reportedly safe in patients with agitated delirium (Tesar and Stern 1988) and is reportedly efficacious in combination with benzodiazepines in managing patients with IABPs (Sanders et al. 1992). In individuals with a history of dilated cardiomyopathy and alcohol abuse, haloperidol therapy may present a risk of arrhythmia (Metzger and Friedman 1993) and must therefore be used with care. Most acutely ill cardiac patients occupy monitored beds, and following conduction intervals with routine electrocardiograms is thus possible and is recommended (Rosenbaum 1980).

Perioperative Issues

Confusion and agitation. In the immediate postoperative period, the majority of patients who have undergone cardiothoracic surgery are placed in an intensive care unit for close observation of vital signs and continuing assessment for blood loss. During recovery, anesthesia gradually wears off and members of the staff observe the patient for evidence of alertness. Depending on the surgery and the patient's condition, extubation is usually performed a relatively short time after surgery. It is during this perioperative period that postanesthesia confusion may develop. In patients who have undergone major cardiac procedures, this state may persist to and may extend beyond the third postoperative day and may progress to postcardiotomy delirium (PCD).

Dubin and colleagues (1979) concluded that "cardiac status, the severity of physical illness, the complexity of the surgical procedure, and preoperative organic brain disease are the determining factors in PCD" (p. 586). These same factors guide assessment today.

Delirium is reported in up to 70% of postcardiotomy patients (Hazan 1966; Mravinac 1991). As expected, the risk of delirium is increased among elderly patients undergoing valve replacement (Heller et al. 1970). Breuer and colleagues (1983) reported that use of postoperative IABP and pressor agents was significantly associated with prolonged PCD.

During assessment for PCD, all of the following should be examined: the patient, vital signs, laboratory data (preoperative and postoperative), and drug regimens. Medications such as midazolam and morphine—often given in the intensive care unit to quiet restless patients—can perpetuate and exacerbate the delirium. As noted earlier, high-potency neuroleptics are safe, effective agents for controlling agitation and do not contribute to the confusion (Sos and Cassem 1980; Tesar and Stern 1986, 1988). As in any patient in the intensive care unit, reorientation, reassurance, and explanation of procedures sometimes help to limit behavioral problems in patients who have undergone cardiotomy (P.D. Sadler 1981). These measures may also limit the need for pharmacotherapy.

Cardiac assist devices. Assist devices are sometimes necessary during the perioperative period until the heart resumes adequate functioning. It is often difficult for family members to see these devices in use, having expected their loved one to come out of surgery with marked improvement in function. Patients may respond with social withdrawal and a sense of alienation, both of which are risk factors for major depressive disorder (Petrucci et al. 1999).

Substance withdrawal. During the perioperative period, observation for substance withdrawal is imperative. Withdrawal from substances of abuse such as alcohol, benzodiazepines, narcotics, and barbiturates can cause hyperthermia, hypertension or hypotension, seizures,

hallucinations, changes in respiratory rate, and delirium. These symptoms are sometimes misdiagnosed as surgical complications, and their occurrence may increase morbidity (e.g., when a confused patient pulls out an IABP). Patients often deny or minimize their substance use, making a diagnosis of substance withdrawal more difficult than would otherwise be the case. It is usually necessary to obtain collateral information from family members about a patient's possible history of substance abuse or dependence. Prompt recognition and treatment of substance withdrawal can prevent unnecessary and expensive testing and harm or death.

Pain control. It is important to remember the principles of acute pain management outlined by the American Pain Society (1992) (see Table 27–5). Analgesia must be individually tailored because patients do not respond uniformly to pain medication. It is imperative to assess the patient's underlying mental state; delirium with associated agitation in an intubated patient is sometimes mistaken for pain and treated incorrectly. Similarly, anxiety should be treated with appropriate reassurance and anxiolytics.

A common problem in thoracic surgery patients is ensuring adequate pain management. Surgical procedures involving thoracotomy are especially painful if an anesthetic block is not used; also, significant discomfort is associated with respiration, which can adversely affect clearing of secretions and weaning from ventilatory support.

TABLE 27–5. Clinician management of acute pain

Treat patients as individuals.

Provide medication around the clock, especially during the immediate postoperative period (this is when pain is usually severe).

Know the potency and period of action of the analgesics used.

Assess the patient frequently, especially when initiating or changing the route of administration of analgesics.

Recognize and treat side effects.

Remember that commonly used medications, such as meperidine, may accumulate and cause symptoms from anxiety to seizures. *Note:* normeperidine, meperidine's primary metabolite, is highly deliriogenic.

Observe for the development of tolerance, and adjust dose appropriately.

Be aware that narcotic-dependent or narcotic-tolerant patients will likely require higher doses of medication for adequate pain control.

Prescribe anxiolytics if the patient has anxiety in addition to pain.

Source. Adapted from American Pain Society: *Principles of Analgesic Use in the Treatment of Acute and Cancer Pain,* 3rd Edition. Skokie, IL, American Pain Society, 1992, pp. 10–27.

Ventilator weaning. Psychiatric consultation is sometimes requested to assist in weaning an individual from ventilatory support. Weaning causes dyspnea, which may result in anxiety, fear, helplessness, loss of vitality, and preoccupation with shortness of breath (DeVito 1990). Dyspnea is characterized by an individual's perception of difficult labored breathing and his or her response to it (Carrieri et al. 1984). Air hunger, during mechanical ventilation or not, is exacerbated by anxiety and fear. The outward manifestations of fear can lead to overmedication with sedatives and narcotics, contributing to difficulties in maintaining an airway and preventing adequate oxygenation. Assessment for anxiety and delirium and recommendations for appropriate pharmacotherapy are of invaluable help in these cases.

There are several prerequisites for successful weaning. Respiratory factors include adequate respiratory muscle strength, oxygenation, ventilatory demand, and work of breathing. Other important factors are adequate cardiac function, oxygen transport capacity, metabolic parameters, fluid balance, nutritional status, mental state, and psychological readiness (Henneman 1991; Knebel 1991). Psychological readiness relates to fears and concerns that result from weaning trials (such as when a patient tires during a trial and, as a consequence, cannot complete the weaning process).

There are a variety of pharmacological approaches to decreasing anxiety during weaning. These include use of low-dose benzodiazepines or neuroleptics (Cassem and Hackett 1978). Progressive relaxation and focused biofeedback (Acosta 1988; Holliday and Hyers 1990) and hypnosis (Bowen 1989) are alternatives. Often neglected during evaluation is inquiry into sleep hygiene. Disturbed sleep can leave the patient exhausted and ill-equipped to handle the physical and emotional challenge of weaning.

A multimodal approach to weaning is generally recommended. Consultation with nursing staff can help nurses manage some patients' emotional lability. Pharmacological intervention is necessary, especially for individuals who are excessively anxious or even terrified about the weaning process (Mendel and Khan 1980). In some cases, successful weaning requires a significant amount of time and patience, commodities that are sometimes in short supply in the fast-paced world of the cardiothoracic intensive care unit. Reassurance of the patient and staff members is helpful, and tracking performance using a wall chart or other means serves to highlight daily progress for both patient and staff. Intervention to educate the family regarding the process may be needed if family members are putting undue pressure on the patient.

Family support. The crisis precipitated by a major surgical procedure affects family members as well as patients. Many families describe the time their loved one is in the operating room and recovery room as the most stressful. In one study, investigators found that the primary need of spouses and relatives during this period was to have accurate information provided and to have questions answered honestly (Norheim 1989).

When the functional equilibrium of a family unit is interrupted by illness, or when the potential for death exists, erratic behavior can result. Families in turmoil often need assistance to interact appropriately with the treatment team. In addition, setting limits regarding the frequency of visits and number of visitors is sometimes necessary to allow the patient to recuperate. With large families, it is helpful to identify one individual who will talk with the team and disseminate information to the rest of the family. This prevents misperceptions and allows the nursing staff to spend time caring for the patient instead of interacting with numerous family members.

Postoperative Issues

Neuropsychological changes. Possible neurological complications during the postoperative period range from a catastrophic cerebrovascular accident to subtle cognitive changes. Risk factors for impairment are similar to those for PCD and include a poor baseline condition, certain intraoperative factors, and a slow rate of recovery. Some patients report preoperative cognitive disturbances; these may result from microemboli caused by a diseased valve or chronic atrial fibrillation (Kimball 1972; Middlekauff et al. 1991). Long-standing cardiac dysfunction such as arrhythmia, hypotension, congestive failure, and asystolic arrest may also cause subtle central nervous system dysfunction.

The incidence of postsurgical neuropsychological impairment reported in the 1970s varied from 0% to 100% (Freyhan et al. 1993; Lee et al. 1971). More recent work revealed that impairment is present in 24%–79% of coronary artery bypass patients, depending on the criteria selected (Hammeke and Hastings 1988; Shaw et al. 1986, 1987). The frequency of neuropsychological impairment varies according to study design and the patient population selected. Frequent reference was made in the early literature to the role of cardiopulmonary bypass techniques in neuropsychological dysfunction and delirium. The technology has dramatically improved over the last 20 years, which may explain some of the decrease in rates of postoperative neuropsychological impairment.

Attention, concentration, and psychomotor speed are all potentially affected by cardiac surgery (Adrian et al. 1988; Blumenthal et al. 1991; Hammeke and Hastings 1988; Strauss et al. 1992). Patients undergoing single or multiple valve repair are at higher risk for cognitive decline (Blumenthal et al. 1991; Kornfeld et al. 1965; Lee et al. 1971). Resolution of cognitive deficits usually occurs within 6 weeks to 6 months (Hammeke and Hastings 1988; Klonoff et al. 1989; Savageau et al. 1982a, 1982b). Smith and colleagues (1986) found that neuropsychological deficits were present in about one-third of all patients 8 weeks after surgery.

Theories about causes of cognitive impairment remain controversial. The pulsatile method of cardiopulmonary bypass (versus nonpulsatile) affects hypothalamic and pituitary axes and is postulated to play a role in postoperative cognitive impairment (Hammeke and Hastings 1988; Taylor et al. 1978a, 1978b). Vik et al. (1991) examined a small group of patients with coronary artery bypass grafts (CABGs) and found no magnetic resonance imaging (MRI) evidence of new cerebral lesions 1 month postoperatively. This suggests that deficits either resolved over the month or were imperceptible on magnetic resonance images. Microemboli may account for a high proportion of cases of neurological impairment among individuals with no head MRI abnormalities (Shaw et al. 1985).

Depression and return to function. The prevalence of depression among patients who have undergone CABG surgery is around 25%. Lindal (1990) found that 33% of CABG surgery patients were depressed according to scores on the Minnesota Multiphasic Personality Inventory, administered 3 months after surgery. More recently, Shapiro et al. (1998) found that during the 6 months after CABG surgery, 38% of patients met criteria for major depressive disorder as estimated by Beck Depression Inventory scores. The presence of depressive symptoms immediately after surgery strongly predicted ongoing depression 6 months later. Folks and colleagues (1988) found that sexual dysfunction is associated with preoperative depression and confers greater risk of postoperative depression and maladjustment. Over a period of 3 months following surgical intervention, Rankin (1990) noted decreasing scores on Profile of Mood States scales, except for the anger scale, on which scores remained constant.

Although there is some agreement among physicians about depression after open heart surgery, there is little agreement regarding etiology. Major cardiac surgery often causes a significant disruption of an individual's view of self and the future. The need to make dietary and lifestyle changes may be an additional perturbing factor. Given the prevalence of subtle cognitive impairment postoperatively and the evidence of electroencephalographic changes postoperatively—changes that seem lateralized to the left hemisphere—postcardiotomy depression is likely attributable to subtle brain injury in a susceptible individual (Witoszka et al. 1973; Zeitlhoffer et al. 1988). An association between reduced cerebral blood flow during cardiac surgery and postoperative central nervous system dysfunction has also been reported (Henriksen 1984). Finally, there is increasing evidence to suggest that mood disorders may share elements of underlying pathophysiology with coronary artery disease, especially dysregulation of the autonomic nervous and serotonin neurotransmitter systems (Musselman et al. 1998).

The 5-year follow-up results of the Veterans Affairs Cooperative Study and the Coronary Artery Surgery Study indicated that compared with medical therapy alone, CABG surgery improved quality of life (i.e., resulted in decreased use of medications, improved subjective status, and elimination of chest pain). This improvement was sustained for 3–5 years after surgery (Booth et al. 1991; "Coronary Artery Surgery Study [CASS]" 1983).

Despite patient reports of being better physically (90% of patients) and emotionally (67% of patients), researchers in one study found that both CABG surgery patients and valve replacement patients experienced decreases in active social participation. These patients spent increasing amounts of time in passive activities such as watching television and listening to music on the radio (Bunzel and Eckersberger 1989).

Predictors for return to work after cardiotomy have been identified. An individual's expectations are strong predictors of return-to-work rates. Educational level and family income were determined to be stronger predictors than occupation or level of physical exertion required (Stanton et al. 1983).

There is some evidence that cardiac rehabilitation may improve daily functioning and decrease emotional distress (Dracup et al. 1991). When patients participating in group cardiac rehabilitation were compared with individuals who were not, the members of the rehabilitation group were found to have significantly less depression and anxiety and more satisfaction with their marriages.

Valve replacement. Chief among the complaints of individuals who have undergone mechanical valve replacement is the noise. Mechanical valves reportedly cause annoyance, disrupt sleep of both the patient and his or her partner, disrupt concentration, and are a source of social embarrassment for some individuals (Limb et al. 1992). These difficulties are described as more troublesome for younger individuals and women. One group of researchers found that these complaints are related to the audibility of the measured sounds from the valves (Moritz et al. 1992). Other individuals described a feeling of comfort from or being soothed by the regular monotonous tones but acknowledged alarm when skipped beats or an accelerated heart rate occurred.

Implantation of an automatic implantable cardioverter-defibrillator. Individuals with sustained ventricular tachycardia unresponsive to pharmacotherapy or ablation are often advised to undergo implantation of an automatic implantable cardioverter-defibrillator (AICD). This device contains a computer that senses the heart rate and delivers an electric shock when the heart rate reaches a preset level. The device is intended to prevent sudden death by providing immediate defibrillation—before extensive damage is done to the myocardium by the abnormal rhythm. The frequency and number of shocks delivered depend on the individual.

Implantation of these devices is associated with generalized anxiety and adjustment disorder, as well as with depression and sexual dysfunction. Morris et al. (1991) found that 30% of patients who underwent implantation of AICDs experienced a transient psychiatric disturbance, and 20% had a major psychiatric disorder. Patients with more frequent AICD discharges appear to have lessened work confidence and increased feelings of dependency and thoughts of dying (Heller et al. 1997). A recent case series highlighted the fact that patients with AICDs may be vulnerable to PTSD because of the firing of their devices (Hamner et al. 1999). Several of these patients showed improvement when treated with antidepressants and/or psychotherapy.

ORTHOPEDIC SURGERY

Patients who undergo orthopedic surgery fall into three primary problem groups: 1) patients with congenital problems, 2) patients with problems associated with accident-related injuries, and 3) patients with problems related to aging. Patients in the first category are usually children. In addition to the issues of pain and immobility, the developmental stage of the child is a significant factor in the treatment plan. For instance, issues of understanding, control, and dependence versus independence may seriously impede recovery. Patients who require orthope-

dic surgery as a result of an accident-related injury may be any age. These patients must also deal with the shock of the event and the unanticipated disruption of their daily lives. In addition, they may need to deal with the injury or loss of friends or family in the same accident, and they may also have feelings of guilt or blame about the cause of the accident. Elderly patients with orthopedic problems must face the seemingly inevitable demons of aging: loss of mobility, function, and independence. Orthopedic injury, especially hip fracture, appears to add to these demons by conferring a significantly increased risk of psychiatric morbidity. A recent large study documented a prevalence of psychiatric disorder (including depression, anxiety, and dementia) after hip fracture of nearly 50% (Bond et al. 1998).

Psychiatric consultation with hospitalized orthopedic patients has a demonstrably positive impact. After consultation, patients report improvement in their sense of well-being, the quality of their medical care, and their physical outcome. Psychiatric consultation also reduces orthopedic care costs. In one study involving 363 hospitalized medical-surgical patients, 18% of the hospital days were due to psychosocial rather than medical factors (Glass et al. 1978). On the basis of these data, Strain and colleagues (1991) examined whether psychiatric screening of elderly patients with hip fractures would shorten the average length of hospital stay and increase the proportion of patients who returned home after discharge. These authors studied 452 patients age 65 or older at two hospitals. During a baseline year, patients underwent traditional referral (i.e., whenever the regular staff asked) for psychiatric consultation. During the experimental year, patients were systematically screened for the need for psychiatric consultation. Patients who underwent systematic screening had a higher consultation rate than those who underwent traditional referral. The rates of DSM-III (American Psychiatric Association 1980) disorders in the experimental year were 56% at one hospital and 60% at the other. The mean length of stay was reduced from 20.7 to 18.5 days at hospital 1 and from 15.5 to 13.8 days at hospital 2, which resulted in a significant reduction in hospital costs. Therefore, admission screening of elderly patients with hip fractures resulted in early detection of psychiatric morbidity, better psychiatric care, earlier discharge, and substantial cost savings to the hospital (Strain et al. 1991).

In addition to the general issues discussed here, several specific areas of concern to psychiatric consultants emerge in dealing with orthopedic patients: delirium, chronic pain, and substance abuse.

Delirium

Delirium is extensively described in this book. Regardless of patient age, delirium has been scientifically linked to a high mortality rate. Weddington (1982) reviewed the records of 116 medical-surgical inpatients who had undergone psychiatric consultations. Among patients with a diagnosis of depression ($n = 43$), only 1 died. Of 15 patients with a diagnosis of delirium, 5 died within 3 months.

Postoperative delirium has been identified as a significant problem in elderly patients undergoing total hip replacement, with the prevalence reaching 25% among these patients (Millar 1981; Sheppeard et al. 1980; Titchener et al. 1958). Multiple etiologies for postoperative delirium, including older age, preoperative cognitive deficits, anesthesia, sleep deprivation, sensory deprivation, and increasing magnitude of surgery, have been postulated. A number of preoperative and postoperative interventions—short therapeutic sessions, education or information about what might happen, relaxation exercises, and even discussion of the possibility of postoperative delirium—seemed to decrease the incidence or at least the effect of the delirium (Rogers and Reich 1986).

Chronic Pain

There is a positive correlation between pain perception and levels of depression and anxiety. Patients with chronic orthopedic pain present an exceptionally complex and difficult management challenge because of the psychological aspects of such pain. Compared with patients who do not have recurring pain, patients who have chronic pain often present with an increase in neuroticism, anxiety, depression, and hysteria. Response to surgical treatment is worse in this patient population (Crown 1978). A psychiatric consultation may be quite helpful in assisting the patient to deal with the depression and anxiety stemming from the unrelenting pain. Antianxiety and antidepressant medications have also been demonstrated to act synergistically with pain medications, often permitting reduction in doses of pain medication.

Narcotic analgesics are often included in standard treatment regimens, and a consultant should determine whether the patient has any history of substance abuse or other addictive behavior before such drugs are given. Alternative pain management methods should be considered for all patients with pain but may be especially important for the patient with chronic orthopedic pain who abuses substances. Such alternative methods are frequently quite effective and may be used in combination with each other and with administration of pain medication. Manual or electrical massage and transcutaneous electrical nerve stimulation may be used to stimulate mechanoreceptors, which release a synaptic transmitter (an endorphin). These techniques may produce pain relief for up to 6 hours. Massage may also increase blood flow, relax muscles, and improve muscle tone (Paterson and Burn 1985). Other alternative methods include applications of moist or dry heat, cold applications, injection of lidocaine at trigger points, injection of steroids in some joints, supports or braces, acupuncture, traction, physical therapy, and corrective surgery. Behavioral techniques include relaxation exercises, guided imagery, hypnosis, and biofeedback. These techniques may also serve to give patients some sense of control over their situation, thereby further decreasing levels of depression and anxiety, which again may decrease patients' perception of pain.

Although it is difficult, the numerous psychological and physiologic symptoms of pain can be effectively managed by using the pain management expertise of the anesthesiologist, the orthopedic surgeon, and the psychiatrist. (For additional information on management of chronic pain, see Chapter 43.)

Substance Abuse

Burton et al. (1991) found that 20%–40% of inpatients admit to having substance problems, as opposed to 15%–18% of the general population. This higher prevalence is especially likely in orthopedic units. Although psychiatric consultation and referrals are often readily available to medical-surgical patients, there is evidence that substance abuse often goes undetected and that even when such a problem is recognized, a consultation is not always requested. Often, significant complications confound the medical management of patients who abuse substances, especially if the substance abuse is related to the medical condition (as in the case of patients with chronic pain). The importance of a psychiatric intervention in such cases cannot be overestimated.

Burton et al. (1991) also found that patients with substance abuse problems were often referred to aftercare programs, whereas nonabusing patients were more likely to receive social support, environmental manipulations, or referral to a chaplain or social worker. Although no significant differences were found between the substance-abusing and substance-nonabusing groups in the average timing of the consultation, follow-up visits were made to nonabusing patients more often than to abusing patients, and these visits lasted longer. Overall, patients who abused substances were not successfully cared for, despite the psychiatric intervention.

Orthopedic patients found to have substance abuse problems need careful evaluation to determine etiological factors. Did the substance abuse predate the orthopedic injury, or did it result from a chronic pain syndrome? Preexisting conditions should be dealt with in the same manner used with any other substance-abusing patient. Patients with chronic pain conditions require a more aggressive approach to pain management, utilizing alternative pain control methods (e.g., relaxation, hypnosis, acupuncture, nerve blocks), as noted earlier. However, significant attention must be paid to rehabilitation with regard to the substance abuse.

OPHTHALMOLOGY

Emotional stress is known to accompany ophthalmic disorders. A number of articles in the literature deal with "psychosomatic ophthalmology," although few are geared toward aiding the practicing ophthalmologist or psychiatrist. Usually there is no hesitation in referring to the psychiatric consultant patients who have an obvious disturbance, such as psychotic episodes and delirium (sometimes agitated by sensory deprivation or "black patch psychosis"), or who experience a loss of vision in the absence of a recognizable organic disease. However, the ophthalmologist may not know when to refer a patient who has sustained acute, partial, or total loss of vision. Moreover, the psychiatrist may have trouble offering meaningful and relevant advice when he or she is asked to consult with such patients (G.L. Adams and Pearlman 1970).

Vision Loss in Children

Children who experience vision loss manifest two common responses. The first is a neurobehavioral reaction that is best interpreted as a behavioral adaptation to poor vision. The second response affects personality development by limiting social and cognitive growth. The neurobehavioral reaction is often misinterpreted by adults as a conscious attempt to misbehave. However, many behaviors are specific to disease states and can be addressed as such. Developmental disturbances such as delayed mobility and confusion of the pronouns *I* and *you* have been noted in vision-impaired children. Often, children experience a combination of symptoms. For example, patients whose vision loss accompanies hearing loss require special rehabilitation and attention. A grieving process will sometimes continue for a long time as the child and his or her parents compare abilities—in the many developmental stages of life—with those of children with normal sight.

Acute Vision Loss in Adults

The loss, or even the threat of loss, of visual function is inevitably accompanied by serious emotional stress, although the stress is not always immediately evident. The way in which a patient handles this stress can benefit or harm his or her physical and mental health. It is the role of the psychiatric physician to help the patient cope with the various forms of stress engendered by visual loss, to help the patient evaluate the relevance and severity of the symptoms, and to aid in the patient's management (G.L. Adams and Pearlman 1972).

Acute vision loss often results in a full grieving process. Long-standing or permanent blindness may lead to depression and social isolation. Indeed, depression is more common among blind persons than among persons who are deaf (Abolfotouh and Telmesani 1993). Paradoxically, however, several studies have shown that compared with total blindness, the threat of vision loss or partial vision loss may be more productive of psychiatric pathology, including suicide (De Leo et al. 1999). Similarly, restoration of sight is often a highly stressful experience, and rates of depression are also high among these patients (Firlik 1992). A patient may experience personality changes, low motivation (in the case of an otherwise highly motivated person), and communication problems (with the patient having lost the ability to note the emotional facial expressions of others). Good (1993) suggested that immediate interventions can minimize the impact of vision loss—for example, the provision of reading machines, Seeing Eye dogs, low-vision aids, braille instruction, or companionship. Introducing these aids as soon as possible reduces the amount of social isolation, desperation, and depression felt by these patients.

Visual hallucinations, although more common in visually impaired patients, should be carefully monitored in any patient with an ophthalmological problem because such hallucinations could be signs of a mental illness or of an organic brain disease. Perceptual disorders (such as a distortion of size and shape) or palinopsia (a visual hallucination that is characterized by the persistence of an image after its removal) may occur.

Lifestyle changes almost always accompany loss of vision; these changes, which may include loss of work and social activities, can be quite devastating for patients and in fact may be of more importance than the disease process itself. Generally, children cope better than adults with lifestyle changes because children are more open to learning compensatory strategies.

When treatment involves full restitution of vision (e.g., cataract surgery), the decision to go ahead with treatment is usually based on the patient's medical history and level of dissatisfaction with his or her reduced vision. When treatment cannot restore or even improve vision, the patient must be supported and assisted in coping with this new disability and with the inevitable grief process that is involved.

Patients can be taught to adapt to decreased vision through use of other senses to compensate for vision failure, stand magnifiers to enlarge print, a cane, and a guide dog; through use of a closed-circuit television; and through instruction in braille and in mobility. Many national organizations have services available to assist sight-impaired persons.

So much of human communication involves eye contact that loss of sight has a great psychological effect on both patient and caregiver. Compared with other types of wounds, eye injuries often cause countertransference and transference reactions in people (patient, caregiver, attending physician), with the characteristics of these responses determined by the specific personalities involved.

Neuropsychiatric Aspects of Blindness

The neuropsychiatric (functional) form of vision loss is usually diagnosed when sight failure occurs in the absence of a physical explanation. Psychiatric consultation is often requested to define the etiology of the vision loss. Usually this request is phrased in the form of determining the "functional overlay." A neuropsychiatric vision loss may occur for many different reasons. Physical examples are a medical history of amblyopia, cone dystrophy, retinitis pigmentosa, and end-stage glaucoma. Psychiatric examples include sociopathy or malingering, depression, tunnel vision (in conversion disorder patients), hysteria, child abuse, and other affective disturbances.

Trauma to the eye can also alert an ophthalmologist to the need for a psychiatric consultation. Childhood situations such as poorly supervised play, abuse, sports-related injuries, and low socioeconomic status are considered risk factors for eye trauma. More dramatic examples include suicide attempts (involving gunshot wounds, for example), when precautions and psychiatric care become paramount, and shaken baby syndrome, which may cause retinal blood vessels to rupture. Attempts at self-enucleation (removal of one's own eye) are almost always associated with schizophrenia or severe psychiatric disorders and must be addressed as carefully as the eye injury (Good 1993).

Various topical ophthalmic medications, when absorbed systemically, may cause psychiatric problems. For instance, β-blockers used to treat glaucoma may cause depression (with symptoms ranging from mild dysphoria to anergia to suicidal ideation), hallucinations, lethargy, confusion, or impotence. Administration of topical anticholinergics, used to dilate pupils, can result in diminished salivation, increased heart rate, GI disturbances, and changes in activity levels (ranging from drowsiness to transient attention deficit with hyperactivity); transient delirium may even occur. These reactions are more likely to occur in children; yet in this population they are also more likely to be missed or ignored because children may not complain of these symptoms.

Dementia, preoperative anxiety, preoperative anesthesia, and the use of medicines to prepare the eyes for surgery (resulting in blurred vision) can all result in confusion, fear, and agitation. Adequate preoperative assessment and an individual treatment plan are essential (e.g., a patient with dementia may do better with general rather than local anesthesia).

The psychiatrist must be aware of ophthalmic complications of various psychotropic medications. Some drugs with anticholinergic effects, such as tricyclic antidepressants and neuroleptics, may produce acute angle-closure glaucoma. An ophthalmic consultation is required for any psychiatric patient with a glaucoma history who is a candidate for treatment with these medications.

Blindness can occur in patients who take more than 800 mg of thioridazine daily. Dosages at this level should be avoided, and patients who take 600 mg/day should undergo eye examinations every 6 months. Chlorpromazine can cause anterior cataracts. Initial concern, based on results of testing in animals, that the new atypical antipsychotic quetiapine (Seroquel) may cause cataracts led the manufacturer to recommend slit-lamp examinations before initiation of therapy, shortly thereafter, and then every 6 months. More recent data from human trials, however, suggest that the rate of cataract development with quetiapine therapy is not different from the rate with haloperidol therapy (Brown et al. 1999). Given these conflicting results, it is unclear whether eye examination is indicated in patients beginning treatment with quetiapine, and the current standard of practice varies among physicians. Lithium toxicity can cause gaze-evoked nystagmus and occasionally downbeat nystagmus, fast eye movements, oculogyric crisis, and opsoclonia. Neuroleptic drugs may also cause oculogyric crisis, which can be treated with anticholinergic medications; however, use of anticholinergics may in turn result in blurred vision.

Some potential drug interactions should be noted. Ophthalmic β-blockers (such as timolol and betaxolol) may react with phenothiazines. The simultaneous use of propranolol and chlorpromazine or thioridazine results in increases in serum levels of the β-blocker and the neuro-leptic. When calcium-channel blockers are used with topical β-blockers, conduction defects, heart failure, and hypotension may result.

BURN UNITS

The role of the consultation psychiatrist in the burn unit and after hospitalization can be linked to three important phases in the care and management of the patient who has sustained burns: 1) the acute phase, 2) the reconstructive phase, and 3) the long-term adjustment phase (Welch 1987). The interventions of the psychiatrist are closely linked to the issues that emerge in these phases.

Acute Phase

In the first 24–72 hours after the burn occurs, the patient experiences a period of initial lucidity. This period offers the psychiatric consultant an opportunity to assess the patient's history, personality dynamics, and coping patterns. A high percentage of burn patients have important predisposing factors for burn injuries, such as alcoholism, cognitive degeneration or dementia (in elderly patients), chronic mental illness, family dysfunction, or, in the case of burned children, frank neglect. In one study, Mac-Arthur and Moore (1975) showed that 59% of men and 38% of women with burn injuries have a combination of such factors. A recent study demonstrated a similarly high prevalence of psychiatric disorders among burn patients, with depression and alcoholism being especially common (Fauerbach et al. 1996). Patients with a pre-morbid psychiatric history show poorer postburn adjustment and a higher rate of postburn psychiatric symptoms than do burn patients without a premorbid psychiatric history (Fauerbach et al. 2001). The issue of self-inflicted burns should be an obvious red flag for the psychiatric consultant. In one study of self-immolation, 73% of patients had a psychiatric history and 55% had previously attempted suicide (Sonneborn and Vorstraelen 1992). Even in cases in which the burn injury is not related to psychiatric illness, the presence of premorbid psychiatric pathology predicts poor long-term adjustment and increased rates of postburn psychiatric symptoms (Fauerbach et al. 1996, 1997).

After the initial phase of lucidity, between 30% and 70% of burn patients develop delirium, presumably caused by stress and burn-induced metabolic disturbances (Andreasen et al. 1977). Both chlorpromazine and haloperidol have been recommended for treating burn patients with delirium. Haloperidol is usually adminis-

tered in doses of 1–5 mg iv as a bolus, with a total dose as high as 185 mg over a 24-hour period (Cassem and Sos 1980). Chlorpromazine is also given intravenously, with 100 mg administered in 100 mL of normal saline infused over 15–30 minutes. With either drug, the initial loading dose should be given at 30-minute intervals until sedation is achieved. To maintain sedation, half the total induction dose is given every 12 hours (Welch 1987).

Pain management is a crucial area of intervention for the consultation psychiatrist. Although pain is a chronic issue for the patient with a burn injury, it becomes most acute during dressing changes and debridement. In a provocative editorial, Perry (1984) described the psychodynamics of undermedication for pain in burn units. Although staff insensitivity, mistaken ideas about analgesics, and fears of iatrogenic addiction may play a role, Perry did not believe that these adequately explain the continuing problem of undermedication. The most commonly used intravenous analgesics include morphine, meperidine, methadone, and fentanyl. Each of these agents has advantages and disadvantages; dosages vary widely from patient to patient. Because of its fast onset and short duration of action, fentanyl is recommended before dressing changes and debridement (Welch 1987).

Two major psychological issues must be addressed during this period: denial and education. Psychiatrists who are experienced in burn unit work attest to the rapid alteration between a patient's request for more information and profound denial. This rapid shifting between the two poles often confuses the family and confounds the staff. Experience has shown that it is not wise, nor kind, to attempt to dispel denial, especially early on. On the other hand, direct questions should be answered kindly but directly. This includes answering the question "Will I die?" even if the patient is in extremis.

Reconstructive Phase

The reconstructive phase extends from the end of acute surgical intervention and delirium up to discharge from the unit. Thus, this period may last for weeks or months, depending on the extent of the burn and the pace of the recovery. Because the patient is now able to face the implications of the event with clear cognitive acuity, this phase is the most psychologically difficult. However, the patient's physical problems, including the pain associated with physical therapy and dressing changes, also continue. During this phase, the psychiatrist must be prepared to deal with grief, facilitate affective expression, and intervene in the management of regression. Bilowitz et al. (1980) argued for significant liaison activities with the staff of the burn unit in the form of team meetings, work rounds, and informal meetings with individual staff members as needed. These authors described how physical immobilization, forced passive dependency, and bodily disfigurement lead to regression in many patients. Regressive behavior is frequently followed by negative countertransference reactions in staff.

Long-Term Adjustment Phase

Studies of long-term adjustment of patients with burn injuries have shown satisfactory outcomes ranging from 20% to 70% (Andreasen and Norris 1972; Woodward 1959). However, despite significant emotional distress in this phase, patients often have difficulty engaging in psychotherapy or communicating with their families. The psychological goal is to encourage good coping.

On the basis of the work of Weisman and Sobel (1979), we suggest that clinicians use the following approach for patients with burn injuries:

1. Identify the primary feelings about the burn experience without making this the exclusive focus of therapy.
2. Define a hierarchy of problems facing the patient.
3. Define a hierarchy of desired goals and solutions using a problem-solving or cognitive approach.
4. Continue to work with flexibility on these goals while addressing other issues that worry or concern the patient.

We believe that this confrontational, problem-solving approach is an active ingredient in prevention of depression.

When PTSD occurs, it is of significant importance for the patient, the staff, and the consulting psychiatrist. Diagnosis should be made at the earliest possible time, and treatment should be started as soon as the diagnosis is made. In one study, 35.3% of burn patients met DSM-III-R (American Psychiatric Association 1987) criteria for PTSD at 2 months postinjury, 40% met criteria at 6 months, and 45.2% met criteria at 12 months postinjury (Perry et al. 1992). In a second study, 7% of patients with burn injuries met PTSD criteria at the time of hospital discharge, and 22% met criteria at follow-up 4 months later (Roca et al. 1992). Although the rates of PTSD in these two studies differ, both studies illustrated the increasing incidence of PTSD over time. We urge that psychiatric follow-up be provided for all patients with burn injuries. The consultant should be prepared to offer expressive-emotive, grief-oriented, and problem-solving or cognitive therapy. Management of sleep disorder symptoms is essential for this population as well.

COSMETIC SURGERY

As with patients with burn injuries, psychiatric consultation with patients undergoing cosmetic surgery is related to the stages of surgery and to recovery. Pruzinsky (1988) outlined five stages in elective cosmetic surgery: 1) the decision to seek consultation, 2) the initial consultation, 3) the preoperative and intraoperative periods, 4) the immediate postoperative period, and 5) the long-term postoperative period.

Initial Psychiatric Consultation

The psychiatrist usually is asked to see the patient after an informed discussion with the surgeon. The initial consultation has two primary objectives: prevention of adverse psychiatric sequelae and provision of direct services, if required. Perhaps the most important aspect of prevention is careful patient selection (Correa et al. 1999; Pruzinsky 1988). This can be done only after extensive patient interviewing, careful documentation of the patient's history, and formal psychological testing, if needed. Two findings warrant special care: major depressive disorder and body dysmorphic disorder (Phillips et al. 2000). Patients with either of these diagnoses may expect the surgery to cure the underlying psychiatric disorder. According to DSM-IV-TR (American Psychiatric Association 2000), one feature of body dysmorphic disorder is "preoccupation with an imagined defect in appearance. If a slight physical anomaly is present, the person's concern is markedly excessive" (p. 510).

Another red flag is a history of multiple surgeries, especially elective cosmetic surgeries whose results were unsatisfactory to the patient. Provision of services can involve clarification of the patient's motivation and expectations, as well as formation of a working alliance in the event that surgery is actually performed.

Preoperative and Intraoperative Periods

In stage 3, the preoperative and intraoperative periods, the consulting psychiatrist has three objectives: 1) reduction of anxiety, 2) management of traumatic intraoperative reactions, and 3) management of postsurgical delirium. Treatment for preoperative anxiety is usually a combination of psychotherapy and psychopharmacology. If the patient experiences a panic attack, a delay of surgery, with further exploration of the diagnostic and personality issues, is warranted. In some patients, cosmetic surgery may be an unconscious or even conscious antecedent to a significant life change, such as separation or divorce. This decision may be laden with more conflict than the patient realizes.

Interventions for traumatic intraoperative reactions usually are focused on the myriad of minor but routine surgical sequelae that frighten or alarm the patient. Usually, swelling and discoloration cause the most concern. Patients often complain, "I never imagined that I would look so bad. I only imagined that I would look better." Sometimes the problem is complicated by an unsympathetic surgeon, who is pleased with the results and hopes for appreciation from the patient. In these situations, the psychiatrist should be prepared to spend some time with the patient, providing realistic reassurance and support. Benzodiazepines and sleep medications may be very helpful during this period as well.

Immediate Postoperative Period

Treatment for postsurgical delirium should follow the same lines as those suggested for burn patients, but with doses substantially reduced. The psychological reactions, however, may be more difficult to diagnose and treat in the population of patients who have undergone cosmetic surgery. During the postoperative period, the full extent of what was beginning to occur during the preoperative and intraoperative periods may be experienced by the patient, who may feel acutely traumatized and very disappointed. Affective responses ranging from severe depression to anxiety and panic may ensue. Often, the patient feels very isolated and withdrawn, not wishing to be visited by family or friends because of the presence of bleeding, swelling, and discoloration. This provokes further feelings of depression and phobic anxiety (Goin and Goin 1986). Management requires substantial reassurance plus empathy. A visit by the surgeon may be more anxiety-reducing for the patient at this stage than any psychotherapy or pharmacotherapy (Pruzinsky 1988).

Long-Term Postoperative Period

In stage 5, the long-term postoperative period, psychiatric intervention is focused on treatment of the negative psychiatric sequelae, regardless of whether the surgical outcome was positive or negative. Adverse psychological reactions to a technically positive surgery range from dissatisfaction to loss of identity. The sources of patient dissatisfaction can be based on the reemergence of previous psychological problems that were not solved by the surgery, lack of understanding of realistic outcome of the surgery, or failure to obtain external approval for surgical changes (Macgregor 1981). Usually these dissatisfied patients require intensive psychotherapy that moves well

beyond the supportive efforts of most consultation-liaison psychiatrists. Patient dissatisfaction with a technically positive surgery may indicate an "insatiable" cosmetic surgery patient, one who repeatedly asks for reoperation on a particular body part to "get it right" (Knorr et al. 1967). These patients have been described as having borderline personality disorder (Groenman and Soner 1983). Rhinoplasty appears to be the major type of cosmetic surgery that attracts this particular kind of patient (Book 1971; Ness 1978). Another warning of "insatiability" should be sounded when a patient, usually female, requests repeat blepharoplasty (Goin and Goin 1986).

HEAD AND NECK SURGERY

Psychiatric Contraindications to Surgery

Most head and neck cancer patients adjust to and cope very well with severely disfiguring surgeries performed to save their lives. However, in one study, 18% of patients reported that the disadvantages outweighed the advantages (Gamba et al. 1992). These patients responded with statements such as "I no longer recognize myself" and "I look like a monster." For this group, surviving cancer was less important than having a certain appearance. This finding led the authors to propose that the best way to help a patient prepare for surgery is through education. This should include discussion about how daily life functions—such as swallowing, tasting, hearing, smelling, seeing, and eating—may be altered. In addition, information about expected energy level and psychological reactions, such as depression and anxiety, should be included. Finally, presurgery education should include preparing the patient for the possibility of a psychosis or delirium.

It is very helpful for the patient to meet a person who is well adjusted after undergoing a similar operation. This makes the important point that people can adjust well to the procedure in question; in fact, in one study, more than 86% of head and neck patients adjusted functionally to their disfigurement (West 1977). One-third of these patients had visible disfigurement as a result of surgical treatment. A crucial ingredient in preventing untoward emotional reactions is the support that the patient receives from the family and the treatment team, both preoperatively and postoperatively.

Primary Psychiatric Disorders

A patient who has previously had a psychiatric disorder is at increased risk of developing a psychiatric illness after disfiguring surgery. Psychopathology also affects the patient's ability to cope with surgery. Breitbart and Holland (1988) noted that a preexisting anxiety disorder constituted a major impediment to treatment and rehabilitation for patients with head and neck cancer.

Secondary Psychiatric Disorders

Several psychiatric disorders are likely to develop as a result of disfiguring surgery. It is not unusual for patients to experience mild depression and/or anxiety; however, a major depression or an anxiety disorder may develop. David and Barrit (1982) defined an "expectable pattern" of severe postoperative depression that can persist over time. Morton et al. (1984) found that 40% of patients with oropharyngeal cancer met DSM-III criteria for depression 6 months after treatment.

Diagnosing depression is complicated when a patient already has difficulty with sleep and appetite; these are key vegetative signs of depression. Other signs to look for, specifically in patients who will undergo or who have undergone surgery for head and neck cancer, include

- Excessive dependency
- Anger
- Social withdrawal (demonstrated, for example, by very little eye contact or by avoidance of family gatherings)
- Feelings of hopelessness and helplessness
- Excessive pain complaints
- Noncompliance with treatment

The psychiatrist should also watch for subtle, nonverbal cues (gestures and expressions) to determine the patient's mood after disfiguring surgical procedures.

The etiology of depression in head and neck surgery patients is multifactorial (Baile et al. 1992a). There are tumor-related factors, individual differences in coping resources, and preexisting psychopathology. The severity of depression is often correlated with pain and with family or marital problems (Andreasen and Norris 1972). Patients must adjust to and learn to cope with changes in movement, speech, swallowing, vision, smell, taste, hearing, and, most of all, face and body disfigurement.

Although the causes of the depression are multifactorial, effective treatment exists. Antidepressant medications are very effective in treating depressed patients with head and neck cancer (Fernandez and Adams 1986). Supportive psychotherapy and cognitive therapy help to mobilize the patient and help the patient to develop healthy coping strategies. Family support and support from the medical treatment team are very important factors as well.

Anxiety is also a significant problem in patients who are disfigured. Many factors contribute to anxiety in patients adjusting to disfigurement. If a patient was involved in an accident, an anxiety reaction to that specific trauma usually occurs, as well as anxiety about the patient's appearance. In a study at Memorial Sloan-Kettering Cancer Center involving patients with head and neck cancer, half of the patients had adjustment disorders with anxious mood (Breitbart and Holland 1988).

Many symptoms besides feeling anxious or feeling as if one were "falling apart" are associated with anxiety. Patients may not realize that they are anxious but may have other related symptoms (Table 27–6). Anxiety can lead to distortion of body image, especially in the context of disfigurement. Patients can perceive disfigurement as much worse than it is, which can cause further isolation, depression, and anxiety.

There are several helpful interventions for anxiety. Early interventions in the postoperative period include relaxation training, guided imagery, and desensitization. A combination of imagery plus desensitization can help the patient to master fears and learn how to relax. Cognitive restructuring is another way to reduce anxiety. With this intervention, patients measure their cognitions to determine whether they are accurate and, if they are not, restructure them so that they are less stress-inducing. Pharmacological interventions are helpful for patients who are too anxious to engage in these exercises or for patients who are sleepless and unable to concentrate because of their anxiety symptoms.

TABLE 27–6. Anxiety symptoms commonly encountered in disfigured patients

Difficulty falling asleep
Nightmares
Restlessness
Tremulousness
Sweating
Dry mouth
Pressured speech
Frequent urination
Tachycardia
Light-headedness
Fear of fainting
Palpitations
Generalized fatigue
Vague aches and pains
Shortness of breath
Paresthesias

Source. Data from Lucente et al. 1987.

Altered mental status is a common postoperative occurrence in patients who have undergone head and neck surgery. Mild disorientation, confusion, illusions, or hallucinations may represent functional conditions caused by sensory overload, sensory deprivation, sleep deprivation, or the shock of extremely threatening events. F. Adams et al. (1984), using bedside testing, found that a high percentage of patients who had been labeled as "depressed" by surgeons had substantial neuropsychological deficits.

Patients with delirium may present with apathy, withdrawal, poor cooperation with self-care, agitation, excessive fatigue, weakness, and subdued affect, as well as disorganized and uncontrolled emotional and motor discharge. Assessment with the Mini-Mental State Exam (Folstein et al. 1975) is helpful for diagnosing neuropsychological deficits, although it is insensitive to subtle or right-hemisphere deficits. In the case of a patient who cannot speak or write, having him or her draw a clock showing a specific time is a way to evaluate mental status. The Bender-Gestalt Test (Bender 1938), which involves copying geometric figures, is also used to assess neuropsychological deficits.

The first step in treatment of delirium in patients who have undergone head and neck surgery, as in patients with burn injuries and patients who have undergone cosmetic surgery, is to find the biomedical etiology of the problem. Patients with head and neck cancer are prone to aspiration pneumonia and wound infections, which can cause mental status changes. Length of surgery also correlates with risk of postsurgical delirium. Low-dose, high-potency antipsychotic medications are very helpful in the management of patients with agitation secondary to delirium (Shapiro and Kornfeld 1987).

Comorbid psychiatric disorders complicate treatment and subsequent adjustment to disfigurement. Patients with a history of depression are at higher risk for postoperative depression (Breitbart and Holland 1988). The coping ability of patients with a preexisting psychiatric diagnosis is often poor; therefore, a new stress such as disfigurement or a diagnosis of cancer is difficult for such patients. The psychiatrist should also look for alcohol and drug abuse or dependence. Healthy coping strategies may not exist for such patients and are not readily instilled. Given these difficulties, such patients can tax the treatment team and family resources.

There are many psychological reactions to illness and hospitalization, but a particularly common one in disfigured patients is the feeling of helplessness. Patients struggle with complete dependency on family members, friends, and nurses. Things that were once done easily are now difficult or impossible and require assistance.

Humiliation, shame, and anger are common reactions to this enforced dependency and loss of control. Fear, as with any other illness, is also common; fears in this patient population relate to medical procedures, disfigurement, loss of function, pain, and death. Reactions and meanings of sickness and disfigurement are unique. It is important to give each patient an opportunity to express those unique feelings.

Reactions to Loss and Body Image Problems

Patients who undergo disfiguring surgery experience multiple losses. There are losses of function and abilities and of specific body parts, but most important, such patients experience losses of identity and self-image. The face is crucial to an individual's identity and self-image, and so surgery that disfigures the facial area carries the greatest risk of emotional devastation and subsequent depression. The fear of social reaction to a facial disfigurement may lead, at times, to social isolation, which further perpetuates depression. Shame underlies such self-isolation, which also worsens depression. Disfiguring surgery can give rise as well to anxiety related to fears of separation, abandonment, or a damaged, disintegrated self (Bronheim et al. 1991). Patients can feel an increased vulnerability because they do not have the "equipment" to deal with the world the way they once did.

Sexuality is also seriously affected by alterations in body image. Although not writing specifically about persons with head and neck cancer, Grinker (1976) stated that the "dread of exposing oneself to one's spouse as crippled, damaged, incomplete or dying may cause sexual inhibition or abstinence" (p. 131). Intimacy and sexual bodily functions are also affected by shame and embarrassment (Grinker 1976). Open communication with the treatment team about sexuality, both before and after surgery, is usually helpful. Effective communication among team members about the validity and importance of a patient's sexuality is essential; otherwise, members of the treatment team will "pass the buck," expecting others to deal with the topic.

Often, patients believe that they can no longer function sexually because of disfigurement. We encourage patients to experiment with their sexual behavior to achieve some satisfaction. Communication is an important tool in overcoming changes in body image and sexuality. We also encourage patients to speak with partners and physicians about questions or concerns.

One of the main factors that influences patients' adjustment to changes in body is how accepted they feel. Perceived absence of social support undermines recovery.

Orr et al. (1989) found that patients who perceived more social support (friends more than family) had a more positive body image, greater self-esteem, and less depression than did those who had less social support. The patient's first "social exposure" after surgery or trauma is to the treatment team. Thus, social support and communication about sensitive patient issues, such as sexuality or shame related to body image, begin in the hospital. Patient acceptance begins with staff members comfortably and effectively communicating within the staff-patient relationship.

Substance Withdrawal

Patients with head and neck cancer have high rates of alcoholism and drug abuse (Shapiro and Kornfeld 1987). When alcohol intake is abruptly interrupted by trauma or surgery, withdrawal often occurs.

Family Problems

Family members also go through a major adjustment when a relative becomes disfigured. Sometimes a family has a fixed idea regarding how much the patient should know about his or her prognosis; this idea is usually related to the family members' own difficulties with the diagnosis and prognosis. The family's misguided attempt at protection of the patient in this way creates difficulties for the treatment team. The family members' discomfort is sometimes reduced when they understand that they are not responsible for telling the patient bad news (Lucente et al. 1987). It is important that family members have an outlet to discuss feelings, either in a group or with a physician, therapist, or social worker. Failure to provide this opportunity can lead to increased family-patient difficulties.

Staff Issues

A difficult aspect of working with disfigured patients is the reactions of the hospital staff. These patients may look grotesque, exude secretions constantly, and smell repulsive and are sometimes hard to understand because of extensive facial bandaging. It is often difficult for staff members to remember that behind the tubes, the unattractive exterior, and the excretions lies a human being (Bronheim et al. 1991). Thus, it is all too easy to reduce contact and communication with such patients, setting up a cycle of avoidance. The psychiatric consultant is not immune to these feelings. More frequent therapeutic interviews of shorter duration help to prevent therapist burnout. Human contact is of vital importance to disfig-

ured patients; they need to express and process feelings and to be reassured that they are not abandoned because of their disfigurement. The liaison with staff is a vital part of the consultant's mandate. Prevention of nursing burnout is another important aspect of the psychiatrist's liaison role.

CONCLUSION

One of the psychiatrist's major tasks in working with surgical patients is establishing a relationship with the referring surgeon, who may or may not be knowledgeable about psychiatric issues. Surgeons vary considerably in their sensitivity to these factors. Some are exquisitely aware of the psychological dimensions of patient care. Others, often at the beginning of their careers, are less likely to regard these issues as sufficiently important to take up valuable time. Thus, the first rule of consultation to surgery is "Know your surgeon."

REFERENCES

Abolfotouh MA, Telmesani A: A study of some psycho-social characteristics of blind and deaf male students in Abha City, Asir region, Saudi Arabia. Public Health 107:261–269, 1993

Acosta F: Biofeedback and progressive relaxation in weaning the anxious patient from the ventilator: a brief report. Heart Lung 17:299–301, 1988

Adams F, Larson DL, Goeptert H: Does the diagnosis in head and neck cancer mask organic brain disease? Otolaryngol Head Neck Surg 92:618–624, 1984

Adams GL, Pearlman JT: Emotional response and management of visually handicapped patients. Psychiatry in Medicine 1:233–240, 1970

Adams GL, Pearlman JT: Prevention of mental disorders in ophthalmic patients. Annals of Ophthalmology 4:555–560, 1972

Adrian J, Crankshaw DP, Tiller JWG, et al: Affective, cognitive and subjective changes in patients undergoing cardiac surgery: a preliminary report. Anaesth Intensive Care 16:144–149, 1988

Agency for Health Care Policy and Research: Acute pain management: operative or medical procedures and trauma, part 2. Clin Pharm 11:391–414, 1992

American Pain Society: Principles of Analgesic Use in the Treatment of Acute and Cancer Pain, 3rd Edition. Skokie, IL, American Pain Society, 1992, pp 1–41

American Psychiatric Association: Diagnostic and Statistical Manual of Mental Disorders, 3rd Edition. Washington, DC, American Psychiatric Association, 1980

American Psychiatric Association: Diagnostic and Statistical Manual of Mental Disorders, 3rd Edition, Revised. Washington, DC, American Psychiatric Association, 1987

American Psychiatric Association: Diagnostic and Statistical Manual of Mental Disorders, 4th Edition, Text Revision. Washington, DC, American Psychiatric Association, 2000

Andreasen NJ, Norris AS: Long term adjustment and adaptation mechanisms in severely burned adults. J Nerv Ment Dis 154:352–362, 1972

Andreasen NJ, Hartford CE, Knott JR, et al: EEG changes associated with burn delirium. Diseases of the Nervous System 38:27–31, 1977

Appelbaum PS, Grisso T: Assessing patient's capacities to consent to treatment. N Engl J Med 319:1635–1638, 1989

Argenziano M, Oz MC, Rose EA: The continuing evolution of mechanical ventricular assistance. Curr Probl Surg 34: 317–386, 1997

Baile WF, Biertini M, Scott L, et al: Depression and tumor stage in cancer of the head and neck. Psychooncology 1:15–24, 1992a

Baile WF, Kuehn CV, Straker D: Factitious cancer. Psychosomatics 33:100–105, 1992b

Beliles K, Stoudemire A: Psychopharmacologic treatment of depression in the medically ill. Psychosomatics 39:S2–S19, 1998

Bender L: A visual motor Gestalt test and its clinical use. Research Monograph No 3. Albany, NY, American Orthopsychiatric Association, 1938

Berlin RM: Management of insomnia in hospitalized patients. Ann Intern Med 100:398–404, 1984

Bilowitz A, Friedson W, Schubert DSP: Liaison psychiatry on a burn unit. Gen Hosp Psychiatry 2:300–306, 1980

Blumenthal JA, Madden DJ, Burker EJ, et al: A preliminary study of the effects of cardiac procedures on cognitive performance. International Journal of Psychosomatics 38:13–16, 1991

Bohets H, Lavrijsen K, Hendrickx J: Identification of the cytochrome P-450 enzymes involved in the metabolism of cisapride: in vitro studies of potential co-medication interactions. Br J Pharmacol 129:1655–1667, 2000

Bond J, Gregson B, Smith M, et al: Outcomes following acute hospital care for stroke or hip fracture: how useful is an assessment of anxiety or depression for older people? Int J Geriatr Psychiatry 13:601–610, 1998

Book HE: Psychiatric assessment for rhinoplasty. Archives of Otolaryngology 94:51–55, 1971

Booth DC, Deupree RH, Hultgren HN, et al: Quality of life after bypass surgery for unstable angina. Circulation 83:87–95, 1991

Bostwick JM, Masterson BJ: Psychopharmacological treatment of delirium to restore mental capacity. Psychosomatics 39:112–117, 1998

Bovill JG: Adverse drug interactions in anesthesia. J Clin Anesth 9:3S–13S, 1997

Bowen DE: Ventilator weaning through hypnosis. Psychosomatics 30:449–450, 1989

Breitbart W, Holland J: Psychosocial aspects of head and neck cancer. Semin Oncol 15:61–69, 1988

Breuer AC, Furlan AJ, Hanson MR, et al: Central nervous system complications of coronary artery bypass graft surgery: prospective analysis of 421 patients. Stroke 14:682–687, 1983

Bronheim H, Strain JA, Biller HF: Psychiatric aspects of head and neck surgery, part II: body image and psychiatric intervention. Gen Hosp Psychiatry 13:225–232, 1991

Brown CS, Markowitz JS, Moore TR, et al: Atypical antipsychotics, part II: adverse effects, drug interactions and costs. Ann Pharmacother 33:210–217, 1999

Bunzel B, Eckersberger F: Changes in activities performed in leisure time after open heart surgery. Int J Cardiol 23:315–320, 1989

Burton RW, Lyons JS, Devens M, et al: Psychiatric consultations for psychoactive substance disorders in the general hospital. Gen Hosp Psychiatry 13:83–87, 1991

Caley CF, Silvia RJ: Cytochrome P-450 drug interactions and the selective serotonin reuptake inhibiting antidepressants. Connecticut Medicine 64:721–724, 2000

Carrieri P, Orefice G, Fioretti A, et al: Effects of long-term ticlopidine treatment on platelet function and its tolerability in cerebrovascular disease. J Int Med Res 12:286–291, 1984

Cassem NH, Hackett TP: The setting of intensive care, in Massachusetts General Hospital Handbook of General Hospital Psychiatry. Edited by Hackett TP, Cassem NH. St. Louis, MO, CV Mosby, 1978, pp 319–341

Cassem NH, Sos J: The intravenous use of haloperidol for acute delirium in intensive care settings, in Psychic and Neurological Dysfunctions After Open-Heart Surgery. Edited by Speidel H, Rodewald G. Stuttgart, Germany, Theime, 1980, pp 196–199

Castor B, Ursin J, Aberg M, et al: Infected wounds and repeated septicemia in a case of factitious illness. Scand J Infect Dis 22:227–232, 1990

Caumo W, Schmidt AP, Schneider CN, et al: Risk factors for preoperative anxiety in adults. Acta Anesthesiol Scand 45:298–307, 2001

Chapman CR: Psychological aspects of postoperative pain control. Acta Anaesthiol Belg 43:41–52, 1992

Coronary Artery Surgery Study (CASS): A randomized trial of coronary artery bypass surgery: quality of life in patients randomly assigned to treatment groups. Circulation 68: 951–960, 1983

Correa AJ, Sykes JM, Ries WR: Considerations before rhinoplasty. Otolaryngol Clin North Am 32:7–14, 1999

Crown S: Psychological aspects of low back pain. Rheumatology Rehabilitation 17:114–123, 1978

David JD, Barrit JA: Psychosocial implications of surgery for head and neck cancer. Clin Plast Surg 9:327–336, 1982

De Leo D, Hickey PA, Meneghel G, et al: Blindness, fear of sight loss, and suicide. Psychosomatics 40:339–344, 1999

DeVito AJ: Dyspnea during hospitalizations for acute phase of illness as recalled by patients with chronic obstructive airway disease. Heart Lung 19:186–191, 1990

Dilsaver SC, Kronfol Z, Sackelaves JC: Antidepressant withdrawal syndrome: evidence supporting the cholinergic over-drive hypothesis. J Clin Psychopharmacol 3:157–164, 1983

DiMartini A: Short gut syndrome, tricyclic antidepressants and prolonged QT interval syndromes. Psychosomatics 38:401–402, 1997

DiMartini A, Fitzgerald MG, Magill J, et al: Psychiatric evaluations of small intestine transplantation patients. Gen Hosp Psychiatry 18:25S–29S, 1996

Dracup K, Moser DK, Marsden C, et al: Effects of a multidimensional cardiopulmonary rehabilitation program on psychosocial function. Am J Cardiol 68:31–34, 1991

Dubin WR, Field HL, Gastfriend DR: Postcardiotomy delirium: a critical review. J Thorac Cardiovasc Surg 77:586–594, 1979

Fauerbach JA, Lawrence J, Haythornthwaite J, et al: Preinjury psychiatric illness and postinjury adjustment in adult burn survivors. Psychosomatics 37:547–555, 1996

Fauerbach JA, Lawrence J, Haythornthwaite J, et al: Preburn psychiatric history affects posttrauma morbidity. Psychosomatics 38:374–385, 1997

Fauerbach JA, Engrav L, Kowalske K, et al: Barriers to employment among working-aged patients with major burn injury. Journal of Burn Care and Rehabilitation 22:26–34, 2001

Fernandez F, Adams F: Methylphenidate treatment of patients with head and neck cancer. Head & Neck Surgery 8:296–300, 1986

Fiore MC, Jorenby DE, Baker TB, et al: Tobacco dependence and the nicotine patch: clinical guidelines for effective use. JAMA 268:2687–2694, 1992

Firlik AD: A piece of my mind. What we fail to see. JAMA 267:1328, 1992

Folks DG, Blake DJ, Freeman AM, et al: Persistent depression in coronary bypass patients reporting sexual maladjustment. Psychosomatics 29:387–391, 1988

Folstein MF, Folstein SE, McHugh PR: "Mini-mental state": a practical method for grading the cognitive state of patients for the clinician. J Psychiatr Res 12:189–198, 1975

France RD, Krishnan KRR: Psychotropic drugs in chronic pain, in Chronic Pain. Edited by France RD, Krishnan KRR. Washington, DC, American Psychiatric Association, 1988, pp 322–375

Freyhan FA, Giannelli S, O'Connell RA, et al: Psychiatric complications following open heart surgery. Compr Psychiatry 12:181–195, 1993

Gamba A, Romano M, Grosso IM, et al: Psychosocial adjustment of patients surgically treated for head and neck cancer. Head & Neck Surgery 14:218–223, 1992

Gattaz WF, Dressing H, Hewer W: Munchhausen syndrome: psychopathology and management. Psychopathology 23:33–39, 1990

Gil KM, Ginsburg B, Muir M, et al: Patient-controlled analgesia in postoperative pain: the relation of psychological factors to pain and analgesic use. Clin J Pain 6:137–142, 1990

Glass R, Mulvihill M, Smith H, et al: The 4 score: an index for predicting a patient's nonmedical hospital days. Am J Public Health 8:751–755, 1978

Goin MK, Goin JM: Psychological effects of aesthetic facial surgery. Adv Psychosom Med 15:84–108, 1986

Golinger RC: Delirium in the surgical patient. Am Surg 55:549–551, 1989

Good WV: Ophthalmology, in Surgical Subspecialties and Trauma. Edited by Stoudemire A. New York, Oxford University Press, 1993, pp 829–838

Grinker RR: Sex and cancer. Medical Aspects of Human Sexuality 10:130–139, 1976

Groenman NH, Soner HC: Personality characteristics of the cosmetic surgery insatiable patient. Psychother Psychosom 40:241–245, 1983

Grosso-Haacker M: Coping with an ostomy. Ostomy/Wound Management 33:43–46, 1991

Hackett TP, Weisman AD: Psychiatric management of operative syndromes—the therapeutic consultation and the effect of noninterpretive intervention. Operative Syndromes 22:267–282, 1960

Hall MA, Ellman IM: The patient lacking decision-making capacity, in Health Care Law and Ethics. Edited by Hall MA, Ellman IM. Minneapolis, MN, West Publishing, 1990, pp 236–311

Hammeke TA, Hastings JE: Neuropsychologic alterations after cardiac operation. J Thorac Cardiovasc Surg 96:326–331, 1988

Hamner M, Hunt N, Gee J, et al: PTSD and automatic implantable cardioverter defibrillators. Psychosomatics 40:82–85, 1999

Hazan SJ: Psychiatric complications following cardiac surgery. J Thorac Cardiovasc Surg 51:307–319, 1966

Heller SS, Frank KA, Malm JR, et al: Psychiatric complications of open-heart surgery: a re-examination. N Engl J Med 283:1015–1020, 1970

Heller SS, Ormont MA, Lidagoster LC, et al: Psychiatric aspects of the cardiac defibrillator. Psychosomatics 38:200–201, 1997

Henneman EA: The art and science of weaning from mechanical ventilation. Focus on Critical Care 18:490–501, 1991

Henriksen L: Evidence suggestive of diffuse brain damage following cardiac operations. Lancet 1:816–820, 1984

Holliday JE, Hyers TM: The reduction of weaning time from mechanical ventilation using tidal volume and relaxation biofeedback. Am Rev Respir Dis 141:1214–1220, 1990

Holmes J, House A: Psychiatric illness predicts poor outcome after surgery for hip fracture: a prospective cohort study. Psychol Med 30:921–929, 2000

Hravnak M, George E: Nursing considerations for the patient with a total artificial heart. Critical Care Nursing Clinics of North America 1:495–513, 1989

Jacobsen P, Holland JC: Psychological reactions to surgery, in Handbook of Psychooncology: Psychological Care of the Patient With Cancer. Edited by Holland JC, Rowland JH. New York, Oxford University Press, 1989, pp 117–133

Jelicic M, Bonke B: Preoperative anxiety and motives for surgery. Psychol Rep 68:849–850, 1991

Johnston M: Anxiety in surgical patients. Psychol Med 10:145–152, 1980

Jolly D, Finegan BA, Beach J, et al: Preoperative anxiety and myocardial ischemia: is there a relationship? (abstract) Can J Anaesth 37:77, 1990

Katz M, Abbey S, Rydall A, et al: Psychiatric consultations for competency to refuse medical treatment. Psychosomatics 36:33–34, 1995

Kimball CP: The experience of open heart surgery. Arch Gen Psychiatry 27:57–63, 1972

King TC, Smith CR: Chest wall, pleura, lung and mediastinum, in Principles of Surgery, 5th Edition. Edited by Schwartz SI, Shires GT, Spencer FC. New York, McGraw-Hill, 1989, pp 627–770

Klonoff H, Clark C, Kavanaugh-Gray D, et al: Two-year follow-up of coronary surgery: psychologic status, employment status, and quality of life. J Thorac Cardiovasc Surg 97:78–85, 1989

Knebel AR: Weaning from mechanical ventilation: current controversies. Heart Lung 20:321–334, 1991

Knorr NJ, Edgerton MT, Hoopes JE: The "insatiable" cosmetic surgery patient. Plast Reconstr Surg 40:285–289, 1967

Kornfeld DS, Zimberg S, Malm JR: Psychiatric complications of open-heart surgery. N Engl J Med 273:287–292, 1965

Lawrence JM: Reactions to withdrawal of antidepressants, antiparkinsonian drugs, and lithium. Psychosomatics 26:869–874, 877, 1985

Lazarus HR, Hagens JH: Prevention of psychosis following open-heart surgery. Am J Psychiatry 124:1190–1195, 1968

Lee WH, Brady MP, Rowe JM, et al: Effects of extracorporeal circulation upon behavior, personality, and brain function, part II: hemodynamic, metabolic, and psychometric correlations. Ann Surg 173:1013–1023, 1971

Levenson JL, Olbrisch ME: Psychosocial evaluation of organ transplant candidates: a comparative survey of process, criteria, and outcomes in heart, liver, and kidney transplantation. Psychosomatics 34:314–323, 1993

Limb D, Kay PH, Murday AJ: Problems associated with mechanical heart valves. Eur J Cardiothorac Surg 6:618–620, 1992

Lindal E: Post-operative depression and coronary surgery. International Disability Studies 12:70–74, 1990

Lipowski ZJ: Update on delirium. Psychiatr Clin North Am 15:335–346, 1992

Lucente FE, Strain JJ, Wyatt DA: Psychological problems of the patient with head and neck cancer, in Comprehensive Management of Head and Neck Tumors. Edited by Thawley SE, Panje WR. Philadelphia, PA, WB Saunders, 1987, pp 69–78

Lyons JS, Hammer JS, Strain JJ, et al: The timing of psychiatric consultation in the general hospital and length of hospital stay. Gen Hosp Psychiatry 8:159–162, 1986

MacArthur JD, Moore FD: Epidemiology of burns. JAMA 231:259–263, 1975

Macgregor FC: Patient dissatisfaction with results of technically satisfactory surgery. Aesthetic Plast Surg 5:27–32, 1981

McKegney FP, Schwartz BJ, O'Dowd MA: Reducing unnecessary psychiatric consultations for informed consent by liaison with administration. Gen Hosp Psychiatry 14:15–19, 1992

Mendel JG, Khan FA: Psychological aspects of weaning from mechanical ventilation. Psychosomatics 6:465–471, 1980

Metzger E, Friedman R: Prolongation of the corrected QT and torsades de pointes cardiac arrhythmia associated with intravenous haloperidol in the medically ill. J Clin Psychopharmacol 13:128–132, 1993

Middlekauff HR, Stevenson WG, Stevenson WL: Prognostic significance of atrial fibrillation in advanced heart failure. Circulation 84:40–48, 1991

Millar HR: Psychiatric morbidity in elderly surgical patients. Br J Psychiatry 138:17–20, 1981

Moritz A, Steinseifer U, Kobinia G, et al: Closing sounds and related complaints after heart valve replacement with St. Jude Medical, Duromedics Edwards, Bjork-Shiley Monostrut, and Carbomedics prostheses. Br Heart J 67:460–465, 1992

Morris PL, Badger J, Chmielewski C, et al: Psychiatric morbidity following implantation of the automatic implantable cardioverter defibrillator. Psychosomatics 32:58–64, 1991

Morton RP, Davies ADM, Baker J, et al: Quality of life in treated head and neck cancer patients: a preliminary report. Clin Otolaryngol 9:181–185, 1984

Mravinac CM: Neurologic dysfunctions following cardiac surgery. Critical Care Nursing Clinics of North America 3:691–698, 1991

Mumford E, Schlesinger HJ, Glass GV: The effects of psychological intervention on recovery from surgery and heart attacks: an analysis of the literature. Am J Public Health 72:141–151, 1982

Musselman DL, Evans DL, Nemeroff CB: The relationship of depression to cardiovascular disease. Arch Gen Psychiatry 55:580–592, 1998

Ness RG: "Change me": the request for rhinoplasty, in Contemporary Models in Liaison Psychiatry. Edited by Faguet RA, Fawzy F, Wellisch D, et al. Jamaica, New York, SP Medical & Scientific Books, 1978, pp 103–111

Neukam FW, Strauss J, Schliephake H, et al: Preoperative blood alcohol levels in patients hospitalized for prolonged surgical procedures. Klinik und Poliklinik fur Mund-, Kiefer- und Gesichtschirurgie, Medizinische Hochschule Hannover 47:53–55, 1992

Norheim C: Family needs of patients having coronary artery bypass graft surgery during the intraoperative period. Heart Lung 18:622–626, 1989

Orr DA, Reznikoff M, Smith GM: Body image, self-esteem, and depression in burn-injured adolescents and young adults. J Burn Care Rehabil 10:454–461, 1989

Pairolero PC, Trastek VF, Payne WS: Esophagus and diaphragmatic hernias, in Principles of Surgery, 5th Edition. Edited by Schwartz SI, Shires GT, Spencer FC. New York, McGraw-Hill, 1989, pp 1103–1156

Paterson JK, Burn L: General considerations, in An Introduction to Medical Manipulation. Edited by Paterson JK, Burn L. Boston, MA, MTP Press Limited, 1985, pp 1–7

Perloff JK: Congenital heart disease in adults: a new cardiovascular subspecialty. Circulation 84:1881–1890, 1991

Perry SW: Undermedication for pain on a burn unit. Gen Hosp Psychiatry 6:308–316, 1984

Perry S[W], Difede J, Musngi G, et al: Predictors of posttraumatic stress disorder after burn injury. Am J Psychiatry 149:931–935, 1992

Petrucci R, Kushon D, Inkles R, et al: Cardiac ventricular support: considerations for psychiatry. Psychosomatics 40:298–303, 1999

Phillips EH, Carroll BJ, Fallas MJ: Laparoscopically guided cholecystectomy: a detailed report of the first 453 cases performed by one surgical team. Am Surg 59:235–242, 1993

Phillips KA, Dufresne RG Jr, Wilkel CS, et al: Rate of body dysmorphic disorder in dermatology patients. J Am Acad Dermatol 42:436–441, 2000

Pollock BG, Perel JM, Nathan RS, et al: Acute antidepressant effect following pulse loading with intravenous and oral clomipramine. Arch Gen Psychiatry 46:29–35, 1989

Porter KA, Rosenthal SH: Postoperative mania: a case report and review of the literature. Psychosomatics 34:171–173, 1993

Pruzinsky IT: Collaboration of plastic surgeon and medical psychotherapist: elective cosmetic surgery. Medical Psychotherapy 1:1–13, 1988

Psychiatric drug use and surgery. J Psychosoc Nurs Ment Health Serv 37:9, 1999

Rankin SH: Differences in recovery from cardiac surgery: a profile of male and female patients. Heart Lung 19:481–485, 1990

Redelmeier DA, Rozin P, Kahneman D: Understanding patients' decisions: cognitive and emotional perspectives. JAMA 270:72–76, 1993

Reynaud M, Malet L, Facy F, et al: Hospital morbidity of alcohol use disorders in the center of France. Alcohol Clin Exp Res 24:1057–1062, 2000

Richelson E: Pharmacology of antidepressants. Mayo Clin Proc 76:511–527, 2001

Roca RP, Spence RJ, Munster AM: Posttraumatic adaptation and distress among adult burn survivors. Am J Psychiatry 149:1234–1238, 1992

Rogers M, Reich P: Psychological intervention with surgical patients: evaluation outcome. Adv Psychosom Med 15:23–50, 1986

Rosenbaum JF: Psychotropic drugs and the cardiac patient. Drug Therapeutics 10:111–121, 1980

Ruzevich SA, Swartz MT, Reedy JE, et al: Retrospective analysis of the psychologic effects of mechanical circulatory support. Journal of Heart Transplantation 9:209–212, 1990

Sadler JZ: Ethical and management considerations in factitious illness: one and the same. Gen Hosp Psychiatry 9:31–36, 1987

Sadler PD: Incidence, degree, and duration of post cardiotomy delirium. Heart Lung 10:1084–1092, 1981

Sanders KM, Stern TA, O'Gara PT, et al: Delirium during intra-aortic balloon pump therapy: incidence and management. Psychosomatics 33:35–44, 1992

Savageau JA, Stanton BA, Jenkins CD, et al: Neuropsychological dysfunction following elective cardiac operation, I: early assessment. J Thorac Cardiovasc Surg 84:585–594, 1982a

Savageau JA, Stanton BA, Jenkins CD, et al: Neuropsychological dysfunction following elective cardiac operation, II: a six-month reassessment. J Thorac Cardiovasc Surg 84:595–600, 1982b

Schlesinger RD, Daniel DG, Rabin P, et al: Factitious disorder with physical manifestations: pitfalls of diagnosis and management. South Med J 82:210–214, 1989

Schor JD, Levkoff SE, Lipsitz LAZ, et al: Risk factors for delirium in hospitalized elderly. JAMA 267:827–831, 1992

Sedgwick JV, Lewis IH, Linter SP: Anesthesia and mental illness. Int J Psychiatry Med 20:209–225, 1990

Seymour DG, Vaz FG: A prospective study of elderly general surgical patients, II: post-operative complications. Age Ageing 18:316–326, 1989

Shader RJ, Greenblatt DJ: Use of benzodiazepines in anxiety disorders. N Engl J Med 328:1398–1405, 1993

Shapiro PA, Kornfeld DS: Psychiatric aspects of head and neck cancer surgery. Psychiatr Clin North Am 10:87–100, 1987

Shapiro PA, DePena M, Lidagoster L, et al: Depression after coronary artery bypass graft surgery: effect on six-month outcome. Psychosomatics 39:224–225, 1998

Shaw PJ, Bates D, Cartlidge NEF, et al: Early neurological complications of coronary artery bypass surgery. BMJ 291:1384–1387, 1985

Shaw PJ, Bates D, Cartlidge NEF, et al: Early intellectual dysfunction following coronary bypass surgery. Quarterly Journal of Medicine 58:59–68, 1986

Shaw PJ, Bates D, Cartlidge NEF, et al: Neurologic and neuropsychological morbidity following major surgery: comparison of coronary artery bypass and peripheral vascular surgery. Stroke 18:700–707, 1987

Sheppeard H, Cleak DK, Ward DJ, et al: A review of early mortality and morbidity in elderly patients following Charnley total hip replacement. Arch Orthop Trauma Surg 97:243–248, 1980

Shipley RH, Butt JH, Horwitz B: Preparation for a stressful medical procedure: effect of amount of stimulus pre-exposure and coping style. J Consult Clin Psychol 46:499–507, 1978

Smith PLC, Treasure T, Newman SP, et al: Cerebral consequences of cardiopulmonary bypass. Lancet 1:823–825, 1986

Sonneborn CK, Vorstraelen PM: A retrospective study of self-inflicted burns. Gen Hosp Psychiatry 14:404–407, 1992

Sos J, Cassem NH: Managing post-operative agitation. Drug Therapeutics 10:103–106, 1980

Spacek A, Neiger FX, Krenn CG, et al: Rocuronium-induced neuromuscular block is affected by chronic carbamazepine therapy. Anesthesiology 90:109–112, 1999

Spencer FC: Congenital heart disease, in Principles of Surgery, 5th Edition. Edited by Schwartz SI, Shires GT, Spencer FC. New York, McGraw-Hill, 1989, pp 771–842

Spencer FC, Culliford AT: Acquired heart disease, in Principles of Surgery, 5th Edition. Edited by Schwartz SI, Shires GT, Spencer FC. New York, McGraw-Hill, 1989, pp 843–908

Stanton BA, Jenkins CD, Denlinger P, et al: Predictors of employment status after cardiac surgery. JAMA 249:907–911, 1983

Stengrevics S, Sirois C, Schwartz CE, et al: The prediction of cardiac surgery outcome based upon preoperative psychological factors. Psychol Health 11:471–477, 1996

Strain JJ: The surgical patient, in Psychiatry, Vol 2. Edited by Michels R, Cazenar JO. Philadelphia, PA, JB Lippincott, 1985, pp 1–11

Strain JJ, Lyons JS, Hammer JS, et al: Cost offset from a psychiatric consultation-liaison intervention with elderly hip fracture patients. Am J Psychiatry 148:1044–1049, 1991

Strauss B, Paulsen G, Strenge H, et al: Preoperative and late postoperative psychosocial state following coronary artery bypass grafting. Thorac Cardiovasc Surg 40:59–64, 1992

Surman OS: The surgical patient, in Massachusetts General Hospital Handbook of General Hospital Psychiatry, 2nd Edition. Edited by Hackett TP, Cassem NH. Littleton, MA, PSG Publishing, 1987, pp 69–83

Surman OS, Hackett TP, Silverberg EL, et al: Usefulness of psychiatric intervention in patients undergoing cardiac surgery. Arch Gen Psychiatry 30:830–835, 1974

Taylor KM, Wright GS, Reid JM, et al: Comparative studies of pulsatile and nonpulsatile flow during cardiopulmonary bypass, II: the effects on adrenal secretion of cortisol. J Thorac Cardiovasc Surg 75:574–578, 1978a

Taylor KM, Wright GS, Bain WH, et al: Comparative studies of pulsatile and nonpulsatile flow during cardiopulmonary bypass, III: response of anterior pituitary gland to thyrotropin-releasing hormone. J Thorac Cardiovasc Surg 75:579–584, 1978b

Tesar GE, Stern TA: Evaluation and treatment of agitation in the intensive care unit. Journal of Intensive Care Medicine 1:137–148, 1986

Tesar GE, Stern TA: Rapid tranquilization of the agitated intensive care unit patient. Journal of Intensive Care Medicine 3:195–201, 1988

Thomas RI, Cameron DJ, Fahs MC: A prospective study of delirium and prolonged hospital stay: exploratory study. Arch Gen Psychiatry 45:937–940, 1988

Thompson D, DiMartini A: Nonenteral routes of administration for psychiatric medications. Psychosomatics 40:185–192, 1999

Titchener J, Zwerling I, Gottschalk L, et al: Psychological reactions of the aged in surgery. Archives of Neurological Psychiatry 79:63–73, 1958

Van Sweden B: Rebound antidepressant cardiac arrhythmia. Biol Psychiatry 24:360–369, 1988

Verboskey LA, Franco KN, Zrull JP: The relationship between depression and length of stay in the general hospital patient. J Clin Psychiatry 54:177–181, 1993

Vieta E, De Pablo J, Cirera E, et al: Rapidly cycling bipolar II disorder following liver transplantation. Gen Hosp Psychiatry 15:129–131, 1993

Vik A, Brubakk AO, Rinck PA, et al: MRI: a method to detect minor brain damage following coronary bypass surgery. Neuroradiology 33:396–398, 1991

Vingerhoets G: Perioperative anxiety and depression in open-heart surgery. Psychosomatics 39:30–37, 1998

Voulgari A, Lykouras L, Papnikolaou M, et al: Influence of psychological and clinical factors on postoperative pain and narcotic consumption. Psychother Psychosom 55:191–196, 1991

Wade TC: Patients may not recall disclosure of death risk: implications for informed consent. Med Sci Law 30:259–262, 1990

Weddington WW: The mortality of delirium: an underappreciated problem? Psychosomatics 23:1232–1235, 1982

Weisman AD, Sobel HJ: Coping with cancer through self instruction: a hypothesis. Human Stress 5:3–8, 1979

Welch CA: Psychiatric care of the burn victim, in Massachusetts General Hospital Handbook of General Hospital Psychiatry, 2nd Edition. Edited by Hackett TP, Cassem NH. Littleton, MA, PSG Publishing, 1987, pp 438–447

Wellisch DK, Gritz ER, Schain W, et al: Psychological functioning of daughters of breast cancer patients, part I: daughters and comparison subjects. Psychosomatics 32:324–336, 1991

Wellisch DK, Gritz ER, Schain W, et al: Psychological functioning of daughters of breast cancer patients, part II: characterizing the distressed daughter of the breast cancer patient. Psychosomatics 33:171–179, 1992

West DW: Social adaptation patterns among cancer patients with facial disfigurements resulting from surgery. Arch Phys Med Rehabil 58:473–479, 1977

Witoszka MM, Tamura H, Ideglia R, et al: Electroencephalographic changes and complications in open heart surgery. J Thorac Cardiovasc Surg 66:855–864, 1973

Woodward JM: Emotional disturbances of burned children. BMJ 1:1009–1013, 1959

Zatzick DF, Kang SM, Kim SY, et al: Patients with recognized psychiatric disorders in trauma surgery: incidence, inpatient length of stay, and cost. J Trauma 49:487–495, 2000

Zeitlhoffer J, Saletu B, Anderer P, et al: Topographic brain mapping of EEG before and after open-heart surgery. Neuropsychobiology 20:51–56, 1988

Zisselman MH: Recognition and management of delirium in medical-surgical patients. New Dir Ment Health Serv 57:29–37, 1993

28

Solid Organ Transplantation

Christine E. Skotzko, M.D.

Thomas B. Strouse, M.D.

Bone marrow and solid organ transplantation are among the triumphs of twentieth-century medicine, resting on great advances in surgery, medical management of organ failure, and the clinical science of immunosuppression. Transplantation also is one of the most complex of all current medical interventions; it depends on efficient communication and transportation systems, on a national system of organ procurement and distribution, and on the coordinated activities of large multidisciplinary organ transplant teams at individual transplant centers.

Clinically successful and widely used bone marrow and solid organ transplantation developed rapidly during the 1970s and 1980s. Future biomedical developments will likely extend the clinically useful role of transplantation to organs for which transplantation is still experimental or rarely used (e.g., small bowel transplantation, multiple organ transplantation) and will help further extend the lives of patients with severe cardiac, lung, renal, and liver disease.

Counterbalancing the extraordinary advances in immunology and clinical transplantation, the potential limits to the role of organ transplantation in the health care system in the United States were increasingly clear in the early 1990s. Widespread use of solid organ transplantation is complicated by the relatively stable yearly number of donor organs available for transplantation, despite rapidly growing numbers of patients on organ transplant waiting lists (Belle et al. 1996). In addition, the competition for health care dollars among organ transplantation and other health care services has restricted the growth of organ transplantation, and third-party payers are taking more proactive roles in setting their own criteria for paying for transplantation. Public interest and patient advocacy groups are increasingly strident participants in the ethical debates surrounding organ allocation and distribution (Neuberger et al. 1998).

In this chapter, we provide an overview of the psychiatric aspects of organ transplantation. Full-spectrum—pretransplant candidate evaluation, perioperative psychiatric care, and long-term follow-up—organ transplant psychiatry (OTP) is a critical component of university/tertiary care hospital consultation-liaison clinical activity and research (Freeman et al. 1995). Clinically, the OTP specialist functions both as a provider of patient care and as a transplant team member. Clinical research opportunities in OTP are extensive, and important basic scholarly work now routinely appears in peer-reviewed journals. Today's OTP specialist needs specific knowledge and skills beyond those of the general consultation-liaison psychiatrist in order to optimally fulfill the clinical and transplant team membership roles.

The critical patient care roles of the OTP clinician include the diagnosis and treatment of psychiatric disorders in organ transplant candidates and recipients. OTP specialists also participate in the transplant candidate evaluation and selection process. This participation raises for the psychiatrist multiple ethical, legal, scientific, and public policy concerns. OTP specialists are called on to assess past, current, and predicted future transplant candidate medical treatment regimen adherence and to help manage other interpersonal and social behaviors that may interfere with optimal patient–transplant team relationships. The psychiatric assessment and management of patients with dysfunctional personality traits or formal personality disorders, patients with substance abuse histories or ongoing patterns of substance abuse, and patients with acute liver failure after drug overdose (usually with acetaminophen) are common challenges faced by the OTP specialist. Among the many psychiatric and psychosocial issues that are commonly directed to the OTP clinician for attention are transplant candidate or recipient neuropsychiatric disorders, treatment regimen nonadherence, and issues related to adaptation to post-transplant life.

The OTP specialist is also called on to fulfill many formal or informal functions as a member of the organ transplant team. The degree to which the psychiatrist is accepted as a member of the transplant team depends on his or her

- Ability to communicate psychiatric concepts effectively and succinctly to other team members
- Clinical judgment and the extent to which it is trusted
- Ability to effectively diffuse serendipitous or arbitrary adverse reactions of transplant team members to particular patients in order to permit optimal team decision making or patient care
- Ability to work collaboratively and effectively with other psychosocial services team members (e.g., medical social workers, psychologists)
- Effectiveness in providing informal support to distressed transplant team members

The broad goal of this chapter is to enhance the reader's clinical knowledge of current clinical practice issues and the research literature in OTP.

BIOPSYCHOSOCIAL ASSESSMENT OF TRANSPLANT CANDIDATES AND LIVING RELATED DONORS

Team Concept

The complexity of solid organ transplantation requires that a multidisciplinary team participate in caring for transplant applicants, candidates, and recipients as well as for living donors. In the assessment phase, persons with life-threatening illnesses are screened for appropriateness to enter the transplant candidate pool. The composition of the transplant selection team varies among centers. Almost all programs include internists and surgeons with specialization in the relevant organ system(s)—nephrologists and urologists, hepatologists and hepatic surgeons, cardiologists and cardiac surgeons, and pulmonologists and thoracic surgeons. Members of this group typically serve as gatekeepers, controlling the flow of patients into the evaluation phase.

Psychosocial data are important and are generally reviewed before an individual is accepted as a transplant candidate (Wolcott 1991) or living related donor. Exceptions occur when a transplant is performed on an emergent basis, which does not allow time for psychosocial

assessment. Interest in the use of psychosocial screening criteria has existed since the inception of organ transplantation with renal cadaveric and living donor transplantation (Eisendrath et al. 1969; Fellner 1971; Vidt 1971). The degree and extent of psychosocial evaluation varies among transplant centers and by organ system (Levenson and Olbrisch 1993b)

After a patient has undergone a general screening by the appropriate specialist, transplant centers commonly rely heavily on nursing coordinators to facilitate the patient's entry into the formal assessment phase. Coordinators ensure that all of the necessary medical and psychosocial assessments are performed. They also gather valuable information about patient and family motivation, understanding of transplantation, and potential for adherence to a complex posttransplant regimen. Because of the frequency of contacts, transplant nurse coordinators frequently provide significant support and reassurance to patients and family members during this very stressful time.

Social work assessment of the patient's home environment, support system, disposition, and housing needs is common to most programs (Levenson and Olbrisch 1993b). With the changing nature of health care services, many individuals seek treatment in areas that are geographically distant from their homes. It is not unusual for an insurance carrier to send a patient to a distant regional transplant center, which creates social upheaval for the transplant patient and his or her family. In addition, transplant programs often expect patients to temporarily relocate to minimize transportation delays when an organ becomes available and to facilitate follow-up. These factors underscore the importance of stable marital relationships, availability of involved others, and financial and geographic resources in considering transplant candidacy.

As adept as these providers are at recognizing distress, the involvement of a psychiatrist or psychologist with significant experience in working with severely medically compromised individuals is essential. Somatic symptoms of chronic illness may mimic symptoms of psychiatric illness, and accurate diagnosis is essential to ensure appropriate treatment (Mai 1987). Additionally, competence is required in the assessment of substance abuse (including abstinence and relapse risk), character disorder, and the potential for unacceptable or undesirable psychosocial outcomes. Consultation-liaison psychiatrists are exceptionally well suited to lead the clinical psychosocial assessment of applicants for transplantation. In addition to diagnosis, assessment, and case formulation, the organ transplant psychiatrist should be skilled at formulating and implementing individualized treatment programs (Surman et al. 1987a, 1987b; Wolcott 1991).

Evaluation of Living Donors

Whole or partial organs, sometimes donated by relatives and acquaintances, are an increasingly important source of tissue grafts (Spital 1994, 1997). For a variety of immunological and technical reasons, donation of kidneys by relatives has been a common practice for more than two decades, and living donors now account for about 20% of the kidneys transplanted in the United States. Despite such progress, inequities related to sex and race persist: in a study of trends from 1983 to 1990, Ojo and Port (1993) found that a greater percentage of white male potential recipients received kidneys from living related donors than did white women or persons of color of either sex.

The donation of partial organ segments, from both paired and single organ systems (lung, liver)—primarily by parents to children—is a growing transplant practice (Broelsch et al. 1990; Goldman 1993). For pediatric patients younger than 1 year, Sindhi et al. (1999) documented that live donor grafts are associated with superior graft and patient outcomes. Unique ethical and psychological issues often accompany consideration of related donation and have attracted a great deal of public attention.

No standardized criteria are available for the assessment of potential living related organ donors. Nevertheless, many transplant centers involve psychiatrists in prospective patient screening. Potential donors should be assessed for the same standard ingredients of informed consent that apply in any other presurgical situation. However, in assessing potential donors, a variety of other areas are also important, including

- The potential for coercion of the individual donating
- Any implied obligation of the recipient of the "gift" to his or her donor
- Evolving family relationships and the potential for the donor to have overvalued beliefs that long-standing interpersonal problems will be healed by the donation
- Personal, cultural, or religious concerns on the part of the donor about consequences of organ donation
- Potential for underlying donor psychopathology to be exacerbated by the psychobiological stress of donation

Most of the data on psychosocial consequences of organ donation concern kidney donors. Smith et al. (1986) reported that 97% of 536 kidney donors said that they would make the same decision again, despite the fact that a significant proportion (23%) attributed financial hardship to their choice to donate a kidney. Fellner and Marshall (1968) followed up a cohort of 12 donors for 10 years and reported similarly high rates of willingness to "do it over again." More recently, Toronyi et al. (1998) surveyed 78 living donors who were all in favor of living related donation; 63% would be willing donate to a friend, but fewer approved donation to a stranger (46%). None of these donors, who had a mean time since donation of 8.9 years, had personal health concerns.

In the only available study of psychiatric outcomes in donors of partial liver segments, Goldman (1993) described 20 patients from the University of Chicago. All recipients were children; 19 of the 20 donors were parents, and 1 donor was a grandmother. Preoperatively, families tended to make summary decisions to donate and tended to minimize risks to the donors. Parents presented idealized versions of their relationships and greatly played down personal factors, such as psychopathology, that might jeopardize their candidacy as donors. Psychological outcomes appeared to parallel findings from the literature on kidney donors. Donors of partial liver segments tended to do psychologically well in the immediate posttransplant period, with increased self-esteem and expressed satisfaction. One marriage dissolved; no major psychopathology ensued. The UCLA experience with a pilot program in parent-to-child partial segment donation confirmed these findings (Stuber 2000).

Rating Scales in Candidate Assessment

Two formalized rating scales are currently available for the clinical assessment of psychosocial factors in transplant candidates: the Psychosocial Assessment of Candidates for Transplant (PACT), developed by Olbrisch et al. (1989), and the Transplantation Evaluation Rating Scale (TERS), developed by Twillman et al. (1993). Both scales include weighted ratings for psychiatric diagnoses, substance abuse, health behaviors, adherence, social support, prior coping, and disease-specific coping. The TERS also rates affective and mental states.

These scales were developed in an attempt to quantify what many nonpsychiatric physicians believe is an inexact science: predicting risk of nonadherence. The use of rating scales encourages standardization of psychosocial data collection, promotes continuity for transplant services staffed by rotating consultants, and enriches the research base (Riether and Libb 1991). Eventually, such rating scales may have sufficient predictive power to drive selection criteria and to guide clinical psychosocial interventions.

Both the PACT and the TERS have good interrater reliability and predictive power, with similar conceptual items being fairly highly correlated with one another (Presberg et al. 1995). The PACT also has shown good interrater reliability and concurrent validity with other standard measures, such as the Minnesota Multiphasic

Personality Inventory and the Beck Depression Inventory (Olbrisch et al. 1989). In a comparison of the PACT and the TERS in a cohort of patients with liver transplants, the TERS had superior interrater reliability and correlated better with clinical outcomes (Twillman et al. 1993). Neither instrument can be said to have validity in and of itself because each requires an astute clinician to gather the necessary information to accurately complete the tools.

TRANSPLANTATION ISSUES THAT FREQUENTLY LEAD TO PSYCHIATRIC CONSULTATION

Ethical Considerations

Despite annual increases in the numbers of organ transplants performed in the United States, potential recipients still outnumber donors (Surman 1989). Transplant selection committees provide local gatekeeping for the precious resource of donor organs and are thus inherently involved in a selection process based on ethical, psychosocial, and biomedical factors (Freeman et al. 1992; Jonsen 1989; Orentlicher 1996).

Both clinicians and observers of the transplant field are increasingly aware of the intertwining nature of medical, psychiatric, psychosocial, and ethical issues in the assessment of organ transplant candidates (Craven and Rodin 1992; R.C. Fox and Swazey 1992; Surman and Cosimi 1996). This observation is not surprising because the tasks of psychosocial assessment require careful judgments about a patient's coping style, illness behavior, ability to form an alliance with the medical team, needs for emotional support, and financial and other material resources (Freeman et al. 1992) (Table 28–1). Beyond these tasks, psychosocial teams are called on to make complex predictions about posttransplant quality of life, the adequacy of family support systems, the effect of transplantation on preexisting psychiatric illness, and future adherence. It is generally agreed that psychosocial assessment should promote fairness and equal access and should emphasize the avoidance of harm to and discrimination against the patient (Lowy and Martin 1992; Orentlicher 1996). Frequently, however, mental health clinicians are aware of conflicts between the stated wishes or overt best interests of the patient (e.g., life extension, receiving transplant) and the reasonable needs of the transplant program (e.g., for adherence, solid sobriety, or enthusiastic participation by the patient in treatment) (Gellman 1989; Murray 1989).

Are there ethical remedies to these inherent problems? Most authors conclude that psychosocial selection

TABLE 28–1. Psychosocial screening criteria for solid organ transplantation

Absolute contraindications
  Active substance abuse
  Psychosis significantly limiting informed consent or compliance
  Refusal of transplant and/or active suicidal ideation
  Factitious disorder with physical symptoms
  Noncompliance with the transplant system
  Unwillingness to participate in necessary psychoeducational and psychiatric treatment

Relative contraindications
  Dementia or other persistent cerebral dysfunction, if
  • Adequate psychosocial resources to supervise compliance cannot be arranged OR
  • Of a type known to correlate with high risk of adverse posttransplant neuropsychiatric outcome (e.g., alcohol dementia, frontal lobe syndromes)
  Treatment-refractory psychiatric illness, such as intractable, life-threatening mood disorder, schizophrenia, eating disorder, character disorder

processes should include at minimum "informed consent" for patients—that is, a clear accounting of the purpose and use by the selection committee of psychosocial data (Lowy and Martin 1992). Surman and Purtillo (1992), Wolcott (1990), and Olbrisch and Levenson (1995) stressed the importance of developing scientifically valid, data-based criteria for exclusion. Loewy (1987) argued that committees should take care to avoid "social worth" considerations. Based in part on potential applications of the Americans With Disabilities Act to transplant candidate selection, Merrikin and Overcast (1987), Orentlicher (1996), and others discourage generic disqualification of patients because of mental conditions. Instead, they emphasize practical, case-by-case determinations based on more specific issues such as capacity to consent, previous health behaviors, previous participation in treatment for psychiatric disorders, and patient response to the direct provision of psychiatric care within the transplant program.

PSYCHIATRIC DISORDERS IN CANDIDATES FOR TRANSPLANTS

Patients With Cardiac Disease

Etiologies of cardiac disease warranting transplantation can be divided into two categories: congenital and acquired. Transplantation for congenital defects may occur in infancy or at any time during later adolescence or adulthood. Acquired cardiac disease, including ischemic and idiopathic cardiomyopathy, can be associated with severe congestive heart failure (CHF), ventricular arrhythmias, and pulmonary edema.

With rates of depression ranging from a point prevalence of 20% (Frasure-Smith et al. 1993) to 45% (Schleifer et al. 1989) in heart disease, depression is a significant comorbid factor. The relation between depression and cardiovascular disease is well documented in ischemic heart disease (Frasure-Smith et al. 1995; Westin et al. 1997). Evidence indicates that dysphoria and major depressive disorder increase the risk of myocardial infarction (Pratt et al. 1996) and mortality (Barefoot and Schroll 1996; Frasure-Smith et al. 1995). There is conflicting evidence on the effect of depression in individuals with CHF. Koenig (1998) evaluated elderly hospitalized patients with CHF and reported a 36.5% rate of major depressive disorder and a 21.5% rate of minor depression. Murberg et al. (1998a) reported a relatively low prevalence of depression; 13% had moderate to severe symptoms of depression, and an additional 27% had mild symptoms. Poor social support, social disability, and neuroticism were associated with depression (Murberg et al. 1998b).

Anxiety symptoms are often directly related to a patient's cardiac status. Kahn et al. (1987) reported that 83% of the individuals with idiopathic cardiomyopathy had probable panic disorder compared with 16% of the individuals with postinfarction heart failure, rheumatic heart disease, or congenital heart disease. Wells et al. (1989) found a significantly greater degree of lifetime and recent anxiety disorders in persons with heart disease compared with a group of individuals with no chronic medical condition.

The development of implantable cardiac defibrillators has resulted in salvation for many patients with uncontrollable arrhythmias but at a significant cost. Rates of significant anxiety and depression of 30% at implantation increase to 40%–63% over 1 year's time (Hegel et al. 1997). The number of shocks (device discharges) has been associated with increased health concerns, fatigue, sadness, and nervousness (Heller et al. 1998).

Kuhn et al. (1990) and Freeman et al. (1988b) reported adjustment disorders in 19%–25% of the individuals who were seen before heart transplantation. Dysthymia and neuropsychiatric syndromes accounted for an additional 4%–12% of the disorders in this population. Despite the relatively low rate of frank delirium reported, there is convincing evidence of the adverse neuropsychiatric effect of cardiac surgery (Barbut and Caplan 1997; Gokgoz et al. 1997; Hofste et al. 1997; Nollert et al. 1995; Vingerhoets et al. 1997; Walzer et al. 1997),

which many patients have undergone before being considered as candidates for cardiac transplantation. These data support those of Schall et al. (1989), who found evidence of cognitive difficulties in pretransplant patients with CHF. As impaired individuals decompensate medically, their underlying deficits are often more apparent. After cardiac transplantation, delirium and mood disorders are frequently seen in individuals with preoperative difficulties.

Patients With Pulmonary Disease

Patients who are candidates for single or double lung transplantation have serious limitations in daily functioning that are directly related to their underlying disease. Wells et al. (1989) examined the recent and lifetime prevalence of psychiatric disorders in a group of individuals with self-reported chronic lung disease and found that their lifetime risk for mood disorder, substance-related disorders, and anxiety disorder was significantly higher than that of a control group with no chronic medical condition. Kellner and co-workers (1992) found that the degree of dyspnea in patients with chronic pulmonary conditions was positively correlated with the degree of depression and anxiety.

Not surprisingly, Craven (1990b) found that 50% of a consecutive series of applicants for lung transplantation reported a history of psychiatric disorder. These disorders included organic brain syndrome (19%), major depressive disorder (16%), panic or anxiety disorder not otherwise specified (11%), and alcohol or other substance abuse (11%). Despite the significant degree of psychiatric symptoms found in chronic lung disease, there is little science that defines specific decision-making and treatment algorithms. Although lung transplants offer a survival advantage for individuals with cystic fibrosis and pulmonary fibrosis, no advantage has been shown for lung transplants for emphysema patients (Hosenpud et al. 1998). Clinical improvement in anxiety symptoms related to air hunger is generally seen with good graft function.

Patients With Liver Disease

Delirium, including hepatic encephalopathy, is the most common psychiatric disorder found in patients with liver disease both before and after transplantation. Trzepacz et al. (1989) found rates of hepatic encephalopathy approaching 20% in prospectively studied candidates for liver transplant at the University of Pittsburgh. "Subclinical" encephalopathy probably occurs at much higher rates (Trzepacz et al. 1988), although large-scale prospective studies that would document the incidence are not available. During the posttransplant period, the prevalence of delirium is also high. Although it is widely accepted that liver transplantation is associated with improvement in neuropsychological (Tarter et al. 1992) and neuropsychiatric functioning, secondary neuropsychiatric syndromes are diagnosed postoperatively in up to 33% of liver recipients (DeGroen and Craven 1992; DeGroen et al. 1987; Tollemar et al. 1988). Some patients have prolonged delirium that progresses to syndromes resembling dementia (DeGroen and Craven 1992).

Several primary psychiatric disorders have been reported in candidates for liver transplant. In the series described above, Trzepacz et al. (1989) found that 20% of candidates had current adjustment disorders, 4.5% had major depressive disorder, 9% met the criteria for alcohol abuse or alcohol dependence, and 2% met the criteria for abuse of other substances.

Patients With Renal Disease

Current major depressive disorder has been described in as few as 5% (Smith et al. 1985) and as many as 22% (Lowry 1979) of the patients undergoing dialysis. Robins et al. (1981) use the Diagnostic Interview Schedule to diagnose major depressive disorder in 8.1% of an unselected sample of 99 patients undergoing renal dialysis. Of these depressed patients, 50% had a history of major depressive disorder (Rodin and Voshart 1987); another 12% of the patients met the criteria for past major depressive disorder only. Cognitive problems and syndromes resembling dementia have been reported to be associated with chronic renal disease and dialysis (Alter et al. 1989; Nissenson et al. 1987). These disorders may reverse after renal transplantation, but definitive research in this area has not been done.

Patients With Diabetes

Major depressive disorder is common in individuals with diabetes (Carney 1998). Dissatisfaction with quality of life is more frequent in individuals with comorbid depression (Kohen et al. 1998), and nonadherence to dietary and exercise guidelines is common among individuals with comorbid psychological distress. The generally debilitating nature of diabetic complications, including painful nephropathy (Goodnick et al. 1997) and visual loss, has devastating consequences (Cox et al. 1998). Lustman et al. (1998) reported that cognitive-behavioral therapy is effective in treating depression when compared with a control intervention. Simulta-

neous pancreas-kidney transplantation is accepted treatment for type 1 diabetes mellitus and diabetic nephropathy (Freise et al. 1999). As this procedure becomes more accepted, it offers hope for diminished chronic consequences of hyperglycemia. There are sparse published data regarding the psychological effect of pancreatic or simultaneous pancreas-kidney transplantation beyond gross descriptions of "improved" quality of life (Milde et al. 1995; Zehrer and Gross 1994).

Patients With Chronic Intestinal Dysfunction

Patients who require small bowel transplantation are children or adults who have had a catastrophic insult to their bowel resulting in short gut syndrome (Pirenne 1996). Many of these individuals develop secondary hepatic failure as a result of prolonged total parenteral nutrition. The psychological effects of this illness are significant because of the inability to eat normally and debilitating diarrhea. These symptoms can have a devastating effect on family dynamics (Tarbell and Kosmach 1998). The propensity for malabsorption makes the likelihood of secondary (organic) mood disorders high. Small bowel transplantation originally was thought to potentially offer significant relief, but 1-year survival rates of 50% for small bowel transplantation alone and of 40% for small bowel transplantation in combination with liver transplantation are not encouraging (Brook 1998).

PSYCHIATRIC DISORDERS, THEIR RELATION TO SELECTION CRITERIA, AND PREDICTION OF OUTCOME

Table 28–1 shows proposed absolute and relative biopsychosocial contraindications for organ transplantation. In this table, current standards of practice are combined with provisionally data-based predictors of poor outcomes in the domains of graft survival, perioperative medical and psychological morbidity, and quality of life (Dew et al. 2000; House and Thompson 1988; Kuhn et al. 1988a, 1988b, 1988c; Levenson and Olbrisch 1987, 1993a; Surman 1992; Wolcott 1990).

Earlier surveys (Levenson and Olbrisch 1993b; Olbrisch and Levenson 1991) documented that 100% of responding liver transplant programs and high percentages of other organ transplant programs use psychosocial assessments in candidate selection. General consensus is lacking among the medical community about absolute and relative psychosocial contraindications to transplantation, with the exception of active or recent substance abuse, addressed below (see section "Substance-Related Disorders"). This disparity is reflected in minimal listing criteria conference summary papers published in *Transplantation* ("Consensus conference" 1998; Lucey et al. 1998; Maurer et al. 1998; Miller 1998) (Table 28–2).

When queried by Olbrisch and Levenson (1991) more than a decade ago, more than 70% of the heart transplant programs reported excluding patients with dementia, "active" schizophrenia, current suicidal ideation, history of multiple suicide attempts, severe mental retardation, current heavy alcohol use, and current use of addictive drugs. Other authors have proposed similar criteria (House and Thompson 1988; Kuhn et al. 1988a, 1988b, 1988c). Ethicists, legal scholars, and clinicians, however, have worried about the potential for prejudicial application of selection standards (Lowy and Martin 1992; Merrikin and Overcast 1987; Orentlicher 1996), particularly to underserved, medically ill psychiatric patients.

The imperfect consensus about psychosocial selection criteria for transplant candidates engenders valid criticism from outside the field. Questions are raised about the power of psychosocial variables to predict "good" and "bad" transplant outcomes. The field clearly lacks agreement about what "good" and "bad" or "acceptable" and "unacceptable" outcomes are (Olbrisch and Levenson 1995; Surman and Cosimi 1996; Wolcott 1990). Most transplant psychiatrists embrace the view that psychosocial factors should not be taken as immutable or as definitively precluding candidacy, a priori (Surman 1989, 1992). Instead, factors once rigidly considered as absolute contraindications to transplant are best viewed as risk factors and as targets for aggressive intervention. Treatable psychiatric illness remains frequently unrecognized and undertreated in the United States (Regier et al. 1993) and is probably more prevalent among potential transplant recipients.

The lack of coherent, uniform screening and acceptance procedures across transplant programs makes the comparative evaluation of outcome data across centers unwise. Availability of experienced transplant psychiatry support and longitudinal, comprehensive mental health services allows for successful transplantation in many individuals who might otherwise have significant morbidity (Skotzko et al., in press). The reality is that few transplant programs have this degree of integration with mental health services. As a result, outcome data across centers need to be viewed with caution because of the variable mental health services offered to individuals undergoing transplants.

TABLE 28–2. Summary of published listing criteria for solid organ transplantation

Organ system	Psychosocial criteria included	Compliance addressed	Psychiatric issues	Substance abuse
Heart[a]	Yes	Yes	Yes	Yes
Lung[b]	Yes	Yes	Yes	Yes
Liver[c]	No	No	No	Yes
Kidney[d]	No	No	No	No

[a]Miller LW: Listing criteria for cardiac transplantation. Transplantation 66:956–962, 1998.
[b]Maurer JR, Frost AE, Estenne M, et al: International guidelines for the selection of lung transplant candidates. Transplantation 66:956–962, 1998.
[c]Lucey MR, Brown KA, Everson TG, et al: Minimal criteria for placement of adults on the liver transplantation waiting list. Transplantation 66:956–962, 1998.
[d]Consensus conference on standardized listing criteria for renal transplant candidates. Transplantation 66:962–967, 1998.

Substance-Related Disorders

Alcohol causes major health problems in the United States, and its abuse accounts for approximately one-third of the patients with end-stage liver disease who present for transplant evaluation and one-half of all patients with end-stage liver disease (Loewy 1987). Additionally, alcohol-related cardiomyopathy is a common reason for heart transplantation, accounting for a significant, although unknown, measure of the 30% of patients with "idiopathic" cardiomyopathy who are evaluated for transplants (Burdine et al. 1990). Lucey and colleagues (1990; Lucey and Beresford 1992) pioneered an approach to the assessment of alcoholic patients for organ transplantation based in part on the seminal work of George Vaillant (1983). The Beresford Algorithm (Beresford et al. 1990) emphasizes careful diagnosis, the importance of recognition by the patient and family of alcoholism as a disease, assessment of social stability factors, and evaluation for the attainment of commonly accepted predictors of long-term abstinence from alcohol. Data from this group (Lucey and Beresford 1992) confirm that positive identification with a nondrinking person, good social support systems, effective time-structuring, and a smooth medical course are highly associated with abstinence in liver transplant recipients who are alcohol abusers. Rigid predetermined periods of sobriety for patients with end-stage liver disease are correlated with high degrees of mortality during the period in which they wait to complete the time requirement (Currie and Jones 1991).

The University of Michigan reported outcomes for 99 carefully selected alcoholic liver transplant candidates, of whom 45 received transplant: 5 relapsed, and of these, 2 had episodes of uncontrolled drinking (Lucey et al. 1992). In 1988, the University of Pittsburgh program reported good surgical outcomes and "low" rates of relapse drinking in short analysis (11.5%) (Starzl et al. 1988) and in extended analysis (11.5%) (Kumar et al. 1990). Most patients drank "socially" rather than in an uncontrolled manner. The University of Wisconsin group reported satisfactory surgical clinical outcomes in a group of alcoholic patients with end-stage liver disease, some of whom were drinking until the time of transplant (Knechtle et al. 1992). This suggests that family commitment to successful transplantation and medical variables were much more robust predictors of outcomes, including relapse drinking, than was duration of pretransplant sobriety.

Along similar lines, the University of Pittsburgh Liver Transplantation Program has continued to provide follow-up data on clinical outcomes among its alcoholic patients, confirming the finding that pretransplant duration of sobriety has little to do with medical-surgical survival outcomes or redrinking rates. Tringali et al. (1996) reported on 108 alcoholic liver recipients, showing no significant predictive relation of pretransplant duration of sobriety or participation in alcohol rehabilitation to clinical outcomes or relapse drinking. DiMartini et al. (1998) recently reanalyzed a larger cohort of Pittsburgh patients with similar results. Prospectively, DiMartini et al. (2001) found that 38% of individuals who had received transplants for alcoholic liver disease continued to drink alcohol. Overall, reported relapse drinking rates vary from 11% to 38%.

Although the results from the United States are reassuring, in the United Kingdom, Tang et al. (1998) reported alcohol recidivism rates approaching 50% in a retrospective case-controlled study of all patients who received transplants for alcoholic liver disease at their center. Most patients had been psychiatrically cleared and sober for a minimum of 6 months before transplantation. In the authors' confidential interviews with individuals surviving more than 3 months after transplantation, 28 of 56 individuals (3 were not assessed) had resumed drinking. Nineteen (32%) reported moderate use with a median relapse time of 8 months, and 9 (15%) reported heavy use with a median relapse time of 6 months. Patient recall of abstinence advice was unreliable, and most relapsed within the first year posttransplantation. Tang et al. (1998) made a rational case for ongoing posttransplant treatment of the underlying addictive disorder as the primary treatment focus rather than looking to preoperative abstinence for individuals with alcoholic liver disease who receive transplants.

This approach makes sense because accumulating outcomes data fail to support a significant relation between duration of pretransplant sobriety and successful posttransplant abstinence or medical-surgical results. Many programs have adopted 6-month sobriety rules (Lucey et al. 1997). After much uproar (Ferguson and Ferguson 1997), the United Network for Organ Sharing recently enacted guidelines (C.E. Fox 1998) that mandate 6 months of sobriety for eligibility for transplantation and liver allocation.

This trend, in part, emerges from extreme pressures brought to bear on the transplantation community by governmental agencies, the United Network for Organ Sharing, health insurers, the media, and the public to produce standardized selection criteria, particularly in the wake of highly publicized solid organ transplants for celebrities perceived by the public to have received special treatment or privileged access to organs. Such criteria may reflect a necessary although relatively unscientific pragmatic solution to the pressures of third-party payers, transplant advocacy groups concerned with morale among potential donors, and a candidate population increasingly representing persons with significant substance abuse histories.

Abuse of substances other than alcohol receives much less attention in the transplant literature. Gastfriend et al. (1989) convincingly showed that substance abuse in transplant recipients is highly correlated with nonadherence and graft loss. Additionally, immunocompromised transplant recipients are vulnerable to fungal, bacterial, and viral infections; lung injury; and multiple other medical complications of exposure to inhaled, injected, and orally administered recreational drugs. Even as consensus statements sponsored by the National Institutes of Health confirm the overall efficacy of long-term methadone maintenance programs for opioid-dependent patients (Office of Medical Applications of Research, National Institutes of Health 1998), many solid organ programs appear to arbitrarily require detoxification from maintenance opioids before consideration for transplant.

Psychotic Illness

Only a small, anecdotal literature exists about transplantation performed in patients with schizophrenia or other chronic psychotic illnesses. DiMartini and Twillman (1994) described successful liver and bone marrow transplants in two schizophrenic men. Sills and Popkin (1992) reported on a case of elective removal of a transplanted kidney from a patient who had recurrent organic psychosis, nonadherence, antisocial behavior, and alcohol abuse after his transplant. They also described a pancreas transplant recipient who reversed his request for removal of his graft after treatment of psychotic major depressive disorder. Riether and Libb (1991) described a patient with schizotypal personality disorder who psychotically decompensated before liver transplant, rapidly responded to hospital psychiatric treatment, and committed suicide a few months after his transplant. Most recently, Krahn and colleagues (1998) reported on a schizophrenic male who received a cadaveric renal transplant but who became nonadherent to his immunosuppressive regimen a few months after transplant. Graft rejection was managed medically, and it became clear that the patient's affiliational needs, previously met by thrice-weekly dialysis, had not been sufficiently replaced after his transplant. Psychosocial interventions and more frequent clinic appointments provided a satisfactory alternative and a good clinical outcome. Efforts are now under way to compile a registry of solid organ experience among North American programs offering transplantation to recipients with chronic major psychiatric illnesses (K.L. Coffman, C. Crone, personal communication, November 1998).

Kidney transplantation provides a unique alternative to the life-sustaining technology of chronic dialysis; other transplanted organs sustain life without durable "fall-back" technologies. With its attendant freedom from the logistical difficulties of chronic dialysis, Surman (1989) suggests that kidney transplant is almost always a better alternative for psychiatrically ill patients.

Suicidal Ideation and/or Transplant Refusal

It is uncommon for transplant teams to encounter actively suicidal candidates, inasmuch as impending or recently attempted suicide plans are typically associated with refusal by patients to consider transplant. Passive suicidality or hopeless resignation to death on the waiting list may occur in candidates who have unrecognized or untreated mood disorders related to their underlying organ failure, and such patients may benefit significantly from treatment for their depressions.

Some transplant candidates who are or have recently been suicidal, however, present acutely with fulminant organ failure caused by suicide attempts (e.g., acetaminophen-induced hepatic necrosis). These situations warrant consideration of complex ethical and clinical factors and are among the most challenging cases. Profound dynamic and countertransference factors such as rescue fantasies and the importations of desperate, guilt-ridden families often drive the group process of candidate evaluations by transplant programs, frequently with only minimal data directly available from the patient. Should

transplant be performed, for example, after an effectively lethal acetaminophen overdose in a comatose 18-year-old who has no other chance of awakening?

Transplant programs have neither the mandate nor the special ethical or legal authority to perform involuntary procedures on protesting patients. Patients who would likely benefit from a transplant but who competently refuse should be permitted to make such decisions. Desperately ill patients, whose mental status may preclude participation in decision making, may not protest but also frequently cannot provide meaningful consent. The posttransplant medication regimen and a perpetual patient role, which are epiphenomena of transplantation, impose a very different set of demands on the incompletely assenting patient than a discrete intervention such as cardioversion. These maintenance requirements may tip the scale of ethical considerations away from performing transplants on incompletely assenting or highly ambivalent patients (Lowy and Martin 1992).

Dementia and Mental Retardation

As mentioned earlier in this chapter, ethical and legal trends, including the Americans With Disabilities Act, increasingly charge gatekeepers of organ transplantation with a responsibility for decision making that does not discriminate against those with mental impairments (Lowy and Martin 1992; Merrikin and Overcast 1987; Orentlicher 1996). Candidates with certain kinds of dementia or mental retardation may have few risk factors for premature demise other than organ failure; to exclude them, a priori, on the basis of mental impairments is potentially discriminatory.

A preferable approach recognizes the possible adherence problems associated with dementia and retardation, seeks to characterize current functioning (particularly in the domains critical to successful self-care after organ transplant), and attempts to organize resources necessary for posttransplant care. With this approach, Benedetti et al. (1998) found 100% graft survival at 1 and 5 years in mentally retarded individuals who underwent renal transplantation. Extra scrutiny is warranted in cases in which the dementia syndrome has a progressive course (e.g., Alzheimer's or human immunodeficiency virus related) or in which transplantation and immune suppression have a high probability of exacerbating the dementia (e.g., alcohol dementia with chronic encephalopathy).

Treatment-Refractory Psychiatric Illness

No prospective studies have been done on outcomes in transplant recipients who had pretransplant treatment-refractory psychiatric illnesses. Surman and Purtilo (1992) and Surman and Cosimi (1996) wrote thoughtful reviews of a series of patients who had been judged "borderline acceptable" transplant candidates for reasons of age, malignancy, human immunodeficiency virus status, mental retardation, or extensive prior treatment for mood, character, and substance abuse problems. The authors emphasized the variable, and sometimes biased, ethical models that selection committees tend to apply to the anticipation of medical and psychiatric risks. They noted the lack of standardized ethical guidelines to determine selection policies among treatment-refractory patients with psychiatric disorders.

In the past, decisions to exclude transplant candidates with nonpsychotic psychiatric illnesses were often based on worries about posttransplant adherence. Reports from the cardiac transplant literature cast doubt on whether patients with prior nonpsychotic psychiatric diagnoses have more medical or psychological morbidity than do other transplant patients (Frierson and Lippmann 1987; Maricle et al. 1991; Skotzko et al. 1994; Surman 1989). Personality disorders, however, especially those that coexist with mood disorders or substance abuse, were found to predict postoperative surgical and psychiatric complications (Freeman et al. 1988a; Gastfriend et al. 1989; Kuhn et al. 1988c). Although the presence of a treatable recurrent nonpsychotic psychiatric illness should not exclude patients from transplant candidacy, a patient's refusal of necessary psychiatric treatment generally warrants refusal by a transplant program.

Adherence to Medical Regimen (Compliance)

The complex demands for adherence made on transplant recipients include strict adherence to a medication regimen, active participation in medical surveillance and follow-up regimens, abstinence from substances of abuse, and scrupulous record keeping.

A history of significant medical nonadherence raises valid concerns about future compliance. Two inferential lines of reasoning support this view: 1) that past compliance best predicts future behavior and 2) that nonadherence causes significant morbidity in organ transplant recipients. The latter point is well demonstrated: nonadherence contributed to graft loss in renal transplant recipients (DeLong et al. 1989; Didlake et al. 1988; Rovelli et al. 1989; Schweizer et al. 1990) and accounted for up to 26% of the deaths in a series of heart transplant recipients (Cooper et al. 1984). Fewer reports have been published of nonadherence in liver transplant recipients (Surman et al. 1987a, 1987b), which may reflect the

imperatives faced by patients whose organ failure cannot be managed by artificial means. Some investigators have shown that past adherence or nonadherence reliably predicts posttransplant behavior. Didlake and colleagues (1988) concluded that reliable predictors of compliance are unavailable for kidney transplant recipients, but other investigators have shown high correlations between pretransplant and posttransplant nonadherence (Rodriguez et al. 1991). Gastfriend and associates (1989) correlated substance abuse history, age younger than 30 years, mood disorder, and socioeconomic duress with nonadherence and graft loss. Other work supports the view that adults have fewer compliance difficulties than do children or adolescents (Hesse et al. 1990; Rovelli et al. 1989; Schweizer et al. 1990). Numbers of prescribed medications, mood state, employment status, perceived social support, and lower socioeconomic status correlate with increased risk for nonadherence (Kiley et al. 1993). Lower socioeconomic status may affect access to health care, perceived locus of control, health beliefs, feelings of relatedness to health care providers, and other important issues.

SELECTION COMMITTEE

The selection process varies from center to center. Most have a chartered working group that meets regularly and follows at least informal rules of operation. Individual candidates are presented, and the medical and surgical indications and contraindications are discussed. Strengths and weaknesses observed in the psychiatric and social work assessments are also presented. Generally, the group arrives at a consensus decision, which may include preconditions for acceptance such as "trials of compliance" or referrals for substance abuse treatment. The assessment, treatment, and monitoring of individuals with chemical dependence requires specific expertise (Stowe and Kotz 2001).

Stuber (1992) presented observational data from several different organ-specific pediatric transplant groups, noting the prominence of the transplant surgeon and primary pediatric transplant specialist in decision making. Information provided by various team members had variable weight in decision making.

The psychiatric liaison to a transplant selection committee can perform a valuable function by knowing as much as possible about the personalities, seats of authority, decision-making styles, recent triumphs and disappointments, and other elements of the program's culture. Such a familiarity with the selection committee cannot generally be attained by brief patient-centered consultation and requires a longitudinal role as a team member. When internal conflicts, bias, or irrelevant facts distort rational decision making, the effective psychiatrist–team member can provide observations to the group that help to free up impasses or redirect interpersonal frictions (R.C. Fox and Swazey 1992; Phipps 1991). Education about psychiatric disorders also helps the team understand difficult patients (Phipps 1991).

TRANSPLANT WAITING PERIOD

Patients expect less distress once they have been accepted for organ transplantation (Kuhn et al. 1988a, 1988b). However, increasing numbers of candidates are awaiting fewer available organs, and the waiting period continues to grow (Dec et al. 1991). It is estimated that nonemergent cardiac transplantation has essentially become a relic of the past (Mudge et al. 1993). Under the status quo, emergent cardiac transplant candidates may wait many months in an intensive care unit (ICU) to receive a donor organ, facing death and progression of their illness, which might make transplantation impossible. These events are often devastating for the patient, caregivers, and treatment team; they signal failure in the agreed-on goal of return to function and a relatively "normal" life.

The uncertain timing of transplantation stresses individuals (Freeman et al. 1988a) and, at times, entire families. Anxiety is a common complaint (Craven 1990b; Mai et al. 1986; Surman et al. 1987a, 1987b; Weems and Patterson 1989). Behavioral manifestations of anxiety include restlessness, irritability, insomnia, aggression, increasing somatic complaints, substance abuse, marital discord, and nonadherence; risk of suicide also is increased. Recognition of anxiety by treating physicians is important and can prompt referral for psychiatric assessment and treatment. Maricle et al. (1991) found that preoperative psychological distress did not negatively affect postoperative medical outcome in a population of heart transplant patients. This report warrants cautious interpretation because a support system that is ultimately unable to contain and manage distress preoperatively can result in life-threatening nonadherence postoperatively.

Coping is influenced by personality, previous experience, available support, and severity of illness. Zumbrunnen (1989) and Kuhn et al. (1988b) outlined the adaptive tasks that are necessitated by transplantation, including the knowledge that, in most instances, another human must die to become an organ donor. As a result, a morbid preoccupation with weather and television news

reports of shootings and accidents is relatively common (Weems and Patterson 1989).

Although it is relatively uncommon for renal and lung transplant candidates to await transplantation in the hospital, candidates for heart and liver transplants often require extended hospitalization because of medical decompensation. The incidence of delirium in this group varies widely and may complicate medical and supportive management. Milder forms of delirium are frequently overlooked and require careful inquiry and observation to allow treatment as needed (Surman 1989).

Frustration and demoralization also are commonly seen while an individual awaits transplantation. Patients' personality traits and ambivalence regarding transplantation may result in pathological behavior (Kuhn et al. 1988a; Phipps 1991). The patient and medical team need encouragement, support, and reassurance to work together effectively. Periodic reevaluation regarding continued commitment to transplantation is important. Some individuals may decide that transplantation, or the quality of life afforded by an inpatient wait for transplantation, is unacceptable (Collins et al. 1990). In the absence of delirium or imminently treatable psychiatric illness, their wishes should be respected.

Artificial organs function as a bridge to transplantation that increases the number of critically ill patients in the hospital and, ultimately, the number of candidates who can survive until transplantation. Renal dialysis prolongs life in patients with kidney failure, and bioartificial liver technology continues to progress, making "hepatic dialysis" as a bridge to liver transplantation increasingly viable (Dixit and Gitnick 1998; Wiles 1999). Cardiac assist devices allow many patients to ambulate and live outside the ICU for extended periods until a suitable donor is found (Hravnak and George 1989); these devices are becoming more common and may someday provide primary treatment for most patients.

The potential for psychological and medical complications associated with an artificial organ is great. These complications include loss of control, adjustment difficulties, delirium, infection, bleeding, and death (Levenson and Glocheski 1991; Levy 1981; Reedy et al. 1990; Ruzevich et al. 1990). Bridging technology is still primarily experimental, and availability is quite limited; the questions of eligibility and access are largely unanswered.

Support groups provide benefit to individuals awaiting transplantation and their families (Buchanan 1978; Suszycki 1986). Regional organ procurement associations welcome participation of patients and family members. Active involvement in public organ procurement activities can help patients and their families feel less helpless during the waiting period. The Transplant Recipient

International Organization (TRIO) provides a forum in which candidates can learn from transplant recipients, hear physicians address topics pertinent to transplantation, and help promote organ donation in the community. It also serves as an advocacy group that informs government and insurers about the needs of transplant recipients. For many transplant candidates, the opportunity to meet with a transplant recipient is a valuable experience that provides reassurance and peace of mind that professional intervention may not.

Although not extensively investigated, "beeper" and "telephone" anxiety are often encountered. Beepers and telephones, signaling a possible summons to the hospital, can raise expectations of imminent transplantation. Individuals may develop a sense of dread or foreboding associated with further beeps or calls. Some become homebound and strictly curtail all activity because they are concerned that they will miss "the call" to their transplant. Treatment interventions aimed at alleviating anxiety are sometimes necessary.

Aggressive treatment of psychiatric symptoms present during the waiting period is essential. Many individuals die of their underlying disease or its complications; improving quality of life during a patient's remaining months is a reasonable treatment goal. Table 28–3 delineates common issues in the psychotherapy of patients who are entering the realm of organ transplantation.

TABLE 28–3. Common psychotherapeutic issues for transplant patients

Transplant evaluation
 Acceptance versus rejection by the transplant team
 Acceptance of seriousness of illness
 Motivation for transplantation
 Expectations for future
 Death and dying

Transplant candidate
 Timing of transplantation
 Death and dying
 Preoccupation with donor organ availability
 Aggressiveness of care (assist devices)
 Quality of life
 Family expectations
 Dependency

Transplant recipient
 Graft rejection
 Dependency
 Changing roles
 Return to work
 Quality of life
 Death and dying
 Curse or cure?

Treatment Issues

A variety of feeling states and psychopathological conditions are part of the transplant waiting period. Symptom-oriented behavioral interventions, relaxation techniques, supportive psychotherapy, and psychopharmacological treatment can all be useful (Surman et al. 1987a, 1987b). Religion has long assisted humankind in understanding what might otherwise be experienced as overwhelming uncertainty. Faith plays an important role in well-being among some transplant recipients (Harris and Dew 1992).

Transplant candidates have significant constitutional symptoms of end-organ failure, which include psychophysiological symptoms. Examples are anxiety and air hunger among lung candidates; diffuse fatigue, anxiety, and heightened sensitivity to cardiac activity among heart candidates; profound circadian disruptions, fatigue, and depression among liver candidates; and depression and organic mental disorders among dialysis-dependent kidney transplant candidates (Rodin and Voshart 1987). Additionally, some transplant candidates have preexisting primary psychiatric disorders and will require management of these problems in the face of organ failure.

Psychologists can provide ongoing support and assistance with stress management and behavioral techniques. These interventions provide patients and families with alternatives to pharmacotherapy to cope with the anxiety of chronic disease states, the evaluation process, and waiting. Psychiatric nurses also may provide patients with reassurance and play a valuable role in educating nursing staff in the general hospital who come in contact with transplant applicants. Teaching methods are based on the individual's cognitive and affective state.

Psychopharmacological Considerations

The major classes of psychopharmacological agents and special considerations in patients with organ dysfunction and failure are reviewed in Table 28–4. Further discussions are available in Stoudemire and Fogel (1987), Trzepacz et al. (1991, 1993a, 1993b), and Beliles and Stoudemire (1998).

When close follow-up is feasible, we advocate efforts to provide relief for psychiatric symptoms whenever safely possible. The side effects of conventional tricyclic antidepressants are often not tolerated in candidates for organ transplant. In addition, new data (Beliles and Stoudemire 1998; Glassman and Preudhomme 1993; Glassman et al. 1993b) suggest that tricyclic use in any patient with heart disease is potentially problematic. Newer agents such as the selective serotonin reuptake inhibitors

TABLE 28–4. Psychopharmacological considerations in organ failure

Agent	Liver	Heart	Kidney	Lung
Mood stabilizers				
Lithium	1. No effect on clearance or drug levels 2. Ascites associated with lower lithium levels (new fluid compartment) 3. Diuretics will raise lithium levels	1. Rare conduction effects at toxic levels (which can follow lower cardiac output and decreased renal perfusion) 2. Rare sinus node effects limit treatment	May be used as necessary in patients with CRF and in those who are dialysis dependent; monitor levels, oral dosing after dialysis, and lithium in dialysate[a,b]	Unknown
Carbamazepine	1. Delayed metabolism, elevated levels 2. 5% of patients with normal liver function develop benign transaminasemia[c] 3. Risk of acute hepatic necrosis is 1:10,000 4. Known liver disease may increase risk; a relative contraindication to use[a]	Tricyclic antidepressant structure of carbamazepine: conduction effects possible; orthostasis	1. Conjugated OH metabolites accumulate, with tricyclic antidepressants 2. SIADH sometimes occurs in healthy patients; risk in patients with renal disease is unclear[d]	Unknown
Valproate	1. Slight risk of acute hepatic failure 2. Routinely elevated ammonia[e,f] may be intolerable in patients with chronic liver disease			
Gabapentin	Like lithium, no hepatic pathways involved in biotransformation and excretion		Identical to lithium	Unknown
Lamotrigine	No available data for liver failure or chronic liver disease	N-methyl metabolite may be cardiotoxic but typically not found at relevant levels in humans	Delayed clearance of glucuronidated metabolite	Unknown
Anxiolytics				
Benzodiazepines	1. Delayed metabolism, active metabolites, potential oversedation, and exacerbation of encephalopathy 2. Agents requiring only hepatic glucuronidation (oxazepam, temazepam, lorazepam) less affected than those requiring oxidation[g]	Cardiac depressant effects only in overdose	1. At physiologic pH, all are lipid-soluble, associated with low dialysance 2. Higher-than-normal levels of glucuronidated metabolites are often found, but these metabolites are often inactive 3. In patients with normal liver function, careful dosing is generally safe[h]	Respiratory suppression is a theoretical concern
Buspirone	Delayed clearance in patients with cirrhosis[i]		Clearance also delayed up to 50% in renal disease[j]	May have respiratory stimulant effects[k,l]

TABLE 28–4. Psychopharmacological considerations in organ failure (*continued*)

Agent	Liver	Heart	Kidney	Lung
Antipsychotics				
Butyrophenones	1. Delayed metabolism 2. Increased free fractions with hypoproteinemia	In high-dose boluses, may be arrhythmogenic[m]	Rare reports of toxicity[h]	Apparently tolerated and effective in patients with agitation
Phenothiazines	1. Delayed metabolism; anticholinergic delirium 2. 1%–2% risk of cholestatic jaundice with chlorpromazine	1. Orthostasis and tachycardia not tolerated 2. Generally benign ECG changes	Rare reports of toxicity[h]	
Clozapine	Delayed metabolism	Orthostasis and tachycardia not tolerated		
Risperidone	Delayed metabolism; 35% increase, 60% decrease in clearance in free fraction with hypoalbuminemia; dose decrease indicated	Possible Q-Tc prolongation; orthostasis	CRF associated with >50% decrease in clearance; dose decrease needed	
Olanzapine	Childs Pugh A/B cirrhosis only minimally alters clearance	No conduction effects; rare orthostasis	CRF has minimal or no effects on clearance	
Antidepressants				
Conventional tricyclic antidepressants	Impaired hepatic oxidative capacity, shunting, and hypoalbuminemia may lead to elevated free blood levels of parent compounds[n]	Quinidine associated with excess arrhythmic morbidity and mortality.[o] Because of quinidine-like action, tricyclic antidepressants are probably contraindicated in all patients with ischemic disease or history of ventricular arrhythmias[p]	Elevated serum levels of conjugated OH metabolites, which may be psychoactive and organotoxic[q,r]	1. Decreased tissue oxygenation may affect receptor affinity[s] 2. Protriptyline may have unique efficacy in patients with chronic lung disease to increase wake and sleep oxygenation[t,u]
MAOIs	1. Impaired liver function associated with slower clearance 2. Rarely hepatotoxic; hepatotoxicity is more likely with hydrazines (phenelzine and isocarboxazid) than with nonhydrazines (tranylcypromine and pargyline)[v]	1. No known contractility or conduction effects, but orthostasis may not be tolerable 2. Interaction with pressor agents used for surgery or resuscitation may cause severe hypertensive crisis		May be logistically impossible because of need for β-adrenergic bronchodilators
SSRIs	1. Fluoxetine and norfluoxetine half-life tripled in patients with cirrhosis[w] 2. Paroxetine levels elevated in patients with liver disease[x]	No known conduction effects; however, levels elevated and clearance delayed when hemodynamic compromise leads to hepatic congestion	1. Fluoxetine half-life and serum levels reported unchanged in patients with renal disease[y] 2. Elevated paroxetine levels reported in patients with renal disease[x]	
Bupropion	Delayed metabolism	Generally safe with regard to lack of adverse effects on ECG, preexisting arrhythmias, orthostasis, or pulse[z]	Metabolites may accumulate in patients with renal insufficiency and have been associated with delirium, seizure risks, and movement disorders[aa]	

TABLE 28–4. Psychopharmacological considerations in organ failure (*continued*)

Agent	Liver	Heart	Kidney	Lung
Trazodone/ nefazodone	Delayed metabolism in elderly patients;[bb] mCPP metabolite may cause paradoxical effects[cc]	Metabolite accumulates with left ventricular dysfunction;[cc] ECG effects rare[dd]	mCPP clearance depends on renal function[cc]	
Venlafaxine	Significant delays in elimination half-life with cirrhosis[ee]		Elimination half-life prolonged 50% in patients with renal impairment; elimination half-life increased up to 180% in patients on dialysis[ee]	
Mirtazapine	Clearance delayed c. 30% in cirrhotics	Like SSRIs, remarkably safe; dose reductions recommended	30%–50% decrease in oral clearance in CRF	
Psychostimulants				
Methylphenidate/dextroamphetamine	Delayed metabolism	Tachyarrhythmias		

Note. CRF = chronic renal failure; ECG = electrocardiogram; MAOI = monoamine oxidase inhibitor; mCPP = m-Chlorophenylpiperazine; OH = hydroxide; SIADH = syndrome of inappropriate (secretion of) antidiuretic hormone; SSRI = selective serotonin reuptake inhibitor.

Source. [a]Stoudemire and Fogel 1987; [b]Das Gupta and Jefferson 1990; [c]Jeavons 1983; [d]Viewig and Godleski 1988; [e]Eadie et al. 1988; [f]Cotariu and Zaidman 1988; [g]Howden et al. 1989; [h]Sellers and Bendayan 1987; [i]Dalhoff et al. 1987; [j]Gammans et al. 1988; [k]Rapoport 1988; [l]Kiev and Domantay 1988; [m]Metzger and Friedman 1993; [n]Leipzig 1990; [o]Glassman and Preudhomme 1993; [p]Glassman et al. 1993; [q]Lieberman et al. 1985; [r]McCue et al. 1989; [s]Series et al. 1989; [t]Simonds et al. 1986; [u]Trzepacz et al. 1993a, 1993b; [v]Schenker et al. 1988; [x]Tulloch and Johnson 1992; [y]Aronoff et al. 1984; [z]Roose et al. 1991; [aa]Strouse et al. 1993; [bb]von Moltke et al. 1993; [cc]Caccia et al. 1981; [dd]Spar 1987; [ee]Troy et al. 1994.

(SSRIs), bupropion, venlafaxine, nefazodone, or mirtazapine are generally well tolerated by persons with end-organ disease. Special considerations are addressed in Table 28–4.

Profoundly fatigued patients often benefit remarkably from treatment with psychostimulants such as methylphenidate or dextroamphetamine. Time-limited treatment (with the end point often defined by transplant) with 5–10 mg twice daily can vastly improve patients' functioning in and experience of the waiting period.

Clinically significant pretransplant anxiety states can be quite difficult to treat, particularly in individuals who have had intermittent delirium. Typically, psychiatrists have invoked the safety of the benzodiazepines oxazepam, temazepam, and lorazepam, which have no active metabolites and are glucuronidated to water-soluble compounds (Greenblatt and Shader 1987). However, benzodiazepines are minimally dialyzable and may worsen confusion in individuals with hepatic encephalopathy (Surman 1992, 1994) and low perfusion states associated with cardiac failure. Some reports implicate endogenous γ-aminobutyric acid (GABA)-ergic compounds in the encephalopathy of liver failure (Basile et al. 1991, 1994; Pomier-Layrargues et al. 1994). Alternatives to careful benzodiazepine dosing include buspirone, which may have special efficacy in the chronic anxiety associated with lung disease (Rapoport 1988); high-potency neuroleptics such as haloperidol and droperidol; and novel compounds such as risperidone and olanzapine. Diphenhydramine should be avoided whenever possible because its anticholinergic effects may exacerbate delirium.

PERIOPERATIVE ISSUES: ACUTE CLINICAL SYNDROMES AND THEIR MANAGEMENT

Medical and psychiatric complications that manifest in the ICU after transplantation depend on several factors, including procedure performed, length of surgery, intraoperative complications, metabolic disruption, physiologic state, and medications. Extubation is generally performed in the first 24–48 hours after transplantation, assuming no complications interfere; this allows for easier communication with the patient and assessment of cognitive state. Delirium in the transplant ICU is relatively common and should be high on the differential diagnosis in agitated and "depressed" recipients.

Procedures vary among transplant programs regarding the nature and extent of isolation during the post-transplant period. Strict isolation is relatively uncommon. When used, it can leave mildly delirious recipients feeling paranoid, isolated, and alone. Most recipients understand the risk of infection and admonish staff entering their rooms without appropriate attention to isolation procedures.

Donor Information

Questions often arise after transplantation about the individual who donated his or her organ; recipients or their families may inquire about the age, race/ethnicity, sex, nature of death, and geographic location of the donor. Some programs provide limited information about the donor, such as age and sex. Overall, the anonymity of donor and recipient has been maintained by transplant and procurement programs as a fundamental aspect of the transplantation process. Recipient families are encouraged to write an anonymous letter thanking the donor family, which is passed through the organ procurement association for anonymous delivery to the donor family. This is done to prevent unsolicited contact between the donor family and the recipient.

A movement is under way to legislate increased communication between donor families and recipients (Youngner et al. 1998). This grassroots movement is being pursued by families of organ donors. Despite their claims of support from the general transplant community, the consensus among mental health care providers in transplantation appears at odds with the loss of anonymity and the potential for unlimited discourse between transplant recipients and donor families. Many transplant programs have clinical experience with donor–recipient "accidental" acquaintances, which have had associated boundary violation issues. Clinical vignettes of these boundary violations include a donor's mother wanting to celebrate the donor's birthday annually with the recipient, requests for cash and other tangible goods that the donor had previously provided to their family, and frequent intrusive visits by donor family members to recipient's home.

Medication Regimen

The task of learning a new, complex medication regimen begins immediately after recovery from anesthesia. Patients are presented with new medications that may be given intravenously or orally. Many unfamiliar tablets of various sizes, to be taken at different times of the day, begin to appear. Indoctrination into the appropriate form of record keeping generally begins early, with lists of medications that the recipient and family are expected to commit to memory by name and appearance. Intravenous medication may be required even after hospital discharge, and families may be expected to manage intravenous lines and drains with only occasional nursing supervision. Vital signs, including weight, heart rate, blood pressure, and temperature, will need to be checked.

Education about warning signs of impending rejection and infection is given with admonitions to "call with any problems." The focus of these efforts is to provide the recipient and family with the tools necessary to understand the treatment regimen, cooperate with care, and remain compliant (Merz 1998). Attempts to use less personnel-intensive teaching tools have included videotapes, which were found to be effective when used in conjunction with other media (Steinberg et al. 1996).

At discharge, many individuals experience anxiety. Surman et al. (1987a, 1987b) and Freeman et al. (1988a, 1988b) noted adjustment difficulties in liver and heart transplant recipients before discharge. The expectation that recipients will be responsible and responsive to a team of nurses and physicians with very specific agendas is sometimes overwhelming to the patient. This may be at least partially related to a sense of unfamiliarity with the new organ, a feeling of being overwhelmed with the new, frequently changing medication regimen, and a sense of uncertainty about the potential for possible life-threatening infection and rejection episodes. Potential etiologies may include low-grade delirium and the relatively large doses of steroids and high levels of immunosuppressants at discharge. These agents are associated with significant neuropsychiatric side effects, which are addressed later in this chapter.

Rejection

The concept of rejection is explained early and often to transplant candidates and recipients. The potential for the individual's own body to attack and damage the much-desired organ can carry great symbolic meaning. Although mild rejection is a normal part of the posttransplant course, many recipients convince themselves that they will not have such problems. This reaction usually represents fear and resultant denial. Sutton and Murphy (1989) cited fear of rejecting a transplanted kidney as a major stressor reported at 2- and 4-year follow-up assessments.

Routine surveillance is intended to detect rejection before it becomes severe. Frequent follow-up and routine laboratory assessments attempt to uncover early evidence of mild asymptomatic rejection. When detected, rejection is sometimes met with disbelief and fear by the recipient. Surman (1989) noted that allograft rejection was generally associated with withdrawal, depression, and reactivation of feelings associated with previous illness. Symptoms suggestive of severe rejection are sometimes ignored or not reported by patients until the recipient is no longer able to function independently. Recipients who have had prolonged difficult hospitalizations preceding or as a result of the transplant surgery may develop a posttraumatic stress disorder that results in this life-threatening avoidance (Dew et al. 1998).

Collusion between recipient and family in denying symptoms results from many factors, including fatigue resulting from transplantation after an extended wait for a donor organ or a prolonged postoperative course; ambivalence resulting from the realization that transplantation was not a "cure"; interpersonal discord, altering how couples communicate; and lack of financial resources, arising from geographic relocation and the expense of immunosuppressant medications.

Adjustment to Medical Complications or Retransplantation

Despite careful preparation by transplant teams, many candidates approach transplantation with high hopes that they will have a smooth medical course. Such hopes can represent defenses to ward off overwhelming anxiety. For some patients, however, the inability to imagine a less-than-perfect course conceals a lack of preparation for a prolonged medical stay and the anxieties that go with medical uncertainty. Such patients are at high risk for becoming overwhelmingly anxious, regressed, uncooperative, depressed, and noncompliant.

The need for retransplantation may arise within days to years of the first surgery and can be caused by primary graft failure, vascular occlusion, chronic or acute rejection, nonadherence, and other factors. Survival rates vary by organ system for retransplantation. Emergent retransplantation has poor results and is not pursued in most cases. Survival rates for nonemergent retransplantation generally are less favorable than for the initial procedure (Bryan et al. 1998; John et al. 1999; Markmann et al. 1999; U.K. National Transplant Database 1997).

Patients react to the possibility of retransplantation in many ways. Some are delirious or obtunded, and decisions must be made on the basis of prior discussions or by proxies. Decisions to decline a retransplantation procedure should be supported, unless frank, quickly treatable psychiatric difficulty exists. Significant primary and secondary mood and anxiety symptoms often accompany graft failure and its treatment. These can affect critical decision making by the patient. Longitudinal psychiatric intervention is very important. A psychotherapeutic relationship and competent somatic treatment are often necessary to support a patient who is facing retransplantation.

When rejection and/or retransplantation are largely the result of noncompliance or substance abuse relapse, or when other behavioral factors have jeopardized the patient's—and the graft's—survival, a crisis ensues for the patient, his or her family, and the transplant service (Surman and Purtillo 1992). Transplant teams invest extraordinary effort and resources in their patients. It is often very difficult for the transplant team not to offer retransplantation, even with behavior that might have precluded a first transplant. Refusal of third-party payers to subsidize repeat transplantation may diffuse some of the team's sense of responsibility for the recipient's immediate clinical situation.

NEUROPSYCHIATRIC PROBLEMS IN THE PERIOPERATIVE PERIOD

Delirium and Disorders of Consciousness

Acute secondary mental disorders are common in the perioperative period among recipients of all types of solid organs. In view of the reported prevalence rate of 20%–30% for clinically evident hepatic encephalopathy before liver transplant (Trzepacz et al. 1989), it is not surprising that up to one-third of all liver transplant recipients have an acute neuropsychiatric syndrome in the perioperative period (Craven 1991; DeGroen and Craven 1992; DeGroen et al. 1987; Strouse et al. 1998; Surman 1994; Tollemar et al. 1988). A recent report on clinical outcomes in nine liver recipients who were sustained until transplant by the bioartificial liver found minimal permanent neurological sequelae but did not comment on acute postoperative delirium (Coffman et al. 1996). As many as 70% of lung transplant recipients may experience postoperative delirium (Craven 1990a). Heart and kidney transplant recipients have acute delirium less frequently. Opportunistic infections of the central nervous system (CNS) are often heralded in transplant recipients by delirium or other mental status changes (Boon et al. 1990; Conti and Tubin 1988; Surman 1994; Surman and Purtillo 1992). Common etiological factors for delirium in transplant recipients include the consequences to the brain of chronic organ failure, residua of general anesthesia, lengthy transplant surgeries, volume and electrolyte shifts associated with reperfusion of the new organ, cyclosporine/tacrolimus/corticosteroid loading, postoperative opiate treatment, early graft dysfunction, fever,

coagulopathy, infection, and other processes (Abbasoglu et al. 1998; Dubin et al. 1979; Plevak et al. 1989). Psychoactive substance withdrawal must also be considered.

A growing body of literature links cyclosporine, tacrolimus, and other elements of the transplant pharmacopoeia with postoperative delirium and neurotoxicity (Adams et al. 1987; Belli et al. 1993; Berden et al. 1985; Bhatt et al. 1988; Craven 1991; De Bruijn et al. 1989; DeGroen and Craven 1992; DeGroen et al. 1987; DiMartini et al. 1997; European FK-506 Multicentre Liver Study Group 1994; Frank et al. 1993; Fryer et al. 1996; Kabeer et al. 1995; Laubenberger et al. 1996; Lee et al. 1996; Lopez et al. 1991; Palmer and Toto 1991; Strouse 1996; C.B. Thompson et al. 1984; Tollemar et al. 1988; U.S. Multicenter FK506 Liver Study Group 1994; Vogt et al. 1988; Wilczek et al. 1984; Winnock et al. 1993). Among patients who have received organ transplants, recipients of liver transplants are most susceptible to these adverse events (Bennett and Norman 1986; Boon et al. 1990; Conti and Tubin 1988; Craven and Rodin 1992; De Bruijn et al. 1989; DeGroen et al. 1987; Lopez et al. 1991; Plevak et al. 1989; Surman and Purtillo 1992; Tollemar et al. 1988; Trzepacz et al. 1993a, 1993b), with large centers reporting some degree of cyclosporine or tacrolimus neurotoxicity in 25%–40% of liver recipients in the postoperative phase. There are fewer case series describing these syndromes in recipients of donor hearts (Cooper et al. 1989; Lane et al. 1988; McManus et al. 1992) or kidneys (Palmer and Toto 1991).

The first signs of immunosuppressant neurotoxicity are often seen in the ICU. Patients may be lethargic or confused and may require reintubation despite previously adequate respiratory functioning (Craven 1991). Variable symptoms are seen; they include seizures, cortical blindness, aphasia, paresthesia, neuropathy, delusions, and agitation (Bennett and Norman 1986; DeGroen et al. 1987; Strouse et al. 1998). Obtundation, deeper coma, status epilepticus, and neurological death rarely occur (Adams et al. 1987). Diffuse white matter changes are seen on magnetic resonance imaging (MRI), accompanied by symmetric electroencephalographic (EEG) dysrhythmia. Cyclosporine holidays have been associated with symptom remission and normalization of white matter changes in some patients (DeGroen et al. 1987).

Although it is generally seen as an acute postoperative complication, immunosuppressant neurotoxicity sometimes occurs months after organ transplant (De Bruijn et al. 1989; Strouse et al. 1998). New-onset cyclosporine-related delirium, complex partial seizures, cortical blindness, frontal lobe syndromes, and secondary mood syndromes have been observed 3–6 months after liver transplant. A scholarly review of the possible mechanisms of cyclosporine neurotoxicity is found in DeGroen and Craven (1992). Table 28–5 summarizes cyclosporine and tacrolimus toxicity symptoms.

Despite early enthusiasm to the contrary, prospective trials have concluded that tacrolimus may be associated with greater, rather than less, neurotoxicity when compared with cyclosporine (Eidelman et al. 1991; Frank et al. 1993; Lopez et al. 1991). A prospective 1-year randomized trial of tacrolimus and cyclosporine in liver recipients showed nearly twice the rates of neurotoxicity in the tacrolimus group (Mueller et al. 1995). A consecutive series of 100 liver recipients treated with tacrolimus and prospectively followed up by Burkhalter and colleagues (1994) had equally high rates of "severe" posttransplant neurotoxicity (34%), including central pontine myelinolysis.

Other agents used commonly in organ transplantation that are associated with delirium include corticosteroids (Kershner and Wang-Cheng 1989; Lewis and Smith 1983) and OKT3 (Coleman and Norman 1990).

Although the general principles of assessing and managing delirium (see Chapter 15, this volume) pertain to patients with organ transplants, some special considerations are warranted. For example, benzodiazepines may worsen hepatic encephalopathy or lead to further behavioral disinhibition, presumably via increased GABAergic activity (Basile and Jones 1988; Basile et al. 1991). The benzodiazepine antagonist flumazenil can temporarily reverse the impaired level of consciousness found in advanced hepatic encephalopathy and benzodiazepine intoxication in some patients (Basile et al. 1994; Grimm et al. 1988; Pomier-Layrargues et al. 1994). Heart recipients with delirium may have new CNS vascular insults associated with cardiopulmonary bypass (Shaw et al. 1985).

TABLE 28–5. Some neuropsychiatric syndromes associated with solid organ transplantation and with immune suppression by cyclosporine and tacrolimus

---

Delirium

Seizures

Headache/visual symptoms

Cortical blindness

Isolated visual hallucinations

Dementia-like syndromes

Frontal lobe syndromes

Secondary mood, anxiety, thought disorders

Movement disorders

Central pontine myelinolysis

Impaired taste sensation

Incontinence

Sexual dysfunction

High-potency neuroleptic agents such as haloperidol and droperidol are effective in treating agitation or posttransplant delirium; however, patients who have received liver transplants may have special vulnerability to extrapyramidal symptoms because of the effects of chronic liver disease on the basal ganglia (Neiman et al. 1990). Heart recipients are possibly sensitive to butyrophenone-induced hypotension or arrhythmias (Metzger and Friedman 1993). Kast's (1989) theoretical concern that cyclosporine's immunosuppressive benefits might be opposed by dopamine-blocking agents (i.e., neuroleptics, including metoclopramide) is unconfirmed by clinical observations. The novel antipsychotic olanzapine has been increasingly used by consultation psychiatrists to treat psychotically agitated delirious patients; it has efficacy equal to that of haloperidol and few extrapyramidal side effects (Sipahimalani and Masand 1998). Olanzapine is also helpful because it is strongly sedating and thus induces sleep in agitated delirious patients, for whom resetting sleep-wake patterns may provide immense benefit.

The practice of combining moderate dosages of butyrophenones (haloperidol 2–4 mg iv every 6–8 hours, droperidol 2–4 mg iv every 2–4 hours, or olanzapine 2.5–5.0 mg po twice a day) with benzodiazepines that do not have active metabolites (lorazepam 1–4 mg iv every 4–6 hours) often provides sufficient management of the acute symptoms of delirium. The Massachusetts General Hospital group has reported use of 250–2,000 mg/24 hours of intravenous haloperidol in the treatment of patients with postcardiotomy delirium without ill effects (Tesar et al. 1985). Lung recipients also appear to tolerate large cumulative amounts of haloperidol without adverse side effects (Craven 1990a). An extensive review of the differential diagnosis and pharmacological treatment of delirium in transplant recipients is available in reviews by Trzepacz and associates (1991, 1993a, 1993b).

Seizures

At some centers, generalized tonic-clonic seizures and complex partial seizures are the most commonly reported neuropsychiatric complications of transplant; liver recipients may be the most likely to be afflicted (Adams et al. 1987; Estol et al. 1989a, 1989b; C.B. Thompson et al. 1984; Vogt et al. 1988). Seizures also were reported in 10% of the patients in a series of lung transplant recipients (Craven 1990a). Cyclosporine is often implicated (Craven 1991; Estol et al. 1989a, 1989b), directly or indirectly; associated CNS lesions, including white matter changes, microinfarcts, central pontine myelinolysis, and edema, are commonly found

(Estol et al. 1989a, 1989b). In early studies, both seizure frequency and the severity of the neuropathology appeared to be less with tacrolimus (FK-506) than with cyclosporine (Eidelman et al. 1991). Unfortunately, contrary data were published more recently (Frank et al. 1993). OKT3, a drug that is used to prevent rejection, also has been associated with posttransplant seizures (Coleman and Norman 1990), as have acyclovir and ganciclovir (Trzepacz et al. 1993a, 1993b).

Both generalized and partial complex status epilepticus have been described in transplant recipients. These dramatic complications have generally occurred within 2 weeks of transplantation (Surman 1989; C.B. Thompson et al. 1984; Vogt et al. 1988) and occasionally may be refractory to conventional treatment with benzodiazepines and standard antiepileptic agents. Cyclosporine holidays are sometimes necessary to bring seizures under control, in part because correction of magnesium imbalances can be impossible with continued cyclosporine therapy.

Headache and Visual Symptoms

Severe headache is a common complaint among transplant recipients who are taking cyclosporine (Adams et al. 1987). The headache may wax and wane with peak blood levels, and medication adherence can be threatened if this complication is left unattended. Headache occurs less commonly among patients who are taking tacrolimus. In our experience, cyclosporine headache can resemble classical migraine, with scotomata and symptoms mimicking transient ischemic attacks, but the pain does not respond to ergot alkaloids, opiates, or sumatriptan.

Severe headache may signal other neurological problems in patients who have received organ transplant. The most dramatic among these is transient cortical blindness, a known complication of cyclosporine therapy (Ghalie et al. 1990; Rubin and Kang 1987; Wilson et al. 1988). After liver transplant, at the peak of headache crisis, we have seen cortical blindness associated with complex partial seizure activity and bilateral occipital abnormalities visible on brain MRI. Hinchey and colleagues (1996) characterized this as a "reversible posterior leukoencephalopathy syndrome." Seizures, blindness, and edema generally resolve with a cyclosporine holiday. Because cyclosporine is known to induce hypertension, severe headache also may herald a hypertensive crisis.

Isolated visual hallucinations are also attributed to cyclosporine in patients who do not have delirium following transplant (Noll and Kulkarni 1984) and are reported with ganciclovir antiviral therapy (Faulds and Heel 1990; M.N. Thompson and Jeffries 1989) as well as with many of the antibiotics used to treat patients posttransplantation (Trzepacz et al. 1993a, 1993b). Blurred vision is another common complaint; maintenance of lower cyclosporine levels is sometimes helpful.

Secondary Mood, Anxiety, and Thought Disorders

Uncontrolled studies report that the incidence of secondary ("organic") mood syndromes (depressed or manic/hypomanic) and major depressive disorder is 68% among recipients of heart transplants (Shapiro and Kornfeld 1989) and 25% among recipients of liver transplants (Surman et al. 1987a, 1987b). Rates among recipients of kidney transplants have not been reported using contemporary criteria.

A variety of case reports and small series describe the full syndrome of mania (Wamboldt et al. 1984), racing thoughts and dense insomnia suggesting hypomania (DeGroen and Craven 1992), and depressive syndromes (Craven 1991; DeGroen and Craven 1992; C.B. Thompson et al. 1984). Many reports temporally link mood symptoms to the initiation of cyclosporine or tacrolimus therapy following organ transplantation, with symptom remission after cyclosporine or tacrolimus holidays, dose decrements, or primary immunosuppressant switches (Strouse et al. 1998).

Our group has observed transient mania that evolved into fixed frontal lobe syndromes as part of the clinical presentation of late-onset cyclosporine neurotoxicity in recipients of liver transplants. Mania and depression have been linked to high-dose steroid treatment (Kershner and Wang-Cheng 1989; Lewis and Smith 1983; Ling et al. 1981) and to the prodrome of CNS infection with cytomegalovirus (Surman 1992). Tacrolimus is associated with "mood changes" (Eidelman et al. 1991), and acyclovir is associated with psychotic major depressive disorder (Sirota et al. 1988).

We have also observed new-onset and recurrent anxiety disorders. A few patients have manifested clear-cut panic disorder, and we have seen two patients develop apparently new-onset obsessive-compulsive disorder with ego-alien intrusive thoughts and rituals. These disorders responded well to standard pharmacological and behavioral treatment. A few case reports described transient paranoid psychoses in patients without delirium following liver transplant (Adams et al. 1987). These psychotic states were attributed to cyclosporine (Adams et al. 1987), tacrolimus (Eidelman et al. 1991), a variety of antibacterial and antifungal agents (Trzepacz et al. 1993a, 1993b), steroids, sleep deprivation, opiates, and "stress reactions."

Whether primary or secondary, mood and anxiety disorders warranting pharmacological interventions are increasingly recognized in solid organ recipients. No placebo-controlled or head-to-head trials are intended to measure the efficacy of antidepressant medications in transplantation. Recognition of the theoretical potential for drug interactions between contemporary antidepressant compounds and the immunosuppressant pharmacopeia, however, has led to basic trials examining safety and pharmacokinetics. Strouse et al. (1996) found no evidence that fluoxetine altered serum state cyclosporine levels in a group of 13 depressed mixed solid organ recipients compared with similar patients who received desipramine or nortriptyline and matched control subjects. Markowitz et al. (1998) prospectively followed up six depressed heart or lung recipients treated with either fluoxetine, sertraline, or paroxetine and found no evidence of significant alterations in cyclosporine blood levels after initiation of antidepressant medication therapy. Helms-Smith et al. (1996) reported a single case of significant elevation of cyclosporine steady-state blood levels by coadministration of nefazodone; this is a predictable interaction because nefazodone is a potent inhibitor of the P450 3A3/4 isoenzyme system, which is primarily responsible for the biotransformation of cyclosporine.

Movement Disorders

Gross tremor is a common problem in organ transplant recipients. High serum immunosuppressant levels are often associated with extreme symptoms, although tremor occurs in many patients with normal and low-normal levels. OKT3 also can cause or exacerbate tremor (Coleman and Norman 1990). The chronic brain effects of alcohol may predispose transplant recipients to postsurgical tremor (Neiman et al. 1990). Other potentiating factors may include hypomagnesemia or hypocalcemia (Adams et al. 1987; C.B. Thompson et al. 1984) or the concomitant administration of other drugs that are known to elevate cyclosporine and tacrolimus levels, including erythromycin, oral contraceptives, methylprednisolone, ketoconazole, fluconazole, cimetidine, and verapamil (Trzepacz et al. 1993a, 1993b). Some patients experience fasciculations or myoclonic jerking, which may be worse at night and may interrupt sleep. No controlled treatment data exist. When immunosuppressive dosing changes and careful attention to drug interactions are ineffective, clonazepam successfully manages tremor and myoclonic jerking.

Various symptoms of cerebellar dysfunction, such as ataxia, nystagmus, weakness, and dysarthria, are also described in patients following organ transplantation (Adams et al. 1987; Belli et al. 1993; C.B. Thompson et al. 1984; Vogt et al. 1988). As with many of these neuropsychiatric problems, patients who have received livers seem more vulnerable than other solid organ recipients. These symptoms, most often described as acute neurotoxic states, can improve or clear entirely despite unclear etiologies but may persist and can become quite disabling. Transient limb paresis, hemiplegia, and spasticity also have been reported (DeGroen and Craven 1992; DeGroen et al. 1987; Martinez et al. 1988). One case report described improvement in chronic hepatocerebral degeneration during the first posttransplant year in a patient who had a liver transplant (Powell et al. 1990).

A syndrome of akinetic mutism, orofacial dyskinesias, pseudobulbar palsy, and MRI-confirmed central pontine myelinolysis in patients following liver transplantation has been described at several centers (Bird et al. 1990; Burkhalter et al. 1994; Estol et al. 1989a, 1989b; Fryer et al. 1996; Kabeer et al. 1995; Laubenberger et al. 1996; Lee et al. 1996; Martinez et al. 1988; Strouse et al. 1998). A possibly related syndrome of diffuse white matter lesions associated with movement abnormalities and altered consciousness has been described in patients who have undergone heart transplantation (Lane et al. 1988). The dramatic pontine syndrome in patients with donor livers has been convincingly linked to cyclosporine and tacrolimus. The syndrome has been reported to clear with primary immunosuppressant holidays, empirical switches, or dose reductions, a finding confirmed by the UCLA experience, in which both clinical symptoms and MRI findings have substantially improved or normalized in some of these patients (Strouse et al. 1998). The risk of recurrence with cyclosporine or tacrolimus rechallenge remains unclear; some liver grafts may have intrinsic P450 IIIA isoenzymes, which compromise cyclosporine metabolism and predispose to neurotoxicity (Lucey et al. 1990) even at normal serum levels.

Other Constitutional Symptoms

Impaired taste sensation is a common complaint after organ transplantation. Hypersensitivity to olfactory inputs is also frequently reported, as are hyperacusis and hypoacusis. Incontinence (DeGroen et al. 1987) and male and female sexual dysfunction also have been reported. Liver transplantation is believed to restore reproductive endocrine function in women (Cundy et al. 1990), and there are reports of term pregnancies following liver transplant. Depression, postoperative body image concerns, relationship issues, and self-esteem are also of critical importance to postoperative sexual adjustment.

Some patients endure subtle but persistent subjective cognitive problems, experience fatigue, and have demonstrable neuropsychological deficits (DiMartini et al. 1991) after transplant, all in the absence of conventionally defined mood disorder or detectable metabolic abnormality. Whether these states represent the brain consequences of chronic preoperative end-organ failure or some new equilibrium state potentiated by the CNS effects of immunosuppressive medications is unclear (DiMartini et al. 1991). Psychostimulants (such as methylphenidate) and activating antidepressants (including fluoxetine and desipramine) are empirically useful (Craven 1989) for the malaise, psychomotor slowing, and struggles with motivation.

Staff Stress

Significant stress is associated with membership on a transplant team; it affects physicians and nursing staff. Early postoperative care is fast-paced and requires close surveillance of the patient for evidence of organ dysfunction and acute physiologic decompensation. There are grave consequences for misinterpretation of signs and symptoms, including permanent organ dysfunction and death.

Surgical ICU staff members are generally accustomed to patients who present in a relatively unstable condition, receive urgent interventions, and move to a less acute care setting for a brief length of stay. When complications arise that preclude successful recovery and eventual discharge from the hospital, questions about aggressive future care must be considered. Members of the nursing staff may feel ill-prepared for the management issues that arise, including dealing with multisystem organ failure and working collaboratively with family members.

Courageous treatment decisions and courageous patients are responsible for the development of the transplantation field. At times, this courage is viewed as a disregard for individual suffering. When these issues arise, it is often helpful to bring nursing and physician staff together to discuss concerns, treatment options, and likely outcomes. Such meetings allow discussion and development of rational and projected treatments.

Appointing a surrogate decision maker well in advance of the actual transplantation surgery is essential to assist in communication with family members. It is exceedingly important to keep the family apprised of the likely outcomes of life-threatening complications. Information may decrease unrealistic expectations or premature requests to terminate care. A formal family meeting may be necessitated by quarreling family factions, inter-

ruption of the staff's ability to care for the patient, and the development of fatal complications.

Nursing coordinators have highly stressful roles. Their responsibilities include screening calls regarding possible organ donors, summoning appropriate candidates to the transplant center, serving as liaison to the medical and surgical wards, ensuring that appropriate treatment protocols are followed, providing focused feedback to floor nursing staff, teaching patients and families about medication and follow-up procedures, and providing continuity of care and access to the medical teams after discharge. Duties after discharge often include follow-up telephone calls with the results of laboratory tests and biopsies and instructions about immunosuppressant medication dose changes or the need for a patient to come to the clinic or hospital.

Stress and burnout are common to the fields of medicine (Fawzy et al. 1983; McDermott 1984) generally and transplantation specifically. The presence of a consultation-liaison psychiatrist on the transplant team may allow team members to seek out assistance early and informally. Brief supportive interactions with various team members can diminish feelings of frustration and isolation. Referral to other mental health care providers or employee assistance programs should be pursued if necessary.

Group support for a transplant team may at times include inviting the chaplaincy service to hold a memorial service for a particularly compelling patient. Annual retreats to review the purpose and goals of the transplant program also may prove helpful in maintaining a cohesive working group.

POSTOPERATIVE COURSE AND LIFE AFTER TRANSPLANTATION

Adherence

As noted previously in this chapter (see section "Adherence to Medical Regimen [Compliance]"), some patients' adherence problems may be anticipated. Siegal and Greenstein (1998) offered increased insight into nonadherence with their survey of more than 1,400 renal transplant recipients. They found that partial adherence with medical care was associated with the denial of physical symptoms and the attempt to self-manage the renal graft, compared with the compliant individuals who worked with the transplant team. Although this research used renal transplant recipients, the issues delineated are applicable to all organ systems.

The same authors (Greenstein and Siegal 1998) described three distinct profiles of posttransplant noncompliers: accidental noncompliers, invulnerables, and decisive noncompliers. The accidental noncompliers simply forgot to adhere to the regimens because of the complexity. As a result, the authors proposed that this group would benefit from education programs that focus on improving cues to take medication. Meanwhile, the invulnerables were not convinced that strict adherence to an immunosuppressive regimen was required. The relative youth and frequency of living related donation that characterized this group were proposed to foster invincibility and the belief that their grafts were more compatible and less dependent on medication adherence. This group also had a low education level, and ongoing continuing education via verbal and written materials on the necessity of long-term medication adherence was advocated.

The decisive noncompliers presented a different problem. They were highly educated and accustomed to making independent work-related decisions. Most had retained graft function over time and believed that they could relax their vigilance. Many had had infections that they attributed to the immunosuppressive drugs, which may have decreased adherence. This group requires recognition of their independent decision-making style and collaborative environment with the team so that they feel that they are involved in decision making.

Postoperative Adjustment

There is increasing interest in the return of the transplant recipient to a reasonable quality of life. Successful readjustment to life after transplantation generally requires several months or longer. Kuhn et al. (1988b) found that the first anniversary after cardiac transplantation was a major milestone and that full readjustment did not occur until after this point.

Tasks after transplantation and discharge include readjustment to family and vocational roles, changing body image, coping with the persistent fear of rejection and infection, tolerating side effects of immunosuppressant medications, meeting the expectations of the medical staff, and coping with continued disability and cost (Craven 1990b). All transplant recipients face these difficulties, which can become the source of major disability. Jones and colleagues (1988) found that individuals were more anxious 4 and 12 months after transplant than they were at the time of discharge posttransplant, underscoring the stress associated with being a convalescing transplant recipient.

Increased autonomy and independence are cited by many transplant recipients as among the reasons for initially seeking transplantation. Actual outcome often falls far short of expectations for immediate recovery and return to health (Stevenson et al. 1990; Walden et al. 1989). This may contribute to distress because the recipient must rely on others for transportation and other tangible needs. Adverse neurological events, or other complications such as renal failure, can leave individuals with significant unanticipated disability and long-term dependency needs. When these events occur, they inevitably disrupt the social network.

Many barriers exist to the return of patients to gainful employment following organ transplant surgery (Thomas 1996). Loss of health insurance associated with recovery from disability is among the most pressing issues. To date, there are no good options for transplant recipients who recover from their illness only to be faced with the high cost of health care, understanding that they will require a lifetime of follow-up visits and expensive immunosuppressant medications. Employers are often unwilling to hire an individual with such an unusual medical condition. In addition, employers fear that the recipient is a potential liability to the company health insurance policy. If hired, a transplant recipient may be disqualified from participating in the company health insurance plan because of his or her preexisting condition.

Lobbying for legislation at federal and local levels that may assuage some of these concerns is under way. The savvy transplant recipient must carefully review options when choosing health insurance coverage at open enrollment periods and when given choices regarding Medicare and Medicaid health maintenance organizations to ensure that he or she will be able to follow up with the transplant providers.

Data on early outcome are mixed; some individuals cite marked improvement in almost all spheres (Bunzel et al. 1991; Jones et al. 1988), whereas others acknowledge significant difficulties (Baumann et al. 1992; Niset et al. 1988). Niset et al. (1988) noted that emotional behavior, social interaction, alertness, and communication were diminished after surgery in a group of heart transplant recipients. These variables took weeks to months to normalize, whereas physical dimensions were likely to respond earlier. Fortunately, 4 months after transplant, 71% of the individuals who had worked 6 months before their transplant surgery had returned to work.

Results for rehabilitation and return to employment for various transplant groups vary. Williams et al. (1987) examined the socioeconomic cost of hepatic transplantation and found that it produced high quality of life in a predictable and cost-effective way, with 82% of 1-year survivors fully rehabilitated (work or housekeeping) and returned to preillness activity. Craven (1990b) found that 82% of the lung transplant survivors had resumed full- or part-time roles as homemakers, volunteers, or employees. Paris et al. (1998) documented that only 37% of the lung transplant recipients who were able to work returned to the work force. Factors associated with successful transition back to the work force included prior employment, feeling physically able to work, and functional improvement after the procedure.

Paris et al. (1993) examined a large group of surviving heart transplant recipients and found that 45% were employed, 36% were unemployed, 13% were medically disabled, and 6% were retired. These data do not recognize housekeeping as a potential site of employment, unless it was a pretransplant role. Molzahn et al. (1997) reported a 67% employment rate 5 years after cardiac transplant, but the number of patients surveyed was extremely low.

Return to employment for recipients of donor kidneys was also low. Markell et al. (1997) examined unemployment in inner-city renal transplant recipients and found that 58% were unemployed despite a pretransplant employment rate of 81%. Frisk and associates (1987) found that 72% of the individuals 10 years posttransplant had returned to full- or part-time employment. At 15-year follow-up, the percentage had declined to 64%.

Paris et al. (1993) documented six predictors for return to employment:

1. Feeling physically able to work
2. No risk of losing health insurance
3. Longer length of time since transplant
4. Education beyond high school
5. Maintenance of disability income
6. Shorter period of pretransplant disability

An additional factor that plays an important role in recipient status posttransplantation is that of immunosuppressant medication. Although these medications allow the graft to survive in the host, they have significant side effects that affect quality of life. As allograft rejection is most likely to occur soon after transplantation, dosing of medications is generally higher at this time, and the likelihood of side effects during this period is increased. The long-term consequences of these medications are only beginning to be understood.

CONCLUSION

In this chapter, we have reviewed the literature and shared current clinical experiences of the organ transplant psychiatrist as a clinician and transplant team member. Although OTP has made impressive early progress,

and the scope and sophistication of the OTP research literature has advanced, many challenges remain to the continued growth and vitality of OTP.

Among the greatest challenges is the relatively small number of individuals transplanted at each center. The small numbers and varying psychosocial selection policies at each center make powerful aggregate analysis difficult. Comparison of quality of life, medical outcomes, compliance, and return to employment data must be done cautiously because center-specific selection criteria and values differ widely and have a great effect on these factors.

The clinical activities of practitioners of consultation-liaison psychiatry in general, and in OTP settings in particular, are driven by the treatment team more than by patient request. Therefore, the demand for OTP services and programs fundamentally depends on the judgments of organ transplant program directors that psychiatric services are a necessary, effective, and cost-effective component of the organ transplant program. In the current organ transplant professional services reimbursement environment, it is essential that OTP services be highly effective in meeting the clinical patient care needs and transplant team membership role expectations discussed earlier in this chapter. This professional role competence and success are essential to the long-term economic survival of any OTP program. To be successful, the consultation-liaison psychiatrist doing organ transplant work must have highly developed and specific organ transplant knowledge and skills beyond the realm of general consultation-liaison training.

In addition to fostering specialized clinical competence in its practitioners (which ultimately may require the development of a small number of formal fellowship training programs in OTP), developing sophisticated strategies to ensure its long-term economic survival must be addressed. OTP as a field faces significant research challenges. Table 28–6 summarizes several areas in which further knowledge is needed.

OTP is a dynamically developing field of clinical and research activity. It provides profound personal and professional rewards to its practitioners because they see the many individuals whose lives are greatly extended by the application of modern technology. Psychiatrists, along with psychologists, social workers, and other mental health care professionals who may be team members, need to work closely and effectively with the wide variety of health care professionals who compose the organ transplant team. This collaborative spirit and the specific skills that psychiatrists and other mental health care professionals bring to organ transplant programs make critically important contributions to successful transplant recipient outcomes.

TABLE 28–6. Areas of organ transplant psychiatry in which further research is needed

Neuropsychiatric sequelae and neuropsychiatric management of patients who develop end-stage organ failure and who undergo organ transplantation

Indications for, safety of, and efficacy of psychopharmacological treatments of psychiatric disorders in patients in this population

Efficacy of specific psychiatric interventions, including psychotherapy, in targeted or high-risk transplant recipients

Cost offset of psychiatric/mental health treatment for high-risk transplant recipients

Pretransplantation predictors of important psychiatric, behavioral, and psychosocial outcomes among patients who receive organ transplants

Assessment and management of patients with substance-related disorders who are candidates for and recipients of transplants

Pretransplantation psychosocial variables that may predict critical medical (as opposed to psychiatric) outcomes in patients who receive transplants (e.g., survival status or duration)

Predictors of critical transplant recipient rehabilitation, adaptation, and quality-of-life outcomes

Effects of organ donation on living donors

Effects of bridging technology on candidates awaiting transplantation

REFERENCES

Abbasoglu O, Goldstein RM, Vodapaly MS, et al: Liver transplantation in hyponatremic patients with emphasis on central pontine myelinolysis. Clin Transplant 12:263–269, 1998

Adams DH, Ponsford S, Gunson B, et al: Neurological complications following liver transplantation. Lancet 1:949–951, 1987

Alter M, Favero MS, Miller JK: National surveillance of dialysis-associated diseases in the United States. Transactions of the American Society of Artificial Internal Organs 35:820–831, 1989

Aronoff GR, Bergstrom RF, Pottratz ST, et al: Fluoxetine kinetics and protein binding in normal and impaired renal function. Clin Pharmacol Ther 36:138–144, 1984

Barbut D, Caplan LR: Brain complications after cardiac surgery. Curr Probl Cardiol 22:449–480, 1997

Barefoot JC, Schroll M: Symptoms of depression, acute myocardial infarction, and total mortality in a community sample. Circulation 93:1976–1980, 1996

Basile AS, Jones E: Hepatic encephalopathy and the GABA/benzodiazepine receptor chloride ionophore complex: an update. J Gastroenterol Hepatol 3:387–398, 1988

Basile AS, Hughes RD, Harrison PM, et al: Elevated concentration of 1,4 benzodiazepines in fulminant liver failure. N Engl J Med 327:473–478, 1991

Basile AS, Harrison PM, Hughes RD, et al: Relationship between plasma benzodiazepine receptor ligand concentration and severity of hepatic encephalopathy. Hepatology 19:112–121, 1994

Baumann LJ, Young CJ, Egan JJ: Living with a heart transplant: long term adjustment. Transpl Int 5:1–8, 1992

Beliles K, Stoudemire A: Psychopharmacologic treatment of depression in the medically ill. Psychosomatics 39 (suppl 3):S2–S19, 1998

Belle SH, Beringer KC, Detre KM: Recent findings concerning liver transplantation in the United States. Clin Transplant 10:15–29, 1996

Belli LS, De Carlis L, Romani F, et al: Dysarthria and cerebellar ataxia: late occurrence of severe neurotoxicity in a liver transplant recipient. Transpl Int 6:176–178, 1993

Benedetti E, Asolati M, Dunn T, et al: Kidney transplantation in recipients with mental retardation: clinical results in a single-center experience. Am J Kidney Dis 31:509–512, 1998

Bennett WM, Norman DJ: Action and toxicity of cyclosporine. Annu Rev Med 37:215–224, 1986

Berden JHM, Hoitsma AJ, Merx JL, et al: Severe central nervous system toxicity associated with cyclosporine. Lancet 1:219–220, 1985

Beresford TP, Turcotte JP, Merion R, et al: A rational approach to liver transplantation for alcoholic candidates. Psychosomatics 31:241–254, 1990

Bernstein JG: Monoamine oxidase inhibitors, in Handbook of Drug Therapy in Psychiatry. Edited by Bernstein JG. Littleton, MA, PSG Publishing, 1988, pp 161–188

Bhatt BD, Meriano FV, Buchwald D: Cyclosporine associated central nervous system toxicity (letter). N Engl J Med 318:788, 1988

Bird FLA, Meadows J, Goka J, et al: Cyclosporin-associated akinetic mutism and extrapyramidal syndrome after liver transplantation. J Neurol Neurosurg Psychiatry 53:1068–1071, 1990

Boon AP, Adams DH, Buckels J, et al: Cerebral aspergillosis in liver transplantation. J Clin Pathol 43:114–118, 1990

Broelsch CE, Whitington PF, Edmond JC: Evolution and future perspectives for reduced-size hepatic transplantation. Surg Gynecol Obstet 171:353–360, 1990

Brook G: Quality of life issues: parenteral nutrition to small bowel transplantation—a review. Nutrition 14:813–816, 1998

Bryan CF, Baier KA, Nelson PW, et al: Long term graft survival is improved in cadaveric renal retransplantation by flow cytometric crossmatching. Transplantation 66:1827–1832, 1998

Buchanan DC: Group therapy for chronic physically ill patients. Psychosomatics 19:425–431, 1978

Bunzel B, Grundbock A, Laczkovics A, et al: Quality of life after orthotopic heart transplantation. J Heart Lung Transplant 10:455–459, 1991

Burdine J, Fischel RJ, Bolman RM: Cardiac transplantation. Crit Care Clin 6:927–945, 1990

Burkhalter EL, Starzl TE, Van Thiel DH: Severe neurological complications following orthotopic liver transplant in patients receiving FK-506 and prednisone. J Hepatol 21:572–577, 1994

Caccia S, Ballabio M, Samanin R, et al: m-Chlorophenyl-piperazine, a central 5-hydroxytryptamine agonist, is a metabolite of trazodone. J Pharm Pharmacol 33:477–478, 1981

Carney C: Diabetes mellitus and major depressive disorder: an overview of prevalence, complications, and treatment. Depress Anxiety 7:149–157, 1998

Coffman KL, Hoffman A, Rosenthal P, et al: Neurological and psychological sequelae in transplant recipients after bridging with the bioartificial liver. Gen Hosp Psychiatry 18 (suppl):20S–24S, 1996

Coleman AE, Norman DJ: OKT3 encephalopathy. Ann Neurol 28:837–838, 1990

Collins JA, Skidmore MA, Melvin DB, et al: Home intravenous dobutamine therapy in patients awaiting heart transplantation. J Heart Lung Transplant 9:205–208, 1990

Conti DJ, Tubin RH: Infection of the central nervous system in organ transplant recipients. Neurosurg Clin N Am 6:241–260, 1988

Cooper DKC, Lanza RP, Barnard CN: Noncompliance in heart transplant recipients: the Cape Town experience. Heart Transplantation 3:248–253, 1984

Cooper DK, Novitzky D, Davis L, et al: Does central nervous system toxicity occur in transplant patients with hypocholesterolemia receiving cyclosporine? J Heart Lung Transplant 8:221–224, 1989

Cotariu D, Zaidman JL: Valproic acid and the liver. Clin Chem 34:890–897, 1988

Cox DJ, Kiernan BD, Schroeder BD, et al: Psychosocial sequelae of visual loss in diabetes. Diabetes Educator 24:481–484, 1998

Craven JL: Methylphenidate for cyclosporin-associated organic mood disorder (letter). Am J Psychiatry 146:553, 1989

Craven JL: Postoperative organic mental syndromes in lung transplant recipients: the Toronto Lung Transplant Group. J Heart Lung Transplant 9:129–132, 1990a

Craven J: Psychiatric aspects of lung transplant: the Toronto Lung Transplant Group. Can J Psychiatry 35:759–764, 1990b

Craven JL: Cyclosporine-associated organic mental disorders in liver transplant recipients. Psychosomatics 32:94–102, 1991

Craven J, Rodin G: Introduction, in Psychiatric Aspects of Organ Transplantation. Edited by Craven J, Rodin GJ. Oxford, England, Oxford University Press, 1992, pp 1–5

Cundy TF, O'Gracy JG, Williams R: Recovery of menstruation and pregnancy after liver transplantation. Gut 31:337–338, 1990

Currie KO, Jones DL: Orthotopic liver transplantation for alcohol-related end-stage liver disease (abstract). Book of abstracts presented at the annual meeting of the Academy of Psychosomatic Medicine, Atlanta, GA, October 1991

Dalhoff K, Poulsen HE, Garrard P, et al: Buspirone pharmacokinetics in patients with cirrhosis. Br J Pharmacol 24:547–550, 1987

Das Gupta K, Jefferson JW: The use of lithium in the medically ill. Gen Hosp Psychiatry 12:83–97, 1990

De Bruijn KM, Klompmaker IJ, Slooff MJH, et al: Cyclosporine neurotoxicity late after liver transplantation. Transplantation 47:575–576, 1989

Dec GW, Semigran MJ, Vlahakes GJ: Cardiac transplantation: current indications and limitations. Transplant Proc 23:2095–2106, 1991

DeGroen P, Craven J: Organic brain syndromes in transplant patients, in Psychiatric Aspects of Organ Transplantation. Edited by Craven J, Rodin G. Oxford, England, Oxford University Press, 1992, pp 67–88

DeGroen P, Aksamit AJ, Rakela J, et al: Central nervous system toxicity after liver transplantation: the role of cyclosporine and cholesterol. N Engl J Med 317:861–866, 1987

DeLong P, Trollinger JH, Fox N, et al: Noncompliance in renal transplant recipients: methods for recognition and intervention. Transplant Proc 21:3982–3984, 1989

Dew MA, DiMartini A, Griffith BP, et al: Mental health and compliance-related predictors of morbidity and mortality in the long-term after heart transplantation. Presentation at the 5th Biennial Conference on Psychiatric, Psychosocial, and Ethical Issues After Transplantation, Cleveland, OH, October 2, 1998

Didlake RH, Dreyfus K, Kerman RH, et al: Patient noncompliance: a major cause of late graft failure in cyclosporine treated renal transplant. Transplant Proc 20:63–69, 1988

DiMartini A, Twillman R: Organ transplantation and paranoid schizophrenia. Psychosomatics 35:159–160, 1994

DiMartini A, Pajer K, Trzepacz P, et al: Psychiatric morbidity in liver transplant patients. Transplant Proc 23:3179–3180, 1991

DiMartini AF, Trzepacz PT, Pajer KA, et al: Neuropsychiatric side effects of FK-506 vs. cyclosporine A. Psychosomatics 38:565–569, 1997

DiMartini A, Jain A, Irish W, et al: Outcome of liver transplantation in critically ill patients with alcoholic cirrhosis: survival according to medical variables and sobriety. Transplantation 66:298–302, 1998

Dixit V, Gitnick G: The bioartificial liver: state of the art. Eur J Surg Suppl 582:71–76, 1998

Dubin WR, Field HL, Gastfriend DR: Postcardiotomy delirium: a critical review. J Thorac Cardiovasc Surg 77:586–594, 1979

Eadie MJ, Hooper WD, Dickinson RG: Valproate-associated hepatotoxicity and its biochemical mechanisms. Medical Toxicology and Adverse Drug Experience 3:85–106, 1988

Eidelman B, Abu-Elmagd K, Wilson J, et al: Neurologic complication of FK-506. Transplant Proc 23:3175–3178, 1991

Eisendrath RM, Guttmann RD, Murray JE: Psychologic considerations in the selection of kidney transplant donors. Surg Gynecol Obstet 129:243–248, 1969

Estol CJ, Faris AA, Martinez AJ, et al: Central pontine myelinolysis after liver transplantation. Neurology 39:493–498, 1989a

Estol CJ, Lopez O, Brenner RP, et al: Seizures after liver transplantation: a clinicopathologic study. Neurology 39:1297–1301, 1989b

European FK 506 Multicentre Liver Study Group: Randomized trial comparing tacrolimus to cyclosporine in prevention of liver allograft rejection. Lancet 344:423–428, 1994

Faulds D, Heel RC: Ganciclovir: a review of its antiviral activity, pharmacokinetic properties, and therapeutic efficacy in cytomegalovirus infections. Drugs 39:597–638, 1990

Fawzy FI, Wellisch DK, Pasnau RO, et al: Preventing nursing burnout: a challenge for liaison psychiatry. Gen Hosp Psychiatry 5:141–149, 1983

Fellner CH: Selection of living kidney donors and the problem of informed consent. Seminars in Psychiatry 3:79–85, 1971

Fellner CH, Marshall JR: Twelve kidney donors. JAMA 206:2703–2707, 1968

Ferguson ME, Ferguson RM: Rescuing Prometheus: a policy proposal to alleviate excess demand for liver transplantation. Clin Transplant 11:49–55, 1997

Fox CE: Building a more equitable system of organ sharing and increasing donation: consonant goals. Presentation at the 5th Biennial Conference on Psychiatric, Psychosocial, and Ethical Issues After Transplantation, Cleveland, OH, October 2, 1998

Fox RC, Swazey JP: Leaving the field. Hastings Cent Rep 22:9–15, 1992

Frank B, Perdrizet GA, White HM, et al: Neurotoxicity of FK-506 in liver transplant recipients. Transplant Proc 25:1887–1888, 1993

Frasure-Smith N, Lesperance F, Talajic M: Depression following myocardial infarction: impact on 6-month survival. JAMA 270:1819–1825, 1993

Frasure-Smith N, Lesperance F, Talajic M: Depression and 18-month prognosis after myocardial infarction. Circulation 91:999–1005, 1995

Freeman AM, Folks DG, Sokol RS, et al: Cardiac transplantation: clinical correlates of psychiatric outcome. Psychosomatics 29:47–54, 1988a

Freeman AM, Sokol RS, Folks DG, et al: Psychiatric characteristics of patients undergoing cardiac transplantation. Psychiatr Med 6:8–23, 1988b

Freeman A, Davies L, Libb JW, et al: Assessment of transplant candidates and prediction of outcome, in Psychiatric Aspects of Organ Transplantation. Edited by Craven J, Rodin G. Oxford, England, Oxford University Press, 1992, pp 9–19

Freeman AM, Westphal JR, Davis LL, et al: The future of organ transplant psychiatry. Psychosomatics 36:429–437, 1995

Freise CE, Narumi S, Stock PG, et al: Simultaneous pancreas-kidney transplantation: an overview of indications, complications, and outcomes. West J Med 170:11–18, 1999

Frierson RL, Lippmann SB: Heart transplantation patients rejected on psychiatric indication. Psychosomatics 28:347–355, 1987

Frisk B, Persson H, Wedel N, et al: Study of 172 patients at 10 to 21 years after renal transplantation. Transplant Proc 19:3769–3771, 1987

Fryer JP, Fortier MV, Metrakos P, et al: Central pontine myelinolysis and cyclosporine neurotoxicity following liver transplantation. Transplantation 61:658–661, 1996

Gammans PE, Mayoe RF, La Budde SA: Metabolism and disposition of buspirone. Am J Med 80 (suppl):S41–S51, 1988

Gastfriend DR, Surman OS, Gaffey G, et al: Substance abuse and compliance in organ transplantation. Substance Abuse 10:149–153, 1989

Gellman RN: Divided loyalties: a physician's responsibility in an information age. Soc Sci Med 23:817–826, 1989

Ghalie R, Fitzsimmons WE, Bennette D, et al: Cortical blindness: a rare complication of cyclosporine therapy. Bone Marrow Transplant 6:147–149, 1990

Glassman AH, Preudhomme XA: Review of the cardiovascular effects of heterocyclic antidepressants. J Clin Psychiatry 54 (suppl):16–22, 1993

Glassman AH, Rose SP, Bigger JT: The safety of tricyclic antidepressants in cardiac patients: risk benefit reconsidered. JAMA 269:2673–2675, 1993

Gokgoz L, Gunaydin S, Sinci V, et al: Psychiatric complications of cardiac surgery postoperative delirium syndrome. Scand Cardiovasc J 31:217–222, 1997

Goldman LS: Liver transplantation using living donors: preliminary donor psychiatric outcomes. Psychosomatics 34:235–240, 1993

Goodnick PJ, Jimenez I, Kumar A: Sertraline in diabetic neuropathy: preliminary results. Ann Clin Psychiatry 9:255–257, 1997

Greenblatt DJ, Shader R: Pharmacokinetics of antianxiety agents, in Psychopharmacology: The Third Generation of Progress. Edited by Meltzer HY. New York, Raven, 1987, pp 387–401

Greenstein S, Siegal B: Compliance and noncompliance in patients with a functioning renal transplant: a multicenter study. Transplantation 66:1718–1726, 1998

Grimm G, Ferenci P, Katzenschlager R, et al: Improvement of hepatic encephalopathy treated with flumazenil. Lancet 2:1392–1394, 1988

Harris RC, Dew MA: The association of religious beliefs and behaviors with the well being of heart transplant recipients (abstract). Proceedings of the Psychiatric, Psychosocial, and Ethical Issues in Organ Transplantation Conference, September 1992, p 61

Hegel MT, Griegel LE, Black C, et al: Anxiety and depression in patients receiving implanted cardioverter-defibrillators: a longitudinal investigation. Int J Psychiatry Med 27:57–69, 1997

Heller SS, Ormont MA, Lidagoster RR, et al: Psychosocial outcome after ICD implantation: a current perspective. Pacing Clin Electrophysiol 21:1207–1215, 1998

Helms-Smith KM, Curtis SL, Hatton RC: Apparent interactions between nefazodone and cyclosporine (letter). Ann Intern Med 125:424, 1996

Hesse UJ, Roth B, Knuppertz G, et al: Control of patient compliance in outpatient steroid treatment of nephrologic disease and renal transplant recipients. Transplant Proc 22:1405–1406, 1990

Hinchey J, Chavbes C, Appignani B, et al: A reversible posterior leukoencephalopathy syndrome. N Engl J Med 34:494–500, 1996

Hofste WJ, Linssen CA, Boezeman EH, et al: Delirium and cognitive disorders after cardiac operations: relationship to pre- and intraoperative quantitative electroencephalogram. International Journal of Clinical Monitoring Computers 14:29–36, 1997

Hosenpud JD, Bennett LE, Keck BM, et al: Effect of diagnosis on survival benefit of lung transplantation for end stage lung disease. Lancet 35:24–27, 1998

House R, Thompson RL: Psychiatric aspects of organ transplantation. JAMA 260:535–539, 1988

Howden CW, Birnie GG, Brodie MJ: Drug metabolism in liver disease. Pharmacol Ther 40:439–474, 1989

Hravnak M, George E: Nursing considerations for the patient with a total artificial heart. Critical Care Nursing Clinics of North America 1:495–513, 1989

Jeavons PM: Hepatotoxicity in antiepileptic drugs, in Chronic Toxicity of Antiepileptic Drugs. Edited by Oxley J, Janz D, Meinardi H. New York, Raven, 1983, pp 1–46

John R, Chen JM, Weinberg A, et al: Long-term survival after cardiac retransplantation: a twenty-year single-center experience. J Thorac Cardiovasc Surg 117:543–555, 1999

Jones BM, Chang VP, Esmore D, et al: Psychological adjustment after cardiac transplantation. Med J Aust 149:118–122, 1988

Jonsen AR: Ethical issues in organ transplantation, in Medical Ethics. Edited by Veatch RM. Boston, MA, Jones & Bartless, 1989, pp 181–204

Kabeer MH, Filo RS, Milgrom ML, et al: Central pontine myelinolysis following liver transplant: association with cyclosporine toxicity. Postgrad Med J 71:239–241, 1995

Kahn JP, Drusin RE, Klein DF: Idiopathic cardiomyopathy and panic disorder: clinical association in cardiac transplant candidates. Am J Psychiatry 144:1327–1330, 1987

Consensus conference on standardized listing criteria for renal transplant candidates. Transplantation 66:962–967, 1998

Kast R: Blocking of cyclosporine immune suppression by neuroleptics (letter). Transplantation 47:1095–1096, 1989

Kellner R, Samet J, Pathak D: Dyspnea, anxiety, and depression in chronic respiratory impairment. Gen Hosp Psychiatry 14:20–28, 1992

Kershner P, Wang-Cheng R: Psychiatric side effects of steroid therapy. Psychosomatics 30:135–139, 1989

Kiev A, Domantay AG: A study of buspirone coprescribed with bronchodilators in 82 anxious ambulatory patients. J Asthma 25:281–284, 1988

Kiley DJ, Lam CS, Pollak R: A study of treatment compliance following kidney transplantation. Transplantation 55:51–56, 1993

Knechtle SJ, Fleming MF, Barry KL, et al: Liver transplantation for alcoholic liver disease. Surgery 112:694–701, 1992

Koenig HG: Depression in hospitalized older patients with congestive heart failure. Gen Hosp Psychiatry 20:29–43, 1998

Kohen D, Burgess AP, Catalan J, et al: The role of anxiety and depression in quality of life and symptom reporting in people with diabetes mellitus. Qual Life Res 7:197–204, 1998

Krahn LE, Santoscoy G, Van Loon JA: A schizophrenic patient's attempt to resume dialysis following renal transplantation. Psychosomatics 39:470–473, 1998

Kuhn WF, Myers B, Davis MH: Ambivalence in cardiac transplantation candidates. Int J Psychiatry Med 18:305–314, 1988a

Kuhn WF, Davis MH, Lippmann SB: Emotional adjustment to cardiac transplantation. Gen Hosp Psychiatry 10:108–113, 1988b

Kuhn WF, Myers B, Brennan AF, et al: Psychopathology in heart transplant candidates. J Heart Transplant 7:223–226, 1988c

Kuhn WF, Brennan AF, Lacefield PK, et al: Psychiatric distress during stages of the heart transplant protocol. J Heart Lung Transplant 9:25–29, 1990

Kumar S, Stauber RE, Gavaler JS, et al: Orthotopic liver transplantation for alcoholic liver disease. Hepatology 11:159–164, 1990

Lane RJ, Roche SW, Leung AA, et al: Cyclosporin neurotoxicity in cardiac transplant recipients. J Neurol Neurosurg Psychiatry 51:1434–1437, 1988

Laubenberger J, Schneider B, Ansorge O, et al: Central pontine myelinolysis: clinical presentation and radiologic findings. Eur Radiol 6:177–183, 1996

Lee YJ, Lee SG, Kwon TW, et al: Neurologic complications after orthotopic liver transplantation incline central pontine myelinolysis. Transplant Proc 28:1674–1675, 1996

Leipzig RM: Psychopharmacology in patients with hepatic and gastrointestinal disease. Int J Psychiatry Med 202:109–139, 1990

Levenson JL, Glocheski S: Psychological factors affecting end-stage renal disease: a review. Psychosomatics 32:382–389, 1991

Levenson JL, Olbrisch ME: Shortage of donor organ and long waits. Psychosomatics 28:399–403, 1987

Levenson JL, Olbrisch ME: Psychiatric aspects of heart transplantation. Psychosomatics 34:114–123, 1993a

Levenson JL, Olbrisch ME: Psychosocial evaluation of organ transplant candidates: a comparative survey of process, criteria, and outcomes in heart, liver, and kidney transplantation. Psychosomatics 34:314–323, 1993b

Levy NB: Psychological reactions to machine dependency: hemodialysis. Psychiatr Clin North Am 4:351–363, 1981

Lewis DA, Smith RE: Steroid-induced psychiatric syndromes. J Affect Disord 5:319–332, 1983

Lieberman JA, Cooper TB, Suckow RF, et al: Tricyclic antidepressant and metabolite levels in chronic renal failure. Clin Pharmacol Ther 37:301–307, 1985

Ling MHM, Perry PJ, Tsuang MT: Side effects of corticosteroid therapy: psychiatric aspects. Arch Gen Psychiatry 38:471–477, 1981

Loewy EH: Drunks, livers, and values: should social value judgments enter into liver transplant decisions? J Clin Gastroenterol 9:436–441, 1987

Lopez OL, Martinez AJ, Torre-Cisneros J: Neuropathologic cyclosporine and FK-506. Transplant Proc 23:3181–3182, 1991

Lowry MR: Frequency of depressive disorder in patients entering home hemodialysis. J Nerv Ment Dis 167:199–204, 1979

Lowy F, Martin D: Ethical consideration in transplantation, in Psychiatric Aspects of Organ Transplantation. Edited by Craven J, Rodin G. Oxford, England, Oxford University Press, 1992, pp 212–230

Lucey MR, Beresford TP: Alcoholic liver disease: to transplant or not to transplant. Alcohol Alcohol 27:103–108, 1992

Lucey MR, Kolars JC, Merion RM, et al: Cyclosporin toxicity, therapeutic blood levels and cytochrome P-450 IIIA. Lancet 335:11–15, 1990

Lucey M, Merion R, Henley KS, et al: Selection for and outcome of liver transplantation in alcoholic liver disease. Gastroenterology 102:1736–1741, 1992

Lucey MR, Brown KA, Everson TG, et al: Minimal criteria for placement of adults on the liver transplant waiting list: a report of a national conference organized by the American Society of Transplant Physicians and the American Association for the Study of Liver Diseases. Liver Transpl Surg 3:628–637, 1997

Lucey MR, Brown KA, Everson TG, et al: Minimal criteria for placement of adults on the liver transplantation waiting list. Transplantation 66:956–962, 1998

Lustman PJ, Griffith LS, Freedland KE, et al: Cognitive behavioral therapy for depression in type 2 diabetes mellitus: a randomized, controlled trial. Ann Intern Med 129:613–621, 1998

Mai FM: Liaison psychiatry in the heart transplant unit. Psychosomatics 28:44–46, 1987

Mai FM, McKenzie FN, Kostuk WJ: Psychiatric aspects of heart transplantation: preoperative. BMJ 292:311–313, 1986

Maricle RA, Hosenpud JD, Norman DJ, et al: The lack of predictive value of preoperative psychologic distress for postoperative medical outcome in heart transplant recipients. J Heart Lung Transplant 10:942–947, 1991

Markell MS, DiBenedetto A, Maursky V, et al: Unemployment in inner city renal transplant recipients: predictive and sociodemographic factors. Am J Kidney Dis 29:881–887, 1997

Markmann JF, Gornbein J, Markowitz JS, et al: A simple model to estimate survival after retransplantation of the liver. Transplantation 67:422–430, 1999

Markowitz JS, Gill HS, Hunt NM, et al: Lack of antidepressant-cyclosporine pharmacokinetic interactions. J Clin Psychopharmacol 18:91–93, 1998

Martinez AJ, Estol C, Faris A: Neurologic complication of liver transplantation. Neurol Clin 6:327–348, 1988

Maurer JR, Frost AE, Estenne M, et al: International guidelines for the selection of lung transplant candidates. Transplantation 66:956–962, 1998

McCue RE, Georgotas A, Suckow RF, et al: 10-Hydroxy nortriptyline and treatment effects in elderly depressed patients. J Neuropsychiatry Clin Neurosci 1:176–180, 1989

McDermott D: Professional burnout and its relation to job characteristics, satisfaction, and control. Journal of Human Stress 10:79–85, 1984

McManus RP, O'Hair DP, Schweiger J, et al: Cyclosporine-associated central neurotoxicity after heart transplantation. Ann Thorac Surg 53:326–327, 1992

Merrikin KJ, Overcast TD: Patient selection for heart transplantation: when is a discriminating choice discrimination? Journal of Politics, Policy, and the Law 10:7–32, 1987

Merz DA: Nursing issues related to post-transplant patients and their families. J Psychosoc Nurs Ment Health Serv 36:32–36, 1998

Metzger E, Friedman R: Prolongation of the corrected QT and torsades de pointes cardiac arrhythmia associated with intravenous haloperidol in the medically ill. J Clin Psychopharmacol 13:128–132, 1993

Milde FK, Hart LK, Zehr PS: Pancreatic transplantation: impact on the quality of life of diabetic renal transplant recipients. Diabetes Care 18:93–95, 1995

Miller LW: Listing criteria for cardiac transplantation. Transplantation 66:956–962, 1998

Molzahn AE, Burton JR, McCormick P, et al: Quality of life of candidates for and recipients of heart transplants. Can J Cardiol 13:141–146, 1997

Mudge GH, Goldstein S, Addonizio LJ, et al: 24th Bethesda conference: cardiac transplantation. Task Force 3: Recipient guidelines/prioritization. J Am Coll Cardiol 22:21–31, 1993

Mueller AR, Platz KP, Blumhardt G, et al: The optimal immunosuppressant after liver transplantation according to diagnosis: cyclosporine A or FK506. Clin Transplant 9:176–184, 1995

Murberg TA, Bru E, Aarsland T, et al: Functional status and depression among men and women with congestive heart failure. Int J Psychiatry Med 28:273–291, 1998a

Murberg TA, Bru E, Aarsland T, et al: Social support, social disability and their role as predictors of depression among patients with congestive heart failure. Scand J Soc Med 26(2):87–95, 1998b

Murray TH: Divided loyalties for physicians: social context and moral problems. Soc Sci Med 23:827–832, 1989

Neiman J, Lang AE, Fornazzari L, et al: Movement disorders in alcoholism: a review. Neurology 40:741–746, 1990

Neuberger J, Adams D, MacMacter P, et al: Assessing priorities for allocation of donor liver grafts: survey of public and clinicians. BMJ 317:172–175, 1998

Niset G, Coustry-Degre C, Degre S: Psychosocial and physical rehabilitation after heart transplantation: 1-year follow-up. Cardiology 75:311–317, 1988

Nissenson AR, Levin ML, Klawans HL, et al: Neurological sequelae of end stage renal disease. Journal of Chronic Disease 30:705–733, 1987

Noll RB, Kulkarni R: Complex visual hallucination and cyclosporine. Arch Neurol 41:329–330, 1984

Nollert G, Mohnle P, Tassini-Prell P, et al: Postoperative neuropsychological dysfunction and cerebral oxygenation during cardiac surgery. Thorac Cardiovasc Surg 43:260–264, 1995

Office of Medical Applications of Research, National Institutes of Health: Effective medical treatment of opiate addictions: National Consensus Panel on Effective Medical Treatment of Opiate Addiction. JAMA 280:1936–1943, 1998

Ojo A, Port FK: Influence of race and gender on related donor renal transplantation rates. Am J Kidney Dis 22:835–841, 1993

Olbrisch ME, Levenson JL: Psychosocial evaluation of heart transplant candidates: an international survey of process, criteria, and outcomes. J Heart Lung Transplant 10:948–955, 1991

Olbrisch ME, Levenson JL: Psychosocial assessment of organ transplant candidates: current status of methodological and philosophical issues. Psychosomatics 36:236–243, 1995

Olbrisch ME, Levenson J, Hamer R: The PACT: a rating scale for the study of clinical decision-making in psychosocial screening criteria for organ transplant candidates. Clin Transplant 3:164–169, 1989

Orentlicher D: Psychosocial assessment of organ transplant candidates and the Americans With Disabilities Act. Gen Hosp Psychiatry 18 (suppl):5S–12S, 1996

Palmer BF, Toto RD: Severe neurologic toxicity induced by cyclosporine A in three renal transplant patients. Am J Kidney Dis 1:116–121, 1991

Paris W, Woodbury A, Thompson S, et al: Returning to work after heart transplantation. J Heart Lung Transplant 12:46–53, 1993

Paris W, Diercks M, Bright J, et al: Return to work after lung transplantation. J Heart Lung Transplant 17:430–436, 1998

Phipps L: Psychiatric aspects of heart transplantation. Can J Psychiatry 36:563–568, 1991

Pirenne J: Short bowel syndrome: medical aspects and prospect of intestinal transplantation. Acta Chir Belg 96:150–154, 1996

Plevak DJ, Southorn PA, Narr BJ, et al: Intensive care unit experience in the Mayo Liver Transplantation Program: the first 100 cases. Mayo Clin Proc 64:433–445, 1989

Pomier-Layrargues G, Giguere JF, Lavoie J, et al: Flumazenil in cirrhotic patients in hepatic coma: a randomized double-blind placebo-controlled crossover trial. Hepatology 19:32–37, 1994

Powell EE, Pender MP, Chalk JB, et al: Improvement in chronic hepatocerebral degeneration following liver transplantation. Gastroenterology 98:1079–1082, 1990

Pratt LA, Ford DE, Crum RM, et al: Depression, psychotropic medication, and risk of myocardial infarction: prospective data from the Baltimore ECA follow-up. Circulation 94:3123–3129, 1996

Presberg BA, Levenson JL, Olbrisch AM, et al: Rating scales for psychosocial evaluation of organ transplant candidates: comparison of the PACT and TERS with bone marrow transplant patients. Psychosomatics 36:458–461, 1995

Rapoport DM: Buspirone: anxiolytic treatment with respiratory implications. Fam Pract Res J 11:32–37, 1988

Reedy JE, Swartz MT, Termuhlen DF, et al: Bridge to heart transplantation: importance of patient selection. J Heart Lung Transplant 9:473–480, 1990

Regier DA, Narrow WE, Rae DS, et al: The de facto US mental and addictive disorders services system. Arch Gen Psychiatry 50:85–94, 1993

Riether AM, Libb JW: Heart and liver transplantation, in Medical Psychiatric Practice, Vol 1. Edited by Stoudemire A, Fogel BS. Washington, DC, American Psychiatric Press, 1991, pp 309–346

Robins LN, Helzer JE, Croughan J, et al: National Institute of Mental Health Diagnostic Interview Schedule: its history, characteristics, and validity. Arch Gen Psychiatry 38:381–389, 1981

Rodin G, Voshart K: Depressive symptoms and functional impairment in the medically ill. Gen Hosp Psychiatry 9:251–258, 1987

Rodriguez A, Diaz M, Colon A, et al: Psychosocial profile of noncompliant transplant patients. Transplant Proc 23:1807–1809, 1991

Roose SP, Dalack GW, Glassman AH, et al: Cardiovascular effects of bupropion in depressed patients with liver disease. Am J Psychiatry 148:512–516, 1991

Rovelli M, Palmeri D, Vossler E, et al: Noncompliance in organ transplant recipients. Transplant Proc 21:833–834, 1989

Rubin AN, Kang H: Cerebral blindness and encephalopathy with cyclosporin A toxicity. Neurology 37:1072–1076, 1987

Ruzevich SA, Swartz MT, Reedy JE, et al: Retrospective analysis of the psychologic effects of mechanical circulatory support. J Heart Lung Transplant 9:209–212, 1990

Schall RR, Petrucci RJ, Brozena SC, et al: Cognitive function in patients with symptomatic dilated cardiomyopathy before and after cardiac transplantation. J Am Coll Cardiol 14:1666–1672, 1989

Schenker S, Bergstrom RF, Wolen RL, et al: Fluoxetine disposition and elimination in cirrhosis. Clin Pharmacol Ther 44:353–359, 1988

Schleifer SJ, Macari-Hinson MM, Coyle DA, et al: The nature and course of depression following myocardial infarction. Arch Intern Med 149:1785–1789, 1989

Schweizer RT, Rovelli M, Palmeri D, et al: Noncompliance in organ transplant recipients. Transplantation 49:374–377, 1990

Sellers EM, Bendayan R: Pharmacokinetics of psychotropic drugs in selected patient populations, in Psychopharmacology: The Third Generation of Progress. Edited by Meltzer HY. New York, Raven, 1987, pp 1397–1406

Series F, Cormier Y, Laforge J: Changes in day and night time oxygenation with protriptyline in patients with chronic obstructive pulmonary disease. Thorax 44:275–279, 1989

Shapiro PA, Kornfeld DS: Psychiatric outcome of heart transplantation. Gen Hosp Psychiatry 11:352–357, 1989

Shaw PJ, Bates D, Cartlide NEF: Early neurological complication of coronary artery bypass surgery. BMJ 291:1384–1386, 1985

Siegal B, Greenstein SM: Differences between compliers and partial compliers: a multicenter study. Transplant Proc 30:1310–1311, 1998

Sills LM, Popkin MK: Elective removal of a transplanted organ. Psychosomatics 33:461–465, 1992

Simonds AK, Parker RA, Branthwaite MA: Effects of protriptyline on sleep-related disturbances of breathing in restrictive chest wall disease. Thorax 41:586–590, 1986

Sindhi R, Rosendale J, Mundy D, et al: Impact of segmental grafts on pediatric liver transplantation—a review of the United Network for Organ Sharing Scientific Registry data (1990–1996). J Pediatr Surg 34:107–111, 1999

Sipahimalani A, Masand PS: Olanzapine in the treatment of delirium. Psychosomatics 39:422–430, 1998

Sirota P, Stoler M, Meshulam B: Major depressive disorder with psychotic features associated with acyclovir therapy. Drug Intelligence and Clinical Pharmacy 22:306–308, 1988

Skotzko CE, Brownfield E, Kobashigawa J, et al: Non-psychotic DSM-III-R Axis I psychiatric disorders and the outcome after cardiac transplantation (abstract). Psychosomatics 35:200, 1994

Smith MD, Hong BA, Robson AM: Diagnosis of depression in patients with end-stage renal disease: comparative analysis. Am J Med 79:160–166, 1985

Smith MD, Kappell DF, Provience MA, et al: Living-related kidney donors: a multicenter study of donor education, socioeconomic adjustment, and rehabilitation. Am J Kidney Dis 8:223–233, 1986

Spar JE: Plasma trazodone concentration in elderly depressed inpatients: cardiac effects and short-term efficacy. J Clin Psychopharmacol 7:406–409, 1987

Spital A: Unrelated living kidney donors: an update of attitudes and use among US transplant centers. Transplantation 27:1722–1726, 1994

Spital A: Ethical and policy issues in altruistic living and cadaveric organ donation. Clin Transplant 11:77–87, 1997

Starzl TE, Van Thiel D, Tzakis AG, et al: Orthotopic liver transplantation for alcoholic cirrhosis. JAMA 260:2542–2544, 1988

Steinberg TG, Diercks MJ, Millspaugh J: An evaluation of the effectiveness of a videotape for discharge teaching of organ transplant recipients. Journal of Transplant Coordination 6:59–63, 1996

Stevenson LW, Sietsema K, Tillisch JH, et al: Exercise capacity for survivors of cardiac transplantation or sustained medical therapy for stable heart failure. Circulation 81:78–85, 1990

Stoudemire A, Fogel BS: Psychopharmacology in the medically ill, in Principles of Medical Psychiatry. Edited by Stoudemire A, Fogel BS. Orlando, FL, Grune & Stratton, 1987, pp 79–112

Strouse TB: Neuropsychiatric outcomes in liver transplantation, in Transplantation of the Liver. Edited by Busuttil RW, Klintmalm GW. Philadelphia, PA, WB Saunders, 1996, pp 659–664

Strouse TB, Salehmoghaddam S, Spar JE: Acute delirium and parkinsonism in a bupropion-treated liver transplant recipient (letter). J Clin Psychiatry 54:489–490, 1993

Strouse TB, Fairbanks LA, Skotzko CE, et al: Fluoxetine and cyclosporine in organ transplantation: failure to detect significant drug interactions or adverse clinical events in depressed organ recipients. Psychosomatics 37:23–30, 1996

Strouse TB, El-Saden SM, Glaser NEM, et al: Immunosuppressant neurotoxicity in liver transplant recipients. Psychosomatics 39:124–133, 1998

Stuber M: Structural issues in selecting pediatric transplant candidates (abstract). Psychiatric, Psychosocial, and Ethical Issues in Organ Transplantation 4:23, 1992

Stuber M: Paper presented at the annual meeting of the Academy of Psychosomatic Medicine, Palm Springs, CA, November 17, 2000

Surman OS: Psychiatric aspects of organ transplantation (published erratum appears in Am J Psychiatry 146:1523, 1989). Am J Psychiatry 146:972–982, 1989

Surman OS: Liver transplantation, in Psychiatric Aspects of Organ Transplantation. Edited by Craven J, Rodin G. Oxford, England, Oxford University Press, 1992, pp 177–188

Surman OS: Psychiatric aspects of liver transplantation. Psychosomatics 35:297–307, 1994

Surman OS, Cosimi AB: Ethical dichotomies in organ transplantation: a time for bridge building. Gen Hosp Psychiatry 18 (suppl):13S–19S, 1996

Surman OS, Purtillo R: Reevaluation of organ transplantation criteria: allocation of scarce resources to borderline candidates. Psychosomatics 33:202–212, 1992

Surman OS, Dienstag JL, Cosimi AB, et al: Liver transplantation: psychiatric considerations. Psychosomatics 28:615–618, 621, 1987a

Surman OS, Dienstag JL, Cosimi AB, et al: Psychosomatic aspects of liver transplantation. Psychother Psychosom 48:26–31, 1987b

Suszycki LH: Social work groups on a heart transplant program. J Heart Lung Transplant 5:166–170, 1986

Sutton TD, Murphy SP: Stressors and patterns of coping in renal transplant patients. Nurs Res 38:46–49, 1989

Tang H, Boulton R, Grunson B, et al: Patterns of alcohol consumption after liver transplantation. Gut 43:140–145, 1998

Tarbell SE, Kosmach B: Parental psychosocial outcomes in pediatric liver and/or intestinal transplantation: pretransplantation and early postoperative period. Liver Transpl Surg 4:378–387, 1998

Tarter RE, Switala J, Plail J, et al: Severity of hepatic encephalopathy before liver transplantation is associated with quality of life after transplantation. Arch Intern Med 152:2097–2101, 1992

Tesar GE, Murray GB, Cassem NH: Use of high-dose intravenous haloperidol in the treatment of agitated cardiac patients. J Clin Psychopharmacol 5:344–347, 1985

Thomas DJ: Returning to work after liver transplant: experiencing the roadblocks. Journal of Transplant Coordination 6:134–138, 1996

Thompson CB, June CH, Sullivan KM, et al: Association between cyclosporin neurotoxicity and hypomagnesemia. Lancet 2:1116–1120, 1984

Thompson MN, Jeffries DJ: Ganciclovir therapy in iatrogenically immunosuppressed patients with cytomegalovirus disease. J Antimicrob Chemother 23:61–70, 1989

Tollemar J, Ringden O, Ericzon BG, et al: Cyclosporin associated central nervous system toxicity. N Engl J Med 318:788–789, 1988

Toronyi E, Alfoldy F, Jaray J, et al: Attitudes of donors towards organ transplantation in living related kidney transplantations. Transpl Int 11S(1):481–483, 1998

Tringali RA, Trzepacz PT, DiMartini A, et al: Assessment and follow-up of alcohol-dependent liver transplantation patients: a clinical cohort. Gen Hosp Psychiatry 18 (suppl):70S–77S, 1996

Troy SM, Schultz RW, Parker VD, et al: The effect of renal disease on the disposition of venlafaxine. Clin Pharmacol Ther 56:14–21, 1994

Trzepacz PT, Brenner RP, Coffman G, et al: Delirium in liver transplantation candidates: discriminant analysis of multiple test variables. Biol Psychiatry 24:3–14, 1988

Trzepacz PT, Brenner R, Van Thiel DH: A psychiatric study of 247 liver transplantation candidates. Psychosomatics 30:147–153, 1989

Trzepacz PT, Levenson JL, Tringali RA: Psychopharmacology and neuropsychiatric syndromes in organ transplantation. Gen Hosp Psychiatry 13:233–245, 1991

Trzepacz PT, DiMartini A, Tringali R: Psychopharmacologic issues in organ transplantation, part I: pharmacokinetics in organ failure and psychiatric aspects of immunosuppressants and anti-infectious agents. Psychosomatics 34:199–207, 1993a

Trzepacz PT, DiMartini A, Tringali RD: Psychopharmacologic issues in organ transplantation, part II: psychopharmacologic medications. Psychosomatics 34:290–298, 1993b

Tulloch IF, Johnson AM: The pharmacologic profile of paroxetine, a new serotonin-specific reuptake inhibitor. J Clin Psychiatry 53 (no 2, suppl):7–12, 1992

Twillman RK, Manetto C, Wolcott DL: The Transplant Evaluation Scale: a revision of the psychosocial levels system for evaluating organ transplant candidates. Psychosomatics 34:144–153, 1993

U.K. National Transplant Database: Retransplantation in the UK and Republic of Ireland, 1987–1996: UKTSSA National Transplant Database. Clin Transplant 11:81–86, 1997

U.S. Multicenter FK506 Liver Study Group: A comparison of tacrolimus and cyclosporine for immunosuppression in liver transplantation. N Engl J Med 331:1110–1115, 1994

Vaillant GE: The Natural History of Alcoholism. Cambridge, MA, Harvard University Press, 1983

Vidt DG: Selection and preparation of patients for renal transplantation. Surg Clin North Am 51:1105–1121, 1971

Viewig WVR, Godleski LS: Carbamazepine and hyponatremia. Am J Psychiatry 145:1323–1324, 1988

Vingerhoets G, Van Nooten G, Jannes C: Neuropsychological impairment in candidates for cardiac surgery. J Int Neuropsychol Soc 3:480–484, 1997

Vogt DP, Lederman RJ, Carey WD, et al: Neurologic complication after liver transplantation. Transplantation 45:1057–1061, 1988

von Moltke LL, Greenblatt DJ, Shader RI: Clinical pharmacokinetics of antidepressants in the elderly: therapeutic implications. Clin Pharmacokinet 24:141–160, 1993

Walden JA, Stevenson LW, Dracup K, et al: Heart transplantation may not improve quality of life for patients with stable heart failure. Heart Lung 18:497–506, 1989

Wamboldt FW, Weiler SV, Kalin NH: Cyclosporin-associated mania (letter). Biol Psychiatry 19:1161–1162, 1984

Weems J, Patterson ET: Coping with uncertainty and ambivalence while awaiting a cadaveric renal transplant. ANNA J 16:27–31, 1989

Wells KB, Golding JM, Burnam MA: Affective, substance use, and anxiety disorders in persons with arthritis, diabetes, heart disease, high blood pressure, or chronic lung conditions. Gen Hosp Psychiatry 11:320–327, 1989

Westin L, Carlsson R, Israelsson B, et al: Quality of life in patients with ischaemic heart disease: a prospective controlled study. J Intern Med 242:239–247, 1997

Wilczek H, Rigden O, Tyden G: Cyclosporine associated central nervous system toxicity after renal transplantation (letter). Transplantation 39:110, 1984

Wiles CE: Critical care apheresis: hepatic failure. Therapeutic Apheresis 3:31–33, 1999

Williams JW, Vera S, Evans LS: Socioeconomic aspects of hepatic transplantation. Am J Gastroenterol 82:1115–1119, 1987

Wilson SE, DeGroen PC, Aksamit AJ, et al: Cyclosporine A induced reversible cortical blindness. Clinical Neuro-Ophthalmology 8:215–220, 1988

Winnock S, Janvier G, Parmentier F, et al: Pontine myelinolysis following liver transplantation: a report of two cases. Transpl Int 6:26–28, 1993

Wolcott DL: Organ transplant psychiatry: psychiatry's role in the second gift of life. Psychosomatics 1:388–394, 1990

Wolcott DL: Psychiatric aspects of renal dialysis and organ transplantation. Psychiatric Medicine 9:623–640, 1991

Youngner SJ, Coolican MB, Corr C: Should donor families and transplant recipients communicate? Presentation at the 5th Biennial Conference on Psychiatric, Psychosocial, and Ethical Issues After Transplantation, Cleveland, OH, October 3, 1998

Zehrer CL, Gross CR: Patient perceptions of benefits and concerns following pancreas transplantation. Diabetes Educator 20:216–220, 1994

Zumbrunnen R: Coping with heart transplantation: a challenge for liaison psychiatry. Psychother Psychosom 52:66–73, 1989

29

Oncology and Psychooncology

Fawzy I. Fawzy, M.D.

Mark E. Servis, M.D.

Donna B. Greenberg, M.D.

Advances in the diagnosis and treatment of cancer, and an increasingly sophisticated understanding of psychiatric illness in cancer patients, have led to the development of psychooncology as a formal discipline. Psychooncology concerns the phenomenology, prevention, and treatment of psychiatric illness in cancer patients and the role of psychological factors in the onset and progression of cancer. The tasks of clinicians in psychooncology include facilitating life after a cancer diagnosis, helping patients adapt to the many effects of cancer on their lives and their functioning, and managing psychiatric complications in patients and families. A life-threatening disease such as cancer interrupts a forward life trajectory, disrupting an individual's assumptive world (Fawzy and Fawzy 1982; Fawzy and Natterson 1994; Holland and Rowland 1989). Patients who are in great distress may seek out a psychiatrist as they adjust their assumptions, find adaptive and maladaptive coping strategies, and move forward. The psychiatrist's task is 1) to make diagnoses and treat patients who have syndromes that impair psychological function, 2) to help patients build on their strengths and improve their ability to adapt, and 3) to help patients identify and access useful family and community resources (Breitbart 1995).

The experience of cancer includes distinct chronological phases: prediagnosis, diagnosis, initial treatment, posttreatment, recurrence, progressive disease, and the terminal or palliation phase. These phases are accompanied by adaptive and maladaptive responses (Table 29–1). In the prediagnostic phase, when the question of cancer is first pursued medically, patients face fears of pain, disfigurement, dependence, disability, isolation, and death. The oncologist or primary physician guides the patient through diagnostic tests and evaluation decisions. Ideally, in the diagnostic phase, the physician delivers the news of cancer in an unhurried and honest manner, with realistic hope and a commitment to stand by the patient. The physician communicates at the patient's level of understanding and, if necessary, offers information over several visits. In this early phase, the patient faces his or her own mortality, and most often he or she adjusts to the tasks at hand with hope for the future. Frequently, however, repetition of clinical information is necessary because anxiety blocks complete comprehension and assimilation of information. Sleep may be disrupted; shock and disbelief come with the normal defense of denial.

Psychiatric referral during the prediagnostic and diagnostic phases takes place when a patient's psychiatric signs and symptoms cause severe distress and interfere with a management plan. It is not necessary to tamper with denial unless it interferes with the best care for the patient. Fatalistic treatment refusal may prompt a consultation. When the patient's anger regarding the diagnosis is aimed at the physician, family, friends, or a deity, the distress and conflict of these confrontations may also lead to consultation. Patients may blame themselves or feel persecuted. Anxiety and grief are typical; however, persistent depressive symptoms for more than 2 weeks are another common reason for referral. The psychiatric consultant takes the time to explore coping strategies for specific problems, to hear out the anguish, and to listen to the patient's fears and expectations, armed with medical knowledge that will permit dispelling of fears that are unfounded.

Patients must come to terms with the reality of a limited life span and the inevitability of their death. These two issues are often dealt with separately. The first is a

TABLE 29–1.   Psychological responses to cancer

Phase	Normal, adaptive	Abnormal, maladaptive
Prediagnosis	Concern about the possibility of having cancer	Hypervigilance Inappropriate preoccupation Development of cancer symptoms without having the disease
Diagnosis	Shock Disbelief Initial, partial denial Anger, hostility, persecutory feelings Anxiety Depression	Complete denial, with treatment refusal Fatalistic treatment refusal on the grounds that death is inevitable Clinical depression Search for alternative (quack) cures
Initial treatment		
Surgery	Fear of pain and death Fear of anesthesia Grief reaction to changes in body image	Postponement of surgery Search for nonsurgical alternatives Postoperative reactive depression
Radiation therapy	Fear of X-ray equipment and of side effects Fear of abandonment	Psychotic-like delusions/hallucinations
Chemotherapy	Fear of side effects Anxiety, mild depression Changes in body image Isolation Altruistic feelings	Residual drug-induced psychoses Severe isolation-induced psychotic disturbances Organic brain syndrome/delirium
Posttreatment	Return to normal coping patterns Fear of recurrence Posttreatment anxiety and depression	Severe posttreatment anxiety and depression
Recurrence	Shock Disbelief Initial, partial denial Anger, hostility, persecutory feelings Anxiety Depression	Severe reactive depression with insomnia, anorexia, restlessness, anxiety, and irritability
Progressive disease	Frenzied search for new information, other consultants, and quack cures	Depression
Terminal/palliation	Fear of abandonment Fear of loss of composure and dignity Fear of pain Unfinished business Personal mourning with anticipation of death and a degree of acceptance Fear of the unknown	Depression Acute delirium

problem that both patient and physician can more easily address with the development of practical solutions and responses. The second is an existential dilemma (Weisman and Worden 1976–1977) that may require obtaining a spiritual history, spiritual assessment, and interventions that include religious personnel. Religious faith and spirituality in cancer patients have been the focus of recent studies and have been positively correlated with psychological adjustment and quality of life (Cotton et al. 1999;

Feher and Maly 1999; Mytko and Knight 1999). Eventually, most patients come to an ambivalent acceptance of death. The task of the psychiatrist is to recognize this stage and assist families and staff to recognize and accept it as well. Treatment brings fears of surgical pain, death, or loss of control and vulnerability. Patients may grieve the loss of a breast, uterus, arm, or leg. They may lose the activities of the healthy world of work, social contact, sexuality, and the ability to move easily. Physical changes such as weight gain and hair loss come with chemotherapy. Sexual function and fertility are at risk. Neuropsychiatric complications of treatment must be identified, treated, and, if possible, prevented.

When initial treatment has been completed, patients face the threat of recurrence of the cancer. Just when it seems as if a patient could be rejoicing at the completion of treatment, the anxiety of the posttreatment phase becomes prominent. Many patients fear that cancer will recur while doctors are not watching as closely and while the treatment is not actively killing the tumor. With that fear, the patient may feel that he or she must become the guardian over every ache and pain. When symptoms recur, it is helpful to the patient if the physician is readily available. For many patients who proceed through a schedule of the checkups that structure life in remission, each visit and each follow-up scan provoke significant anticipatory anxiety.

Recurrent cancer produces great distress and disappointment, especially when recurrence signals that the tumor is not be curable. The adaptive cycle, with its attendant denial, anger, and anxiety, may be experienced many times, with more psychological difficulty each time. With progressive disease, patients still seek rescue and may search desperately for new information, new doctors, and alternative therapies. The terminal or palliation phase signals the patient's awareness of the irreversible nature of the illness. He or she fears abandonment, loss of dignity, and pain. Concerns include unfinished business, children left without caregivers, and grief over losses.

PSYCHIATRIC ILLNESS IN CANCER PATIENTS

Undoubtedly because of the severe nature of the stressor, the incidence of psychiatric illness may be as high as 51% among patients with cancer, with most of the psychiatrically ill patients having anxiety and mood disorders (Berard et al. 1998; Hardman et al. 1989; McCartney et al. 1989). Assessment of psychiatric illness in cancer patients involves a comprehensive assessment of biological and psychosocial factors. The psychiatrist must evaluate the patient in the context of his or her coping style, developmental history, phase of illness, and psychiatric history and must know the natural course of the illness and the common complications of treatment. Treatment should be characterized by therapeutic activism, with the use of effective psychopharmacological and brief psychotherapeutic modalities to relieve symptoms rapidly and prevent complications due to preventable psychological trauma.

ANXIETY

Anxiety is often a response to the existential plight and to the threat of deformity, abandonment, loss of control, and loss of dignity that may come with the diagnosis of cancer. However, there are also specific anxiety syndromes that are likely to occur in the course of treatment that significantly disrupt patient functioning.

Anticipatory Nausea and Vomiting

Side effects of chemotherapy often include profound nausea and vomiting, a vivid visceral memory that may result in classical conditioning to associated stimuli in up to 75% of all patients (Ellis et al. 1979). Patients who vomit with chemotherapy frequently develop an aversion to the hospital, nurses, or the sight and smell of medical implements. Nausea or vomiting may be the most obvious manifestation, but the entire array of anticipatory symptoms is mediated by the severity of anxiety before treatment, and the conditioned anxiety is linked to these memories (Andrykowski 1990). Patients who are younger, have a history of motion sickness, have higher trait anxiety, or have undergone a greater number of emetic treatments are more prone to this anticipatory response (Jacobsen et al. 1993; Kvale et al. 1994; Stockhorst et al. 1993). Older patients and those with alcoholism are less prone (Morrow 1989). The anxiety may enlarge its realm, presenting as insomnia, transient feelings of dread, pervasive anxiety, dysphoria, increasing areas of avoidance, and subsequent depression. Paradoxically, the patient is trapped by visceral dread of the very treatment that may preserve his or her life (Greenberg 1991).

There are several ways to manage this clinical phenomenon. The first strategy is to prevent this condition by optimal antiemetic treatment, blocking or decreasing the initial episode and conditioned response. Mild nausea is sometimes ignored, although with more treatments the conditioning can take hold and anticipatory anxiety may subsequently develop (Stefanek et al. 1988). The second strategy is to minimize anxiety just before treatment, by use of benzodiazepines such as alprazolam or lorazepam (Greenberg 1991; Holland et al. 1991; Razavi et al. 1993; Triozzi et al. 1988). Behavior therapies may also be useful. Systematic desensitization that extinguishes the conditioned response (Morrow and Morrell 1982), or cognitive distraction that blocks the perception of the conditioned stimulus, may successfully eliminate anxiety that has arisen due to classical conditioning. Even patients who have persistent nausea after the treatment due to direct anticancer drug toxicity also have a component of conditioned anxiety (Greenberg et al. 1987; Stefanek et al. 1988). When the aversion reaches phobic proportions, the site of treatment may be changed and antidepressants may be added to the patient's treatment regimen.

Treatment with benzodiazepines should continue through the period of nausea after chemotherapy, but with an end point for their use agreed on in advance by physician and patient. The use of highly specific, centrally acting antiemetics such as ondansetron, in combination with dexamethasone and lorazepam, has revolutionized chemotherapy, and most patients today do not experience the nausea and vomiting that those in years past did. The amnestic effect of lorazepam often prevents future anticipatory anxiety if any emesis does occur. Benzodiazepines may be used strategically in patients with cancer to relieve reactive anxiety, insomnia, claustrophobia, anticipatory nausea, posttreatment nausea, muscle spasm, and neuropathic pain. With chemotherapy, benzodiazepines cause sedation and suppress recall but limit vomiting and are seen as desirable agents by patients (Greenberg 1991). Addiction potential is minimal when psychiatric follow-up is adequate.

Claustrophobia

Patients with clinical anxiety in closed spaces have great difficulty with magnetic resonance imaging equipment (Meléndez and McCrank 1993) and occasionally with other diagnostic tests. Antianxiety premedication helps, as does having the patient come to the laboratory with a significant other. Special attention by the technicians is helpful as well. Pain management should be maximized; staying supine for a prolonged period is difficult, but the experience is made worse by pain and anxiety. If the phobia is recognized as a problem in advance, the physician may be able to tailor and shorten the test by, for example, obtaining magnetic resonance images of the section of the patient's body that poses the most immediate diagnostic question. Commitment to performing a more complete study may be worthless if the patient's anticipation of a long study prevents his or her cooperation.

Alcoholism

Patients with alcoholism, who are dealing with substance dependence as well as anxiety, may be leaving for a drink when they appear to be noncompliant or phobic. Alcohol withdrawal is always in the differential diagnosis of anxiety. The link between alcohol consumption and certain types of cancer is well documented, and effective assessment and

management of alcoholism are crucial to improving treatment adherence and quality of life in cancer patients (Lundberg and Passik 1997).

Akathisia

The restlessness and need to walk around that is associated with neuroleptics—akathisia—can be mistaken for anxiety in the oncology setting. Restlessness, insomnia, and inner discomfort may be mistaken for agitated depression. Because phenothiazines such as perphenazine and prochlorperazine are commonly used to prevent nausea, patients may not even report their use of them when asked about drug intake. Usually one of the phenothiazines or metoclopramide is the hidden culprit. Drug elimination resolves the problem. Other drugs frequently used in cancer patients that can cause akathisia and anxiety include bronchodilators (in lung cancer patients), steroids, and interferon.

Complex Partial Seizures

Complex partial seizures, like generalized seizures, occur more commonly in patients with cancer than in the general population. Cerebral metastases, cerebral injury due to chemotherapy (Gilliam et al. 1993), leptomeningeal disease (Dexter et al. 1990), or an electrolyte imbalance such as hypomagnesemia (Schilsky and Anderson 1979) may be the cause. Fear is the emotion most often associated with complex partial seizures (Gloor et al. 1982; McNamara and Fogel 1990), and so autonomous episodes of anxiety, such as panic attacks, should arouse suspicion of complex partial seizures. Intermittent confusion that is associated with tremor, odd hallucinations, and syncope may be clues to diagnosis.

Pulmonary Embolus or Pulmonary Edema

Pulmonary edema and, in particular, pulmonary embolus are medical causes of anxiety due to hypoxia; these conditions should cross a consultant's mind in the first moments of anxiety symptom evaluation. Emboli are commonly seen with many types of cancer.

Acute and Posttraumatic Stress Disorder

Both the diagnosis and the treatment of cancer may be intense stressors capable of traumatizing patients and inducing symptoms of acute and posttraumatic stress disorder (PTSD). A recent study examined the empiric evidence for cancer's inclusion as a traumatic stressor and found PTSD in both adults and children who survived cancer (Smith et al. 1999). The diagnosis of acute stress disorder can allow for early intervention to prevent later PTSD. The stressor of a life-threatening illness such as cancer can kindle memories of earlier trauma and dormant PTSD symptoms in patients.

DEPRESSION

Depressive disorders in cancer patients may be a response to the psychosocial stress of cancer, a medical symptom of cancer or its treatment, or unrelated to cancer and coincidental. Whatever their cause, depressive disorders are common: the prevalence of major depression is approximately 8%–14% (Berard et al. 1998; Lansky et al. 1985; Payne et al. 1999; Sellick and Crooks 1999; Valente et al. 1994) and the prevalence of adjustment disorder is higher, perhaps 25% (Derogatis et al. 1983). Those with a history of depression, panic disorder, or bipolar disorder are at greater risk. Patients with chronic pain are also more likely to have associated depressive features, including suicidality. Pancreatic cancer has been associated with a disproportionate incidence of dysphoria (Holland et al. 1986). Steroids and biological agents such as interferon are the anticancer medications most commonly associated with affective instability. Patients who are generally more vulnerable to distress (see Table 29–2) and susceptible to depression have more physical symptoms, more financial and marital problems, and lower ego strength.

The diagnosis of depression in medically ill patients is always confounded by similar neurovegetative or physical symptoms in both depression and somatic illness (McDaniel et al. 1995). The unrelenting awareness of the diagnosis, the inability to concentrate, guilt about being a burden, suicidal thoughts, insomnia not due to pain, and awakening in the morning with dread all argue differentially in favor of primary depression. Comparisons of different formalized criteria by Kathol et al. (1990) showed that the Brief Symptom Inventory (Derogatis and Spencer 1982) was a fair screening device and that the Beck Depression Inventory (Beck 1978) was overly sensitive. The Zung Self-Rating Depression Scale has recently been proven effective and reliable as a screening tool for depression in cancer patients (Dugan et al. 1998). Endicott's (1984) technique of replacing some physical with some cognitive symptoms identified a population of depressed patients that was similar to, but somewhat larger than, that identified by DSM-III-R (American Psychiatric Association 1987) criteria alone.

There has been intense debate and study about the possible etiological links between depression and cancer.

The American tradition to believe in the power of positive thinking has a strong appeal to patients with cancer. Positive thinking offers hope and implies a means to directly control the course of the cancer. Depression and cancer were linked by Galen, and patients who learn of the growing field of psychoneuroimmunology sometimes have the impression that negative thoughts or admission of demoralization has the power to make tumor cells grow (Greenberg 1989). The search for a cancer-prone personality has not confirmed the existence of traits associated with a greater risk of developing cancer (Wellisch and Yager 1987). Pessimism, low self-esteem, the tendency to blame oneself, and the depression scale of the Minnesota Multiphasic Personality Inventory (Hathaway and McKinley 1943) have all been studied in hopes of finding a link to cancer (Fox 1982; Shekelle et al. 1975). The rate of cancer among 5,000 British widows and 800 hospitalized depressed patients was no higher than that among subjects in the general population (Jones et al. 1984). Any emotional predisposition to cancer is likely to be embedded in other strong biological factors that account for most of the variance (Fox 1982). In psychotherapy, the task may be to put a patient's negative thoughts, anger, and sadness in perspective and to clarify that these thoughts do not correlate simply with tumor growth.

Suicide

Suicide is rare among patients with cancer. Only 8% of psychiatry consultations at Memorial Sloan-Kettering Cancer Center were for evaluation of suicidal ideation (Breitbart 1987). Half of these patients had diagnosable personality disorder, half had adjustment disorder with depressed mood, and one-third had a major depressive disorder. Suicidal thoughts may occur at the time of diagnosis (10% of cases), at recurrence (14%) (Weisman 1976), with chronic pain, or if major depression is present (Kugaya et al. 1999). Epidemiologic studies in Finland (Louhivuori and Hakama 1979) and Connecticut (Fox et al. 1982), as well as studies of death certificates, demonstrated an only slightly higher suicide rate among patients with cancer compared with the general population. Men with head and neck cancer may be at greater risk (Farberow et al. 1963, 1971). This risk may relate more to the higher risk for isolated men with a history of alcoholism than to the consequences of the tumor or to the location of the tumor. Table 29–3 lists some of the important risk factors for suicide in cancer patients.

Some patients hold onto the option of suicide—which they regard as an escape from the specter of unremitting pain—and in this way preserve the sense that they

TABLE 29–2.   Correlates of vulnerability

Higher emotional stress	Lower emotional stress
Pessimistic, including about outcome of illness	Optimistic attitudes in general
Regrets about past	Fewer regrets, if any
History of psychiatric treatment or suicidal ideation	Less extensive psychiatric treatment, if any
High anxiety; low ego strength (MMPI)	Low anxiety; high ego strength
Marital problems before cancer	Few marital problems, if any
Lower socioeconomic status	Higher socioeconomic status
More alcohol abuse	Abstinence or use, not abuse
Little or no church attendance	Church attendance
More physical symptoms	Fewer physical symptoms
Cancer at advanced stage	Less-advanced cancer stage
Expects little support from others	Expects adequate support from others
Doctor seen as less helpful	Doctor's help is adequate at least
More current concerns of all types	Fewer current concerns
Feels more like giving up	Feels less like giving up
Poor problem resolution	Better problem resolution

Note.   MMPI = Minnesota Multiphasic Personality Inventory. Not significant: age, marital status, lag time until diagnosis, life stress events (Holmes-Rahe scale).
Source.   Adapted from Weisman AD: *Coping With Cancer.* New York, McGraw-Hill, 1979, p. 67.

TABLE 29–3.   Suicide risk factors in cancer patients

Advanced stage of disease
Alcohol abuse
Chemotherapy
Delirium
Depression[a]
Financial problems
Head and neck cancer
Physical and emotional exhaustion
Poorly controlled pain
Poor prognosis
Social isolation

can be in control. Paradoxically, the possibility of ending their lives and their suffering may be the one thing that keeps them going. Cancer patients have figured prominently in the debates about physician-assisted suicide and euthanasia. While society wrestles with the complex ethical and legal issues of physician-assisted suicide, psychiatrists need to remember that even dying patients whose physical, emotional, and spiritual needs are being met rarely pursue the option of suicide. Most patients wish to receive continuing care and symptomatic relief even if their disease is progressing (Massie et al. 1994).

Psychopharmacological Treatment

In general, antidepressant choice depends on target symptoms and the need to avoid undesirable side effects in a given patient. In the patient with cancer, the choice depends on interactions with other medications; toler-

ance of postural hypotension, urinary retention, and constipation; and individual sensitivities. In patients without cardiac conduction defects, tricyclic antidepressants may be beneficial, especially if effects on sleep and pain are sought. However, because many patients with cancer—including those with breast cancer, for example, who are undergoing adjuvant chemotherapy—will gain weight (Demark-Wahnefried et al. 1993), the tendency for patients receiving tricyclic medication to crave sweets may be an undesirable side effect. A trial of a psychostimulant, such as dextroamphetamine (Fernandez et al. 1987), methylphenidate, or pemoline (Breitbart and Mermelstein 1992), is appropriate for a rapid effect in patients who are systemically ill and who are depressed, apathetic, and not eating. A course of treatment lasting 1–2 months has been shown to provide lasting benefit in patients with cancer.

Trazodone is widely used among medically ill patients, including patients with cancer. This drug has the distinct advantage of addressing the troublesome target symptoms of insomnia and appetite disturbance. Unfortunately, the potential adverse effects include nausea and orthostatic hypotension. Nevertheless, the lack of anticholinergic side effects makes trazodone an attractive agent to use alone or in combination with selective serotonin reuptake inhibitors (SSRIs).

SSRIs are commonly used in medical-surgical populations because of their favorable adverse-effect profile. Fluoxetine, paroxetine, sertraline, and citalopram do not have the disadvantage of anticholinergic and sedative side effects. However, all of the SSRIs can increase anorexia, jitteriness, and agitation, and, as with the tricyclic medications, the antidepressant response is usually delayed by several weeks (Massie et al. 1991; Shuster et al. 1992). Fluoxetine and paroxetine both significantly inhibit metabolism by cytochrome P450 enzymes, with lesser inhibition seen with sertraline and citalopram. It is fortunate, however, that competitive cytochrome P450 enzyme inhibition is unlikely to affect most chemotherapy regimens (Kalash 1998). The initial appetite-suppressant effect of SSRIs, along with occasional nausea, diarrhea, and agitation, can also cause problems in some debilitated patients. Nevertheless, SSRIs are the most widely prescribed antidepressants in cancer patients and have proven equal in antidepressant efficacy to tricyclics (Holland et al. 1998; Bruera and Neumann 1998). Combination pharmacotherapy and psychotherapy has proven more effective than either treatment alone for most anxiety and depressive disorders in cancer patients (Twillman and Manetto 1998).

Neither tricyclic medications nor SSRIs typically interact with chemotherapeutic agents. However, procarbazine, a mild monoamine oxidase inhibitor and a disulfiram-like drug that is used primarily for Hodgkin's disease, delays metabolism of other psychotropic medications. Most oncologists proscribe alcohol but not tyramine-containing foods when prescribing procarbazine. Fortunately, a hypertensive crisis is unlikely to occur, even if the patient is concurrently given a tricyclic antidepressant (De Vita et al. 1965); hypertensive crisis has never been reported. However, use of procarbazine with SSRIs should probably be avoided.

MANIA

Mania is rarely related to cancer itself. Although in rare cases diencephalic tumors and cerebral metastases have led to secondary mania, corticosteroids are the most frequent cause of syndromes resembling mania among patients with cancer (Greenberg and Brown 1985).

As cancer treatment progresses, lithium and valproic acid therapy remain appropriate for patients with primary bipolar disorder (Greenberg et al. 1993a). Lithium favorably increases the patient's white blood cell count by stimulating production of granulocyte colony-stimulating factor and interleukin-6.

Lithium should be withheld on days that the patient receives chemotherapy. Lithium may expose more than the desired number of bone marrow cells to cell death at the time of chemotherapy; therefore, in chemotherapy protocols that have included lithium, lithium has been withheld for 2 days before chemotherapy. The nausea, vomiting, hypercalcemia, and relative dehydration that may occur on days of chemotherapy make lithium toxicity both more likely to occur and more difficult to recognize.

Lithium may be continued during radiation treatment. White blood cell death is not more likely for the patient taking lithium during radiation treatment, because radiation-induced cell death is not cell-cycle specific. During cranial irradiation, it is best to stop lithium therapy because of the risk of neurotoxicity and seizures from the tumor or edema, making possible lithium toxicity more difficult to monitor.

The consultation-liaison psychiatrist should remain alert for renal compromise or brain injury that would increase the risk of lithium toxicity in a patient who is otherwise stable when taking the medication. Bipolar patients receiving maintenance valproic acid therapy need to be closely monitored for signs of liver toxicity with liver function tests. Alternatives to lithium and valproic acid include carbamazepine and neuroleptics. Carbamazepine may also be useful for its anticonvulsant effect. The mild leukopenia that can occur early in treatment with carbamazepine must be evaluated in light of bone marrow reserves.

DELIRIUM

Delirium is a frequent result of cancer and its treatment and is a significant cause of morbidity and mortality in patients. Agitation and hyperalertness are the most common behavioral symptoms in cancer patients with delirium (Olofsson et al. 1996). Haloperidol has proven effective in cancer patients with delirium (Akechi et al. 1996).

PSYCHOTHERAPEUTIC TREATMENTS

In systematic studies, individual psychotherapy (Massie et al. 1989; Watson 1983; Weisman 1976), behavioral treatment, and group therapy (Bloch and Kissane 2000) have been shown to reduce distress in patients with cancer. Behavioral programs and hypnosis have resulted in decreased anxiety, pain, nausea, and vomiting (Trijsburg et al. 1992). Researchers have evaluated not only the role of psychotherapy in reducing distress in patients with cancer but also whether psychotherapy can prolong life in these patients (Fawzy et al. 1995). In one study, women with metastatic breast cancer were randomized to 1 year of weekly support group sessions (Spiegel et al. 1981,

1989). The intervention group had less mood disturbance, fewer phobic responses, and half the pain compared with the control group. The treated group also lived an average of 36.6 months, compared with 18.9 months for the control group. In contrast, a longer-term, 10-year follow-up study involving 34 women with breast cancer who had participated in the Exceptional Cancer Patients program of psychosocial support did not show prolonged survival compared with patients whose tumor data had been entered in the Connecticut Tumor Registry (Gellert et al. 1993).

Another study looked at the effects of group cognitive-behavioral therapy on patients with metastatic breast cancer and demonstrated no effects on survival time (Edelman et al. 1999). The idea that psychosocial interventions may have an effect on cancer progression is seductive to both patients and researchers. The link between immunological function and psychological states such as bereavement, depression, and stress suggests a possible mechanism. Although the positive benefits of psychotherapeutic intervention on a patient's emotional health, relationships, and functioning are well established (Baider 1995; Edelman et al. 1999; Edmonds et al. 1999; Kissane et al. 1997; Moorey et al. 1998), the field of psychoneuroimmunology remains in its infancy. In a study designed to look at psychosocial interventions, cancer survival, and immune function, newly diagnosed patients with stage I or II malignant melanoma who were randomized to a 6-week psychoeducational intervention experienced less turmoil than did the control group after diagnosis (Fawzy et al. 1990a, 1990b, 1993). At 6 years, significantly fewer patients who had received psychiatric intervention had died. The depths of the original lesions in the two groups did not account for the difference in prognosis. Ironically, more distress at the time of diagnosis was associated with increased survival. The relation to immune parameters such as natural killer cell activity was complex and was not simply predictive of longer survival.

In summary, the benefit of psychosocial intervention for the reduction of distress is clear; the benefits of psychiatric intervention for increased immunity or longer life are more modest, complex, and preliminary. Psychotherapy and psychosocial interventions are more likely to contribute to quality than to quantity of life in oncology patients.

COMMON NEUROLOGICAL COMPLICATIONS OF CANCER

Metastatic Brain Tumors

When a psychiatric consultant evaluates a patient with cancer for change in mental status, he or she considers the possibility that a tumor might have metastasized to the brain (Cascino 1993) (Table 29–4). Lung cancer, both small cell and non–small cell, metastasizes to the brain most frequently and accounts for a majority of metastatic brain tumors. Ten percent of lung cancer patients have brain metastases at the time of diagnosis, and as many as 30% develop them later. Breast cancer metastasizes to the brain in 6%–20% of patients. In patients with metastatic melanoma, metastases to the central nervous system (CNS) are also common. Kidney cancer, typically a tumor with a very variable course, metastasizes to the brain in 11%–13% of patients. Other tumors—thyroid, pancreatic, ovarian, uterine, prostate, testicular, and bladder tumors, as well as sarcomas—metastasize to the brain more rarely. The most acute management issues are treatment of brain edema with dexamethasone and treatment of seizures with anticonvulsants. Metastatic brain lesions are identified best by computed tomography (CT) with high doses of iodinated contrast material and delayed scanning. When a metastatic tumor appears to be isolated, surgical resection is considered. Otherwise, the treatment is whole-brain irradiation.

TABLE 29–4. Interval between diagnosis of cancer and occurrence of brain metastases

Tumor	Patients with brain metastases (%)			
	At diagnosis of primary tumor	Sometime during course of tumor growth	At autopsy	After given interval from diagnosis of primary tumor
Lung tumor	10–15	22–30	30–50	90 after 3 months
Breast tumor	1	6–20	15–30	90 after 1 year
Melanoma	6	20	20–30	80 after 1 year
Renal tumor	4	11–13	8–20	90 after 1 year
Colorectal tumor	1	—	1	75 after 2 years
Sarcoma	1	10–15	15–20	90 after 1 year

Leptomeningeal Disease

Leptomeningeal disease should be considered when mental status changes are associated with normal CT findings (Wasserstrom 1982). Cytological examination of cerebrospinal fluid may reveal malignant cells. This finding is most likely in patients with non-Hodgkin's lymphoma, leukemia, melanoma, or adenocarcinoma of the lung, breast, or gastrointestinal system. In addition to mental status changes, patients usually have cranial nerve deficits or radicular signs. The nonspecific signs that may prompt psychiatric referral include headache, balance difficulty, and seizures.

Complex Partial Seizures

Patients with cancer are prone to seizures not only because of brain tumors but also because of leptomeningeal carcinomatosis, treatment-related brain injury, hyponatremia, hypomagnesemia, hyperviscosity syndrome (Gilbert and Armstrong 1995; Stern et al. 1985), and infections (in immunocompromised hosts). Patients without motor symptoms but with primary psychiatric manifestations may be referred to the psychiatrist. Delirium, catatonia, transient focal symptoms, minor tremors, vocalization and speech arrest, simple hallucinations, tingling, light flashes, buzzing, episodic autonomic changes, epigastric sensations, distortions of time, strong emotions, dreamy states, panic attacks, illusions, and the pathognomonic symptom of bad smells should suggest partial seizures. Of note, phenytoin levels decrease in patients receiving chemotherapy (Grossman et al. 1989).

Paraneoplastic Syndromes

Delirium in patients with cancer may be related to distant, nonmetastatic effects of tumors. Subacute cerebellar degeneration, encephalomyopathy, and Eaton-Lambert syndrome form a spectrum of neurological insults that are frequently associated with delirium and dementia. Limbic encephalopathy results in a prominent memory defect, anxiety, depression, and seizures. The mechanism is thought to be autoimmune and to be associated with antineuronal antibodies (Cornelius et al. 1986; Moll et al. 1990; Newman et al. 1990; Posner 1989).

Ectopic production of hormone by tumors can alter mental status by 1) increasing antidiuretic hormone production and causing low sodium levels, 2) increasing parathyroid hormone production and causing high calcium levels, or 3) increasing adrenocorticotropic hormone production and causing Cushing's syndrome, characterized by excess cortisol production that is often associated with affective change. Paraneoplastic phenomena are most common in patients with small cell carcinoma of the lung; however, breast, stomach, uterine, renal, testicular, thyroid, and colon cancers may also be associated with paraneoplastic syndromes (Minotti et al. 1994; Peterson et al. 1994; Schiller and Jones 1993).

Other Causes of Delirium

Delirium secondary to hypercalcemia is an oncological emergency and is often secondary to bone metastases. The treatment is rehydration, administration of diphosphonates (specific anticalcium agents), and possibly a change in antitumor regimen. Subtle signs of hypercalcemia, such as fatigue, nausea, or cognitive impairment, may be mistaken for depression. Calcium is bound to albumin, and total serum calcium values that are within normal limits may be significant if the albumin level is low.

Hypomagnesemia in patients with cancer is most commonly due to impaired nutrition or to the tubular defect caused by cisplatin therapy (Schilsky and Anderson 1979). Hypomagnesemia has been associated with lethargy and depression, hypocalcemia, hypokalemia, and increased risk of seizures.

Hyperviscosity syndrome, with a sudden onset of confusion or seizures, occurs in patients with lymphoma, Waldenström's macroglobulinemia, or myeloma (Crawford et al. 1985). Paraproteins increase blood viscosity and impair circulation in the brain. A level above 4.0 centipoise (cp) (normal is between 1.56 and 1.68 cp) has been associated with symptoms. Classic symptoms of hyperviscosity syndrome are bleeding, visual signs and symptoms, and delirium. Plasmapheresis, along with primary anticancer treatment, may be indicated.

COMPLICATIONS OF TREATMENT

Complications of Radiation Treatment

An anticancer radiation regimen usually requires a treatment for several minutes each day, sometimes twice a day, Monday through Friday, until the intended dose of radiation has been administered at a specific site. Sometimes focused boosts are given. The treatment plan usually requires an average of 6–9 weeks. In addition to skin inflammation and bone marrow suppression, patients may develop fatigue or nausea. Side effects are related to the volume irradiated, and nausea is related to irradiation over viscera. Fatigue tends to increase after about 4 weeks, and then time spent sleeping increases even in those who undergo irradiation of the breast or prostate (Greenberg 1991; Greenberg et al. 1992, 1993c). After the course of treatment is complete, fatigue diminishes over several weeks. Patients in whom radiation is delivered to the CNS take dexamethasone to reduce swelling. The required dose of dexamethasone is commonly associated with insomnia and agitation. Brain irradiation causes much more profound fatigue than does irradiation of other sites. Changes in mental status that occur during brain irradiation may also be related to seizures that occur as edema increases or anticonvulsant levels change. Radiation treatment near the neck presents the risk of hypothyroidism. Brain irradiation may also affect pituitary function.

Neuropsychiatric Side Effects of Anticancer Agents

Neuropsychiatric side effects are among the most important potential clinical complications of treatment with anticancer agents. Table 29–5 describes some of the important side effects that consultation-liaison psychiatrists may encounter.

Treatment-Related Dementia

Cancer treatment sometimes causes a late dementia. The most common etiology is disseminated necrotizing leukoencephalopathy. The accompanying white matter lesions, seen better on magnetic resonance images than on CT scans, may be transient or progressive. Ataxia, confusion, somnolence, spasticity, and dementia may mark the onset of this disease. Gray matter and basal ganglia are spared. The subtle losses of neuropsychological function that are noted in survivors of childhood acute lymphocytic leukemia are related to disseminated necrotizing leukoencephalopathy. Rarely, treatment causes mineralizing microangiopathy—small-vessel damage in areas of gray matter and putamen. Cerebral atrophy is common after brain irradiation but correlates poorly with neurological function and may be reversible (Frytak et al. 1985; Lee et al. 1986; Rottenberg 1991). Delayed cerebral radiation necrosis is an infrequent consequence of brain irradiation and is more likely to occur in the setting of microvascular disease due to hypertension or diabetes. Identifying symptoms include headache, personality change, focal neurological deficits, seizures, and symptoms mimicking those of a brain tumor. The treatment—steroid therapy—has limited benefit; surgery is sometimes recommended to remove the area of necrosis (DeAngelis et al. 1989).

Anorexia

When patients with cancer lose their appetite, their refusal to eat often becomes a focus for family conflict (Holland et al. 1977). Some appetite loss may be due to chemotherapy, irradiation, or progression of a systemic tumor. Major depressive disorder, conditioned taste aversion (Bernstein 1978), and anxiety about pain or diarrhea that will follow food intake may also contribute. Gastritis, gastroparesis, and liver disease may contribute to anorexia as well. In the setting of medical illness, appetite may be stimulated by increasing the patient's energy with agents such as dextroamphetamine. Megestrol acetate (Loprinzi 1995; Loprinzi et al. 1990, 1994b), cyproheptadine, prednisone, and cannabinoids have all been used to foster weight gain (Nelson et al. 1994). All of the drugs commonly used to prevent nausea on oncology wards and in cancer clinics (see Table 29–6) have psychiatric effects (Gralla 1992).

Sexual Dysfunction and Infertility

Cancer can cut life short. Initially, mortality eclipses all other issues, but as the hope for survival increases, younger patients consider their sexual attractiveness, sexual function, and ability to have children. In women who have ovarian cancer or endometrial cancer, which requires surgical resection of reproductive organs, the loss of fertility is immediate (Flay and Matthews 1995). After breast cancer, the hormones of pregnancy may promote micrometastases, so a woman must feel confident of cure as she faces pregnancy. The impact of surgical mastectomy for breast cancer on sexual behavior and marital relationships may need to be addressed through marital counseling (Baider 1995). Issues related to sexuality may delay a patient's decision to consult a physician in the cases of testicular cancer and ovarian cancer (Gascoigne et al. 1999; Hallowell 1998) and may guide a woman's decision making regarding breast cancer surgery (Reaby 1998). Procarbazine and alkylating agents are the chemotherapeutic agents most apt to cause infertility (Thachil et al. 1981), but many regimens do not affect fertility. Men with Hodgkin's disease or testicular cancer may have low sperm counts at the time of diagnosis. With regard to procarbazine and alkylating agents, men become sterile as treatment progresses but may become fertile again years later. Some men may choose to preserve sperm before chemotherapy treatment. In women, these same drugs shorten the reproductive life span. How soon menopause occurs depends on the drug dosage and the age of the woman at the time of treatment. For patients who have undergone chemotherapy

TABLE 29–5. Neuropsychiatric side effects of chemotherapeutic agents

Hormones

Tamoxifen[a]
1. Syndrome mimics menopausal symptoms: hot flashes, sleep disorder, irritability
2. Occasionally associated with hypercalcemia early in treatment
3. One report of confusion that began after 2 days and remitted in 7–10 days

Aminoglutethimide
1. Initial syndrome of rash, malaise, fatigue
2. Congener of glutethimide
3. Symptoms minimized with gradual dose increases

Megestrol acetate[b]
1. Progestogen
2. Increases appetite; useful in patients with cachexia; weight gain and side effects are dose related
3. Low doses (20 mg qid) are useful for hot flashes[c]

Fluoxymesterone
1. Androgen
2. Irritability, increased libido, hirsutism

Corticosteroids[d]
1. Graded by Rome and Braceland (1952): grade I, mild to more severe; grade II, hyperactivity and insomnia; grade III, lability, anxiety, agitation; grade IV, psychosis with prominent affective features
2. Dose related; more common with equivalent of ≥60 mg of prednisone per day
3. Manic and depressive features prominent
4. History of psychosis apparently does not increase risk
5. In repeated cycles of chemotherapy, affective response may vary
6. Cessation of steroid therapy may be associated with muscle aching and letdown
7. If a major organic affective syndrome has occurred, remission does not occur immediately with stopping of steroid therapy and patient should be treated with psychotropic medication
8. Treatment for hyperactivity and insomnia is with major tranquilizers, such as perphenazine and haloperidol; clonazepam may also be helpful
9. Lithium has been used prophylactically in the setting of steroid treatment in patients with multiple sclerosis

Chemotherapeutic agents

Procarbazine[e]
1. Mechanism unclear; likely inhibits DNA, RNA, and protein synthesis
2. Causes somnolence, psychosis, and delirium with immediate onset, rapid resolution
3. Weak MAO effect: no clinical reports of drug interaction leading to hypertensive crisis; most oncologists do not recommend a tyramine-restricted diet; no reports of hypertensive crisis
4. One case of mania reported
5. Delays metabolism of barbiturates and phenothiazines
6. Disulfiram-like effect; do not mix with alcohol

L-Asparaginase[f]
1. Mechanism: deprives acute lymphocytic leukemia cells of aspartate, a required amino acid that these cells cannot synthesize
2. Somnolence, lethargy, delirium, of immediate onset and rapid resolution; not dose related, common
3. Rare, late-onset (day 8) delirium; may be related to lack of asparagine

Pyrimidine analogues (inhibit DNA synthesis)

Cytosine arabinoside[g]
1. High dose causes delirium; dose related, age related
2. Onset on days 2–4, lasting a week
3. May be due to toxic metabolite, uracil arabinoside
4. Leukoencephalopathy may result from high dose: syndrome of personality change, drowsiness, dementia, psychomotor retardation, ataxia
5. Periventricular white matter signal densities on MR images: discrete, multifocal, coagulative necrosis in periventricular white matter and centrum semiovale bilaterally; demyelination occurs
6. Cerebellar syndrome

5-Fluorouracil[h]
1. Fatigue
2. Rare delirium or seizure (especially with break in blood-brain barrier or aberrant metabolic pathway)
3. Cerebellar syndrome

Folate antagonists

Methotrexate[i,j]
1. Inhibits reduction of dihydrofolate and thereby inhibits DNA, RNA, and protein synthesis
2. More neurological toxicity with high-dose or intrathecal regimens
3. More toxicity with concomitant radiation treatment
4. Transient delirium—days 10–13
5. High-dose or intrathecal administration may cause leukoencephalopathy

TABLE 29–5.   Neuropsychiatric side effects of chemotherapeutic agents *(continued)*

Metaphase inhibitors[k]

Vincristine, vinblastine

1. Dysphoria, lethargy
2. Dose related
3. Consider risk of seizures, inappropriate ADH (low sodium) levels
4. Vincristine inhibits dopamine hydroxylase; more dysphoria in small cell lung cancer protocol when added to complex regimen
5. Myelotoxic effects of vinblastine are more limited, so neurotoxicity is less common than with vincristine

Alkylating agents[l]

Ifosfamide

1. Related to cyclophosphamide, which is not associated with neurotoxicity
2. Urinary toxicity related to metabolite acrolein-related hemorrhagic cystitis; now toxicity is blocked by concomitant use of mesna, which binds acrolein, so ifosfamide can be used at higher doses
3. CNS toxicity ranges from lethargy to seizures, coma, and death; includes delirium, cerebellar signs, weakness, and cranial nerve deficit
4. EEG shows delta rhythmic slowing consistent with metabolic or toxic syndrome
5. Usually patients return to normal in 3 days
6. Attributed to chloracetaldehyde (metabolite of ifosfamide) but not to cyclophosphamide
7. Degraded by alcohol dehydrogenase
8. Renal impairment (e.g., from nephrectomy, previous DDP toxicity) is a risk factor for CNS toxicity
9. Mimics alcohol intoxication
10. Ifosfamide associated with inappropriate ADH levels, so check sodium levels

Biologicals

Interferon[m]

1. Most patients develop flulike syndrome, with fever, myalgias, malaise, which dissipates
2. Diffuse encephalopathy noted at high doses
3. Syndrome of fatigue, difficulty in concentration, psychomotor retardation, and general disinterest at 3 million units/day; affective changes not prominent
4. Two reports of patients with psychotic reactions, two reports of patients with manic symptoms; four other cases of psychosis reported in patients receiving more than 20 million units/day
5. Among 58 patients treated with interferon for chronic viral hepatitis: 4 had marked irritability and short temper (organic personality syndrome); 3 had tearfulness, depression, and hopelessness (organic affective syndrome); 3 had delirium (delirium occurred in those with a history of brain injury or more severe liver disease)

Interleukin-2 (IL-2) and lymphokine-activated killer cells[n]

1. Delirium is dose related
2. Mostly at end of course of IL-2 or several days after onset of combined treatment
3. Delirium in IL-2 phases did not predict delirium in next phase
4. Recovery in 2–3 days
5. Other factors such as hypoxia or sepsis can contribute to delirium
6. Most patients have flulike syndrome, with malaise, chills, anorexia, fatigue with treatment (fever and chills are effectively treated with meperidine 50 mg iv)
7. Affective changes other than delirium not prominent
8. Hypothyroidism posttreatment (mostly in women with preexisting antibodies suggesting autoimmune thyroiditis)

Note.   ADH = antidiuretic hormone; CNS = central nervous system; DDP = diamminedichloroplatinum (cisplatin); DNA = deoxyribonucleic acid; EEG = electroencephalogram; iv = intravenously; MAO = monoamine oxidase; MR = magnetic resonance; qid = four times a day; RNA = ribonucleic acid.
Source.   [a]Pluss and DiBella 1984; [b]Loprinzi et al. 1990; [c]Loprinzi et al. 1994a; [d]Ling et al. 1981; [e]De Vita et al. 1965; [f]Holland et al. 1974; [g]Lazarus et al. 1981; [h]Lynch et al. 1981; [i]Mulhern et al. 1987; [j]Walker et al. 1986; [k]Silberfarb et al. 1983; [l]Zalupski and Baker 1988; [m]Adams et al. 1984; [n]Denicoff et al. 1987.

and who later become pregnant, the rate of congenital abnormality appears to be similar to that in the general population (Green et al. 1991; Reichman and Green 1994).

Loss of the ovaries by irradiation or chemotherapy leads to the symptoms of early menopause and a range of psychological responses (Hamilton 1999). In men, testosterone production is usually not affected, so libido and secondary masculine characteristics are not altered (unless there is hypothyroidism or hyperprolactinemia). Irradiation of the pelvis gradually causes small-vessel disease, which may prevent normal congestion or erections

(Goldstein et al. 1984), so loss of potency in men and vaginal stenosis and decreased lubrication in women may be a delayed complication of chemotherapy. Lymphadenectomy for testicular cancer has been associated with retrograde ejaculation; fortunately, surgical procedures have been developed to limit this complication (Presti et al. 1993; Schover 1987). Occasionally, sexual function is diminished after brain injury or persistent physical illness.

When sexual and procreative functions are still intact, clinical depression or fear of recurrence may affect the patient's sexual interest. Some survivors of child-

TABLE 29–6. Psychiatric aspects of antiemetic drugs used with chemotherapy

Haloperidol

High-potency, dopamine-blocking butyrophenone antipsychotic

Half-life 12 hours with intravenous administration, 24 hours with oral dosing

Risk of extrapyramidal symptoms, akathisia

Droperidol

Antipsychotic similar to haloperidol in mechanism of action

Half-life 90 minutes; administered intravenously only

Greater risk of hypotension than with haloperidol

Risk of extrapyramidal side effects similar to that of haloperidol

Perphenazine

High-potency, dopamine-blocking phenothiazine antipsychotic

Administered at 6-hour intervals

Risk of sedation

Fewer extrapyramidal side effects than with haloperidol and droperidol

Prochlorperazine

High-potency, dopamine-blocking phenothiazine antipsychotic

Available in long-acting suppository form

High risk of agitation, extrapyramidal side effects

Indicated for, but less commonly used in, patients with psychosis; principal use is as antiemetic

Metoclopramide

In low doses, cholinergic effect fosters gastric emptying; in high doses, has cholinergic, dopamine-blocking, and serotonin-blocking activity

Risk of akathisia, extrapyramidal side effects, diarrhea

Ondansetron[a]

Serotonin-receptor blocker; acts on receptors primarily in gastrointestinal tract but also in chemoreceptor trigger zone

Headache is most common side effect[b]

In much lower, continuous doses, ondansetron is under study as a drug for anxiety and for dementia

Granisetron

Longer half-life than ondansetron; otherwise similar to ondansetron

Scopolamine[c]

Anticholinergic medication

Available as slow-release transdermal patch

May be effective in patients with vestibular disorders and nausea due to visceral stimulation

Reverses extrapyramidal side effects of other antiemetics

Mild hypnotic action

Potential culprit in anticholinergic delirium

Patch may be difficult to find on physical examination because of its color and variable locations

Diphenhydramine

Antihistaminic, but with anticholinergic action similar to that of scopolamine; blocks allergic reaction

For use in patients with nausea, can be administered intravenously; oral form is also available over the counter

Lorazepam

Sedative-hypnotic benzodiazepine antianxiety agent

Exerts antiemetic effect by unclear mechanism

Can be administered orally, sublingually, intravenously

Blocks anticipatory anxiety and anticipatory nausea

Elicits amnestic response

Effective in patients with akathisia

Alprazolam

Antianxiety agent

Short acting; oral and perhaps sublingual absorption

Effective in patients with anticipatory anxiety and anticipatory nausea

Dexamethasone[c]

Corticosteroid that exerts antiemetic effect, by unclear mechanism, alone or in combination with ondansetron

May be used as an adjunct to ondansetron therapy

May be beneficial in patients with delayed vomiting after cisplatin treatment

Psychiatric side effects of agitation or insomnia usually related to repeated use rather than one-time use

[a]Cubeddu et al. 1990.

[b]Serotonin is released from the gastrointestinal tract during treatment with antineoplastic agents.

[c]Gralla 1992.

hood cancer attribute their not wanting children to the fact that they had cancer (Greenberg et al. 1993b). Partners may withdraw emotionally because of depression, anticipatory grief, resentment at the partner's illness, fear of abandonment, or fear of hurting the sick partner. On the other hand, the diagnosis of cancer may also increase the expression of affection (Lieber et al. 1976).

SITE-SPECIFIC BIOPSYCHOSOCIAL ISSUES

Lung Cancer

Oncologists distinguish small cell carcinoma of the lung from other types because non–small cell cancers are more likely to be resected surgically if they are limited. Small cell cancer is more typically a systemic disease that is responsive to chemotherapy. Small cell cancers are associated with high rates of brain metastases, paraneoplastic syndromes, and ectopic hormonal effects. By contrast, the decision to perform surgery is made after the initial evaluation of non–small cell lung cancer. Irradiation is often used for residual disease. Some patients receive chemotherapy as well. The brain is a common site for the spread of disease. The relation between lung cancer and smoking gives the patient an external reason for feeling guilty and responsible for the tumor. Those who have not smoked but who acquire the disease anyway may particularly feel the unfairness of their lot (Bernhard and Ganz 1995).

Breast Cancer

Historically, breast cancer was a taboo subject. Today, by law, women must be presented with treatment options and information about prognosis. With this information, however, comes the stress of evaluating a variety of choices: simple mastectomy, lumpectomy, irradiation, breast reconstruction (Clifford 1979; Lewis and Bloom 1978–1979; Meyerowitz 1980; Schain et al. 1984), adjuvant chemotherapy, and bone marrow transplantation (Stefanek 1993). The prognosis is initially defined by the number of positive nodes and the size of the tumor. The decisions about mastectomy or reconstruction are affected by the patient's familial or previous concerns about breast cancer and by the patient's coping style (Reaby 1998). Coping styles in women with breast cancer can be predictive of positive adjustment to the disease (McCaul et al. 1999; Schnoll et al. 1998). Adjuvant chemotherapy is associated with alopecia, fatigue, and weight gain. Many women with metastatic breast cancer live with bone scans showing abnormalities, variable bone pains, the risk of fracture, and progression. Depressed mood augments bone pain (Spiegel and Bloom 1983); the tricyclic antidepressant side effect of postural hypotension should be monitored more closely in patients with metastatic bone disease, for whom a fall is associated with an increased risk of fracture (Front et al. 1979). Pericarditis, pleural effusion, and lung, liver, and brain metastases define the visceral progression of disease (Rowland and Holland 1989).

Head and Neck Cancer

Patients with head and neck cancer may have highly visible and often disfiguring changes in facial appearance. They may lose the ability to speak and have to learn esophageal or mechanized speech. Taste, smell, and eating dysfunction may follow radiation treatment. Alcohol dependence and cigarette smoking, both of which occur at a high rate among these patients, may complicate care (Breitbart and Holland 1989; Rapoport et al. 1993). The high risk of metastases to the CNS with head and neck cancer should always be considered when evaluating patients with psychiatric symptoms.

Colon and Rectal Cancer

Colon and rectal cancer that is detected early can be resected, leaving intact bowel. Some patients, however, must adjust to a permanent colostomy, which may cause self-consciousness, feelings of decreased attractiveness, and avoidance of social life for fear of accidental spillage, noise, or odor. Metastases are most likely to occur in the liver.

Pancreatic Cancer

Pancreatic cancer is the cancer possibly most likely to present or to be associated with psychiatric changes. Because pancreatic cancer often causes pain, malaise, and weight loss, dysphoria often precedes the diagnosis. Some researchers have suspected that the neurotransmitters of the pancreas have systemic effects that increase the likelihood of depression, anxiety, and psychosis (Green and Austin 1993; Holland et al. 1986).

Testicular Cancer

Testicular cancer, now often curable, predominantly affects men between ages 20 and 40 years. The discovery of testicular cancer produces emotional responses that include embarrassment and fear of castration (Gascoigne et al. 1999). Those who undergo retroperitoneal lymphadenectomy are at risk for difficulty in ejaculating sperm. Fertility and perception of sexual attractiveness are jeopardized. Men often choose to bank sperm before treatment. Survivors have concerns about sexual function (Bloom et al. 1993; Gritz et al. 1989; Rieker et al. 1989; Schover and von Eschenbach 1985; Tross 1989).

Prostate Cancer

With wider screening for prostate cancer, some men become aware of low-grade tumors at an early stage when the benefits of treatment are not definitely known. The anxiety related to knowledge of an untreated low-grade tumor must be balanced against the morbidity of treatment. Impotence occurs in 20%–50% of those who undergo nerve-sparing surgery (Gittes 1991). With irradiation, delayed impotence may develop in 50% of patients after 7 years, the result of vascular injury (Bagshaw et al. 1988). Elimination of testosterone by orchiectomy or medication leads to loss of libido and sometimes to hot flashes, gynecomastia, and female fat distribution (Herr 1987). Metastases occur most often in bone; the clinical challenge is pain management.

Hodgkin's Disease, Non-Hodgkin's Lymphoma, and Leukemia

Chemotherapy begins immediately in patients with acute leukemia. Treatment is divided into three phases (induction, consolidation, and maintenance) that span approximately 2–3 years. Both induction and consolidation require a 4- to 6-week hospitalization; maintenance treatments are outpatient procedures (Lesko 1989; Mumma et al. 1992). The treatment of lymphoma depends on the type and the stage of the disease. Limited disease may be treated with irradiation alone, but many cases require chemotherapy. Bone marrow transplantation is a consideration for both illnesses.

Patients with markers for chronic leukemia can now be identified from incidentally noted increased white blood cell counts. Patients are usually anxious as they adjust to the diagnosis at a time when treatment is not yet appropriate. As the white blood cell count increases, systemic fatigue may complicate assessment of anxiety and depression. Those with Hodgkin's disease or non-Hodgkin's lymphoma have fatigue, decreased libido, depression, anxiety, and irritability during treatment (Devlen et al. 1987a, 1987b). Those treated with procarbazine and alkylating agents are particularly prone to infertility. Patients with high paraprotein levels, especially from myeloma or Waldenström's macroglobulinemia, are at risk for hyperviscosity syndrome. Survivors of Hodgkin's disease are at high risk for problems in psychosocial adaptation; some have reported that their energy levels did not return to normal (Bloom et al. 1993; Cella and Tross 1986; Fobair et al. 1986; Kornblith et al. 1992).

Malignant Bone Tumors

Osteosarcoma and Ewing's sarcoma, the most common bone tumors, occur at any age but predominately during adolescence. Patients must make the difficult choice between amputation or limb salvage surgery followed by chemotherapy and, often, radiation treatment. Slow-growing metastases to the lung may be resected repeatedly. Normal adolescent issues, such as control, identity,

and acceptance, are heightened by the onset of cancer (Greenberg et al. 1993c, 1993b; Heiligenstein and Holland 1989; Zelter 1980). Fortunately, data suggest that those patients who undergo amputation tend to make career and marital adjustments comparable to those made by their healthy siblings (S.G. Lundberg and Guggenheim 1986; Nicholson et al. 1992). With allografts, there is a risk of secondary fracture or infection, especially during chemotherapy. When treated with current chemotherapy regimens, survivors are often able to preserve fertility.

FAMILIES OF PATIENTS WITH CANCER

Longer survival times for patients with cancer bring greater demands for families. The course of cancer involves many emotional ups and downs that still, in some cases, end in loss. The manner in which a family deals with this turmoil depends on the ages and number of family members, their coping resources, their stability before the patient's diagnosis, their ethnic and cultural background, and the roles and responsibilities of each family member (Lewis 1993).

In the best scenarios, the cohesiveness and emotional closeness of the family actually increase, creating a sense of joy and appreciation of home life and life in general. In such cases, the family communicates openly with both the patient and the physician throughout the patient's illness. The patient's ability to discuss feelings openly with the physician and family, and to participate in family plans, gives meaning and continuity to all concerned (Fawzy et al. 1983b). Family and social support have been positively correlated with patients' psychological adjustment to cancer (Akechi et al. 1998).

However, emotional and financial drains may disrupt families. Family caregivers must deal with their own emotional distress while also meeting the needs of the patient and other family members, whose needs usually increase as well. Often, caregivers must take on the regular roles of the now sick member and cope with increasing monetary, physical, and psychological demands at a time when resources are decreasing. All of this is usually done in varying states of sleep deprivation (Rait and Lederberg 1989). Some caregivers perceive the care as a burden, whereas others consider it a challenge (Nijboer et al. 1998). Caregivers can benefit from being informed that they need not feel guilty about taking time away from the patient to meet their own needs for food, rest, and relaxation. They may require help to set priorities and to share time effectively among the patient and other family members, especially children. Caregivers need to know that they can and should ask for help from staff members, from other family members, and from friends. Rather than viewing requests as an imposition, many family members and friends are relieved and grateful to be able to do something to help (Rait and Lederberg 1989). The patient with cancer and his or her partner often hide their feelings of helplessness and fear in an effort to appear optimistic and reassuring. Studies suggest that a conspiracy of silence is not helpful but that expression of feelings and shared involvement in decision making improve adjustment (Baider et al. 1998). Support groups are an excellent resource for partners and are appearing at many medical centers.

Cancer in a child invariably results in a high level of stress on the parents. Because family disintegration, substance abuse, and serious psychopathology are common among parents of seriously ill or dying children, early psychiatric referral may be offered even in the absence of overt symptoms. When a parent is the patient, preschool and school-age children often act out their emotional distress at school. The child should know what is happening to his or her parent; the explanation should match the child's level of understanding. Older children and adolescents often experience role reversal as they become caregivers (Fawzy and Natterson 1994). As children who survive cancer reach adulthood, a number of serious long-term physical and psychiatric health issues emerge (Stevens et al. 1998).

Some specific problems signal the need for psychiatric consultation for a family member. Preexisting psychopathology and intrafamily conflicts often become worse when someone in the family has cancer. Major differences in how family members process information about the illness can fuel hostility and emotional chaos. Family exhaustion and abandonment occur in the setting of frustration, anger, and guilt. Families may withdraw physically and emotionally from the patient or demand inappropriately that the patient start to take care of himself or herself, eat better, and cheer up. A terminal crisis could occur when the patient dies before the family has faced the progression of illness. Guilt and scapegoating are then more likely to occur among the survivors (Massie et al. 1989).

The turmoil felt in the family may be vented at the physician or medical staff. The family may idealize the doctor as omnipotent, the one controlling the beloved patient's fate, or family members may become irritable and extremely sensitive to real or imagined slights to the patient by the staff or physician.

Many family members will appreciate the physician's letting them know or confirming their impression that the patient's death is near. The death of a loved one may often be met with relief, both personal and projected, and with the rationalization that at least the suffering is over. The physician can offer a close family member the opportunity to visit the office a few weeks after the patient's death to ask questions about the course of the illness or autopsy results. This meeting often gives the family member a chance to discuss guilt or anxiety over something that he or she believes may have contributed to the patient's discomfort or early death. Talking with a physician who knew and respected the patient, who assisted the patient and family during the final days of the illness, can help to resolve familial grief (Fawzy et al. 1983b). Family grief therapy may be initiated during palliative care and has been effective in promoting healthier family functioning during the struggle to care for a terminally ill patient (Kissane et al. 1998).

ONCOLOGY STAFF

Often, the psychiatric consultant to the oncology center will be asked to help medical and other center staff cope with the stresses of caring for patients with cancer. For instance, being a target of a patient's rage can be a strain on the oncology nurse. When family members are absent, patients tend to direct their rage primarily toward nurses, who not only are seen as maternal figures but are unconsciously viewed perhaps as more expendable than physicians and hence as more appropriate objects of anger. The consultation psychiatrist may help staff members to see that the patients' rage is at the illness, not at the staff for perceived inadequacy. In research units, the staff members may not understand the role of protocols and may feel that things are done to patients rather than for them. Both education of the staff about the significance of ongoing research protocols and the provision of follow-up information on patients and families add to staff satisfaction.

The physical and emotional responses and ineffective coping mechanisms associated with burnout are summarized in Table 29–7 (Fawzy et al. 1983a, 1991). Multidisciplinary staff meetings are successful vehicles for helping physicians and other medical staff members become a team that provides high-quality comprehensive care. These meetings are most often instituted as a forum for consideration of psychological and behavioral problems in patient management. Meetings typically begin with a discussion and review of each patient's clinical course and

TABLE 29–7. Symptoms of burnout in medical staff

Physical symptoms
>   Headaches
>   Intestinal disorders
>   Chronic fatigue
>   Sleep disorders

Emotional symptoms
>   Depression
>   Detachment
>   Guilt
>   Hopelessness
>   Powerlessness

Maladaptive coping mechanisms
>   Altered work patterns (absenteeism, arriving late or leaving early, clock watching)
>   Excessive death watch
>   Negativism/cynicism
>   Withdrawal from patients and co-workers
>   Uncontrollable crying
>   Family conflicts
>   Substance abuse (caffeine, nicotine, alcohol, other drugs)

psychosocial condition. This process leads to an atmosphere that permits discussion of conflicts among staff. As psychosocial needs become more readily accepted as critical aspects of care, the consulting psychiatrist can expand his or her role. Such programs have a threefold objective: 1) to help physicians gain a better understanding of how to deal with severely ill patients, 2) to allow staff members to admit more openly to the emotional stresses they face, and 3) to help staff members discover more effective ways to deal with these stresses. The more successful meetings focus initially on patients rather than on staff concerns. In one hospital-based oncology program (Fawzy et al. 1977), the psychiatric consulting group identified some problems and set up group meetings. After some initial resistance by physicians, the meeting became a forum to explore feelings, to communicate openly, and to mourn patients. As a result, nursing absenteeism and the number of transfers decreased sharply, house staff began spending more time in the unit, and patient morale improved.

Some hospitals employ a clinical psychologist or psychiatrist whose primary assignment is to help physicians and nurses to cope with the anguish of cancer patients that the staff members are exposed to daily. The National Cancer Institute's Pediatric Oncology Branch requires new oncology fellows to attend weekly social psychiatry seminars.

One method to help oncology staff to deal with the stresses of working with cancer patients is to have clearly identified goals for each patient and then to strive to meet those goals. Patients fall into one of three categories: 1) those for whom treatment will result in a cure or long-term, disease-free survival; 2) those for whom the goal is long-term control and good quality of life (patients who need good supportive symptom therapy, including pain control); and 3) those for whom death is fairly imminent. Patients in the third group need to know that they will not be abandoned. They need increased human contact. Recognition that the needs of each group of patients are of equal importance can go a long way toward helping staff members to feel a sense of helpfulness and satisfaction with their work.

REFERENCES

Adams R, Quesada JR, Gutterman JU: Neuropsychiatric manifestations of human leukocyte interferon therapy in patients with cancer. JAMA 252:938–941, 1984

Akechi T, Uchitomi Y, Okamura H, et al: Usage of haloperidol for delirium in cancer patients. Support Care Cancer 4:390–392, 1996

Akechi T, Kugaya A, Okamura H, et al: Predictive factors for psychological distress in ambulatory lung cancer patients. Support Care Cancer 6:281–286, 1998

Akechi T, Okamura H, Yamawaki S, et al: Why do some cancer patients with depression desire an early death and others do not? Psychosomatics 42:141–145, 2001

American Psychiatric Association: Diagnostic and Statistical Manual of Mental Disorders, 3rd Edition, Revised. Washington, DC, American Psychiatric Association, 1987

Andrykowski MA: The role of anxiety in the development of anticipatory nausea in cancer chemotherapy: a review and synthesis. Psychosom Med 52:458–475, 1990

Bagshaw MA, Cox RS, Ray GR: Status of Radiation Treatment of Prostate Cancer at Stanford University. NCI Monographs No 7 (NIH Publ No 88-3005). Washington, DC, National Institutes of Health, 1988, pp 127–131

Baider L: Psychological intervention with couples after mastectomy. Support Care Cancer 3:239–243, 1995

Baider L, Koch U, Esacson R, et al: Prospective study of cancer patients and their spouses: the weakness of marital strength. Psychooncology 7:49–56, 1998

Beck AT: Depression Inventory. Philadelphia, PA, Philadelphia Center for Cognitive Therapy, 1978

Berard RM, Boermeester F, Viljoen G: Depressive disorders in an outpatient oncology setting: prevalence, assessment, and management. Psychooncology 7:112–120, 1998

Bernhard J, Ganz PA: Psychosocial issues in lung cancer patients. Cancer Treat Res 72:363–390, 1995

Bernstein IL: Learned taste aversions in children receiving chemotherapy. Science 200:1302–1303, 1978

Bloch S, Kissane D: Psychotherapies in psycho-oncology: an exciting new challenge. Bj J Psychiatry 177:112–116, 2000

Bloom JR, Fobair P, Gritz E, et al: Psychosocial outcomes of cancer: a comparative analysis of Hodgkin's disease and testicular cancer. J Clin Oncol 11:979–988, 1993

Breitbart W: Suicide in cancer patients. Oncology 1:49–53, 1987

Breitbart W: Identifying patients at risk for, and treatment of, major psychiatric complications of cancer. Support Care Cancer 3:45–60, 1995

Breitbart W, Holland JC: Head and neck cancer, in Handbook of Psychooncology: Psychological Care of the Patient With Cancer. Edited by Holland JC, Rowland JH. New York, Oxford University Press, 1989, pp 232–239

Breitbart W, Mermelstein H: Pemoline: an alternative psychostimulant in the management of depressive disorders in cancer patients. Psychosomatics 33:352–356, 1992

Bruera E, Neumann CM: The uses of psychotropics in symptom management in advanced cancer. Psychooncology 7:346–348, 1998

Cascino TL: Neurologic complications of systemic cancer. Med Clin North Am 77:265–278, 1993

Cella DF, Tross S: Psychological adjustment to survival from Hodgkin's disease. J Consult Clin Psychol 54:618–622, 1986

Clifford E: The reconstruction experience: the search for restitution, in Breast Reconstruction Following Mastectomy. Edited by Georgiade NG. London, CV Mosby, 1979, pp 22–34

Cornelius JR, Soloff PH, Miewald BK: Behavioral manifestations of paraneoplastic encephalopathy. Biol Psychiatry 21:686–690, 1986

Cotton SP, Levine EG, Fitzpatrick CM, et al: Exploring the relationships among spiritual well-being, quality of life, and psychological adjustment in women with breast cancer. Psychooncology 8:429–438, 1999

Crawford J, Cox EB, Cohen HJ: Evaluation of hyperviscosity in monoclonal gammopathies. Am J Med 79:13–22, 1985

Cubeddu LX, Hoffmann IS, Fuenmayor NT, et al: Efficacy of ondansetron (GR 38032F) and the role of serotonin in cisplatin-induced nausea and vomiting. N Engl J Med 322:810–816, 1990

DeAngelis LM, Delattre JY, Posner JB: Radiation-induced dementia in patients cured of brain metastases. Neurology 39:789–796, 1989

Demark-Wahnefried W, Winer EP, Rimer BK: Why women gain weight with adjuvant chemotherapy for breast cancer. J Clin Oncol 11:1418–1429, 1993

Denicoff KD, Rubinow DR, Papa MZ, et al: The neuropsychiatric effects of treatment with interleukin-2 and lymphokine-activated killer cells. Ann Intern Med 107:293–300, 1987

Derogatis LR, Spencer MS: The Brief Symptom Inventory (BSI): Administration, Scoring, and Procedures Manual. Baltimore, MD, Clinical Psychometric Research, 1982

Derogatis LR, Morrow RG, Fetting J, et al: The prevalence of psychiatric disorders among cancer patients (abstract). JAMA 249:751, 1983

De Vita VT, Hahn MA, Oliverio VT: Monoamine oxidase inhibition by a new carcinostatic agent, N-isopropyl-a-(2-methylhydrazino)-p-toluamide (MIH). Proc Soc Exp Biol Med 120:561–565, 1965

Devlen J, Maguire P, Phillips P, et al: Psychological problems associated with diagnosis and treatment of lymphomas, I: retrospective study. British Medical Journal (Clinical Research Edition) 295:953–954, 1987a

Devlen J, Maguire P, Phillips P, et al: Psychological problems associated with diagnosis and treatment of lymphomas, II: prospective study. British Medical Journal (Clinical Research Edition) 295:955–957, 1987b

Dexter DD, Westmoreland BF, Cascino TL: Complex partial status epilepticus in a patient with leptomeningeal carcinomatosis. Neurology 40:858–859, 1990

Dugan W, McDonald MV, Passik SD, et al: Use of the Zung Self-Rating Depression Scale in cancer patients: feasibility as a screening tool. Psychooncology 7:483–493, 1998

Edelman S, Kidman AD: Description of a group cognitive behavior therapy program with cancer patients. Psychooncology 8:306–314, 1999

Edelman S, Bell DR, Kidman AD: A group cognitive behavior therapy programme with metastatic breast cancer patients. Psychooncology 8:295–305, 1999

Edmonds CV, Lockwood GA, Cunningham AJ: Psychological response to long-term group therapy: a randomized trial with metastatic breast cancer patients. Psychooncology 8:74–91, 1999

Ellis HC, Bennett TC, Daniel TC, et al: Psychology of Learning and Memory. Monterey, CA, Brooks Cole Publishing, 1979, pp 33–34

Endicott J: Measurement of depression in patients with cancer. Cancer 53:2243–2249, 1984

Farberow NL, Schneidman EW, Leonard CV: Suicide among general medical and surgical hospital patients and those with malignant neoplasms. Medical Bulletin of the Veterans Administration 9:1–16, 1963

Farberow NL, Ganzler S, Cutter F, et al: An eight-year survey of hospital suicides. Life Threatening Behavior 1:184–201, 1971

Fawzy FI, Fawzy NW: Psychosocial aspects of cancer, in Diagnosis and Management of Cancer. Edited by Nixon D. Menlo Park, NJ, Addison-Wesley, 1982, pp 111–123

Fawzy FI, Natterson B: Psychological care of the cancer patient, in Clinical Oncology: A Lange Clinical Manual. Edited by Cameron R. San Mateo, CA, Simon and Schuster Higher Education Group, 1994, pp 40–44

Fawzy FI, Wellisch DK, Yager J: Psychiatric liaison to the bone-marrow transplant project, in The Family in Mourning. Edited by Hollingsworth CE, Pasnau RO. New York, Grune & Stratton, 1977, pp 181–189

Fawzy FI, Wellisch DK, Pasnau RO, et al: Preventing nursing burnout: a challenge for liaison psychiatry. Gen Hosp Psychiatry 5:141–149, 1983a

Fawzy FI, Pasnau RO, Wolcott DL, et al: Psychosocial management of cancer. Psychiatric Medicine 1:165–180, 1983b

Fawzy FI, Cousins N, Fawzy NW, et al: A structured psychiatric intervention for cancer patients, I: changes over time in methods of coping and affective disturbance. Arch Gen Psychiatry 47:720–725, 1990a

Fawzy FI, Kemeny ME, Fawzy NW, et al: A structured psychiatric intervention for cancer patients, II: changes over time in immunological measures. Arch Gen Psychiatry 47:729–735, 1990b

Fawzy FI, Fawzy NW, Pasnau RO: Burnout in the health professions, in Handbook of Studies on General Hospital Psychiatry. Edited by Judd FK, Burrows GD, Lipsett DR. New York, Elsevier Science, 1991, pp 119–130

Fawzy FI, Fawzy NW, Hyun CS, et al: Malignant melanoma: effects of an early structured psychiatric intervention, coping, and affective state on recurrence and survival 6 years later. Arch Gen Psychiatry 50:681–689, 1993

Fawzy FI, Fawzy NW, Arndt LA, et al: Critical review of psychosocial interventions in cancer care. Arch Gen Psychiatry 52:100–113, 1995

Feher S, Maly RC: Coping with breast cancer in later life: the role of religious faith. Psychooncology 8:408–416, 1999

Fernandez F, Adams F, Holmes VF, et al: Methylphenidate for depressive disorders in cancer patients. Psychosomatics 28:455–461, 1987

Flay LD, Matthews JH: The effects of radiotherapy and surgery on the sexual function of women treated for cervical cancer. Int J Radiat Oncol Biol Phys 31:399–404, 1995

Fobair P, Hoppe RT, Bloom J, et al: Psychosocial problems among survivors of Hodgkin's disease. J Clin Oncol 4:S805–S814, 1986

Fox BH: A psychological measure as a predictor in cancer, in Psychosocial Aspects of Cancer. Edited by Cohen J, Cullen JW, Martin LR. New York, Raven, 1982, pp 275–296

Fox BH, Stanek EJ, Boyd SC, et al: Suicide rates among cancer patients in Connecticut. Journal of Chronic Disease 35:85–100, 1982

Front D, Schneck SO, Franketl A, et al: Bone metastases and bone pain in breast cancer (letter). JAMA 242:1747, 1979

Frytak S, Earnest F 4th, O'Neill BP, et al: Magnetic resonance imaging for neurotoxicity in long-term survivors of carcinoma. Mayo Clin Proc 60:803–812, 1985

Gascoigne P, Mason MD, Roberts E: Factors affecting presentation and delay in patients with testicular cancer: results of a qualitative study. Psychooncology 8:144–154, 1999

Gellert GA, Maxwell RM, Siegel BS: Survival of breast cancer patients receiving adjunctive psychosocial support therapy: a 10 year follow up study. J Clin Oncol 11:66–69, 1993

Gilbert MR, Armstrong TS: Management of seizures in the adult patient with cancer. Cancer Practice 3:143–149, 1995

Gilliam F, Simonian N, Chiappa K: Complex partial status epilepticus associated with ifosfamide infusion (abstract). Epilepsia 33 (suppl):3, 1993

Gittes RF: Carcinoma of the prostate. N Engl J Med 324:236–245, 1991

Gloor P, Olivier A, Quesney LF, et al: The role of the limbic system in experiential phenomena of temporal lobe epilepsy. Ann Neurol 12:129–144, 1982

Goldstein I, Felman MI, Deckers PJ, et al: Radiation-associated impotence: a clinical study of its mechanism. JAMA 251:903–910, 1984

Gralla RJ: Antiemetic drugs for chemotherapeutic support: current treatments and rationale for development of newer agents. Cancer 70:1003–1006, 1992

Green AI, Austin CP: Psychopathology of pancreatic cancer: a psychobiologic probe. Psychosomatics 34:208–221, 1993

Green DM, Zevon MA, Lowrie G, et al: Congenital anomalies in children of patients who received chemotherapy for cancer in childhood and adolescence. N Engl J Med 325:141–146, 1991

Greenberg DB: Depression and cancer, in Depression and Coexisting Disease. Edited by Robinson RG, Rabins PV. New York, Igaku-Shoin Medical Publishers, 1989, pp 103–115

Greenberg DB: Strategic use of benzodiazepines in cancer patients. Oncology 5:83–88, 1991

Greenberg DB, Brown GL: Mania resulting from brain stem tumor. J Nerv Ment Dis 173:434–436, 1985

Greenberg DB, Surman OS, Clarke J, et al: Alprazolam for phobic nausea and vomiting related to cancer chemotherapy. Cancer Treatment Reports 71:549–550, 1987

Greenberg DB, Sawicka J, Eisenthal S, et al: Fatigue syndrome due to localized radiation. J Pain Symptom Manage 7:38–45, 1992

Greenberg DB, Younger J, Kaufman SD: Management of lithium in patients with cancer. Psychosomatics 34:388–394, 1993a

Greenberg DB, Goorin A, Gebhardt M, et al: Quality of life in osteosarcoma survivors (abstract). Proceedings of the American Society of Clinical Oncology 12:456, 1993b

Greenberg DB, Gray JL, Mannic CM, et al: Treatment related fatigue and serum interleukin 1 levels in patients during external beam irradiation for prostate cancer. J Pain Symptom Manage 8:196–199, 1993c

Gritz ER, Wellisch DK, Wang HJ, et al: Long-term effects of testicular cancer on sexual functioning in married couples. Cancer 64:1560–1567, 1989

Grossman SA, Sheidler VR, Gilbert MR: Decreased phenytoin levels in patients receiving chemotherapy. Am J Med 87:505–510, 1989

Hallowell N: Women's perceptions of prophylactic surgery as a cancer risk management option. Psychooncology 7:263–275, 1998

Hallowell N: Women's perceptions of prophylactic surgery as a cancer risk management option. Psychooncology 7:263–275, 1999

Hamilton AB: Psychological aspects of ovarian cancer. Cancer Invest 17:335–341, 1999

Hardman A, Maguire P, Crowther D: The recognition of psychiatric morbidity on a medical oncology ward. J Psychosom Res 33:235–239, 1989

Hathaway SR, McKinley JC: Minnesota Multiphasic Personality Inventory. Minneapolis, MN, University of Minnesota, 1943

Heiligenstein E, Holland JC: Malignant bone tumors, in Handbook of Psychooncology: Psychological Care of the Patient With Cancer. Edited by Holland JC, Rowland JH. New York, Oxford University Press, 1989, pp 250–253

Herr HW: Strategies for the management of recurrent and advanced urologic cancers: quality of life. Cancer 60 (suppl 3):623–630, 1987

Holland JC, Rowland JH (eds): Handbook of Psychooncology: Psychological Care of the Patient With Cancer. New York, Oxford University Press, 1989

Holland J[C], Fasanello S, Ohnuma T: Psychiatric symptoms associated with L-asparaginase administration. J Psychiatr Res 10:105–113, 1974

Holland JC, Rowland J, Plumb M: Psychological aspects of anorexia in cancer patients. Cancer Res 37:2425–2428, 1977

Holland JC, Korzun AH, Tross S, et al: Comparative psychological disturbance in patients with pancreatic and gastric cancer. Am J Psychiatry 143:982–986, 1986

Holland JC, Morrow G, Schmale A, et al: A randomized clinical trial of alprazolam versus progressive muscle relaxation in cancer patients with anxiety and depressive symptoms. J Clin Oncol 9:1004–1011, 1991

Holland JC, Romano SJ, Heiligenstein JH, et al: A controlled trial of fluoxetine and desipramine in depressed women with advanced cancer. Psychooncology 7:291–300, 1998

Jacobsen PB, Bovbjerg DH, Redd WH: Anticipatory anxiety in women receiving chemotherapy for breast cancer. Health Psychol 12:469–475, 1993

Jones DR, Goldblatt PO, Leon DA: Bereavement and cancer: some data on deaths of spouses from the longitudinal study of Office of Population Censuses and Surveys. British Medical Journal (Clinical Research Edition) 289:461–464, 1984

Kalash GR: Psychotropic drug metabolism in the cancer patient: clinical aspects of management of potential drug interactions. Psychooncology 7:307–320, 1998

Kathol RG, Mutgi A, Williams J, et al: Diagnosis of major depression in cancer patients according to four sets of criteria. Am J Psychiatry 147:1021–1024, 1990

Kissane DW, Bloch S, Miach P, et al: Cognitive-existential group therapy for patients with primary breast cancer—techniques and themes. Psychooncology 6:25–33, 1997

Kissane DW, Bloch S, McKenzie M, et al: Family grief therapy: a preliminary account of a new model to promote healthy family functioning during palliative care and bereavement. Psychooncology 7:14–25, 1998

Kornblith AB, Anderson J, Cella DF, et al: Hodgkin disease survivors at increased risk for problems in psychosocial adaptation. The Cancer and Leukemia Group B. Cancer 70:2214–2224, 1992

Kugaya A, Okamura H, Nakano T, et al: Suicidal thoughts in cancer patients: clinical experience in psycho-oncology. Psychiatry Clin Neurosci 53:569–573, 1999

Kvale G, Psychol C, Hugdahl K: Cardiovascular conditioning and anticipatory nausea and vomiting in cancer patients. Behav Med 20:78–83, 1994

Lansky SB, List MA, Herrman CA, et al: Absence of major depressive disorder in female cancer patients. J Clin Oncol 3:1553–1560, 1985

Lazarus HM, Herzig RH, Herzig GP, et al: Central nervous system toxicity of high-dose systemic cytosine arabinoside. Cancer 48:2577–2582, 1981

Lee Y, Nauert C, Glass JP: Treatment related white matter changes in cancer patients. Cancer 57:1473–1482, 1986

Lesko LM: Hematological malignancies, in Handbook of Psychooncology: Psychological Care of the Patient With Cancer. Edited by Holland JC, Rowland JH. New York, Oxford University Press, 1989, pp 218–231

Lewis FM: Psychosocial transitions and the family's work in adjusting to cancer. Semin Oncol Nurs 9:127–129, 1993

Lewis FM, Bloom JR: Psychosocial adjustment to breast cancer: a review of selected literature. Int J Psychiatry Med 9:1–17, 1978–1979

Lieber L, Plumb MM, Gerstenzang M, et al: The communication of affection between cancer patients and their spouses. Psychosom Med 38:379–389, 1976

Ling MHM, Perry PJ, Tsuang MT: Side effects of corticosteroid therapy: psychiatric aspects. Arch Gen Psychiatry 38:471–477, 1981

Loprinzi CL: Management of cancer anorexia/cachexia. Support Care Cancer 3:120–122, 1995

Loprinzi CL, Ellison NM, Schaid DJ, et al: Controlled trial of megestrol acetate for the treatment of cancer anorexia and cachexia. J Natl Cancer Inst 82:1127–1132, 1990

Loprinzi CL, Michalak JC, Quella SK, et al: Megestrol acetate for the prevention of hot flashes. N Engl J Med 331:347–352, 1994a

Loprinzi CL, Bernath AM, Schaid DJ, et al: Phase III evaluation of 4 doses of megestrol acetate as therapy for patients with cancer anorexia and/or cachexia. Oncology 51 (suppl 1):2–7, 1994b

Louhivuori KA, Hakama J: Risk of suicide among cancer patients. Am J Epidemiol 109:59–65, 1979

Lundberg JC, Passik SD: Alcohol and cancer: a review for psycho-oncologists. Psychooncology 6:253–266, 1997

Lundberg SG, Guggenheim FG: Sequelae of limb amputation. Adv Psychosom Med 15:199–210, 1986

Lynch HT, Droszcz CP, Albano WA, et al: Organic brain syndrome secondary to 5-fluorouracil toxicity. Dis Colon Rectum 24:130–131, 1981

Massie MJ, Holland JC, Straker N: Psychotherapeutic interventions, in Handbook of Psychooncology: Psychological Care of the Patient With Cancer. Edited by Holland JC, Rowland JH. New York, Oxford University Press, 1989, pp 455–469

Massie MJ, Heiligenstein E, Lederberg MS: Psychiatric complications in cancer patients, in American Cancer Society Textbook of Clinical Oncology. Edited by Holleb AI, Fink DJ, Murphy GP. Atlanta, GA, American Cancer Society, 1991, pp 576–586

Massie MJ, Gagnon P, Holland JC: Depression and suicide in patients with cancer. J Pain Symptom Manage 9:325–340, 1994

McCartney CF, Cahill P, Larson DB, et al: Effect of a psychiatric liaison program on consultation rates and on detection of minor psychiatric disorders in cancer patients. Am J Psychiatry 146:898–901, 1989

McCaul KD, Sandgren AK, King B, et al: Coping and adjustment to breast cancer. Psychooncology 8:230–236, 1999

McDaniel JS, Musselman DL, Porter MR, et al: Depression in patients with cancer: diagnosis, biology, and treatment. Arch Gen Psychiatry 52:89–99, 1995

McNamara ME, Fogel BS: Anticonvulsant-responsive panic attacks with temporal lobe EEG abnormalities. J Neuropsychiatry Clin Neurosci 2:193–196, 1990

Meléndez JC, McCrank E: Anxiety-related reactions associated with magnetic resonance imaging examinations. JAMA 270:745–747, 1993

Meyerowitz BE: Psychosocial correlates of breast cancer and treatment. Psychol Bull 8:108–131, 1980

Minotti AM, Kountakis SE, Stiernberg CM: Paraneoplastic syndromes in patients with head and neck cancer. Am J Otolaryngol 15:336–343, 1994

Moll JWB, Henzen-Logmans SC, Splinter TAW, et al: Diagnostic value of anti-neuronal antibodies for paraneoplastic disorders of the nervous system. J Neurol Neurosurg Psychiatry 53:940–943, 1990

Moorey S, Greer S, Bliss J, et al: A comparison of adjuvant psychological therapy and supportive counseling in patients with cancer. Psychooncology 7:18–28, 1998

Morrow GR: Clinical characteristics associated with the development of anticipatory nausea and vomiting in cancer patients undergoing chemotherapy. J Clin Oncol 2:1170–1175, 1989

Morrow GR, Morrell C: Behavioral treatment for the anticipatory nausea and vomiting induced by cancer chemotherapy. N Engl J Med 307:1476–1480, 1982

Mulhern RK, Ochs J, Fairclough D, et al: Intellectual and academic achievement status after CNS relapse: a retrospective analysis of 40 children treated for acute lymphoblastic leukemia. J Clin Oncol 5:933–940, 1987

Mumma GH, Mashberg D, Lesko LM: Long-term psychosocial adjustment of acute leukemia survivors. Gen Hosp Psychiatry 14:43–55, 1992

Mytko JJ, Knight SJ: Body, mind and spirit: towards the integration of religiosity and spirituality in cancer quality of life research. Psychooncology 8:439–450, 1999

Nelson K, Walsh D, Deeter P, et al: A phase II study of delta-9-tetrahydrocannabinol for appetite stimulation in cancer-associated anorexia. J Palliat Care 10:14–18, 1994

Newman NJ, Bell IR, McKee AC: Paraneoplastic limbic encephalitis: neuropsychiatric presentation. Biol Psychiatry 27:529–540, 1990

Nicholson HS, Mulvihill JJ, Byrne J: Late effects of therapy in adult survivors of osteosarcoma and Ewing's sarcoma. Med Pediatr Oncol 20:6–12, 1992

Nijboer C, Tempelaar R, Sanderman R, et al: Cancer and caregiving: the impact on the caregiver's health. Psychooncology 7:3–13, 1998

Olofsson SM, Weitzner MA, Valentine AD, et al: A retrospective study of the psychiatric management and outcome of delirium in the cancer patient. Support Care Cancer 4:351–357, 1996

Payne DK, Hoffman RG, Theodoulou et al: Screening for anxiety and depression in women with breast cancer: psychiatry and medical oncology gear up for managed care. Psychosomatics 40:64–69, 1999

Peterson K, Forsyth PA, Posner JB: Paraneoplastic sensorimotor neuropathy associated with breast cancer. J Neurooncol 21:159–170, 1994

Pluss JL, DiBella NJ: Reversible central nervous system dysfunction with tamoxifen in a patient with breast cancer (letter). Ann Intern Med 101:652, 1984

Posner JB: Central nervous system synthesis of autoantibodies in paraneoplastic syndromes. Neurology 39 (suppl 1):244–245, 1989

Presti JC, Herr HW, Carroll PR: Fertility and testis cancer. Urol Clin North Am 20:173–179, 1993

Rait D, Lederberg M: The family of the cancer patient, in Handbook of Psychooncology: Psychological Care of the Patient With Cancer. Edited by Holland JC, Rowland JH. New York, Oxford University Press, 1989, pp 585–597

Rapoport Y, Kreitler S, Chaitchik S, et al: Psychosocial problems in head-and-neck cancer patients and their change with time since diagnosis. Ann Oncol 4:69–73, 1993

Razavi D, Delvaux N, Fravacques C, et al: Prevention of adjustment disorders and anticipatory nausea secondary to adjuvant chemotherapy: a double-blind, placebo-controlled study assessing the usefulness of alprazolam. J Clin Oncol 11:1384–1390, 1993

Reaby LL: The quality and coping patterns of women's decision-making regarding breast cancer surgery. Psychooncology 7:252–262, 1998

Reichman BS, Green KB: Breast cancer in young women: effect of chemotherapy on ovarian function, fertility, and birth defects. J Natl Cancer Inst Monogr 1994:125–129, 1994

Rieker PP, Fitzgerald EM, Kalish LA, et al: Psychosocial factors, curative therapies and behavioral outcomes. Cancer 64:2399–2407, 1989

Rome HP, Braceland PJ: Psychological response to corticotropin, cortisone, and related steroid substances. JAMA 148:27–30, 1952

Rottenberg DA: Acute and chronic effect of radiation therapy on the nervous system, in Neurological Complications of Cancer Treatment. Edited by Rottenberg DA. Boston, MA, Butterworth-Heinemann, 1991, pp 3–19

Rowland JH, Holland JC: Breast cancer, in Handbook of Psychooncology: Psychological Care of the Patient With Cancer. Edited by Holland JC, Rowland JH. New York, Oxford University Press, 1989, pp 188–207

Schain WS, Jacobs E, Wellisch DK: Psychosocial issues in breast reconstruction: intrapsychic, interpersonal, and practical concerns. Clin Plast Surg 11:237–251, 1984

Schiller JH, Jones JC: Paraneoplastic syndromes associated with lung cancer. Curr Opin Oncol 5:335–342, 1993

Schilsky RL, Anderson T: Hypomagnesemia and renal magnesium wasting in patients receiving cisplatin. Ann Intern Med 90:929–931, 1979

Schnoll RA, Harlow LL, Stolbach LL, et al: A structural model of the relationships among stage of disease, age, coping, and psychological adjustment in women with breast cancer. Psychooncology 7:69–77, 1998

Schover LR: Sexuality and fertility in urologic cancer patients. Cancer 60:553–558, 1987

Schover LR, von Eschenbach AC: Sexual and marital relationships after treatment for nonseminomatous testicular cancer. Urology 25:251–255, 1985

Sellick SM, Crooks DL: Depression and cancer: an appraisal of the literature for prevalence, detection, and practice guideline development for psychological interventions. Psychooncology 8:315–333, 1999

Shekelle RB, Raynor JW, Ostfeld AM, et al: Psychological depression and 17-year risk of death from cancer. Psychosom Med 19:147–153, 1975

Shuster JL, Stern TA, Greenberg DB: Pros and cons of fluoxetine for the depressed cancer patient. Oncology 6:45–56, 1992

Silberfarb PM, Holland JCB, Anbar D, et al: Psychological response of patients receiving two drug regimens for lung carcinoma. Am J Psychiatry 140:110–111, 1983

Smith MY, Redd WH, Peyser C, et al: Post-traumatic stress disorder in cancer: a review. Psychooncology 8:521–537, 1999

Spiegel D, Bloom J: Pain in metastatic breast cancer (letter). Cancer 52:341, 1983

Spiegel D, Bloom JR, Yalom I: Group support for patients with metastatic cancer. Arch Gen Psychiatry 38:527–533, 1981

Spiegel D, Bloom JR, Kraemer HC, et al: Effect of psychosocial treatment on survival of patients with metastatic breast cancer. Lancet 2:888–891, 1989

Stefanek ME: Psychosocial aspects of breast cancer. Curr Opin Oncol 5:996–1000, 1993

Stefanek ME, Sheidler VR, Fetting JH: Anticipatory nausea and vomiting: does it remain a significant clinical problem? Cancer 62:2654–2657, 1988

Stern TA, Purcell JJ, Murray GB: Complex partial seizures associated with Waldenström's macroglobulinemia. Psychosomatics 26:890–892, 1985

Stevens MC, Mahler H, Parkes S: The health status of adult survivors of cancer in childhood. Eur J Cancer 34:694–698, 1998

Stockhorst U, Klosterhalfen S, Klosterhalfen W, et al: Anticipatory nausea and vomiting in cancer patients receiving chemotherapy: classical conditioning etiology and therapeutical implications. Integr Physiol Behav Sci 28:177–181, 1993

Thachil JV, Jewitt MAS, Rider WD: The effects of cancer and cancer therapy on male fertility. J Urol 126:141–145, 1981

Trijsburg RW, van Knippenberg FCE, Rijpma SE: Effects of psychological treatment on cancer patients: a critical review. Psychosom Med 54:489–517, 1992

Triozzi PL, Goldstein D, Laszlo J: Contributions of benzodiazepines to cancer therapy. Cancer Invest 6:103–111, 1988

Tross S: Psychological adjustment in testicular cancer, in Handbook of Psychooncology: Psychological Care of the Patient With Cancer. Edited by Holland JC, Rowland JH. New York, Oxford University Press, 1989, pp 240–245

Twillman RK, Manetto C: Concurrent psychotherapy and pharmacotherapy in the treatment of depression and anxiety in cancer patients. Psychooncology 7:285–290, 1998

Valente SM, Saunders JM, Cohen MZ: Evaluating depression among patients with cancer. Cancer Practice 2:65–71, 1994

Walker RW, Allen JC, Rosen G, et al: Transient cerebral dysfunction secondary to high-dose methotrexate. J Clin Oncol 4:1845–1850, 1986

Wasserstrom WR: Diagnosis and treatment of leptomeningeal metastases from solid tumors: experience with 90 patients. Cancer 49:759–763, 1982

Watson M: Psychosocial intervention with cancer patients: a review. Psychol Med 13:839–846, 1983

Weisman AD: Early diagnosis of vulnerability in cancer patients. Am J Med Sci 271:187–196, 1976

Weisman A[D], Worden W: The existential plight in cancer: significance of the first 100 days. Int J Psychiatry Med 7:1–15, 1976–1977

Wellisch DK, Yager J: Is there a cancer-prone personality? CA Cancer J Clin 33:145–153, 1987

Zalupski M, Baker LH: Ifosfamide. J Natl Cancer Inst 80:556–566, 1988

Zelter LK: The adolescent with cancer, in Psychological Aspects of Childhood Cancer. Edited by Kellerman J. Springfield, IL, Charles C Thomas, 1980, pp 70–99

30

Neurology and Neurosurgery

Gregory Fricchione, M.D.

Zeina el-Chemali, M.D.

Jeffrey B. Weilburg, M.D.

George B. Murray, M.D.

In this chapter, we focus on the consultative evaluation, diagnosis, and management of neurological and neurosurgical disorders in patients who also have psychiatric or neurobehavioral signs and symptoms. These patients may have primary or secondary psychiatric disorders that account for their problems.

EPIDEMIOLOGY AND CLINICAL FEATURES

In a study of the referral patterns of a university hospital psychiatric consultation-liaison service, Craig (1982) found that 12.1% of consultation requests came from the neurology service. The most common reasons for these consultations included management of behavioral problems (21.6%), depression (18.9%), diagnosis or evaluation (13.5%), psychosis (5.4%), suicide attempt (5.4%), and history of psychiatric disorder (5.4%). Psychiatric diagnoses included depression (29.7%), personality disorder or situational reaction (27%), "organic brain syndrome" (21.6%), schizophrenia (10.8%), alcohol or drug abuse (2.7%), and other diagnoses (8.1%). In another survey of general hospitals, Wallen and colleagues (1987) found that 4.5% of 2,374 psychiatric consultations were with patients with central nervous system (CNS) diseases.

A knowledge of disease frequency is essential to the psychiatric consultant to the neurology and neurosurgery service. Tables 30–1 and 30–2 summarize the prevalence and incidence rates of certain neuropsychiatric disorders.

Structural Lesions

Cerebrovascular Disease

Cerebrovascular disease is the most common neurological disorder in the world and the third leading cause of morbidity and mortality in the United States, after cardiac disease and cancer (Hachinski and Norris 1985; Starkstein and Robinson 1992). Ischemia accounts for 85% of cerebrovascular disease cases. Hemorrhagic phenomena account for the remaining 15%. Atherosclerotic thrombosis and cerebral embolism are responsible for about one-third of all strokes. Among the intraparenchymal hemorrhages, primary hypertension-related intracerebral hemorrhage is most common. Subdural and epidural hematomas usually occur in the context of head trauma.

Poststroke depression (PSD). The major psychiatric sequela of cerebrovascular disease is depression. Wiart (1997) reported that PSD occurs in 30%–50% of hemiplegic patients in the first 2 years after a cerebrovascular accident. He added that the clinical picture can range from minor or masked depression (75%–95% of cases) to melancholia (5%–25%). His findings were similar to those of Robinson et al. (1983), Eastwood et al. (1989), and Ebrahim et al. (1987), obtained in various treatment settings.

Follow-up longitudinal natural history studies suggest that the average duration of major PSD is approximately 1 year. Dysthymia may last longer, often more than 2 years (Robinson et al. 1983, 1987). A longitudinal

Table 30–1. Prevalence of neuropsychiatric disorders in the general population

Disease	Population prevalence per 100,000
Dyslexia	5,000–10,000
Dementia (Alzheimer's disease)	7,700
Major depression	2,200
Seizure disorder	650–1,700
Schizophrenia	600–900
Brain injury	800
Cerebrovascular accident	600
Panic disorder	500
Bipolar illness	500
Parkinson's disease	133–200
Narcolepsy	10–100
CNS tumors (primary and secondary)	80
Persistent postconcussive syndrome	80
Multiple sclerosis	60
Subarachnoid hemorrhage	50
Transient postconcussive syndrome	50
Tourette's syndrome	28.7
Dementia (Pick's disease)	24
Huntington's disease	19
Lesch-Nyhan syndrome	10
Wilson's disease	10
Myotonic dystrophy	5.5
Metachromatic leukodystrophy	2.5
Acute intermittent porphyria	2
Acquired immunodeficiency syndrome (AIDS)	
Prevalence of CNS dysfunction in AIDS population	30%–75%[a]
Prevalence of AIDS dementia complex in AIDS population	16%–33%[b]

Note. CNS = central nervous system.
Data obtained from [a]Levy and Bredesen 1988; [b]Portegies et al. 1993.
Source. Adapted from Black DW, Yates WR, Andreasen NC, et al.: "Schizophrenia, Schizophreniform Disorder, and Delusional (Paranoid) Disorders," in *The American Psychiatric Press Textbook of Psychiatry.* Edited by Talbott JA, Hales RE, Yudofsky SC. Washington, DC, American Psychiatric Press, 1988, pp. 357–402; Kurtzke JF: "Neuroepidemiology." *Annals of Neurology* 16:265–277, 1984. Copyright 1984, Little, Brown; Malaspina D, Quitkin HM, Kaufmann CA: "Epidemiology and Genetics of Neuropsychiatric Disorders," in *The American Psychiatric Press Textbook of Neuropsychiatry*, 2nd Edition. Edited by Yudofsky SC, Hales RE. Washington, DC, American Psychiatric Press, 1992, pp. 187–226; Regier DA, Boyd JH, Burke JD Jr, et al.: "One-Month Prevalence of Mental Disorders in the United States." *Archives of General Psychiatry* 45:977–986, 1988. Copyright 1988, American Medical Association. Used with permission.

study by Morris and colleagues (1990) confirmed the average 1-year duration of major depression but found a more variable, shorter duration for dysthymia.

Table 30–2. Incidence of neuropsychiatric disorders in the general population

Disease	Annual incidence per 100,000
Brain injury	200
Cerebrovascular accident	150
Transient postconcussive syndrome	150
Schizophrenia	11–70
Seizure disorder	50
Dementia	50
Brain tumors (benign, metastatic, malignant)	30
Parkinson's disease	30
Persistent postconcussive syndrome	20
Subarachnoid hemorrhage	15
Multiple sclerosis	3

Source. Adapted from Black DW, Yates WR, Andreasen NC, et al.: "Schizophrenia, Schizophreniform Disorder, and Delusional (Paranoid) Disorders," in *The American Psychiatric Press Textbook of Psychiatry.* Edited by Talbott JA, Hales RE, Yudofsky SC. Washington, DC, American Psychiatric Press, 1988, pp. 357–402; Kurtzke JF: "Neuroepidemiology." *Annals of Neurology* 16:265–277, 1984. Copyright 1984, Little, Brown; Malaspina D, Quitkin HM, Kaufmann CA: "Epidemiology and Genetics of Neuropsychiatric Disorders," in *The American Psychiatric Press Textbook of Neuropsychiatry*, 2nd Edition. Edited by Yudofsky SC, Hales RE. Washington, DC, American Psychiatric Press, 1992, pp. 187–226; Regier DA, Boyd JH, Burke JD Jr, et al.: "One-Month Prevalence of Mental Disorders in the United States." *Archives of General Psychiatry* 45:977–986, 1988. Used with permission.

Possible etiologies of PSD include the depletion of intracerebral neurotransmitters in the first few months poststroke and attempts to cope with the various physical and cognitive losses. In addition, baseline subcortical atrophy and a family or personal history of affective illness increase the predisposition to PSD (Starkstein et al. 1988a, 1988b, 1989).

Whereas some studies have not found a relationship between left- versus right-hemisphere stroke location and risk of depression (Agrell and Dehlin 1994; Ebrahim et al. 1987; Sinyor et al. 1986), other studies support the contention that the risk of depression is higher the closer the lesion is to the left frontal (and right posterior) pole, with left anterior frontal lesions being most highly associated with depression (Robinson and Starkstein 1990; Robinson et al. 1984). There is also evidence that left frontal cortical and left basal ganglia strokes produce depression to a greater degree than do lesions elsewhere in the brain (Robinson and Starkstein 1990). More recently, Harvey and Black (1996) studied the response to the dexamethasone suppression test as a marker for PSD.

In addition, it appears that peak prolactin responses are attenuated in stroke patients, compared with healthy elderly individuals, suggesting a role for serotonergic responsiveness in stroke patients (Ramasubbu et al. 1998).

Psychiatric consultants are sometimes called to see patients who are thought to be depressed but who actually have aprosodia. Prosody (the melodic line that lends attitudinal and emotional meaning to speech) and gesturing appear to be functions of the nondominant hemisphere (Ross and Mesulam 1979). Aprosodia is a disorder of the affective components of language, and it can be classified in the same manner as aphasia. In aprosodia, a group of assessments analogous to those used to assess dysphasia are used to observe spontaneous prosody, prosodic repetition, prosodic comprehension, and comprehension of emotional gesturing (Ross 1981). Deficits in spontaneous prosody and prosodic repetition suggest a motor aprosodia, whereas faulty comprehension of prosody and emotional gesturing are characteristic of sensory aprosodia. Some patients, who at first appear to have PSD, may simply have aprosodia and be unable to mount appropriate affective responses to the treatment team. A helpful marker for depression in the poststroke patient population is lack of motivation in physical therapy (Ross and Rush 1981).

There are also psychiatric sequelae of lacunar strokes and infarcts. Lacunar infarcts are small lesions, often the result of hypertension, that occur in the deeper subcortical parts of the cerebrum and in the brain stem (Fisher 1982). They result from occlusion of the small penetrating branches of the large cerebral arteries. A wide range of mood changes may occur after lacunar strokes, including emotional incontinence and depression.

Poststroke mania. Poststroke mania is rather rare. Starkstein and Robinson (1992) saw only 3 cases in a series of 300 consecutive patients who had had a stroke. Nevertheless, poststroke mania can be seen with orbitofrontal, basotemporal, basal ganglia, and thalamic lesions, especially in the right hemisphere (Robinson and Starkstein 1990). It has been suggested that limbically connected basotemporal cortex, when damaged, may be especially critical for the development of secondary mania (Robinson and Starkstein 1990). Genetic vulnerability, suggested by family history of mood disorder, and subcortical atrophy may also increase the risk of poststroke mania.

Poststroke anxiety. In a series of 98 patients with acute first stroke, only 6 met adapted criteria for generalized anxiety disorder. On the other hand, almost half (23 of 47) of one series of patients with PSD had comorbid anxiety symptoms (Starkstein et al. 1990).

Brain Tumors

Brain neoplasms account for almost 10% of nontraumatic neurological disease (Silver et al. 1990). Table 30–3 lists the frequencies of common primary CNS tumors and common metastatic tumor types.

TABLE 30–3. Tumor types and relative frequencies

Tumor type	Frequency (%)
Primary	75–85
Gliomas	40–50
Astrocytomas	10–15
Glioblastomas	20–25
Others	10–15
Meningiomas	10–20
Pituitary adenomas	10
Neurilemmomas (mainly acoustic neuromas)	5–8
Medulloblastomas and pinealomas	5
Other primary tumors	5
Metastatic	15–25
Lung	35–45
Breast	10–20
Kidney	5–10
Gastrointestinal tract	5–10
Melanoma	2–5
Other	25–30

Source. Reprinted from Lohr JB, Cadet JL: "Neuropsychiatric Aspects of Brain Tumors," in *The American Psychiatric Press Textbook of Neuropsychiatry.* Edited by Hales RE, Yudofsky SC. Washington, DC, American Psychiatric Press, 1987, pp. 351–364. Used with permission.

Unrecognized brain cancer is sometimes responsible for psychotic and other psychiatric syndromes. Between 1% and 2% of patients with a psychiatric disorder may actually have unrecognized brain neoplasms (Price et al. 1992). The posterior fossa is the site of 30% of CNS tumors, 22% are found in both the frontal and temporal regions, 12% are located in the parietal area, 10% are found in the pituitary, and 4% are found in the occipital lobes (Lohr and Cadet 1987).

Several factors may determine psychiatric disturbance in patients with CNS tumors (Price et al. 1992). Increased intracranial pressure related to brain neoplasms may change the level of consciousness and cause mood and behavior changes. Tumor growth rate may affect symptom severity. Premorbid personality and functioning may have an impact on psychiatric morbidity associated with tumors. Anatomic location of the tumor may be associated with specific neuropsychiatric findings.

Frontal lobe neoplasms are especially likely to be associated with neuropsychiatric symptoms; the association was noted up to 90% of the time in one survey of 85 subjects (Strauss and Keschner 1935). Three types of frontal lobe dysfunction have been suggested (Cummings 1985a, 1985b, 1985c):

1. *Orbitofrontal syndrome* is characterized by disinhibition, impulsivity, emotional lability with inappropriate jocularity and euphoria, and inattention with poor insight and judgment.
2. The hypothesized *frontal convexity syndrome* is characterized by apathy, indifference and psychomotor retardation, angry outbursts, motor perseveration, impersistence, lack of congruity between motor and verbal behavior, deficits in motor programming, concreteness, and poor categorization.
3. *Medial frontal syndrome* is associated frequently with akinetic presentations. There is loss of spontaneous gesturing, decreased speech production, leg weakness, sensation loss, and incontinence in medial frontal syndrome (Cummings 1985a, 1985b, 1985c). The akinetic mutism seen with anterior cingulate lesions is sometimes considered a medial frontal syndrome.

Unfortunately, strong clinical data are lacking to support the existence of these potentially useful specific clinical entities.

Many patients with frontal lobe tumors have a mixture of symptoms because the tumor directly and/or indirectly affects several frontal regions. Mood syndromes, depressive or manic, are frequently seen (63% of cases in the Strauss and Keschner [1935] series). Belyi (1987) hypothesized that manic symptoms predominate in right frontal lesions, whereas depressive symptoms are more frequently related to left frontal lesions.

Emotional alterations noted in patients with temporal lobe tumors include depression, irritability, apathy, or elation. Episodic dyscontrol and affective lability may also be present.

Parietal and occipital lobe neoplasms are more likely to cause psychiatric symptoms than are tumors in other locations. However, visual hallucinations, usually unformed, occur in patients with occipital tumors (Lohr and Cadet 1987). Agitation, paranoid trends, and affective disturbances can also occur.

Midline diencephalic tumors involve subcortical, limbically related structures, such as thalamus, hypothalamus, and periventricular regions. Schizophreniform psychoses have been reported in patients with such tumors (Malamud 1967). Mood and personality changes and akinetic mutism have also been reported (Burkle and Lipowski 1978; Cairns and Mosberg 1951). Hypothalamic neoplasms may cause eating disorders and hypersomnia,

including excessive daytime sleepiness (Climo 1982; Coffey 1989); problems with thirst and temperature regulation may also be seen. Up to 90% of corpus callosum tumors cause neurobehavioral abnormalities (Selecki 1964).

Pituitary tumors, such as craniopharyngiomas, can affect diencephalic function, including that of the hypothalamus, through direct tumor growth. A panorama of psychiatric disturbance is seen with pituitary tumors. In one series, one-third of patients' presentations were dominated by psychiatric symptoms (Russell and Pennybacker 1961). Sanders and Murray (1992) reported that in a woman who was being treated for depression and who had a craniopharyngioma, all signs and symptoms of depression remitted after surgery. In addition, pituitary tumors are responsible for endocrinopathies associated with psychiatric sequelae. Basophilic pituitary adenomas can lead to Cushing's syndrome, which can cause depression and other secondary psychiatric syndromes. Acidophilic pituitary adenomas can present with acromegaly, which is associated with depression and anxiety (Price et al. 1992). The combination of a visual field loss such as bitemporal hemianopsia and a mental status change is indicative of a pituitary or hypothalamic lesion.

Paraneoplastic processes affect the CNS as a consequence of the remote effects of a tumor. CNS paraneoplastic syndromes often result from an immune reaction directed against antigens shared by the underlying neoplasm and certain neurons. One example is the autoimmune mechanism for Eaton-Lambert myasthenic syndrome found with small cell lung cancer (Newsom-Davis 1985). Autoimmunity against neuronal antigens is also found in paraneoplastic cerebellar degeneration and in paraneoplastic sensory neuropathy encephalomyelitis (Furneaux et al. 1990). Brown and Paraskevas (1982) proposed that "antiidiotypic antibodies" directed against both tumor tissue proteins and CNS serotonin receptors reduce serotonin function and contribute to the depressive symptoms seen in paraneoplastic syndrome. The cancer most commonly associated with CNS paraneoplastic disease is small cell lung cancer. Other associated cancers include breast, stomach, uterine, renal, testicular, thyroid, and colon cancers (Skuster et al. 1992).

Limbic encephalitis is a rare complication of cancer, one that most commonly affects middle-aged men and women (Newman et al. 1990). It is associated with small cell lung cancer in 70% of cases. The neurological symptomatology can precede the tumor appearance by up to 2 years. The course is insidious; cancer patients with limbic encephalitis have been admitted to psychiatry units for a syndrome that includes depression, anxiety, personality disturbances, hallucinations, catatonia, and memory impairment with or without delirium. A severe impairment of recent memory is the most striking feature of limbic encephalitis (Bakheit et al. 1990).

Even when findings from early neurological and cerebrospinal fluid (CSF) examinations are negative and when early computed tomography (CT) scans of the head and electroencephalograms show no abnormalities, the psychiatrist should strongly consider a diagnosis of a CNS paraneoplastic syndrome when psychiatric signs and symptoms occur in a patient with cancer.

Seizure Disorder

The incidence rate of new epilepsy diagnoses in the United States is estimated to be 48.7 per 100,000 annually (Hauser and Kurland 1975). Given the number of patients treated for epilepsy in the United States (estimated to be more than 2 million), the lifetime prevalence of epilepsy is at least 1% (Locharernkul et al. 1992; Mesulam 1985).

The original definition of epilepsy by John Hughlings Jackson remains current: Epilepsy is an "occasional, excessive and disorderly electrical discharge of nerve tissue" (quoted in Browne et al. 1983, p. 414). The electroencephalogram may corroborate the seizure activity with spikes, spike and wave complexes, or other findings (Mendez et al. 1984). Focal sharp and slow waves suggest seizure activity in patients with a clinical picture of epilepsy. It should be noted, however, that of the more than 2 million Americans who have epilepsy, 60% have nonconvulsive seizures free of any body motor symptoms and signs that otherwise herald the end of a seizure (Goldensohn 1983). As Murray (1985) pointed out, the majority of patients with nonconvulsive epilepsy have partial seizures, and 40% of these patients do not show focal spiking on their electroencephalograms. Electroencephalograms from patients in the latter group are often considered to show no abnormalities (Klass 1975; Murray 1985). Seizure is a clinical and not primarily an electroencephalographic (EEG) diagnosis. Table 30–4 summarizes the most recent International League Against Epilepsy classification of epileptic seizure syndromes.

Generalized seizures are characterized by simultaneous involvement of both cerebral hemispheres. In partial seizures, focal signs and symptoms emerge from excitation in a limited site in one hemisphere. Simple partial seizures occur without impaired consciousness and usually originate from primary motor, sensory, or visual cortical regions. Complex partial seizures are associated with impairment of consciousness and most often originate from limbic system foci in the medial temporal lobe. This may explain why psychiatric signs and symptoms—

including cognitive auras (depersonalization, forced thinking, déjà vu), affective auras (fear, depression, pleasure), perceptual changes (illusions, hallucinations), and memory dysfunction (amnesia)—are so common (Mendez et al. 1984). Complex partial status epilepticus appears to have two separate behavioral phases. A continuous twilight state with partial and amnestic responsiveness, partial speech, and reactive complex automatisms cycles with the other phase of total unresponsiveness, speech arrest, staring, and stereotyped automatisms (Treiman and Delgado-Escueta 1983).

Psychiatric consultants may be called by neurologists to evaluate patients with possible pseudoseizures. A significant number of patients have both true seizures and pseudoseizures (or nonepileptic seizures) (Blumer 1997; van Merode et al. 1997). In one series of 27 patients referred for pseudoseizure evaluation, 11 had pseudoseizures, 7 had epilepsy, and 2 cases were unclear. Of the 7 epileptic patients, 3 were found to have coexisting pseudoseizures (Ramchandani and Schindler 1993).

In a study of 62 reported cases, van Merode et al. (1997) found that the prevalence of nonepileptic seizures was greater among women than among men; sexual abuse was cited as a possible reason for this difference. These investigators also noted that certain types of attacks were sex specific; men usually had generalized tonic-clonic seizures (80% of cases), whereas equal numbers of generalized tonic-clonic and complex partial seizure attacks occurred in women.

Blumer (1997) reported that 50% of all patients with chronic epilepsy have an intermittent and polysymptomatic affective disorder. Ten percent have interictal psychosis, which tends to develop in patients with severe affective disorders who respond poorly to treatment. Mendez et al. (1986) suggested that depression in some epileptic patients may be due to a specific epileptic psychosyndrome secondary to limbic dysfunction. Compared with 7% of control subjects in their study, 30% of patients with epilepsy had a history of suicide attempts. The suicide rate in one series of patients with epilepsy was five times that in the general population (Barraclough 1981). In patients with temporal lobe epilepsy, the incidence of suicide is 25 times that in the general population (M.M. Robertson and Trimble 1983).

A schizophreniform psychosis is also described in patients with epilepsy, usually in those with temporal lobe epilepsy (McKenna et al. 1985; Mendez et al. 1984). Symptoms may include thought disorder, paranoid ideations, hallucinations, and mood changes in the context of preserved affect. Brief psychotic episodes in epilepsy unrelated to the delirium seen in ictal and postictal states have also been recognized (Tsopelas et al. 2001) and have been hypothesized

TABLE 30–4.   Epileptic seizure classification of the International League Against Epilepsy

I. Partial seizure disorder (localized origin)

    A. Simple partial seizures (no impairment of consciousness)

    B. Complex partial seizures (impairment of consciousness)
        EEG findings
            Ictal type: unilateral or frequently bilateral discharge, diffuse or focal in temporal or frontotemporal regions
            Interictal expression: unilateral or bilateral asynchronous focus in temporal or frontal areas

    C. Partial seizures progressing to secondary generalized seizures (tonic, clonic, or tonic-clonic)

        1. Simple partial to generalized

        2. Complex partial to generalized

        3. Simple partial to complex partial generalized

II. Generalized seizures

    A. Absence seizures

        1. Typical absence seizures ("petit mal seizures")
            Ictal type: 2–4 Hz, regular, synchronous, symmetrical, bilateral, 3/sec spike, and slow-wave complexes
            Interictal expression: usually normal, although paroxysmal spike or spike and slow-wave complexes can occur

        2. Atypical absence seizures
            Ictal type: more heterogeneous than typical absence seizures, irregular, and asymmetric bilateral paroxysmal activity
            Interictal expression: background usually abnormal, with irregular, asymmetrical, paroxysmal activity

    B. Myoclonic seizures: jerking movement, single or multiple; "minor motor seizures"
        EEG findings
            Ictal type: polyspike and wave
            Interictal expression: same as ictal

    C. Clonic seizures

    D. Tonic seizures

    E. Tonic-clonic seizures: "grand mal epilepsy," "major motor seizures"

    F. Atonic (astatic) seizures: "minor motor seizures," "drop attacks"

III. Unclassified epileptic seizures (all that cannot be classified because of lack of data or unusual type [e.g., some neonatal seizures])

IV. Addendum

    A. *Status epilepticus* refers to prolonged or repetitive seizures that do not permit recovery between attacks

    B. Repeated epileptic seizures occur as

        1. fortuitous attacks without provocation

        2. cyclic attacks (e.g., in relation to menstrual or sleep-wake cycle)

        3. provoked attacks caused by

            a. nonsensory factors such as fatigue, emotion, substances

            b. sensory factors such as those that occur in "reflex seizures"

Note.   EEG = electroencephalographic.

Source.   Adapted from Commission on Classification and Terminology of the International League Against Epilepsy: "Proposal for Revised Clinical and Electroencephalographic Classification of Epileptic Seizures." *Epilepsia* 22:489–501, 1981. Copyright 1981, Raven Press. Used with permission.

to be related to subictal temporal lobe dysrhythmias. Persistent psychoses are well-known concomitants of epilepsy, again often attributed to subictal temporal lobe dysrhythmias. Incidence studies suggest that the psychosis risk among patients with epilepsy is 6–12 times greater than in the population without epilepsy (McKenna et al. 1985).

Episodic dyscontrol syndrome, a controversial entity, is characterized by recurrent attacks of uncontrollable rage that are out of character for the patient and that occur with minimal provocation (Elliot 1984; Fedio 1986). In one series of 286 cases of episodic dyscontrol, 37.4% of patients received a diagnosis of complex partial seizures or temporal lobe epilepsy (Elliot 1984). Abnormal aggression in patients with this type of seizure disorder is more than just an ictal or subictal event. Although related to early seizure onset and psychosis, aggression is also associated with psychosocial and educational problems, diminished intelligence, poverty, family turmoil, and a history of abuse (Fedio 1986). Purposeful acts of directed violence are not ictal events (Delgado-Escueta et al. 1981).

Bear and Fedio (1977) wrote about so-called interictal behavioral syndrome (humorless sobriety, dependence, obsessionalism), seen in patients with temporal lobe epilepsy. Hyperreligiosity, hypergraphia, and hyposexuality are associated with the temporal lobe epileptic interictal personality (Waxman and Geschwind 1975), although these associations are controversial (Rodin and Schmaltz 1984). Indeed, the whole notion of a characteristic epileptic personality is controversial, especially because inconsistencies have been found when controlled studies employing structured diagnostic testing have been reviewed (Benson 1991). However, there does seem to be a clear and distinctive verbosity in patients with complex partial seizures that gives them a viscous interpersonal quality (Hoeppner et al. 1987). This can prevent an interviewer from completing afternoon rounds expeditiously.

Complex partial seizure disorder can present with panic disorder symptoms (Weilberg et al. 1987), as well as with bradycardia and other cardiac arrhythmias (Constantin et al. 1990; Gilchrist 1985).

Head Trauma

Head trauma is an important public health problem, with 750,000 to 3 million cases occurring each year in the United States (Jennett and Teasdale 1981; Kwentus et al. 1985). More than 500,000 of these traumatic brain injuries are classified as severe (Frankowski et al. 1986). Many patients with head trauma are plagued by the neuropsychiatric aftermath of their injuries, which is often long-lasting (Silver et al. 1990). Even individuals with mild head trauma can have persistent cognitive and psychiatric dysfunction that may be the greatest source of stress for the patient and family and the greatest source of overall psychosocial disability.

Alcohol intoxication at the time of injury is predictive of poorer outcome and higher mortality (Ruff et al. 1990; Silver et al. 1992). Posttraumatic seizures occur in 7% of patients within the first year and 11.5% within the first 5 years after severe closed head trauma (Annegers et al. 1980). Head trauma can also produce significant changes in personality, when neuropsychological test results indicate frontal lobe damage (A.J. Mattson and Levin 1990). Whether there is damage to frontal lobes or whether these structures remain unharmed, psychiatric consultants may encounter frontal lobe syndrome, which is characterized by lability, irritability, shallowness, and inappropriateness. Patients may have diminished ability to use language, calculation skills, and logical analysis, as well as reduced ability to concentrate and abstract (Silver et al. 1990). Temporal lobe damage may lead to complex partial seizure disorder.

Premorbid mood disorders are often worsened by brain injuries, but depression or mania can emerge after head injury without any prior personal or family history (Robinson et al. 1988). Significant head injury before a first psychotic episode has been found in up to 15% of patients with schizophrenia (Lishman 1987).

Perhaps the most difficult clinical problem in patients with head injuries is irritability or aggressiveness. Irritability or aggressiveness may be a major source of disability for the victim and of strife in the victim's family (Silver et al. 1990). In one series, for example, up to 70% of patients with head trauma exhibited irritable or aggressive behaviors (McKinlay et al. 1981).

Symptoms of *postconcussion syndrome* include headache, dizziness, tiredness, and insomnia. Patients may exhibit memory dysfunction, lack of concentration, perceptual changes, dysthymia, anxiety, irritability, and personality changes (Lishman 1988; Silver et al. 1990). Postconcussion syndrome is not correlated with head injury severity or degree of loss of consciousness. It can occur even after milder traumas and with brief loss of consciousness (Silver et al. 1990). The psychiatric consultant is sometimes called on in the midst of a compensation case to comment on the degree of psychopathology present, often in the face of a normal neurological workup, including normal imaging studies.

There may be long-term psychiatric sequelae of head injury. H.S. Levin et al. (1987) reported that in 57 patients who had concussions, 22% had persistent anergy and dizziness and 47% had continuing headaches. In another study involving patients with minor head injury, 54% had irritability, 47% had memory complaints, and 39% were depressed after 1 year (Schoenhuber and Gentil 1988). In general, degree of recovery does not appear to be altered by compensation claims or litigation (Bornstein et al. 1988).

Degenerative Diseases

A wide variety of degenerative diseases cause neuropsychiatric signs and symptoms. *Parkinson's disease* is a degenerative disorder with high psychiatric comorbidity (Fogel 1993): 65% of patients with Parkinson's disease develop an associated dementia by age 85 (Mayeux et al. 1990). About 40% of patients with Parkinson's disease can expect to eventually have at least one major depressive syndrome (Cummings 1992). This degree of comorbidity and the added risk of psychiatric dysfunction as a result of treatment with antiparkinsonian medications suggest the need for psychiatric as well as neurological management for optimal patient care.

Patients with Parkinson's disease have tremor, bradykinesia, rigidity, gait dysfunction, and/or postural unsteadiness. Presentations of Parkinson's disease are heterogeneous, and early on, diagnosis may be made difficult by the presence of only two of these signs (Fogel 1993). Patients often report prodromal symptoms such as mild tremors, apathy, micrographia, and muscle stiffness. Drugs are a frequent cause of parkinsonism; neuroleptics are the most common offenders. Metoclopramide (Albibi and McCallum 1983) and fluoxetine (Bouchard et al. 1989), as well as amoxapine and lithium, may also cause extrapyramidal syndromes.

The selective monoamine oxidase inhibitor selegiline has been shown to delay the need for L-dopa treatment in patients with early Parkinson's disease (Tetrud and Langston 1989). As Fogel (1993) pointed out, it is controversial whether the physician should add L-dopa to selegiline in the further treatment of patients with Parkinson's disease or rely on direct dopamine agonists, such as bromocriptine or pergolide, for as long as possible until L-dopa is needed. Any of these agents may be helpful in activating the frontal lobes, enhancing the treatment of accompanying depressive symptoms. Anticholinergics and amantadine continue to have a place in the management of mild Parkinson's disease. Later in the course of the disease, the psychiatric side effects of antiparkinsonian medications, such as psychosis and confusion, often lead to treatment alterations. If slow withdrawal of one antiparkinsonian medication at a time does not resolve psychotic symptoms, then clozapine can be tried (Fogel 1993). (For more information about drug treatment, see the section "Psychopharmacology" later in this chapter.)

Depression in patients with Parkinson's disease appears to be associated with more anxiety and less self-recrimination than are seen in patients with primary depression (Cummings 1992). Depression also seems to be more common in patients with Parkinson's disease who have more severe bradykinesia and gait disturbance than in those who have a more dominant tremor presentation. Fogel (1993) pointed out, however, that depression in patients with Parkinson's disease is not merely a reaction to degree of disability, given the association between depression and the neurological and biochemical features of Parkinson's disease, as well as the inconsistent relation between depression and Parkinson's disease severity and duration. On the other hand, diagnosis of Parkinson's disease is complicated by the presence of physical signs (apathy, bradykinesia, rigidity) that mimic the psychomotor and vegetative symptoms of depression. Focusing on the psychological symptoms of depression can help with diagnosis of a depressive syndrome.

Huntington's disease is an autosomal-dominant, degenerative, basal ganglia disease in which psychiatric issues are often dominant until the late stages of illness (Maricle 1993). Patients with Huntington's disease make involuntary choreic movements and abnormal voluntary movements and have cognitive deficits and psychiatric dysfunction. Common psychiatric syndromes in patients with Huntington's disease include conduct disorder, antisocial personality disorder, other personality syndromes, mood disorder (in more than 50%), schizophrenia-like conditions (with more negative than positive symptoms), and alcoholism (Maricle 1993). Suicidal behavior is exhibited by 30% of patients, with 2%–7% completing suicide (Maricle 1993). A subcortical dementia eventually affects all those with Huntington's disease and progresses at a variable rate. In addition to pharmacological management of psychiatric syndromes associated with Huntington's disease, consultation-liaison psychiatrists are also often involved in providing individual, marital, and family therapies. More recently, with the advent of predictive testing based on the Huntington's disease genetic marker on chromosome 4 (Gusella et al. 1983), consultation-liaison psychiatrists have become more involved in helping patients and doctors decide about testing and in helping patients adjust to the results.

The most important example of a demyelinating degenerative disease is *multiple sclerosis*. The etiology of multiple sclerosis remains unknown, but recent discoveries seem to point to an autoimmune component. Multiple sclerosis is diagnosed most often in young women, with onset between ages 20 and 40 years. At least early on, neuropsychiatric symptoms tend to remit and recur. Lesions most commonly affect the optic nerve, cerebellum, brain stem, and long tracts of the spinal cord, causing ataxic gait, intention tremor, dysarthria, dissociation of lateral conjugate gaze, paraparesis, sensory loss in limbs, and urinary incontinence. Surridge (1969) published an extensive study of the psychiatric aspects of 108 patients with multiple sclerosis, using a control group of patients with muscular dystrophy. Some psychiatric disturbance was noted in 75% of the patients with multiple sclerosis but in less than 50% of the patients with muscular dystrophy. Intellectual decline was found in 61% of the patients with multiple sclerosis and was moderately severe in at least 20%. None of the patients with muscular dystrophy had intellectual decline. Compared with 13% of the control subjects, 53% of the patients with multiple sclerosis exhibited mood disorder during their illness: 27% were depressed, 26% were euphoric, and 10% showed emotional exaggeration. Personality change occurred in 43% of the multiple sclerosis cohort, usually marked by irritability.

The most frequent abnormalities are abnormalities in abstraction, recent memory, attentional tasks, and processional speed (Rao et al. 1991, 1993). The total lesion load as shown by magnetic resonance imaging (MRI) correlates with the neuropsychiatric impairment (Swirsky-Sacchetti et al. 1992). This research has also confirmed that there is discernible psychopathology in up to two-thirds of multiple sclerosis patients, most commonly depression. Some studies suggest a physiologic basis for depression in patients with multiple sclerosis. In one study comparing 30 patients with multiple sclerosis with equally disabled neurologically ill control subjects, patients with multiple sclerosis were more likely to be depressed before they showed signs of their disease, as well as during the illness phase (Whitlock and Suskind 1980). Depression can be severe in patients with multiple sclerosis. In a study of multiple sclerosis cases in Israel, the suicide rate in the disease group was 14 times higher than in the general population (Kahana et al. 1971).

The consultation-liaison psychiatrist is sometimes asked by the neurologist to consult with patients who have multiple sclerosis and pseudoneurological symptoms that are nonanatomic in presentation (Lishman 1987). Many clinicians have long believed that conversion symptoms coexist with multiple sclerosis more often than with any other neurological disease (Brain 1930). Others believe that the "hysterical" symptoms represent a "pre-disseminated" subjective symptom stage of multiple sclerosis (Wilson 1940).

Amyotrophic lateral sclerosis (ALS) is a degenerative motor neuron disease characterized by loss of strength and muscle atrophy. It is sometimes associated with dementia (Wikstrom et al. 1982). In 2%–3% of ALS patients, personality changes occur before the onset of motor neuron disease, sometimes in association with frontotemporal atrophy. Positron emission tomography studies have shown reduced activation in the frontolimbic systems of ALS patients. Motor neuron disease with dementia can also be seen in patients with *Creutzfeldt-Jakob disease*. However, Creutzfeldt-Jakob disease usually has a rapid onset, and patients die within 1 year. Patients with ALS may show impaired memory, judgment, abstraction, and calculation skills. They may also have hallucinations (Whitehouse and Rabins 1992). Recent work has shown that quality-of-life measures in ALS patients are independent of physical function decline (Robbins et al. 2001).

Cerebellar degenerative diseases include the olivo-pontocerebellar atrophies, which present with progressive ataxias. In at least one type of olivopontocerebellar atrophy (type V), dementia, parkinsonism, ophthalmoplegia, and ataxia occur. Friedreich's ataxia, an autosomal recessive disease of cerebellar degeneration, presents with an early slow onset of progressive ataxia. In addition to ataxia, patients with Friedreich's ataxia exhibit inten-

tion tremor, past pointing, dysarthria, and poor rapid alternating movements (Whitehouse and Rabins 1992); 25% may have neuropsychiatric syndromes. Personality disorder may be prominent, and psychoses are also sometimes noted.

Other degenerative conditions, such as Steele-Richardson-Olszewski syndrome, present with prominent frontal lobe dysfunction. In young adults and adolescents, Lafora's myoclonic epilepsy and Hallervorden-Spatz disease also present with cognitive impairment and frontal lobe dysfunction.

CNS Infections

CNS infections, although part of the potential differential diagnosis any consultation-liaison psychiatrist will consider, are usually managed by a neurologist or internist. The psychiatric consultant is frequently called in later regarding issues of management (Lishman 1987).

Human immunodeficiency virus (HIV) infection is among the greatest mimics of all diseases. HIV is a neurotropic virus. HIV dementia is of great concern to consultation-liaison psychiatrists. Prior to the introduction of today's highly active antiretroviral therapy, the cumulative prevalence of HIV dementia during the course of acquired immunodeficiency syndrome (AIDS) could be expected to be 21%–25% (McArthur et al. 1993). More recent estimates of the HIV dementia prevalence rate in the United States are much lower: 7%–10% (Goodkin et al. 2001). Patients exhibit bradyphrenia, diminished facial expression, hypophonia, abnormal eye pursuits, impaired coordination and balance, and postural tremor (Navia et al. 1986). There is evidence to suggest that HIV dementia relates to viral load in serum and CSF (K. Robertson et al. 1998).

Neurosyphilis is becoming more common because of immunodeficiency related to HIV infection (Gliatto and Caroff 2001). Neurosyphilis may start with headache, lethargy, poor concentration, forgetfulness, and poor judgment. Early on, the nonspecific and vague complaints can lead to misdiagnosis of a primary psychiatric disorder. Early neuropsychiatric evidence of neurosyphilis may include ophthalmoplegia, pupillary abnormalities, and, rarely, Argyll Robertson pupils (small irregular pupils reacting normally to convergence but not at all to light and only partially to mydriatic agents). CSF examination reveals moderate leukocytosis (200 cells/mL) of mostly mononuclear cells. The clinical picture may, over time, deteriorate to a dementia. Alternatively, there can be the waxing and waning picture of a delirious process.

Hooshmand and colleagues (1972) suggested that a firm diagnosis of neurosyphilis can be made 1) when results of the blood fluorescent treponemal antibody-absorption (FTA-ABS) test are positive and ocular or neurological signs consistent with neurosyphilis are present, 2) when results of both blood and CSF FTA-ABS tests are positive and examination of the CSF reveals leukocytosis in the absence of another meningitis, or 3) when results of blood and CSF FTA-ABS tests are positive and there are unexplained neurological symptoms.

Acute bacterial, fungal, and *viral meningitis* may sometimes be seen in hospitalized medical-surgical patients. Immunocompromised individuals in hospital units serving patients with AIDS or in oncology units, as well as patients who have indwelling ventriculoperitoneal shunts, sometimes develop acute meningitis. Headache, meningismus, and CSF abnormalities are associated with a wide variety of mental status changes in patients with meningitis (Coyle 1999).

Chronic meningitis is a syndrome marked by the signs and symptoms of meningoencephalitis accompanied by CSF changes (usually pleocytosis), which persist for more than 4 weeks (Coyle 1999). Clinical features include headache, fever, stiff neck, cranial nerve palsies and other focal deficits, seizures, and mental status changes. Psychiatric sequelae include prominent behavioral symptoms, cognitive dysfunction, and confusion (Skuster et al. 1992). *Mycobacterium tuberculosis* is the most common cause of chronic meningitis (Coyle 1999). In one series, 40% of cases of chronic meningitis were induced by *M. tuberculosis* (Coyle 1999). Neoplasms were the second leading cause, at 8%, and *Cryptococcus* was the third, at 7%. In one-third of the cases, no etiology could be documented (Anderson and Willoughby 1987; Swartz 1987). The increasing immunosuppressed population, swelled by the AIDS epidemic and by organ transplantation, has led to an increased incidence of chronic meningitis. Chronic meningitis is distinguished from recurrent meningitis; in the latter, patients return to baseline and have normal CSF findings.

Encephalitis is a generalized CNS infection that usually has an acute onset and presents with fever, meningeal signs, focal neurological findings, and delirium, sometimes progressing to stupor (Skuster et al. 1992). The most frequently encountered focal encephalitis is caused by herpes simplex virus, which has a predilection for temporal lobes and the inferomedial portions of the frontal lobes. Associated findings may include anosmia, olfactory or gustatory perceptual changes, simple or complex partial seizures, personality changes, and psychosis. Unless encephalitis is treated early with antiviral agents such as acyclovir, there is significant morbidity and mortality. Long-standing sequelae of encephalitis include personality alteration, affective lability, cognitive dysfunction, and hallucinations (Baker 1988).

DIFFERENTIAL DIAGNOSIS

Etiologies of Neuropsychiatric Disorders

A host of neurological diseases can present as or cause psychiatric syndromes. Skuster et al. (1992) assembled an impressive listing. Disorders such as Tourette's syndrome, juvenile Huntington's disease, and acute intermittent porphyria may present as psychiatric disorders first diagnosed in childhood or adolescence. Multiple sclerosis, epilepsy, porphyria, infections, and metabolic diseases can sometimes be mistaken for substance abuse disorders. Schizophrenia-like disorders can be caused by lupus cerebritis, temporal lobe epilepsy, Huntington's disease, Wilson's disease, neurosyphilis, HIV encephalopathy, and Wernicke's aphasia. Extrapyramidal disorders, CNS infections, demyelinating diseases, epilepsy, CNS neoplastic disease, cerebrovascular disease, and degenerative diseases all can be mistaken for paranoid delusional disorders (Cummings 1986). Frontal lobe disorders, multiple sclerosis, Huntington's disease, Parkinson's disease, vitamin B_{12} deficiency, HIV encephalopathy, cerebrovascular disease, neoplastic and paraneoplastic syndromes, and metabolic diseases all can present with major depressive and manic symptoms (Cummings 1986; Skuster et al. 1992). A large number of these neurological conditions also present as anxiety disorders.

For example, Salloway and White (1997) described paroxysmal limbic disorder, characterized by acute onset of severe anxiety. They ascribed this syndrome in many cases to partial complex epilepsy. Often, patients with multiple sclerosis, lupus, porphyria, neurosyphilis, or epilepsy are thought to have somatoform disorder, especially early in the course of their disease. The diagnosis of conversion disorder versus neurological illness can, therefore, be quite challenging.

Examination for Conversion Disorder and Somatoform Pain Disorder

Conversion disorder is often diagnosed prematurely (Boffeli and Guze 1992). In one 10-year follow-up study, 10 of 40 men who originally received a diagnosis of conversion disorder were later found to have recognizable neurological disease, most commonly a CNS degenerative disease (Watson and Buranen 1979). In another provocative study, Gould and colleagues (1986) found at least one nonphysiologic sensory examination feature, such as nonanatomic anesthesia or a midline split of pain or vibration, in 29 of 30 neurology inpatients with documented CNS injury, 25 of whom had had acute strokes.

Delirium versus conversion disorder. In conversion disorder, orientation is usually preserved, or when "disorientation" occurs, it often includes person as well as place and time. Cognition is also usually intact, but if poor, it commonly is out of proportion to alertness and responsiveness. Hallucinations are rare in patients who have conversion delirium.

Stupor versus conversion stupor. In conversion stupor, variable awareness is possible. For example, the patient is often motionless but can respond to command or pain. He or she is completely mute (usually a sign of conversion stupor) or may utter monosyllabic or short phrases. He or she may swallow or may require tube feeding and suctioning.

"Focal" findings versus conversion disorder. Psychogenic ptosis usually fails to have accompanying frontalis muscle overcompensation. The patient with psychogenic hemiplegia will not adduct the weak arm or leg when asked; however, if these limbs are placed in the adducted position bilaterally and tested against resistance, adductor contraction on both sides is present. In psychogenic paraplegia, sphincter dysfunction is not found. Hoover's sign is often present in cases of conversion weakness. Normally, when a supine individual flexes his or her thigh to lift his or her leg, there is downward leg movement contralaterally, which is easily appreciated by the examiner who has placed his or her hand beneath that heel or leg. A patient with psychogenic hemiparesis has no downward movement in the contralateral normal leg when attempts are made to raise the "paretic" leg (Wells and Duncan 1980).

Patients with somatoform disorders may complain of sensory deficits. Suspicion of somatization is aroused when there is a well-defined, abrupt border between an area of sensory loss and another of normal sensation. Unilateral sensory loss with a midline border is highly unusual, especially if it is persistent along the nose and genitalia. Similarly, a midline loss of vibration sense over the skull or sternum has no physiologic etiology. Conversion disorders often coincide with neurological illnesses, so they are by no means mutually exclusive (Wells and Duncan 1980).

Movement disorders versus conversion movement disorder. Asterixis and multifocal myoclonus are usually not conversion symptoms. On the other hand, conversion myoclonus, consisting of atypical movements responsive to distraction or suggestion, is the most frequent somatoform symptom in a movement disorder clinic population (Monday and Jankovic 1993).

Seizures versus conversion seizures (pseudoseizures). Several useful diagnostic approaches are available to differentiate actual seizures from conversion seizures (pseudoseizures). Conversion seizures should be suspected when seizures are unusual or variable in presentation, when ictal EEG monitoring reveals no epileptic activity and postictal EEG monitoring shows no slowing of activity, and when seizure frequency does not change despite decreased plasma concentration of anticonvulsants (Desai et al. 1982). Provocative tests using suggestion can sometimes initiate or terminate a conversion "spell." Weeping has recently been suggested as a common element of pseudoseizures, but it is an extremely rare ictal phenomenon, except in dacrystic epilepsy (a type of epilepsy with profuse, sudden weeping as the predominant sign) (Bergen and Ristanovic 1993). Video-EEG monitoring of patients with intractable seizures has been helpful in uncovering "psychogenic fits" (King et al. 1982). Of patients with seizures, 20%–25% have both seizures and pseudoseizures (Ramani et al. 1980).

It is sometimes diagnostically helpful to study serum prolactin levels in patients after a seizure. A twofold or greater increase in serum prolactin concentration is usually seen in generalized and complex partial seizure patients 15–20 minutes postictus, but no such increase is seen in patients with pseudoseizures (Dana-Haeri and Trimble 1984; Pritchard et al. 1985; Trimble 1978).

Syncope versus conversion syncope. Conversion disorder is a possible explanation for "syncope," which occurs more often in women. Conversion syncope usually occurs in the presence of witnesses, is dramatic in presentation, may carry some sexual association, and is rarely associated with personal injury or with autonomic changes.

Suggestions for the management of conversion disorders can be found in Table 30–5.

Laboratory Evaluation

In addition to ordering routine blood and urine studies, consultation-liaison psychiatrists evaluating patients with neurological and neurosurgical problems often recommend additional laboratory data collection, especially CSF examination (Adams et al. 1997).

CSF does not normally contain more than five lymphocytes or monocytes per milliliter. An increase in white blood cells reflects an inflammation brought on by bacteria, viruses, other infectious agents, blood, chemicals, or neoplastic disease. Bacterial and fungal CNS infection may precipitate CSF polymorphonuclear cell

TABLE 30–5. Management of conversion disorder in neurology and neurosurgery settings

Abreaction and positive suggestion

Engage in one-to-one discussion—alone without family, friends; discuss experience and events surrounding onset of symptoms. Use sympathetic, patient, supportive encouragement of emotion.

Allow for saving face in explaining diagnosis; avoid statements such as "It's all in your head" and "There's nothing wrong."

Avoid confrontation; use direct, nonthreatening explanation of role of emotional difficulties in physical symptoms.

Make use of patient's characteristic suggestibility by suggesting reasonable timetable for improvement of patient's particular condition.

Conduct an interview with patient under influence of amobarbital, pentobarbital, a benzodiazepine, or hypnosis, which may be useful in uncovering conflict and leading to abreaction.

Behavioral approaches

Teach simple behavioral coping techniques that are more appropriate as a response in dealing with emotional problems than having physical symptom (e.g., seizure). Can be done in individual or group sessions.

Use behavioral approach aimed at rewarding "well behavior" in some patients with chronic problem.

Family involvement

Demonstrate appropriate "well behavior" to family and friends.

Minimize, through education, convenient sources of secondary gain in the family.

Begin family therapy, which may be helpful, especially in patients with chronic problem.

Chronically ill patient care

Employ systematic, reeducative type of psychotherapy based on personality profile and psychosocial variables.

Use behavioral therapy.

Use family therapy.

Require (infrequently) inpatient hospitalization to prevent consequences of conversion disorder (e.g., muscle atrophy).

response, whereas tuberculosis sparks lymphocytic pleocytosis. A white blood cell count less than 50 cells/mL suggests a noninfectious etiology, such as sarcoidosis, vasculitis, or meningeal carcinoma.

The protein content of CSF is normally 45 mg/dL or less. CSF protein levels are typically increased in bacterial meningitis and to a lesser extent in viral meningitis, brain and spinal cord tumors, diabetes mellitus, syphilis, multiple sclerosis, Guillain-Barré syndrome, lupus cerebritis, myxedema, and Cushing's syndrome. CSF protein levels can be low (less than 15 mg/dL) in meningismus

and in hyperthyroidism. The normal range of CSF glucose concentrations is 45–80 mg/dL. Abnormal CSF glucose levels, usually less than 40 mg/dL, occur in the presence of pleocytosis and usually signify a pyogenic, tubercular, or fungal meningitis. The CSF glucose concentration is usually also low in sarcoidosis, subarachnoid hemorrhage, and widespread neoplastic meningeal infiltration. Monocytic pleocytosis with increased protein and decreased glucose levels is typically seen in chronic meningitis and is also seen in meningeal carcinoma.

Cytology can be diagnostic in meningeal carcinoma, with 45%–75% of cases diagnosed after the first lumbar puncture and 80%–90% after three lumbar punctures (Coyle 1999).

Imaging and Electrophysiology

Computed Tomography of the Head

With the widespread use and high resolution of MRI, head CT is not used as universally as in the past. It has lost its importance in the diagnosis of arteriovenous malformations, hydrocephalus, herpes encephalitis, parasitic infestations, and progressive neurodegenerative diseases; MRI and other diagnostic measures are generally used in such cases. However, head CT continues to be very useful in the diagnosis of acute CNS bleeds and subarachnoid hemorrhages. It is also sometimes of benefit in the search for causes of partial or focal seizure disorders (Goodstein 1985). If contrast media is used, CT can reveal a small primary brain neoplasm. Metastatic tumors of the brain can also be visualized. Up to 95% of brain tumors can be seen on CT scans. CT can also distinguish between ischemic and hemorrhagic cerebrovascular lesions. Decreased density is seen on a CT scan when there is an infarct. Use of contrast with CT can increase the number of cerebrovascular lesions found. Goodstein (1985) reviewed indications for ordering a head CT scan in hospital psychiatry. Table 30–6 lists neuropsychiatric indications.

Magnetic Resonance Imaging

MRI provides greater contrast between gray and white matter than does CT (Gilman 1992). In addition, there is increased sensitivity, especially with T2-weighted images (for a detailed review of imaging, see Chapter 5, this volume), to white matter lesions that occur in demyelinating diseases such as multiple sclerosis. Particularly when contrast (gadolinium) is used, visualization of certain tumors such as meningiomas and acoustic neuromas is improved. Arteriovenous malformations, gliomas, and cerebral anomalies, on the other hand, are well delin-

TABLE 30–6. Computed tomography of the head: suggestions for use in neuropsychiatry

Atypical presentations (such as late-onset psychosis)

Abrupt mental status changes and rapid deteriorations

Refractory responses to treatment

Neurological complaints and findings
Ataxia
Electroencephalographic changes
Focal neurological signs
Incontinence
Seizures
Unusual headaches
Vertigo

Neuropsychiatric conditions
Dementia and pseudodementia
Gross head trauma
Mental retardation
Persistent central nervous system symptoms (in a patient in an alcoholic stupor)
Unexplained delirium

Other conditions
Anticoagulation and associated symptomatology
Ear pain with drainage
Immunosuppression and associated symptomatology

eated with noncontrast MRI. MRI is particularly effective in showing posterior fossa pathology of brain stem and cerebellar lesions. MRI requires that the patient be placed in a tightly confining receptacle; claustrophobia is a significant problem in approximately 5% of patients who undergo MRI.

MRI is superior to CT in evaluating most cerebral parenchymal lesions. Nevertheless, CT is preferable in certain situations, such as when patients have equipment needs, are unable to remain immobile, have head or spine injuries that require rapid evaluation, are uncooperative, or have pacemakers, mechanical valves, or intracranial clips.

Electroencephalography

Although electroencephalography generally lacks diagnostic specificity, it is still helpful in certain clinical states. An electroencephalogram with generalized slowing can help establish the diagnosis of delirium. A patient with paroxysmal spells of behavioral symptoms in whom the diagnosis of epilepsy is being considered should undergo electroencephalography. Electroencephalograms may be considered to show no abnormalities in a high percentage of patients with complex partial seizure disorder; that diagnosis ultimately rests on clinical findings. Specific clinical conditions have specific EEG patterns.

For example, Creutzfeldt-Jakob disease is associated with triphasic waves every 0.5–1.5 seconds.

Neuropsychological Testing

Cognition and associated behaviors are measured in a standardized fashion through the use of neuropsychological testing (Tranel 1992). Neuropsychological testing can help delineate suspected neurological illnesses that are not detected by other neurodiagnostic procedures; help differentiate "organic" from "functional" illness; be used to monitor mental status after medical or surgical treatment; assess cognitive capacities of the brain-injured patient to determine needs for rehabilitation, placement, or competence; and help identify learning disorders and guide remediation efforts. (For a detailed review of neuropsychological testing, see Chapter 7, this volume.)

TREATMENT AND MANAGEMENT

Psychopharmacology

General information about psychopharmacological treatment of psychiatric syndromes in neurology and neurosurgical patients can be found in the overview by Dubovsky (1992) and in Chapter 42 in this volume. However, the practical use of psychopharmacological agents for some neuropsychiatric syndromes and their target symptoms requires additional specific knowledge (Silver et al. 1990).

Neuroleptics

When psychotic thought and behavior occur in the neurology or neurosurgical patient and offending factors such as antiparkinsonian drugs cannot be removed or diminished, patients can be treated with neuroleptic medications (Silver et al. 1990). However, neuroleptics have sedative, anticholinergic, and hypotensive side effects that must be carefully monitored (Dubovsky 1992).

Neurological side effects must also be considered, including extrapyramidal symptoms such as akathisia, dystonia, parkinsonism, neuroleptic malignant syndrome, perioral tremor, tardive dystonia, and tardive dyskinesia. In general, higher-potency neuroleptics carry a higher risk for these side effects. Thus, patients with Parkinson's disease are not likely to tolerate haloperidol or fluphenazine, whereas they may do well when administered clozapine or thioridazine in low doses. The atypical neuroleptic clozapine controls psychotic symptoms without worsening parkinsonism signs (Fogel 1993). Clozapine is usually started at a low dosage, such as 25 mg/day, with the patient being monitored closely for sedation, anticholinergic side effects, and blood dyscrasia, especially agranulocytosis. Patients often respond to dosages as low as 25 mg/day (Kahn et al. 1991). Results with risperidone in patients with Parkinson's disease have been mixed. One study compared the response of six patients with Parkinson's disease and other akinetic rigid syndromes to risperidone therapy with response to clozapine therapy (Rich et al. 1995). Five of six had worsening motor symptoms and two of six developed encephalopathy while taking risperidone. When risperidone was replaced with clozapine, the patients' symptoms improved. However, a pilot study of risperidone use in nine inpatients with Parkinson's disease, dementia, and psychosis found the drug to be safe and effective, with minimal to mild impacts on parkinsonian symptoms (Workman et al. 1997). In patients with Huntington's disease, treatment with potent dopamine antagonists such as haloperidol can be helpful in reducing choreiform movements as well as in managing psychosis and aggression (Maricle 1993). Haloperidol can be started at 0.5–1.0 mg and titrated slowly; a total daily dosage of 2–15 mg is usually sufficient.

Psychotic symptoms can occur interictally in epileptic patients. Anticonvulsants may not control these symptoms, so neuroleptics must be used. Molindone and fluphenazine may be best because they have the lowest potential for lowering seizure threshold (Silver and Yudofsky 1988). Clinicians should keep seizure potential in mind in patients with agitated delirium secondary to brain dysfunction. Anticonvulsant medications are sometimes necessary when psychotropics that lower seizure threshold must be used (Ojemann 1987).

Neurologically ill psychotic patients are unusually susceptible to neuroleptic side effects, so low doses are used when possible. Patients must be closely monitored for neuroleptic malignant syndrome, a disorder characterized by autonomic hyperactivity, hyperpyrexia, rigidity, and mutism. This disorder has significant mortality.

In certain cases, however, neuropsychiatric emergencies—sometimes in the context of severe head injury, coupled with spinal fracture—still require aggressive treatment. Wise and Rundell (1988) presented suggested guidelines for the use of intravenous haloperidol and lorazepam in the treatment of agitation.

Psychostimulants and Dopaminergics

Methylphenidate and dextroamphetamine have been used successfully in medically ill depressed patients without causing anorexia or worsening confusion, even in patients with dementia or other primary brain disorders (Woods et al. 1986). Patients with PSD frequently respond to psychostimulants (Masand et al. 1991). Average daily dosages required are about 10–15 mg for methylphenidate and about 10 mg for dextroamphetamine. Psychostimulants also improve attention, concentration, and performance on neuropsychological testing in some patients with AIDS, and decrease depression as well (Fernandez et al. 1988). Bromocriptine, a direct dopamine agonist, has been anecdotally associated with improvement in abulia and akinetic mutism (Barrett 1991; Ross and Stewart 1981).

Antidepressants

The literature on the use of antidepressants in patients with major depression accompanying neurological illness is rather sparse (Silver et al. 1990). Treatment of patients with PSD has been studied. Therapeutic levels of nortriptyline are effective in relieving PSD (Lipsey et al. 1984). Silver et al. (1990) suggested that a patient with "clinically significant depressed mood," motivation, apathy, poor compliance, and impaired progress in physical rehabilitation therapy should be strongly considered for a trial of an antidepressant, usually a selective serotonin reuptake inhibitor (SSRI) (Dam et al. 1996; Lane et al. 1994). If a cyclic antidepressant is used, one with the most favorable risk-benefit ratio should be chosen. Among the tricyclic antidepressants, secondary amines are generally preferred. Tricyclic antidepressant therapies remain first-line treatments for chronic pain, fibromyalgia, migraine, sleep disorders, and severe depressions (Stahl 1998). Nortriptyline, which has relatively little anticholinergic activity and is the least likely to cause orthostatic hypotension, is often the tricyclic chosen; it is started at the lowest possible dose—10 mg orally at night. This dose is increased by 10 mg every 3 days or so, until a therapeutic level is reached. Elderly patients sometimes respond to lower doses. Oversedation, hypotension, confusion and worsening cognition, other anticholinergic effects, cardiotoxicity, and a lowered seizure threshold sometimes require discontinuation of cyclic antidepressant therapy.

Trazodone has also been reported to benefit patients with PSD (Reding et al. 1986). Maprotiline at dosages greater than 225 mg/day and bupropion at dosages greater than 450 mg/day appear to be particularly prone to lowering seizure threshold in predisposed patients. Patients with brain tumors, bulimia, and EEG abnormalities are at the greatest risk for problems related to bupropion's potential to lower seizure threshold. Amoxapine should also be used with special caution.

SSRIs have gained popularity in the treatment of mood disorders related to epilepsy. In a study by Blumer

(1997), patients with chronic epilepsy who had treatment-unresponsive mood disorders were treated again with a double antidepressant regimen of an SSRI plus a tricyclic antidepressant. After 20 months of treatment, 68% of previously unresponsive patients had responded favorably. Careful use of trazodone, monoamine oxidase inhibitors, SSRIs, or secondary amine tricyclic antidepressants can be justified in this population (McNamara 1993).

For patients with Parkinson's disease and depression, some clinicians still favor the use of the tricyclic antidepressants (e.g., nortriptyline and imipramine), especially if anxiety or panic symptoms are present. However, anticholinergic effects can be problematic, given that most of these patients are elderly (Dubovsky 1992; Fogel 1993). Bupropion is theoretically a good choice because of its dopaminergic action, especially if apathy and anhedonia are prominent (Fogel 1993). However, experience with bupropion in this clinical setting is limited, especially in combination with L-dopa (leading to an increased risk of psychosis) or selegiline. Amoxapine should be avoided because it may worsen extrapyramidal side effects (Dubovsky 1992). Trazodone and SSRIs (e.g., fluoxetine, sertraline, and paroxetine) may be useful, especially when the patient has a prominent negative affect. However, a worsening of parkinsonian symptoms may occur, especially with fluoxetine (Fogel 1993). For some patients, selegiline is an effective antidepressant, at least at higher doses. It selectively inhibits monoamine oxidase B at a dose of 10 mg, but at doses greater than 30–40 mg, it also inhibits monoamine oxidase A, and therefore, diet and drug restrictions must be observed.

Antidepressants have a number of specific uses in particular neurological patient groups (Table 30–7). Tricyclic antidepressants and SSRIs have been used with some success to reduce the depression associated with Huntington's disease. The same can be said about the use of antidepressants in patients with multiple sclerosis. Patients with chronic pain syndromes or fibromyalgias may benefit from treatment with antidepressants such as amitriptyline, nefazodone, doxepin, and the anticonvulsant gabapentin. SSRIs are also used for pain management, sometimes in combination with tricyclic antidepressants. Mirtazapine may also have a role in chronic pain and fibromyalgia management (Stahl 1998). Tinnitus may be improved with nortriptyline therapy. Amitriptyline and nortriptyline have been anecdotally reported to be effective in reducing pathological laughing and crying, as have SSRIs such as citalopram and fluoxetine (Andersen et al. 1993; Schiffer et al. 1985; Sloan et al. 1992). Amitriptyline has been used widely in headache management, especially for migraine prophylaxis. Nefazodone

TABLE 30–7. Antidepressants to consider when specific neurological disorders coexist with depression

Brain injury or disease-related agitation: *trazodone*

Brain tumors: *SSRIs, trazodone*

Chronic pain syndrome: *amitriptyline, desipramine, doxepin, gabapentin, SSRIs*

Huntington's disease: *SSRIs, tricyclic antidepressants*

Migraine headaches: *amitriptyline, doxepin*

Multiple sclerosis: *SSRIs, trazodone*

Neurogenic bladder with retention: *bupropion, methylphenidate, SSRIs, trazodone*

Parkinson's disease: *bupropion, imipramine, nortriptyline, SSRIs, trazodone*

Pathological laughing and crying: *amitriptyline, nortriptyline, SSRIs*

Seizure disorder: *MAOIs, secondary amine tricyclic antidepressants, SSRIs, trazodone*

Stroke: *methylphenidate, nortriptyline, SSRIs, trazodone*

Tinnitus: *nortriptyline*

Note. MAOI = monoamine oxidase inhibitor; SSRI = selective serotonin reuptake inhibitor.

and possibly mirtazapine may also prove helpful (Stahl 1998). Trazodone has been used to control agitation in patients with brain injury or brain disease. Neurogenic bladder with urinary retention, common in several neurological illnesses, is a challenge when treatment of depression is required. Drugs that are low in anticholinergic potency, such as sertraline, paroxetine, fluoxetine, trazodone, bupropion, and methylphenidate, are reasonable choices for patients who have urinary retention (Dubovsky 1992).

In a study that may have significance for our understanding of depression in neuropsychiatric illness, Malberg and colleagues (2000) showed that chronic antidepressant treatment increased cell proliferation and neuronal number in adult rat hippocampus. Electroconvulsive therapy also increases hippocampal neurogenesis, reversing the stress-induced atrophy and loss of hippocampal neurons that may contribute to the pathophysiology of depression.

Anticonvulsants (Including Benzodiazepines)

Carbamazepine is an anticonvulsant known to be effective for generalized and partial seizures. With the kindling hypothesis of bipolar syndromes came the idea of using carbamazepine for bipolar disorder (Post 1989). Carbamazepine appears to have antimanic efficacy, especially in patients who are more severely manic at onset, are more dysphoric, are cycling more rapidly, and have less genetic predisposition for the disease. Nevertheless, with regard to efficacy in treating acute mania, there is more evidence in favor of lithium than of carbamazepine (Bauer et al. 1999). Secondary manias may be responsive to carbamazepine therapy, especially if they are due to a seizure disorder. (For further information about the treatment of manic disorders, see Chapter 18, this volume.)

Carbamazepine is also effective for aggression and violence related to neuropsychiatric illnesses such as complex partial seizure disorder and head trauma. It can be given in divided doses of 600–1,200 mg/day to maintain serum levels at 4–12 μg/nL (Silver et al. 1990). Carbamazepine, as well as gabapentin, is also beneficial in paroxysmal neuropathic pain syndromes such as trigeminal neuralgia.

Sodium valproate is as effective as carbamazepine in treating generalized seizures but is less effective for complex partial seizure disorder (R.H. Mattson et al. 1992). Nevertheless, valproate has clinically important acute and prophylactic effects in manic and depressive illness (Post 1989). Valproate may block mania more than depression.

Experience with newer anticonvulsants such as gabapentin and particularly lamotrigine in the management of bipolar disorders is limited but increasing (Calabrese et al. 1996; Schaffer and Schaffer 1997; Stanton et al. 1997).

These newer medications make it possible to treat a patient's epilepsy and mood disorder with the same drug. Simplifying the drug regimen enhances medical compliance. Drug-drug interactions should always be kept in mind (Freeman and Stoll 1998). For example, SSRIs and nefazodone can decrease hepatic clearance of carbamazepine.

Clonazepam is a benzodiazepine anticonvulsant that has antimanic and limited antidepressant properties. Clonazepam is helpful in the management of manic breakthroughs and for sleep hygiene in the patient with mania (Post 1989). Lorazepam has been found to be a useful agent in the treatment of patients who are in catatonic states (Fricchione 1989).

Lithium Carbonate

There is some evidence that lithium can reduce aggressive, impulsive, and destructive behaviors in patients with mood lability secondary to brain syndromes (Silver and Yudofsky 1988).

When a patient with an underlying CNS disorder who is taking lithium becomes delirious, lithium therapy, sometimes even at therapeutic levels, is often the cause. Thus, lithium must be withheld and the clinician must search for other potential contributors. Lithium can also worsen secondary psychiatric disorders. Lithium-induced hypothyroidism may cause mental status changes and may also exacerbate lithium toxicity. Lithium may occasionally lower seizure threshold and initiate seizure activity, even in nonepileptic patients (Massey and Folger 1984). Patients with epilepsy may require increased anticonvulsant doses when taking lithium. Extrapyramidal side effects sometimes occur with lithium therapy.

Neurotoxicity syndromes have been reported with combinations of lithium and neuroleptics, carbamazepine, calcium-channel blockers, and clonazepam. The use of lithium should be limited to patients with mania and recurrent depressions that preceded brain disease (Silver et al. 1990) and to patients with aggression related to mania. When a decision is made to administer lithium to a patient with CNS disease, a strategy that is used with elderly patients seems reasonable: the dose should be started low and increased slowly, and lower therapeutic levels should be a focus. Neurological status should be monitored closely.

β-Blockers

Anecdotal evidence indicates that β-blockers, including propranolol, nadolol, pindolol, and metoprolol, are effective in the treatment of aggression related to neurological illnesses such as epilepsy, head trauma, Huntington's disease, Wilson's disease, and dementia (Silver et al. 1990). Silver et al. (1990) recommended a test dose of propranolol of 20 mg/day, especially if there are concerns about hypotension or bradycardia. The dose can be increased by 20 mg/day every 3 days. Dose increases should be stopped when the pulse rate falls below 50 beats/minute or when systolic blood pressure is less than 90 mm Hg. β-Blockers may take 4–6 weeks at maximum doses to work, a major drawback when acute agitation requires control.

Electroconvulsive Therapy

In addition to its well-known efficacy in mania and primary major depression, electroconvulsive therapy is an effective treatment for PSD (Murray et al. 1986; Wiart 1997) and for major depression associated with epilepsy, Parkinson's disease, or multiple sclerosis (Dubovsky 1986). In addition, it is the most powerful treatment for catatonic states (Fink and Taylor 1991). Confusional states and short-term memory dysfunction are the main neurological side effects of electroconvulsive therapy (Weiner 1984).

Psychotherapy

Most neurologically ill patients do not initiate their own psychiatric referrals (Minden 1992). Depression, lack of motivation, overelaborated symptomatology, or family discord may prompt the neurologist or neurosurgeon to seek a psychiatric consultation. These patients vary in their willingness to go to a psychiatrist. For this reason, one of the chief goals of the evaluation is to establish a therapeutic alliance (Minden 1992). A related goal is to pay attention to the patient's skepticism about psychiatry, typically coupled with a lack of "psychological-mindedness."

The psychiatrist must make the patient's comfort a priority during the examination. If anxiety emerges, the topic should be changed gently or a question's purpose should be explained. The psychiatrist's role as a medical consultant is likely to put the patient at ease. The psychiatrist should use a medical consultation model, gathering detailed medical data regarding neurological function and pain, while in an easygoing and natural way inquiring about the psychological concomitants of illness. "How has this illness affected your life?" is often a successful question, and asking it is a way of improving compliance and participation in the process. Psychological jargon should be avoided, and the patient's emotional experience should be validated, with normality emphasized. Common themes in the therapy include self-image, sexual function, employment problems, marital problems, and change in number and quality of relationships (R. Levin et al. 1988).

The psychotherapy evaluation should end with a simple, clear summary of the patient's problems and the factors that may be contributing (Minden 1992). A discussion of available effective treatments can then follow. If the neurologically ill patient does not want to enter psychotherapy, it is best to react neutrally and to offer help in the future.

Couples, family, group, and behavioral psychotherapies are helpful for many patients with neurological disorders (Forrest 1992; Minden 1992). Such therapies help foster compliance and provide support. Patients with a degenerative disease such as multiple sclerosis often benefit from the shared experience of others with the disease in a support or educational group setting. Family approaches can establish healthy communication between the patient and family members involved in the patient's care. Caregiver groups help reduce caregiver burnout syndromes.

Ward Management

Environmental management is important for many neuropsychiatric patients. Patients with delirium require close observation. Restraints are sometimes required for patient protection. The need should be reevaluated every few hours. Patients who have lost independence because of their neurological illness can gain some sense of control if they are permitted to schedule activities and request medications and are taught autohypnosis or deep relaxation techniques to control anxiety. Firm structure consistently applied by all staff members is frequently required for patients with impulsive behaviors and low frustration tolerance (e.g., patients with frontal lobe syndromes).

Staff members who work in neurological and neurosurgical units, particularly where there are a substantial number of chronic care patients, sometimes have a tendency to become demoralized and discouraged by the lack of patient progress or the degree of functional loss. Group support enables the staff to ventilate these feelings and to make constructive suggestions. An excellent model is a group meeting led by a consultation-liaison nurse and supervised by a consultation-liaison psychiatrist.

REFERENCES

Adams RD, Victor M, Ropper AH: Principles of Neurology, 6th Edition. New York, McGraw-Hill, 1997, pp 120–140

Agrell B, Dehlin O: Depression in stroke patients with left and right hemisphere lesions: a study in geriatric rehabilitation inpatients. Aging (Milano) 6:49–56, 1994

Albibi R, McCallum RW: Metoclopramide: pharmacology and clinical application. Ann Intern Med 98:86–95, 1983

Andersen G, Vestergaard K, Riis JO: Citalopram for post-stroke pathological crying. Lancet 342:837–839, 1993

Anderson NE, Willoughby EW: Chronic meningitis without predisposing illness—a review of 83 cases. Quarterly Journal of Medicine 63:283–295, 1987

Annegers JF, Grabow JD, Groove RV, et al: Seizures after head trauma: a population study. Neurology 30:683–689, 1980

Baker AB: Viral encephalitis, in Clinical Neurology. Edited by Baker AB. Philadelphia, PA, JB Lippincott, 1988, pp 1–147

Bakheit AM, Kennedy PG, Behan PO: Paraneoplastic limbic encephalitis: clinicopathological correlations. J Neurol Neurosurg Psychiatry 53:1084–1088, 1990

Barraclough B: Suicide and epilepsy, in Epilepsy and Psychiatry. Edited by Reynolds EH, Trimble MR. New York, Churchill Livingstone, 1981, pp 72–76

Barrett K: Treating organic abulia with bromocriptine and lisuride: four case studies. J Neurol Neurosurg Psychiatry 54:718–721, 1991

Bauer MS, Callahan AM, Jampala C, et al: Clinical practice guidelines for bipolar disorder from the Department of Veterans Affairs. J Clin Psychiatry 60:9–21, 1999

Bear DM, Fedio P: Quantitative analysis of interictal behavior in temporal lobe epilepsy. Arch Neurol 34:454–467, 1977

Belyi BI: Mental impairment in unilateral frontal tumors: role of the laterality of the lesion. Int J Neurosci 32:799–810, 1987

Benson DF: The Geschwind syndrome. Adv Neurol 55:411–412, 1991

Bergen D, Ristanovic R: Weeping as a common element of pseudoseizures. Arch Neurol 50:1059–1060, 1993

Blumer D: Antidepressant and double antidepressant treatment for the affective disorder of epilepsy. J Clin Psychiatry 58:3–11, 1997

Boffeli TJ, Guze SB: The simulation of neurologic disease. Psychiatr Clin North Am 15:301–310, 1992

Bornstein RA, Miller HB, Van Schoor T: Emotional adjustment in compensated head injury patients. Neurosurgery 23:622–627, 1988

Bouchard RH, Pourcher E, Vincent P: Fluoxetine and extrapyramidal side effects. Am J Psychiatry 146:1352–1353, 1989

Brain WR: Critical review: disseminated sclerosis. Quarterly Journal of Medicine 34:65–85, 1930

Brown JH, Paraskevas F: Cancer and depression: cancer presenting with depressive illness: an autoimmune disease? Br J Psychiatry 141:227–232, 1982

Browne TR, Feldman RG, Buchanan RA, et al: Methsuximide for complex partial seizures: efficacy, toxicity, clinical pharmacology, and drug interactions. Neurology 33:414–418, 1983

Burkle FM, Lipowski ZJ: Colloid cyst of the third ventricle presenting as psychiatric disorder. Am J Psychiatry 135:373–374, 1978

Cairns H, Mosberg WH: Colloid cysts of the third ventricle. Surgical Gynecology and Obstetrics 92:545–570, 1951

Calabrese JR, Fatemi SH, Woyshville MJ: Antidepressant effects of lamotrigine in rapid cycling bipolar disorder (letter). Am J Psychiatry 153:1236, 1996

Climo LH: Anorexia nervosa associated with hypothalamic tumor: the search for clinical-pathological correlations. Psychiatric Journal of the University of Ottawa 7:20–25, 1982

Coffey RJ: Hypothalamic and basal forebrain germinoma presenting with amnesia and hyperphagia. Surg Neurol 31:228–233, 1989

Constantin L, Martins JB, Fincham RW, et al: Bradycardia and syncope as manifestations of partial epilepsy. J Am Coll Cardiol 15:900–905, 1990

Coyle PK: Overview of acute and chronic meningitis. Neurol Clin 17:691–710, 1999

Craig TJ: An epidemiological study of a psychiatric liaison service. Gen Hosp Psychiatry 4:131–137, 1982

Cummings JL: Clinical Neuropsychiatry. Orlando, FL, Grune & Stratton, 1985a

Cummings JL: Organic delusions: phenomenology, anatomical correlations and review. Br J Psychiatry 146:184–197, 1985b

Cummings JL: Psychosomatic aspects of movement disorders. Adv Psychosom Med 13:111–132, 1985c

Cummings JL: Organic psychoses: delusional disorders and secondary mania. Psychiatr Clin North Am 9:293–311, 1986

Cummings JL: Depression and Parkinson's disease. Am J Psychiatry 149:443–454, 1992

Dam MP, Tonin P, DeBoni A, et al: Effects of fluoxetine and maprotiline on functional recovery in post-stroke hemiplegic patients undergoing rehabilitation therapy. Stroke 27:1211–1214, 1996

Dana-Haeri J, Trimble MR: Prolactin and gonadotrophin changes following partial seizures in epileptic patients with and without psychopathology. Biol Psychiatry 19:329–336, 1984

Delgado-Escueta AV, Mattson RH, King L, et al: The nature of aggression during epileptic seizures: a special report. N Engl J Med 305:711–716, 1981

Desai BT, Porter RJ, Kiffin-Penry J: Psychogenic seizures. Arch Neurol 39:202–209, 1982

Dubovsky SL: Using electroconvulsive therapy for patients with neurological disease. Hospital and Community Psychiatry 37:819–825, 1986

Dubovsky SL: Psychopharmacological treatment in neuropsychiatry, in The American Psychiatric Press Textbook of Neuropsychiatry, 2nd Edition. Edited by Yudofsky SC, Hales RE. Washington, DC, American Psychiatric Press, 1992, pp 663–701

Eastwood MR, Rifat SL, Nobbs H, et al: Mood disorder following cerebrovascular accident. Br J Psychiatry 154:195–200, 1989

Ebrahim S, Barer D, Nouri F: Affective illness after stroke. Br J Psychiatry 151:52–56, 1987

Elliot FA: The episodic dyscontrol syndrome and aggression. Neurol Clin 2:113–125, 1984

Fedio P: Behavioral characteristics of patients with temporal lobe epilepsy. Psychiatr Clin North Am 9:267–280, 1986

Fernandez F, Adams F, Levy JK, et al: Cognitive impairment due to AIDS-related complex and its response to psychostimulants. Psychosomatics 29:38–46, 1988

Fink M, Taylor MA: Catatonia: a separate category in the DSM-IV? Integrative Psychiatry 7:2–7, 1991

Fisher CM: Lacunar strokes and infarcts: a review. Neurology 32:871–876, 1982

Fogel BS: Parkinson's disease: recent developments of psychiatric interest, in Medical-Psychiatric Practice, Vol 2. Edited by Stoudemire A, Fogel BS. Washington, DC, American Psychiatric Press, 1993, pp 447–469

Forrest DV: Psychotherapy of patients with neuropsychiatric disorders, in The American Psychiatric Press Textbook of Neuropsychiatry, 2nd Edition. Edited by Yudofsky SC, Hales RE. Washington, DC, American Psychiatric Press, 1992, pp 703–739

Frankowski RF, Annegers JF, Whitman S: Epidemiological and descriptive studies, part 1: the descriptive epidemiology of head injury in the United States. Adv Psychosom Med 16:153–172, 1986

Freeman M, Stoll A: Mood stabilizer combinations: a review of safety and efficacy. Am J Psychiatry 155:12–21, 1998

Fricchione GL: Catatonia: a new indication for benzodiazepines? Biol Psychiatry 26:761–765, 1989

Furneaux HF, Reich L, Posner JB: Autoantibody synthesis in the central nervous system of patients with paraneoplastic syndromes. Neurology 40:1085–1091, 1990

Gilchrist JM: Arrhythmogenic seizures: diagnosis by simultaneous EEG/ECG recording. Neurology 35:1503–1506, 1985

Gilman S: Advances in neurology (1). N Engl J Med 326:1608–1616, 1992

Goldensohn ES: Symptomatology of nonconvulsive seizures: ictal and postictal. Epilepsia 24 (suppl 1):S5–S21, 1983

Gliatto MF, Caroff SN: Neurosyphilis: a history and clinical review. Psychiatric Annals 31:153–161, 2001

Goodstein RK: Guide to CAT scanning in hospital psychiatry: overview of clinical practice and criteria for use. Gen Hosp Psychiatry 7:367–376, 1985

Goodkin K, Baldewicz TT, Wilkie FL, et al: HIV-1 Infection of the brain: a region-specific approach to its neuropathophysiology and therapeutic prospects. Psychiatric Annals 31:182–192, 2001

Gould R, Miller BL, Goldberg MA, et al: The validity of hysterical signs and symptoms. J Nerv Ment Dis 174:593–597, 1986

Gusella JF, Wexler NS, Conneally PM, et al: A polymorphic DNA marker genetically linked to Huntington's disease. Nature 306:234–238, 1983

Hachinski V, Norris JW: The Acute Stroke. Philadelphia, PA, FA Davis, 1985

Harvey SA, Black KJ: The dexamethasone suppression test for diagnosing depression in stroke patients. Ann Clin Psychiatry 8:35–39, 1996

Hauser WA, Kurland LT: The epidemiology of epilepsy in Rochester, Minnesota, 1935 through 1967. Epilepsia 16:1–66, 1975

Hoeppner JB, Garron DC, Wilson RS, et al: Epilepsy and verbosity. Epilepsia 28:35–40, 1987

Hooshmand H, Escobar MR, Kopf SW: Neurosyphilis: a study of 241 patients. JAMA 219:721–729, 1972

Jennett B, Teasdale J: Management of Head Injuries. Philadelphia, PA, FA Davis, 1981

Kahana E, Liebowitz U, Alter M: Cerebral multiple sclerosis. Neurology 21:1179–1185, 1971

Kahn N, Freeman A, Juncos JL, et al: Clozapine is beneficial for psychosis in Parkinson's disease. Neurology 41:1699–1700, 1991

King DW, Gallagher BB, Murvin AJ, et al: Pseudoseizures: diagnostic evaluation. Neurology 32:18–23, 1982

Klass DW: Electroencephalographic manifestations of complex partial seizures, in Complex Partial Seizures and Their Treatment (Advances in Neurology Series, Vol 2). Edited by Penry JK, Daly DD. New York, Raven, 1975, pp 113–140

Kwentus JA, Hart RP, Peck ET, et al: Psychiatric complications of closed-head trauma. Psychosomatics 26:8–15, 1985

Lane RM, Sweeney M, Henry JA: Pharmacotherapy of the depressed patient with cardiovascular and/or cerebrovascular illness. Br J Clin Pract 48:256–262, 1994

Levin HS, Mattis S, Ruff RM, et al: Neurobehavioral outcome following minor head injury: a three-center study. J Neurosurg 66:234–243, 1987

Levin R, Banks S, Berg B: Psychosocial dimensions of epilepsy: a review of the literature. Epilepsia 29:805–816, 1988

Levy R, Bredesen DE: Central nervous system dysfunction in acquired immunodeficiency syndrome. J Acquir Immune Defic Syndr 1:46–64, 1988

Lipsey JR, Robinson RG, Pearlson GD, et al: Nortriptyline treatment of post-stroke depression: a double blind study. Lancet 1:297–300, 1984

Lishman WA: Organic Psychiatry: The Psychological Consequences of Cerebral Disorder, 2nd Edition. Oxford, UK, Blackwell Scientific, 1987

Lishman WA: Physiogenesis in the "post-concussional syndrome." Br J Psychiatry 153:460–469, 1988

Locharernkul C, Primrose D, Pilcher WH, et al: Update in epilepsy, part I: diagnosis and treatment of epilepsy. New York State Medical Journal 92:14–17, 1992

Lohr JB, Cadet JL: Neuropsychiatric aspects of brain tumors, in The American Psychiatric Press Textbook of Neuropsychiatry. Edited by Hales RE, Yudofsky SC. Washington, DC, American Psychiatric Press, 1987, pp 351–364

Malamud N: Psychiatric disorder with intracranial tumors of the limbic system. Arch Neurol 17:113–123, 1967

Malberg JE, Eisch AJ, Nestler EJ, et al: Chronic antidepressant treatment increases neurogenesis in adult rat hippocampus. J Neurosci 20:9104–9110, 2000

Maricle RA: Psychiatric disorders in Huntington's disease, in Medical-Psychiatric Practice, Vol 2. Edited by Stoudemire A, Fogel BS. Washington, DC, American Psychiatric Press, 1993, pp 471–512

Masand P, Murray GB, Pickett P: Psychostimulants in post-stroke depression. J Neuropsychiatry Clin Neurosci 3:23–27, 1991

Massey EW, Folger WN: Seizures activated by therapeutic levels of lithium carbonate. South Med J 77:1173–1175, 1984

Mattson AJ, Levin HS: Frontal lobe dysfunction following closed head injury: a review of the literature. J Nerv Ment Dis 178:282–291, 1990

Mattson RH, Cramer JA, Collins JF, et al: A comparison of valproate with carbamazepine for the treatment of complex partial seizures and secondarily generalized tonic-clonic seizures in adults. N Engl J Med 327:765–771, 1992

Mayeux R, Chen J, Mirabello E, et al: An estimate of the incidence of dementia in idiopathic Parkinson's disease. Neurology 40:1513–1517, 1990

McArthur JC, Hoover DR, Bacellar H, et al: Dementia in AIDS patients: incidence and risk factors. Multicenter AIDS Cohort Study. Neurology 43:2245–2252, 1993

McKenna PJ, Kane JM, Parrish K: Psychotic syndromes in epilepsy. Am J Psychiatry 142:895–904, 1985

McKinlay WW, Brooks DN, Bond MR, et al: The short-term outcome of severe blunt head injury as reported by the relative of the injured person. J Neurol Neurosurg Psychiatry 44:527–533, 1981

McNamara ME: Clinical neurology, in Psychiatric Care of the Medical Patient. Edited by Stoudemire A, Fogel BS. New York, Oxford University Press, 1993, pp 455–483

Mendez MF, Cummings JL, Benson DF: Epilepsy: psychiatric aspects and use of psychotropics. Psychosomatics 25:883–894, 1984

Mendez MF, Cummings JL, Benson DF: Depression in epilepsy: significance and phenomenology. Arch Neurol 43:766–770, 1986

Mesulam MM: Principles of Behavioral Neurology. Philadelphia, PA, FA Davis, 1985, pp 41–58

Minden SL: Psychotherapy for people with multiple sclerosis. J Neuropsychiatry Clin Neurosci 4:198–213, 1992

Monday K, Jankovic J: Psychogenic myoclonus. Neurology 43:349–352, 1993

Morris PLP, Robinson RG, Raphael B: Prevalence and course of post-stroke depression in hospitalized patients. Int J Psychiatry Med 20:349–364, 1990

Murray GB: Psychiatric disorders secondary to complex partial seizures. Drug Therapy 4:21–26, 1985

Murray GB, Shea V, Conn DK: Electroconvulsive therapy for post-stroke depression. J Clin Psychiatry 47:258–260, 1986

Navia BA, Jordan BD, Price RW: The AIDS dementia complex: clinical features. Ann Neurol 19:517–524, 1986

Newman NJ, Bell IR, McKee AC: Paraneoplastic limbic encephalitis: neuropsychiatric presentation. Biol Psychiatry 27:529–542, 1990

Newsom-Davis J: Lambert-Eaton myasthenic syndrome. Springer Semin Immunopathol 8:129–140, 1985

Ojemann R: Effect of psychotropic medication on seizure control in patients with epilepsy. Neurology 37:1525–1527, 1987

Portegies P, Enting RH, de Gans J, et al: Presentation and cause of AIDS dementia complex: 10 years of follow up in Amsterdam, The Netherlands. AIDS 7:669–675, 1993

Post RM: Use of anticonvulsants in the treatment of manic-depressive illness, in Clinical Use of Anticonvulsants in Psychiatric Disorders. Edited by Post RM, Trimble MR, Pippenger CE. New York, Demos, 1989, pp 113–152

Price TRP, Goetz KL, Lovell MR: Neuropsychiatric aspects of brain tumors, in The American Psychiatric Press Textbook of Neuropsychiatry, 2nd Edition. Edited by Yudofsky SC, Hales RE. Washington, DC, American Psychiatric Press, 1992, pp 473–497

Pritchard PB III, Wannamaker BB, Sagel J, et al: Serum prolactin and cortisol levels in evaluation of pseudoepileptic seizures. Ann Neurol 18:87–89, 1985

Ramani SV, Quesney LF, Olson D, et al: Diagnosis of hysterical seizures in epileptic patients. Am J Psychiatry 137:705–709, 1980

Ramasubbu R, Flint A, Brown G, et al: Diminished serotonin-mediated prolactin responses in nondepressed stroke patients compared with healthy normal subjects. Stroke 29:1293–1298, 1998

Ramchandani D, Schindler B: Evaluation of pseudoseizures: a psychiatric perspective. Psychosomatics 34:70–79, 1993

Rao SM, Leo GJ, Bernardin L, et al: Cognitive dysfunction in multiple sclerosis, I: frequency, patterns, and prediction. Neurology 41:685–691, 1991

Rao SM, Reingold SC, Ron MA, et al: Workshop on Neurobehavioral Disorders in Multiple Sclerosis: Diagnosis, underlying disease, natural history, and therapeutic intervention, Bergamo, Italy, June 25–27, 1992. Arch Neurol 50:658–662, 1993

Reding MJ, Orto LA, Wanter SW, et al: Antidepressant therapy after stroke: a double blind trial. Arch Neurol 43:763–765, 1986

Rich SS, Friedman JH, Ott BR: Risperidone versus clozapine in the treatment of psychosis in six patients with Parkinson's disease and other akinetic-rigid syndromes. J Clin Psychiatry 56:556–559, 1995

Robbins RA, Simmons Z, Bremer BA, et al: Quality of life in ALS is maintained as physical function declines. Neurology 56:442–444, 2001

Robertson K, Fiscus S, Kapoor C, et al: CSF, plasma viral load and HIV-associated dementia. J Neurovirol 4:90–94, 1998

Robertson MM, Trimble MR: Depressive illness in patients with epilepsy: a review. Epilepsia 24 (suppl 2):S109–S116, 1983

Robinson RG, Starkstein SE: Current research in affective disorders following strokes. J Neuropsychiatry Clin Neurosci 2:1–14, 1990

Robinson RG, Starr LB, Kubos KL, et al: A two-year longitudinal study of post-stroke mood disorders: findings during the initial evaluation. Stroke 14:736–741, 1983

Robinson RG, Kubos KL, Starr LB, et al: Mood disorders in stroke patients: importance of lesion location. Brain 107:81–93, 1984

Robinson RG, Bolduc PL, Price TR: Two-year longitudinal study of post-stroke mood disorders: diagnosis and outcome at one and two years. Stroke 18:837–843, 1987

Robinson RG, Boston JD, Starkstein SE: Comparison of mania and depression after brain injury: causal factors. Am J Psychiatry 145:172–178, 1988

Rodin E, Schmaltz S: The Bear-Fedio personality inventory and temporal lobe epilepsy. Neurology 34:591–596, 1984

Ross ED: The aprosodias: functional-anatomic organization of the affective components of language in the right hemisphere. Arch Neurol 38:561–569, 1981

Ross ED, Mesulam MM: Dominant language functions of the right hemisphere: prosody and emotional gesturing. Arch Neurol 36:144–148, 1979

Ross ED, Rush AJ: Diagnosis and neuroanatomical correlates of depression in brain damaged patients. Arch Gen Psychiatry 38:1344–1354, 1981

Ross ED, Stewart RM: Akinetic mutism from hypothalamic damage: successful treatment with a dopamine agonist. Neurology 31:1435–1439, 1981

Ruff RM, Marshall LF, Klauber MR, et al: Alcohol abuse and neurological outcome of the severely head injured. J Head Trauma Rehabil 5:21–31, 1990

Russell RW, Pennybacker JB: Craniopharyngioma in the elderly. J Neurol Neurosurg Psychiatry 24:1–13, 1961

Salloway S, White J: Paroxysmal limbic disorders in neuropsychiatry. J Neuropsychiatry Clin Neurosci 9:403–419, 1997

Sanders KM, Murray GB: Immediate resolution of depression after surgery for craniopharyngioma. Neuropsychiatry Neuropsychol Behav Neurol 5:56–59, 1992

Schaffer CB, Schaffer LC: Gabapentin in the treatment of bipolar disorder (letter). Am J Psychiatry 154:291–292, 1997

Schiffer RB, Herndon RM, Rudick RA: Treatment of pathologic laughing and weeping with amitriptyline. N Engl J Med 312:1480–1482, 1985

Schoenhuber R, Gentil M: Anxiety and depression after mild head injury: a case control study. J Neurol Neurosurg Psychiatry 51:722–724, 1988

Selecki BR: Cerebral mid-line tumors involving the corpus callosum among mental hospital patients. Med J Aust 2:954–960, 1964

Silver JM, Yudofsky SC: Psychopharmacology and electroconvulsive therapy, in The American Psychiatric Press Textbook of Psychiatry. Edited by Talbott JA, Hales RE, Yudofsky SC. Washington, DC, American Psychiatric Press, 1988, pp 767–853

Silver JM, Hales RE, Yudofsky SC: Psychiatric consultation to neurology, in The American Psychiatric Press Review of Psychiatry, Vol 9. Edited by Tasman A, Goldfinger SM, Kaufmann CA. Washington, DC, American Psychiatric Press, 1990, pp 433–465

Silver JM, Hales RE, Yudofsky SC: Neuropsychiatric aspects of traumatic brain injury, in The American Psychiatric Press Textbook of Neuropsychiatry, 2nd Edition. Edited by Yudofsky SC, Hales RE. Washington, DC, American Psychiatric Press, 1992, pp 363–395

Sinyor D, Jacques P, Kaloupek DA, et al: Post-stroke depression and lesion location: an attempted replication. Brain 109:537–546, 1986

Skuster DZ, Digre KB, Corbett JJ: Neurologic conditions presenting as psychiatric disorders. Psychiatr Clin North Am 15:311–333, 1992

Sloan RL, Brown KW, Pentland B: Fluoxetine as a treatment for emotional liability after brain injury. Brain Inj 6:315–319, 1992

Stahl SM: Selecting an antidepressant by using mechanism of action to enhance efficacy and avoid side-effects. J Clin Psychiatry 59 (suppl 18):23–29, 1998

Stanton SP, Keck PE Jr, McElroy SL: Treatment of acute mania with gabapentin (letter). Am J Psychiatry 154:287, 1997

Starkstein SE, Robinson RG: Neuropsychiatric aspects of cerebral vascular disorders, in The American Psychiatric Press Textbook of Neuropsychiatry, 2nd Edition. Edited by Yudofsky SC, Hales RE. Washington, DC, American Psychiatric Press, 1992, pp 449–472

Starkstein SE, Robinson RG, Price TR, et al: Comparison of patients with and without post-stroke major depression matched for size and location of lesion. Arch Gen Psychiatry 45:247–252, 1988a

Starkstein SE, Robinson RG, Price TR: Comparison of spontaneously recovered versus non-recovered patients with post-stroke depression. Stroke 19:1491–1496, 1988b

Starkstein SE, Robinson RG, Honig MA, et al: Mood changes after right-hemisphere lesions. Br J Psychiatry 155:79–85, 1989

Starkstein SE, Cohen BS, Federoff P, et al: Relationship between anxiety disorders and depressive disorders in patients with cerebrovascular injury. Arch Gen Psychiatry 47:246–251, 1990

Strauss I, Keschner M: Mental symptoms in cases of tumor of the frontal lobe. Archives of Neurology and Psychiatry 33:986–1005, 1935

Surridge D: An investigation into some psychiatric aspects of multiple sclerosis. Br J Psychiatry 115:749–764, 1969

Swartz MN: "Chronic meningitis"—many causes to consider. N Engl J Med 317:957–959, 1987

Swirsky-Sacchetti T, Mitchell DR, Seward J, et al: Neuropsychological and structural brain lesions in multiple sclerosis: a regional analysis. Neurology 42:1291–1295, 1992

Tetrud JW, Langston JW: The effect of deprenyl (selegiline) on the natural history of Parkinson's disease. Science 245:519–522, 1989

Tranel D: Neuropsychological assessment. Psychiatr Clin North Am 15:283–299, 1992

Treiman DM, Delgado-Escueta AV: Complex partial status epilepticus, in Advances in Neurology, Vol 34: Status Epilepticus. Edited by Delgado-Escueta AV, Wasterlain CG, Treiman DM, et al. New York, Raven, 1983, pp 69–81

Trimble MR: Serum prolactin in epilepsy and hysteria (letter). British Medical Journal 2:1682, 1978

Tsopelas ND, Saintfort R, Fricchione GL: The relationship of psychiatric illnesses and seizures. Curr Psychiatry Rep 3:235–242, 2001

van Merode T, de Krom MC, Knottnerus JA: Gender-related differences in non-epileptic attacks: a study of patients' cases in the literature. Seizure 6:311–316, 1997

Wallen J, Pincus HA, Goldman HH, et al: Psychiatric consultations in short-term general hospitals. Arch Gen Psychiatry 44:163–168, 1987

Watson CG, Buranen C: The frequency and identification of false positive conversion reactions. J Nerv Ment Dis 167:243–247, 1979

Waxman SG, Geschwind N: The interictal behavior syndrome of temporal lobe epilepsy. Arch Gen Psychiatry 32:1580–1586, 1975

Weilberg JB, Bear DM, Sachs G: Three patients with concomitant panic attacks and seizure disorder: possible clues to the neurology of anxiety. Am J Psychiatry 144:1053–1056, 1987

Weiner RD: Does ECT cause brain damage? Behav Brain Sci 7:1–53, 1984

Wells CE, Duncan GW: Neurology for Psychiatrists. Philadelphia, PA, FA Davis, 1980

Whitehouse PJ, Rabins PV: Quality of life and dementia. Alzheimer Dis Assoc Disord 6:135–137, 1992

Whitlock FA, Suskind MM: Depression as a major symptom of multiple sclerosis. J Neurol Neurosurg Psychiatry 43:861–865, 1980

Wiart L: Post-cerebrovascular stroke depression. Encephale 3:51–54, 1997

Wikstrom J, Paetau A, Palo J, et al: Classic amyotrophic lateral sclerosis with dementia. Arch Neurol 39:681–683, 1982

Wilson SAK: Neurology. London, Edward Arnold, 1940

Wise MG, Rundell JR: Concise Guide to Consultation Psychiatry. Washington, DC, American Psychiatric Press, 1988

Woods S, Tesar G, Murray GB, et al: Psychostimulant treatment of depressive disorders secondary to medical illness. J Clin Psychiatry 47:12–15, 1986

Workman RH, Orengo CA, Bakey AA, et al: The use of risperidone for psychosis and agitation in demented patients with Parkinson's disease. J Neuropsychiatry Clin Neurosci 9:594–597, 1997

31

Obstetrics and Gynecology

Nada L. Stotland, M.D., M.P.H.

Obstetrician/gynecologists work with the most affect-laden processes, situations, and interventions in medicine: sexuality, sexual assault, fertility frustrated or unwanted, birth, malignancy, and loss. They must manipulate highly complex physiologic processes and master an ever-increasing variety of surgical and other technical skills. They have little time to spend with each patient. They are acutely aware of their vulnerability to malpractice suits (American College of Obstetricians and Gynecologists 1985).

Obstetrician/gynecologists also find themselves embroiled in social changes and discontent surrounding women's roles and women's health care (Stotland 1988). These changes differ from subculture to subculture and patient to patient. One patient, mindful of the questions about the high rate of cesarean deliveries or hysterectomies in the United States, regards a well-founded recommendation for a procedure with suspicion. The next patient demands a surgical delivery or hysterectomy that is not medically advisable. One patient is incensed by the practitioner's failure to explain some aspect of a proposed treatment; the next refuses information, insisting, "You are the doctor; just tell me what I should do."

Medical school and residency training in obstetrics and gynecology offer little information about psychological, cultural, social, and psychiatric issues (Weissberg 1990). The risk is that the physician who is poorly trained to handle anxiety evoked by affect-laden situations will react by blaming or stigmatizing patients for their psychological needs or psychiatric illnesses, by overgeneralizing from his or her own experiences, by imposing his or her own values, and/or by ignoring clinically significant findings.

Psychiatrists and other mental health professionals are often unfamiliar and uncomfortable with obstetrics and gynecology. Psychiatrists may neglect to inquire or counsel about Papanicolaou tests, contraception, sexual function, sexual side effects of medications, sexual concerns, and protection against sexually transmitted diseases (Lesko et al. 1982). Mental health professionals may fail to take an adequate sexual and reproductive history that would alert them to anniversary reactions and the relations between psychiatric symptoms and recent reproductive events. Psychiatrists may be unaware of recent developments in obstetrics and gynecology—for example, the discovery of biological causes for most cases of infertility, the physical and emotional demands of diagnostic and treatment protocols for infertility, and the psychiatric aspects of hormones used for contraception and at menopause.

REPRODUCTIVE PHYSIOLOGY AND PSYCHOLOGY THROUGH THE LIFE CYCLE

So much is now known about the physiology of reproduction that vital aspects of it can be manipulated in vivo and duplicated in vitro. Hormonal concomitants of the menstrual cycle are mapped not only in daily but also in hourly detail. However, vexing physiologic mysteries remain. The physiologic control of the onset of labor is not understood, and there is still no effective intervention for premature labor. Little is known about the relations between physiologic and psychosocial factors in symptoms related to the reproductive system. What causes some women to experience psychiatric symptoms during a particular phase of the menstrual cycle? What makes most women want to become mothers, and how do we draw the line between a healthy and an exaggerated desire for parenthood in a patient who is seeking infertility treatment? By what mechanisms do maternal anxiety, preparation, and interpersonal support affect the course and outcome of labor? There is a growing literature on reproductive psychology, as well as psychiatric diagnoses, situations, and treatments specific to obstetrics and gynecology.

Gender identity is closely linked to the capacity for sexual relationships and reproduction (Notman 1991). The assignment of gender at—or before—birth has a significant effect on virtually every aspect of the child's experience. Names are assigned by gender; parental expectations and behaviors are shaped by gender. Because gender is determined for most people by genitalia, conditions, illnesses, and treatments affecting the genitalia impinge on an individual's core identity and roles in society. A cholecystectomy does not carry the same emotional valence or interpersonal implications as does a hysterectomy, although the emotional meaning of the latter surgery varies extensively from woman to woman and from context to context.

More recent studies seem to have invalidated Freud's assertion that very young girls are unaware of their internal genitalia and therefore experience themselves as castrated males (Chodorow 1989; Freud 1931/1961; Russo 1991). Recent child observation studies and psychological theory stress the social rather than the anatomic experience of being female. Compared with male children, female children do not have prominent sexual organs, but they can look forward to developing breasts and gestating and breast-feeding their infants.

Women's lives are defined not only by reproductive stages but also by graduations, jobs, and other non-gender-related events. However, reproductive milestones define the boundaries of some of the most important stages for women. Women's reproductive lives are marked by distinct milestones: menarche, first intercourse, conception, first and subsequent deliveries, and menopause. Most cultures mark some of the milestones with rituals and/or changes in status, roles, and responsibilities. The age at which menarche occurs has decreased over centuries and decades, from the middle to late teenage years to a current average in the United States of about age 13 years (Eveleth and Tanner 1976). Physiologically, menarche marks the beginning of fertility. In some societies, first menstruation makes a girl marriageable. At the same time, menstruation is associated with taboos and a sense of shame in many cultures. Not infrequently referred to as "the curse," menstruation is considered polluting and disabling. In at least some societies with stringent menstrual taboos, females are depressed during each menstrual period, from menarche to menopause (Ullrich 1987).

Like menstruation, first intercourse tends to evoke mixed feelings (Lewis and Volkmar 1990). Because girls' genitalia are internal, casual visual inspection cannot evoke either competition or reassurance of normality as it does in boys. Even women who have successfully borne children are anecdotally reported to have doubts about the normality of their external genitalia. Anticipation of first intercourse evokes fear of physical pain and of the revelation of defectiveness. Conflicts about having engaged in intercourse may therefore complicate the prospect of gynecological examination. However, the ability to engage in coitus confirms anatomic normality and is a symbol of maturity.

The desire to conceive, gestate, bear, and raise one or more children is not precisely the same as the desire to know that one is capable of doing so. Some women report becoming pregnant to prove their fertility, with no intention of carrying the pregnancy to term. The gynecologist may assume that a woman who has a certain number of children, has reached a certain age, and/or has expressed a desire to curtail further childbearing will have little or no emotional reaction to a medical or surgical intervention resulting in sterility. These assumptions can result in serious miscommunication, psychological turmoil, adverse psychiatric reactions, and malpractice suits. Similarly, the tendency of gynecologists to assume that all women are heterosexual has resulted in a general unwillingness of lesbians to obtain gynecological care (Valanis 2000).

The cessation of monthly bleeding signifies entry of a woman into the "older" category. Powerful and pervasive social influences shape the individual woman's experience of menopause and confound scientific research into the relation between physiologic menopause and psychiatric symptoms. Several generations of psychiatrists were taught that menopause frequently precipitated a developmental crisis or psychiatric illness. More recent studies indicate that there is no association between clinical depression and menopause as a physiologic event (Matthews et al. 1990; McKinlay et al. 1987).

The hormonal changes that occur during the climacteric (see Table 31–1) are associated with vasomotor episodes commonly referred to as "hot flashes" and with changes in vaginal lubrication and other functions. For some women, hot flashes may be so frequent and severe as to interfere with sleep, secondarily leading to decreased energy and concentration, depressed mood, and anxiety (MacLennan et al. 2001; Sherwin 1993). Changes in sexual physiology may necessitate changes in sexual technique. On the one hand, little has been written about the natural course of menopause, and little information is available to women wondering how long the symptoms will last or to inform their choices. On the other hand, a great deal has been written about the medical "management" of menopause.

TABLE 31–1. Hormonal changes during the climacteric

Estrogen production is decreased.
Progesterone levels are unchanged.
Follicle-stimulating hormone production is increased.
Luteinizing hormone levels are unchanged.
Prolactin levels are decreased.
Androgen production is unchanged.

Source. Adapted from Droegemueller et al. 1987.

Many gynecologists now believe that the prescription of hormones is the single most beneficial intervention they have to offer their patients. The use of unopposed estrogen necessitates periodic uterine biopsies; the addition of progesterone causes periodic bleeding that is inconvenient and experienced as age-inappropriate (Pilon et al. 2001; Sturdee 2000). Advertisements aimed at physicians and at consumers convey the message that "replacement" therapy will prolong youth and sexual attractiveness (Apfel and Palmund 1992). It is perhaps not surprising, given these realities and those discussed in the next paragraph, that only 25% or less of women who are prescribed hormones are still taking them after 1 year.

The ubiquitous term *replacement* is not apt, because there is no hormone deficiency; different levels of hormones are normative at different stages of life. A postmenopausal woman is no more deficient in hormones than a prepubertal girl. The unquestioning use of the term *replacement* in nearly every scientific paper, lay article, and advertisement reifies this inaccurate and psychologically damaging concept of deficiency. Years of studies claiming crucial cardiovascular and bone benefits were found to have suffered from confounding variables not evident in surface demographics; apparently, women who took hormones took better care of themselves or simply enjoyed better health than those who did not take hormones. Cardiovascular effects are currently being reexamined. Protection against osteoporosis can be achieved with "designer" estrogens and, better still, with exercise and a calcium-rich diet beginning in childhood. Research is now focused on cognitive and affective effects. Hormones do not restore cognitive abilities to those who have already lost them. They may affect the cognitive abilities of postmenopausal women, but only those whose menopause is symptomatic (LeBlanc et al. 2001). The effects of estrogen on mood are also controversial. Progesterone can provoke depressive symptoms. Each patient responds differently; treatment is empirical at this point.

Rates of depression in menopausal and postmenopausal women are linked to the psychological and social implications of aging and the loss of fertility (Holte 1992). Women whose chief gratification and status were derived from their youthful attractiveness and their ability to bear children, as well as women who desired but were not able to achieve gratifying childbearing and mothering, are both vulnerable to depression at menopause (Apfel and Handel 1993). When women's resources and environment allow them to make a gratifying and acknowledged contribution to society after parenting tasks have ended, menopause is usually experienced as a relief from the inconvenience of monthly bleeding, the fear and pain of childbearing, and the demands of child rearing, as well as an opportunity for the expression of other interests and talents. Nevertheless, negative images of menopause persist not only among psychiatrists but also among gynecologists, who often view menopause as a deficiency state.

WOMEN'S HEALTH AND HEALTH CARE: TRADITION AND CHANGE

Women's health care has recently become a legislative, marketing, and research focus (Cotton 1992a, 1992b). The government and other major social institutions, including foundations and health care managers, have highlighted the need for increased numbers and availability of primary care—rather than specialty and subspecialty—providers. Faced with the prospect of financial and other incentives for training and practice in primary care, obstetrician/gynecologists, whose training focuses on the aggressive management of labor and of disease, successfully lobbied to be considered primary care physicians. This designation recognized the primary role many gynecologists have played for their patients, but it also placed an additional, and arguably unrealistic, burden on gynecological training, continuing medical education, and practice.

The significance of psychological factors in obstetrics and gynecological care begins at the level of education and preventive care. Women who are asked to draw diagrams of their reproductive systems commonly confuse and combine orifices and tracts. Many women experience pelvic examinations as embarrassing, awkward, and uncomfortable, if not frankly painful. Only a minority of women in the United States obtain regular gynecological care, and almost a quarter of all pregnant women receive no first trimester prenatal care (Muller 1990).

Many women lack the language to explain and locate their symptoms. These problems lead to social and health problems. Contraceptive care is not obtained; diaphragms are incorrectly placed. Sexually transmitted diseases are pandemic. Breast masses and cervical lesions are not diagnosed when still treatable (Ciotti 1992; Rimer and King 1992). There are additional reasons that women need information and the ability to advocate for their own health care. Women are overrepresented among the poor, and nearly one-quarter of the women in the United States lack health insurance. Women's health care is partitioned among several medical specialties; not all internists are experts at pelvic examination, and gynecologists may not be best trained to handle nonpelvic complaints. Many women describe frightening health care experiences during which the not uncommon problem of lower abdominal symptoms caused them to be shunted between care providers. Consultation-liaison psychiatrists can reinforce the need for patient education and improve obstetrician/gynecologists' empathy and communication. Communication barriers can lead not only to avoidance but also to clashes between patient and doctor. Psychiatric consultation may be requested when the obstetrician/gynecologist and the patient cannot agree on a course of action (Stotland and Garrick 1990).

CLINICAL PRESENTATIONS

The belief that female reproductive events are associated with psychopathology is related to the designation of specific nosological entities specific to women, including postpartum depression, postpartum psychosis, premenstrual syndrome, and involutional melancholia. These complaints can present to either mental health or obstetrician/gynecologist practitioners. Some disorders, such as pseudocyesis and hyperemesis gravidarum, are unique to the obstetrics and gynecology setting.

Research in these areas is fraught with methodological problems. Inequities in access to care result in difficulty in obtaining representative, heterogeneous population samples. Discontinuities in care and in record keeping make it very difficult to track responses to episodic reproductive events and interventions. Patients may receive only perfunctory care after a brief hospitalization for surgery or delivery.

Like most requests for psychiatric consultation, those generated by obstetrician/gynecologists are usually precipitated by the patient's gross behavioral derangements, the patient's failure to accept or comply with medical recommendations, symptoms that are unresponsive to first-line diagnosis and treatment, medical-legal questions, or conflicts between patient and staff. In the outpatient setting, more subtle problems such as sexual dysfunction, relational difficulties, and mood disorders may be referred to a mental health practitioner (not necessar-

ily a psychiatrist). Some outpatient obstetrics and gynecology specialty clinic staffs include a mental health practitioner who provides patient screening, support, and treatment and who may conduct or assist in research. The consulting psychiatrist needs to know what mental health interventions have already been undertaken and to discuss the situation with the practitioner. When an ongoing consultation and/or liaison relationship is contemplated, the psychiatrist should work with the obstetrician/gynecologist, and the mental health staff, if any, to demarcate areas of responsibility and criteria and mechanisms for referral and collaboration.

STERILITY, FERTILITY, AND INFERTILITY

Voluntary Sterilization

Female sterilization is an extremely common form of birth control in the United States and in several other countries. Psychiatric consultation related to voluntary sterilization usually involves issues of competency to consent. Some individual practitioners and/or institutions impose criteria including the patient's age and number of living children (Wilcox et al. 1991). Anxieties about "irreversible" sterilization are somewhat relieved by the increasing availability of relatively reversible procedures. However, reversibility is never guaranteed. In addition, there are questions about connections between tubal ligation and later health complications (Alderman and Gee 1989).

Barriers to voluntary sterilization often derive from the assumption that other, effective and reversible, forms of contraception are available to the patient. However, factors such as lack of knowledge and/or the presence of significant psychological, interpersonal, and medical complications can render them ineffective. Sterilization frees women from concern that an unplanned pregnancy will force them into a choice between abortion and undesired motherhood. The consultant psychiatrist should be alert to the possibility that a male partner has pressured the patient into requesting tubal ligation. Women also may accept or press for hysterectomy in order to be sterilized without articulating that purpose. This is especially true for women who belong to religious faiths that prohibit voluntary sterilization. In some situations, the possibility of conception is the only motivation for the use of condoms, which protects both partners against infection with sexually transmitted diseases.

Gynecologists often request psychiatric consultation when a patient with a major psychiatric illness requests sterilization. They may assume that a psychotic illness, per se, renders a patient incompetent to consent. The psychiatrist determines whether the patient understands the nature of, risks and benefits of, and alternatives to the procedure. However, patients who are in the throes of depression or labor may request or agree to sterilization and regret it afterward. The liaison psychiatrist can help the obstetrician/gynecologist recognize the complexities of these situations. Both psychiatrist and obstetrician/gynecologist need to be aware of their own prejudices; is it their wish that a patient be sterilized or hers?

Infertility and Infertility Treatment

Infertility is believed to affect approximately 10% of the couples in the United States (Kraft et al. 1980). Infertility is no longer thought to have an unconscious psychodynamic basis. In most cases, anatomic and physiologic etiologies are identified (Green et al. 2001). In two clinical situations, psychiatric factors play an etiological role: 1) infertility in patients with amenorrhea related to eating disorders, and 2) infertility in patients whose sexual practices (or lack of them) are responsible for the failure to conceive. Generally, psychiatric consultants now focus on helping patients with the reactions to, not the causes of, infertility.

The inability to conceive or to carry a pregnancy to term is a narcissistic injury and a profound psychosocial loss. Infertile patients complain that they do not feel like "real" men or women. Tensions arise in the relationship as members of a couple, and members of their families, may blame one partner for the problem. Discovery of an anatomic or physiologic problem may exacerbate or reverse these dynamics—or may have no effect on mistaken attribution. In some subcultures, men complain that intercourse with an infertile woman, including a woman who has had a hysterectomy, is "like putting a coin in an empty vending machine." This feeling often secondarily affects sexual behavior; patients may withdraw or may overcompensate by engaging in frenzied activity.

Men are more likely to want to keep infertility secret, and women are more likely to talk about it with friends and relatives (Myers 1990). Both women and men report that infertility is stressful; however, women are more likely to describe it as the worst life crisis they have experienced. Strain is often compounded when the partners misinterpret each other's behaviors, feeling that the other is unavailable. Office counseling can be helpful in opening lines of communication.

Media coverage of new reproductive technologies has raised expectations beyond what technologies can safely provide. Patients are uncertain about when to seek treatment and what provider to see. Care at a center offering the latest infertility treatment may necessitate repeated trips or interim geographic relocation. Infertility treatment centers are not always forthcoming about their outcomes. Treatments such as in vitro fertilization are unsuccessful more often than not. Diagnosis and treatment are extremely expensive, intense, and intrusive. Sexual intercourse must be performed according to a prescribed regimen, the menstrual cycle and ovulation are manipulated with exogenous hormones, ova are surgically retrieved from women after intense hormonal stimulation, semen must be produced from men by masturbation, and gametes and embryos are obtained from individuals outside the couple.

At times, the infertile patient may experience the world as being filled with pregnant women and happy parents. Awareness of women who undergo elective abortions or become unwilling, unloving, or incapable parents is particularly galling. Exposure to others' infants may provoke jealousy and rage, emotions that, in turn, provoke guilt and make previously enjoyable gatherings of friends and family painful. The couple must decide how much time, energy, emotion, and money to expend before discontinuing efforts to achieve biological parenthood.

The consultation-liaison psychiatrist may assist the infertility team in dealing with patients—or staff members—who are unwilling to discontinue treatments despite repeated failures.

Brief bedside or office counseling can enhance patients' abilities to communicate with and use their own sources of psychosocial support; support groups are particularly helpful (Stewart 1992). It should be noted that patients whose infertility is secondary to ablative treatment for malignancy or other medical disorders cannot regain their fertility through treatment. Their loss of fertility may not be attended to during the acute stages of diagnosis and lifesaving treatment; in fact, they may be implicitly or explicitly criticized for any concern about it "when your life is at stake," but it must be mourned.

Unmarried heterosexual women and lesbians face additional frustrations because of the powerful social constraints, varying from subculture to subculture, on their reproduction. The quest for parenthood may entail the establishment of new family constellations. Mothers may gestate embryos for their daughters, women may gestate pregnancies and donate ova for unrelated couples, and some divorcing couples fight for "custody" of frozen embryos. Mental health professionals are sometimes consulted and asked to serve as gatekeepers in the context of these risky and unorthodox avenues to parenthood. Unfortunately, very little scientific literature is available to guide consultations; criteria for the identification of candidates at risk are not available, and long-term studies are rare. Until more information is available, common sense would indicate that the consultant should determine whether the patient has any condition interfering with her ability to make an informed decision, facilitate access to all relevant information, and help the patient to review her options, values, and circumstances.

ABORTION

There is no evidence that most women who make decisions about and who undergo induced abortion—including those under the age of majority—need psychiatric services or experience adverse psychiatric sequelae (Russo and Zierk 1992; Stotland 1992). Nevertheless, both counseling and psychiatric referral should be available, and women should be offered sufficient information to give informed consent. A woman may experience a sense of loss despite the fact that an abortion is her informed choice. Women who experience paralyzing ambivalence, are subjected to outside pressure, have a history of and/or experience ongoing psychiatric disorders, or have abortions because of genetic or other medical indications are at increased risk for postabortion psychiatric illness (Blumenthal 1991; Major et al. 2000). That is not to say that the abortion itself caused the illness, and, in fact, the incidence of psychiatric sequelae is 8–10 times higher after term delivery than after first-trimester abortion.

Second-trimester abortion is associated with increased psychiatric risk as well because abortion is generally delayed because of ignorance, family and social chaos, and poverty. Preabortion consultation, in addition to the assurance of informed consent and the evaluation of psychiatric vulnerability, should assist the patient in reviewing the faith and values with which she was raised and those she currently considers her own. Additional consultation questions include her current life circumstances and her most realistic estimation of what her feelings and circumstances would be 3 months, 6 months, 1 year, and 5 years from now if she has the baby and if she terminates the pregnancy.

It is normal for women to experience a wide range of feelings after having an abortion: transient guilt and sadness, anger at the man involved, and, most often, relief. Sadness should not be confused with clinical depression. When there is an ongoing relationship with the man involved, he may appreciate the opportunity for counseling as well.

PSYCHIATRIC COMPLICATIONS OF PREGNANCY

Pseudocyesis

Pseudocyesis, which was described by Hippocrates, is a condition characterized by a nonpregnant woman's conviction that she is pregnant, with signs and symptoms of pregnancy, including nausea and vomiting, increasing abdominal girth, amenorrhea, and objective changes in the appearance of the breasts and cervix. There are no other associated delusions or hallucinations and no single characteristic psychiatric diagnosis or patient population. Findings are consistent, in some cases, with the persistence of a corpus luteum, as in pregnancy (i.e., gonadotropin, luteinizing hormone, and prolactin levels may be elevated). Unconscious psychodynamic factors may play a role as well. The obstetrics staff and psychiatric consultant must empathically share with the patient the negative results of pregnancy tests and ultrasound examinations; abrupt confrontations may simply lead her to seek care elsewhere (Whelan and Stewart 1990).

Hyperemesis Gravidarum

The older psychoanalytic literature is replete with references to the nausea and vomiting of pregnancy as manifestations of ambivalence about motherhood. In the absence of methodologically adequate, prospective studies, it is difficult to know whether negative feelings about pregnancy cause nausea and vomiting or vice versa. Vomiting associated with electrolyte changes and inability to maintain adequate hydration and nutrition is characterized as *hyperemesis* and may require hospitalization and parenteral administration of fluids and electrolytes. It is now believed that neurohormonal and emotional factors are involved and interrelated in this condition. Supportive psychotherapy, relaxation techniques, and symptomatic treatment of somatic deficits usually are helpful (Cohen and Rosenbaum 1998; Hod et al. 1994).

Noncompliance With Obstetric Advice

Complicated pregnancies can pose substantial maternal risks, which patients misunderstand or deny. Their decisions or behavior may seem bizarre or self-destructive to care providers. It is emotionally and medically difficult to provide care for a woman whose behavior may threaten the well-being of her fetus. The clinician is sometimes tempted to coerce a patient into interventions on these grounds. In one well-publicized case, a woman dying of a malignancy was forced to undergo a cesarean delivery, prior to term and against her will. She and the premature infant soon died. Obstetrics services may try to pressure the psychiatric consultant to hospitalize patients involuntarily on fetal, rather than maternal, grounds. The right of an individual to refuse a procedure necessary to the health or even life of another has been upheld in court.

Professional specialty organizations, including the American College of Obstetricians and Gynecologists and the American Psychiatric Association, have developed carefully reasoned positions addressing conflicts between fetal and maternal rights in the medical care setting. Both organizations advise practitioners that a woman's autonomy must not be violated because she is pregnant (Brown et al. 1991). In more than one state, women have been incarcerated and criminally charged for their use of illicit substances during pregnancy. The American Psychiatric Association has adopted an official position urging therapeutic, rather than punitive, approaches to substance abuse during pregnancy. The punitive approach seems particularly misguided as social policy because more patients are interested in treatment than there are treatment programs to accommodate them, and punitive responses have been shown to decrease women's likelihood of seeking prenatal care. Psychiatric consultants may be called in as enforcers rather than as diagnosticians and therapists.

Morbid Anxieties Associated With Pregnancy

Given the tendency of contemporary middle- and upper-class Western society to overvalue thinness in women, it is not surprising that some women fear the bodily expansion of pregnancy. Taken to an extreme, this fear can interfere with a woman's ingestion of a nourishing diet. Patients with a history of or with current eating disorders are at higher risk for this complication. Patients with severe anxiety may require psychotherapy or treatment for an eating disorder, including hospitalization, if normal weight gain cannot be achieved.

Noncompliance or paralyzing anxiety during pregnancy also can result from a morbid fear of the process of childbirth. Although childbirth preparation courses are useful in reducing the fear of helplessness through active mastery (Walcher 1992), the realities of labor and delivery may precipitate acute anxiety in the vulnerable patient. Traumatic medical or obstetric experiences in the past often play a role. Relaxation techniques and hypnosis are helpful. Childbirth preparation courses have actually been shown to result in a decrease in obstetric morbidity.

Acute Psychiatric Decompensation in the Gravid Patient

Psychiatric histories are seldom elicited in the obstetrics and gynecology setting. Psychiatric syndromes often "erupt" as emergencies—pregnant patients stab themselves in the abdomen, patients in labor become psychotic and combative, or mothers are unable to assume the care of their newborns. Problems are sometimes exacerbated by the tendency of obstetricians to discontinue psychotropic medications—without psychiatric consultation or the use of alternative means of management—for fear of teratogenicity.

A consultation-liaison psychiatrist can avert many such disasters by convincing obstetrics and gynecology staff to include in the initial workup a brief series of psychiatric screening questions: Have you or a member of your family ever seen a psychiatrist? Taken medications for your emotions or thinking? The possibility of identifying a problem without the resources to manage it discourages practitioners from asking the questions; therefore, they must be aware of mental health resources (Miller and Finnerty 1996).

Decisions about the use of psychoactive medications during pregnancy (see Table 31–2) must be made in consultation with the patient, and her partner, should she wish to include him or her. The risks of medication and the untreated psychiatric illness are weighed against the benefits of treatment. Psychotic, mood, and anxiety disorders themselves have significant effects on fetal development and obstetric outcome (Chang and Renshaw 1986); they influence maternal nutrition, sleep, circulation, substance abuse, adherence to medical advice, exercise, and other physiologic and behavioral parameters (Apfel and Handel 1993).

The debacle with thalidomide, which left thousands of children with grossly deformed limbs, terrified physicians and patients. To protect fetuses and neonates, new medications were not tested on lactating or pregnant women or women who might become pregnant, causing a major gap in knowledge about the use of drugs in all women of childbearing age.

However, many women took psychotropic medications before realizing that they were pregnant or decided not to discontinue them because of the severity of their psychiatric symptoms. Over the last 10 years, observational studies of these patients have provided a great deal of reassuring evidence. Carbamazepine can cause neural tube defects, and lithium can cause Ebstein's anomaly, although the latter effect is very rare and can be detected by cardiac ultrasound before viability. Diazepam was thought at one time to cause cleft palate. Although

Table 31–2.   Psychotropic drug use in pregnancy: risks of selected agents

Agent	FDA risk factor	Comments
Antidepressants		
Lithium	D	Suspected teratogen in first trimester, especially cardiovascular abnormalities, including Ebstein's anomaly
		Self-limited toxicity in newborn
		Avoid during first trimester, near term
		Contraindicated during lactation
Fluoxetine	ND	?Increased risk of miscarriage
		No reported risk of major malformations
Amitriptyline	D	No reported teratogenicity
		?Withdrawal in neonate
		Avoid in first trimester
Imipramine	D	Few rare malformations reported
		Neonate withdrawal
		Avoid in first trimester
Clomipramine	D	Neonatal toxic morbidity
Phenelzine (MAOI)	C	Increased risk of malformations
		Avoid in pregnancy because of possibility of hypertensive crises
Neuroleptics		
Chlorpromazine (phenothiazine)	C	No conclusive evidence of teratogenicity
		Avoid during labor; possible hypotension
		Avoid near term; neonatal withdrawal
		Safe if used occasionally in small doses
		Not recommended in first trimester
Haloperidol (butyrophenone)	C	Reported use without negative effects
Sedative-hypnotics		
Diazepam (benzodiazepine)	D	May be teratogenic; two major syndromes
		1. Floppy baby syndrome (hypotonia, lethargy, sucking difficulties)
		2. Withdrawal syndrome (tremors, irritability, vigorous sucking, hypertonicity)
		Not recommended during lactation

Note.   MAOI = monoamine oxidase inhibitor; ND = not designated.
FDA risk factors (A, B, C, D, X) are assigned by the U.S. Food and Drug Administration (FDA) to all drugs based on the risks posed to a fetus.
Category C indicates that animal studies show an adverse effect on the fetus or that no studies in animals or women are available. Drug should only be used if potential benefit justifies the potential risk to the fetus.
Category D indicates that there is evidence of human risk, but the benefits may be worth the risk in some situations.
Source.   Briggs et al. 1990; Mortola 1989; Pastuszak et al. 1993.

cohort and case-control studies have not confirmed this finding, administration near term may lead to a withdrawal syndrome or cardiorespiratory instability in the infant after birth. The tricyclic antidepressants, older selective serotonin reuptake inhibitors, and antipsychotics have not been associated with risks to the fetus or newborn. Confounding variables in long-term studies and the lack of prospective, randomized, double-blind studies mean that we cannot be completely confident that there are no subtle sequelae, but it is fairly clear that there are no gross effects. This is especially reassuring because many women taking psychotropic medications do not realize that they are pregnant until the crucial early weeks of embryogenesis are over.

Some patients or their physicians may insist on continuing or discontinuing medication; most will prefer a plan that combines a minimum of medication with an enhancement of other treatment modalities, including careful attention by family members, frequent outpatient visits, and hospitalization if necessary. Another compromise is to taper medication as delivery is anticipated and to begin again immediately afterward. A 1998 review in the *New England Journal of Medicine* (Koren et al. 1998) listed the tricyclic antidepressants, fluoxetine, lithium (with the caveat above), chlorpromazine, and haloperidol as drugs that can be used safely during pregnancy.

Patients who decompensate during labor often have received no prenatal care, or the prenatal record contains no information about mental status and psychiatric history. Table 31–3 contains guidelines for psychiatric consultation during labor. The patient's fear and perception of pain may be intensified by a cognitive or sensory limitation such as mental retardation or deafness or by a personality disorder associated with impulsivity, dependence, entitlement, and/or rage. The patient may not understand or speak English. She or a woman close to her may have experienced a traumatic birth experience in the past. Some patients misinterpret the powerful sensations of normal labor as symptoms of serious complications, or they overhear and misinterpret discussions about themselves or other patients. Even under the stress of labor, it is usually possible to "reach" and calm a patient by looking at her directly; speaking calmly, softly, confidently, and reassuringly; asking what she is upset about; offering information; and making meaningful concessions to her preferences.

The Unacknowledged Pregnancy

The consulting psychiatrist is occasionally called to see women who present in labor, or who deliver outside the hospital, without themselves or their families having recognized that they were pregnant. No single psychiatric diagnosis explains this phenomenon (Spielvogel and Hohener 1995). Some patients are psychotic, but others are perimenopausal women who "didn't think I could get pregnant" and adolescents perhaps so overwhelmed by the difficulties posed by a pregnancy that they deny it altogether, as do their families. In some such cases, the young woman kills the newborn. If she delivers in the bathroom, having mistaken her labor contractions for an urge to defecate, she may drown the neonate; if not, she may discard it in the trash. The response of the system tends to be quite punitive, and the police generally arrive before the psychiatrist. Psychiatric follow-up is uncommon.

ADOLESCENT PREGNANCY

Approximately 10% of the women in the United States conceive during their high school years (Children's Defense Fund 1988; Hayes 1987). This is the highest frequency of adolescent pregnancy in the developed world. Although in some other societies, pregnancy in adolescents is normative and supported, in the United States, it demands psychological and material resources that the environment seldom provides. The most effective preventive interventions are school health clinics that include gynecological and contraceptive care and programs that provide information and teach assertiveness techniques. Few adolescents have access to such programs,

TABLE 31–3. Keys to psychiatric consultation during labor

1. Determine the patient's premorbid level of intelligence, psychological health, and psychosocial functioning.
2. Observe the interaction between the patient and staff.
   Is the patient being left alone, physically or psychologically?
   Are others focused only on monitoring devices?
   Has the patient's behavior provoked irritation in staff?
   Have the patient's coping mechanisms been overwhelmed?
3. Evaluate for signs and symptoms of acute intoxication or withdrawal from psychoactive substances.
4. Help the patient to focus on one calm, consistent care provider.
   Stand or sit in the direct line of vision of the patient.
   Hold the patient's hand, if indicated.
   Speak using a soft, soothing cadence.
   Ask her to state what is bothering her and what help she needs.
   Perform a simple, formal mental status examination if the patient does not seem to understand.
5. Ascertain from the obstetrics staff the stage of labor, complications, treatment plan, and prognosis.
   Make sure the patient understands this information.

and few use contraceptives regularly before the first conception. School-based child care programs also have been highly successful in reducing the rate of subsequent pregnancies and increasing the rate of high school graduation. Both of these factors are extremely important in determining the socioeconomic fate of the adolescent mother and her children (Maynard 1997).

In all states, pregnant minors may obtain obstetric care and make decisions about that care without parental notification or consent. This is not true for decisions to terminate pregnancies; those laws vary from state to state and over time. Decisions should be informed by knowledge about the risks of pregnancy in adolescence. The consultation-liaison psychiatrist who sees a young pregnant woman should work with her to decide how to proceed and whether it is in her best interest to involve her parents or guardian. Often, the parents will respond more constructively than the patient had anticipated, but sometimes she appropriately fears abuse or exile from the family home. Approximately half of all adolescent pregnancies end in spontaneous or therapeutic abortion, 45% result in the birth of a child that the mother will raise, and 5% result in the birth of a child who is adopted out (Hayes 1987).

THE POSTPARTUM PATIENT

Psychiatric treatment in the critical peripartum period can have a significant effect on mother-child attachment, behavior, and outcome. Mothers who have experienced medical or obstetric complications are at increased risk for postpartum psychiatric sequelae. The medical problems may have separated the mother from her newborn. These mothers may fear that irreparable psychic damage has been done. They can be reassured that healthy, strong mother-child relationships can flourish even under these circumstances.

Current medical practices complicate the identification and treatment of postpartum disorders. Obstetricians practice in groups, lessening the opportunity for any one of them to become familiar with a patient and for a patient to get to know her doctor. Hospital stays are minimal, and postpartum checkups can be somewhat perfunctory. Medical staff, family, and friends tend to dismiss postpartum sleeplessness, loss of energy, and loss of appetite as normal and often exacerbate the mother's guilt by reminding her that she is lucky to have a healthy baby.

Up to 80% of postpartum women develop a mild, self-limited mood disturbance often called "baby blues" (Bagedahl-Strindlund 1992; Rosenthal and O'Grady 1992). Tearfulness, emotional lability, and anxiety begin approximately 3 days postpartum and usually abate by the seventh day. No hormonal risk marker or effective hormonal treatment has been identified (Hendrick et al. 1998).

Approximately 10% of parturients experience a major depressive episode during the postpartum period (Apfel and Handel 1993). Opinions differ as to whether postpartum psychiatric illness is a distinct entity (Hamilton 1992). Women with premenstrual dysphoric disorder or previous depressions and especially women with previous postpartum depressions are at considerably increased risk for postpartum depression. Hormonal and psychosocial stresses of the puerperium play an etiological role, and patients' symptoms often center on maternal concerns and affect maternal functions (Miller 2000).

Treatment of postpartum depression does not differ in substance from the treatment of any other depression, except that the decision to use antidepressant medication and the choice among medications may be affected by breast-feeding. Evidence to date indicates that the more established selective serotonin reuptake inhibitors reach breast milk in very small concentrations; no adverse outcomes have been noted (Gelenberg 1997; Llewellyn and Stowe 1998; Wisner et al. 1996). Still, there may be unknown risks, and parents should be aware of this when making their decisions. Mild to moderate cases can be primarily approached psychotherapeutically. For some women, a recommendation to forgo breast-feeding is so upsetting as to exacerbate the depression. Untreated maternal depression represents a risk to the infant. Acute maternal psychosis, especially with hostile or fearful delusions about the infant, is a medical emergency. Infanticide is a real possibility. No significant deleterious effects of maternal antipsychotics or anxiolytics on the nursing infant have been noted.

PREGNANCY LOSS

Women may have complicated grief after complex and/or operative deliveries, the birth of a child with a congenital defect, or the death of an embryo, a fetus, or a newborn. Emphasis on the quality of the childbirth experience may leave some mothers—those whose conditions required significant, unanticipated interventions—with grief over the "natural childbirth" experiences they did not have. Postpartum grief is sometimes complicated by a sense that the woman's body did not function normally or by rage at the infant for causing emotional and physical suffering. The delivery of a defective, dead, or dying child, at any gestational age, also precipitates feelings of disgust, failure, guilt, and shame (Leon 1995).

The support offered by health care providers at the time of a perinatal death is a key factor in helping the mother and father adjust to the loss (Benfield et al. 1978; Knapp and Peppers 1979; Murray and Callan 1988). A physician may complicate the emotional situation by asking questions about family history and prenatal behaviors, compounding the patient's sense of responsibility. Unless this information is vital to the care of a sick infant, it can be sought at a later date. Care providers, particularly obstetricians, may feel responsible and unsure how to behave with the disappointed parents. The obstetrician and the consulting psychiatrist can review the events of the delivery with the family to absorb the family's emotional responses without defensiveness and to elicit the patient's preferences: Does she wish to be left alone, to have visitors and family excluded, or to have someone with her? Would she like to see a member of the clergy and to make funeral arrangements? Religious patients are sometimes upset by their own rage at God and are reassured to hear that God understands and accepts their anger (Zeanah et al. 1995).

Parents and grandparents should be allowed and even encouraged to see and hold a dead or dying baby. The infant can be draped in such a way as to emphasize its most normal features, and the parents may unwrap the infant if they wish. A knowledgeable professional should be present at all times to explain the physical findings and to point out areas of normalcy but not to intrude on the family's own assimilation of the event. Parents find that holding and speaking to their baby, even one who is dead, fulfills some of their sense of parental obligation. If they do not do so, they may feel that they have abandoned their child. They can be reminded that their prenatal preparations, which they may feel were in vain, represented their parenting of the lost child. Photographs of the infant, dressed and undressed, should be taken and made available. Counseling at the time of the loss and at intervals of 6 weeks, 6 months, and 1 year later enhances communication and recovery and facilitates the identification of psychological complications.

Parents of a "defective" child must grieve the perfect child they had hoped for and must live with and constantly be reminded of their "reproductive failure," however minor or major. The degree of distress this imposes depends on their religion, their financial and social resources, their personal coping skills, their relationships, and the nature of the child's defect and treatment.

CUSTODY ISSUES

Postpartum psychiatric consultations are frequently sought when a patient's history or behavior raises questions about her ability to provide adequate care for the newborn. Quality foster care is in short supply in most areas of the United States and is likely to disrupt the child's attachment to parental figures (American Academy of Pediatrics, Committee on Early Childhood, Adoption, and Dependent Care 1993). For these reasons, the psychiatric consultant must make every effort to enlist resources to enhance maternal confidence, competence, and investment. The existence of a psychiatric disorder, even a severe one, does not in and of itself preclude adequate mothering.

In addition to the standard psychiatric history and mental status examination, the consultation must focus on an assessment of the patient's ability to recognize her newborn's needs and provide for them. Unless there is evidence of immediate danger to the child, mother-child interaction in the hospital should be maximized, closely observed, and carefully documented by the obstetrics and pediatric nursing staff as well as by the psychiatrist (Jacobsen et al. 1997). If the mother seems to provide adequate care, every effort should be made to mobilize social, psychiatric, and medical support for the mother-infant dyad after discharge. The psychiatric consultant may recommend care by a visiting nurse, general household helper, or mobile psychiatric treatment team and may advise the gynecologist and pediatrician about parameters to be assessed on outpatient visits. In the event that the mother's verbal statements or behavior consti-

tutes a threat to the child's safety, the psychiatrist is required to advocate forcefully for the removal of custody. Hospitals have legal authority to assume protective custody in cases of suspected child abuse.

OTHER REASONS FOR CONSULTATION

Psychiatrists are probably not called often enough to the acute care setting by obstetrician/gynecologists; unless a patient manifests grossly disturbed behavior, the demands of the emergency situation distract clinicians' attention from the psychiatric issues. A patient's allusion to suicide is sometimes the only cue for an emergency psychiatric referral; no further exploration is usually attempted. For example, a woman in her late teens delivered her second child and was informed that the new baby, like her first, had a genetic defect that invariably results in demise within the first months of life. Deeply grieved, but not suicidal, she responded by saying "I wish I were dead." The psychiatrist, urgently summoned, had to assess the patient's suicidal intent before she was able to help the patient and family cope with their tragedy.

RAPE AND DOMESTIC VIOLENCE

Many cases of victimization, rape, abuse, and violence appear in the outpatient or emergency room setting. Consultation-liaison psychiatrists can play a vital liaison function in this setting. Until very recently, the care that rape victims received exacerbated their psychological injuries; many were disbelieved, interrogated, and overexamined. Data indicate that relatively few unfounded accusations of rape are made (Hursch 1977). The risk of false accusation, although real, is far less than the risk of retraumatizing the victims by insinuating that the accusation is unfounded.

Many health care settings now have improved systems for dealing with rape. These approaches may include a trained patient advocate who accompanies the patient (if she wishes) throughout the procedures, regardless of the time of day or night. The advocate is available to the patient afterward, and referral for professional counseling is made if necessary. The advocate helps the patient to understand the examination process; medical care must include the systematic gathering of forensic information such as samples of fluids present in the genitalia, pubic hairs of victim and assailant, and documentation of injuries. The process, even if sensitively carried out, is unpleasant to the traumatized patient but is vital to the subsequent identification and prosecution of the perpetrator. Screening for infection with human immunodeficiency virus (HIV) and other sexually transmitted diseases is also a painful reminder of the terrifying possible infectious sequelae of the assault.

Care providers' misconceptions and insensitivities are related to the widespread lack of knowledge about the typical behavior of assault victims. Emotional shock and desperate attempts at self-control, such as the patient's reluctance to undergo examination, are sometimes misinterpreted as evidence that no trauma took place. Medical and law enforcement professionals may be visibly annoyed by the loss of evidence when victims bathe, douche, or destroy clothing and other objects bearing stigmata of the assault. Victims' tendency to blame themselves—for past sexual behavior, for being "in the wrong place at the wrong time," for failing to take safety precautions, for allowing themselves to be alone with the perpetrator—is synergistic with some care providers' denial and tendency to believe that the victim "asked for it." All of these factors may conspire to distort the historical evidence and to compound the adverse psychiatric sequelae.

Rape victims are at significant risk for leading constricted, isolated lives. Psychotherapy can forestall severe complications (Rose 1993). All female patients seen by consultation-liaison psychiatrists should be sensitively queried about the history of sexual abuse/rape. The history may not emerge until weeks, months, or even years of therapy have enabled the patient to trust the therapist. That is not possible in systems in which the length of treatment is drastically curtailed.

Victims of sexual, psychological, and/or physical abuse may present in the acute care setting with symptoms of pelvic inflammatory disease, other gynecological infections, or seemingly unrelated injuries. There may also be vague somatic complaints, often involving headaches or gastrointestinal or gynecological dysfunction. Most often, abusers severely limit victims' social contacts. The medical care setting is often one of the few outside contacts allowed. Several studies have found that emergency care providers frequently fail to ask about domestic violence (Kurz and Stark 1988; Warshaw 1989). Some may accept proffered explanations for injuries, no matter how unlikely. Lacerations are stitched, bones are set, and the patient is sent back to the abusive environment, which puts her at significant risk for further injury and even death. Of particular importance in the obstetrics setting is the counterintuitive fact that the incidence of domestic violence increases during pregnancy.

The consultation-liaison psychiatrist must work with the obstetrics and gynecology staff to ensure that all patients, and especially those who present with injuries of dubious origin, are interviewed in privacy—away from the partner suspected of abuse, who typically hovers as close as possible—by an empathic care provider who asks specifically about violence and offers information about shelters and other resources for battered women. Medical staff ought not confront the abuser because this significantly increases the risk to the patient. The past medical record should be obtained, and current injuries and statements should be carefully documented; photographs of wounds may be helpful at a later date, such as when the abuser attempts to gain custody of children. Many such women frustrate care providers by denying the violence and refusing the help at first, although they are able to free themselves from the abusive situation at a later date. The interest and information provided can be lifesaving (Resnick et al. 2000).

HIV/AIDS AND OTHER SEXUALLY TRANSMITTED DISEASES

Aside from their implications in the emergency setting, HIV and other sexually transmitted diseases may occasion psychiatric consultation because of the anxiety they engender. Most of the early and ongoing research into the transmission, prevention, and treatment of HIV infection and acquired immunodeficiency syndrome (AIDS) concerned homosexual men and intravenous substance abusers. Although women constitute the fastest-growing group with HIV infection, relatively little is known about the differential manifestations and natural courses between the sexes. Current data show that women, in general, die sooner after diagnosis than do men (American College of Obstetricians and Gynecologists 1992; Mocroft et al. 1996). This may be accounted for by the fact that women tend to be diagnosed later in the course of illness, have decreased access to antiviral therapy, are older at the time of infection, or have other concurrent risk factors (Lemp et al. 1992). Gynecological presentations have recently been added to the definition of AIDS but are frequently unrecognized. AIDS, and to a lesser extent pre-AIDS HIV infection, may also present with neuropsychiatric symptoms.

Because women with HIV infection are at risk for transmitting the virus to their unborn children, they are sometimes treated as vectors rather than as patients. This discourages some women from seeking prenatal care that would greatly benefit them and their unborn children.

Society's efforts to discourage HIV-infected men and women from childbearing may conflict with their psychological need to enjoy the normal pleasures of parenthood and to produce offspring who will survive after they are gone. However, pregnant women infected with HIV are often impoverished and abused and may find it difficult to obtain birth control or abortion services when they desire them (Laurence 1999). Consultation-liaison psychiatrists can work, or prepare others to work, with HIV-infected women and their partners who are faced with decisions about fertility under these especially difficult conditions. Patients and care providers, including the consultation-liaison psychiatrist, may experience feelings of rage, resentment, longing, and despair precipitated by the ravages of HIV disease.

Transmission of HIV infection to women generally occurs through the sharing of intravenous needles and through heterosexual contact with bisexual and/or intravenous substance–abusing men. Although clean needles and condoms can help to prevent physical transmission, their use presupposes not only knowledge but also access and psychological assertiveness, which many susceptible women lack. The woman who is addicted to crack cocaine frequently resorts to prostitution to support herself and her habit and is in no position to demand the use of condoms by her drug-supplying sexual partners. It is equally frustrating to discover that many women who are well educated, well informed, and well off find themselves unable to insist that their sexual partners use condoms. When appropriate to the clinical situation, it is incumbent on the practicing consultation-liaison psychiatrist to ask sexually active female patients about their means of contraception and protection from sexually transmitted diseases and to work with them to develop understanding and mastery of any reluctance to protect themselves.

GYNECOLOGICAL ONCOLOGY

Gynecological neoplasms range in lethality and incidence from the common, benign myomata of the uterus to rare teratomas and ovarian carcinomas. Patients react with the usual responses to cancer: fear, denial, anger, shame, and mustering of social supports and psychological coping skills. Neoplasms of the reproductive organs provoke guilt and shame about past sexual behavior and about current sexual and reproductive dysfunction. Ignorance and uncertainty compound decisions about treatments such as ablative surgery. Medical inattention to the psychological significance of individual organs is reflected in the use of terms such as *total hysterectomy;* the fact that the ovaries and fallopian tubes are also removed is not always clear to patients.

Gynecological cancer treatment is complicated by a sense of mutilation and loss of gender identity. Sexual dysfunction is common and should be inquired about because patients may be reluctant to complain about it. Involvement of the sexual partner in counseling is advised; often, patients are surprised at their partners' understanding and generosity, especially as enhanced by their access to accurate information and support. They must be reassured that cancer is not contagious and taught alternative sexual skills for the recovery period (Schover 1997).

EATING DISORDERS

Patients with a history of eating disorders may present in the obstetrics and gynecology setting, either because the obstetrician/gynecologist is their primary physician or because the eating disorder affects the reproductive system. A classic presentation is the amenorrheic patient in the gynecological endocrinology/infertility clinic. Of course, most patients in the acute phases of anorexia and bulimia deny that they are ill. Given the societal pressures on women to become and remain slim, even physicians may fail to notice that patients are wasting away until the situation becomes emergent. It is important to include eating disorders in liaison case conferences and grand rounds. As with other conditions, obstetrician/gynecologists particularly want to know what questions should be included on standard diagnostic screening and when and how to refer a patient to a psychiatrist.

CONCLUSION

Psychiatric consultation and liaison with obstetrics and gynecology encompasses a fascinating array of ethical, scientific, educational, and clinical challenges. Issues literally range from birth to death. The central psychological significance of sexuality and reproduction heightens the emotional response of every aspect of gynecological and obstetric care. Several allied organizations and publications can serve as resources to the consultant, consultee, and patient. Obstetrician/gynecologists learn and practice under extreme pressures of time, legal liability, and impending medical emergency, in addition to the psychological demands of their patients. Consultation-liaison psychiatrists, who are knowledgeable about the medical and psychological aspects of obstetrics and gynecology and empathic to the situations of both the obstetrician/gynecologist and the patient, can forestall crises, relieve suffering and disability, and enhance the health of future generations.

REFERENCES

Alderman PM, Gee EM: Sterilization: Canadian choices. Can Med Assoc J 140:645–649, 1989

American Academy of Pediatrics, Committee on Early Childhood, Adoption, and Dependent Care: Developmental issues in foster care for children. Pediatrics 91:1007–1009, 1993

American College of Obstetricians and Gynecologists: Professional Liability Insurance and Its Effects: Report of a Survey of ACOG's Membership. Washington, DC, American College of Obstetricians and Gynecologists, 1985

American College of Obstetricians and Gynecologists: Issues in Women's Health: Media Kit. Washington, DC, American College of Obstetricians and Gynecologists, 1992

Apfel RJ, Handel MH: Madness and Loss of Motherhood: Sexuality, Reproduction, and Long-Term Mental Illness. Washington, DC, American Psychiatric Press, 1993

Apfel RJ, Palmund I: Medical advertising images of menopausal women. Paper presented at the 10th International Congress of Psychosomatic Obstetrics and Gynecology, Stockholm, Sweden, June 1992

Bagedahl-Strindlund M: Postpartum mental illness: cross-cultural and social anthropological aspects—a review, in Reproductive Life: Advances in Research in Psychosomatic Obstetrics and Gynecology. Edited by Wijma K, von Schoultz B. Park Ridge, NJ, Parthenon Publishers, 1992, pp 121–140

Benfield DG, Leib SA, Vollman JH: Grief response of parents and parental participation in deciding care. Pediatrics 62:171–177, 1978

Blumenthal SJ: Psychiatric consequences of abortion: overview of research findings, in Psychiatric Aspects of Abortion. Edited by Stotland NL. Washington, DC, American Psychiatric Press, 1991, pp 17–37

Briggs GG, Freeman RK, Yaffe SJ: Drugs in Pregnancy and Lactation: A Reference Guide to Fetal and Neonatal Risk, 3rd Edition. Baltimore, MD, Williams & Wilkins, 1990

Brown D, Andersen HF, Elkins TF: An analysis of the ACOG and AAP ethics statements on conflicts in maternal-fetal care. J Clin Ethics 2:19–24, 1991

Carlson KJ, Miller BA, Fowler FJ Jr, et al: The Maine Women's Health Study, 1: outcomes of hysterectomy. Obstet Gynecol 83:556–565, 1994

Chang S, Renshaw D: Psychosis and pregnancy. Compr Ther 12:36–41, 1986

Children's Defense Fund: Teenage Pregnancy: Advocate's Guide to the Numbers. Washington, DC, Children's Defense Fund, 1988

Chodorow NJ: Feminism and Psychoanalytic Theory. New Haven, CT, Yale University Press, 1989

Ciotti MC: Screening for gynecologic and colorectal cancer: is it adequate? Womens Health Issues 2(2):83–93, 1992

Cohen LS, Rosenbaum JF: Psychotropic drug use during pregnancy: weighing the risks. J Clin Psychiatry 59 (suppl 2):18–28, 1998

Cotton P: Women's health initiative leads way as research begins to fill gender gaps. JAMA Medical News and Perspectives 267:469–473, 1992a

Cotton P: Women scientists explore more ways to smash through the "glass ceiling." JAMA Medical News and Perspectives 268:173, 1992b

Droegemueller W, Herbst AL, Mishell DR Jr, et al: Comprehensive Gynecology. St. Louis, MO, CV Mosby, 1987

Eveleth P, Tanner J: Worldwide Variation in Human Growth. New York, Cambridge University Press, 1976

Freud S: Female sexuality (1931), in The Standard Edition of the Complete Psychological Works of Sigmund Freud, Vol 21. Translated and edited by Strachey J. London, England, Hogarth Press, 1961, pp 57–79

Furstenberg FF, Brooks-Gunn J, Morgan SP: Adolescent Mothers in Later Life. New York, Cambridge University Press, 1987

Gelenberg AJ: Antidepressants during pregnancy and lactation. Biological Therapies in Psychiatry Newsletter 20:41–43, 1997

Green JA, Robins JC, Scheiber M, et al: Racial and economic demographics of couples seeking infertility treatment. Am J Obstet Gynecol 184:1080–1082, 2001

Hamilton JA: The issue of unique qualities, in Postpartum Psychiatric Illness: A Picture Puzzle. Edited by Hamilton JA, Harberger PN. Philadelphia, PA, University of Pennsylvania Press, 1992, pp 135–162

Hayes C: Risking the Future: Adolescent Sexuality, Pregnancy and Childbearing, Vol 1. Washington, DC, National Academy Press, 1987

Hendrick V, Altshuler LL, Suri R: Hormonal changes in the postpartum and implications for postpartum depression. Psychosomatics 39:93–101, 1998

Hod M, Orvieto R, Kaplan B, et al: Hyperemesis gravidarum: a review. J Reprod Med 39:605–612, 1994

Holte A: The search for a climacteric mood disorder: methodological problems and recent results, in Reproductive Life: Advances in Research in Psychosomatic Obstetrics and Gynecology. Edited by Wijma K, von Schoultz B. Park Ridge, NJ, Parthenon Publishers, 1992, pp 214–233

Hursch CJ: The Trouble With Rape. Chicago, IL, Nelson-Hall, 1977

Jacobsen T, Miller LJ, Kirkwood KP: Assessing parenting competency in individuals with serious mental illness: a comprehensive service. Journal of Mental Health Administration 24:189–199, 1997

Knapp RJ, Peppers LG: Doctor-patient relationships in fetal/infant death encounters. Journal of Medical Education 54:775–780, 1979

Koren G, Pastuszak A, Ito S: Drugs in pregnancy. N Engl J Med 338:1128–1137, 1998

Kraft AD, Palombo J, Mitchell D, et al: The psychological dimensions of infertility. Am J Orthopsychiatry 50:618–628, 1980

Kurz D, Stark E: Not-so-benign neglect: the medical response to battering, in Feminist Perspectives on Wife Abuse. Edited by Yllo K, Bograd M. Newbury Park, NJ, Sage, 1988, pp 54–72

Laurence J: Women and AIDS. AIDS Patient Care STDS 13:77–79, 1999

LeBlanc ES, Janowsky J, Chan BK, et al: Hormone replacement therapy and cognition: systematic review and meta-analysis. JAMA 285:1489–1499, 2001

Lemp GF, Hirozawa AM, Cohen JB, et al: Survival for women and men with AIDS. J Infect Dis 166:74–79, 1992

Leon IG: Pregnancy termination due to fetal anomaly: clinical considerations. Infant Mental Health Journal 16:112–126, 1995

Lesko LM, Stotland NL, Seagraves RT: Three cases of female anorgasmia associated with MAOIs. Am J Psychiatry 139:1353–1354, 1982

Lewis M, Volkmar FR: Clinical Aspects of Child and Adolescent Development: An Introductory Synthesis of Developmental Concepts and Clinical Experience, 3rd Edition. Philadelphia, PA, Lea & Febiger, 1990

Llewellyn A, Stowe ZN: Psychotropic medications in lactation. J Clin Psychiatry 59 (suppl 2):41–52, 1998

MacLennan A, Lester S, Moore V: Oral estrogen replacement therapy versus placebo for hot flushes: a systematic review. Climacteric 4:58–74, 2001

Major B, Cozzarelli C, Cooper ML, et al: Psychological responses of women after first-trimester abortion. Arch Gen Psychiatry 57:785–786, 2000

Matthews KA, Wing RR, Kuller LH, et al: Influences of natural menopause on psychological characteristics and symptoms of middle-aged healthy women. J Consult Clin Psychol 58:345–351, 1990

Maynard RA: The study, the context, and the findings in brief, in Kids Having Kids: Economic Costs and Social Consequences of Teen Pregnancy. Edited by Maynard RA. Washington, DC, Urban Institute Press, 1997, pp 57–71

McKinlay JB, McKinlay SM, Brambilla DJ: Health status and utilization behavior associated with menopause. Am J Epidemiol 125:110–121, 1987

Miller LJ: Postpartum Mood Disorders. Washington, DC, American Psychiatric Press, 2000

Miller LJ, Finnerty M: Sexuality, pregnancy, childbearing among women with schizophrenic-spectrum disorders. Psychiatr Serv 47:502–506, 1996

Mocroft A, Johnson MA, Phillips AN: Factors affecting survival in patients with the acquired immunodeficiency syndrome. AIDS 10:1057–1065, 1996

Mortola J: The use of psychotropic agents in pregnancy and lactation. Psychiatr Clin North Am 12:69–87, 1989

Muller C: Health Care and Gender. New York, Russell Sage Foundation, 1990

Murray J, Callan V: Predicting adjustment to perinatal death. Br J Med Psychol 61:237–244, 1988

Myers MF: Male gender-related issues in reproduction and technology, in Psychiatric Aspects of Reproductive Technology. Edited by Stotland NL. Washington, DC, American Psychiatric Press, 1990, pp 25–35

Notman MT: Gender development, in Women and Men: New Perspectives on Gender Differences. Edited by Notman MT, Nadelson CC. Washington, DC, American Psychiatric Press, 1991, pp 117–127

Pastuszak A, Schick-Boschetto B, Zuber C, et al: Pregnancy outcome following first trimester exposure to fluoxetine (Prozac). JAMA 269:2246–2248, 1993

Pilon D, Castilloux AM, LeLorier J: Estrogen replacement therapy: determinants of persistence with treatment. Obstet Gynecol 97:97–100, 2001

Resnick H, Acierno R, Holmes M, et al: Emergency evaluation and intervention with female victims of rape and other violence. J Clin Psychol 56:1317–1333, 2000

Rimer BK, King E: Why aren't older women getting mammograms and clinical breast exams? Womens Health Issues 2:94–101, 1992

Rose DS: Sexual assault, domestic violence, and incest, in Psychological Aspects of Women's Health Care: The Interface Between Psychiatry and Obstetrics and Gynecology. Edited by Stewart DE, Stotland NL. Washington, DC, American Psychiatric Press, 1993, pp 447–483

Rosenthal M, O'Grady JP: Affective and anxiety disorders, in Obstetrics: Psychological and Psychiatric Syndromes. Edited by O'Grady JP, Rosenthal M. New York, Elsevier, 1992, pp 109–138

Russo NF: Reconstructing the psychology of women: an overview, in Women and Men: New Perspectives on Gender Differences. Edited by Notman MT, Nadelson CC. Washington, DC, American Psychiatric Press, 1991, pp 43–61

Russo NF, Zierk KL: Abortion, childbearing and women's well-being. Professional Psychology, Research and Practice 23:269–280, 1992

Schover LR: Sexuality and Fertility After Cancer. New York, Wiley, 1997

Sherwin BB: Menopause: myths and realities, in Psychological Aspects of Women's Health Care: The Interface Between Psychiatry and Obstetrics and Gynecology. Edited by Stewart DE, Stotland NL. Washington, DC, American Psychiatric Press, 1993, pp 227–248

Spielvogel AM, Hohener HC: Denial of pregnancy: a review and case reports. Birth 22:220–226, 1995

Stewart DE: A prospective study of the effectiveness of brief professionally led infertility support groups, in Reproductive Life: Advances in Research in Psychosomatic Obstetrics and Gynecology. Edited by Wijma K, von Schoultz B. Park Ridge, NJ, Parthenon Publishers, 1992, pp 151–165

Stotland NL: Social change and women's reproductive health care, in Psychiatric Aspects of Reproductive Technology. Edited by Stotland NL. New York, Praeger, 1988, pp 89–104

Stotland NL: The myth of the abortion trauma syndrome (commentary). JAMA 268:2078–2079, 1992

Stotland NL, Garrick TR: Manual of Psychiatric Consultation. Washington, DC, American Psychiatric Press, 1990

Sturdee DS: The importance of patient education in improving compliance. Climacteric 3 (suppl 2):9–13, 2000

Ullrich HE: A study of change and depression among Havik Brahmin women in a south Indian village. Cult Med Psychiatry 11:261–287, 1987

Valanis BG, Bowen DJ, Bassford T, et al: Sexual orientation and health: comparisons in the women's health initiative sample. Arch Fam Med 9:843–853, 2000

Walcher W: Results of holistic childbirth preparation, in Reproductive Life: Advances in Research in Psychosomatic Obstetrics and Gynecology. Edited by Wijma K, von Schoultz B. Park Ridge, NJ, Parthenon Publishers, 1992, pp 101–119

Warshaw C: Limitations of the medical model in the care of battered women. Gender and Society 3(4):506–517, 1989

Weissberg M: The meagerness of physicians' training in emergency psychiatric intervention. Acad Med 65:747–750, 1990

Whelan CI, Stewart DE: Pseudocyesis: a review and report of six cases. Int J Psychiatry Med 20:97–108, 1990

Wilcox LS, Chu SY, Eaker ED, et al: Risk factors for regret after tubal sterilization: 5 years of follow-up in a prospective study. Fertil Steril 55:927–933, 1991

Wisner KL, Findling RL, Perel JM: Antidepressant treatment during breast-feeding. Am J Psychiatry 153:1132–1137, 1996

Zeanah CH, Danis B, Hirshberg L, et al: Initial adaptation in mothers and fathers following perinatal loss. Infant Mental Health Journal 16:80–93, 1995

32

Pediatrics

Gregory K. Fritz, M.D.

Larry K. Brown, M.D.

Child psychiatrists have worked in the pediatric arena for many years. Consultation-liaison in child psychiatry has developed as a distinct area, and at a different pace, from adult consultation-liaison psychiatry. Work (1989) reviewed the history of child consultation-liaison psychiatry in an article aptly titled, "The 'Menace of Psychiatry' Revisited: The Evolving Relationship Between Pediatrics and Child Psychiatry." His report documents how this evolutionary process was shaped by individuals in both disciplines who were concerned about the mental health of pediatric patients. As summarized in a review (Fritz 1990), input of pediatric experts into the process has been prominent from the beginning, marked early on by contributions from pediatricians such as Carouthers, Spock, and Richmond. For many years, child psychiatrists have written about conceptual issues in liaison child psychiatry (Bergman and Fritz 1985; Rothenberg 1979), the establishment and organization of child consultation-liaison services (Ahsanuddin and Adams 1982; Lewis 1978), pediatricians' use of consultation-liaison services (Froese 1976–1977; Schowalter and Lord 1971), the incidence of particular clinical disorders encountered in the pediatric setting (Sack et al. 1977; Stocking et al. 1972), interdisciplinary collaboration (Greene 1984), financial aspects of pediatric consultation work (Wright et al. 1987), and child psychiatrists' training in consultation-liaison work (Fritz and Bergman 1984).

Child psychiatrists' involvement in the medical setting is historically complicated by the fact that child psychiatry as a subspecialty grew out of the child guidance–juvenile justice system rather than evolving from pediatrics. There has, therefore, always been a degree of ambivalence on the part of many child psychiatrists about their place in consultation-liaison work, which affects the pediatricians' responses to psychiatric input. The status

of child consultation-liaison psychiatry was described in a monograph by Fritz et al. (1993), which is still a useful reference for those who seek a more complete discussion of the relevant issues.

Although sometimes consulted to evaluate pediatric patients, adult psychiatrists are generally unfamiliar with contributions and unique aspects of pediatric consultation-liaison psychiatry, at least as reflected in the articles referenced in the general psychiatry consultation-liaison literature. In fact, a considerable amount of literature and a reasonable amount of accumulated experience exist pertaining to child and adolescent consultation-liaison psychiatry. The theoretical perspectives that underlie the field and the emerging research base for pediatric consultation activities are summarized in detail elsewhere (Knapp and Harris 1998a, 1998b).

This information is important to the many general psychiatrists who find themselves in the position to provide consultation and who may even act as a liaison resource for children and adolescents in the general hospital. This situation occurs in part because of the relative scarcity of child and adolescent psychiatrists in the United States. (There are approximately 5,200 child psychiatrists, and fewer than 200 are estimated to be involved in consultation-liaison work on a full-time or part-time basis.) Furthermore, adolescents are frequently hospitalized on adult wards in general hospitals, either because of privilege limitations of physicians or because of bed availability. It is essential that the general psychiatrist who is involved in consultation work with children or adolescents not simply equate child and adolescent consultation-liaison psychiatry with the adult process. Several important differences in the characteristics of pediatric practice, the children's hospital medical system, and the process of consulting must be considered before a physician begins consulting in pediatrics. We discuss these issues in the first part of this chapter and then provide examples of content areas that are unique to the pediatric setting.

PEDIATRICS AS A SPECIALTY

In a series of studies exploring physician characteristics, Enzer and co-workers (1986) described the differences in views of childhood held by pediatricians and child psychiatrists both before and after training. Pediatricians tended to have an upbeat, optimistic attitude toward childhood; on average, they viewed it as a happy, carefree period. In contrast, child psychiatrists were more likely to see childhood as a time of struggle, powerlessness, and conflict. These attitudinal differences were present at the outset of training (suggesting that pediatricians and psychiatrists self-select by their choice of discipline) and were magnified by the end of training (suggesting that residency training reinforces the different worldviews). The optimistic, positive orientation toward childhood is associated with another important characteristic of pediatricians: the ability—and even the need—to reassure patients and families effectively in order to decrease anxiety. Reassurance is a staple of pediatric practice, one that is usually a helpful and efficient intervention. However, when reassurance is not appropriate or effective, pediatricians are considerably less comfortable in dealing with anxiety and other strong emotions than are child psychiatrists.

It is not coincidental that pediatrics and internal medicine have evolved as separate specialties—they are remarkably different from each other. Pediatrics has always emphasized a preventive, public health perspective in care, stemming from the significant positive effect of immunizations and nutritional improvement. Promoting normal development has traditionally been a primary value for most pediatricians, one which requires a greater baseline level of interest in psychosocial issues than is generally encountered among internists. For example, almost 75% of a national sample of pediatricians believed that they were adequately trained to treat psychosocial problems (Fritz and Bergman 1985). The dramatic reduction in the incidence of infectious diseases, which previously accounted for a large portion of pediatric morbidity, has resulted in a major change in pediatric practice. Addressing the "new morbidity," shorthand for psychosocial and developmental problems, is increasingly seen as a central part of general pediatric care. This trend has evolved to the point at which a new pediatric subspecialty has emerged, called *developmental and behavioral pediatrics*, with its own professional society, journal, and fellowship programs. Thus, the psychiatrist responding to a consultation request on a pediatric unit may be working in conjunction with a developmental pediatrician, who has also been called as a consultant. It is not uncommon to encounter a very sophisticated pediatric group with substantial psychosocial interest and knowledge; failure to recognize this expertise will impair the consultant's effectiveness.

DEVELOPMENTAL PERSPECTIVE

A primary difference between work with children and work with adults is the need to maintain a developmental perspective with regard to children. Pediatricians and child psychiatrists are imbued with this central principle and may even take it for granted. A developmental perspective implies recognition that the rapid physical and psychological changes taking place in a child or an adolescent alter the manifestations of disease, the effect of illness on the patient's life, and the patient's coping capacities. Therefore, developmental landmarks, age-appropriate behavior, changes in cognitive abilities, Tanner staging, and so forth are variables that are routinely considered by pediatricians and should be well known to the psychiatric consultant. It is true that adults have developmental stages, but these are more subtle and gradual compared with those that pertain to childhood and adolescence. Nowhere are developmental factors more salient than in the assessment of somatoform disorders, a frequent reason for psychiatric consultation. A comprehensive review has delineated the problems associated with applying adult somatoform criteria to children and summarized the current empirical evidence regarding these disorders in children (Fritz et al. 1997). The fact that known developmental steps (based on previous steps) exist for each stage of childhood and adolescence presents a major complicating variable to the consultant who seeks to assess the meaning of a symptom or a behavior. At the same time, this push toward healthy development constitutes a powerful, resilient force promoting growth and recovery. The stress of an illness and hospitalization frequently leads to regression, in which a child temporarily loses some of the cognitive, emotional, or behavioral advances previously achieved and appears much less mature. Such regression is disconcerting for parents, difficult for caregivers, and often uncomfortable to the child. The assessment and management of regressive behavior is a common reason for pediatricians to request psychiatric consultation.

FAMILY FOCUS

Related to the developmental perspective and equally essential in pediatric consultation is a concern with the family. In contrast to what occurs with many adult consultations, the medical history and psychiatric history are virtually never obtained only from the pediatric patient; a parent or an adult caregiver must be interviewed for even the briefest assessment. Children's fundamental reliance on their parents for care requires that every intervention on behalf of the child also include the parents. As an extreme example, although an infant with failure to thrive is the identified patient, it is impossible to treat the infant without involving the primary caregiver to an equal or greater degree. A concrete result of this family awareness is that a consultation that would take approximately an hour and a half with an adult in the nongeriatric population may take three times that long when the patient is a child.

PEDIATRIC UNITS

Psychiatric consultants must be familiar with every aspect of the medical system in which they are working. Pediatric services exist as either one or more defined wards within a general hospital or as part of a freestanding children's hospital. In either case, certain characteristics distinguish them from corresponding adult medical or surgical wards. First, in keeping with the emphasis on a developmental perspective, unless the total number of beds is extremely small, children are hospitalized in units designated by age. Typically, infants and toddlers are in one unit, school-aged children in another, and adolescents in a third, although variations in the scheme are common. Nurses self-select based on the age group they like to work with, and even within pediatrics there is little overlap in skills between a nurse who is comfortable with adolescent medicine and a nurse who is skilled in caring for infants. Nurses typically function as surrogate parents for hospitalized children, and their attachment to their young patients may become very intense, especially to children who are hospitalized for a prolonged time. The experienced pediatric consultation-liaison psychiatrist recognizes this proprietary interest and even the healthy protective role that nurses may assume in regard to the children. However, when this attitude leads to competition with or displacement of the child's actual parents, the consultant must recognize the problem and intervene effectively.

Children's hospitals vary in their psychological sophistication in meeting the needs of hospitalized children and adolescents as well as their families. Many of the components of a state-of-the-art children's hospital are unparalleled in the adult medical setting. For example, rooming-in for parents, with facilities for sleeping and an encouraging attitude by ward staff, is now recognized as almost essential when a toddler or a young child is hospitalized. Medical inns, such as the Ronald McDonald Houses in many pediatric centers, provide convenient lodging for those parents who do not room-in but who must spend considerable time in the hospital. Such resources mitigate the separation problems associated with hospitalization and promote more effective coping by both the child and the family.

Family support services, including pediatric social workers, parent advocates, groups for parent support and education, and resource counseling, are considered essential in a modern pediatric facility. Child life workers are professionals whose job is to normalize the hospital environment to allow children and their parents to continue functioning and to promote development despite the stresses of hospitalization. Skillful child life workers do psychological preparation for hospitalization and medical procedures, hold ward meetings for children, organize age-appropriate recreational activities, and develop individualized programs for children who have particular problems. Child life workers have no counterparts on adult wards, and a psychiatric consultant must be aware of their existence and the significant potential for effective psychological intervention that these workers offer. For children who are hospitalized more than a few days, an in-hospital school experience or a tutor should be provided to maintain the normalizing structure of a child's life and to prevent the child from falling too far behind in schoolwork.

When all of these components of progressive pediatric care are available, the consultant must be aware of them and encourage their appropriate use. When one or more is lacking, the consultant must help staff to creatively devise a plan for the particular patient that fills the void while still advocating for improvements within the institution. Volunteers in the hospital, school personnel from the child's home institution, community charitable agencies, and existing ward staff can be organized to provide any of the necessary services described above. The consultant's creativity and leadership skills can be used to implement individualized plans for "normalizing" the hospitalization and result in a major improvement in hospital adjustment and psychological functioning for the young patient.

PROCESS OF CONSULTATION

Broadly speaking, the process of providing psychiatric consultation in pediatrics is similar to consultation with adult patients. However, several aspects are unique in the pediatric setting, and the general consultation-liaison psychiatrist who is new to pediatric consultation should be aware of these differences and give them due consideration.

In preparing for the consultation, it is not sufficient to inform only the young patient. The parents must be aware that the consultation is taking place and should understand the referring physician's reasons for it. Some parents feel that psychiatric evaluation of their child will reflect poorly on them and are more resistant than the child is to participating in the consultation. Most pediatricians have solid, ongoing relationships with the families of patients they care for, and family involvement in preparing for the consultation is important. The experienced consultant advises the referring pediatrician, gently and early, how to prepare both the patient and the parents for psychiatric consultation.

Involvement of the parents continues beyond preparation for the consultation. The first direct contact is usually made with the parents. The consultant expects that the parents of a sick child will want to maintain their decision-making and protective roles but also recognizes that they may feel threatened by multiple, variably intrusive authority figures that they encounter in the hospital environment. The detailed history of a child's illness, as well as his or her developmental history and the family background, is obtained from the parents in most consultations. Perhaps because the seriousness of a hospitalization changes everyone's schedule, fathers are frequently as available as mothers; in any case, the expectation is that both parents will participate in the consultation. Occasionally, the focus of a consultation is entirely on parental concerns or the parents' own difficulties. In such cases, the consultant can make a useful contribution without direct involvement of the child.

In addition to obtaining information from parents, data from outside the family are often needed. A child's schoolteacher, caseworker, probation officer, or therapist may be able to provide important information that will help in the evaluation. Although this information is sometimes difficult to obtain under the pressure of time, the consultant should use the authority of the children's hospital and communicate a degree of urgency to obtain facts rapidly from these important outside sources. Standardized self-report questionnaires, although typically underused in pediatric consultation, are readily available and can provide efficient sources of data when they are completed by the patient, the parents, or a ward observer. Examples of appropriate standardized instruments suitable for pediatric consultation are included in Table 32–1.

TABLE 32–1. Examples of assessment instruments for children

Child Behavior Checklist (Achenbach and Edelbrock 1983)
Wide-range, parent-reported scale of behavior problems; available forms for children from preschool through adolescence

Children's Depression Inventory (Kovacs and Beck 1977)
Brief, widely used self-report measure of depressive symptoms

Eating Attitudes Test (Rosen et al. 1988)
Test of adolescent norms for attitudes and behavior associated with eating disorders

Revised Children's Manifest Anxiety Scale (Reynolds and Richman 1978)
Self-report measure of trait anxiety; includes lie scale

Child Somatization Inventory (Walker and Greene 1989)
Quantifies common somatic symptoms in children

Kidcope (Spirito et al. 1988)
10-item checklist for assessment of common coping strategies in children

Perceived Competence Scale for Children (Harter 1982)
Scale for assessment of competence and self-esteem in multiple domains

CHILD ASSESSMENT

In an individual evaluation of a child, the consultant should arrange for a private, nonregressed setting. This means, for example, that a private office or a playroom is preferable to a ward room, with the patient being out of bed or sitting up instead of lying down and dressed or modestly covered rather than exposed. Few pediatric wards provide the ideal setting as a matter of course, but the consultant should use creativity, flexibility, and a reasonable amount of energy to establish the best environment for assessment.

Establishing an alliance is essential in any psychiatric evaluation, but hospitalized children are especially wary of adult professionals. For younger children, a small collection of carefully selected toys (such as safe medical equipment, a family of dolls, a deck of cards, a space gun to express aggression) are useful icebreakers. In some cases, all the important information from the child is communicated through the medium of play. The consultant must make clear an interest in the whole child, assessing strengths, interests, preferences, and life outside the hospital as well as problems and difficulties. Because of children's cognitive immaturity, the consultant should make a special effort to assess the child's understanding of his or her medical situation (cause, symptoms, treatment, and prognosis) as well as to evaluate associated fears and expectations.

The consultant should bear in mind that although cognitive maturity and knowledge of disease state are often related, frequently a dissociation exists. For example, young adolescents who are just beginning to experience the world with abstract thinking may be overwhelmed by anxiety resulting from the hospitalization and may process information about their condition more like a concrete-thinking, elementary school child. Conversely, a 10-year-old with a chronic illness who has been hospitalized repeatedly may have a more sophisticated understanding of the nuances of his or her illness than the average medical student does.

The mental status examination is as important in pediatric consultations as it is with adults. Table 32–2 contains an outline for the child mental status examination.

Normal responses vary dramatically among preschoolers, latency-aged children, preteens, young adolescents, and mid- to older adolescents. For example, use of language is as good an indicator of intelligence in children as it is in adults. However, the normal speech of an 8-year-old is precocious when it occurs in a 5-year-old, and it may suggest borderline retardation when it characterizes the language of a 12-year-old. Regressive symptoms during hospitalization (e.g., immature behavior, clinging,

enuresis) are extremely common in preschoolers, but the same behavior in a young adolescent is a cause for more concern. A thorough description of the normal responses and differences in mental status examination for each age group is beyond the scope of this chapter but is provided by Call (1985) and Lewis and Volkmar (1990).

The elements of the mental status examination may be elicited in a formal series of questions for adolescents, but usually the data are obtained as the opportunity arises within the flow of the interview. Regardless of how or in what order the material is obtained, a concise baseline description of mental functioning is always essential. In addition to elements that are well known to every adult psychiatrist (including affect, thought processes, and cognition), the consultant will observe and describe the quality of the child's relationship with parents and other caregivers. Ward staff are often unable to articulate what they have observed in the child's mental functioning, especially regarding younger children; the consultant's mental status description can serve as a useful model.

A DSM-IV-TR (American Psychiatric Association 2000) diagnosis is an important part of the consultant's report. However, epidemiologic evidence has underlined the prognostic importance of symptoms associated with psychosocial impairment, even when the children do not meet DSM criteria for any well-defined disorder (Angold et al. 1999).

TABLE 32–2. Outline for child mental status examination

I. Appearance
  A. Build (in relation to age, pubertal status)
  B. Clothing (signs of neglect, T-shirt messages, fastidiousness)
  C. Mannerisms (autistic stereotypies, tics, or habits)

II. Interpersonal relationships
  A. Interaction with parent (informally together, separation response, parental limit setting)
  B. Interaction with examiner (level of trust, activity vs. passivity, cooperation, change in relationship over time)

III. Capacities
  A. Intelligence (estimated from vocabulary, fund of age-appropriate knowledge, understanding of illness, imagination, orientation)
  B. Affects (range, appropriateness, somatic expressions)
  C. Motor (large and small motor movements, hyperactivity, inhibition)
  D. Speech (clarity of diction, defects, spontaneity)
  E. Attention span, distractibility, curiosity

IV. Content (attitudes, feelings, ideas)
  A. Toward illness, hospitalization, and the reasons for the consultation
  B. Toward self (appearance, body, behavior, preoccupations, suicidality)
  C. Toward others (parents, siblings, medical staff, peers)
  D. Toward things (pets, possessions, interests, school)

V. Play and fantasy
  A. Play (approach to and interest in toys; hospital play; character of play—disorganized, repetitious, distractible, etc.)
  B. Fantasy (three wishes, dreams, stories)

VI. Interviewer's subjective response to the child

ADMINISTRATIVE ISSUES

Certain administrative procedures are different in the pediatric realm than in an adult setting, and a consultant who is new to a children's hospital should seek orientation in regard to the existing policy on commitment, restraint, use of constant observation, and rules for discharge against medical advice. The fact that minors legally are dependents of their parents (unless a social agency has custody) means that, in general, decisions about hospitalization are made with parents rather than with the patients themselves. When both the patient and the parents are resistant to needed psychiatric hospitalization—such as after an adolescent's suicide attempt—the possibility of involuntary commitment for the patient exists, but the process is extremely complicated in most states. The administration and staff on most pediatric wards are less comfortable with the use of physical restraints than are the personnel who run a comparable adult medical ward; four-point restraint equipment may not even be available in the pediatric setting. The consultant should not assume that the pediatric staff has any expertise or comfort with restraining an agitated patient. The fact that the patients are typically smaller and less dangerous does not mean that the staff's comfort level is higher.

The number of pediatric patients who intentionally harm themselves in the hospital is small. Thus, the routine use of one-to-one constant observation is less common on pediatric units than on adult wards and is usually difficult to arrange on short notice. In general, privacy is less easily obtained on most pediatric units than on adult units, a fact that has its benefits in making routine observation more possible in the pediatric unit. A general psychiatrist who is called to do an emergency pediatric consultation on a children's ward who feels that he or she is in unfamiliar territory should seek a nursing supervisor who can clarify these policy issues.

The issue of confidentiality is never simple when one is dealing with children or adolescents and their parents. It is even more complicated in consultation work. As in consultation with adults, the consultant is involved in the case at the request of the attending physician. Therefore, it must be clear that the consultant will provide an expert opinion to the requesting physician. This report will become part of the medical record and, as such, will be available to everyone who reads the chart. These facts should be made clear to both the parents and the child at the outset of the consultation. At the same time, the consultant's clinical judgment should allow for the determination of what information is or is not useful to the primary physician and the ward staff. The consultant is justified in keeping information confidential that is not relevant to the pediatric care of the child. However, care must be taken not to be backed into an untenable position in which the data that form the basis for the consultant's recommendations cannot be shared with the staff. A more common problem is a request by a child that particular information be kept secret from the parents. Adolescents in particular may request confidentiality as a condition for candor. In most cases, this confidentiality is appropriate and must be explained to the parents. The age at which informed consent and the right to refuse treatment become the prerogative of the patient rather than the parent varies from state to state and may not be explicitly established. From mid-adolescence on, a consultant should err in the direction of assuming that the patient has the same legal rights and need for informed consent as an adult.

PSYCHOPHARMACOLOGY IN PEDIATRIC PATIENTS

All classes of psychopharmacological agents have a role in the psychiatric treatment of children and adolescents on a pediatric service. More comprehensive reviews of these medications and their indications, adverse effects, interactions with medical conditions, and interactions with other medications can be found in two special issues of the *Journal of Child and Adolescent Psychopharmacology* (1990), Green (1991, 1995), Wagner and Ambrosini (2001), and Riddle et al. (2001). Table 32–3 indicates the forms and suggested dose ranges for the most commonly used medications, although it is not totally inclusive of all drugs and forms in each category. Many medications are not universally approved by the U.S. Food and Drug Administration for use in either adolescents or children, so particular attention must be paid to the potential risks and benefits in individual patients. Psychotropic medications can cause inhibitions in the cytochrome enzyme systems in children, as in adults (Oesterheld and Shader 1998). This inhibition can result in interactions with multiple drugs commonly prescribed by pediatricians, such as antibiotics, antiepileptics, and antiarrhythmics. Knowledge of these systems and their importance for children is beginning to emerge. It is evident that by age 2 years, children possess cytochrome systems similar to those of adults but with greater metabolic activity.

Stimulants are used for children with attention-deficit/hyperactivity disorder (ADHD), which may be encountered in those with a variety of neurological disor-

TABLE 32–3. Psychopharmacology for children in a medical setting

Medications	Forms	Dosage
Stimulants		
Methylphenidate	5 mg, 10 mg, 20 mg (tablets); 20 mg (sustained-release tablet); 18 mg, 36 mg (extended 12-hour release tablets)	5 mg bid to start; can increase to 1 mg/kg/day
Antidepressants		
Citalopram	20 mg, 40 mg (tablets)	10 mg as single dose, to a maximum of 40 mg/day
Paroxetine	10 mg, 20 mg, 30 mg, 40 mg (tablets); 10 mg/5 mL (liquid)	Children: 10 mg/day to start Adolescents: 20 mg/day to start, to a maximum of 40 mg/day
Sertraline	25 mg, 50 mg, 100 mg (tablets); 20 mg/1 mL (liquid)	Children: 25 mg/day to start Adolescents: 50 mg/day to start, to a maximum of 150 mg/day
Fluoxetine	10 mg (tablets); 20 mg, 40 mg (pulvules); 20 mg/5 mL (liquid)	10 mg/day initially, given as a single daily dose in the morning; can increase to 60 mg/day in adolescents
Imipramine	10 mg, 25 mg, 50 mg (tablets)	25 mg/day to start, given in divided doses; can increase gradually to a maximum of 2.5–3.0 mg/kg/day
Neuroleptics		
Haloperidol	0.5 mg, 1 mg, 2 mg, 5 mg, 10 mg, 20 mg (tablets); 2 mg/1 mL (liquid)	Children: 0.5 mg to start; can increase to 0.15 mg/kg/day Adolescents: 0.5–5 mg bid or tid
Anxiolytics		
Lorazepam	0.5 mg, 1 mg, 2 mg (tablets); 2 or 4 mg/mL (injectable)	0.5–1 mg every 4–6 hours for short-term treatment of agitation
Diphenhydramine	25 mg, 50 mg (tablets or capsules); 12.5 mg/5 mL (liquid); 10 and 50 mg/mL (injectable)	25 mg bid or tid; can increase to a maximum of 5 mg/kg/day or 300 mg/day (whichever is lower)

ders, including head injury. Common side effects of stimulants include loss of appetite, irritability, abdominal pain, and insomnia (avoid late-afternoon doses). Pemoline is the most likely to cause chemical hepatitis, so liver function tests must be monitored, and overall the use of pemoline should be avoided in favor of safer drugs (Safer et al. 2001). Despite the common parental worry, stimulants do not increase seizure frequency. They are, however, associated with an increase in blood levels of several anticonvulsants and antidepressants when these drugs are given concomitantly.

Antidepressants are indicated for the treatment of a wide range of psychiatric disorders. Selective serotonin reuptake inhibitors (SSRIs) have been found to be useful in the treatment of major mood disorders, anxiety disorders, and posttraumatic stress disorders. In addition, they are also used as adjuvant therapy for children with chronically painful medical conditions, regardless of the level of depression. The SSRIs have few adverse effects (mainly nausea) and are commonly used in children and adolescents. The mechanisms of action and side effect profiles are similar for all drugs in this class but only sertraline has received U.S. Food and Drug Administration approval specifically for use in children and adolescents. Tricyclic antidepressants, such as imipramine, have been used for the treatment of enuresis and ADHD as well as

mood and anxiety disorders. Similar to the adverse effects noted in adults, the most common effects of tricyclic antidepressants in children are anticholinergic effects and a quinidine-like action on the heart. An electrocardiogram (ECG) should be performed and vital signs should be documented before treatment, and these procedures should be repeated frequently during treatment. Although investigators in several studies have not found clinically significant ECG changes in children (Wilens et al. 1993), four cases of sudden death in children taking desipramine have been reported (Riddle et al. 1993). A long–Q-T syndrome is one proposed explanation, although considerable uncertainty remains. Tricyclic antidepressants also lower the seizure threshold and interact with many commonly used medications. Selective serotonin reuptake inhibitors (SSRIs) have few adverse effects (mainly nausea), but their safety in children has not yet been established.

Neuroleptics are indicated for the treatment of psychotic disorders and severe agitation associated with primary brain disorders in children. Important adverse effects in children are similar to those seen in adults and include sedation, parkinsonism, dystonia, and neuroleptic malignant syndrome. Their potential for inducing serious orthostatic hypotension or respiratory depression may be particularly troublesome for children who are medically compromised. Anxiolytics are used primarily in children with chronic anxiety disorders or for those with anticipatory anxiety (preceding painful medical procedures). Sedation and blunting of cognition are especially common in children who take anxiolytic medications. Behavioral disinhibition and dependence are serious but rare side effects.

Analgesics are often underused in pediatric settings. Table 32–4 contains the relative potencies of common analgesics. Inadequate doses are most likely to be administered when a switch is made from injectable to oral forms of medications. Analgesics may be underused because of inappropriate concerns about addiction, ill-founded beliefs that infants and children do not feel pain to the same degree as adults, and unrealistic expectations of the resiliency of children.

CLINICAL ISSUES IN PEDIATRIC CONSULTATION

The clinical problems that confront the consultation psychiatrist in pediatrics may differ substantially from those seen in the adult realm. For example, depression may be as common a problem for the consultant on a pediatric unit as on an adult ward, but as thoroughly discussed in a recent review, the conceptualization, presentation, assessment, and treatment are distinct in children (Burke and Elliott 1999). Certain clinical problems have no equivalent in internal medicine. For example, technological advances in the intensive care nursery have made it the rule, rather than the exception, for premature infants weighing more than 800 g (1.75 lb) to survive, giving rise to a number of immediate and long-term psychological complications for the child and his or her family. Although cancer occurs in both children and adults, the characteristics and prognoses associated with most pediatric malignancies are dramatically different (usually

much better) from those associated with the most common malignancies in adults. Thus, most pediatric cancer is appropriately seen as a chronic rather than fatal illness that has more in common with certain congenital disorders and cystic fibrosis than with adult malignancies. At the same time, many disorders that are commonly encountered by psychiatric consultants who treat adults—such as Alzheimer's disease, symptoms of alcohol withdrawal, coronary artery disease, and infertility—are rarely or never encountered by the pediatric psychiatric consultant. A thorough discussion of the problems and interventions common in pediatric consultation-liaison psychiatry is beyond the scope of this chapter. Nevertheless, to convey the flavor of such work, we have included four examples of consultation problems that are typically encountered in pediatric settings.

The Suicide Attempt

As a matter of policy, a consultation was requested for a 15-year-old girl who was hospitalized after her deliberate ingestion of a large quantity of acetaminophen, aspirin, and a nonprescription sleep aid. The next morning, the girl was disheveled but coherent and revealed that the attempt was made impulsively and without premeditation in response to rejection by her boyfriend. She was no longer suicidal and could "contract" for safety in the hospital. Thus, her "sitter" was discontinued, which had been the nursing staff's prime question for the consultant. Developmentally appropriate questions did not identify any evidence of major mood disorder, anxiety disorder, psychosis, or personality disorder. The consultant noted that the patient's schoolwork had declined in the past year following her parents' divorce but that she had many close friends and several nonacademic interests. Brief, separate interviews with the young woman's parents confirmed the historical information and all parties' willingness for further outpatient evaluation. The consultant's initial tasks were to decrease the intensity of nursing supervision in a safe, predictable manner and to arrange for outpatient psychiatric care.

TABLE 32–4. Narcotic analgesics used in pediatric settings

Medication	Duration of action (hours)	Route	Equianalgesic dose (mg)	Dosage
Morphine	4–5	im/iv	10	0.1–0.2 mg/kg/dose
		Oral	60	0.5 mg/kg q6h
Meperidine	2–4	im/iv	75	1 mg/kg/dose to 100 mg/dose q4h
		Oral	300	
Oxycodone	4–5	Oral	30	0.05–0.15 mg/kg/dose to 10 mg/dose q4h
Codeine	4–6	Oral	200	0.5 mg/kg/dose to 5 mg/dose q4h

Note. im = intramuscular; iv = intravenous.

Source. Adapted from LeBel-Schwartz A: "Pain Management in Children," in *Psychiatric Aspects of General Hospital Pediatrics.* Edited by Jellinek MS, Herzog DB. St. Louis, MO, Mosby-Year Book, 1990, pp. 312–331. Used with permission.

After an uneventful course of therapy for the acetaminophen overdose during the next 2 days, the mother arrived for the patient's discharge. A nurse detected alcohol on the mother's breath and urgently paged the consultant. During the emergent reconsultation, the psychiatrist evaluated the mother's current level of impairment, reviewed her drug and psychiatric history (not disclosed on first evaluation), and postponed the discharge despite the protests of mother and child. A family meeting the next day, when the mother was sober, resulted in provision of additional information that supported the rationale for discharge to the mother's care, beginning of a separate therapeutic plan for the mother, and involvement of local social support agencies.

Exaggerated Pain

An orthopedic surgeon requested a consultation for a 6-year-old boy because of "exaggerated pain complaints" 3 days after the child sustained a femur fracture. The leg had been pinned and placed in traction. On rounds, the surgeons noted that the boy was tearful and irritable; his mother reported that he was "inconsolable." The consultant found him straining against the traction and whimpering while his mother held his hand. The boy said little spontaneously, had no interest in the toys he was invited to play with, and grimaced while he talked briefly about his injured leg. He seemed sensitive to any bodily movement. There was no history of unexplained somatic complaints, prior behavior disorder, or recent family stresses. A chart review indicated that his medication had been changed abruptly 24 hours earlier from analgesics administered intravenously to oral acetaminophen. Nursing staff noted that he had had few pain complaints immediately postoperatively and also that he cried more when his mother was present.

In an individual interview, the boy was more verbal and engaging but was still in obvious pain. The patient's mother confided to the consultant that she was quite worried that her son would never walk properly because his injury reminded her of an uncle who had had a significant limp from a foreshortened leg. Her fear about her son's incomplete recovery was exacerbated by his crying. The consultant's tasks were to 1) provide adequate oral analgesics (analgesics are often underused in pediatric settings because of inappropriate concerns about addiction, ill-founded beliefs that children do not feel as much pain as adults, and unrealistic expectations of children's resiliency); 2) decrease the mother's anxiety by clear, repeated explanations from the surgeons that included reviewing with her the X rays of the child's healing bone; and 3) help the nursing staff to understand that the mother was not "poor at coping," because although her anxiety made her less able to console the boy, she was still the adult who was most able to correctly interpret the child's cues that he was in pain. The child's subsequent recovery was uneventful.

Compliance With a Medical Regimen

Consultation was requested for a 2-year-old boy who was hospitalized repeatedly with poorly controlled asthma. The pediatric staff determined that his medication regimen was not being followed effectively and sought psychiatric help for the patient. The child's mother readily admitted that she could not get her son to swallow his oral medications. She described fruitless games, bribes, and battles. Her lack of success was reflected in low levels of the medication in the serum and poor asthma control. The consultant arrived at the child's bed at the same time as the father, who was reported to be unhelpful and uninvolved with the child's care. The consultant quickly elicited from the father (who was audibly wheezing himself) his belief that his son did not have asthma and did not need medication any more than he, the father, did. Moreover, he thought that his wife and the female pediatrician, with their emphasis on asthma and medicine, would make the child view himself as sickly. He refused to help his wife in the management of a disease whose existence he denied in his son (and in himself). He was a caring father and involved with his son in other areas, however. The pediatrician and the consultant worked together to help the father to confront his fears and his misinformation as the critical step in improving the child's asthma treatment.

Behavioral Intervention in a Patient With a Medical Illness

Billy was a 2-year-old boy with severe atopic dermatitis. His constant, deep scratching led to superficial infection and continued itching. A week of baseline monitoring showed that the scratching was particularly pronounced at bedtime. Scratching also escalated after Billy was reprimanded by his parents or when he was bored. Billy's concerned—and usually quite competent—parents typically responded in the following sequence: they asked him to stop scratching, tried to distract Billy from the scratching, reprimanded him, and, finally, spanked him.

The first intervention involved instructing Billy's parents to pay less attention to him when he was scratching and to greatly increase the amount of attention they paid to Billy when he did not scratch. For example, the parents were instructed to turn their heads away until Billy stopped scratching if he began to scratch when they were playing with him (extinction); they were told to redirect their attention to Billy when he stopped scratching. In addition, the parents were told to praise (reinforce) Billy for scratch-free periods ("I really like it when you don't scratch your skin when we're playing"). At bedtime, it was necessary to rearrange the contingencies in order to get some control over the scratching—that is, Billy's bedtime story was delayed until he showed several minutes of not scratching. This period was gradually lengthened, so that eventually Billy did not scratch in bed for a half-hour before he was read his bedtime story. This treatment approach, conducted over a 6-week period, resulted in almost complete cessation of scratching.

CONCLUSION

Until the national shortage of child and adolescent psychiatrists is alleviated, consultation-liaison psychiatrists who have been trained to work with adults will continue to be called on to provide psychiatric expertise to medical professionals who treat youngsters. The general consultation-liaison psychiatrist can make a useful contribution as a consultant to individuals in the pediatric health care system if adequate thought is given to the differences between adult and child consultation-liaison work before undertaking a consultation. Unique characteristics of pediatricians and the practice of pediatrics, essential consideration of the developmental and family perspective, organization and staffing of pediatric units, specific aspects of the consultation process, and a different set of clinical problems common to pediatrics all distinguish child and adolescent consultation-liaison work from its adult counterpart (Table 32–5). Ignoring the differences and proceeding as one would consult to an adult medical unit will result in frustration for all involved. A degree of preparation and appropriate recognition of the "cultural" differences, however, will allow general consultation-liaison psychiatrists to extend their range and provide a service that is clinically useful as well as professionally satisfying.

TABLE 32–5. Key characteristics of pediatric consultation

Pediatrics versus internal medicine
  Developmental perspective
  Family focus

Consultation process in pediatrics
  Consultation normally takes longer
  Parents as well as patient should be prepared and involved
  Multiple sources of information should be used
  Standardized instruments may be helpful

Examination process
  Alliance critical; toys, drawings, television characters, etc., should be used
  Interactions should be tailored to level of cognitive maturity
  Child's understanding, fears, expectations need to be assessed
  Confidentiality must be maintained

Clinical highlights
  Medical problems may be unique to pediatrics (e.g., cancer is less often fatal, dementia is uncommon)
  Analgesics are often underused for children
  Behavioral treatments are especially effective
  Intervention to children often extends to family

REFERENCES

Achenbach TM, Edelbrock C: Manual for the Child Behavior Checklist and Revised Child Behavior Profile. Burlington, University of Vermont, Department of Psychiatry, 1983

Ahsanuddin KM, Adams JE: Setting up a pediatric consultation-liaison service. Psychiatr Clin North Am 5:259–270, 1982

American Psychiatric Association: Diagnostic and Statistical Manual of Mental Disorders, 4th Edition, Text Revision. Washington, DC, American Psychiatric Association, 2000

Angold A, Costello EJ, Farmer EMZ, et al: Impaired but undiagnosed. J Am Acad Child Adolesc Psychiatry 38:129–137, 1999

Bergman AS, Fritz GK: Pediatricians and mental health professionals: patterns of collaboration and utilization. Am J Dis Child 139:155–159, 1985

Burke P, Elliott M: Depression in pediatric chronic illness: a diathesis-stress model. Psychosomatics 40:5–17, 1999

Call JD: Psychiatric evaluations of the infant and child, in Comprehensive Textbook of Psychiatry, 4th Edition. Edited by Kaplan LI, Sadock BJ. Baltimore, MD, Williams & Wilkins, 1985, pp 1614–1624

Enzer NG, Singleton DS, Snellman LA, et al: Interferences in collaboration between child psychiatrists and pediatricians: a fundamental difference in attitude toward childhood. J Dev Behav Pediatr 7:186–193, 1986

Fritz GK: Consultation-liaison in child psychiatry and the evolution of pediatric psychiatry. Psychosomatics 31:85–90, 1990

Fritz GK, Bergman AS: Consultation-liaison training for child psychiatrists: results of a survey. Gen Hosp Psychiatry 6:25–29, 1984

Fritz GK, Bergman AS: Child psychiatrists seen through pediatricians' eyes: results of a national survey. J Am Acad Child Adolesc Psychiatry 24:81–86, 1985

Fritz GK, Mattison RE, Nurcombe B, et al (eds): Child and Adolescent Mental Health Consultation in Hospitals, Schools, and Courts. Washington, DC, American Psychiatric Press, 1993

Fritz GK, Fritsch S, Hagino O: Somatoform disorders in children and adolescents: a review of the past 10 years. J Am Acad Child Adolesc Psychiatry 36:1329–1338, 1997

Froese AP: Pediatric referrals to psychiatry, I: comparison of referrals and nonreferrals. Int J Psychiatry Med 7:241–247, 1976–1977

Green WH: Child and Adolescent Clinical Psychopharmacology. Baltimore, MD, Williams & Wilkins, 1991

Green WH: Child and Adolescent Clinical Psychopharmacology, 2nd Edition. Baltimore, MD, Williams & Wilkins, 1995

Greene CM: Mutual collaboration between psychiatry and pediatrics: resistance and facilitation. J Dev Behav Pediatr 5:315–318, 1984

Harter S: The Perceived Competence Scale for Children. Child Dev 53:87–97, 1982

Knapp P, Harris E: Consultation-liaison in child psychiatry: a review of the past 10 years, part I: clinical findings. J Am Acad Child Adolesc Psychiatry 37:17–25, 1998a

Knapp P, Harris E: Consultation-liaison in child psychiatry: a review of the past 10 years, part II: research on treatment approaches and outcomes. J Am Acad Child Adolesc Psychiatry 37:139–146, 1998b

Kovacs M, Beck AT: An empirical approach towards a definition of childhood depression, in Depression in Children: Diagnosis, Treatment and Conceptual Models. Edited by Schulterbrandt JG, Raskin A. New York, Raven, 1977, pp 1–26

LeBel-Schwartz A: Pain management in children, in Psychiatric Aspects of General Hospital Pediatrics. Edited by Jellinek MS, Herzog DB. St. Louis, MO, Mosby-Year Book, 1990, pp 312–331

Lewis M: Child psychiatric consultation in pediatrics. Pediatrics 62:359–364, 1978

Lewis M, Volkmar FR: The psychiatric evaluation of the infant, child and adolescent, in Clinical Aspects of Child and Adolescent Development: An Introductory Synthesis of Developmental Concepts and Clinical Experience, 3rd Edition. Philadelphia, PA, Lea & Febiger, 1990

Oesterheld J, Shader R: Cytochrome: a primer for child and adolescent psychiatrists. J Am Acad Child Adolesc Psychiatry 37:447–451, 1998

Reynolds CR, Richman BO: What I think and feel: a revised measure of children's manifest anxiety. J Abnorm Child Psychol 6:271–280, 1978

Riddle MA, Geller B, Ryan N: Case study: another sudden death in a child treated with desipramine. J Am Acad Child Adolesc Psychiatry 32:792–797, 1993

Riddle MA, Kastelic EA, Frosch E: Pediatric psychopharmacology. J Child Psychol Psychiatry 42:73–90, 2001

Rosen JC, Silberg NT, Gross J: Eating Attitudes Test and Eating Disorders Inventory: norms for adolescent girls and boys. J Consult Clin Psychol 56:305–308, 1988

Rothenberg MB: Child psychiatry-pediatrics consultation-liaison services in the hospital setting: a review. Gen Hosp Psychiatry 1:281–286, 1979

Sack W, Cohen S, Grout C: One year's survey of child psychiatry consultations in a pediatric hospital. J Am Acad Child Adolesc Psychiatry 16:716–727, 1977

Safer DJ, Zito JM, Gardner JF: Pemoline hepatotoxicity and postmarketing surveillance. J Am Acad Child Adolesc Psychiatry 40:622–629, 2001

Schowalter J, Lord RD: The utilization of child psychiatry on a pediatric adolescent ward. J Am Acad Child Adolesc Psychiatry 10:685–699, 1971

Special Issues: The safe and effective use of psychotropic medications in adolescents and children. Journal of Child and Adolescent Psychopharmacology, Vol 1 and 2, 1990

Spirito A, Stark LJ, Williams C: Development of a brief coping checklist for use with pediatric populations. J Pediatr Psychol 13:555–574, 1988

Stocking M, Rothney W, Grosser G, et al: Psychopathology in the pediatric hospital: implications for community health. Am J Public Health 62:551–556, 1972

Wagner KD, Ambrosini PJ: Childhood depression: pharmacological therapy/treatment. J Clin Child Psychol 30:88–97, 2001

Walker LS, Greene JW: Children with recurrent abdominal pain and their parents: more somatic complaints, anxiety and depression than other patient families? J Pediatr 14:231–243, 1989

Wilens T, Biederman J, Baldessarini RJ, et al: Electrocardiographic effects of desipramine and 2-hydroxydesipramine with children, adolescents and adults treated with desipramine. J Am Acad Child Adolesc Psychiatry 32:798–804, 1993

Work H: The "menace of psychiatry" revisited: the evolving relationship between pediatrics and child psychiatry. Psychosomatics 30:86–93, 1989

Wright HH, Eaton JS, Butterfield PT, et al: Financing of child psychiatry pediatric consultation-liaison programs. J Dev Behav Adolesc Pediatr 8:221–226, 1987

33

Physical Medicine and Rehabilitation

Duane S. Bishop, M.D.

L. Russell Pet, M.D.

Life is short, the art long
Opportunity fleeting
Experience treacherous
Judgment difficult—
But the rewards are superb!

After Hippocrates/Goethe/Gunther
(Group for the Advancement of Psychiatry, Committee on Handicaps 1993, p. 122)

Rehabilitation medicine is a rapidly expanding area of medicine that requires effective and efficient attention by consultation-liaison psychiatrists. Inpatient rehabilitation admissions increased by 17% and outpatient visits by 29% between 1980 and 1990 (AHA News 1993). Forty million Americans have some physical impairment, disability, or handicap (Hahn 1983). The rate of disability increases with age and is higher among ethnic minorities (Group for the Advancement of Psychiatry, Committee on Handicaps 1993). Contrary to common belief, disability benefits generally are going to the right people (i.e., people with genuine disabilities) (International Center for the Disabled 1986). A disabled person is likely to receive one-quarter of the income of nondisabled individuals, and only 40% of the individuals who are disabled are employed (Group for the Advancement of Psychiatry, Committee on Handicaps 1993). Unfortunately, only one-quarter of disabled people will receive some type of rehabilitation (Group for the Advancement of Psychiatry, Committee on Handicaps 1993). In this chapter, we focus on consultation-liaison psychiatry issues that are salient to inpatient and related outpatient rehabilitation treatment settings.

Psychiatry in rehabilitation medicine is a challenge. Rehabilitation medicine is not acute medicine, and consultation-liaison psychiatry in rehabilitation settings demands a different conceptualization and approach. Rehabilitation staff are intensely invested in their patients, remain motivated despite daunting situations, and may receive little immediate return for their efforts. When they ask for psychiatric assistance, they want more than a diagnosis from DSM-IV-TR (American Psychiatric Association 2000) and medication recommendations. Members of the staff have detailed observations and knowledge they wish to share and a need to understand behavior in the context of their interventions. They want feedback, and most of all they demand an integrated, consistent team plan for patient problems. Psychiatric credibility is gained only by addressing these expectations.

DEFINITIONS

The terms *impairment, disability,* and *handicap* (World Health Organization 1980) have specific meanings in rehabilitation. *Impairment* is defined as loss of psychological, physiologic, or anatomic structure or function. *Disability* refers to a loss in ability to perform activities of daily living such as walking, talking, dressing, and feeding.

Handicap is defined as the sum of social and environmental disadvantage arising out of disease, impairment, or disability. A direct relation among the three does not always exist, and interventions are different for each. Rehabilitation addresses the problems of patients who have a medical condition that is likely to become chronic and result in a disability. Rehabilitation focuses on minimizing disability and handicap.

CONTEXT OF REHABILITATION

Effective psychiatric consultation on rehabilitation units requires considering many contextual issues so that psychiatric care is well integrated into the overall treatment plan. Extra care and attention are necessary to avoid well-intentioned but inappropriate action.

Diagnostic Groups and Problems

Patients in a variety of diagnostic groups and with a variety of medical problems receive rehabilitation medicine care. Table 33–1 summarizes diagnoses among rehabilitation patients.

Rehabilitation Versus Acute Medicine and Surgery

In acute medical-surgical settings, patients are acutely ill and are relatively passive recipients of care. During rehabilitation, patients and their families assume more and more responsibility for patient progress. Rehabilitation assists patients and families to prepare for life in the community; the period of treatment is one of transition.

As in all of medicine, changes in regulations as well as pressure from government and insurers have all combined to trigger changes in rehabilitation. Much of the acute rehabilitation for joint replacement, hip fracture surgery, some strokes, and other traditional inpatient rehabilitation care has moved to "subacute" rehabilitation units in nursing homes (Murray et al. 1999). The population found on inpatient rehabilitation units has changed. More recently, the introduction of the prospective payment system has changed nursing home approaches, and it is as yet unclear how this will influence the flow of patients with complex medical problems to both nursing homes and inpatient rehabilitation programs.

Referring Source

Internists and physiatrists may share responsibility for care on inpatient rehabilitation units. One or both may have

TABLE 33–1. Diagnoses among patients undergoing rehabilitation

Potential diagnostic groups
  Amputation
  Arthritis
  Brain tumor
  Deconditioning from prolonged catastrophic medical illness
  Degenerative neurological disorders
  Guillain-Barré syndrome
  Hemophilia
  Multiple sclerosis
  Multiple trauma
  Muscular dystrophy
  Neuropathies and myopathies
  Polio
  Postpolio syndrome
  Spinal cord injury
  Stroke
  Traumatic brain injury

Potential underlying and associated diagnoses[a]
  Cardiovascular disease
  Diabetes
  Gastrointestinal disorders
  Hypertension
  Respiratory disorders
  Seizures
  Skin problems

[a]Older patients are more likely to have a combination of these disorders.

physician assistants or nurse practitioners working with them who provide direction for primary care. Distinctions among all these providers can become blurred. The consultation-liaison psychiatrist can then run into difficulty if one of the four refers for a consultation, two "do not mind" the consult, and the fourth thinks that the referral was inappropriate. This complexity is increased if nurses or therapists and not physicians were the initial source of the request.

Time and Patient Stability

Rehabilitation generally involves a longer stay than is required for acute inpatient medical-surgical care. Patients referred for rehabilitation are also usually medically stable and physically active. This facilitates both initial psychiatric consultation and follow-up care.

Three-Hour Rule

To meet admission criteria for inpatient rehabilitation units, most patients must be able to tolerate and receive 3 hours a day of any combination of physical therapy, occupational therapy, and speech therapy. Therapists usually are assigned to a patient for the entire rehabilitation period, and the patient is usually seen a minimum of 5–6 days per week. Such consistent contact provides reliable information about behavior, mood, and cognition.

Psychiatric comorbidity, especially depression and cognitive deficits, can make meeting the 3-hour rule difficult and can jeopardize continued rehabilitation. Psychiatric consultation and treatment in such situations may prevent premature discharge. Consultation-liaison psychiatrists may find that patient availability for consultation and follow-up appointments is limited by the primacy of therapy time. Fortunately, however, most programs have formal scheduling systems that can assist the psychiatric consultant in advance booking for the most efficient time for consultation.

Rehabilitation Teams

The rehabilitation staff members function in interdisciplinary teams that are divided into core and extended components (Browne and Bishop 1980). The core team for any given patient is usually larger than an inpatient psychiatry treatment team and includes a physiatrist, a nurse, a physical therapist, an occupational therapist, a speech therapist, and a social worker. This core team, which is adequate for most patients, may be expanded when clinically appropriate to include psychologists, recreational therapists, or vocational rehabilitation counselors. The extended component includes consultants in psychiatric, medical, and surgical specialties, as well as dietary counselors, pastoral counselors, and others. Teams also vary in their ability to efficiently integrate all of these various players. Differences in expectations can occur between members of the core team and the extended components.

Extended team members such as consultation-liaison psychiatrists should try to schedule consultation visits and/or follow-up visits in order to meet briefly with the core team. This approach provides a better picture of the consultation problem and improves feedback and treatment planning. If this is not possible, the psychiatrist may ask the team to designate an individual who will serve as liaison with the psychiatrist for a given patient.

Rehabilitation teams often schedule meetings with the family for goal setting, monitoring, and discharge planning. When patients have complex problems, attending such meetings frequently provides more direct and effective feedback.

Comprehensive Evaluation

Good assessment is good management. Careful review of the record for medical history, multidisciplinary assessment data, physical examination findings, hospital course, surgical procedures, laboratory data, and medications is a must. The psychiatric examination must include a thorough evaluation of mood syndrome psychological and vegetative signs and symptoms, as well as a comprehensive mental status examination. Psychiatrically significant vegetative signs and symptoms must be differentiated from signs and symptoms of concurrent medical conditions. During the evaluation, patients may indicate medical symptoms to the psychiatrist that have not been previously noted. This information must be passed on to the consulting physiatrist and/or primary care physician.

Management Protocols

Rehabilitation staff traditionally use a number of protocols for bowel control, safety, and assistive devices. These protocols focus on pragmatic action to improve function, and protocols often fit best with the cognitive set of rehabilitation staff. Psychiatric interventions often may be most effectively delivered in rehabilitation settings if presented in protocol form.

Cultural Sensitivity

Cultural values play a significant role in rehabilitation (Group for the Advancement of Psychiatry, Committee on Handicaps 1993). Cultures vary in their values and views regarding issues such as dependence/independence, pain, acceptance of body deformities, sexuality, and caregiving expectations that influence course and outcome. At times, members of the rehabilitation staff underestimate the importance of cultural issues, and rehabilitation programs also can be structured in ways that are culturally inappropriate. Consultation-liaison psychiatrists who are asked to consult on rehabilitation units must ensure that cultural issues are addressed.

Functional Assessment

Psychiatric consultants should become familiar with functional capacity assessment methods used in rehabilitation. Maximal functioning is a central goal, and all programs document detailed assessments of functioning at admission and at regular intervals thereafter. These functional measures provide crucial information, point to areas of discrepancy between expected and observed functioning, and suggest when psychosocial factors may be affecting a patient's progress. For example, staff can tell the consultant what a patient with quadriplegia from an injury at the level of C-6/C-7 should be able to do, what assistive devices he or she needs, and what he or she is not able to do.

If the patient is not achieving expected improvement goals, this may signal that undetected medical and/or significant psychosocial factors are involved. Changes in functional capacity scores can provide an outcome measure of the effectiveness of psychiatric interventions.

Functional recovery is also important because findings indicate a direct relation between functional capacity scores and the amount of direct caregiver assistance that a patient will require (Granger et al. 1993). Although the consultation-liaison psychiatrist may be asked to see patients for traditional reasons, the question of how the intervention will affect functional treatment outcomes will be central for staff.

Multidisciplinary Focus

Practitioners of each discipline involved in rehabilitation provide formal, quantified assessment information. Speech therapists provide detailed evaluations of language comprehension and expression as well as assessments of other cognitive factors. They can indicate whether a language-impaired patient can reliably point to or in some other way indicate "Yes" and "No" responses to questions. In particularly difficult cases, it is helpful for the consultation-liaison psychiatrist to see the patient with the speech therapist.

On some units, speech therapists or other clinicians record standardized mental status evaluations for all patients. Occupational therapists evaluate activities of daily living, upper-extremity function, fine motor control, and visual-perceptual functions. Nurses' assessments provide information about medications, treatment compliance, lifestyle issues (e.g., dieting, exercise), and 24-hour observations of behavior. Social workers provide detailed social histories and coordinate postdischarge psychosocial issues. Discharge planners help with placement issues. Vocational rehabilitation counselors assess the patient's preferred interests and work history. Recreation therapists detail leisure activities and interests. Psychologists and neuropsychologists can provide information about cognitive functioning, intelligence, mood, and personality factors as well as cognitive rehabilitation interventions (Caplan 1987; Diller 1980; Gordon et al. 1985; Rosenthal 1987). In contrast to what is usually found in acute settings, the medical record in the rehabilitation setting often provides psychiatric consultants with a rich description of the patient and his or her background.

REASONS FOR PSYCHIATRIC CONSULTATION

The most frequent problems that consultation-liaison psychiatrists are asked to address in rehabilitation include depression, cognitive changes, adjustment problems, and behavioral difficulties. It is important to define the reason for the consultation at the outset. It is not unusual for the psychiatric consultant to be asked to see a patient for a problem that staff members identify as depression or adjustment disorder and to make a diagnosis that is quite different—for example, mental disorder resulting from a toxic or medical condition. The consultation-liaison psychiatrist must then help the staff to accept and respond appropriately to this changed mind-set.

Depression

Depression is one of the most frequent reasons for psychiatric consultation in rehabilitation medicine. In one study, the diagnosis of depression was overlooked in 70%–80% of depressed inpatients in acute medical settings and in up to 68% of depressed patients in rehabilitation settings (Schubert et al. 1992a). Major depression is associated with longer duration of inpatient rehabilitation (Kennedy and Rogers 2000), functional capacity (Loon et al. 1995; Malec and Neimeyer 1983; Mossey et al. 1990; Schubert et al. 1992b; Tiller 1992), and delay in resumption of premorbid social activities (Tiller 1992). However, one research team (Starkstein and Robinson 1989) found that depression does not appear to be related to severity of neurological impairment in patients who have had a stroke. Another study found no relation between depression and functional capacity or neurological impairment in spinal cord injury (Fuhrer et al. 1993). The reported incidences of depression and dysthymia in rehabilitation-related disorders are outlined in Table 33–2. Depression can continue from early onset or arise and become a significant factor years later in both spinal cord injury (Craig et al. 1994; Scivoletto et al. 1997) and stroke (Lofgren et al. 1999) patients. It is therefore important that follow-up be arranged for these patients. Others have reported less depression in community samples of stroke patients than in inpatient rehabilitation or general hospital settings (Burvill et al. 1995a).

Depression syndromes have many etiologies that include but are not limited to 1) primary major depression; 2) dysthymia; 3) exacerbation of dysthymic and/or depressive personality features under the stress of events leading to rehabilitation; 4) adjustment disorder with depressed mood; 5) the general malaise of being ill; 6) a

TABLE 33–2. Rates of depression in rehabilitation diagnostic groups

Diagnostic group	Rate of depression (%)
Amputation	35–58[a,b,c]
Chronic pain	28 dysthymia[d]
	8–87 major depression[d,e]
Multiple sclerosis	6–27[f]
Oncology	6–25[g,h]
Rheumatoid arthritis	19–50[i]
Spinal cord injury	2–48[j,k,l,m]
Stroke	25–30[n]
Traumatic brain injury	25[o]

Source. [a]Gerhardt et al. 1984; [b]Rybarczyk et al. 1992; [c]Shukla et al. 1982; [d]Large 1986; [e]Lindsay and Wyckoff 1981; [f]Lishman 1987; [g]Holland 1987; [h]Massie and Holland 1990; [i]Beckham et al. 1992; [j]MacDonald et al. 1987; [k]Fullerton et al. 1981; [l]Krause et al. 2000; [m]Kennedy and Rogers 2000; [n]Tiller 1992; [o]Federoff et al. 1992.

secondary disorder resulting from medical conditions such as hypothyroidism and Addison's disease (Robinson et al. 1999); 7) a side effect of medications such as propranolol, reserpine, and metoclopramide; and 8) central nervous system (CNS) deficits resulting from stroke, brain tumor, or head injury (Bishop 1980; Robinson et al. 1999). Depression is often the result of a mixture of at least two or three of these etiologies in rehabilitation settings. Therapists who have daily contact with the patient are crucial sources of information. It has been shown that clinicians in some rehabilitation disciplines (e.g., occupational therapists) may be more accurate in their assessment of depression than those in other disciplines (Caplan 1983; Dijkers and Cushman 1990; Guilmette et al. 1992).

The principles of assessment for the rehabilitation patient do not vary significantly from those that apply to patients in any other medical-surgical setting. However, the ongoing neurobehavioral impairment seen in many patients on rehabilitation units can interfere with accurate diagnosis. Reports of depressed mood by the patient may be misleading because of cognitive deficits, lack of awareness, or aphasia. Depressed mood also must be differentiated from organic labile affect (Caplan and Shechter 1987), which is reported to occur in 10% of multiple sclerosis (Feinstein et al. 1997) and stroke patients. The short form of the Geriatric Depression Scale (Yesavage et al. 1982/1983), despite its title, is appropriate for all age groups in rehabilitation settings because it uses dichotomous choice, which is better in cognitively problematic cases (Caplan 1987), and does not contain potentially confounding somatic symptoms. It has demonstrated value in patients undergoing rehabilitation (Guilmette et al. 1992).

The suicide rate is higher among patients in rehabilitation settings than among individuals in the general population and among patients with other types of medical illness (Table 33–3). Missel (1978) reported that concerns about suicide risk led to 15% of the requests for psychiatric consultation in one series of patients undergoing rehabilitation. Suicidal patients undergoing rehabilitation may not always have traditional suicide risk factors, such as active alcoholism or current major depression. Suicidal thinking and behaviors can also be a reaction to life circumstances in patients who have no concurrent active psychiatric disorder (Sakinofsky 1980; Whitlock 1986). Some patients choose to die when quality of life or burden on others reaches a critical personal threshold.

TABLE 33–3. Suicide prevalence among patients with illnesses compared with general population

Diagnosis	Suicide prevalence
Cancer	15–20 times greater
Cerebrovascular accident	2–6 times greater
Multiple sclerosis	14 times greater
Musculoskeletal diseases (excluding rheumatoid arthritis)	No greater prevalence
Rheumatoid arthritis	2–3 times greater
Spinal cord injury	15 times greater

Source. Adapted from Whitlock 1986.

Mania

Patients with previous diagnoses of bipolar disorder are at greatest risk for developing mania or hypomania after a CNS event or injury. Mania is relatively rare in patients with head injury (Jorge et al. 1993; Reiss et al. 1987; Starkstein et al. 1987), stroke (Fujikawa et al. 1995), and other CNS disorders, with the exception of early classic reports of euphoric mood or manic syndromes in patients with multiple sclerosis (e.g., Cottrell and Wilson 1926). This has been substantiated by more recent studies suggesting a prevalence of 6%–26% (Lishman 1987). Schiffer et al. (1986) found a prevalence of bipolar disorder in patients with multiple sclerosis that was twice that of individuals in the general population, but this study did not control for the use of steroids. Steroids often precipitate or exacerbate mania in patients with multiple sclerosis (S. Minden, personal communication, July 1990).

Cognitive and Neurobehavioral Problems

Cognitive and neurobehavioral deficits occur in 25%–64% of patients undergoing rehabilitation (Caplan 1987; Luxenberg and Feigenbaum 1986). Indeed, many rehabilitation programs have special protocols for the rehabilitation of patients with traumatic brain injury with accompanying neurobehavioral problems. Neuropsychiatric disorders such as delirium, dementia, and secondary personality disorder are seen. Delirium is less common in rehabilitation than in acute care settings because delirium is usually an exclusion criterion for admission except for patients with head injury. Cognitive problems encountered in rehabilitation medicine include problems with memory, vision, intellect, neglect, apraxia, aprosody, aphasia, agnosia, distractibility, impulsivity, poor judgment and safety awareness, and orientation difficulties. Unrecognized cognitive and neurobehavioral problems may be mislabeled as poor motivation (Goodstein 1984).

Careful assessment of cognitive factors is essential (Caplan 1987; Gordon et al. 1985). The need is obvious following head injury and stroke but also should be considered in patients with other disorders. For example, occult head injury occurs in up to 50% of the patients with spinal cord injury (Wilmot et al. 1985), and cognitive deficits are related to a significant number of outcome variables in spinal cord injury (Davidoff et al. 1992). Although neuropsychologists should, ideally, be a part of a psychiatric consultation-liaison team, such positions are seldom paid for (Lipowski 1991). Fortunately, in rehabilitation medicine, diagnosis-related group (DRG)–exempt, CARF (Certified Acute Rehabilitation Facility), and CORF (Certified Outpatient Rehabilitation Facility) accreditations all require adequate neuropsychology services for both assessment and cognitive rehabilitation efforts.

Adjustment and Coping Problems

Most patients in rehabilitation settings cope well, even when they have major and disfiguring injuries (Bowden et al. 1980). Nevertheless, consultation-liaison psychiatrists are commonly asked to see patients whom staff members designate as having adjustment problems. These difficulties may represent a number of clinical entities and situations: 1) DSM-IV-TR adjustment disorder; 2) major depression, clinical anxiety disorder, or other major psychiatric disorders that have been misidentified by staff as adjustment problems; 3) cognitive problems (e.g., receptive aphasia or aprosody); 4) reactions by staff to the particular problem the patient is facing; and 5) adjustment problems because the disability prevents the use of personally preferred coping strategies. For example, a patient who had previously exercised to cope with stress will be prevented from doing so if he or she has quadriplegia. This patient then faces both the stress of his or her condition

and the need to establish new coping mechanisms. Conversely, a patient who is paraplegic who exercised before the injury may adapt well, actively engage in physical therapy, and build compensatory upper body strength.

Differences in personality, temperament, and coping vary in the ways that they affect rehabilitation outcome. Skarin (K. Skarin, personal communication, December 1981) showed that ego strength, self-assurance, self-sufficiency, and internal control are each associated with better stroke rehabilitation outcomes.

Etiology differences—congenital, trauma, medical disorder, or cancer—as well as course, prognosis, and age at onset of the disability can affect physical, emotional, social, and occupational adjustment in unique ways. Congenital impairments that are present very early in life require different clinical approaches by the rehabilitation team. Never having walked is very different from suddenly losing the ability to so do, for example (Featherstone 1980).

Conditions seen in rehabilitation have varying clinical courses. Some are associated with fluctuating activity (e.g., arthritis), some are associated with progression (e.g., amyotrophic lateral sclerosis, multiple sclerosis), and some are life-threatening (e.g., aggressive brain tumor). The patient's and family's understanding, experience, and perceptions of and reactions to expected course and prognosis all must be assessed.

Many patients struggle with the need to use assistive devices. Concerns include operation, utility, social contexts, consequences, and cultural meanings (Gitlin et al. 1998). Effective rehabilitation requires that families and other support systems be involved. Improvement is not always obvious, and progress is sometimes followed by steps backward. Patients can have difficulty maintaining the commitment and drive required of them, or the pace of the rehabilitation program may be much faster than a given individual is used to. Adjustment may entail stress for the individual and family beyond that associated specifically with physical limitations. The financial stress of health care costs, loss of work, and changes in contribution to household management can be stressful and require active family involvement during the rehabilitation process.

Body Image Changes

The report from the Group for the Advancement of Psychiatry (1993) entitled *Caring for People With Physical Impairment: The Journey Back* noted that conditions with body disfigurement require considerable adjustment of "body image." We all have a body image, a highly individualized, subjective, and integrated sense of what we look like and what we feel about ourselves (Group for the Advancement of Psychiatry, Committee on Handicaps 1993). Rehabilitation staff and psychiatric consultants may be confronted by malformed bodies, which can trigger strong and painful reactions. These reactions must be monitored because they provide information and so that inappropriate responses to the patient can be prevented.

Changes in body image and other emotional aspects of catastrophic events can trigger significant boundary and vulnerability issues and lead to primitive, unrealistic patient fantasies about how caregivers should relate. For example, patients can split staff into "good" and "bad." Families can be divided and compete with staff to be the "good" caregiver. These regressive, splitting, boundary, responsibility, powerlessness, and "whose life is it anyway?" issues are well described in the Group for the Advancement of Psychiatry (1993) report. Disabled patients are acutely aware of their bodies and their disorders. Many legitimately complain of not being listened to or of being written off as hypochondriacs or somatizers. For example, many patients with postpolio syndrome have inappropriately received a previous diagnosis of hypochondriasis (Halstead and Wiechers 1985).

Three particular body image changes frequently seen in rehabilitation deserve special consideration. First, 30%–70% of the patients with amputations will experience a phantom limb syndrome (Ehde et al. 2000; Gerhardt et al. 1984; Katz 1992), which persists in some patients for up to 25 years (Katz 1992). Etiological mechanisms are not well understood, and treatments have a low success rate (Katz 1992). Second, in our experience, patients with hand and finger amputations present special problems. These patients present with anxiety, apprehension, and obsessive ruminations that can be significantly out of proportion to the circumstance. They have difficulty when others look at their hands and often have sexual difficulties related to loss of, or changes in, touch. Patients with hand amputations following mangling injuries are especially likely to have psychological complications and pain from neuronal damage. Third, "hemineglect" is a neurologically based body image problem seen particularly in patients after a nondominant parietal stroke. In severe cases, these patients do not recognize the left side of their body, have major problems with safety (e.g., they will allow their arm to dangle in wheelchair spokes), do not recognize their deficits, are impulsive, and have anosognosia. This combination can be easily misinterpreted as a psychiatric symptom.

Nonadherence to Treatment

One manifestation of poor adjustment is nonadherence to treatment. Bradley (1985) reported nonadherence rates of 22%–67% for medications and 38%–66% for physical therapy instructions in patients with rheumatoid arthritis, for example. Factors predicting lack of adherence in this study included type of medication, duration of illness, disease severity, and patient beliefs about efficacy. Similar patterns are seen in patients with other disorders.

Loss and Mourning

Loss, mourning, and stages of recovery are historically important concepts in rehabilitation medicine (Group for the Advancement of Psychiatry, Committee on Handicaps 1993; Krueger 1984; Wortman and Silver 1989). However, disability is not death! Disabling conditions provide a different set of challenges, and every step of recovery poses new challenges. Research indicates that specific stages do not occur in adjustment to spinal cord injury (Craig et al. 1994; S. Harasymin, personal communication, August 1981). We have argued that although the "staff may be motivated to seek staged mourning models by their desire to have specific interventions to handle difficult situations, the application of stages of mourning in the context of disability can lead to premature closure and a failure to fully appreciate the course of any given individual with a disability" (Bishop 1980, p. 7).

Consultation-liaison psychiatrists are sometimes asked to see patients who are "in denial." Individuals undergoing rehabilitation at times must cope with overwhelming anxiety. Especially during early stages of rehabilitation, a balance between denial and reality is required (Caplan and Shechter 1987; Group for the Advancement of Psychiatry, Committee on Handicaps 1993). Unfortunately, the term *denial* has been neither clearly operationalized nor well studied in rehabilitation, although it has been applied in a number of ways (Table 33–4).

TABLE 33–4. Presentations of denial in patients undergoing rehabilitation

In the rehabilitation setting, denial may present as

The patient's unconscious defense mechanism to contain and bind significantly threatening conflict

A disagreement occurring when the patient is consciously and clearly aware of circumstances and consequences but chooses a course that is different from what staff members believe is best

The patient's failure to appreciate left-sided deficits and left "hemi-neglect," as can occur when the patient has right-hemisphere insult

Noncompliant and difficult behavior

Behavior Problems

Behavior problems seen include aggression, yelling out, and inappropriate sexual behavior. These behaviors can be expressions of depression, cognitive dysfunction, adjustment problems, anxiety, or personality problems. A few disruptive individuals can use up resources and disturb therapeutic alliances. In general, fewer problems occur on units that have an experienced staff and a well-integrated psychosocial program that includes consultation-liaison psychiatry.

Gallagher (1980) noted that aggression is not a diagnosis but rather a part of the human condition and is often a symptom of a more serious problem. Aggressive behavior can be categorized as active or passive. Active aggression may lead staff to 1) punish the patient, 2) capitulate to the patient's demands, or 3) withdraw from important aspects of care. Unfortunately, however, these staff reactions may paradoxically escalate the aggressive behavior. Passive forms of aggression include inaction, interfering actions, dependency, displacement, and projections. Passive aggression also can lead to a variety of unhelpful staff responses.

Some patients undergoing rehabilitation may be identified by staff as splitting, noncompliant, unmotivated, dependent, needy, or otherwise "difficult." Crewe (1980a) cautioned that 1) these labels are often based on the values and perceptions of health care providers and not the behaviors of the patient; 2) the range of behaviors shown by patients is quite broad; 3) the same behavior may elicit different reactions and descriptions from different health care personnel; and 4) a person may behave one way in an acute care setting, another way in a rehabilitation unit, and still another way in an outpatient setting. Vanderpool (1984) described six concepts that are useful in addressing behavior problems among "difficult" patients (Table 33–5).

There are many conceptual approaches to rehabilitation unit behavior problems, including team processes, special interviewing techniques, and psychological assessment methods (Group for the Advancement of Psychiatry, Committee on Handicaps 1993; Guenther et al. 1993; Vanderpool 1984). Psychiatric consultants can most effectively address character and behavior problems by assisting rehabilitation staff 1) to operationally define the "difficult behavior"; 2) to know when, where, and in whose presence it is most likely to occur; and 3) to clarify expected responses to specific staff and family interventions. This approach works best when it incorporates all staff members who work regularly with the patient; a careful and integrated behavioral analysis; and consideration of adjustment, personality, defense mechanism, and cultural contributions to the problem (Brooks 1984; Crewe and Krause 1987; Rosenthal 1987; Trieschman 1980).

TABLE 33–5. Concepts for managing rehabilitation in "difficult patients"[a]

Recognize neuropsychiatric syndromes early.[a]

Make a careful, complete, and inclusive diagnosis.[a]

Know what may or may not work.[a]

Ask "Can the patient be helped?" (Is status quo all that may be expected?)[a]

Know the patient mix on the unit and the effect on staff working with them.[a]

Avoid inappropriate "overhelping" that may do more harm than good for the patient or treatment team.[a]

Work toward prevention—primary, secondary, and tertiary.[b]

Staff members should strive for an understanding of
- Themselves
- Their specific treatment center
- The effect of program on different types of patients[b]

Source. [a]Vanderpool 1984; [b]Crewe 1980a.

A range of troublesome externalized (seductiveness, obscene language, and aggression) and internalized (denial and repression) sexual behavior problems may occur among patients undergoing rehabilitation (Crewe 1980b). These difficulties should be addressed in an open manner, and firm limits should be set with patients. Sexual issues should be addressed with all patients. Treatment should be offered to patients and partners who desire it.

Anxiety

Although anxiety in rehabilitation settings has not been well studied, it is common. Clinically significant anxiety syndromes have been reported in 21% of rheumatoid arthritis patients (Chandarana et al. 1987; Kennedy and Rogers 2000), 16% of spinal cord injury patients (Scivoletto et al. 1997), 10%–37% of stroke patients (Bond et al. 1998; Castillo et al. 1995; Gustafson et al. 1995), hip fracture patients (Bond et al. 1998, Burvill et al. 1995b), and traumatic brain injury patients. The paucity of information about anxiety in rehabilitation is surprising because, in our experience, aspects of anxiety, fears, apprehension, and worry are very common, are underrecognized, and are the underlying cause of many behavior difficulties. Assessment of anxiety requires a careful formulation; the challenge is to understand the patient and to assess her or his situation.

Anxiety may present as a symptom or a disorder. DSM-IV-TR primary anxiety disorders—including phobias, panic disorders, obsessive-compulsive disorder, social phobia, general anxiety disorder, posttraumatic stress disorder (PTSD), and acute stress disorder—are all seen. DSM-IV-TR anxiety disorder resulting from toxic or general medical conditions may follow traumatic brain injury, stroke (Starkstein et al. 1990), and brain tumor. The serious falls, accidents, and gunshot wounds that cause multiple trauma, head injuries, and spinal cord injuries can lead to acute stress disorder or PTSD. The use of benzodiazepines for anxiety disorders must be weighed against the potential effects on ability to function. Catastrophic accidents or falls following stroke can lead to phobias concerning heights, falling, or closed spaces. Apprehension of falling is common. It becomes apparent when patients are learning to transfer from bed to wheelchair or are beginning to learn to walk and is seldom associated with the levels of avoidance or physiologic symptoms required to warrant a diagnosis of phobia. However, this apprehension frequently does interfere with rehabilitation therapies. Patients also may have unrecognized claustrophobic responses to closed bedside curtains, halos, traction devices, and wheelchairs.

Despite their significant personal distress, it is surprising that patients often do not easily volunteer information about anxiety and phobias. Patients seem to talk about these issues only if they are brought up by others and if it is suggested that these are "normal" reactions. In general, these problems respond well to appropriate and brief supportive psychotherapy and relaxation training.

Patients with Guillain-Barré syndrome also may develop anxiety, especially when progression of the other disease leads to respirator use. Patients with Guillain-Barré syndrome often develop a "terror" associated with the progressive loss of function, their sense of impending death, and the slow recovery. They become hypervigilant for any symptoms that may indicate a returning paralysis, and this can be reinforced by the unpredictable myalgic pain that frequently occurs during recovery. Generally, they resist use of medications because they fear that it may upset their recovery. They respond well to reframing their experience as "normal," to imagery, and to relaxation and pain control techniques that improve their sense of autonomy.

Pervasive anxiety also may be seen in patients who have coronary artery bypass graft or carotid endarterectomy surgery and sustain an unexpected intraoperative or postoperative stroke. Patients with cognitive deficits can experience catastrophic anxiety when their deficits are confronted; this anxiety may initiate avoidance behavior (e.g., patients with aphasia may attempt to avoid speech therapy). Family members' personal anxieties and/or responses to the patient can also escalate the patient's anxiety.

Physical, occupational, and speech therapists see patients daily and can help to identify increasing anxiety and the specific situations in which it occurs. Anxiety occurring in only one therapy setting is likely to be related to a particular staff member or specific aspects of the therapy. Anxiety that occurs across all therapies suggests an anxiety syndrome. Input from family members is also important in both the assessment of anxiety and the identification of responses that typically calm the patient.

Substance-Related Problems

The epidemiology of alcohol and drug abuse among patients in rehabilitation settings has not been well studied. This is surprising because alcohol and drug abuse can cause and/or be disabling conditions and/or be a maladaptive adjustment to such disabilities (Greenwood 1984). Premorbid alcohol and drug abuse are major contributors to accidents resulting in traumatic brain injury. Alcohol abuse is also a significant premorbid risk factor for hemorrhagic stroke. Among patients with spinal cord injuries, 24% report missing prescription medications (Roth et al. 1992), 21%–60% have a history of alcohol use disorder, and 30%–60% have a history of drug abuse (O'Donnell et al. 1981/1982; M.E. Young et al. 1995). In addition, marijuana may decrease spasticity after spinal cord injury, reinforcing its use (J. Malec, personal communication, October 1981). It is perhaps surprising then that two studies reported that marijuana use in patients with spinal cord injury is lower than in the general population (Kirubakaran et al. 1986; M.E. Young et al. 1995). It has been reported that 78% of the patients undergoing rehabilitation who have a history of premorbid drug or alcohol use resume use late in rehabilitation or a few months after discharge (Donahue et al. 1986; Gorelick and Kelly 1992; O'Donnell et al. 1981/1982). However, a more recent report suggested a potential window of readiness to change maladaptive substance use behaviors an average of 5 weeks after spinal cord injury (Bombardier and Rimmele 1998). Pain medication abuse and dependence are most likely to occur among patients who are already predisposed. These patients may arrive in the rehabilitation setting receiving large quantities of narcotics after major surgical procedures and require a tapering of their medication regimen.

Accurate identification of premorbid substance use is crucial, especially in patients with trauma, head injury, spinal cord injury, or hemorrhagic stroke. Patients admit drug abuse more easily to physicians and psychologists than to professionals in other disciplines (W. Bilkey, M. Hove, S. Brake, personal communication, October 1981). Traditional alcohol and drug abuse programs have difficulty handling patients with a major disability and, to an even greater extent, patients with cognitive deficits. Fortunately, some rehabilitation programs are beginning to develop specialized substance disorders treatment programs.

Sleep Problems

Sleep problems are common among patients undergoing rehabilitation (Kryger et al. 1989). Hypersomnia is usually the result of problems of arousal or neuropsychiatric effects of medications. Insomnia is often caused by a primary or secondary psychiatric disorder, neurological disorder, or exacerbation of long-standing primary insomnia. Stroke patients have an increase in apnea and fragmented sleep (Mohsenin and Valor 1995). The same is true for traumatic brain injury (Webster et al. 2001) and spinal cord injury (Burns et al. 2000). Several other problems, including pain, opioid dependence, nighttime opioid withdrawal symptoms, sedative-hypnotic tolerance, the activating quality of some antidepressants, urinary tract problems, and incontinence, also may interfere with sleep. As a group, patients with spinal cord injury have proportionately less Stage IV sleep than do other persons. This lack of sleep may contribute to spasticity problems, possibly triggered by pathophysiologic mechanisms similar to those seen in patients with fibromyalgia (Bishop 1980).

Sleep charts, detailed sleep histories, and sleep monitoring systems are all helpful. In cases in which a diagnosis is difficult, 24-hour portable encephalographic (EEG) monitoring should be considered. This technology can help differentiate among sleep deprivation, brain syndromes, seizures, and other neuropsychiatric disorders.

Nonpharmacological nursing interventions incorporating back rubs, warm drinks, and relaxation tapes assist older patients with sleep (McDowell et al. 1998).

Pain

Pain of various types is common among patients in rehabilitation settings (Fey and Williamson-Kirkland 1987; Kennedy et al. 1997; Steger and Brockway 1980; Steger et al. 1980; Tunks and Merskey 1980; Turner et al. 2001). Pain during rehabilitation occurs for many reasons, including postoperative pain, painful procedures, central pain, frozen shoulders from stroke, neuropathies, myalgias, phantom pain, and sore and tender muscles from physical therapy workouts.

Patients who are dependent on narcotic analgesics pose special problems. It is useful to have the patient rate his or her pain on an open 10-point scale (0 = no pain and

10 = worst possible pain imaginable). Sidney Schnoll (personal communication, 1998) suggested that the goals of pain management be reframed by using the scale to determine the number for the level of pain that the patient can live with yet function. A patient might say that his or her pain is 8 now but that he or she could tolerate and function with a level of 5. In other words, the pain treatment goal is reframed for the patient to decrease perceived pain to a tolerable level that allows adequate function rather than to eliminate pain completely. Reaching a goal of improved function is more practical and has a higher likelihood of success. It is also helpful at times to have the patient keep 24-hour diaries of major pain episodes and circumstances. Charting for a few days is usually sufficient to establish an understanding of the pain pattern. The patient's medication use should not be challenged immediately. Most patients are surprised to learn that pain itself can be a medication withdrawal symptom. The process of education and reframing helps to develop an active collaboration for a tapering and detoxification program.

Sexual Dysfunction

Although sexual activity is a vital part of normal life, society tends to ignore the sexuality of both elderly and disabled individuals. From 25% to 55% of men with spinal cord injury cannot achieve an erection (Ducharme 1987; Trieschman 1980). When a patient with a spinal cord injury does have an erection, it may not be sufficient to engage in intercourse, or those who are capable of having intercourse may not attempt it (Vrey and Henggeler 1987). Ejaculation and conception are possible for most men with spinal cord injuries with the assistance of special techniques. In women, spinal cord injury may result in an inability to experience orgasm; women with such injuries may see themselves as less attractive and desirable to their partners (Vrey and Henggeler 1987). Women with spinal cord injuries respond to audiovisual stimulation in a manner similar to that of able-bodied women but require manual stimulation for reflex genital vasocongestion (Sipski et al. 1995). They report more dysfunction postinjury, but their feelings about sex and its importance are unaffected (Harrison et al. 1995).

Sexual dysfunction also may occur in patients with other rehabilitation diagnoses. For example, sexual activity decreased in 46% of the patients with rheumatoid arthritis after disease onset (Deyo et al. 1982). Sexual dysfunction is reported in 50% of women and 75% of men with multiple sclerosis, regardless of mobility (Valleroy and Kraft 1984). Studies also have documented a decline in sexual activity after stroke (Bray et al. 1981;

Fugl-Meyer and Jaasko 1980). Although sexual activity in patients with stroke is approximately half as frequent in those who were active before the stroke, drive and desire remain relatively unaffected (Bray et al. 1981). As dependence on others for assistance increases, sexuality decreases. Fugl-Meyer and Jaasko (1980) reported that touch sensation impairment is more of a factor than motor dysfunction. A report that there is no association between sexual and hormonal dysfunction in patients with stroke (Sjogren et al. 1983) also is applicable for most other disabilities and suggests that problems are more often neurological, vascular, urological, or psychological in origin.

Despite these findings, patients undergoing rehabilitation and their partners generally do not receive sexual counseling (Sjogren et al. 1983). Ironically, however, patients and partners usually welcome frank and open discussion about their sexuality and report feeling better after these discussions. They may prefer that a physician rather than some other type of health professional (e.g., nurse, psychologist) do the counseling, if possible (Florian 1983). This neglected area should always be part of a psychiatric consultation in rehabilitation units. Clinicians should encourage patients to discuss sexuality issues and offer sexuality teaching and counseling (Ducharme 1987). Staff and patients can benefit from Sexuality Attitude Reassessment (SAR) programs. Information about these and related issues can be obtained from several sexuality and disability centers listed by Ducharme (1987, p. 436), as well as in a special issue of *NeuroRehabilitation* (Sipski 2000).

FAMILIES AND CAREGIVERS

Managed care and fiscal pressures cause patients to return home from hospitals sooner than ever before, which increases pressure on families and caregivers. Indeed, the family home has become an unfunded second step-down rehabilitation unit. Families and caregivers are affected by disabling conditions in a family member and significantly affect the outcome. Most patients have one primary person who provides most of the assistance for them (i.e., their primary caregiver). Caregivers can provide a great deal of information and can assist by following through on instructions, particularly when care reverts to the outpatient setting. Families and caregivers provide information that is crucial for accurate diagnosis, notice changes in behavior, and often have an intuitive sense of why the patient has a response to a particular situation. Caregivers appear to experience similar degrees of burden and similar levels of psychological morbidity

whether dealing with disabilities or dementias (Gwyther and George 1986; Lichtenberg and Gibbons 1993). Attention must be paid, therefore, to caregiver mood, function, family life, and health. Consultation for a patient undergoing rehabilitation often involves psychiatric assessment and treatment of a spouse, partner, or other caregiver.

Most home care for disabled patients is in fact provided by partners or adult children (Lichtenberg and Gibbons 1993). Partners who serve as caregivers generally receive less structural assistance (e.g., skilled nursing care workers, homemakers) than do adult children caregivers (Pruchno 1990); they also have poorer health (Cantor 1983). As many as 50% of caregivers can expect to develop major depression (Schulz et al. 1990). Many employed caregivers must quit their jobs to provide care (Brocklehurst et al. 1981). Cultural caregiving expectations are different based on gender. For example, a man's reluctance to assist a disabled female partner with toileting is likely to be respected; a woman's reluctance to assist a male partner is likely to be scorned (Lichtenberg and Gibbons 1993). Optimal care in the home is more likely when there is a significant-other relationship that functions effectively and when a partner/caregiver is knowledgeable about the disorder and is not depressed (R.L. Evans et al. 1991). Screening the family caregiver for psychiatric problems is, therefore, a crucial part of psychiatric consultation with a patient undergoing rehabilitation (Bishop and Miller 1988).

Unfortunately, most families have had at least one bad experience with a health care team, and the families may take offers of psychosocial assessment and assistance as an indication of deficiencies on their part (Gonzalez et al. 1989). Each patient's family is unique and requires an individualized approach. The literature on families and caregivers is more extensive and helpful than is generally appreciated. Table 33–6 summarizes research findings on how families function following the onset of disability in one of its members. After the onset of a disability, families tend to lock onto a fixed pattern for adapting that they later find difficult to change. This pattern results in developmental and other family issues being "put on the shelf." As a result, the "disability" becomes a member of the family and "takes over," much like a "2-year-old tyrant" (Gonzalez et al. 1989).

COMPETENCY

The issues of competency are addressed elsewhere in this text. In rehabilitation, the therapists and nursing staff usually have a much clearer view of the patient's capacity

---

TABLE 33–6.   Summary of family functioning and disability research findings

In the general population, 25% of families function at a level that places them at risk for significant family problems if a family member becomes disabled.[a]

Many families function well despite a member's disability.[a]

Family functioning during the acute crisis does not predict later functioning, which is similar to what is found in nonclinical community samples.[b]

The relations between family functioning and other variables in one diagnostic group do not necessarily apply in another diagnostic group (i.e., findings and observations cannot be generalized).[a]

Families have more difficulty dealing with cognitive dysfunction than with the loss of other functions.[a]

The presence of a family, the patient's perception of a significant family role to return to, and the family's support of the rehabilitation process positively affect outcomes.[b]

Families require education and follow-up.[c] Families who receive education have reduced anxiety and cooperate better with the health care team.[b]

Families with a disabled member face changes in roles, leisure, activities, and health statuses of other members.[b]

Depression is common among patients undergoing rehabilitation. Depression has a negative effect on rehabilitation patients' families, which is worsened if patients also have a medical disorder.[d,e]

Source.   [a]Bishop and Miller 1988; [b]Bishop et al. 1984; [c]R.L. Evans et al. 1988; [d]Keitner et al. 1989; [e]Keitner et al. 1991.

---

to function independently and the risk factors depending on different areas and the areas in which they cannot. An occupational therapist may have assessed the patient's kitchen safety and observed him or her burning items on the stove; the therapist also may have seen the patient getting up from a wheelchair that is not locked or being unsafe on stairs. The psychiatrist does not determine the patient's physical safety but rather the patient's appreciation of risks, options, and the consequences of each.

STAFF PROBLEMS

In general, staff problems arise out of situations that confront and threaten a staff member's sense of professional and personal self (Crewe 1980a; Gans 1987; Group for the Advancement of Psychiatry, Committee on Handicaps 1993; Gunther 1987; Romano 1984). Professionals in rehabilitation are dedicated, motivated, effective, and committed to maximizing recovery even though it is slow and uncertain. As a result, they need to experience a sense of effectiveness and competency from the help that they provide in order to preserve their professional identities. Staff problems often arise when events, circumstances, colleagues, and especially patients lead them to feel inefficient or ineffective. It is within the intimacy of the staff-patient relationship and the need to be successful that the greatest staff problems arise. Staff members may sometimes respond to perceptions of real or

anticipated failure with behaviors that escalate the very problems that concern them. When consultation-liaison psychiatrists are well known and respected by the rehabilitation team, they have the opportunity to help staff members to better understand their own reactions and those of their patients, as well as to develop a better repertoire of adaptive interventions.

TREATMENT AND MANAGEMENT

Medical Interventions

Medical interventions include the usual attention to diagnosis and management of electrolyte imbalance, sequelae of surgical procedures, infections, medication side effects, and other correctable medical causes for primary and secondary psychiatric symptoms and syndromes. Rehabilitation-related guidelines from the Agency for Health Care Policy and Research cover urinary incontinence, pain, pressure sores, stroke rehabilitation, depression in primary care, and other topics.[1]

Clinical Psychopharmacology

Psychotropic medications can effectively treat primary and secondary psychiatric disorders in patients undergoing rehabilitation, and new approaches are advancing rapidly (Cook 1984; McLean et al. 1993; Murray 1987; Silver and Yudofsky 1993). However, medication can be a

---

[1] Each guideline is provided as a book, a physician's guide, and a consumer pamphlet. These books provide a succinct update in each area and are available from the Department of Health and Human Services, Public Health Service, Agency for Health Care Policy and Research, Executive Office Center, 2101 East Jefferson Street, Suite 501, Rockville, MD 20852.

double-edged sword. Just as in other consultation-liaison settings, some side effects can worsen specific functions in patients who are already compromised. A report suggested that impaired motor recovery is seen in stroke patients who receive commonly used medications (e.g., haloperidol, α_1- and α_2-receptor antagonists, and benzodiazepines) that have been shown to impair recovery in animal stroke models (Goldstein 1995). Interactions between psychiatric and other medications must be monitored (Norman and Burrows 1991). These interactions are particularly important because rehabilitation patients are often taking several medications. Table 33–7 shows various medications and their beneficial uses and potential adverse effects in rehabilitation settings.

Most psychotropic medications should be used in lower-than-usual dosages in patients with brain injuries (Finklestein et al. 1987; Goodstein 1984). For example, Finklestein and associates (1987) suggested that dosages equivalent to 70 mg/day of imipramine are effective for treating major depression in patients who have a CNS disorder. There are no recommendations for the use of selective serotonin reuptake inhibitors (SSRIs), but our experience is that lower-than-usual dosages are effective and that "usual" doses can be associated with an increased incidence of side effects in patients with CNS dysfunction.

Studies on the treatment of depression in stroke are opening new horizons and are worthy of special attention. In a study comparing the effects of nortryptiline, fluoxetine, and placebo on poststroke recovery, Robinson et al. (2000) treated both depressed and nondepressed subjects to assess whether activities of daily living (ADLs), levels of cognition, social functioning, or mood were improved. Nortryptiline outperformed fluoxetine and placebo in treating poststroke depression, anxiety, and ADLs. Neither medication had an effect on cognition or social functioning. The authors correctly pointed out that the titration of nortryptiline from 25 to 100 mg/day and of fluoxetine from 10 to 40 mg/day may have influenced the results. In a subsequent report, Kimura et al. (2000) indicated that nortyptiline produced improvements in cognition for poststroke patients if they were depressed and their depression remitted with treatment. The authors posited that poststroke depression leads to a "dementia of depression."

Patients undergoing rehabilitation may have been taking narcotic analgesics for weeks or months. Consultation-liaison psychiatrists may be asked to help taper patients off their pain medications. A calculated and gradual narcotic withdrawal protocol is essential. The psychiatrist establishes baseline data, describes the protocol to the patient, obtains his or her agreement to initiate it, and carefully briefs the treatment team. Narcotic medication doses are totaled for the preceding 24–48 hours and converted to morphine sulfate equivalents (for patients who are not allergic to morphine, in whom liquid hydromorphone can be used). Morphine dosages are given every 3–4 hours around the clock. Some clinicians use methadone instead of morphine. The patient should be informed that it is necessary to stay ahead of the pain and to prevent nighttime rebound. Whenever possible, morphine sulfate concentrate is used and given in 60 cc of a caffeine-free cola beverage to mask the dosage volume and color. The psychiatrist should explain that this is necessary because counting pills is part of the problem and that decreasing by one pill decreases the dose substantially, whereas the concentrate can be decreased by very small amounts spread out over time. After pain is controlled, the dosage should be slowly tapered, at a rate of about 10%/day. It is essential that the patient not be told the details of the taper schedule. If a patient refuses the tapering protocol, significant addiction, cognitive disorder, primary psychiatric disorder, and personality disorder should be considered.

Patients require a great deal of emotional support from staff and family, especially toward the end of the tapering process. Relaxation and imagery pain control techniques are potentially effective. There should be agreement with other treating physicians that the psychiatrist will control all pain medication orders during the protocol. The caffeine-free cola beverage is continued at regular dosing times (including nighttime) for up to 48 hours after the final morphine dose. At the end of the tapering period, the patient should be congratulated and the implications processed. Relaxation techniques and biofeedback should be continued. Sometimes pain does not abate with narcotic tapering or will increase slightly near the end of the taper. Other forms of treatment such as ibuprofen and other nonnarcotic analgesics, as well as antidepressants or anticonvulsants when appropriate, are then useful (see Table 33–7). (For further information on psychopharmacology, see Chapter 42, this volume.)

Psychotherapy

Psychotherapy during rehabilitation must consider the patient's cognitive, attention, and concentration limitations; the patient's personal adjustment; the ward milieu; staff issues; and the patient's schedule. The consultation-liaison psychiatrist must coordinate and integrate psychotherapy with other aspects of the rehabilitation team's treatment plan.

TABLE 33–7. Psychopharmacological medications: unique indications, benefits, and risks in patients undergoing rehabilitation

Medication	Unique indications	Specific benefits	Risks in patients undergoing rehabilitation
Analgesics			
Methadone	Pain; opiate tapering	Long half-life	Anticholinergic effects; tolerance; withdrawal; sedation
Morphine sulfate concentrate	Pain; opiate tapering	Can be given via nasogastric tube; can be mixed with juices to disguise dosage	Anticholinergic effects; tolerance; withdrawal; sedation
NSAIDs	Inflammation and bone pain	No tolerance, withdrawal, sedation, or anticholinergic effects	Gastrointestinal distress
Anticonvulsants			
Carbamazepine	Seizure disorder; trigeminal neuralgia[a], peripheral neuropathy pain[b], rapid-cycling mood syndrome; secondary mania[b]	Partial seizures; seizure treatment and prophylaxis	Bone marrow suppression; sedation for some patients; hepatic enzyme induction
Phenytoin	Seizure disorder	Seizure treatment and prophylaxis	Ataxia with drug toxicity; hepatic enzyme induction
Valproic acid	Same as carbamazepine except for peripheral neuropathic pain[b]	Partial seizures; seizure treatment and prophylaxis	Hepatotoxicity[b]
Gabapentin	Chronic pain in spinal cord injury[c]	No metabolism/processing; medication passed directly; minimal/no risk of drug-drug interaction	Sedation in some patients
Antidepressants	Aggression[b], primary or secondary depression (e.g., poststroke depression)[d]		
Amitriptyline	Insomnia; peripheral neuropathic pain[e], mood lability[b], cancer pain[a], fibrositis pain[a], poor appetite	Helps with sleep; stimulates appetite; effective with patients who are incontinent	Anticholinergic effects[b]; oversedation; lowered seizure threshold; paradoxical agitation in patients with CNS disorders; hypotension; heart block; tachycardia
Desipramine	Pain,[a] including neuropathic pain[e]	Secondary amine tricyclic	Lowers seizure threshold; heart block
Doxepin	Pain; insomnia; poor appetite	Helps with sleep; stimulates appetite; effective analgesic[a]; H$_2$-receptor blockade in patients with gastrointestinal distress	Anticholinergic effects; oversedation; lowers seizure threshold; hypotension; heart block; tachycardia
Imipramine	Spasticity	Secondary amine tricyclic	Lowers seizure threshold; heart block
MAOIs	Pain[a]	No anticholinergic activity	Hypotension; hypertensive crisis
Nortriptyline	Labile affect; pathological laughing and crying[f]; poststroke depression[g], pain[a], ADLs[h], cognition[i]	As a secondary amine, tricyclic is not overly sedating and has minimal anticholinergic effects	Lowers seizure threshold; heart block
SSRIs	Mood lability[b], pain[a], body dysmorphia	Lack of anticholinergic activity; not sedating; sertraline metabolized by conjugation	Potential for extrapyramidal side effects, dystonia, and sexual dysfunction; may be associated with a discontinuation syndrome
Trazodone	Insomnia; agitation; pain[a]	No anticholinergic activity	Sedation; priapism; hypotension
Antiparkinsonian medications			
Amantadine	Parkinson's disease; fatigue in patients with multiple sclerosis[b,j]	No anticholinergic effects	Anxiety; agitation; psychosis
Benztropine	Parkinson's disease	Not as likely as amantadine to cause agitation or psychosis	Memory and mood changes, especially in elderly patients[j]

TABLE 33–7. Psychopharmacological medications: unique indications, benefits, and risks in patients undergoing rehabilitation (*continued*)

Medication	Unique indications	Specific benefits	Risks in patients undergoing rehabilitation
Benzodiazepines			
Clonazepam	Myoclonus; partial seizure disorder	Can be used for tapering patients off alprazolam	Tolerance; withdrawal; impaired short-term memory; sedation
Diazepam	Aggression[b], muscle tension; spasticity	Muscle relaxant; antispasticity effect	Tolerance; withdrawal; impaired short-term memory; sedation; paradoxical rage[b]
Lorazepam	Aggression[b], acute agitation in delirium	Short-acting; metabolized by hepatic conjugation (can be used for alcohol withdrawal in patients with hepatic impairment)	Tolerance; withdrawal; impaired short-term memory; sedation; accumulation in patients with renal impairment
β-Blockers	Chronic or recurrent agitation[b,k,l]	May help patients with chronic anxiety	4–6 weeks' latency of response for agitation[b]; hypotension; depression[a]
Buspirone	Anxiety[b], agitation in patients with closed-head injury[m,n], agitation in patients with major depression[b]	No tolerance or withdrawal; lacks benzodiazepines' memory effects; nonsedating	3–4 weeks' latency of response[b]
Lithium	Mania[b]; aggression[b]	Does not induce hepatic enzymes	Tremor; gastrointestinal symptoms; ataxia
Neuroleptics	Psychosis and psychosis-related aggression[b]		Extrapyramidal signs; dystonia; akathisia; tardive dyskinesia
Haloperidol	Agitation following head injury[o], experience with intravenous use	Little anticholinergic activity; effective analgesic adjuvant	Possible impaired recovery following stroke[b,p]
Thioridazine	Agitation; delirium; insomnia	Helps agitated patients sleep	Oversedation; anticholinergic effects; hypotension; short-term memory impairment; must be used in very small doses
Atypical neuroleptics	Agitation[q]	Reduced EPS, TD, motor side effects (may differ with individual and medication)	Sedation weight gain, decreased seizure threshold; with clozapine, agranulocytosis
Stimulants	Disorders of attention, concentration, arousal, and memory[r,s,t]	May diminish anger[r,t]	Agitation; anxiety; psychosis[b]
Other			
Bromocriptine	Antimotivational states resulting from nondominant parietal stroke[u,v], nonfluent aphasia[w,x]	May improve "hemi-neglect" in patients with nondominant-hemisphere stroke[u]	Psychotic symptoms
Clonidine	Mania[b]; spasticity[y]	Can be used in patients with substance withdrawal syndromes	Hypotension
Physostigmine	Arousal disorder following traumatic head injury[j]	Improves memory following head injury in conjunction with other medications and memory training	Nausea; vomiting; salivation; can precipitate cholinergic crisis in overdose
Experimental			
CDP-choline	Closed-head trauma[j]	Reduced neuropsychiatric signs and symptoms	
Gangliosides	Spinal cord injury; stroke[j]	Improved recovery potential	
Pramiracetam	Head injury	Enhanced memory recovery with and without memory training	

Note. ADLs = activities of daily living; CNS = central nervous system; MAOIs = monoamine oxidase inhibitors; NSAIDs = nonsteroidal anti-inflammatory drugs; SSRIs = selective serotonin reuptake inhibitors; EPS = extrapyramidal symptoms; TD = tardive dyskinesia.

Source. [a]Block 1993; [b]Silver and Yudofsky 1993; [c]Kapadia and Harden 2000; [d]Finklestein et al. 1987; [e]Max et al. 1992; [f]Robinson et al. 1993; [g]Lipsey et al. 1984; [h]Robinson et al. 2000; [i]Kimura et al. 2000; [j]McEvoy 1987; [k]Greendyke et al. 1986; [l]Petrie et al. 1982; [m]McLean et al. 1993; [n]Gualtieri 1991; [o]Rao et al. 1985; [p]Feeney et al. 1982; [q]R. W. Evans et al. 1987; [s]Brooke et al. 1992; [t]Mooney and Haas 1993; [u]Fleet et al. 1987; [v]Passler and Riggs 2001; [w]Gupta Sudha and Milcoch 1992; [x]Raymer et al. 2001; [y]Nance et al. 1985.

Brief and Supportive Psychotherapy

Brief psychotherapy is best suited for patients in acute medical and surgical situations (Blacher 1991). It is also helpful for patients in rehabilitation with physical trauma and illness (Murdaugh 1984). However, the efficacy of brief or supportive psychotherapy has not been well defined for patients in rehabilitation settings. This area deserves more rigorous attention and research. Brief and supportive psychotherapy may be helpful in dealing with a defined focal problem, such as limited or inappropriate coping strategies, lifestyle or body image change, death and dying, or feelings of guilt, punishment, and revenge. Brief psychiatric treatment can often be completed within a single rehabilitation inpatient program and not require additional sessions in the outpatient setting. Frieden and Cole (1984) have provided an approach to creative problem solving that is also useful in brief psychotherapy.

Behavior and Cognitive Therapies

Several behavior and cognitive therapy approaches are useful (Ince 1980). These treatments are outlined in Table 33–8. Social skills training (Dunn 1987) is useful when patients need assistance in asserting themselves in the contexts of wheelchairs, access problems, stairs, and other barriers to maximal functioning. Group cognitive-behavioral therapy has been reported to beneficially affect 2-year outcomes for both anxiety and depression (Craig et al. 1998). Studies report cognitive therapy's beneficial effect on decreasing health care use (L. D. Young et al. 1995) but not on decreasing pain and coping (Kraaimaat et al. 1994) in rheumatoid arthritis. Stress management training has been shown to improve pain, coping, and health status (Parker et al. 1995). Biofeedback (Brucker 1980; Gianutsos and Eberstein 1987; Harris 1980; Sachs 1980) is widely used in muscle retraining by both physical and occupational therapists. Interviewing patients who are already wearing biofeedback apparatus provides a visual display of muscle tension changes as various topics are covered. This technique can be used to identify conflicts that are closely tied to disability-related physiologic responses. It is surprising but helpful to learn that some minor issues have substantial physiologic significance whereas some major issues do not. Treatment can then be focused on the most physiologically relevant content.

Operant conditioning (Friedlander 1980; Guenther et al. 1993; Levenkron 1987; Rapoff et al. 1984) has been widely used in the rehabilitation of patients with chronic pain and for those with a variety of other behavior problems. Targeting problematic behaviors, goal setting, and

TABLE 33–8. Psychiatric treatments used in rehabilitation

Biofeedback
Brief psychotherapy
Cognitive therapy
Family therapy
Group therapy
Operant conditioning
Psychodynamic psychotherapy
Psychoeducation
Psychopharmacology
Relaxation and imagery
Social skills training
Supportive therapy

rewarding techniques are often required to resolve "difficult patient" and staff-patient problems. However, these interventions require a high degree of integration and consistency by all staff members if they are to be effective.

Relaxation and imagery techniques are widely used in group formats for stress management on rehabilitation units. The outcomes of relaxation techniques for chronic pain have been recently reviewed (Carroll and Seers 1998). They are also helpful with speech therapy (Marshall and Watts 1976), anxiety, spasticity, increased muscle tone, and pain management. Many generic relaxation tapes and standard group approaches do not work as well as individualized regimens because they decrease the patient's perceived control and may tell a subject to focus on an impaired body part. Once an individualized program has been devised, the procedures can be taped for repeated use, and appropriate patients can be brought together for group applications.

Cognitive therapy (Larcombe and Wilson 1984), cognitive restructuring, and attribution-altering techniques are effective for treating patients with depression or anxiety, for those who are adjusting to major life changes, and for some inpatients with personality disorders.

Many professionals in rehabilitation have experience in various behavior therapy techniques. The psychologist working on a rehabilitation unit or on the consultation-liaison psychiatry service can provide significant leadership in this area.

Cognitive Rehabilitation and Retraining

Patients with traumatic brain injury, stroke, brain tumor, or other CNS insult require neuropsychological assessment. This establishes baseline data and clear outcomes. Cognitive rehabilitation and retraining can "maximize recovery of the individual's abilities in the areas of intellectual functioning, visual processing, language and…memory" (Lovell and Starratt 1992, p. 742). The focus of cognitive rehabilitation varies depending on the presentation of neuropsychiatric disorders in specific individuals (Gualtieri 1988, 1993; Kikmen et al. 1986; Levin et al. 1982; Lovell and Starratt 1992). For example, cognitive rehabilitation for memory deficits may range from teaching specific mnemonic strategies (e.g., association tasks using visual imagery) to using external aids (memory logs or memory cuing strategies). Patients with stroke with hemispatial neglect may benefit from training in techniques for visual scanning to the neglected side (Diller and Weinberg 1977). Computers are also being used in cognitive rehabilitation, although demonstrations of effectiveness are still needed.

Family Treatment

The consultation-liaison psychiatrist should involve and work with the family. Family members are sometimes the outsiders in the rehabilitation team system. They need to be actively involved in the rehabilitation process as early as possible. The family and caregivers should be asked at each contact if there are any particular issues that they want to see addressed. Staff members may need education about how to talk to families and how to deal with difficult family situations. Families respond well to structure and to formalized assessments. Open, loosely defined meetings lead families to feel "under the microscope" and defensive about perceived interpretations. Problems must be clarified and agreed on and action plans developed that are consistent with the given family's structure, usual approach, and culture. Family education is crucial (R.L. Evans and Held 1984). R.L. Evans and co-workers (1988) found that follow-up counseling sessions focusing on key elements in an education program led to more sustained benefits than did the education alone. Families also require assistance and advocacy.

Patients and caregivers face many challenges in making the transition to the home and community. Designating a primary physician to coordinate care and a care coordinator (often the patient and/or significant caregiver) to coordinate plans with the primary physician, all other health professionals, and agencies is essential. These roles must be established early in the course of rehabilitation. The psychiatric consultant should learn who these individuals are, and if individuals have not been designated to fill these roles, the consultation-liaison psychiatrist can insist that such designations be made. Table 33–9 provides a checklist of possible issues that must be considered by the rehabilitation team for effective community transition.

TABLE 33–9. Services and patient needs for effective community transition

Adult day centers
Caregiver home health care training
Caregiver respite care
Driver training and evaluation
Education and information
Emergency alerting services
Equipment and supplies
Financial and estate planning
Health insurance issues
Home health care services
Homemaker assistance
Leisure activities
Meals
Psychological counseling
Support groups
Transportation
Travel assistance
Vocational guidance

Group Psychotherapy

Group psychotherapy approaches used in rehabilitation settings include 1) ward groups, to deal with the issues arising on the unit; 2) predischarge groups; 3) education groups (R.L. Evans and Held 1984); 4) sexuality groups; 5) family groups (Gonzalez et al. 1989; Rohrer et al. 1980); 6) peer counseling and self-help groups; 7) support groups in the community; and 8) specific intervention groups (Salhoot 1984). Occupational therapists increasingly use groups for their therapy.

The psychiatrist who provides consultation on a rehabilitation unit should be aware of the type, focus, and frequency of groups. It is often appropriate to recommend and/or reinforce attendance at these groups. Unfortunately, the functioning of some groups may precipitate some of the problems that the psychiatrist is being asked to address. Psychiatric consultants may be called on to supervise or consult regarding groups, their process, and their effects on unit functioning.

Ward Management

Ward management issues include milieu staff problems, transfers to a psychiatric ward, and restraints for safety. Romano (1984) and Stewart and Shields (1985) believe that the overall rehabilitation ward environment plays a central role in assisting patients to reestablish their sense of self-worth. Problems in this environment can occur as a result of team or staff issues. Consultation-liaison psychiatrists may be asked to assess patients and to intervene when major safety issues arise. In these cases, a systems approach (Terrell and Mohl 1991) and thorough knowledge about organizations, rehabilitation, and rehabilitation teams are important.

At times, the psychiatric condition of the patient will require transfer to a psychiatric unit, but this is rare. It usually happens at the end of the physical rehabilitation phase when a psychiatric condition contraindicates discharge, yet inpatient rehabilitation can no longer be justified. This is frequently the result of unremitting depression occurring late in rehabilitation.

In general, the treatment of most suicidal patients can be managed on a rehabilitation unit. Close and constant observation, contracting for safety, and the other procedures that are used on inpatient psychiatric units can be implemented in rehabilitation settings (see Chapter 9, this volume, for further information). If the suicidality continues for longer than a few days and interferes with rehabilitation, then transfer to a psychiatric ward or medical-psychiatric unit should be considered.

Cognitive deficits, including problems with attention, concentration, judgment, orientation, and impulsivity, all lead to the need for appropriate safety precautions. These precautions can include use of mechanical restraints for patients who are confined to a wheelchair or bed. Electronic surveillance and warning systems are used on many neurorehabilitation units so that patients are free to move about the unit, but staff members are alerted if they attempt to leave unaccompanied. Medication restraint is rarely needed and usually is not helpful in rehabilitation settings because it may sedate the patient to the point that he or she is no longer able to be actively involved in rehabilitation.

OUTPATIENT CONSULTATION-LIAISON PSYCHIATRY AND REHABILITATION

As with virtually all other medical specialties, more and more rehabilitation is being provided on an outpatient basis. With this development, the need for outpatient rehabilitation consultation-liaison psychiatrists is growing. The chronic and disabling nature of many of the conditions that bring patients to the attention of rehabilitation increases the risks for medical and psychosocial difficulties as outpatients.

Patients and families describe two nodal time periods that are most likely to be associated with psychosocial problems. The first is the initial period after the patient returns home. Patients and families are often, despite education, shocked by the effect of the disability.

The burden of care shifts and falls almost totally on them. These early transition difficulties can arise in almost any rehabilitation case, and it is at this time that active, if not urgent, outpatient needs may surface.

The second risk period usually occurs some time later and is in response to those situations in which patients and caregivers are faced with the reality that "this is it, and it may not get a whole lot better." This problem is seldom seen, therefore, in those who make a steady return to full recovery. Many patients leave inpatient rehabilitation with a strong sense of hope that once they get home, life will eventually return to normal. Problems occur when functional, health, cognitive, and other improvements plateau or—in some cases—begin to fall off, and psychiatric syndromes can be part of this.

Outpatient follow-up appointments, therefore, must extend through the expected recovery curves for any given disorder (e.g., 6–12 months for functional improvement in stroke and longer for aphasia). The general principles of careful assessment and treatment outlined in this chapter and the rest of the book apply equally well to outpatient work. Consultation-liaison psychiatrists also may be asked to provide special outpatient assessments relating to long-term disability, driving, and return to work or to perform independent medical evaluations in workers' compensation and other cases. Most outpatients in rehabilitation also are likely to be seeing many other physician specialists and combinations of occupational, speech, and physical therapists. Many will actively and regularly attend formal outpatient rehabilitation programs and follow-up services. Findings, plans, and goals must be effectively communicated to these care providers in a manner that ensures coordinated care. Much more work is needed to develop efficient and effective multidisciplinary models for outpatient consultation-liaison psychiatric care for patients undergoing rehabilitation and for those with chronic illness.

CONSULTATION-LIAISON PSYCHIATRY TRAINING IN REHABILITATION

Medical students as well as consultation-liaison psychiatry residents and fellows can gain exposure to unique educational experiences in rehabilitation medicine. Nowhere else in medicine—with the possible exception of inpatient psychiatry—is there such a substantial focus on multidisciplinary team functioning, functional outcomes, and integration of multiple issues and interventions. As a result, rehabilitation medicine presents special opportunities for experience and training in liaison work that are not found elsewhere. This training also affords an increased appreciation of the skills of occupational, physical, and speech therapies and how their work can influence behavior. The diagnostic mix and problems presented in rehabilitation units are different from those found in general medicine and surgery units. Patients undergoing rehabilitation are in the hospital longer than most other patients, and psychiatrists can be actively engaged in the type of ongoing care that other consultation-liaison service experiences cannot offer. Rehabilitation cases are ideal for learning how to formulate therapy based on multiple models (e.g., behavioral, psychodynamic, systems, biological), as well as how to integrate multimodality interventions. There is also a wide variety of patients with interesting neuropsychiatric phenomena to observe, assess, and treat.

SUMMARY

Rehabilitation is a rapidly expanding area that benefits from a close relationship with consultation-liaison psychiatrists. Work with patients undergoing rehabilitation is both challenging and rewarding.

> The complex array of factors and the ways in which they interact; the diagnostic tasks of both patient and system; the uncovering of hidden issues that no one else recognizes; the task of designing an intervention strategy of appropriate effectiveness—these are the challenges. And the rewards? The exciting opportunity to accompany and identify with a fellow human being's struggle to overcome adversity in the journey back is a reward that does not need much elaboration. (Group for the Advancement of Psychiatry, Committee on Handicaps 1993, p. 122)

REFERENCES

AHA News: Rehab inpatient admissions, outpatient visits up, AHA survey finds. AHA News 29(13):4, 1993

American Psychiatric Association: Diagnostic and Statistical Manual of Mental Disorders, 4th Edition, Text Revision. Washington, DC, American Psychiatric Association, 2000

Beckham JC, D'Amico CJ, Rice JR, et al: Depression and level of functioning in patients with rheumatoid arthritis. Can J Psychiatry 37:538–543, 1992

Bishop D: Behavior and disability: challenges for assessment and management, in Behavior Problems and the Disabled: Assessment and Management. Edited by Bishop D. Baltimore, MD, Williams & Wilkins, 1980, pp 1–16

Bishop DS, Miller IW: Traumatic brain injury: empirical family assessment techniques. J Head Trauma Rehabil 3:16–30, 1988

Bishop DS, Baldwin LM, Epstein NB, et al: Assessment of family functioning, in Functional Assessment in Rehabilitation Medicine. Edited by Granger C, Gresham G. Baltimore, MD, Williams & Wilkins, 1984, pp 305–323

Blacher R: Brief psychotherapy for medical and surgical patients, in Handbook of Studies on General Hospital Psychiatry. Edited by Judd F, Burroughs G, Lipsitt D. Amsterdam, The Netherlands, Elsevier, 1991, pp 149–162

Block B: Antidepressants in the treatment of pain. Resident and Staff Physician 39(2):49–52, 1993

Bombardier CH, Rimmele CT: Alcohol use and readiness to change after spinal cord injury. Arch Phys Med Rehabil 79: 1110–1115, 1998

Bond J, Gregson B, Smith M, et al: Outcomes following acute hospital care for stroke or hip fracture: how useful is an assessment of anxiety or derpression for older people? Int J Geriatr Psychiatry 13:601–610, 1998

Bowden ML, Feller I, Tholen D, et al: Self-esteem of severely burned patients. Arch Phys Med Rehabil 61:449–452, 1980

Bradley LA: Psychological aspects of arthritis. Bull Rheum Dis 35:1–12, 1985

Bray GP, DeFrank RS, Wolfe TL: Sexual functioning in stroke survivors. Arch Phys Med Rehabil 62:286–288, 1981

Brocklehurst JC, Morris P, Andrews K, et al: Social effects of stroke. Soc Sci Med 15:35–39, 1981

Brooke M, Patterson D, Questad K, et al: The treatment of agitation during initial hospitalization after traumatic brain injury. Arch Phys Med Rehabil 73:917–921, 1992

Brooks N: Head injury and the family, in Closed Head Injury: Psychological, Social, and Family Consequences. Edited by Brooks N. New York, Oxford University Press, 1984, pp 123–147

Browne J, Bishop D: Team functioning: a professional versus lay perspective, in Behavior Problems and the Disabled: Assessment and Management. Edited by Bishop D. Baltimore, MD, Williams & Wilkins, 1980, pp 378–400

Brucker B: Biofeedback and rehabilitation, in Rehabilitation Medicine. Edited by Ince L. Baltimore, MD, Williams & Wilkins, 1980, pp 188–217

Burnett DM, Kennedy RE, Cifu DX, et al: Using atypical neuroleptic drugs to treat agitation in patients with a brain injury: a review. NeuroRehabilitation 13:165–172, 1999

Burns SP, Little JW, Hussey JD, et al: Sleep apnea syndrom in chronic spinal cord injury: associated factors and treatment. Arc Phys Med Rehabil 81:1334–1339, 2000

Burvill PW, Johnson GA, Jamrozik KD, et al: Prevalence of depression after stroke: the Perth Community Stroke Study. Br J Psychiatry 166:320–327, 1995a

Burvill PW, Johnson GA, Jamrozik KD, et al: Anxiety disorders after stroke: results from the Perth Community Stroke Study. Br J Psychiatry 166:328–332, 1995b

Cantor M: Strain among caregivers: a study of experience in the United States. Gerontologist 23:597–604, 1983

Caplan B: Staff and patients perception of patient mood. Rehabilitation Psychology 28:67–77, 1983

Caplan B: Neuropsychological assessment in rehabilitation, in Rehabilitation Psychology Desk Reference. Edited by Caplan B. Rockville, MD, Aspen, 1987, pp 247–280

Caplan B, Shechter J: Denial and depression in disabling illness, in Rehabilitation Psychology Desk Reference. Edited by Caplan B. Rockville, MD, Aspen, 1987, pp 133–170

Carroll D, Seers K: Relaxation for the relief of chronic pain: a systemic review. J Adv Nurs 27(3):467–487, 1998

Castillo CS, Schultz SK, Robinson RG: Clinical correlates of early onset and late onset poststroke generalized anxiety. Am J Psychiatry 152:1174–1179, 1995

Chandarana PC, Eals M, Steingart AB, et al: The detection of psychiatric morbidity and associated factors in patients with rheumatoid arthritis. Can J Psychiatry 32:356–361, 1987

Cook L: Psychopharmacology in rehabilitation medicine, in Rehabilitation Psychology: A Comprehensive Textbook. Edited by Krueger D. Rockville, MD, Aspen, 1984, pp 139–147

Cottrell S, Wilson S: The affective symptomatology of disseminated sclerosis: a study of 100 cases. Journal of Neurology and Psychopathology 7:1–30, 1926

Craig AR, Hancock KM, Dickson HG: A longitudinal investigation into anxiety and depression in the first 2 years following a spinal cord injury. Paraplegia 32:675–679, 1994

Craig A, Hanock K, Chang E, et al: The effectiveness of group psychological intervention in enhancing perceptions of control following spinal cord injury. Aus N Z J Psychiatry 32:112–118, 1998

Crewe N: The difficult patient, in Behavior Problems and the Disabled: Assessment and Management. Edited by Bishop D. Baltimore, MD, Williams & Wilkins, 1980a, pp 98–119

Crewe N: Sexually inappropriate behavior, in Behavior Problems and the Disabled: Assessment and Management. Edited by Bishop D. Baltimore, MD, Williams & Wilkins, 1980b, pp 120–141

Crewe N, Krause J: Spinal cord injury: psychological aspects, in Rehabilitation Psychology Desk Reference. Edited by Caplan B. Rockville, MD, Aspen, 1987, pp 3–36

Deyo RA, Inui TS, Leininger J, et al: Physical and psychosocial function in rheumatoid arthritis: clinical use of a self-administered health status instrument. Arch Intern Med 142:879–882, 1982

Davidoff GN, Roth EJ, Richards JS: Cognitive deficits in spinal cord injury: epidemiology and outcome. Arch Phys Med Rehabil 73:275–284, 1992

Dijkers MP, Cushman LA: Differences between rehabilitation disciplines in views of depression in spinal cord injury patients. Paraplegia 28:380–391, 1990

Diller L: The development of a perceptual-remediation program in hemiplegia, in Behavioral Psychology in Rehabilitation Medicine: Clinical Applications. Edited by Ince L. Baltimore, MD, Williams & Wilkins, 1980, pp 200–224

Diller L, Weinberg J: Hemi-inattention in rehabilitation: the evolution of a rational remediation program. Adv Neurol 18:63–82, 1977

Donahue RP, Abbott RD, Reed DM, et al: Alcohol and hemorrhagic stroke: the Honolulu heart program. JAMA 255:2311–2314, 1986

Ducharme S: Sexuality in physical disability, in Rehabilitation Psychology Desk Reference. Edited by Caplan B. Rockville, MD, Aspen, 1987, pp 419–436

Dunn M: Social skills in rehabilitation, in Rehabilitation Psychology Desk Reference. Edited by Caplan B. Rockville, MD, Aspen, 1987, pp 345–359

Ehde DM, Czerniecki JM, Smith DG, et al: Chronic phantom sensations, phantom pain, residual limb pain and other regional pain after lower limb amputation. Arch Phys Med Rehabil. 81:1039–1044, 2000

Evans RL, Held S: Evaluation of family stroke education. Int J Rehabil Res 7:47–51, 1984

Evans RL, Matlock A, Bishop D, et al: Family intervention after stroke: does counseling or education help? Stroke 19:1243–1249, 1988

Evans RL, Bishop DS, Haselkorn JK: Factors predicting satisfactory home care after stroke. Arch Phys Med Rehabil 72:144–147, 1991

Evans RW, Gualtieri CT, Patterson D: Single case study: treatment of chronic closed head injury with psychostimulant drugs: a controlled case study and an appropriate evaluation procedure. J Nerv Ment Dis 175:106–110, 1987

Featherstone H: A Difference in the Family: Life With a Disabled Child. New York, Basic Books, 1980

Federoff JP, Starkstein SE, Forrester AW, et al: Depression in patients with acute traumatic brain injury. Am J Psychiatry 149:918–923, 1992

Feeney D, Gonzalez A, Law W: Amphetamine, haloperidol, and experience interact to affect rate of recovery after motor cortex injury. Science 217:855–857, 1982

Feinstein A, Feinstein K, Gray T, et al: Prevalence and neurobehavioral correlates of pathological laughing and crying in multiple sclerosis. Arch Neurol 54:1116–1121, 1997

Fey S, Williamson-Kirkland TE: Chronic pain: psychology and rehabilitation, in Rehabilitation Psychology Desk Reference. Edited by Caplan B. Rockville, MD, Aspen, 1987, pp 247–280

Finklestein SP, Weintraub RJ, Karmouz N, et al: Antidepressant drug treatment for poststroke depression: retrospective study. Arch Phys Med Rehabil 68:772–776, 1987

Fleet WS, Valenstein E, Watson RT, et al: Dopamine agonist therapy for neglect in humans. Neurology 37:1765–1770, 1987

Florian V: Sex counseling: comparison of attitudes of disabled and nondisabled subjects. Arch Phys Med Rehabil 64:81–84, 1983

Frieden L, Cole J: Creative problem solving, in Rehabilitation Psychology: A Comprehensive Textbook. Edited by Krueger D. Rockville, MD, Aspen, 1984, pp 69–80

Friedlander B: Automated operant methods for assessment and treatment in physical rehabilitation, in Rehabilitation Medicine. Edited by Ince L. Baltimore, MD, Williams & Wilkins, 1980, pp 25–63

Fugl-Meyer A, Jaasko L: Post stroke hemiplegia and sexual intercourse. Scand J Rehabil Med Suppl 7:158–166, 1980

Fuhrer MJ, Rintala DH, Hart KA, et al: Depressive symptomatology in persons with spinal cord injury who reside in the community. Arch Phys Med Rehabil 74:255–260, 1993

Fullerton DT, Harvey RF, Klein MH, et al: Psychiatric disorders in patients with spinal cord injuries. Arch Gen Psychiatry 38:1369–1371, 1981

Gallagher R: Aggressive behavior in the disabled, in Behavior Problems and the Disabled: Assessment and Management. Edited by Bishop D. Baltimore, MD, Williams & Wilkins, 1980, pp 71–97

Gans J: Facilitating staff/patient interaction in rehabilitation, in Rehabilitation Psychology Desk Reference. Edited by Caplan B. Rockville, MD, Aspen, 1987, pp 185–218

Gerhardt F, Florin I, Knapp T: The impact of medical, reeducational, and psychological variables on rehabilitation outcome in amputees. Int J Rehabil Res 7:379–388, 1984

Gianutsos J, Eberstein A: Computer-augmented feedback displays: treatment of hemiplegic motor deficits as a paradigm, in Rehabilitation Psychology Desk Reference. Edited by Caplan B. Rockville, MD, Aspen, 1987, pp 241–264

Goldstein LB: Common drugs may influence motor recovery after stroke. The Sygen In Acute Stroke Study Investigators. Neurology 45:865–871, 1995

Gonzalez S, Steinglass P, Reiss D: Putting the illness in its place: discussion groups for families with chronic medical illnesses. Fam Process 28:69–87, 1989

Goodstein R: Cerebrovascular accident: a multidimensional clinical problem, in Emotional Rehabilitation of Physical Trauma and Disability. Edited by Krueger D. New York, Spectrum Publications, 1984, pp 111–140

Gordon WA, Hibbard MR, Egelko S, et al: Perceptual remediation in patients with right brain damage: a comprehensive program. Arch Phys Med Rehabil 66:353–359, 1985

Gorelick PB, Kelly MA: Alcohol as a risk factor for stroke. Heart Disease and Stroke 1:255–258, 1992

Granger CV, Cotter AC, Hamilton BB, et al: Functional assessment scales: a study of persons after stroke. Arch Phys Med Rehabil 74:133–138, 1993

Greendyke RM, Kanter DR, Schuster DB, et al: Propranolol treatment of assaultive patients with organic brain disease: a double-blind crossover, placebo-controlled study. J Nerv Ment Dis 174:290–294, 1986

Greenwood W: Alcoholism: a complicating factor in the rehabilitation of disabled individuals. Journal of Rehabilitation 7:51–52, 72, 1984

Group for the Advancement of Psychiatry, Committee on Handicaps: Report #135: Caring for People With Physical Impairment: The Journey Back. Washington, DC, American Psychiatric Press, 1993

Gualtieri CT: Pharmacotherapy and the neurobehavioral sequelae of traumatic brain injury. Brain Inj 2:101–109, 1988

Gualtieri CT: Buspirone for the behavior problems of patients with organic brain disorders. J Clin Psychopharmacol 11:280–281, 1991

Gualtieri CT: Traumatic brain injury, in Psychiatric Care of the Medical Patient. Edited by Stoudemire A, Fogel BS. New York, Oxford University Press, 1993, pp 517–535

Gupta Sudha R, Milcoch AG: Bromocriptine treatment of nonfluent aphasia. Arch Phys Med Rehabil 73:373–376, 1992

Guenther R, Frank R, McAdams C: Management of behavior on a spinal cord injury unit. NeuroRehabilitation 3:50–59, 1993

Guilmette TJ, Snow MG, Grace J, et al: Emotional dysfunction in a geriatric population: staff observations and patients' reports. Arch Phys Med Rehabil 73:587–593, 1992

Gunther M: Catastrophic illness and the caregiver: real burdens and solutions with respect to the role of behavioral sciences, in Rehabilitation Psychology Desk Reference. Edited by Caplan B. Rockville, MD, Aspen, 1987, pp 219–240

Gustafson Y, Nilsson I, Mattsson M, et al: Epidemiology and treatment of psot-stroke depression. Drugs Aging 7:298–309, 1995

Gwyther LP, George LK: Caregivers of dementia patients: complex determinants of well-being and burden. Gerontologist 26:245–247, 1986

Hahn H: Paternalism and public policy. Society 20:36–46, 1983

Halstead LS, Wiechers DO (eds): Late Effects of Poliomyelitis. Bloomington, IL, Accent Books, 1985

Harris F: Exteroceptive feedback of position and movement in remediation for disorders of coordination, in Rehabilitation Medicine. Edited by Ince L. Baltimore, MD, Williams & Wilkins, 1980, pp 87–156

Harrison J, Glass CA, Owens RG, et al: Factors associated with sexual functioning in women following spinal cord injury. Paraplegia 33:687–692, 1995

Holland JC: Managing depression in the patient with cancer. CA Cancer J Clin 37:366–371, 1987

Ince L (ed): Behavioral Psychology in Rehabilitation Medicine. Baltimore, MD, Williams & Wilkins, 1980

International Center for the Disabled: ICD Survey of Disabled Americans: Bringing Disabled Americans Into the Mainstream. New York, ICD-International Center for the Disabled (in cooperation with the National Council on the Handicapped), 1986

Jorge RE, Robinson RG, Starkstein SE, et al: Secondary mania following traumatic brain injury. Am J Psychiatry 150:916–921, 1993

Kapadia NP, Harden N: Gabapentin for chronic pain in spinal cord injury: a case report. Arch Phys Med Rehabil 81:1439–1441, 2000

Katz J: Psychophysiological contributions to phantom limbs. Can J Psychiatry 37:282–298, 1992

Keitner GI, Miller IW, Ryan CE, et al: Compounded depression and family functioning during the acute episode and 6-month follow-up. Compr Psychiatry 30:512–521, 1989

Keitner GI, Ryan CE, Miller IW, et al: 12-Month outcome of patients with major depression and comorbid psychiatric or medical illness (compound depression). Am J Psychiatry 148:345–350, 1991

Kennedy P, Rogers BA: Anxiety and depression after spinal cord injury: a longitudinal analysis. Arch Phys Med Rehabil 81: 932–937, 2000

Kennedy P, Frankel H, Gardner B, et al: Factors associated with acute and chronic pain following traumatic spinal cord injuries. Spinal Cord 35:814–817, 1997

Kikmen S, McLean A, Temkin N: Neuropsychological and psychosocial consequences of minor head injury. J Neurol Neurosurg Psychiatry 49:1227–1232, 1986

Kimura M, Robinson RG, Kosier JT: Treatment of cognitive impairment after poststroke depression: a double-blind treatment trial. Stroke 31:1482–1486, 2000

Kirubakaran VR, Kumar VN, Powell BJ, et al: Survey of alcohol and drug misues in spinal cord injure veterans. J Stud Alcohol 47:223–227, 1986

Kraaimaat FW, Brons MR, Geenen R, et al: The effect of cognitive behavior therapy in patients with rheumatoid arthritis. Behav Res Ther 33:487–495, 1995

30 Krause JS, Kemp B, Coker J: Depression after spinal cord injury: relation to gender, ethnicity, aging, and socioeconomic indicators. Arch Phys Med Rehabil 81:1099–1109, 2000

Krueger D: Psychological rehabilitation of physical trauma and disability, in Rehabilitation Psychology: A Comprehensive Textbook. Edited by Krueger D. Rockville, MD, Aspen, 1984, pp 3–14

Kryger M, Roth T, Dement W (eds): Principles of Sleep Medicine. Philadelphia, PA, WB Saunders, 1989

Larcombe NA, Wilson PH: An evaluation of cognitive-behaviour therapy for depression in patients with multiple sclerosis. Br J Psychiatry 145:366–371, 1984

Large RG: DSM-III diagnoses in chronic pain: confusion or clarity? J Nerv Ment Dis 174:295–303, 1986

Levenkron J: Behavior modification in rehabilitation: principles and clinical strategy, in Rehabilitation Psychology Desk Reference. Edited by Caplan B. Rockville, MD, Aspen, 1987, pp 383–416

Levin HS, Benton AL, Grossman RG: Neurobehavioral Consequences of Closed Head Injury. New York, Oxford University Press, 1982

Lichtenberg PA, Gibbons TA: Geriatric rehabilitation and the older adult family caregiver: stages of caregiving. NeuroRehabilitation 3:62–71, 1993

Lindsay PG, Wyckoff M: The depression-pain syndrome and its response to antidepressants. Psychosomatics 22:571–577, 1981

Lipowski Z: Consultation-liaison psychiatry, in Handbook of Studies on General Hospital Psychiatry. Edited by Judd F, Burroughs G, Lipsitt D. Amsterdam, The Netherlands, Elsevier, 1991, pp 30–49

Lipsey J, Robinson R, Pearlson G, et al: Nortriptyline treatment of post-stroke depression: a double-blind study. Lancet 1(8372): 297–300, 1984

Lishman WA: Other disorders affecting the nervous system, in Organic Psychiatry: The Psychological Consequences of Cerebral Disorder, 2nd Edition. Boston, MA, Blackwell Scientific, 1987, pp 588–650

Lofgren B, Nyberg L, Mattsson M, et al: Three years after inpatient stroke rehabilitation: a follow-up study. Cerebrovascular Dis 9:163–170, 1999

Loong CK, Kenneth NKC, Paulin ST: Post-stroke depression: outcome following rehabilitation. Aust N Z J Psychiatry 29:609–614, 1995

Lovell MR, Starratt C: Cognitive rehabilitation and behavior therapy of neuropsychiatric disorders, in The American Psychiatric Press Textbook of Neuropsychiatry, 2nd Edition. Edited by Yudofsky SC, Hales RE. Washington, DC, American Psychiatric Press, 1992, pp 741–754

Luxenberg J, Feigenbaum L: Cognitive impairment on a rehabilitation service. Arch Phys Med Rehabil 67:796–798, 1986

MacDonald MR, Nielson WR, Cameron MGP: Depression and activity patterns of spinal cord injured persons living in the community. Arch Phys Med Rehabil 68:339–343, 1987

Malec J, Neimeyer R: Psychologic prediction of duration of inpatient spinal cord injury rehabilitation and performance of self-care. Arch Phys Med Rehabil 64:359–363, 1983

Marshall RC, Watts MT: Relaxation training: effects on the communicative ability of aphasic adults. Arch Phys Med Rehabil 57:464–467, 1976

Massie M, Holland J: Depression and the cancer patient. J Clin Psychiatry 51 (suppl 7):12–17, 1990

Max M, Lynch S, Muir J, et al: Effects of desipramine, amitriptyline, and fluoxetine on pain in diabetic neuropathy. N Engl J Med 326:1250–1256, 1992

McDowell JA, Mion LC, Lydon TJ, et al: A nonpharmacologic sleep protocol for hospitalized older patients. J Am Geriatr Soc 46:700–705, 1998

McEvoy JP: A double-blind crossover comparison of antiparkinson drug therapy: amantadine versus anticholinergics in 90 normal volunteers, with an emphasis on differential effects on memory function. J Clin Psychiatry 48 (suppl 9):20–23, 1987

McLean A, Cardenas D, Haselkorn J, et al: Cognitive psychopharmacology. NeuroRehabilitation 3:1–14, 1993

Missel JL: Suicide risk in the medical rehabilitation setting. Arch Phys Med Rehabil 59:371–376, 1978

Mohsenin V, Valor R: Sleep apnea in patients with hemispheric stroke. Arch Phys Med Rehabil 76:71–76, 1995

Mooney GF, Haas L: Effect of methylphenidate on brain injury-related anger. Arch Phys Med Rehabil. 74:153–160, 1993

Mossey JM, Knott K, Craik R: The effects of persistent depressive symptoms on hip fracture recovery. J Gerontol 45: M163–M168, 1990

Murdaugh J: Psychotherapeutic intervention in physical trauma and illness, in Rehabilitation Psychology: A Comprehensive Textbook. Edited by Krueger D. Rockville, MD, Aspen, 1984, pp 37–42

Murray P: Clinical pharmacology in rehabilitation, in Rehabilitation Psychology Desk Reference. Edited by Caplan B. Rockville, MD, Aspen, 1987, pp 501–526

Murray PK, Singer ME, Fortinsky R, et al: Rapid growth of rehabilitation services in traditional community-based nursing homes. Arch Phys Med Rehabil 80:372–328, 1999

Nance P, Shears A, Nance D: Clonidine in spinal cord injury. Can Med Assoc J 133:41–43, 1985

Norman TR, Burrows GD: Psychotropic drugs: potential drug reactions, in Handbook of Studies on General Hospital Psychiatry. Edited by Judd F, Burroughs G, Lipsitt D. Amsterdam, The Netherlands, Elsevier, 1991, pp 53–178

O'Donnell J, Cooper J, Gessner J, et al: Alcohol, drugs, and spinal cord injury. Alcohol Health Res World 3:27–29, 1981/1982

Parker JC, Smarr KL, Buckelew SP, et al: Effects of stress management on clinical outcomes in rheumatoid arthritis. Arthritis Rheum 38:1807–1818, 1995

Passler MA, Riggs RV: Positive outcomes in traumatic brain injury—vegetative state: patients treated with bromocriptine. Arch Phys Med Rehabil 82:311–315, 2001

Petrie WM, Maffucci RJ, Woosely RL: Propranolol and depression (letter). Am J Psychiatry 129:92, 1982

Pruchno R: The effects of help patterns on the mental health of spouse caregivers. Research on Aging 12:57–71, 1990

Rao N, Jellinek H, Woolston D: Agitation in closed head injury: haloperidol effects on rehabilitation outcome. Arch Phys Med Rehabil 66:30–33, 1985

Rapoff MA, Lindsley CB, Christophersen ER: Improving compliance with medical regimens: case study with juvenile rheumatoid arthritis. Arch Phys Med Rehabil 65:267–269, 1984

Raymer AM, Bandy D, Adair JC, et al: Effects of bromocriptine in a patient with crossed nonfluent aphasia: a case report. Arch Phys Med Rehabil 82:139–144, 2001

Reiss H, Schwartz CE, Klerman GL: Manic syndrome following head injury: another form of secondary mania. J Clin Psychiatry 48:29–30, 1987

Robinson RG, Parikh RM, Lipsey JR, et al: Pathological laughing and crying following stroke: validation of a measurement scale and a double-blind treatment study. Am J Psychiatry 150:286–293, 1993

29 Robinson RG, Chemerinski E, Jorge R: Pathophysiology of secondary depression in the elderly. J Geriatr Psychiatry Neurol 12:128–136, 1999

Robinson RG, Schultz SK, Castillo C, et al: Nortryptiline versus fluoxetine in the treatment of depression and in short-term recovery after stroke: a placebo-controlled, double-blind study. Am J Psychiatry 157:351–359, 2000

Rohrer K, Adelman B, Puckett J, et al: Rehabilitation in spinal cord injury: use of a patient-family group. Arch Phys Med Rehabil 61:225–229, 1980

Romano M: The therapeutic milieu in the rehabilitation process, in Rehabilitation Psychology: A Comprehensive Textbook. Edited by Krueger D. Rockville, MD, Aspen, 1984, pp 43–50

Rosenthal M: Traumatic head injury: neurobehavioral consequences, in Rehabilitation Psychology Desk Reference. Edited by Caplan B. Rockville, MD, Aspen, 1987, pp 37–64

Roth EJ, Lovell L, Heinemann AW, et al: The older adult with a spinal cord injury. Paraplegia 30:520–526, 1992

Rybarczyk BD, Nyenhuis DL, Nicholas JJ, et al: Social discomfort and depression in a sample of adults with leg amputations. Arch Phys Med Rehabil 73:1169–1173, 1992

Sachs D: Behavioral feedback techniques for rehabilitation of motor problems, in Rehabilitation Medicine. Edited by Ince L. Baltimore, MD, Williams & Wilkins, 1980, pp 157–187

Sakinofsky I: Depression and suicide in the disabled, in Behavior Problems and the Disabled: Assessment and Management. Edited by Bishop D. Baltimore, MD, Williams & Wilkins, 1980, pp 17–51

Salhoot J: Group therapy in rehabilitation, in Rehabilitation Psychology: A Comprehensive Textbook. Edited by Krueger D. Rockville, MD, Aspen, 1984, pp 61–68

Schiffer RB, Wineman NM, Weitkamp LR: Association between bipolar affective disorder and multiple sclerosis. Am J Psychiatry 143:94–95, 1986

Schubert DSP, Taylor C, Lee S, et al: Detection of depression in the stroke patient. Psychosomatics 33:290–294, 1992a

Schubert DSP, Burns R, Paras W, et al: Increase of medical hospital length of stay by depression in stroke and amputation patients: a pilot study. Psychother Psychosom 57:61–66, 1992b

Schulz R, Visintainer P, Williamson G: Psychiatric and physical morbidity effects of caregiving. J Gerontol 45:181–191, 1990

Scivoletto G, Petrelli A, DiLucente L, et al: Psychological investigation of spinal cord injury patients. Spinal Cord 35:516–520, 1997

Shukla GD, Sahu SC, Tripathi RP, et al: A psychiatric study of amputees. Br J Psychiatry 141:50–53, 1982

Silver J, Yudofsky S: Pharmacologic treatment of neuropsychiatric disorders. NeuroRehabilitation 3:15–25, 1993

35 Sipski M (ed): Sexuality in Neurologic Disability (special issue). NeuroRehabilitation 15(2), 2000

Sipski ML, Alexander CJ, Rosen RC: Physiological parameters associated with psychogenic sexual arousal in women with complete spinal cord injuries. Arch Phys Med Rehabil 76:811–818, 1995

Sjogren K, Damber J, Liliequist B: Sexuality after stroke with hemiplegia: I. Scand J Rehabil Med 4:80–87, 1983

Starkstein SE, Robinson RG: Affective disorders and cerebral vascular disease. Br J Psychiatry 154:170–182, 1989

Starkstein SE, Pearlson GD, Boston J, et al: Mania after brain injury: a controlled study of causative factors. Arch Neurol 44:1069–1073, 1987

Starkstein SE, Cohen BS, Federoff P, et al: Relationship between anxiety disorders and depressive disorders in patients with cerebrovascular injury. Arch Gen Psychiatry 47:246–251, 1990

Steger H, Brockway J: Management of chronic pain in the disabled, in Behavior Problems and the Disabled: Assessment and Management. Edited by Bishop D. Baltimore, MD, Williams & Wilkins, 1980, pp 272–301

Steger H, Fox C, Fienberg S: Behavioral evaluation and management of chronic pain, in Behavior Problems and the Disabled: Assessment and Management. Edited by Bishop D. Baltimore, MD, Williams & Wilkins, 1980, pp 302–336

Stewart T, Shields CR: Grief in chronic illness: assessment and management. Arch Phys Med Rehabil 66:447–450, 1985

Terrell C, Mohl P: Systems approach to consultation-liaison psychiatry, in Handbook of Studies on General Hospital Psychiatry. Edited by Judd F, Burroughs G, Lipsitt D. Amsterdam, The Netherlands, Elsevier, 1991, pp 98–115

Tiller J: Post-stroke depression. Psychopharmacology 106 (suppl): S130–S133, 1992

Trieschman R: Spinal Cord Injuries: The Psychological, Social, and Vocational Adjustment. Elmsford, NY, Pergamon, 1980

Tunks E, Merskey H: Psychiatric treatment in chronic pain, in Behavior Problems and the Disabled: Assessment and Management. Edited by Bishop D. Baltimore, MD, Williams & Wilkins, 1980, pp 195–217

Turner JA, Cardenas DD, Warms CA, et al: Chronic pain associated with spinal cord injuries: a community survey. Arch Phys Med Rehabil 82: 501–508, 2001

Valleroy ML, Kraft GH: Sexual dysfunction in multiple sclerosis. Arch Phys Med Rehabil 65:125–128, 1984

Vanderpool J: Stressful patient relationships and the difficult patient, in Rehabilitation Psychology: A Comprehensive Textbook. Edited by Krueger D. Rockville, MD, Aspen, 1984, pp 167–174

Vrey JR, Henggeler SW: Marital adjustment following spinal cord injury. Arch Phys Med Rehabil 68:69–74, 1987

Webster JB, Bell KR, Hussey JD, et al: Sleep apnea in adults with traumatic brain injury: a preliminary investigation. Arch Phys Med Rehabil 82:316–321, 2001

Whitlock FA: Suicide and physical illness, in Suicide. Edited by Roy A. Baltimore, MD, Williams & Wilkins, 1986, pp 151–170

Williams S: The impact of aphasia on marital satisfaction. Arch Phys Med Rehabil 74:361–367, 1993

Wilmot CB, Cope DN, Hall KM, et al: Occult head injury: its incidence in spinal cord injury. Arch Phys Med Rehabil 66:227–231, 1985

World Health Organization: International Classification of Impairments, Disabilities, and Handicaps: A Manual of Classification Relating to the Consequences of Disease. Geneva, Switzerland, World Health Organization, 1980

Wortman CB, Silver RC: The myths of coping with loss. J Consult Clin Psychol 57:349–357, 1989

Yesavage JA, Brink TL, Rose TL, et al: Development and validation of a geriatric depression screening scale: a preliminary report. J Psychiatr Res 17:37–49, 1982/1983

Young LD, Bradley LA, Turner RA: Decreases in health care resource utilization in patients with rehumatoid arthritis following a cognitive behavioral intervention. Biofeedback Self Regul 20:259–268, 1995

Young ME, Rintala Dh, Rossi CD, et al: Alcohol and marijuana use in a community-based sample of persons with spinal cord injury. Arch Phys Med Rehabil 76:525–532, 1995

34

Intensive Care Units

John L. Shuster Jr., M.D.

Theodore A. Stern, M.D.

Physicians who work in the intensive care unit (ICU) often request psychiatric consultation for their patients. Some patients are seen in consultation because of psychiatric reactions to serious medical illnesses, some are seen because of neuropsychiatric complications of medical illness or its treatment, and some are seen because management of long-term psychiatric disorders is required or because management of the untoward consequences of a psychiatric disorder and/or its treatment is necessary. Consultation-liaison psychiatry in the critical care setting is a challenging and rewarding activity that forces the psychiatrist to manage a wide variety of clinical problems under the pressure of time and to make decisions about and implement biological, psychological, and behavioral interventions at a rapid pace.

In this chapter, we focus on several topics. In the following sections, we

- Review aspects of the psychiatric evaluation unique to patients in ICUs
- Provide a general discussion of treatment recommendations for critically ill patients
- Review some of the psychiatric and behavior problems that commonly lead to a request for psychiatric consultation
- Discuss the stresses frequently encountered by staff in the ICU

PSYCHIATRIC EVALUATION OF THE CRITICALLY ILL PATIENT

General Approach

Few, if any, of the skills required to perform effective psychiatric consultation in the ICU are unique to this setting.

The effective consultant in the ICU applies the same principles of evaluation and treatment used by general psychiatrists and by good consultation-liaison psychiatrists in any other area. Psychiatrists in the ICU must use their skills and knowledge of psychopharmacology, behavioral interventions, and psychotherapy (including individual, family, and group treatments). However, because patients in the ICU are seriously ill, are less able to cooperate with or tolerate an extended evaluation, and are cared for in an environment where the time pressure to produce results is greater than in other settings, psychiatric consultation in the critical care setting is especially challenging. Much like having one's skills in the game of golf tested by a difficult new course, psychiatric consultation in the ICU is often very satisfying and can provide an opportunity to hone one's clinical skills; however, it is the same "game" that consultation-liaison psychiatrists "play" on other "courses." Delivering helpful and effective consultation in a setting in which mental health is usually an afterthought casts a favorable light on the entire field of psychiatry.

When called on to see a patient in the ICU, the psychiatric consultant often assumes the role of medical detective. Performing a consultation in the ICU usually requires piecing together scattered clues. Patients in the ICU are often too ill to provide detailed history or to participate in a complete mental status examination. Psychiatric evaluation in the ICU is complicated by lack of privacy and by noises, distractions, and interruptions created by the provision of intensive medical care. Physical barriers (e.g., placement of an endotracheal tube) or pharmacological barriers (e.g., use of paralytic agents or sedatives) to psychiatric evaluation are frequently present. Family members, when available, are sometimes too emotionally overwhelmed to contribute much to the history. ICU staff members are typically so focused on treatment of the patient's critical illness that they have a limited awareness of the patient's affect, behavior, or cognition. Medical records of ICU patients often contain massive amounts of data, only a portion of which is pertinent to the psychiatric evaluation. One important task of the psychiatric consultant is to determine which information is relevant. Consultation-liaison psychiatrists who are comfortable playing the role of medical detective are effective in the ICU.

Gathering Historical Information

As with any medical evaluation, the patient's history is the most helpful guide to diagnosis. Unfortunately, the patient in the ICU is often unable to provide an extensive history. Thus, collateral history, obtained from family, ICU staff, and consulting physicians, is of greater importance in the ICU than it is in other settings. At the time of initial assessment and recommendations, little reliable history may be known. Persistence often pays off; additional history is often obtained from the patient as he or she becomes more alert, family members can provide additional data after the consultation is initiated, and staff members can refine the physical diagnoses and provide ongoing history.

The ICU chart is unrivaled in the hospital as a source of information. The consultant should review the physicians' and nurses' progress notes, especially admission, consultation, and summary notes. The ICU flowsheet, with graphic representations of many physiologic parameters (including vital signs), pertinent laboratory values, medications administered, and notes about patient behavior, will often help to establish temporal relations between interventions and symptoms. Laboratory sheets should be reviewed to identify electrolyte, metabolic, hematological, or infectious disturbances that may contribute to or cause neuropsychiatric symptoms. Medication orders for the patient should be reviewed—with special attention given to medications recently discontinued or prescribed, as well as all medications currently administered. In patients who have undergone surgery, the operation records also should be reviewed for adverse intraoperative events such as reactions to intraoperatively administered medications, prolonged intraoperative hypoxia, or hypotension; these events can lead to behavioral symptoms in the postoperative phase. The anesthesia record provides thorough moment-to-moment documentation of important events that can alter central nervous system (CNS) function.

Patient Examination

In the alert and cooperative patient in the ICU, conventional psychiatric examination techniques are used. However, the consultation-liaison psychiatrist must adapt his or her interview technique to a variety of situations. The psychiatric examination in the ICU relies heavily on neuropsychiatric evaluation (Strub and Black 1985).

The evaluation of patients who are intubated poses a problem for many clinicians. Although verbal responses to open-ended questions are obviously impossible, a full examination is possible. The first step is an assessment of the patient's level of alertness and concentration. Inquiry into a patient's subjective sense of confusion and an assessment of his or her ability to follow commands gives the interviewer a chance to assess alertness. If intubation is the only obstacle to the interview, the patient usually is able to write answers out on paper and to convey information with facial expressions. If the patient cannot write, information is obtained by asking a series of binary (yes or no) questions aimed at symptom identification or by using nonverbal techniques to facilitate communication—for example, having patients point to letters on a letter board or reading the patients' lips.

Assessing Cognitive Function

A formal assessment of cognitive function is necessary for every patient evaluated in the ICU. Although a formal battery of neuropsychological tests is seldom indicated (and would be extremely difficult for an ICU patient to tolerate), administration of a brief, structured test is helpful. The Mini-Mental State Exam (MMSE; Folstein et al. 1975) is commonly used for this purpose and allows rapid assessment of orientation, registration of information, attention, calculation ability, recall, language functions, reading, writing, and design construction. The chief advantages of the MMSE are its ease of use, brevity, and usefulness for serial examinations. Its chief drawbacks are its low sensitivity (patients with mild to moderate impairment may score well on the test) and its unfortunate name (many nonpsychiatrists confuse the test with the full mental status examination).

Making a Diagnosis

Given the sketchy information about psychiatric history and current psychiatric symptoms that is often available to the ICU psychiatrist, a definitive psychiatric diagnosis is sometimes difficult to establish. It is best to label diagnoses as provisional when incomplete information is available. As soon as a diagnosis is possible, the psychiatrist should communicate it clearly and without jargon in the chart. The dynamic state of the patient in the ICU necessitates frequent diagnostic reassessments and revisions. Figure 34–1 (Wool et al. 1991) illustrates a general

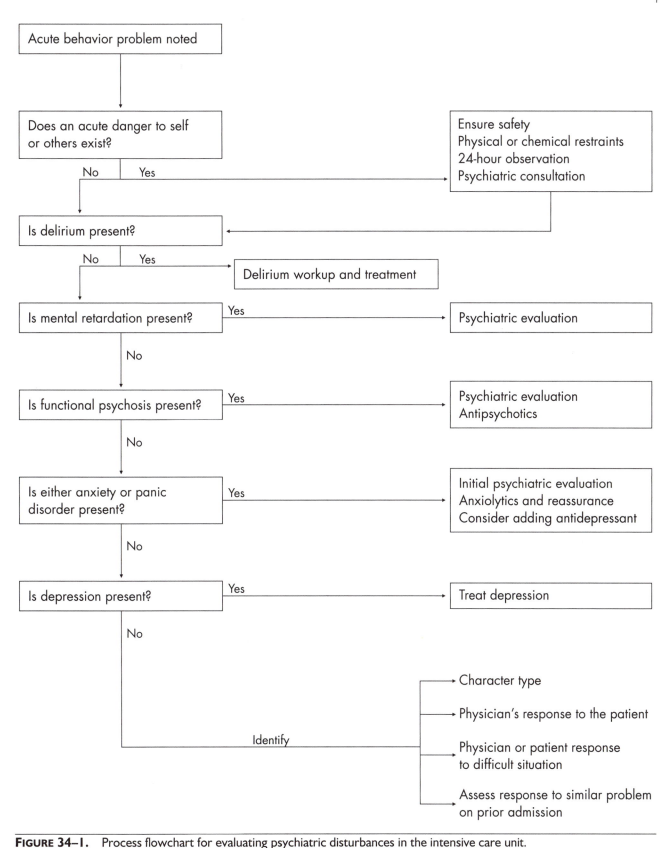

FIGURE 34–1. Process flowchart for evaluating psychiatric disturbances in the intensive care unit.

Source. Reprinted from Wool C, Geringer ES, Stern TA: "The Management of Behavioral Problems in the ICU," in *Intensive Care Medicine*, 2nd Edition. Edited by Rippe JM, Irwin RS, Alpert JS, et al. Boston, MA, Little, Brown, 1991, pp 1906–1916. Copyright 1991, Little, Brown and Company. Used with permission.

scheme for evaluating patients with psychiatric disturbances in the ICU.

Affective, behavioral, and cognitive disturbances in patients in the ICU are often secondary to physical problems or their treatment. Thus, mental disorders resulting from medical or substance-induced disorders (particularly delirium), mood disorders, and anxiety disorders are frequently diagnosed in critically ill patients. These disorders were reclassified as disorders due to a general medical condition in DSM-IV (American Psychiatric Association 1994). Substance-related disorders, drug withdrawal states, major depression, and personality disorders are commonly seen in patients in the ICU, especially in those patients admitted to the ICU after a suicide attempt (Reich and Kelly 1976; Shuster and Stern 1991; Stern et al. 1984).

PSYCHIATRIC TREATMENT OF THE CRITICALLY ILL PATIENT: GENERAL CONCEPTS

Changes in Medical-Surgical Management

All patients in ICUs have serious physical illnesses. A large proportion of the psychiatric symptoms and disorders seen in the ICU setting are secondary to these medical disorders and/or their treatments. Consequently, the first step in the management of psychiatric disorders in the ICU setting is the consideration of whether changes in the medical management of a disorder would alleviate or treat the psychiatric symptoms. For example, it is not logical (and will not be effective) to treat delirium that is caused by hypoxia or hypoglycemia with neuroleptics alone. Whenever possible, delirium should be treated specifically (e.g., reversal of hypoxia with oxygen or hypoglycemia with glucose). A physical cause for mental symptoms in the patient in the ICU must always be considered first. A useful framework for remembering the life-threatening causes of delirium in patients in ICUs is the WWHHHIMP mnemonic (Tesar and Stern 1986), found in Table 34–1 (see also Chapter 15, this volume).

Temporal correlations between the onset of mental symptoms and changes in the medical-surgical management of the patient are important to detect. The ICU flowchart or laboratory summary sheet may reveal a metabolic or infectious problem that accounts for an altered mental status. The medication list should be reviewed for medications added just before symptom onset or discontinued long enough before symptom onset to induce a withdrawal reaction. These and other temporal correlations are often the primary (or only) clues available to help identify the

TABLE 34–1. Life-threatening causes of delirium (WWHHHIMP)

Wernicke's encephalopathy
Withdrawal states
Hypertensive encephalopathy
Hypoglycemia
Hypoxia/hypoperfusion of the brain
Intracranial processes (bleeding, tumors, edema)
Meningitis/encephalitis or metabolic imbalances
Poisons (or drug side effects)

Source. Adapted from Tesar GE, Stern TA: "Evaluation and Treatment of Agitation in the Intensive Care Unit." *Journal of Intensive Care Medicine* 1:137–148, 1986. Copyright 1986, Little, Brown and Company. Used with permission.

cause of psychiatric symptoms in ICU patients.

When a physical problem (e.g., hypoxia, intracranial hemorrhage, medication side effect) is suspected as a cause of psychiatric symptoms, recommendations for changes in the medical-surgical management of the patient are included in the consultation report. Missing a physical problem is potentially embarrassing for the referring physician, so the consultant's note is best written in a direct, helpful manner, without gloating or being critical. In such cases, a telephone call to the referring physician is often more appreciated (and better tolerated) than an extensive note with a remedial tone. Clinical one-upmanship or hurt feelings should not supersede or jeopardize the provision of excellent patient care.

Psychopharmacological Treatments

Psychotropic drugs are often indicated for critically ill patients, but the consultation-liaison psychiatrist must consider the individual patient's physical condition. As Townsend and Reynolds (1991) pointed out, the dynamic physiologic state of the critically ill patient can lead to rapid changes in pharmacokinetic parameters. Most pharmacodynamic and pharmacokinetic data for psychotropic agents are derived from studies of patients without serious physical illness. Decrements in hepatic or renal function brought on by the patient's illness (or its treatment) may adversely affect drug clearance. Serious physical illness also may render the patient more sensitive to drug side effects (Stoudemire et al. 1990).

The guidelines proposed by Jenike (1989) for prescription of psychotropic drugs to the elderly are useful for critically ill patients (Table 34–2). These guidelines also remind us to make every effort to achieve an accurate diagnosis before the initiation of treatment. Symptomatic treatment alone may not solve the targeted problem; it may even create new problems.

TABLE 34–2. Guidelines for prescription of psychotropic drugs to critically ill patients

1. Take a careful psychiatric history (do not base treatment on assumptions).
2. Diagnose before initiation of treatment.
3. Optimize the patient's environment.
4. Know the pharmacology of the drugs prescribed (consider effects of the alterations in hepatic or renal function, interactions with other drugs, side effects in light of patient's current illness).
5. Use a low dosage initially and advance dosage slowly (if the clinical situation warrants it).
6. Avoid polypharmacy whenever possible.
7. Monitor drugs and response to target symptoms on a regular basis (remember that physiologic parameters in the critically ill patient may change rapidly).
8. Observe for drug side effects.
9. Evaluate potential for noncompliance in both the patient and the referring physician.
10. Do not avoid the use of psychotropic agents simply because the patient is critically ill.

Source. Adapted from Jenike MA: *Geriatric Psychiatry and Psychopharmacology.* Chicago, IL, Year Book Medical, 1989. Used with permission.

A thorough knowledge of the pharmacological properties of psychotropic agents is crucial to successful use of these drugs in the intensive care setting. Most psychotropics are metabolized in the liver; most are cleared through the liver or kidneys. Therefore, alteration in hepatic or renal function clearly influences the choice and dosing of psychotropic drugs. Before administering a psychotropic drug, the clinician must consider known or potential drug interactions (Dec and Stern 1990; Lipson and Stern 1991; Shuster et al. 1992; Stoudemire et al. 1990, 1991). (Drugs that interact with antidepressants, neuroleptics, lithium, benzodiazepines, psychostimulants, and carbamazepine are outlined in Chapter 42, this volume.) In addition, the side-effect profile of the psychotropic drug must be considered in light of the patient's physical problems. For example, patients in a cardiac care unit who have cardiac conduction system abnormalities may have difficulty with the quinidine-like effects of tricyclic antidepressants and low-potency neuroleptics. Because the kinetic and dynamic behavior of psychotropic drugs in critically ill patients is somewhat unpredictable, low doses are, in general, initially appropriate. Unless the clinical situation requires prompt treatment, doses should be advanced slowly to maximize patient tolerance. Clinical experience shows that doses below the standard therapeutic range are often effective in patients with medical illnesses. This is particularly true

when drug interactions or renal or hepatic impairment slows drug clearance. Some critically ill patients, however, require doses similar to or higher than those required in healthy adults. Higher doses are safely achieved by titrating beneficial effects to side effects.

The consultation-liaison psychiatrist must monitor medications given to the patient in the ICU because nonpsychiatric physicians may have ordered psychotropics before consultation, and additional medications are sometimes ordered by cross-covering physicians. A particular problem that is often seen with many medications, including psychotropics, is delirium. For example, delirium is a common result of the additive effects of individual anticholinergic medications (Sunderland et al. 1987; Tune et al. 1981).

As for any patient given psychotropic medications, consultation-liaison psychiatrists should monitor side effects and response of target symptoms in patients in the ICU. Given the potential for a critically ill patient's clinical condition and his or her overall pharmacological regimen to change rapidly, frequent checks—at least daily—are necessary in most cases.

Drug side effects are sometimes troublesome to critically ill patients and can complicate the diagnostic picture. For example, neuroleptic-induced akathisia can cause restlessness and agitation that is in some cases extreme. In patients for whom the neuroleptic was initially prescribed to treat agitation, this creates a vexing clinical problem. It is best not to neglect the common side effects of psychotropics in the setting of critical illness, even when low doses are used.

It is unwise to avoid the use of psychotropic drugs simply because the patient is critically ill. At times, it might seem that using psychiatric medications in critically ill patients is not worth the trouble. However, when used appropriately, psychotropic drugs are generally well tolerated and effective. The presence of psychiatric symptoms adds to the suffering of critically ill patients; it is inconsistent with excellent clinical care to neglect these symptoms and/or disorders when effective treatments are available.

Nonpharmacological Measures

Nonpharmacological measures also may help reduce the patient's suffering. For example, patients with confusion, delirium, or dementia can benefit from efforts to provide a calming environment, with frequent reassurance and reorientation. Anxious or fearful patients are often reassured by frequent visits from trusted relatives or friends. Although confusional states in the ICU are sometimes attributed to exposure to a stressful and noisy environment (so-called ICU psychosis), severe psychiatric symptoms are much more commonly caused by brain dysfunction related to the patient's physical disorder(s) and/or treatment. Environmental manipulations are helpful in such patients, but they do not address the cause of the symptoms.

Psychotherapeutic Treatments

Psychotherapy in the ICU sounds almost absurd at first. Indeed, most patients who are physically well enough to participate in and benefit from standard psychotherapeutic treatments are well enough to be medically managed outside the ICU. However, knowledge of psychodynamic theories is helpful in the evaluation of many patients in the ICU. Maladaptive behaviors and personality traits are often amplified under the stress of severe physical illness.

Psychotherapeutic interventions are woven into the treatment of most psychiatric problems in the ICU (Stein et al. 1969). Occasionally, a patient's stay in the ICU is long enough for a course of brief psychotherapy. Treatment of a patient's family, when indicated and possible, almost always involves psychodynamic issues that are activated by the critical illness.

Ward Management

Treatment recommendations sometimes include changes in the way patients are managed in the ICU. Such interventions are often effective in reducing psychiatric symptoms. For example, provision of as much calm, quiet, and protection from interruptions in sleep as possible, in combination with reassurance and reorientation, may help to calm a patient with delirium. Patients who are depressed or fearful usually are reassured by more frequent contact with ICU staff. Patients who are anxious or confused can benefit from having a supportive friend or relative nearby.

Use of Restraints

When a patient is agitated or threatening or is at risk for causing injury to himself or herself or to others, appropriate measures must be taken to ensure the safety of the individual and the staff. Mechanical restraint is required when explosive outbursts of agitation or a serious threat to self or others is present. Some staff members, who are fearful of litigation, may object to the use of physical restraint. Mechanical restraints are associated with injuries in some reports (Francis 1989). However, when indicated for the prevention of injury and used with appropri-

ate safety measures and close supervision, use of mechanical restraint is consistent with the goal of excellent medical care. It is much easier to defend an ICU staff member against charges of battery resulting from restraint when restraint is indicated for safety than to defend him or her against charges of negligence resulting from failure to protect a patient or bystander from harm (Hackett and Stern 1991).

Restraints are typically used in combination with sedatives or neuroleptics as a means of controlling dangerous behavior until the medications begin to take effect. However, sometimes it may be necessary to leave the restraints in place for an extended time during a patient's stay in the ICU. Keys to the proper use of restraints in the ICU are thorough documentation of the current need for such safety measures and close clinical supervision of the patient while he or she is in restraints. Implementation of these principles is facilitated by development of a restraint protocol, which outlines the intensity of clinical supervision by ward staff, the frequency of examination used to prevent injury resulting from restraint, and the frequency of reassessment for continued restraint.

Involuntary Treatment

When a mental disorder renders a patient dangerous to himself or herself or to others, or unable to care for himself or herself, involuntary psychiatric treatment is sometimes indicated (depending on the specifics of the law in a given state). In the ICU setting, this situation most commonly arises when the patient in question has attempted suicide (Shuster and Stern 1991; see also Chapter 9, this volume). When evaluation reveals that the patient is at persistent risk for injury to himself or herself or to others, procedures for involuntary psychiatric treatment should be initiated to facilitate transfer to a psychiatric facility once the problem that led to the ICU admission has been stabilized or resolved.

Frequent Follow-Up Visits

For the reasons already described, frequent follow-up is a key to effective psychiatric consultation in the ICU. Ongoing medical evaluation may reveal new clues to the etiology and proper treatment of the mental disorder that were not initially available to the consultant. Improvements in the patient's condition may allow a more thorough examination. As previously discussed, the condition of a patient in the ICU may change dramatically; factors affecting the safety, effectiveness, and tolerability of recommended treatments often vary. Even without rapid changes in a patient's overall condition, treatment response is less predictable in a patient with severe medical illness, thereby necessitating close monitoring. Finally, referring physicians appreciate the consultant's diligence and availability to assist in the ongoing care of critically ill patients.

PSYCHIATRIC DISTURBANCES IN THE CRITICALLY ILL PATIENT

Anxiety

Anxiety, discussed in detail in Chapter 20 of this volume, is a common symptom or complaint of patients in the ICU (Pollack and Stern 1991; Strain et al. 1981). It can present as fearfulness, dread, nervous tension, paniclike symptoms, or full-blown agitation. The anxious patient is typically unable to describe a cause of his or her anxiety. It may interrupt sleep or interfere with the patient's ability to comply with treatment in the ICU. Anxiety can also have adverse physiologic consequences for the critically ill patient because anxiety and stress are associated with sympathetic arousal, elevated catecholamine levels, and electrical and ischemic cardiac events (Charney and Redmond 1983; Hickam et al. 1948; Jewitt et al. 1969; Reich et al. 1981).

The differential diagnosis of anxiety in the patient in the ICU leans heavily toward medical and substance-induced causes (MacKenzie and Popkin 1983; Strain et al. 1981), especially in patients with no personal or family history of anxiety disorders. Common causes include hypoxia (often associated with confusion and agitation), metabolic abnormalities, sepsis, and medication side effects. Intoxication and drug withdrawal states always should be considered, including iatrogenically induced intoxication and withdrawal. Because a complete history is often unavailable in ICU patients, a history of substance use is often not identified until symptoms of drug withdrawal appear. Neurological disorders, such as complex partial seizures, can also present with anxiety symptoms. Patients with preexisting anxiety disorders or a predisposition to anxiety disorders may have an exacerbation of such symptoms under the stress of critical illness. Experiences in the ICU also can place the patient at risk for development of posttraumatic stress disorder (Schelling et al. 1998; Stoll et al. 1999). Fear is differentiated from anxiety primarily in that it is a reaction to an identifiable—and, in the ICU, an often understandable—stressor. Fear can present in a manner identical to anxiety and may range in severity from mild worry (not evident unless the patient is directly questioned) to extreme emotional upset, agitation, or irrational behavior (e.g., refusing needed medical treatment).

Fear also implies a different diagnosis and prognosis. When fear is the primary symptom, it is much more likely that the patient is manifesting a time-limited, reasonable response to a severe stressor, an adjustment disorder, or a maladaptive reaction to the stress of serious illness resulting from limited or inflexible coping skills rather than a true anxiety disorder. Anecdotal evidence based on clinical experience suggests that a trial of low-dose neuroleptic medication may be especially helpful in treating patients who have severe fearfulness.

Treatment of anxiety in the ICU setting (Table 34–3) begins with correction of any underlying physical disorder or imbalance that is producing the symptom, if possible. Anxiety is reduced as these symptomatic treatments progress, but this is not a substitute for addressing the primary problem. This approach is not always feasible; if the physical problem does not respond to treatment or if the putative offending agent (e.g., corticosteroids in patients who have undergone transplantation, parenteral antibiotics in patients being treated for sepsis) cannot safely be discontinued, symptomatic treatment should be initiated to reduce the patient's suffering.

Anxiety caused by primary anxiety disorders should be treated according to accepted guidelines, taking the patient's physical condition into account. Education about the nature of the symptoms, suspected causes, treatments, and expected responses is often quite therapeutic. Benzodiazepines and neuroleptics are the mainstays of anxiolytic therapy for patients in the ICU. These agents are typically underprescribed and are given in inadequate doses when they are ordered for anxiety relief in the medical setting. In the ICU, providing anxiolytics on an as-needed basis, rather than scheduled dosing, is usually inadequate for treatment of anxiety because as-needed anxiolytics are not reliably administered by ICU staff (Stern et al. 1987).

Benzodiazepines are generally the medications of choice for the treatment of anxiety in the ICU. Although all benzodiazepines are effective anxiolytics, lorazepam is often favored because it is available in oral and injectable forms, is reliably absorbed by the intramuscular route, and is more rapidly and simply metabolized. Lorazepam is not oxidatively metabolized, but it is conjugated and then excreted without the formation of active metabolites.

If anxiety or fearfulness is severe or is complicated by psychotic symptoms or confusion, time-limited use of a neuroleptic is usually effective. Additionally, some patients have paradoxical disinhibitory reactions to benzodiazepines (common in elderly individuals or in those who are brain injured). These patients also tend to res-

TABLE 34–3.   Treatment of patients with anxiety in the intensive care unit

Correct any underlying physical disorders, if possible

Discontinue anxiogenic medications, if possible

Pharmacological interventions
    Benzodiazepines
    Neuroleptics

Nonpharmacological interventions
    Education
    Support
    Behavioral techniques
        Hypnosis
        Relaxation techniques
        Imagery
    Cognitive therapy
    Family therapy

Source. Adapted from Pollack MH, Stern TA: "Recognition and Treatment of Anxiety in the ICU Patient," in *Intensive Care Medicine,* 2nd Edition. Edited by Rippe JM, Irwin RS, Alpert JS, et al. Boston, MA, Little, Brown, 1991, pp. 1875–1887. Copyright 1991, Little, Brown and Company. Used with permission.

pond preferentially to neuroleptics. In the ICU, high-potency agents such as haloperidol are preferred over low-potency agents because the higher-potency agents cause less sedation, have fewer anticholinergic and adverse cardiac effects, and have a long history of use in the ICU setting (Settle and Ayd 1983).

Therapeutic support, relaxation treatments, hypnosis, and cognitive therapy are sometimes helpful as primary treatments or as adjuncts to use of medication for anxiety and fearfulness. These nonpharmacological measures are also sometimes sufficient for relief of fear.

Depression

Depression (see also Chapter 17, this volume) can present in patients in the ICU as apathy, withdrawal, help-lessness, tearfulness, decreased cooperation with treatment, or suicidal ideation or behavior (Cassem 1990; Cohen-Cole and Stoudemire 1987; Geringer and Stern 1991; Kathol et al. 1990; Rodin and Voshart 1986). Discouragement and worry about medical problems are very frequently seen in patients in the ICU, and these are often mistaken as symptoms of a formal depressive disorder. Anger, fear, apathetic states, and nonagitated delirium are at times misdiagnosed as depression. Depression is usually the result of major depressive disorder, dysthymia, or a medically or substance-induced mood disorder. ICU admission frequently results when depressed mood leads to a suicide attempt or extreme inattention to self-care.

Some patients who appear depressed may not meet diagnostic criteria for one of the disorders listed in DSM-IV-TR (American Psychiatric Association 2000). Feelings of despondency cause suffering and can lead to a consultation request. Patients may become despondent for several reasons. It is important to remember that the stresses that predispose to despondency can also lead to depression.

Depressive symptoms, even when they do not meet criteria for a major depressive syndrome, are a significant cause of morbidity and disability (Wells et al. 1990). Depression, especially if untreated, increases mortality in general and mortality from cardiac causes in particular (Avery and Winokur 1976; Malzberg 1937; Murphy et al. 1987; Rabins et al. 1985).

Some patients in ICUs who feel they are dying (regardless of whether they really are) have catastrophic responses. In cases in which this perception is inaccurate, simple education about the true clinical situation can provide great relief. Sadness and despondency that do not resolve with such reassurance should prompt the psychiatrist to consider a diagnosis of depression. In cases in which the patient's illness truly is life-threatening or terminal, an open, empathic, and supportive attitude often helps. Interventions that address concerns about comfort, autonomy, availability of loved ones, and feared abandonment by medical caregivers usually will lead to relief (Cassem 1991).

Another cause of depressed mood among patients in the ICU is grief. Many patients have visited an ICU before, usually during the critical (often terminal) illness of a relative or friend—possibly during a past personal episode of illness. If the ICU setting reminds the patient of past experience, feelings of dread or grief are sometimes aroused. This is especially true if the grief was not dealt with appropriately at the time.

Critical illness may be perceived as a narcissistic injury. Particularly when the illness necessitating admission to the ICU is sudden in onset (e.g., myocardial infarction), the resultant change in self-perception is sometimes devastating. Stern (1985) described a modification of the Draw-a-Person Test, in which the patient is asked to draw a picture of a person and a picture of what the patient thinks is wrong, as a useful technique to access and monitor such changes in self-perception.

Treatment of major depression usually includes pharmacological agents. In the ICU, the selective serotonin reuptake inhibitors (SSRIs) and psychostimulants are used more often than tricyclic antidepressants and monoamine oxidase inhibitors (MAOIs). The SSRIs have fewer side effects and a better safety profile in critically ill patients compared with the tricyclic antidepressants (which can cause cardiac arrhythmias, constipation, orthostasis, and anticholinergic delirium) or the MAOIs (which can cause significant hypotension and require strict dietary and pharmacological restrictions to prevent hypertensive crisis). SSRIs, including fluoxetine, sertraline, and paroxetine, are generally well tolerated, even by critically ill patients. Common side effects of the SSRIs include headache, nausea, jitteriness, insomnia, and sedation. Awareness of drug interactions is important (Shuster et al. 1992), particularly the inhibitory effect that SSRIs have on the cytochrome P450 system. Levels of drugs metabolized via these pathways are commonly raised by the concomitant administration of an SSRI. Psychostimulants are generally safe and useful in the treatment of depression in medically ill patients (Kaufman et al. 1982; Woods et al. 1986). The ICU setting allows close monitoring of the response to psychostimulant administration. The chief advantages of stimulants for depression in the ICU are rapid therapeutic response, rapid clearance of the drug if side effects emerge, and safety and tolerability at the low doses usually required. Initially, dosing begins with 2.5–5.0 mg of dextroamphetamine in the morning or 5.0 mg of methylphenidate in the morning and early afternoon, with an increase of 2.5 mg/dose/day until the desired therapeutic benefit is achieved, intolerable side effects emerge, or a dose of 15–20 mg/day of dextroamphetamine or 15–20 mg/dose with twice-daily dosing of methylphenidate is reached. Side effects that may limit psychostimulant treatment include hypertension, tachycardia, arrhythmia, agitation, confusion, insomnia, and appetite suppression. Low doses of stimulants often increase appetite in medically ill patients with depression. The clinician should screen for each of these side effects before each dose increase.

Confusion

Critically ill patients commonly experience confusion or agitation (Engel and Romano 1959; Lipowski 1989; Tesar and Stern 1991; Wise and Brandt 1992). Although confused or agitated behavior in the ICU can have several etiologies (e.g., anger, pain, severe anxiety, psychosis, personality disorder under stress), most confusional states experienced by patients in the ICU are secondary to medical and substance-induced causes (e.g., delirium, dementia, secondary personality disorder). (For further discussion, please refer to Chapters 15 and 16, this volume.) As noted throughout this chapter, the high rate of secondary mental disorders in ICU patients is largely related to the severity of physical problems necessitating ICU care.

The presentation of confusional states among patients in the ICU varies. Delirium often goes unrecog-

nized in the ICU (Eden and Foreman 1996). Confusion is so common in the ICU that psychiatric consultation is often not requested unless the patient is also agitated. The quietly confused patient is often mistakenly referred by his or her physicians for depression, anxiety, or an unpleasant personality. At the other extreme, when patients become agitated, combative, or otherwise uncooperative, psychiatric assistance is urgently required. Confusion with agitation is often misdiagnosed by the nonpsychiatrist as functional psychosis.

All instances of confusion in the ICU merit attention and evaluation because a confusional state is usually a sign of an underlying medical complication. Moreover, because alert and cognitively intact patients are better able to cooperate with treatment and comply with specific instructions (e.g., use of incentive spirometers, ambulation), aggressive screening and treatment of delirium are cost-effective in that they reduce the length of ICU stay and use of resources (Levenson et al. 1990).

Treatment of delirium in the ICU, as outlined in Table 34–4 (Lipowski 1990), begins with a thorough search for causative medical or substance-induced problems (e.g., infections, head trauma, metabolic abnormalities). Medications, as listed in Table 34–5, or interactions between drugs also should be considered, and any offending agents should be discontinued whenever possible. Withdrawal states, particularly those related to alcohol and sedative-hypnotic medications, are always possible, even when the admitting history indicates no problem with substance use—patients typically underreport substance-use patterns (Hackett et al. 1991; Khantzian and McKenna 1979). Sensory overstimulation should be minimized to help patients sleep, although adequate interpersonal contact and stimulation should be maintained—admittedly a difficult task in the ICU. General supportive care with frequent reassurance and reorientation is very helpful to the patient who is recovering from delirium.

Medications used to treat agitation in the ICU include neuroleptics, benzodiazepines, narcotics, and paralytic agents (Sos and Cassem 1980; Tesar and Stern 1988; Thompson and Thompson 1983). The pharmacological properties of medications commonly used to treat confusion and agitation in patients in the ICU are outlined in Table 34–6.

Neuroleptics usually are the drugs of first choice in the ICU setting, although benzodiazepines are commonly used alone or in combination with neuroleptics (Breitbart et al. 1996; Salzman et al. 1986). Haloperidol, a high-potency butyrophenone, is the most commonly used neuroleptic agent in the ICU setting because of its long record of safety and utility (Cameron 1978; Donlon et al.

TABLE 34–4.   Guidelines for treatment of delirium in the intensive care unit

1. Monitor the patient's mental state and behavior closely.
2. Search for causative physical problems and correct them when possible.
   Consider adverse effects of medications.
   Consider interactions between medications.
   Consider withdrawal states.
3. Use medications (e.g., neuroleptics, benzodiazepines) to treat agitation and psychotic symptoms.
4. Structure the patient's environment to provide adequate contact with others, without overstimulation.
5. Maintain nutrition, fluid and electrolyte balance, and vitamin intake.
6. Provide general nursing care aimed at reorienting the patient, observing and reporting his or her behavior, and providing emotional support.
7. Provide supportive psychotherapy at the bedside, which may help calm the patient and aid adaptation after resolution of delirium.

Source. Adapted from Lipowski ZJ: *Delirium: Acute Confusional States.* New York, Oxford University Press, 1990. Copyright 1990, Oxford University Press. Used with permission.

TABLE 34–5.   Common delirium-inducing drugs used in the intensive care unit

Group	Agent
Antiarrhythmics	Lidocaine
	Mexiletine
	Procainamide
	Quinidine
Antibiotics	Penicillin
	Rifampin
Anticholinergics	Atropine
Antihistamines	Nonselective
	Diphenhydramine
	Promethazine
	H$_2$-blockers
	Cimetidine
	Ranitidine
β-Blockers	Propranolol
Narcotic analgesics	Meperidine
	Morphine
	Pentazocine

Source. Adapted from Tesar GE, Stern TA: "Evaluation and Treatment of Agitation in the Intensive Care Unit." *Journal of Intensive Care Medicine* 1:137–148, 1986. Copyright 1986, Little, Brown and Company. Used with permission.

1979; Settle and Ayd 1983). Another feature of haloperidol that makes it appealing for use in the ICU is its safety and efficacy when it is administered intravenously (Cassem and Hackett 1991; Fernandez et al. 1988). Pharmacological treatments for delirium can usually be safely discontinued once the patient is symptom-free for 24–48 hours, unless habituating agents such as benzodiazepines were used long enough to induce tolerance and withdrawal, in which case drug tapering is appropriate.

When sedation of the agitated ICU patient is a primary treatment goal, agents such as benzodiazepines, narcotics, and paralytics are often used. Recently, the short-acting intravenous anesthetic propofol has also come into wide use for this indication in the ICU. The advantages of propofol include rapid onset, easy titration, and more rapid emergence from sedation after discontinuation as compared with midazolam and other similar gents (Barrientos-Vega et al. 1997; Chamorro et al. 1996; Harvey 1996). Propofol has been safely and effectively used for short-term (1 day to a few days) and long-term (greater than 1 week) sedation in the ICU (Miller and Wiles-Pfeifler 1998; Treggiari-Venzi et al. 1996; Weinbroum et al. 1997). Potential adverse effects include hyperlipidemia, depression of cardiovascular function, and zinc deficiency (due to the chelating agent ethylenediaminetetraacetic acid [EDTA] added for bacteriostasis) (Marinella 1997).

Psychosis

The ICU is potentially a frightening and distressing place for patients with psychosis. Patients with schizophrenia or other psychotic disorders, delusional disorder, bipolar disorder, or psychotic depression can have problems adapting to the stress of critical illness and ICU treatment (Goff et al. 1991). This is particularly true if the patient has paranoia or active psychotic symptoms.

A diagnosis (or even the suggestion) of schizophrenia may strike fear in the hearts of referring physicians and ICU staff. In addition to assessment of the patient and provision of treatment recommendations, effective management of the patient with psychosis in the ICU requires close cooperation with the unit staff (Goff et al. 1991). Staff members may require instruction or coaching regarding the behavior management of patients with psychosis and the opportunity to discuss the feelings aroused by a patient whose behavior is bizarre, paranoid, or hostile. Otherwise, the discomfort of staff members may compromise excellent clinical care by leading them to be less attentive to the patient's physical problems (e.g., recommending premature transfer out of the ICU).

The patient with psychosis is treated in the ICU much as he or she would be treated in other settings. Neuroleptic agents are the mainstays of treatment. If the

TABLE 34–6. Pharmacology of drugs used to treat confusion and agitation

Drug	Route	Onset (minutes)	Peak effect (minutes)	Starting dosage	Comments
Neuroleptics					
Haloperidol	iv,[a] im	5–20	15–45	Mild agitation: 0.5–2.0 mg	Generally considered the first line of
	po	30–60	120–240	Moderate agitation: 5–10 mg	treatment, especially when confusion is
				Severe agitation: ≥10 mg	prominent
Droperidol	iv, im	3–10	15–45	2.5–10.0 mg	
Chlorpromazine	im, iv[b]	5–40	10–30	25 mg	
Benzodiazepines					
Diazepam	iv	2–5	5–30	2–5 mg	Useful alone or in combination with
	po	10–60	30–180		neuroleptics; especially useful when
					symptoms of anxiety predominate
Lorazepam	iv, im	2–20	60–120	1–2 mg	
	sl	2–20	20–60	0.5–1.0 mg	
	po	20–60	20–120	0.5–1.0 mg	
Midazolam	im, iv	1–2	30–40	0.05–0.15 mg/kg	
Narcotic					
Morphine	im, iv	1–2	20	4–10 mg	ICU staff familiar with use; reversible with naloxone if necessary; very useful if pain is prominent
Paralytic agents					
Metocurine	iv	1–4	2–10	0.2–0.4 mg/kg	Generally considered treatment of last resort to prevent patient self-injury; requires intubation
Pancuronium	iv	0.5–1	5	0.04–0.10 mg/kg	
Alkylphenol anesthetics					
Propofol	iv	0.5–1	5	1–2 mg/kg	Easy titration, rapid clearance of sedative effects; requires intubation

Note. ICU = intensive care unit; im = intramuscular; iv = intravenous; po = per os (orally); sl = sublingual.
[a]Intravenous haloperidol is not approved for routine use by the U.S. Food and Drug Administration; permission for its use should be requested from the hospital's formulary.
[b]Intravenous administration of chlorpromazine is more likely to cause cardiovascular disturbance (e.g., hypotension) than intramuscular administration.
Source. Adapted from Tesar GE, Stern TA: "Rapid Tranquilization of the Agitated Intensive Care Unit Patient." *Journal of Intensive Care Medicine* 3:195–201, 1988. Copyright 1988, Little, Brown and Company. Used with permission.

patient takes a neuroleptic that has proven effective as outpatient therapy, this medication is generally continued if the patient can tolerate it while critically ill. In some cases, low-potency neuroleptics are discontinued and high-potency agents (e.g., haloperidol) are substituted at equivalent doses. Depot preparations are almost always avoided in the ICU. Benzodiazepines (e.g., lorazepam, clonazepam) are helpful adjuncts to neuroleptics for psychosis. The patient in the ICU with psychotic agitation may be treated with a range of agents, listed in Table 34–6.

Personality

Most patients in the ICU who are alert enough to interact with staff members tolerate their stay without major interpersonal conflicts. The typical patient is very ill but does not exhibit behavior that impedes medical care or alienates the ICU staff. Unfortunately, patients with maladaptive personality traits or full-blown personality disorders rely on familiar maladaptive patterns of behavior when challenged by stressors such as severe illness (Groves 1975; Wool et al. 1991). In fact, personality styles usually are amplified in the ICU because these traits are the patient's best or only defense against such stress (e.g., the paranoid person becomes more hostile, withdrawn, and suspicious when admitted to the cardiac care unit after a myocardial infarction). Obviously, such patterns of behavior impede the delivery of care by rendering the patient less able to cooperate with ICU staff in a mature and appropriate manner and by rendering the staff less able (and sometimes less willing) to deliver needed care.

As in other general hospital settings, such patterns of behavior in the ICU frequently lead to requests for psychiatric consultation. (The relation between personality and response to medical illness is more fully discussed in Chapter 8, this volume.) An outline of the manifestations, etiologies, characteristic staff responses, and management strategies for these behaviors is presented in Table 34–7.

TABLE 34–7. Problematic acute behaviors among patients in the intensive care unit and their manifestations, etiologies, staff responses, and management

Behavior	Manifestations	Etiologies	Staff responses	Management
Frightened	Screaming Crying Threatening Litigiousness	Pain Psychosis Terror Delirium Anxiety	Fear Aggression Avoidance	Restraints Sedatives Antipsychotics Narcotics Reassurance
Self-destructive	Secret smoking Pulling lines Suicidal actions	Character Psychosis Anxiety Depression Delirium Mania	Anger Repulsion Helplessness Withholding	Team communication Limits Restraints Sedatives
Inappropriate	Bizarre behavior Seductiveness Rejecting help	Psychosis Narcissism Hysteria	Avoidance Fear Anger	Antipsychotics Team communication Restraints Limits Sedatives Keeping appropriate distance
Helpless	Inconsolable crying Depression fantasies	Character Futile condition	Avoidance Rescue	Antidepressants
Infantile	Depression Whining	Helplessness Family conflict Culture	Reassurance Support Anger	Exploration of feelings Family meeting Encouragement of independence
Noncompliant	Leaving AMA Spitting up pills	Character Depression Sociopathy Psychosis Dementia Retardation	Fury Collusion Denial	Paradoxical approach Psychiatric evaluation Antidepressants Strict limits Determination of incompetence; if so, find guardian
Uncooperative	Rudeness Refusing procedures	Psychosis Depression Anxiety Mania Malingering	Annoyance Revenge Avoidance	Limits Recognition of own limits Psychiatric evaluation
Obnoxious	Insulting Self-righteousness	Character Anxiety Family conflict Culture Psychosis Delirium	Anger "Yes 'em"	Limits Team communication Treatment of anxiety Treatment of depression

Note.   Within each behavior group, each column should be read down, not across. AMA = against medical advice.
Source.   Adapted from Wool C, Geringer ES, Stern TA: "The Management of Behavioral Problems in the ICU," in *Intensive Care Medicine*, 2nd Edition. Edited by Rippe JM, Irwin RS, Alpert JS, et al. Boston, MA, Little, Brown, 1991, pp. 1906–1916. Copyright 1991, Little, Brown and Company. Used with permission.

In general, patients who have maladaptive, irrational, uncooperative, or irritating behavior in the ICU are evaluated according to the protocol illustrated in Figure 34–1. Before such behavior is attributed to personality, a careful evaluation of substance-induced and medical causes (e.g., confusion, delirium) should be performed. Confusional states may render the patient irritable, paranoid, combative, or unable to cooperate with treatment, although this behavior is not intentional, and the patient may have little awareness of or control over the behavior. The consulting psychiatrist should next screen for other Axis I disorders (e.g., severe anxiety, psychosis), as well as physical problems (e.g., pain) and interpersonal difficulties (e.g., anger at staff or family members). If this search for other explanations of maladaptive behavior is unrevealing, characterological problems should be considered. A life-threatening illness often causes regressive behaviors in many patients; this behavior does not necessarily reflect baseline (premorbid) functioning.

Kahana and Bibring (1965) described the characteristic patterns of response to medical illness and hospitalization for several personality types: dependent (oral), obsessive, histrionic, masochistic, paranoid, narcissistic, and schizoid. Most of these behavior patterns roughly correspond to formal personality disorders of the same name, but the correlation is not absolute. For purposes of patient management in the ICU, it is useful to classify personality types by the behavior exhibited. Table 34–8 provides an overview of the response to illness of these seven personality types, along with some simple management suggestions.

CLINICAL SITUATIONS UNIQUE TO THE INTENSIVE CARE UNIT

Clinical situations or procedures unique to the ICU setting and worth special mention include mechanical ventilation, placement of an intra-aortic balloon pump (IABP), and cardiac surgery.

Respirators

Mechanical ventilation poses special challenges for the psychiatric evaluation, as described earlier in this chapter (Feeley 1976). In addition to impediments to assessment, placement of a patient on a respirator is associated with anxiety, depression, agitation, and delirium.

Anxiety is very commonly associated with mechanical ventilation. In addition, the underlying respiratory problems often produce sufficient hypoxia to produce or exacerbate anxiety symptoms. Although ventilatory support usually resolves such anxiety by correcting hypoxia, patients are at times made more anxious by intubation and ventilation. The endotracheal tube is often uncomfortable, and ventilation is sometimes suboptimal even with aggressive respiratory therapy. In addition, the constant rhythmic noise of the respirator can serve as a nerve-wracking reminder to the patient of his or her critical state. Alert patients may worry about their prognosis or may feel helpless and out of control.

Anxiety is particularly common when the patient is weaned from the ventilator. Several factors can play a role in the anxiety: patients may experience at least brief periods of relative hypoxia during weaning trials; prolonged ventilation usually leads to deconditioning of muscles of respiration, so patients become frightened by the unfamiliar difficulty they experience with breathing until these muscles are reconditioned; and patients often become psychologically dependent on the ventilator and fearful when the device is disconnected.

Depression and confusional states are commonly seen in patients who are mechanically ventilated, probably because ventilation is associated with severe medical illness. Depression (and severity of depression) correlates with severity of concurrent medical illness. As noted throughout this chapter, secondary mental disorders are commonly seen in patients with serious medical illnesses. Patients who require mechanical ventilation often have infections, metabolic imbalances, and side effects of multiple medications in addition to their respiratory insufficiency; all of these conditions contribute to the development of delirium.

Intra-aortic Balloon Pumps and Cardiac Surgery

Delirium is a common complication of cardiac procedures in the critically ill patient. An association between placement of the IABP and delirium occurred in 34% of 198 patients undergoing this procedure at Massachusetts General Hospital (Sanders et al. 1992). Delirium usually developed acutely—on the first or second day after IABP insertion—and resolved rapidly after the IABP was removed. Although in-hospital mortality was nearly identical between patients with delirium and those without delirium, the patients who became delirious had significantly longer hospital stays and a greater likelihood of developing residual neuropsychiatric deficits.

Cardiac surgery is also associated with a high rate of delirium during the postoperative phase, estimated at 32% in a literature review and meta-analysis by Smith and Dimsdale (1989). Factors that contribute to delirium following cardiac surgery are outlined in Table 34–9. Preexisting brain dysfunction and the duration and complex-

TABLE 34–8.   Impact of seven personality types on response to critical illness

Personality type	Leading traits	Response to stress or illness	Suggested management
Dependent	Craves special attention Urgently demands services Naively expects total care at all times Constantly seeks reassurance that others care	Fears total abandonment and subsequent helplessness Increased anxiety leads to increased demands	Express willingness to care for patient as completely as possible Set limits, give thoughtful explanation of limits Make small concessions when possible
Obsessive/overly orderly	Excessive attention to order and detail Ambiguity, unknowns, surprises increase anxiety Keeps tight rein on expression of emotion, pain, and fear	Illness seen as threat to self-control Double-bind: inner control prevents acknowledgment of confusion, hence unable to ask questions, hence ambiguity and anxiety increase	Use scientific medical approach; give enough information Help patient to establish intellectual control over anxiety Allow patient to participate in decisions of care and management (e.g., monitoring diet, exercise)
Histrionic/dramatic	Trusting person, often forms sexualized relationships Deals with anxiety by denying, avoiding, repressing, or "forgetting" Dramatic presentations May have phobias	Illness experienced as an attack on femininity or masculinity	Appreciate attractiveness, physical prowess, and courage Give general reassurance (not detailed) if anxiety is high Provide opportunity to discuss fears
Masochistic/long-suffering/martyrlike	History of repeated suffering Steadfast and self-sacrificing Feels he or she is unappreciated	Illness experienced as deserved punishment May be "good" patient if illness feels like yet another burden to shoulder May have increased noncompliance if suffering is not acknowledged	Appreciate difficulties being endured Do not attempt to comfort or placate Present treatment as task that will help others
Paranoid/guarded	Wary, suspicious Hypersensitive to slights, real or imagined Can be quarrelsome when feeling persecuted	Illness experienced as assault from the outside Feels unconsciously betrayed by himself or herself for being ill Medical procedures may lead to increased suspiciousness and fear of being harmed	Keep patient thoroughly informed of diagnostic and treatment strategies Listen to complaints and appreciate how hard things are to endure in the light of illness and hospitalization
Narcissistic/superior feelings	Difficulty asking for or accepting help Must appear strong, competent, knowledgeable Fears dependence on others	Illness experienced as attack on perfection Increases efforts to show strength (e.g., excessive exercise) and independence (e.g., signing out AMA)	Make patient an active partner in proceedings Acknowledge strengths Expect omissions in history (illness = weakness)
Schizoid/aloof	Distant, unsociable, uninvolved with daily events Lives and works with minimum contact with others required (this protects against expected disappointments)	Illness forces closeness Can feel intolerable because protection against expected rejection has been removed Leads to more aloofness and withdrawal Illness is experienced as intrusion	Accept and respect unsociability and insulation Continue interested, caring, and nonintrusive stance

Note.   Table should read down, not across, each column. AMA = against medical advice.
Source.   Adapted from Kahana RJ, Bibring GL: "Personality Types in Medical Management," in *Psychiatry and Medical Practice in a General Hospital.* Edited by Zinberg NE. New York, International Universities Press, 1965, pp. 108–123; Wool C, Geringer ES, Stern TA: "The Management of Behavioral Problems in the ICU," in *Intensive Care Medicine,* 2nd Edition. Edited by Rippe JM, Irwin RS, Alpert JS, et al. Boston, MA, Little, Brown, 1991, pp. 1906–1916. Copyright 1991, Little, Brown and Company. Used with permission.

ity of the surgical procedure are the most important factors. The type of oxygenator used in the bypass device also may have a great deal to do with the patient's postoperative neuropsychiatric outcome. Investigators in one study reported a markedly lower and statistically significant prevalence of postoperative retinal microemboli when a membrane-type oxygenator was used as compared with a bubble-type oxygenator (Blauth et al. 1989).

STAFF STRESS

The task of providing intensive care for patients with critical illness is very stressful (Gonzales and Stern 1991). Patients in ICUs are very ill. Treatment of acute and often rapidly changing illnesses puts pressure on the ICU staff to produce good clinical results in very difficult sit-

TABLE 34–9. Factors contributing to the development of delirium following cardiac surgery

Time course	Factor
Preoperative	History of MI
	Preexisting CNS dysfunction
	Psychiatric disorders and factors
	Panic-level anxiety
	Major depression
	Alcohol or drug abuse
	Poor understanding of or reluctance to undergo planned procedure
	Severe physical illness
Intraoperative	Body temperature ≤28°C
	Complexity of surgical procedure
	Systolic blood pressure ≤50–60 mm Hg
	Total anesthesia time
	Type of oxygenator used in the bypass device (?)
Postoperative	Complications during recovery
	Environment (e.g., sensory overload or deprivation)
	Intra-aortic balloon pump (?)
	Medications administered (e.g., excess anticholinergic agents, narcotics, sedative-hypnotics)

Note. CNS = central nervous system; MI = myocardial infarction.
Source. Adapted from Tesar GE, Stern TA: "Evaluation and Treatment of Agitation in the Intensive Care Unit." *Journal of Intensive Care Medicine* 1:137–148, 1986. Copyright 1986, Little, Brown and Company. Used with permission.

uations under great time pressure. Family members, themselves burdened by concern about their critically ill loved one, may express fears and frustrations to or at ICU staff members. Some members of the treatment team, who are also under pressure, can withdraw, be less supportive, or inappropriately direct feelings of frustration, anger, or helplessness toward one another or toward the patient or his or her family. Clearly, intensive care is aptly named from the perspective of the caregiver. The intensity, the fast pace, and the action inherent in ICU medicine are part of the appeal of this field for those who choose it. These same factors, however, place clinicians who work in the ICU at great risk for burnout.

Unless the factors that predispose to stress and burnout are addressed, ICU staff members are likely to disengage and withdraw from the intense and often daunting work they face daily. Problems with quality of care, increased staff turnover, adverse health effects and absenteeism, and adverse effects on the personal lives of affected personnel can result.

Prevention or intervention measures require recognition of the potential sources of stress related to provision of intensive care. Table 34–10 lists some stresses for ICU staff. Some stresses are related to staffing shortages, common in ICUs, which are addressed by recruiting additional staff or otherwise reducing workload. Other sources of stress are related to training and education deficits, which are best addressed by supervision or in-service training. Feelings aroused by constantly dealing with death and severe morbidity, or by responding to the needs of critically ill patients and their families, are more difficult to address because these factors are integral to the provision of critical care. When stress leads to symptoms of depression, an anxiety disorder, or another psychiatric disorder, psychiatric evaluation is helpful to treat a disorder (if present), help the staff member to examine his or her situation objectively, and improve his or her skills for coping with the stressful environment of the ICU.

Group interventions for ICU physicians, nurses, and other staff members are very effective in reducing work stress in the ICU (Cassem and Hackett 1975; Siegal and Donnelly 1978; Simon and Whitely 1977; Weiner et al. 1983). Stern et al. (1993) reported on autognosis rounds, a group stress reduction and self-knowledge intervention that has been an ongoing part of the medical house staff's experience in the medical ICU at Massachusetts General Hospital for more than 15 years. The goals for the house staff participants are

> to 1) identify their subjective reactions to clinical situations, 2) learn to use their emotions in clinical practice, 3) learn how to minimize possible disruptive effects of their reactions to patients (e.g., manage their angry feelings toward patients so they can be expressed during the rounds and not interfere with patient care), and 4) share their reactions with each other and thereby learn that they are not alone with their feelings. (Stern et al. 1993, p. 2)

Stern has also maintained The Red Book, a sort of community journal, as an adjunct to autognosis rounds. Participants are invited to contribute as they see fit. The Red Book, now in its twentieth year, contains an impressive and often enlightening collection of jokes, reflections, slogans, and even impromptu essays. These interventions are valued and well attended by the medical house staff.

CONCLUSION

Although consultation-liaison psychiatry in the ICU is challenging and intense, it is not qualitatively different from other areas of consultation psychiatry. Compared

TABLE 34–10.   Common stresses for intensive care unit staff

Physician stressors	Nurse stressors
Being sleep-deprived	Having an excessive workload (high patient-to-nurse ratio)
Having long on-duty assignments	Having too little time to deal with patients' or their families' emotional needs
Providing high-technology care	
Dealing with chronically and/or severely ill patients	Dealing with death
Feeling a responsibility to patients' families	Dealing with the unnecessary prolongation of life
Having limited training in ethics	Providing high-technology care
Being exposed to contagious and/or deadly diseases (e.g., AIDS)	Having unpredictable schedules
Performing complex or invasive procedural tasks	Being subjected to environmental disturbances (e.g., noise)
Being overloaded with information	Having administrative conflicts
Having a large financial debt	Feeling powerless or insecure
Anxiety about malpractice	

Note.   AIDS = acquired immunodeficiency syndrome.
Source.   Reprinted from Gonzales JJ, Stern TA: "Recognition and Management of Staff Stress in the ICU," in *Intensive Care Medicine*, 2nd Edition. Edited by Rippe JM, Irwin RS, Alpert JS, et al. Boston, MA, Little, Brown, 1991, pp. 1916–1922. Copyright 1991, Little, Brown, and Company. Used with permission.

with other settings, the patients to be treated are sicker, the pace is faster, and the stress level is higher. The same mental disorders that are seen in other settings are seen in the ICU, especially the secondary mental disorders, but these are complicated by the severity and dynamic state of the patients' physical problems. The consultation-liaison psychiatrist can offer help by focusing efforts on clinical care of ICU patients and by focusing liaison efforts on helping members of the ICU staff care for the critically ill while preventing burnout.

REFERENCES

American Psychiatric Association: Diagnostic and Statistical Manual of Mental Disorders, 4th Edition. Washington, DC, American Psychiatric Association, 1994

American Psychiatric Association: Diagnostic and Statistical Manual of Mental Disorders, 4th Edition, Text Revision. Washington, DC, American Psychiatric Association, 2000

Avery D, Winokur G: Mortality in depressed patients treated with electroconvulsive therapy and antidepressants. Arch Gen Psychiatry 33:1029–1037, 1976

Barrientos-Vega R, Mar Sanchez-Soria M, Morales-Garcia C, et al: Prolonged sedation of critically ill patients with midazolam or propofol: impact on weaning and costs. Crit Care Med 25:33–40, 1997

Blauth CI, Smith PL, Arnold JV, et al: Influence of oxygenator type on the incidence and extent of microembolic retinal ischemia during cardiopulmonary bypass: assessment by digital image analysis (abstract). Paper presented at the annual meeting of the American Association for Thoracic Surgery, Boston, MA, May 8, 1989

Breitbart W, Marotta R, Platt MM, et al: A double-blind trial of haloperidol, chlorpromazine, and lorazepam in the treatment of delirium in hospitalized AIDS patients. Am J Psychiatry 153:231–237, 1996

Cameron OG: Safe use of haloperidol in a patient with cardiac dysrhythmia (letter). Am J Psychiatry 135:1244, 1978

Cassem NH: Depression and anxiety secondary to medical illness. Psychiatr Clin North Am 13:597–612, 1990

Cassem NH: The dying patient, in Massachusetts General Hospital Handbook of General Hospital Psychiatry, 3rd Edition. Edited by Cassem NH. St. Louis, MO, CV Mosby, 1991, pp 343–371

Cassem NH, Hackett TP: Stress on the nurse and therapist in the intensive care unit and the coronary care unit. Heart Lung 4:252–259, 1975

Cassem NH, Hackett TP: The setting of intensive care, in Massachusetts General Hospital Handbook of General Hospital Psychiatry, 3rd Edition. Edited by Cassem NH. St. Louis, MO, CV Mosby, 1991, pp 373–399

Chamorro C, deLatorre FJ, Montero A, et al: Comparative study of propofol versus midazolam in the sedation of critically ill patients: results of a prospective, randomized, multicenter trial. Crit Care Med 24:932–939, 1996

Charney DS, Redmond DE Jr: Neurobiological mechanisms in human anxiety: evidence supporting noradrenergic hyperactivity. Neuropharmacology 22:1531–1536, 1983

Cohen-Cole S, Stoudemire A: Major depression and physical illness. Psychiatr Clin North Am 10:1–17, 1987

Dec GW, Stern TA: Tricyclic antidepressants in the intensive care unit. Journal of Intensive Care Medicine 5:69–81, 1990

Donlon PT, Hopkin J, Schaffer CB, et al: Cardiovascular safety of rapid treatment with intramuscular haloperidol. Am J Psychiatry 136:233–234, 1979

Eden BM, Foreman MD: Problems associated with underrecognition of delirium in critical care: a case study. Heart Lung 25:388–400, 1996

Engel GL, Romano J: Delirium: a syndrome of cerebral insufficiency. Journal of Chronic Diseases 9:260–277, 1959

Feeley TW: Problems in weaning patients from ventilators. Resident and Staff Physician 22:291–298, 1976

Fernandez F, Holmes VF, Adams F, et al: Treatment of severe, refractory agitation with a haloperidol drip. J Clin Psychiatry 49:239–241, 1988

Folstein MF, Folstein SE, McHugh PR: Mini-Mental State, a practical method for grading the cognitive state of patients for the clinician. J Psychiatr Res 12:189–198, 1975

Francis J: Using restraints in the elderly because of fear of litigation (letter). N Engl J Med 320:870, 1989

Geringer ES, Stern TA: Recognition and treatment of depression in the ICU, in Intensive Care Medicine, 2nd Edition. Edited by Rippe JM, Irwin RS, Alpert JS, et al. Boston, MA, Little, Brown, 1991, pp 1887–1902

Goff DC, Manschreck TC, Groves JE: Psychotic patients, in Massachusetts General Hospital Handbook of General Hospital Psychiatry, 3rd Edition. Edited by Cassem NH. St. Louis, MO, CV Mosby, 1991, pp 217–236

Gonzales JJ, Stern TA: Recognition and management of staff stress in the ICU, in Intensive Care Medicine, 2nd Edition. Edited by Rippe JM, Irwin RS, Alpert JS, et al. Boston, MA, Little, Brown, 1991, pp 1916–1922

Groves JE: Management of the borderline patient on a medical surgical ward: the psychiatric consultant's role. Int J Psychiatry Med 6:337–348, 1975

Hackett TP, Stern TA: Suicide and other disruptive states, in Massachusetts General Hospital Handbook of General Hospital Psychiatry, 3rd Edition. Edited by Cassem NH. St. Louis, MO, CV Mosby, 1991, pp 281–307

Hackett TP, Gastfriend DR, Renner JA: Alcoholism: acute and chronic states, in Massachusetts General Hospital Handbook of General Hospital Psychiatry, 3rd Edition. Edited by Cassem NH. St. Louis, MO, CV Mosby, 1991, pp 9–22

Harvey MA: Managing agitation in critically ill patients. Am J Crit Care 5:7–16, 1996

Hickam JB, Cargill WH, Golden A: Cardiovascular reactions to emotional stimuli: effect on the cardiac output, arteriovenous oxygen difference, arterial pressure, and peripheral resistance. J Clin Invest 27:290–298, 1948

Jenike MA: Geriatric Psychiatry and Psychopharmacology. Chicago, IL, Year Book Medical, 1989

Jewitt DE, Mercer CJ, Reid D, et al: Free noradrenaline and adrenaline excretion in relation to the development of cardiac arrhythmias and heart failure in patients with acute myocardial infarction. Lancet 1:635–641, 1969

Kahana RJ, Bibring GL: Personality types in medical management, in Psychiatry and Medical Practice in a General Hospital. Edited by Zinberg NE. New York, International Universities Press, 1965, pp 108–123

Kathol RG, Noyes R, Williams J, et al: Diagnosing depression in patients with medical illness. Psychosomatics 31:434–440, 1990

Kaufman MW, Murray GB, Cassem NH: Use of psychostimulants in medically ill depressed patients. Psychosomatics 23:817–819, 1982

Khantzian EJ, McKenna GJ: Acute toxic and withdrawal reactions associated with drug use and abuse. Ann Intern Med 90:361–372, 1979

Levenson JL, Hamer RM, Rossiter LF: Relation of psychopathology in general medical inpatients to use and cost of services. Am J Psychiatry 147:1498–1503, 1990

Lipowski ZJ: Delirium in the elderly patient. N Engl J Med 320:578–582, 1989

Lipowski ZJ: Delirium: Acute Confusional States. New York, Oxford University Press, 1990

Lipson RE, Stern TA: Management of monoamine oxidase inhibitor-treated patients in the emergency and critical care setting. Journal of Intensive Care Medicine 6:117–125, 1991

MacKenzie TB, Popkin MK: Organic anxiety syndrome. Am J Psychiatry 140:342–344, 1983

Malzberg B: Mortality among patients with involution melancholia. Am J Psychiatry 93:1231–1238, 1937

Marinella MA: Propofol for sedation in the intensive care unit: essentials for the clinician. Respir Med 91:505–510, 1997

Miller LJ, Wiles-Pfeifler R: Propofol for the long-term sedation of a critically ill patient. Am J Crit Care 7:73–76, 1998

Murphy JM, Monson RR, Oliver DC, et al: Affective disorders and mortality. Arch Gen Psychiatry 44:473–480, 1987

Pollack MH, Stern TA: Recognition and treatment of anxiety in the ICU patient, in Intensive Care Medicine, 2nd Edition. Edited by Rippe JM, Irwin RS, Alpert JS, et al. Boston, MA, Little, Brown, 1991, pp 1875–1887

Rabins PV, Harvis K, Koven S: High fatality rates of late-life depression associated with cardiovascular disease. J Affect Disord 9:165–167, 1985

Reich P, Kelly MJ: Suicide attempts by hospitalized medical and surgical patients. N Engl J Med 294:298–301, 1976

Reich P, deSilva RA, Lown B, et al: Acute psychological disturbances preceding life-threatening ventricular arrhythmias. JAMA 246:233–235, 1981

Rodin G, Voshart K: Depression in the medically ill: an overview. Am J Psychiatry 143:696–705, 1986

Salzman C, Green AI, Rodriguez-Villa F, et al: Benzodiazepines combined with neuroleptics for management of severe disruptive behavior. Psychosomatics 27 (suppl):17–22, 1986

Sanders KM, Stern TA, O'Gara PT, et al: Delirium during intraaortic balloon pump therapy: incidence and management. Psychosomatics 33:35–44, 1992

Schelling G, Stoll C, Haller M, et al: Health-related quality of life and posttraumatic stress disorder in survivors of the acute respiratory distress syndrome. Crit Care Med 26:651–659, 1998

Settle EC, Ayd FJ: Haloperidol: a quarter century of experience. J Clin Psychiatry 44:440–448, 1983

Shuster JL, Stern TA: Suicide, in Intensive Care Medicine, 2nd Edition. Edited by Rippe JM, Irwin RS, Alpert JS, et al. Boston, MA, Little, Brown, 1991, pp 1902–1906

Shuster JL, Stern TA, Greenberg DB: Pros and cons of fluoxetine for the depressed cancer patient. Oncology 6:45–50, 1992

Siegal B, Donnelly JC: Enriching personal and professional development: the experience of a support group for interns. Journal of Medical Education 53:908–914, 1978

Simon NM, Whitely S: Psychiatric consultation with MICU nurses: the consultation conference as a working group. Heart Lung 6:497–504, 1977

Smith LW, Dimsdale JE: Postcardiotomy delirium: conclusions after 25 years? Am J Psychiatry 146:452–458, 1989

Sos J, Cassem NH: Managing postoperative agitation. Drug Therapeutics 10:103–106, 1980

Stein EH, Murdaugh J, MacCleod JA: Brief psychotherapy of psychiatric reactions to physical illness. Am J Psychiatry 125:1040–1047, 1969

Stern TA: The management of depression and anxiety following myocardial infarction. Mt Sinai J Med 52:623–633, 1985

Stern TA, Mulley AG, Thibault GE: Life-threatening drug overdoses: precipitant and prognosis. JAMA 251:1983–1985, 1984

Stern TA, Caplan RA, Cassem NH: Use of benzodiazepines in a coronary care unit. Psychosomatics 28:19–23, 1987

Stern TA, Prager LM, Cremens MC: Autognosis rounds for medical house staff. Psychosomatics 34:1–7, 1993

Stoll C, Kapfhammer HP, Rothenhausler HB, et al: Sensitivity and specificity of a screening test to document traumatic experiences and to diagnose post-traumatic stress disorder in ARDS patients after intensive care treatment. Intensive Care Med 25:697–704, 1999

Stoudemire A, Moran MG, Fogel BS: Psychotropic drug use in the medically ill: part I. Psychosomatics 31:377–391, 1990

Stoudemire A, Moran MG, Fogel BS: Psychotropic drug use in the medically ill: part II. Psychosomatics 32:34–44, 1991

Strain JJ, Leisowitz MR, Klein DF: Anxiety and panic attacks in the medically ill. Psychiatr Clin North Am 4:333–350, 1981

Strub RL, Black FW: The Mental Status Examination in Neurology, 2nd Edition. Philadelphia, PA, FA Davis, 1985

Sunderland T, Tariot PN, Cohen RM, et al: Anticholinergic sensitivity in patients with dementia of the Alzheimer type and age-matched controls: a dose-response study. Arch Gen Psychiatry 44:418–426, 1987

Tesar GE, Stern TA: Evaluation and treatment of agitation in the intensive care unit. Journal of Intensive Care Medicine 1:137–148, 1986

Tesar GE, Stern TA: Rapid tranquilization of the agitated intensive care unit patient. Journal of Intensive Care Medicine 3:195–201, 1988

Tesar GE, Stern TA: The diagnosis and treatment of agitation and delirium in the ICU patient, in Intensive Care Medicine, 2nd Edition. Edited by Rippe JM, Irwin RS, Alpert JS, et al. Boston, MA, Little, Brown, 1991, pp 1865–1875

Thompson TL, Thompson WL: Treating postoperative delirium. Drug Therapeutics 13:30–43, 1983

Townsend PL, Reynolds JR: Applied pharmacokinetics: an overview, in Intensive Care Medicine, 2nd Edition. Edited by Rippe JM, Irwin RS, Alpert JS, et al. Boston, MA, Little, Brown, 1991, pp 1695–1707

Treggiari-Venzi M, Borgeat A, Fuchs-Buder T, et al: Overnight sedation with midazolam or propofol in the ICU: effects on sleep quality, anxiety and depression. Intensive Care Med 22:1186–1190, 1996

Tune LE, Damlouji NF, Holland A, et al: Association of postoperative delirium with raised serum levels of anticholinergic drugs. Lancet 2:651–653, 1981

Weinbroum AA, Halpern P, Rudick V: Midazolam versus propofol for long-term sedation in the ICU: a randomized prospective comparison. Intensive Care Med 23:1258–1263, 1997

Weiner MF, Caldwell T, Tyson J: Stresses and coping in ICU nursing: why support groups fail. Gen Hosp Psychiatry 5:179–183, 1983

Wells KB, Stewart A, Hays RD, et al: The functioning and well-being of depressed patients: results from the Medical Outcomes Study. JAMA 262:914–919, 1990

Wise MG, Brandt GT: Delirium, in the American Psychiatric Press Textbook of Neuropsychiatry, 2nd Edition. Edited by Yudofsky SC, Hales RE. Washington, DC, American Psychiatric Press, 1992, pp 291–310

Woods SW, Tesar GE, Murray GB, et al: Psychostimulant treatment of depressive disorders secondary to medical illness. J Clin Psychiatry 47:12–15, 1986

Wool C, Geringer ES, Stern TA: The management of behavioral problems in the ICU, in Intensive Care Medicine, 2nd Edition. Edited by Rippe JM, Irwin RS, Alpert JS, et al. Boston, MA, Little, Brown, 1991, pp 1906–1916

35

Psychiatric Issues in the Care of Dying Patients

William Breitbart, M.D.

Kathleen Lintz, B.A.

The British singer-composer Sting wrote the lyrics to his song "Let Your Soul Be Your Pilot," from his album *Mercury Falling* (A&M Records, 1996), shortly after visiting a friend who was dying from acquired immunodeficiency syndrome (AIDS) in a New York City hospital. The lyrics include such lines as "When the doctors fail to heal you . . . When no medicine chest can make you well . . . Let your soul be your pilot." They reflect a growing realization that medical technology does in fact have limits and that ultimately, perhaps, one must embrace a more spiritual perspective in life and, especially, in the face of death. One of the most challenging roles of the consultation-liaison psychiatrist is to guide terminally ill patients physically, psychologically, and spiritually through the dying process.

As a member of the palliative care team, the consultation-liaison psychiatrist must gain an understanding of the complexity of their dying patients' problems and anxieties and must be able to guide them in the management of their illnesses and their subsequent psychiatric problems. In addition to experiencing fear of the suffering that usually accompanies death, each individual has different medical and psychological issues during the dying process. A physician should strive to help each patient to achieve a personal death that is consistent with his or her own beliefs and values. To assist a patient in achieving a "good death," the consultation-liaison psychiatrist must be knowledgeable about the psychological aspects of care, be familiar with the principles of symptom control, and be comfortable in dealing with issues surrounding mortality. The task of caring for a dying patient can be complex, especially when the cultural, religious, and spir-

itual dimensions of the patient are taken into account. The patient must be treated holistically, with consideration given to the patient's individual attributes, family and social supports, psychological strengths, and spiritual and religious values as interventions are planned (Stjernsward and Papallona 1998).

Historically, medical textbooks have placed little emphasis on end-of-life care. Carron et al. (1999) evaluated medical textbook coverage of clinical management of patients in advanced stages of fatal illnesses and found that general medical textbooks contain little information that would aid a physician in caring for a dying patient. Carron and colleagues (1999) concluded that "time while dying and near death should be comfortable, supportive of independence and function, enhancing of family relationships, and meaningful" (p. 86). The results of the study indicate the need for new information, practices, and care systems that will improve outcomes for patients and their families. Enhancement of textbooks will be part of that endeavor (Carron et al. 1999).

In an attempt to improve the care of terminally ill patients and their families, we will address the complete care of the dying patient in this chapter. We will first discuss the state of dying in America today, the definition of a good death, the changing role of palliative care in the treatment of dying patients, the importance of doctor-patient communication, and cultural perspectives on dying. We will then focus on the role of the consultation-liaison psychiatrist in the care of dying patients, outline the major factors contributing to adaptation to illness and death, and review the management of anxiety, depression, suicidal ideation, delirium, and pain in dying patients.

771

DYING IN AMERICA

To die of old age is a death rare, extraordinary, and singular…a privilege rarely seen.

Montaigne

Although the average American's life expectancy today is markedly longer than that of a European during the sixteenth century, few people die at home of old age, the supposedly ideal death. To understand and treat psychiatric issues in the dying patient today, physicians must have an appreciation of why, when, and where Americans die.

Why do Americans die? Whereas communicable diseases were the number one killers of Americans a century ago, heart disease, cancer, and stroke are the top three causes of death in the United States today. In 1995, approximately 62% of all deaths and 67% of deaths among individuals older than 65 years were caused by either heart disease, cancer, or stroke (Rosenberg et al. 1996). The leading causes of death among children (ages 1–14 years) are unintentional injuries, cancer, congenital abnormalities, and homicide (Field and Cassel 1997). Causes of death also vary across cultural and racial backgrounds. For example, homicide, AIDS, and accidents were the third, fourth, and fifth leading causes of death among black males in 1993 (U.S. Public Health Service 1996). Whereas some common causes of death can be sudden (e.g., myocardial infarction, stroke, gunshot wound), others, such as cancer and human immunodeficiency virus (HIV) disease, have become chronic diseases, with a prolonged dying process that may necessitate psychiatric intervention and treatment.

When do Americans die? Today the average American can expect to die at an old age. This year, less than 1% of Americans will die, but that 1% constitutes more than two million people, many of whom will require psychiatric care during the dying process (Field and Cassel 1997). Because of today's increased population and decreased infant mortality rate, more Americans die per year than ever before. In 1980, the number of Americans who died was 1,989,841 (National Center for Health Statistics 1985); in 1990, that number was 2,148,463 (National Center for Health Statistics 1994); and in 1995, an even greater number died (2,312,180) (Rosenberg et al. 1996). This increase in the number of deaths per year has drawn attention to the need for and the deficiencies in end-of-life care.

Americans are dying older. Whereas life expectancy was less than 50 years in 1900, by 1995 the average American life expectancy was 79 years for women and 73 years for men, an average of 76 years (Rosenberg et al. 1996). Today, Americans older than 65 years constitute a greater proportion of the population than ever before. In 1994, one in eight was older than 65 years (13% of the population); by the year 2030, one in five Americans will be in that age group (20% of the population) (Hobbs and Damon 1996). These statistics highlight the importance of care for elderly and dying individuals.

Where do Americans die? Centuries ago, most Americans died at home, surrounded by family and friends. Today, the majority of Americans die in institutions. In 1949, 49.5% of Americans died in institutions; by 1958, that percentage was 60.9%; and by 1980, the percentage was 74% (Brock and Foley 1996). Since the early 1980s, Medicare coverage changes have slightly shifted the place of death. In 1992, a total of 57% of Americans died in hospitals, 17% died in nursing homes, 20% died at home, and 6% died elsewhere (Field and Cassel 1997). Although two Gallup polls, conducted in 1992 and 1996, found that 9 of 10 terminally ill patients with less than 6 months to live would prefer to die at home (Foreman 1996; National Hospice Organization 1996; Seidlitz et al. 1995), today most Americans die in institutions, surrounded by medical caregivers. Therefore, health care workers should be well educated in and practiced in approaching end-of-life issues, including psychiatric issues.

WHAT IS A GOOD DEATH?

Dying is both "a biological process and a psychological and social experience that occurs in a cultural context" (Field and Cassel 1997, p. 2). The Study to Understand Prognoses and Preferences for Outcomes and Risks of Treatments (SUPPORT; "A Controlled Trial to Improve Care" 1995) and other studies have suggested that a technological imperative characterizes Western medical practice, including care of the dying. SUPPORT found substantial shortcomings in the care of seriously ill hospitalized patients—shortcomings including poor communication between physicians and dying patients and implementation of overly aggressively treatment, often against patients' wishes ("A Controlled Trial to Improve Care" 1995). The findings of this study emphasize the need for greater skills and education in end-of-life issues, as well as increased communication with and support of dying patients. Perhaps the most perturbing conclusion from this study is that in general, Americans are dying not good deaths but bad deaths, characterized by needless suffering and disregard for patients' or families' wishes or values.

Clearly, each individual has his or her own definition of a good death. However, regardless of individual preferences, a good death must involve a good dying process. A meaningful dying process is one throughout which the patient is physically, psychologically, spiritually, and emotionally supported by his or her family, friends, and caregivers. In 1997, the World Health Organization (WHO) offered this statement: "Inevitably, each human life reaches its end. Ensuring that it does so in the most dignified, caring and least painful way that can be achieved deserves as much priority as any other. This is a priority not merely for the medical profession, the health sector or social services. It is a priority for each society, community, family and individual" (p. 26).

According to WHO (World Health Organization 1997), a good death is one "free from avoidable distress and suffering for patient, family and caregivers, in general accord with patient's and family's wishes, and reasonably consistent with clinical, cultural, and ethical standards" (p. 2). Weisman (1972) described four criteria for what he called an "appropriate death":

1. Internal conflicts, such as fears about loss of control, should be reduced as much as possible.
2. The individual's personal sense of identity should be sustained.
3. Critical relationships should be enhanced or at least maintained; conflicts should be resolved, if possible.
4. The person should be encouraged to set and attempt to reach meaningful goals—even though limited—such as attending a graduation, a wedding, or the birth of a child, as a way to provide a sense of continuity into the future.

These four criteria and the aforementioned considerations for achieving a good death can serve as general guidelines for the consultation-liaison psychiatrist in caring for terminally ill patients.

PALLIATIVE CARE TODAY

To cure sometimes
To relieve often
To comfort always

Anonymous

As expressed by a sixteenth-century anonymous author, the most important roles of a doctor, beyond that of curing, are to relieve and to comfort. These two roles define palliative care.

What is palliative care? The term *palliation* is derived from the Latin word *palliare,* which means "to cloak" or "to conceal." This derivation suggests that although some illnesses cannot be cured, their physical and psychological symptoms can still be treated—the illness can be "concealed." Throughout this century, palliative care has evolved, expanding beyond the concept of comfort care for the dying to include palliative care from the very beginning of a life-threatening illness.

The Palliative Care Foundation (1981) defined palliative care as "active compassionate care of the terminally ill at a time that their disease is no longer responsive to traditional treatment aimed at cure or prolongation of life, and when the control of symptoms is paramount." According to this definition, palliation is comfort care, only to be implemented once treatment of the disease has ceased. In 1990, the World Health Organization defined palliative care as "the active total care of patients whose disease is not responsive to curative treatment. Control of pain, of other symptoms, and of psychological, social and spiritual problems, is paramount. The goal of palliative care is achievement of the best quality of life for patients and their families. Many aspects of palliative care are also applicable earlier in the course of the illness in conjunction with anti-cancer treatment" (Canadian Palliative Care Association 1995). Like the 1981 definition of palliative care, this definition suggests that palliation should be provided to patients only when aggressive or potentially curative treatment has ceased, although some mention of earlier use of palliative care is made in the later statement. These early-stage definitions of palliative care are graphically represented in Figure 35–1.

More recently, the term *palliative care* refers to palliation from the very beginning of a life-threatening illness. Such a definition suggests that palliative care and aggressive treatment are not mutually exclusive. This progressive definition of palliative care is graphically represented in Figure 35–2.

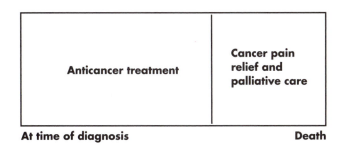

Anticancer treatment	Cancer pain relief and palliative care
At time of diagnosis	Death

FIGURE 35–1. Early concept of palliative care.

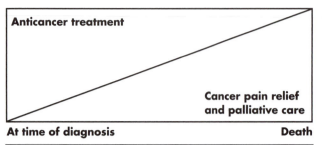

FIGURE 35–2.   Progressive concept of palliative care.

What are the goals of palliative care? According to WHO (World Health Organization 1990), palliative care

- Affirms life, with dying regarded as a normal process
- Neither hastens nor postpones death
- Provides relief from pain and other symptoms
- Integrates psychological and spiritual care
- Offers a support system to help patients live as actively as possible until death
- Helps family cope with illness and bereavement
- Is multidisciplinary

Well-established palliative care programs also include home care, consultation service, day care, inpatient care, and bereavement support. The aim of palliative care today is to treat the whole patient—and his or her family—physically, psychologically, and spiritually throughout his or her illness.

The growing need for palliative care programs has gained recognition in the past several years. As mentioned earlier, SUPPORT emphasized the need for improved end-of-life care ("A Controlled Trial to Improve Care" 1995). This study documented shortcomings in communication, frequency of aggressive treatment, and the characteristics of hospital death ("A Controlled Trial to Improve Care" 1995). SUPPORT investigators found that only 47% of the time did doctors know whether their patients wished to be resuscitated, and the researchers also noted that 46% of do-not-resuscitate (DNR) orders were written within the last 2 days of a patient's life. The study also found that 38% of patients who died spent at least 10 days in the intensive care unit, and in the case of 50% of patients who died in the hospital, the family reported that the ill relative was in moderate to severe pain at least half of the time. SUPPORT clearly demonstrated the need for improved end-of-life care and improved communication between doctors and patients.

A second study of end-of-life care (Hanson et al. 1997) had similar findings. According to statements by bereaved family members, 9% of related patients underwent cardiopulmonary resuscitation, 11% had ventilatory

support, and 24% received intensive care during the last month of life. Twenty-three percent of family members could not recall a discussion about treatment decisions, and the presence or absence of a living will did not influence whether a treatment discussion occurred. Eighteen percent advocated for more care to relieve pain or other symptoms. To compensate for these end-of-life care deficiencies, family members recommended better communication (44% recommended this), greater access to doctors' time (17%), and improved pain management (10%).

In addition to these studies, a number of other factors appear to be contributing to increased interest in palliative care in the United States (Billings and Block 1997):

- Growing interest in death and dying
- Development of hospice programs and their increasing integration into conventional care
- Concern about the high cost of dying
- Increased national focus on pain management and incorporation of questions about pain and palliative care in licensing examinations
- Greater attention to the role of medicine in caring rather than curing
- National debates on physician-assisted suicide and euthanasia

Given apparent insufficiencies in the care of dying patients, improved education in palliative care is imperative. Billings and Block (1997) found that most medical schools provide some training in end-of-life care but the exposure is inadequate, especially in the clinical years. The investigators' report revealed the following shortcomings in the teaching of palliative care: curricular offerings are not well integrated; the predominant teaching format is lectures; formal teaching is mostly preclinical; and home care, hospice, and nursing home care are largely neglected. However, Billings and Block (1997) did find that students are receptive to learning about palliative care and that such education positively influences their attitudes and enhances their communication skills.

Meier et al. (1997) found similar shortcomings in the teaching of end-of-life care. These investigators discussed "barriers to achieving a peaceful death, including inadequate medical professional education on palliative care, and public and professional uncertainty about the difference between forgoing life-sustaining treatment and active euthanasia, and health professionals' difficulty recognizing when patients are dying and the associated sense that death is a professional failure" (Meier et al. 1997, p. 227). Both of these reports emphasized the importance of recognizing the obstacles to end-of-life care and the necessity of implementing improved palliative care programs to ensure complete, compassionate care of the dying patient.

DOCTOR-PATIENT COMMUNICATION

Doctor-patient communication is an essential component in caring for a dying patient (Baile and Beale 2001; Buckman 1993; Parker et al. 2001; Smith 2000). Several studies have focused on doctor-patient communication during the dying process. A study of the connection between cancer patients' predictions regarding outcome and the treatments they chose revealed misinterpretations by dying patients due to lack of adequate communication with their physicians (Weeks et al. 1996). Patients with terminal lung and colon cancer overestimated their probability of surviving 6 months, and these overestimations influenced their treatment decisions. Patients who believed that they were going to live more than 6 months were more likely to choose aggressive, life-extending therapy than were patients who believed that they had a less than 10% chance of living beyond 6 months; the latter patients were more likely to choose comfort care. The survival rate for those who opted for aggressive treatment was not higher than the survival rate for those who chose comfort care.

Despite the recognized importance of caregiver-patient communication, many physicians are not adequately trained in communication. In a study of oncologists' communication skills, less than 35% of oncologists reported having received any previous communication training (Fallowfield et al. 1998). However, this study did find that most oncologists desire to learn better communication techniques and are willing to sacrifice the necessary time to do so. Improved training in doctor-patient communication can help ease anxiety on both sides and improve health outcomes (Simpson et al. 1991). Suchman et al. (1997) found that improving physicians' empathic responses to patients in medical interviews can improve the doctor-patient relationship, improve quality of care, and increase both physician and patient satisfaction. On the basis of their findings, Suchman et al. (1997) defined basic empathic skills, necessary for meaningful communication with patients, as "recognizing when emotions may be present but not directly expressed, inviting exploration of these unexpressed feelings, and effectively acknowledging these feelings so that the patient feels understood" (p. 680).

Buckman (1993) proposed a guide for communication and empathy in caring for the dying patient. He declared that the important elements of communication in palliative care are basic listening skills, the breaking of bad news, therapeutic dialogue, and communicating with the family and with other professionals. He acknowledged several sources of difficulty in communicating with a dying patient, including the social denial of death, a lack of experience of death in the family, high expectations of health and life, materialism, and the changing role of religion. The patient's fear of dying also contributes, as do factors originating in the health care professional, such as sympathetic pain, fear of being blamed, fear of the untaught, fear of expressing emotions, and fear of one's own illness and death. However, Buckman (1993) emphasized the importance of teaching and practicing listening skills, using comforting body language, responding empathically to patients, and engaging in therapeutic and supportive dialogue. He also advocated improved communication with patients' families and friends and among medical caregivers.

CULTURAL PERSPECTIVES ON DYING

Ethnicity and culture strongly influence a person's attitude toward death and dying. Although there is a "universal fear of cancer [and other terminal diseases] that results from its [cancer's] association with images of extreme debility and pain and the fear of death" (Butow et al. 1997, p. 320), every culture approaches and expresses this fear differently. Blackhall et al. (1995) studied ethnic attitudes toward patient autonomy regarding disclosure of the diagnosis and prognosis of a terminal illness and toward end-of-life decision making. They found that different cultures have distinct opinions about how much information physicians should provide concerning diagnoses and prognoses. The investigators determined that African Americans (88%) and European Americans (87%) are significantly more likely than Mexican Americans (65%) or Korean Americans (47%) to believe that a patient should always be informed of a diagnosis of metastatic cancer. They also found that African Americans (63%) and European Americans (69%) are more likely than Korean Americans (35%) and Mexican Americans (48%) to believe a patient should be informed of a terminal prognosis and be actively involved in decisions concerning use of life-sustaining technology. Blackhall and colleagues (1995) concluded that physicians should ask their patients whether they wish to be informed of their diagnoses and prognoses and whether they wish to be involved in treatment decisions or prefer to let family members or caregivers handle such matters.

A similar study of Navajo Indian beliefs concerning autonomy in patient diagnosis and prognosis found that in the Navajo culture, physicians and patients must speak in only a positive way, avoiding any negative thought or speech (Carrese and Rhodes 1995). Because Navajos believe that language can "shape reality and control events," informing patients of a negative diagnosis or prognosis is considered disrespectful and physically and emotionally dangerous (Carrese and Rhodes 1995). As these two studies show, physicians must be careful to respect their patients' cultural beliefs in disclosing the diagnosis and prognosis of a terminal illness.

SPIRITUALITY AND DYING

To help a terminally ill patient achieve a personally meaningful death, the consultation-liaison psychiatrist must respectfully explore and assess the patient's individual belief system and the role religion and spirituality play in the patient's ability to cope with illness and dying. When a patient is confronted with a life-threatening illness, spirituality assumes greater importance in the patient's life and affects his or her attitude toward life and death and ability to cope with hardship. In a national survey on spiritual beliefs and the dying process, individuals were asked which worried them the most when thinking about their own deaths: practical, emotional, medical, or spiritual matters ("Spiritual Beliefs and the Dying Process" 1997). A total of 42% selected spirituality as their main concern, whereas only 38% chose medical concerns as their main worry. Thirty-nine percent of those interviewed also reported that having a doctor who was spirituality attuned to them was "very important."

Brady et al. (1999) examined the importance of including spirituality in the assessment of quality of life in cancer patients and determined that spirituality plays a unique and important role in a dying patient's quality of life. This study found that spirituality is as significant a determinant of quality of life as physical well-being. Furthermore, Brady et al. (1999) discovered that spiritual well-being is related to the ability to enjoy life even during illness and in the midst of pain. Patients with a higher sense of spiritual well-being were able to endure significant pain and symptoms, while still enjoying life. Forty-eight percent of patients with high pain levels and high levels of meaning or peace reported themselves still able to "enjoy life very much," whereas only 9% of patients with high levels of pain and low levels of meaning or

peace were able to do so. Likewise, 66% of patients with high levels of fatigue but also high levels of meaning or peace reported themselves able to enjoy life very much. In comparison, only 11% of those with high levels of fatigue and low levels of meaning or peace reported themselves able to enjoy life very much.

That meaning or peace might preserve well-being in the midst of symptoms is consistent with the theorizing of Cassell (1991), Fife (1994), and Taylor (1983), who stressed that people require a meaning context in which to understand and cope with life's difficulties. Meaning is thought to bring a unified order to a person's experience (Csikszentmihalyi 1990; Frankl 1963; Yalom 1980). Such order can help an individual achieve an "inner hold on life" (Frankl 1963), enabling him or her to function "even in the worst of circumstances" (Brady et al. 1999).

In their study, Brady and colleagues (1999) used a new method of assessment, the Functional Assessment of Chronic Illness Therapy–Spiritual Well-Being scale. This scale measures important aspects of spirituality, such as meaning in one's life, harmony, peacefulness, and the sense of strength and comfort drawn from one's faith. Several other instruments have been created to measure spirituality as a factor in health outcomes. Holland et al. (1999) used the newly validated Systems of Belief Inventory in a study of the role of religious and spiritual beliefs in coping with malignant melanoma. A measure designed by Stoddard and Burns-Haney (1990) focuses on the concept of God, the subjective meaning of illness, the approach to hoping, and the relationship to support systems. Rather than assessing specific beliefs, Kuhn's (1988) descriptive, multidimensional model examines how an individual creates meaning in life. Chaplain Gary Berg (1994) designed a computer program to measure organizational religious activity, nonorganizational activity, intrinsic religiousness, and spiritual injury. And finally, Fitchett (1993) developed a model for spiritual assessment that investigates both how a person finds meaning and purpose in life and the emotions, behavior, relationships, and practices associated with that meaning and purpose.

Few studies have been conducted on specific effects of spirituality on the dying process, but several studies concluded that spirituality can greatly enhance the life of terminally ill people. Musick et al. (1998) described four specific ways that cancer patients can draw strength from their religious or spiritual views: secondary control, provision of a spiritual worldview, participation in a spiritual community, and dealing with death and dying.

In designating secondary control, patients transfer control of their illnesses to God or whatever higher power they believe in. One study on spirituality and cancer patients found that patients who believed God was in control of their fate had lower levels of psychological distress and higher self-esteem than those who did not (Jenkins and Pargament 1988). Likewise, patients with a strong spiritual or religious worldview are more likely to find meaning in their illnesses and to have less psychological stress. Acklin et al. (1983) reported that cancer patients with higher levels of transcendent meaning had a greater sense of mental well-being than did a control group. Furthermore, participation in a religious community can instill a sense of belonging and closeness, which can be comforting to the dying patient. Yates and colleagues (1981) found that although only 37% of cancer patients studied had attended church in the past month (presumably many patients were unable to attend because of physical limitations), those who did were substantially more satisfied with life, were happier, and had a more positive affect and better pain control. Lastly, and for the terminally ill patient perhaps most importantly, spirituality and religion can directly help a patient to cope with dying and death. Religion and spirituality can provide a framework in which to explore and give meaning to the dying process. Because death is a very personal, intimate, final event, each individual must decide how he or she desires to exit this world. As everyone lives his or her own unique life, everyone must die his or her own unique death. The spiritually attuned physician places value on every patient's personal views on life, death, and existence and weaves these views into the patient's care, enabling him or her to die a meaningful and personal death.

Because spirituality is a crucial determinant of the way in which many dying patients cope with and give meaning to their last days, the physician should make every effort to be attuned to his or her patient's spiritual beliefs and practices in order to help the patient achieve a good death, one that is consistent with his or her own personal beliefs and meanings. "If indeed spirituality is a factor that enables a person to derive deep satisfaction from life despite symptom load, and we fail to measure it, we are in danger of miscalculating the actual perceived 'burden' of the disease, and perhaps severely underestimating the true 'quality' of a person's life" (Brady et al. 1999, p. 428).

ROLE OF THE CONSULTATION-LIAISON PSYCHIATRIST

The traditional role of the psychiatrist is broadened in several ways in the care of the dying patient (Table 35–1). Consultation-liaison psychiatrists have participated in

TABLE 35–1. Role of the consultation-liaison psychiatrist in treating patients with terminal illnesses

Assistance to patient and family in dealing with the existential crisis
Control of comorbid psychiatric disorders (anxiety, depression, delirium), pain, and physical symptoms
Advocacy for patient
Conflict management: patient, family, staff
Psychotherapy for anticipatory bereavement and bereavement of survivors
Teaching of medical staff about psychological issues regarding dying patients
Dealing with the ethical issues in end-of-life decisions
 Resuscitation
 Withdrawal or withholding of life support
 Evaluation of requests for physician-assisted suicide

the movement toward better care of dying patients and have, more recently, taken an active role in teaching the management of depression, anxiety, delirium, and pain in terminally ill patients (Breitbart and Holland 1993). Anticipatory grief and management of social, psychological, ethical, legal, and spiritual issues that complicate the care of dying patients are areas in which the consultation-liaison psychiatrist can also play an important role.

The psychiatrist must provide assistance in dealing with the existential crisis posed by a terminal diagnosis. Through discussions with the primary care physician, the patient and family may have begun to confront the reality that the disease is no longer curable or controllable. The psychiatrist can help the patient to deal with the prognosis and to explore treatment options, including palliative care. Some patients prefer to seek alternative treatments, others choose to participate in experimental clinical trials, and still others choose maximal comfort care only. At times, the family disagrees with the patient regarding his or her desires, especially when the patient chooses minimal intervention. The patient, family, and caregivers must collaborate, however, to decide whether treatment is to be given at home or in a hospice, nursing home, or hospital. The appointment of a health care proxy should be encouraged if it has not been done previously. Decisions about wishes for resuscitation and life support should be made early on; these issues usually arise in an emergency situation, when circumstances are less than optimal for making such decisions. Hospice care ensures that the focus is on comfort and that pain control is well managed. Studies by several groups showed that more and more families are choosing to have their loved ones die at home despite the stresses that such home care brings (Ferrell et al. 1991; Hileman et al. 1992; Sankar 1991; Siegel et al. 1991).

The psychiatrist's unique role in the care of the dying patient is to diagnose and treat comorbid psychiatric disorders that may complicate the course of illness. Intolerable, uncontrolled symptoms are risk factors for suicide attempts during terminal illness. Furthermore, fear that the physician will not or cannot control distressing symptoms is a major force behind the public's current drive for legalization of physician-assisted suicide and euthanasia.

The psychiatrist must often advocate on behalf of the patient as questions about insurance, coverage of home health aides, and eligibility for home care services arise. The psychiatrist helps resolve conflicts among patient, family, and staff by opening lines of communication and helping families to deal with the strong emotions that surround the imminent death of a loved one. Conflicts with the physician and staff are common because the clinicians are also stressed; resolution of these conflicts is a critical intervention for the patient's physical and psychological well-being.

Psychotherapeutic interventions for patients and families who are experiencing anticipatory grief are important to provide. During the bereavement period, the family often turns to the psychiatrist who participated in the patient's care and who shares memories of the patient. This role as a continuing support for the bereaved can be important.

The consultation-liaison psychiatrist's role includes teaching the medical staff about the psychological issues involved in care of dying patients. Physical and psychological symptom management must be emphasized. In addition, however, members of the house staff usually have had little experience in or education regarding talking with dying patients or conducting a discussion concerning DNR orders. This lack of experience and knowledge often leads to avoidance of discussions with the patient out of fear of questions the patient may ask about his or her prognosis. Also, discomfort with having the DNR discussion to determine the patient's wishes about withholding resuscitation leads to delaying of the discussion until the patient's clinical condition precludes his or her participation; the discussion is often then held with the relatives alone (Misbin et al. 1993).

The psychiatrist also has an ethical role in the issue of encouraging discussion of end-of-life decisions—decisions regarding treatment, withholding resuscitation, and life support. The capacity of the patient to make rational judgments and the proxy's ability to make an appropriate decision for the patient often require psychiatric evaluation. The decision to withdraw life support is highly emotional and may require psychiatric consultation for maximal comfort (Subcommittee on Psychiatric Aspects of Life-Sustaining Technology 1996).

FACTORS IN ADAPTATION TO TERMINAL ILLNESS AND DEATH

Factors that influence the way an individual adapts to impending death are the sociocultural environment, the individual's personal attributes, and the medical illness and the variables associated with it (Table 35–2).

TABLE 35–2. Factors in adaptation to terminal illness

Sociocultural
- Attitudes of society about illness and death
- Socioeconomic resources
- Social supports

Personal
- Personality, strength of coping, level of maturity
- Psychiatric history
- Spiritual, religious, and philosophical views about death and the meaning of life and death
- Prior experiences with loss and death

Medical
- Diagnosis, nature of symptoms (e.g., pain, dyspnea)
- Skills and knowledge of caregivers in palliative and supportive care
- Place where terminal care is given (home, hospital, nursing home, hospice)

Sociocultural Factors

The social environment and culture contribute to how a person faces death. Views of illness, dying, and death differ across cultural groups and also across historical periods, as revealed in religious writings, classical literature, poetry, and music. Historically, religion has played a central role in the decision about whether the patient is told that he or she is dying. In the Middle Ages, the Catholic Church required that persons receive extreme unction before death, to save their souls. During that same time, Jewish physicians placed more emphasis on the patient's individual comfort during the process of dying. As the Catholic Church declined in power, the custom in Europe of telling white lies became common. The patient was not told of a poor prognosis or of a fatal diagnosis such as cancer (Weil et al. 1993). This custom in Europe is still prevalent, although there is a slow trend toward greater candor with regard to a poor prognosis or fatal disease.

In the United States during the 1970s, increasing numbers of patients were told their diagnoses; this change coincided with the rise of the consumers' and patients' rights movement, which questioned the authority of all institutions, including medicine. In the past 10 years, prognosis has also been more candidly discussed as decisions about resuscitation and life-sustaining measures have been discussed with patients. A federal law now requires that patients be told about the need to appoint a proxy who can give a substituted judgment about their wishes.

Individual economic resources and access to compassionate palliative care are also important factors. There is limited reimbursement for hospice care, and home care services are often poorly reimbursed as well. Because of costs, some economically disadvantaged patients are not easily managed at home. Many patients die in acute care facilities where less attention is given to the humanistic aspects of care.

Personal Factors

There is an adage that people die as they have lived. Personality and previously used coping strategies do not change when an individual is facing death. The psychiatrist who conducts a life review with the patient can help him or her to identify his or her strengths in coping. In addition, the person's philosophy of life, religion, and understanding of the meaning of death are important. Individuals with strong religious beliefs have a framework for dealing with suffering and death. For this reason, clergy should be a part of a palliative care team and should work closely with the psychiatrist. The patient's reaction to impending death is also colored by his or her prior experiences with death and loss. Relatives who have cared for the patient during a lengthy terminal illness may have definite ideas about what he or she wants or wishes to avoid, such as ventilatory support or heroic measures.

Medical Factors

The disease and associated symptoms determine the physical problems the person is facing. Pain, dyspnea, weakness, fatigue, and loss of appetite and weight produce secondary anxiety. Distressing symptoms should be treated aggressively. Symptom relief depends to a large extent on the expertise of the physician and nurses in charge, especially their knowledge and willingness to use narcotic analgesics and psychotropic medications. The psychiatrist can be helpful in providing expertise in the use of psychotropic drugs.

PSYCHOLOGICAL ISSUES AND MANAGEMENT

Patients who face death, especially when it entails a slow downhill course, experience anticipatory grief. This grief is manifested differently by individual patients. For example, some patients maintain strong denial and do not wish to discuss their feelings; others are relieved to talk about their situations. It is the psychiatrist's task to discern the best strategy for each patient.

The primary psychological issues in anticipatory grieving are those of facing losses brought on by illness and anticipated losses related to death (Barton 1977). A sense of loss of control is experienced with worsening of illness and with increasing symptoms that do not remit. Hope that control of the illness will be reestablished diminishes. The impending loss of life and continuity with the future and with those who will live on becomes painfully real. The sense of being isolated and alone, despite closeness of others, adds to distress. Continuing evidence of affection from others may mitigate some of the pain of loss (Lieber et al. 1976).

Psychotherapy with terminally ill patients differs in significant ways from therapy provided in traditional settings (Sourkes 1982). The psychiatrist must be willing to visit the patient at home or in the hospital, clinic, or nursing home. The visits may need to be shortened to accommodate the patient's medical condition, and they may need to be more frequent, providing an opportunity for the patient to explore the feelings of loss.

The primary psychological issues for the family are similar in that family members are responding to the changes in the patient's physical condition and, at the same time, beginning anticipatory grieving. Questions in their minds are "When and how will the loved one die?" "What will the moment of death be like?" and "How will I be able to manage it?" As more patients, especially those with cancer and AIDS, choose to die at home, the family caregiver must be prepared to handle an increasingly heavy burden of care and the terminal event itself. Support for the family as well as the patient is important (Schachter 1992).

Home and hospice programs need the consultation of a consultation-liaison psychiatrist who can help in management of the psychiatric disorders that are common in patients who are dying and in monitoring family members' responses to signs of distress that may require intervention (Chochinov and Holland 1989).

PSYCHIATRIC DISORDERS

Patients with advanced disease, such as advanced cancer, are particularly vulnerable to psychiatric disorders and complications (Breitbart et al. 1995, 1998). The incidences of pain, depression, and delirium increase with higher levels of physical debilitation and advanced illness.

Approximately 25% of all cancer patients experience severe depressive symptoms, with the prevalence increasing to 77% among those with advanced illness. The prevalence of what DSM-III-R (American Psychiatric Association 1987) called organic mental disorders (for a discussion of terms, see "Cognitive Impairment Disorders" later in this chapter, such as delirium among cancer patients, ranges from 25% to 40% and is as high as 85% among patients in terminal stages of the illness.

Minagawa and colleagues (1996) used the Structured Clinical Interview for DSM-III-R to evaluate the incidence of psychiatric disorders in a sample of 109 terminally ill cancer patients admitted to a palliative care unit (90% died within 6 months of admission; the mean survival time from admission was 54.7 days). In this sample of cancer patients approaching death, 53.7% met criteria for a specific psychiatric disorder. (This incidence is similar to the incidence of 47% found in a much earlier study of psychiatric disorders in a general cancer population [Derogatis et al. 1983].) The most common psychiatric disorders among terminally ill cancer patients were delirium (28%), dementia (10.7%), adjustment disorder (7.5%), amnestic disorder (3.2%), major depression (3.2%), and generalized anxiety disorder (1.1%). This most recent study dramatically underestimated the prevalence of depression among patients with advanced disease. The sample studied consisted of patients who were admitted to hospice and were only days or weeks away from death. Organic mental disorders were therefore overrepresented.

Recent evidence suggests that as patients with cancer or AIDS become more ill, entering advanced stages of illness, the burden of both physical and psychological symptoms becomes staggering. Perhaps most compelling is the fact that physical symptoms such as pain, dyspnea, and constipation are not the most prevalent symptoms of patients with advanced cancer or AIDS. In fact, psychological symptoms such as worrying, nervousness, lack of energy, insomnia, and sadness are among the most prevalent and distressing in these populations (Portenoy et al. 1994). Symptoms and syndromes of a neuropsychiatric nature, such as mood disorders (depression), cognitive impairment disorders (delirium), anxiety, insomnia, and suicidal ideation, must be treated in patients with advanced disease. Neuropsychiatric symptoms and syndromes coexist with many other physical and psychological symptoms and interact with each other, negatively affecting quality of life. Psychological symptoms and psychiatric disorders must be understood in the context of the patient and family as the unit of concern. Prompt recognition and effective treatment of both psychiatric and physical symptoms is critically important to the well-being of the patient with advanced disease and to the well-being of his or her family. Physicians caring for terminally ill patients must develop their skills in assessment and management of psychiatric symptoms and disorders.

There are two strategies for treating psychiatric disorders in dying patients. Psychiatric symptom control in patients with advanced disease can be understood and approached in a fashion similar to physical symptom control. Just as a physical symptom can be approached from the perspective of management, either as a nonspecific symptom (e.g., pain) or as a specific syndrome (e.g., HIV-related peripheral neuropathy), so can psychological and psychiatric symptoms be approached (Breitbart et al. 1995). A management approach focusing on symptoms as opposed to syndromes often involves nonspecific treatment for a symptom (e.g., opioids for pain or benzodiazepines for insomnia) but more specific treatment for an identifiable syndrome (e.g., adjuvant analgesics for neuropathic pain or antidepressants for major depression). The second strategy for treating psychiatric disorders in dying patients, based on a specific syndrome, requires diagnostic assessment of psychiatric symptoms and is extraordinarily challenging, partly because the origin of such symptoms is often unclear. Psychiatric symptoms may be due to advanced medical illness, medical treatments, or a psychiatric syndrome. The consultation-liaison psychiatrist must incorporate both approaches, depending on the specific clinical presentation. In this section, we describe the assessment and management of common psychiatric disorders in patients with advanced disease.

Anxiety Disorders

As outlined in Table 35–3, anxiety occurs in terminally ill patients as 1) an adjustment disorder with anxious mood alone or in combination with depressed mood, 2) a disease-related or treatment-related condition, or 3) an exacerbation of a preexisting anxiety disorder (Kerrihard et al. 1999; Massie 1989). Adjustment disorder with anxiety is related to adjusting to the existential crisis and the uncertainty of the prognosis and the future (Holland 1989). Anxiety related to medical causes is frequently a consequence of poorly controlled pain. The patient who is in pain appears restless and tense and may be agitated. Once the pain is controlled, the secondary anxiety most likely subsides. Metabolic abnormalities such as hypoxia, sepsis with fever, and delirium can produce anxiety and restlessness. A sudden onset of anxiety with respiratory distress or chest pain may signal pulmonary embolism or an acute cardiac event. Corticosteroids occasionally

TABLE 35–3. Common causes of anxiety in dying patients

Types of anxiety	Causes
Reactive anxiety/adjustment disorder	Awareness of terminal condition
	Fears and uncertainty about death
	Conflicts with family or staff
	DNR discussion
Disease- and treatment-related anxiety	Poor pain control
	Related metabolic disturbances
	Hypoxia
	Hypoglycemia
	Delirium
	Sepsis
	Bleeding
	Pulmonary embolus
Substance-induced anxiety	Anxiety-producing drugs
	Corticosteroids
	Dexamethasone
	Prednisone
	Antiemetic neuroleptics
	Metoclopramide
	Prochlorperazine
	Bronchodilators
	Withdrawal
	Opioids
	Benzodiazepines
	Alcohol
Preexisting anxiety disorders	Exacerbation of symptoms related to fears and distressing medical symptoms
General anxiety disorder	
Panic	
Phobias	
Posttraumatic stress disorder	

Note. DNR = do not resuscitate.

cause anxiety. Antiemetic neuroleptics, such as metoclopramide and prochlorperazine, often cause profound akathisia and anxiety. Bronchodilators used for dyspnea can produce tremulousness and anxiety. Withdrawal from opioid analgesics, benzodiazepines, alcohol, and barbiturates produces anxiety and agitation. Use of short-acting benzodiazepines, such as lorazepam and alprazolam, may be associated with rebound anxiety.

When faced with terminal illness, patients with preexisting anxiety disorders are at risk for reactivation of symptoms. A generalized anxiety disorder or panic disorder is apt to recur, especially in the presence of shortness of breath or pain. Persons with histories of phobias, especially fear of death, will have anxiety symptoms that will require medication and necessitate reassurance. Posttraumatic stress disorder may be activated in dying patients as they relate their situation to some prior near-death experience, such as the Holocaust or a combat experience, and the terror associated with it.

Prevalence of anxiety disorders among terminally ill cancer patients ranges from 15% to 28%. Studies suggest that anxiety disorders are common and that adjustment disorder with anxious mood is the most prevalent psychiatric manifestation of psychological distress. In a study involving 215 cancer patients and the use of DSM-III-R, the Psychological Collaborative Oncology Group determined that 53% of patients evaluated were adjusting normally to the stresses of cancer, with no diagnosable psychiatric disorder, whereas 47% presented with clinically apparent disorders (Derogatis et al. 1983). Of the latter group, 68% had reactive anxiety and depression (adjustment disorders with depressed or anxious mood). However, different studies have found different prevalences. Moorey et al. (1991) found that 28% of patients at a British cancer hospital had anxiety syndromes, Sensky et al. (1989) found a rate of 15%, and Bergman et al. (1991) reported a rate of 9%.

The prevalence of anxiety disorders in HIV disease and AIDS has also been addressed by a variety of researchers, and reported prevalences range from 0% to 39% (Kerrihard et al. 1999). As individuals progress from HIV infection to AIDS, their anxiety may include fears about the disease process, the clinical course, possible treatment outcomes, and death. In addition, anxiety may result from fear of increasing social stigma as medical illness becomes more evident, as well as from fear of increasing financial consequences of treatments. Research study findings have often differed with regard to time since notification, stage of disease, gender, and sexual orientation. Most commonly, studies have attempted to identify the prevalence of anxiety disorders among patients at different stages of illness, including patients waiting to be notified of their HIV status, patients just notified of their HIV status, asymptomatic HIV-positive patients, and patients with AIDS-related complex or AIDS. Anxiety associated with adjustment disorders is the most common manifestation of anxiety in HIV-positive patients; among patients with newly diagnosed HIV infection, the prevalence is as high as 37%. Generalized anxiety disorder is also commonly identified in HIV-positive populations; the prevalence is approximately 15%. Not as well studied are the prevalences of panic and posttraumatic stress disorder, which generally occur less frequently (G.R. Brown et al. 1992; Kerrihard et al. 1999).

Management of significant anxiety in dying patients is likely to require pharmacological treatment, given along with psychological support or behavioral interventions. Pharmacotherapy primarily involves the use of benzodiazepines, neuroleptics (Table 35–4), antidepressants, and opioid analgesics. Short-acting benzodiazepines, such as lorazepam and alprazolam, are used most often. Lorazepam is metabolized by conjugation in the liver and is therefore safer to use in patients with hepatic disease. Alprazolam is metabolized through oxidative mechanisms in the liver and can exacerbate liver damage. Midazolam, a very-short-acting benzodiazepine, is administered intravenously to achieve rapid sedation in patients who are agitated or anxious. In an intensive care setting, midazolam is most often administered intravenously; it is also useful and safe when administered subcutaneously (Bottomley and Hanks 1990). Starting doses should be low (i.e., 10–60 mg, given over 24 hours), and the patient should be carefully monitored (DeSousa and Jepson 1988). Clonazepam, a longer-acting benzodiazepine, is used in patients who experience breakthrough anxiety when treated with short-acting drugs. It is also useful when tapering alprazolam. Diazepam can be administered rectally, when oral administration is not possible, to control anxiety and restlessness (Twycross and Lack 1984).

Neuroleptics such as haloperidol or thioridazine, given in low doses, are used when benzodiazepines are contraindi-

TABLE 35–4. Anxiolytic medications useful in patients with terminal illnesses

Drug	Approximate daily dose range (mg)	Route[a]
Benzodiazepines		
Very-short-acting		
Midazolam	10–60 (over 24 hours)	im, iv, sc
Short-acting		
Alprazolam	0.25–2 (tid–qid)	po, sl
Lorazepam	0.5–2 (tid–qid)	im, iv, po, sl
Long-acting		
Clonazepam	0.5–2 (bid–qid)	po
Diazepam	5–10 (bid–qid)	im, iv, po, pr
Neuroleptics		
Chlorpromazine	12.5–50 (every 4–12 hours)	po
Haloperidol	0.5–5 (every 2–12 hours)	im, iv, po, sc
Thioridazine	10–25 (tid–qid)	po
Olanzapine	2.5–10 (bid)	po

Note. bid = twice a day; im = intramuscular; iv = intravenous; po = per os (orally); pr = per rectum; qid = four times a day; sc = subcutaneous; sl = sublingual; tid = three times a day.
[a]Parenteral doses are generally twice as potent as oral doses.
Source. Adapted from Breitbart W, Passik S: "Psychiatric Aspects of Palliative Care," in *Oxford Textbook of Palliative Medicine*. Edited by Doyle D, Hanks GWC, MacDonald N. New York, Oxford University Press, 1993, pp. 607–626. Copyright 1993, Oxford University Press. Used with permission.

cated or do not control anxiety. Haloperidol (0.5–5 mg given orally, intravenously, subcutaneously or intramuscularly every 2–12 hours) controls anxiety without causing sedation. The combination of haloperidol and a benzodiazepine is often used to control the anxiety and agitation associated with delirium. Thioridazine and chlorpromazine, both low-potency neuroleptics, are effective anxiolytics that also promote sedation. Thioridazine should be administered orally at doses of 10–25 mg three to four times a day; 12.5–50 mg of chlorpromazine should be given orally every 4–12 hours. Because of the side effects of hypotension and anticholinergic symptoms, these drugs must be used with caution. Neuroleptics can have extrapyramidal side effects, and the development of neuroleptic malignant syndrome is possible with the use of such drugs. New atypical neuroleptics such as olanzapine have fewer such side effects and may be effective anxiolytics (Sipahimalani and Massand 1998).

Tricyclic antidepressants, which are effective in treating anxiety with accompanying depression and panic attacks, have limited utility in patients who are dying, because of delayed onset of action and anticholinergic effects; however, the sedative effects of these medications are useful.

Narcotic analgesics, primarily used for pain management, are extremely effective in relieving dyspnea and the anxiety associated with it. Continuous intravenous infusion of morphine is particularly useful in dying patients who have respiratory distress accompanied by anxiety. The dose is titrated to achieve optimal comfort. Buspirone, a nonbenzodiazepine anxiolytic, has limited usefulness in terminally ill patients, because of its delayed onset of action. Hydroxyzine is an antihistamine that has mild anxiolytic, sedative, and analgesic effects when given orally, intravenously, or subcutaneously at doses of 25–50 mg every 4–6 hours.

For providing psychological support, supportive, crisis-oriented psychotherapy is the best model. The consultation-liaison psychiatrist must be able to discuss the meaning of information about the medical condition and treatment plan, listen to the patient's fears and concerns, and support adaptive ways of coping. Cognitive-behavioral techniques are used to reduce anxiety through providing information and teaching self-monitoring techniques, distraction, and relaxation. Cognitive approaches focus on thought processes and perceptions; behavioral approaches focus on modifying behavior. The behavioral techniques most often use elements of muscular relaxation and cognitive distraction, passive breathing followed by passive or active muscle relaxation, and pleasant imagery (Mastrovito 1989).

Depression

Prevalence rates for major depressive syndromes among patients with cancer range from 4.5% to 58%, according to psychiatric consultation database studies (Hinton 1972; Levine et al. 1978; Massie and Holland 1987; Massie et al. 1979) and research-based prevalence studies (Bukberg and Holland 1980; Bukberg et al. 1984; Chochinov et al. 1994; Dean 1987; Derogatis et al. 1983; Evans et al. 1986; Kathol et al. 1990; Lansky et al. 1985; Morton et al. 1984; Plumb and Holland 1977; Weddington et al. 1986). Only a limited number of these studies examined the prevalence of depression among patients with greatly advanced disease (Bukberg and Holland 1980; Bukberg et al. 1984; Chochinov et al. 1994; Derogatis et al. 1983; Hinton 1972; Kathol et al. 1990), and the data from these studies suggested that depression is more common in later stages of the disease, ranging in prevalence from 23% to 58%. A family history of depression and a history of previous depressive episodes lend support to a diagnosis of depression. Evaluation of cancer-related organic factors that can present as depression must precede initiation of treatment. These factors include effects of administration of corticosteroids (Stiefel et al. 1989), chemotherapeutic agents (including vincristine, vinblastine, asparaginase, intrathecal methotrexate, interferon, and interleukin-2) (Adams et al. 1984; Denicoff et al. 1987; Holland et al. 1974; Young

1982), and amphotericin B (Weddington 1982); effects of whole-brain irradiation (DeAngelis et al. 1989); central nervous system (CNS) metabolic-endocrine complications (Breitbart 1989a); and paraneoplastic syndromes (Patchell and Posner 1989; Posner 1988).

Assessment of Depression in Terminally Ill Patients

Depressed mood and sadness can be appropriate responses as the terminally ill patient faces death. These emotions can be manifestations of anticipatory grief over loss of life, health, loved ones, and autonomy. Therefore, diagnosis of a major depressive syndrome in a patient who is terminally ill can be problematic (Endicott 1983; Massie and Holland 1990; Plumb and Holland 1977).

The first difficulty in diagnosing depression in terminally ill patients is determining which diagnostic classification system to use. Use of different diagnostic classification systems such as DSM-III (American Psychiatric Association 1980), DSM-III-R, DSM-IV (American Psychiatric Association 1994), DSM-IV-TR (American Psychiatric Association 2000), and the Research Diagnostic Criteria (RDC; Spitzer et al. 1978) often leads to widely varying rates of detection of depression in patients with cancer. Kathol and colleagues (1990) found as much as a 13% difference in rates of major depression when using DSM-III criteria (38%), DSM-III-R criteria (29%), and the RDC (25%).

A second critical difficulty in diagnosing depression in patients who are terminally ill is determining how best to utilize and interpret the physical and somatic symptoms of depression. Knowledge of the presence of neurovegetative signs and symptoms of depression, such as fatigue and loss of energy, is often not helpful in establishing a diagnosis of depression in this population. Terminal illness itself can produce many of the physical symptoms that are characteristic of major depression in physically healthy people.

Four approaches to diagnosis of major depression in the cancer patient with advanced disease have been described (Cohen-Cole et al. 1993; McDaniel and Nemeroff 1993):

1. The *inclusive approach*, which includes all physical symptoms, whether or not they may be the result of cancer illness or treatment
2. The *etiological approach*, in which the clinician attempts to determine whether the physical symptom is due to cancer and treatment or to a depressive disorder
3. The *exclusive approach*, which eliminates all physical symptoms from consideration
4. The *substitutive approach*, in which physical symptoms of uncertain etiology are replaced by other nonsomatic symptoms. The substitutive approach is best exemplified by the Endicott Substitution Criteria (Endicott 1983), listed in Table 35–5.

TABLE 35–5.   Endicott Substitution Criteria for measurement of depression

Physical/somatic symptom	Psychological symptom substitute
1. Change in appetite, weight	1. Tearfulness, depressed appearance
2. Sleep disturbance	2. Social withdrawal, decreased talkativeness
3. Fatigue, loss of energy	3. Brooding, self-pity, pessimism
4. Diminished ability to think or concentrate, indecisiveness	4. Lack of reactivity

Source.   Adapted from Endicott J: "Measurement of Depression in Patients With Cancer." *Cancer* 53:2243–2245, 1983. Used with permission.

Chochinov and colleagues (1994) studied the prevalence of depression in a terminally ill cancer population and compared low and high diagnostic thresholds as well as Endicott Substitution Criteria. Interestingly, identical rates of 9.2% for major depression and 3.8% for minor depression (a total of 13%) were found using high-threshold RDC and Endicott criteria. More recently, Chochinov and colleagues (1997) compared the accuracy of a simple single-item screening method (answering Yes or No to the question "Have you been depressed most of the time for the past 2 weeks?") to more extensive assessments. The single-item screening identified 100% of patients with major depression.

The strategy of relying on the psychological or cognitive signs and symptoms of depression for diagnostic specificity (the exclusive approach) is also not without pitfalls. How is the clinician to interpret feelings of hopelessness in the dying patient when there is no hope of cure or recovery? Our practice is to explore feelings of hopelessness, worthlessness, or suicidal ideation in some detail. Although many dying patients lose hope of a cure, they are able to maintain hope regarding aspects such as pain control. Hopelessness that is pervasive and that is accompanied by despair or despondency is more likely to represent a symptom of a depressive disorder (Massie and Holland 1990). Similarly, patients often state that they feel they are burdening their families unfairly, causing them great pain and inconvenience. Those beliefs are less likely to represent a symptom of depression than is the belief by a patient that his or her life has never had any worth or that he or she is being punished for evil things done in the past. Suicidal ideation, even mild and passive forms, is very likely to be associated with significant degrees of depression in terminally ill cancer patients (Breitbart 1987, 1990).

Management of Depression in Terminally Ill Patients

Depression in patients with advanced disease is optimally managed with a combination of supportive psychotherapy, cognitive-behavioral techniques, and antidepressant medications (Block 2000; Massie and Holland 1990). Psychotherapy and cognitive-behavioral techniques are useful in the management of psychological distress in patients with cancer and have been applied to the treatment of depressive and anxious symptoms related to cancer and cancer pain. Psychotherapeutic interventions, in the form of either individual or group counseling, have been shown to reduce psychological distress and depressive symptoms in patients with cancer (Massie et al. 1989; Spiegel and Bloom 1983; Spiegel et al. 1981). Cognitive-behavioral interventions, such as relaxation and distraction with pleasant imagery, have been shown to decrease depressive symptoms in patients with mild to moderate levels of depression (Holland et al. 1987). However, psychopharmacological interventions such as treatment with antidepressant medications (see Table 35–6) are the mainstay of treatment of terminally ill patients with severe depressive symptoms who meet criteria for a major depressive episode (Massie and Holland 1990). The efficacy of antidepressants in the treatment of depression in patients with cancer has been established (Costa et al. 1985; Massie and Holland 1990; Popkin et al. 1985; Purohit et al. 1978; Rifkin et al. 1985). However, few controlled studies of antidepressant drug therapy have focused on the treatment of patients who are terminally ill (Mermelstein and Lesko 1992).

Pharmacological Treatment of Depression in Terminally Ill Patients

Tricyclic and heterocyclic antidepressants as well as the psychostimulants have roles in the pharmacological treatment of the terminally ill patient who is depressed (Massie and Holland 1990). Factors such as prognosis and the time frame for treatment may be important in determining the type of pharmacotherapy that is chosen for depression. A patient with depression whose life expectancy is several months can afford to wait the 10–14 days it may take to respond to a tricyclic antidepressant. The dying patient with depression who has less than 3 weeks to live may do best with a rapid-acting psychostimulant (Breitbart 1988). Patients who are within hours or days of death and who are in distress are likely to benefit most from the use of sedatives or narcotic analgesic infusions.

TABLE 35–6. Antidepressants used in patients with advanced disease

Drug	Therapeutic oral daily dose (mg)
Benzodiazepines	
Alprazolam	0.75–6
Heterocyclic antidepressants	
Amoxapine	100–150
Maprotiline	100–200
Monoamine oxidase inhibitors	
Isocarboxazid	20–40
Moclobemide[a]	100–600
Phenelzine	30–60
Tranylcypromine	20–40
Psychostimulants	
Dextroamphetamine	5–30
Methylphenidate	5–30
Pemoline	37.5–150
Second-generation antidepressants	
Bupropion	200–450
Trazodone	50–200
Selective serotonin reuptake inhibitors	
Citalopram	10–40
Fluoxetine	10–60
Fluvoxamine	50–300
Paroxetine	10–60
Sertraline	25–200
Tricyclic antidepressants	
Amitriptyline	25–125
Clomipramine	25–125
Desipramine	25–125
Doxepin	25–125
Imipramine	25–125
Nortriptyline	25–125
Other agents	
Mirtazapine	15–45
Nefazodone	100–500

[a]Available in Canada and Europe; not yet available in the United States.
Source. Adapted from Massie MJ, Holland JC: "Depression and the Cancer Patient." *Journal of Clinical Psychiatry* 51:12–17, 1990. Used with permission.

Tricyclic antidepressants. The tricyclic antidepressants are frequently used to treat patients with cancer who have depression. Treatment should be initiated at low dosages (10–25 mg at bedtime), especially in patients who are debilitated and have advanced disease; the doses should be increased slowly, by increments of 10–25 mg every 1–2 days, until a beneficial effect is achieved. Patients with cancer who have depression often have a therapeutic response at much lower dosages (25–125 mg/day orally) than are usually required in patients who do not have medical illness (150–300 mg/day) (Massie and Holland 1990). It is often useful to monitor plasma levels of tricyclics (desipramine, nortriptyline, amitriptyline, imipramine), because patients who are medically ill, and patients with advanced cancer in particular, are often found to have therapeutic plasma levels at modest doses (Stoudemire and Fogel 1987). Moreover, typical regimens of the tricyclics (100–250 mg/day) can cause toxic effects in medically ill, debilitated patients, and plasma levels obtained on a serial basis can guide the physician in effective and safe administration. The anticholinergic, orthostatic, and cardiac side effects of the tricyclics are often troubling and are occasionally serious. Monitoring of plasma levels can ensure adequate treatment while minimizing the risk of side effects or toxicity (Preskorn and Jerkovich 1990).

The selection of a tricyclic depends on the side-effect profile, the existing medical problems, the nature of the depressive symptoms, and past response to specific antidepressants. Sedating tricyclics such as amitriptyline or doxepin are prescribed to patients with agitation and depression accompanied by insomnia. Desipramine or nortriptyline have relatively low anticholinergic potential and thus are useful when one must avoid exacerbating urinary retention, decreased intestinal motility, or stomatitis. Patients who are receiving multiple drugs with anticholinergic properties (e.g., meperidine, atropine, diphenhydramine, phenothiazines) are at risk for an anticholinergic delirium; therefore, tricyclics with potent anticholinergic properties should be avoided in these patients.

Most tricyclics are also available as rectal suppositories. Outside the United States, certain tricyclics are given by intravenous infusion (Massie and Holland 1984). Amitriptyline, imipramine, and doxepin can be given intramuscularly (Breitbart 1988; Massie and Holland 1990).

Second-generation antidepressants. If a patient does not respond to a tricyclic antidepressant or cannot tolerate its side effects, a second-generation antidepressant such as trazodone or bupropion can be used. The second-generation antidepressants are generally considered less cardiotoxic than the tricyclic antidepressants (Glassman 1984). Trazodone is strongly sedating and in low doses (50–100 mg at bedtime) is helpful in the treatment of depression in patients with insomnia. Trazodone is highly serotonergic, and its use should be considered when the patient requires analgesia in addition to antidepressant effects. Trazodone has been associated with priapism and therefore should be used with caution in male patients (Sher et al. 1983).

At present, bupropion is not the drug of first choice for depressed patients in a medical setting; however, we would consider prescribing bupropion to patients who have a poor response to a reasonable trial of other antidepressants. Bupropion may have a role in the treatment of the terminally ill patient with psychomotor retardation, because this drug has energizing effects similar to those of the psychostimulant drugs (Peck et al. 1983; Shopsin 1983). However, because bupropion therapy is associated with an increased incidence of seizures among patients with CNS disorders, this drug has a limited role in cancer patients with brain tumors or CNS metastases.

Heterocyclic antidepressants. The heterocyclic antidepressants have side-effect profiles similar to those of the tricyclic antidepressants. Maprotiline should be avoided in patients with brain tumors and in patients who are at risk for seizures, because the incidence of seizures is increased with use of this medication (Lloyd 1977). Amoxapine has mild dopamine-blocking activity. Patients who are taking other dopamine blockers (e.g., antiemetics) as well as amoxapine have an increased risk of extrapyramidal symptoms and dyskinesia (Ayd 1979). Mianserin (which is not available in the United States) is a serotonergic antidepressant with adjuvant analgesic properties that is used widely in Europe and Latin America. Costa et al. (1985) showed mianserin to be a safe and effective drug for the treatment of depression in patients with cancer.

Selective serotonin reuptake inhibitors. Fluoxetine, a selective inhibitor of neuronal serotonin uptake, has fewer sedative cardiac and autonomic effects than the tricyclic antidepressants (Cooper 1988). This aspect of its side-effect profile has made fluoxetine an attractive antidepressant for use in patients who are medically ill. However, certain other common side effects of fluoxetine may limit its usefulness in patients with cancer who are terminally ill. Fluoxetine can cause mild nausea and a brief period of increased anxiety, as well as appetite suppression that usually lasts for several weeks. Some of our patients have experienced transient weight loss, but weight usually returns to baseline level. Furthermore, fluoxetine and its active metabolite, norfluoxetine, have long half-lives. The half-life of the parent compound averages 1–4 days; that of the metabolite, 7–14 days. Also, since fluoxetine went on the market, there have been several reports of significant drug-drug interactions (Ciraulo and Shader 1990; Pearson 1990). Until it has been further studied in patients who are medically ill, we suggest cautious use of fluoxetine, particularly in patients who are debilitated and dying.

Two newer selective serotonin reuptake inhibitors (SSRIs)—sertraline and paroxetine—have shorter half-lives, and their metabolites are not significantly active (Boyer and Feighner 1991). They have been useful additions to the list of choices of antidepressants for patients who are terminally ill. Paroxetine may have the additional benefit of being a potent analgesic agent for the management of neuropathic pain (Sindrup et al. 1990). Fluvoxamine is a newly released SSRI, but there is little clinical experience with it in patients who are medically ill. Similarly, venlafaxine, a serotonin and norepinephrine reuptake inhibitor, is newly available, and reports of its use in patients who are medically ill are appearing in the literature (Feighner 1994; Khan et al. 1991). Because of its mild side-effect profile (nausea, somnolence, insomnia, increase in blood pressure), venlafaxine might prove useful in medical settings.

Psychostimulants. Treatment with psychostimulants (dextroamphetamine, methylphenidate, and pemoline) is an alternative and effective pharmacological approach to depression in terminally ill patients (Chiarello and Cole 1987; Fernandez et al. 1987; Fisch 1985–1986; Katon and Raskind 1980; Kaufmann et al. 1982; Satel and Nelson 1989; Woods et al. 1986). These drugs have a more rapid onset of action than do the tricyclics, and they are often energizing. They are most helpful in the treatment of depression in patients with advanced disease and in those in whom dysphoric mood is associated with severe psychomotor slowing and even mild cognitive impairment. Psychostimulants have been shown to improve attention, concentration, and overall performance on neuropsychological tests in patients who are medically ill (Fernandez et al. 1988). At relatively low doses, psychostimulants improve appetite, promote a sense of well-being, and counteract feelings of weakness and fatigue.

Treatment with dextroamphetamine or methylphenidate usually begins with a dose of 2.5 mg at 8:00 A.M. and at noon. The dose is slowly increased over several days, until a desired effect is achieved or side effects (overstimulation, anxiety, insomnia, paranoia, confusion) become intolerable. Typically, a dosage greater than 30 mg/day is not necessary, although patients occasionally require up to 60 mg/day. Patients usually are treated with methylphenidate for 1–2 months, and approximately two-thirds can discontinue methylphenidate therapy without recurrence of depressive symptoms. Patients whose symptoms do recur can be treated with a psychostimulant for up to 1 year without significant abuse problems. Tolerance will develop, and adjustment of dose may be necessary. Stimulants such as methylphenidate and dextroamphetamine have also been shown to reduce sedation secondary to opioid analgesics, and stimulants provide adjuvant analgesia in patients with cancer

(Bruera et al. 1987). Common side effects of these drugs include nervousness, overstimulation, mild increases in blood pressure and pulse rate, and tremor. Less common side effects include dyskinesia and motor tics as well as paranoid psychosis and exacerbation of an underlying and unrecognized confusional state.

Pemoline is a unique psychostimulant that is chemically unrelated to amphetamine. Pemoline is a less potent stimulant that has little abuse potential (Chiarello and Cole 1987). The advantages of pemoline as a psychostimulant in patients with advanced illness include the near lack of abuse potential, the lack of federal regulations requiring special triplicate prescriptions, the drug's mild sympathomimetic effects, and the fact that the drug comes in a chewable tablet form that can be absorbed through the buccal mucosa and be used by patients who have difficulty swallowing or who have intestinal obstruction. In our clinical experience, pemoline is as effective as methylphenidate or dextroamphetamine in the treatment of depressive symptoms in patients who are terminally ill (Breitbart and Mermelstein 1992). Pemoline can be started at a dose of 18.75 mg in the morning and at noon and can be increased gradually over days. Typically, patients require 75 mg or less per day for adequate symptom relief. Pemoline should be used with caution in patients with liver impairment, and liver function tests should be performed periodically with longer-term treatment regimens (Stein et al. 1980). Modafinil is a new psychostimulant, unrelated to the amphetamines, that may have utility as an antidepressant augmenting agent (Menza et al. 2000).

Monoamine oxidase inhibitors. Monoamine oxidase inhibitors (MAOIs), if considered, must be used with great caution. Instructions to avoid tyramine-containing foods during MAOI treatment are poorly received by severely ill patients who already have dietary and nutritional restrictions. One must be extremely cautious when using narcotic analgesics for patients taking MAOIs, because myoclonus and delirium have been reported with such combinations (Breitbart 1988). The concomitant use of meperidine and an MAOI is absolutely contraindicated and can lead to hyperpyrexia and cardiovascular collapse. Sympathomimetic drugs and other less obvious MAOIs, such as the chemotherapeutic agent procarbazine, can cause a hypertensive crisis in patients taking an MAOI. If a patient has responded well in the past to an MAOI given for depression, its continued use is warranted, but again caution must be taken. The reversible inhibitors of monoamine oxidase subtype A, such as clorgyline and moclobemide (available in Canada and Europe), may have important applications in treating depression in patients with advanced disease. Controlled

trials of these new agents for the treatment of depression in patients with advanced disease are necessary.

Lithium carbonate. Patients who were taking lithium before their illnesses should continue lithium therapy, if necessary, with close monitoring in the preoperative and postoperative periods when fluids and salt may be restricted. Maintenance doses of lithium may need to be reduced in patients who are seriously ill. Lithium should be prescribed with caution to patients receiving cisplatin, because of the potential nephrotoxicity of both drugs. Several authors have reported that lithium can transiently stimulate leukocyte production in leukopenic cancer patients. It is unclear, however, whether such lithium-stimulated leukocytes function normally. No mood changes have been noted in such patients (Stein et al. 1980).

Benzodiazepines. The triazolobenzodiazepine alprazolam has been shown to be a mildly effective antidepressant as well as an anxiolytic. In patients with mixed symptoms of anxiety and depression, the starting dose is 0.25 mg, given three times a day; effective doses are usually in the range of 4–6 mg/day (Holland et al. 1987).

Electroconvulsive Therapy

Occasionally, it is necessary to consider electroconvulsive therapy for patients who have depression with psychotic features or in whom treatment with antidepressants poses unacceptable side effects. The safe, effective use of electroconvulsive therapy in patients who are medically ill has been reviewed by others (Massie and Holland 1990).

Nonpharmacological Treatment of Depression in Terminally Ill Patients

Supportive psychotherapy is a useful treatment approach to depression in the patient who is terminally ill. Psychotherapy with the dying patient consists of active listening with supportive verbal interventions and occasional interpretation (Cassem 1987). Despite the seriousness of the patient's plight, it is not necessary for the psychiatrist or psychologist to appear overly solemn or emotionally restrained. Often it is only the psychotherapist, of all the patient's caregivers, who is comfortable enough to converse lightheartedly and allow the patient to talk about his or her life and experiences rather than to focus solely on impending death. The dying patient who wishes to talk or ask questions about death should be allowed to do so freely, with the therapist maintaining an interested, interactive stance. It is not uncommon for the dying patient to benefit from pastoral counseling. If a chaplaincy service is available, it should be offered to the patient and family.

SUICIDE AND TERMINALLY ILL PATIENTS

Patients in terminal stages of illness with multiple complications such as pain, depression, delirium, and deficit symptoms are at increased risk for suicide compared with the general population. Listed in Table 35–7 are factors associated with increased risk of suicide in patients with advanced disease (Breitbart 1987, 1990). Psychiatric disorders are frequently present in hospitalized medically ill patients who are suicidal. A review of psychiatric consultation data at Memorial Sloan-Kettering Cancer Center (MSKCC) showed that about 33% of suicidal patients with cancer had major depression, about 20% had delirium, and 50% were diagnosed with an adjustment disorder with both anxious and depressed features at the time of evaluation (Breitbart 1987, 1990).

Patients with cancer are more likely to commit suicide in advanced stages of disease (Bolund 1985; Farberow et al. 1963; Fox et al. 1982; Louhivuori and Hakama 1979). A reported 86% of suicides studied by Farberow et al. (1963) occurred in the preterminal or terminal stages of illness, despite patients' greatly reduced physical capacities. Poor prognosis and advanced illness usually go hand in hand, so it is not surprising that a study found that patients who were expected to die within a matter of months were the most likely to commit suicide (Bolund 1985). In that study, of the 88 patients with cancer who committed suicide, 14 patients had uncertain prognoses and 45 patients had poor prognoses. Uncontrolled pain is a dramatically important risk factor for suicide. Several studies have shown that the vast majority of patients with cancer who commit suicide had severe pain that was often inadequately controlled and poorly tolerated (Bolund 1985; Farberow et al. 1971).

TABLE 35–7. Risk factors for suicide among patients with terminal illnesses

Depression and hopelessness
Debilitating illness
Uncontrolled pain
Delirium and disinhibition
Previous depression or suicide attempts
Family history of depression
Lack of social supports
History of substance abuse
Feeling of being a burden on others
Recent loss or bereavement

Depression is a factor in 50% of all suicides. Patients with depression are at 25 times greater risk of suicide than the general population (Guze and Robins 1970; Robins et al. 1950). The role that depression plays in suicide because of cancer is equally significant. Among patients with advanced illness and progressively impaired physical function, symptoms of severe depression increase to 77% (Bukberg et al. 1984). Hopelessness is the key variable that links depression and suicide in the general population. Furthermore, hopelessness is a significantly better predictor of completed suicide than is depression alone (Beck et al. 1975; Kovacs et al. 1975). In Scandinavia, the highest incidence of suicide was found among cancer patients who were offered no further treatment and no further contact with the health care system (Louhivuori and Hakama 1979). Being left to face illness alone creates a sense of isolation and abandonment that is conducive to the development of hopelessness. Chochinov and colleagues (1998) demonstrated that major depression and hopelessness were highly correlated with suicidal ideation in terminally ill cancer patients. In fact, hopelsssness appears to be a critical mediation between depression and suicidal ideation. In our clinical experience, we have also found delirium to be a major contributing factor in impulsive suicide attempts, especially in the hospital setting.

Loss of control and a sense of helplessness in the face of terminal illness are important factors in suicide susceptibility. *Loss of control* refers to the helplessness induced by symptoms or deficits resulting from disease or treatments. In addition, some patients have an excessive need to be in control of all aspects of living or dying and may experience a loss of control in another sense. Farberow et al. (1963) noted that patients who were accepting and adaptable were much less likely to commit suicide than patients who exhibited a need to be in control of even the most minute details of their care (Fox et al. 1982). Most distressing to patients, especially those who are confused or sedated by medications, is the sense that they are losing control of their minds. The risk of suicide is increased in patients with physical impairments, especially when accompanied by psychological distress and disturbed interpersonal relationships (Farberow et al. 1971).

Fatigue, in the form of exhaustion of physical, emotional, spiritual, financial, familial, communal, and other resources, increases the risk of suicide in the patient with a terminal illness (Breitbart 1987). Symptom control becomes a prolonged process, with frequent advances and setbacks. The dying process also can become extremely long and arduous for all concerned. It is not uncommon for both family members and health care providers to withdraw prematurely from the dying patient under these circumstances. A suicidal patient can thus feel even more isolated and abandoned. The existence of a strong support system for the patient that may act as an external control of suicidal behavior reduces the risk of suicide significantly.

Holland (1993) advised that it is extremely rare for a patient with cancer to commit suicide without some degree of premorbid psychopathology that places him or her at increased risk. Farberow et al. (1963) described a large group of patients with cancer who committed suicide as the "dependent dissatisfied." These patients were immature, demanding, complaining, irritable, hostile, and difficult to manage. Staff members often felt manipulated by these patients and became irritable because of what they saw as excessive demands for attention. Suicide attempts or threats were often seen as "hysterical" or manipulative. Our consultation data on suicidal patients with cancer showed that half had a diagnosable personality disorder (Breitbart 1987). This finding is consistent with the statistics on suicide in general, which show that a previous suicide attempt greatly increases the risk of completed suicide (Dubovsky 1978; Murphy 1977). A family history of suicide increases suicide risk.

Thoughts of suicide probably occur quite frequently, particularly in the setting of advanced disease, and seem to act as a steam valve for feelings often expressed by patients as "If it gets too bad, I always have a way out." It has been our experience in working with patients with cancer that once a trusting and safe relationship develops, patients almost universally reveal that they have had occasionally persistent thoughts of suicide as a means of escaping the threat of being overwhelmed by cancer. However, published reports suggest that suicidal ideation is relatively infrequent in patients with cancer and is limited to those who are significantly depressed. Silberfarb et al. (1980) found that only 3 of 146 patients with breast cancer had suicidal thoughts, and none of the 100 cancer patients interviewed in a Finnish study expressed suicidal thoughts (Achte and Vanhkouen 1971). In a study conducted at St. Boniface General Hospice in Winnipeg, Canada, only 10 of 44 terminally ill patients with cancer were suicidal or desired an early death, and all 10 had clinical depression (J.H. Brown et al. 1986). At MSKCC, suicide risk evaluation accounted for 8.6% of psychiatric consultations, usually requested by staff in response to a patient's verbalizing suicidal wishes (Breitbart 1987). Breitbart (1990) studied 185 cancer patients with pain at MSKCC and found that suicidal ideation occurred in 17% of the study population. The discrepancy between clinical impression and research conclusions may be the result of limitations of the research interview with regard to eliciting reports of suicidal thinking.

Euthanasia and Physician-Assisted Suicide

In 1997, Slome and colleagues conducted a survey of AIDS physicians in the San Francisco, California, area. Ninety-eight percent of respondents reported having received requests for physician-assisted suicide. More than half admitted to having granted at least one patient's request for assistance with his or her suicide. Today, requests for physician-assisted suicide are abundant and real. What is the appropriate response to such a request? Medical training reinforces the view of suicide as a manifestation of psychiatric disturbance to be prevented at all costs. However, many people view suicide in those who face the distress of a fatal and painful disease as rational and a means to regain control and achieve a dignified death.

The term *euthanasia* encompasses a number of concepts, all of which have become controversial but important issues in the care of patients with terminal illnesses. *Active euthanasia* refers to the intentional termination of a patient's life by a physician. *Physician-assisted suicide* is the provision by a physician of the means by which a patient can end his or her own life. *Passive euthanasia* refers to the withholding or withdrawal of life-sustaining measures and is viewed as acceptable in many societies (Pellegrino 1991). Active euthanasia and physician-assisted suicide, however, are perhaps the most intensely and bitterly debated issues in medical ethics today.

Active euthanasia has been taking place in The Netherlands since the 1980s (de Wachter 1989; van der Maas et al. 1991). Although it is still illegal there, active termination of a patient's life by a physician is tolerated under the conditions that 1) the patient's consent is explicit and freely, consciously, and persistently given; 2) the patient and physician agree that the suffering is intolerable; 3) other measures for relief have been exhausted; 4) a second physician concurs; and 5) these facts are documented. A best estimate is that 1.8% of deaths in The Netherlands are the result of euthanasia with physician involvement (van der Maas et al. 1991). Common reasons for requesting euthanasia included loss of dignity (57% of cases), pain (46%), "unworthy dying" (46%), dependence on others (33%), and "tiredness of life" (23%) (van der Maas et al. 1991) (Table 35–8). California and Washington have considered initiatives that would allow for active euthanasia along the lines of the Netherlands model. The case of "Debbie," reported on in the *Journal of the American Medical Association* ("A Piece of My Mind" 1988) in 1988, forced a debate, still ongoing, on active euthanasia in the United States (Gaylin et al. 1988; Singer 1990; Wanzer et al. 1989).

TABLE 35–8. Factors associated with requests for physician-assisted suicide and euthanasia in patients with terminal illnesses

Depression and hopelessness
Feeling of helplessness
Exhaustion and weakness
Uncontrolled pain
Feelings of being a burden (financial, physical, emotional)
Recent loss or bereavement

Physician-assisted suicide has also become a topic of public debate, following the dramatic case in 1990 of a woman with Alzheimer's disease who used Dr. Jack Kevorkian's "suicide machine." Kevorkian was acquitted by a Michigan court of any wrongdoing. Dr. Timothy E. Quill, a physician who helped a patient with leukemia commit suicide, was not indicted by a Rochester, New York, grand jury in July 1991. Quill's account of his participation in the patient's suicide was published in the *New England Journal of Medicine* (Quill 1991) and sparked debate regarding the physician's role in aiding patients to die. In interviews conducted after publication of the article, Quill said that he had decided to go public in order to present an alternative to Kevorkian's approach. Kevorkian had used a machine to assist in the death of a patient whom he did not know well. In contrast, Quill had been treating the patient with leukemia for 8 years and knew her quite well. In his article, Quill described the process that he and the patient undertook, in which they explored her choice to actively end her life. He also described recommending that the patient contact the Hemlock Society and prescribing barbiturates for sleep 1 week later at the patient's request.

The Humane and Dignified Death Act, which would have freed physicians from criminal and civil liability if they participated in active voluntary euthanasia, did not appear on the 1988 California ballot, because the sponsoring group, Americans Against Human Suffering, barely failed to obtain the required number of signatures. That group, an affiliate organization of the National Hemlock Society, did however undertake a survey of California physicians as part of its efforts to build support for the act; the results are revealing (Helig 1988). Of the physicians who responded, 70% agreed that patients should have the option of active euthanasia in cases of terminal illness. More than 50% of the respondents said that they would practice active voluntary euthanasia if it were legal, and 23% revealed that they already had practiced active euthanasia at least once in their careers. Of the 60% of physicians who indicated that they had been asked by patients with terminal illness to hasten death,

nearly all agreed that such requests from patients could be described as rational. Public support for the "right to die" has been growing as well; 65%–85% of the general population supports a change in the law to permit physicians to help patients die, and there is greater acceptance by the public of suicide when pain and suffering coexist with terminal illness. Results of recent surveys conducted in Oregon indicated high rates of public support for legalized physician-assisted suicide, as well as relatively significant rates of endorsement and even performance of assisted suicide among medical professionals (Howard et al. 1997; Meier et al. 1998; Suarez-Almazor et al. 1997).

Clinicians who provide care for cancer patients with pain and advanced illness are sympathetic to the goals of symptom control and relief of suffering and are also obviously influenced by those who view suicide and active voluntary euthanasia as rational alternatives for patients who are already dying and are in distress. There is a danger that suicidal ideation or a request to hasten death in the patient with cancer may be prematurely assumed to be a "rational act" unencumbered by psychiatric disturbance. Accepted criteria for "rational suicide" (Siegel 1982; Siegel and Tuckel 1984) include the following: 1) the person must have clear mental processes that are unimpaired by psychological illness or severe emotional distress, such as depression; 2) the person must have made a realistic assessment of the situation; and 3) the motives for the decision of suicide are understandable to most uninvolved observers. Clearly, some suicides that occur in the cancer setting do meet these criteria for rationality, but a significant percentage—possibly the majority—do not, by virtue of the fact that significant psychiatric comorbidity exists. By reviewing the current research data on suicide in cancer patients and the role of factors such as pain, depression, and delirium, we hope to provide a factual framework on which to base guidelines for managing this vulnerable group of patients. (For further discussion, see Chapter 9.)

Studies have shown that special attention must be directed toward depression, social support, and other psychosocial issues, in addition to pain and physical symptom control, in the treatment of suicidal terminally ill patients. In their studies involving ambulatory patients with AIDS, Rosenfeld and colleagues (1996) found that although pain itself, and more severe pain, appeared to heighten psychological distress and depression, there was no direct relationship between pain and interest in assisted suicide (Breitbart et al. 1996a). Interest in assisted suicide appeared to be more a function of psychological and social factors (e.g., depression, social support, fear of becoming a burden to one's friends) than of physical factors (e.g., pain, symptom distress, disease status). The strongest predictors of interest in physician-assisted suicide were high levels of depressive symptoms, hopelessness, overall psychological distress, and current suicidal ideation. Other strong predictors included perceived lack of social support, death of a family member or friend, race (whites greater than nonwhites), and religious practice (nonreligious greater than religious). Interest in assisted suicide was not related to the presence or severity of pain, physical symptoms, or extent of HIV disease. Rosenfeld et al. (1998) found cognitive impairment to be significantly associated with the desire for death in a sample of hospitalized terminally ill patients with AIDS. Thus, cognitive impairments (which are quite common in terminally ill patients) may lead to diminished ability to perceive long-term risks and benefits (versus immediately apparent ones) and therefore adversely influence end-of-life decision making and suicidal ideation. Breitbart and colleagues (2000) recently demonstrated that depression and hopelessness were the most powerful predictors of desire for hastened death in terminally ill cancer patients. Depression and hopelessness contributed uniquely as well as synergistically to desire for death. Social support and spiritual well-being were other important factors.

Unfortunately, several studies have demonstrated inadequate recognition and treatment of both psychological and physical symptoms (Passik et al. 1998), with symptoms such as depression and anxiety going largely unrecognized in many medically ill patients. Also disturbing is a finding of the study by Meier and colleagues (1998) of physician responses to requests for assisted suicide or euthanasia: only 2% of physicians who received requests for assisted suicide referred their patients for psychiatric consultation. Similarly, in a recent survey conducted by the American Society of Clinical Oncology Task Force on End-of-Life Care, oncologists estimated that 40% of their terminally ill patients had untreated depression (R. Mayer, personal communication, October 1998). Because of the strong influence of psychiatric, psychological, and social influences on the desire to die in terminally ill patients, psychiatric assessment of these patients and subsequent appropriate treatment are crucial.

Management of Problems in Terminally Ill Suicidal Patients

Assessment of suicide risk and appropriate intervention for suicidal patients with terminal illnesses are critical. A careful evaluation includes a search for the meaning of suicidal thoughts as well as an exploration of the seriousness of the risk. The clinician's ability to establish rapport and elicit a patient's thoughts is essential as he or she assesses history, degree of intent, and quality of internal and external controls. The clinician must listen sympathetically and not appear critical nor state that such thoughts are inappropriate. Allowing the patient to discuss suicidal thoughts often decreases the risk of suicide. The myth that asking about suicidal thoughts puts the idea of suicide in the patient's head is one that should be dispelled, especially with regard to patients with cancer (McKegney and Lange 1971). Patients often reconsider and reject the idea of suicide when the physician acknowledges the legitimacy of the option and the need to retain a sense of control over aspects of their deaths.

A new standardized measure of desire for death, entitled the Schedule of Attitudes Toward Hastened Death, was recently created by Rosenfeld and colleagues (1999) to assist physicians in psychiatric assessment of suicidal terminally ill patients. This measure has proven a reliable, valid measure of desire for death among patients with HIV disease or AIDS.

Analgesic, neuroleptic, or antidepressant medications should be used when appropriate to treat pain, agitation, psychosis, or major depression. Underlying causes of depression, delirium, or pain should be addressed specifically, when possible. Pharmacological interventions (i.e., antidepressant drug therapy) may play an important role in the treatment of suicidal terminally ill patients. Initiation of a crisis intervention–oriented psychotherapeutic approach, mobilizing as much of the patient's support system as possible, may also be important. A close family member or friend should be involved to support the patient, provide information, and assist in treatment planning.

Psychiatric hospitalization can sometimes be helpful; however, it is usually not desirable for the patient who is terminally ill. Thus, the medical hospital or home is the setting in which management most often takes place. Although it is appropriate to intervene when medical or psychiatric factors are clearly the driving force behind suicidal ideation, in some circumstances usurping control from the patient and his or her family with overly aggressive intervention may be less helpful. This is most evident in patients with advanced illness, for whom comfort and control of symptoms are the primary concerns.

The goal of the intervention should be to prevent suicide that is driven by desperation, rather than to prevent suicide at all cost. Prolonged suffering because of poorly controlled symptoms leads to such desperation, and it is the consultant's job to provide effective management of such problems as an alternative to suicide in the patient who is terminally ill.

AIDS and Suicide

Persons with AIDS are at increased risk for suicide (Marzuk et al. 1988). A study of the rate of suicide in 1985 among New York City residents with AIDS revealed that the relative risk of suicide among men with AIDS ages 20–59 years was 36 times that among men without AIDS in the same age group and 66 times that in the general population (Marzuk et al. 1988). Patients with AIDS who commit suicide generally do so within 9 months of diagnosis and usually die as a result of falling from heights or hanging. In the study by Marzuk et al. (1988), about 25% of the AIDS patients who committed suicide had made a previous suicide attempt, half had reportedly been severely depressed, and 40% saw a psychiatrist within 4 days before committing suicide. Poor prognosis, delirium, depression, hopelessness, helplessness, loss of control, preexisting psychopathology, a history of substance abuse or alcohol abuse, prior suicide attempts, social isolation, and perceived lack of social support are all factors that help to identify and seem to contribute to increased risk of suicide.

In addition, the rate of suicidal ideation among patients with HIV disease or AIDS is increased among those with more advanced disease and those with physical and psychiatric symptoms such as pain and depression. Our group at MSKCC found that pain, depressed mood, low T4-lymphocyte counts, and a diagnosis of AIDS increased rates of suicidal ideation (Sison et al. 1991). For instance, more than 40% of those with pain reported suicidal ideation, whereas only 20% of ambulatory patients with HIV infection who were pain free reported suicidal ideation. Clinicians must be alert to this increased risk of suicide among patients with AIDS and must promote early intervention for psychiatric complications such as delirium and depression, as well as for social isolation.

COGNITIVE IMPAIRMENT DISORDERS

Cognitive failure is very common in patients with advanced illness. DSM-IV-TR does not use the term *organic mental disorders*. The class of organic mental disorders has been replaced by three categories: 1) delirium, dementia, and amnestic and other cognitive disorders; 2) mental disorder due to a general medical condition; and 3) substance-induced disorders. Although virtually all of these conditions can be seen in the patient with advanced disease, the most common include delirium, dementia, and mood and anxiety disorders due to a general medical condition. For instance, in a patient with mood disturbance meeting criteria for major depression who is severely hypothyroid or taking high-dose corticosteroids, the most accurate diagnosis is mood disorder with a major depression–like episode resulting from hypothyroidism or induced by corticosteroids.

Delirium and Dementia

Delirium has been characterized as an etiologically nonspecific, global cerebral dysfunction, with concurrent disturbances in consciousness, attention, thinking, perception, memory, psychomotor behavior, emotion, and the sleep-wake cycle. Disorientation, fluctuation, and waxing and waning of the aforementioned symptoms, as well as acute or abrupt onset of such disturbances, are other critical features of delirium. Unlike dementia, delirium is often reversible, even in the patient with advanced illness; however, it may not be reversible in the last 24–48 hours of life, most likely because irreversible processes such as multiple organ failure are occurring during that time. In the palliative care literature, delirium in these last days of life is often referred to as *terminal restlessness* or *terminal agitation*.

At times, it is difficult to differentiate delirium from dementia, because the two conditions frequently share common clinical features such as disorientation and impaired memory, thinking, and judgment. Dementia appears in relatively alert individuals with little or no clouding of consciousness. The onset of symptoms in dementia is more subacute or is progressive, and the sleep-wake cycle seems less impaired. Most prominent in dementia are impaired short- and long-term memory, impaired judgment, and disturbances of abstract thinking, as well as disturbed higher cortical functions (e.g., aphasia, apraxia). Occasionally, the clinician will encounter a patient with delirium superimposed on an underlying dementia, such as in the case of an elderly patient, a patient with AIDS, or a patient with a paraneoplastic syndrome.

Clinicians often use a number of scales or instruments in making diagnoses of delirium, dementia, and cognitive failure. The Delirium Rating Scale (DRS), developed by Trzepacz et al. (1988), is a 10-item, clinician-rated symptom rating scale for delirium. The DRS is based on DSM-III-R diagnostic criteria for delirium and is designed to be used by the clinician to identify delirium and to reliably distinguish delirium from dementia and other neuropsychiatric disorders. Each item is scored by choosing one best rating and carries a numerical weight chosen to distinguish the phenomenology characteristic of delirium. A score of 12 or greater is diagnostic of delirium. The Mini-Mental State Exam (MMSE; Folstein et al. 1975) is also useful in screening for cognitive failure, but it does not distinguish between delirium and dementia. The MMSE permits quantitative assessment of cognitive performance and capacity and measures severity of cognitive impairment. It is most sensitive to cortical dementias such as Alzheimer's disease and is less sensitive to subcortical deficits such as those found in AIDS dementia. The MMSE assesses five general cognitive areas: orientation, registration, attention and calculation, recall, and language.

Delirium is highly prevalent in patients with advanced cancer or AIDS, especially in the last few weeks of life; prevalence ranges from 25% to 85% (Breitbart and Sparrow 1998). Delirium can result from either direct effects of cancer on the CNS or indirect CNS effects of the disease or treatments (medications, electrolyte imbalance, failure of a vital organ or system, infection, vascular complications and preexisting cognitive impairment, or dementia). Early symptoms of delirium can be misdiagnosed as anxiety, anger, depression, or psychosis. A diagnosis of delirium should be considered in any patient with acute onset of agitation, impaired cognitive function, altered attention span, or a fluctuating level of consciousness (Lipowski 1987).

Because of the large number of drugs that patients with cancer require and the fragile state of physiologic functioning of these patients, even routinely ordered hypnotics are enough to cause delirium. Narcotic analgesics such as levorphanol, morphine sulfate, and meperidine are common causes of confusional states, particularly in elderly and terminally ill patients (Bruera et al. 1989). Chemotherapeutic agents known to cause delirium include methotrexate, fluorouracil, vincristine, vinblastine, bleomycin, carmustine, cisplatin, asparaginase, procarbazine, and the glucocorticosteroids (Adams et al. 1984; Denicoff et al. 1987; Holland et al. 1974; Stiefel et al. 1990; Weddington 1982). Most patients receiving these agents, steroids excepted, do not develop prominent CNS effects. The spectrum of mental disturbances related to treatment with steroids includes minor mood lability, affective disorders (mania or depression), cognitive impairment (reversible dementia), and delirium (steroid psychosis). The incidence of these disorders ranges from 3% to 57% in populations of patients without cancer, and they occur most commonly with higher doses. Symptoms usually develop within the first 2 weeks of steroid therapy but can occur at any time, at any dose, even during the tapering phase. Prior psychiatric illness and prior disturbance during treatment with steroids are not good predictors of susceptibility to or the nature of men-

tal disturbance with steroid therapy. These disorders are often rapidly reversible with dose reduction or discontinuation of the medication (Stiefel et al. 1989). However, Bruera et al. (1992) reported that in less than 50% of cases is the etiology of terminal delirium determined. Yet, not knowing the cause of the delirium does not preclude treatment or reversal of the disorder. Bruera and colleagues (1992) also found that the condition of 68% of delirious cancer patients could be improved.

Management of Delirium in Terminally Ill Patients

A standard approach to managing delirium includes a search for underlying causes, correction of those factors, and management of the symptoms of delirium. The treatment of delirium in the dying patient is unique, however, because 1) most often, the etiology of terminal delirium is multifactorial or may not be determined; 2) when a distinct cause is found, that cause is often irreversible (e.g., hepatic failure or brain metastases); 3) the workup may be limited by the setting (home, hospice); and 4) the consultant's focus is usually on the patient's comfort, and ordinarily helpful diagnostic procedures that are unpleasant or painful (e.g., computed tomography scan, lumbar puncture) may be avoided. When delirium is present in a cancer patient who is terminally ill or dying, a differential diagnosis should always be formulated; however, studies should be performed only when a suspected factor can be identified easily and treated effectively.

In addition to seeking out and addressing the underlying cause of delirium, one must consider administering symptomatic and supportive therapies (Lipowski 1987). In fact, in the dying patient, these therapies may be the only steps taken. Maintenance of fluid and electrolyte balance, nutritional support, and administration of vitamins may be helpful. Factors that may help reduce anxiety and disorientation include a quiet, well-lit room with familiar objects, a visible clock or calendar, and the presence of family. Judicious use of physical restraints, along with one-to-one nursing observation, may also be necessary and useful. Often these supportive techniques alone are not effective, and symptomatic treatment with neuroleptic or sedative medications is necessary (Table 35–9).

Haloperidol, a neuroleptic agent that is a potent dopamine blocker, is the drug of choice in the treatment of delirium in the medically ill patient (Levine et al. 1978; Lipowski 1987; Murray 1987). Haloperidol in low doses (i.e., 1–3 mg) is usually effective against agitation, paranoia, and fear. Although up to about 85% of terminally ill patients have delirium, only 17% of dying patients receive an antipsychotic for their agitation or

TABLE 35–9.   Medications useful in managing delirium in patients with terminal illness

Drug	Approximate daily dose range (mg)	Route[a]
Traditional antipsychotics		
Haloperidol	0.5–2 (every 1–2 hours)	po, iv, sc, im
Chlorpromazine	2 (every 24 hours)	po, iv
Thioridazine	10–75 (every 2–12 hours)	po
Methotrimeprazine	12.5–50 (every 4–8 hours)	iv, sc
Molindone	10–50 (every 8–12 hours)	po
Droperidol	0.5–5 (every 12 hours)	im, iv
Novel antipsychotics		
Risperidone	1–6 (every 24 hours)	po
Olanzapine	2.5–5 (every 12 hours)	po
Sedatives		
Lorazepam	0.5–2 (every 1–4 hours)	po, iv, im
Midazolam	30–100 (every 2–4 hours)	iv, sc
Propofol	10–70 mg/hour infusion, titrated up to 200–400 mg/hour	iv

Note.   im = intramuscular; iv = intravenous; po = per os (orally); sc = subcutaneous.

[a]Parenteral doses are generally twice as potent as oral doses; intravenous infusions or bolus injections should be administered slowly; intramuscular injections should be avoided if repeated use becomes necessary; oral forms of medication are preferred; subcutaneous infusions are generally accepted modes of drug administration in patients who are terminally ill.

psychological distress (Goldberg and Mor 1985; Jaeger et al. 1985). Typically, 0.5–1.0 mg of haloperidol is administered orally or parenterally, with repeat doses (titrated as needed) given every 45–60 minutes (Breitbart 1988, 1989b; Massie et al. 1983). Intravenous administration is preferable because it facilitates rapid onset of the drug's effects. If an intravenous line is unavailable, we suggest starting with intramuscular or subcutaneous administration and switching to the oral route when possible. Oral dosing can be used in the majority of patients with delirium. Parenteral doses are approximately twice as potent as oral doses. Many palliative care practitioners deliver haloperidol by the subcutaneous route (Fainsinger and Bruera 1992; Twycross and Lack 1983). We have generally found that it is not necessary to exceed 20 mg of haloperidol in a 24-hour period; however, some clinicians advocate high dosages (up to 250 mg/24 hours, usually given intravenously) for selected patients (Adams et al. 1986; Fernandez et al. 1989; Murray 1987).

A common strategy in the management of symptoms related to delirium is to add parenteral lorazepam to a regimen of haloperidol (Adams et al. 1986; Fernandez et al. 1989; Murray 1987). Lorazepam, given orally or intravenously at a dose of 0.5–1.0 mg every 12 hours along with haloperidol, may be more effective than haloperidol alone in rapidly sedating the agitated patient with delirium. In a double-blind, randomized, comparison trial of haloperidol versus chlorpromazine versus lorazepam, Breitbart et al. (1996b) demonstrated that lorazepam alone, in doses up to 8 mg in a 12-hour period, was inef-

fective in the treatment of delirium and contributed to worsening delirium and cognitive impairment. However, both neuroleptic drugs, in low doses (approximately 2 mg of haloperidol equivalent per 24 hours), were highly effective in controlling the symptoms of delirium—resulting in a dramatic improvement in DRS scores—and in improving cognitive function, as demonstrated by dramatic improvement in scores on the MMSE. Low doses of thioridazine, 10–75 mg every 2–12 hours, are sometimes useful; however, caution is recommended because of thioridazine's high anticholinergic potency.

Methotrimeprazine, given intravenously or subcutaneously, is often used to control confusion and agitation in patients with terminal delirium (Oliver 1985). Doses range from 12.5 to 50 mg every 4–8 hours, up to 300 mg/day for most patients. Hypotension and excessive sedation are problematic limitations of this drug. Midazolam, given by subcutaneous or intravenous infusion in doses ranging from 30 to 100 mg/day, is also used to control agitation related to delirium in the terminal stages of disease (Bottomley and Hanks 1990). The goal of midazolam therapy, and to some extent methotrimeprazine therapy, is quiet sedation only. In contrast to neuroleptic drugs such as haloperidol, midazolam does not clear a sensorium or improve cognition in patients with delirium. These clinical differences may be due to the underlying pathophysiology of delirium. One hypothesis is that an imbalance of central cholinergic and adrenergic mechanisms underlies delirium, and so a dopamine-blocking drug may initiate a rebalancing of these systems (Itil and

Fink 1966). Although neuroleptic drugs such as haloperidol are most effective in diminishing agitation, clearing the sensorium, and improving cognition in the patient with delirium, achievement of these goals is not always possible in the last days of life. Processes causing delirium may be ongoing and irreversible during the active dying phase. Ventafridda et al. (1990) and Fainsinger et al. (1991) reported that a significant proportion (10%–20%) of terminally ill patients experience delirium that can be controlled only by sedation to the point of a significantly decreased level of consciousness.

The use of neuroleptics in the management of delirium in the dying patient remains controversial in some circles. Some have argued that pharmacological interventions with neuroleptics or benzodiazepines are inappropriate in the dying patient. Delirium is viewed as a natural part of the dying process that should not be altered. Another rationale that is often presented is that these patients are so close to death that aggressive treatment is unnecessary. Use of parenteral neuroleptics or sedatives may be mistakenly avoided because of fears that these drugs might hasten death through hypotension or respiratory depression. Many clinicians are unnecessarily pessimistic about the possible results of neuroleptic treatment for delirium. They argue that because the underlying pathophysiologic process (such as hepatic or renal failure) often continues unabated, no improvement can be expected in the patient's mental status. Physicians may be concerned that neuroleptics or sedatives may worsen delirium by making the patient more confused or sedated.

However, our clinical experience in managing delirium in patients with cancer who are dying suggests that the use of neuroleptics to treat agitation, paranoia, hallucinations, and altered sensorium is safe, effective, and quite appropriate. Management of delirium on a case-by-case basis seems most wise. The agitated patient with delirium who is dying should probably be given neuroleptics to help restore calm. A wait-and-see approach regarding use of neuroleptics may be most appropriate with patients who have lethargic or somnolent presentations of delirium. When deciding whether to use pharmacological interventions in a dying patient who presents with delirium, the consultant must educate staff, the patient, and the patient's family and weigh each of the issues discussed here. The clinician caring for patients with life-threatening illnesses is likely to encounter delirium as a common major psychiatric complication of advancing illness—particularly in the last weeks of life, when up to 85% of patients may develop delirium. Proper assessment, diagnosis, and management are needed to minimize morbidity and improve quality of life.

Cognitive Impairment Disorders in Patients With AIDS

The spectrum of psychiatric disorders seen in patients with AIDS is similar to that seen in patients with other terminal illnesses (with the exception of dementia associated with HIV disease) and includes delirium, dementia (AIDS dementia complex [ADC]), mood disorder, anxiety disorder, personality disorder, hallucinosis, and delusional disorders due to HIV disease (Perry 1990). HIV is neurotropic: it invades the CNS early in the course of infection and can result in ADC.

ADC is a very common neurological complication of AIDS (Brew et al. 1988). The syndrome of ADC is characterized by disturbances in motor performance, cognition, and behavior. It is estimated that two-thirds of AIDS patients will develop clinical dementia during the course of their illness. Patients with ADC clinically exhibit a triad of cognitive, motor, and behavioral disturbances. Cognitive and intellectual impairment is typically both subtle in onset and progressive. Progression can be rapid or gradual and is quite variable. Initially, the presentation is one of memory impairment, mental slowing, and impaired concentration. This can progress to global cognitive impairment with disorientation, confusion, psychosis, and mutism. Motor disturbances can begin with clumsiness, unsteady gait, tremor, and impaired handwriting and lead to ataxia, paraplegia, myoclonus, incontinence, and seizures. Early behavioral symptoms include apathy, withdrawal, depression, and anxiety. Late behavioral changes include paranoia, agitation, confusion, psychosis, hallucinations, and affective disturbances (i.e., mania or depression) (Breitbart et al. 1988).

The earliest symptoms of AIDS dementia are often mistaken for functional psychiatric disturbance such as reactive depression or anxiety. As dementia progresses, the nature of the psychiatric symptoms becomes more obvious. Many of the psychiatric symptoms that develop after a diagnosis of AIDS or AIDS-related complex are similar to those reported in patients with cancer (American Psychiatric Association 2000; Perry 1990). Patients often react with disbelief, denial, numbness, anxiety, depression, feelings of hopelessness, and, occasionally, suicidal ideation. Differentiating early ADC from a functional psychiatric disorder can be quite difficult. Early behavioral changes seen in ADC include irritability, anxiety, and depression. These symptoms are common in patients with major depression, anxiety disorders, and adjustment disorders and are easily misconstrued as an understandable reaction to the diagnosis of a life-threatening illness rather than seen as signs of early encephalopathy (American Psychiatric Association 2000; Perry 1990).

Formal neuropsychological testing can be helpful in diagnosing ADC and distinguishing it from depression or adjustment disorder. The pattern of neuropsychological abnormalities conforms to what has been termed *subcortical dementia*. Characteristic abnormalities include impaired fine and rapid motor movement, difficulty with complex sequencing, reduced verbal fluency, impaired short-term memory, diminished visual-motor and visual-spatial abilities, and impaired integrated sequential problem solving. Patients typically have the greatest difficulty, and deficits are most obvious, when tasks are timed, requiring rapid processing and reaction (Tross and Hirsch 1988). Notably, in many patients a discrepancy is found between their perceived frequent forgetfulness and their (relatively good) performance on formal memory testing. Although depression may mimic ADC clinically, the pattern of impaired performance on neuropsychological tests that is seen in patients with ADC is somewhat distinctive and is not reproduced in patients with depression.

The use of pharmacotherapy in patients with AIDS must be prudent and cautious because it is becoming increasingly clear that patients with neurological complications of AIDS are quite sensitive to the adverse side effects of psychoactive medications. For this reason, nonpharmacological treatments, such as relaxation techniques, hypnosis, and cognitive coping techniques, should be used whenever possible.

PAIN

From 60% to 90% of patients with advanced cancer experience pain (Foley 1985). Pain is also frequent in patients with advanced AIDS (Breitbart 1998). Pain usually symbolizes advancing disease and is therefore experienced with more dread and suffering. Depression and anxiety also increase the experience of pain. In the evaluation of pain, the first step is to assess the quality of pain, the time course, fluctuations, and factors that exacerbate or relieve the pain. A mental status examination and medical and neurological evaluations are performed. Pain is also assessed repeatedly because the analgesic dose is adjusted according to the level of pain and level of alertness (Elliott and Foley 1990).

Management of Pain in Terminally Ill Patients

Pharmacological therapy is central to the management of physiologically based pain. Nonnarcotic analgesics, opi-

oids, and adjuvant analgesic drugs have specific indications. Nonopioid analgesics (i.e., nonsteroidal antiinflammatory drugs) are prescribed for mild to moderate pain. Opioid analgesics are prescribed for moderate to severe pain. Opioids are a diverse group of compounds that bind to specific opioid receptors. They are subdivided into agonists, antagonists, and agonist-antagonists (drugs in this last group have both analgesic and antagonist properties). The narcotic agonists morphine, hydromorphone, and levorphanol are the preferred analgesics for moderate to severe pain (Table 35–10).

To treat pain adequately, clinicians should observe the following principles (Portenoy and Foley 1989):

1. Choose a specific drug for the specific level of pain—for example, codeine or oxycodone for moderate pain or morphine or a morphine-like agonist for moderate to severe pain.
2. Know the duration of effect and the pharmacokinetics of the drug chosen—for example, morphine and hydromorphone have short half-lives, and methadone and levorphanol have long half-lives.
3. Prescribe analgesics around the clock. As-needed dosing, which requires the patient's request, results in considerable time loss, anxiety, and increased pain.
4. Remember that combinations of drugs, such as opioids and nonnarcotic analgesics, have additive effects.
5. Treat patients who have analgesic-induced sedation with low doses of stimulants, and use high-potency neuroleptics for delirium.

Adjuvant analgesics are often used in managing pain. Tricyclic antidepressants are widely used for this purpose and are especially effective against neuropathic pain, which is common in patients with advanced AIDS. Amitriptyline is commonly used. Paroxetine is also effective (Sindrup et al. 1990). Psychostimulants, neuroleptics, and anxiolytics are used to enhance analgesic properties as well. Behavioral and cognitive-restructuring techniques are also applied in pain treatment. Using these techniques, the clinician attempts to change the meaning of pain; relaxation techniques reduce tension and anxiety and thereby reduce pain (Strain et al. 1981).

STAFF ISSUES IN THE CARE OF DYING PATIENTS

Working with a dying patient produces a range of painful emotions in caregivers: fear, guilt, anger, intolerance, vulnerability, overattachment, ambivalence, frustration, and

TABLE 35–10. Narcotic analgesics for moderate to severe pain in advanced illness

Analgesic	Route	Equianalgesic dose (mg)	Analgesic onset (hours)	Analgesic duration (hours)	Plasma half-life (hours)	Comments
Immediate-release morphine	po im, iv, sc	30–60 10	1–1½ ½–1	4–6 4–6	2–4 3–4	Standard of comparison for the narcotic analgesics. Now available in long-acting, oral, sustained-release preparations.
Sustained-release morphine	po	30–60	1–1½	8–12	12–16	Cannot be broken or chewed. Supplement with "rescue doses" of shorter-acting agent for breakthrough pain.
Hydromorphone	po im, iv	7.5 1.5	½–1 ¼–½	3–4 3–4	2–3 2–3	Short half-life may be preferable for elderly patients. Available in rectal suppository form and high-potency injectable forms.
Methadone	po im, iv	20 10	½–1 ½–1	4–8 —	15–30 15–30	Long half-life; tends to accumulate and cause sedation with initial dosing, requiring careful titration. Good oral potency.
Levorphanol	po im	4 2	1–1½ ½–1	4–6 4–5	12–16 12–16	Long half-life; requires careful dose titration in first week. Note that analgesic duration is considerably less than plasma half-life.
Meperidine	po im	300 75	1–1½ ½–1	4–6 4–5	3–4 3–4	Active toxic metabolite, normeperidine, tends to accumulate (plasma half-life is 12–16 hours), especially with renal impairment and in elderly patients, causing delirium, myoclonus, and seizures.
Fentanyl	Transdermal	0.1	12–18[a]	48–72	72	Transdermal patch useful for improved compliance and as alternative to oral or parenteral routes.

Note. im = intramuscular; iv = intravenous; po = per os (orally); sc = subcutaneous.

[a]12–18 hours to onset of analgesia with first application of transdermal patch. Once blood levels of fentanyl reach therapeutic levels, analgesic effect is continuous with continued use of transdermal patch.

Source. Adapted from Breitbart W, Holland JC (eds): *Psychiatric Aspects of Symptom Management in Cancer Patients.* Washington, DC, American Psychiatric Press, 1993. Used with permission.

feelings of helplessness, inadequacy, and lack of control (Barton 1977). These negative emotions are increased when a staff member experiences a personal loss, an illness, or a significant conflict or crisis. In one study, Kash and Holland (1990) found that the stress was buffered by three primary factors: a personal system of beliefs about life and death, a high level of peer support, and a supportive supervisor. Nurses and doctors who had the responsibility of taking care of patients dying from cancer and who considered themselves to be religious scored lower on the measures of burnout, suggesting that an existential perspective helped them to handle the stress of caring for many dying patients. The data also underscore the importance of social support derived from a cohesive staff with adequate supervision. A consultation-liaison psychiatrist is often able to identify problems that arise from poor cohesion and poor delineation of lines of authority.

The psychiatrist should monitor staff responses and be prepared to serve as a person with whom professional issues can be raised when the care of dying patients produces troublesome distress. Regular support meetings help promote discussion of problems and interdisciplinary conflicts; a special meeting for staff should be arranged when a particularly difficult management problem or the death of a special patient occurs. For all caregivers, providing support can be draining at times. In evaluating a caregiver, the staff member's loss history should be obtained because overinvolvement or inappropriate underinvolvement most often reflects an unrecognized countertransference (Sourkes 1982). Teaching of medical and psychiatric team members should include admonitions to monitor self and colleagues for stress. The value of sharing experiences with colleagues, including seeking psychiatric consultation, must be stressed.

SUMMARY

Palliative care for terminally ill patients must include not only control of pain and symptoms but also assessment of and intervention for psychiatric and psychosocial complications. Existential and spiritual issues must be taken into account as well. As part of a multidisciplinary team, the consultation-liaison psychiatrist can play an important role in the provision of comprehensive care.

REFERENCES

Achte KA, Vanhkouen ML: Cancer and the psyche. Omega 2:46–56, 1971

Acklin M, Brown E, Mauger P: The role of religious values in coping with cancer. Journal of Religion and Health 22:322–333, 1983

Adams F, Quesada JR, Gutterman JU: Neuropsychiatric manifestations of human leukocyte interferon therapy in patients with cancer. JAMA 252:938–941, 1984

Adams F, Fernandez F, Andersson BS: Emergency pharmacotherapy of delirium in the critically ill cancer patient. Psychosomatics 27:33–37, 1986

American Psychiatric Association: Diagnostic and Statistical Manual of Mental Disorders, 3rd Edition. Washington, DC, American Psychiatric Association, 1980

American Psychiatric Association: Diagnostic and Statistical Manual of Mental Disorders, 3rd Edition, Revised. Washington, DC, American Psychiatric Association, 1987

American Psychiatric Association: Diagnostic and Statistical Manual of Mental Disorders, 4th Edition. Washington, DC, American Psychiatric Association, 1994

American Psychiatric Association: Diagnostic and Statistical Manual of Mental Disorders, 4th Edition, Text Revision. Washington, DC, American Psychiatric Association, 2000

A piece of my mind. It's over, Debbie (case report). JAMA 259:272, 1988

Ayd F: Amoxapine: a new tricyclic antidepressant. International Drug Therapy Newsletter 14:33–40, 1979

Baile W, Beale E: Giving bad news to cancer patients: matching process and content. J Clin Oncol 19(9):2575–2577, 2001

Barton D: The dying person, in Dying and Death: A Clinical Guide for Caregivers. Edited by Barton D. Baltimore, MD, Williams & Wilkins, 1977, pp 41–58

Beck AT, Kovacs M, Weissman A: Hopelessness and suicidal behavior: an overview. JAMA 234:1146–1149, 1975

Berg GE: The use of the computer as a tool for assessment and research in pastoral care. J Health Care Chaplain 6:11–25, 1994

Bergman B, Sullivan M, Sorenson S: Quality of life during chemotherapy for small cell lung cancer, I: an evaluation with generic health measures. Acta Oncol 30:947–957, 1991

Billings JA, Block S: Palliative care in undergraduate medical education. JAMA 278:733–738, 1997

Blackhall LJ, Murphy ST, Frank G, et al: Ethnicity and attitudes toward patient autonomy. JAMA 274:820–825, 1995

Block SD: Assessing and managing depression in the terminally ill patient. Ann Intern Med 132(3):209–218, 2000

Bolund C: Suicide and cancer, II: medical and care factors in suicide by cancer patients in Sweden. Journal of Psychosocial Oncology 3:17–30, 1985

Bottomley DM, Hanks GW: Subcutaneous midazolam infusion in palliative care. J Pain Symptom Manage 5:259–261, 1990

Boyer WF, Feighner JP: Side effects of the selective serotonin reuptake inhibitors, in Selective Serotonin Reuptake Inhibitors. Edited by Feighner JP, Boyer WF. Chichester, UK, Wiley, 1991

Brady MJ, Peterman AH, Fitchett G, et al: A case for including spirituality in quality of life measurement in oncology. Psychooncology 8:417–428, 1999

Breitbart W: Suicide in cancer patients. Oncology (Huntingt) 1:49–55, 1987

Breitbart W: Psychiatric complications of cancer, in Current Therapy in Hematology, 3rd Edition. Edited by Brain MC, Carbone PP. Philadelphia, PA, Marcel Dekker, 1988, pp 268–274

Breitbart W: Endocrine-related psychiatric disorders, in Handbook of Psychooncology: Psychological Care of the Patient With Cancer. Edited by Holland JC, Rowland JH. New York, Oxford University Press, 1989a, pp 356–368

Breitbart W: Psychiatric management of cancer pain. Cancer 63:2336–2342, 1989b

Breitbart W: Cancer pain and suicide, in Advances in Pain Research and Therapy, Vol 16. Edited by Foley K, Bonica JJ, Ventafridda V, et al. New York, Raven, 1990, pp 399–412

Breitbart W: Pain in AIDS: an overview. Pain Review 5:279-304, 1998

Breitbart W, Holland JC (eds): Psychiatric Aspects of Symptom Management in Cancer Patients. Washington, DC, American Psychiatric Press, 1993

Breitbart W, Mermelstein H: Pemoline: an alternative psychostimulant for the management of depressive disorders in cancer patients. Psychosomatics 33:352–356, 1992

Breitbart W, Sparrow B: Management of delirium in the terminally ill. Progress in Palliative Care 6:107–113, 1998

Breitbart W, Marotta RF, Call P: AIDS and neuroleptic malignant syndrome. Lancet 2:1488–1489, 1988

Breitbart W, Levenson JA, Passik SD: Terminally ill patients, in Psychiatric Aspects of Symptom Management in Cancer Patients. Edited by Breitbart W, Holland JC. Washington, DC, American Psychiatric Press, 1993, pp 173–230

Breitbart W, Bruera E, Chochinov H, et al: Neuropsychiatric syndromes and psychological symptoms in patients with advanced cancer. J Pain Symptom Manage 10:131–141, 1995

Breitbart W, Rosenfeld BD, Passik SD: Interest in physician-assisted suicide among ambulatory HIV-infected patients. Am J Psychiatry 153:238–242, 1996a

Breitbart W, Marotta R, Platt MM, et al: A double-blind comparison trial of haloperidol, chlorpromazine, and lorazepam in the treatment of delirium in hospitalized AIDS patients. Am J Psychiatry 153:231–237, 1996b

Breitbart W, Chochinov H, Passik S: Psychiatric aspects of palliative care, in Oxford Textbook of Palliative Medicine, 2nd Edition. Edited by Doyle D, Hanks GWC, MacDonald N. New York, Oxford University Press, 1998, pp 933–954

Breitbart W, Rosenfeld B, Pessin H, et al: Depression, hopelessness, and desire for death in terminally ill patients with cancer. JAMA 284:2907–2911, 2000

Brew BJ, Sidtis JJ, Petito CK, et al: The neurologic complications of AIDS and human immunodeficiency virus infection. Archives of Contemporary Neurology 149:1–49, 1988

Brock DB, Foley DJ: Demography and epidemiology of dying in the U.S., with emphasis on deaths of older persons, in A Good Dying: Shaping Health Care for the Last Months of Life. Briefing book for a symposium sponsored by the George Washington University Center to Improve Care of the Dying and by the Corcoran Gallery of Art, Washington, DC, April 30, 1996

Brown GR, Rundell JR, McManis SE, et al: Prevalence of psychiatric disorders in early stages of HIV infection. Psychosom Med 54:588–601, 1992

Brown JH, Henteleff P, Barakat S, et al: Is it normal for terminally ill patients to desire death? Am J Psychiatry 143:208–211, 1986

Bruera E, Chadwick S, Brenneis C, et al: Methylphenidate associated with narcotics for the treatment of cancer pain. Cancer Treat Rep 71:67–70, 1987

Bruera E, Macmillan K, Hanson J, et al: The cognitive effects of the administration of narcotic analgesics in patients with cancer pain. Pain 39:13–16, 1989

Bruera E, Miller L, McCallion J, et al: Cognitive failure in patients with terminal cancer: a prospective study. J Pain Symptom Manage 7:192–195, 1992

Buckman R: How to Break Bad News—A Guide for Healthcare Professionals. London, Macmillan Medical, 1993

Bukberg J, Holland JC: A prevalence study of depression in a cancer hospital population (abstract). Proceedings of the American Association for Cancer Research 21:382, 1980

Bukberg J, Penman D, Holland J: Depression in hospitalized cancer patients. Psychosom Med 46:199–212, 1984

Butow P, Tattersall M, Goldstein D: Communication with cancer patients in culturally diverse societies. Ann N Y Acad Sci 809:317–329, 1997

Canadian Palliative Care Association: Palliative Care: Towards a Consensus in Standardized Principles of Practice. Ottawa, ON, Canadian Palliative Care Association, 1995

Carrese J, Rhodes L: Western bioethics on the Navajo reservation. JAMA 274:826–829, 1995

Carron A, Lynn J, Keaney P: End-of-life care in medical textbooks. Ann Intern Med 130:82–86, 1999

Cassell E: The Nature of Suffering and the Goals of Medicine. New York, Oxford University Press, 1991

Cassem NH: The dying patient, in Massachusetts General Hospital Handbook of General Hospital Psychiatry, 2nd Edition. Edited by Hackett TP, Cassem NH. Littleton, MA, PSG Publishing, 1987, pp 332–352

Chiarello RJ, Cole JO: The use of psychostimulants in general psychiatry: a reconsideration. Arch Gen Psychiatry 44:286–295, 1987

Chochinov HM, Holland JC: Bereavement: a special issue in oncology, in Handbook of Psychooncology: Psychological Care of the Patient With Cancer. Edited by Holland JC, Rowland JH. New York, Oxford University Press, 1989, pp 612–631

Chochinov HM, Wilson KG, Enns M, et al: Prevalence of depression in the terminally ill: effects of diagnostic criteria and symptom threshold judgments. Am J Psychiatry 151(4):537–540, 1994

Chochinov H, Wilson K, Enns M, et al: "Are You Depressed?" screening for depression in the terminally ill. Am J Psychiatry 154(5):674–676, 1997

Chochinov H, Wilson K, Enns M, et al: Depression, hopelessness, and suicidal ideation in the terminally ill. Psychosomatics 39(4):366–370, 1998

Ciraulo DA, Shader RI: Fluoxetine drug-drug interactions, I: antidepressants and antipsychotics. J Clin Psychopharmacol 10:48–50, 1990

Cohen-Cole SA, Brown FW, McDaniel S: Diagnostic assessment of depression in the medically ill, in Principles of Medical Psychiatry, 2nd Edition. Edited by Stoudemire A, Fogel B. New York, Oxford University Press, 1993, pp 53–70

A controlled trial to improve care for seriously ill hospitalized patients: the Study to Understand Prognoses and Preferences for Outcomes and Risks of Treatments (SUPPORT). JAMA 274:1591–1598, 1995

Cooper GL: The safety of fluoxetine: an update. Br J Psychiatry 153:77–86, 1988

Costa D, Mogos I, Toma T: Efficacy and safety of mianserin in the treatment of depression of women with cancer. Acta Psychiatr Scand Suppl 320:85–92, 1985

Csikszentmihalyi M: Flow: The Psychology of Optimal Experience. New York, Harper & Row, 1990

Dean C: Psychiatric morbidity following mastectomy: preoperative predictors and types of illness. J Psychosom Res 31:385–392, 1987

DeAngelis LM, Delattre J, Posner JB: Radiation-induced dementia in patients cured of brain metastases. Neurology 39:789–796, 1989

Denicoff KD, Rubinow DR, Papa MZ, et al: The neuropsychiatric effects of treatment with interleukin-2 and lymphokine-activated killer cells. Ann Intern Med 107:293–300, 1987

Derogatis LR, Morrow GR, Fetting J, et al: The prevalence of psychiatric disorders among cancer patients. JAMA 249:751–757, 1983

DeSousa E, Jepson A: Midazolam in terminal care. Lancet 1:67–68, 1988

de Wachter MAH: Active euthanasia in The Netherlands. JAMA 262:3316–3319, 1989

Dubovsky SL: Averting suicide in terminally ill patients. Psychosomatics 19:113–115, 1978

Elliott K, Foley KM: Pain syndromes. Journal of Psychosocial Oncology 8:11–45, 1990

Endicott J: Measurement of depression in patients with cancer. Cancer 53:2243–2245, 1983

Evans DL, McCartney CF, Nemeroff CB, et al: Depression in women treated for gynecological cancer: clinical and neuroendocrine assessment. Am J Psychiatry 143:447–452, 1986

Fainsinger R, Bruera E: Treatment of delirium in a terminally ill patient. J Pain Symptom Manage 7:54–56, 1992

Fainsinger R, MacEachern T, Hanson J, et al: Symptom control during the last week of life in a palliative care unit. J Palliat Care 7:5–11, 1991

Fallowfield L, Lipkin M, Hall A: Teaching senior oncologists communication skills: results from phase I of a comprehensive longitudinal program in the United Kingdom. J Clin Oncol 16:1961–1968, 1998

Farberow NL, Schneidman ES, Leonard CV: Suicide Among General Medical and Surgical Hospital Patients With Malignant Neoplasms (Medical Bulletin 9). Washington, DC, U.S. Veterans Administration, 1963

Farberow NL, Ganzler S, Cutter F, et al: An eight-year survey of hospital suicides. Suicide Life Threat Behav 1:984–201, 1971

Feighner JP: The role of venlafaxine in national antidepressant therapy. J Clin Psychiatry 55:62–68, 1994

Fernandez F, Adams F, Holmes VF, et al: Methylphenidate for depressive disorders in cancer patients. Psychosomatics 28:455–461, 1987

Fernandez F, Adams F, Levy J, et al: Cognitive impairment due to AIDS related complex and its response to psychostimulants. Psychosomatics 29:38–46, 1988

Fernandez F, Levy JK, Mansell PWA: Management of delirium in terminally ill AIDS patients. Int J Psychiatry Med 19:165–172, 1989

Ferrell BR, Ferrell BA, Rhiner M, et al: Family factors influencing cancer pain management. J Postgrad Med 67:564–569, 1991

Field M, Cassel C (eds): Approaching Death: Improving Care at the End of Life. Washington, DC, National Academy Press, 1997

Fife BL: The conceptualization of meaning in illness. Soc Sci Med 38:309–316, 1994

Fisch R: Methylphenidate for medical inpatients. Int J Psychiatry Med 15:75–79, 1985–1986

Fitchett G: Assessing Spiritual Needs: A Guide for Caregivers. Minneapolis, MN, Augsburg, 1993

Foley KM: The treatment of cancer pain. N Engl J Med 313:84–95, 1985

Folstein MF, Folstein SE, McHugh PR: "Mini-Mental State": a practical method for grading the cognitive state of patients for the clinician. J Psychiatr Res 12:189–198, 1975

Foreman J: 70% would pick hospice, poll finds. Boston Globe, October 4, 1996

Fox BH, Stanek EJ, Boyd SC, et al: Suicide rates among cancer patients in Connecticut. J Chronic Dis 35:89–100, 1982

Frankl V: Man's Search for Meaning. New York, Washington Square Press, 1963

Gaylin W, Kass LR, Pellegrino ED, et al: Doctors must not kill. JAMA 259:2139–2140, 1988

Glassman AH: The newer antidepressant drugs and their cardiovascular effects. Psychopharmacol Bull 20:272–279, 1984

Goldberg G, Mor V: A survey of psychotropic use in terminal cancer patients. Psychosomatics 26:745–751, 1985

Guze S, Robins E: Suicide and primary affective disorders. Br J Psychiatry 117:437–438, 1970

Hanson LC, Danis M, Garrett J: What is wrong with end-of-life care? Opinions of bereaved family members. J Am Geriatr Soc 45:1339–1344, 1997

Helig S: The San Francisco Medical Society euthanasia survey: results and analysis. San Francisco Medicine 61:24–34, 1988

Hileman JW, Lackey NR, Hassanein RS: Identifying the needs of home caregivers of patients with cancer. Oncol Nurs Forum 19:771–777, 1992

Hinton J: Psychiatric consultation in fatal illness. Proceedings of the Royal Society of Medicine 65:1035–1038, 1972

Hobbs FB, Damon BL: Sixty-Five Plus in the U.S. (Current Population Reports, series P234-190). Washington, DC, U.S. Census Bureau, 1996

Holland JC: Anxiety and cancer: the patient and the family. J Clin Psychiatry 50 (suppl):20–25, 1989

Holland JC: Principles of psychooncology, in Cancer Medicine, 3rd Edition. Edited by Holland JC, Frei E. Philadelphia, PA, Lea & Febiger, 1993, pp 1017–1033

Holland JC, Fasanello S, Ohnuma T: Psychiatric symptoms associated with L-asparaginase administration. J Psychiatr Res 10:105–113, 1974

Holland JC, Morrow G, Schmale A, et al: Reduction of anxiety and depression in cancer patients by alprazolam or by a behavioral technique (abstract). Proceedings of the American Society of Clinical Oncology 6:258, 1987

Holland JC, Passik S, Kash KM, et al: The role of religious and spiritual beliefs in coping with malignant melanoma. Psychooncology 8:14–26, 1999

Howard OM, Fairclough DL, Daniels ER, et al: Physician desire for euthanasia and assisted suicide: would physicians practice what they preach? J Clin Oncol 15:428–432, 1997

Itil T, Fink M: Anticholinergic drug-induced delirium: experimental modification, quantitative EEG and behavioral correlations. J Nerv Ment Dis 143:492–507, 1966

Jaeger H, Morrow G, Brescia F: A survey of psychotropic drug utilization by patients with advanced neoplastic disease. Gen Hosp Psychiatry 7:353–360, 1985

Jenkins RA, Pargament KI: Cognitive appraisals in cancer patients. Soc Sci Med 26:625–633, 1988

Kash KM, Holland JC: Reducing stress in medical oncology house officers: a preliminary report of a prospective intervention study, in Educating Competent and Humane Physicians. Edited by Hendrie HC, Lloyd C. Bloomington, IN, Indiana University Press, 1990, pp 183–195

Kathol RG, Mutgi A, Williams J, et al: Diagnosis of major depression in cancer patients according to four sets of criteria. Am J Psychiatry 147:1021–1024, 1990

Katon W, Raskind M: Treatment of depression in the medically ill elderly with methylphenidate. Am J Psychiatry 137:963–965, 1980

Kaufmann MW, Murray GB, Cassem NH: Use of psychostimulants in medically ill depressed patients. Psychosomatics 23:817–819, 1982

Kerrihard T, Breitbart W, Dent K, et al: Anxiety in patients with cancer and human immunodeficiency virus. Semin Clin Neuropsychiatry 4(2):114–132, 1999

Khan A, Fabre LF, Rudolph R: Venlafaxine in depressed outpatients. Psychopharmacol Bull 27:141–144, 1991

Kovacs M, Beck AT, Weissman A: Hopelessness: an indication of suicidal risk. Suicide 5:98–103, 1975

Kuhn CC: A spiritual inventory of the medically ill patient. Psychiatr Med 6:87–100, 1988

Lansky SB, List MA, Herrmann CA, et al: Absence of major depressive disorder in female cancer patients. J Clin Oncol 3:1553–1560, 1985

Levine PM, Silberfarb PM, Lipowski ZJ: Mental disorders in cancer patients: a study of 100 psychiatric referrals. Cancer 42:1385–1391, 1978

Lieber L, Plumb MM, Gerstenzang ML, et al: The communication of affection between cancer patients and their spouses. Psychosom Med 38:379–389, 1976

Lipowski ZJ: Delirium (acute confusional states). JAMA 285:89–92, 1987

Lloyd AH: Practical considerations in the use of maprotiline (Ludiomil) in general practice. J Int Med Res 5:122–138, 1977

Louhivuori KA, Hakama J: Risk of suicide among cancer patients. Am J Epidemiol 109:59–65, 1979

Marzuk PM, Tierney H, Tardiff K, et al: Increased risk of suicide in persons with AIDS. JAMA 259:1333–1337, 1988

Massie MJ: Anxiety, panic, phobias, in Handbook of Psychooncology: Psychological Care of the Patient With Cancer. Edited by Holland JC, Rowland JH. New York, Oxford University Press, 1989, pp 300–309

Massie MJ, Holland JC: Diagnosis and treatment of depression in the cancer patient. J Clin Psychiatry 42:25–28, 1984

Massie MJ, Holland JC: The cancer patient with pain: psychiatric complications and their management. Med Clin North Am 71:243–248, 1987

Massie MJ, Holland JC: Depression and the cancer patient. J Clin Psychiatry 51:12–17, 1990

Massie MJ, Gorzynski JG, Mastrovito R, et al: The diagnosis of depression in hospitalized patients with cancer (abstract). Proceedings of the American Society of Clinical Oncology 20:432, 1979

Massie MJ, Holland JC, Glass E: Delirium in terminally ill cancer patients. Am J Psychiatry 140:1048–1050, 1983

Massie MJ, Holland JC, Straker N: Psychotherapeutic interventions, in Handbook of Psychooncology: Psychological Care of the Patient With Cancer. Edited by Holland JC, Rowland JH. New York, Oxford University Press, 1989, pp 455–469

Mastrovito R: Behavioral techniques: progressive relaxation and self regulatory therapies, in Handbook of Psychooncology: Psychological Care of the Patient With Cancer. Edited by Holland JC, Rowland JH. New York, Oxford University Press, 1989, pp 492–501

McDaniel JS, Nemeroff CV: Depression in the cancer patient: diagnostic, biological and treatment aspects, in Current and Emerging Issues in Cancer Pain: Research and Practice. Edited by Chapman CR, Foley KM. New York, Raven, 1993, pp 1–19

McKegney PP, Lange P: The decision to no longer live on chronic hemodialysis. Am J Psychiatry 128:47–55, 1971

Meier DE, Morrison RS, Cassel CK: Improving palliative care. Ann Intern Med 127:225–230, 1997

Meier DE, Emmons CA, Wallenstein S, et al: A national survey of physician-assisted suicide and euthanasia in the United States. N Engl J Med 338:1193–1201, 1998

Mermelstein HT, Lesko L: Depression in patients with cancer. Psychooncology 1:199–215, 1992

Menza M, Kaufman K, Castellanos A: Modafinil augmentation of antidepressant treatment in depression. J Clin Psychiatry 61(5):378-381, 2000

Minagawa H, Uchitomi Y, Yamawaki S, et al: Psychiatric morbidity in terminally ill cancer patients. Cancer 78:1131–1137, 1996

Misbin RI, O'Hare D, Lederberg MS, et al: Compliance with New York State's do-not-resuscitate law at Memorial Sloan-Kettering Cancer Center: a review of patient deaths. N Y State J Med 93:165–168, 1993

Moorey S, Greer S, Watson M, et al: The factor structure and factor stability of the hospital anxiety and depression scale in patients with cancer. Br J Psychiatry 158:255–259, 1991

Morton RP, Davies ADM, Baker J, et al: Quality of life in treated head and neck cancer patients: a preliminary report. Clin Otolaryngol 9:181–185, 1984

Murphy GE: Suicide and attempted suicide. Hospital Practice 12:78–81, 1977

Murray GB: Confusion, delirium, and dementia, in Massachusetts General Hospital Handbook of General Hospital Psychiatry, 2nd Edition. Edited by Hackett TP, Cassem NH. Littleton, MA, PSG Publishing, 1987, pp 84–115

Musick M, Koenig H, Larson D: Religion and spiritual beliefs, in Psycho-Oncology. Edited by Holland JC. New York, Oxford University Press, 1998, pp 780–789

National Center for Health Statistics: Vital Statistics of the United States, 1980, Vol II: Mortality, Part A (DHHS Publ No [PHS] 85-1101). Washington, DC, U.S. Government Printing Office, 1985

National Center for Health Statistics: Vital Statistics of the United States, 1990, Vol II: Mortality, Part B (DHHS Publ No [PHS] 94-1102). Washington, DC, U.S. Government Printing Office, 1994

National Hospice Organization: New findings address escalating end-of-life debate (press release). Arlington, VA, National Hospice Organization, October 3, 1996

Oliver DJ: The use of methotrimeprazine in terminal care. Br J Clin Pract 39:339–340, 1985

Palliative Care Foundation: Palliative Care Services in Hospitals, Guidelines. Report of the Working Group on Special Services in Hospitals, Ottowa, Ontario. Toronto, Canada, National Health and Welfare, Palliative Care Foundation, 1981

Parker B, Baile W, deMoor C, et al: Breaking bad news about cancer: patients' preferences for communication. J Clin Oncol 19(7):2049–2056, 2001

Passik SD, Dugan W, McDonald MV, et al: Oncologists' recognition of depression in their patients with cancer. J Clin Oncol 16:1594–1600, 1998

Patchell RA, Posner JB: Cancer and the nervous system, in Handbook of Psychooncology: Psychological Care of the Patient With Cancer. Edited by Holland JC, Rowland JH. New York, Oxford University Press, 1989, pp 327–341

Pearson HJ: Interaction of fluoxetine: an update. Br J Psychiatry 153:77–86, 1990

Peck AW, Stern WC, Watkinson C: Incidence of seizures during treatment with tricyclic antidepressant drugs and bupropion. J Clin Psychiatry 44:197–201, 1983

Pellegrino ED: Ethics. JAMA 265:3118–3199, 1991

Perry SW: Organic mental disorders caused by HIV: update on early diagnosis and treatment. Am J Psychiatry 147:696–710, 1990

Plumb MM, Holland JC: Comparative studies of psychological function in patients with advanced cancer, II: interviewer-rated current and past psychological symptoms. Psychosom Med 39:264–276, 1977

Popkin MK, Callies AL, MacKenzie TB: The outcome of antidepressant use in the medically ill. Arch Gen Psychiatry 42:1160–1163, 1985

Portenoy R[K], Foley KM: Management of cancer pain, in Handbook of Psychooncology: Psychological Care of the Patient With Cancer. Edited by Holland JC, Rowland JH. New York, Oxford University Press, 1989, pp 369–382

Portenoy RK, Thaler HT, Kornblith AB, et al: The Memorial Symptom Assessment Scale: an instrument for the evaluation of symptom prevalence, characteristics, and distress. Eur J Cancer 30A:1326–1336, 1994

Posner JB: Nonmetastatic effects of cancer on the nervous system, in Cecil's Textbook of Medicine, 8th Edition. Edited by Wyngaarden JB, Smith LH. Philadelphia, PA, WB Saunders, 1988, pp 1104–1107

Preskorn SH, Jerkovich GS: Central nervous system toxicity of tricyclic antidepressants: phenomenology, course, risk factors, and role of therapeutic drug monitoring. J Clin Psychopharmacol 10:88–95, 1990

Purohit DR, Nevlakha PL, Modi RS, et al: The role of antidepressants in hospitalized cancer patients. J Assoc Physicians India 26:245–248, 1978

Quill TE: Death and dignity: a case of individualized decision making. N Engl J Med 324:691–694, 1991

Rifkin A, Reardon G, Siris S, et al: Trimipramine in physical illness with depression. J Clin Psychiatry 46:4–8, 1985

Robins E, Murphy G, Wilkinson RH Jr, et al: Some clinical considerations in the prevention of suicide based on 134 successful suicides. Am J Public Health 49:888–889, 1950

Rosenberg HM, Ventura SJ, Maurer JD, et al: Births and Deaths, United States, 1995. Hyattsville, MD, National Center for Health Statistics, 1996 (Monthly Vital Statistics Report 45 [suppl 2]:31, 1996)

Rosenfeld B, Breitbart W, McDonald MV, et al: Pain in ambulatory AIDS patients, II: impact of pain on psychological functioning and quality of life. Pain 68:323–328, 1996

Rosenfeld B, Galieta M, Breitbart W, et al: Interest in physician-assisted suicide among terminally ill AIDS patients: measuring and understanding desire for death. Paper presented at the biennial conference of the American Psychology-Law Society, Redondo Beach, CA, March 1998

Rosenfeld B, Breitbart W, Stein K, et al: Measuring desire for death among patients with HIV/AIDS: the schedule of attitudes toward hastened death. Am J Psychiatry 156:94–100, 1999

Sankar A: Dying at Home: A Family Guide for Caregivers. Baltimore, MD, Johns Hopkins University Press, 1991

Satel SL, Nelson CJ: Stimulants in the treatment of depression: a critical overview. J Clin Psychiatry 50:241–249, 1989

Schachter S: Quality of life for families in the management of home care patients with advanced cancer. J Palliat Care 8:61–66, 1992

Seidlitz L, Duberstein PR, Cox C, et al: Attitudes of older people toward suicide and assisted suicide: an analysis of Gallup poll findings. J Am Geriatr Soc 43:993–998, 1995

Sensky T, Dennehy M, Gilbert A, et al: Physicians' perceptions of anxiety and depression among their outpatients: relationships with patients and doctors' satisfaction with their interviews. J R Coll Physicians Lond 23:33–38, 1989

Sher M, Krieger JN, Juergen S: Trazodone and priapism. Am J Psychiatry 140:1362–1364, 1983

Shopsin B: Bupropion: a new clinical profile in the psychobiology of depression. J Clin Psychiatry 44:140–142, 1983

Shuster JL, Breitbart W, Chochinov HM: Psychiatric aspects of excellent end-of-life care: position statement of the Academy of Psychosomatic Medicine. Psychosomatics 40:1–3, 1999

Siegel K: Rational suicide: considerations for the clinician. Psychiatr Q 54:77–83, 1982

Siegel K, Tuckel P: Rational suicide and the terminally ill cancer patient. Omega 15:263–269, 1984

Siegel K, Raveis VH, Houts P, et al: Caregiver burden and unmet patient needs. Cancer 68:1131–1140, 1991

Silberfarb PM, Maurer LH, Crouthamel CS: Psychosocial aspects of neoplastic disease, I: functional status of breast cancer patients during different treatment regimens. Am J Psychiatry 137:450–455, 1980

Simpson M, Buckman R, Stewart M, et al: Doctor-patient communication: the Toronto consensus statement. BMJ 303: 1385–1387, 1991

Sindrup SH, Gram LF, Brosen K, et al: The selective serotonin reuptake inhibitor paroxetine is effective in the treatment of diabetic neuropathy symptoms. Pain 42:135–144, 1990

Singer PA: Euthanasia: a critique. N Engl J Med 322:1881–1883, 1990

Sipahimalani A, Massand P: Olanzapine in the treatment of delirium. Psychosomatics 39:422–430, 1998

Sison A, Keller K, Segal J, et al: Suicidal ideation in ambulatory HIV infected patients: the roles of pain, mood, and disease status (abstract). Paper presented at Current Concepts in Psychooncology IV, New York, October 10–12, 1991

Slome LR, Mitchell TF, Charlebois E, et al: Physician-assisted suicide and patients with human immunodeficiency virus disease. N Engl J Med 336:417–421, 1997

Smith TJ: Tell it like it is. J Clin Oncol 18:3441–3445, 2000

Sourkes BM: The Deepening Shade: Psychological Aspects of Life Threatening Illness. Pittsburgh, PA, University of Pittsburgh Press, 1982

Spiegel D, Bloom JR: Group therapy and hypnosis reduce metastatic breast carcinoma pain. Psychosom Med 4:333–339, 1983

Spiegel D, Bloom JR, Yalom ID: Group support for patients with metastatic cancer: a randomized prospective outcome study. Arch Gen Psychiatry 38:527–533, 1981

Spiritual Beliefs and the Dying Process: A Report on a National Survey Conducted for the Nathan Cummings Foundation and Fetzer Institute. Princeton, NJ, Gallup Institute, 1997

Spitzer RL, Endicott J, Robins E: Research diagnostic criteria: rationale and reliability. Arch Gen Psychiatry 35:773–782, 1978

Stein RS, Flexner JH, Graber SE: Lithium and granulocytopenia during induction therapy of acute myelogenous leukemia: update of an ongoing trial. Adv Exp Med Biol 127: 187–197, 1980

Stiefel FC, Breitbart W, Holland JC: Corticosteroids in cancer: neuropsychiatric complications. Cancer Invest 7:479–491, 1989

Stiefel FC, Kornblith AB, Holland JC: Changes in the prescription patterns of psychotropic drugs for cancer patients during a 10 year period. Cancer 65:1048–1053, 1990

Sting: Let Your Soul Be Your Pilot, in Mercury Falling, CD/album, A&M Records, London, England, 1996

Stjernsward J, Papallona S: Palliative medicine—a global perspective, in Oxford Textbook of Palliative Medicine, 2nd Edition. Edited by Doyle D, Hanks GWC, MacDonald N. New York, Oxford University Press, 1998, pp 1227–1245

Stoddard G, Burns-Haney J: Developing an integrated approach to spiritual assessment: one department's experience. Caregiver Journal 7:63–86, 1990

Stoudemire A, Fogel BS: Psychopharmacology in the medically ill, in Principles of Medical Psychiatry. Edited by Stoudemire A, Fogel BS. Orlando, FL, Grune & Stratton, 1987, pp 79–112

Strain JJ, Liebowitz MR, Klein DF: Anxiety and panic attacks in the medically ill. Psychiatr Clin North Am 4:333–350, 1981

Suarez-Almazor ME, Belzile M, Bruera E: Euthanasia and physician-assisted suicide: a comparative survey of physicians, terminally ill cancer patients, and the general population. J Clin Oncol 15:418–427, 1997

Subcommittee on Psychiatric Aspects of Life-Sustaining Technology: The role of the psychiatrist in end-of-life treatment decisions, in Caring for the Dying: Identification and Promotion of Physician Competency. (Educational Resource Document.) Philadelphia, PA, American Board of Internal Medicine, 1996, pp 61–67

Suchman AL, Markakis K, Beckman HB, et al: A model of empathic communication in the medical interview. JAMA 277:678–681, 1997

Taylor S: Adjustment to threatening events: a cognitive theory of adaptation. Am Psychol 38:1161–1173, 1983

Tross S, Hirsch DA: Psychological distress and neuropsychological complications of HIV infection and AIDS. Am Psychol 43:929–934, 1988

Trzepacz PT, Baker RW, Greenhouse J: A symptom rating scale of delirium. Psychiatry Res 23:89–97, 1988

Twycross RG, Lack SA: Symptom Control in Far Advanced Cancer: Pain Relief. London, Pitman, 1983

Twycross RG, Lack SA: Therapeutics in Terminal Disease. London, Pitman, 1984, pp 99–103

U.S. Public Health Service: Health, United States, 1995 (DHHS Publ No [PHS] 96-1232). Hyattsville, MD, U.S. Public Health Service, 1996

van der Maas PJ, van Delden JJM, Pijnenborg L, et al: Euthanasia and other medical decisions concerning the end of life. Lancet 338:669–674, 1991

Ventafridda V, Ripamonti C, De Conno F, et al: Symptom prevalence and control during cancer patients' last days of life. J Palliat Care 6:7–11, 1990

Wanzer SH, Federman DD, Edelstein ST, et al: The physician's responsibility toward hopelessly ill patients: a second look. N Engl J Med 320:844–849, 1989

Weddington WW: Delirium and depression associated with amphotericin B. Psychosomatics 23:1076–1078, 1982

Weddington WW, Segraves KB, Simon MA: Current and lifetime incidence of psychiatric disorders among a group of extremity sarcoma survivors. J Psychosom Res 30:121–125, 1986

Weeks JC, Cook EF, O'Day SJ, et al: Relationship between cancer patients' predictions of prognosis and their treatment preferences. JAMA 279:1709–1714, 1996

Weil M, Khayat D, Smith M: Truth-telling to cancer patients in the western European context. Journal of Psychooncology 3:21–27, 1993

Weisman AD: On Dying and Denying: A Psychiatric Study of Terminality. New York, Behavioral Publications, 1972

Woods SW, Tesar GE, Murray GB, et al: Psychostimulant treatment of depressive disorders secondary to medical illness. J Clin Psychiatry 47:12–15, 1986

World Health Organization: Cancer Pain Relief and Palliative Care: Report of a WHO Expert Committee (Technical Bulletin 804). Geneva, World Health Organization, 1990

World Health Organization: Cancer Pain Relief and Palliative Care: Report of a WHO Expert Committee (Technical Bulletin 804). Geneva, World Health Organization, 1997

Yalom I: Existential Psychotherapy. New York, Basic Books, 1980

Yates J, Chalmer B, St. James P, et al: Religion in patients with advanced cancer. Med Pediatr Oncol 9:121–128, 1981

Young DF: Neurological complications of cancer chemotherapy, in Neurological Complications of Therapy: Selected Topics. Edited by Silverstein A. New York, Futura, 1982, pp 57–113

Appendix

Psychiatric Aspects of Excellent End-of-Life Care

The Academy of Psychosomatic Medicine (A.P.M.) is the organization of Consultation-Liaison (C-L) Psychiatry. Its international membership includes many of the leading clinicians and researchers in the field of C-L Psychiatry, a discipline which focuses on the psychiatric care of the medically ill. This clinical focus includes the psychiatric problems of catastrophically ill and dying patients. Prepared by the A.P.M.'s Ad Hoc Committee on End-of-Life Care, this Position Statement has been approved by the A.P.M. Executive Council in the method described in the constitution and bylaws of the A.P.M. This document is the A.P.M.'s Position Statement regarding psychiatric aspects of care provided to patients nearing the end of life.

1. Psychiatric morbidity at the end of life is significant and causes substantial, potentially remediable suffering to dying patients and their families. Further, we believe that quality care for the psychiatric complications of terminal illness is and should be an integral component of excellent, comprehensive end-of-life care.
2. The most basic challenge at the end of life which stresses patients and families is loss, which is related to both the disabilities of the illness with their threats to self-esteem, and the patient's death, which ruptures the direct relationship with the family. Psychiatric problems and issues commonly seen at the end of life include anxiety symptoms and anxiety disorders, depressive symptoms and depressive disorders, delirium and other cognitive disorders, suicidal ideation, consequences of low perceived family and other social support, personality disorders or personality traits that cause problems in the setting of extreme stress, questions of capacity to make informed decisions, grief and bereavement, and general and health-related quality of life. Spiritual and religious issues, including both personal faith and relationship to a community of believers, are important for most people. Good end-of-life care requires explicit attention to these matters.
3. Studies show that psychiatric morbidity in the setting of terminal illness is exceptionally high. The prevalence of delirium in terminal cancer and AIDS patients ranges from 30–85%, and the prevalence of clinically significant depression ranges from 20–50%. The prevalence of depression among terminally ill patients with a desire for death is eight times higher than in those without a significant desire for death. Depression is the strongest determinant of suicidal ideation and desire for death in those with serious or terminal illness.
4. Psychiatric complications at the end of life are treatable, but often go unrecognized and untreated. Several factors or barriers contribute to the underrecognition and undertreatment of psychiatric problems at the end of life. These include:

   - Difficulty in diagnosing psychiatric disorders (e.g. anxiety, delirium, depression) in the setting of sig-

Reprinted from Shuster et al. 1999, with permission by the Academy of Psychosomatic Medicine.

nificant physical illness, owing to the overlap in the symptoms caused by the psychiatric disorder and the comorbid physical problems.

- Beliefs held by many patients, family members, physicians, and hospice and palliative care providers whereby psychiatric symptoms, especially depression, are viewed as normal parts of the dying process.

- The fact that many patients and physicians do not understand that patients who suffer from mental disorders at the end of life can respond to treatment. This therapeutic nihilism prevents the search for treatable mental disorders at the end of life.

- The presence of structural barriers to coordinated care of dying patients. Psychiatrists may not be readily available to care for terminally ill patients and consult with physicians providing end-of-life care for a variety of reasons. Among these are limited geographic access (most C-L psychiatrists are affiliated with academic medical centers in urban areas), psychiatrists who feel inadequately prepared to assess and treat dying patients, healthcare insurance carve-outs (which may limit or exclude access to and coverage for psychiatric care), and logistical obstacles to formal addition of a psychiatrist to a hospice care team.

- The stigma experienced by patients and families due to psychiatric evaluations or the assignment of a psychiatric diagnosis. Physicians and other caregivers may share this feeling.

- The occurrence of countertransference of hopelessness on the part of families and healthcare providers that may discourage seeking assessment of suffering from psychiatric causes in dying patients and weaken the commitment to helping maintain morale at the end of life.

- The fact that treatment based on formal diagnosis (as opposed to symptomatic treatment) is not sufficiently emphasized in palliative care.

1. We believe that the current enthusiasm for legalized assisted suicide and euthanasia at least partly reflects public concern that suffering (including suffering due to psychiatric causes) and distress at the end of life may elude or exceed our best current treatment efforts, making death seem preferable. Appropriately, aggressive treatment for psychiatric complications of terminal illness is the best way to address this fear and should reduce requests for assisted suicide and euthanasia.

2. We maintain that laws and regulations must allow physicians to provide appropriately aggressive care for psychiatric complications of terminal illness and must provide protection for qualified physicians who provide this care. For example, excellent treatment of depression at the end of life often requires the use of psychostimulants, most of which are Schedule II controlled substances. Appropriate use of these agents to control depression at the end of life should be viewed as analogous to the use of opiate analgesics to treat pain in this setting. Similarly, appropriate treatment of agitated and delirious patients who are dying may require sufficient sedation to relieve the suffering of the patient and family. When clinically indicted and acceptable to the patient or surrogate, such sedation is the standard of care and should be employed even if it hastens death. Such treatment is ethically sound and is not an act of assisted suicide or euthanasia.

3. In response to the above, the A.P.M. believes that remedial efforts must be encouraged. These include:

- Education about the prevalence and morbidity of psychiatric complications of terminal illness. Target audiences should include the general public, students and trainees in all healthcare professions, and healthcare providers in hospice and palliative care, primary care, and medical specialties (including psychiatry).

- Education and other efforts to reduce or remove barriers to excellent psychiatric end-of-life care, as outlined in Section 4 above.

- Education and advocacy efforts to insure that legal or regulatory barriers do not hinder or prevent excellent psychiatric care at the end of life.

- Clinical (and, where appropriate, basic science) research into psychiatric complications of terminal illness, their effects on suffering and quality of life in dying patients and their families; interactions with other comorbid conditions such as pain, fatigue, shortness of breath, anorexia and nausea; and reliably effective treatment strategies used at the end of life. Collaboration with governmental funding agencies and private foundations should be encouraged to develop research in these areas. Particular attention should be paid to training young investigators in research related to the psychiatric complications of terminal illness.

36

HIV Disease/AIDS

Mark H. Halman, M.D., F.R.C.P.C.

Philip Bialer, M.D.

Jonathan L. Worth, M.D.

Sean B. Rourke, Ph.D., C.Psych.

Psychiatrists have been involved in the comprehensive care of persons with human immunodeficiency virus (HIV) infection since the beginning of the epidemic. The pace of change in the understanding and treatment of HIV disease has been rapid, and the demands on psychiatrists working in this field have changed as the epidemic has progressed. Recent advances in care have resulted in dramatic successes in managing the immunological deterioration associated with HIV infection. New treatments have also highlighted the issues of access to care, both locally and globally. Epidemiologically, new risk factor groups have emerged in the second decade, including young gay men, persons who use injection drugs, low-income urban residents, homeless individuals, immigrants, and persons with severe and persistent mental illness.

Antiretroviral regimens and technologies to monitor progression of infection and disease have been introduced so rapidly that much may change between the time of the writing of this chapter and its publication. There have certainly been dramatic changes since the writing of this chapter for the first edition of this book. Acquired immune deficiency syndrome (AIDS)–defining clinical conditions happen much less frequently, and attention has shifted from treatment of opportunistic conditions that constitute AIDS to management of HIV infection and disease. Despite the advances, HIV disease remains a progressive illness, resulting from infection with HIV. It is marked by progressive immunological and often neurological and neurocognitive deterioration. Management is an attempt to preserve the host immune system by shutting down viral replication while minimiz-

ing toxicities associated with treatments. When the treatments can no longer contain the virus, because of viral resistance or intolerable side effects, immunological deterioration leads to opportunistic infections and tumors that eventually lead to death. There is no curative treatment, and a prophylactic vaccine has not been identified to date. Effective primary prevention programs, which stress risk-reduction behaviors, remain the cornerstone to limiting the spread of this disease.

Mental health issues have been central to overall management. Psychological distress resulting from news of a recent seroconversion, a decrease in $CD4^+$ count, or an increase in viral load needs to be processed and integrated into one's life. Facing early death and loss was the focus of many in affected communities in the first decade of the epidemic. More recently, facing living, after psychologically preparing to die, has been a theme for many. The psychiatric treatment and management of HIV disease must take into consideration a wide range of ongoing etiological factors, including premorbid primary psychiatric disorders, disorders secondary to HIV central nervous system (CNS) infection, and neuropsychiatric side effects of medications used to manage HIV disease. Advanced systemic disease and drug interactions can constrain the pharmacotherapeutic options available to the consultation-liaison psychiatrist. Psychiatrists treating persons with HIV disease must determine when a theoretical interaction is clinically meaningful, in order to bring the full range of psychopharmacological options to a patient. Clinicians must also understand and appreciate the more complex and salient features of how people cope with illness and infection. Psychotherapy and counseling have been essential features of care. Clinicians must consider the perspectives of patients who come from communities that have often been stigmatized, socially disenfranchised, and impoverished. Cooperation and liaison with community-based HIV/AIDS service organizations, interactions with care advocates and activists, and meeting the needs of highly diverse social and family support groups have all brought important aspects of community and social psychiatry into the realm of the consultation-liaison psychiatrist.

For optimum psychiatric treatment of adult patients with HIV disease, consultation-liaison psychiatrists must understand 1) the epidemiology and transmission of HIV infection, 2) the natural course of systemic HIV disease and the general principles of its treatment, 3) HIV CNS infection and related neurological and neurocognitive complications, 4) the diagnosis and management of psychiatric syndromes associated with HIV disease, 5) aspects of pharmacotherapy that are unique to patients with HIV disease, and 6) psychosocial factors that affect the illness course and the implications of such factors for psychotherapeutic intervention. In addition, with the increased numbers of persons with HIV disease and severe and persistent mental illness, HIV and consultation-liaison psychiatrists must apply skills of the general psychiatrist in providing care for patients with these interfacing conditions.

EPIDEMIOLOGY OF HIV/AIDS

Since the publication of the first edition of this book, the epidemiology of HIV/AIDS in the United States has changed dramatically. The cumulative number of reported cases of AIDS since 1981 is now greater than 650,000, and more than 400,000 of these people have died (Centers for Disease Control and Prevention 1998a). However, in 1996, the estimated incidence of AIDS decreased (by 6%) for the first time since the beginning of the epidemic. The number of deaths from AIDS decreased by 25% in 1996 (Centers for Disease Control and Prevention 1997) and 42% in 1997 (Centers for Disease Control and Prevention 1998a). Among persons ages 25–44 years, HIV disease changed from being the leading cause of death in 1995 to being the third leading cause in 1996 and the fifth leading cause in 1997 (Ventura et al. 1998). These changes are most likely due to the effectiveness of highly active antiretroviral therapy (HAART). Although these statistics sound encouraging, at least 40,000 new HIV infections occur every year. The decreasing death rate combined with continued infections has resulted in an increasing prevalence of living

with HIV/AIDS. In 1997, there were an estimated 271,000 people living with AIDS (Centers for Disease Control and Prevention 1998a) and between 650,000 and 900,000 infected with HIV in the United States.

The demographics of HIV/AIDS in the United States have also shifted in recent years. The majority (54%) of cumulative AIDS cases have been reported among African Americans and Hispanics, and these ethnic groups accounted for 67% of AIDS cases reported between July 1, 1997, and June 30, 1998 (Centers for Disease Control and Prevention 1998a). Women accounted for 22% of AIDS cases reported during this period and now make up 16% of the cumulative total. In addition, cases of heterosexual exposure to HIV have been reported as the most rapidly increasing subset of AIDS cases (Wortley and Fleming 1997) and account for more than half the cases among women younger than 25 years. Alarmingly, 15% of new HIV infections in 1997 occurred in individuals ages 13–24 years (Centers for Disease Control and Prevention 1997).

Men who have sex with men remain the single largest exposure category among reported cases of AIDS and HIV infection. This group accounted for 45% of reported cases of AIDS and 39% of reported cases of HIV infection among men in 1997–1998. After several years of decreasing rates of HIV/AIDS among men who have sex with men, HIV infection appears to be on the rise in this group. A study in San Francisco found that between 1994 and 1997, the proportion of these men reporting anal sex increased from 57.6% to 61.2%, and consistent condom use decreased from 69.6% to 60.8%. In addition, the proportion of men reporting multiple sex partners and unprotected anal intercourse increased, with the largest increase among those < 25 years old (22%–32%) (Centers for Disease Control and Prevention 1999). Recent reports confirm increasing rates of high-risk sexual behaviors and increasing rates of new HIV infections among gay and bisexual men in several cities, including Toronto (Calzavara et al. 2000), Vancouver (Martindale et al. 2001), San Francisco (Ekstrand et al. 2001), London (Elford et al. 2001), and Paris (Adam et al. 2001) in the year 2000. These reports highlight the need for renewed and sustained HIV prevention strategies targeted to gay and bisexual men.

The proportion of persons with AIDS whose exposure risk is parenteral transmission through injection drug use increased from 17.4% in 1985 to 26% in 1998. HIV infection rates among users of injection drugs who enter drug treatment programs are highly variable, with wide regional differences; rates range from 3% in the West to 29% in the Northeast (Prevots et al. 1995).

Infants and children represent 1.2% of all reported AIDS cases, with an accumulated 8,289 cases reported by mid-1998. Untreated, perinatal transmission of HIV infection occurs at a rate of about 33% (Blanche 1989). Breast milk and intrauterine exposure are both established modes of transmission of HIV infection from mother to newborn. Antiretroviral treatments, including short courses of zidovudine (AZT; Connor et al. 1994), nevirapine (Guay et al. 1999), and established HAART regimens, along with strategies to decrease exposure through the breast-feeding period, have been able to dramatically reduce mother-to-infant transmission rates (Fowler et al. 2000). Implementation of these strategies on a global basis is an essential component of reducing the spread of HIV infection.

Before HIV serological screening of blood products became available in 1985, transfusion recipients, including patients with hemophilia, were at risk for parenteral infection from infected blood products. Transfusion recipients and persons with hemophilia each represent 1% of all AIDS cases (Centers for Disease Control and Prevention 1997), and it is estimated that 64%–90% of patients with hemophilia are HIV infected.

Patients with major mental illness in urban areas with high AIDS prevalence appear to be at increased risk for HIV infection. Studies in New York City demonstrated an estimated 6%–8% HIV seroprevalence in this population, based on the serological testing of patients who were consecutively admitted to two public psychiatric hospitals (Cournos et al. 1991) and a private, voluntary psychiatric hospital (Sacks et al. 1992), as well as a population of homeless mentally ill patients committed to an inpatient psychiatric facility (Empfield et al. 1993). Schizophrenia or schizoaffective disorder was diagnosed in 54%–92% of these patients, and a majority of these patients engaged in frequent sexual activity involving behavior that put them at high risk for HIV infection (Cournos et al. 1994).

Homeless persons also appear to be a group with increased prevalence of HIV infection. Prevalence varies depending on sampling methodology and geographic location. Studies involving representative adult homeless populations found HIV prevalences of 8.5% in San Francisco (Zolopa et al. 1994) and 1.8% in Toronto (Halman et al. 1998). In both samples, HIV infection was associated with high-risk drug use behaviors, including crack use.

In this chapter, we focus on HIV/AIDS in the United States and Canada, but the epidemic is a global one. Approximately 33.5 million people worldwide are living with HIV/AIDS, and 95% of these people live in the developing world. HIV prevention and care issues highlight the global differences in health care access and the importance of social determinants of health. Developing countries in the new millennium are facing the financial challenges of drug access to fight HIV disease and infrastructure implementation to ensure that those in need can have access to care. There are encouraging signs in 2001 that developing and developed nations are committing to working together to ensure a global response to HIV disease.

COURSE OF HIV DISEASE

HIV is a ribonucleic acid (RNA) virus that can cause slowly progressive immunodeficiency, progressive neurodegeneration, or both. HIV is composed of an outer envelope and an inner core. The envelope is made up of knoblike glycoproteins (gp120s), which bind to the CD4 molecules of susceptible host cells. The viral core contains components that are necessary for the integration of the viral genome into the human host's genome, including viral RNA, the reverse transcriptase enzyme, and coding for other enzymes necessary to generate new virions. The virus uses the host cell's machinery to transcribe, translate, and make copies of itself. Copies of the virus are made and host cells are destroyed, resulting in immunological deterioration. HIV disease is the resulting dynamic interplay between virus replication and host attempts, including natural immune responses and antiretroviral medications, to limit that replication.

Initial infection commonly produces an acute seroconversion illness that often goes undiagnosed. During this period there are high levels of replicating virus, and a vigorous virus-specific immune response is mounted by the host. Emerging from the acute seroconversion period is a viral set point, representing a balance between virus and host. The viral set point has value in terms of predicting disease progression, with a high viral set point being associated with more rapid progression (Kahn and Walker 1998; Mellors et al. 1996). It is unclear what determines an individual's viral set point, but factors likely include genetic differences in host immune response and coreceptors and differences in strain virulence.

The course of HIV disease was originally understood as involving acute seroconversion followed by a long latent period wherein the virus was essentially dormant. It was thought that after an average of 7–10 years, the dormant virus became activated, leading to progressive immunosuppression as indicated by decreasing CD4[+] counts and the presence of symptomatic conditions of immunosuppression (Fauci 1993; Pantaleo et al. 1993). More recently, it has been determined that there is no latent period; rather, early on, HIV infection leads to a dynamic battle between actively replicating virus and the host immune response. The host immune response keeps viral replication in check at the expense of host immune cells, which are destroyed (Ho et al. 1995). Clinical deterioration results when the host immune response is overtaxed and can no longer limit viral replication. Signs and symptoms of disease occur with immune suppression (Figure 36–1). In general, as CD4$^+$ counts fall below 500 cells/mL, patients become at risk for symptomatic but non-AIDS-defining conditions associated with decreased immunological function. These conditions include fatigue, weight loss, minor cognitive decline, and thrush (oral candidiasis). At CD4$^+$ counts < 200 cells/mL, AIDS-defining conditions—that is, opportunistic infections, neoplasms, and HIV-related dementia—begin to occur (Brookmeyer 1991; Muñoz et al. 1989). At counts < 50 cells/mL, patients are at increased risk for fatal HIV-related illness (Yarchoan et al. 1991). The 1993 Centers for Disease Control and Prevention (1992) revised case definition for AIDS among adolescents and adults uses both clinical presentation and CD4$^+$ count in disease staging (Table 36–1).

TREATMENT OF HIV DISEASE

At the beginning of the epidemic, treatment consisted primarily of managing opportunistic conditions as they arose and preventing their development with prophylactic strategies when significant immune suppression had occurred. Treating and preventing opportunistic conditions became coupled with treatments directed against HIV itself in the mid-1980s. AZT was the first antiretroviral agent to be used. It inhibits viral reverse transcriptase, thereby decreasing viral replication. AZT was shown to reduce morbidity and prolong life among patients with symptomatic HIV disease (Fischl et al. 1987), but the response was short-lived and the impact on virus replication was not durable. The compromised quality of life associated with high doses of AZT often outweighed the benefits (Gelber et al. 1992; Lenderking et al. 1994), leading patients to consider discontinuing treatment. Many additional therapeutic interventions brought hope when short-term data were analyzed but then produced disappointment when longer-term efficacy and side effect data were examined.

In the mid-1990s, several important changes occurred. The dynamics of HIV infection became better understood, which shifted the principles of treatment from treating only when symptomatic conditions had begun (on the understanding that this represented the end of the latent phase) to treating early and aggressively, to suppress viral replication from the outset and preserve the integrity of the host's immune system (Ho 1996). Technologies to quantitatively measure viral load copies enhanced the ability to monitor viral activity and gained widespread clinical use in the mid-1990s. Viral load determination and the CD4$^+$ count are the standard laboratory measures for monitoring disease progression. Each measure independently has predictive value when assessing disease stage and outcome (Mellors et al. 1997).

During the 1990s, several new drugs were introduced in efforts to fight HIV replication (Table 36–2). These drugs inhibit either the reverse transcriptase enzyme or the protease enzyme. Initially, drugs were introduced as monotherapies and each produced short-lived decreases in viral load followed by a rebound in viral activity. Increases in CD4$^+$ counts were also short-lived, with a parallel decrease as viral load rebounded. The breakthrough in attaining a durable suppression of the virus came with the introduction of combinations of antiretroviral drugs—agents used together to fully suppress the virus and minimize the development of viral resistance. HAART is the current mainstay of treatment and has been shown to be far superior to sequential introduction of single antiretroviral agents (Gulick et al. 1998). Since the introduction of these drug combinations, morbidity and mortality associated with HIV infection have dramatically decreased (Hogg et al. 1998; Palella et al. 1998).

Currently, intervention is aimed at aggressively suppressing viral replication with combination therapies, in an effort to stop deterioration of immune function, allow immune reconstitution with an increase in CD4$^+$ count, and enable the host immune system to ward off opportunistic conditions. The optimum time to initiate HAART and the optimum regimens to be used have been widely debated. Consensus guidelines have been published and have been updated frequently as new data and new drugs have emerged (BHIVA Guidelines Co-ordinating Committee 1997; Carpenter et al. 1996, 1997, 1998). Initial enthusiasm over the theory that prolonged suppression of virus would lead to viral eradication has given way to the understanding that despite prolonged suppression, a latent reservoir of HIV remains (Finzi et al. 1997; J. K.

TABLE 36–1. Centers for Disease Control and Prevention revised classification system for HIV infection

CD4$^+$ count (cells/mL)	Clinical categories		
	(A) Asymptomatic, 1° HIV infection or PGL	(B) Symptomatic, not (A) or (C) conditions	(C) AIDS-indicator conditions
≥500	A1	B1	C1
200–499	A2	B2	C2
≤200	A3	B3	C3

Note. 1° = first-degree; PGL = persistent generalized lymphadenopathy.
Source. Adapted from Centers for Disease Control and Prevention 1992.

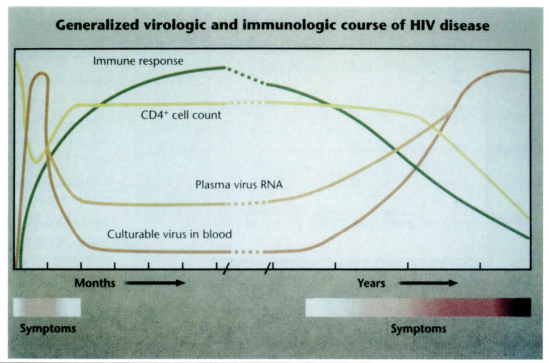

Figure 36–1. Generalized virologic and immunologic course of HIV disease.

Left side of the graph = earlier course of the disease (in months); right side = later course (in years); Months and Years portions are separated by two slashes (bottom horizontal axis) and dotted lines (within graphed solid lines). Darker shading = increased severity of symptoms (in graphed lines and wide bars below lines). Left-hand portion of the graphed lines shows that shortly after initial infection there are symptoms associated with the new infection and with seroconversion. These symptoms then decrease after the first few weeks to a month; there are then no symptoms until later in the disease process (the right-hand portion of the graphed lines), when the CD4 count begins to decrease and the viral count begins to increase.
Source. Reprinted from Saag MS, Holodniy M, Kuritzkes DR, et al: "HIV Viral Load Markers in Clinical Practice." *Nature Medicine* 2:625–629, 1996. Used with permission.

TABLE 36–2. Currently available antiretroviral agents

Nucleoside reverse transcriptase inhibitors	Nonnucleoside reverse transcriptase inhibitors	Protease inhibitors
Abacavir (Ziagen)	Delavirdine (Rescriptor)	Amprenavir (Agenerase)
Didanosine (DDI, Videx)	Efavirenz (Sustiva)	Indinavir (Crixivan)
Lamivudine (3TC)	Nevirapine (Viramune)	Nelfinavir (Viracept)
Zalcitabine (ddC)		Ritonavir (Norvir)
Zidovudine (AZT, Retrovir)		Saquinavir (Invirase, Fortovase)
Stavudine (d4T, Zerit)		Lopinavir/ritonavir (Kaletra)

Wong et al. 1997) that gives rise to active viral replication if HAART is discontinued or even replaced with less intensive regimens (Havlir et al. 1998; Pialoux et al. 1998). HAART is a long-term and likely lifelong venture, and patients must be prepared for that reality before beginning treatment (L. Zhang et al. 1999).

Patients begin HAART with a backbone of two nucleoside transcriptase inhibitors (NRTIs) and one or two protease inhibitors (PIs) or one nonnucleoside transcriptase inhibitor (NNRTI). All the drugs are initiated together, and strict regimen adherence is necessary for durable viral suppression. Efficacy of HAART is measured by CD4$^+$ count, determination of viral load, and determination of tolerability. In clinical trials, represent-

ing optimum conditions and motivated subjects, roughly 80% of subjects (range for 17 trials, 57%—97%) who have never been previously treated with antiretroviral agents will have a decrease in viral load to < 500 copies/ mL at 24 weeks (for examples, see Gulick et al. 1997; Hammer et al. 1997). With improved technologies that can measure lower limits of detection down to < 20 copies/mL, it has been shown that greater viral suppression is associated with more durable long-term suppression (Kempf et al. 1998; Raboud et al. 1998). This lower limit of detection has become the target of viral suppression. When lower limits of detection (<50 copies/mL) are used and clinical trial data are interpreted more conservatively, particularly accounting for subject dropouts, the mean response rate for HAART trials decreases to 52% (range, 30%–78%) and more likely represents the overall effectiveness in community samples (Hill 1999).

Side effects of HAART have significant bearing on quality of life and psychological distress. Common side effects include nausea, headache, diarrhea, asthenia, weakness, rash, insomnia, neuropsychiatric disturbances, and neuropathy. Lipodystrophy, a redistribution of fat, is as-sociated with HAART use and is characterized as wasting of fat in the face, buttocks, arms, and legs and concurrent abdominal obesity and breast enlargement. It can be associated with impaired glucose control and increased triglyceride levels. Lipodystrophy may emerge after months of HAART therapy and can have a profound impact on quality of life (Aboulafia and Bundow 1998; ; Carr and Cooper 1998; Collins et al. 2000) (see Figure 36–2).

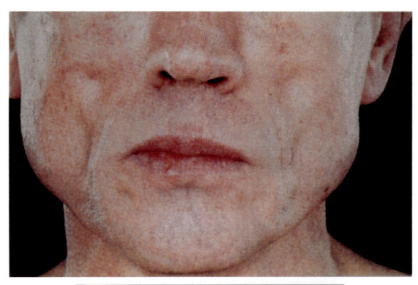

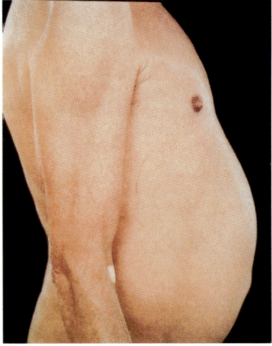

FIGURE 36–2.   Lipodystrophy.

(Top) Typical lipoatrophy.   *(Bottom)* Typical central fat redistribution. Lipodystrophy includes not only changes in shape of parts of the body, but changes in skin quality and coloration, as shown. Lipodystrophy is the current most important psychological issue facing these patients, and practitioners need to be familiar with lipodystrophy and with the appearance produced by it in order to discuss it with patients and with other medical professionals.

Source.   Reprinted from Carr A, Cooper DA: "Images in Clinical Medicine: Lipodystrophy Associated With an HIV-Protease Inhibitor." *New England Journal of Medicine* 339:1296, 1998.

Perhaps the greatest obstacle in HAART is resistance. When suppression with antiretroviral treatment is suboptimal, viral replication occurs in the presence of antiretroviral agents. This process results in changes in amino acid sequences in the viral protease and reverse transcriptase enzyme systems. This process in turn reduces the sensitivity of the virus to those agents and eventually leads to drug resistance (Wainberg 1998; Wainberg and Friedland 1998). Achieving complete viral suppression is highly emphasized to avoid conditions that foster mutagenesis and viral resistance. Some agents (e.g., lamivudine, NNRTIs) develop high-level resistance with only single mutations, whereas others (e.g., AZT, abacavir, PIs) require three or more mutations to render high-level resistance. Cross-resistance develops within classes of medications so that resistance to one NNRTI, for example, may lead to resistance to all other NNRTIs.

Patients who were treated over the years with sequentially added monotherapies (the standard of care in the early 1990s) are likely to have developed resistance to successive agents in the face of sequential suboptimal suppression of virus. These patients may benefit from HAART but are less likely to attain full viral suppression (Hirsch et al. 1998; Wainberg and Friedland 1998). Many of these patients are running out of options as they become resistant to all available drugs and are unable to stop immunological deterioration.

To minimize the emergence of resistance and maintain viral suppression, there must be maintenance of therapeutic blood levels of the HAART agents. Individual variations in drug absorption and metabolism, the impact of drug-drug interactions on metabolism and drug levels, and individual differences in adherence to regimens can all affect regimen success. Many of the drugs require strict adherence in terms of not only taking the pills at specific intervals but also accepting dietary constraints to ensure that absorption is not impeded. In many patients, the need to maintain strict adherence and the uncertainty and anxiety that go along with maintaining nondetectable viral loads compound the stress of managing HIV disease.

Managing viral resistance has become a key therapeutic challenge in HIV disease. New genotypic testing assays have been developed that can detect specific codon mutations, and phenotypic assays have been developed that measure viral susceptibility to different drugs. At the time of writing, the optimum use of these technologies remains unclear, but these tests will likely be the next major laboratory tools for monitoring HIV disease and guiding antiretroviral treatment choices (Hirsch et al. 1998).

Although HAART is a great advance, its limited effectiveness (particularly in pretreated patients), its side effects, resistance concerns, and the need for strict adherence to complex regimens indicate that HAART is neither a cure for HIV disease nor a sign of the end of AIDS, as has sometimes been depicted in the popular press (Sullivan 1996). With increased experience, patients and caregivers are rethinking the optimum time to start therapy, and the most recent guidelines for the use of antiretroviral agents reflect a more conservative approach to the timing of the initiation of HAART (Fauci et al. 2001). Access and high drug costs are also significant obstacles. There is a growing recognition of the limitations of HAART, and despite its benefits, some patients still experience AIDS-related illnesses and clinical deterioration (Garrett 1999). The realities of the medical course of HIV disease and the associated treatment issues are the backdrop against which much of the psychiatric work with these patients occurs.

Drug Regimen Adherence

Given that poor adherence is an important independent predictor of lack of viral suppression in patients receiving HAART, understanding the determinants of regimen adherence has become an integral part of HIV care. One study found that 80% of subjects who self-reported adherence levels exceeding 95% had undetectable viral loads. By contrast, only 65% of those with adherence levels between 80% and 95% and only 50% reporting levels <80% had undetectable viral loads (Hecht et al. 1998). A study using Medication Event Monitoring Systems (MEMSCaps) found similar associations between viral suppression and adherence (Paterson et al. 1999). It is a challenge for clinicians to emphasize the need for adherence levels exceeding 95% while not making the patient anxious about failure, virologic nonsuppression, or loss of suppression. With the extensive emphasis on adherence, patients who experience viral breakthrough or do not achieve complete suppression may feel responsible for the lack of response, generating complex reactions of sadness, anger, or shame.

Surveys of HIV-positive subjects yielded a wide range of reasons for missed doses, including forgetting to take one's medications (52%), being away from home or out of one's routine (34%–42%), sleeping through the time for taking medications (37%), changing one's routine (27%), being depressed (9%–23%), and experiencing side effects (10%) (Chesney and Ickovics 1997; Gifford et al. 1998). Determinants of adherence include patient demographics, regimen characteristics, care relationships, disease factors, barriers to treatment, and neuropsychiatric factors. In a self-report study of adherence, better adherence was associated with older age, male sex, white race, and possession of health insurance. Better adherence was predicted by better perception by the patient of how the regimen could be fit into his or her daily schedule, and better adherence was also associated with perception of regimen effectiveness. Importantly for psychiatrists, poor adherence was predicted by active alcohol- and drug-related problems (Wenger et al. 1999). In the MEMSCaps study, poor adherence was associated with active depression and active alcoholism (Paterson et al. 1999). In another study, mild HIV-related neuropsychological impairments were associated with poor adherence to drug regimens (Albert et al. 1998).

Psychiatrists have a role to play in identifying and treating psychiatric conditions that may affect adherence and virologic outcomes. This role may include not only treatment of psychiatric conditions (mood disorders, substance-related disorders, cognitive disorders) but also application of principles of cognitive and behavior therapies, cognitive rehabilitation, and psychotherapy targeting issues of perceived efficacy in order to improve adherence.

Drug-Drug Interactions

The potential for drug-drug interactions is of particular concern for patients with HIV/AIDS, given the multiple medications they may be taking as part of their ongoing treatment of HIV infection. Before the introduction of PIs, the only interaction between an AIDS medication and a psychotropic that appeared to be of any concern was methadone's mild inhibition of AZT metabolism, leading to potential AZT toxicity (Schwartz et al. 1992). However, with the release of newer antiretrovirals, including PIs and NNRTIs, clinicians have been cautioned about an increasing number of potential drug-drug interactions, with the result that some psychiatrists are very hesitant to prescribe psychotropics to patients with HIV disease (Shader and Greenblatt 1996). In part, this hesitancy is due to a better understanding of the cytochrome P450 oxidative enzyme system, which consists of more than 30 isoforms found mainly in the hepatic endoplasmic reticulum (Callahan et al. 1996; Ereshefsky et al. 1996; Nemeroff et al. 1996). P450 3A3/3A4 and P450 2D6 are the enzymes most involved in potential interactions between AIDS medications and psychotropics, and it is the inhibition and/or induction of these enzymes that can cause problems. However, many medications are metabolized by more than one enzyme; therefore, the overall effect of enzyme inhibition may be lessened.

In general, use of agents that inhibit metabolism will lead to drug interactions that cause increases in drug levels, with increased potential for toxicity and side effects.

Starting with lower doses and increasing more slowly may offset worrisome side effects. Agents that induce metabolism are of most concern, because these drugs may cause subtherapeutic serum levels of antiretroviral medications, resulting in loss of viral suppression during HAART.

All the PIs are metabolized primarily by P450 3A3/3A4 and can competitively inhibit this enzyme (Deeks et al. 1997). However, only ritonavir (Norvir) has demonstrated significant inhibition of P450 3A3/3A4, which can result in clinically important drug-drug interactions. This enzyme makes up approximately 50% of the P450 system and is involved in the metabolism of many medications. Inhibition of P450 3A3/3A4 can therefore result in increased serum levels of some medications, as well as toxicity. Examples of psychotropic medications metabolized primarily by P450 3A3/3A4 include the triazolobenzodiazepines and some other benzodiazepines (i.e., triazolam, alprazolam, midazolam, clonazepam, diazepam), zolpidem, some antidepressants (i.e., tertiary amine tricyclics, nefazodone, fluoxetine, sertraline), and some neuroleptics (i.e., clozapine, pimozide, quetiapine). Ritonavir also inhibits P450 2D6, though to a lesser degree. Psychotropic medications potentially affected include most neuroleptics, tricyclic antidepressants (TCAs), and the selective serotonin reuptake inhibitors (SSRIs). See Table 36–3 for a list of psychotropic medications contraindicated for patients taking ritonavir. Of note is bupropion, which was thought to be primarily metabolized by P450 3A3/3A4 at the time ritonavir was released but which is now believed to be metabolized by P450 2B6. Until the safety of the combination of bupropion and ritonavir has been determined, clinicians should remain cautious about using these two drugs together.

Of the NNRTIs, delavirdine (Rescriptor) is an inhibitor of P450 3A3/3A4 and can cause some of the same interactions as ritonavir. Nevirapine (Viramune) induces P450 3A3/3A4 and may produce decreased serum levels of psychotropics metabolized by this enzyme. Efavirenz (Sustiva) is both an inducer and an inhibitor of 3A3/3A4. Clinically, induction predominates, but predicting interactions is difficult (A. Tseng, M. Foisy, and D. Fletcher, "Handbook of HIV Drug Therapy," unpublished document, 1999, pp 137–149).

The potential for drug-drug interactions is also a function of the effects psychotropics can have on the P450 system. For instance, nefazodone and fluvoxamine demonstrate significant competitive inhibition of P450 3A3/3A4; if either drug is given in combination with a PI, toxicity due to increased serum levels of the psychotropic and/or the PI may result. Most importantly, barbiturates, carbamazepine, phenytoin, and St. John's wort have all been shown to induce P450 3A3/3A4. Administration of

TABLE 36–3. Psychotropics that interact with ritonavir

Contraindicated for patients taking ritonavir	Possibly toxic in patients taking ritonavir
Anxiolytics/Sedatives	**Antidepressants**
Alprazolam	Fluvoxamine
Clorazepate	Nefazodone
Diazepam	Trazodone
Estazolam	Tricyclic antidepressants
Flurazepam	**Neuroleptics**
Midazolam	**Analgesics**
Triazolam	Fentanyl
Zolpidem	Methadone
Antidepressants	Oxycodone
Bupropion	**Anticonvulsants**
Neuroleptics	Carbamazepine
Clozapine	Clonazepam
Pimozide	
Analgesics	
Meperidine	
Propoxyphene	

these medications to patients taking PIs could result in subtherapeutic serum levels of these crucial AIDS drugs. Theoretically, such changes could lead to inadequate viral suppression and promotion of viral resistance.

Patients may also be taking medications other than antiretrovirals, and drug-drug interactions may result. In particular, some antifungals (e.g., fluconazole, ketoconazole) can inhibit P450 3A3/3A4, and rifampin may induce enzymatic metabolism of some psychotropics.

A recent retrospective chart review revealed that although combinations of PIs and psychotropics may produce an increased incidence of side effects, this increase rarely is clinically important enough to cause discontinuation of use of the medications (Bialer et al. 1998). Psychopharmacological treatment of disorders such as depression, mania, and psychosis is discussed in other sections of this chapter, and clinicians are advised to consult package inserts for specific medication contraindications.

NEUROPSYCHIATRIC SYNDROMES

One of the unique challenges of HIV psychiatry is the interface of mind, brain, and body. HIV exerts its effect not only on the immune system, causing systemic disease, but also on the brain, leading to neuropsychiatric syndromes. With progression of HIV disease, patients are at high risk for secondary neuropsychiatric disorders, and any change in mental status in a person with HIV infection must be considered to have an organic cause until it

is proven otherwise. The neuropsychiatric differential diagnosis must broadly include the following causes: HIV CNS infection and associated neurocognitive disorders; CNS opportunistic infections and tumors; metabolic consequences of systemic HIV disease; primary psychiatric disorders, including psychoactive substance–related disorders; other neurological-medical complications of HIV disease; and medication side effects. The differential diagnosis of mental status changes in an individual with HIV infection is outlined in Table 36–4.

An organic neuropsychiatric syndrome is most likely to occur in a patient with later-stage systemic HIV disease. In the pre-HAART era, CNS-related opportunistic conditions were seen almost exclusively in patients with $CD4^+$ counts <200 cells/mL. Today, because of HAART, many patients who previously had nadir $CD4^+$ counts <200 cells/mL have experienced a rebound in $CD4^+$ counts. On rare occasions, some of these patients may still develop CNS opportunistic conditions because of incomplete immune function reconstitution. Therefore, the clinician must ask about not only the current $CD4^+$ count but also the nadir count when assessing for CNS opportunistic conditions.

The most common CNS opportunistic conditions that present with change in mental status include HIV dementia (discussed later in this chapter), toxoplasmosis, CNS lymphoma, cryptococcal meningitis, and progressive multifocal leukoencephalopathy. All these conditions usually also present with neurological signs or signs of systemic illness. Figure 36–3 illustrates the brain magnetic resonance image (MRI) of a brain of a man with then-unknown HIV status who presented with neuropsychiatric and neurological signs and was found to have cerebral toxoplasmosis as an AIDS-defining condition. A good history, a mental status examination, a neurological examination, and ancillary laboratory testing including brain imaging are essential in patients presenting with new-onset mental status changes, particularly in patients with signs of systemic illness, nadir $CD4^+$ counts <200 cells/mL, and neurological signs (Simpson and Tagliati 1994). In the HAART era, there has been a clear decrease in incidence of all these CNS opportunistic conditions. One HIV center reported a decrease in incidence, from 1993 to 1997, of toxoplasmosis (–71%), HIV dementia (–43%), and progressive multifocal leukoencephalopathy (–45%) (Moore et al. 1998).

As the incidence of CNS opportunistic conditions has decreased with HAART, the rate of mental status changes being caused by medication side effects has increased. In more systemically ill patients, with more vulnerable brains, the use of more medications, with an increased potential for drug interactions, raises the likeli-

TABLE 36–4. Differential diagnosis of HIV-related mental status changes

CNS opportunistic infections

Fungi	*Cryptococcus, Histoplasma, Candida, Aspergillus*
Parasites	*Toxoplasma*, ameba, others (endemic)
Viruses	Progressive multifocal leukoencephalopathy, CMV,[a] herpes simplex, herpes zoster, human herpesvirus 6[b]
Bacteria	*Mycobacterium avium-intracellulare, Mycobacterium tuberculosis,* gram-negative bacteria, *Treponema pallidum*[c]

Neoplasms

Primary CNS lymphoma[d]

Metastatic Kaposi's sarcoma[e]

Others

Drug-related neurotoxicities

Medication side effects and toxicities

Endocrinopathies and specific nutrient deficiencies

Addison's disease (secondary to HIV, CMV, ketoconazole therapy)

Hypothyroidism

Vitamin B_6 or B_{12} deficiency[f,g]

Hypogonadism

Anemia

Metabolic abnormalities including abnormal liver function

Hypoxic encephalopathy

Vasculitis

First-degree Axis I psychiatric disorders

Major depressive episode

Bipolar disorder

Schizophrenia

Psychoactive substance intoxication or withdrawal

Non-HIV-related medical or neurological illness

Note. CMV = cytomegalovirus; CNS = central nervous system.
Source. [a]Wiley and Nelson 1988; [b]Knox and Carrigan 1995; [c]Berger 1991; [d]R.M. Levy and Bredesen 1988; [e]Y. Chang et al. 1994; [f]Beach et al. 1992; [g]Kieburtz et al. 1991a.

hood of delirium secondary to use of medications, particularly benzodiazepines, anticholinergics, narcotics, and illicit drugs. In addition, many antiretroviral agents may have neuropsychiatric side effects (Table 36–5). The prevalence of these side effects is hard to determine, since clinical trials tend to underestimate psychiatric side effects that are of only limited severity, and estimating true prevalences relies on postmarketing reporting by physicians. Despite these limitations, it is clear that many patients experience subclinical mood symptoms, most commonly anxiety, sleep disturbance, and sadness. In addition, most of the antiretrovirals may cause weakness and lethargy. The more dramatic side effects—new-onset mania or psychosis, intense anxiety, and exacerbation of preexisting major depression—likely occur with most of the antiretrovirals at a rate of < 1% and have been reported in specific case reports and in reports of serious adverse events. Patients with prior psychiatric histories may be at the greatest risk for these severe psychiatric, medication-related, adverse events.

One of the newer NNRTIs, efavirenz, which has recently become popular in HAART because of good antiviral efficacy, good CNS penetration, and convenient once-a-day dosing, appears to have problematic neuropsychiatric side effects in approximately 50% of patients beginning therapy. These effects, which include insomnia, disorientation, depression, and vivid dreams, occur primarily in the first 1–4 months of treatment in the majority of patients. Patients should be alerted to the potential side effects, and supports should be made available during the initiation phase of treatment. In the majority of patients, emergent psychiatric side effects may be managed by

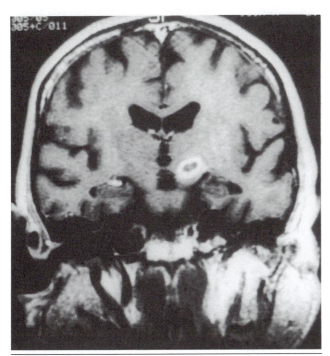

FIGURE 36–3. Magnetic resonance image of a 60-year-old man who presented with a 3-week history of fever, headache, and a change in personality, with disinhibition and grandiosity.

The patient sought medical attention only when he developed hemiballismus. A magnetic resonance image showed atrophy and a ring-enhancing lesion. HIV test results were positive, and he was treated empirically for toxoplasmosis. Antiretroviral therapy was then started.

using standard psychiatric interventions. Dose adjustment and dose splitting are not recommended. Approximately 3% of patients need to discontinue efavirenz therapy because of neuropsychiatric side effects (Moyle 1999).

From a practical point of view, the approach to neuropsychiatric symptoms secondary to antiretroviral therapy must be individualized. Stopping a regimen, or removing a single drug from a regimen and then reintroducing it to find out whether the symptoms are temporally related to administration of the antiretroviral drug, is not a simple or benign intervention, given the importance of viral suppression and concerns over mutation. Close consultation with the patient and the treating internist is essential to determine whether the optimum treatment will be to discontinue the antiretroviral regimen, provide supportive care in the expectation that side effects will diminish over time, or introduce a psychotropic agent to treat the side effects (Halman 2001).

HIV-ASSOCIATED NEUROCOGNITIVE DISORDERS

Neurocognitive impairment related to HIV disease is due to HIV in the brain and the indirect effects on the brain of host immune factors liberated in response to brain and systemic HIV infection. The risk of neurocognitive impairment due to HIV infection is increased at each successive stage of HIV infection (Centers for Disease Control and Prevention 1992; Heaton et al. 1995), and the nature and severity of the impairment are best delineated using neuropsychological (psychometric) testing (Butters et al. 1990; Grant and Martin 1994; Heaton et al. 1995, 1996; Miller et al. 1990, 1991; D. A. White et al. 1995). Relatively recent reviews from the pre-HAART era suggest that 35% of asymptomatic patients (CDC stage A; see Table 36–1), 44% of patients who are mildly symptomatic (CDC stage B), and 55% of patients with AIDS (CDC stage C) exhibit neurocognitive impairments, particularly in the areas of attention, speed of information processing, learning efficiency, and psychomotor skills (Heaton et al. 1995; A. White et al. 1995), with frontal lobe executive deficits developing mostly in later stages (Bornstein et al. 1993; Law et al. 1994; Marcotte et al. 1996; Sahakian et al. 1995; R. A. Stern et al. 1996; Y. Stern et al. 1995). The pattern of neurocognitive impairment associated with HIV infection is typical of other "subcortical" or frontostriatal disorders (e.g., multiple sclerosis, Huntington's disease, Parkinson's disease) (see Cummings 1990; Grant and Adams 1996; Parks et al. 1993). Neurocognitive impairment, even when mild, is known to affect work functioning (Albert et al. 1995; Heaton et al. 1994, 1996) and adherence to HIV medication regimens (Albert et al. 1998) and to lead to reduced quality of life (R. M. Kaplan et al. 1995).

The cardinal feature of an HIV-associated neurocognitive disorder is neurocognitive impairment that is severe enough to interfere with everyday functioning. In 1991, the American Academy of Neurology AIDS Task Force published nomenclature and criteria for two neurocognitive disorders (Table 36–6), HIV-associated dementia complex (HADC)[1] and HIV-associated minor cognitive-motor disorder (MCMD). The Memorial Sloan-Kettering Clinical Staging System for AIDS Dementia Complex (Price and Brew 1992; Table 36–7)

---

[1] Previously referred to as *subacute encephalitis*, *HIV encephalopathy*, *HIV dementia*, and *AIDS-related dementia*; DSM-IV-TR (American Psychiatric Association 2000) classification: dementia due to other general medical conditions (294.1x—dementia due to HIV disease).

TABLE 36–5. Neuropsychiatric side effects of medications frequently used for HIV/AIDS

Drug	Side effect(s)
Abacavir	Asthenia
	Insomnia
Acyclovir	Visual hallucinations
	Depersonalization
	Tearfulness
	Confusion
	Hyperesthesia
	Hyperacusis
	Thought insertion
	Insomnia
	Agitation
Amphotericin B	Delirium
	Peripheral neuropathy
	Diplopia
	Anorexia
Co-trimoxazole	Depression
	Loss of appetite
	Insomnia
	Apathy
	Headache
Didanosine (ddI)	Insomnia
	Peripheral neuropathy
	Mania
Efavirenz	Disorientation
	Confusion
	Depression
	Insomnia
	Nightmares
Ganciclovir	Mania
	Psychosis
	Agitation
	Delirium
	Irritability
Interferon-α	Depression
	Weakness (dose-dependent)
Isoniazid	Depression
	Agitation
	Hallucinations
	Paranoia
	Impaired memory
Lamivudine (3TC)	Mania
Pentamidine	Hypotension
Protease inhibitors	Asthenia
	Depression
	Insomnia
Stavudine (d4T)	Mania
Steroids	Depression
	Euphoria
	Mania
	Psychosis

TABLE 36–5. Neuropsychiatric side effects of medications frequently used for HIV/AIDS *(continued)*

Drug	Side effect(s)
Vinblastine	Depression
	Anorexia
	Headache
Vincristine	Depression
	Hallucinations
	Headache
	Ataxia
	Sensory loss
	Agitation
Zidovudine (AZT)	Headache
	Restlessness
	Agitation
	Insomnia
	Mania
	Depression
	Irritability

also stages HIV-associated neurocognitive disorder according to level of functional impairment. Patients with minimal or mild deficits (MSK stage 0.5 or 1) experience cognitive and motor deficits that do not adversely affect basic activities of daily living but that may affect work function; these stages are analogous to MCMD. HADC is comparable to MSK stages 2–4.

HADC, which is sufficient for a diagnosis of AIDS, is characterized by moderate to severe neurocognitive impairments that markedly interfere with day-to-day functioning (e.g., work, home, life, social activities). HADC is usually diagnosed in patients with other concurrent AIDS-defining illnesses. The annual incidence of HADC in the pre-HAART era was 7%–14% (Day et al. 1992; McArthur et al. 1993); approximately 4% of patients with HIV infection presented with HADC as their first AIDS-defining diagnosis. Risk factors for HADC include anemia, wasting syndrome, a higher number of constitutional symptoms that occur before AIDS diagnosis, and older age (McArthur et al. 1993).

HADC is characterized by cognitive, affective, behavioral, and motor dysfunction. Cognitive deficits affect a range of neuropsychological domains, including memory and new learning, concentration and attention, and executive function. Clinically, patients describe short-term memory loss, word-finding difficulties, and difficulty with sequential tasks. They may report that activities that were once automatic now require concentration for successful completion. Behaviorally, patients commonly report apathetic or depressed mood, social withdrawal, and decreased energy. Disinhibition, poor judgment, and impaired modulation of mood occur, but less

TABLE 36–6. American Academy of Neurology criteria for HIV-associated cognitive-motor disorder

1. Acquired abnormality in at least two of the following cognitive abilities (present for ≥1 month):

   Attention/concentration   Speed of processing
   Abstraction/reasoning   Visuospatial skills
   Memory learning   Speech/language

   a. Decline verified by history and mental status examination; when possible, history should be obtained by an informant, and examination supplemented by neuropsychological testing

   b. Cognitive dysfunction causing impairment of work or activities of daily living; impairment not attributable solely to severe systemic illness

2. At least one of the following:

   a. Acquired abnormality in motor function or performance verified by physical examination, neuropsychological tests, or both

   b. Decline in motivation or emotional control or change in social behavior, characterized by any of the following:

   Apathy
   Inertia
   Irritability
   Emotional lability
   New-onset impaired judgment, characterized by socially inappropriate behavior or disinhibition

3. Absence of clouding of consciousness during a period long enough to establish the presence of #1

4. Evidence for another etiology—including active CNS opportunistic infections or malignancy, psychiatric disorders (e.g., depressive disorders), active substance abuse, or acute or chronic substance withdrawal—must be ruled out by history, physical and psychiatric examination, and appropriate laboratory and radiological tests

HIV-associated dementia complex: deficits markedly interfere with day-to-day function
HIV-associated minor cognitive-motor disorder: deficits cause only mild functional impairment

Note. CNS = central nervous system.
Source. Adapted from American Academy of Neurology AIDS Task Force 1991.

TABLE 36–7. Memorial Sloan-Kettering Clinical Staging System for AIDS Dementia Complex

Stage	Degree of severity	Characteristic
0	Normal	Normal mental and motor function.
0.5	Equivocal	Either minimal or equivocal symptoms of cognitive or motor dysfunction characteristic of HIV-associated cognitive-motor disorder, or mild signs (snout response, slowed extremity movements), but without impairment of work or capacity to perform ADLs. Gait and strength are normal.
1	Mild	Unequivocal evidence (symptoms, signs, neuropsychological test performance) of functional intellectual or motor impairment characteristic of HIV-associated cognitive-motor disorder, but able to perform all but the more demanding aspects of work or ADLs. Can walk without assistance.
2	Moderate	Cannot work or maintain the more demanding ADLs, but able to perform basic self-care ADLs. Ambulatory, but may require a single prop.
3	Severe	Major intellectual incapacity (cannot follow news or personal events, cannot sustain complex conversation, considerable slowing of all output) or motor disability (cannot walk unassisted, requiring walker or personal support, usually with slowing and clumsiness of arms as well).
4	End stage	Nearly vegetative. Intellectual and social comprehension and output are at a rudimentary level. Nearly or absolutely mute. Paraparetic or paraplegic with double incontinence (urinary and bowel).

Note. ADL = activity of daily living.
Source. Adapted from Price and Brew 1992.

commonly than apathy and withdrawal. Mania, hypomania (Halman et al. 1993a; Kieburtz et al. 1991b), and new-onset psychosis (Sewell et al. 1994) are rare but have been reported and are associated with advanced systemic HIV disease. Motorically, patients describe slowing of their movements, clumsiness, gait unsteadiness, and a decline in handwriting. The reporting of deficits can be affected by many factors, including mood symptoms, and needs corroboration by neurocognitive testing (discussed later in this chapter). The deficit complex and longitudinal course of HADC vary, with some patients showing progressive deterioration and others continuing at unchanged severity. During periods of intercurrent infection or metabolic disturbances, the severity of cognitive dysfunction is often increased.

MCMD, in contrast, is not sufficient for an AIDS diagnosis, although it is often present in patients with AIDS. The major difference between HADC and MCMD is the degree of impairment in activities of daily living (i.e., in MCMD, only the most demanding activities of daily living are mildly impaired) (American Academy of Neurology AIDS Task Force 1991). Recent estimates suggest that 5% of patients with CDC stage A, 27% with CDC stage B, and 21%–24% with CDC stage C disease (Heaton and Grant 1995) meet criteria for MCMD. In the pre-HAART era, HADC was the neurocognitive syndrome that was the primary focus of both research and clinical concern. With the introduction of HAART, understanding MCMD is emerging as an important focus as it is increasingly appreciated how these neurocognitive deficits affect quality of life.

Both MCMD and HADC are associated with increased risk of morbidity (Y. Stern et al. 1998) and mortality (Ellis et al. 1997; Marder et al. 1998). It is still unclear whether MCMD and HADC vary only in severity of neurocognitive impairments and disruption in activities of daily living or also in clinical course and underlying pathogenesis (M. D. Kelly et al. 1996). Current consensus is that in most patients with MCMD, that disorder does not progress to HADC. In a recent follow-up study, the DANA Consortium on Therapy for HIV Dementia and Related Cognitive Disorders (1996) found that only 17% of patients with MCMD developed HADC (Marder et al. 1998). It will be important to evaluate the effectiveness of HAART in terms of preventing the onset of any neurocognitive disorders in persons newly infected with HIV. It will also be important to determine whether, in patients who already have MCMD or HADC, stabilization or improvement in neurocognitive status can occur with maximal HAART.

Diagnostic Issues

The diagnosis of HIV-associated neurocognitive disorder is based on a suggestive history and on findings of psychiatric, neuropsychological, and neurological examinations. Further evaluation should be performed to gather data both to support the diagnosis of HIV-associated neurocognitive disorder and to exclude other causes of CNS dysfunction. There is no single investigation by which the diagnosis of HIV-associated neurocognitive disorder can be made. Supportive investigations include neuropsychological testing, brain imaging, and blood tests, including measurement of hemoglobin, glucose, electrolyte, vita-

min B_{12}, thyroid-stimulating hormone, and total and free testosterone levels and screening for syphilis. Cerebrospinal fluid (CSF) examination is important particularly if there is clinical suspicion of a contributing CNS opportunistic condition. Research is being conducted on the sensitivity and utility of several surrogate measures, including brain imaging, CSF examination, and neuropsychological testing, to help refine the understanding of and the ability to monitor and treat HIV-related cognitive disorders.

Neuropsychological Testing

Neuropsychological testing permits objective documentation of neurocognitive deficits and provides clinical information about the degree to which cerebral dysfunction will affect the patient's everyday functioning. Longitudinal follow-up testing is a way to monitor the patient for progression of neurocognitive dysfunction and to evaluate response to treatment interventions. Testing can also assist the clinician in planning neurocognitive rehabilitation or behavioral interventions. (For descriptions of and aid in selecting tests, see Butters et al. 1990; Ginzburg et al. 1988; Heaton et al. 1996; Hirsch 1988; M.D. Kelly et al. 1996; McArthur et al. 1989; and Miller et al. 1990, 1991.) Screening for risk of neurocognitive impairment is best accomplished through use of the HIV Dementia Scale (Power et al. 1995) or a combination of the Symbol Digit Modalities Test and the Trail Making Test (Sacktor et al. 1996). The Mini-Mental State Exam (Folstein et al. 1975) is not sensitive to HIV-associated neurocognitive deficits, particularly in the less severe MCMD stage, and is not a useful screening tool in this disorder (Power et al. 1995).

Up to 52% of patients with HIV infection report a variety of subjective cognitive complaints (Mehta et al. 1996), which may include increased distractibility, short-term memory loss, word-finding difficulties, reduced reading comprehension, motor incoordination, and difficulty with multitasking, problem solving, and sustained concentration. Subjective cognitive complaints correlate significantly with mood symptoms (Claypoole et al. 1998; Hinkin et al. 1996; Rourke et al. 1999a) but not consistently with neuropsychological test performance (Claypoole et al. 1998; Hinkin et al. 1996; Rourke et al. 1999b; van Gorp et al. 1991). During decision making about the presence of HIV-associated neurocognitive disorders, referral for neuropsychological testing can help to minimize the number of false-positive results. HIV-infected patients meeting criteria for a mood disorder who respond well to antidepressant treatment can be expected to show significant reductions in their subjective cognitive complaints (Claypoole et al. 1998; Halman et al. 2001b).

Failure to report cognitive complaints may not necessarily reflect normal cerebral functioning. A recent study demonstrated that HIV-positive patients with extensive disruption of frontal executive processing skills documented through neuropsychological testing minimized or "underreported" the extent and severity of their cognitive impairments (Rourke et al. 1999b). These patients often are unable to appreciate the nature of their deficits, which leaves them vulnerable to safety hazards and often poses challenges for them and their caregivers.

Cerebrospinal Fluid Examination

CSF examination is used primarily to rule out contributing CNS opportunistic conditions. In HADC alone, CSF examination may show nonspecific findings including pleocytosis, increased protein levels, and oligoclonal banding (McArthur et al. 1988). Patients with HADC have no or only a few white blood cells in the CSF. Significant numbers of white blood cells in the CSF should prompt assessment for a brain opportunistic condition other than HADC. Although measurement of CSF viral load is an important research tool in investigating the neuropathogenesis of HIV-related neurocognitive disorders (Enting et al. 1998), it is not yet useful for establishing the diagnosis of such disorders or monitoring the progression of HADC. In general, CSF viral load is usually less than plasma viral load. In neurologically symptomatic patients, CSF viral load, but not plasma viral load, correlates with neuropsychological impairment severity (Brew et al. 1997; Cinque et al. 1998; McArthur et al. 1997; Pratt et al. 1996; Sei et al. 1996). Preliminary evidence suggests that in patients with HADC, CSF viral load also correlates with brain viral load (McArthur et al. 1997).

Brain Imaging

Anatomic brain imaging techniques used to enhance the clinical examination should be sensitive to early changes secondary to CNS HIV infection, show correlation with clinical disease severity, and provide a marker for change by which to measure effects of therapeutic interventions. Computed tomography is useful for detecting atrophy, masses, or vascular lesions of secondary opportunistic conditions that may complicate the course of HIV disease, and this technique is particularly useful for screening for these complications when a patient presents with a new, acute change in mental status. Computed tomography is not reliably sensitive to subtle changes associated

with neuronal dysfunction or injury or to subtle neurocognitive deficits associated with HIV brain infection. Magnetic resonance imaging (MRI) is more sensitive to changes associated with HADC, including cerebral atrophy, ventricular enlargement, and multifocal or diffuse hyperintense signal abnormalities in the periventricular white matter regions (see Figure 36–4 for typical MRI findings associated with HIV dementia) (Kieburtz et al. 1990; Post et al. 1991). Radiological correlation with neuropsychological performance has been limited (Brouwers et al. 1995; Hestad et al. 1993) because of confounding effects of clinical staging and $CD4^+$ count, but regional studies have shown correlations between subcortical volume reductions and severity of cognitive impairment in HIV-positive subjects with $CD4^+$ counts < 200 cells/mL (DiSclafani et al. 1998). A recent study suggests that MRI changes may be useful markers by which to measure the benefit of HAART to patients with HIV-related brain disease (Filippi et al. 1998).

Magnetic resonance spectroscopy appears to be sufficiently sensitive to detect brain changes that correlate with early neuropsychological impairments in HIV disease. Although still a research tool, it may prove to be a noninvasive means of determining HIV-related brain involvement. Magnetic resonance spectroscopy measures metabolic alterations in selected brain regions. Studies have found increased levels of myoinositol (a marker of glial proliferation) in frontal white matter of neurologically asymptomatic patients and patients with MCMD, as well as increased levels of choline (a marker of cell membrane injury) in patients with MCMD. In patients with HADC, increases in myoinositol and choline concentrations have been found in frontal white matter, frontal cortex, and basal ganglia; in patients with the most severe forms of dementia, decreases in levels of *N*-acetyl compounds, a marker of neuronal injury, have been noted (L. Chang et al. 1999; Lenkinski et al. 1998).

Single photon emission computed tomography and positron emission tomography, measures of regional brain perfusion and metabolism, are research tools whose clinical usefulness in HIV disease has not been demonstrated (Harris et al. 1994; Holman et al. 1992). Electroencephalography may indicate mild, nonspecific slowing but usually contributes little to the diagnostic evaluation unless a seizure component is clinically suspected—for example, in cases of new-onset psychosis, atypical panic attacks, or mania. The prevalence of abnormal electroencephalographic findings increases with systemic disease severity, in concert with increased prevalence of neurological dysfunction, decreased neuropsychological function, and MRI abnormalities (Harrison et al. 1998).

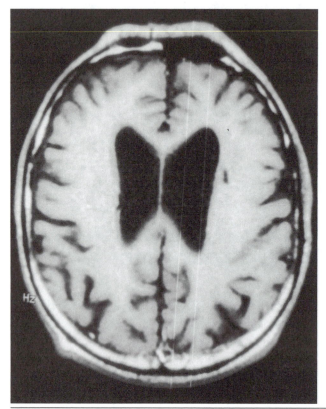 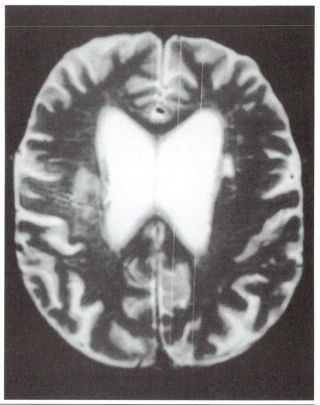

FIGURE 36–4. Magnetic resonance images of a man with HIV-associated dementia complex.

(Left) T1-weighted image showing atrophy and a small infarct. *(Right)* T2-weighted image. Note the periventricular white matter signal abnormalities.

Neuropathophysiology

The neuropathophysiology of CNS HIV infection and how such infection leads to HIV-related neurocognitive abnormalities are active areas of basic science research that inform clinical management strategies. HIV is thought to enter the CNS shortly after primary infection (Davis et al. 1992), being carried to the CNS via infected macrophages (Peudenier et al. 1991). Brain HIV replication in monocyte-macrophage-microglia cell lines occurs with disease progression, activated by decreasing CD4[+] counts, increasing systemic viral load, and opportunistic conditions (Tan and Guiloff 1998). Active brain HIV replication is considered a driving factor in the development of HIV-related neurocognitive disorders, and decreasing the propensity for the brain to be a sanctuary for HIV is a cornerstone to treatment.

Although actively replicating HIV in the brain is necessary for HIV-related neurocognitive disorders, it is not sufficient for development of HADC. Certain viral quasi species may be more neurovirulent (Jozwiak et al. 1998), and certain host factors may render an individual more susceptible to HIV-related neurocognitive disorders (Corder et al. 1998). Further work is needed to understand how these host and virus factors intersect to make certain patients vulnerable to HIV-related neurocognitive disorders.

Many theories about how active brain HIV replication leads to CNS disease are also being investigated. Proposed mechanisms focus on several pathways and include cytokine dysregulation, which can lead to astrocyte proliferation and gliosis (Tyor et al. 1995; Wesselingh et al. 1994); production of excitotoxins and free radicals, such as quinolinic acid and nitric oxide, that lead to neurotoxicity and neuronal dysfunction and loss (Lipton 1992b); and impairments of host repair mechanisms such as S-adenosylmethionine (Tan and Guiloff 1998) that may be necessary to counterbalance neurotoxic effects.

In advanced cases of HADC, pathological studies show cerebral atrophy, neuronal loss, multinucleated giant cells, diffuse myelin pallor, microgliosis, astrocytosis, and productive brain HIV infection in macrophage lineage cells (Masliah et al. 1997; Tan and Guiloff 1998). Dendritic injury and dendritic simplification have been shown to correlate with clinically significant HIV-related neurocognitive abnormalities, including MCMD (Masliah et al. 1997) and may be a neurobiological correlate of HIV-related neurocognitive impairment (Grant et al. 1998).

Treatment and Management

Pharmacotherapy

The pharmacological management of patients with HIV dementia should consider three main goals: 1) suppression of the virus in the brain as well as systemically; 2) protection of neurons, optimization of their environment, and enhancement of their function; and 3) symptomatic treatment of the consequences of HIV dementia. Pharmacotherapy is also important in preventing the onset and progression of HIV-related neurocognitive impairment, with particular goals of 1) suppressing virus to prevent development of cognitive disorders related to HIV, 2) stopping the progression of MCMD to a more severe dementing illness, and 3) halting the progression and reversing impairments of the dementing illness. Despite the many unknowns about the pathophysiology of HIV-related cognitive disorders, most researchers agree that the pathophysiology is driven by the presence of HIV in the brain and the neurotoxic impact of immune system factors that are released in response to central and systemic infection. Antiretroviral therapies that reduce viral burden systemically and centrally are currently the treatment of choice for HIV-related cognitive disorders. In considering the evidence for the use of antiretrovirals, one must consider whether 1) the agent in question has been shown to be effective against HIV systemically; 2) the drug has been shown to effectively penetrate the CNS at levels known to inhibit viral replication; 3) the agent has been demonstrated to reduce central viral replication, as measured by viral loads in the CSF; and 4) treatment with the agent has been associated with improvement in neuropsychological test results, quality of life, and patient function.

Levels of evidence differ regarding the impact of various antiretrovirals on the brain.

AZT is the most widely investigated of the antiretrovirals. One early placebo-controlled trial demonstrated improved neuropsychological outcomes in patients taking AZT (Schmitt et al. 1988). In a later, 4-month placebo-controlled trial of high-dose AZT (1,000 vs. 2,000 mg/day), cognitive function improved in patients receiving 2,000 mg/day, although the effect plateaued after 3 months (Sidtis et al. 1993). High doses were the first choice in the pre-HAART era, the assumption being that higher doses would mean better CNS penetration. Clinically, these doses were intolerable for most patients, and sufficient CSF penetration is achieved at normal daily dosing (300–600 mg/day). The plateau of effect on neuropsychological function is likely due to the development of viral resistance and loss of durable efficacy, the hallmark limitation of any monotherapy treatment. In a 10-year longitudinal population study, Portegies et al. (1993) observed less cognitive dysfunction in patients with HIV dementia who were treated with AZT.

Many agents have now been assessed for adequate penetration of the CSF and achievement of levels necessary to inhibit viral replication (Enting et al. 1998). Evidence exists for good penetration of AZT, stavudine (Haas et al. 1999), abacavir (Brew et al. 1998), nevirapine (Kearney et al. 1999), indinavir (Letendre et al. 1999; Polis et al. 1999), and efavirenz (Tashima et al. 1998). Reduction of CSF viral load has been demonstrated with AZT, stavudine (Haas et al. 1999), abacavir (Brew et al. 1998), lamivudine (Foudraine et al. 1998), indinavir (Polis et al. 1999), and efavirenz (Tashima et al. 1998). A recent double-blind, placebo-controlled trial examined the impact of adding abacavir versus placebo to the current stable regimen of patients with HIV dementia (Brew et al. 1998). Abacavir achieved sufficient CSF penetration and was well tolerated. Both the group of patients receiving abacavir and the control group showed improved neuropsychological function over 12 weeks, but the difference between the groups was not statistically significant. The study indicates that adding a single antiretroviral agent, even one that penetrates the CSF well, has little benefit in terms of improvement of cognitive function.

Overall, HAART has been the most effective strategy for treating HIV-related brain disorders. Since the introduction of HAART, the incidence of HIV dementia has decreased (Moore et al. 1998). Several studies have found that patients receiving HAART exhibit fewer neurocognitive impairments than do patients treated with less potent regimens (Ferrando et al. 1998a; Galgani et al. 1998; Letendre et al. 1998; Martin et al. 1998; Sacktor et al. 1998). The improvement appears to be due primarily to the reduction in systemic viral burden and the concomitant reduction in neurotoxic factors associated with immune activation (e.g., quinolinic acid, tumor necrosis factor, and nitric oxide) (Gendelman et al. 1998). Even regimens containing agents that do not penetrate the CSF well have been associated with CSF viral load reduction (Aweeka et al. 1999) and improved neurocognitive function. In a study involving subjects with HIV dementia, improvements in neurocognitive function and as shown by MRI were demonstrated in subjects receiving HAART with PIs, but not in subjects receiving only double NRTIs (Filippi et al. 1998). Many of the subjects were taking ritonavir and/or saquinavir, both of which have been shown not to penetrate the CSF well (Gisolf et al. 1999), and these patients still showed improvement in cognition, presumably because of improved systemic status. To date, no studies have compared different HAART regimens with respect to reversing cognitive symptoms, and although it makes intuitive sense to use brain-penetrating antiretrovirals, there are no data to suggest that regimens that better penetrate the CSF have an advantage in terms of either reversing dementia or preventing its onset or progression.

Although antiretroviral therapy is the first-line treatment for HIV-related cognitive impairment, agents that protect the neurons or enhance the function of neurons may have an important adjunctive role. These agents may work by affecting the neuropathophysiologic mechanisms set into motion by brain viral replication and thought to underlie the cognitive impairment. Evidence for efficacy of any of these agents is sparse (Vitiello 1998), and none are used routinely in clinical care at present. Peptide T is thought to protect neurons by blocking binding of gp120 and has been reported to inhibit gp120-induced neuronal killing in vitro (Pert et al. 1988). A 6-month double-blind, placebo-controlled study of peptide T (2 mg tid intranasally) conducted in the pre-HAART era found no significant difference between peptide T and placebo in terms of improvement in neurocognitive function (Heseltine et al. 1998). Post hoc analyses suggested that peptide T had some advantage in the most cognitively impaired subjects. Its benefit in patients treated with HAART is unclear, and peptide T has not found its way into widespread routine clinical care for HIV dementia. The calcium-channel antagonist nimodipine has in vitro activity against gp120-mediated neuronal toxicity (Dreyer et al. 1990), and nimodipine therapy has also been evaluated as a potential treatment for HIV dementia. A Phase I/II study of nimodipine versus placebo found that nimodipine had no significant impact on neuropsychological function (Navia et al. 1998). Memantine, an N-methyl-D-aspartate (NMDA)–glutamate antagonist that also exhibits in vitro activity against gp120-mediated neuronal toxicity (Lipton 1992a), is currently being evaluated in a clinical trial (Lenkinski et al. 1998). Cholinesterase inhibitors (e.g., donepezil) used to enhance cognitive function in patients with Alzheimer's disease may have a theoretical benefit in HIV dementia, but as of yet, no data are available to support their clinical use.

Symptomatic treatment with psychopharmacological medications is an important aspect of management. Specific syndromes, including delirium, psychosis, depression, and manic disorders, warrant specific evaluation and management, with attention paid to the possible direct contribution attributable to CNS HIV infection. Cognitive symptoms—particularly poor concentration and attention, but also dysphoria, apathy, and anergia—may improve with administration of a stimulant, either dextroamphetamine or methylphenidate (Fernandez et al. 1988). A recent single-blind, placebo-controlled study of methylphenidate 30 mg/day found that methylphenidate improved cognitive slowing associated with HIV disease (Hinkin et al. 1999). The effect on cognitive slowing was seen only in patients with more severe slowing or affective symptomatology.

Behavior Therapy and Psychotherapy

Although HAART has decreased the incidence of new HIV dementia, it has also increased the prevalence of living with HIV dementia. Many HIV dementia patients receiving HAART have experienced immune reconstitution with only partial improvement of brain function. To continue to benefit from HAART, these patients often need high levels of home care—for their safety, for help with cognitive retraining, and for enhancement of adherence to HAART. Psychosocial interventions and support for the patient and caregivers (Green and Kocsis 1988; Taylor and Lavallee 1989) are crucial. Behavioral management and cognitive retraining may be helpful (J. Levy and Fernandez 1993) and must become better developed. Strategies include developing cues to maintain and redirect attention, developing skills to monitor behavior and reduce stimulation when necessary, and using tasks that maintain mental activity but are limited in complexity to avoid frustration. In situations in which the HIV-related cognitive impairment has had substantial impact on executive function, external structures will need to be put in place to ensure patient safety, and transfer to supervised housing may be necessary (Clarke et al. 1993).

DELIRIUM

Delirium is the neuropsychiatric complication that occurs most frequently in hospitalized patients with AIDS (Bialer et al. 1996; Fernandez et al. 1989). Patients with advanced systemic disease and HIV dementia are at high risk for delirium, the cause of which is often multifactorial (Table 36–8). A sudden change in mental status should not be ascribed to HIV dementia alone and is more frequently the result of other "organic" causes superimposed on a brain vulnerable to insult. In the management of delirium, the primary goal is identification and treatment of the underlying factors. In patients who are in more advanced stages of immunosuppression, including those in long-term care facilities, there must be a high index of suspicion for opportunistic infections, both systemic and intracranial, as well as metabolic derangements. These patients are often being treated with multiple medications, which may complicate the picture. Specific medications associated with delirium include narcotics, benzodiazepines, anticholinergics, antihistamines, and steroids (Uldall and Berghuis 1997). The need for ancillary investigations, including anatomic brain imaging, electroencephalography, CSF examination, and laboratory blood tests, is guided by clinical examination.

Symptomatic treatment with neuroleptics may be necessary to control agitation and help resolve confusion. Patients generally respond to daily doses of neuroleptic drugs equivalent to 0.5–5.0 mg of haloperidol. Patients with HIV disease are at increased risk for neuroleptic-induced extrapyramidal side effects (Hriso et al. 1991); hence, the minimum neuroleptic dose necessary to control target symptoms should be used. Newer atypical antipsychotic agents, including olanzapine (2.5–10 mg), may be very helpful in managing delirium while limiting extrapyramidal side effects. In a double-blind study in which hospitalized patients with AIDS were given haloperidol, chlorpromazine, or lorazepam for delirium, low doses of neuroleptics (either haloperidol or chlorpromazine) helped reduce symptoms of delirium; treatment with lorazepam had to be discontinued because of worsening symptoms (Breitbart et al. 1996a). Benzodiazepines should not be used as single agents in the treatment of patients with delirium, except in the case of alcohol or sedative/hypnotic withdrawal delirium. Lorazepam may also be a useful adjunct to treatment with neuroleptics, particularly in very agitated patients in whom sedation is desirable. Because the symptoms of delirium can be frightening or disturbing for patients, their friends, and family, a brief clarifying explanation can be very reassuring to all parties.

MOOD DISORDERS

Mania

An acute manic episode in a patient with HIV infection may be the result of primary bipolar disorder, or it may be a medication side effect or an HIV CNS effect or be due to a metabolic insult or a CNS opportunistic condition associated with severe immunosuppression. Reported precipitants of HIV-related mania include HIV dementia (Halman et al. 1993a; Kieburtz et al. 1991b; Smith et al. 1992); CNS opportunistic infections such as toxoplasmosis cerebritis, or cryptococcal meningitis; CNS opportunistic tumors from non-Hodgkin's lymphoma (Halman et al. 1993a; Johannessen and Wilson 1988); and side effects of medications, including antiretroviral agents such

TABLE 36–8. Differential etiologies of delirium in the patient with HIV infection

Anemia

Drug intoxication
  Alcohol
  Antibiotics
  Anticholinergics, including antidepressants
  Anticonvulsants
  Antineoplastics
  Cocaine
  Opiates
  Phencyclidine
  Sedative-hypnotics

Endocrine disorders and vitamin deficiencies
  Addison's disease
  Thyroid disease
  Vitamin B_{12} insufficiency

Head trauma

Hypoglycemia (of particular concern in patients receiving systemic pentamidine or in patients with new-onset impaired glucose control or diabetes)

Hypotension

Infections
  Systemic
  Bacteremia
    Disseminated herpes zoster, *Mycobacterium avium-intracellulare*, and candidiasis
    Pneumonia
    Septicemia
    Subacute bacterial endocarditis
  Intracranial
    CMV encephalitis
    Cryptococcal meningitis
    Neurosyphilis
    Progressive multifocal leukoencephalopathy
    Toxoplasmosis
    Tubercular meningitis

Intracranial neoplasms
  Metastatic Kaposi's sarcoma (rarely)
  Primary lymphoma

Metabolic encephalopathies
  Acidosis
  Alkalosis
  Dehydration
  Hepatic, renal, pulmonary, adrenal, and pancreatic insufficiency
  Hypernatremia, hyponatremia
  Hypocalcemia
  Hypomagnesemia
  Hypoxia
  Water intoxication

Psychoactive substance withdrawal syndromes

Seizure disorder

Note. CMV = cytomegalovirus.

as AZT and lamivudine (see Table 36–5). Periods of irritability and hypomania have been associated with HIV dementia (Smith et al. 1992), and patients with HIV dementia and significant frontal lobe disruption may present with some features of a manic episode, including behavioral disturbances, impulsivity, disinhibition, mood instability, and poor judgment.

The prevalence of mania in HIV disease has been estimated to be 1.4% (Lyketsos et al. 1993b), and the prevalence increases with HIV disease progression. Patients with new-onset mania at more advanced stages of systemic disease often have evidence of comorbid HIV dementia (Mijch et al. 1998), often have no personal or family history of a mood disorder, and are more likely to have a secondary or organic manic syndrome. By contrast, patients presenting with a manic syndrome early in HIV disease are likely to have a personal and/or family history of mood disorders, are less likely to have comorbid neuropsychological impairments of HIV dementia, and more closely resemble patients with a primary bipolar illness (Lyketsos et al. 1993b). New-onset mania in an HIV-infected patient should be considered secondary mania until proven otherwise, and the evaluation must include anatomic brain imaging and, particularly in the immunosuppressed patient (CD4$^+$ count ≤200 cells/mL), CSF examination, to exclude CNS opportunistic conditions.

Treatment and Management

In many respects, the most important parts of management are an awareness that a manic episode is a treatable condition and the recognition that a severe manic episode may necessitate aggressive psychiatric interventions, including treatment with medication and application of restraints, to establish safety for the patient and his or her surroundings and permit completion of appropriate organic evaluations. In a recent study, psychiatric hospitalization was found to be common for this group of patients, but survival did not differ from that of a nonmanic HIV-positive control group (Mijch et al. 1998). Dialogue between the patient and medical and psychiatric treatment teams is essential as complex issues including restraint, consent, and aggressivity of intervention are negotiated.

Standard treatment with neuroleptics and lithium can be effective, but the usefulness of these agents may be restricted by the development of dose-limiting adverse side effects, particularly in patients with advanced HIV disease and CNS involvement. In one study, failure to respond to standard treatment with lithium and haloperidol was predicted by MRI abnormalities, but all treatment-resistant or treatment-intolerant patients re-

sponded to anticonvulsants (Halman et al. 1993a). Lithium toxicity, including encephalopathy, may develop despite normal therapeutic blood levels (Tanquary 1993). Dehydration, diarrhea, and poor oral intake necessitate careful monitoring of lithium levels, and extra caution must be exercised when indinavir is prescribed; patients taking this PI must drink large volumes of water to prevent drug crystallization in the kidneys. Neuroleptics are often necessary in the acute treatment of patients with manic syndromes. Because patients with advanced HIV disease or evidence of brain pathology are sensitive to extrapyramidal side effects (Halman et al. 1993a; Hriso et al. 1991) and are sensitive to hypotension and sedation associated with low-potency agents (Breitbart 1993), low daily doses of high- to medium-potency neuroleptics should be used (e.g., haloperidol 0.5–1.0 mg, perphenazine 4–24 mg, risperidone 1–2 mg). Olanzapine at doses as low as 2.5–5 mg may be very useful for reducing agitation with fewer problematic side effects.

Anticonvulsants are useful in patients with mania and may have a particular advantage in patients with advanced HIV disease. Divalproex sodium is generally effective and well tolerated (Halman et al. 1993a; Rach-Beisel and Weintraub 1997). A starting dose of 250–500 mg orally at bedtime is used, with increases of 250 mg/day every 2–4 days until symptomatic control is achieved, titrated against the emergence of side effects, using blood levels for seizure control as an approximate guideline. Liver function and hematological parameters, particularly platelets, need to be monitored. Valproic acid has been used safely with antiretrovirals, may raise AZT levels (Lertora et al. 1992), and does not appear to meaningfully alter metabolism of PIs or NNRTIs. Although carbamazepine can be effective for mania, its safe use in patients with HIV disease remains to be clarified, because these patients are at increased risk for hematological and dermatological complications. Through induction of hepatic P450 enzymes, carbamazepine decreases serum levels of coadministered drugs, including PIs, and may lead to subtherapeutic PI levels and loss of viral suppression. If carbamazepine is used with PIs or NNRTIs, consultation with the HIV medical treatment team and a pharmacist is imperative in order to determine whether PI dose alteration is necessary. Case reports have indicated that clonazepam and gabapentin can also be effective.

No studies have specifically addressed the length of time to continue mood-stabilizing treatment in HIV-infected patients presenting with a manic episode. Clinically, if a patient appears to have a primary bipolar disorder, he or she is encouraged to consider long-term prophylactic mood stabilization with tight control of mood symptoms. The patient must receive both psychoeducation about the nature of bipolar disorder and education about the safe use of antiretrovirals and mood-stabilizing agents. The impact of future manic episodes on adherence to antiretroviral therapy should also be explored, and strategies should be put in place to help maintain adherence even in the face of mood decompensation. Patients with organic manic syndromes should be stabilized and started on appropriate antiretroviral therapies. Antipsychotic medications may be tapered after the first 2–4 weeks of stable mood; anticonvulsants may be tapered after 6 months. Patients with HIV dementia complicated by mood symptoms and behavioral disturbance may need to continue taking anticonvulsants indefinitely.

In vitro studies have demonstrated that valproic acid stimulates an increase in HIV viral replication. The clinical relevance of this discovery remains uncertain, but the finding is a concern for patients with HIV infection and bipolar disorder and illustrates the complexity of drug interactions in this field. A recent retrospective analysis found that in patients receiving HAART with full viral load suppression, the addition of divalproex sodium did not lead to viral breakthrough and loss of suppression (Maggi and Halman 2001). A prospective study is currently under way to determine the clinical relevance of the in vitro findings and confirm the observations of the retrospective study.

Major Depression

Depressed mood occurs frequently in patients with HIV disease, and depression is a common reason for psychiatric consultation. An accurate diagnosis is essential, given the wide range of diagnostic possibilities and the wide range of effective therapeutic options, including conventional and adjuvant antidepressant pharmacotherapy, correction of physiologic parameters that may contribute to organic mood disorders, and psychotherapies.

The stage of HIV disease should be considered when evaluating a patient for depression. As HIV disease progresses, the clinician's index of suspicion for secondary mood disorders should increase. Many patients are at increased risk for major depression at various nodal points throughout their illness, but major depression is not a natural consequence of HIV disease. The consultation-liaison psychiatrist may frequently observe health care workers rationalizing depression as a reasonable response to developing a fatal illness, identifying with a patient's nihilism, and failing to accurately diagnose or to offer treatment. Withholding treatment for depression may add to a patient's suffering and emotional pain. The differential diagnosis of depression is outlined in Table 36–9.

TABLE 36–9. Differential diagnosis of depressed mood

Adjustment disorder with depressed mood
Anger
Apathy and fatigue due to advanced systemic disease
Apathy due to HIV-associated dementia
Bipolar disorder, depressed phase
Despondency/Demoralization
Dysthymic disorder
Major depressive episode, unipolar; single or recurrent
Psychoactive substance use disorder
Secondary mood disorder (CNS or systemic disease, drug therapy)
Unresolved grief and bereavement

Note. CNS = central nervous system.

Epidemiology

Major depression is diagnosed in 1.4%–15% of hospitalized patients with HIV/AIDS seen by consultation-liaison psychiatrists (Bialer et al. 1996; Buhrich and Cooper 1987; Dilley et al. 1985; O'Dowd and McKegney 1990) and in 8%–33% of ambulatory patients referred for psychiatric evaluation (Hintz et al. 1990; O'Dowd et al. 1993; Worth et al. 1993). In one study involving 37 ambulatory patients who consented to a structured interview at the time of their initial medical evaluation, major depression or dysthymia was diagnosed in 44% (McDaniel et al. 1995). Community-based cohort studies in the United States have shown rates of current major depression at 4%–18% among gay or bisexual men in early stages of HIV disease (Atkinson et al. 1988; Brown et al. 1992; Williams et al. 1991) and 9%–35% among HIV-infected patients who use injection drugs (Kosten 1993; Rabkin et al. 1997). Many studies based in the United States may underestimate the prevalence of major depression and other Axis I disorders because self-selected samples of well-educated, middle-class, primarily white men are used (Maj et al. 1994b). Some groups at high risk for HIV disease, including gay or bisexual men, also appear to have a high premorbid risk of major depression (Atkinson et al. 1988; Perkins et al. 1994; Williams et al. 1991) and individuals who use injection drugs (Kosten 1993). A recent meta-analysis reports that rates of major depression are at least twice the rates seen in the general population (Ciesla and Roberts 2001).

Contributing factors to major depression may include psychosocial stressors related to HIV disease, the effects of systemic HIV disease on the CNS, and HIV CNS infection. Psychosocial factors found to be associated with major depression in HIV-infected patients include unemployment (Hoover et al. 1992), lower level of education (Bornstein et al. 1993; Lyketsos et al.

1993a), unresolved grief and multiple losses (Gluhoski et al. 1997; Sciolla et al. 1992), history of mood disorders (Atkinson et al. 1994; Lyketsos et al. 1996), and psychoactive substance–related disorders.

Systemic HIV disease and its treatments, particularly as the disease progresses, may also contribute to major depression. Several medications used in the treatment of HIV disease may cause depression (see Table 36–5). In a large-scale longitudinal study, Lyketsos et al. (1996) observed a significant increase in depressive symptoms as HIV disease progressed to AIDS, and several studies have found depression to be associated with HIV-related symptoms (Hays et al. 1992; Lyketsos et al. 1993a; Maj et al. 1994a). Depression and HIV-associated cognitive disorders often coexist and, like other disorders with subcortical pathology, often involve affective disturbances, including apathy, anergia, and dysphoria. Apathy independent of major depression is common in late-stage HIV disease, is associated with working memory impairment, and may be an indicator of CNS HIV involvement (Castellon et al. 1998).

Endocrinological and metabolic disturbances may complicate advanced stages of HIV disease and contribute to depressive symptomatology. These disturbances include adrenocortical insufficiency (Abbott et al. 1993), thyroid function abnormalities (Bélec et al. 1993; Grunfeld et al. 1993), vitamin B_{12} deficiency (Beach et al. 1992), hypogonadism and low testosterone levels (Grinspoon and Bilezikian 1992), and protein and calorie malnutrition (Süttmann et al. 1993).

Diagnosis

As systemic HIV disease progresses, symptoms of depression, including insomnia and poor appetite (Hintz et al. 1990; Williams et al. 1991), that occur may be due to the mood disorder or to HIV disease or its treatments. Determining whether a symptom is due to depression or to HIV disease is often impossible, even after examining temporal relationships of symptom onset. An inclusive attribution system, wherein a symptom is counted as a criterion for major depression even in the presence of a medical disorder, will allow most cases of major depression to be detected and is usually the most pragmatic approach.

Bereavement and Unresolved Grief

Many persons with HIV/AIDS live in socially circumscribed communities (Woodhouse et al. 1994) with a high prevalence of HIV disease and as such have experienced multiple losses because of HIV disease. Repeated bereavement has psychiatric and social implications for patients with HIV disease and at-risk communities. Mul-

tiple and frequent bereavements may not allow time for adequate grieving, and the risk of unresolved grief appears to be increasing among homosexual men with HIV disease (Gluhoski et al. 1997). Compared with those with resolved grief, men with unresolved grief had higher rates of major depression and panic disorder, higher levels of depression and anxiety, and lower levels of social support. Addressing issues of grief, bereavement, and multiple loss is an important component of treating major depression in this population.

Treatment and Management

Pharmacotherapy. Pharmacotherapy is effective for most patients with HIV-related major depression and is well tolerated. In more systemically advanced patients, there is greater need to start at low doses and increase doses slowly, but it is also important not to undertreat because of systemic illness. Whereas psychotherapy and pharmacotherapy may be equally effective in mild to moderate major depression, pharmacotherapy is superior in severe major depression and should be strongly recommended (Rabkin et al. 1999). In all treatments, a combination of pharmacotherapy and psychotherapy may prove most effective in reducing symptoms, limiting relapse, and fostering psychological adaptation to illness.

Laboratory tests. Before antidepressant therapy is initiated, baseline blood tests should be performed. They include a complete blood count; determination of electrolyte, fasting glucose, thyroid-stimulating hormone, vitamin B_{12}, and free testosterone levels; liver function tests; and, if tricyclics are being considered, electrocardiography.

Selective serotonin reuptake inhibitors. The SSRIs fluoxetine (Hintz et al. 1990; Levine et al. 1990; Rabkin et al. 1999), paroxetine (Elliot et al. 1998), and sertraline (Rabkin et al. 1994b) are generally effective for HIV-related major depression and are well tolerated in patients with advanced HIV disease (Ferrando et al. 1997). In an 8-week double-blind, placebo-controlled trial, Rabkin et al. (1999) found a 57% rate of response to fluoxetine therapy in an intent-to-treat analysis and a 74% response rate among those who completed treatment (vs. rates of 41% and 47%, respectively, for subjects receiving placebo). Elliot et al. (1998) demonstrated the effectiveness of both paroxetine and imipramine compared with placebo in a randomized study; however, paroxetine appeared to be better tolerated.

Although drug interactions can occur between SSRIs (particularly fluvoxamine) and some antiretrovirals because of competition for P450 3A3/3A4 metabolism (Ereshefsky et al. 1996), these interactions appear to be clinically insignificant (Bialer et al. 1998). SSRIs should be given at low doses at first. Fluoxetine and paroxetine should be started at dosages of 10 mg/day and increased to standard doses after 7–10 days. Citalopram has little interaction with P450 3A3/3A4 and may also be a useful choice, starting at 10 mg/day. Side effects and potential drug interactions should be explained, and dose increases should be titrated to balance antidepressant effect against side effects. In general, HIV-positive patients can be treated at standard dose ranges. Decreased libido, difficulty maintaining an erection, and difficulty achieving an orgasm are dose-dependent side effects of all SSRIs and can be intolerable or dose-limiting for many. Gastrointestinal side effects, dry mouth, headache, and anxiety are also frequently reported and generally subside 7–10 days after a dose increase. Because of good antidepressant effect and good tolerability, SSRI therapy has emerged as a first-line antidepressant treatment in depressed HIV-positive patients.

Tricyclic antidepressants. TCAs have been found to be effective in patients with HIV infection. In a double-blind, placebo-controlled trial, Rabkin et al. (1994a) noted a 74% response rate among patients with HIV infection who received imipramine, compared with a response rate of 26% among placebo-treated control subjects. Imipramine had no adverse effects on studied aspects of immune function (Rabkin et al. 1991). In more systemically advanced patients, the hypotension, sedation, and anticholinergic side effects (including confusion) associated with TCA therapy can be problematic. Treatment should be initiated at the lowest dose available, with titration upward every 2–3 days as tolerated, until normal therapeutic doses are reached. Serum levels of tricyclics should be monitored when they are coadministered with ritonavir. Increased serum levels of desipramine have been reported in patients taking ritonavir and may be related to inhibition of P450 2D6. If ritonavir is being added to a stable regimen of desipramine (or, theoretically, other TCAs, including amitriptyline, clomipramine, doxepin, imipramine, and nortriptyline), reduction of the TCA dose by one-third to one-half should be considered, to avoid TCA-related toxicity. There appear to be no clinically meaningful drug interactions between the tricyclics and other antiretrovirals, although in theory, interactions may occur to a lesser degree with other PIs and NNRTIs.

Other antidepressants. Venlafaxine appears to interact little with HIV medications and may be a good choice in

this population (Ereshefsky 1996). Nausea is a common and potentially problematic side effect in patients with HIV/AIDS, so administering starting doses of 37.5 mg once daily with sustained-release formulation is recommended. Nefazodone is also a useful choice. It has less impact on sexual function and has sedating properties, which make it appealing for many HIV-positive patients. It is, however, a potent inhibitor of P450 3A3/3A4 and may have clinically significant interactions with the PIs and other antivirals that are metabolized by this enzyme, so close attention to dosing and side effects is needed. Bupropion may be particularly helpful for patients with significant apathy and fatigue (Fernandez and Levy 1991) and is appealing because its use is associated with less sexual dysfunction. Because of theoretical concerns over inhibition of P450 enzymes involved in metabolism of bupropion and the relative ease with which toxic levels of bupropion are reached, there is considerable concern over the coadministration of ritonavir and bupropion. The clinical impact of this interaction is unclear. Currently, the ritonavir product monograph lists this combination as a contraindication, whereas the buproprion monograph lists it as a precaution. Bupropion has been used successfully with other antiviral agents.

Adjuvant treatments, including stimulants. Stimulants are not first-line agents for major depression, but at low doses in open trials, both dextroamphetamine (Holmes et al. 1989) and methylphenidate were effective for HIV-related major depression, as primary agents (Fernandez and Levy 1991; Holmes et al. 1989) or adjuvant agents (Rabkin 1993). The response rate associated with these agents has been shown to be up to 80%. Stimulants are especially effective for anergia and apathy, but some patients also report improvement in mood, attention, and concentration. Stimulants may be particularly helpful in patients with a predominance of apathy versus sadness and in patients who are unable to tolerate the side effects of conventional antidepressants. A recent study has demonstrated the benefit of stimulants for fatigue in patients with HIV/AISDS (Breitbart et al. 2001).

Stimulants have short half-lives and rapid onsets of action, allowing quick assessment of efficacy and tolerability. Treatment should begin with a morning dose of 5 mg, and the dose should be increased by 5 mg every 1–2 days until a good response is achieved or until dose-limiting side effects occur. A second midday dose, usually half the morning dose, may be needed to sustain a clinical effect throughout the afternoon, or the sustained-release formulation can be used. The usual daily dose range is 20–40 mg, and higher doses are unlikely to elicit a greater response. At low doses, stimulants are generally well tolerated and may stimulate appetite. Some patients experience a dose-dependent feeling of being "wired" or "nervous," and doses taken later than 1:00 P.M. may interfere with nighttime sleep.

Stimulant abuse is uncommon in patients who have no history of substance-related disorders. A history of substance dependence does not contraindicate the use of stimulants but does present the need for increased caution in their use and necessitates an open exploration of the psychological impact on the patient of taking a controlled substance. It is beneficial to establish a clear contract for usage so that the patient is aware of the parameters of safe, therapeutic uses and to prevent the unlimited and escalating drug use that is characteristic of abuse patterns.

Decreased serum testosterone levels can also produce depressive symptoms and may explain some cases of treatment-resistant depression in patients with HIV disease. At least one study has demonstrated improved mood in men with HIV receiving testosterone replacement therapy (Rabkin et al. 1995). Other conventional augmentation strategies, including cytomel, lithium, and SSRI-TCA combinations used in treating major depression, may also be used in HIV-positive patients. Psychiatrists should consider the relatively unique contributions that standard, augmentation, and adjuvant antidepressant strategies can bring to the treatment regimen (Wagner et al. 1996).

Electroconvulsive therapy.   Schaerf et al. (1989) reported the successful use of electroconvulsive therapy (ECT) in four patients: three with asymptomatic HIV infection and one with AIDS. Organic contributions and CNS HIV disease must be ruled out before ECT is performed. Because of the potential impact of ECT on cognitive function, pre-ECT neurocognitive test results should be assessed.

Psychotherapy.   Psychotherapy is widely used for treatment of depression and psychological distress. Research has been limited in this area, in part because of the complexity of psychotherapy studies and the high dropout rates in these studies. All psychotherapies are used clinically, and success is dependent on patient-therapist and patient-modality fits.

In a 16-week study, 101 ambulatory patients with HIV disease and depressive symptoms received interpersonal therapy, imipramine with supportive therapy, supportive therapy alone, or cognitive-behavioral therapy (Markowitz et al. 1998). The dropout rate was 32%, highlighting the importance of good patient-modality fit. Interpersonal therapy and imipramine plus supportive

therapy resulted in greater symptom reduction on Hamilton and Beck depression inventories than did supportive therapy alone and cognitive-behavioral therapy. The authors hypothesized that interpersonal therapy, with its connection to the impact of life events, may have a particular advantage, given the losses incurred by many patients with HIV disease. Although these findings need replication, particularly in the era of HAART, the study is important in that the findings challenge psychiatrists to discern which modalities and aspects of psychotherapy are most advantageous to which patients, and what works best in helping patients recover from depression.

SUICIDE

Suicidal ideation is a frequent reason for psychiatric consultation for the hospitalized patient with HIV/AIDS (Alfonso et al. 1994). In general, patients with AIDS are at increased risk for suicide. Coté et al. (1992) reported that in 1987–1989, suicide was 7.4 times more likely among men with AIDS than among demographically similar men without AIDS. These rates have decreased over time, possibly reflecting changing community attitudes and a greater sense of hope that comes with treatment advances. Two recent studies indicated that HIV seropositivity in and of itself (as opposed to clinical AIDS) may be associated with a risk of suicide that is approximately two times that in the general population (Dannenberg et al. 1996; Marzuk et al. 1997). In the study by Marzuk et al. (1997), 25% of all black or Hispanic men between ages 35 and 44 years who committed suicide during the study period were HIV-seropositive, as were 19% of all black or Hispanic women ages 25–44 years who committed suicide during that time.

Factors such as age, ethnicity, psychiatric disorders, comorbid substance-related disorders, systemic HIV disease, social support, and coping styles must all be considered in the evaluation of suicidal ideation. Populations at highest risk for HIV disease may also have increased rates of suicidal ideation and suicide. It is unclear whether gay or bisexual men have increased rates of suicidal ideation or suicide, but gay youths appear to be at high risk (Department of Health and Human Services 1990; Remafedi and Farrow 1991). B. Kelly et al. (1998) reported lifetime suicide attempt rates of 29.1% and 21.4%, respectively, in a sample of HIV-negative and HIV-positive gay and bisexual men interviewed between 1989 and 1992. Similarly, individuals who use injection drugs, regardless of HIV status, have high rates of both suicide and accidental drug overdose (Smythe et al. 1992).

HIV disease stage and the personal experience the patient has had with HIV disease as an epidemic should be evaluated. In a study involving HIV-infected military personnel who attempted suicide, Rundell et al. (1992) identified several risk factors for suicide attempts (see Table 36–10). Of the population studied, 44% used alcohol during an attempt, 44% made an attempt in the first 6 months after positive HIV serological test results had been obtained, and 22% made a second suicide attempt, all within 6 months of the first attempt. Uncertainty of illness course, anxiety over prognosis (Marzuk et al. 1988), and grief and bereavement (Gorman et al. 1992) may contribute to suicidal ideation (Chuang et al. 1989; O'Dowd et al. 1993). In the study by B. Kelly et al. (1998), current suicidal ideation among HIV-positive men was associated with greater hopelessness, with having a greater number of current AIDS diagnoses, and with lower fighting spirit. Highest suicidal ideation scores were associated with current major depression and current anxiety disorder diagnoses.

Treatment and Management

Patients with underlying Axis I disorders must receive treatment for those disorders, because depression and substance-related disorders are key treatable factors associated with suicide. Understanding the breakdown in a patient's ability to cope and to effectively use social supports is essential to processing suicidal ideation, as is understanding the patient's loss of hope and his or her feeling of disconnection from the human world. Illness factors including pain, fatigue, nausea, and loss of autonomy need to be addressed. Complex feelings of sadness, fear, and anger may be overwhelming for some patients as they consider the reality of their lives with HIV disease or anticipate the future. Treatment must ensure patient safety, support the processing of complex feelings, keep fears within realistic contexts, and foster reconnection with natural supports. Psychotherapy and pharmacotherapy, legal and social services, home health services, and community-based AIDS service agencies may all have a role in relieving a patient's underlying pain and suffering and enhancing his or her autonomy. Ensuring patient safety and contracting with the patient to use crisis services and emergency departments as needed are essential first steps in management.

Treatment refusal, end-of-life decisions, and physician-assisted suicide are complex issues that are associated with HIV/AIDS, and contributing psychiatric factors, particularly depression, must be assessed in HIV/AIDS patients. The prevalence of physician-assisted suicide among these patients is unclear, but in one study,

TABLE 36–10.   Risk factors for suicide in HIV-infected persons

Social isolation
Perception of poor social support
HIV-related occupational problems
Abandonment
Stigmatization
Financial difficulty
Comorbidity: psychiatric disorders and substance abuse

55% of HIV-infected patients surveyed considered this as an option for themselves (Breitbart et al. 1996b). A survey of gay men whose partners had died from AIDS indicated that 12.1% of the patients had received an increase in their medications with the intention of hastening death (Cooke et al. 1998). Euthanasia and physician-assisted suicide account for 13%–21% of all AIDS deaths in the Netherlands (see Starace and Sherr 1998 for a review of suicide and euthanasia in AIDS). Thinking about suicide as an option commonly represents issues of fear and anger about the patient's projected quality of life rather than true suicidal ideation. Psychotherapy allows the patient to talk about these fears, which helps to dissipate feelings of isolation and abandonment and allows the processing of incurred losses.

ADJUSTMENT DISORDERS AND COPING

Coping with HIV disease—that is, managing aspects of HIV disease cognitively, behaviorally, and affectively—is an important variable in overall health management. Several factors, including psychological distress, psychiatric disorders, personality variables, the ability to express affects, social support, and interpersonal ties, interact and influence how people cope (Grassi et al. 1998). Patients with adjustment disorders often present to their primary care physicians or to counselors or peer supports at community AIDS service organizations, but a sizable number are also referred for psychiatric consultation. Between 29% and 69% of ambulatory patients referred for psychiatric evaluation have adjustment disorders (O'Dowd et al. 1993; Worth and Halman 1993), and screening for adjustment and coping should become a routine part of HIV care.

During the course of their illness, patients with HIV disease encounter many crisis points that may provoke an adjustment disorder (Dilley and Forstein 1990; Nichols 1985). These include HIV serological testing (S. Perry et al. 1990, 1991), disclosure of serological status to sexual partners and friends (Hays et al. 1993; Marks et al. 1991), initiation of antiretroviral treatment, progression of disease and symptoms (Atkinson et al. 1988; Chuang et al. 1989; Hays et al. 1992), and diagnosis of the first AIDS-defining condition (Joseph et al. 1993). Disease-specific themes affecting coping that are more recent include stresses surrounding medication regimen adherence, fear over losing viral suppression, distress over side effects, distress over failure to attain viral suppression, and distress that comes with accepting the uncertainties that still exist in the management of HIV disease.

Although much of the variance in depressive symptoms and distress can be explained by mood disorders and HIV-related symptoms, a significant amount of variance can be explained by coping styles (Atkinson et al. 1993; Folkman et al. 1993). Active behavioral coping has been found to be associated with lower mood disturbance (Namir et al. 1987), and avoidant coping has been found to be associated with higher distress (Krikorian et al. 1995). Personality factors have important bearing on coping. An Axis II disorder may increase the risk of poor psychological adaptation (Perkins et al. 1993). The inability to manage affects, particularly the inability to manage anger, has been associated with poorer coping and increased depressive symptoms (Grassi et al. 1998). Finally, social support and the patient's perception of his or her supports and interpersonal connections affect adjustment to HIV disease (Packenham et al. 1994).

Enhancing coping and adjustment has importance on many levels. From a psychoimmunological perspective, severe stress has been associated with disease progression and poorer immunological function in patients with depressive symptoms and poor coping (Evans et al. 1997; Goodkin et al. 1992). From a risk-reduction perspective, the risk of unprotected anal intercourse among gay men was found in one study to be positively associated with a coping style that involved keeping one's feelings to oneself (Folkman et al. 1992). Drug regimen adherence has been found to be negatively associated with depressive symptoms and distress (Chesney and Ickovics 1997). Finally, with respect to suicidal ideation, B. Kelly et al. (1998) found higher suicidal ideation to be associated with poorer coping as defined by greater hopelessness and lower fighting spirit, independent of HIV-related illness factors and personality characteristics.

Treatment

Many patients will be able to identify the important psychosocial stressors that have precipitated an adjustment disorder, although some patients will present simply as

being overwhelmed and not knowing where to turn. Provision of information about HIV disease, treatments, and community resources and provision of psychoeducation are integral to helping patients cope. Shame, fear of stigmatization, and discomfort in dealing with negative affects such as depression or anger can lead some patients to turn inward and withdraw from natural support systems, avoid using community support services, or become avoidant in the management of their illness. It is often helpful to patients with newly diagnosed disease to emphasize the need to allow time for healing and to be clear that this span of time may be a year or more, as pieces fall into place and these patients start to believe that they can in fact live with HIV infection.

Despite changes in illness course, medical advances, and changing mental health care systems, the backbone of adjusting to HIV disease and supporting coping is still counseling, peer support, and psychotherapies. Finding the right fit for each patient remains integral to providing support, and using an array of services and an eclectic range of interventions is necessary because individuals and circumstances differ so widely. Referral to appropriate community resources may help the patient obtain information and gain access to activities and new social supports such as the "buddy system" (Velentgas et al. 1990). In a community-based study involving gay men with HIV disease, Hays et al. (1992) found that satisfaction with social supports, including emotional, informational, and practical supports, correlated with lower levels of depression. For symptomatic patients, informational support—that is, provision of information about HIV disease and available treatments—appeared to be the most effective form of social support for buffering against depression.

Beyond provision of information, interventions should help patients reconnect with supports, manage intense affects, and work through often long-standing dynamic issues that may affect their disease and health management. HIV disease frequently stimulates old feelings of guilt, humiliation, and shame and prompts reexamination of old conflicts over identity and self-esteem. Similarly, the threat of illness might intensify the desire to resolve issues that to that point have been barriers to the formation of satisfactory intimate relationships. Intense affects of anger and sadness experienced over the course of the disease may be processed within the safety of a consistent, empathic, and trusting psychotherapeutic relationship; such processing will help patients avoid burning out friends and family on whom they may feel that they are becoming a burden. Psychotherapy may help to ease feelings of abandonment and isolation and help patients to maintain confidence in their interpersonal connections. Finally, psychotherapy may help patients examine important existential issues precipitated by the threat of illness.

Group psychotherapies and peer support groups have been extensively used since the beginning of the AIDS epidemic. Rapid development of group cohesion appears to be achieved when the group is demographically homogeneous, particularly with respect to exposure risk factor and gender (Beckett and Rutan 1990). Universality, group cohesiveness, and instillation of hope have been rated as the most potent therapeutic factors in different groups (Halman et al. 1993b; Prager et al. 1992). Countertransference issues can be marked (G. Bernstein and Klein 1995), and clinical supervision or consultation can be very helpful. Sikkema et al. (1992) and Summers et al. (1993) reported that short-term cognitive-behavioral group psychotherapy effectively reduced psychological distress and depression in individuals with AIDS-related bereavement, and Goodkin et al. (1998) found that 10 weeks of participation in a bereavement support group had a beneficial impact on CD4 count in gay men who had lost a partner or close friend in the past 6 months. In a randomized study involving patients with asymptomatic HIV disease and mild to moderate depressive symptoms, Targ et al. (1994) found that short-term, structured group therapy plus treatment with fluoxetine or with placebo resulted in similar reductions in levels of depression.

Family and Caregiver Support

The psychosocial demands on the domestic caregivers of patients with HIV disease can be significant, leading to burnout and depression (Folkman et al. 1994; van den Bloom and Gremmen 1992). Compared with patients, families may be less informed about the availability of support services, leading to even greater isolation and distress. Families often receive dual disclosures from patients—the diagnosis of HIV disease and the patients' HIV-risk behaviors—and are forced to confront their own fears and prejudices. Acceptance is often best predicted by the quality of the premorbid relationship. Persistent fears and intolerance may prevent families from effectively using available services and information. Other sources of support, such as religious advisers, may be easier for them to access than counselors at AIDS service organizations.

Family therapy interventions (Walker 1987) include 1) providing accurate information about HIV disease and about access to resource centers; 2) assisting families in processing a wide range of affects, including guilt, shame, fear, betrayal, anger, and sadness; 3) diminishing isolation by working through feelings of stigmatization, often through the use of peer support groups; 4) supporting healthy forms of self-protective denial and encouraging hopefulness when appropriate; and 5) doing grief work. Often, the crisis raised by the threat of illness intensifies the family members' commitment to psychotherapy in an effort to resolve long-standing family conflicts.

Couples Psychotherapy

Partners and spouses of HIV-positive patients experience a multitude of feelings, including an overwhelming fear of relationship breakdown and family dissolution, as well as anticipation of loss. The initial acuity of illness may overshadow the degree of relationship conflict, but over time, communication blockages, feelings of betrayal, and an erosion of intimacy are common (Myers 1991). A couple's adaptation to HIV disease may be more complicated if one person is HIV-positive and the other is not, particularly if the noninfected partner thinks that he or she is at risk for infection (Dew et al. 1991). The goals of couples psychotherapy include improved communication about feelings such as fear, sadness, and anticipated bereavement and a return to a satisfying and safe intimate relationship. Models of therapy must acknowledge differences between homosexual and heterosexual couples (Friedman 1991). With the improvements in health status that have been brought about by HAART, some couples have shifted their focus from dealing with illness and preparing for early death to living with a chronic disease—a situation permitting longer-term goals and challenges in a relationship.

Pharmacotherapy

Short-term trials of anxiolytics can be very helpful while the patient initially engages in psychotherapy and begins to reestablish his or her psychological equilibrium. Judicious use of benzodiazepines to manage stress and anxiety is common and important. Close monitoring of prescriptions, psychoeducation about risks of tolerance, and reinforcement of the benefit of concomitant psychotherapeutic or support programs make it possible for anxiolytics to be used in most patients to diminish distress.

ANXIETY DISORDERS

Patients with HIV/AIDS can present with a range of anxiety syndromes, from short-term anxious mood accompanying an adjustment disorder to more severe anxiety states such as panic disorder, acute stress disorder, posttraumatic stress disorder, or obsessive-compulsive disorder. In community studies, the prevalence of anxiety disorders in HIV-infected individuals ranged from 2% (Williams et al. 1991) to 18% (Atkinson et al. 1988) in asymptomatic patients and was 38% in patients with symptomatic but non-AIDS-defining conditions (Atkinson et al. 1988) and 27% in patients with AIDS (Atkinson et al. 1988).

The overlap between anxiety disorders, adjustment disorders, and mood disorders is great. Many patients report that unpredictability of illness progression, preoccupation with viral loads and CD4$^+$ counts, uncertainty surrounding the investigations of new symptoms, and fears of isolation and abandonment provoke anxious feelings. Obsessive preoccupation with symptoms and laboratory markers of disease progression may occur, as may compulsive checking of the body. Rumination is a particularly common manifestation of psychological distress and may suggest an underlying mood disorder.

Treatment and Management

Psychotherapy and pharmacotherapy as discussed in the sections on adjustment disorders and mood disorders apply here. Cognitive and behavioral therapies, biofeedback, self-relaxation techniques, and acupuncture can be very useful. Judicious use of benzodiazepines is helpful when used acutely, and buspirone may be considered as a nonbenzodiazepine alternative, particularly when the patient has a history of a psychoactive substance–related disorder. When treating with benzodiazepines, the clinician should consider agents with short to intermediate half-lives at low daily doses: lorazepam 0.5–1 mg, temazepam 15 mg, clonazepam 0.5–1 mg, or oxazepam 15 mg. Agents that require metabolism by P450 3A3/3A4, such as diazepam or alprazolam, need to be used with caution when coadministered with PIs such as ritonavir, which is a potent inhibitor of P450 3A3/3A4; their coadministration can result in increased levels of the anxiolytic. High doses or increased plasma levels of benzodiazepines may place patients at risk for depressive symptoms, fatigue, and cognitive and motor side effects, particularly if patients have coexistent HIV dementia, MCMD, intracranial lesions, or delirium (Breitbart 1993). Patients should be informed of the risk of tolerance to and dependence on benzodiazepines, and patients' use of these agents should be closely monitored.

SSRIs are highly effective in managing anxiety disorders and should be used as first-line agents for treating panic disorder, obsessive-compulsive disorder, social phobia, and mixed anxiety and depression disorders. If the anxiety symptoms being treated are not simply temporary problems associated with adjustment, SSRIs

should be considered, particularly if symptoms are not fully resolving with psychotherapy or if benzodiazepine use is becoming prolonged.

SLEEP DISORDERS

Sleep complaints are reported by up to 70%–80% of patients with HIV disease (Prenzlauer et al. 1993; Rubinstein and Selwyn 1998). In addition to insomnia, fatigue is also a common problem in HIV disease. Management includes identification of coexistent psychiatric disorders, delineation of potential contributing organic factors, and inclusion of secondary causes of sleep disorder. Frequently, physiologic and psychological factors coexist and contribute to sleep difficulties.

Primary Sleep Disorders

Norman et al. (1988, 1990) reported alterations in sleep architecture in asymptomatic patients who were HIV-seropositive compared with matched control subjects who were HIV-seronegative. Alterations included a decreased sleep efficiency index, increased stage 1 shifts, and increased amounts of slow-wave sleep. Subsequent studies replicated sleep structure alterations in asymptomatic HIV-infected individuals, finding that slow-wave sleep was increased in the second half of the night (Norman et al. 1992; J.L. White et al. 1995). This alteration in sleep architecture may result from HIV CNS infection or may be secondary to inflammatory factors such as tumor necrosis factor–α that are liberated as part of the host immune response to HIV infection (Darko et al. 1998).

Secondary Sleep Disorders

Other psychiatric disorders, including major depression, delirium, psychosis, substance-related disorders, and pain disorder, can cause sleep complaints (Prenzlauer et al. 1993). A number of medications used in patients with HIV disease can cause sleep disturbances, including AZT, didanosine, abacavir, and efavirenz (see Table 36–5).

Diagnosis and Treatment

The diagnosis of a sleep disorder is made by obtaining a detailed sleep history and conducting a general psychiatric interview, followed by a polysomnographic examination if indicated. Management includes treatment or correction of secondary causes, behavioral interventions, and pharmacotherapy. Behavioral interventions include improving sleep hygiene, regulating sleep-wake cycles, self-hypnosis, relaxation techniques, and elimination of psychoactive substances, including caffeine, nicotine, alcohol, and other drugs of abuse. Low doses of sedating antidepressants such as trazodone are useful in treating patients with sleep disorders. Male patients taking trazodone should be advised of the risk of priapism. Sedative-hypnotics, both benzodiazepine- and nonbenzodiazepine-based, can be useful for management of sleep disorders. Although the goal is to use hypnotics for a short time only, for many patients fatigue and insomnia are chronic difficulties that significantly affect quality of life. Often the physiologic contributors to insomnia cannot be corrected, or the medication that causes insomnia cannot be removed from the regimen of a patient receiving HAART. In such cases, more chronic hypnotic use is often necessary, and a well-discussed, judicious plan is needed to manage sleep without development of dependence.

SEXUAL DISORDERS

Sexual complaints are frequent among patients with HIV disease. In a study involving HIV-positive gay men and HIV-positive hemophiliac men, ejaculatory difficulties were more common in HIV-positive men than in HIV-negative control subjects (Jones et al. 1994). In a study involving predominantly minority, inner-city women, HIV-positive women had higher rates of sexual dysfunction, even at early stages of HIV disease, than did the matched HIV-negative control group (Meyer-Bahlberg et al. 1993). A second study involving HIV-positive women found that 39% met criteria for hypoactive sexual desire disorder (the Structured Clinical Interview for DSM-III-R was administered) and 48% had deficient testosterone levels (Goggin et al. 1998). Sexual dysfunction was not related to the presence of a mood disorder or endocrinological abnormalities but was associated with depressive symptoms. In an open-label study involving men with advanced HIV disease and low levels of serum testosterone, Rabkin et al. (1995) found that testosterone replacement therapy was effective in increasing sexual desire, decreasing sexual dysfunction, and diminishing depressed mood.

When evaluating sexual disorders, the clinician must consider both physiologic and psychological factors. Distress, psychosocial stressors, guilt, fear of transmitting virus, psychoactive substance–related disorders, and mood disorders such as major depression may contribute to sexual dysfunction at all stages of HIV disease. At more advanced stages of HIV disease, neurological and endocrinological factors may play an increasing etiological role in sexual dysfunction (Welby et al. 1991). Antiretrovirals, particularly protease inhibitors, are increasingly recognized as associated with sexual dysfunction (Schrooten et al. 2001). Side effects of psychotropic medications must be considered in evaluating sexual dysfunction, particularly ejaculatory delay associated with SSRI therapy.

Treatment should include assessment for endocrinological and metabolic abnormalities, with the recognition that sexual dysfunction in this population is usually multifactorial. Sexual dysfunction as a side effect of SSRI therapy may be a significant difficulty and lead to poor compliance, necessitating a switch to an antidepressant with fewer sexual side effects. Strategies to enhance sexual function include biological interventions such as testosterone replacement therapy and the use of sildenafil citrate (Viagra) for erectile dysfunction. Because sildenafil requires metabolism by P450 enzymes, its metabolism is inhibited by PIs such as ritonavir; therefore, treatment with sildenafil should be initiated at the lowest available dose. Couples psychotherapy can be helpful in facilitating open discussion about sexual issues, nonpenetrative sexual practices, and physical intimacy and in resolving feelings of guilt and shame about the couple's fears and reactions.

PAIN SYNDROMES

The prevalence of pain among patients with HIV disease has been reported to range from 30% to 80% (Breitbart 1996). The evaluation of pain and adequate treatment and management of pain are essential in the care of patients with HIV/AIDS. Pain, rather than death, is often what patients fear most (Lenderking et al. 1994), and the experience of pain may be influenced by anxiety, anger, depression, and psychological defenses. Although pain is subjective, visual and numeric analogues can be used to assess pain intensity and treatment effectiveness. Pain syndromes, including neuropathy, myopathies, and headache, are common among patients with HIV/AIDS (see Table 36–11). Reports indicate that pain is undertreated in this population (Breitbart et al. 1996c; McCormack et al. 1993), particularly in those with a history of psychoactive substance–related disorders—health care providers may inadequately treat a pain syndrome when they fail to distinguish between management of problems associated with a patient's addiction and adequate treatment of his or her pain. Patients from racial and ethnic minority groups may also receive inadequate treatment for pain (Todd et al. 1993). The approach to pain man-

TABLE 36–11.   Pain syndromes in AIDS patients

Pain related to HIV/AIDS
   HIV neuropathy
   HIV myelopathy
   Kaposi's sarcoma
   Opportunistic infections (intestines, skin)
   Organomegaly
   Arthritis/Vasculitis
   Myopathy/myositis

Pain related to HIV/AIDS therapy
   Antiretrovirals, antivirals
   Antimycobacterials, PCP prophylaxis
   Chemotherapy (vincristine)
   Radiation
   Surgery
   Procedures (bronchoscopy, biopsies)

Pain unrelated to AIDS
   Spinal disk disease
   Diabetic neuropathy

Note. PCP = *Pneumocystis carinii* pneumonia.
Source. Reprinted from Breitbart W: "Pharmacotherapy of Pain in AIDS," in *A Clinical Guide to AIDS and HIV*. Edited by Wormser G. Philadelphia, PA, Lippincott-Raven, 1996, pp. 359–378.

agement should include consideration of use of anti-inflammatory drugs, analgesics, opiates, adjunctive pain management medications, and nonmedication technologies. Attention should also be paid to reducing concomitant psychological distress that may be contributing to the illness and pain experience (Breitbart and McDonald 1996).

Peripheral Neuropathy

Peripheral neuropathy is the most common pain syndrome in patients with HIV disease, affecting up to 35%–40% of patients with AIDS (Breitbart 1996; So et al. 1988). Most commonly, it presents as a distal symmetric polyneuropathy that can be caused by HIV infection and exacerbated or triggered by use of antiretroviral agents such as didanosine, zalcitabine, and stavudine. The diagnosis is based on findings from a neurological examination, electromyelographic findings, and results of nerve conduction studies. It is often difficult to determine the etiology of the neuropathy in patients with advanced HIV disease. Treatment may include alteration of the antiretroviral regimen, although drug discontinuation may not result in resolution of neuropathy. Acupuncture may be useful in some patients. Opiates may be beneficial, although the goals of pain control must be weighed

against the possibility of development of tolerance and dependence. Regular dosing is preferable to as-needed dosing, to avoid development of pain and to reduce associations between developing pain and taking analgesic medication. A history of substance-related disorders does not preclude the use of opiates for analgesia, but careful monitoring for unusual escalation of dose is required. For the entire treatment team to provide optimum care, open discussion of apparent excessive use is essential.

TCAs, either alone or in combination with opiates, can be effective for neuropathic pain. Amitriptyline, nortriptyline, desipramine, and imipramine may all be helpful adjunctive agents, although anticholinergic side effects, hypotension, and sedation may be dose-limiting. Paroxetine may have analgesic properties and may be used as an adjunctive pain medication.

In low doses, anticonvulsants—either alone or in combination with opiates—can also be effective for neuropathic pain. Both carbamazepine and valproic acid are effective, but hematopoietic and hepatic side effects are possible, as are drug interactions. Clonazepam can be effective for hyperpathic pain, and gabapentin has been shown to be effective for postherpetic and diabetic neuropathies (Backonja et al. 1998; Rowbotham et al. 1998) and may be a useful agent for HIV-positive patients.

Some antiarrhythmics have local anesthetic properties and may be useful for some types of pain syndromes. The oral antiarrhythmic drug mexiletine has been studied as a possible agent for treating HIV-related peripheral neuropathy; however, it has not been shown to be effective (Kemper et al. 1998; Kieburtz et al. 1998) and cannot be recommended at this time. Other strategies, including the use of L-carnitine therapy, are under investigation.

Terminal Stages of HIV Disease

During the terminal stages of HIV disease, adequate analgesia is often the mainstay of palliative care. The goal is to eliminate the patient's pain and associated suffering. Doses should be titrated to achieve this goal. All the analgesic agents mentioned above can cause or worsen delirium, adding to the patient's suffering. A trial of a low-dose neuroleptic, typical or atypical, as tolerated, may reduce the delirium and allow maintenance of adequate analgesic doses for pain relief. Stimulants such as methylphenidate can also be useful to counteract sedation and allow adequate analgesic dosing. Nonoral administration of drugs, including transdermal administration of narcotic analgesics, can be helpful in attaining pain relief goals.

SUBSTANCE-RELATED DISORDERS

Prevalence

Substance-related disorders occur frequently in patients with HIV disease. Individuals using injection drugs accounted for 24% of cases of AIDS reported in men and 47% of those in women in 1997 (Centers for Disease Control and Prevention 1998a). The prevalence of substance-related disorders among hospitalized patients with HIV/AIDS referred for psychiatric consultation has been reported to range from 35% to 63% (Bialer et al. 1996; O'Dowd and McKegney 1990). Among ambulatory patients with HIV/AIDS who are referred for psychiatric evaluation, the prevalence of substance-related disorders has been reported to be 42%–45% (O'Dowd et al. 1993; Worth and Halman 1993). Estimates of the rates of current noninjection substance–related disorders among gay and bisexual men with HIV disease range from 2% to 11% (Atkinson et al. 1988; Brown et al. 1992; Ferrando et al. 1998b; Williams et al. 1991). High rates of depression and psychological distress have been reported among HIV/AIDS patients with substance-related disorders (Rabkin et al. 1997), although this cohort showed no evidence of psychiatric or psychosocial decline over the course of 3 years.

Increased risk-taking behaviors have been associated with both injection and noninjection substance–related disorders (Centers for Disease Control and Prevention 1996). Noninjection psychoactive drugs may impair the user's judgment and contribute to higher-risk behaviors. Some (Hauth et al. 1993) but not all (M. J. Perry et al. 1994; Weatherburn et al. 1993) studies have shown an association between recidivism from risk-reduction behaviors and alcohol use. Crack cocaine use (Edlin et al. 1994, 1995; Word and Bowser 1997; Zanis et al. 1997) and inhalant abuse (Ostrow et al. 1990, 1993) are consistently associated with high-HIV-risk behaviors. A study involving African American women demonstrated an association between recent alcohol consumption and inconsistent condom use and an association between crack use and having multiple sexual partners (Wingwood and DiClemente 1998). Amphetamine, inhalant, and crack or cocaine use were shown to increase the relative risk of seroconversion in a large cohort of gay men in San Francisco (Chesney et al. 1998).

Treatment and Management

Treatment and management of the patient who uses injection drugs are dictated by several factors, including the degree of social integration, ethnic and cultural iden-

tification, socioeconomic status, usage patterns, and the individual's choice of drug or drugs (O'Connor et al. 1994). Up to 72% of individuals with HIV who use injection drugs use drugs other than heroin (Diaz et al. 1994). The diagnosis of antisocial personality disorder (Brooner et al. 1993) and the presence of increased psychiatric symptoms (Woody et al. 1997) in persons who use injection drugs have been shown to be associated with a significantly higher rate of HIV infection. Benzodiazepine use among individuals who use injection drugs may be associated with higher rates of additional Axis I disorders (Darke et al. 1993). Active injection drug use may enhance the progression of HIV disease (Phillips et al. 1994; Ronald et al. 1994) and may be related to overall nonadherence to medical treatment. It is unclear how noninjection substance–related disorders affect HIV, but at least one study showed no association between use of marijuana, inhalants, stimulants, or psychedelics and progression of HIV disease (DiFranco et al. 1996).

The management of substance-related disorders and HIV disease follows the concept of harm reduction (Brettle 1991). This model is based on a pragmatic approach to social and individual problems associated with substance-related disorders, which recognizes that these disorders, by natural history, have a chronic course characterized by relapses. For a program to be effective, it must provide not only information about HIV transmission but also access to drug abuse treatment programs and the means for behavior change in both drug use and sexual behavior. If drug use cannot be eliminated, treatment should be aimed at minimizing the consequences of the drug use—the harm reduction approach. This includes reducing HIV-transmission risk, minimizing social stigmatization, and facilitating access to treatment and educational programs. The goals of harm reduction prevention programs for patients in this population include stopping all drug use, switching from injection drugs to other types, decreasing frequency of drug use, improving safer needle practices, and increasing safer sexual behavior. Individuals who enter and remain in drug treatment engage in less drug-related risk behavior, resulting in fewer HIV infections (Metzger et al. 1998).

For users of injection drugs who use heroin, therapy with methadone maintenance is the most effective treatment, having been shown to reduce risk behavior and decrease the rate of infection (Cooper 1989; Drucker et al. 1998; Hartel and Schoenbaum 1998). In addition, primary HIV care has been provided through some methadone maintenance programs, with beneficial effects on health and quality of life. Although politically controversial, needle and syringe exchange programs have also been successful in decreasing rates of HIV infection among individuals who use injection drugs, while providing additional education about risk behaviors and referrals to drug treatment (Centers for Disease Control and Prevention 1998b; DesJarlais et al. 1996; Drucker et al. 1998; Vlahov and Junge 1998). For needle exchange to be most successful, it must have sufficient resources to meet users' needs and must be part of an integrated HIV, mental health, and addiction treatment program.

It must be noted that initiation of methadone maintenance in the patient with HIV disease can result in drug interactions. Methadone has been shown to inhibit glucuronidation of AZT, resulting in increased serum levels (McCance-Katz et al. 1998; Schwartz et al. 1992; Trapnell et al. 1998). This can lead to increased AZT toxicity, which may contribute to decreased treatment adherence. Methadone is primarily metabolized by P450 3A3/3A4, so use of medications that induce or inhibit P450 3A3/3A4 can lead to clinically significant interactions (Iribarne et al. 1997; Moody et al. 1997). Efavirenz, nevirapine, and rifampin, which all induce P450 3A4, can increase methadone metabolism, potentially precipitating acute opiate withdrawal. In such cases, the patient's daily methadone dose must be increased. Conversely, ritonavir, which inhibits P450 3A4, may increase serum levels of methadone, resulting in oversedation (Iribarne et al. 1998). In either case, close contact with the patient's methadone maintenance program is of paramount importance, and the need for methadone titration is assessed on the basis of the patient's subjective report of symptom control. In addition to methadone maintenance, nonpharmacological treatments such as acupuncture may be helpful during periods of opiate withdrawal (Washburn et al. 1993) and in the early phases of addiction recovery.

For the hospitalized patient who is still abusing psychoactive drugs, the aim of treatment is to prevent morbidity and mortality associated with withdrawal syndromes and to provide the patient with the opportunity to start on a path to addiction recovery, with referral to a comprehensive addiction treatment program. The diagnosis of HIV disease may induce the patient to seek both medical and psychiatric care, and such action may include entry into a recovery program. Close cooperation between treatment team members, including the patient's primary care physician, and his or her addiction treatment program is essential. It is useful to give the patient clear treatment explanations, as well as to delineate the patient's responsibilities for his or her own care. Often, a written contract helps to minimize conflicts over prescription of opiates, amphetamines, and benzodiazepines, which predictably raises concerns among treatment teams.

Because many patients using psychoactive drugs are stigmatized, poor, and socially disenfranchised, recovery efforts may be hampered by limited ambulatory treatment options and a social environment that may foster continued use. Some community-based HIV/AIDS organizations have recovery programs that provide outreach, connecting the community with the general hospital. Integrated programs that address HIV care and addiction care together may help streamline health management and foster drug regimen adherence. Evaluation of strategies to enhance antiretroviral therapy adherence among persons with substance-related disorders is currently under way.

HIV DISEASE, CHRONIC AND PERSISTENT MENTAL ILLNESS, AND PSYCHOTIC DISORDERS

Many physicians, including psychiatrists, believe that individuals with chronic and persistent mental illness are not at risk for HIV disease. However, reviews of seroprevalence studies conducted in this population indicate that rates range from 5% to 22.9%, higher than in the general population (Cournos 1996; Gottesman and Groome 1997). Although the assumption that persons with chronic and persistent mental illness are either asexual or too disorganized to inject drugs has been shown to be false (Cournos and McKinnon 1997), lack of appreciation of risk remains one of the main obstacles in the diagnosis and management of HIV disease in this group of patients.

Risk-taking behaviors, both sexual and drug use behaviors, are highly prevalent among these patients. A review of published studies of sexual behavior among individuals with severe mental illness revealed that approximately half of such patients have been sexually active in the past 12 months (McKinnon 1996). Homosexual and bisexual activity may be higher than in control groups, multiple sex partners have been reported by up to 62% of these patients, and the rate of condom use is generally poor. The lifetime prevalence of injection drug use among patients with chronic and persistent mental illness is as high as 25% (McKinnon 1996). Horwath et al. (1996) reported that 20% of a cohort of adult patients with chronic mental illness had injected drugs at least once since 1978.

Psychosocial variables such as homelessness may also be associated with HIV risk among persons with chronic and persistent mental illness. One study found a seroprevalence rate of 19% in a group of homeless mentally ill men (Susser et al. 1993). Further evaluation by Susser et al. (1995, 1996) of risk behaviors in this cohort revealed that the majority of the men having sex usually were doing so with nonmonogamous partners and without condoms and that 23% reported a history of injecting drugs mainly by sharing needles or in shooting galleries.

Other factors that may place individuals with chronic and persistent mental illness at high risk for HIV infection include poor knowledge of HIV and its associated risk behaviors (Aruffo et al. 1990; J. A. Kelly et al. 1992); impaired social interactions (Kalichman et al. 1994); lower levels of assertiveness in negotiating safer sex (Susser et al. 1998); exacerbation of the underlying psychiatric disorder, resulting in impaired judgment (Carmen and Brady 1990); low socioeconomic status, which may promote trading sex for food, money, lodging, or drugs (Otto-Salaj et al. 1998); and institutionalization. In this population, seroprevalence appears to be equal among men and women (Cournos 1996).

New-onset psychosis in HIV disease is a rare occurrence that may be related to HIV CNS infection, seizure disorder, adverse drug side effects, or other CNS complications of HIV disease. In one study involving 20 patients with HIV and new-onset psychosis, 100% had delusions and 90% reported hallucinations (Sewell et al. 1994); 65% had substantial mood symptoms. Complex partial seizures in patients with HIV disease may present with new-onset, episodic symptoms, including formed visual hallucinations, visual perceptual distortions, panic attacks, and racing thoughts. M.C. Wong et al. (1990) found that among inpatients with HIV infection and new-onset seizure disorders, 46% had seizures because of HIV CNS infection alone, without evidence of other secondary opportunistic infections or tumors. Symptoms of new-onset psychosis often overlap with delirium, new-onset mania, drug-induced psychosis, or a primary psychotic disorder. Management includes diagnostic clarification, removal of offending agents that may be etiologically associated with new-onset psychosis, and targeted symptom control through the of antipsychotic and anticonvulsant agents.

Management

The management of chronic and persistent mental illness may be crucial in helping these patients adhere to proper medical treatment of their HIV illness. Neuroleptics remain the drugs of choice for the treatment of psychosis. Caution must be exercised, however; Hriso et al. (1991) reported a higher-than-expected rate of extrapyramidal side effects with use of typical neuroleptic medications in patients with HIV, and cases of neuroleptic

malignant syndrome have been reported as well (W. B. Bernstein and Scherokman 1986; Breitbart and Knight 1989). The use of clozapine in patients with HIV infection has not been systematically studied, but theoretical concerns include an increased potential for myelosuppression when clozapine is used with antiretrovirals and other myelosuppressive agents and an increased risk of seizures in patients with CNS complications of HIV disease. Other atypical neuroleptics, such as risperidone or olanzapine, may be effective and well tolerated in this population. Quetiapine should be used with caution in patients who are taking medications that either inhibit or induce P450 3A4. Most other neuroleptics are primarily metabolized by P450 2D6 and can be safely given to patients taking PIs and other antiretroviral medications.

When psychosis is attributable to a seizure disorder, anticonvulsants remain the drugs of choice. However, when these drugs are used, careful attention must be paid to hematopoietic and hepatic parameters, which may be altered because of the presence of other myelosuppressive or hepatotoxic drugs and/or medical sequelae of HIV disease. Carbamazepine and phenytoin must be used with caution; they are inducers of P450 enzymes, and their use can lead to subtherapeutic antiretroviral levels. Gabapentin may be a good choice given that it has few side effects and is metabolized by glucuronidation, making it safer in terms of potential drug-drug interactions.

Nonpharmacological management of chronic mental illness should focus on risk-reduction strategies and adherence to medical treatment in addition to alleviation of psychiatric symptoms. Psychoeducational and cognitive-behavioral interventions have been shown to be helpful in patients with chronic and persistent mental illness (M. Kaplan and Herman 1996; Katz et al. 1996; Susser et al. 1998). Day treatment programs for HIV-positive patients with mental illness have been developed. Intensive case management, directly observed treatment, and assertive community treatment strategies may all have a role to play in ensuring stabilization of severe mental illness and optimizing treatment for HIV disease.

CONCLUSION

With the introduction of HAART in 1996, there have been rapid changes in the treatment of HIV disease. For psychiatrists in the field, these changes has brought many exciting challenges and experiences. They have brought the opportunity to witness dramatic recoveries of people certain to have died of HIV disease just months earlier. The site of care delivery has changed from medical and palliative care units to ambulatory clinics, community mental health agencies, and AIDS service organizations. There has been a dramatic change in focus in the lives of many with HIV disease as these individuals have moved from a psychological state of preparing to die into a state of learning again to live. Access to care has become a central issue because HIV disease increasingly affects members of marginalized and impoverished communities, who may not be able to take advantage of the technological advances. Discrepancies in medication availability and infrastructure support between developed and developing countries highlight access issues on a global level.

Staying current with new technologies to monitor disease progression, new medications and drug interactions, and new understandings of the pathophysiology of HIV disease is challenging and stimulating, and at times dizzying. This field affords an opportunity to use a true biopsychosocial model and challenges psychiatrists to draw on a wide knowledge base and skill set. Psychiatrists' own struggle to make sense of it all gives them insight into the uncertainties and the hurdles facing their patients. Ultimately, the ability to listen to and appreciate the importance of patients' experiences becomes integral to the overall healing process.

REFERENCES

Abbott M, Khoo SH, Wilkins EGL, et al: Adrenocortical deficiency common in late HIV. Scientific Program and Abstracts (PO-B01-0907), 9th International Conference on AIDS, Berlin, Germany, June 1993

Aboulafia DM, Bundow D: Images in clinical medicine: Buffalo hump in a patient with the acquired immunodeficiency syndrome (photograph). N Engl J Med 339:1297, 1998

Adam P, Hauet E, Caron C, et al: Increase in unprotected anal intercourse with casual partners among readers of the gay press in France and its association with age (Abstract 39.1). AIDS Impact: Biopsychosocial Aspects of HIV Infection Fifth International Conference, Brighton, UK, July 9, 2001, p 114

Albert SM, Marder K, Dooneief G, et al: Neuropsychologic impairment in early HIV infection: a risk factor for work disability. Arch Neurol 52:525–530, 1995

Albert SM, Weber C, Todak G, et al: An observed performance test of medication management ability in HIV: relation to neuropsychological status and adherence (abstract). J Neurovirol 4:338, 1998

Alfonso CA, Cohen MA, Aladjem AD, et al: HIV seropositivity as a major risk factor for suicide in the general hospital. Psychosomatics 35:368–373, 1994

American Academy of Neurology AIDS Task Force: Nomenclature and research case definitions for neurological manifestations of human immunodeficiency virus type-1 (HIV-1) infection. Neurology 41:778–785, 1991

American Psychiatric Association: Diagnostic and Statistical Manual of Mental Disorders, 4th Edition, Text Revision. Washington, DC, American Psychiatric Association, 2000

Aruffo JF, Coverdale JH, Chacko RC, et al: Knowledge about AIDS among women psychiatric outpatients. Hospital and Community Psychiatry 41:326–328, 1990

Atkinson JH, Grant I, Kennedy CJ, et al: Prevalence of psychiatric disorders among men infected with human immunodeficiency virus. Arch Gen Psychiatry 45:859–864, 1988

Atkinson JH, Patterson T, Heaton R, et al: Psychological subgroups in HIV: correlates and interventions. Scientific Program and Abstracts (PO-D22-4097), 9th International Conference on AIDS, Berlin, Germany, June 1993

Atkinson JH, Patterson TL, Chandler JL, et al: Predicting depression in HIV disorders, in 1994 New Research Program and Abstracts: American Psychiatric Association 150th Annual Meeting, Philadelphia, PA, May 1994. Washington, DC, American Psychiatric Association, 1994

Aweeka F, Jayewardene A, Staprans S, et al: Failure to detect nelfinavir in the cerebrospinal fluid of HIV-1-infected patients with and without AIDS dementia complex. Journal of Acquired Immune Deficiency Syndromes and Human Retrovirology 20:39–43, 1999

Backonja M, Beydoun A, Edwards KR, et al: Gabapentin for the symptomatic treatment of painful neuropathy in patients with diabetes mellitus: a randomized controlled trial. JAMA 280:1831–1836, 1998

Beach RS, Mantero-Atienza E, Shor-Posner G, et al: Specific nutrient abnormalities in asymptomatic HIV-1 infection. AIDS 6:701–708, 1992

Beckett A, Rutan SJ: Treating persons with ARC and AIDS in group psychotherapy. Int J Group Psychother 40:19–29, 1990

Bélec L, Meillet D, Vohito MD, et al: High serum levels of TNF-α in HIV-1-infected patients with euthyroid sick syndrome. Scientific Program and Abstracts (PO-A13-0246), 9th International Conference on AIDS, Berlin, Germany, June 1993

Berger JR: Neurosyphilis in human immunodeficiency virus-type 1-seropositive individuals. Arch Neurol 48:700–702, 1991

Bernstein G, Klein R: Countertransference issues in group psychotherapy with HIV-positive and AIDS patients. Int J Group Psychother 45:91–99, 1995

Bernstein WB, Scherokman B: Neuroleptic malignant syndrome in a patient with acquired immunodeficiency syndrome. Acta Neurol Scand 73:636–637, 1986

BHIVA Guidelines Co-ordinating Committee: British HIV Association guidelines for antiretroviral treatment of HIV seropositive individuals. Lancet 349:1086–1092, 1997

Bialer PA, Wallack JJ, Prenzlauer SL, et al: Psychiatric comorbidity among hospitalized AIDS patients vs. non-AIDS patients referred for psychiatric consultation. Psychosomatics 37:469–475, 1996

Bialer PA, Bluestine SL, Termine AW, et al: Psychiatric implications for AIDS patients taking protease inhibitors. Psychosomatics 39:183–184, 1998

Blanche S, Rouzioux C, Moscato MG, et al: A prospective study of infants born to women seropositive for human immunodeficiency virus type 1. N Engl J Med 320:1643–1648, 1989

Bornstein RA, Nasrallah HA, Para MF, et al: Neuropsychological performance in symptomatic and asymptomatic HIV infection. AIDS 7:519–524, 1993

Breitbart W: HIV-1 and delirium: psychopharmacology and HIV-1 infection. Paper presented at Clinical Challenges and Research Directions, National Institute of Mental Health, Washington, DC, April 27–28, 1993

Breitbart W: Pharmacotherapy of pain in AIDS, in A Clinical Guide to AIDS and HIV. Edited by Wormser G. Philadelphia, PA, Lippincott-Raven, 1996, pp 359–378

Breitbart W, Knight RT: AIDS and neuroleptic malignant syndrome. Lancet 2:1488–1489, 1989

Breitbart W, McDonald MV: Pharmacologic pain management in HIV/AIDS. Journal of the International Association of Physicians in AIDS Care 2:17–26, 1996

Breitbart W, Marotta R, Platt MM, et al: A double-blind trial of haloperidol, chlorpromazine, and lorazepam in the treatment of delirium in hospitalized AIDS patients. Am J Psychiatry 153:231–237, 1996a

Breitbart W, Rosenfeld BD, Passik SD: Interest in physician-assisted suicide among ambulatory HIV-infected patients. Am J Psychiatry 153:238–242, 1996b

Breitbart W, Rosenfeld BD, Passik SD, et al: The undertreatment of pain in ambulatory AIDS patients. Pain 65:243–249, 1996c

Breitbart W, Rosenfeld B, Kaim M, et al: A randomized, double-blind, placebo-controlled trial of psychostimulants for the treatment of fatigue in ambulatory patients with human immunodeficiency virus disease. Arch Int Med 161(3):411–420, 2001

Brettle RP: HIV and harm reduction for injection drug users. AIDS 5:125–136, 1991

Brew BJ, Pemberton L, Cunningham P, et al: Levels of human immunodeficiency virus type 1 RNA in cerebrospinal fluid correlate with AIDS dementia stage. J Infect Dis 175:963–966, 1997

Brew BJ, Brown SJ, Catalan J, et al: Safety and efficacy of abacavir (ABC, 1592) in AIDS dementia complex (study CNAB 3001) (abstract 561/32192). International Conference on AIDS 12:559, 1998

Brookmeyer R: Reconstruction and future trends of the AIDS epidemic in the United States. Science 253:37–42, 1991

Brooner RK, Greenfield L, Schmidt CW, et al: Antisocial personality disorder and HIV infection among intravenous drug abusers. Am J Psychiatry 150:53–58, 1993

Brouwers P, DeCarli C, Civitetto L, et al: Correlation between computed tomographic brain scan abnormalities and neuropsychological function in children with symptomatic HIV disease. Arch Neurol 52:39–44, 1995

Brown GR, Rundell JR, McManis SE, et al: Prevalence of psychiatric disorders in early stages of HIV infection. Psychosom Med 54:588–601, 1992

Buhrich N, Cooper DA: Requests for psychiatric consultation concerning 22 patients with AIDS and ARC. Aust N Z J Psychiatry 21:346–353, 1987

Butters N, Grant I, Haxby J, et al: Assessment of AIDS-related cognitive changes: recommendations of the NIMH Workshop on Neuropsychological Assessment Approaches. J Clin Exp Neuropsychol 12:963–978, 1990

Callahan AM, Marangell LB, Ketter TA: Evaluating the clinical significance of drug interactions: a systematic approach. Harv Rev Psychiatry 4:153–158, 1996

Calzavara L, Burchell A, Major C, et al: Increasing HIV incidence among MSM repeat testers in Ontario, Canada 1992-1998 (Abstract ThOrC718). Paper presented at the 13th Annual AIDS Conference, Durban, South Africa, July 9–14, 2000

Carmen E, Brady SM: AIDS risk in the mentally ill: clinical strategies for prevention. Hospital and Community Psychiatry 41:652–657, 1990

Carpenter CCJ, Fischl MA, Hammer SM, et al: Antiretroviral therapy for HIV infection in 1996: recommendations of an international panel. JAMA 276:146–154, 1996

Carpenter CCJ, Fischl MA, Hammer SM, et al: Antiretroviral therapy for HIV infection in 1997: updated recommendations of the International AIDS Society–USA panel. JAMA 277:1962–1968, 1997

Carpenter CCJ, Fischl MA, Hammer SM, et al: Antiretroviral therapy for HIV infection in 1998: updated recommendations of the International AIDS Society–USA panel. JAMA 280:78–86, 1998

Carr A, Cooper DA: Images in clinical medicine. Lipodystrophy associated with an HIV-protease inhibitor (photograph). N Engl J Med 339:1296, 1998

Castellon SA, Hinkin CH, Wood S, et al: Apathy, depression, and cognitive performance in HIV-1 infection. J Neuropsychiatry Clin Neurosci 10:320–329, 1998

Centers for Disease Control and Prevention: 1993 revised classification system for HIV infection and expanded surveillance case definition for AIDS among adolescents and adults. MMWR Morb Mortal Wkly Rep 41:1–19, 1992

Centers for Disease Control and Prevention: Continued sexual risk behavior among HIV-seropositive, drug-using men—1993. MMWR Morb Mortal Wkly Rep 45:151–153, 1996

Centers for Disease Control and Prevention: Update: trends in AIDS incidence, deaths and prevalence—United States, 1996. MMWR Morb Mortal Wkly Rep 46:165–173, 1997

Centers for Disease Control and Prevention: HIV/AIDS surveillance report. MMWR Morb Mortal Wkly Rep 10:1–40, 1998a

Centers for Disease Control and Prevention: Update: syringe exchange programs—United States, 1997. MMWR Morb Mortal Wkly Rep 47:652–655, 1998b

Centers for Disease Control and Prevention: Increases in unsafe sex and rectal gonorrhea among men who have sex with men—San Francisco, California, 1994–1997. MMWR Morb Mortal Wkly Rep 48:45–48, 1999

Chang L, Ernst T, Leonido-Yee M, et al: Cerebral metabolite abnormalities correlate with clinical severity of HIV-1 cognitive motor complex. Neurology 52:100–108, 1999

Chang Y, Cesarman E, Pessin MS, et al: Identification of herpesvirus-like DNA sequences in AIDS-associated Kaposi's sarcoma. Science 266:1865–1869, 1994

Chesney M[A], Ickovics J: Adherence to combination therapy in AIDS clinical trials. Paper presented at the annual meeting of the AIDS Clinical Trials Group, Washington, DC, July 1997

Chesney MA, Barrett DC, Stall R: Histories of substance use and risk behavior: precursors to HIV seroconversion in homosexual men. Am J Public Health 88:113–116, 1998

Chuang HT, Devins GM, Hunsley J, et al: Psychosocial distress and well-being among gay and bisexual men with human immunodeficiency virus infection. Am J Psychiatry 146:876–880, 1989

Ciesla JA, Roberts JE: Meta analysis of the relationship between HIV infection and risk for depressive disorders. Am J Psychiatry 158:725-730, 2001

Cinque P, Vago L, Ceresa D, et al: Cerebrospinal fluid HIV-1 RNA levels: correlation with HIV encephalitis. AIDS 12:389–394, 1998

Clarke JA, Harris H, Ostrow D, et al: Assessing a new model: inpatient subacute care for HIV-related dementia. Scientific Program and Abstracts (WS-B32-1), 9th International Conference on AIDS, Berlin, Germany, June 1993

Claypoole KH, Elliott AJ, Uldall KK, et al: Cognitive functions and complaints in HIV-1 individuals treated for depression. Appl Neuropsychol 5:74–84, 1998

Collins E, Wagner C, Walmsley S: Psychosocial impact of the lipodystrophy syndrome in HIV infection. AIDS Reader 10(9):546–550, 2000

Connor EM, Sperling RS, Gelber R, et al: Reduction of maternal-infant transmission of human immunodeficiency virus type 1 with zidovudine treatment. N Engl J Med 331: 1173–1180, 1994

Cooke M, Gourlay L, Collette L, et al: Informal caregivers and the intention to hasten AIDS-related death. Arch Intern Med 158:69–75, 1998

Cooper JR: Methadone treatment and acquired immunodeficiency syndrome. JAMA 262:1664–1668, 1989

Corder EH, Robertson K, Lannfelt L, et al: HIV-infected subjects with the E4 allele for APOE have excess dementia and peripheral neuropathy. Nat Med 4:1182–1184, 1998

Coté TR, Biggar RJ, Dannenberg AL: Risk of suicide among persons with AIDS: a national assessment. JAMA 268:2066–2068, 1992

Cournos F: Epidemiology of HIV, in AIDS and People With Severe Mental Illness. Edited by Cournos F, Bakalar N. New Haven, CT, Yale University Press, 1996, pp 3–16

Cournos F, McKinnon K: HIV seroprevalence among people with severe mental illness in the United States: a critical review. Clin Psychol Rev 3:259–269, 1997

Cournos F, Empfield M, Horwath E, et al: HIV seroprevalence among patients admitted to two psychiatric hospitals. Am J Psychiatry 148:1225–1230, 1991

Cournos F, Guido JR, Coomaraswamy S, et al: Sexual activity and risk of HIV infection among patients with schizophrenia. Am J Psychiatry 151:228–232, 1994

Cummings JL: Subcortical Dementia. New York, Oxford University Press, 1990

DANA Consortium on Therapy for HIV Dementia and Related Cognitive Disorders: Clinical confirmation of the American Academy of Neurology algorithm for HIV-1-associated cognitive/motor disorder. Neurology 47:1247–1253, 1996

Dannenberg AL, McNeil JG, Brundage JF, et al: Suicide and HIV infection: mortality follow-up of 4147 HIV-seropositive military service applicants. JAMA 276:1743–1746, 1996

Darke S, Swift W, Hall W, et al: Drug use, HIV risk-taking and psychosocial correlates of benzodiazepine use among methadone maintenance clients. Drug Alcohol Depend 34:67–70, 1993

Darko DF, Mitler MM, Miller JC: Growth hormone, fatigue, poor sleep, and disability in HIV infection. Neuroendocrinology 67:317–324, 1998

Davis LE, Hjelle BL, Miller VE, et al: Early viral brain invasion in iatrogenic human immunodeficiency virus infection. Neurology 42:1736–1739, 1992

Day JJ, Grant I, Atkinson JH, et al: Incidence of AIDS dementia in a two-year follow-up of AIDS and ARC patients on an initial phase II AZT placebo-controlled study: San Diego cohort. J Neuropsychiatry Clin Neurosci 4:15–20, 1992

Deeks SG, Smith M, Holodny M, et al: HIV-1 protease inhibitors: a review for clinicians. JAMA 277:145–153, 1997

Department of Health and Human Services: Report of the Secretary's Task Force on Youth Suicide. Washington, DC, U.S. Government Printing Office, 1990

DesJarlais DC, Marmor M, Paone D, et al: HIV incidence among injecting drug users in New York City syringe-exchange programs. Lancet 348:987–991, 1996

Dew MA, Ragni MV, Nimorwicz P: Correlates of psychiatric distress among wives of hemophilic men with and without acquired immune deficiency syndrome. Am J Psychiatry 148:1016–1022, 1991

Diaz T, Chu SY, Byers RH Jr, et al: The types of drugs used by HIV-infected injection drug users in a multistate surveillance project: implications for intervention. Am J Public Health 84:1971–1975, 1994

DiFranco MJ, Sheppard HW, Hunter DJ, et al: The lack of association of marijuana and other recreational drugs with progression to AIDS in the San Francisco Men's Health Study. Ann Epidemiol 6:283–289, 1996

Dilley JW, Forstein M: Psychosocial aspects of the human immunodeficiency virus (HIV) epidemic, in American Psychiatric Press Review of Psychiatry, Vol 9. Edited by Tasman A, Goldfinger SM, Kaufmann C. Washington, DC, American Psychiatric Press, 1990, pp 631–655

Dilley JW, Ochitill HN, Perl M, et al: Findings in psychiatric consultations with patients with acquired immune deficiency syndrome. Am J Psychiatry 142:82–86, 1985

DiSclafani V, Chung B, Tolou-Shams M, et al: Volume reductions of subcortical nuclei in HIV+ subjects are correlated with the severity of cognitive impairments (abstract 32215). Scientific Proceedings, International Conference on AIDS 12:563, 1998

Dreyer EB, Kaiser PK, Offermann JT, et al: HIV-1 coat protein neurotoxicity prevented by calcium channel antagonists. Science 248:364–367, 1990

Drucker E, Lurie P, Wodak A, et al: Measuring harm reduction: the effects of needle and syringe exchange programs and methadone maintenance on the ecology of HIV. AIDS 12 (suppl A):S217–S230, 1998

Edlin BR, Irwin KL, Faruque S, et al: Intersecting epidemics: crack cocaine use and HIV infection among inner-city young adults. N Engl J Med 331:1422–1427, 1994

Edlin BR, Word CO, McCoy CB, et al: HIV incidence among young urban street-recruited crack cocaine smokers. Program and abstracts, 2nd National Conference on Human Retroviruses, Washington, DC, January–February 1995

Ekstrand M, Crosby GM, Stall R: High Levels of sexual risk taking among HIV positive individuals on HAART (Abstract 25.4). AIDS Impact: Biopsychosocial Aspects of HIV Infection, Fifth International Conference, Brighton, UK, July 9, 2001, p 84

Elford J, Bolding G, Sherr L: The recent increase in high risk sexual behaviour among London gay men can not be explained by HIV optimism (Abstract 25.8). AIDS Impact: Biopsychosocial Aspects of HIV Infection, Fifth International Conference, Brighton, UK, July 9, 2001, p 84

Elliot AJ, Uldall KK, Bergram K, et al: Randomized, placebo-controlled trial of paroxetine versus imipramine in depressed HIV-positive outpatients. Am J Psychiatry 155:367–372, 1998

Ellis RJ, Deutsch R, Heaton RK, et al: Neurocognitive impairment is an independent risk factor for death in HIV infection. Arch Neurol 54:416–424, 1997

Empfield M, Cournos F, Meyer I, et al: HIV seroprevalence among homeless patients admitted to a psychiatric inpatient unit. Am J Psychiatry 150:47–52, 1993

Enting RH, Hoetelmans RMW, Lange JMA, et al: Antiretroviral drugs and the central nervous system. AIDS 12:1941–1955, 1998

Ereshefsky L: Drug-drug interactions involving antidepressants: focus on venlafaxine. J Clin Psychopharmacol 16 (suppl 2):37S–49S, 1996

Ereshefsky L, Riesenman C, Lam YWF: Serotonin selective reuptake inhibitor drug interactions and the cytochrome P450 system. J Clin Psychiatry 57 (suppl 8):17–25, 1996

Evans DL, Leserman J, Perkins DO, et al: Severe life stress as a predictor of early disease progression in HIV infection. Am J Psychiatry 154:630–634, 1997

Fauci AS: Multifactorial nature of human immunodeficiency virus disease: implications for therapy. Science 262:1011–1018, 1993

Fauci AS, Bartlett JG, et al: Guidelines for the Use of Antiretroviral Agents in HIV-Infected Adults and Adolescents. Rockville, MD, U.S. Department of Health and Human Services/Henry J. Kaiser Family Foundation, February 2001

Fernandez F, Levy JK: Psychopharmacotherapy of psychiatric syndromes in asymptomatic and symptomatic HIV infection. Psychiatr Med 9:377–394, 1991

Fernandez F, Adams F, Levy JK, et al: Cognitive impairment due to AIDS-related complex and its response to psychostimulants. Psychosomatics 29:38–46, 1988

Fernandez F, Levy JK, Mansell PWA: Management of delirium in terminally ill AIDS patients. Int J Psychiatry Med 19:165–172, 1989

Ferrando SJ, Goldman JD, Charness WE: Selective serotonin reuptake inhibitor treatment of depression in symptomatic HIV infection and AIDS. Gen Hosp Psychiatry 19:89–97, 1997

Ferrando S, van Gorp W, McElhiney M, et al: Highly active antiretroviral treatment in HIV infection: benefits for neuropsychological function. AIDS 12:F65–F70, 1998a

Ferrando S, Goggin K, Sewell M, et al: Substance use disorders in gay/bisexual men with HIV and AIDS. Am J Addict 7:51–60, 1998b

Filippi CG, Sze G, Farber SJ, et al: Regression of HIV encephalopathy and basal ganglia signal intensity abnormality at MR imaging in patients with AIDS after the initiation of protease inhibitor therapy. Radiology 206:491–498, 1998

Finzi D, Hermankova M, Pierson T, et al: Identification of a reservoir for HIV-1 in patients on highly active antiretroviral therapy. Science 278:1295–1300, 1997

Fischl MA, Richman DD, Grieco MH, et al: The efficacy of azidothymidine (AZT) in the treatment of patients with AIDS and AIDS-related complex: a double-blind, placebo-controlled trial. N Engl J Med 317:185–191, 1987

Folkman S, Chesney MA, Pollack L, et al: Stress, coping, and high-risk sexual behavior. Health Psychol 11:218–222, 1992

Folkman S, Chesney M, Pollack L, et al: Stress, control, coping, and depressive mood in human immunodeficiency virus-positive and -negative gay men in San Francisco. J Nerv Ment Dis 181:409–416, 1993

Folkman S, Chesney MA, Cooke M, et al: Caregiver burden in HIV-positive and HIV-negative partners of men with AIDS. J Consult Clin Psychol 62:746–756, 1994

Folstein MF, Folstein SE, McHugh PR: "Mini-mental state": a practical method for grading the cognitive state of patients for the clinician. J Psychiatr Res 12:189–198, 1975

Foudraine NA, Hoetelmans RM, Lange JMA, et al: Cerebrospinal fluid HIV-1 RNA and drug concentrations after treatment with lamivudine plus zidovudine or stavudine. Lancet 351:1547–1551, 1998

Fowler MG, Simonds RJ, Roongpisuthipong A: Update on perinatal HIV transmission. Pediatr Clin North Am 47(1):21–38, 2000

Friedman RC: Couple therapy with gay couples. Psychiatric Annals 21:485–490, 1991

Galgani S, Balestra P, Tozzi V, et al: Comparison of efficacy of different antiretroviral regimens on neuropsychological performance in HIV-1 patients (abstract). J Neurovirol 4:350, 1998

Garrett L: The virus at the end of the world. Esquire Magazine, March 1999

Gelber RD, Lenderking WR, Cotton DJ, et al: Quality of life evaluation in a clinical trial of zidovudine therapy in patients with mildly symptomatic HIV infection. Ann Intern Med 116:961–966, 1992

Gendelman HE, Zheng J, Coulter CL, et al: Suppression of inflammatory neurotoxins by highly active antiretroviral therapy in human immunodeficiency virus-associated dementia. J Infect Dis 178:1000–1007, 1998

Gifford AL, Shively MJ, Bormann JE, et al: Self-reported adherence to combination antiretroviral medication (ARV) regimens in a community-based sample of HIV-infected adults. Paper presented at the 12th World AIDS Conference, Geneva, Switzerland, July 1998

Ginzburg HM, Fleming PL, Miller KD: Selected public health observations derived from Multicenter AIDS Cohort Study. J Acquir Immune Defic Syndr 1:2–7, 1988

Gisolf E, Jurriaans S, Van der Ende M, et al: The Prometheus Study: double protease inhibitor (PI) treatment only is unable to suppress detectable viral load in the CSF (abstract 403). Paper presented at the 6th Conference on Retroviruses and Opportunistic Infections, Chicago, IL, February 1999

Gluhoski VL, Fishman B, Perry S: The impact of multiple bereavement in a gay male sample. AIDS Educ Prev 9:521–531, 1997

Gonorrhea among men who have sex with men—selected sexually transmitted diseases clinics, 1993–1996. MMWR Morb Mortal Wkly Rep 46:889–892, 1997

Goggin K, Engelson ES, Rabkin JG, et al: The relationship of mood, endocrine, and sexual disorders in human immunodeficiency virus positive (HIV+) women: an exploratory study. Psychosom Med 60:11–16, 1998

Goodkin K, Blaney NT, Feaster D, et al: Active coping style is associated with natural killer cell cytotoxicity in asymptomatic HIV-1 seropositive homosexual men. J Psychosom Res 36:635–650, 1992

Goodkin K, Feaster DJ, Asthana D, et al: A bereavement support group intervention is longitudinally associated with salutary effects on the CD4 cell count and number of physician visits. Clin Diag Lab Immunol 5:382–391, 1998

Gorman M, Wiley J, Winkelstein W, et al: Suicide as the leading cause of non-AIDS mortality in a cohort of men in San Francisco. Scientific Program and Abstracts, 8th International Conference on AIDS, Amsterdam, The Netherlands, July 1992

Gottesman II, Groome CS: HIV/AIDS risks as a consequence of schizophrenia. Schizophr Bull 23:675–684, 1997

Grant I, Adams KM (eds): Neuropsychological Assessment of Neuropsychiatric Disorders. New York, Oxford University Press, 1996

Grant I, Martin A: Neuropsychology of HIV Infection. New York, Oxford University Press, 1994

Grant I, Heaton RK, Ellis RO, et al: Neurocognitive complications in HIV (abstract 32208). Inf Conf AIDS 12:562, 1998

Grassi L, Righi R, Sighinolfi L, et al: Coping styles and psychosocial-related variables in HIV-infected patients. Psychosomatics 39:350–359, 1998

Green J, Kocsis A: Counseling patients with AIDS-related encephalopathy. J R Coll Physicians Lond 22:166–168, 1988

Grinspoon S, Bilezikian J: AIDS and the endocrine system. N Engl J Med 327:1360–1365, 1992

Grunfeld C, Pang M, Doerrler W, et al: Indices of thyroid function and weight loss in HIV infection and AIDS. Metabolism 42:1270–1276, 1993

Guay LA, Musoke P, Fleming T, et al: Intrapartum and neonatal single-dose nevirapine compared with zidovudine for prevention of mother-to-child transmission of HIV-1 in Kampala, Uganda: HIVNET 012 randomized trial. Lancet 354 (9181):795-802, 1999

Gulick RM, Mellors JW, Havlir D, et al: Treatment with indinavir, zidovudine, and lamivudine in adults with human immunodeficiency virus infection and prior antiretroviral therapy. N Engl J Med 337:734–739, 1997

Gulick RM, Mellors JW, Havlir D, et al: Simultaneous vs sequential initiation of therapy with indinavir, zidovudine, and lamivudine for HIV-1 infection: 100-week follow-up. JAMA 280:35–41, 1998

Haas DW, Spearman P, Johnson B, et al: Discordant HIV-1 RNA decay in CSF versus plasma following initiation of antiretroviral therapy: a prospective ultra-intensive CSF sampling study (abstract 405). Paper presented at the 6th Conference on Retroviruses and Opportunistic Infections, Chicago, IL, February 1999

Halman MH: Management of depression and related neuropsychiatric symptoms associated with HIV/AIDS and antiretroviral therapy. Can J Infect Dis (suppl C):9C-19C, 2001

Halman MH, Worth JL, Sanders KM, et al: Anticonvulsant use in the treatment of manic syndromes in patients with HIV-1 infection. J Neuropsychiatry Clin Neurosci 5:430–434, 1993a

Halman MH, Sanders KM, Lenderking WR, et al: Short-term group psychotherapy for long-term AIDS survivors. Scientific Program and Abstracts, annual meeting of the Academy of Psychosomatic Medicine, New Orleans, LA, November 1993b

Halman MH, Tolomiczenko G, Goering P, et al: HIV prevalence in the adult homeless population of Toronto. Paper presented at the 151st annual meeting of the American Psychiatric Association, Toronto, ON, Canada, May 30–June 4, 1998

Halman MH, Sota T, Rourke SB: Paroxetine for HIV-related depression: impact on mood, quality of life and cognition (abstract). Can J Infect Dis 12(suppl B):52B, 2001

Hammer SM, Squires KE, Hughes MD, et al: A controlled trial of two nucleoside analogues plus indinavir in persons with human immunodeficiency virus infection and CD4 cell counts of 200/μL or less. N Engl J Med 337:725–733, 1997

Harris GJ, Pearlson GD, McArthur JC, et al: Altered cortical blood flow in HIV-seropositive individuals with and without dementia: a single photon emission computed tomography study. AIDS 8:495–499, 1994

Harrison MJ, Newman SP, Hall-Craggs MA, et al: Evidence of CNS impairment in HIV infection: clinical, neuropsychological, EEG, and MRI/MRS study. J Neurol Neurosurg Psychiatry 65:301–307, 1998

Hartel DM, Schoenbaum EE: Methadone treatment protects against HIV infection: two decades of experience in the Bronx, New York City. Public Health Rep 113 (suppl 1):107–117, 1998

Hauth AC, Perry MJ, Solomon LJ, et al: Alcohol use is strongly associated with continued risky sex among gay men: risk behavior patterns and alcohol-sex attributions. Scientific Program and Abstracts (PO-C23-3172), 9th International Conference on AIDS, Berlin, Germany, June 1993

Havlir DV, Marschner IC, Hirsch MS, et al: Maintenance antiretroviral therapies in HIV-infected subjects with undetectable plasma HIV RNA after triple-drug therapy. N Engl J Med 339:1261–1268, 1998

Hays RB, Turner H, Coates TJ: Social support, AIDS-related symptoms, and depression among gay men. J Consult Clin Psychol 60:463–469, 1992

Hays RB, McKusick L, Pollack L, et al: Disclosing HIV seropositivity to significant others. AIDS 7:425–431, 1993

Heaton RK, Grant I: Neurobehavioral Progress Report/Preliminary Studies (Research Plan presented to NIMH, Office on AIDS). Edited by Grant I. San Diego, CA, HIV Neurobehavioral Research Center, 1995

Heaton RK, Velin RA, McCutchan JA, et al: Neuropsychological impairment in human immunodeficiency virus-infection: implications for employment (HNRC Group, HIV Neurobehavioral Research Center). Psychosom Med 56:8–17, 1994

Heaton RK, Grant I, Butters N, et al: The HNRC 500: neuropsychology of HIV infection at different disease stages. J Int Neuropsychol Soc 1:231–251, 1995

Heaton RK, Marcotte TD, White DA, et al: Nature and vocational significance of neuropsychological impairment associated with HIV infection. Clin Neuropsychol 10:1–14, 1996

Hecht FM, Colfax G, Swanson M, et al: Adherence and effectiveness of protease inhibitors in clinical practice. Paper presented at the 5th Conference on Retroviruses and Opportunistic Infections, Chicago, IL, February 1998

Heseltine PNR, Goodkin K, Atkinson JH, et al: Randomized double-blind placebo-controlled trial of peptide T for HIV-associated cognitive impairment. Arch Neurol 55:41–51, 1998

Hestad K, McArthur JH, Del Pan GJ, et al: Regional brain atrophy in HIV-1 infection: association with specific neuropsychological test performance. Acta Neurol Scand 88:112–118, 1993

Hill AM: Different analyses lead to highly variable estimates of HIV-1 RNA undetectability in clinical trials (abstract 394). Paper presented at the 6th Conference on Retroviruses and Opportunistic Infections, Chicago, IL, February 1999

Hinkin CH, van Gorp WG, Satz P, et al: Actual versus self-reported cognitive dysfunction in HIV-1 infection: memory-metamemory dissociations. J Clin Exp Neuropsychol 18:431–443, 1996

Hinkin CH, Castellon SA, Farinpour R, et al: Methylphenidate improves HIV-associated cognitive slowing (abstract). J Int Neuropsychol Soc 5:97, 1999

Hintz S, Kuck J, Peterkin JJ, et al: Depression in the context of human immunodeficiency virus infection: implications for treatment. J Clin Psychiatry 51:497–501, 1990

Hirsch MS: Antiviral drug development for the treatment of human immunodeficiency virus infections: an overview. Am J Med 85:182–185, 1988

Hirsch MS, Conway B, D'Aquila RT, et al: Antiretroviral drug resistance testing in adults with HIV infection: implications for clinical management. JAMA 279:1984–1991, 1998

Ho DD: Viral counts in HIV infection. Science 272:1124–1125, 1996

Ho DD, Neumann AU, Perelson AS, et al: Rapid turnover of plasma virions and CD4 lymphocytes in HIV-1 infection. Nature 373:123–126, 1995

Hogg RS, Heath KV, Yip B, et al: Improved survival among HIV-infected individuals following initiation of antiretroviral therapy. JAMA 279:450–454, 1998

Holman BL, Gerada B, Johnson KA, et al: A comparison of brain perfusion SPECT in cocaine abuse and AIDS dementia complex. J Nucl Med 33:1312–1315, 1992

Holmes VF, Fernandez F, Levy JK: Psychostimulant response in AIDS-related complex patients. J Clin Psychiatry 50:5–8, 1989

Hoover DR, Saah A, Bacellar H, et al: The progression of untreated HIV-1 infection prior to AIDS. Am J Public Health 82:1538–1541, 1992

Horwath E, Cournos F, McKinnon K, et al: Illicit drug injection among psychiatric patients without a primary substance abuse diagnosis: implications for HIV risk. Psychiatr Serv 47:181–185, 1996

Hriso E, Kuhn T, Masdeu JC, et al: Extrapyramidal symptoms due to dopamine-blocking agents in patients with AIDS encephalopathy. Am J Psychiatry 148:1558–1561, 1991

Iribarne C, Dreano Y, Bardou LG, et al: Interaction of methadone with substrates of human hepatic cytochrome P450 3A4. Toxicology 117:13–23, 1997

Iribarne C, Berthou F, Carlhant D, et al: Inhibition of methadone and buprenorphine N-dealkylations by three HIV-1 protease inhibitors. Drug Metab Dispos 26:257–260, 1998

Johannessen DJ, Wilson LG: Mania with cryptococcal meningitis in two AIDS patients. J Clin Psychiatry 49:200–201, 1988

Jones M, Klimes I, Catalan J: Psychosexual problems in people with HIV infection: controlled study of gay men and men with hemophilia. AIDS Care 6:587–593, 1994

Joseph JG, Eshlemann S, Lackner J, et al: Psychological functioning across the course of HIV-1 illness and AIDS diagnosis: a 6 year longitudinal study. Scientific Program and Abstracts (PO-D20-4009), 9th International Conference on AIDS, Berlin, Germany, June 1993

Jozwiak R, Ng T, Osborn R, et al: Molecular and biological characteristics of HIV-1 strains from patients with AIDS dementia complex (abstract 21110). International Conference on AIDS 12:260–261, 1998

Kahn JO, Walker BD: Acute human immunodeficiency virus type 1 infection. N Engl J Med 339:33–39, 1998

Kalichman SC, Kelly JA, Johnson JR, et al: Factors associated with risk for HIV infection among chronic mentally ill adults. Am J Psychiatry 151:221–227, 1994

Kaplan M, Herman R: Cognitive-behavioral risk reduction groups for teaching safer sex, in AIDS and People With Severe Mental Illness. Edited by Cournos F, Bakalar N. New Haven, CT, Yale University Press, 1996, pp 125–135

Kaplan RM, Anderson JP, Patterson TL, et al: Validity of the Quality of Well-Being Scale for persons with human immunodeficiency virus infection (HNRC Group, HIV Neurobehavioral Research Center). Psychosom Med 57:138–147, 1995

Katz RC, Westerman C, Beauchamp K, et al: Effects of AIDS counseling and risk reduction training on the chronic mentally ill. AIDS Educ Prev 8:457–463, 1996

Kearney B, Price R, Sheiner L, et al: Estimation of nevirapine exposure within the cerebrospinal fluid using CSF: plasma area under the curve ratios (abstract 406). Paper presented at the 6th Conference on Retroviruses and Opportunistic Infections, Chicago, IL, February 1999

Kelly B, Raphael B, Judd F, et al: Suicidal ideation, suicide attempts, and HIV infection. Psychosomatics 39:405–415, 1998

Kelly JA, Murphy DA, Bahr G, et al: AIDS/HIV risk behavior among the chronic mentally ill. Am J Psychiatry 149:652–657, 1992

Kelly MD, Grant I, Heaton RK, et al: Neuropsychological findings in HIV infection and AIDS, in Neuropsychological Assessment of Neuropsychiatric Disorders. Edited by Grant I, Adams KM. New York, Oxford University Press, 1996, pp 403–422

Kemper CA, Kent G, Burton S, et al: Mexiletine for HIV-infected patients with painful peripheral neuropathy: a double blind, placebo-controlled, crossover treatment trial. Journal of Acquired Immune Deficiency Syndromes and Human Retrovirology 19:367–372, 1998

Kempf DJ, Rode RA, Xu Y, et al: The duration of viral suppression during protease inhibitor therapy for HIV-1 infection is predicted by plasma HIV-1 RNA at the nadir. AIDS 12:F9–F14, 1998

Kieburtz KD, Ketonen L, Zettelmaier AE, et al: Magnetic resonance imaging findings in HIV cognitive impairment. Arch Neurol 47:643–645, 1990

Kieburtz KD, Giang DW, Schiffer RB, et al: Abnormal vitamin B_{12} metabolism in human immunodeficiency virus infection. Arch Neurol 48:312–314, 1991a

Kieburtz K[D], Zettelmaier AE, Ketonen L, et al: Manic syndromes in AIDS. Am J Psychiatry 148:1068–1070, 1991b

Kieburtz K[D], Simpson D, Yiannoutsos C, et al: A randomized trial of amitriptyline and mexiletine for painful neuropathy in HIV infection. AIDS Clinical Trial Group 242 Protocol Team. Neurology 51:1682–1688, 1998

Knox KK, Carrigan DR: Active human herpesvirus-6 infection of the CNS in patients with AIDS. Program and abstracts, 2nd National Conference on Human Retroviruses, Washington, DC, January–February 1995

Kosten T: Treatment of substance abusing AIDS patients: psychopharmacology and HIV-1 infection. Paper presented at Clinical Challenges and Research Directions, National Institute of Mental Health, Washington, DC, April 27–28, 1993

Krikorian R, Kay J, Liang WM: Emotional distress, coping, and adjustment in human immunodeficiency virus infection and acquired immune deficiency syndrome. J Nerv Ment Dis 183:293–298, 1995

Law WA, Martin A, Mapou RL, et al: Working memory in individuals with HIV infection. J Clin Exp Neuropsychol 16:173–182, 1994

Lenderking WR, Gelber RD, Cotton DJ, et al: Evaluation of the quality of life associated with zidovudine treatment in asymptomatic human immunodeficiency virus infection. N Engl J Med 330:738–743, 1994

Lenkinski R, Navia B, Lee L, et al: In vivo proton MRS studies of HIV brain injury and HIV dementia (abstract 32204). Scientific Proceedings, International Conference on AIDS 12:561, 1998

Lertora J, Akula S, Rege A, et al: Valproic acid inhibits zidovudine glucuronidation in patients with HIV infection. Scientific Program and Abstracts, 8th International Conference on AIDS, Amsterdam, The Netherlands, July 1992

Letendre S[L], Ellis R, Heaton RK, et al: Change in CSF RNA level correlates with the effects of antiretroviral therapy on HIV-1 associated neurocognitive disorder (abstract). J Neurovirol 4:357, 1998

Letendre SL, Caparelli E, Ellis RJ, et al: Levels of serum and cerebrospinal fluid (CSF) indinavir (IDV) and HIV RNA in HIV-infected individuals (abstract 407). Paper presented at the 6th Conference on Retroviruses and Opportunistic Infections, Chicago, IL, February 1999

Levine S, Anderson D, Bystritsky A, et al: A report of eight HIV-seropositive patients with major depression responding to fluoxetine. J Acquir Immune Defic Syndr 3:1074–1077, 1990

Levy J, Fernandez F: Memory rehabilitation in HIV encephalopathy (abstract). Clin Neuropathol 12:S27, 1993

Levy RM, Bredesen DE: Central nervous system dysfunction in acquired immunodeficiency syndrome. J Acquir Immune Defic Syndr 1:41–64, 1988

Lipton SA: Memantine prevents HIV coat protein-induced neuronal injury in vitro. Neurology 42:1403–1405, 1992a

Lipton SA: Models of neuronal injury in AIDS: another role for the NMDA receptor? Trends Neurosci 15:75–79, 1992b

Lyketsos CG, Hoover DR, Guccione M, et al: Depressive symptoms as predictors of medical outcomes in HIV infection. JAMA 270:2563–2567, 1993a

Lyketsos CG, Hanson AL, Fishman M, et al: Manic syndrome early and late in the course of HIV. Am J Psychiatry 150:326–327, 1993b

Lyketsos CG, Hoover DR, Guccione M, et al: Changes in depressive symptoms as AIDS develops. Am J Psychiatry 153:1430–1437, 1996

Maggi J, Halman M: The effect of divalproex sodium on HIV replication in-vivo: a retrospective study of patients with HIV-mania. Paper presented at the 152nd annual meeting of the American Psychiatric Association, Washington, DC, May 15–20, 1999

Maggi JD, Halman MH: The effect of divalproex sodium on viral load: a retrospective review of HIV positive patients with manic syndromes. Can J Psychiatry 46:359–362, 2001

Maj M, Janssen R, Starace F, et al: WHO Neuropsychiatric AIDS study, cross-sectional phase I: study design and psychiatric findings. Arch Gen Psychiatry 51:39–49, 1994a

Maj M, Satz P, Janssen R, et al: WHO Neuropsychiatric AIDS study, cross-sectional phase II: neuropsychological and neurological findings. Arch Gen Psychiatry 51:51–61, 1994b

Marcotte TD, Heaton RK, Masliah E, et al: The relationship between midfrontal dendritic complexity and pre-agonal neuropsychological functioning in HIV. J Int Neuropsychol Soc 2:57, 1996

Marder K, Albert SM, McDermott M: Prospective study of neurocognitive impairment in HIV (DANA cohort): dementia and mortality outcomes. DANA Consortium on Therapy for HIV Dementia and Related Disorders. J Neurovirol 4:358, 1998

Markowitz JC, Kocsis JH, Fishman B, et al: Treatment of depressive symptoms in human immunodeficiency virus-positive patients. Arch Gen Psychiatry 55:452–457, 1998

Marks G, Richardson JL, Maldonado N: Self-disclosure of HIV infection to sexual partners. Am J Public Health 81:1321–1322, 1991

Martin EM, Pitrak DL, Pursell KJ, et al: Information processing and antiretroviral therapy in HIV-1 infection. J Int Neuropsychol Soc 4:329–335, 1998

Martindale S, Craib K, Chan K, et al: Increasing rate of new HIV infections among young gay and bisexual men in Vancouver, 1995-99 vs. 2000 (Abstract 7.1). AIDS Impact: Biopsychosocial Aspects of HIV Infection, Fifth International Conference, Brighton, UK, July 9, 2001, p 41

Marzuk PM, Tierney H, Tardiff K, et al: Increased risk of suicide in persons with AIDS. JAMA 259:1333–1337, 1988

Marzuk PM, Tardiff K, Leon AC, et al: HIV seroprevalence among suicide victims in New York City, 1991–1993. Am J Psychiatry 154:1720–1725, 1997

Masliah E, Heaton RK, Marcotte TD, et al: Dendritic injury is a pathological substrate for human immunodeficiency virus-related cognitive disorders (HNRC Group, HIV Neurobehavioral Research Center). Ann Neurol 42:963–972, 1997

McArthur JC, Cohen BA, Farzedegan H, et al: Cerebrospinal fluid abnormalities in homosexual men with and without neuropsychiatric findings. Ann Neurol 23 (suppl):S34–S37, 1988

McArthur JC, Cohen BA, Selnes OA, et al: Low prevalence of neurological and neuropsychological abnormalities in otherwise healthy HIV-1–infected individuals: results from the Multicenter AIDS Cohort Study. Ann Neurol 26:601–611, 1989

McArthur JC, Hoover DR, Bacellar H, et al: Dementia in AIDS patients: incidence and risk factors. Multicenter AIDS Cohort Study. Neurology 43:2245–2252, 1993

McArthur JC, McClernon DR, Cronin MF, et al: Relationship between human immunodeficiency virus-associated dementia and viral load in cerebrospinal fluid and brain. Ann Neurol 42:689–698, 1997

McCance-Katz EF, Rainey PM, Jatlow P, et al: Methadone effects on zidovudine disposition. Journal of Acquired Immune Deficiency Syndromes and Human Retrovirology 18:435–443, 1998

McCormack JP, Li R, Zarowny D, et al: Inadequate treatment of pain in ambulatory HIV patients. Clin J Pain 9:279–283, 1993

McDaniel SJ, Fowlie E, Summerville MB, et al: An assessment of rates of psychiatric morbidity and functioning in HIV disease. Gen Hosp Psychiatry 17:346–352, 1995

McKinnon K: Sexual and drug-use risk behavior, in AIDS and People With Severe Mental Illness. Edited by Cournos F, Bakalar N. New Haven, CT, Yale University Press, 1996, pp 17–46

Mehta P, Gulevich SJ, Thal LJ, et al: Neurological symptoms, not signs, are common in early HIV infection. Journal of Neuro-AIDS 1:67–85, 1996

Mellors JW, Rinaldo CR Jr, Gupta P, et al: Prognosis in HIV-1 infection predicted by the quantity of virus in plasma. Science 272:1167–1170, 1996

Mellors JW, Muñoz A, Giorgi JV, et al: Plasma viral load and CD4+ lymphocytes as prognostic markers of HIV-1 infection. Ann Intern Med 126:946–954, 1997

Metzger DS, Navaline H, Woody GE: Drug abuse treatment as AIDS prevention. Public Health Rep 113 (suppl 1):97–106, 1998

Meyer-Bahlburg HFL, Dolezal C, Stern Y, et al: Sexual dysfunction in homosexual HIV+ men: association with immune function, endocrine, neurologic, and psychiatric factors. Scientific Program and Abstracts, 9th International Conference on AIDS, Berlin, Germany, June 1993

Mijch A, Judd FK, Ellen S, et al: HIV-associated mania and risk of AIDS dementia complex (abstract 32257). Scientific Proceedings, International Conference on AIDS 12:571, 1998

Miller EN, Selnes OA, McArthur JC, et al: Neuropsychological performance in HIV-1-infected homosexual men: the Multicenter AIDS Cohort Study (MACS). Neurology 40:197–203, 1990

Miller EN, Satz P, Visscher B: Computerized and conventional neuropsychological assessment of HIV-1 infected homosexual men. Neurology 41:1608–1616, 1991

Moody DE, Alburges ME, Parker RJ, et al: The involvement of cytochrome P450 3A4 in the N-demethylation of L-alpha-acetylmethadol (LAAM), norLAAM, and methadone. Drug Metab Dispos 25:1347–1353, 1997

Moore R, Keruly JC, Gallant J, et al: Decline in mortality rates and opportunistic disease with combination antiretroviral therapy (abstract 22374). Scientific Proceedings, International Conference on AIDS 12:338–339, 1998

Moyle GJ: Efavirenz: shifting the HAART paradigm in adult HIV-1 infection. Expert Opinion on Investigational Drugs 8:1–14, 1999

Muñoz A, Wang MC, Bass S, et al: Acquired immunodeficiency syndrome (AIDS)-free time after human immunodeficiency virus type 1 (HIV-1) seroconversion in homosexual men. Multicenter AIDS Cohort Study Group. Am J Epidemiol 130:530–539, 1989

Myers MF: Marital therapy with HIV-infected men and their wives. Psychiatric Annals 21:466–470, 1991

Namir S, Wolcott D, Fawzy FI, et al: Coping with AIDS: psychological and health implications. Journal of Applied Social Psychology 17:309–328, 1987

Navia BA, Dafni U, Simpson D, et al: A phase I/II trial of nimodipine for HIV-related neurologic complications. Neurology 51:221–228, 1998

Nemeroff CB, DeVane L, Pollock BG: Newer antidepressants and the cytochrome P450 system. Am J Psychiatry 153: 311–320, 1996

Nichols SE: Psychosocial reactions of persons with the acquired immunodeficiency syndrome. Ann Intern Med 103:765–767, 1985

Norman SE, Resnick L, Cohn MA, et al: Sleep disturbances in HIV-seropositive patients. JAMA 260:922–923, 1988

Norman SE, Chediak AD, Kiel M, et al: Sleep disturbances in HIV-infected homosexual men. AIDS 4:775–781, 1990

Norman SE, Chediak AD, Freeman C, et al: Sleep disturbances in men with asymptomatic human immunodeficiency (HIV) infection. Sleep 15:150–155, 1992

O'Connor PG, Selwyn PA, Schottenfeld RS: Medical care for injection-drug users with HIV infection. N Engl J Med 331:450–459, 1994

O'Dowd MA, McKegney FP: AIDS patients compared with others seen in psychiatric consultation. Gen Hosp Psychiatry 12:50–55, 1990

O'Dowd MA, Biderman DJ, McKegney FP: Incidence of suicidality in AIDS and HIV-positive patients attending a psychiatry outpatient program. Psychosomatics 34:33–40, 1993

Ostrow DG, VanRaden MJ, Fox R, et al: Recreational drug use and sexual behavior change in a cohort of homosexual men. Chicago Multicenter AIDS Cohort Study (MACS)/Coping and Change Study. AIDS 4:759–765, 1990

Ostrow DG, Beltran ED, Joseph JG, et al: Recreational drugs and sexual behavior in the Chicago MACS/CCS cohort of homosexually active men. J Subst Abuse 5:311–325, 1993

Otto-Salaj LL, Heckman TG, Stevenson LY, et al: Patterns, predictors and gender differences in HIV risk among severely mentally ill men and women. Community Ment Health J 34:175–190, 1998

Packenham KI, Dadds MR, Terry DJ: Relationships between adjustment to HIV and both social support and coping. J Consult Clin Psychol 62:1194–1203, 1994

Palella FJ, Delaney KM, Moorman AC, et al: Declining morbidity and mortality among patients with advanced human immunodeficiency virus infection. N Engl J Med 338:853–860, 1998

Pantaleo G, Graziosi C, Fauci AS: The immunopathogenesis of human immunodeficiency virus infection. N Engl J Med 328:327–335, 1993

Parks RW, Zec RF, Wilson RS (eds): Neuropsychology of Alzheimer's Disease and Other Dementias. New York, Oxford University Press, 1993

Paterson D, Swindells S, Mohr J, et al: How much adherence is enough? A prospective study of adherence to protease inhibitor therapy using MEMSCaps (abstract 92). Paper presented at the 6th Conference on Retroviruses and Opportunistic Infections, Chicago, IL, February 1999

Perkins DO, Davidson EJ, Leserman J, et al: Personality disorder in patients infected with HIV: a controlled study with implications for clinical care. Am J Psychiatry 150:309–315, 1993

Perkins DO, Stern RA, Golden RN, et al: Mood disorders in HIV infection: prevalence and risk factors in a nonepicenter of the AIDS epidemic. Am J Psychiatry 151:233–236, 1994

Perry MJ, Solomon LJ, Winett RA, et al: High risk sexual behavior and alcohol consumption among bar-going gay men. AIDS 8:1321–1324, 1994

Perry S, Jacobsberg L, Fishman B: Suicidal ideation and HIV testing. JAMA 263:679–682, 1990

Perry S, Fishman B, Jacobsberg L, et al: Effectiveness of psychoeducational interventions in reducing emotional distress after human immunodeficiency virus antibody testing. Arch Gen Psychiatry 48:143–147, 1991

Pert CB, Ruff MR, Ruscetti F, et al: HIV receptor in brain and deduced peptides that block viral infectivity, in Psychological, Neuropsychiatric, and Substance Abuse Aspects of AIDS. Edited by Bridge TP. New York, Raven, 1988, pp 110–134

Peudenier S, Hery C, Montagnier L, et al: Human microglial cells: characterization in cerebral tissue and in primary culture, and study of their susceptibility to HIV-1 infection. Ann Neurol 29:152–161, 1991

Phillips AN, Sabin CA, Mocroft A: Active drug injecting and progression of HIV infection. AIDS 8:385–386, 1994

Pialoux G, Raffi F, Brun-Vezinet F, et al: A randomized trial of three maintenance regimens given after three months of induction therapy with zidovudine, lamivudine, and indinavir in previously untreated HIV-1-infected patients. N Engl J Med 339:1269–1276, 1998

Polis M, Yoder C, Mican J, et al: More than 2 months of an aggressive 4-drug antiretroviral regimen is required to suppress CSF HIV viral burden in previously antiretroviral naive patients (abstract 404). Paper presented at the 6th Conference on Retroviruses and Opportunistic Infections, Chicago, IL, February 1999

Portegies P, Enting RH, de Gans J, et al: Presentation and course of AIDS dementia complex. AIDS 7:669–675, 1993

Post JM, Berger JR, Quencer RM: Asymptomatic and neurologically symptomatic HIV-seropositive individuals: prospective evaluation with cranial MR imaging. Radiology 178:131–139, 1991

Power C, Selnes OA, Grim JA, et al: HIV Dementia Scale: a rapid screening test. Journal of Acquired Immune Deficiency Syndromes and Human Retrovirology 8:273–278, 1995

Prager M, Nichols S, Schaffner B: Therapeutic factors in a support group for non-IVDU HIV(+) women. Scientific program and Abstracts (PoB 3810), 8th International Conference on AIDS, Amsterdam, The Netherlands, July 1992

Pratt RD, Nichols S, McKinney N, et al: Virologic markers of human immunodeficiency virus type 1 in cerebrospinal fluid of infected children. J Infect Dis 174:288–293, 1996

Prenzlauer SL, Bogdonoff L, Tiamson MLA, et al: Sleep and HIV illness. Scientific Program and Abstracts (PO-B16-1752), 9th International Conference on AIDS, Berlin, Germany, June 1993

Prevots R, Allen D, Lehman S, et al: Trends in seroprevalence among injection drug users entering drug treatment. Program and abstracts, 2nd National Conference on Human Retroviruses, Washington, DC, January–February 1995

Price RW, Brew BJ: The AIDS dementia complex. J Infect Dis 158:1079–1083, 1992

Rabkin JG: Psychostimulant medication for depression and lethargy in HIV illness: a pilot study. Progress Notes 4:1–4, 1993

Rabkin JG, Williams JBW, Remien RH, et al: Depression, distress, lymphocyte subsets, and human immunodeficiency virus symptoms on two occasions in HIV-positive homosexual men. Arch Gen Psychiatry 48:111–119, 1991

Rabkin JG, Rabkin R, Harrison W, et al: Effect of imipramine on mood and enumerative measures of immune status in depressed patients with HIV illness. Am J Psychiatry 151:516–523, 1994a

Rabkin JG, Wagner G, Rabkin R: Effects of sertraline on mood and immune status in patients with major depression and HIV illness: an open trial. J Clin Psychiatry 55:433–439, 1994b

Rabkin JG, Rabkin R, Wagner G: Testosterone replacement therapy in HIV illness. Gen Hosp Psychiatry 17:37–42, 1995

Rabkin JG, Johnson J, Lin SH, et al: Psychopathology in male and female HIV-positive and negative injecting drug users: longitudinal course over 3 years. AIDS 11:507–515, 1997

Rabkin JG, Wagner GJ, Rabkin R: Fluoxetine treatment for depression in patients with HIV and AIDS: a randomized, placebo-controlled trial. Am J Psychiatry 156:101–107, 1999

Raboud JM, Montaner JS, Conway B, et al: Suppression of plasma viral load below 20 copies/ml is required to achieve a long-term response to therapy. AIDS 12:1619–1624, 1998

RachBeisel JA, Weintraub E: Valproic acid treatment of AIDS-related mania. J Clin Psychiatry 58:406–407, 1997

Remafedi G, Farrow JA: Risk factors for attempted suicide in gay and bisexual youth. Pediatrics 87:869–875, 1991

Ronald PJM, Robertson JR, Elton RA: Continued drug use and other cofactors for progression to AIDS among injecting drug users. AIDS 8:339–343, 1994

Rourke SB, Halman MH, Bassel C: Neurocognitive complaints in HIV-infection and their relationship to depressive symptoms and neuropsychological functioning. J Clin Exp Neuropsychol 21:737–756, 1999a

Rourke SB, Halman MH, Bassel C: Neuropsychiatric correlates of memory-metamemory dissociations in HIV-infection. J Clin Exp Neuropsychol 21:757–768, 1999b

Rowbotham M, Harden N, Stacey B, et al: Gabapentin for the treatment of postherpetic neuralgia: a randomized controlled trial. JAMA 280:1837–1842, 1998

Rubinstein ML, Selwyn PA: High prevalence of insomnia in an outpatient population with HIV infection. Journal of Acquired Immune Deficiency Syndromes and Human Retrovirology 19:260–265, 1998

Rundell JR, Kyle KM, Brown GR, et al: Risk factors for suicide attempts in a human immunodeficiency virus screening program. Psychosomatics 33:24–27, 1992

Sacks M, Dermatis H, Looser-Ott S, et al: Seroprevalence of HIV and risk factors for AIDS in psychiatric inpatients. Hospital and Community Psychiatry 43:736–737, 1992

Sacktor NC, Bacellar H, Hoover DR, et al: Psychomotor slowing in HIV infection: a predictor of dementia, AIDS and death. J Neurovirol 2:404–410, 1996

Sacktor N[C], Skolasky C, Lyles RL, et al: Highly active antiretroviral therapy (HAART) improves cognitive impairment in HIV+ homosexual men (abstract). J Neurovirol 4:365, 1998

Sahakian BJ, Elliott R, Low N, et al: Neuropsychological deficits in tests of executive function in asymptomatic and symptomatic HIV-1 seropositive men. Psychol Med 25:1233–1246, 1995

Schaerf FW, Miller RR, Lipsey JR, et al: ECT for major depression in four patients infected with human immunodeficiency virus. Am J Psychiatry 146:782–784, 1989

Schmitt FA, Bigley JW, McKinnis R, et al: Neuropsychological outcome of zidovudine (AZT) treatment of patients with AIDS and AIDS-related complex. N Engl J Med 319:1573–1578, 1988

Schrooten W, Colebunders R, Youle M, et al: Sexual dysfunction associated with protease inhibitor containing highly active antiretroviral treatment. AIDS 15(8):1019–1023, 2001

Schwartz EL, Brechbuhl AB, Kahl P, et al: Pharmacokinetic interactions of zidovudine and methadone in intravenous drug-using patients with HIV infection. J Acquir Immune Defic Syndr 5:619–626, 1992

Sciolla A, Patterson T, Atkinson J, et al: Psychosocial characteristics of grief in HIV-infected men. Scientific Program and Abstracts, 8th International Conference on AIDS, Amsterdam, The Netherlands, July 1992

Sei S, Stewart SK, Farley M, et al: Evaluation of human immunodeficiency virus (HIV) type 1 RNA levels in cerebrospinal fluid and viral resistance to zidovudine in children with HIV encephalopathy. J Infect Dis 174:1200–1206, 1996

Sewell DD, Jeste DV, Atkinson JH, et al: HIV-associated psychosis: a study of 20 cases. Am J Psychiatry 151:237–242, 1994

Shader RI, Greenblatt DJ: Protease inhibitors and drug interactions—an alert. J Clin Psychopharmacol 16:343–344, 1996

Sidtis JJ, Gatsonis C, Price RW, et al: Zidovudine treatment of the AIDS dementia complex: results of a placebo-controlled trial. Ann Neurol 33:343–349, 1993

Sikkema KJ, Kelly JA, Bahr GR, et al: Mental health intervention to help persons cope with AIDS-related bereavement. Scientific Program and Abstracts, 8th International Conference on AIDS, Amsterdam, The Netherlands, July 1992

Simpson DM, Tagliati M: Neurologic manifestations of HIV infection. Ann Intern Med 121:769–785, 1994

Smith J, Craib KJB, Wales PW: Mood elevation/irritability in patients with AIDS dementia complex. Scientific Program and Abstracts, 4th International Conference on the Neuroscience of HIV Infection, Amsterdam, The Netherlands, July 1992

Smythe W, Frischer M, Bloor M, et al: Mortality among injecting drug users in Glasgow. Scientific Program and Abstracts, 8th International Conference on AIDS, Amsterdam, The Netherlands, July 1992

So YT, Holtzman DM, Abrams DI, et al: Peripheral neuropathy associated with acquired immunodeficiency syndrome. Arch Neurol 45:945–948, 1988

Starace F, Sherr L: Suicidal behaviors, euthanasia and AIDS. AIDS 12:339–347, 1998

Stern RA, Silva SG, Chaisson N, et al: Influence of cognitive reserve on neuropsychological functioning in asymptomatic human immunodeficiency virus-1 infection. Arch Neurol 53:148–153, 1996

Stern Y, Liu X, Marder K, et al: Neuropsychological changes in a prospectively followed cohort of homosexual and bisexual men with and without HIV infection. Neurology 45:467–472, 1995

Stern Y, Marder K, Albert SM, et al: The DANA cohort: predictors of HIV dementia (abstract). DANA Consortium on Therapy for HIV Dementia and Related Disorders. J Neurovirol 4:367, 1998

Sullivan A: When AIDS ends. The New York Times Magazine, November 10, 1996

Summers J, Robinson R, Zisook S, et al: The efficacy of short-term group therapy in men with unresolved grief at high risk for HIV. Scientific Program and Abstracts (PO-B35-2330), 9th International Conference on AIDS, Berlin, Germany, June 1993

Susser E, Valencia E, Conover S: Prevalence of HIV infection among psychiatric patients in a New York City men's shelter. Am J Public Health 83:568–570, 1993

Susser E, Valencia E, Miller M, et al: Sexual behavior of homeless mentally ill men at risk for HIV. Am J Psychiatry 152:583–587, 1995

Susser E, Miller M, Valencia E, et al: Injection drug use and risk of HIV transmission among homeless men with mental illness. Am J Psychiatry 153:794–798, 1996

Susser E, Valencia E, Berkman A, et al: Human immunodeficiency virus sexual risk reduction in homeless men with mental illness. Arch Gen Psychiatry 55:266–272, 1998

Süttmann U, Selberg O, Melzer A, et al: Nitrogen balance in HIV-infected patients during total parenteral nutrition. Scientific Program and Abstracts (WS-B34-4), 9th International Conference on AIDS, Berlin, Germany, June 1993

Tan SV, Guiloff RJ: Hypothesis on the pathogenesis of vacuolar myelopathy, dementia, and peripheral neuropathy in AIDS. J Neurol Neurosurg Psychiatry 65:23–28, 1998

Tanquary J: Lithium neurotoxicity at therapeutic levels in an AIDS patient. J Nerv Ment Dis 18:518–519, 1993

Targ EF, Karasic DH, Diefenbach PN, et al: Structured group therapy and fluoxetine to treat depression in HIV-positive persons. Psychosomatics 35:132–137, 1994

Tashima KT, Caliendo AM, Ahmad MA, et al: Cerebrospinal fluid HIV-1 RNA levels and efavirenz concentrations in patients enrolled in clinical trials (abstract 32202). Scientific Proceedings, International Conference on AIDS 12:561, 1998

Taylor K, Lavallee D: Neuropsychiatric management of AIDS. AIDS Patient Care 2:22–29, 1989

Todd KH, Samaroo N, Hoffman JR: Ethnicity as a risk factor for inadequate emergency department analgesia. JAMA 269:1537–1539, 1993

Trapnell CB, Klecker RW, Jamis-Dow C, et al: Glucuronidation of 3′-azido-3′-deoxythymidine (zidovudine) by human liver microsomes: relevance to clinical pharmacokinetic interactions with atovaquone, fluconazole, methadone, and valproic acid. Antimicrob Agents Chemother 42:1592ñ1596, 1998

Tyor WR, Wesselingh SL, Griffin JW, et al: Unifying hypothesis for the pathogenesis of HIV-associated dementia complex, vacuolar myelopathy, and sensory neuropathy. Journal of Acquired Immune Deficiency Syndromes and Human Retrovirology 9:379–388, 1995

Uldall KK, Berghuis JP: Delirium in AIDS patients: recognition and medication factors. AIDS Patient Care STDS 11:435–441, 1997

van den Bloom F, Gremmen AW: AIDS and grief. Scientific Program and Abstracts (POB 3814), 8th International Conference on AIDS, Amsterdam, The Netherlands, July 1992

van Gorp WG, Satz P, Hinkin C, et al: Metacognition in HIV-1 seropositive asymptomatic individuals: self-ratings versus objective neuropsychological performance. J Clin Exp Neuropsychol 13:812–819, 1991

Velentgas P, Bynum C, Zierler S: The buddy volunteer commitment in AIDS care. Am J Public Health 80:1378–1380, 1990

Ventura SJ, Anderson RN, Martin JA, et al: Births and deaths: preliminary data for 1997. Natl Vital Stat Rep 47:1–44, 1998

Vitiello B: Research on possible treatments of HIV-associated cognitive impairment (abstract 60804). International Conference on AIDS 12:1148, 1998

Vlahov D, Junge B: The role of needle exchange programs in HIV prevention. Public Health Rep 113 (suppl 1):75–80, 1998

Wagner GJ, Rabkin JG, Rabkin R: A comparative analysis of standard and alternative antidepressants in the treatment of human immunodeficiency virus patients. Compr Psychiatry 37:402–408, 1996

Wainberg MA, Friedland G: Public health implications of antiretroviral therapy and HIV drug resistance. JAMA 279:1977–1983, 1998

Walker G: AIDS and family therapy. Family Therapy Today 26:1–7, 1987

Washburn AM, Fullilove RE, Fullilove MT, et al: Acupuncture heroin detoxification: a single-blind clinical trial. J Subst Abuse Treat 10:345–351, 1993

Weatherburn P, Davies PM, Hickson FCI, et al: No connection between alcohol use and unsafe sex among gay and bisexual men. AIDS 7:115–119, 1993

Welby SB, Rogerson SJ, Beeching NJ: Autonomic neuropathy is common in human immunodeficiency virus infection. J Infect 23:123–128, 1991

Wenger N, Gifford A, Liu H, et al: Patient characteristics and attitudes associated with antiretroviral (AR) adherence (abstract 98). Paper presented at the 6th Conference on Retroviruses and Opportunistic Infections, Chicago, IL, February 1999

Wesselingh SL, Glass J, McArthur JC, et al: Cytokine dysregulation in HIV-associated neurological disease. Adv Neuroimmunol 4:199–206, 1994

White A, Eldridge R, Andrews E, et al: Birth outcomes following zidovudine exposure in pregnancy: the Antiretroviral Pregnancy Registry. Scientific Program and Abstracts, 2nd National Conference on Human Retroviruses, Washington, DC, January–February 1995

White DA, Heaton RK, Monsch AU, et al: Neuropsychological studies of asymptomatic human immunodeficiency virus-type-1 infected individuals. J Int Neuropsychol Soc 1:304–315, 1995

White JL, Darko DF, Brown SJ, et al: Early central nervous system response to HIV infection: sleep distortion and cognitive-motor decrements. AIDS 9:1043–1050, 1995

Wiley CA, Nelson JA: Role of human immunodeficiency virus and cytomegalovirus in AIDS encephalitis. Am J Pathol 133:73–81, 1988

Williams JBW, Rabkin JG, Remien RH, et al: Multidisciplinary baseline assessment of homosexual men with and without human immunodeficiency virus infection. Arch Gen Psychiatry 48:124–130, 1991

Wingwood GM, DiClemente RJ: The influence of psychosocial factors, alcohol, drug use on African-American women's high-risk sexual behavior. Am J Prev Med 15:54–59, 1998

Wong JK, Hezareh M, Günthard HF, et al: Recovery of replication-competent HIV despite prolonged suppression of plasma viremia. Science 278:1291–1295, 1997

Wong MC, Suite NDA, Labar DR: Seizures in human immunodeficiency virus infection. Arch Neurol 47:640–642, 1990

Woodhouse DE, Rothenberg RB, Potterat JJ, et al: Mapping a social network of heterosexuals at high risk for HIV infection. AIDS 8:1331–1336, 1994

Woody GE, Metzger D, Navaline H, et al: Psychiatric symptoms, risky behavior, and HIV infection. NIDA Res Monogr 172:156–170, 1997

Word CO, Bowser B: Background to crack cocaine addiction and HIV high-risk behavior: the next epidemic. Am J Drug Alcohol Abuse 23:67–77, 1997

Worth JL, Halman MH: Nine-month experience of an HIV/AIDS psychiatry clinic: demographics, diagnoses, and outcome. Poster presented at the 146th annual meeting of the American Psychiatric Association, San Francisco, CA, May 22–27, 1993

Worth JL, Savage C, Baer L, et al: Computer-based screening for AIDS dementia complex. AIDS 7:677–681, 1993

Wortley PM, Fleming PL: AIDS in women in the United States: recent trends. JAMA 2787:911–916, 1997

Yarchoan R, Venzon DJ, Pluda JM, et al: CD4 count and the risk for death in patients infected with HIV receiving antiretroviral therapy. Ann Intern Med 115:184–189, 1991

Zanis DA, Cohen C, Myers K, et al: HIV risks among homeless men differentiated by cocaine use and psychiatric distress. Addict Behav 22:287–292, 1997

Zhang L, Ramratnam B, Tenner-Racz K, et al: Quantifying residual HIV-1 replication and decay of the latent reservoir in patients on seemingly effective combination antiretroviral therapy (abstract 495). Paper presented at the 6th Conference on Retroviruses and Opportunistic Infections, Chicago, IL, February 1999

Zolopa AR, Hahn JA, Gorter R, et al: HIV and tuberculosis infection in San Francisco's homeless adults. JAMA 272:455–461, 1994

37

Geriatric Medicine

Jürgen Unützer, M.D., M.P.H.

Gary W. Small, M.D.

Ibrahim Gunay, M.D.

The vast majority of older adults with mental disorders receive their care for physical and mental disorders in general medical settings and have little access to providers with special expertise in geriatric psychiatry. Consultation-liaison psychiatrists in general hospitals or primary care settings are in an ideal position to provide such expertise, and in this chapter, we review issues that arise in evaluating and treating elderly patients in a consultation-liaison setting.

NORMAL AGING AND QUALITY OF LIFE

The consultation-liaison psychiatrist must distinguish changes that are seen in normal aging from pathological changes, often a subtle distinction in persons in the oldest age groups. Aging, a sine qua non of life, is a process that affects biological, psychological, and social functioning. Normal aging is defined as a decline in the number of active cells and overall reserve for biological systems. People older than 65 years were first considered "old" in the late nineteenth century, when Otto von Bismarck selected 65 years as the starting age for social welfare benefits. Increased illness survival rates have led to many more people living beyond age 65 years than during Bismarck's time. *Young-old* and *old-old* are newer terms that describe the population between ages 65 and 75 years and 75 years or older, respectively. The emphasis on chronological age in our approach to normal aging is potentially misleading, however, because psychological and biological aging progress at varying rates.

Proponents of numerous biological theories, based on observations in animals and in humans, attempt to explain cellular biological aging, but the basic mechanisms of aging remain poorly understood (Rowe 1985). Both intrinsic factors (i.e., genetic and constitutional makeup of the organism) and extrinsic factors (i.e., environment, nutrition) determine biological aging (Rowe and Kahn 1998).

Because medical and scientific advances have diminished the prevalence of infectious diseases and other acute illnesses, chronic illnesses are now highly prevalent among elderly persons (Department of Health and Human Services 1990; World Health Organization 1992). For the psychiatrist, comorbid medical illness is the single most important difference between younger and older patients. The combination of chronic medical illnesses and the resulting disability can cause significant psychological distress and result in secondary psychiatric syndromes (Ormel et al. 1997), and acute exacerbations of these chronic illnesses often lead to hospitalization. Thus, it is not surprising that the percentage of elderly inpatients with mental disorders in the general hospital population is high. Patients older than 65 account for 30% of all acute hospital admissions and 42% of all days of hospital care; 80% of elderly individuals have at least one chronic medical illness (e.g., arthritis, heart disease, hypertension, urinary incontinence, diabetes mellitus, hearing or visual impairment). Coexisting medical illnesses, or their treatments, often mask an elderly patient's psychiatric symptoms. Psychiatric diagnosis becomes a further challenge because secondary psychiatric disorders resulting from substances or medical conditions can mimic the entire spectrum of primary psychiatric disorders. Moreover, some symptoms of primary psychiatric disorders in older patients differ from those in younger patients.

Diagnosis is further complicated by normal age-associated changes. Although most people in their 60s and older complain of forgetfulness, the prognostic implications of such age-associated memory complaints remain a question for current research (Small et al. 1994, 1995). As people age, they sleep less. This normal age-related change must be distinguished from insomnia secondary to depression or anxiety or from primary sleep disorders such as apnea. Sensory deprivation from hearing and visual impairment can lead to social isolation and can exacerbate or cause psychotic symptoms.

Although people live longer, physical, psychological, and social losses may diminish the quality of life, especially during the sixth, seventh, and eighth decades. Improving functional independence, not just the length of life, is crucial. Social support and network characteristics that contribute to depression among patients in the geriatric population include loss of a spouse, inadequate emotional support, loss of a confidant, and fewer children making weekly visits (Oxman et al. 1992). One indicator of quality of life is ability to perform required activities of daily living (ADLs). Approximately 6 million elderly persons require some form of long-term assistance with basic activities such as eating, bathing, dressing, and toileting. Cohen and colleagues (1992) found that a person's ability to perform ADLs is a stronger predictor of mortality following hospitalization than is their medical diagnosis.

DEMOGRAPHIC TRENDS AND EPIDEMIOLOGY

Elderly persons constitute the fastest-growing segment of the population in the United States and in all advanced industrial societies (Department of Health and Human Services 1990; World Health Organization 1992). In 1900, people age 65 or older made up only 4% of the total population; by the year 2000, this group represented 13%. The subgroup of elderly persons age 85 years or older is growing at an even faster pace, accounting for 10% of the 65 or older age group in 1990 and a predicted 22% in 2050. This older group has the greatest frequency of chronic physical illnesses, dependency, and long-term care. Although the general elderly population will double between 1990 and 2050, the elderly Hispanic American population will increase sevenfold, and the number of African Americans age 65 and older is expected to increase threefold.

Large epidemiologic surveys designed to determine prevalence rates of mental disorders among medically ill elderly patients are unavailable. There are, however, some studies of psychiatric disorders among elderly patients receiving psychiatric consultations in general hospital settings (Table 37–1). Most frequently, consultants diagnose mood disorder (17%–55%) or organic mental disorder (36%–46%). Such diagnostic rates differ from those observed among younger patients in comparable clinical settings (Figure 37–1) (Levitte and Thornby 1989; Popkin et al. 1984; Small and Fawzy 1988). Older patients are more likely to have dementia or delirium but less likely to be given diagnoses of personality disorders than are younger consultation-liaison patients. Younger and older groups in the general hospital, however, have similar rates of mood disorders. Subsyndromal or syndromal depressive disorders occur in 50% of all patients seen in consultation, regardless of a patient's age (Small and Fawzy 1988).

Thirty percent of the older adults seen in primary care settings have at least one active psychiatric diagnosis, including 10%–20% with clinically significant depressive syndromes (Gurland et al. 1996).

PSYCHIATRIC CONSULTATION REQUESTS FOR GERIATRIC PATIENTS

Despite the high prevalence of psychiatric disorders among elderly hospitalized patients, psychiatric consultations are less frequently requested for such patients than for their younger counterparts (Rabins et al. 1983). Moreover, the referral rate for hospitalized inpatients age 65 or older is remarkably lower than the estimated prevalence of psychiatric problems in the same population (Folks and Ford 1985; Koenig et al. 1988b; Popkin et al. 1984). Ageism, therapeutic nihilism, and the false assumption that mental impairment is a normal aspect of aging could contribute to this low referral rate.

Several research groups have examined psychiatric consultation request patterns for elderly patients in general hospitals (Grossberg et al. 1990; Levitte and Thornby 1989; Mainprize and Rodin 1987; Popkin et al. 1984; Ruskin 1985; Small and Fawzy 1988); 34%–78% of the referrals are from medical services, and only 15%–25% are from surgical services. In general, evaluations for depression or cognitive impairment are the most frequent reasons for such requests. Other reasons for consultation requests include mental status evaluation, agitation, suicidal and other disturbing behaviors, and medication

TABLE 37–1. Primary psychiatric diagnoses for elderly patients receiving psychiatric consultations in general hospitals

		Disorder frequency (%)			
Study	N	Dementia/ delirium	Mood disorder	Adjustment disorder	Psychotic disorder
Grossberg et al. 1990	147	37	28	26	2
Levitte and Thornby 1989	384	37	25	—	5
Mainprize and Rodin 1987	238	51	17	15	7
Popkin et al. 1984	166	46	23	9	—
Ruskin 1985	67	37	24	—	16
Small and Fawzy 1988	88	47	55	22	16

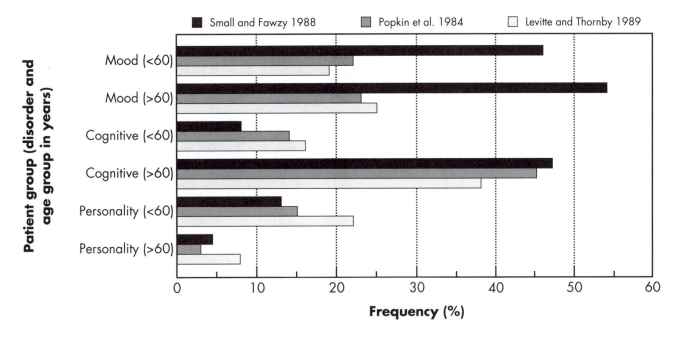

FIGURE 37–1. Differences in primary psychiatric diagnosis between younger and older patients.

management. When consultants are called for such problems, they must address a variety of age-related issues that color the diagnostic presentation and treatment approach.

MODELS OF CARE FOR GERIATRIC CONSULTATION-LIAISON PSYCHIATRY

With recognition of the special needs of the geriatric patient, several models of care have been proposed to improve care for older adults with comorbid medical and psychiatric disorders. In a randomized controlled trial, Levitan and Kornfeld (1981) found that elderly patients hospitalized with a hip fracture who received psychiatric consultations spent 12 fewer days in the hospital and

were more likely to be discharged to their home rather than to a nursing home when compared with patients who did not receive such consultation. Strain and colleagues (1991) showed that routine psychiatric screening of elderly patients admitted with hip fractures resulted in earlier discharge and significant cost savings when compared with traditional referrals for consultations. Cole and associates (1991) evaluated the effectiveness of geriatric psychiatry consultation in diminishing confusion, anxiety, and other behavioral disturbances in patients in a primary acute care hospital. They used a randomized clinical trial design and showed only modest improvement in psychiatric symptoms and functional status. The most effective consultation services seem to be targeted at high-risk patients likely to benefit from psychiatric intervention, such as patients with hip fractures. Most geriatric psychiatrists encourage educational programs along with consultation services to enhance acceptance of recommendations made by consultants and to improve the consultee's psychiatric skills. In an ideal situation, the hospitalized elderly patient would receive consultation from a specially trained geriatric psychiatrist. However, the shortage of such specialists (Small 1993) makes this model more utopian than realistic. The burden of caring for the psychiatric needs of elderly patients in the general hospital currently falls most frequently on consultation-liaison psychiatrists.

A model developed by Lipowski (1983) bases psychogeriatric consultations, research, and teaching on existing consultation-liaison services, which eliminates the need to create new services. This approach requires special training in geriatric psychiatry for consultation-liaison psychiatrists. Lipowski also has recommended establishing postresidency fellowships that combine consultation-liaison and geriatric psychiatry. Others have suggested variations of this model (e.g., Schneider and Plopper 1984; Shulman et al. 1986).

In recent years, several systematic approaches have been developed to improve the treatment of common mental disorders such as depression or anxiety in general medical settings (Katon et al. 1997; Klinkman and Okkes 1998; Unützer et al. 1999, 2001). Such interventions include systematic case finding with simple screening instruments such as the Prime-MD (Spitzer et al. 1994), patient and family education, clinician education and support, systematic assessment and treatment matching, proactive outcomes tracking, and, most important, the integration of primary care and specialty mental health services. These models may use physician extenders such as geriatric nurse specialists who work in collaboration with primary care providers and consulting psychiatrists. Examples of such integrated systems of care have been shown to be cost-effective in mixed-aged primary care populations (Katon et al. 1997), and they are currently being evaluated in several large randomized controlled trials that focus on older adults (Mulsant et al. 2001; Unützer et al. 2001).

CLINICAL SYNDROMES AND CONSULTATION ISSUES

Delirium

Structural brain disease, age-related central nervous system (CNS) changes, sensory deprivation, diminished hearing and vision, chronic medical illness, age-related changes in pharmacokinetics and pharmacodynamics, and decreased resistance to physical stress make elderly persons particularly vulnerable to delirium. If delirium is not recognized and treated promptly, 20%–80% of affected patients die (Curyto et al. 2001; Lipowski 1989). A study (Francis and Kapoor 1992) of medical inpatients age 70 years and older showed a 2-year mortality of 39% for patients who had had an episode of delirium during hospitalization compared with 23% for those who had not developed delirium. Although the most recent four editions of the *Diagnostic and Statistical Manual of Mental Disorders* (American Psychiatric Association 1980, 1987, 1994, 2000) have traditionally specified the need for evidence of a specific medical or toxic factor judged to be etiologically related to the disturbance, surveys indicate that a specific cause is never detected in up to 20% of cases.

Early clinical features of delirium in elderly persons are similar to those in younger patients and include malaise, agitation, headache, sleep disturbance, irritability, disorientation, impaired short-term memory, perceptual disturbance, anxiety, and depression or decreased interests. As the illness progresses, disordered attention and concentration are prominent. Many medical illnesses can cause delirium, and medications are an important cause in elderly patients. Delirium occurs in approximately 40% of elderly patients after orthopedic surgeries such as bilateral knee replacement (Williams-Russo et al. 1992).

Dementia

Both delirium and dementia are prevalent in medically ill elderly persons. It is difficult to determine whether a patient with delirium also has dementia, but it is not so difficult to determine whether a patient with dementia also has delirium. Prominent fluctuations in the level of consciousness are indicative of a delirium, with or without an underlying dementia. Patients with dementia are particularly vulnerable to acute insults to brain metabolism, which often result in a superimposed acute confusional state. Patients with dementia remain as medical inpatients significantly longer and require more daily nursing care than their counterparts without dementia (Erkinjuntti et al. 1986). Erkinjuntti and colleagues (1986) reported that 40% of dementia patients age 55 and older had delirium on admission to a general hospital and that 25% of elderly patients with delirium also have dementia.

Surveys of elderly patients with dementia suggest that 10%–30% have a medical illness that further impairs cognition. Patients with progressive dementias and their relatives often deny the cognitive decline early in its course, and patients first may be seen by the physician when the illness is moderately severe. Psychosocial stresses (e.g., death or illness of a spouse) also may cause an acute worsening and prompt recognition of the dementia by family members and clinicians.

The results of a national consensus conference on the diagnosis and treatment of Alzheimer's disease and related disorders were recently published by Small and colleagues (1997). Small et al. (1998) also reported on an economic analysis of treatment with donepezil, a new cholinesterase inhibitor indicated for the treatment of cognitive symptoms associated with mild to moderate Alzheimer's disease. They concluded that at the end of a 6-month treatment period, the overall costs in the group receiving donepezil were not significantly higher than the costs in comparison subjects who were not receiving this form of drug therapy. Despite the higher drug costs, the group receiving donepezil had a lower rate of institutionalization during the 6-month observation period. In addition to cognitive impairments, elderly patients with dementia may have psychosis and agitation (Wragg and Jeste 1989) or other behavioral symptoms of their underlying dementia, and the clinical picture in such patients can mimic that of delirium. Borson and Raskind (1997) reviewed the treatment of such behavioral symptoms, which includes environmental and judicious pharmacological management strategies.

The stress of taking care of a patient with dementia predisposes family members or other caregivers to a spectrum of emotional disturbances such as anxiety, depression, frustration, guilt, sleep disturbances, and irritability (Baumgarten et al. 1992; Russo et al. 1995). The consulting psychiatrist often finds that evaluation and treatment of caregivers is an important aspect of intervention.

Depression

Late-life depression is common in primary care settings (Gurland et al. 1996; Lebowitz et al. 1997) and general medical hospitals (Koenig et al. 1988a, 1988b, 1993) but often is not diagnosed or treated (Unützer et al. 2000). Such depression may present differently from depression in young adults (Addonizio and Alexopoulos 1993; National Institutes of Health Consensus Development Panel on Depression in Late Life 1992; Small 1991). For example, elderly depressed patients may be less likely to express guilt feelings than are their younger counterparts (Small et al. 1986). In addition, elderly patients are known to minimize or even to deny their depressed mood and instead become preoccupied with somatic symptoms. Conwell et al. (1990a) reported that six of one series of eight persons older than 65 who committed suicide had somatic delusions of having cancer and presented to their primary physicians with this concern before their deaths. Family members and even health care providers may also minimize the importance of geriatric depression and assume, incorrectly, that depression is the result of physical and social problems associated with "normal" aging. Symptoms such as loss of appetite, anhedonia, anergy, and insomnia are more prominent than depressed mood in elderly patients. The term *masked* is often used to describe the depressed condition of the patient who focuses on physical rather than affective complaints. Such patients frequently have neutral affects but complain about constipation, back pain, or some other physical symptom. A trial of antidepressant medication may help the clinician to determine whether somatic complaints reflect depression rather than an underlying physical illness.

Symptoms of depression and dementia frequently overlap in elderly patients, resulting in complex clinical syndromes (Small 1989). Some elderly patients with depression have cognitive complaints and present with a dementia syndrome of depression. The term *depressive pseudodementia* is no longer considered to be accurate by many clinicians because the cognitive dysfunction is real, albeit reversible. Complaints of memory problems tend to exceed actual memory impairment observed during neuropsychological testing. Such patients also are more likely to have an acute onset of symptoms and predominant affective complaints compared with patients with progressive dementias. Moreover, cognitive complaints usually improve with antidepressant treatment in the patient with depression. Evidence suggests, however, that depressed patients with significant cognitive impairments that respond to depression treatment are at increased risk for developing irreversible dementia over the long run (Alexopoulos et al. 1993). To complicate the situation, patients with primary progressive dementias (e.g., Alzheimer's disease, multi-infarct dementia) frequently develop depression, especially when the dementia is of mild to moderate severity. Among such patients with chronic dementia, subsyndromal depressive syndromes are more common than full-blown major depression. Patients with Alzheimer's disease who have major depression are more likely to have a family history of mood disorders than are patients with dementia who are not depressed (Pearlson et al. 1990). Sometimes such depressive symptoms appear to be a psychological reaction to cognitive losses, but evidence also exists for organic causes (Zubenko and Moosy 1988).

Geriatric depression often accompanies cerebrovascular disease, the third leading cause of death in the United States (Department of Health and Human Services 1990). Studies comparing patients with orthopedic conditions and those with stroke who had comparable physical disabilities found higher rates of depression in patients with stroke, suggesting a mechanism involving direct brain injury. Thus, depression following stroke is not just a psychological reaction to disability. Approximately half of the patients with acute stroke develop clinically significant depression. Patients with cortical or subcortical lesions in the left anterior hemisphere show a high frequency of depression compared with patients with lesions in other locations (Starkstein et al. 1988). Robinson and associates (1984), who studied 103 patients between ages 20 and 80 during the 6 months following a stroke, reported a 34% prevalence of major depression and a 26% prevalence of dysthymia. Lipsey and colleagues (1984) also showed that depressive symptoms significantly improved in patients who had a stroke and were given the tricyclic antidepressant nortriptyline.

Depressive symptoms are observed in approximately 40% of the patients with Parkinson's disease (Cummings 1992). Major depression occurs in nearly one-third of these patients; depressive episodes may predate the movement disorder. The depression associated with Parkinson's disease is not solely a reaction to the stress of physical disability and is associated with low levels of 5-hydroxyindoleacetic acid (5-HIAA), a serotonin metabolite in cerebrospinal fluid (CSF) (Cummings 1992).

Koenig and colleagues (1988a) found major depression in 12% and other depressive syndromes in 23% of 130 men age 70 and older who were hospitalized for medical illnesses. Studies of elderly patients attending medical outpatient clinics have reported rates of depression ranging from 10% to 20%. In general, health care providers are less likely to recognize major depression in hospitalized medically ill elderly patients than in younger hospitalized patients. In a study of 53 hospitalized elderly men with medical illness and major depression, 44% of the medical records contained no mention of depression (Koenig et al. 1992). The high frequency of affective symptoms in medically ill elderly patients and failure to recognize such symptoms present arguments in favor of routine depression screening in this patient population.

A significant public health problem related to depression is the high suicide rate, especially for elderly white men (Blazer et al. 1986; Rabins 1992). The suicide rate continues to be higher among men age 65 and older than among any other age group in the United States. The number of widowers who commit suicide is higher among older age groups and increases with age; highly lethal methods of suicide are more prevalent in older age groups as well (Conwell et al. 1990b). Approximately 90% of the elderly people who commit suicide have depression; therefore, early recognition and treatment of major depression would likely result in decreased suicide rates (Rabins 1992).

Anxiety

Hospitalized elderly patients often worry about medical illnesses and the accompanying pain, disability, and death. Severely ill elderly patients also must contend with acute physical illness that compromises quality of life and threatens existence. The loss of function and the possibility of death are difficult to deny and result in anxiety. Elderly patients hospitalized with an acute medical illness can become increasingly helpless, dependent, and isolated—consequently, their fears and anxiety escalate. Some elderly persons have an undiagnosed anxiety disorder, which is unmasked by the exacerbation of a physical illness, hospital admission, or surgery. A variety of physical and substance-related conditions can cause a secondary anxiety disorder; thyroid disease and medication effects are common causes of anxiety in elderly patients. Somatic anxiety symptoms, such as palpitations, dyspnea, and dizziness, can result from either underlying anxiety disorders or worsening physical illness, which complicates the differential diagnosis.

Phobic disorders are relatively common in old age, with 1-month prevalence rates ranging from 5% to 10% (Lindesay 1991; Regier et al. 1988). Agoraphobic fears in elderly persons are often precipitated by an episode of physical illness or other traumatic event (Lindesay 1991).

Late-Life Psychosis

Although DSM-III (American Psychiatric Association 1980) criteria indicated that the onset of schizophrenic symptoms must occur before age 45, schizophrenia with onset after age 45 identified as late-onset schizophrenia was recognized in subsequent DSM editions. An important change in DSM-IV (American Psychiatric Association 1994) was the absence of an age-at-onset criterion for the diagnosis of schizophrenia. Jeste et al. (1988), in their comparison of patients with early-onset and late-onset schizophrenia, described similarities in the degree of psychopathology and positive symptoms among the two groups. However, they reported a lower frequency of negative symptoms in the late-onset group.

Patients with dementias often develop psychotic symptoms. Patients with Alzheimer's disease often have simple persecutory delusions and visual hallucinations (Wragg and Jeste 1989). Zubenko and co-workers (1991) found associations between the presence of psychosis and densities of senile plaques and neurofibrillary tangles in the brains of patients with Alzheimer's disease. Jeste et al. (1992) reported that patients with Alzheimer's disease and psychosis show greater cognitive impairment than do their counterparts without psychosis. Psychotic symptoms also occur in patients with delirium, so careful diagnostic assessment is required. Regardless of whether the psychiatric disorder is a dementia with psychotic symptoms or a primary psychosis, neuroleptic agents offer effective treatment (Lohr et al. 1992).

Substance Dependence, Abuse, and Misuse

Although alcoholism is recognized as a major health and social problem in society, only recently has its effect on the geriatric population received attention. Elderly persons often underreport their alcohol consumption and related problems (Atkinson 1990), and clinicians fail to recognize alcohol-related problems in elderly patients (Curtis et al. 1989). In the absence of liver disease, hepatic metabolism of alcohol remains relatively unchanged with age. However, decreased lean body mass and total body water cause the total volume of distribution for alcohol to decline with age. Cognitive and cerebellar functions after a standard alcohol load worsen with age. Such effects make distinctions between "heavy" and "problem" drinking less meaningful for elderly persons, and in elderly patients, all heavy drinking is problem drinking. Heavy alcohol consumption for 5 or more years at some time in life is associated with current psychiatric diagnosis (e.g., major depression) in elderly persons (Saunders et al. 1991). By contrast, light to moderate alcohol consumption (less than 1 ounce/day) in elderly persons is associated with lowered cardiovascular mortality (Scherr et al. 1992).

Elderly persons sometimes abuse more than one substance at a time. Finlayson et al. (1988) reported that 14% of 216 alcoholic inpatients who were age 65 years or older also were abusing narcotic analgesics and anxiolytics. A useful and simple screen for alcohol consumption in elderly persons is the CAGE questionnaire (Buchsbaum et al. 1992). Depressive symptoms also are common in older persons with alcoholism, as are cognitive impairment and diseases of other organ systems—for example, occult cardiovascular disease, hypertension, osteoporosis, diabetes mellitus, hypoglycemia, and hyperuricemia (Atkinson 1990). Elderly persons may medicate themselves for conditions such as arthritis and other medical problems, insomnia, anxiety, or depression. Although over-the-counter (OTC) medications are considered safe by many doctors and patients, sometimes these medications are psychoactive and can cause adverse effects in elderly patients. For example, many OTC preparations for colds and allergies have anticholinergic side effects. These agents, as well as prescribed medications with anti-

cholinergic side effects, increase the risk for delirium. Therefore, consultation-liaison psychiatrists must review OTC drug use routinely during diagnostic evaluations.

Cohort Effects and Ageism

Elderly persons often consider psychiatric intervention as a last resort for "crazy people." They are reluctant to accept psychiatric referral and sometimes have psychiatric disorders that are overlooked or are inadequately treated. Ageism or age-related prejudice also complicates intervention, clouds decision making, and can result in improper treatment. Psychiatrists are not immune to ageist attitudes, which may involve fears of death, the belief that psychiatric symptoms are somehow "appropriate" in the elderly, and the inaccurate belief that elderly people do not respond to treatment (Ford and Sbordone 1980).

Elder Abuse

Although both victims and perpetrators deny and minimize the frequency and severity of elder abuse, an estimated 10% of Americans older than 65 are abused (Council on Scientific Affairs 1987). The abuser is often a relative who lives with the victim, and the abuse is generally recurring. Physical, sexual, or psychological abuse can take a variety of forms (Table 37–2). A typical victim is a physically or mentally impaired 75-year-old widow whose limited finances force her to move in with a younger relative (Taler and Ansello 1985). Clinicians should consider the possibility of elder abuse when a caregiver 1) expresses frustration in providing care, 2) shows signs of psychological distress, 3) has a history of committing abuse or violence, or 4) has a history of alcohol or drug abuse.

DIAGNOSTIC EVALUATION

Clinical Examination

In consultation-liaison settings, attention to physical problems and the medical history is as important as obtaining detailed information about the patient's psychiatric history. This is even more crucial in evaluating geriatric patients, in whom the likelihood of multiple medical conditions is high and symptoms of medical and psychiatric disorders overlap. Obtaining the history and performing a mental status examination are sometimes tedious because of the many years patients have lived, complications from multiple illnesses, and brain dysfunction. A reliable collateral source can save time and contribute important clinical information; this is essential when the patient has cognitive impairment.

TABLE 37–2. Types of elder abuse

Physical or sexual abuse
Bruises (bilateral; at different stages of healing)
Welts
Lacerations
Punctures
Fractures
Evidence of excessive drugging
Burns
Physical constraints (e.g., tying to beds)
Malnutrition and/or dehydration
Lack of personal care
Inadequate heating
Lack of food and water
Unclean clothes or bedding
Pain or itching, bruises, or bleeding of external genitalia, vaginal area, or anal area

Psychological abuse[a]
Threats
Insults
Harassment
Withholding of security and affection
Harsh orders
Caregiver refusal to allow travel, visits, church attendance

Exploitation
Misuse of vulnerable person's income or other financial resources (victim is best source of information, but in most cases has turned management of financial affairs over to another person; as a result, there may be some confusion about finances)

Medical abuse
Withholding or improper administration of medications or necessary medical treatments for a condition
Withholding of aids the person would medically require (e.g., false teeth, glasses, hearing aids)

Neglect
Conduct causing deprivation of care necessary to maintain physical and mental health; may be manifested by malnutrition, poor personal hygiene, or any of the indicators for medical abuse

[a]Vulnerable adults react by exhibiting resignation, defeat, depression, mental confusion, anger, ambivalence, and/or insomnia.
Source. Adapted from Council on Scientific Affairs: "Elder Abuse and Neglect." *Journal of the American Medical Association* 257:968, 1987. Copyright 1987, American Medical Association. Originally published by Washington State Medical Association. Used with permission.

Physical Examination

Patients usually are examined by their primary physicians before the psychiatrist is consulted. The consultant should review the medical record to gather details of history, diagnosis, and management of the present illness.

Sometimes the consultation-liaison psychiatrist must perform a limited physical examination, particularly an examination of vital signs or a screening neurological examination. Consultants occasionally will discover a physical sign overlooked by the primary physician. For example, the patient who is agitated and disturbed (e.g., a frail elderly patient with psychosis) can make the primary physician anxious and thus cloud clinical assessment. (For a detailed review of history-taking and the initial physical examination, the reader is referred to a geriatric medicine text [e.g., Brocklehurst et al. 1992; Kane et al. 1989].)

Mental Status Examination

Certain aspects of the mental status examination deserve special attention in elderly patients. Depressed elderly patients who minimize dysphoria may demonstrate it nonverbally through facial expressions and sighs. A careful investigation of suicidal thinking and intent is essential because of the lethal methods chosen by this age group. Cognitive assessment of geriatric patients is particularly important. A comprehensive cognitive examination usually includes examination of attention and concentration, language functions (e.g., spontaneous speech, comprehension, repetition, naming), orientation, memory functions, constructional ability, praxis, and frontal lobe function. The Mini-Mental State Exam (MMSE; Folstein et al. 1975) provides a brief, yet reliable and valid, measure of cognition that includes tests of orientation, memory, concentration, language, and conceptual ability. Although the MMSE does not identify patients with subtle cognitive dysfunction and the language items have low sensitivity, the memory item, attention-concentration items, and constructional item have adequate sensitivity and specificity in many clinical settings and correlate significantly with scores on neuropsychological tests (Feher et al. 1992). Administration of the MMSE is easily taught to other health professionals, which increases their awareness of cognitive function in elderly patients. Another simple cognitive screening tool that has been validated in a general hospital setting is the 10-point clock test (Manos 1997, 1998).

Laboratory Findings

A clinical chemistry screen is routine for almost all hospital admissions and for most initial outpatient visits. Such screens are essential in diagnostic evaluations of patients with cognitive impairment. Abnormal sodium and chloride levels can warn of dehydration that may, if untreated, progress to delirium, lethargy, or convulsions.

This screen also will detect respiratory or metabolic acidosis, which can lead to drowsiness and weakness that may be mistakenly diagnosed as depression.

Decreased protein intake and decreased muscle mass in older patients lead to an overestimate of renal function because blood urea nitrogen (BUN) and creatinine levels decrease. Therefore, normal serum levels for BUN and creatinine may indicate decreased renal function, and minor elevations may represent significant dysfunction. Liver function typically remains adequate throughout life, despite some decrease in the speed of drug metabolism.

CSF examinations are indicated for patients with suspected CNS infection, trauma, or bleeding. In degenerative CNS diseases, CSF proteins are usually high.

The electrocardiogram (ECG) is used to screen for cardiovascular disease and to identify the presence of conduction defects that would complicate the use of tricyclic antidepressants or electroconvulsive therapy (ECT). It also reveals the presence of cardiovascular disease that can have psychiatric manifestations.

Brain Imaging Studies

Structural Imaging

Developed about 25 years ago, computed tomography (CT) is still widely used in geriatric psychiatry. Both abnormal anatomic and pathological structural alterations are identified by CT scanning. Routine scans are often performed without contrast media; however, use of contrast media for scans in patients with suspected intracranial malignancy or bleeding may help to diagnose these conditions. CT is the imaging modality of choice for the evaluation of acute head trauma and stroke. Magnetic resonance imaging (MRI) offers greater resolution of structural images than does CT. The disadvantages of MRI include greater cost and greater discomfort (i.e., some patients become claustrophobic during the procedure). The procedure is contraindicated in patients with ferrous metal implants.

Functional Imaging

Positron-emission tomography (PET) is the most advanced functional imaging modality available and provides measures of regional blood flow and metabolism. Its main clinical application in geriatric psychiatry is in the diagnosis and differential diagnosis of the dementias (Small 1991). Single photon emission computed tomography (SPECT) provides measures of cerebral blood flow. Although it has less resolution than PET, SPECT is sometimes less expensive and is generally more available.

The electroencephalogram (EEG) and quantitative EEG (QEEG) can be useful in evaluating patients with possible seizure disorders or mental disorders resulting from a general medical condition or substance use. This test may help when the course of psychiatric disorder is unusual, when the disorder is refractory to treatment, or when diagnosing and following up patients with delirium.

TREATMENT AND MANAGEMENT

Treatment of Medical Problems

The treatment of medical problems in elderly patients is especially crucial. Most psychiatric problems in this population occur either because of or concurrently with medical illnesses. Although the attending physician controls the medical treatment, the consultant occasionally must suggest additional diagnostic evaluations or alternative medical treatments.

Psychopharmacological Treatment

Age-Related Pharmacokinetic and Pharmacodynamic Factors

Interactions of drugs with the brain and the rest of the body change with age (Abernethy 1992) (Table 37–3). Gastrointestinal function alterations include increased gastric pH, diminished splanchnic blood flow, and diminished intestinal motility, yet drug absorption generally does not diminish as people age. Most psychotropic medications are highly lipid-soluble and protein-bound. Aging causes a relative decrease in total body water, reduction in lean body mass, and increase in body fat. With the resultant larger volume of distribution, more time is required for drugs to reach steady-state levels, and plasma levels are lower at any given dose. Moreover, liver disease can impair protein synthesis, leading to decreased protein availability for binding to psychotropics in plasma. Thus, more unbound or active drug is present, causing greater clinical effect at any given plasma level. In addition, reduced hepatic blood flow and function diminish the metabolism of psychotropics (e.g., chlordiazepoxide, diazepam) that undergo phase I biotransformation. Hepatic metabolism of cyclic antidepressants forms water-soluble hydroxy metabolites; such metabolites are cardiotoxic and depend on renal clearance. Renal function often decreases with age, and thus the risk of cardiotoxicity from such agents increases. Lithium also requires careful monitoring in elderly patients because of predominant renal elimination and potentially serious toxicity.

TABLE 37–3.   Pharmacokinetic changes associated with aging

Factor	Age effect	Consequence
Absorption	Decreased gastric acidity	In absence of gastric pathology or drug-drug interactions, absorption of psychotropic drugs not significantly altered
	Decreased motility	
	Decreased blood flow	
	Decreased GI surface area	
Hepatic function	Decreased hepatic blood flow	Increased circulating, unmetabolized, and partially metabolized psychotropic drug
	Decreased first-pass effect	Prolonged time required for psychotropic drug elimination
	Decreased hepatic enzyme activity	Prolonged exposure to unmetabolized drug
	Decreased demethylation	
	Decreased hydroxylation	
Protein binding	Decreased albumin	Increase in active drug (unclear effects)
	Increased (?) α_1 glycoprotein	Unclear effect on pharmacokinetics
Renal excretion	Decreased renal blood flow	Decreased lithium clearance and increased risk of toxicity
	Decreased GFR	Decreased antidepressant hydroxy metabolite clearance
		Increased cardiotoxicity
	Decreased tubular excretory capacity	Decreased benzodiazepine clearance
		Prolonged elimination half-life

Note.   GFR = glomerular filtration rate; GI = gastrointestinal.
Source.   Wise MG, Tierney J: "Psychopharmacology in the Elderly." *Journal of the Louisiana State Medical Society* 144:471–476, 1992. Used with permission.

Pharmacodynamics also change with age. Neurotransmitter synthesis and turnover, receptor binding, and synaptic neurotransmission change in many brain areas as people age. The precise clinical significance of such changes is unknown, but available evidence suggests that elderly persons have greater receptor-site sensitivity for many drugs, particularly benzodiazepines (e.g., diazepam). By contrast, changes in β-adrenergic function result in lower sensitivity to β-adrenergic stimulation and blockade.

Plasma drug levels are sometimes used to monitor antidepressant medications in younger adults. In geriatric patients, particularly those with multiple medical illnesses, the clinical value of plasma levels is unclear. Georgotas et al. (1986) adjusted nortriptyline dosage so that serum levels remained in the therapeutic window of 50–180 ng/mL and found a robust response for the nortriptyline group. Studies of other antidepressants have not consistently shown a significant correlation between plasma levels and clinical response. Antidepressant plasma levels, particularly levels of tricyclic antidepressants, may be most useful if patients experience side effects at low doses, do not respond to an adequate trial of an antidepressant, or are taking other drugs that may increase antidepressant blood levels.

Polypharmacy

The use of multiple drugs affects all pharmacokinetic processes. Because elderly persons are likely to use more than one medication, drug-drug interactions are a critical issue in management. The metabolism of psychotropic drugs is often complicated by chronic medical illnesses and medications that alter gastrointestinal, hepatic, or renal functions. Potential combinations of various drugs and diseases are too numerous to study systemically, so data to guide clinicians are unavailable. Some recent reviews outlined common and clinically significant interactions of psychotropic medications in late life (Lebowitz et al. 1998; Salzman 1998). Fait et al. (Chapter 42 in this volume) review the metabolism of the most commonly used psychotropic drugs by the P450 isoenzyme system in the liver, and the resulting drug-drug interactions are particularly relevant for older adults who may be taking several medications metabolized by the same isoenzyme systems. In most situations, clinical guidelines generalize from data derived from patients that only partially resemble the complicated geriatric patient. Educational programs that target health care providers can reduce polypharmacy (Avorn et al. 1992).

All psychotropic medications have been used to treat medically ill geriatric patients (Table 37–4). Unfortunately, however, data from controlled studies in this patient population are limited. Thus, clinicians should use caution and conservative guidelines (see "Follow Conservative and Rational Pharmacological Guidelines" later in this chapter) and consult recent references on the use of psychotropic medications in late life when prescribing psychotropic drugs for elderly patients (Lebowitz et al. 1998; Salzman 1998).

TABLE 37–4. Some psychotropic drugs and treatment recommendations in the elderly

Drug type	Recommended drug	Approximate daily dose range (mg)	Comments/common side effects
Typical neuroleptics	Haloperidol	0.25–4.00	EPS common; risk of TD
	Thiothixene	1–15	EPS common; risk of TD
	Thioridazine	10–200	Sedation; hypotension; anticholinergic side effects; risk of TD
Atypical neuroleptics	Clozapine	10–100	Sedation; anticholinergic side effects; risk of agranulocytosis
	Risperidone	0.25–4.00	EPS at higher doses
	Olanzapine	2.5–10.0	Sedation; weight gain
Heterocyclic antidepressants	Desipramine	10–150	Affects cardiac conduction; hypotension; anticholinergic side effects
	Nortriptyline	10–75	Affects cardiac conduction; hypotension; anticholinergic side effects
Selective serotonin reuptake inhibitors	Fluoxetine	5–40	GI distress; insomnia; excess activation
	Fluvoxamine	50–150	GI distress; insomnia; excess activation
	Paroxetine	5–30	GI distress; anticholinergic side effects
	Sertraline	12.5–150.0	GI distress
	Citalopram	10–30	GI distress
New/atypical antidepressants	Bupropion	75–100 bid–tid	Twice-daily dosing with sustained-release preparation; increased risk of seizures at high doses
	Nefazodone	50–100 bid	Sedation; serious drug-drug interactions with other drugs
	Venlafaxine	12.5–125 bid	Once-daily dosing with XR preparation; nausea; elevated blood pressure at high doses
	Trazodone	25–50	Orthostatic hypotension and sedation at higher doses; frequently used in low doses as a hypnotic; some use for behavioral agitation in dementia
	Mirtazapine	15–30	Increased appetite/weight gain, sedation
Anxiolytics	Alprazolam	0.25–0.50	Sedation; short half-life can cause rebound and withdrawal; cognitive impairment at higher doses; risk of falls
	Lorazepam	0.5–1.0	Sedation; cognitive impairment at higher doses; risk of falls
	Oxazepam	10–30	Sedation; cognitive impairment at higher doses; risk of falls
	Buspirone	5–60	
Hypnotics	Temazepam	7.5–20.0	Cognitive impairment at higher doses; risk of falls
	Triazolam	0.125–0.250	Short half-life may cause rebound insomnia; cognitive impairment at higher doses; risk of falls
	Zolpidem	5–10	Short half-life; insufficient data about cognitive impairment at higher doses
Mood stabilizers	Lithium	150–1,500	Renal excretion; narrow therapeutic window, especially in older adults; delirium at high doses
	Carbamazepine	100–1,200	May cause agranulocytosis; induces its own metabolism and that of other drugs
	Divalproex sodium	250–1,800	Ataxia; GI distress; weight gain; cognitive impairment (?)

Note. EPS = extrapyramidal side effects; GI = gastrointestinal; TD = tardive dyskinesia; XR = extended release.

Antidepressant Medications

More than 30 randomized controlled trials of antidepressants found that physically healthy depressed elderly patients respond to a variety of agents, including cyclic antidepressants and selective serotonin reuptake inhibitors (SSRIs) (Schneider 1996; Small and Salzman 1998). Fluoxetine has been shown to be safe and effective for geriatric depression (Tollefson et al. 1995), but newer SSRIs such as paroxetine, sertraline, fluvoxamine, and citalopram are also reasonable choices and offer the advantage of shorter elimination half-lives (Bump et al. 2001). The lack of anticholinergic and cardiac side effects with SSRIs offers a marked advantage for geriatric use, and these drugs have become the antidepressant of first choice over the past few years in the treatment of depression in older adults. One recent study by Schneider and co-workers (1997) suggested that in depressed older women, estrogen replacement therapy may augment the response to fluoxetine and that this should be considered as a factor in future clinical trials with elderly women.

Other newer agents such as nefazodone, bupropion, mirtazapine, and venlafaxine have also been used successfully in older adults (Small and Salzman 1998). Among tricyclic antidepressants, secondary amine compounds (e.g., nortriptyline, desipramine) are preferred to tertiary amines (e.g., amitriptyline, imipramine) because of their favorable side-effect profile. The observation that monoamine oxidase activity increases with age (Bridge et al. 1985) suggests a place for monoamine oxidase inhibitors (MAOIs) in the treatment of geriatric depression. Initial reports indicate efficacy in patients with Alzheimer's disease and major depression (Jenike 1985). Unfortunately, the potential for MAOIs to produce orthostatic hypotension, especially in predisposed individuals, limits their usefulness for many geriatric patients.

Psychostimulants

Limited data on psychostimulants suggest their usefulness in treating medically ill withdrawn elderly patients who cannot tolerate adverse effects (e.g., cardiac conduction abnormalities) that are associated with other antidepressants (Katon and Raskind 1980). Psychostimulants also have been used in combination with noradrenergic antidepressant drugs. The antidepressant effects of psychostimulants may result from catecholamine reuptake blockage that prolongs effects of synaptically released norepinephrine (Chiarello and Cole 1987).

Mood-Stabilizing Medications

Lithium can be used safely and effectively in medically ill elderly patients, but some caution is needed (Foster 1992). In general, elderly patients require lower lithium doses and blood levels. Consultation-liaison psychiatrists must recognize and appreciate the potentially serious adverse interactions between lithium and other drugs such as diuretics, nonsteroidal anti-inflammatory drugs, cardiovascular drugs, anticonvulsants, antidepressants, and neuroleptics. Newer mood stabilizers such as valproic acid, carbamazepine, lamotrigine, and gabapentin have been found useful in younger populations and have been used clinically in older adults but have not been tested in clinical trials involving large samples of older subjects.

Benzodiazepines

Benzodiazepines are recommended for anxiety and agitation, especially when the elderly patient's medical condition poses a risk of toxicity from other psychotropics (e.g., tricyclic antidepressants or antipsychotic drugs). Short-acting benzodiazepines are preferred. Benzodiazepines with long elimination half-lives and active metabolites (e.g., diazepam) are more likely to cause ataxia and confusion and are best avoided in older patients.

Neuroleptic Medications

A limited number of studies indicates that neuroleptic medications are useful in treating psychotic symptoms in elderly patients with dementia, schizophrenia, psychotic depressions, or delirium. Traditionally, high-potency compounds such as haloperidol have been the agents of first choice because of fewer cardiovascular and anticholinergic effects. Side effects of concern include parkinsonian symptoms, akathisia, and tardive dyskinesia. Caution is appropriate because neuroleptic discontinuation studies show that up to 50% of chronically medicated elderly patients with dementia show less agitation once the neuroleptic is stopped. Several studies documented the high vulnerability of elderly patients to tardive dyskinesia; incidences of 31% were reported after 43 weeks of neuroleptic treatment (Saltz et al. 1991; Yassa et al. 1992). Side effects from neuroleptic medications sometimes call for alternative and adjunctive treatments such as benzodiazepines, β-blockers, carbamazepine, lithium, and trazodone (Lacro et al. 1993). Initial clinical and research experience with novel antipsychotic medications (e.g., risperidone, olanzapine, and quetiapine) suggests that these medications will likely become the agents of first choice in treating psychosis in elderly patients because of their lower risk of acute side effects and long-term complications such as tardive dyskinesia.

Electroconvulsive Therapy

ECT is generally the safest and most effective treatment for severe depression in elderly patients and is the treatment of choice for those with psychotic depression. Although patients with multiple medical problems and those older than 75 are at increased risk for adverse effects, modification of treatment can minimize risks. Although temporary memory effects are common in elderly patients, overall cognitive dysfunction actually improves after ECT (Stoudemire et al. 1991).

Psychotherapy and Related Nonpharmacological Approaches

Psychotherapy is effective in the treatment of depression in geriatric patients, especially when a patient's cognitive impairment or severity of illness does not interfere with talk therapy. In geriatric patients, depression has been treated successfully with individual psychodynamic, cognitive, and behavioral approaches, as well as group psychotherapy (Arean et al. 1993; Niederehe 1996; Weiss and Lazarus 1993). In a medical inpatient setting, psychotherapeutic interventions are often supportive and time-limited.

Many elderly patients receive care from spouses, adult children, and other relatives (Jarvik and Small 1990). Caregivers experience considerable stress and are prone to depression and health problems (Baumgarten et al. 1992; Russo et al. 1995). Psychological support for caregivers may lessen their emotional burden and, in the final analysis, benefit the older patient.

Environmental Management

Modifications of the environment help to minimize confusion in hospitalized elderly patients. Prominent clocks, night-lights, and personal items from home can assist orientation. Frequent visits and reorientation from relatives and friends are also helpful. Finally, clinicians should consider bright-light treatment for patients with seasonal mood disorders (Kripke et al. 1992). Phototherapy also has been used to treat patients with Alzheimer's disease who have behavioral and sleep disturbances (Satlin et al. 1992).

STRATEGIES FOR PSYCHIATRIC CONSULTATION FOR GERIATRIC PATIENTS

Table 37–5 summarizes several strategies for psychiatric consultation for geriatric patients that are discussed in the following sections.

Collect Data From Multiple Sources

Many elderly patients rely on family members or other caregivers for assistance with ADLs; thus, the consultant must obtain comprehensive histories from the caregivers and maintain close contact with them. For cognitively impaired patients, caregivers' and collateral histories are essential. The complexity and multiplicity of medical problems also warrant careful review of previous medical records and detailed discussions with the patient's primary physicians and consultants.

Recognize Unique Clinical Presentations of Geriatric Syndromes

Geriatric depression often differs from depression in young adults. Physical and memory complaints are more

TABLE 37–5. Suggested strategies for psychiatric consultation for geriatric patients

Collect data from multiple sources
Recognize unique clinical presentations of geriatric syndromes
Search for medical and toxic causes of psychiatric syndromes
Reduce polypharmacy
Follow conservative and rational pharmacological guidelines
Identify adverse drug effects sooner rather than later
Emphasize nonpharmacological interventions

prominent in elderly patients. In unclear clinical situations, a therapeutic trial of an antidepressant medication may resolve the question. The presence of dementia may overshadow an underlying delirium; the reverse is also true. Multiple medical and psychiatric conditions require a systematic approach to these problems.

Search for Medical Causes of Psychiatric Syndromes

Patients with medical illnesses should be treated so that the illness or its treatment does not cause or exacerbate psychiatric symptoms. Although a psychiatric disorder may present with characteristic clinical features, the high prevalence of medical illness in elderly patients frequently requires an aggressive search for medical and toxic causes. A comprehensive history, a physical examination, and laboratory tests usually identify underlying physical illnesses that cause psychiatric symptoms. Close collaboration among medical colleagues is essential.

Reduce Polypharmacy

Elderly patients with physical illnesses generally take numerous medications. A relative should bring all medication bottles for initial evaluation. When possible, one medication at a time should be eliminated, especially drugs that are likely to cause adverse effects.

Follow Conservative and Rational Pharmacological Guidelines

"Start low and go slow" is the recommended strategy. Many elderly patients respond to relatively low dosages; however, some will need the full adult dosage. Medications should be selected according to side-effect profile. For example, sedating antidepressants may be best for patients with agitated depressions. In patients who are at high risk for relapse or recurrence, maintenance antidepressant or antipsychotic medications should be given according to existing treatment guidelines. Reynolds and colleagues (1999) recently reported that maintenance therapy with antidepressant medications and/or interpersonal therapy was significantly more effective in preventing depression recurrence than was placebo.

Identify Adverse Drug Effects Sooner Rather Than Later

Close monitoring of patients for side effects is crucial. For example, agitation in a patient with dementia may initially improve with a neuroleptic, then worsen after weeks of treatment (i.e., akathisia). Benzodiazepines with long elimination half-lives and active metabolites will accumulate over time and cause confusion and ataxia.

Emphasize Nonpharmacological Interventions

Physically ill geriatric patients are often sensitive to medication side effects and may not initially tolerate psychotropic medications. These situations call for nonpharmacological approaches. ECT, psychotherapy, phototherapy, and environmental interventions may help facilitate later pharmacological interventions, which can benefit the patient.

CONCLUSION

Providing expert evaluation and treatment for elderly medically ill patients can be both a challenging and a rewarding experience for the consultation-liaison psychiatrist. A practical, systematic approach to diagnostic and treatment decision making is essential. The medical illnesses will, of course, often complicate accurate diagnosis, but the consultant also must consider complications from dementia syndromes, cohort effects, ageism, and heterogeneity of patient populations. Age-related pharmacokinetic changes tend to increase an elderly person's sensitivity to medications. Various psychotropic drugs have been found to be safe and effective in elderly patients with psychiatric and physical conditions, but some modification in their use is suggested. A systematic approach is provided to assist the clinician when confronted with this often complex and challenging patient population.

REFERENCES

Abernethy DR: Psychotropic drugs and the aging process: pharmacokinetics and pharmacodynamics, in Clinical Geriatric Psychopharmacology, 2nd Edition. Edited by Salzman C. Baltimore, MD, Williams & Wilkins, 1992, pp 61–76

Addonizio G, Alexopoulos GS: Affective disorders in the elderly. Int J Geriatr Psychiatry 8:41–47, 1993

Alexopoulos GS, Meyers BS, Young RC, et al: The course of geriatric depression with "reversible dementia": a controlled study. Am J Psychiatry 150:1693–1699, 1993

American Psychiatric Association: Diagnostic and Statistical Manual of Mental Disorders, 3rd Edition. Washington, DC, American Psychiatric Association, 1980

American Psychiatric Association: Diagnostic and Statistical Manual of Mental Disorders, 3rd Edition, Revised. Washington, DC, American Psychiatric Association, 1987

American Psychiatric Association: Diagnostic and Statistical Manual of Mental Disorders, 4th Edition. Washington, DC, American Psychiatric Association, 1994

American Psychiatric Association: Diagnostic and Statistical Manual of Mental Disorders, 4th Edition, Text Revision. Washington, DC, American Psychiatric Association, 2000

Arean PA, Perri MG, Nezzu AM, et al: Comparative effectiveness of social problem solving therapy and reminiscence therapy as treatments for depression in older adults. J Consult Clin Psychol 61:1003–1010, 1993

Atkinson RM: Aging and alcohol use disorders: diagnostic issues in the elderly. Int Psychogeriatr 2:55–70, 1990

Avorn J, Soumerai SB, Everitt DE, et al: A randomized trial of a program to reduce the use of psychoactive drugs in nursing homes. N Engl J Med 327:168–173, 1992

Baumgarten M, Battista RN, Infante-Rivard C, et al: The psychological and physical health of family members caring for an elderly person with dementia. J Clin Epidemiol 45:61–70, 1992

Blazer DG, Bachar JR, Manton KE: Suicide in late life: review and commentary. J Am Geriatr Soc 34:519–525, 1986

Borson S, Raskind MA: Clinical features and pharmacological treatment of behavioral symptoms of Alzheimer's patients. Neurology 5:S17–S24, 1997

Bridge TP, Soldo BJ, Phelps BY, et al: Platelet monoamine oxidase activity: demographic characteristics contribute to enzyme activity variability. J Gerontol 40:23–28, 1985

Brocklehurst JC, Tallis RC, Fillit HM (eds): Textbook of Geriatric Medicine and Gerontology, 4th Edition. New York, Churchill Livingstone, 1992

Buchsbaum DG, Buchanan RG, Welsh J, et al: Screening for drinking disorders in the elderly using the CAGE questionnaire. J Am Geriatr Soc 40:662–665, 1992

Bump GM, Mulsant BH, Pollock BG, et al: Paroxetine versus nortriptyline in the continuation and maintenance treatment of depression in the elderly. Depress Anxiety 13:38–44, 2001

Chiarello RJ, Cole JO: The use of psychostimulants in general psychiatry: a reconsideration. Arch Gen Psychiatry 44:286–296, 1987

Cohen HJ, Saltz CC, Samsa G, et al: Predictors of two-year post-hospitalization mortality among elderly veterans in a study evaluating a geriatric consultation team. J Am Geriatr Soc 40:1231–1235, 1992

Cole MG, Fenton FR, Engelsmann F, et al: Effectiveness of geriatric psychiatry consultation in an acute care hospital: a randomized clinical trial. J Am Geriatr Soc 39:1183–1188, 1991

Conwell Y, Caine ED, Olsen K: Suicide and cancer in late life. Hospital and Community Psychiatry 41:1334–1339, 1990a

Conwell Y, Rotenberg M, Caine ED: Completed suicide at age 50 and over. J Am Geriatr Soc 38:640–644, 1990b

Council on Scientific Affairs: Elder abuse and neglect. JAMA 257:966–971, 1987

Cummings JL: Depression and Parkinson's disease. Am J Psychiatry 149:443–454, 1992

Curtis JR, Geller G, Stokes EG, et al: Characteristics, diagnosis and treatment of alcoholism in elderly patients. J Am Geriatr Soc 37:310–316, 1989

Curyto KJ, Johnson J, TenHave T, et al: Survival of hospitalized elderly patients with delirium: a prospective study. Am J Geriatr Psychiatry 9:141–147, 2001

Department of Health and Human Services, Public Health Service: Healthy People 2000: National Health Promotion and Disease Prevention Objectives. Washington, DC, Department of Health and Human Services, 1990

Erkinjuntti T, Wikstrom J, Palo J, et al: Dementia among medical inpatients: evaluation of 2000 consecutive admissions. Arch Intern Med 146:1923–1926, 1986

Feher EP, Mahurin RK, Doody RS, et al: Establishing the limits of the Mini-Mental State: examination of "subtests." Arch Neurol 49:87–92, 1992

Finlayson ER, Hurt RD, Davis LJ, et al: Alcoholism in elderly persons: a study of the psychiatric and psychosocial features of 216 inpatients. Mayo Clin Proc 63:761–768, 1988

Folks DG, Ford CV: Psychiatric disorders in geriatric medical/surgical patients, part I: report of 195 consecutive consultations. South Med J 78:239–241, 1985

Folstein MF, Folstein SE, McHugh PR: Mini-Mental State: a practical method for grading the cognitive state of patients for the clinician. J Psychiatr Res 12:189–198, 1975

Ford CV, Sbordone RJ: Attitudes of psychiatrists toward elderly patients. Am J Psychiatry 137:571–575, 1980

Foster JR: Use of lithium in elderly psychiatric patients: a review of the literature. Lithium 3:77–93, 1992

Francis J, Kapoor WN: Prognosis after hospital discharge of older medical patients with delirium. J Am Geriatr Soc 40:601–606, 1992

Georgotas A, McCue RE, Hapworth W, et al: Comparative efficacy and safety of MAOIs versus TCAs in treating depression in the elderly. Biol Psychiatry 21:1155–1166, 1986

Grossberg GT, Zimny GH, Nakra BRS: Geriatric psychiatry consultations in a university hospital. Int Psychogeriatr 2:161–168, 1990

Gurland BJ, Cross PS, Katz S: Epidemiologic perspectives on opportunities for treating depression. Am J Geriatr Psychiatry 4:S7–S13, 1996

Jarvik L, Small G: Parentcare. New York, Bantam, 1990

Jenike MA: MAO inhibitors as treatment for depressed patients with primary degenerative dementia (Alzheimer's disease). Am J Psychiatry 142:763–764, 1985

Jeste DV, Harris MJ, Pearlson GD, et al: Late-onset schizophrenia: studying clinical validity. Psychiatr Clin North Am 11:1–13, 1988

Jeste DV, Wragg RE, Salmon DP, et al: Cognitive deficits of Alzheimer's disease patients with and without delusions. Am J Psychiatry 149:184–189, 1992

Kane RL, Ouslander JB, Abrass IB: Essentials of Clinical Geriatrics, 2nd Edition. New York, McGraw-Hill, 1989

Katon W, Raskind M: Treatment of depression in the medically ill elderly with methylphenidate. Am J Psychiatry 137:963–965, 1980

Katon WJ, Von Korff M, Lin E, et al: Population-based care of depression: effective disease management strategies to decrease prevalence. Gen Hosp Psychiatry 19:169–178, 1997

Klinkman MS, Okkes I: Mental health problems in primary care: a research agenda. J Fam Pract 47:379–384, 1998

Koenig HG, Meador KG, Cohen HJ, et al: Depression in elderly hospitalized patients with medical illness. Arch Intern Med 148:1929–1936, 1988a

Koenig HG, Meador KG, Cohen HJ, et al: Detection and treatment of major depression in older medically ill hospitalized patients. Int J Psychiatry Med 18:17–31, 1988b

Koenig HG, Goli V, Shelp F, et al: Major depression in hospitalized medically ill older men: documentation, management, and outcome. Int J Geriatr Psychiatry 7:255–334, 1992

Koenig HG, O'Connor CM, Cuarisco SA, et al: Depressive disorder in older medical inpatients on general medicine and cardiology services at a university teaching hospital. Am J Geriatr Psychiatry 1:197–210, 1993

Kripke DF, Mullaney DJ, Klauber MR, et al: Controlled trial of bright light for nonseasonal major depressive disorders. Biol Psychiatry 31:119–134, 1992

Lacro JP, Harris MJ, Jeste DV: Late life psychosis. Int J Geriatr Psychiatry 8:49–57, 1993

Lebowitz BD, Pearson JL, Schneider LS: Diagnosis and treatment of depression in late life: consensus statement update. JAMA 278:1186–1190, 1997

Lebowitz BD, Person JL, Cohen GD: Clinical Geriatric Psychopharmacology. Baltimore, MD, Williams & Wilkins, 1998

Levitan S, Kornfeld D: Clinical and cost benefits of liaison psychiatry. Am J Psychiatry 138:790–793, 1981

Levitte SS, Thornby JI: Geriatric and non-geriatric psychiatry consultation: a comparison study. Gen Hosp Psychiatry 11:339–344, 1989

Lindesay J: Phobic disorders in the elderly. Br J Psychiatry 159:531–541, 1991

Lipowski ZJ: The need to integrate liaison psychiatry and geropsychiatry. Am J Psychiatry 140:1003–1005, 1983

Lipowski ZJ: Delirium in the elderly patient. N Engl J Med 320:578–582, 1989

Lipsey JR, Robinson RG, Pearlson GD, et al: Nortriptyline treatment of post-stroke depression: a double blind study. Lancet 2:298–300, 1984

Lohr JB, Jeste DV, Harris MJ, et al: Treatment of disordered behavior, in Clinical Geriatric Psychopharmacology, 2nd Edition. Edited by Salzman C. Baltimore, MD, Williams & Wilkins, 1992, pp 79–113

Mainprize E, Rodin G: Geriatric referrals to a psychiatric consultation-liaison service. Can J Psychiatry 32:5–9, 1987

Manos PJ: The utility of the ten-point clock test as a screen for cognitive impairment in general hospital patients. Gen Hosp Psychiatry 19:439–444, 1997

Manos PJ: Monitoring cognitive disturbance in delirium with the ten-point clock test. Int J Geriatr Psychiatry 13:646–648, 1998

Mulsant BH, Alexopoulos GS, Reynolds CF 3rd, et al: Pharmacological treatment of depression in older primary care patients: the PROSPECT algorithm. Int J Geriatr Psychiatry 16:585–592, 2001

National Institutes of Health Consensus Development Panel on Depression in Late Life: Diagnosis and treatment of depression in late life. JAMA 268:1018–1024, 1992

Niederehe G: Psychosocial treatments with depressed older adults. Am J Geriatr Psychiatry 4:S66–S78, 1996

Ormel J, Kempen GIJM, Penninx BWJH, et al: Chronic medical conditions and mental health in older people: disability and psychosocial resources mediate specific mental health effects. Psychol Med 27:1065–1077, 1997

Oxman TE, Berkman LF, Kasl S, et al: Social support and depressive symptoms in the elderly. Am J Epidemiol 135:356–368, 1992

Pearlson GD, Ross CA, Lohr WD, et al: Association between family history of affective disorder and the depressive syndrome of Alzheimer's disease. Am J Psychiatry 147:452–456, 1990

Popkin MK, MacKenzie TB, Callies AL: Psychiatric consultation to geriatric medically ill inpatients in a university hospital. Arch Gen Psychiatry 41:703–707, 1984

Rabins PV: Prevention of mental disorder in the elderly: current perspectives and future prospects. J Am Geriatr Soc 40:727–733, 1992

Rabins P, Lucas MJ, Teitelbaum M, et al: Utilization of psychiatric consultation for elderly patients. J Am Geriatr Soc 31:581–584, 1983

Regier DA, Boyd JH, Burke JD, et al: One-month prevalence of mental disorders in the United States. Arch Gen Psychiatry 45:977–986, 1988

Reynolds FE, Frank E, Kupfer DJ, et al: Nortriptyline and interpersonal psychotherapy as maintenance therapies for recurrent major depression: a randomized controlled trial in patients older than 59 years. JAMA 281:39–45, 1999

Robinson RG, Kubos KL, Storr LB, et al: Mood disorders in stroke patients. Brain 107:81–93, 1984

Rowe JW: Health care of the elderly. N Engl J Med 312:827–835, 1985

Rowe JW, Kahn RL: Successful Aging. New York, Pantheon Books, 1998

Ruskin PE: Geriatric consultation in a university hospital: a report on 67 referrals. Am J Psychiatry 142:333–336, 1985

Russo J, Vitaliano PP, Brewer DD, et al: Psychiatric disorders in spouse-caregivers of care recipients of Alzheimer's disease and matched controls: a diathesis-stress model of psychopathology. J Abnorm Psychol 104:197–204, 1995

Saltz BL, Woerner MG, Kane JM, et al: Prospective study of tardive dyskinesia incidence in the elderly. JAMA 266:2402–2406, 1991

Salzman C: Clinical Geriatric Psychopharmacology, 3rd Edition. Baltimore, MD, Williams & Wilkins, 1998

Satlin A, Volicer L, Ross V, et al: Bright light treatment of behavioral and sleep disturbances in patients with Alzheimer's disease. Am J Psychiatry 149:1028–1032, 1992

Saunders PA, Copeland JRM, Dewey ME, et al: Heavy drinking as a risk factor for depression and dementia in elderly men: findings from the Liverpool Longitudinal Community Study. Br J Psychiatry 159:213–216, 1991

Scherr PA, LaCroix AZ, Wallace RB: Light to moderate alcohol consumption and mortality in the elderly. J Am Geriatr Soc 40:651–657, 1992

Schneider LS: Pharmacologic considerations in the treatment of late life depression. Am J Geriatr Psychiatry 4:S51–S65, 1996

Schneider L, Plopper M: Geropsychiatry and consultation-liaison services. Am J Psychiatry 141:721–722, 1984

Schneider LS, Small GW, Hamilton SH, et al: Estrogen replacement and response to fluoxetine in a multicenter geriatric depression trial. Am J Geriatr Psychiatry 5:97–106, 1997

Shulman KI, Silver IL, Hershberg RI, et al: Geriatric psychiatry in the general hospital: the integration of services and training. Gen Hosp Psychiatry 8:223–228, 1986

Small GW: Behavioral disorders in Alzheimer disease: depression is common. Bull Clin Neurosci 54:2–7, 1989

Small GW: Recognition and treatment of depression in the elderly. J Clin Psychiatry 52 (suppl):11–22, 1991

Small GW: Geriatric psychiatry fellowship recruitment: crisis or opportunity? Am J Geriatr Psychiatry 1:67–73, 1993

Small GW: Positron emission tomography scanning for the early diagnosis of dementia. West J Med 171:293–294, 1999

Small GW, Fawzy FI: Psychiatric consultation for the medically ill elderly in the general hospital: need for a collaborative model of care. Psychosomatics 29:94–103, 1988

Small GW, Salzman C: Treatment of depression with new and atypical antidepressants, in Clinical Geriatric Psychopharmacology, 3rd Edition. Edited by Salzman C. Baltimore, MD, Williams & Wilkins, 1998, pp 245–261

Small GW, Komanduri R, Gitlin M, et al: The influence of age on guilt expression in major depression. Int J Geriatr Psychiatry 1:121–126, 1986

Small GW, Okonek A, Mandelkern MA, et al: Subjective and objective age-associated memory loss: initial neuropsychological, family history, and brain metabolic findings of a longitudinal study. Int Psychogeriatr 6:23–44, 1994

Small GW, Mazziotta JC, Collins MT, et al: Apolipoprotein E type 4 allele and cerebral glucose metabolism in relatives at risk for familial Alzheimer disease. JAMA 273:942–947, 1995

Small GW, Rabins PV, Barry PP, et al: Diagnosis and treatment of Alzheimer disease and related disorders: consensus statement of the American Association for Geriatric Psychiatry. JAMA 278:1363–1371, 1997

Small GW, Donohue JA, Brooks RL: An economic evaluation of donepezil in the treatment of Alzheimer's disease. Clin Ther 20:838–850, 1998

Spitzer R, Williams J, Kroenke K, et al: Utility of a new procedure for diagnosing mental disorders in primary care. JAMA 272:1749–1756, 1994

Starkstein SE, Robinson RG, Price TR: Comparison of patients with and without post-stroke major depression matched for size and location of lesion. Arch Gen Psychiatry 45:247–252, 1988

Stoudemire A, Hill CD, Morris R, et al: Cognitive outcome following tricyclic and electroconvulsive treatment of major depression in the elderly. Am J Psychiatry 148:1336–1340, 1991

Strain JJ, Lyons JS, Hammer JS, et al: Cost offset from a psychiatric consultation-liaison intervention with elderly hip fracture patients. Am J Psychiatry 148:1044–1049, 1991

Taler G, Ansello EF: Elder abuse. Am Fam Physician 32:107–114, 1985

Tollefson GD, Bosomworth JC, Heiligenstein JH, et al: A double-blind placebo-controlled clinical trial of fluoxetine in geriatric patients with major depression. Int Psychogeriatr 7:89–104, 1995

Unützer J, Katon WJ, Sullivan M, et al: Treating depressed older adults in primary care: narrowing the gap between efficacy and effectiveness. Milbank Q 77:225–256, 1999

Unützer J, Simon G, Belin TR, et al: Care for depression in HMO patients aged 65 and older. J Am Geriatr Soc 48:871–878, 2000

Unützer J, Katon W, Williams JW Jr, et al: Improving primary care for depression in late life: the design of a multicenter randomized trial. Med Care 39:785–799, 2001

Weiss LJ, Lazarus LW: Psychosocial treatment of the geropsychiatric patient. Int J Geriatr Psychiatry 8:95–100, 1993

Williams-Russo P, Urquhart BL, Sharrock NE, et al: Post-operative delirium: predictors and prognosis in elderly orthopedic patients. J Am Geriatr Soc 40:759–767, 1992

Wise MG, Tierney J: Psychopharmacology in the elderly. J La State Med Soc 144:471–476, 1992

World Health Organization: World Health Statistics: Demographic Trends, Aging and Noncommunicable Disease. Geneva, Switzerland, World Health Organization, 1992

Wragg R, Jeste DV: Overview of depression and psychosis in Alzheimer's disease. Am J Psychiatry 146:577–587, 1989

Yassa R, Nastase C, Dupont D, et al: Tardive dyskinesia in elderly psychiatric patients: a 5-year study. Am J Psychiatry 149:1206–1211, 1992

Zubenko GS, Moosy J: Major depression in primary dementia. Arch Neurol 45:1182–1186, 1988

Zubenko GS, Moosy J, Martinez AJ, et al: Neuropathologic and neurochemical correlates of psychosis in primary dementia. Arch Neurol 48:619–624, 1991

38

Strategic Integration of Inpatient and Outpatient Medical-Psychiatry Services

Roger G. Kathol, M.D., C.P.E.

Alan Stoudemire, M.D.[†]

Health care is in the midst of major ongoing change. The idealized goal of these changes is to curb medical costs while preserving the quality of patient care. Before these changes in health care, integrated inpatient medical and psychiatric programs (medical-psychiatric units) were rare and primarily located in academic medical centers (Fava et al. 1985; Fogel 1985; Fogel and Stoudemire 1986; Fogel et al. 1985; Goldberg and Fogel 1989; Goldberg and Stoudemire 1996; Goodman 1985; Hall and Kathol 1992; Harsch et al. 1989, 1991; Kathol 1994; Stoudemire and Fogel 1986; Summergrad 1994). Clinicians knew that patients with combined medical and psychiatric illness were common, but effective treatment programs to address *both* physical and psychiatric illness simultaneously and efficiently were generally unavailable. Most health care systems still do not enjoy the advantages of concurrent medical and psychiatric care in either inpatient or outpatient settings (Kathol et al. 1992a, 1992b; Stoudemire 1996a, 1996b, 1997).

The literature now documents the high prevalence of psychiatric comorbidity in medical settings (Table 38–1) (Academy of Psychosomatic Medicine 1997; Ormel et al. 1994; Regier et al. 1993; Smith 1991; Spitzer et al. 1994). Perhaps more important, the common mental disorders seen in medical patients (i.e., mood, anxiety, somatoform, and substance use disorders and delirium) contribute substantially to the financial health care burden of our nation (Table 38–2) (Francis and Kapoor 1992; Francis et al. 1990; Goetzel et al. 1998; Holder and Blose 1991; Mayou et al. 1988; Miller et al. 1998; Olfson et al. 1999; Rost et al. 1994; Salvador-Carulla et al. 1995; Saravay 1996; Simon et al. 1995; Smith et al. 1986, 1995; Unützer et al. 1997; Wells 1994). Research studies also indicate that when these psychiatric disorders are effectively treated, both clinical and economic outcomes generally improve (Holder and Blose 1991; Olfson et al. 1999; Salvador-Carulla et al. 1995; Smith et al. 1986, 1995; Von Korff et al. 1992). In fact, in one study, employer-sponsored active case finding via an employee assistance program coupled with psychiatric treatment for patients with psychiatric illness resulted in a healthier, less costly, and more productive work force (Figure 38–1) (McDonnell Douglas Corporation 1989).

If, on average, more than 20% of medical outpatients and 30% of medical inpatients have clinically significant, potentially treatable psychiatric illness (Table 38–1) and these patients increase the average cost of medical care approximately 40% annually (Table 38–2), then what steps are necessary to change the suffering that these patients experience, the effect that these illnesses have on our health care economy, and the stress that these illnesses impose on patients' families and employers? Studies report that traditional approaches, which separate medical and psychiatric treatment and apply interven-

---

[†] Deceased.

TABLE 38–1. Prevalence ranges for mental disorders in different populations

	Community	Primary care	General hospital
Depressive disorder	2%–6%	5%–14%	>15%
Panic disorder	1%	11%	5%
Somatization disorder	0.1%–0.5%	3%–5%	2%–9%
Substance dependence/abuse	3%	10%–30%	20%–50%
Any psychiatric disorder	16%	21%–26%	30%–60%

Source. Adapted from Academy of Psychosomatic Medicine 1997.

TABLE 38–2. Estimates of annual health care costs per medical patient with comorbid medical-psychiatric illness

Disorder	Annual costs/patient	Source
No psychiatric illness	$2,500	Simon et al. 1995
Distress	$2,600 (4% increase)	Scott and Robertson 1996
Depression	$3,500 (40% increase)	Goetzel et al. 1998; Simon et al. 1995; Unützer et al. 1997
Anxiety	$3,000 (20% increase)	Salvador-Carulla et al. 1995; Wells 1994
Somatization	$3,750 (50% increase)	Rost et al. 1994; Smith et al. 1986, 1995
Substance abuse	$3,325 (33% increase)	Holder and Blose 1991; Miller et al. 1998
Mixed	$3,750 (50% increase)	Mayou et al. 1988; Saravay 1996
Delirium[a]	100% increase in length of stay	Francis and Kapoor 1992; Francis et al. 1990
Psychiatric comorbidity	$3,500 (40% average increase)	

[a]Inpatient only.

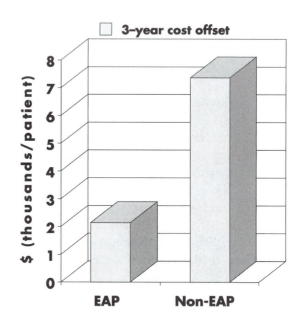

- **20,000 employees**
- **1,000 with substance abuse and/or psychiatric illness (5%)**
- **3–year claims and productivity assessment**

No effect on life circumstance problems.

Estimated $8 million in savings (patient and family).

3-year cost offset

–1985–1988 (McDonnell Douglas 1989)

FIGURE 38–1. McDonnell Douglas cost offset.

Note. EAP = employee assistance program.

Source. McDonnell Douglas Corporation: "Employee Assistance Program Financial Offset Study 1985–1988." Bridgeton, MO, Alexander & Alexander Consulting Group, 1989.

tions without monitoring compliance or outcome, may have limited long-term therapeutic effects (Carr et al. 1997; Levenson 1998).

To maximize improvement of clinical and financial outcomes, several critical components in an outpatient care program are required: 1) ready availability of psychiatric assessment in the medical setting; 2) active screening of identified high-risk patients for psychiatric illnesses, especially mood, anxiety, substance-related, and somatoform disorders; 3) application of proven pharmacological, psychotherapeutic, and psychosocial interventions (i.e., use of treatments that improve outcome); 4) coordination of medical and psychiatric care among clinicians through improved communication; and 5) availability of case management for patients with chronic, complicated illnesses to improve compliance. Few of these elements are found in traditional outpatient approaches to psychiatric treatment for medical patients (Table 38–3). In the inpatient setting, high-acuity medical and psychiatric assessment capabilities should be added.

The *horizontal* integration of inpatient and outpatient treatment programs (i.e., the concurrent treatment of medical and psychiatric conditions) incorporates these components and has the potential to transform the process of care. The chapter titled "Medical-Psychiatric Units" in the first edition of this textbook targeted inpatient services (Stoudemire 1996a). In this update, we describe how health care systems can provide comprehensive, versatile, and flexible models of care that span all levels of illness acuity and include all locations in which medical patients requiring integrated medical and psychiatric services are encountered. Whereas inpatient programs often form the cost-saving cornerstone, *vertical* integration, in which the intensity of care required (inpatient, transitional, and outpatient services) is coordinated into a seamless treatment continuum, usually will decrease the length of time required for more costly inpatient treatment.

In this chapter, we review why traditional "standalone" outpatient psychiatry and inpatient consultation, by themselves, address only a portion of the needs of patients with comorbid medical and psychiatric illness. A biopsychosocial approach to care is practiced, with emphasis on the application of biological, psychotherapeutic, and social interventions that are in proportion to the clinical needs of the patient. We describe outpatient and inpatient programs that consistently change outcomes while potentially decreasing the cost of care and improving the patient's ability to function at home and at work. Such programs do not just happen, however, by the reassignment of a few personnel in traditional clinical settings. A change in the conceptual model of care is re-

TABLE 38–3. Critical components necessary for outcome improvement in the care of patients with medical-psychiatric comorbidity

Readily available psychiatric assessment in the primary care setting

Active screening in the primary care setting to identify high-risk patients with psychiatric illnesses/disorders

Ability to apply pharmacotherapeutic, psychotherapeutic, and psychosocial interventions that have proven effective through well-designed studies

Coordination and integration of medical and psychiatric care among clinicians

Case management for patients with chronic and/or complicated illness

quired (i.e., an integration paradigm). The steps used to accomplish this goal are summarized.

Although this chapter provides a comprehensive view of integrated care, we do not intend to cover all clinical aspects of the concurrent treatment of medical and psychiatric illness. For instance, we do not specifically address the important role of integrated care in disease prevention and health maintenance (such as smoking cessation, obesity, and cardiac rehabilitation). It is not possible to review all, or even most, of the common problems seen at the interface of medicine and psychiatry, such as psychiatric side effects of prescription drugs, fibromyalgia, chronic fatigue syndrome, and neuroleptic malignant syndrome. Finally, we do not focus on interventions for patient distress, problems in living, or personality disorders. Comprehensive textbooks on integrated medical-psychiatric care covering all these conditions, and others, are available (Brown and Stoudemire 1998; Stoudemire et al. 2000).

The areas not covered in this chapter are obviously important components of integrated care and should be discussed and included in the context of program development. They do, however, flow naturally into the programs described in this chapter, which emphasize the diagnosis and treatment of the most common psychiatric illnesses seen in primary care settings.

CASE EXAMPLES

Most clinicians can easily remember patients who would be better served in an integrated medical-psychiatric care program, but it is helpful to have representative examples of how treatment in an integrated model differs from that provided through traditional practice. The critical elements involve the geographical and physical setting, the skills of the integrated care team members, and communication and coordination of care between primary or specialty care physicians and psychiatrists. The following are examples of patients who would benefit from outpatient and inpatient integrated treatment.

Outpatient

Ms. A, a 28-year-old woman, arrived, unscheduled, at the primary care clinic for evaluation of persistent headaches. The patient was taking multiple medications for headaches and other somatic complaints. She was the wife of an influential businessman and had been admitted to the hospital several times by different physicians for vague, unexplained, persistent, and varied physical complaints. Previous headache evaluations, including computed tomography, were unremarkable. Nonaddicting analgesic medications were tried without success. Ms. A pleaded for symptom relief.

Ms. A had seen many internists and surgeons because her problems were "physical." She, however, conceded that all her medical problems made her very discouraged. This opened the door to a quick assessment by the psychiatrist who worked in the primary care clinic. A diagnosis of somatization disorder was confirmed. Intermittent episodes of major depression were another problem. Ms. A had undergone three inadequate antidepressant medication trials.

The internist and the psychiatrist discussed with the patient the risks of doctors and their treatments (iatrogenic disease). She was informed that her current medications actually could be contributing to her headaches. A thorough history was taken during a comprehensive clinic visit a week later. With this information, it was possible to taper and stop 13 of the 18 medications Ms. A was using. She was scheduled for more frequent but nonemergent clinic appointments and encouraged to seek all medical services through her internist's office. Creative reassurance (Kathol 1997), the mainstay of treatment and a form of supportive psychotherapy, was provided by medical and psychiatric personnel. With this approach, symptoms decreased, clinic visits became less frequent, hospitalizations stopped, and the patient returned to work. Family sessions were held to address how her chronic illness had affected the family and marriage. She and her husband decided to enter marital therapy.

Ms. B, a 47-year-old woman with type 1 diabetes mellitus, presented at the primary care clinic with fatigue, insomnia, a 10-pound weight loss, nonspecific abdominal complaints, and constipation. The physical examination did not identify any abnormal abdominal findings or diabetic complications. A 2-hour postprandial blood glucose level was 275 mg%, and a glycosylated hemoglobin was 8.6%. Stool guaiac results were negative, as were urine ketones. Ms. B was given a stool softener and an antacid and was encouraged to moni-

tor her blood sugar more carefully. As she dressed to leave the clinic, her family approached the family physician who had examined her and indicated that Ms. B was having another depressive episode (new information). The patient refused to go to a mental health clinic. The family was worried that she might be suicidal.

After Ms. B finished dressing, the physician took her into the examination room and asked her whether personal concerns were contributing to her poor diabetic control. She admitted that she was depressed but denied suicidal thoughts. The psychiatrist who worked in the primary care clinic agreed to see the patient briefly before she left the clinic. The psychiatrist confirmed that Ms. B had major depression that was exacerbated by long-standing marital problems. Antidepressant medication was started immediately, and she was referred to a marital therapist for further assessment. Because the patient could see both medical and psychiatric practitioners in the primary care clinic, diabetic checks were coordinated with psychiatric follow-up visits. Blood sugar levels stabilized as depressive symptoms resolved. The patient's insulin requirements decreased during treatment for depression, suggesting that compliance might have been a factor contributing to poor glucose control. Within 4 months, the patient's glycosylated hemoglobin was 5.2%. As a result of marital therapy, she reported a happier family and sexual life.

Inpatient

Mr. C, a 58-year-old man with Parkinson's disease taking high-dose dopaminergic agents, was admitted to the hospital in a very agitated state for treatment of delusions. He thought that two male talk show hosts were trying to harm him and his family. He knew this because they were sending special messages to him via the radio, even when the radio was not turned on. He had called the police for protection on several occasions. Police asked family members to have the patient evaluated.

After admission to the inpatient integrated medicine and psychiatry unit, Mr. C's antiparkinsonian medication dosages were adjusted and supportive measures initiated (Inouye et al. 1999). His psychotic symptoms persisted despite medication adjustments and the addition of a low-dose atypical antipsychotic agent—quetiapine. Electroconvulsive therapy (ECT), an effective treatment for refractory dopaminergic-agent-induced psychoses, was offered to the patient and family; they agreed. ECT was started and had the added benefit of transiently reducing antiparkinsonian medication requirements (Moellentine et al. 1998). After two treatments, Mr. C's psychotic symptoms resolved and he adjusted to his new antiparkinsonian medication regimen. He was discharged after four ECT sessions with recommendations to consider prophylactic quetiapine if antiparkinsonian medication requirements increased.

Mr. D, a 38-year-old man with chronic agitation and alcoholism, was admitted 18 hours after his last drink for treatment of melanotic stools and a hematocrit that decreased from 42% 3 days earlier (emergency room visit) to 29% now. He had numerous prior admissions for alcohol detoxification, often complicated by alcohol withdrawal delirium. He wanted to sign out against medical advice but was too confused to understand the potential dangers associated with that decision (i.e., he lacked the capacity to make an informed decision).

Mr. D was placed on involuntary hold on the integrated medicine and psychiatry unit because he had an emergent medical problem (severe anemia with gastrointestinal bleeding) and was delirious (mental illness). After a through medical evaluation, his agitation and delirium were controlled with aggressive benzodiazepine administration and physical restraints. He was closely monitored to prevent injury to self or others. Gastroscopy detected an active bleeding ulcer that stopped oozing with cold lavage. Because the patient remained hemodynamically stable, transfusion was deemed unnecessary. Benzodiazepines were tapered over the following 7 days. Visits from friends were monitored to prevent access to alcohol while he was in the hospital.

Mr. D agreed to try naltrexone prophylaxis (Garbutt et al. 1999) and, after discussion with the substance abuse counselor, to restart participation in Alcoholics Anonymous. Referral to a halfway house was arranged. Regular follow-up with the substance abuse counselor also was arranged.

LIMITATIONS OF TRADITIONAL APPROACHES IN THE CARE OF PATIENTS WITH CONCURRENT MEDICAL AND PSYCHIATRIC ILLNESS

Outpatient

There is no such thing as "usual care" for psychiatrically ill medical patients. However, three common models are used in the United States to address the needs of medical outpatients with comorbid psychiatric conditions:

1. Self- or physician referral to stand-alone mental health practitioners and clinics is the most prevalent model.
2. Placement of nonmedical therapists in primary or specialty care clinics with nonpsychiatric physicians is a model commonly used by managed care companies and some health maintenance organizations. It also relies on patients, the staff, or physicians to identify the clinical need for psychiatric care; however, access

to basic mental health personnel is usually improved.
3. Primary or specialty care physicians are expected to assume therapeutic responsibility for the identification and treatment of common psychiatric problems, such as mood disorders.

Table 38–3 summarizes the critical components required for outcome change in patients with medical-psychiatric comorbidity. The self- or physician referral model is far from optimal because it contains *none* of the critical components necessary for effective and cost-efficient care for medical-psychiatric patients. In fact, for common illnesses in primary care settings, such as major depression, it creates an environment in which only a small fraction of patients are likely to have symptom resolution. The literature makes it possible to quantify the process variables that lead to marginal success. Only about 50% of the patients with mood and anxiety disorders are appropriately identified by primary care physicians (Higgins 1994; Linden et al. 1999), and only 50% of these show up for their stand-alone psychiatric clinic visit when referred (Chen 1991; Henk et al. 1996; Krulee and Hales 1988; Perez and Silverman 1983; Weddington 1983). Twenty-five percent of these receive appropriate care (Linden et al. 1999; Wells et al. 1988; Williams et al. 1999), and, generously, 75% of those who receive evidence-based care respond (U.S. Department of Health and Human Services 1993a, 1993b). This is known as the "50, 50, 25, 75 = 5% rule" ($0.50 \times 0.50 \times 0.25 \times 0.75 = 5\%$ of patients with psychiatric illness are effectively treated).

The on-site therapist intervention and primary care physician intervention models would theoretically improve the number of patients exposed to potentially effective treatment because they obviate the need for patients to enter a formal mental health treatment setting. The primary care physician intervention model might do even better than the on-site therapist model because a well-trained physician who knows basic psychiatric assessment should understand how psychiatric conditions affect the patient's medical symptomatology and treatment. The literature, however, suggests that recovery rates for disorders, such as major depression, do not improve when these models are used instead of the self- or physician referral model (Katon et al. 1995; Schulberg et al. 1997). This is probably because the models are not organized to allow the practitioner time to make psychiatric diagnoses or deliver appropriate care (assuming adequately trained physicians and on-site therapists). Data do indicate that within the same health care system, close concurrent primary care physician–psychiatrist comanagement improves outcome over primary care physician only care for depression (Katon et al. 1995). Given that primary care physicians receive minimal psychiatric training compared with psychiatrists, it is not surprising that a primary care–psychiatrist comanagement model has the best evidence for improved outcome in primary care settings.

Inpatient

Although psychiatric liaison services exist in the private sector, they are relatively uncommon. The main way that psychiatrically ill medical-surgical inpatients receive psychiatric assistance in the private sector is through "single consultation." If the same critical components (Table 38–3) are used to assess the likelihood for improved patient outcomes through inpatient consultation, again, serious limitations are found.

In most hospitals, psychiatrists for the medically ill (*psychiatry in the medically ill* is the terminology adopted by the Academy of Psychosomatic Medicine to replace consultation-liaison psychiatry) are available to come to the patient's bedside, but even this solitary critical component has limited utility. Assessment and treatment by psychiatrists for the medically ill are crisis-oriented rather than long-term-outcome–oriented. These psychiatrists are rarely reimbursed for seeing a patient more than once. Such inadequate payment discourages active ongoing treatment. "Treatment initiation" with careful follow-up rarely occurs (France et al. 1978). Most psychiatric assistance given is, therefore, through recommendations to the referring physician, with the expectation that they will be implemented. Unfortunately, medical personnel usually are unfamiliar with and untrained in the treatment of psychiatric illness. In addition, the

time to initiate treatment programs by nonpsychiatrist physicians is limited. Therapy is started in only one-half of patients and then in ways that are unlikely to continue after discharge (Freyne et al. 1992; Huyse et al. 1993; Perez and Silverman 1983). In short, treatment results are poor unless longer-term treatment is provided.

It is no wonder that some (Carr et al. 1997; Levenson 1998), but not all (Levitan and Kornfeld 1981; Strain et al. 1991), short-term psychiatry in the medically ill intervention outcome studies fail to document improvement after inpatient consultation. When one considers that patients with psychiatric disorders in the medical setting have significantly longer lengths of stay—on average, 2 days longer than patients without psychiatric illness (Fulop et al. 1987; Saravay and Levin 1994)—the additional cost of care for these patients is substantial (Table 38–2). Even with shorter lengths of stay found in our health care environment, psychiatric comorbidity still adds 2 days to a hospital admission (Table 38–4). Psychiatrists for the medically ill often do not have time to effectively institute treatment in the hospital and monitor patient responses. Furthermore, outpatient follow-up care for these patients has not traditionally been seamless and contiguous with inpatient care.

If traditional models used to treat medical patients with psychiatric illness fail to reduce suffering and the economic burden imposed, what are some alternative models of conjoint medical-psychiatric care that might have better results? In the remainder of this chapter, we discuss a practical treatment model for medical and psychiatric integration through comprehensive mental health psychiatry in the medically ill teams and medical-psychiatric units.

TABLE 38–4.   Average length of stay for medical patients with and without psychiatric comorbidity admitted to a general hospital

		Patients with medical illness only		Patients with comorbid psychiatric illness		Delta	Patients with comorbid
		Admissions	ALOS (days)	Admissions	ALOS (days)	ALOS[a] (days)	psychiatric illness
Site 1	Missouri	19,791	5.60	2,496	7.40	1.6	12.6
Site 2	California	9,016	4.06	1,131	5.96	1.9	12.5
Site 3	New York	19,176	8.01	1,641	10.77	2.7	8.6
Site 4	Indiana	4,277	3.65	970	4.88	1.2	22.7
Site 5	Georgia	25,803	4.06	1,197	6.40	2.4	4.6
Site 6	Michigan	5,264	5.53	681	6.58	1.1	12.9
Total		83,327	5.15	8,116	7.00	1.82	9.7

Note.   ALOS = average length of stay.
[a]Difference in ALOS: medical illness only vs. psychiatric comorbidity.
Source.   Benchmarking data, courtesy of *Cartesian Solutions*, 1999.

IMPROVEMENT IN PATIENT OUTCOMES THROUGH INTEGRATION OF MEDICAL-PSYCHIATRIC CARE

The frustration among medical staff generated by medical patients with psychiatric comorbidity is legend. These patients have more complaints, demand more attention, interfere with intervention attempts, and respond to treatment less well than do those without psychiatric problems (Hahn et al. 1996; Kroenke et al. 1997). Nonetheless, medical personnel do the best they can, given the limited time, knowledge and skills in psychiatry, and resources available. As mentioned previously, traditional psychiatric consultation and referral does little to change the outcomes for these patients. Patients, therefore, are seen three times more often (Katon and Schulberg 1992), require more tests (Simon et al. 1995), are admitted to the hospital more frequently (Baez et al. 1998; Simon et al. 1995), and have longer lengths of stay in the hospital (Fulop et al. 1987; Saravay and Levin 1994; Table 38–4). Even the type of insurance program can influence outcome (Rogers et al. 1993). Integration of psychiatric care into the medical setting is a way to alter these outcomes.

Integrated Outpatient Programs

The actual percentage of medical outpatients referred to mental health professionals for psychiatric problems is not precisely known. Despite the fact that at least 20% of medical outpatients have active psychiatric comorbidity (Table 38–1), indirect evidence from research protocols suggests that referral rates from inpatient settings are between 0.1% and 11%, with a median rate of 1% or less. Higher rates of referral are associated with active screening protocols for psychiatric problems (W. Katon and P. Nutting, personal communication, 1999).

Only about 40% of the patients referred have a formal DSM psychiatric illness (Katon et al. 1990). Most are distressed and in need of the "psychological" and "social" components of the biopsychosocial approach but do not need intense psychotherapy. Of the psychiatric disorders seen in medical outpatients, depression, anxiety, substance abuse or dependence, and somatization are among the most common problems identified (Spitzer et al. 1995). All patients deserve attention, regardless of whether they are distressed or have formally diagnosed disorders, but those with serious clinical psychiatric disorders have the best clinical and economic outcomes with evidence-based treatment (Holder and Blose 1991;

Krulee and Hales 1988; McDonnell Douglas Corporation 1989; Olfson et al. 1999; Salvador-Carulla et al. 1995; Smith et al. 1986, 1995; Von Korff et al. 1992).

Table 38–3 summarizes the critical components of care that are likely to improve patient outcomes; they are missing from traditional outpatient treatment programs. Thoughtful incorporation of these components does several things. First, it increases the number of patients who gain access to psychiatric treatment. In fact, the patient's primary or specialty care physician participates in the treatment process. Second, it improves the likelihood, regardless of which professional treats the patient, that effective interventions are administered. Finally, to maximize the chance of sustained improvement in patients with chronic, more complicated diseases, case management can contribute to outcome improvement in an integrated treatment by a mental health team model (Figure 38–2). Case management helps patients comply with diagnostic and therapeutic recommendations, attend follow-up appointments, identify sources of funds for medication refills, access community resources, or obtain prompt emotional support during crisis.

The outpatient model used for the treatment of medical-psychiatric patients has significant implications for the health care system. For instance, traditional practice (model 1) that uses self- or physician referral to stand-alone psychiatric services (Bronheim et al. 1998) is hampered by the unwillingness of referring physicians and/or patients to initiate mental health contact (Perez and Silverman 1983). By using existing psychiatric services, however, it is actually still possible to decrease the excess use of medical services and thus the number of health care dollars spent annually (Table 38–2).

When looking for better models of psychiatric care in medical patients, one of the first steps is to explore ways in which existing models can add value to patient care. For instance, patients with depression could be identified by screening high-risk individuals who would then receive treatment with well-established techniques, such as cognitive-behavioral therapy, from on-site nonmedical therapists (model 2). This could increase the number of patients treated as much as fourfold. Unfortunately, the annual cost of treatment of these depressed patients would also increase by approximately $22 per patient per month, largely because two therapists are needed to treat the patients of each physician. Trials with psychotherapy for somatization disorder, as yet, have not changed outcomes. Substance abuse or dependence requires formal substance abuse treatment programs, Alcoholics Anonymous, and perhaps preventive medications, such as naltrexone (Garbutt et al. 1999), to change outcome.

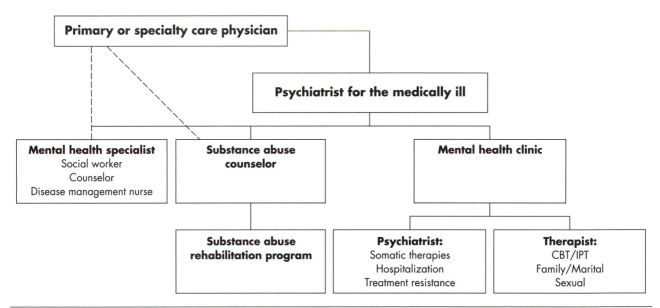

FIGURE 38–2.   Mental health team[a] (model).

Dashed lines represent direct communication between mental health caregiver and referring physician, with coordination and supervision by psychiatrist. CBT = cognitive-behavioral therapy; IPT = interpersonal therapy.

[a]The primary or specialty care physician retains ultimate responsibility for patients for whom a consultation is requested; however, he or she works closely with members of the mental health team who are coordinated and supervised by a psychiatry in the medically ill psychiatrist. This ensures that effective therapy is provided. The primary or specialty care physician communicates with the psychiatrist for the medically ill, the nurse clinician, the social worker, or other team member directly involved in evaluating and treating a specific patient. The mental health team members maintain close communication with other psychiatric service providers in their region and, thus, facilitate the assistance of other mental health caregivers and programs not associated with the mental health team. Only chronic, nonresponsive, and/or complicated patients or patients with special psychiatric needs (e.g., cognitive-behavioral therapy or treatment for substance dependence) would be sent to the psychiatric sector (e.g., mental health clinic) for continued care.

Even if primary or specialty care physicians serve as the patients' primary psychiatric caregivers (model 3), the net cost of care remains high. The real drawback of primary- or specialty-care-physician–directed psychiatric treatment relates to the commitment of time required and the physician's lack of expertise in psychiatry. Physicians who take on this task decrease their medical illness treatment productivity by more than one-third, an unacceptable level for most nonpsychiatrists.

If these two new integration models have significant drawbacks, then the question is whether another approach exists with a greater likelihood of clinical and economic success. The answer comes from the research literature, which documents that 1) evidence-based treatment of psychiatric illness is actually less expensive than the incremental cost of health care services; 2) cost savings are directly related to the number of patients who receive effective treatment, not those just "exposed" to treatment; 3) clinical and economic outcome is influenced by which intervention is applied and who applies it; and 4) steps taken to ensure compliance in treatment-resistant or difficult patients also can improve outcome (Holder and Blose 1991; Krulee and Hales 1988; McDonnell Douglas Corporation 1989; Salvador-Carulla

et al. 1995; Smith et al. 1986, 1995; Von Korff et al. 1992). This information can be used to devise a core model of integrated outpatient psychiatric care for medical patients.

Integrated Treatment by a Mental Health Team

The model that adds the greatest psychiatric value in the medical outpatient setting is integrated treatment by a mental health team (Figure 38–2). Such a team is specifically designed to be responsive to the needs of the primary or specialty care physician and to minimize the effect of psychiatric illness on medical utilization. As such, it must include 1) immediate access to mental health services, 2) co-location of medical and psychiatric personnel, 3) improved communications, and 4) quick intervention with effective therapies. The composition of the mental health team depends on the goals and objectives of the clinical service, the targeted population, and the clinical skills/knowledge base and availability of various types of mental health professionals. Core members of the team will necessarily be psychiatrists, nurse clinicians and/or physician assistants, and social workers. The numbers of each are determined by the population served, the frequency of various presenting illnesses, and the division of responsibilities among team members.

Under the direction of a psychiatrist for the medically ill, who ensures appropriate assessment and accurate diagnosis, patients are matched by diagnosis or problem to the mental health professional most likely to provide cost-effective benefit (Bronheim et al. 1998). For instance, patients with conditions requiring medications, such as major mood and anxiety disorders, are treated by team members with medical and/or nursing backgrounds. Those with mild to moderate levels of situational distress, in the absence of a psychiatric disorder, are treated by a counselor or social worker with time-limited crisis intervention and supportive psychotherapy. Patients with somatization disorder are seen initially by a psychiatrist because they require examination before reassurance is given (Kathol 1997). Therapeutic response is primarily determined by patient and referring physician compliance and the patient's response to a given treatment modality.

Formal psychotherapy, such as cognitive-behavioral therapy or other short-term therapies, is not provided in the primary or specialty care clinic because therapists become inaccessible as patients accumulate over time. Patients who need these forms of therapy are referred to stand-alone mental health clinics. If a patient is a likely responder to short-term therapy, such as problem-oriented therapy (Mynors-Wallis et al. 1997), such treatments are occasionally used as first-line therapy after appropriate evaluation and exclusion of significant psychiatric disorders.

The mental health team works together to ensure that patients are exposed to effective treatment provided by a competent professional whose skills and therapeutic abilities are appropriate. For instance, medications are, and will likely remain, a widely used intervention for major depressive and anxiety disorders in primary or specialty care patients. These medications may be initiated under the direction of the psychiatrist after the diagnosis has been confirmed and the need for psychotherapy has been assessed, but the patient may be followed up by a physician assistant or nurse clinician until symptoms resolve. If symptoms do not or only partially resolve, diagnostic reassessment is essential, and adjunctive pharmacotherapy and/or psychotherapy should be considered. Because logistical problems prevent ready access to formal psychotherapies in the primary care setting, effective psychotherapies, such as cognitive-behavioral therapy or interpersonal psychotherapy, will be prescribed for patients who prefer not to take medication or who require the combination of medication and psychotherapy.

While acute substance abuse treatment is provided in substance abuse programs, the mental health team facilitates referral by working with the patient and the patient's family in the primary care setting. Because substance abuse is a chronic, debilitating problem, many patients are assigned a caseworker to improve compliance. A medically trained mental health team member also may assist the substance abuse program with adjunctive medications, such as naltrexone prophylaxis (Garbutt et al. 1999).

Although no curative psychological interventions are available for the nondepressed, nonanxious somatizing patient, inappropriate medical use is controllable. The mental health team can provide the primary or specialty care physicians with an appropriate diagnosis, assist them in limiting aggressive medical workups and treatments, and administer supportive forms of psychotherapy, such as reassurance therapy (Kathol 1997). Because many of these patients also have chaotic personal lives, they often benefit from comprehensive case management so that compliance with their prescribed treatment plan is followed as closely as possible.

Stand-Alone Psychiatric Clinics

Integrated outpatient programs in primary or specialty care clinics do not replace stand-alone psychiatric outpatient programs; they enhance access to these specialized services. For instance, alcohol rehabilitation programs are necessarily located outside the medical setting. Formal evidence-based psychotherapy also should be located in a stand-alone location. If the integrated program personnel are occupied with psychotherapy or formal substance abuse treatment programs, then mental health team access is curtailed, substantially decreasing their availability to the referring physicians.

This does not mean that most patients are merely triaged and referred. Most patients with subthreshold and threshold stress-related somatic complaints can be given supportive reassurance (Kathol 1997) in the medical setting. Patients with uncomplicated major depression and anxiety are easily shepherded through initiation and follow-up pharmacotherapy in medical-surgical clinics. Patients with substance abuse disorders can be supported in primary care clinics through encouragement to pursue ongoing substance abuse treatment (e.g., Alcoholic Anonymous, monitor naltrexone). Finally, mildly distressed patients are often best supported in the primary care setting because it is an acceptable venue for treatment of patients without a formally defined psychiatric disorder. Furthermore, the distress is often, but not always, related to medical factors (e.g., recent notification of life-threatening disease, poor treatment response, lifestyle-altering illness).

Integrated Inpatient Programs

Approximately 30% of general medical patients will have comorbid psychiatric illness (Table 38–1) complicating their admitting medical condition; between 2% and 5% of all patients admitted to the hospital would benefit from an integrated inpatient program that facilitates more appropriate care and potentially a shorter length of stay. The remaining patients could be managed via the coordinated efforts of a mental health consultation team similar to that described for the outpatient setting (Kishi and Kathol 1999, 2000).

In general, the more acute a patient's medical and psychiatric illness, the more value is added to patient care through the creation of an integrated medical-psychiatric unit. For instance, it is much easier to handle an acutely agitated (delirious) patient undergoing cancer chemotherapy in a location where nurses and physicians can control infections *and* manage disruptive behavior. Other common examples include patients who are depressed after a serious suicide attempt, patients who are delirious and demented, patients who are acutely intoxicated or medically unstable and in withdrawal, patients who are actively manic or psychotic and have other acute medical illnesses, patients who require involuntary treatment in a medical setting, and patients who are noncompliant with medical treatment because of a personality disorder.

The objective of an integrated program is to supply concurrent rather than consecutive medical-psychiatric care, thus possibly reducing the length of stay while improving both medical and psychiatric symptoms before discharge. All integrated inpatient medical-psychiatric programs (medical-psychiatric units) must have three core features in order to do this: 1) a medically and psychiatrically safe environment that includes clinical programming in both disciplines; 2) professional staff trained in both medical and psychiatric illnesses, procedures, and treatments; and 3) physician coverage from both medicine and psychiatry, which allows the unit to deal with emergent and nonemergent clinical problems.

Admission Criteria

Admission criteria depend on the target population, such as general medical, substance abuse, geriatric, eating disorders, or renal disease. It is preferable to admit only patients who have active combined medical and psychiatric illness. Prevalence studies indicate that such patients are not difficult to find once the service capabilities of the unit become apparent and are readily accessible to medi-

cal and psychiatric clinicians in the region. If beds are licensed as medical, the referral base is large because admission privileges are open to the primary or specialty care clinicians as well as psychiatrists. Reimbursement for services is determined by the patient's insurance carrier.

The target population drives decisions about how the unit is organized, the types of training professional staff receive, and the level and type of physician coverage required (Kathol et al. 1992a). These factors determine which patients can be safely admitted and adequately treated. Patients with acuity higher than the unit can handle are necessarily diverted to a medical or psychiatric setting capable of treating sicker patients until factors restricting admission have resolved. Then, if the patients still require concurrent medical and psychiatric care, they are transferred to the medical-psychiatric unit.

Integrated medical-psychiatric units are, and should be recognized as, the medical resource facility for complicated patients who have failed therapy in other locations. Some may even describe them as the "dump" units. Combined medical and psychiatric treatments often lead to remarkable transformations in these difficult patients. It is important to strike a balance between overly restrictive and excessively lenient admission policies. Overly restrictive admission policies prevent access to these services. Excessively lenient policies can tie up beds if untreatable, chronically debilitated patients are admitted and placement cannot be found. Requiring referring nursing facilities to agree to accept back-referred patients on discharge appears to be a logical solution to many disposition problems. However, this does not always work because illness severity, such as the need for a long-term urinary catheter, may prevent readmission to the facility of origin.

To maximize value to patients, physicians, the health care center, and those who pay for care, clear written admission policies should be delineated in advance and fine-tuned through communication among the medical director, head nurse, and admission personnel. Appropriate admission criteria should be defined (e.g., delirium, medically unstable eating disorders, medical or medication-induced psychosis). Exclusion criteria also must be defined (e.g., uncomplicated dementia). Exceptions always arise and are adjudicated via discussion and consensus. The central principle in admitting patients is to add value by focusing on the admission of patients most likely to benefit from the special care provided within safety constraints. Based on experience, admission authority must rest with the medical director and head nurse to prevent inappropriate admissions and the admission of patients whose medical problems exceed what the unit can provide.

Some integrated inpatient programs are set up to address the problems of select populations, such as geriatric patients, patients with behavior disorders and delirium, medically compromised patients with eating disorders, neuropsychiatric patients (such as those with head trauma), and medically unstable substance-dependent patients who require acute detoxification. Such subspecialty integrated units meet the unique needs of the personnel and/or system in which clinical service occurs. These units serve the targeted population, but they also exclude patients who fall outside target patient parameters but are still commonly seen within the health care network. For this reason, as inpatient programs are organized, inclusion of as many comorbid patients as possible should be considered. A diversely trained physician and nursing staff provides the greatest degree of flexibility in admissions.

Unit Organization

Features of the unit are driven by the target population and include the level of illness acuity, the administrative structure, the unit licensure, the payer mix, the availability of postcare services, and the mission and objectives of the institution. All of these are factored into a customized operational plan that serves as the guidebook from which specific decisions are made (Table 38–5). Although each integrated inpatient program is different, all type III (moderate medical acuity, moderate to high psychiatric acuity) and type IV (high medical and psychiatric acuity) programs (Kathol et al. 1992a) should include certain core elements (Table 38–6) that differentiate them from medical units with psychiatric consultation-liaison coverage (type II) or psychiatric units that provide only very basic, low-acuity medical services (type I).

Patients who are admitted to type III and type IV units are different from patients admitted to general psychiatry units (Kishi and Kathol 1999). They require individualized conjoint medical-psychiatric care. For instance, many bedridden medically ill psychiatric patients cannot attend group therapy sessions or ward meetings. Often patients are too cognitively impaired, even if not bedridden, to participate in psychotherapeutic discussions. On the medical side, life-sustaining medical interventions, such as nasogastric feeding tubes, intravenous therapy lines, or postoperative drainage tubes, may necessitate the use of physical or chemical restraints. This requires flexible, rather than rigid, nursing staff and daily programs to maximize patient improvement.

Admission criteria should *not* restrict access to patients who cannot attend group therapy. Activities and occupational therapy should offer both unitwide and individualized therapeutic interventions. Nurses should

TABLE 38–5. Integrated medicine and psychiatry program operational plan

Institutional mission and goals
Needs assessment and market analysis
Current practice patterns
   Clinical
   Financial
Target population
Financial effect
Implementation plan
Conclusions

TABLE 38–6. Core elements of a type III[a] or type IV[b] inpatient integrated care program

Reformulated physical structure with medical and psychiatric safety features
General medical hospital location
Professional staff specifically hired because of their desire to care for comorbid patients
Professional staff training in medical and psychiatric policies and procedures
Emergency cardiopulmonary resuscitation
Clinical programming that includes both medical and psychiatric features
Daily review and supervision of patients by medical and psychiatric physicians

[a]Type III = moderate medical acuity, moderate to high psychiatric acuity.
[b]Type IV = high medical and psychiatric acuity.

have time to provide one-to-one support and reassurance and even offer assertiveness training and/or relaxation therapy. This is all done along with medical procedures, hygiene, assistance with nutrition, and medical-surgical interventions.

With changes in reimbursement, therapies that were once provided in the inpatient setting are now initiated there and continued after discharge. For instance, formal psychotherapy such as cognitive-behavioral therapy for depression or alcohol rehabilitation is started as inpatient therapy, and then the patient is transferred to a day or partial hospital or an outpatient program for completion. The same is true for some medical interventions, such as intermittent long-term intravenous chemotherapy or antibiotic therapy or postoperative wound care. Unit programs must take these changing medical practices into consideration as units are established.

Vertical Integration of Medical-Psychiatric Care

Both outpatient and inpatient integrated medical-psychiatric programs are currently available in only a few locations. As these programs develop during the next decade, it will be important to directly connect the services provided (vertical integration). This ensures that benefits experienced by patients in an integrated inpatient setting are consolidated and maintained by coordinated medical and psychiatric care after discharge. Properly configured outpatient services should decrease the need for initial hospitalization and/or rehospitalization, further reducing costs.

Unfortunately, many of the patients served by these programs experience chronic debilitation. In such cases, transitional and/or partial programs also are used as cost-conserving measures. Patients who no longer require intensive treatment but who are too ill to live independently are placed in transitional day-hospital programs. Medical and psychiatric needs are met, which helps the patient progress more rapidly to a self-supporting environment.

ECONOMICS OF INTEGRATED CARE

Although inertia, professional autonomy, and space limitations are barriers to the development of integrated programs, perhaps the greatest perceived barrier is economic. Despite their inherent cost-saving potential, integrated programs in our current health care environment are at significant risk for fiscal insolvency if not properly organized. Mental health benefits are "carved out" of most medical coverage contracts. Therefore, patients with comorbid medical and psychiatric illness fall between two budgets, with both parties intent on minimizing expenses.

Competition results to determine who is the "most successful" at *not* paying for services. Such arrangements are often not fair, effective, or ethical. The result is very evident when care is provided by psychiatrists for the medically ill. Many "carved out" behavioral health managed care companies do not have written into their contracts provisions (or are unwilling) to pay for psychiatric consultations or for psychiatric services provided in a nonpsychiatric setting. On the medical side, budget managers consider psychiatric consultation a mental/behavioral health service that is appropriately reimbursed from the mental/behavioral health fund pool. The result is that psychiatrists for the medically ill often do not get paid unless consultation and payment are preapproved.

It is little wonder that individuals interested in a psychiatry in the medically ill practice do not stay long, or they must generate their income through other clinical activities. Even academic psychiatry departments may limit psychiatry in the medically ill activities because they are (or appear to be) a drain on departmental resources. At the same time, primary and specialty care physicians wonder why they can never get a psychiatrist to see their patients.

Similar problems arise for psychiatric patients needing medical care. Some insurers raise premiums to unrealistic/unaffordable levels if a patient has a psychiatric history, because actuarial tables indicate that such individuals are at risk for more medical problems (i.e., they are likely to cost the insurance company more money). Psychiatric patients who do have medical coverage find care difficult to access because many plans require that medical care be provided only by an approved health plan physician in an approved medical facility. The problem can become critical for psychiatric inpatients who develop concurrent acute medical problems. It is often too dangerous or difficult to transfer a patient to the medical setting under these circumstances. In this situation, patients may be billed for medical services provided while under formal psychiatric care. More often, medical services are delayed or neglected because the subcontractor for behavioral health care services does not want to bear the cost of medical procedures. Managed care companies that do not limit expenses or that exceed capitation limits are destined to lose their contract. Hence, every incentive exists to deny care or to sanction care only when provided by the least expensive provider. The way to circumvent these problems is through the development of integrated services that meet licensure requirements for both medical and psychiatric billing. Thereafter, denials should be aggressively challenged with formal complaints to the insurance commissioner if necessary.

A recent survey (Westerman and Kunkel 1999) indicated that payment problems for services to patients with concurrent medical and psychiatric illness do not receive much attention from most managed care organizations and indemnity insurers, perpetuating reimbursement difficulties. They mistakenly consider it too "small" a population on which to expend their resources. However, this underdiagnosed and inadequately treated patient population is responsible for 30% or more of our health care expenditures (Katon et al. 1990).

Outpatient Integration of Medical-Psychiatric Services

The mechanics of setting up an integrated outpatient medical-psychiatry program can be complicated. It is not possible to add a person or two to existing traditional service programs and expect a truly integrated program to exist and be successful. Furthermore, each health care system has individual objectives, target populations, payer mixes, and personnel availability. These all influence the components included in the program, patients treated, team members involved, and so forth. For these reasons, the best way to initiate an integrated outpatient program is to develop an operational plan, starting with the mission and goals of the institution (Table 38–5). This plan formally assesses the value that an integrated program would bring to medical-surgical clinics and its relation to other services. Such a plan must consider cost efficiency and cost benefits to the population served.

Substantial research data now show that effective treatments for mood, anxiety, substance use, and somatization disorders can actually reduce total costs. This is best accomplished if the critical components found in Table 38–3 are used in the integrated treatment by a mental health team model (Figure 38–2). As previously discussed, a problem arises in allocating resources from medical and behavioral health budgets. Recognizing that a problem exists is half the battle, because then one can develop strategies to address the problem. If behavioral health care coverage is not already combined with medical coverage, then an agreement among medical and behavioral health budget managers and providers is needed. Such cooperation should become commonplace during the next several years, because the National Committee for Quality Assurance (1999a, 1999b) 1999 Standards for the Accreditation of Managed Care Organizations and the American Medical Association (1999) now have policies that mandate communication, access, and reimbursement for medical and psychiatric care coordination. Momentum for federal regulation of the health care industry is likely to increase as public dissatisfaction grows with health care plans that maximize profits through denial of care.

Ultimately, resources saved from decreased medical utilization will fund increased psychiatric service capabilities and lead to a net reduction in the total number of dollars spent for patient care. Furthermore, reduction in disability related to psychiatric illness will lead to a decrease in the indirect society burden of illness (Murray and Lopez 1996), an increase in workplace productivity (McDonnell Douglas Corporation 1989), and an improved quality of life for patients with medical-psychiatric illnesses.

Inpatient Integration of Medical-Psychiatric Services

As noted earlier in this chapter, the "Medical-Psychiatric Units" chapter in the first edition of this textbook was entirely devoted to inpatient integration. That chapter strongly emphasized the development of type III integrated care programs (Kathol et al. 1992a). These programs usually are administered through psychiatry to take advantage of federal guidelines for diagnosis-related-group–exempt TEFRA (Tax Equity and Fiscal Responsibility Act) rates. At the time, this was an economically viable way to support the acute care of patients with concurrent medical and psychiatric illness (Fogel and Stoudemire 1986).

During the past 5 years, a transformation has occurred in strategies to set up integrated inpatient services. TEFRA reimbursement rates have declined, the acuity of admitted patients has increased, and the economic burden these patients place on health centers that provide primary or specialty care services has been better defined (Goldberg and Stoudemire 1995; Goldberg et al. 1994). As a result, in the past few years, several psychiatrically based integrated care units closed because the cost exceeded payments under highly restrictive psychiatric reimbursements. The same phenomenon has occurred with general psychiatric hospitals, which, almost universally, have reduced beds, closed programs, or closed completely.

One solution that has worked in several locations is the development of integrated inpatient programs under medical licensure, but with psychiatric care capabilities also meeting psychiatric licensure requirements. Some states recognize joint licensure as long as both medical-surgical and psychiatric code requirements are met. This serves several purposes. First, it makes the *medical* managed care organization accountable for the reimbursement of most admissions. This ensures reimbursement rates sufficient to cover medical tests and procedures but also leaves the door open to bill behavioral health companies when days are denied. Second, it ensures active medical staff participation in unit operations. Third, it increases the level of medical acuity while maintaining high psychiatric acuity. Fourth, it broadens the referral base because both nonpsychiatric and psychiatric practitioners now have admitting privileges. Furthermore, when a co-attending model (psychiatrist is responsible for the psychiatric illness and nonpsychiatrist for the medical-surgical illness) is used, it even solves the problem of reimbursement for psychiatrists because insurance companies can legitimately be billed daily by both physicians. Finally, it allows the treatment of patients who benefit the most from integrated services and are the greatest economic burden on the health care system.

Using medical beds to provide integrated services does not mean just changing the sign on the door of a general medical unit. It entails incorporation of the psychiatric space requirements and services, psychiatric safety features, cross-trained nursing staff, and psychiatric coverage. Only when licensure requirements for both medical and psychiatric care are met can one feel assured that both medical and psychiatric payers can be held responsible to reimburse the hospital and professional services.

With integrated care transplanted from the psychiatric to the medical setting, some circumstances may change. All patients will require an admitting medical condition or a combination of illnesses that makes it difficult or dangerous to treat in the psychiatric setting. Psychiatric programming (e.g., unit milieu, one-to-one interaction between patient and staff, unit activities) may receive less attention unless staff levels allow appropriate attention to both medical and psychiatric nursing needs. Psychiatrists may find themselves poorly paid consultants unless a co-attending model of care is adopted.

SUMMARY

Inpatient and outpatient integrated medical and psychiatric treatment programs include five components: 1) combined medical and psychiatric services, usually in the nonpsychiatric setting; 2) active case finding in high-risk targeted populations; 3) use of treatments that have been proven effective in systematic studies; 4) clinical outcomes orientation, and 5) long-term disease management of complicated, chronic illnesses. In the inpatient setting, high-acuity medical and psychiatric capabilities can be added. By instituting an integrated approach, it is possible to achieve greater medical and psychiatric symptom reduction by providing concurrent, collaborative care.

Outpatient programs are composed of an alliance between primary or specialty care physicians and a mental health team with an appropriate skill mix so that patients can receive guidelines-based intervention and cost-effective care. Currently, inpatient programs have a better chance of financial success under medical unit licensure, but only when psychiatric safety features, dually trained nursing personnel, and active participation by psychiatrists are included and reimbursed fairly. When properly developed, and managed well clinically and fiscally, type III units under psychiatric administration remain viable. Type IV units are at greater financial risk if only under psychiatric licensure.

Integrated programs will become highly desirable in the future as the American model of health care matures. Medical-psychiatric programs introduce cost saving mainly by delivering cost-effective, cost-beneficial treatment in both inpatient and outpatient settings. They do this by providing concurrent rather than sequential care

and by selecting treatment providers matched to the needs of the patient and the system. Perhaps most important, outcomes will improve.

Although integrated care allows treatment of numerous patients neglected in the current system, it will not replace outpatient mental health clinics, substance abuse programs, inpatient psychiatry in the medically ill (consultation) services, or inpatient psychiatry units. Patients with more severe or chronic psychiatric disorders will continue to need specialized longitudinal outpatient psychiatry programs and inpatient psychiatric treatment. Psychiatrists for the medically ill will continue to provide acute care for most patients in medical inpatient settings, reserving transfer to integrated medical-psychiatric programs for patients requiring ongoing and persistent combined nursing and physician capabilities.

Intangible benefits of integrated care also occur as programs develop. Communication between mental health professionals and medical-surgical personnel improves. Alliances among these individuals lead to fewer treatment conflicts, adverse events, and treatment delays. Academic medical centers can provide better training to medical students and residents for the 25% or more of patients in clinical practice with comorbid medical-psychiatric illness (Stoudemire 1996b). Patients are more satisfied with the integrated and coordinated approach to their health needs, treatment in a nonpsychiatric setting, and increased convenience and less frustration. Employers who pay for health care coverage benefit from a healthier and more productive work force with fewer complaints about the disjointed care available in traditional health plans.

Medical-psychiatric programs have great educational and fiscal value in academic settings (tertiary care, state-of-the-art interventions, reduced cost for indigent and capitated patients), in county and state hospitals (higher quality and lower cost for nonpaying patients, reduced lengths of stay), in private hospitals (unique quality-enhancing service capabilities), and in veterans affairs hospitals (high-end primary care psychiatry initiative). They enhance the clinical capabilities of primary or specialty care physicians and psychiatrists. They reduce costs to indemnity insurers at "total risk" for patients and also reduce the cost to at-risk health care systems or organizations providing capitated reimbursement contracts. Finally, they improve the quality of life for many patients.

As psychiatric problems appear to escalate, family structures become more fragmented, and rates of substance dependency and abuse rise, integrated care is one improvement that helps individuals and society cope. Unfortunately, integrated programs do not just happen. They take careful planning and diligent long-term commitment.

REFERENCES

Academy of Psychosomatic Medicine: Mental disorders in general medical practice: adding value to healthcare through consultation-liaison psychiatry, in Primary Care Meets Mental Health. Edited by Haber JD, Mitchell GE. Tiburon, CA, CentraLink Publications, 1997, pp 255–292

American Medical Association: Medical, surgical, and psychiatric service integration and reimbursement (table). Primary Psychiatry 6(7):45, 1999

Baez K, Aiarzaguena JM, Grandes G, et al: Understanding patient-initiated frequent attendance in primary care: a case-control study. Br J Gen Pract 48:1824–1827, 1998

Bronheim HE, Fulop G, Kunkel EJ, et al: The Academy of Psychosomatic Medicine practice guidelines for psychiatric consultation in the general medical setting. The Academy of Psychosomatic Medicine. Psychosomatics 39:S8–S30, 1998

Brown TM, Stoudemire A: Psychiatric Side Effects of Prescription and Over the Counter Medications. Washington, DC, American Psychiatric Press, 1998

Carr VJ, Lewin TJ, Reid AL, et al: An evaluation of the effectiveness of a consultation-liaison psychiatry service in general practice. Aust N Z J Psychiatry 31:714–727, 1997

Chen A: Noncompliance in community psychiatry: a review of clinical interventions. Hospital and Community Psychiatry 42:282–287, 1991

Fava GA, Wise TN, Molnar G, et al: The medical-psychiatric unit: a novel psychosomatic approach. Psychother Psychosom 43:194–201, 1985

Fogel BS: A psychiatric unit becomes a psychiatric-medical unit: administrative and clinical implications. Gen Hosp Psychiatry 7:26–35, 1985

Fogel BS, Stoudemire A: Organization and development of combined medical-psychiatric units: part 2. Psychosomatics 27:417–420, 425–428, 1986

Fogel BS, Stoudemire A, Houpt JL: Contrasting models for combined medical and psychiatric inpatient treatment. Am J Psychiatry 142:1085–1089, 1985

France RD, Weddington WW Jr, Houpt JL: Referral of patients from primary care physicians to a community mental health center. J Nerv Ment Dis 166:594–598, 1978

Francis J, Kapoor WN: Prognosis after hospital discharge of older medical patients with delirium. J Am Geriatr Soc 40:601–606, 1992

Francis J, Martin D, Kapoor WN: A prospective study of delirium in hospitalized elderly. JAMA 263:1097–1101, 1990

Freyne A, Buckley P, Larkin C, et al: Consultation liaison psychiatry within the general hospital: referral pattern and management. Ir Med J 85(3):112–114, 1992

Fulop G, Strain JJ, Vita L, et al: Impact of psychiatric comorbidity on length of hospital stay for medical/surgical patients: a preliminary report. Am J Psychiatry 144:878–882, 1987

Garbutt JC, West SL, Carey TS, et al: Pharmacological treatment of alcohol dependence: a review of the evidence. JAMA 281:1318–1325, 1999

Goetzel RZ, Anderson DR, Whitmer RW, et al: The relationship between modifiable health risks and health care expenditures. J Occup Environ Med 40:843–854, 1998

Goldberg RJ, Fogel BS: Integration of general hospital psychiatric services with freestanding psychiatric hospitals. Hospital and Community Psychiatry 40:1057–1061, 1989

Goldberg RJ, Stoudemire A: The future of consultation-liaison psychiatry and medical-psychiatric units in the era of managed care. Gen Hosp Psychiatry 17:268–277, 1995 [Published erratum appears in Gen Hosp Psychiatry 18:209, 1996]

Goldberg RJ, Daly J, Golinger RC: The impact of psychiatric comorbidity on Medicare reimbursement for inpatient medical care. Gen Hosp Psychiatry 16:16–19, 1994

Goodman B: Combined psychiatric-medical inpatient units: the Mount Sinai model. Psychosomatics 26:179–182, 185–186, 189, 1985

Hahn SR, Kroenke K, Spitzer RL, et al: The difficult patient: prevalence, psychopathology, and functional impairment. J Gen Intern Med 11:1–8, 1996 [Published erratum appears in J Gen Intern Med 11:191, 1996]

Hall RC, Kathol RG: Developing a level III/IV medical/psychiatry unit: establishing a basis, design of the unit, and physician responsibility. Psychosomatics 33:368–375, 1992

Harsch HH, LeCann AF, Ciaccio S: Treatment in combined medical psychiatry units: an integrative model. Psychosomatics 30:312–317, 1989

Harsch HH, Koran LM, Young LD: A profile of academic medical-psychiatric units. Gen Hosp Psychiatry 13:291–295, 1991

Henk HJ, Katzelnick DJ, Kobak KA, et al: Medical costs attributed to depression among patients with a history of high medical expenses in a health maintenance organization. Arch Gen Psychiatry 53:899–904, 1996

Higgins ES: A review of unrecognized mental illness in primary care: prevalence, natural history, and efforts to change the course. Arch Fam Med 3:908–917, 1994

Holder HD, Blose JO: The reduction of health care costs associated with alcoholism treatment: a 14-year longitudinal study. J Stud Alcohol 53:293–302, 1991

Huyse FJ, Lyons JS, Strain JJ: The sequencing of psychiatric recommendations: concordance during the process of a psychiatric consultation. Psychosomatics 34:307–313, 1993

Inouye SK, Bogardus ST Jr, Charpentier PA, et al: A multicomponent intervention to prevent delirium in hospitalized older patients. N Engl J Med 340:669–676, 1999

Kathol RG: Medical psychiatry units: the wave of the future. Gen Hosp Psychiatry 16:1–3, 1994

Kathol RG: Reassurance therapy: what to say to symptomatic patients with benign or non-existent medical disease. Int J Psychiatry Med 27:173–180, 1997

Kathol RG, Harsch HH, Hall RCW, et al: Categorization of types of medical/psychiatry units based on level of acuity. Psychosomatics 33:376–386, 1992a

Kathol RG, Harsch HH, Hall RCW, et al: Quality assurance in a setting designed to care for patients with combined medical and psychiatric disease. Psychosomatics 33:387–396, 1992b

Katon W, Schulberg H: Epidemiology of depression in primary care. Gen Hosp Psychiatry 14:237–247, 1992

Katon W, Von Korff M, Lin E, et al: Distressed high utilizers of medical care: DSM-III-R diagnoses and treatment needs. Gen Hosp Psychiatry 12:355–362, 1990

Katon W, Von Korff M, Lin E, et al: Collaborative management to achieve treatment guidelines: impact on depression in primary care. JAMA 273:1026–1031, 1995

Kishi Y, Kathol R: Integrating medicine and psychiatry treatment in an inpatient medical setting: the type IV program. Psychosomatics 40:345–355, 1999

Kishi Y, Kathol RG: Integrating medical and psychiatric treatment in an inpatient medical setting (reply to letter by Alan Stoudemire). Psychosomatics 41:367–369, 2000

Kroenke K, Jackson JL, Chamberlin J: Depressive and anxiety disorders in patients presenting with physical complaints: clinical predictors and outcome. Am J Med 103:339–347, 1997

Krulee DA, Hales RE: Compliance with psychiatric referrals from a general hospital psychiatry outpatient clinic. Gen Hosp Psychiatry 10:339–345, 1988

Levenson LJ: The ability of psychiatric consultation to change outcome. Paper presented at the annual meeting of the Academy of Psychosomatic Medicine, Orlando, FL, November 1998

Levitan SJ, Kornfeld DS: Clinical and cost benefits of liaison psychiatry. Am J Psychiatry 138:790–793, 1981

Linden M, Lecrubier Y, Bellantuono C, et al: The prescribing of psychotropic drugs by primary care physicians: an international collaborative study. J Clin Psychopharmacol 19:132–140, 1999

Mayou R, Hawton K, Feldman E: What happens to medical patients with psychiatric disorder? J Psychosom Res 32:541–549, 1988

McDonnell Douglas Corporation: Employee assistance program financial offset study 1985–1988. Bridgeton, MO, Alexander & Alexander Consulting Group, 1989

Miller NS, Swift RM, Gold MS: Health care economics for integrated addiction treatment in clinical settings. Psychiatric Annals 28:682–689, 1998

Moellentine C, Rummans T, Ahlskog JE, et al: Effectiveness of ECT in patients with parkinsonism. J Neuropsychiatry Clin Neurosci 10:187–193, 1998

Murray CJL, Lopez AD. The Global Burden of Disease. Boston, MA, Harvard School Public Health, World Health Organization and the World Bank, 1996

Mynors-Wallis L, Davies I, Gray A, et al: A randomized controlled trial and cost analysis of problem-solving treatment for emotional disorders given by community nurses in primary care. Br J Psychiatry 170:113–119, 1997

National Committee for Quality Assurance: Quality management and improvement QI 6. Primary Psychiatry 6(7):46, 1999a

National Committee for Quality Assurance: Quality management and improvement QI 9. Primary Psychiatry 6(7):46, 1999b

Olfson M, Sing M, Schlesinger HJ: Mental health/medical care cost offsets: opportunities for managed care. Health Aff (Millwood) 18:79–90, 1999

Ormel J, VonKorff M, Ustun TB, et al: Common mental disorders and disability across cultures: results from the WHO Collaborative Study on Psychological Problems in General Health Care. JAMA 272:1741–1748, 1994

Perez EL, Silverman M: Utilization pattern of a Canadian psychiatric consultation service. Gen Hosp Psychiatry 5:185–190, 1983

Regier DA, Narrow WE, Rae DS, et al: The de facto US mental and addictive disorders service system: Epidemiologic Catchment Area prospective 1-year prevalence rates of disorders and services. Arch Gen Psychiatry 50:84–94, 1993

Rogers WH, Wells KB, Meredith LS, et al: Outcomes for adult outpatients with depression under prepaid or fee-for-service financing. Arch Gen Psychiatry 50:517–525, 1993

Rost K, Kashner TM, Smith RG Jr: Effectiveness of psychiatric intervention with somatization disorder patients: improved outcomes at reduced costs. Gen Hosp Psychiatry 16:381–387, 1994

Salvador-Carulla L, Seguí J, Fernández-Cano P, et al: Costs and offset effect in panic disorders. Br J Psychiatry 166 (suppl 27):23–28, 1995

Saravay SM: Psychiatric interventions in the medically ill: outcomes and effectiveness research. Psychiatr Clin North Am 19:1–14, 1996

Saravay SM, Levin M: Psychiatric comorbidity and length of stay in general hospital: a critical review of outcome studies. Psychosomatics 35:233–252, 1994

Schulberg HC, Block MR, Madonia MJ, et al: The 'usual care' of major depression in primary care practice. Arch Fam Med 6:334–339, 1997

Scott JC, Robertson BJ: Kaiser Colorado's Cooperative Health Clinic: a group approach to patient care. Managed Care Quarterly 4(3):41–45, 1996

Simon GE, VonKorff M, Barlow W: Health care costs of primary care patients with recognized depression. Arch Gen Psychiatry 52:850–856, 1995

Smith GR Jr: Effectiveness of treatment for somatoform disorder patients. Psychiatr Med 9:545–558, 1991

Smith GR Jr, Monson RA, Ray DC: Psychiatric consultation in somatization disorder: a randomized controlled study. N Engl J Med 314:1407–1413, 1986

Smith GR Jr, Rost K, Kashner TM: A trial of the effect of a standardized psychiatric consultation on health outcomes and costs in somatizing patients. Arch Gen Psychiatry 52:238–243, 1995

Spitzer RL, Williams JB, Kroenke K, et al: Utility of a new procedure for diagnosing mental disorders in primary care. The PRIME-MD 1000 study. JAMA 272:1749–1756, 1994

Spitzer RL, Kroenke K, Linzer M, et al: Health-related quality of life in primary care patients with mental disorders: results from the PRIME-MD 1000 study. JAMA 274:1511–1517, 1995

Stoudemire A: Medical-psychiatric units, in The American Psychiatric Press Textbook of Consultation-Liaison Psychiatry. Edited by Rundell JR, Wise MG. Washington, DC, American Psychiatric Press, 1996a, pp 900–913

Stoudemire A: Psychiatry in medical practice: implications for the education of primary care physicians in the era of managed care: part 1. Psychosomatics 37:502–508, 1996b

Stoudemire A: Psychiatry in medical practice: implications for the education of primary care physicians in the era of managed care: part 2. Psychosomatics 38:1–9, 1997

Stoudemire A, Fogel BS: Organization and development of combined medical-psychiatric units: part 1. Psychosomatics 27:341–345, 1986

Stoudemire A, Fogel BS, Greenberg D (eds): Psychiatric Care of the Medical Patient, 2nd Edition. New York, Oxford University Press, 2000

Strain JJ, Lyons JS, Hammer JS, et al: Cost offset from a psychiatric consultation-liaison intervention with elderly hip fracture patients. Am J Psychiatry 148:1044–1049, 1991

Summergrad P: Medical psychiatry units and the roles of the inpatient psychiatric service in the general hospital. Gen Hosp Psychiatry 16:20–31, 1994

Unützer J, Patrick DL, Simon G, et al: Depressive symptoms and the cost of health services in HMO patients aged 65 years and older: a 4-year prospective study. JAMA 277:1618–1623, 1997

U.S. Department of Health and Human Services, Agency for Health Care Policy and Research, Public Health Service, Depression Guideline Panel: Clinical Practice Guideline for the Detection and Diagnosis of Depression in Primary Care (AHCPR Publ No 93-0550). Rockville, MD, U.S. Department of Health and Human Services, April 1993a

U.S. Department of Health and Human Services, Agency for Health Care Policy and Research, Public Health Service, Depression Guideline Panel: Clinical Practice Guideline for the Treatment of Major Depressive Disorder in Primary Care (AHCPR Publ No 93-0551). Rockville, MD, U.S. Department of Health and Human Services, April 1993b

Von Korff M, Ormel J, Katon W, et al: Disability and depression among high utilizers of health care: a longitudinal analysis. Arch Gen Psychiatry 49:91–100, 1992

Weddington WW Jr: Adherence by medical-surgical inpatients to recommendations for outpatient psychiatric treatment. Psychother Psychosom 39:225–235, 1983

Wells KB: Depression in general medical settings: implications of three health policy studies for consultation-liaison psychiatry. Psychosomatics 35:279–296, 1994

Wells KB, Goldberg G, Brook R, et al: Management of patients on psychotropic drugs in primary care clinics. Med Care 26:645–656, 1988

Westerman P, Kunkel E: Consultation-liaison psychiatry: traditional inpatient integrated psychiatric services in a managed care world. Primary Psychiatry 6(7):47–48, 67–70, 1999

Williams JW Jr, Mulrow CD, Kroenke K, et al: Case-finding for depression in primary care: a randomized trial. Am J Med 106:36–43, 1999

39

The Emergency Department

George E. Tesar, M.D.

Joseph A. Locala, M.D.

PSYCHIATRIC EMERGENCY SERVICES

Psychiatric emergency services were established in Great Britain as early as the 1920s (Wellin et al. 1987) and in the United States in the late 1950s and early 1960s (Chafetz et al. 1966; J. V. Coleman and Errera 1963; M. D. Coleman and Zwerling 1959). The release of patients from publicly funded psychiatric hospitals and the scarcity of community and general hospital mental health services contributed to the demand for psychiatric care in emergency facilities in the United States. Emergency psychiatric evaluation continues to be provided on a consultative basis (Chafetz et al. 1962; Wellin et al. 1987); however, as the need for psychiatric consultation increased in large, academic training centers, distinct and self-contained psychiatric emergency services evolved (Chafetz et al. 1966; J. V. Coleman and Errera 1963; M. D. Coleman and Zwerling 1959). In these autonomous services, psychiatric residents and supervising staff, social workers, nurses, mental health workers, and psychologists collaborate to provide onsite crisis intervention, evaluation of substance abuse disorders, and referral for psychiatric hospitalization.

PSYCHIATRIC CONSULTATION IN THE EMERGENCY DEPARTMENT

Hospitals that are unable to sustain separate psychiatric emergency services continue to rely on consultation-liaison psychiatrists or on-call psychiatrists in the emergency department (ED). This is not an ideal approach because the request for an emergency consultation is typically added onto the schedule of a busy clinician. In addition, the consultant generally has little help with arrangement of the patient's disposition. Based on the paucity of available inpatient and outpatient psychiatric resources in most communities, disposition planning is often the most challenging part of an emergency psychiatric assessment.

This chapter addresses important issues in emergency psychiatric consultation. Because safety is a special concern, discussion is devoted to weapons management, the use of seclusion, and the use of mechanical restraints. Patient evaluation begins in the ED's triage area. Accurate assessment depends on acquisition of reliable information and careful consideration of requests made by both the referring physician and the patient. Special attention is devoted to life-endangering psychiatric emergencies (e.g., acute psychosis, suicide, violence, the severely agitated or disruptive patient, sedative-hypnotic withdrawal) and to specific populations of emergency psychiatric patients (e.g., those with substance abuse disorders, sociopathic or borderline personality disorders, or mood or anxiety disorders; homeless individuals; and repeat users of emergency services). Mobile crisis services are addressed. In addition, the important and often time-consuming task of arranging for a clinically sound disposition is addressed.

SAFETY

Case Example 1

The police brought a 35-year-old woman to the ED from the airport after she exhibited inappropriate behavior. She was placed in a seclusion room pending the psychiatrist's evaluation. Toward the end of the evaluation, she pulled a penknife from the pocket of her jeans and pointed it at the psychiatrist before handing it to him. The psychiatrist was surprised because he assumed that the patient had been thoroughly searched, and then he became angry about being exposed to potential danger.

Case Example 2

A 43-year-old man with alcohol use disorder, well known by the ED staff, arrived at the ED in a state of acute intoxication. He was admitted to the seclusion room, searched, and then placed in two-point restraints. Some time later, he pulled himself outside the seclusion room door toward his belongings. He was returned to the seclusion room, and two more restraints were applied.

"Fire, fire!" was then heard from the seclusion room. Assuming further provocation, ED personnel ignored the yelling. Ultimately, however, the smell of smoke and the fire alarm captured the staff's attention. They found the patient's mattress aflame and a cigarette lighter on the floor.

Weapons Screening and Initial Management of Violent or Potentially Violent Patients

Contrary to what might be expected, it is not unusual for psychiatric patients to carry weapons into the ED. In studies performed at the Langley Porter Psychiatric Institute Emergency Service in San Francisco, 4%–8% of patients had weapons (McCulloch et al. 1986; McNiel and Binder 1987a). Traditionally, psychiatrists either underestimate the number of psychiatric patients who carry weapons or overestimate their ability to detect weapon-carrying patients. McNiel and Binder (1987a) found that male gender and history of substance abuse were the only distinctive features among those who carried weapons and were seen for psychiatric assessment in an ED.

Some clinicians may object to routine weapons screening on grounds that patients might disapprove, that routine screening might provoke violence, or that routine screening might violate the patient's right to privacy. A study by McCulloch et al. (1986) suggested that these concerns, although potentially relevant in selected cases, are unfounded. Responding to self-report questionnaires, the vast majority of patients and staff agreed that weapons screening was a good idea (84% and 88%, respectively) and that it did not violate the patients' civil rights (85% and 89%, respectively). Although 69% of staff anticipated that weapons screening would upset the patients, only 15% of patients who were screened acknowledged being upset by the procedure, and none of the patients were uncooperative.

The consulting psychiatrist must know the ED's policy regarding weapons screening and patient violence (see "Patients Who Are Violent" section, later in this chapter). A written policy is mandatory. The policy must require either that patients are searched or that they wear a standard hospital gown. Violation of the psychiatric patient's civil liberties and unnecessary intrusiveness are potential arguments against such a policy. Admittedly, disrobing of patients is unnecessary in some instances, and a few patients may refuse to disrobe. Maintenance of safety, however, favors such a policy. Also, a physical examination is more likely to occur when a patient wears a hospital gown.

The requirement that psychiatric emergency patients wear a hospital gown significantly reduces the risk of concealed weapons. It is essential to remember, however, that the ED is filled with potentially dangerous instruments (e.g., needles, scalpels, glass objects, razors, tourniquets)—patient access to these objects must be restricted. Most states mandate continuous observation of dangerous patients in publicly funded hospitals. Although general hospital EDs do not, as a rule, fall within the state's jurisdiction, compliance with the state's policies and regulations regarding care of dangerous psychiatric patients is recommended.

The ED must also address the management of the patient's belongings. In Case Example 2, the partially restrained patient retrieved his cigarette lighter from a plastic bag left outside the seclusion room door. The ED staff should place all personal belongings in a secure area that is inaccessible to the patient. Staff should also remember to segregate personal belongings from the patient during transfer to another facility.

When the patient has a weapon, it is recommended that the clinician not take it directly. Instead, the clinician should instruct the patient to place the weapon on a flat surface and then call security staff to confiscate it. Accepting the weapon directly poses a risk of accidental injury to either the clinician or the patient. Moreover, if there is any chance that the weapon was used to commit a crime, all hospital personnel should avoid touching it or handling it in a way that would contaminate legal evidence.

Seclusion and Mechanical Restraint

All EDs must have a written policy for the seclusion and mechanical restraint of threatening, disruptive, or agitated patients. The policy must address 1) the indications for seclusion or mechanical restraint (e.g., the threat or occurrence of danger to oneself or others), 2) technical issues (e.g., the appropriate use and application of mechanical restraints, requirements for the monitoring and care of the restrained or secluded patient by medical and nursing staff), and 3) facility requirements (e.g., a safe, adequately soundproofed seclusion room that has an unbreakable window offering a full view of the room).

The standard of least restrictive treatment must be applied. A verbal attempt to calm a threatening or agitated patient must be documented before seclusion or restraint is used (Soloff 1987). The clinician should speak softly, move slowly, and behave deferentially during the evaluation procedure. An offer of food or liquids or oral medication may encourage the patient's cooperation. A show of force by hospital security guards demonstrates that adequate force is available to control unruly behavior if necessary. If these measures do not help the patient to achieve self-control, or if agitation is intense or rapidly escalating, then mechanical restraint is appropriate until the safety of the patient and the staff is ensured.

TRIAGE AND EVALUATION

Triage

Case Example 3

A disheveled, malodorous, and intoxicated man stumbled into the ED and uttered slurred expletives at the triage nurse. In response to the nurse's opening inquiry, the man mumbled something about assailants and then fell to the floor. Because of his inappropriate behavior, presumed paranoia, and intoxication, psychiatric consultation was urgently requested.

The psychiatrist was able to discern from the semistuporous patient that he had been struck on the head with a baseball bat. A computed tomography (CT) scan of the patient's head revealed a right frontal subdural hematoma.

The job of the triage nurse is challenging, especially in a busy, multispecialty urban ED. Rapid decision making is necessary and often with little history available, as in Case Example 3. A patient's uncooperative, disagreeable, or inappropriate behavior not only interferes with obtaining important information but also typically alienates triage personnel. The patient's behavior can precipitate a cycle of animosity (e.g., the psychiatrist receives the nurse's displaced anger and frustration and transmits it back to the patient). It can help if the consulting psychiatrist knows triage personnel and has a comfortable working relationship with them.

In selected cases, the psychiatrist must learn exactly what happened during the triage process. Case Example 3 can be viewed pessimistically as an example of the emergency psychiatrist's misfortune or, more constructively, as an inevitable occurrence that demands comprehensive evaluation of all patients and a high index of suspicion for underlying medical illness. A policy that all patients be examined first by an emergency physician might theoretically obviate the problem in the case example. However, psychiatric patients typically receive inadequate general medical evaluation (Weissberg 1979). For example, even basic vital sign measurements are sometimes neglected in an agitated or uncooperative psychiatric patient. Either the patient's behavior interferes with the performance of a physical examination or, once identified as a psychiatric patient, the patient's complaints and condition are taken less seriously. As a result, the quality of care is inadequate.

Patient Transfers

The consultant is occasionally asked to triage incoming telephone calls. Interhospital transfer has legal implications. The Consolidated Omnibus Budget Reconciliation Act of 1985 makes "patient dumping" a violation of federal law. The hospital that transfers a patient without first obtaining formal acceptance from the receiving institution is subject to stiff penalties (Frew et al. 1988).

Several important questions must be addressed before a patient is transferred: 1) Is the proposed receiving facility the correct one? 2) Is the patient medically stable for transfer? and 3) Is the patient exhibiting transient symptoms that, if stabilized, could result in another disposition?

Correct Facility

In some states, the patient's address, type of medical insurance coverage, and location of previous psychiatric hospitalization influence the ultimate disposition. Transfer to the wrong hospital can occur if these issues are not considered adequately.

Medically Stable

Federal law requires that all patients be medically stable before transfer from the ED (Frew et al. 1988). As noted previously, medical evaluation of psychiatric patients is often inadequate, particularly when patients are agitated or uncooperative. It is important, therefore, to note vital sign measurements (including respirations), level of consciousness, results of physical examination, and results of specific laboratory studies (e.g., electrolyte levels; toxicology screen; blood alcohol level; and in selected cases, electrocardiogram, chest X ray, and arterial blood gases). It is not appropriate to transfer a patient whose mental status changes are the result of a medical illness, alcohol withdrawal, or a life-threatening drug overdose that requires monitoring or admission to a medical unit (e.g., tricyclic antidepressant, anticholinergic, aspirin, or acetaminophen overdose).

Transient Symptoms

Whether the patient's symptoms are transient is relevant to cases of intoxication. A common example is that of the intoxicated patient who is making suicidal threats or gestures. Often, once sober, the same patient will deny suicidal thoughts, and transfer for psychiatric evaluation will be unnecessary.

Interview and Mental Status Examination

Establishment of the Patient's Request

Successful consultation depends, among other things, on an understanding of the patient's request. The request is often different from the chief complaint. For example, the chief complaint may be anxiety or trouble sleeping, whereas the request is for Xanax. Lazare and Eisenthal (1977) found that 6% of patients entering an emergency psychiatric walk-in clinic had no request (e.g., did not want psychiatric help, did not know why they came to the clinic, or were brought to the clinic against their wishes). However, 94% had one or more requests that fell into 13 categories:

1. Administrative action ("use your role to do something for me")
2. Advice ("tell me what to do")
3. Clarification ("help me put my feelings into perspective")
4. Community triage ("guide me to where I can get the help I want")
5. Confession ("assuage my guilt")
6. Control ("keep me from falling apart")
7. Insight ("help me understand the root of my problem")
8. Medical advice or treatment ("make a diagnosis and treat me")
9. Psychological expertise ("use your skills to help me understand myself better")
10. Reality contact ("help me feel real")
11. Social intervention ("help me deal with some other people")
12. Succor ("fill my void")
13. Ventilation ("listen while I get things off my chest")

The most common requests were for clarification, insight, and psychological expertise; requests for ventilation, control, and medical advice or treatment were less common; and the least common requests were for administrative action and social intervention. These findings by Lazare and Eisenthal have been replicated by others (Gillig et al. 1990; Rapaport and Zisook 1987).

Investigations of the patient's request show that it is highly correlated with patient satisfaction and the negotiation of a treatment strategy. Unlike the chief complaint, the request is often concealed, and the patient may have more than one request; the most important request is often not revealed until later in the interview. Knowledge of the typical kinds of requests made by emergency psychiatric patients can help the consultant elicit them and formulate valid clinical hypotheses and diagnoses.

All requests neither can nor should be fulfilled, but their verbalization can open a process of negotiation that allows for an evaluation of their legitimacy (Lazare 1976; Lazare et al. 1975b). Lazare et al. (1975a) observed that the majority of walk-in patients had a very specific idea of what they wanted. Although the request did not always address the entire problem, it was often appropriate.

Establishment of the Patient's Reason for Now Seeking Help

It is also important to determine why the patient decided to come to the ED now. Many problems surface in the context of chronic illness or smoldering crisis. What has happened or what has changed to make the patient seek help now rather than last week, or yesterday, or next week? It can be productive to ask what the patient thinks would have happened had he or she not come for help now. Also, it is important to ask about expectations: "What do you hope we can do for you?" "What are your wishes?" "What do you want to accomplish before leaving here today?" Such questions quickly focus ambiguous complaints or requests.

Mental Status Examination

The neuropsychiatric interview and mental status examination are discussed in detail in Chapter 6 in this volume. Given the rapid time frame of emergency evaluations, it is neither practical nor always necessary to perform every aspect of a complete neuropsychiatric examination. Several important components, however, warrant special emphasis in emergency psychiatric patients.

The spontaneity of ED presentation affords a unique view of the patient's appearance and behavior that is not usually evident once the patient is admitted to the hospital. The patient's manner of dress (if street clothes are still being worn) and level of hygiene often reveal useful information about the intensity and duration of illness.

The patient's speech and use of language must be examined carefully to avoid mistaking aphasic speech for the illogical, loosely connected thinking of a patient with acute psychosis or schizophrenia (Benson 1973). In addition to the usual investigation for disordered thinking and perceptions, explicit inquiry about hopelessness, suicidal thinking, and command auditory hallucinations is essential. If the clinician is suspicious after the patient denies self-destructive or homicidal thoughts, it is sometimes revealing to ask, "If you did have any suicidal (homicidal) thoughts, would you be able to tell me?" If the presentation suggests a psychotic or borderline disorder, the clinician must ask about auditory hallucinations that command the patient to harm himself or herself or others. Some patients experience chronic command auditory hallucinations and do not act on them; these patients are the only exception to the rule that all those who have command auditory hallucinations should be hospitalized for further investigation and treatment.

Tests of intention or executive function are not included in the Mini-Mental State Exam (Folstein et al. 1975) and are often overlooked in routine clinical examination. Frontal-lobe dysfunction, because it can present without the usual focal, lateralizing findings elicited by routine neurological examination, is easily overlooked. Frontal-lobe dysfunction is not common and probably occurs more frequently in patients with chronic, nonspecific psychoses and in those with a history of head injury or chronic alcoholism. Clock drawing is a good screening test for global cortical dysfunction; evidence of improper placement or duplication of numbers around the face of the clock may be a clue to impaired executive functions and frontal-lobe damage or diffuse cortical dysfunction. Easily performed bedside maneuvers that more specifically check the integrity of the frontal lobes include visual pattern completion tests and Luria hand maneuvers (see Chapter 6 in this volume).

Physical Examination

An unfortunate trend that occurs during the course of psychiatric training and practice is the gradual loss of medical skills learned during internship and medical school. The practice of emergency psychiatry, perhaps more than any other discipline in psychiatry, mandates retention and continued use of one's medical skills. Not all ED patients receive a thorough medical evaluation before seeing the psychiatric consultant (Tintinalli et al. 1994). Not only does the rush and pressure of the emergency setting increase the likelihood that subtle illnesses will be missed, but, as Weissberg (1979) pointed out, "there is the all too common belief that alcoholics, drug abusers, and suicidal individuals create their own diseases and are therefore less entitled than others to sympathetic and thorough care" (p. 788). The psychiatric consultant must be able to integrate relevant physical findings into an overall understanding of the patient's problem.

Weissberg (1979) contends that psychiatrists' abdication of their medical identity and nonpsychiatrists' unfamiliarity and discomfort with clinical psychiatry have contributed to widespread use of the ambiguous term *medical clearance*, which implies the practice of having an internist or emergency physician examine every psychiatric patient to rule out serious or acute medical illness. Indeed, most requests for medical clearance come from community mental health agencies and publicly funded psychiatric hospitals. The reasons for these requests are generally legitimate but often are nonclinical. For example, it may be difficult and possibly dangerous to care for medically ill patients—even those with chronic, stable, or benign medical illness—in understaffed, overcrowded psychiatric hospitals in which the staff are primarily nonphysicians and a shortage of adequate medical services and supplies is typical. Unfortunately, the emergency physician, whose concept of "medically clear" means having no acute or life-threatening medical illness, may perceive the request for medical clearance as superfluous.

It is suggested, therefore, that the term *medical clearance* be dropped and that the emergency psychiatrist accept the responsibility for medical assessment of the emergency psychiatric patient. When medical or surgical consultation is believed to be necessary, rather than referring the patient with a broad request for medical clearance, the emergency psychiatrist must conduct a sufficiently thorough examination to pose a specific question or set of questions to the medical or surgical consultant.

Laboratory Investigation

It is important to perform a battery of routine laboratory tests on the patient who has an acute change in mental status or behavior. The battery (Table 39–1) should include a complete blood count, serum electrolytes, blood glucose, and a toxicology screen. A serum sample is necessary to obtain quantitative measures of medications and other chemical substances (e.g., antidepressants, sedative-hypnotic agents, alcohol), and a sample of the patient's urine is often required to detect rapidly metabolized agents that undergo renal clearance (e.g., cocaine and its metabolites, marijuana, phencyclidine [PCP], opiates) (Table 39–2).

TABLE 39–1. Important laboratory tests to consider in the evaluation of the patient with an acute change in mental status

Test	Potential problem
Arterial blood gases	Hypoxemia, pulmonary embolus
Blood glucose	Hypoglycemia
Blood urea nitrogen	Renal failure, uremic encephalopathy, myoglobinuria
Cerebrospinal fluid	Central nervous system infection, intracranial bleeding
Chest radiograph	Pneumonia, pneumothorax
Computed tomography scan	Mass lesion, stroke, atrophy
Creatine phosphokinase	Rhabdomyolysis, myocardial infarction
Electrocardiogram	Myocardial infarction
Electroencephalogram	Seizure (generalized, complex partial), delirium
Liver function tests	Alcoholic hepatitis, hepatic encephalopathy
Magnetic resonance imaging	Stroke, demyelination
Serum amylase	Pancreatitis, pancreatic encephalopathy
Serum creatinine	Renal failure, uremic encephalopathy, myoglobinuria
Serum electrolyte levels	Hyponatremia or hypernatremia, hypocalcemia or hypercalcemia, hypomagnesemia (delirium tremens)
Toxicological analysis of both serum and urine	Confirmation of neurobehavioral effects of the following medications and other chemical substances: Alcohol; Anticholinergics; Cimetidine; Cocaine; Corticosteroids; Dopamine agonists (amantadine, L-dopa, bromocriptine); Lidocaine; Opiates (e.g., normeperidine); Pentazocine; Phencyclidine (PCP); Sedative-hypnotic drugs; Stimulants
White blood cell count	Infection, stress-induced demargination

Source. Adapted and modified from Tesar GE: "Emergency Psychiatry: The Agitated Patient, Part I: Evaluation and Behavioral Management." *Hospital and Community Psychiatry* 44:329–331, 1993. Used with permission.

It is argued that emergency toxicology screening is overused and is rarely influential in the emergency management and disposition of patients who have taken an overdose (Mahoney et al. 1990; Wiltbank et al. 1974). Furthermore, the reliability of the toxicology screen in patients with a drug overdose has been questioned (Ingelfinger et al. 1981). These limitations are probably not always applicable to psychiatric patients and individuals with substance use disorders, in whom use of toxicology screening may influence the diagnostic formulation (potentially important to providers of subsequent inpatient or outpatient care); also, toxicology results may influence the decision about where to admit a patient (e.g., psychiatric hospital versus substance abuse unit).

Other tests are optional and depend on the clinical circumstances. Liver function tests should be ordered if the patient appears acutely ill, if hepatitis is suspected, if hepatic encephalopathy is suspected, or if it is important

to document hepatic injury secondary to alcohol abuse. The results of liver function testing, however, are usually not available for hours and generally do not influence the ultimate disposition of the patient. Results of creatine phosphokinase (CPK) testing can be misleading if the patient has sustained skeletal muscle injury (e.g., because of agitation, prolonged prostration, or intramuscular injection). If CPK is elevated, the clinician is possibly obliged to rule out myocardial damage before discharging the patient from the ED. It is best to order CPK analysis in patients who have a history of coronary artery disease or an abnormal electrocardiogram or in whom acute myocardial damage is suspected.

Clinicians should consider imaging studies of the head (i.e., magnetic resonance imaging or computed tomography scan), as well as cerebrospinal fluid analysis and electroencephalograph (EEG), if a metabolic, traumatic, or infectious cause of an abnormal mental state is

TABLE 39–2. Approximate duration of detectability of drugs in urine

Drug	Retention time
Amphetamine and methamphetamine	48 hours
Barbiturates	
Short-acting (e.g., secobarbital, pentobarbital)	24 hours
Intermediate-acting (e.g., amobarbital, butalbital, butabarbital)	48–72 hours
Long-acting (e.g., phenobarbital)	2–3 weeks
Benzodiazepines (at therapeutic doses)	3 days
Cannabinoids	
Moderate smoker (4 times/week)	3 days
Daily smoker	10 days
Daily heavy smoker	3–4 weeks
Cocaine	6–8 hours
Cocaine metabolites	2–4 hours
Ethyl alcohol	7–12 hours
Methaqualone	7 days
Narcotics	
Codeine	48 hours
Heroin (as morphine)	36–72 hours
Hydrocodone	24 hours
Hydromorphone	48 hours
Methadone	3 days
Morphine	48–72 hours
Oxycodone	24 hours
Propoxyphene	6–48 hours
Phencyclidine (PCP)	8 days

Source. Reprinted from Hyman SE, Tesar GE (eds): *Manual of Psychiatric Emergencies*, 3rd Edition. Boston, MA, Little, Brown, 1994, p 334. Copyright 1994, Little, Brown and Company. Used with permission.

suspected or if other tests have not revealed a cause. Neurological literature suggests that scanning techniques have a low diagnostic yield in patients who lack focal neurological findings. However, it is prudent to regard an acute change of mental status as a focal finding. The EEG is useful to differentiate delirium from primary psychosis.

LIFE-ENDANGERING PSYCHIATRIC EMERGENCIES

Patients With Acute Psychosis

Acute psychosis, characterized by thought disorganization, delusions, hallucinations, and inappropriate or agitated behavior, is a medical-psychiatric emergency that requires careful evaluation, safety measures, and prompt treatment. Its causes are numerous (Table 39–3), and failure to detect organic or substance-related etiologies can pose a significant medical risk to the patient. Agitation, abnormal thinking, and impaired judgment can interfere with timely evaluation and treatment, as well as threaten the individual's employment, financial stability, and relationships with family and friends. Acute psychosis also carries with it a significant risk of unlawful behavior, inadvertent injury to self or others, and suicide (Hyman 1994c).

Clinical circumstances and ED personnel generate pressure on the consultant to transfer or discharge the patient who has acute psychosis as quickly as possible. Evaluation and emergency management of the psychotic patient, however, are rarely straightforward. Many important causes of psychosis are detectable only by gathering history and performing a careful physical examination. Because the patient is usually incapable of providing coherent and reliable information, it is important to gather as much information as possible, either directly or by telephone, from family, friends, and associates of the patient. This takes time and requires persistence. Although it is prudent to avoid sedating the patient until a diagnosis is made, it is also inappropriate to permit yelling and agitation to escalate.

Identifying the most likely cause(s) of psychosis is important so that specific treatment can be administered and the most appropriate disposition effected. A diagnosis of delirium, particularly its life-threatening causes, should not be overlooked. The life-threatening causes of delirium can be quickly recalled from the mnemonic WWHHHIMP: withdrawal from drugs (especially barbiturates), Wernicke's encephalopathy, hypoxia, hypoglycemia, hypertensive encephalopathy, infection, meningitis/encephalitis, and poisoning (overdose). Evidence of generalized slowing on the EEG is consistent with a diagnosis of delirium. Although it is often inconvenient to perform an EEG in the ED, an abnormal recording should help convince a skeptical attending physician that the patient is not "just psychotic."

The principles of treatment of psychosis are similar to those for any acute change in mental status: the clinician must correct metabolic and systemic abnormalities (e.g., hypoglycemia, hypoxia, hypertensive encephalopathy), eliminate drug toxicity (e.g., alcohol, PCP, cocaine, or anticholinergic intoxication), treat drug withdrawal, and, if necessary, administer tranquilizing medication.

The preferred route for administration of tranquilizing medication depends on the intensity of accompanying agitation (Hyman 1994a; Tesar 1993). Elixir preparations are indicated for patients who prefer them or for

TABLE 39–3.   Diagnostic possibilities for patients with psychosis

Psychiatric
- Episodic dyscontrol
- Ganser's syndrome
- Bipolar disorder, manic or depressed
- Personality disorder (e.g., borderline)
- Schizophrenia
- Stress (reactive) disorders (e.g., posttraumatic stress disorder)

Neurological
- Delirium or dementia
- Head trauma
- Narcolepsy
- Seizure disorders (especially psychomotor seizures)
- Space-occupying lesions (e.g., tumors, hydrocephalus)
- Vascular lesions (e.g., infarcts, hemorrhages)

Endocrine
- Adrenal dysfunction
- Diabetes mellitus
- Parathyroid disorders
- Pituitary dysfunction
- Thyroid disorders

Metabolic
- Adult phenylketonuria
- Cardiac failure
- Fluid and electrolyte imbalance
- Folate-responsive homocystinuria
- Hepatic failure
- Hypoglycemia, hyperglycemia, ketoacidosis
- Periodic catatonia
- Porphyria
- Renal failure
- Respiratory failure
- Wilson's disease

Intoxications
- Alcohol (e.g., hallucinosis, pathological intoxication)
- Anticholinergic compounds
- Barbiturates
- Bromide
- Carbon disulfide, other industrial agents
- Carbon monoxide
- Hallucinogens (e.g., LSD, mescaline, THC, and PCP)
- Heavy metals
- Opiates
- Organic phosphates (insecticides)
- Stimulants (e.g., amphetamines, cocaine, and caffeine)

Unwanted effects of medication
- Analgesics (narcotics, pentazocine)
- Anticonvulsants
- Antidepressants
- Antihypertensive agents (especially those containing reserpine and methyldopa)
- Anti-inflammatory agents (indomethacin, phenylbutazone)
- Antipsychotics ("psychotoxic" or "paradoxical" reactions, akathisia)
- Antitubercular drugs (isoniazid, cycloserine)
- Cardiac drugs (digitalis, procainamide, propranolol)
- Disulfiram
- Idiosyncratic reactions to almost any medication
- Lithium carbonate
- Sedative-hypnotics
- Steroids

Deficiency states
- Beriberi
- Pellagra
- Pernicious anemia
- Pyridoxine deficiency
- Wernicke-Korsakoff syndrome

Postoperative states
- Postoperative delirium
- Postoperative depression
- Postoperative psychosis

Systemic illnesses
- Carcinomatosis
- Collagen and autoimmune diseases
- Infections (bacterial, fungal, HIV, parasitic)
- Starvation, dehydration, exposure, heatstroke
- Viral syndromes, hepatitis, mononucleosis

Abstinence phenomena
- Alcohol withdrawal, delirium tremens
- Barbiturate withdrawal

Note.   HIV = human immunodeficiency virus; LSD = lysergic acid diethylamide; PCP = phencyclidine; THC = Δ^9-tetrahydrocannabinol.
Source.   Reprinted from Goff DC, Manschreck TC, Groves JE: "Psychotic Patients," in *Massachusetts General Hospital Handbook of General Hospital Psychiatry*, 3rd Edition. Edited by Cassem NH. St. Louis, MO, CV Mosby, 1991, pp. 217–236. Used with permission.

patients who are known to "cheek" tablets or capsules; peak clinical effectiveness with elixir preparations, however, is achieved no more rapidly than with pill forms (Dubin et al. 1985). Injection into the deltoid muscle ensures rapid absorption of benzodiazepine and neuroleptic

agents (Greenblatt et al. 1983). Intravenous administration of haloperidol is also quite effective, achieves peak blood levels within 10–20 minutes (Tesar and Stern 1988), and is typically safe. Intravenous use of haloperidol, however, is not common in the ED, and intravenous administration of this drug is not approved by the U.S. Food and Drug Administration. Intravenous haloperidol should be avoided in patients who have alcoholic cardiomyopathy or conduction abnormalities (prolonged QT_c interval) because these patients are at risk of developing torsades de pointes (Hunt and Stern 1995). We predict that use of parenteral forms of newer, atypical antipsychotics will become more common in treatment of acute agitation. In preliminary studies, olanzapine intramuscular injection has been found effective in the treatment of patients with acute agitation secondary to dementia, mania, and schizophrenia (Breier et al. 2001; Meehan et al. 2001a, 2001b). This class of medication may play an important future role in the management of acute agitation when parenteral forms of the atypical antipsychotics become more readily available.

For rapid control of acute psychosis, concomitant intramuscular administration of haloperidol, 5 mg, and lorazepam, 1 mg, is superior to the use of either agent alone (Garza-Trevino et al. 1989; Mendoza et al. 1991). The combination can be injected from one syringe. One dose is adequate for most patients, but some patients require a second and, infrequently, a third injection. Although low- or intermediate-potency neuroleptic drugs (e.g., chlorpromazine, thioridazine, perphenazine) are indicated for certain patients, haloperidol is the preferred agent because it has little potential for anticholinergic toxicity and a low hypotensive effect. Lorazepam is the preferred benzodiazepine because its absorption after intramuscular injection is more reliable than that of other benzodiazepines.

When giving haloperidol alone or in combination with a benzodiazepine, coadministration of an anticholinergic agent is recommended to prevent acute dystonia (Goff et al. 1991). Numerous studies indicate that the risk of acute dystonia is substantial when a high-potency neuroleptic is given without anticholinergic prophylaxis (Arana et al. 1988; Goff et al. 1991). Benztropine mesylate, 1–2 mg orally or intramuscularly, is typically used. If neuroleptic medication is continued, the same dose of the anticholinergic agent is given twice daily, and this dosage is continued for at least 1 week, the period of greatest risk for acute dystonic reactions (Ayd 1961). Anticholinergic medications should be avoided in patients with delirium because such medications may increase the patients' level of confusion.

Patients at Risk for Suicide

A major priority of any ED is the evaluation and disposition of patients who are at risk for suicide. Emergency psychiatric patients die by suicide at a significantly higher rate than do individuals in the general population (Hillard et al. 1983, 1985). However, studies by Hillard et al. (1983) and others (Browning et al. 1970; Stern et al. 1984) have demonstrated that eventual death by suicide does not occur immediately, or even within 2 weeks, after an ED visit. This may reflect the skill with which triage decisions are made or the value of emergency intervention in forestalling suicidal behavior.

Despite these encouraging data, evaluation of patients who are at risk for suicide is often anxiety provoking for the clinician and requires a careful assessment of risk factors, as well as attention to the clinician's gut feeling about the patient's impulsivity and intent. Ideally, before the consultant's evaluation, the patient should be kept in a safe place and monitored, and the risk of escape must be minimized. If a potentially suicidal patient threatens to leave the ED, then he or she should be detained until the evaluation is complete; this decision should be carefully documented in the patient's record.

Suicidal patients reach the ED in a number of different situations: 1) having just survived a suicide attempt, 2) complaining of suicidal thoughts or urges, 3) having other complaints but admitting to suicidal thoughts during the evaluation, and 4) denying suicidal thoughts but behaving in ways that suggest potential for suicide. The consultant should consider these circumstances, as well as personal and demographic risk factors for suicide, when evaluating the patient who may be at risk for suicide. For example, if the patient made a suicide attempt, the means, the circumstances, and the patient's regard for death should be assessed. Poor prognostic indicators include a persistent wish for, or ambivalence about, death following a failed attempt and use of lethal means (e.g., a gun) in isolated circumstances (e.g., while alone in an isolated area). The examiner must not minimize the seriousness of a patient's suicidal ideation. Suicidal thoughts should be examined in detail. Is the patient frightened about a wish to die? Does the patient have a specific plan? What means is the patient planning to use? When? Where? How will loved ones and others react if the patient dies? What is the patient's conception of death? What will death accomplish for the patient and for others?

Patients whose behavior is inconsistent with their denial of suicidal impulses are the most difficult to evaluate and treat. Some of these patients have a diagnosis of borderline personality disorder; their ambivalence about death and their manipulative behavior can make it impossible for the clinician to predict their ultimate actions. It is best to hospitalize a patient when the clinician is uncertain about the patient's safety and when an adequate plan for follow-up is not available. The rationale for involuntary hospitalization must be carefully documented in the hospital record.

Young patients with schizophrenia typically do not communicate suicidal impulses directly and therefore require careful evaluation (Breier and Astrachan 1984; Nathan and Rousch 1984). Although it is generally accepted that the usual demographic and clinical predictors for suicide are not reliable when applied to patients with schizophrenia, the examiner must attend to subtle indicators of hopelessness, delusional thinking that could precipitate self-destructive behavior, and auditory hallucinations commanding self-destruction.

Risk factors for suicide among emergency psychiatric patients are listed in Table 39–4. Having a psychiatric disorder usually increases the risk of suicide (see Bostwick, Chapter 9, this volume). Untreated depression is the most common psychiatric diagnosis associated with suicide; the risk is even greater if the individual with depression also has features of psychosis or a family history of suicide. Alcohol use is highly associated with an increased risk for suicide. Acutely, alcohol may facilitate a suicide attempt by disinhibiting the patient who is feeling hopeless and depressed. In the ED, suicidal threats made by the alcoholic patient who is acutely intoxicated commonly prompt requests for immediate psychiatric consultation. All such threats must be regarded as serious while the patient remains intoxicated. However, most clinicians who have worked in the ED are quite familiar with the patient who vehemently threatens suicide while intoxicated only to deny suicidal intent and beg for discharge when he or she is again sober. The common practice is to discharge these patients once they have become sober, although presumably their long-term risk of suicide is relatively great.

TABLE 39–4.   Risk factors for suicide

Major depression

Alcoholism

History of suicide attempts and threats

Male gender

Increasing age (peak incidence for men, age 75; peak incidence for women, ages 55–65)

Widowed or never married

Unemployed and unskilled

Chronic illness or chronic pain

Terminal illness

Guns in the home

Source.   Reprinted from Hyman SE: "The Suicidal Patient," in *Manual of Psychiatric Emergencies*, 3rd Edition. Edited by Hyman SE, Tesar GE. Boston, MA, Little, Brown, 1994, pp. 21–27. Copyright 1994, Little, Brown and Company. Used with permission.

Patients Who Are Violent

Case Example 4

A 24-year-old man came to the ED with a complaint of anxiety and a request for Valium. He was well groomed, tanned, and dressed in a karate uniform. While waiting for the doctor, he practiced karate moves in the empty waiting room. On entering the interviewing office, he demanded a prescription for Valium. He had made similar demands on numerous occasions in the ED. When his request was denied, the angered patient stood up, bared his teeth, and threatened the doctor with a karate chop. He then rapidly exited the office, while claiming ownership of a .357 Magnum with which he intended to kill the doctor later that day.

When confronted by a patient who has committed or is contemplating a violent act, the psychiatrist has four obligations: 1) to ensure the safety of the patient and the staff, 2) to determine whether violent ideation or behavior stems from a specific psychiatric disorder, 3) to effect an appropriate treatment plan and disposition, and 4) to warn third parties if a serious threat of harm is present.

Safety is a priority whenever violence is a concern. In addition to the obvious benefits of a safe, protected environment, the clinician who feels safe and unafraid is more likely to be objective and nonthreatening. The measures taken to ensure safety will depend on the nature and severity of violence. If the patient retains adequate self-control, an interview in an office that permits adequate interpersonal distance and has no potential weapons (e.g., syringes, table lamps, ashtrays, pens, pencils) is possible. The clinician and the patient should sit in a manner that allows both to have easy access to the door; in some instances, the patient and the clinician may feel more comfortable if the door is left open. It is sometimes best to have one or more security guards stand by during the interview. In all instances, the clinician's behavior and interviewing style optimally should be nonthreatening, nonauthoritarian, and nonpunitive. It is always prudent to avoid frustrating the patient or, if necessary, to have adequate means of controlling the patient's behavior. For example, in Case Example 4, the best course of action would have been either to call for security personnel or to honor the patient's request with a small supply of diazepam pending follow-up arrangements with the primary therapist. It is important, particularly with patients who have paranoid delusions, to make intermittent eye contact and avoid staring with a deadpan expression, to position oneself at eye level with the patient, and to move slowly and predictably. The clinician should never turn his or her back to the patient and should always keep his or her hands open and visible. Displaying a helpful and understanding attitude without being judgmental or presumptive is best.

Violence should be prevented before it occurs. If the patient shows signs of escalating anger or agitation (e.g., pacing, visible teeth, jaw clenching, fist formation, staring) or is physically violent and is not responding to verbal intervention, then the rapid involvement of security personnel and the application of mechanical restraints are indicated. Pharmacological measures, similar to those used in the treatment of acute psychosis, are sometimes indicated. Prospective identification (e.g., computerized "flagging"), monitoring, and rapid treatment for patients who are potentially violent or are recurrently violent are reported to result in a significant reduction in hospital-based violence (Drummond et al. 1989).

Violent or potentially violent patients come to the ED for various reasons. Some are brought involuntarily by family members or authorities after committing or threatening to commit a violent act, others come for help in dealing with violent impulses, and others become threatening or aggressive during emergency evaluation. The individuals for whom the psychiatrist is often responsible include those with a primary psychiatric disorder, those who are intoxicated or in an early state of withdrawal, those who have an organic or neurological disorder that results in violence, and those who request psychiatric help because they perceive their violent acts and urges as unwanted (i.e., ego-dystonic) (Hyman 1994c). Other patients who are violent or potentially violent but who have no evidence of a psychiatric disorder are handled more appropriately by legal authorities.

Making these decisions requires a thorough psychiatric evaluation that focuses on 1) the demographics of violence (e.g., male gender, youth, poverty, low educational level, being non-Caucasian, unemployment, lack of social and family roots), 2) the mental status examination, 3) the patient's history of violence (e.g., abuse as a child), 4) the mode of referral, 5) whether there are intended victims, 6) the available means to commit violence, 7) the patient's degree of self-control, 8) the presence of external controls, and 9) a physical examination (Hyman 1994c; Simon 1988). Available studies suggest that psychotic disorders (e.g., schizophrenia, mania, and paranoid states with or without command hallucinations), drug abuse (especially PCP, cocaine, and other central nervous system [CNS] stimulants), and alcohol abuse are the most common psychiatric disorders in psychiatric emergency patients who become violent (Skodol and Karasu 1978; Stern et al. 1991). Stern et al. (1991) also emphasized the etiological role of organic brain syndromes. In several studies, a diagnosis of an organic brain syndrome

was either considered or identified in 7%–28% of patients who were violent, hostile, angry, or agitated (Atkins 1967; Muller et al. 1967; Tischler 1966).

Most violent behavior that is manifested in the ED occurs in the context of family strife (Skodol and Karasu 1978). Psychiatric disorders may contribute directly to family violence, or family conflict may lead to intensified symptoms, resulting in violence. The ability to control violent impulses, as judged by clinicians, is the critical determinant of whether to hospitalize the patient who is violent (Mezzich et al. 1984; Segal et al. 1988).

Crucial to accurate diagnosis, effective treatment, and safe disposition are thorough mental status and physical examinations of the violent patient. Assessment should include answers to the following questions (Simon 1988): Does the patient have a fever or exhibit evidence of autonomic arousal (e.g., hypertension, tachycardia, sweating, mydriasis, hyperreflexia), suggesting either drug or alcohol intoxication or withdrawal? Is there physical evidence of a violent lifestyle (e.g., tattoos, scars from bullet or knife wounds, bruised or disfigured knuckles)? Does the patient exhibit a thought disorder? If the patient has expressed violent fantasies, do these constitute a fear, a wish, or an intent? Is there a specific plan of action? If the thoughts have achieved the level of intention, who is the object of the violent thoughts? When is the violent act to be carried out? Where will the violence occur? What is the motive? For how long have these thoughts been occurring? How imminent is the threat of violence? Does the patient have access to weapons?

The answers to these questions lead to a reasonable treatment plan and disposition. The violent patient who is either acutely agitated or incapable of assuring the staff of his or her own safety or that of others requires immediate treatment with mechanical restraints, medication that targets the underlying problem, or both.

For sedation, either diazepam, 5–10 mg, or lorazepam, 1–2 mg, should be given parenterally (either intramuscularly or intravenously). If the intravenous route is chosen, the benzodiazepine is administered slowly over 1–2 minutes to avoid respiratory depression; resuscitative equipment should always be immediately available. Haloperidol, 2–5 mg intramuscularly or intravenously, may be used alone or may be given in combination with a benzodiazepine if the patient's agitation is intense and uncontrolled (Garza-Trevino et al. 1989).

Once the patient is stabilized, his or her attitude toward further violence should be assessed; the clinician should also evaluate the patient's social network and the presence of external controls at this time. If there is no evidence of a psychiatric disorder and violent intentions persist, then the problem is best handled by legal authorities. In all cases, the final disposition is contingent on 1) evidence that emergency treatment has resulted in control of violent ideation and impulsivity, 2) determination that the patient is not returning to circumstances that are likely to rekindle violent behavior, and 3) a commitment from the patient or family members to return to the ED immediately should the threat of violence recur. If these criteria cannot be met, then the patient should be hospitalized for protection, further evaluation, and treatment. Threatened parties must be notified if a patient's homicidal threats are judged to be significant (Tarasoff v. Regents of the University of California 1976). *Tarasoff* indicates that there is a duty to protect third parties from a dangerous patient. Case law varies in different states regarding the interpretation of the *Tarasoff* ruling, and it would be prudent for the clinician to review the laws for his or her state. Although prediction of violence in the distant future is generally inaccurate (Monahan 1978), short-term predictions (i.e., within 72 hours of evaluation) made in the context of emergency civil commitment are distinctly more reliable (McNiel and Binder 1987b).

Patients With Substance-Related Emergencies

Patients who abuse substances come to the attention of the psychiatric consultant either because they have psychosis (or they are presumed to have psychosis when instead they have delirium) or because they are belligerent and disruptive, suicidal, or in denial of their substance abuse. The consultant may also be summoned to facilitate appropriate treatment and determine if the patient requires inpatient detoxification. Of paramount concern are the patient's immediate safety and the risks associated with further substance abuse.

Patients with some form of substance abuse or its complications require immediate medical treatment: 1) patients who have overdosed require prompt medical intervention focusing on airway maintenance, monitoring of vital signs, and elimination of any drug(s) retained in the stomach; 2) patients who have Wernicke's encephalopathy require prompt parenteral administration of thiamine; 3) patients who are in alcohol or sedative-hypnotic withdrawal should be treated with supportive measures, their safety should be attended to, and they should receive adequate doses of the offending or a cross-reactive substance; and 4) patients experiencing cocaine delirium should receive haloperidol. One author states that 80% of patients in treatment had taken two or more substances during their periods of addiction (Winick

1997). Patients who refuse treatment and make suicidal or homicidal threats while under the influence of an intoxicating substance should be detained until they are reevaluated in a sober state; patients should not be discharged from the ED while intoxicated.

Alcohol

As many as one-third of patients seen in general hospital EDs are alcoholic (E. Robins et al. 1977; Rund et al. 1981; Zimberg 1979). Alcohol use is linked with physical trauma, violent death, and psychiatric illness (Teplin et al. 1989). In a prospective study of the relation between blood alcohol level (BAL) and other variables associated with admission to the ED, Teplin et al. (1989) found that psychiatric patients had the highest mean BAL. This finding is consistent with epidemiological data indicating a significant overlap of psychiatric illness and alcoholism (Schuckit 1983).

The acutely intoxicated individual frequently comes to the attention of the psychiatric service because of suicidal or homicidal threats or behavior (e.g., overdose, wrist laceration, gunshot wound) or a history of a comorbid psychiatric illness. In addition to addressing the immediate consultation request, the clinician should carefully evaluate the patient for other sequelae of alcoholism, particularly if no other physician has recently examined the patient. The patient should be evaluated for medical complications of alcoholism (e.g., hypoglycemia, subdural hematoma, other injuries, gastrointestinal bleeding), alcohol withdrawal, Wernicke's encephalopathy, alcohol amnestic disorder (Korsakoff's psychosis), and alcoholic dementia. All intoxicated patients with alcoholism should receive thiamine, 100 mg parenterally, because the signs of Wernicke's encephalopathy (e.g., listlessness or drowsiness, ophthalmoplegia, global confusion, ataxic stance or gait) are difficult to distinguish from the signs of intoxication itself; the classic triad (i.e., ophthalmoplegia, global confusion, and ataxia) is not typically present (Brew 1986; De Keyser et al. 1985). Patients with alcoholism who are agitated or belligerent should be calmed with lorazepam, 1–2 mg intramuscularly, or haloperidol, 2–5 mg intramuscularly. Low-potency neuroleptic drugs should not be used because of their tendency to lower blood pressure and the seizure threshold.

Alcohol withdrawal is potentially lethal if unrecognized and untreated. In general, a high index of suspicion is required because the clinical and laboratory manifestations are nonspecific, and the patient often conceals or is unable to provide the relevant history. The clinician should remember that the intoxicated alcoholic patient can develop early withdrawal as the BAL declines, even though it may be above 100 mg/dL, the legal limit for intoxication.

Early onset withdrawal, characterized by tachycardia, hypertension, sweating, tremor, fever, anxiety, irritability, and occasionally hallucinosis, often begins within 6–8 hours of a substantial decline in the BAL. Physical manifestations of alcohol or sedative withdrawal may be masked by concomitant use of β-blockers or clonidine. Chlordiazepoxide, 25–100 mg orally every 6 hours, is indicated at the first sign of withdrawal, with the initial amount depending on the intensity of symptoms. Often, the appropriate initial dose can be ascertained by asking the patient how anxious he or she feels. Generalized tonic-clonic seizures occur usually within the first 24 hours of the last drink. Inpatient treatment is indicated in the presence of fever above 101°F, seizures, signs of Wernicke's encephalopathy, inability to hold fluids, or a serious underlying medical disorder (Hyman 1994b).

The most severe form of withdrawal, delirium tremens, usually occurs after 24 hours and within 7 days of the last drink. Despite optimal treatment, the mortality associated with delirium tremens is still nearly 5% (Cushman 1987). Delirium tremens is characterized by marked sympathetic overactivity, fever, hallucinosis, agitation, and delirium. It requires treatment in the intensive care unit, including intravenous electrolyte and fluid therapy, acetaminophen and cooling blankets for significant hyperthermia, parenteral thiamine, monitoring for infection and cardiac arrhythmias, and parenteral benzodiazepines (i.e., diazepam, lorazepam, or midazolam). When delirium tremens commences in the ED, diazepam, 10 mg intravenously, is recommended as the initial treatment. Diazepam is preferred because of its rapid onset of effect (Baldessarini 1985). In one study, the average induction dose of diazepam was 89 mg in patients with alcoholism who had intercurrent illnesses and 46 mg in those without illness (Thompson et al. 1980). Total doses ranged from 50 to 780 mg. In one reported case, as much as 2,640 mg of diazepam, administered intravenously over 48 hours, was required to control severe delirium tremens (Nolop and Natow 1985); in another case, an equivalent total dose of midazolam, given intravenously, was necessary (Lineaweaver et al. 1988).

Intensive outpatient detoxification programs have proven successful for patients who have a high degree of motivation and commitment. For patients at higher risk for recidivism, brief inpatient detoxification followed by intensive outpatient or residential treatment, along with the support of Alcoholics Anonymous, is indicated. The practice of giving a patient who is discharged from the ED a single dose of benzodiazepine to prevent seizures or other manifestations of withdrawal is not recommended.

Cocaine and Other Psychostimulants

Approximately 22 million Americans have used cocaine, and nearly 5 million use it regularly (Rich and Singer 1991). Although casual use has declined (Musto 1997), the number of hard-core users and the number of individuals seen in EDs for symptoms related to cocaine use have increased (Rich and Singer 1991). In a study of the frequency of cocaine-related medical, surgical, and psychiatric problems presenting in an urban general hospital ED, psychiatric complaints accounted for most of the presentations (30.6%) (Rich and Singer 1991). Suicidal intent was the most common psychiatric problem. Polysubstance abuse was common; alcohol, opiates, and benzodiazepines were most commonly abused.

Cocaine is mainly used intranasally (snorted), but it is also injected intravenously, freebased, or smoked as crack. The onset of euphoria occurs within seconds to minutes and, depending on the route of administration, may last 15–60 minutes. The euphoria is followed by acute dysphoria (crashing) accompanied, at times, by suicidal thinking and impulses. Prolonged use, particularly of crack cocaine or amphetamine (e.g., dextroamphetamine, methamphetamine), can result in symptoms resembling mania or paranoid schizophrenia. In some instances, acute delirium associated with intense agitation develops after cocaine use.

Urine toxicology, if obtained within 72 hours of use, can help distinguish stimulant abuse from a psychiatric illness such as schizophrenia. The immediate goals in the treatment of stimulant toxicity are to reduce the patient's CNS excitation, sympathetic overactivity, and psychotic symptoms. A dual approach is recommended. Agents to acidify the urine should be used, and haloperidol should be administered to control agitation, delirium, or psychotic symptoms. Clonidine, 0.1–0.3 mg/day, helps to reduce craving and sympathetic arousal in some patients. In one study, subjects who received bromocriptine, 1.25 mg three times daily, had significantly less cocaine use than did a comparable group of patients receiving placebo (Moscovitz et al. 1993). Antidepressants have been used successfully to treat depression resulting from cocaine abstinence (Gawin and Kleber 1984). Because cocaine and other psychostimulants are highly addictive, inpatient treatment is generally indicated to minimize the risk of further drug abuse. Unfortunately, insurers are increasingly reluctant to pay for inpatient care of patients with substance use disorders.

Case Example 5

A 36-year-old man came to the ED complaining of restlessness, insomnia, and headaches. He exhibited paranoid thoughts and was triaged to the emergency psychiatry service. Three days before presentation, he had run out of Fiorinal (butalbital, aspirin, and caffeine capsules), which he had taken for headaches. He had no psychiatric history, and he denied substance abuse.

At the time of admission to the ED, the patient's oral temperature was 98.9°F, his pulse was 92, and his blood pressure was 138/92 mm Hg. Physical examination was remarkable only for restlessness and brisk deep tendon reflexes. He was distractible, mildly confused, and complained that his neighbors had been spying on him.

Within 30 minutes of the initial evaluation, the patient became explosively agitated. Five security guards struggled to restrain him.

He was given intravenous lorazepam, 2 mg; there was no response. Over the next 15 minutes, the patient was given intravenous lorazepam, 12 mg, and intravenous haloperidol, 5 mg; the drugs had no calming effect. Diazepam, 20 mg, was administered in 5-mg intravenous boluses over 15–20 minutes. This resulted in gradual but incomplete calming; respiratory depression necessitated intubation and mechanical ventilation.

The patient was transferred to the intensive care unit, and during the next 24 hours, he received mechanical ventilation and amobarbital sodium, 100 mg intravenously every 2–4 hours, for a presumptive diagnosis of barbiturate withdrawal. It was later established that he had been consuming 12–16 Fiorinal tablets every day for at least 4 months.

Benzodiazepines and Other Sedative-Hypnotics

Sedative-hypnotic drugs are CNS depressants that inhibit central γ-aminobutyric acid (GABA) receptors. Drugs within this class include benzodiazepines, barbiturates, meprobamate, chloral hydrate, ethchlorvynol, glutethimide, and methyprylon (Tables 39–5 and 39–6). Each of these nonbenzodiazepine sedative-hypnotic compounds is capable of producing dependence, tolerance, and potentially fatal toxicity and withdrawal. Familiarity with analgesic compounds that contain the short-lasting barbiturate butalbital is essential for consultation-liaison psychiatrists (see Table 39–6). Sudden discontinuation of these medications, as in Case Example 5, can result in a life-threatening barbiturate withdrawal syndrome.

Barbiturates have a high abuse potential because of their marked euphoriant effect, rapid induction of hepatic microsomal enzymes, and receptor adaptation (i.e., tolerance) (Rall 1990). Additionally, they are more dangerous than the benzodiazepines in overdose (resulting from greater cardiorespiratory and CNS depressant effects), and they have a far lower toxic-to-therapeutic ratio than the benzodiazepines (10 versus more than 100). Tolerance to a barbiturate's hypnotic effect does not result in a proportional increase in the lethal dose. Sudden discontinuation of barbiturates and their analogues can cause a potentially fatal withdrawal syndrome. Fortunately, since the mid-1970s, benzodiazepines have supplanted barbiturates and their analogues as the most widely prescribed sedative-hypnotic agents. However, some patients, particularly older, long-time users, continue to receive barbiturates or one of their analogues (see Table 39–6).

Benzodiazepines are safer and are more widely prescribed than barbiturates. Patients with primary anxiety disorders tend to respond to relatively low, stable doses of high-potency benzodiazepines with little or no tolerance to the anxiolytic effects (Nagy et al. 1989; Pollack 1990). However, benzodiazepine dependence occurs almost universally, especially after 4 months of continuous use. Sudden withdrawal from therapeutic doses of a benzodiazepine may be followed by a fully developed physical withdrawal syndrome (Petursson and Lader 1981). Despite the relative safety of benzodiazepine treatment, certain patient groups and certain benzodiazepine compounds (e.g., alprazolam, diazepam, lorazepam) are associated with a high risk of abuse (Griffiths and Wolf 1990). Although primary benzodiazepine abuse is uncommon (Ladewig and Grossenbacher 1988; Smith and Marks 1985; Woods et al. 1988), Busto et al. (1986) found that 56% of 176 patients who abused benzodiazepines used these agents alone.

Patients who abuse alcohol (Ciraulo et al. 1988a), opiates (Noyes et al. 1988), cocaine, or multiple substances (Kryspin-Exner and Demel 1975) and patients with a diagnosis of borderline personality disorder, many of whom also abuse substances (Dulti et al. 1990), are at high risk for abusing benzodiazepines. Individuals in these groups are also high utilizers of general and psychiatric emergency services. Among the benzodiazepines available in the United States, alprazolam, diazepam, and lorazepam seem to have the greatest abuse liability (Ciraulo et al. 1988b; Griffiths and Wolf 1990; Juergens 1991; Juergens and Morse 1988), presumably because of their very rapid onset of clinical activity. Persons who are addicted to opiates are especially prone to abuse alprazolam, diazepam, and lorazepam. Case reports document the use of 10–300 mg of diazepam or 20–40 mg of alprazolam in a single dose to boost the effect of methadone taken as a maintenance drug (Stitzer et al. 1981; Weddington and Carney 1987). It is estimated that 40% of persons with alcoholism use benzodiazepines and that up to 20% of these individuals abuse benzodiazepines (Ciraulo et al. 1988a). Persons with alcoholism who are

TABLE 39–5. Benzodiazepines available for clinical use in the United States

Drug	Elimination half-life (hours)	Onset	Active metabolites	Approximate dose equivalence (mg)	Possible route(s) of administration[a]
Diazepam[b]	30–60	Very fast	Yes[c]	5	po, im, iv
Chlordiazepoxide	20–50	Slow	Yes[c]	25	po
Clorazepate[d]	30–100	Fast	Yes[c]	7.5	po
Prazepam	50–80	Very slow	Yes	10	po
Flurazepam[e]	50–100	Fast	Yes[f]	15	po
Quazepam	30–100	Intermediate	Yes	15	po
Clonazepam[g]	20–50	Slow	Yes	0.25	po
Lorazepam[h,i]	10–18	Intermediate	No	1	po, im, iv
Temazepam[e]	10–12	Intermediate	No	15	po
Oxazepam[h,i]	6–12	Slow	No	15	po
Alprazolam[b]	8–14	Very fast	Minor[j]	0.5	po
Triazolam[k]	1.5–3	Intermediate	No	0.25	po
Midazolam[l]	1–4	Very fast	No	2.5	im, iv

Note. im = intramuscular; iv = intravenous; po = per os (oral).

[a]For preparations available in the United States.

[b]High abuse liability.

[c]The principal active metabolite is nordiazepam (elimination half-life = 60–100 hours).

[d]Clorazepate itself is inactive but is rapidly converted in gastric acid to its active metabolite, nordiazepam.

[e]Relatively low incidence of rebound insomnia, probably because of relatively long elimination half-life.

[f]Norflurazepam is the principal metabolite, with an elimination half-life similar to that of nordiazepam.

[g]Labeled for the treatment of petit mal epilepsy, but has also been used successfully to treat patients with panic disorder, mania, nocturnal myoclonus, and other sleep-related movement disorders.

[h]Inactivated by glucuronidation, which does not depend on hepatic microsomal activity and remains intact except in the most severe instances of hepatic dysfunction.

[i]Excreted principally in the urine.

[j]It is unclear to what extent metabolites contribute to alprazolam's activity, but judging from its duration of clinical activity (i.e., 4–6 hours), probably not much at all.

[k]Its use is associated with at times profound anterograde amnesia, and its discontinuation with considerable rebound insomnia.

[l]Used principally for induction of anesthesia and sedation during procedures. The most lipophilic and the most potent of benzodiazepines currently available in the United States.

Source. Reprinted from Baldessarini RJ: "Antianxiety Drugs," in *Chemotherapy in Psychiatry: Principles and Practice.* Cambridge, MA, Harvard University Press, 1985, pp. 240–241. Copyright 1986, Harvard University Press. Used with permission.

abstinent apparently derive a significantly greater sense of well-being and euphoria from alprazolam than do control subjects (Ciraulo et al. 1988b).

Based on these data, the psychiatric consultant must maintain a high index of suspicion for sedative-hypnotic abuse among patients who use emergency services. High-risk patients are likely to conceal substance abuse and to complain of anxiety symptoms instead (e.g., panic attacks). If a history or evidence of current substance abuse exists, benzodiazepines should not be prescribed except for patients in established outpatient treatment and then only with the approval of the outpatient psychiatrist. Characteristics of the patient who abuses substances include irritability, insistence, and impatience. The inability to recall the first attack by a patient who reports panic attacks or a history of panic disorder should trigger skepticism about the diagnosis. Substance abuse should be presumed until proven otherwise.

Withdrawal From a Sedative-Hypnotic

Sedative-hypnotic withdrawal is a medical emergency. The symptoms of withdrawal from a sedative-hypnotic drug depend on the type of agent, its elimination half-life ($T_{1/2}$), and the duration of its use. In general, the presentation and course of withdrawal from barbiturates are similar to those of withdrawal from alcohol. Symptoms—including fever, autonomic arousal, sweating, neuromuscular irritability, paranoia, and frightening hallucinations—typically precede the onset of seizures, coma, and death if adequate treatment is not given (Khantzian and McKenna 1979). Withdrawal from benzodiazepines is usually less intense than that from a barbiturate and rarely results in death.

The interval from drug discontinuation to the onset of withdrawal depends on the drug's $T_{1/2}$. For example, withdrawal symptoms may not begin for up to 5 days after stopping diazepam because of the gradual elimina-

TABLE 39–6.   Nonbenzodiazepine sedative-hypnotic agents

Class	Drug	Trade name	Half-life (hours)	Comments
Barbiturates	Amobarbital	Amytal	8–42	
	Butalbital	—	—	Contained in Fiorinal, Fioricet, and other analgesic compounds
	Mephobarbital	Mebaral	11–67	
	Pentobarbital	Nembutal	15–48	Used in barbiturate (pentobarbital) tolerance test
	Phenobarbital	Luminal	80–120	
	Secobarbital	Seconal	15–40	
	Thiopental	Pentothal	3–8	
Propanediol carbamate	Meprobamate	Miltown	6–17	
Chloral derivatives	Chloral hydrate	Noctec	8–10	
	Ethchlorvynol	Placidyl	10–25	
Piperidinediones	Glutethimide	Doriden	5–22	Variable gastrointestinal absorption can cause fluctuating levels of consciousness after overdose
	Methyprylon	Noludar	3–6	

Source.   Adapted from Rall TW: "Hypnotics and Sedatives; Alcohol," in *The Pharmacological Basis of Therapeutics*, 8th Edition. Edited by Gilman GA, Rall TW, Nies AS, et al. New York, Pergamon, 1990, p 357. Copyright 1990, McGraw-Hill, Inc. Used with permission.

tion of the parent compound and its active metabolite, nordiazepam—$T_{1/2} = 100$ hours and can be up to 200 hours in patients with hepatic dysfunction. In contrast, withdrawal occurs within hours of the last dose of a shorter-acting agent such as pentobarbital sodium ($T_{1/2} = 15–48$ hours), butalbital, alprazolam ($T_{1/2} = 8–14$ hours), or lorazepam ($T_{1/2} = 10–18$ hours) (Baldessarini 1985; Rall 1990). Sudden discontinuation of a sedative-hypnotic drug is more likely to result in withdrawal after prolonged use (i.e., more than 4 months) (American Psychiatric Association 1990).

Successful treatment of a patient who has sedative-hypnotic withdrawal syndrome depends on adequate replacement with the drug used or a cross-reactive substance (i.e., one that affects central GABA receptors). If the specific substance is known, resumption should be considered. If the substance is not known or cannot be given by the usual means, parenteral administration of a benzodiazepine or barbiturate is indicated. Adequate respiratory support is essential. Sodium amobarbital, 60–100 mg, or diazepam, 10 mg, given intramuscularly or intravenously, is indicated whenever a rapid response is desired (e.g., in the presence of delirium, intense agitation, or seizures). When the clinical situation permits, it is best to determine the patient's sedative-hypnotic requirement by using the pentobarbital tolerance test, switching to a long-lasting agent (e.g., phenobarbital), and then instituting a gradual taper (see Chapter 21 in this volume). These procedures are particularly effective when the abused agent is a short-lasting barbiturate or benzodiazepine. Clinical experience suggests that alprazolam withdrawal is best treated with alprazolam replacement; this often requires higher than expected doses of cross-reactive agents. Clonazepam is also a suitable alternative. The reason for poor cross-over effect is unknown.

Opioid Dependence and Abuse

Persons who are addicted to and abuse narcotics come to the ED for many reasons, including to request analgesics, because they have overdosed, because they are in a state of withdrawal, or because of a complication of substance abuse (e.g., acquired immunodeficiency syndrome [AIDS], endocarditis, hepatitis) (Weiss et al. 1994). Characteristically, the cloying, irritable, and demanding traits of persons addicted to opioids alienate emergency personnel. Because it is difficult to discern a legitimate request for analgesic medication from drug-seeking behavior, the ED may automatically prohibit prescribing or dispensing narcotic analgesics. As a result, these patients are generally dealt with perfunctorily and with little professional gratification.

The most commonly abused opioid drugs are the semisynthetic derivatives of morphine: heroin, hydromorphone, and oxycodone (found in Percocet and Percodan). Heroin-related admissions to the ED rose from 38,063 in 1988 to 64,221 in 1994, with heroin's rise in popularity attributed to lower price and higher potency. Higher potency permits snorting, which avoids the risk of HIV infection associated with intravenous use (Winick 1997). Heroin is generally purchased in "bags" (small paper envelopes). Intravenous users will solubilize and inject pill forms of oxycodone or hydromorphone when the street supply of heroin is low. Other drugs are usually obtained by prescription or bought on the street and taken orally.

Opiate intoxication is indicated by a depressed level of consciousness, respiratory depression, and narrow pupils. The clinician should examine the patient for injection sites, needle tracks, and venous sclerosis, although these indicators are not often prominent in the inexperienced user. Naloxone, a pure opioid antagonist, is administered intravenously in patients with suspected opioid overdose. The usual adult dosage is 0.4–2 mg every 2–3 minutes until response and 0.1 mg/kg in children who weigh less than 20 kg. Restraints should be placed before naloxone is given because excessive arousal or agitation can occur as intoxication is reversed (precipitated withdrawal). Thorough examination of the patient addicted to opioids includes investigation for pulmonary edema, aspiration pneumonitis, and sources of fever (e.g., AIDS, endocarditis, injection-site cellulitis).

Opioid withdrawal is uncomfortable but not lethal. Typical symptoms include sweating, dilated pupils, gooseflesh, lacrimation, and hyperreflexia. In addition, the patient may experience muscle cramping, abdominal pain, and drug craving. The presence of physical findings indicative of opioid withdrawal helps to differentiate the drug seeker from a patient who is addicted, is withdrawing from opioids, and needs additional narcotics. The usual treatment of narcotic dependence and withdrawal involves methadone maintenance supplemented, as necessary, by clonidine hydrochloride, a presynaptic α_2-adrenergic agonist. The mixed agonist-antagonist buprenorphine may supplant methadone in the future. Outpatient withdrawal using narcotics is not recommended. Instead, 0.1–0.3 mg of clonidine can reduce manifestations of sympathetic overactivity (e.g., tachycardia, hypertension, sweating, gooseflesh) and, in some instances, drug craving. If treatment is effective, the patient can be discharged from the ED with a prescription for clonidine, 0.01–0.02 mg/kg, to be taken daily in three divided doses. Common side effects that complicate this treatment include hypotension and drowsiness. For the majority of patients, opioid detoxification is best accomplished on an inpatient basis.

Anticholinergics

A mild euphoria or dissociative sensation may result from excessive use of anticholinergic medications such as benztropine, trihexyphenidyl hydrochloride, and diphenhydramine. Anticholinergic abuse has been increasing in the population of younger psychiatric patients who are prescribed these agents with their neuroleptic drugs. It has been the clinical observation of one of the authors (JAL) that over-the-counter anticholinergics (e.g., diphenhydramine) have been abused on occasion by patients who have severe personality disorders or posttraumatic stress disorder. Patients who abuse anticholinergic medication may present with confusion and delirium with classic physical manifestations of dilated pupils, dry and warm skin, fever, tachycardia, and urinary retention. Abuse of anticholinergics should be suspected in patients who are prescribed these medications or who admit to over-the-counter use.

Lysergic Acid Diethylamide and Other Hallucinogens

Mescaline, lysergic acid diethylamide (LSD), psilocybin, or 3,4-methylenedioxymethamphetamine (MDMA, or Ecstasy) can produce panic, delirium, or flashbacks that precipitate the need for emergency evaluation (Weiss et al. 1994). The acute effects and recurrent flashbacks are short lived; the only treatment usually required is supportive reassurance and a quiet, comfortable, protected environment until the effects of the drug pass. Diazepam, 10–30 mg orally, is indicated when panic is intolerable. Neuroleptic medication should be avoided except in rare instances of agitation associated with hallucinogen-induced delirium. Before administering neuroleptic medication, the clinician should ensure that the clinical circumstances are not the result of an anticholinergic-induced delirium, because atropine-like substances are often used in the processing of hallucinogenic drugs.

Phencyclidine

PCP, also known as dust or angel dust, is commonly used as a tranquilizer in veterinary medicine (Weiss et al. 1994). Users can experience depressant, stimulant, hallucinogenic, or analgesic effects, depending on the dose and mode of administration. Adverse reactions include delirium, psychosis, agitation, violence, and suicide. Although PCP is usually smoked, it is also taken orally, intranasally, or intravenously. Verification of PCP poisoning generally requires toxicological analysis of the urine, because the $T_{1/2}$ of PCP in serum is short (i.e., 45 minutes).

An overdose of PCP is usually accompanied by increased bronchial and salivary secretions, muscular incoordination, nystagmus, disconjugate gaze, and bizarre behavior (e.g., posturing, catatonia, amnesia for the episode). In extreme cases, seizures, hypertensive crisis, respiratory depression, coma, or death occurs. The goals of treatment include protection of the patient and the staff while the drug effects subside, increasing the rate of the drug's elimination, and treatment of complications. Acidification of the urine helps to speed excretion of the drug. This may be accomplished with ammonium chloride, 2.75 mEq/kg in 60 mL of saline solution administered every 6 hours through a nasogastric tube, along with intravenous administration of ascorbic acid, 2 g in 500 mL of intravenous fluid every 6 hours. Diazepam, 10–30 mg, is the drug of choice for patients who are agitated or restless; however, a high-potency neuroleptic drug (e.g., haloperidol) and hospitalization are sometimes necessary for patients who have persistent psychotic reactions. Note that the use of haloperidol has been reported to be associated with potential for greater muscle damage (Schuckit 1989).

Marijuana and Hashish

The psychoactive component of the cannabinoids, Δ-9-tetrahydrocannabinol (Δ^9-THC), generally produces a state of euphoria, friendliness, relaxation, alteration in time perception, tachycardia, and scleral injection (Weiss et al. 1994). Some individuals develop panic anxiety and some develop full panic disorder (Hillard and Viewig 1983). In some instances, confusion, feelings of depersonalization and derealization, visual and auditory hallucinations, and paranoia develop. These symptoms should be treated with reassurance and close observation until the drug is eliminated (usually 3–5 hours after use). Signs of frontal-lobe dysfunction may be evident in chronic, heavy marijuana smokers (Pope and Yurgelin-Todd 1996).

Inhalants

The fumes of gasoline, glue, paint, paint thinners, spray paints, cleaners, typewriter correction fluid, or spray-can propellants are occasionally inhaled to achieve a state of euphoria similar to that of mild alcohol intoxication (Gillig 1990). Users of inhalants come to the attention of emergency psychiatric personnel when they become aggressive, behave impulsively, or display poor judgment. Infrequent users remain intoxicated usually less than 2 hours, whereas chronic users achieve a more sustained level of intoxication. Moderate to severe intoxication results in delirium, stupor, or coma accompanied by other signs of CNS toxicity (e.g., nystagmus, slurred speech, unsteady gait, psychomotor retardation, depressed reflexes). Chronic abuse can also produce demyelination, myositis, peripheral neuropathy, cardiac arrhythmias, liver failure, and renal failure (Gillig 1990).

COMMON PSYCHIATRIC EMERGENCIES

Patients With Mood Disorders

Symptoms of mood disorders constitute one of the most frequent reasons that individuals seek emergency psychi-

atric intervention (E. Robins et al. 1977). E. Robins et al. (1977) found that the majority (28%) of diagnoses given to psychiatric emergency patients were affective disorders, as determined by Feighner's criteria (Feighner et al. 1972). Half of this group received only an affective disorder diagnosis (usually major depression), one-third received an additional diagnosis, and the rest received two or more additional diagnoses (e.g., mood disorder plus alcoholism, personality disorder, and schizophrenia). Nervousness was the most common complaint made by those with a diagnosis of mood disorder.

Patients who present for acute evaluation of depressive symptoms are a heterogeneous group. Some have a previously diagnosed depressive disorder; some present with a first episode of major depression; and others report depressive symptoms secondary to situational disturbance, grief, personality disorder, substance abuse, or another primary problem. The clinician must evaluate the patient to determine the nature and presumed etiology of the depressive symptoms, to detect the presence of psychotic symptoms and suicide risk, and to decide whether to initiate pharmacological treatment.

Traditionally, antidepressant medication was withheld until the patient underwent evaluation by a second physician, who would see the patient regularly. This approach was justified because of the potential for a life-endangering overdose of tricyclic antidepressant medication, the questionable validity of diagnoses made in the ED, and the delayed response to antidepressant medication. Indeed, if the diagnosis is questionable and inpatient hospitalization is not necessary, it is sometimes prudent to invite the patient for a follow-up visit and further evaluation before committing to a course of antidepressant medication. However, if the patient fulfills the diagnostic criteria for a major depression, the initiation of antidepressant medication is indicated as long as the clinician can arrange for timely follow-up. Prompt reevaluation and follow-up increase the likelihood of compliance; concerns about untoward effects of medication are less relevant with newer antidepressants (e.g., bupropion, selective serotonin reuptake inhibitors, venlafaxine, mirtazapine).

The patient with hypomania or mania who refuses treatment and is not a danger to himself or herself or to others presents a common and difficult management problem. Caught between the competing responsibilities of protecting the patient's civil liberties and of providing appropriate medical care, the clinician must decide whether the patient's judgment is sufficiently impaired to warrant involuntary hospitalization and treatment. Frequently, the information provided by the patient is not reliable. Therefore, the history and the objective input of family members and associates are essential. If family members and associates are not available or the patient refuses to grant permission for the clinician to speak with others, the clinician must weigh the risks versus the benefits of subordinating indicated treatment to the patient's demands for privacy. If there is either inadequate information at the clinician's disposal or insufficient social support to ensure the patient's safety, then involuntary commitment is indicated. The clinician's observations and rationale should be documented in the patient's hospital record.

Patients With Anxiety and Phobic Disorders

Data from the Epidemiologic Catchment Area study indicate that anxiety and phobic disorders are the most prevalent form of psychiatric disturbance in the community (Barlow and Shear 1988); individuals with anxiety and phobias frequently use psychiatric, general medical, and emergency services (Markowitz et al. 1989). In one study, anxiety disorders constituted 36.1% of psychiatric diagnoses made in an ED (Fenichel and Murphy 1985). Only a minority of these patients received psychiatric consultation. Emergency physicians tend not to view anxiety as a disorder that requires specialized treatment and are likely to provide reassurance and small amounts of benzodiazepines or antihistamines to anxious patients who have an underlying medical illness (Schwartz et al. 1987). Based on a retrospective chart review, Schwartz et al. (1987) concluded that anxious patients are referred for emergency psychiatric evaluation only when they have comorbid depression or absence of medical illness or if psychiatrically relevant information is elicited by a triage nurse.

Nearly half of the patients who come to primary care and emergency facilities with somatic complaints (e.g., chest pain, palpitations, choking sensation, respiratory distress, neurological symptoms, gastrointestinal disturbance) for which no organic basis is ultimately identified have panic disorder or depression (Bass and Wade 1984; Beitman et al. 1987, 1990; Lydiard et al. 1986; Rosenbaum 1987; Russell et al. 1991; Wulsin et al. 1991). Special attention should be given to the possibility of panic disorder in patients who present to the ED with complaints of chest pain. Despite high prevalence rates in this population, panic disorder is not frequently diagnosed on initial ED visits. Wulsin et al. (1991) reported that 31% of patients with atypical chest pain presenting to the ED met criteria for panic disorder, and Worthington et al. (1997) identified a 20% prevalence rate in patients with chief complaints of chest pain. In addition to the factors identified by Schwartz et al. (1987), nonfearful panic

attacks (Russell et al. 1991), alexithymia (Jones 1984), and limited-symptom panic attacks (Rosenbaum 1987) may account for failure to diagnose panic disorder in the presence of unexplained somatic symptoms.

Patients who present acutely with a primary complaint of anxiety, nervousness, or panic attacks have a heterogeneous group of disorders, including mood, anxiety, adjustment, and substance-related disorders. Patients already in treatment for these disturbances often present to the ED in crisis or for medications. Requests for benzodiazepines should always arouse suspicion and require careful evaluation. In some instances of suspected drug seeking, urine toxicology screening is helpful (see Table 39–2). If the patient complains of panic attacks, a helpful diagnostic maneuver is to ask for a description of the patient's first (herald) panic attack. An individual with true panic disorder rarely forgets the first attack, which is often the single most upsetting experience in his or her life.

Inability to recall the first attack suggests another disorder, often substance abuse. Given the high incidence of alcohol and substance abuse disorders in the emergency population, it is best to use nonbenzodiazepine medications (e.g., antidepressants) when possible to treat panic disorder, obsessive-compulsive disorder, generalized anxiety disorder, and posttraumatic stress disorder. Antidepressants are not always effective, however, and clinical benefit often is not seen for 2–3 weeks or more; the degree of symptomatic distress and dysfunction often warrants more rapid relief. Buspirone, not useful alone for panic disorder, may help the patient who has generalized anxiety disorder. Behavioral techniques such as deep, diaphragmatic breathing and progressive muscle relaxation are sometimes helpful but are difficult to teach during an emergency visit. Therefore, if the patient is reliable, a small amount of a benzodiazepine drug can be prescribed and the patient advised to return for reevaluation within several days to 1 week. Alprazolam, diazepam, and lorazepam have the highest abuse potential of all benzodiazepines (Griffiths and Wolf 1990), although individuals with addictions (so-called street addicts) also abuse other benzodiazepines (e.g., chlordiazepoxide, clonazepam); in reliable patients, any of these medications is safe for relief of acute anxiety.

Patients With Borderline or Antisocial Personality Disorder

Antisocial and borderline personality disorders—cluster B personality disorders, as classified in DSM-IV-TR (American Psychiatric Association 2000), along with histrionic and narcissistic personality disorders—are the most common types of personality disorders seen among emergency psychiatric patients (Beresin et al. 1994; E. Robins et al. 1977). Because the ED is always open, it attracts individuals with an insatiable appetite for care and attention, as well as those who are impulsive, have a low tolerance for frustration, or have a low threshold for aggression. For some individuals, dealing with unfamiliar caregivers enhances the opportunity for scamming an unwary practitioner. For others, the ED and its personnel become a surrogate extended family.

Individuals with antisocial or borderline personality disorders often seek emergency services during a crisis; both typically respond to crisis by manipulation, deceit, demands, or destructive behavior. Their multifaceted presentations are sometimes diagnostically misleading. In the aftermath of caring for these individuals, members of the ED staff may feel confused, frustrated, and angered. It is important, therefore, that the consulting psychiatrist learn to detect serious personality disorders and to respond effectively and expeditiously.

Antisocial personality disorder is a common diagnosis, surpassed only by depression in the realm of major psychiatric disorders. In the Epidemiologic Catchment Area study, 2%–4% of men and 0.5%–1% of women were diagnosed as antisocial (L. N. Robins et al. 1984). A psychopathy checklist for antisocial personality disorder was proposed for DSM-IV (Table 39–7). Typically, patients with antisocial personality disorder conceal a primary substance abuse disorder. Glib and charming, they ingratiate themselves with the staff, often with the intent of procuring narcotics, benzodiazepines, or an excuse from work or legal obligations. In his book on the subject, Donald Black indicated that "many, if not most, antisocials seem to lack a conscience, feeling little or no empathy for the people whose lives they touch" (Black 1999, p. xiii). These individuals are prone to easy frustration and may present with symptoms suggestive of a mood or anxiety disorder (e.g., major depression or panic disorder).

Vulnerable to either real or perceived abandonment, the patient with borderline personality disorder typically seeks urgent evaluation and care as a result of frustrated expectations or rupture of an important relationship. The patient may be angry and assaultive or helpless and vulnerable, frequently shifting back and forth, which makes it difficult for ED staff members to know how to respond. The patient may idealize certain members of the staff and respond spitefully or ungratefully to others (i.e., splitting). The development of intense feelings (usually negative, sometimes positive) toward the patient, or intense disagreements among the staff about the care of the patient, are clues that the patient has borderline personality disorder.

In general, it is best to minimize waiting time and to employ a direct, problem-solving, and dispassionate approach with patients who have antisocial or borderline personality disorder. The clinician should avoid overreaction to helplessness, seduction, or intimidation. In particular, the clinician should ensure that the patient with borderline personality disorder appreciates the reality of the situation, the practitioner's limitations, and the patient's responsibility in collaborating to help solve the crisis (Beresin et al. 1994). Malingering is common among antisocial individuals who often come to the ED to avoid incarceration or retaliation; thus, effective management requires a high index of suspicion and the examiner's willingness to spend time verifying questionable information. Because patients with antisocial or borderline personality disorders are often threatening or destructive, it is advisable to evaluate them in a safe setting and to ask security guards to stand by, especially if the clinician feels threatened or unsafe. In some instances, security guards can escort uncooperative or inconsolable patients out of the hospital when the physician has determined that there is little risk of harm to either the patient or others.

Domestic Violence and Child Abuse

In the United States, a woman is battered every 7.4 seconds by her husband (Reade 1994). Up to 30% of women who present to the ED with traumatic injury report that it is secondary to battering. Studies have demonstrated that physical abuse increases in frequency and severity over time, and 75% of victims suffer subsequent abuse (McLeer et al. 1989).

Health care professionals, however, commonly fail to identify domestic violence. Roberts et al. (1997) reported that only 50% of cases of domestic violence were identified during ED evaluations when compared with patient self-report. Furthermore, no improvement in detection was observed after an educational program on domestic violence (Roberts et al. 1997). Routine screening for domestic violence has been proven to be of value. Feldhaus et al. (1997) were able to identify 71% of women with a history of partner violence, utilizing a brief screening tool consisting of three basic questions:

1. Have you been hit, kicked, punched or otherwise hurt by someone within the past year? If so, by whom?
2. Do you feel safe in your current relationship?
3. Is there a partner from a previous relationship who is making you feel unsafe now?

Whenever a situation of domestic violence is identified, it is essential to inquire about child abuse or neglect.

TABLE 39–7. Psychopathy checklist

1. *Early behavior problems* (serious behavior problems that begin before age 12, persist through age 17, and are evident in a variety of situations)
2. *Adult antisocial behaviors* (propensity to engage in illicit and illegal behaviors as an adult)
3. *Impulsivity* (frequent engagement in risky behavior; spur-of-the-moment activity without considering consequences, such as frequent changes of sexual partners, employment, or residence)
4. *Poor behavior controls* (e.g., easily angered or frustrated)
5. *Lack of remorse* (e.g., rationalizes, minimizes, or denies negative effects of behavior; statements of remorse are insincere and/or inconsistent with behavior)
6. *Lack of empathy* (callous, cynical, contemptuous, or indifferent to the feelings, rights, or suffering of others)
7. *Deceitful and manipulative behavior* (lies excessively; readily deceives or manipulates to achieve money, sex, power, or other personal gain; engages in fraud, forgery, embezzlement)
8. *Irresponsibility* (consistently fails to meet obligations and commitments or frequently causes others hardship or puts them at risk)
9. *Inflated and arrogant self-presentation* (e.g., opinionated, self-assured, and unconcerned about problems or future)
10. *Glib and superficial personality* (facile, slick, clever, charming)

Source.   Reprinted from Widiger TA, Corbitt EM, Millon T: "Antisocial Personality Disorder," in American Psychiatric Press Review of Psychiatry, Vol 11. Edited by Tasman A, Riba MB. Washington, DC, American Psychiatric Press, 1992, pp. 63–79. Used with permission.

In 1996, more than 3 million children were reported to United States child protective services as having been abused, and almost 1 million of these cases were confirmed (Committee on Child Abuse and Neglect, 1999). Neglect constituted 60% of those cases, physical abuse 23%, sexual abuse 9%, and emotional maltreatment 4%. The federal government and all states have laws that define abuse and require mandatory reporting of suspected cases. The victim may be depressed, withdrawn, hyperactive, anxious, paranoid, or fussy and have difficulty sleeping or be unresponsive to affection (Ostow 1994). Abusers tend to have personality disorders, a personal history of abuse, and drug and alcohol problems.

In cases of domestic violence, child endangerment, or elder abuse, the clinician should conduct a thorough examination and carefully document findings. During psychiatric evaluation, the patient should be assessed for evidence of substance abuse, suicidal or homicidal ideation, mood disorders, and signs or symptoms of stress disorders. Hospitalization should be considered if concerns for safety exist or if the coping skills of those involved are questionable. In the case of domestic violence, victims should be given numbers of emergency hotlines, shelters, and domestic violence agencies. Most institutions have protocols in place to ensure proper management from both a clinical and legal perspective. Physicians and consultants in the ED should review these policies, and in the event that a formal policy does not exist, the ED should develop its own guidelines.

Homeless Patients

Homeless individuals present unique problems and challenges to emergency medical and psychiatric practitioners (Bierer and Tesar 1994). Diagnostic and management problems arise because homelessness produces changes suggestive of primary psychiatric disorders. Difficulty procuring food and trouble finding a safe place to sleep can be mistaken for symptoms of depression, guardedness and suspiciousness can be misconstrued as paranoia, and fighting or stealing may be misinterpreted as evidence of antisocial personality disorder. Comorbid substance abuse occurs in nearly 50% of homeless persons who are mentally ill. The absence of a stable social network complicates disposition planning and possibly contributes to a higher rate of psychiatric hospitalization of these individuals. Negative attitudes toward the homeless person often interfere with delivery of adequate care.

The high concentration of psychiatric illness and substance-related disorders in the homeless population is probably both a cause and an effect of homelessness. In a sample of homeless individuals from Los Angeles with a history of major depression, the first depressive episode preceded homelessness in 71% (Koegel et al. 1988). The stress associated with homelessness can, in turn, precipitate or exacerbate episodes of psychiatric illness in predisposed individuals.

Effective emergency psychiatric evaluation and care of homeless individuals requires attention to several special issues. Perhaps most important are the priorities of the homeless patient. Receiving adequate medical treatment for depression, for example, may not seem as crucial as obtaining food and adequate footwear. If these basic requirements are not addressed, the likelihood of compliance with antidepressant treatment diminishes. Foot care is a major priority in the clinical management of many homeless individuals because podiatric problems are common. Early infections are easily treated, and the consequences (e.g., ulcers, cellulitis) are preventable. Attention to other medical problems is also important, especially in inner-city populations (e.g., pulmonary tuberculosis). It is prudent to ask screening questions about substance abuse and to solicit pertinent information from others (e.g., shelter staff).

Special problems occur in the treatment and disposition of homeless people. In prescribing medications, the physician must consider the high prevalence of substance abuse, the special importance of remaining alert, the problem of finding a safe place to store medications, the likelihood of noncompliance, and the lack of money. The majority of homeless individuals receive treatment on an outpatient basis. However, the chaos of the homeless lifestyle, including its competing demands (e.g., the need to queue up daily for lunch or for a shelter bed, sometimes in distant parts of the city), makes it difficult to keep doctors' appointments and to adhere to a treatment regimen. Moreover, effective coordination of outpatient psychiatric services often requires that the clinician communicate with area shelters, substance abuse treatment facilities, hospital social services, or one of the 110 federally funded Health Care for the Homeless programs in the United States (Bierer and Tesar 1994). These difficulties, the lack of a supportive social network, and the common belief that homelessness itself is evidence of impaired self-care may contribute to the high rate of involuntary psychiatric hospitalization (M. Bierer, unpublished data, May 1990). Important factors that often influence the decision to commit a homeless psychiatric patient include the recent development of homelessness, a history of dangerousness, inadequate social support, and untreated serious or life-threatening medical conditions (Bierer and Tesar 1994).

Psychiatric Emergency Repeaters

Repeat users of emergency services, often glibly referred to as regulars or frequent flyers, constitute 7%–18% of emergency psychiatric patients and account for as many as one-half of total psychiatric emergency visits (Ellison et al. 1986, 1989). Frequent repeaters (i.e., those who return six or more times during a 6-month period) exhibit a predominance of anxiety symptoms and impulsivity (Ellison et al. 1989). During crises, they use frequent emergency visits, self-injury, alcohol, or anxiolytic medication to cope with unbearable affects. Overall, psychiatric emergency repeaters are a diverse group composed of 1) patients in treatment who periodically come to the ED for crisis intervention, 2) patients in need of treatment for a new or recurrent episode of illness, 3) patients not in regular treatment who frequent the ED

during time-limited crises, and 4) patients who use the ED as part of their social network (Ellison et al. 1986; Tesar 1994).

Certain emergency repeaters are best managed in a designated emergency psychiatric facility. An ambulatory crisis clinic has the built-in flexibility to meet the needs of patients who have trouble sticking with a psychotherapist or who episodically require supplemental crisis-oriented evaluation and treatment. The clinician should always investigate whether the emergency visit is related to problems in the psychotherapeutic relationship (e.g., treatment is beginning or terminating, the therapist is away, there is a change in the treatment plan, the treatment is ineffective, or unbearable transference feelings are emerging). It is often necessary for the consultant to speak with the primary therapist in order to clarify the nature of transference or countertransference reactions.

Repeaters who have not successfully engaged in any sustained treatment are perhaps the most troublesome for crisis and emergency clinicians. Often, these individuals have a history of severe interpersonal difficulties, exhibit a pattern of self-destructive behavior (e.g., self-mutilation, low-risk suicide attempts, chronic substance abuse), and were victims of early and severe abuse or deprivation (Bassuk and Gerson 1980). They are usually anxious, impulsive, help-rejecting, and prone to hostile interactions with caregivers, exhausting the caregivers'—and the clinicians'—welcome wherever they go.

Ironically, often little is known about these highly visible patients. Typically, the time spent with the patient is inversely proportional to the frequency of visits. Hesitant to gratify perceived neediness, the clinician is often unwilling to ask questions that engage the patient. The clinician may direct anger or impatience at the patient by arbitrarily limiting the duration of the clinical encounter. In some instances, compliance with a treatment protocol requires that the duration and frequency of visits are limited. Moreover, if multiple clinicians are seeing the patient during repeated visits, the responsibility for knowing and caring for the patient is gradually diffused. "Problem patient rounds" (Santy and Wehmeier 1984) is one way to pool the information of multiple clinicians, familiarizing them with what is and what is not known about the patient and defusing uncomfortable and counterproductive negative reactions to the patient.

Success with repeaters requires patience, a dispassionate attitude, a compulsive commitment to thorough evaluation, and acceptance of limited treatment goals. A mental status examination should be performed that includes tests of cognitive and executive functions, particularly in repeaters who are apathetic or who have difficulty engaging in treatment. In some patients, frontal-lobe dysfunction (e.g., resulting from chronic alcoholism, drug abuse, head injury, or developmental defects) is the cause of impaired attention, diminished mental flexibility, and poor problem-solving skills. In others, severe personality disturbance accounts for a pattern of noncompliance, recidivism, and overuse of emergency facilities. A treatment protocol that specifies the guidelines and limits of treatment is necessary to help shape and modify help-rejecting, abusive, or manipulative behavior. Dialectical behavior therapy, a form of cognitive-behavioral therapy, has been used with some success in psychiatric emergency services for the management of borderline personality disorder. This form of therapy has been shown to reduce number of hospital days, parasuicide attempts, medical risk of parasuicide, and dropout from treatment (Shearin et al. 1994). With this strategy, splitting of staff and fragmentation of care provided by multiple caregivers are less likely to occur. Timely definition and clarification of the type of treatment the patient is to receive should minimize disappointment and frustration (Tesar 1994) and reduce the number of repeat visits (Scesny 1997).

When all available approaches, including hospitalization, treatment protocols, and therapeutic limit setting, have failed to control inappropriate or dangerous behavior, the repeater may have nowhere else to turn but the ED. Adopting an attitude of resignation and acceptance may help caregivers tolerate such patients and provide care for them. The ED is the de facto primary care facility for such individuals. Ironically, in some instances, acceptance of this role by the ED staff defuses the patient's anger and antagonism, resulting in greater compliance and a more comfortable working relationship.

DISPOSITION

The ultimate goal of all emergency work is to effect a safe and clinically sound disposition. Achieving this depends on the quality of the evaluation, attention to the clinically relevant problem(s), and the effectiveness of treatment in the ED. If the evaluation is superficial and treatment is ineffective, then appropriate disposition is more difficult, roadblocks to discharge are more likely to be encountered, and the patient is apt to "bounce back."

The inevitable pressure of time (Gerson and Bassuk 1980), the complexity of the problem(s), and the paucity of clinical and psychosocial information available on most acute psychiatric patients often restrict the ability of the clinician to orchestrate an optimal disposition. An unfortunate tendency, especially when the ED is busy, is for the consultant to focus disproportionately on disposition

and to give comparatively little attention to evaluation and treatment. This ultimately detracts from the satisfaction of emergency psychiatric work and contributes to the devaluation and underrating of emergency psychiatry.

Therefore, the consultant must create sufficient time, not only to perform a thorough medical-psychiatric examination but also to gather historical and psychosocial data that enhance understanding of the case and permit the development of an appropriate disposition. Acquisition of such information often requires communication with therapists, family members, friends, police, ambulance drivers, hospitals where the patient previously stayed, individuals involved with the patient before emergency admission (e.g., the owner of the restaurant where the patient was apprehended by police), or even a pharmacist who has dispensed medication to and may know the patient (the telephone number can be obtained from a prescription bottle).

Studies of the decision to hospitalize psychiatric patients from the ED consistently identify dangerousness as the single most significant criterion (Apsler and Bassuk 1983; Friedman et al. 1983; Gerson and Bassuk 1980; Segal et al. 1988; Tischler 1966). Other important criteria include severity of schizophrenic and psychotic symptoms (Friedman et al. 1983), the years of experience of the admitting clinician (Baxter et al. 1968; Mendel and Rapport 1969; Streiner et al. 1975), the presence of psychosocial supports (Mischler and Waxler 1963; Orleans-Rose et al. 1977), and whether the patient is expected to profit from treatment (Baxter et al. 1968; Orleans-Rose et al. 1977; Shader et al. 1969). Another emerging and important set of variables is the constraints imposed by health maintenance organizations and managed care programs on patient admission (Greenberg et al. 1989; Olfson 1989; Swift 1986). Approval for hospitalization is often contingent on the clinician's ability to document imminent danger to the patient or to others and also on determination that the patient has exhausted all available outpatient resources. In general, third-party payers encourage the use of less costly alternatives to inpatient admission, such as partial hospitalization (e.g., observation in 24-hour holding, transitional, or respite beds), day treatment, or intensive (e.g., daily) crisis-oriented outpatient treatment.

Optimally, discharge from the ED should include a plan that addresses the patient's immediate and longer-term needs. The clinician must assess the patient's ability to obtain food, shelter, and clothing and must also know about available outpatient mental health, substance abuse, and social service resources (Hillard 1990). Satisfaction of the patient's immediate needs often depends on the involvement of family or friends or, if they are not available, on the availability of shelter and homeless services (Pearlmutter 1983). Assuming that the patient's safety and basic needs are ensured, the clinician then recommends follow-up with the patient's therapist, makes a referral for further evaluation and care at an appropriate facility (e.g., hospital outpatient clinic, community mental health center, outpatient substance abuse service), or obtains the patient's agreement to return for follow-up evaluation in the ED. Referral recommendations are more likely to be followed if a specific patient request is identified during the evaluation process, if the patient has a diagnosis of a nonpsychotic disorder (e.g., major depression), and if the patient leaves with clear, written referral recommendations (Blouin et al. 1985; Jellinek 1978).

MOBILE CRISIS PROGRAMS

In the late 1980s, mobile crisis teams emerged as another approach to psychiatric emergency services. These services are typically collaborative efforts of community mental health providers, law enforcement personnel, and ED staff and consulting psychiatrists from the medical center. In a review of the benefits of mobile crisis programs, Zealberg et al (1993) identified advantages to the patients, the community, and the involved EDs and hospitals. For example, patients who do not have access to mental health services receive accurate and efficient evaluations in a setting that is less distressing than a busy ED. Mobile crisis interventions may help lessen the anxiety of law enforcement officials and foster goodwill with members of the community whose lives are disrupted by an individual in crisis. Often, disposition other than an ED evaluation or hospitalization may be facilitated. So-called frequent flyers with chronic illness and repeat assessments may be managed much more efficiently. In some programs, mobile crisis teams will visit the ED in order to provide clinical information and assist with placement of patients requiring psychiatric care.

Some mobile crisis programs function as a central triage unit with the capacity to access all of the mental health facilities and psychiatric units in the region. Kates et al. (1996) described an integrated regional psychiatric emergency service in Canada that has successfully incorporated all of the hospital-run psychiatric emergency services into a single centralized unit. Several cities in the United States have experimented with this model and typically develop services with mobile crisis teams and community mental health centers at the hub of the system. We anticipate that the consulting psychiatrist will increasingly function as a liaison with mobile crisis teams and have a role that extends beyond the confines of the ED walls.

SUMMARY

The job of providing psychiatric consultation to a general hospital ED is both challenging and exciting. Successful crisis intervention with a despondent patient or rapid alleviation of the patient's psychotic symptoms with parenteral neuroleptic medication can be satisfying and personally rewarding for the psychiatric consultant. Also, in a large urban ED, the busy psychiatric consultant has the opportunity to see a wide variety of uncommon neuropsychiatric illnesses and unusual presentations of common illnesses.

Especially for the young or inexperienced psychiatric resident, however, psychiatric consultation in the ED can also be an anxiety-provoking experience. Decisions in the ED must be made rapidly, often with scant historical data, and often with limited available resources to ensure patient safety and well-being. Failure to correctly assess the patient's potential for violence or suicide can result in premature discharge from the ED, with the risk of serious consequences to the patient or others. It is strongly recommended, therefore, that an experienced board-eligible or board-certified psychiatrist supervise all emergency psychiatric evaluations performed by psychiatric residents and nonpsychiatric professionals.

The most important goals of ED psychiatric consultation are to help the patient achieve self-control and to ensure the safety of the patient and others involved with him or her. Accomplishment of these goals requires constant vigilance for threatening behavior or loss of control; comprehensive medical-psychiatric evaluation; and the judicious use of the clinician's medical knowledge, judgment, and skills. The consultant must be prepared to help the ED staff to create circumstances that are safe and that permit thorough patient evaluation. Each evaluation must include a thorough mental status examination and relevant medical evaluation if the consultant suspects medical illness, CNS dysfunction, or substance abuse.

An unfortunate tendency in emergency psychiatric consultation is to revert to what could be called dispositional psychiatry. "Getting rid of the patient" is a phrase often used in this context. The emphasis in dispositional psychiatry is on rapid discharge or transfer of the patient. The decision is generally based on a limited assessment of dangerousness rather than on a thorough assessment of the patient's needs or on a formulation of the presenting problem. Such shortcutting is, to some extent, inevitable and is fostered by busy work schedules and pressure exerted on the consultant to transfer or discharge psychiatric patients as quickly as possible.

An important purpose of this chapter is to discourage cursory, disposition-oriented evaluation and instead to encourage formulation of a treatment plan that addresses the patient's individual needs. Effective treatment planning first requires stabilization of the presenting problem (e.g., agitation, suicidal ideation, depression, substance abuse, panic attacks), assessment of the psychosocial context in which the problem has surfaced, and finally, enlistment of the patient in planning for further treatment beyond the ED.

Rapid stabilization of the patient and development of creative outpatient programs such as mobile crisis intervention are increasingly important as the emphasis on inpatient treatment diminishes and the number of inpatient beds continues to decline.

REFERENCES

American Psychiatric Association: Task Force Report of the American Psychiatric Association: Benzodiazepine Dependence, Toxicity, and Abuse. Washington, DC, American Psychiatric Press, 1990

American Psychiatric Association: Diagnostic and Statistical Manual of Mental Disorders, 4th Edition, Text Revision. Washington, DC, American Psychiatric Association, 2000

Apsler R, Bassuk E: Differences among clinicians in the decision to admit. Arch Gen Psychiatry 40:1133–1137, 1983

Arana GW, Goff DC, Baldessarini RJ, et al: Efficacy of anticholinergic prophylaxis for neuroleptic-induced acute dystonia. Am J Psychiatry 145:993–996, 1988

Atkins RE: Psychiatric emergency services. Arch Gen Psychiatry 17:176–182, 1967

Ayd FJ: A survey of drug-induced extrapyramidal reactions. JAMA 175:1054–1060, 1961

Baldessarini RJ: Chemotherapy in Psychiatry. Cambridge, MA, Harvard University Press, 1985

Barlow DH, Shear MK: Panic disorder, in American Psychiatric Press Review of Psychiatry, Vol 7. Edited by Frances AJ, Hales RE. Washington, DC, American Psychiatric Press, 1988, pp 5–9

Bass C, Wade C: Chest pain with normal coronary arteries: a comparative study of psychiatric and social morbidity. Psychosom Med 14:51–61, 1984

Bassuk E, Gerson S: Chronic crisis patients: a discrete clinical group. Am J Psychiatry 137:1513–1517, 1980

Baxter S, Chodorkoff B, Underhill R: Psychiatric emergencies: dispositional determinants and validity of the decision to admit. Am J Psychiatry 124:1542–1546, 1968

Beitman BD, Basha I, Flaker G, et al: Atypical or nonanginal chest pain: panic disorder or coronary artery disease. Arch Intern Med 147:1548–1552, 1987

Beitman BD, Kushner M, Lamberti JW, et al: Panic disorder without fear in patients with angiographically normal coronary arteries. J Nerv Ment Dis 178:307–312, 1990

Benson DF: Psychiatric aspects of aphasia. Br J Psychiatry 123:555–556, 1973

Beresin EV, Falk WE, Gordon C: Borderline and other personality disorders, in Manual of Psychiatric Emergencies, 3rd Edition. Edited by Hyman SE, Tesar GE. Boston, MA, Little, Brown, 1994, pp 178–193

Bierer M, Tesar GE: Homelessness and psychiatric emergencies, in Manual of Psychiatric Emergencies, 3rd Edition. Edited by Hyman SE, Tesar GE. Boston, MA, Little, Brown, 1994, pp 96–103

Black DW: Bad Boys, Bad Men. New York, Oxford University Press, 1999

Blouin A, Perez E, Minoletti A: Compliance to referrals from the psychiatric emergency room. Can J Psychiatry 30:103–106, 1985

Breier A, Astrachan BM: Characterization of schizophrenic patients who commit suicide. Am J Psychiatry 141:206–209, 1984

Breier A, Wright P, Birkett M, et al: Intramuscular olanzapine: dose-related improvement in acutely agitated patients with schizophrenia (abstract). Syllabus and Proceedings Summary, American Psychiatric Association Annual Meeting, New Orleans, LA, May 5–10, 2001

Brew BJ: Diagnosis of Wernicke's encephalopathy. Aust N Z J Med 16:676–678, 1986

Browning C, Tyson R, Miller J: A study of psychiatric emergencies, part II: suicide. Psychiatr Med 1:359–366, 1970

Busto U, Sellars EM, Naranjo CA, et al: Patterns of benzodiazepine abuse and dependence. British Journal of Addictions 81:87–94, 1986

Chafetz ME, Blane HT, Abram HS, et al: Establishing treatment relations with alcoholics. J Nerv Ment Dis 134:395–409, 1962

Chafetz ME, Blane HT, Muller JJ: Acute psychiatric services in the general hospital, I: implications for psychiatry in emergency admissions. Am J Psychiatry 123:664–670, 1966

Ciraulo DA, Barnhill JG, Greenblatt DJ, et al: Abuse liability and clinical pharmacokinetics of alprazolam in alcoholic men. J Clin Psychiatry 49:333–337, 1988a

Ciraulo DA, Sands BF, Shader RI: Critical review of liability for benzodiazepine abuse among alcoholics. Am J Psychiatry 145:1501–1506, 1988b

Coleman JV, Errera P: The general hospital emergency room and its psychiatric problems. Am J Public Health 53:1294–1301, 1963

Coleman MD, Zwerling I: The psychiatric emergency clinic: a flexible way of meeting community mental health needs. Am J Psychiatry 115:980–984, 1959

Committee on Child Abuse and Neglect: Guidelines for the evaluation of sexual abuse in children: subject review. Pediatrics 103:186–191, 1999

Cushman P: Delirium tremens: update on an old disorder. Postgrad Med 82:117–122, 1987

De Keyser J, Deleu D, Solheid C, et al: Coma as a presenting manifestation of Wernicke's encephalopathy. J Emerg Med 3:361–363, 1985

Drummond DJ, Sparr LF, Gordon GH: Hospital violence reduction among high-risk patients. JAMA 261:2531–2534, 1989

Dubin WR, Waxman HM, Weiss KJ, et al: Rapid tranquilization: the efficacy of oral concentrate. J Clin Psychiatry 46:475–478, 1985

Dulti RA, Fyer MR, Haas GL, et al: Substance use in borderline personality disorder. Am J Psychiatry 147:1002–1007, 1990

Ellison JM, Blum N, Barsky AJ: Repeat visitors in the psychiatric emergency service: a critical review of the data. Hospital and Community Psychiatry 37:37–41, 1986

Ellison JM, Blum N, Barsky AJ: Frequent repeaters in a psychiatric emergency service. Hospital and Community Psychiatry 40:958–960, 1989

Feighner JP, Robins E, Guze SB, et al: Diagnostic criteria for use in psychiatric research. Arch Gen Psychiatry 26:57–63, 1972

Feldhaus KM, Koziol-Mclain J, Amsbury HL, et al: Accuracy of 3 brief screening questions for detecting partner violence in the emergency department. JAMA 277:1357–1361, 1997

Fenichel GS, Murphy JG: Factors that predict consultation in the emergency department. Med Care 23:258–265, 1985

Folstein MF, Folstein SE, McHugh PR: Mini-Mental State, a practical method for grading the cognitive state of patients for the clinician. J Psychiatr Res 12:189–198, 1975

Frew SA, Roush WR, LaGreca K: COBRA: implications for emergency medicine. Ann Emerg Med 17:835–837, 1988

Friedman S, Margolis R, David OJ, et al: Predicting psychiatric admission from an emergency room: psychiatric, psychosocial, and methodological factors. J Nerv Ment Dis 171:155–158, 1983

Garza-Trevino ES, Hollister LE, Overall JE, et al: Efficacy of combinations of intramuscular antipsychotics and sedative-hypnotics for control of psychotic agitation. Am J Psychiatry 146:1598–1601, 1989

Gawin FH, Kleber HD: Cocaine abuse and its treatment: open pilot treatment trial with desipramine and lithium carbonate. Arch Gen Psychiatry 41:903–909, 1984

Gerson S, Bassuk E: Psychiatric emergencies: an overview. Am J Psychiatry 137:1–11, 1980

Gillig P: Drug abuse, in Manual of Clinical Emergency Psychiatry. Edited by Hillard JR. Washington, DC, American Psychiatric Press, 1990, pp 207–227

Gillig PM, Grubb P, Kruger R, et al: What do psychiatric emergency patients really want and how do they feel about what they get? Psychiatr Q 61:189–195, 1990

Goff DC, Arana GW, Greenblatt DJ, et al: The effect of benztropine on haloperidol-induced dystonia, clinical efficacy and pharmacokinetics: a prospective trial. J Clin Psychopharmacol 11:106–112, 1991

Greenberg WM, Seide M, Scimeca MM: The hospitalizable patient as a commodity: selling in a bear market. Hospital and Community Psychiatry 40:184–185, 1989

Greenblatt DJ, Shader RI, Abernathy DR: Current status of benzodiazepines (first of two parts). N Engl J Med 309:354–358, 1983

Griffiths RR, Wolf B: Relative abuse liability of different benzodiazepines in drug abusers. J Clin Psychopharmacol 10:237–243, 1990

Hillard JR: Social treatment principles, in Manual of Clinical Emergency Psychiatry. Edited by Hillard JR. Washington, DC, American Psychiatric Press, 1990, pp 71–77

Hillard JR, Viewig WVR: Marked sinus tachycardia resulting from the synergistic effects of marijuana and nortriptyline. Am J Psychiatry 140:626–627, 1983

Hillard JR, Ramm D, Zung WWK, et al: Suicide in a psychiatric emergency room population. Am J Psychiatry 140:459–462, 1983

Hillard JR, Zung WWK, Ramm D, et al: Accidental and homicidal death in a psychiatric emergency room population. Hospital and Community Psychiatry 36:640–643, 1985

Hunt N, Stern TA: The association between intravenous haloperidol and torsades de pointes. Psychosomatics 36:541–549, 1995

Hyman SE: Acute psychoses and catatonia, in Manual of Psychiatric Emergencies, 3rd Edition. Edited by Hyman SE, Tesar GE. Boston, MA, Little, Brown, 1994a, pp 143–157

Hyman SE: Alcohol-related emergencies, in Manual of Psychiatric Emergencies, 3rd Edition. Edited by Hyman SE, Tesar GE. Boston, MA, Little, Brown, 1994b, pp 294–303

Hyman SE: The violent patient, in Manual of Psychiatric Emergencies, 3rd Edition. Edited by Hyman SE, Tesar GE. Boston, MA, Little, Brown, 1994c, pp 28–37

Ingelfinger JA, Isakson G, Shine D, et al: Reliability of the toxic screen in drug overdose. Clin Pharmacol Ther 29:570–575, 1981

Jellinek M: Referrals from a psychiatric emergency room: relationship of compliance to demographic and interview variables. Am J Psychiatry 135:209–213, 1978

Jones BA: Panic attacks with panic masked by alexithymia. Psychosom Med 25:858–859, 1984

Juergens S: Alprazolam and diazepam: addiction potential. J Subst Abuse Treat 8:43–51, 1991

Juergens S, Morse RM: Alprazolam dependence in seven patients. Am J Psychiatry 145:625–627, 1988

Kates N, Eaman S, Santone J, et al: An integrated regional emergency psychiatry service. Gen Hosp Psychiatry 18:251–256, 1996

Khantzian EJ, McKenna GJ: Acute toxic and withdrawal reactions associated with drug use and abuse. Ann Intern Med 90:361–372, 1979

Koegel P, Burnam MA, Farr RK: The prevalence of specific psychiatric disorders among homeless individuals in the inner city of Los Angeles. Arch Gen Psychiatry 45:1085–1092, 1988

Kryspin-Exner K, Demel I: The use of tranquilizers in the treatment of mixed drug abuse. International Journal of Clinical Pharmacology 12:13–18, 1975

Ladewig D, Grossenbacher H: Benzodiazepine abuse in patients of doctors in domiciliary practice in the Basel area. Pharmacopsychiatry 21:104–108, 1988

Lazare A: The psychiatric examination in the walk-in clinic: hypothesis generation and hypotheses testing. Arch Gen Psychiatry 33:96–102, 1976

Lazare A, Eisenthal S: Patient requests in a walk-in clinic. J Nerv Ment Dis 165:330–340, 1977

Lazare A, Eisenthal S, Wasserman L: The customer approach to patienthood: attending to patient requests in a walk-in clinic. Arch Gen Psychiatry 32:553–558, 1975a

Lazare A, Eisenthal S, Wasserman L, et al: Patient requests in a walk-in clinic. Compr Psychiatry 16:467–477, 1975b

Lineaweaver WC, Anderson K, King DN: Massive doses of midazolam infusion for delirium tremens without respiratory depression. Crit Care Med 16:294–295, 1988

Lydiard RB, Laraia MT, Howell EF, et al: Can panic disorder present as irritable bowel syndrome? J Clin Psychiatry 47:470–473, 1986

Mahoney JD, Gross PL, Stern TA, et al: Quantitative serum toxic screening in the management of suspected drug overdose. Am J Emerg Med 8:16–22, 1990

Markowitz JS, Weissman MM, Oullette R, et al: Quality of life in panic disorder. Arch Gen Psychiatry 46:984–992, 1989

McCulloch LE, McNiel DE, Binder RL, et al: Effects of a weapon screening procedure in a psychiatric emergency room. Hospital and Community Psychiatry 37:837–838, 1986

McLeer SV, Awar AH, Herman S, et al: Education is not enough: a systems failure in protecting battered women. Ann Emerg Med 18:651–653, 1989

McNiel DE, Binder RL: Patients who bring weapons to the psychiatry emergency room. J Clin Psychiatry 48:230–233, 1987a

McNiel DE, Binder RL: Predictive validity of judgments of dangerousness in emergency civil commitment. Am J Psychiatry 144:197–200, 1987b

Meehan KM, Wang H, David SR, et al: Intramuscular olanzapine: efficacy and safety in acutely agitated patients with dementia (abstract). Syllabus and Proceedings Summary, American Psychiatric Association Annual Meeting, New Orleans, LA, May 5–10, 2001a

Meehan KM, Zhang F, David SR, et al: Intramuscular olanzapine: efficacy and safety in acutely agitated patients with mania associated with bipolar disorder (abstract). Syllabus and Proceedings Summary, American Psychiatric Association Annual Meeting, New Orleans, LA, May 5–10, 2001b

Mendel WM, Rapport S: Determinants of the decision for psychiatric hospitalization. Arch Gen Psychiatry 20:321–328, 1969

Mendoza R, Battaglia J, Dubin W, et al: Rapid tranquilization of agitated psychotic patients in the emergency room. Paper presented at the annual meeting of the Association of General Hospital Psychiatrists, Cambridge, MA, November 1991

Mezzich JE, Evanczuk KJ, Mathias RJ, et al: Symptoms and hospitalization decision. Am J Psychiatry 141:764–769, 1984

Mischler EG, Waxler NE: Decision process in psychiatric hospitalization: patients referred, accepted and admitted to a psychiatry hospital. American Sociological Review 28:576–587, 1963

Monahan J: Prediction research and the emergency commitment of dangerous mentally ill persons: a reconsideration. Am J Psychiatry 135:198–201, 1978

Moscovitz H, Brookoff D, Nelson L: A randomized trial of bromocriptine for cocaine users presenting to the emergency department. J Gen Intern Med 8:1–4, 1993

Muller JJ, Chafetz ME, Blane HT: Acute psychiatric services in the general hospital, III: statistical survey. Am J Psychiatry 124:46–56, 1967

Musto DF: Historical Perspectives in Substance Abuse, 3rd Edition. Edited by Lowinson JH, Ruiz P, Millman RB, et al. Baltimore, MD, Williams & Wilkins, 1997, p 14

Nagy LM, Krystal JH, Woods SW, et al: Clinical and medication outcome after short-term alprazolam in behavioral group treatment of panic disorder. Arch Gen Psychiatry 46:993–999, 1989

Nathan RG, Rousch AF: Which patients commit suicide? (letter) Am J Psychiatry 141:1017, 1984

Nolop KB, Natow A: Unprecedented sedative requirements during delirium tremens (letter). Crit Care Med 13:246, 1985

Noyes R, Garvey MJ, Cook BL, et al: Benzodiazepine withdrawal: a review of the evidence. J Clin Psychiatry 49:382–388, 1988

Olfson M: Psychiatry emergency room dispositions of HMO enrollers. Hospital and Community Psychiatry 40:639–641, 1989

Orleans-Rose S, Hawkins J, Apodaca L: Decision to admit: criteria for admission and readmission to a VA hospital. Arch Gen Psychiatry 34:418–421, 1977

Ostow AR: Child abuse, in Manual of Psychiatric Emergencies, 3rd Edition. Edited by Hyman SE, Tesar G. Boston, MA, Little, Brown, 1994

Pearlmutter RA: Family involvement in psychiatry emergencies. Hospital and Community Psychiatry 34:255–257, 1983

Petursson H, Lader MH: Benzodiazepine dependence. British Journal of Addictions 76:133–145, 1981

Pollack MH: Long-term management of panic disorder. J Clin Psychiatry 51 (suppl 5):11–13, 1990

Pope HG, Yurgelin-Todd D: The residual cognitive effects of heavy marijuana use in college students. JAMA 275:521–527, 1996

Rall TW: Hypnotics and sedatives; alcohol, in The Pharmacological Basis of Therapeutics, 8th Edition. Edited by Gilman GA, Rall TW, Nies AS, et al. New York, Pergamon, 1990, pp 359–383

Rapaport MH, Zisook S: Requests by walk-in and scheduled patients at an outpatient clinic. Psychosomatics 28:129–142, 1987

Reade J: Domestic violence, in Manual of Psychiatric Emergencies, 3rd Edition. Edited by Hyman SE, Tesar G. Boston, MA, Little, Brown, 1994, pp 143–157

Rich JA, Singer DE: Cocaine-related symptoms in patients presenting to an urban emergency department. Ann Emerg Med 20:616–621, 1991

Roberts GL, Lawrence J, O'Toole BI: Domestic violence in the emergency department, 2: detection by doctors and nurses. Gen Hosp Psychiatry 19:12–15, 1997

Robins E, Gentry KA, Munoz RA, et al: A contrast of the three more common illnesses with the ten less common in a study and 18-month follow-up of 314 psychiatric emergency room patients, I: characteristics of the sample and methods of study. Arch Gen Psychiatry 34:259–265, 1977

Robins LN, Helzer JE, Weissman MM, et al: Lifetime prevalence of specific psychiatric disorders in three sites. Arch Gen Psychiatry 41:949–958, 1984

Rosenbaum JF: Limited-symptom panic attacks. Psychosom Med 28:407–412, 1987

Rund DA, Summers WK, Levin M: Alcohol use and psychiatric illness in emergency patients. JAMA 245:1240–1241, 1981

Russell JL, Kushner MG, Beitman BD, et al: Nonfearful panic disorder in neurology patients validated by lactate challenge. Am J Psychiatry 148:361–364, 1991

Santy PA, Wehmeier PK: Using "problem patient" rounds to help emergency room staff manage difficult patients. Hospital and Community Psychiatry 35:494–496, 1984

Scesny AM: Measuring the effectiveness of social interventions on health outcomes. Social Work Administration 23:1–12, 1997

Schuckit MA: Alcoholism and other psychiatric disorders. Hospital and Community Psychiatry 34:1022–1027, 1983

Schuckit MA: Drug and Alcohol Abuse. New York, Plenum, 1989, p 180

Schwartz GM, Braverman BG, Roth B: Anxiety disorders and psychiatric referral in the general medical emergency room. Gen Hosp Psychiatry 9:87–93, 1987

Segal SP, Watson MA, Goldfinger SM, et al: Civil commitment in the psychiatric emergency room: mental disorder indicators and three dangerousness criteria. Arch Gen Psychiatry 45:753–758, 1988

Shader RI, Binstock WA, Ohly JI, et al: Biasing factors in diagnosis and disposition. Compr Psychiatry 10:81–89, 1969

Shearin EN, Linehan MM: Dialectical behavior therapy for borderline personality disorder: theoretical and empirical foundations. Acta Psychiatr Scand Suppl 379:61–68, 1994

Simon RI: Clinical Psychiatry and the Law. Washington, DC, American Psychiatric Press, 1988

Skodol AE, Karasu TB: Emergency psychiatry and the assaultive patient. Am J Psychiatry 135:202–205, 1978

Smith DE, Marks J: Abuse and dependency: an international perspective, in The Benzodiazepines: Current Standards for Medical Practice. Edited by Smith DE, Wesson DR. Lancaster, UK, MTP Press, 1985, pp 179–199

Soloff PH: Emergency management of violent patients, in Psychiatry Update: American Psychiatric Association Annual Review, Vol 6. Edited by Hales RE, Frances AJ. Washington, DC, American Psychiatric Press, 1987, pp 510–536

Stern TA, Mulley AG, Thibault GE: Life-threatening drug overdose: precipitants and prognosis. JAMA 251:1983–1985, 1984

Stern TA, Schwartz JH, Cremens MC, et al: The evaluation of homicidal patients by psychiatry residents in the emergency room: a pilot study. Psychiatr Q 62:333–343, 1991

Stitzer ML, Griffiths RR, McLellan AT, et al: Diazepam use among methadone maintenance patients: patterns and dosages. Drug Alcohol Depend 8:189–199, 1981

Streiner DL, Goodman JT, Woodward CA: Correlates of hospitalization decisions: a replicative study. Can J Public Health 66:411–415, 1975

Swift RM: Negotiating psychiatric hospitalization within restrictive admissions criteria. Hospital and Community Psychiatry 37:619–623, 1986

Tarasoff v Regents of the University of California, 118 Cal Rptr 129, 529 P2d 553 (1976)

Teplin LA, Abram K, Michaels SK: Blood alcohol level among emergency room patients: a multivariate analysis. J Stud Alcohol 50:441–447, 1989

Tesar GE: Emergency psychiatry: the agitated patient, part II: pharmacologic treatment. Hospital and Community Psychiatry 44:627–629, 1993

Tesar GE: Psychiatric emergency repeaters, in Manual of Psychiatric Emergencies, 3rd Edition. Edited by Hyman SE, Tesar GE. Boston, MA, Little, Brown, 1994, pp 110–114

Tesar GE, Stern TA: Rapid tranquilization of the agitated intensive care unit patient. Journal of Intensive Care Medicine 3:195–201, 1988

Thompson WL, Johnson AD, Maddrey WL: Diazepam and paraldehyde for treatment of severe delirium tremens: a controlled trial. Ann Intern Med 82:175–180, 1980

Tintinalli JE, Peacock FW, Wright MA: Emergency medical evaluation of psychiatric patients. Ann Emerg Med 23:859–862, 1994

Tischler GL: Decision-making process in the emergency room. Arch Gen Psychiatry 14:69–78, 1966

Weddington WW, Carney AC: Alprazolam abuse during methadone maintenance therapy (letter). JAMA 257:3363, 1987

Weiss RD, Greenfield SF, Mirin SM: Intoxication and withdrawal syndromes, in Manual of Psychiatric Emergencies, 3rd Edition. Edited by Hyman SE, Tesar GE. Boston, MA, Little, Brown, 1994, pp 279–293

Weissberg MP: Emergency room medical clearance: an educational problem. Am J Psychiatry 136:787–790, 1979

Wellin E, Slesinger DP, Hollister CD: Psychiatric emergency services: evolution, adaptation and proliferation. Soc Sci Med 6:475–482, 1987

Wiltbank TB, Sine HE, Brody BB: Are emergency toxicology measurements really used? Clin Chem 20:116–120, 1974

Winick C: Epidemiology, in Substance Abuse: A Comprehensive Textbook, 3rd Edition. Edited by Lowinson J, Ruiz P, Millman R, et al. Baltimore, MD, Lippincott Williams & Wilkins, 1997, p 13

Woods JH, Katz JL, Winger G: Use and abuse of benzodiazepines. JAMA 260:3476–3480, 1988

Worthington JJ, Pollack MH, Otto MW, et al: Panic disorder in emergency ward patients with chest pain. J Nerv Ment Dis 185:274–276, 1997

Wulsin LR, Arnold LM, Hillard JR: Axis I disorders in ER patients with atypical chest pain. Int J Psychiatry Med 21:37–46, 1991

Zealberg JJ, Santos AB, Fisher RK: Benefits of mobile crisis programs. Hospital and Community Psychiatry 44:16–17, 1993

Zimberg S: Alcoholism: prevalence in general hospital emergency room and walk-in clinic. N Y State J Med 79:1533–1536, 1979

40

The Primary Care Clinic

Gregory E. Simon, M.D., M.P.H.

Edward A. Walker, M.D.

The 1990s brought significant changes in the organization and the delivery of health care. Several of these changes reinforce the need to provide psychiatric consultation to physicians and patients in outpatient medical clinics.

One of the most striking changes in health care during the 1990s was the shift from inpatient to outpatient delivery of services. Insurers and government payers have made vigorous attempts to reduce inpatient expenditures through mechanisms such as prospective payment and concurrent utilization review. The proportion of the insured population subject to some type of managed care arrangement has increased steadily. Technological advances have allowed many diagnostic and surgical procedures to move from inpatient wards to outpatient facilities. Together, these cost-control strategies and technological advances have led to dramatic decreases in hospitalization rates and length of stay. The emphasis of hospitalization has shifted toward rapid diagnosis and acute stabilization, with recovery and follow-up relegated to the outpatient clinic. This approach sometimes leads to deferral of psychiatric assessment and treatment until after hospital discharge.

Concern about rising health care costs has led to an increasing focus on the economic impact of psychiatric disorders and the economic value of psychiatric care. Arguments for increased funding of psychiatric services often hinge on the cost-offset effect of mental health treatment. The outpatient medical clinic is one of the principal sites where such an effect could be realized. The influence of psychiatric disorders on health care utilization (Simon et al. 1995; Unutzer et al. 1997), functional disability and lost productivity (Ormel et al. 1994; Spitzer et al. 1995), and mortality (Frasure-Smith et al. 1993; Morris et al. 1993) suggests the potential economic impact of effective psychiatric treatment.

In addition, gatekeeper arrangements designed to manage specialty care costs encourage (or require) initial management of psychiatric conditions by primary care providers. As these arrangements become more prevalent, an increasing portion of the care of anxiety and depressive disorders occurs in medical clinics. Many patients seen in outpatient psychiatric clinics have been filtered through the primary care clinic.

These changes in hospital utilization and outpatient referral patterns are shifting the focus of consultation-liaison psychiatry to the outpatient setting. Both psychiatric and nonpsychiatric physicians will encounter larger numbers of psychiatrically ill patients in primary care clinics, and the burden of care for these patients will require new models of psychiatry–primary care collaboration. In this chapter, we highlight many of the features of effective primary care mental health consultation programs and suggest ways to enhance the development of a collaborative liaison with primary care providers in an outpatient setting. This chapter was written for psychiatrists who are looking for new models of practice in managed care and for primary care providers who are seeking to provide better mental health care by collaborating with psychiatric consultants.

EPIDEMIOLOGY OF PSYCHIATRIC DISORDERS IN PRIMARY CARE

Even before the recent shift from inpatient care, health professionals in primary care clinics were the most frequent providers of outpatient mental health treatment. In community samples, fewer than 25% of patients with psychiatric disorders see specialty mental health providers; the majority of patients are seen in primary care settings (Regier et al. 1993). Epidemiologic surveys in primary care typically show that 10%–15% of primary care patients have well-defined anxiety or depressive disorders

(Spitzer et al. 1994; Ustun and Sartorius 1995). Psychiatric disorders in primary care are associated with a significant burden of disability (Ormel et al. 1994; Spitzer et al. 1995). According to physician surveys, half of physician visits by patients with explicit psychiatric diagnoses occur in primary care clinics (Schurman et al. 1985); this proportion excludes primary care patients who present with physical symptoms. Primary care physicians write the majority of prescriptions for antidepressant (Simon et al. 1993) and anxiolytic medications (Mellinger et al. 1984).

EFFECTIVENESS OF CONSULTATION-LIAISON PROGRAMS

Several randomized trials have examined the effectiveness of primary care–based consultation-liaison programs. Schulberg et al. (1996) studied the effectiveness of organized pharmacotherapy and psychotherapy programs provided in the primary care clinic by consulting specialists (or specially trained primary care providers). Katon et al. (1995, 1996) studied two different models of collaborative care in which primary care physicians and on-site consultants shared responsibility for patient care. Katzelnick et al. (1998) evaluated a stepped-care approach including active psychiatric liaison and direct consultation for patients not responding to initial primary care treatment. When tested in samples of primary care patients with major depression, each of these programs significantly improved both quality of depression treatment and clinical outcomes. It is instructive to contrast these successful consultation-liaison models with other less intensive (and less successful) programs. Examples of these unsuccessful programs include physician training (Lin et al. 1997), academic detailing (Goldberg et al. 1998), and feedback of recommendations based on screening or single-session psychiatric consultation (Callahan et al. 1994; Katon et al. 1992). Considered together, this group of studies suggests that an effective consultation-liaison program must include more than education and advice. Consultants' ongoing involvement in care seems necessary to improve patient outcomes.

OUTPATIENT CONSULTATION-LIAISON PSYCHIATRY SETTINGS

During the 1990s, psychiatric consultation-liaison programs in primary care spread to a broad range of practice settings. Several publications described this increasing diversity. The range of successful programs includes both academic (Camara 1991; Nickels and McIntyre 1996) and community (Kates et al. 1997a, 1997b) practice; urban (Turner and de Sorkin 1997) and rural (Lambert and Hartley 1998) clinics; adult and pediatric (Showalter and Solnit 1998) populations; and programs in Canada (Kates et al. 1997a; Turner and de Sorkin 1997), Israel (Weingarten and Granek 1998), Australia (Carr et al. 1997), and the United Kingdom (Tyrer et al. 1990; Warner et al. 1993). We describe in this section some organizational and clinical issues relevant to specific types of outpatient settings.

Training Clinics

Training clinics for internal medicine or family medicine residents have been among the most common sites for formal outpatient psychiatric consultation-liaison programs. In such programs, consulting psychiatrists typically have both clinical and educational roles. In addition to providing consultation for specific patients, the consultant may also participate in seminars, didactic presentations, or case conferences as part of the residency training curriculum.

Primary Care Group Practices

One consequence of recent consolidation in health care has been the increasing organization of primary care physicians into group practices. Increasingly, these group practices share more than office space; they also share clinical (and possibly financial) responsibility for large, defined patient populations. Primary care group practices are one of the most natural environments for outpatient consultation-liaison programs. Existing referral patterns can eventually develop into true collaborative practice arrangements. The evolution of more formal collaborative practice will depend on the enthusiasm of the participating physicians (from primary care and psychiatry) as well as the development of financial structures that support liaison activities and collaborative practice (see "Financing" section later in the chapter).

Outpatient Medical Specialty Clinics

Some large medical specialty groups may have sufficient need for psychiatric consultation to justify establishing a formal consultation-liaison program. Within tertiary care medical centers, medical and surgical specialists may continue to account for the bulk of outpatient care and the bulk of referrals for outpatient psychiatric consultation (Camara 1991). Although most of the discussion in this chapter refers to primary care clinics and providers, most of the organizational and clinical issues are equally relevant to medical specialty clinic referrals. Some medical specialty populations involve unique clinical issues that are discussed in detail in other chapters of Section III in this volume.

STRUCTURE OF AN OUTPATIENT PSYCHIATRIC CONSULTATION-LIAISON PROGRAM

Location

For patients, availability of psychiatric consultation within the primary care clinic is more than an issue of convenience. Even when the psychiatric clinic is down the hall or up one floor, the psychological distance between the familiar primary care clinic and the often unfamiliar psychiatric clinic can be a real barrier. Patients who view their problems as strictly medical are less likely to resist a referral for psychiatric consultation when it occurs within the medical clinic.

For referring physicians, the presence of a consulting psychiatrist in the clinic, even part time, significantly increases opportunities for communication and follow-up. Consultants' recommendations have much greater clinical and educational impact when delivered face to face. Regular contact in the primary care clinic allows follow-up discussions regarding ongoing management. Personal contact also greatly increases the ease of curbside consultations (brief, informal consultation occurring in person, by telephone, or by electronic mail) and informal discussions regarding patients who may not require a formal consultation.

For consulting psychiatrists, work in the primary care clinic is an immersion in the culture of primary care. Working alongside general medical colleagues leads to a much clearer understanding of the prevalence of psychological problems in primary care patients and the interventions possible in primary care practice. Consulting psychiatrists soon realize the personal understanding and therapeutic leverage that primary care physicians develop when the doctor-patient relationship extends over many years (and sometimes many family members).

Referral

Effective referral involves clear communication with both the patient and the consulting psychiatrist. Patients should understand the reason for psychiatric consultation, the questions to be addressed, and the anticipated plan for continued care. Without this preparation, some patients may misinterpret referral as rejection. Communication with the psychiatric consultant should summarize relevant history, state the question to be addressed by consultation, and indicate the primary care physician's expectations about subsequent management (e.g., will the consultation-liaison psychiatrist or the referring physician maintain primary responsibility for follow-up?). A written referral note is the basic requirement, but personal communication significantly increases the value of the consultation. The consultant's presence in the primary care clinic facilitates face-to-face communication regarding the consultation request.

Consultation Visit

An evaluation visit typically begins with clarification of goals and expectations. The consultant should ask about the patient's understanding of the reason for referral and the expected outcome of the consultation. Any clear conflict between the views of the patient and those of the referring physician should be explored. Such conflicts may involve different explanatory models for the patient's symptoms (e.g., "The doctor thinks it's all in my head") or a conflict about appropriate management (e.g., "The doctor said I had to see you before I could have any more pain pills"). The consultant's role is not to resolve immediately such disagreements but to understand potential sources of difficulty.

The focus of a consultation assessment should be guided by the consultation request. In contrast to the clean slate of a more generic outpatient psychiatric evaluation, the psychiatric consultation requires that the psychiatrist step into an evaluation and treatment already in progress. The consultation assessment is often focused on a specific question. The referring primary care physician may have completed an assessment, initiated a treatment process, and requested help with a particular management decision (e.g., should an antidepressant be prescribed?). In some cases, the consultant may anticipate a relatively circumscribed role. Depending on the referring physician's request, the consultant may anticipate that only one or two visits will be necessary. The consultant must also consider, however, that the referring provider may have been unaware of important issues that will influence treatment. For example, the presence of a personality disorder may strongly influence the treatment of depression. A history of childhood abuse may influence a patient's ability to form a trusting alliance with both medical and psychiatric providers. These and other complicating issues may necessitate a greater intensity of psychotherapeutic treatment.

Conjoint visits involving the patient, primary care physician, and consulting psychiatrist are sometimes quite useful. When consultation involves negotiation around conflict-laden issues (e.g., chronic use of narcotic analgesics), conjoint meetings may be essential. Outside of training settings, however, conjoint visits may be difficult to arrange. Coordination of both providers' schedules is a real logistical hurdle.

Follow-Up

Frequency and duration of psychiatric follow-up will vary widely, depending on patient needs. Many patients benefit from one or two consultation visits followed by management recommendations to the primary care physician. Some patients need a trial period of brief intervention in the primary care clinic followed by either referral back to the primary care physician or transfer of care to the psychiatrist's office. In some cases, the need for transfer to specialty mental health care may be apparent at the initial visit. In a description of the outpatient consultation experience in a tertiary care center, Camara (1991) reported relatively high rates of referral to specialty mental health care. In our experience among primary care patients, the number of patients requiring specialized mental health follow-up is considerably lower. In most cases, the psychiatric specialist can remain in the role of consultant, with the responsibility for ongoing management remaining with the primary care physician.

A period of shared follow-up with the primary care physician allows ongoing psychiatric follow-up while maintaining the involvement of the primary care physician. During the initial phases of treatment (e.g., beginning antidepressant therapy), alternating visits between psychiatrist and primary care physician for 4–6 weeks takes advantage of specialist expertise and the ongoing alliance with the referring physician.

Some patients require chronic but infrequent psychiatric care. Patients with recurring or episodic psychiatric conditions (e.g., recurrent depression of moderate severity) may require brief psychiatric consultation during exacerbations of illness. These patients may return to the referring physician after initial evaluation and stabilization but return to the psychiatric consultant months or years later during another episode of illness. This model of care fits best for patients with medical conditions that require ongoing primary care management. Because such patients already require regular primary care follow-up, monitoring a psychiatric condition (e.g., maintenance antidepressant therapy) can be integrated easily into overall medical care.

The primary care clinic is rarely the best setting for ongoing psychotherapy. Many factors that favor consultation in the primary care setting may conflict with a more

traditional psychotherapeutic relationship: briefer visits, less strict confidentiality, and a less structured treatment frame with respect to scheduling. If ongoing psychotherapy is indicated, transfer to the specialty mental health clinic is usually preferable.

Communication Following Consultation

If possible, the consultant's assessment and recommendations should be communicated in person. A conversation about future management (whether face to face or over the telephone) is far more informative than a written report. Personal communication following the initial visit also establishes a precedent for curbside consultation during subsequent management. In training settings, more detailed discussions about management allow teaching based on clinical experience.

Consultants must remember that the primary care outpatient record is a relatively public document. Compared with the psychiatrist's office record, the primary care record has a relatively broad circulation. Notes about consultation visits are available not only to the referring primary care physician but also to other medical providers involved in the patient's care (including other medical specialists, nurses, and physical therapists). Patients usually prefer that more personal or confidential information revealed during consultation not be widely distributed. If confidential information is relevant to primary care management, the consultant may choose to discuss such issues with the referring physician directly. In some cases, psychiatric consultation records may be maintained separately from the general outpatient record.

Continuity

Much of the cumulative effect of clinic-based consultation comes from ongoing collaboration between the consulting psychiatrist and the referring primary care physician. A continuous collaborative relationship allows primary care physicians to refer patients with greater confidence. Over time, consulting psychiatrists develop a clearer understanding of the skills and interests of individual primary care physicians. In training settings, collaborative work on a series of similar clinical situations allows trainees to learn more subtle tailoring of treatment.

Service Planning

Typical consultation-liaison programs are designed to provide initial evaluation for all patients and brief treatment for many. Some programs may provide longer-term care in the primary care clinic, whereas in others, patients who require longer-term care will be referred to more traditional outpatient psychiatric settings. Staffing levels for an outpatient psychiatric consultation-liaison service directed at shorter-term care should be adequate to provide initial consultation within 1 week of referral as well as an average of one to two follow-up visits for each patient referred. A typical primary care clinic of 10 physicians (15,000–20,000 patients) might generate three to four new consultation requests per week.

Financing

It is not coincidental that primary care consultation-liaison programs have developed most easily in large prepaid health plans or national health systems. Several common attributes of these settings (prepaid financing, salaried physicians, common financial responsibility for general medical and mental health care) facilitate the development of collaborative practice models. Different financial and structural arrangements can complicate the development of consultation-liaison programs. Fee-for-service payment systems create little incentive for providers (psychiatrists or primary care physicians) to spend time in nonbillable activities (e.g., conjoint visits, curbside consultation). Collaborative practice is difficult to establish under carve-out arrangements, which separate general medical and psychiatric care (both clinically and financially). In many settings, a single primary care physician may be responsible for patients from several different managed care organizations, each of which has its distinct panel of psychiatric consultants. Physicians attempting to establish an outpatient consultation-liaison program must assess which elements of such a program are feasible under any specific financing arrangement.

ROLES AND EXPECTATIONS

Consultant

The role of consultant differs significantly from that of sole provider. First, the consulting psychiatrist is expected to respond to the needs and requests of both the patient and the referring physician. Second, the consultant typically has narrow clinical responsibility. Although some patients may receive ongoing specialty mental health care, most will return to the care of the referring physician.

A consultant's satisfaction with outpatient consultation work will be greatly enhanced by flexibility, an eclectic clinical approach, and a willingness to work with a wide range of patients and physicians. Unlike what occurs in most outpatient practices, the outpatient consultant in primary care settings will have little ability to choose referrals that promise the best fit, clinically and interpersonally. Referring physicians typically prefer a single referral destination for the wide range of problems presenting in outpatient clinics. Consultants should also expect that referring providers will differ widely in knowledge about and attitudes toward psychiatric problems.

Consultants should be prepared to adjust the level of service required according to the clinical situation. The consultant may have the greatest overall effect on patients he or she never actually meets. The training effects of consultation-liaison work can magnify the effects of consultation far beyond those produced by direct clinical contact (Carr et al. 1997). In a large number of cases, the primary care physician may request and need nothing more than a telephone or other curbside consultation (Kates et al. 1997b). Most consultation requests can be effectively addressed by a small number of visits. In a significant minority of cases, ongoing specialty management (including transfer to the specialty clinic) is most appropriate.

Working effectively as a consultant in primary care often requires a shift away from the traditional psychiatric treatment paradigm. Consultation more often emphasizes brief and focused intervention. In the majority of cases, the consultant is less focused on developing a long-term therapeutic alliance with the patient than on bolstering his or her alliance with the primary care physician. Effective consultants must translate the concepts of psychiatric diagnosis and treatment into language that is understandable and useful to the primary care provider. In addition, the collaborative nature of consultation occasionally requires a more complex view of confidentiality than is typical of outpatient psychiatric practice (see "Communication Following Consultation" section, earlier).

Primary Care Physician

Effective collaborative management by the primary care provider and the consulting psychiatrist requires active participation from the referring physician. In contrast to the transfer of responsibility that occurs in a traditional referral to a medical or psychiatric specialist, the typical referral to a consultation-liaison psychiatrist in primary care involves the primary care physician sharing in the initial management of the patient's condition and the resumption of full responsibility after brief involvement by the psychiatric consultant. For most primary care physicians, this higher level of involvement is a welcome change. Some primary care physicians, however, may view psychiatric treatment as too complex or may see psychological problems as lying outside the scope of primary care. For those physicians, a more traditional referral for ongoing management by a psychiatrist may be preferable.

Patient

Most primary care patients are more accustomed to a medical treatment model than to a psychotherapeutic treatment model. Patients in medical clinics are more likely to have prior experience with consulting medical specialists than with mental health providers. Structured assessment followed by instruction and advice often fits well with these patients' experiences, desires, and expectations.

Clarity about the time-limited nature of consultation will help avoid misunderstanding or disappointment. The initial visit should establish the goal of assessment and treatment recommendations for the referring physician. In many cases, the primary care physician will be responsible for long-term management. Patients who need or desire ongoing psychotherapy are often best served by referral or transfer to the psychiatric outpatient clinic.

LIAISON ACTIVITIES

Involvement in liaison activities will vary widely, depending on clinical setting and stage of development of the consultation program. Seminars, case conferences, and other activities involving clinic staff are usually part of consultation in training clinics but are variably present in other settings. Outside of training clinics, the initial stages of a consultation-liaison program typically focus on direct clinical service to patients. Broader involvement often comes with the development of collaborative relationships over time. Individual primary care physicians also vary widely in their motivation to participate in liaison activities.

CLINICAL ISSUES

Functional Somatic Symptoms

Medically unexplained physical symptoms are a frequent reason for psychiatric consultation in outpatient clinics. In some cases, such symptoms may be indicators of a well-defined depressive or anxiety disorder (Ormel et al. 1991). Some patients may present with physical symptoms related to major life stresses. In other cases, however, unexplained physical symptoms are part of an overall pattern of repeated physical symptoms without

medical explanation (Barsky 1992). Although most of these patients' conditions would not satisfy diagnostic criteria for somatization disorder, this syndrome of subthreshold somatization is associated with substantial morbidity and use of health services (Escobar et al. 1987; Gureje et al. 1997). These patients appear to have a generalized increase in sensitivity to noxious physical sensations and a tendency to attribute common somatic sensations to medical illness (Barsky 1992).

Outpatient psychiatric consultation for the patient who somatizes should focus on reducing symptoms and restoring function. If a well-defined anxiety or depressive disorder is present, specific treatment is likely to relieve the associated physical symptoms. When physical symptoms accompany major life stresses, support and encouragement are often sufficient. The consulting psychiatrist must acknowledge and legitimize the presenting physical symptoms while gently shifting the agenda to precipitating stresses (Goldberg et al. 1989). For chronically symptom-sensitive patients, treatment includes attention to both physical symptoms and disease fears (Barsky et al. 1988). Relaxation training can reduce anxiety-related symptoms and allow patients to divert attention away from bothersome physical sensations. Regular exercise can help to desensitize patients to somatic sensations by demonstrating that major physical changes (e.g., rapid heart rate, shortness of breath) are usually the result of benign or even desirable causes. Exploration of disease fears can help patients to identify and challenge exaggerated or catastrophic thoughts.

Work in the primary care setting allows the consulting psychiatrist a longitudinal view of symptom-sensitive patients. Review of the medical record often reveals prior episodes with different physical presentations. Effective consultation helps primary care physicians to recognize this pattern. The consultant should also help patients to anticipate symptoms that might occur at times of stress. Patients can learn to see physical symptoms as early warning signs that indicate the need to reactivate the self-care skills learned in consultation visits.

Depressive Disorders

Depression is among the most common psychiatric conditions seen in primary care and is among the most common of all chronic conditions in medical practice. Compared with patients who have depression and are seen in psychiatric clinics, patients who have depression and are seen in primary care settings show less severe illness and may be more likely to present with physical symptoms (Blacker and Clare 1987). Primary care patients with depression are also older and are more likely to have comorbid medical conditions than are psychiatric outpatients with depression.

The research literature suggests significant shortcomings in the current treatment of primary care patients with depression. First, depression in patients who present in a primary care setting may go unrecognized. Surveys using structured interviews and formal diagnostic criteria typically show current major depression in 6%–8% of consecutive primary care patients, with 40%–50% of those not recognized by the treating primary care physician (Ormel et al. 1990; Schulberg et al. 1985; Ustun and Sartorius 1995; VonKorff et al. 1987). In addition, recognition of depression or psychological distress does not always lead to initiation of effective treatment (Katz et al. 1998; Schulberg et al. 1997; Wells et al. 1994). Among patients treated with antidepressant medications, only a minority receive recommended doses of medication for a sufficient period of time (Simon et al. 1993; Wells et al. 1994). As mentioned earlier, clinical trials have demonstrated that appropriate use of psychiatric consultation in primary care can address these shortcomings. Systematic screening for depression can improve patient outcomes—if such screening is followed by appropriate treatment (Katzelnick et al. 1998; Schulberg et al. 1996). Effective consultation programs can improve the quality of pharmacotherapy and the consistency of follow-up care (Katon et al. 1995, 1996). These primary care consultation models can significantly improve patients' outcomes at reasonable cost (Lave et al. 1998; VonKorff et al. 1998). We suggest, however, that consultants take care about criticizing the treatment practices of primary care colleagues. Such criticism certainly will not foster collegial relationships. In fact, available data suggest some similar shortcomings in the management of depression by psychiatrists (Keller et al. 1986; Simon et al. 1993). We suspect that gaps in primary care management of depression are often consequences of the heavy workload and competing demands of primary care practice rather than deficiencies in physicians' knowledge or motivation.

Primary care–based treatment of depression usually emphasizes antidepressant medication over psychotherapy. Given the skills and training of primary care physicians and the time constraints of primary care practice, counseling during the primary care visit is limited to brief support and advice. Even brief visits with the psychiatric consultant, however, typically include limited psychotherapeutic intervention. Advice from the consulting psychiatrist will help primary care physicians to use their limited time more effectively. Brief, focused interventions by primary care staff may offer significant benefit (Klerman et al. 1987; Mynors-Wallis et al. 1995).

Continued coordination with the primary care physician is critical. Primary care patients who begin treatment with antidepressant medication often discontinue treatment during the first few weeks. Advice to both the patient and the primary care physician about managing common side effects may improve adherence to the treatment plan. Patients should be advised to contact the primary care physician or consulting psychiatrist before stopping antidepressant medication. Given the significant risk for recurrence of depressive illness, the consultant must encourage the patient and the primary care physician to develop a plan for responding to signs of recurrence.

Anxiety Disorders

Panic attacks and generalized anxiety are common in all outpatient clinics and are especially prevalent in certain clinical groups. Symptoms of anxiety are easily mistaken for those of cardiac arrhythmia, asthma, coronary disease, vertigo, cerebrovascular disease, or an endocrine disorder. Consequently, patients with anxiety disorders are frequently referred for expensive and unnecessary examinations such as ambulatory electrocardiographic monitoring, cardiac catheterization, or testing for pheochromocytoma. The effect of panic disorder on medical utilization is as great as or greater than the effect of depression (Salvador-Carulla et al. 1995; Simon 1992). The consulting psychiatrist can prevent this unnecessary medical utilization by increasing physicians' sensitivity to anxiety diagnoses.

Because primary care patients with anxiety disorders frequently present with physical complaints, treatment should address physical symptom relief. Breath control and relaxation training are often quite effective in relieving dyspnea, dizziness, or chest pains that accompany anxiety. Enteroceptive exposure exercises (i.e., intentionally recreating the feared physical sensation) can be remarkably effective in desensitizing patients to somatic symptoms such as palpitations or dizziness. For some patients, aerobic exercise is a simple self-administered enteroceptive exposure program. Psychoeducational and cognitive interventions can address the exaggerated disease fears that can accompany anxiety. Behavioral treatments should include efforts to reduce unnecessary health care use (e.g., emergency room visits) as a response to anxiety symptoms. It can be helpful to discuss frequent physician visits as part of an overall pattern of anxiety-related checking behaviors (e.g., pulse taking, frequent blood pressure checks).

Substance Use Disorders

Alcohol is the most common drug of abuse among patients in most primary care settings. Epidemiologic studies show alcohol abuse among 5%–15% of primary care patients, with higher prevalence rates in urban clinics serving patients from lower socioeconomic groups (Johnson et al. 1995). Psychiatric consultants must always consider alcohol abuse or dependence as a possible cause of anxiety or depressive symptoms. Effective treatment or referral of patients with alcoholism requires close collaboration between the consultant and the primary care physician. Both physicians must clearly point out the medical, psychological, and social consequences of continued alcohol use. Brief counseling interventions in the primary care clinic can reduce problematic alcohol use (Fleming et al. 1997).

SUMMARY

Changes in the United States health care system have had far-reaching effects on the delivery of general medical and mental health care. As the site of care has shifted to the outpatient clinic, psychiatrists have increasingly been asked to provide consultative support to primary care and other outpatient medical providers. Consultation-liaison psychiatrists are ideally trained to assist in the evaluation of primary care patients and the development of integrated biopsychosocial treatment in outpatient medical clinics.

For many consultation-liaison psychiatrists, these changes will necessitate a major change in practice and employment of new skills. The emphasis will likely shift from practice based in the hospital ward and psychiatric clinic to a collaborative practice located directly in the primary care clinic. Lengthy diagnostic assessment will be supplanted by rapid, focused assessments. Many patients will have comorbid medical illness that may complicate management. Psychiatric consultants will have to develop treatment plans that are brief and practical and that accommodate the limitations of primary care providers.

REFERENCES

Barsky A: Amplification, somatization, and the somatoform disorders. Psychosomatics 33:28–34, 1992

Barsky A, Geringer E, Wool CA: A cognitive-educational treatment for hypochondriasis. Gen Hosp Psychiatry 10:322–327, 1988

Blacker C, Clare AW: Depressive disorders in primary care. Br J Psychiatry 150:737–751, 1987

Callahan CM, Hendrie HC, Dittus RS, et al: Improving treatment of late life depression in primary care: a randomized clinical trial. J Am Geriatric Soc 42:839–846, 1994

Camara EG: A psychiatric outpatient consultation-liaison clinic. Psychosomatics 32:304–308, 1991

Carr VJ, Faehrmann C, Lewin TJ, et al: Determining the effect that consultation-liaison psychiatry in primary care has on family physician's psychiatric knowledge and practice. Psychosomatics 38:217–219, 1997

Escobar JI, Burnam MA, Karno M, et al: Somatization in the community. Arch Gen Psychiatry 44:713–718, 1987

Fleming MF, Barry KL, Manwell LB, et al: Brief physician advice for problem alcohol drinkers: a randomized controlled trial in community-based primary care practices. JAMA 277:1039–1045, 1997

Frasure-Smith N, Lesperance F, Talajic M: Depression following myocardial infarction: impact on 6-month survival. JAMA 270:1819–1825, 1993

Goldberg D, Gask L, O'Dowd T: The treatment of somatization: teaching techniques of reattribution. J Psychosom Res 33:689–695, 1989

Goldberg HI, Wagner EH, Fihn SD, et al: A randomized controlled trial of academic detailing techniques and continuous quality improvement teams: increasing compliance with national guidelines for the primary care of hypertension and depression. Joint Commission Journal on Quality Improvement 24:130–142, 1998

Gureje O, Simon G, Ustun B: The syndrome of hypochondriasis: a cross-national study in primary care. Psychol Med 27:1001–1010, 1997

Johnson J, Spitzer RL, Williams JB, et al: Psychiatric comorbidity, health status, and functional impairment associated with alcohol abuse and dependence in primary care patients: findings of the PRIME-MD 1000 study. J Consult Clin Psychol 63:133–140, 1995

Kates N, Craven M, Crustolo AM, et al: Integrating mental health services within primary care: a Canadian program. Gen Hosp Psychiatry 19:324–332, 1997a

Kates N, Crustolo AM, Nikolaou L, et al: Providing backup to family physicians by telephone. Can J Psychiatry 42:955–959, 1997b

Katon W, VonKorff M, Lin E, et al: A randomized trial of psychiatric consultation with distressed high utilizers. Gen Hosp Psychiatry 14:86–98, 1992

Katon W, VonKorff M, Lin E, et al: Collaborative management to achieve treatment guidelines: impact on depression in primary care. JAMA 273:1026–1031, 1995

Katon W, Robinson P, VonKorff M, et al: A multifaceted intervention to improve treatment of depression in primary care. Arch Gen Psychiatry 53:924–932, 1996

Katz S, Kessler R, Lin E, et al: Medication management of depression in the United States and Canada. J Gen Intern Med 13:77–85, 1998

Katzelnick DJ, Simon GE, Pearson SD, et al: Randomized trial of a depression management program in high utilizers of medical care. Paper presented at the twelfth annual International National Institute of Mental Health Conference on Mental Health Problems in the General Health Care Sector, Baltimore, MD, July 13–14, 1998

Keller MB, Lavori PW, Klerman GL, et al: Low levels and lack of predictors of somatotherapy and psychotherapy received by depressed patients. Arch Gen Psychiatry 43: 458–466, 1986

Klerman G, Budman S, Berwick D, et al: Efficacy of a brief psychosocial intervention for symptoms of stress and distress among patients in primary care. Med Care 25:1078–1088, 1987

Lambert D, Hartley D: Linking primary care and rural psychiatry: where have we been and where are we going? Psychiatry Serv 49:965–967, 1998

Lave J, Frank R, Schulberg H, et al: Cost-effectiveness of treatments for major depression in primary care practice. Arch Gen Psychiatry 55:645–651, 1998

Lin E, Katon W, Simon G, et al: Achieving guidelines for the treatment of depression in primary care: is physician education enough? Med Care 35:831–842, 1997

Mellinger G, Balter M, Uhlenhuth E: Prevalence and correlates of the long-term regular use of anxiolytics. JAMA 251:375–379, 1984

Morris P, Robinson RG, Samuels J: Depression, introversion, and mortality following stroke. Aust N Z J Psychiatry 24:443–449, 1993

Mynors-Wallis L, Gath DH, Lloyd-Thomas AR, et al: Randomized controlled trial comparing problem solving treatment with amitriptyline and placebo for major depression in primary care. BMJ 310:441–445, 1995

Nickels MW, McIntyre JS: A model for psychiatric services in primary care settings. Psychiatry Serv 47:522–526, 1996

Ormel J, vandenBrink W, Koeter MW, et al: Recognition, management, and outcome of psychological disorders in primary care: a naturalistic follow-up study. Psychol Med 20:909–923, 1990

Ormel J, Koeter MW, vandenBrink W, et al: Recognition, management, and course of anxiety and depression in general practice. Arch Gen Psychiatry 48:700–706, 1991

Ormel J, VonKorff M, Ustun TB, et al: Common mental disorders and disability across cultures: results from the WHO Collaborative Study on Psychological Problems in General Health Care. JAMA 272:1741–1748, 1994

Regier D, Narrow WE, Rae DS, et al: The de facto US mental and addictive disorders service system: Epidemiologic Catchment Area prospective 1-year prevalence rates of disorders and services. Arch Gen Psychiatry 50:85–94, 1993

Salvador-Carulla L, Segui J, Fernandez-Cano P, et al: Costs and offset effect in panic disorder. Br J Psychiatry 166 (suppl 27):23–28, 1995

Schulberg HC, Saul M, McClelland M, et al: Assessing depression in primary medical and psychiatric practices. Arch Gen Psychiatry 42:1164–1170, 1985

Schulberg HC, Block MR, Madonia MJ, et al: Treating major depression in primary care practice: eight-month clinical outcomes. Arch Gen Psychiatry 53:913–919, 1996

Schulberg H, Block M, Madonia M, et al: The "usual care" of major depression in primary care practice. Arch Fam Med 6:334–339, 1997

Schurman RA, Kramer PD, Mitchell JB: The hidden mental health network: treatment of mental illness by nonpsychiatrist physicians. Arch Gen Psychiatry 42:89–94, 1985

Showalter JE, Solnit AJ: Working with the primary care physician. Child Adolesc Psychiatr Clin N Am 7:599–613, 1998

Simon G: Psychiatric disorder and functional somatic symptoms as predictors of health care use. Psychiatr Med 10:49–60, 1992

Simon G, VonKorff M: Somatization and psychiatric disorder in the NIMH Epidemiologic Catchment Area Study. Am J Psychiatry 148:1494–1500, 1991

Simon G, VonKorff M, Wagner EH, et al: Patterns of antidepressant use in community practice. Gen Hosp Psychiatry 15:399–408, 1993

Simon GE, Ormel J, VonKorff M, et al: Health care costs associated with depressive and anxiety disorders in primary care. Am J Psychiatry 152:352–357, 1995

Spitzer RL, Williams JB, Kroenke K, et al: Utility of a new procedure for diagnosing mental disorders in primary care: the PRIME-MD 1000 study. JAMA 272:1749–1756, 1994

Spitzer RL, Kroenke K, Linzer M, et al: Health-related quality of life in primary care patients with mental disorders: results from the PRIME-MD 1000 Study. JAMA 274:1511–1517, 1995

Turner T, de Sorkin A: Sharing psychiatric care with primary care physicians: the Toronto Doctors Hospital experience (1991–1995). Can J Psychiatry 42:950–954, 1997

Tyrer P, Ferguson B, Wadsworth J: Liaison psychiatry in general practice: the comprehensive collaborative model. Acta Psychiatr Scand 81:359–363, 1990

Unutzer JU, Patrick D, Simon G, et al: Depressive symptoms and the use of health services in HMO patients age 65 and over: a four-year prospective study. JAMA 277:1618–1623, 1997

Ustun TB, Sartorius N: Mental Illness in General Health Care. New York: Wiley, 1995

VonKorff M, Shapiro S, Burke JD, et al: Anxiety and depression in a primary care clinic: comparison of Diagnostic Interview Schedule, General Health Questionnaire, and practitioner assessments. Arch Gen Psychiatry 44:152–156, 1987

VonKorff M, Katon W, Bush T, et al: Treatment costs, cost offset, and cost-effectiveness of collaborative management of depression. Psychosom Med 60:143–149, 1998

Warner RW, Gater R, Jackson MG, et al: Effects of a community mental health service on the practice and attitudes of general practitioners. Br J Gen Pract 43:507–511, 1993

Weingarten M, Granek M: Psychiatric liaison with a primary care clinic—14 years' experience. Isr J Psychiatry Relat Sci 35:81–88, 1998

Wells K, Katon W, Rogers B, et al: Use of minor tranquilizers and antidepressant medications by depressed outpatients: results from the Medical Outcomes Study. Am J Psychiatry 151:694–700, 1994

41

Telepsychiatry

Brian J. Grady, M.D.

[T]he first published application of telemedicine in any specialty was in psychiatry.

Baer et al. (1997)

The term *telepsychiatry* was first used by Dwyer (1973) to describe "psychiatric consultation via interactive television." Although telepsychiatry is a novel term for the practice of psychiatric consultation at a distance, Dwyer was neither the first nor the last to integrate communications technologies with psychiatric practice. Today, with the advent of electronic mail (e-mail) and the proliferation of the Internet, the definition of telepsychiatry has expanded. A consultation-liaison psychiatrist must have a good understanding of the benefits, limitations, and risks of these new approaches and their effects on patients. This chapter familiarizes the reader with the history and development, practice, technical aspects, and current applications of information technologies in mental health care.

HISTORY AND DEVELOPMENT OF TELEPSYCHIATRY

The development of telepsychiatry can be divided into three periods. The first period was that of interactive television, from 1959 to the late 1980s. This period included the use of radio transmission, cable, and closed-circuit systems to transmit a two-way television picture. Television, however, required significant equipment and maintenance expenditures to keep the "studio" operational. Not until the 1990s did computer technology and data compression devices become widely available. These developments spurred a second historical period, that of affordable videoconferencing. Equally important in maintaining affordability was the expansion of commercial

telephone company digital communication networks, which improved access and reliability for the business user, the professional user, and the casual user. Although affordable videoconferencing continues to become more accessible, the third and most clinically relevant era of telepsychiatry is just beginning. This period, which parallels traditional medical and mental health care delivery, is most aptly described as evidence-based telepsychiatry. As Sackett and Rosenberg (1995) stated: "The ability to track down, critically appraise (for its validity and usefulness), and incorporate this rapidly growing body of evidence into one's clinical practice has been named 'evidence-based medicine' (EBM)" (p. 620).

Period 1—Interactive Television

The picture telephone had its beginnings in the labs of AT&T in the 1920s as the company merged the technologies of the telephone with the television. In April 1930, from its headquarters in New York City, AT&T provided the first public demonstration of an operational picture telephone. The Picturephone introduced at the 1964 World's Fair was the first digital video telephone. Marketing of the Picturephone was directed at corporate executives, but sales were never realized because executives "had little desire to see one another while using the telephone" (Rosen 1997, p. 16).

In the 1950s, at least one psychiatrist, Cecil Wittson, M.D., became interested in the potential of two-way video technology. Dr. Wittson later headed a pilot project that compared the facilitation of a time-limited psychotherapy group process via two-way television with a traditional face-to-face practice (Wittson et al. 1961). The project, conducted at the Nebraska Psychiatric Institute, consisted of a total of eight groups over a period of six sessions. Four groups were conducted via two-way television, and four were conducted in person. The television picture of the therapists and group members was also broadcast into a third room where Dr. Wittson and others could observe. "Analysis of rating scales and of therapists showed that the choice of therapist and the selection of group members influenced the effectiveness of the therapy more than the use of the TV technique" (Wittson and Benschoter 1972, 136).

In another project, a two-way television link was established between the Nebraska Psychiatric Institute and the Norfolk State Mental Hospital, located 112 miles away. Nursing, psychology, social services, and vocational rehabilitation staff used two-way television for training and education, including weekly grand rounds. Psychiatrists were employed in patient care and ward administration and were thought to contribute to the fall of the inpatient census from 900+ in 1965 to below 500 by the end of 1968. Two-way television was also used to keep patients connected to their families when costs and transportation issues limited travel.

A study by Solow et al. (1971) attempted to reach out to primary care providers in the community. Solow and colleagues established a psychiatric consultative-liaison service with a general hospital located about 26 miles away from Dartmouth Medical School. The purpose of the project was to evaluate "the utility of television as a medium of communication in psychiatric interviewing and consultation at a distance" and "the effectiveness of readily available psychiatric consultation as an educational program for physicians in the community" (Solow et al. 1971). For one year, beginning in December 1968, 12 general practitioners, 1 internist, and 2 psychologists made psychiatric referrals to the medical school. The project called for the referring provider to briefly discuss the case over two-way television with the consultant, who then interviewed the patient alone while the referring provider observed from an adjacent room. After the patient interview, the referring provider returned to the two-way television room to discuss the findings and treatment plan with the consultant. There were 199 consultations, 142 new and 57 follow-up visits. Sixty percent of patients had no prior psychiatric contact, whereas 40% were diagnosed with a psychotic illness. Overall, 90% of patients remained in the community; 70% were managed by their primary care physician and 20% by psychologists at the local mental health clinic. The authors reported high patient acceptance and no significant barrier in establishing rapport. Primary care providers gained knowledge through observation, discussion, and management recommendations that could be generalized to everyday practice.

The period of interactive television demonstrated the potential of two-way television for direct patient care, administration, and education. The principal drawback was cost, which ultimately stalled research and continuing clinical practice of psychiatry from a distance. Maxmen (1978) stated, "Undoubtedly, economic factors are inhibiting the widespread use of telepsychiatry" (p. 452).

Period 2—Affordable Videoconferencing

A technological advance in the 1980s that contributed significantly to the affordability of videoconferencing was the development of real-time digital data compression. Once digitized, audio and video data are compressed (coded) at the originating site and later decompressed (decoded) at the receiving site.

The device that performs the coding and decoding is called a codec. Codecs are ingenious electronic devices designed by engineers to reduce the amount of data (video signal) that needs to be transmitted. One may conceptualize the process this way: once a picture is established, only changes in that picture (e.g., body movement) need be transmitted; the background, provided it is stationary, does not. Similarly, the video picture is made up of columns and rows of data. Each individual data point is called a pixel. Thus, for a blue background, one may collapse a row of blue pixels into a mathematical formula rather than sending the color of each pixel individually—once again reducing the amount of data to be transmitted. Although codecs do a remarkable job, there is a limit to how much the data can be compressed.

The next step is to transmit the signal, via telephone, cable, or satellite networks. The cost of signal transmission depends on the amount of data to be transmitted per unit time, referred to as bandwidth (measured in kbps, kilobits per second). For example, if one uses ISDN (Integrated Services Digital Network) telephone connectivity, bandwidth can be purchased in blocks, starting at 64 kbps. Unfortunately, because of the real-time nature of interactive videoconferencing and the limits of data compression by the codec, any data that cannot fit into the allotted bandwidth is lost, resulting in degradation of the video signal. Currently, as a result of this balance between video quality and cost, telepsychiatry is typically practiced at bandwidths in the range of 128–384 kbps.

In 1994, according to Allen and Wheeler (1998), only 11 telepsychiatry programs were identified: 9 in the

United States and 1 each in Canada and Norway. A 1998 survey revealed 29 active telepsychiatry programs: 25 in the United States and 1 each in Canada, England, Norway, and Australia. The rapid growth of telepsychiatry in the 1990s was made possible by a combination of technological advances and refinements in the telecommunications industry that spurred competition and resulted in improved performance at more reasonable cost. The reduced capital investment and operating costs have, in certain situations, become economically competitive to existing health care delivery systems (B. Grady, "A Comparative Cost Analysis of an Integrated Military TeleMental Healthcare Service," unpublished article, 2001). It is anticipated that continued competition in the telecommunications industry will lead to improvements in the codec and data transmission technology that will continue to make interactive videoconferencing more affordable. Acceptable bandwidths for practicing psychiatry at a distance may also be influenced by the latest period in the development of telepsychiatry, evidence-based telepsychiatry.

Period 3—Evidence-Based Telepsychiatry

With the advent of affordable videoconferencing, telepsychiatry and telepsychiatric literature is flourishing. A new era of telepsychiatry is resulting, one focusing on cost-effective and clinical outcome–based deployment. Research themes include 1) defining the lowest bandwidth necessary to allow accurate psychiatric diagnosis and treatment (the result of the relationship among picture quality, bandwidth, and costs), 2) research into the reliability of rating scales, 3) service delivery, 4) the acceptance of telepsychiatry by patients, providers, and consultants, 5) outcomes, and 6) the patient-provider relationship.

Zarate et al. (1997) investigated bandwidth and its effect on the assessment of three groups of patients with schizophrenia, using the Simultaneous Video Reliability Interview designed by Baer et al. (1995). Group members were interviewed in person, on video at a 128-kbps bandwidth, or on video at a 384-kbps bandwidth. In addition to a standard interview, the researchers used three rating scales—the Brief Psychiatric Rating Scale (BPRS), the Scale for the Assessment of Positive Symptoms (SAPS), and the Scale for the Assessment of Negative Symptoms (SANS). Rater reliability was excellent for the BPRS and the SAPS; however, the reliability of the SANS, though reliable for the in-person group and the higher-bandwidth (384 kbps) group, was poor for the lower-bandwidth (128 kbps) group. The authors hypothesized that negative symptoms of schizophrenia were

more difficult to assess at the lower bandwidth because assessment relies on nonverbal cues. Additionally, they concluded that motion artifact, which is inversely related to bandwidth, may have been interpreted as motor slowing.

Ball et al. (1993) administered the Mini-Mental State Examination (MMSE) over a low-cost videoconferencing system (LCVC), which uses a quarter-screen black-and-white image and high-fidelity sound. The researchers adapted parts of the MMSE for telepsychiatry—for example, having the patient place the paper on his or her head as the final step in the three-step command. They reported a correlation coefficient of 0.89 between the LCVC and face-to-face testing. Montani et al. (1997) assessed the reliability of the MMSE and the Clock Face Test (CFT) in a group of hospitalized elderly patients (mean age of 88 years) via teleconsultation. The mean MMSE scores were 23.7 (for face-to-face examination) and 22.2 (for teleconsultation), resulting in a correlation coefficient of 0.95. The mean CFT scores were 22.4 (face-to-face examination) and 19.8 (teleconsultation), resulting in a correlation coefficient of 0.55. Although the authors were unsure of the effects of interactive video on test performance, their results and those of Ball et al. (1993) appear to indicate that the applicability of the MMSE is greater than than of interactive videoconferencing, whereas the result of the CFT remain inconclusive.

Few clinical outcome studies have examined telepsychiatric practice. Baigent et al. (1997) conducted a controlled study using a semistructured psychiatric interview and various assessment scales. Although the researchers noted differences between face-to-face (FTF) and video teleconference (VTC) interviews (128 kbps), final diagnostic agreement was very good. Zaylor's (1999) retrospective review of telepsychiatry patients (interviewed at 128 kbps) and a control group of face-to-face outpatients noted no significant differences in outcome, based on a statistical analysis of the Global Assessment of Functioning Scale. Elford et al. (2000) conducted a randomized controlled trial of 23 child psychiatric assessments via FTF and VTC. Independent practitioners evaluated each subject by VTC followed by FTF, or by FTF followed by VTC. In 96% of the cases the diagnoses and treatment recommendations were the same in the two groups. Although the psychiatrists preferred FTF evaluation, they felt that the VTC evaluations were adequate and did not affect the diagnoses. Kennedy and Yellowlees (2000) conducted a 2-year evaluation of telepsychiatry in a rural population of Queensland, Australia. The researchers found that there were no significant improvements in well-being or quality of life with VTC augmentation of local services but also concluded that the subjects were no worse off. Ninety-eight percent of the subjects, however, preferred VTC augmentation of onsite services. May et al. (2000) used semistructured informal interviews of 22 patients (with anxiety and depression) and 13 physicians (12 primary care providers and a psychiatrist) for qualitative assessment of a telepsychiatry referral service in northwest England. The interviews were conducted within 3 days following the use of a desktop videoconferencing system (128 kbps) for remote telepsychiatry services. Results indicated a significant amount of ambivalence from patients and general physicians about the use of VTC, particularly in regard to the medium's effect on the interaction and relationship between the patient and the psychiatrist, respectively. Several excellent review articles on the telepsychiatry literature, including evidence-based outcomes, are now available (Baer et al. 1997; Capner 2000; E. A. Miller 2001).

UTILIZATION PATTERNS AND ACCEPTANCE OF TELEPSYCHIATRY

Australia, a country with a significant rural population and limited medical specialty access, has one of the world's most extensive telepsychiatry health systems. Currently, 150 telemedicine sites in Australia are used primarily for mental health (P. Yellowlees, personal communication, December 1999). Norway implemented a video teleconferencing network (at 128–384 kbps) for clinical patient care (Gammon et al. 1996). A survey of this network indicated that only 10% of the sessions were utilized for patient care, whereas meetings (50%), supervision and training (21%), and distant education (10%) made up the majority of sessions. Although these results indicated low utilization for direct patient care, it demonstrated the utility of telepsychiatry to accomplish liaison, supervision, and education, all of which are important to the practicing consultation-liaison psychiatrist.

In the United States, several operational telepsychiatry programs provide a wide range of mental health services. The TelePsychiatry Clinic at the University of Kansas Medical Center provides services to community mental health centers, rural hospitals, schools, group homes, and jails. This clinic has provided treatment to several hundred adults and children, including more than a thousand follow-up visits (Ermer 1999a, 1999b). The Menninger Clinic created a telepsychiatry consultation program to help rural children with serious behavioral problems become engaged in education activities at school (Sargent et al. 1999). Consultants "met" with the

patient, parents, teachers, and other school professionals, resulting in demonstrable benefits. To make the system affordable, and thus readily accessible, the Menninger Clinic used technology that operated over regular telephone services (at approximately 53 kbps). Hilty et al. (1999) described psychiatric consultative models used with primary care providers, as well as the benefits and drawbacks of conducting a primary care consultative service via telepsychiatry.

The U.S. Navy has successfully conducted video telepsychiatric consultations with ships at sea via satellite link (128 kbps). Diagnoses, treatment, and disposition recommendations were discussed after evaluations with the onboard physicians and physician assistants. Significant improvement in the assessment skills of the onboard general physicians was noted with each ensuing consultation request.

The National Naval Medical Center, Bethesda, Maryland, has established a land-based telepsychiatric network, with six medical clinics stateside and one overseas, focusing primarily (more than 90% of VTCs) on direct patient care (Grady 2000a). The telepsychiatry service is a part of the hospital's primary behavioral healthcare service (PBHC), a service emphasizing improved coordination of patient care between primary care providers and mental health professionals. Telepsychiatry services include initial evaluations (including disability evaluations), ongoing medication management, psychotherapy (individual and group), and substance abuse counseling. Regularly scheduled multidisciplinary treatment team planning is conducted between the hospital and community-based primary care and mental health clinics and is a requisite of the service. Psychiatry residents are encouraged to participate in the PBHC/TeleMental HealthCare Service. Noteworthy in this system is the implementation of TeleMental HealthCare standard operating procedures, which include requirements for credentialing, privileging, peer review, patient record maintenance, contingency planning, informed consent, and integrated electronic laboratory and pharmacy ordering and reporting services (Grady 2000b).

Patient, consultee, and consultant perceptions of and satisfaction with telepsychiatry has been frequently studied. For example, residents of rural West Virginia were surveyed about telemedicine ($n = 461$; 54% response rate), and only one-third of respondents had heard of telemedicine (Brick et al. 1997). Respondents who had heard of telemedicine tended to have private health insurance, more education and income, and more contact with medical care. Although most respondents felt it would be less satisfying to see a physician via telemedicine, patients said they would be either somewhat or very willing to use telemedicine for routine or specialist care (75%). For emergency care, 41% said they would be willing if no physician were available locally. In Arkansas, general physicians ($n = 46$) who were about to receive telemedicine equipment were surveyed on their attitudes about its overall usefulness, effectiveness, and expected use and their interest in learning about telemedicine (Tilford et al. 1997). From the survey results (27/46, a 59% response rate), three conclusions were reached: 1) The majority of physicians were not familiar with the potential clinical applications of telemedicine, 2) they were receptive to its application in provider education, and 3) they strongly desired to learn more about telemedicine. These studies point out the need to involve primary care physicians in the planning and implementation phases of this health care delivery system. The consultation-liaison psychiatrist is ideally suited to take the lead in implementing and developing this technology with the primary care provider.

TELEPSYCHIATRY PRACTICE

Considerations in Implementing the Service

One of the major benefits of telepsychiatry may be indirect. In the process of understanding telepsychiatry, one is challenged to look at, and at times to reconsider, communications patterns, patient populations, therapeutic goals, and even the way we furnish our offices. The telepsychiatry session, like a face-to-face session, begins long before the appointment. Both types of session involve setting up the physical arrangements of the ward or office and contain a process for referral, scheduling, and consent. One approach for implementing and maintaining a telepsychiatric practice begins with the seven A's: alliance, assessment, approach, access, accountability, apprehension, and anticipation (Table 41–1).

Alliance consists of the consultant's relationship with the remote site's administrative, support, and provider staff. In my experience, this is the key element in establishing and maintaining a telepsychiatric practice (Grady 2001). When the remote staff is comfortable and confident with the consultant, these positive feelings are passed on to the patient and overshadow preoccupation with the technology. The opposite also appears to be true. If the consultant becomes overly focused or absorbed by the technology, he or she may lose sight of patient and provider needs. The importance of the alliance has also been demonstrated when communication technologies are extended over great distances. My ex-

perience has been that as the distance (i.e., language, culture, and electronic communications reliability) between consultant and patient increases, the consultee needs to take a more active role in caring for the patient (Figure 41–1).

TABLE 41–1. Factors to consider when implementing a telepsychiatry service: The 7 A's

Alliance
　　Administrative staff
　　Support staff
　　Providers

Assessment
　　Needs and resources of satellite site
　　Capabilities and resources of hub site
　　Interest

Approach
　　Clinician driven

Access
　　Patient
　　Remote site
　　Central vs. embedded

Accountability
　　Patient safety
　　Patient records
　　Performance evaluation and improvement/peer review

Apprehension
　　Risk-benefit ratio
　　Outcomes

Anticipation
　　Patient issues
　　Communication interruptions/equipment failure

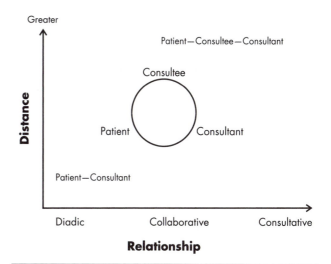

FIGURE 41–1. How distance affects relationships among the telepsychiatry patient, the consultant, and the consultee

The *assessment* consists of identifying the needs and resources of the remote site, the capabilities and resources of the hub site, and the personal investment and commitment of both. In most systems, a consultant, who is usually from an academic or regional hospital, initiates a site visit to assess the needs of the prospective telepsychiatric community. A site visit by the consultant is essential and allows him or her to become familiar with and experience the environment in which the patient lives and works. Having a clear indication and business case analysis for telepsychiatric care renders the program more sustainable in future fiscal budgeting. This approach also keeps the consultant in the business of taking care of patients rather than defending the service delivery system. The consultant's resource assessment must also include the ability of the onsite staff to carry out the plans and recommendations from telepsychiatric consultation (Sederer et al. 1998). Resources of the hub site, such as available consultant time, equipment, and operational funds, are also significant factors affecting the final scope of the teleconsultation system. Finally, but possibly most important, is the level of interest demonstrated by providers, consultants, and even telemedicine directors in establishing a telepsychiatric practice.

Yellowlees (1997) has identified the importance of approaching the clinician as the one who must champion telepsychiatric implementation. Telemedicine systems developed by technically astute professionals have sat idle owing to a lack of clinician interest or champions. Although technical champions are excellent facilitators for implementation, only clinicians can go beyond the stage of intellectualization and develop the appropriate insight into the needs of patients and consultees at the remote sites.

Access in telepsychiatry has multiple meanings. For the patient, the most influential reason for implementing telepsychiatry is improved access to specialty care. Access may also refer to the physical location of the teleconferencing equipment at either the remote or the hub site. A good location in the primary care clinic can favor patient anonymity and foster improved collaboration between primary care provider and consultant. A location in a community mental health clinic may likewise strengthen the relationship with the local therapists and improve care, especially for the severely ill patient. At the hub site, equipment can be centrally located within a telemedicine department or embedded within the consultation-liaison psychiatry department. An embedded model has the benefit of ready availability for the consultant and may help to remove technical phobias among colleagues. The embedded model improves scheduling, is more private, and incorporates personal furnishing of the tele-office.

Accountability includes the physical safety of the patient, patient records, and a plan for performance evaluation and improvement. A plan for the physical safety of the patient is a necessary part of any telepsychiatry standard operating procedures. Safety includes appropriate patient selection, for example, reducing the potential for acting out (violence, self-harm), especially for patients seen alone. An adequate number of appropriately credentialed staff should be present at the remote site to resolve unexpected findings and emergencies. A backup communications plan (e.g., phone and pager numbers of onsite personnel) should exist before the start of any telepsychiatry session. A review of these safety procedures, as well as all other aspects of patient care via telepsychiatry, should be made part of the consulting department's ongoing performance evaluation, improvement program, and peer review.

The statement "First do no harm" is perhaps the source of *apprehension* felt by the medical practitioner whenever a new medication, procedure, or device becomes available. It is no different for the practicing telepsychiatrist, who must remain on constant alert for any untoward or harmful effects of treatment. The American Psychiatric Association (1998) has published guidelines for the practice of telepsychiatry.

A final consideration in the implementation of telepsychiatry is *anticipation*. The consultant should review occurrence and after-action reports and anticipate how these situations will be managed via telepsychiatry. Contingency plans for communications interruptions and equipment failures should also be part of the standard operating procedures.

Preparing for the Session

Telepsychiatry has the capacity to provide quality mental health assessment and care to underserved populations. To effectively care for this population, the consultation-liaison psychiatrist must be familiar with the biological, psychological, and social aspects of each telepsychiatric community. A method or procedure for outpatient referrals should be clearly identified before patient care is initiated and then modified as necessary. The psychiatrist should try to adapt the telepsychiatry referral process to the existing system rather than developing a new one. This approach allows the referral system to fall back on an established process should a significant technical or personnel crisis develop at either the hub or the remote site.

Identification of a single onsite coordinator is of paramount importance, allowing timely resolution of personnel, system, or equipment problems. The consultant should establish consistent telepsychiatry clinic hours, along with a process to arrange for urgent consultations as required. A training program is needed for consultants to prepare them to be on camera, to ensure they have an adequate understanding of the teleconsultation process, and to prepare them thoroughly to respond to a variety of emergency situations that could arise during the session. A readily available training handout that includes the standard operating procedures is invaluable as new consultants prepare to conduct teleconsultation.

The Session

When the psychiatric session begins, the consultant has certain expectations based on the consultation request itself. Factors include the originator of the consultation, where it originated, how urgent it was, and what is the question being asked. If an alliance has developed with the remote site, the consultant may already have some developed hypotheses about the patient.

Although the consultant is unable to greet the patient on the ward or in the clinic waiting area, it is usually possible to observe the patient walk toward the camera and observe his or her interactions with others. Therapists have their own way of greeting patients, some with a handshake, a nod, a smile, or a combination of these approaches. Although there is no substitute for clasping hands, briefly holding the open palm of your hand next to your face appears to have a positive effect; most patients quickly reciprocate. The teleconsultant should then ask the patient if he or she has any questions or concerns about the telesession and then review procedures in case of equipment failure.

The teleconsultation interview itself is very much like a face-to-face interview; however, a delay in the audio portion of the signal invariably occurs in the teleconsultation. A simple explanation and a few minutes of experience usually help everyone accommodate to the delay. Inquiries about posture, voice inflection, expressions, or tears are no different than during a face-to-face interview. For example, if there is a question about weight loss, the consultant can ask the patient to stand and demonstrate the looseness of his or her pants or skirt. Depending on bandwidth, which influences the appearance of the transmitted motion, the patient's gait, tremors, and other physical features may be accessed. When a provider, therapist, or family member accompanies the patient to the session, that individual can also be called on to describe a dermatological lesion, a motor movement, or the like.

Prior planning is imperative if safety concerns arise during the session. The consultant should use a reliable alternate method of communication (e.g., a phone or pager) to notify an onsite attendant or provider that assistance may be necessary. At the conclusion of the session, if the referring provider is readily available, a summary and recommendations may be provided interactively.

Preference for and benefits of telepsychiatry in comparison with the face-to-face encounter are discussed at length in the literature (Bloom et al. 1996; Doze et al. 1999; Zarate et al. 1997). It has been hypothesized that videoconferencing allows increased interpersonal space and a sense of control. It has also been noted that the interaction via videoconferencing appears to bring a measure of equality to the doctor-patient relationship. The color and material of the office furniture, as well as the arrangement of the seating in the office, are far less conspicuous via teleconferencing and may decrease a particular patient's anxiety about the nature of the relationship.

Collins and Sypher (1996) commented on the importance of subtle aspects of the doctor-patient interaction; they made several suggestions about how to convey information that might otherwise be lost during video teleconferencing: "1. Make special effort to communicate personal interest in and concern for the patient. 2. Allow as much time as possible for the patient to ask questions. 3. Make optimal use of the medical professional who is assisting the patient" (p. 42).

TELEPHONE, ELECTRONIC MAIL, AND INTERNET CONSULTATION

Telephone Consultation

Psychiatrists have used the telephone for many years to provide consultation and treatment to consultees and patients. According to a 1973 survey of psychiatrists ($n = 58$) in the San Francisco area, 45% used the telephone in addition to face-to-face contact, and 19% used the telephone as a primary or sole mode of consultation or treatment (Miller 1973). In another survey, psychoanalysts were asked whether they transferred care or continued care via telephone (or written correspondence) when premature interruption of psychotherapy occurred owing to geographical separation (Rosenbaum 1977). Of the 30 respondents, 26 indicated they maintained phone contact or correspondence with certain patients, an average of four patients per analyst.

Telephone consultation has an important role in consultation-liaison psychiatry, even for disorders traditionally thought to require face-to-face examination. Telephone diagnosis of delirium was studied in 41 subjects older than 65 years, 1 month after they had had hip surgery (Marcantonio et al. 1998). Eight patients were diagnosed via telephone as being delirious. When the patients were evaluated in person, six of the eight patients identified via telephone were, in fact, delirious (sensitivity = 1.00; specificity = 0.94). There are other reports of mental health professionals providing psychotherapy via telephone to cancer patients (Mermelstein and Holland 1991) and to blind elderly patients (Evans and Jaureguy 1982), as well as group therapy to visually impaired elderly patients (Evans and Jaureguy 1981).

Electronic Mail Consultation

Although psychiatrists today understand when, how, and with whom they will use the telephone, the benefits and risks of using e-mail with patients or their providers has not been adequately studied. E-mail is similar to voice mail, offering the advantage of access, time efficiency, and conveyance of information, but it is also in a format that can be placed in a patient's record. Although e-mail can contain pictures and audio and video clips, written text is the most common form of communication. Little information on the use and effects of e-mail is available in the literature, although news reporting about its use is abundant. Kane and Sands (1998) published guidelines for the use of e-mail with patients.

Concerns related to the safeguarding of information transmitted via e-mail can be broken down into three areas: security, privacy, and confidentiality. Security refers to the safety of e-mail while in transit. Currently, e-mail transferred over the Internet is subject to interception and, in severe cases, alteration and retransmission to its intended recipient. Methods to improve the security of e-mail include leaving off information that could lead to the identification of the patient, password protection, and the use of encryption software. Privacy refers to the access persons have to the senders' or recipients' computer desktop and/or e-mail client (a program one uses to write e-mail). Unauthorized access can occur when e-mail is left readily available on an unsecured computer desktop, via employer screening, or when messages are not deleted from computer servers. Confidentiality refers to the safeguarding, disposition, and access of patient information and records, including e-mail.

Consultants using e-mail should give patients guidance on what is considered appropriate and inappropriate usage of e-mail. Like voice mail, acute issues related to patient safety are inappropriate. When relatively important but not urgent e-mail is involved, automated e-mail message confirmation or forwarding to the provider's pager or answering service may be an option.

Internet Consultation

The Internet is a network of smaller interconnecting computer networks. Each computer network is made up of two or more computers that are connected so that they can communicate or share information with one another. According to Hahn (1996), today's Internet arose from a late 1960s project called the ARPANET (Advanced Research Projects Agency Network). The ARPANET was a communications network designed to allow vital communications during or following a nuclear event.

Today, the Internet is and will continue to be the focus of controversy regarding the practice of psychiatry or mental health care more generally. From the perspective of the consultation-liaison psychiatrist, the Internet may provide an important liaison function. Physicians can ask for consultation or participate in discussion groups and pose questions on medication, management, or referral to a wide audience of specialists. Some consultation networks are restricted, such as the military's Ask-a-Doc program (Poropatich et al. 1999), through which consultative advice is solicited from a predesignated group of credentialed specialists. Other discussion groups, such as those offered by Physicians Online (http://www.po.com), offer discussion on a variety of topics but allow participants to be involved anonymously. As with any consultation, the patient's attending physician bears the ultimate responsibility for the patient's care.

Whereas the accessibility of information via the Internet is one of its greatest assets, information reliability may be its nemesis. The rapid growth of network technologies and affordable access has created a vast web of lay and non-peer-reviewed literature. The growth of Internet medical information, including mental health information, has outpaced professional organizations' efforts to understand its use, management, or impact. Until a system of peer-reviewed Internet sites is established, the consultation-liaison psychiatrist must adequately assess the origin, completeness, and applicability of the information posted.

Many other questions will be raised about health care delivery via the Internet, including which of these services constitutes medical practice. Possibilities include the completion of on-line diagnostic instruments followed by treatment recommendations and fees for medical information services through various Internet service providers. Answers to questions regarding health information provided over the Internet should come from professional organizations, but legal decisions are expected to influence the practice significantly.

CONCLUSION

Burgeoning new technologies have the potential to revolutionize the way psychiatric consultation is performed. Telemedicine, telephone consultation, e-mail, and the Internet provide substrates for adaptations of current psychiatric consultation practice. Privacy, quality, and safety concerns have yet to be fully addressed, but these technologies are destined to become an increasingly important part of psychiatrists' consultative practices.

REFERENCES

Allen A, Wheeler T: Telepsychiatry background and activity survey. Telemedicine Today, 6(2):34–37, 1998

American Psychiatric Association: APA Resource Document on Telepsychiatry via Teleconferencing. 1998. Available online at http://www.psych.org/pract_of_psych/tp_paper.cfm; accessed September 20, 2001

Baer L, Cukor P, Jenike MA, et al: Pilot studies of telemedicine for patients with obsessive-compulsive disorder. Am J Psychiatry 152:1383–1385, 1995

Baer L, Elford DR, Cukor P: Telepsychiatry at forty: what have we learned? Harv Rev Psychiatry 5:7–17, 1997

Baigent MF, Lloyd CJ, Kavanagh SJ, et al: Telepsychiatry: 'tele' yes, but what about the 'psychiatry'? J Telemed Telecare 3 (suppl 1):3–5, 1997

Ball CJ, Scott N, McLaren PM, et al: Preliminary evaluation of a low-cost videoconferencing (LCVC) system for remote cognitive testing of adult psychiatric patients. Br J Clin Psychol 32:303–307, 1993

Bloom D, Hunter R, Williams ME: The acceptability of telemedicine among healthcare providers and rural patients. Telemedicine Today 4(3):5–8, 1996

Brick JE, Bashshur RL, Brick JF, et al: Public knowledge, perception, and expressed choice of telemedicine in rural West Virginia. Telemed J 3:159–171, 1997

Capner M: Videoconferencing in the provision of psychological services at a distance. J Telemed Telecare 6 (6):311-319, 2000

Collins B, Sypher J: Developing better relationships in telemedicine practice: organizational and interpersonal factors. Telemedicine Today 4(2):159–171, 1997

Doze S, Simpson J, Hailey D, et al: Evaluation of a telepsychiatry pilot project. J Telemed Telecare 5:38–46, 1999

Dwyer TF: Telepsychiatry: psychiatric consultation by interactive television. Am J Psychiatry 130:865–869, 1973

Elford R, White H, et al: A randomized, controlled trial of child psychiatric assessments conducted using videoconferencing. J Telemed Telecare 6 (2):73-82, 2000

Ermer D: Child and adolescent telepsychiatry clinics. Psychiatric Annals 29:409–414, 1999a

Ermer D: Experience with a rural telepsychiatry clinic for children and adolescent. Psychiatr Serv 50(2):260–261, 1999

Evans RL, Jaureguy BM: Group therapy by phone: a cognitive behavioral program for visually impaired elderly. Social Work Health Care 7:79–90, 1981

Evans RL, Jaureguy BM: Phone therapy outreach for blind elderly. Gerontologist 22:32–35, 1982

Gammon D, Bergvik S, Bergmo T, et al: Videoconferencing in psychiatry: a survey of use in northern Norway. J Telemed Telecare 2:192–198, 1996

Grady B: Today: transitioning from contingency support to the sustaining base: using telehealth to expand access to care and "patient encounters." Presentation, U.S. Navy Plenary Session, 107th Annual Meeting of the Association of Military Surgeons of the United States, Las Vegas, NV, November 6, 2000a

Grady B: Standardized operating procedures involving interactive videoconferencing with mental health patients. Poster session, 5th Annual Meeting of the American Telemedicine Association, Phoenix, AZ, May 22, 2000b

Grady B: The capacity to adapt: turning connections into relationships via video teleconferencing. Presentation, 6th Annual Meeting of the American Telemedicine Association, Fort Lauderdale, FL, June 5, 2001

Hahn H: The Internet Complete Reference, 2nd Edition. Berkeley, CA, McGraw-Hill, 1996

Hilty DM, Servis E, Nesbitt TS, et al: The use of telemedicine to provide consultation-liaison service to the primary care setting. Psychiatric Annals 29:421–427, 1999

Kane B, Sands DZ: Guidelines for the clinical use of electronic mail with patients. J Am Med Inform Assoc 5:104–111, 1998

Kennedy C, Yellowlees P: A community-based approach to evaluation of health outcomes and costs for telepsychiatry in a rural population: preliminary results. J Telemed Telecare 6 (suppl 1):155-157, 2000

Marcantonio ER, Michaels M, Resnick NM: Diagnosing delirium by telephone. J Gen Intern Med 13:621–623, 1998

Maxmen J: Telecommunications in psychiatry. Am J Psychother 32:450–456, 1978

May C, Gask L, et al: Telepsychiatry evaluation in the northwest of England: preliminary results of a qualitative study. J Telemed Telecare 6 (suppl 1):20-22, 2000

Mermelstein HT, Holland JC: Psychotherapy by telephone: a therapeutic tool for cancer patients. Psychosomatics 32:407–412, 1991

Miller EA: Telemedicine and doctor-patient communication: an analytical survey of the literature. J Telemed Telecare 7(1):1-17, 2001

Miller WB: The telephone in outpatient psychotherapy. Am J Psychother 27:15–26, 1973

Montani C, Billaud N, Tyrrell J, et al: Psychological impact of a remote psychometric consultation with hospitalized elderly people. J Telemed Telecare 3:140–145, 1997

Poropatich RK, DeWitt D, Sales LY, et al: Ask a Doc—an electronic mail clinical consultative service. Poster session, 4th annual meeting of the American Telemedicine Association, Salt Lake city, UT, April 18–21, 1999

Rosen E: The history of desktop telemedicine. Telemedicine Today, 5(2):16–17, 28, 1997

Rosenbaum M: Premature interruption of psychotherapy: continuation of contact by telephone and correspondence. Am J Psychiatry 134:200–202, 1977

Sackett DL, Rosenberg WM: The need for evidence-based medicine. J R Soc Med 88:620–624, 1995

Sargent J, Maldonado M, Sargent M: School based mental health in rural Kansas: a novel use for telepsychiatry. Poster session, 4th annual meeting of the American Telemedicine Association, April 18–21, 1999

Sederer LI, Ellison J, Keyes C: Guidelines for prescribing psychiatrists in consultative, collaborative, and supervisory relationships. Psychiatr Serv 49:1197–1202, 1998

Solow C, Weiss RJ, Bergen BJ, et al: 24-Hour psychiatric consultation via TV. Am J Psychiatry 127:120–123, 1971

Tilford JM, Garner WE, Strode SW, et al: Rural Arkansas physicians and telemedicine technology: attitudes in communities receiving equipment. Telemed J 3:257–263, 1997

Wittson CL, Benschoter R: Two-way television: helping the medical center reach out. Am J Psychiatry 129:136–139, 1972

Wittson CL, Affleck DC, Johnson V: Two-way television in group therapy. Mental Hospitals 2:22–23, 1961

Yellowlees PM: Successful development of telemedicine systems-seven core principles. J Telemed Telecare 3:215–222, 1997b

Zarate CA, Weinstock L, Cukor P, et al: Applicability of telemedicine for assessing patients with schizophrenia: acceptance and reliability. J Clin Psychiatry 58:22–25, 1997

Zaylor C: Clinical outcomes in telepsychiatry. J Telemed Telecare 5 (suppl 1):59–60, 1999

Treatment

42

Psychopharmacology

Martina L. Fait, M.D.

Michael G. Wise, M.D.

John S. Jachna, M.D.

Richard D. Lane, M.D., Ph.D.

Alan J. Gelenberg, M.D.

INITIATING TREATMENT

The use of any medication involves altering the concentration of a naturally occurring substance or introducing a foreign substance into the body. Therefore, caution is always advised in making decisions about medication use. The promise and the danger of medications are particularly evident when a patient with other medical illnesses develops a psychiatric disorder. Because a patient who is medically ill is typically taking other (often many) medications, the risk of adverse reactions is increased when a psychotropic medication is added (Stoudemire et al. 1990, 1991). In addition, the presence of a psychiatric illness can lengthen the hospital stay of medically ill patients (Ackerman et al. 1988; Fulop et al. 1987; Saravay and Strain 1994; Verbosky et al. 1993). Psychiatric interventions can shorten hospital stays, improve function, and reduce health care costs (Fann 2000; see also Chapter 4 in this volume). For example, the selection of an appropriate antidepressant or stimulant can improve the mood and energy level of a patient who has poststroke depression, whose health is deteriorating, and who is not participating in physical therapy. This single intervention can improve both mental and physical health. The selection of an antidepressant with an inappropriate side-effect profile, however, can render that same patient confused and hypotensive.

The increased number of psychotropic medications made available since the early 1980s has contributed greatly to the effectiveness that consulting psychiatrists have in the treatment of patients' psychological, neurovegetative, and behavioral symptoms. The symptoms associated with many primary and secondary psychiatric disorders are now manageable with medications. Because the exact biochemical mechanisms of psychiatric disorders are not known, disorders are descriptive entities diagnosed by symptom profiles. Therefore, pharmacological interventions are generally directed at ameliorating symptom complexes. Sometimes psychiatrists treat isolated psychiatric symptoms based on empirical responses alone. In some situations, clinicians prescribe other interventions, such as psychotherapy, that have a more general effect on a large variety of receptors. The combination of psychopharmacological and psychotherapeutic interventions is often the most powerful treatment.

Fortunately, psychotropic medications have powerful and dramatic effects and effectively induce remission in many patients. However, like all interventions, whether pharmacological or otherwise, psychotropic drugs can cause unwanted side effects. These side effects are occasionally more distressing than the original disorder. In general, side effects are a significant impediment for patients who are already reluctant to take a psychiatric medication. Thus, the powerful positive and negative effects of these medications demand rigorous evaluation, a reliable diagnosis, patient education, and frequent reevaluation of the patient's symptoms and the medications' side effects.

Formulating a diagnosis for the patient's symptoms provides the context for use of medications. This is the initial step in determining the proper psychopharmacological intervention. This process involves a mental status examination, history, chart review, physical examination, laboratory studies, and the collection of collateral information. Once a diagnosis is made, it provides expectations about medications that might work, an anticipated response, and a prognosis. This hypothetical response is then tested against the patient's reaction to the medications. Because the presentation of a particular disorder can vary widely, the patient's symptoms should be documented clearly. Documenting these target symptoms also allows for comparison of a treatment across time and treatment sites and establishes the basis for evaluating the side effects and the patient's response to medication. The nature of a patient's symptoms, the symptom severity, and the patient's response can be precisely defined with a rating scale, if one is available for the patient's particular psychiatric condition.

TREATMENT PRINCIPLES

Table 42–1 lists treatment principles in the consultation-liaison setting. The clinician should review all medications a patient is taking (including herbal and over-the-counter preparations) in order to make informed medication recommendations. One of the most useful psychopharmacological interventions, especially in the elderly and the medically ill, is to recommend the discontinuation of a medication. The inappropriate use of psychotropic medications can have a significant adverse effect on a patient's physical and mental status. Elderly and medically ill patients are particularly vulnerable to these side effects and often receive medications that interact or potentiate each other's side effects (Ray et al. 1987). If possible, as-needed dosing should be avoided so that the patient's response to a set, regular dose can be established. Failure to do this can result in a confusing and disruptive cycle in which as-needed medication is given, medication side effects occur, doses are withheld, symptoms recur, catch-up (read: excessive) as-needed medications are given, and the cycle is repeated. This cycle can occur in patients with pain, withdrawal syndromes, or delirium. When as-needed dosing is necessary, the frequency of use should be monitored to determine whether a standing dose of medication is appropriate.

Effective medication management also implies using the minimum dose of medication necessary to obtain the desired response and minimize side effects. Knowing common response patterns and monitoring a patient's symptoms help to ensure the prescription of a dose suf-

TABLE 42–1. Psychopharmacological principles in the consultation-liaison setting

Review all medications the patient is taking, including herbal and over-the-counter preparations.

Remember that discontinuing a medication is often a valuable intervention, especially in elderly patients who are taking multiple psychotropic medications.

Avoid prescribing medications on an as-needed basis, particularly for patients with pain, withdrawal syndromes, or delirium.

When as-needed medication is required, monitor frequency of use to determine a standing dosage.

Change one medication at a time, and use the minimum dosage necessary to obtain the desired response.

Keep the medication regimen simple. Whenever possible, use only one medication to treat a symptom or disorder.

Treat prophylactically if a clear rationale exists (e.g., give benztropine to avoid a dystonic reaction from neuroleptics in an anxious young man experiencing his first psychotic break).

Use a medication that was previously effective for the patient or for a family member with a similar disorder.

If treatment fails, reexamine the diagnosis. Always reconsider the possibility of substance abuse.

Remember that serum drug levels are not a certification of efficacy or toxicity.

Be aware that although generic drugs are cost-effective, their bioavailability can vary.

Recognize that social and characterological issues are ever present in influencing treatment and compliance. Psychotherapy is often indicated.

Remember that each patient is unique.

ficient to obtain a complete remission. When a medication change is necessary, it is often best to change one medication at a time. Ideally, a clinician should use only one medication to treat a particular symptom or disorder. In some patients, such as those with refractory depression, carefully planned drug combinations are needed. It is almost never necessary to use more than one medication from the same class at the same time (e.g., two selective serotonin reuptake inhibitors, or SSRIs). In addition, the minimum effective amount of medication should be given so that additional medications are not required to manage side effects. For example, starting a depressed, medically ill patient on the usual SSRI dose often causes insomnia and anxiety, which the physician then treats by adding a sedative and/or an anxiolytic. If the clinician starts the patient on a lower dose, side effects and additional medications are usually avoided. Certain circumstances warrant providing prophylactic treatment. For example, a physician can administer benztropine with an antipsychotic to avoid a frightening dystonic reaction in a young anxious man who is experiencing a psychotic episode. The use of medications with fixed drug combinations should be avoided because they do not allow for adjustments in dosage of the individual medications contained in the combination.

In selecting an appropriate medication from the many that are available, it is usually helpful to use what has previously worked for the individual. Medications that have been effective for first-degree family members with a similar psychiatric disturbance are also more likely to be effective than are other medications. Generic drugs can minimize financial cost, but the bioavailability of these preparations can vary. Most important, the information available on typical responses to all medications is based on statistical analysis, not on clinical experience with an individual patient. Each patient can experience a unique response to medication. If treatment fails, the clinician should reexamine the diagnosis. Substance abuse is a common reason for a poor medication response. In addition, when Dew et al. (1997) looked at predictors for recovery in the depressed elderly receiving antidepressants, they found that the group with a partial or mixed response (including nonresponders) had low levels of social support and high rates of major life stress. In such cases, pharmacotherapy combined with psychotherapy is more likely to be successful than pharmacotherapy alone.

COMPLIANCE

Once a psychotropic medication is prescribed, multiple factors influence the patient's institution and continuation of the medication. Medication cost is often an issue. Factors such as the frequency (i.e., medication administered once versus four times each day) and timing of doses can be important, as are the patient's beliefs about his or her illness and what it means to the patient to take psychotropic medication. Transference feelings toward the physician can affect the patient's use of the medication and the perceived response. The illness itself can impair the patient's ability to take medications. Depressed patients, for example, usually have exaggerated guilt and may not believe they deserve treatment or can afford the cost (Fawcett 1995); cognitive impairment originating from any number of causes can lead to forgetfulness and passive noncompliance. All of these factors can come into play before the patient has taken one pill.

Studies show that compliance with antidepressant medications in the primary care setting is less than optimal. In one study, approximately 28% of patients stopped taking antidepressants during the first month of therapy, and 44% stopped taking the antidepressant by the third

month of therapy (Lin et al. 1995). Patients who received specific educational messages were more likely to comply during the first month of therapy (Table 42–2). Interestingly, medication side effects were associated with early noncompliance only if the side effects were severe. The use of treatment algorithms to find the right medication is likely overemphasized in current practice and the concept of the therapeutic alliance underemphasized. The clinical expertise of the physician prescribing the medication is an important factor influencing compliance. Strategies that involve explaining to the patient his or her illness and the rationale for the use of medications and inquiring into the patient's fears regarding medication use are essential to improve compliance and to ensure the practice of good medicine.

DRUG ACTIONS AND INTERACTIONS

Drug Absorption

A drug can be administered directly into the bloodstream (intravenous administration); by diffusion from a drug depot (intramuscular or subcutaneous administration); or across a mucosal surface such as the stomach, rectum, or sublingual area. Absorption rates differ among these routes, although absorption from different forms of oral medications (i.e., capsule, pill, liquid) is generally similar. Parenteral administration generally results in more rapid effects, although there are some exceptions. Diazepam, for example, is erratically absorbed after intramuscular injection due to its lipophilic properties, paradoxically resulting in a slower and less predictable onset of action. Special preparations, such as long-acting forms of both parenteral and oral drugs, change absorption also. Gastric absorption increases when the stomach is empty because more mucosal surfaces are available; the stomach also empties more rapidly into the jejunum. Many psychotropic drugs are weak bases, which are better absorbed in the jejunum where the pH is higher. There is little overall change in oral absorption of drugs with aging, despite numerous individual changes, such as an increase in gastric pH; a decrease in surface villi; and alterations in gastric motility, gastric emptying, and intestinal perfusion (Altman 1990; Ouslander 1981; Schmucker 1985; Siris and Rifkin 1981; Wise and Tierney 1992).

Drug Distribution

Most psychoactive drugs (except for lithium) are lipophilic and are absorbed preferentially into fatty tissue, including the brain. This means that psychotropic medica-

TABLE 42–2. Important educational messages for patients when starting psychotropic medication

Take the medication each day.

Medications must be used regularly for full effect (e.g., antidepressants must be taken 2–4 weeks, or sometimes longer, particularly in the elderly, before beneficial effects are noticed).

Continue taking the medication even if you are feeling better.

Do not stop taking the medication without checking with your physician.

Give specific instructions about the particular medication prescribed and what to do if a dose is forgotten.

Source. Adapted from Lin et al. 1995.

tions generally have large volumes of distribution. In addition, most psychiatric medications are bound to plasma proteins such as albumin and glycoprotein. When a medication is protein bound, it is not available to tissues such as the brain. Lowering toxic drug levels is more difficult when the medications are highly protein bound. Other medications can alter the amount of protein binding (Table 42–3). With aging and chronic medical illness, albumin decreases and the proportion of unbound (active) drug generally increases. For lipid-soluble drugs, the volume of distribution increases with aging as a result of decreases in total body water and lean body mass and increases in total body fat.

Drug Metabolism

Water-soluble drugs are readily excreted by the kidneys. Active lipid-soluble drugs accumulate unless they are converted to more water-soluble compounds or are metabolized by the liver to less active compounds. Lithium is an exception; it is not metabolized.

Because of the anatomical arrangement of blood flow from the gastrointestinal system, the absorbed drug passes through the liver before entering the systemic circulation. There the drug may be metabolized before the rest of the body is exposed to it. The metabolites are sometimes active psychopharmacological agents. This first-pass effect is sometimes significant. It also helps explain why intramuscular preparations are often more potent than oral equivalents. For example, neuroleptic drugs given intramuscularly have about twice the potency of orally administered drugs, although the potency can vary widely from patient to patient.

Once in the liver, a drug is exposed to two main groups of metabolizing enzymes. This multistep catabolic process of drug elimination involves oxidation and conjugation. The oxidative process occurs via the monooxyge-

nase or cytochrome P450 (CYP) enzyme system. Conjugation is usually the final catabolic enzymatic step (i.e., the drug or its metabolites are coupled with other compounds to form more easily excreted [hydrophilic] compounds). The rate of metabolism, especially the oxidative process, is affected by many factors (Tables 42–4, 42–5, and 42–6) and disease states.

Four CYP enzymes are especially important in the oxidation of medications: CYP2D6, CYP1A2, CYP2C, and CYP3A3/4. The CYP2D6 and CYP2C enzymes are subject to significant genetic variability in contrast to other CYP enzymes such as CYP1A2 and CYP3A4. CYP2D6 is unique in that it cannot be induced (see Table 42–6). Medications usually have a high affinity for metabolism by a particular enzyme, can compete for metabolism with other substrates, or can inhibit an enzyme without being metabolized by it. These CYP-drug interactions are potentially harmful if the substrate has a low therapeutic index, as is the case with tricyclic antidepressants (TCAs) (DeVane 1994).

Drug Elimination

A drug and its metabolites can be excreted by the kidneys as well as into the bile or feces. Small amounts are also lost through sweat, saliva, or tears. Biological or elimination half-life is a measure of the amount of time needed to excrete half of the drug from the body. This measure is usually expressed as plasma half-life, which states how long it takes to remove half of the drug from the plasma. The frequency of drug administration is usually established by the length of its half-life. A steady-state drug level is generally achieved after four to five half-lives; it is at this point that accurate serum drug levels are obtained.

Because the pharmacokinetic properties of some drugs change with extended administration, a maintenance half-life is sometimes defined. For lipophilic, highly bound psychoactive drugs, the maintenance half-life is often much longer after long-term administration. Aging and renal disease also result in decreased renal blood flow and glomerular filtration, slowing renal elimination. Medical and surgical patients usually receive multiple medications; the medications can interact to modify the pharmacokinetic properties of a given psychotropic drug.

Drug Levels

Drug levels are used to monitor compliance, ensure proper dose, and avoid toxicity. The most common causes for low drug levels are pharmacokinetic variation and noncompliance. For example, the lithium level in a patient with acute mania who is disorganized can estab-

TABLE 42–3. Common medications that affect drug levels

Inhibitors of metabolism	Inducers of metabolism	Can displace drugs from protein-binding sites
Acetaminophen	Barbiturates	Aspirin
Allopurinol	Carbamazepine	Phenylbutazone
Chloramphenicol	Chloral hydrate	Phenytoin
Cimetidine	Griseofulvin	Scopolamine
Disulfiram	Phenytoin	Selective serotonin reuptake inhibitors
Erythromycin	Rifampin	Tricyclic antidepressants
Isoniazid		
Itraconazole		
Ketoconazole		
Monoamine oxidase inhibitors		
Methylphenidate		
Oral contraceptives		
Phenothiazines		
Phenylbutazone		
Quinidine		
Valproic acid		

TABLE 42–4. Reported drug interactions with antidepressants (see Table 42–6 for cytochrome P450 effects)

Medication	Interactive effect
Class IA antiarrhythmics (quinidine, procainamide)	TCAs may prolong cardiac conduction time.
Phenothiazines[a]	TCAs may prolong Q-T interval.
Reserpine	May decrease antihypertensive effect.
Guanethidine	
Clonidine	
Prazosin and other α-adrenergic-blocking agents	Antidepressants may potentiate hypotensive effects.
Parenteral: sympathomimetic pressor amines (e.g., epinephrine, norepinephrine, phenylephrine)	Antidepressants may cause slight increases in blood pressure.
Anticholinergic agents	TCAs may potentiate side effects.
Carbamazepine[b]	Additive cardiotoxicity possible.
Digitoxin	Fluoxetine may displace digitoxin from protein-binding sites and increase bioactive levels of digitoxin (converse is also true).

Note. TCAs = tricyclic antidepressants.
[a]May also raise antidepressant levels via cytochrome P450 effects.
[b]May lower tricyclic levels due to cytochrome P450 effects.
Source. Modified from Stoudemire A, Moran MG, Fogel BS: "Psychotropic Drug Use in the Medically Ill, Part I." *Psychosomatics* 31:382, 1990. Copyright 1990, Academy of Psychosomatic Medicine. Used with permission.

lish that noncompliance with drug therapy was an etiological factor in the patient's relapse.

The clinician should remember that a serum drug level is only one indicator; it is not a certification of efficacy or toxicity. It provides a guideline against which the patient's experience is compared. Defined therapeutic drug levels are established for specific circumstances. For example, the therapeutic level for lithium is not the same for a patient with acute mania as it is for a bipolar patient who is clinically stable, nor is it necessarily the same for another use, such as augmentation of antidepressant effect or use in patients with cognitive disorders. Furthermore, ideal drug levels vary among individuals, making

levels for optimum prophylaxis, defined from studies of large populations, difficult to apply in individual cases. For example, the ideal maintenance lithium level for a hospitalized geriatric patient with mania may not be the same as that for a younger, physically healthy person. It is important to modify the dosage of a drug based on previous experience while monitoring signs and symptoms of drug effects and side effects.

Receptor Site Activity

The main target of psychotropic medications is the brain. Psychotropic medications affect, with varying specificity,

TABLE 42–5.   Reported drug interactions with neuroleptics

Medication	Interactive effect
Class IA antiarrhythmics	Chlorpromazine and thioridazine may prolong cardiac conduction.
Gel-type antacids	Neuroleptic absorption may be decreased.
Narcotics	Hypotensive effects of neuroleptics may be potentiated.
Epinephrine	
Enflurane	
Isoflurane	
Prazosin	Neuroleptics may increase hypotensive effect.
Angiotensin-converting enzyme inhibitors (captopril, enalapril)	
Narcotics	Sedative effects of neuroleptics may be increased.
Tricyclic antidepressants	
Barbiturates	
Guanethidine	Neuroleptics may decrease blood pressure control.
Clonidine	

Source.   Adapted from Stoudemire A, Moran MG, Fogel BS: "Psychotropic Drug Use in the Medically Ill, Part II." *Psychosomatics* 32:36, 1991. Copyright 1991, Academy of Psychosomatic Medicine. Used with permission.

a large array of neurotransmitters in this organ. The exact correlation of these effects with the resulting behavioral and emotional changes is unknown. There is also little certainty about the causes of psychiatric disorders themselves. In fact, hypotheses about the etiology of psychiatric disorders are partially based on the responses of these disorders to psychopharmacological agents. Although it had been hoped that cause-and-effect attributions could be made between effects of psychoactive medications and specific neurotransmitters, the actions of these medications are extremely complex, involving multiple effects on a variety of neurotransmitters in many brain pathways, as well as the interactions of these effects.

Medication effects can occur at several points in the life of neurotransmitters. These points include synthesis of the neurotransmitter; transport in the presynaptic neuron; storage of the chemical in vesicles; extrusion of the vesicles' contents; effects on postsynaptic and presynaptic receptors; and disposal of the neurotransmitter through degradation, diffusion, or reuptake. Effects at the receptor depend on the medication's affinity for the receptor, the amount of ligand available, and the presence of competing drugs. A drug's effect at the target receptor is usually mediated by a second messenger in the target cell.

After a ligand binds to the receptor, it can produce a biological response as a full or partial agonist. If it binds without producing the effect, it is an antagonist. Competitive antagonists are displaced by adding higher amounts of ligand, whereas noncompetitive antagonists are not dislodged. After prolonged occupation of a receptor by an antagonist, denervation supersensitivity can develop. This phenomenon involves an increased number of receptors and increased sensitivity to an agonist.

Drug Interactions

Recognition of drug interactions is crucial in consultation-liaison psychiatry. The effect of one drug on another can be pharmacokinetic (i.e., affecting the absorption, distribution, biotransformation, and excretion of the other drug) or pharmacodynamic (i.e., changing the effect of the drug at its point of action). In order to identify these interactions, a complete medication list must be obtained from the patient, including as-needed doses given in the hospital, drugs recently discontinued, over-the-counter medications used, and herbal or other alternative medical preparations used. Families can be extremely helpful in this regard; the family should be asked to bring in all medications found in the patient's home. The clinician should be alert for the so-called shopping bag sign. A positive sign occurs when the family brings in a large bag or container of current and expired medications and over-the-counter and herbal preparations. Also, unless specifically asked, patients may not report medications prescribed by doctors in other specialties, thinking that these other drugs are not of interest to a psychiatrist.

ANTIDEPRESSANTS

Indications

Depression is both overmedicated and underdiagnosed in the medically ill population. Unrecognized depression is a serious problem in medically ill patients and adds significantly to morbidity. At the same time, discouragement,

TABLE 42–6. Cytochrome P450–drug interactions[a]

	Substrates	Inhibitors	Inducers
CYP1A2			
Psychotropic	Caffeine Clozapine Haloperidol Olanzapine Propranolol Tertiary TCAs (amitriptyline, imipramine)	Fluvoxamine	Cigarettes Caffeine
Nonpsychotropic	Phenacetin Theophylline Verapamil Warfarin	Ciprofloxacin Grapefruit juice Tacrine	Cabbage Charbroiled food Omeprazole Rifampin
CYP2C (2C9/2C19)			
Psychotropic	Barbiturates Tertiary TCAs Diazepam Propranolol	Fluoxetine Fluvoxamine Sertraline (?)	
Nonpsychotropic	NSAIDs Phenytoin Tolbutamide Warfarin		Phenobarbital Phenytoin
CYP2D6			
Psychotropic	Clozapine Haloperidol[b] Paroxetine Phenothiazines[c] Quetiapine Risperidone Secondary TCAs (nortriptyline, desipramine) Venlafaxine	Fluoxetine Fluphenazine Fluvoxamine Methylphenidate[d] Norfluoxetine Paroxetine Phenothiazines[c] Sertraline TCAs	Not induced
Nonpsychotropic	Codeine ⇒ morphine β-blockers Class 1C antiarrhythmics (flecainide, propafenone)	Cimetidine Quinidine[e]	
CYP3A3/4			
Psychotropic	Alprazolam Carbamazepine Clozapine Midazolam Nefazodone Pimozide Sertraline Tertiary TCAs Triazolam Venlafaxine	Fluoxetine Fluvoxamine Nefazodone Norfluoxetine Sertraline	Carbamazepine

TABLE 42–6. Cytochrome P450–drug interactions[a] *(continued)*

	Substrates	Inhibitors	Inducers
CYP3A3/4 *(continued)*			
Nonpsychotropic	Anticancer drugs	Cimetidine	Dexamethasone
	Astemizole	Cyclosporine	Phenobarbital
	Calcium-channel blockers	Diltiazem	Primidone
	Cisapride	Erythromycin[e]	Phenytoin
	Cyclosporine	Fluconazole	Rifabutin
	Erythromycin	Grapefruit juice	Rifampin
	Lidocaine	Itraconazole[e]	
	Quinidine	Ketoconazole[e]	
	Steroids	Miconazole	
		Protease inhibitors	

Note.   TCAs are metabolized by CYP2D6, CYP3A, CYP2C, and CYP1A2; (?) denotes incomplete or inconsistent data; CYP = cytochrome P450; NSAIDs = nonsteroidal anti-inflammatory drugs; TCAs = tricyclic antidepressants.
[a]Includes both in vivo and in vitro data.
[b]Complex interaction.
[c]Phenothiazines include chlorpromazine, prochlorperazine, perphenazine, trifluoperazine, fluphenazine, thioridazine, and mesoridazine.
[d]Methylphenidate likely has CYP effects, but particular isoenzymes have not been identified.
[e]Extraordinarily powerful inhibitors of CYP enzymes.
Source.   Data compiled by M.G. Wise and L. Ereshefsky.

unhappiness, and "feeling poorly" are commonly reported by medically ill individuals. Some clinicians try to boost a patient's spirit or appetite by prescribing an antidepressant without first performing an adequate diagnostic assessment (i.e., they do not establish the presence of a mood disorder). Once the diagnosis of major depression is established, full treatment with an antidepressant should be started. Of course, the correct dosage will vary based on factors such as an individual's innate pharmacokinetics, age, other medications, and concurrent medical conditions. In medically ill patients, in whom a clear depressive diagnosis is sometimes difficult to establish, adequate follow-up is essential. It is optimal for the physician who initiated the antidepressant to see the patient for follow-up. Both inpatient and outpatient follow-up by the consultation-liaison psychiatrist is ideal. Barring intolerable side effects, at least 6 weeks of treatment at full antidepressant doses are necessary before a trial of an antidepressant is considered adequate. Longer trials are often needed, especially in the elderly (Dew et al. 1997). One of the most common causes of treatment-resistant depression is failure to use adequate doses or to continue a trial for a sufficient amount of time. Lack of response after 3 weeks may appropriately prompt some clinicians to increase the dosage of the antidepressant to its upper range or to add augmenting agents if dose increases are not possible because of side effects or dose limits. In medically ill patients, the clinician should always prescribe antidepressants with attention to side effects, risks from higher dosages, and drug interactions.

Outward signs of depression generally improve with antidepressant treatment before subjective symptoms improve. Thus, the patient is often the last to recognize the improvement. There is a higher risk of suicide immediately after the initiation of treatment; during this time a patient has increased energy without improved subjective mood. The patient must be monitored closely during this period. Between 9 months and 1 year after an adequate antidepressant response is achieved, the continued use of the antidepressant should be reevaluated and discontinuation of the medication considered. Studies suggest that for patients with recurrent depression, the risk of recurrence warrants continued antidepressant treatment with full-dose therapy (Hall and Wise 1995; Kamlet et al. 1995).

The onset of depression is sometimes tied to a clear emotional stressor, such as development of a severe medical illness, or no obvious stressor may be present. In the consultation-liaison setting, it is always wise to look for organic etiologies of depression even when a clear precipitating event is identified. Antidepressant response rates are best established for major depressive disorder, especially when significant neurovegetative symptoms are present. Predictors of a good response to a particular antidepressant include previous depressive episodes that responded to that antidepressant and family members who have also experienced recurrent depressive episodes that responded to the same medication (Joyce and Paykel 1989). Secondary depressions also respond to antidepressant treatment, although the underlying cause should also be addressed. (For more information on depression, see Chapter 17 in this volume.)

In addition to major depression, antidepressants are often used for patients with other psychiatric diagnoses, such as bipolar disorder, depressed type (observe for cycling); dysthymic disorder; adjustment disorder; grief; eating disorders; substance abuse disorders (especially cocaine dependence and abstinence); and anxiety disorders. They are also used for problems such as incontinence and chronic pain (see Chapter 40 in this volume).

Classes of Antidepressant Drugs

The structure of TCAs, which includes both tertiary and secondary amines, is similar to that of the phenothiazines. The tertiary TCAs include imipramine, amitriptyline, trimipramine, doxepin, and clomipramine. Secondary TCAs are formed when tertiary amines are metabolized; imipramine is demethylated to desipramine, and amitriptyline is demethylated to nortriptyline. Protriptyline is a secondary amine noteworthy for a long half-life and anticholinergic potency. Although maprotiline is a tetracyclic, its pharmacological profile is similar to that of the TCAs (Table 42–7).

Newer antidepressants have distinct structures. Bupropion is a monocyclic phenylbutylamine of the aminoketone type. Trazodone is a triazolopyridine, and nefazodone is a synthetically derived phenylpiperazine. The dibenzoxazepine amoxapine is a metabolite of the neuroleptic loxapine. Venlafaxine, a structurally novel antidepressant, has a tricyclic configuration. Mirtazapine has a tetracyclic structure and belongs to the piperazino-azepine group of compounds. Reboxetine is an α-aryloxy-benzyl derivative that is a mixture of (R,R) and (S,S) enantiomers. The SSRIs include fluoxetine (a straight-chain phenylpropylamine), paroxetine (a phenylpiperidine compound), sertraline (a naphthylamine derivative), fluvoxamine (an aralkylketone), and citalopram (a racemic bicyclic phthalane derivative) (Table 42–8).

Mechanism of Action

The biogenic amine hypothesis holds that depression is associated with decreased levels of the central nervous system (CNS) neurotransmitters norepinephrine (catecholamine) or serotonin (indoleamine). The various cyclic antidepressants were thought to work by blocking reuptake of these neurotransmitters into presynaptic neurons. However, other antidepressants exist that do not have these properties. In addition, because reuptake blockage occurs rapidly, it cannot explain the delayed therapeutic action of antidepressants. Therefore, reuptake blockage alone does not account for the therapeutic effect of antidepressants.

Although the specific mechanisms of action of these varied agents are still undefined, increased norepinephrine and serotonin neurotransmission likely plays some role.

Antidepressant drugs, especially the TCAs, also affect other receptors, such as the cholinergic, CNS histaminic, and α_1 receptors, accounting for many of their side effects (Table 42–9). Most newer antidepressants are more selective and do not cause as many side effects.

Pharmacokinetics

The antidepressants are generally well absorbed orally and are highly protein bound, except for venlafaxine. This means that low serum albumin or displacement of a drug from protein-binding sites by another medication can increase biological effects. Sertraline is more highly protein bound than are fluoxetine or paroxetine.

A large variation exists in antidepressant steady-state levels. Active metabolites are often important in producing therapeutic effects, as well as side effects, particularly with the tertiary amines and fluoxetine. Drug interactions also can occur. For example, several serotonin reuptake inhibitors also inhibit CYP2D6 activity (see Table 42–8). The comparative inhibition among SSRIs is currently debated, but paroxetine appears to be more strongly inhibitory than fluoxetine or sertraline (Crewe et al. 1992). The use of measuring drug levels to achieve efficacy is reasonably well established for imipramine, desipramine, and nortriptyline. For other antidepressants, drug levels offer little more than a loose guide to treatment. Blood levels should be assessed 12 hours after the last dose. For nortriptyline, evidence indicates a therapeutic window between 50 and 150 ng/mL. For this medication, lowering the dose may actually increase efficacy if the blood level is above 150 ng/mL.

Other Indications

SSRIs and TCAs are widely used for treatment of depressive disorders, although SSRIs are usually better tolerated by medical-surgical patients. Patients with psychotic depressions respond better when an antipsychotic is administered concurrently; electroconvulsive therapy (ECT) alone is also effective and is probably the treatment of choice for this disorder (Dubovsky and Buzan 1999). Patients with atypical depressions may respond better to the monoamine oxidase inhibitors (MAOIs), but cyclic antidepressants and SSRIs are more often used by consultation-liaison psychiatrists to avoid drug interactions, hypotension, and the risk of hypertensive crisis. In addition to their use in treating mood disorders, antidepressants are increasingly used to treat anxiety disorders (Feighner 1999; see Table 42–10). The SSRIs are

TABLE 42–7.   Cyclic and related antidepressants

Generic name	Trade name	Alternate modes of administration[d]	Initial dose (mg)[b]	Usual therapeutic dose range (mg)[b]	Effect[a]					
					Norepinephrine reuptake blockade	Serotonin reuptake blockade	Dopamine reuptake blockade	Acetylcholine blockade	Histamine blockade	α_1 blockade
Amitriptyline	Elavil, others	im, iv[c]	25–75	150–300	1	2	1	4	3	3
Amoxapine	Asendin	—	50–150	100–600	3	1	1	1	2	2
Bupropion	Wellbutrin	—	100 bid	200–450	1	0	2	1	1	1
	Wellbutrin SR	—	150 qd	150–400	1	0	2	1	1	1
Citalopram	Celexa	—	20	20–60	1	3	1	1	1	1
Clomipramine	Anafranil	—	25	100–250	2	4	1	2	0	2
Desipramine	Norpramin, others	—	25–75	75–200	4	0	0	2	1	2
Doxepin	Sinequan, others	—	25–75	150–300	2	1	0	3	4	3
Fluoxetine	Prozac	Liquid	20	20–60	1	3	0	1	0	1
Imipramine	Tofranil, others	im, iv[c]	25–75	150–300	2	2	0	3	2	3
Maprotiline	Ludiomil	—	25–75	75–300	4	0	1	2	3	2
Mirtazapine[e]	Remeron	—	15	15–30	2	2	0	2	4	1
Nefazodone	Serzone	—	50 bid	300–600	2	2	1	0	0	2
Nortriptyline	Pamelor, others	—	20–40	50–200	3	1	0	2	2	1
Paroxetine	Paxil	Liquid	20	20–50	1	4	1	2	0	1
Protriptyline	Vivactil	—	10–20	20–60	3	1	0	3	2	2
Reboxetine	Edronax	—	15	15–45	4	0	0	1	1	1
Sertraline	Zoloft	—	50	50–200	0	3	1	1	0	1
Trazodone	Desyrel	—	50	100–600	1	2	0	0	1	3
Venlafaxine	Effexor	—	25 tid	225–375	1	3	0	0	0	1
	Effexor XR	—	75 qd	225–375	1	3	0	0	0	1

Note.   bid = twice daily; im = intramuscularly; iv = intravenously; qd = once daily; tid = three times daily.

[a]0 = least effect; 4 = most effect.

[b]Doses for elderly and medically ill patients are often lower.

[c]Not U.S. Food and Drug Administration approved for iv administration.

[d]Many drugs can be made into rectal suppositories or even lotions by willing pharmacists.

[e]Mechanism not related to reuptake blockade; rather, it increases norepinephrine and serotonin activity by antagonizing the α_2 auto- and heteroreceptors.

TABLE 42–8. Selective serotonin reuptake inhibitors

Generic name	Trade name	Cytochrome P450 effects[a]				Half-life	Other effects
		CYP1A2	CYP2C	CYP2D6	CYP3A4		
Citalopram	Celexa	0	0	0	0	35 hours	
Fluoxetine	Prozac	0	2	3	1	1.9 days	
Norfluoxetine		0	2	3	2	7 days	
Fluvoxamine	Luvox	4	2	0	2	15 hours	
Paroxetine	Paxil	0	0	4	0	15 hours	Cholinergic blockade
Sertraline	Zoloft	0	2	2	2	26 hours	

[a]0 = least effect; 4 = most effect.

Source. Adapted from DeVane 1998 and Shader et al. 1996. Used with permission.

TABLE 42–9. Possible clinical consequences of neurotransmitter blockade

Property	Possible clinical consequences
Blockade of norepinephrine uptake at nerve endings	Alleviation of depression Tremors Tachycardia Erectile and ejaculatory dysfunction Blockade of the antihypertensive effects of guanethidine Augmentation of pressor effects of sympathomimetic amines
Blockade of serotonin uptake at nerve endings	Alleviation of depression and other psychiatric disorders Gastrointestinal disturbance Increase or decrease in anxiety (dose dependent) Sexual dysfunction Extrapyramidal side effects (via indirect dopamine interactions) Interactions with L-tryptophan, monoamine oxidase inhibitors, and fenfluramine
Blockade of dopamine uptake at nerve endings	Psychomotor activation Antiparkinsonian effect Aggravation of psychosis
Blockade of histamine H_1 receptors	Potentiation of central depressant drugs Sedation Weight gain Hypotension
Blockade of muscarinic receptors	Blurred vision Dry mouth Sinus tachycardia Constipation Urinary retention Memory dysfunction
Blockade of α_1-adrenergic receptors	Potentiation of the antihypertensive effect of prazosin, terazosin, doxazosin, and labetalol Postural hypotension, dizziness Reflex tachycardia
Blockade of dopamine D_2 receptors	Extrapyramidal symptoms Endocrine changes (e.g., hyperprolactinemia) Sexual dysfunction (males); infertility, galactorrhea (females)

Source. Reprinted from Richelson E: "The Pharmacology of Antidepressants at the Synapse: Focus on Newer Compounds." *Journal of Clinical Psychiatry* 55 (suppl A):34–39, 1994. Used with permission.

TABLE 42–10. Effects of antidepressants on anxiety disorders

Drug	Panic disorder	General anxiety disorder	Obsessive-compulsive disorder	Social phobia	Posttraumatic stress disorder
Tricyclics	+++	+++	+++[a]	++	++
Selective serotonin reuptake inhibitors	+++	+++	+++	+++	+++
Mirtazapine	0	0	0	0	0
Nefazodone	+	+	0	+	++
Venlafaxine XR	++	+++	0	+	+
Monoamine oxidase inhibitors	+++	++	0	++	++
Reboxetine	0	0	0	0	0

Note. Efficacy as follows: +++ = proven; ++ = strong evidence; + = some evidence; 0 = inconclusive.
[a]Clomipramine is effective in treating obsessive-compulsive disorder.
Source. Adapted from Feighner J: "Overview of Antidepressants Currently Used to Treat Anxiety Disorders." *Journal of Clinical Psychiatry* 60 (suppl 22):18–22, 1999.

also effective in the treatment of eating disorders, particularly bulimia nervosa. Bupropion has proven effective in assisting patients with smoking cessation (Hurt et al. 1997). TCAs are also frequently used to treat chronic pain. The sedative and anticholinergic side effects of TCAs have also prompted clinicians to prescribe these drugs as hypnotics and to treat urinary incontinence.

Dosage and Administration

Treatment with the TCAs is started at a low dose, and the dose is increased gradually every 3–4 days. The initial dose and rate of increase are usually described as "start lower, go slower" for elderly and medically ill patients. To take advantage of the natural hypnotic effect of most TCAs, these drugs are generally taken at bedtime. More activating medications, such as fluoxetine and other SSRIs, are an exception; these should be taken in the morning. Most TCAs produce a response at doses of 150–300 mg in adult outpatients, but lower doses are often used in elderly or medically ill patients. Protriptyline, which has a long half-life, and nortriptyline are more potent than the other TCAs and require lower doses.

Response

A shared disadvantage of all antidepressants is the delay in onset of therapeutic action. At least 10 days to 2 weeks is required for initial response in patients with primary depression, and at least 6 weeks of an adequate dose should be maintained before abandoning a medication. A therapeutic response in elderly patients may take as long as 12 weeks (Dew et al. 1997). Unlike some other psychotropic medications, in which variation in patients' responses generally refers only to side effects, significant individual variation occurs in response to antidepressants,

especially in the context of medical illness. A patient's depression may not respond to one agent but then may respond well to another. If one medication does not improve the patient's depression, we recommend a trial with a drug that has a different neurotransmitter profile. SSRIs are clearly as effective as TCAs in the treatment of mild to moderate depression. Data support their efficacy compared with the TCAs in severely depressed inpatients as well (Anderson and Tomenson 1994). Trazodone appears to achieve a somewhat lower rate of antidepressant response than most antidepressants, but this may be the result of undertreatment. Trazodone's side-effect profile offers some advantages in consultation-liaison settings, such as particular help for patients with prominent sleep disturbance; the drug's disadvantages include priapism in men (rare) and persistent clitoral engorgement in women (even rarer), hypotension, and possible exacerbation of myocardial instability. Nefazodone has a favorable profile in patients who are medically ill because it has few, if any, sexual side effects, has little associated activation, and encourages sleep; it can infrequently cause hypotension.

Side Effects

Tricyclic Antidepressants

Frequent side effects of TCAs include anticholinergic effects (e.g., dry mouth, constipation, urinary retention), sedation, orthostatic hypotension, tachycardia, and weight gain. An increase in pulse rate is a frequent cardiac effect, which rarely interferes with the use of these drugs outside of the setting of the cardiac care unit. Cardiac effects (Jefferson 1989) include electrocardiogram (ECG) abnormalities (such as T-wave flattening or inversion and ST segment depression), conduction delays, and arrhythmias, despite the fact that TCAs are class IA quinidine-like antiarrhythmics. Therefore, for all hospitalized patients, the clinician should review the ECG before beginning treatment with a TCA. Particular caution is required for patients who have atrioventricular blocks, bundle branch blocks, and bradyarrhythmias. Such preexisting cardiac abnormalities can warrant starting the antidepressant in a monitored environment. A cardiologist should be consulted concerning decisions about initiating TCA treatment in such situations.

Treatment with a TCA should not be started immediately after a patient has had a myocardial infarction (MI). The risk of inducing arrhythmias should be carefully evaluated against the need to treat the patient's depression. The Cardiac Arrhythmia Suppression Trial demonstrated that antiarrhythmic drugs, including two class IC antiarrhythmics (encainide and flecainide) and one class IA antiarrhythmic (moricizine), were associated with unexpectedly increased mortality in post-MI patients (Glassman et al. 1993; Roose and Glassman 1994). These results necessitate a reassessment of the potential hazards of TCAs in patients with heart disease. When an antidepressant is needed in a patient immediately post-MI or in a patient who has ischemic heart disease, buproprion or an SSRI, specifically fluoxetine, paroxetine, or sertraline, is recommended (Roose and Spatz 1999).

Other possible side effects are insomnia, confusion (especially in patients with preexisting CNS disease), psychosis, tremor, rash, sweating, and sexual dysfunction. Sedation is a side effect that is often helpful. Sleep disturbance associated with depression resolves over time with successful treatment, and acute sedation from the TCA helps provide some immediate relief. All antidepressants can induce mania in certain individuals.

The anticholinergic effects of the TCAs are particularly important, especially for medical-surgical and elderly patients. Frequent anticholinergic effects are dry mouth, blurred vision, constipation, and urinary retention; the side effect of urinary retention is used to advantage for patients with incontinence. Patients with prostate enlargement, a condition that affects most elderly men, are particularly susceptible to urinary retention. Dry mouth, in addition to significant discomfort, can cause an increase in dental caries and gingivitis. In patients with untreated narrow-angle glaucoma, anticholinergic-induced pupillary dilation can cause an acute attack. This is not a concern in patients with wide-angle glaucoma or in those who have had an iridectomy. Anticholinergic effects may contribute to the sexual dysfunctions often caused by tricyclics. Patients who are medically ill, elderly, or cognitively impaired are at particularly high risk for delirium from drugs with anticholinergic potency.

Orthostatic hypotension is a serious side effect of TCAs, especially for elderly and medically ill patients who are at risk for falls (Thapa et al. 1995). Patients who take TCAs should be instructed to arise slowly from a lying or sitting position to a standing position. Among the tricyclics, imipramine is associated with the highest risk of orthostasis, whereas nortriptyline is associated with the least risk and is preferred when hypotension is a particular concern.

In rare cases, tricyclics can impair cardiac muscle contractility and worsen congestive heart failure (CHF) (Warrington et al. 1989). This concern is based on individual case reports of reproducible worsening of CHF. The evidence for this adverse effect is not strong, however, and should not restrict the use of these medications, except possibly in patients with severely compromised cardiac output in whom a small change in cardiac output is clinically significant (i.e., patients who are candidates for heart transplants who have ejection fractions of 20% or less).

Less frequent antidepressant side effects are hepatic toxicity (probably a hypersensitivity reaction), photosensitivity, and renal failure in overdose. Hematological effects include bone marrow depression, leukopenia and leukocytosis, agranulocytosis, and purpura. Neurological effects include tinnitus, myoclonus, action tremor, peripheral neuropathy, dysarthria, and stuttering. Cyclic antidepressants, especially maprotiline, clomipramine, and bupropion, increase the risk of seizures. They can also lower blood glucose in patients with diabetes. Sexual side effects are not uncommon and include delayed or incomplete orgasm (especially with clomipramine) and erectile failure. Amoxapine can cause extrapyramidal symptoms, tardive dyskinesia, and neuroleptic malignant syndrome (NMS), as well as other symptoms associated with neuroleptics. When TCAs are used during pregnancy, there is no clear evidence of malformations; however, a neonatal withdrawal syndrome may occur.

Selective Serotonin Reuptake Inhibitors

The side-effect profile of the SSRIs differs from that of the TCAs (see Table 42–7). SSRIs are generally considered to be activating, although paroxetine seems less so and can cause sedation (Ayd 1993; Kiev 1992). Frequent side effects include nausea, headache, nervousness, insomnia, decreased libido, and anorgasmia. SSRIs can produce decreased appetite and weight loss acutely, but some studies have indicated that with more chronic use SSRIs may produce weight gain (Fava 2000). Recent placebo-controlled studies indicate that weight gain is most likely related to recovery from depression itself and not a direct medication effect (Michelson et al. 1999). The anxiety-spectrum side effects are generally less common with sertraline and paroxetine than with fluoxetine. The effect of SSRIs on peripheral α_1 receptors appears minimal (Richelson 1994). Because SSRIs do not possess quinidine-like activity, as the TCAs do, cardiac arrhythmias rarely occur. A few reports of SSRI-associated bradycardia exist (Gelenberg 1995; Hussein and Kaufman 1994), although studies show that paroxetine, in particular, does not have a significant effect on heart rate, blood pressure, conduction intervals, or ventricular arrhythmias (Roose et al. 1998).

Other side effects that are less frequent with SSRI than with TCAs include somnolence, rash, fever, arthralgia, alopecia, and elevations in aminotransferase levels. Even more rare are extrapyramidal symptoms (Leo et al. 1995), leukocytosis, respiratory distress, and seizures in patients with preexisting seizure disorder. Hyponatremia is rarely seen with SSRIs. Fluoxetine toxicity, manifested by irritability and increased heart and respiratory rates, is reported in neonates (Spencer 1993).

In the early 1990s the media focused on fluoxetine's purported tendency to produce suicidal ideation or violent and impulsive behavior. Almost every physician, nurse, and patient on medical and surgical services has heard about this risk, even if they know little else about antidepressants; consultation-liaison psychiatrists are frequently asked about these associations. With any depressed patient, a risk of suicide exists, especially immediately after starting an antidepressant while the patient gains energy but still feels a subjective sense of hopelessness and depression. The tendency of SSRIs to produce nervousness or akathisia might add to this risk, although no clear association has been scientifically established.

The SSRIs differ in their effects on the CYP system. In general, paroxetine has the greatest inhibitory effect on the CYP2D6 enzyme, followed by fluoxetine and sertraline, whereas fluvoxamine strongly inhibits CYP1A2 activity. Among the SSRIs, citalopram appears to have no significant effects on the CYP system (see Table 42–8).

Other Antidepressants

Bupropion is stimulating and can produce anxiety, agitation, insomnia, and increased motor activity, along with tremor, nausea, and anorexia. It can also cause headache and rash. Like other cyclic antidepressants, bupropion is associated with a dose-related risk of seizures, especially in patients with bulimia, electrolyte disturbances, or history of significant head trauma. Recent expert consensus guidelines cite bupropion as the antidepressant least likely to cause switches to mania (Frances et al. 1998),

although any somatic treatment with an antidepressant effect, including ECT and sleep deprivation, has this potential. Bupropion causes fewer anticholinergic effects than do the TCAs, little orthostatic hypotension, and few adverse sexual side effects. No significant cardiac effects are associated with bupropion, although increases in blood pressure occur occasionally. In a study with a small sample size, bupropion was found to be safe in patients with depression and CHF, preexisting arrhythmias, and conduction delays (Roose et al. 1991a). Weight gain and sedation are not reported with bupropion. In overdose, bupropion lacks cardiovascular toxicity but does have significant neurological toxicity (Spiller et al. 1994).

Trazodone has significant α_1- and α_2-blocking activity and causes orthostatic hypotension as readily as do the tertiary amine TCAs (see Table 42–7). Rather than a quinidine-like slowing of conduction and suppression of premature ventricular contractions, trazodone—at antidepressant doses—is infrequently associated with an increase in premature ventricular contractions (Warrington et al. 1989). The sedating properties of trazodone are especially helpful for patients who have prominent sleep disturbance. Trazodone is associated with increased libido and has produced priapism rarely in men and persistent clitoral engorgement very rarely in women. This effect is not dose related and is likely caused by the combination of α_1 and α_2 blockade and by the relative absence of anticholinergic effects.

Nefazodone shares some characteristics with trazodone and has some that are distinct. Nefazodone has multiple sites of action, including presynaptic reuptake blockade of serotonin and norepinephrine and antagonism of the 5-hydroxytryptamine type 2 (5-HT_2) serotonin-postsynaptic receptor. It also blocks the α_1 receptor but not the α_2 receptor; it is less likely than trazodone to cause priapism, although cases have been reported (Brodie-Meijer et al. 1999). Because of α_1 blockade, there is potential for orthostasis in frail, medically ill individuals. Nefazodone causes less activation (e.g., insomnia) than do SSRIs (except during rapid switch from SSRI to nefazodone), rapid decrease in anxiety, sexual dysfunction no greater than placebo, and no weight gain or loss.

Venlafaxine is a potent presynaptic reuptake blocker of norepinephrine and serotonin and is less potent for dopamine reuptake blockade. Venlafaxine's major side effects include activation, nausea, high rates of sexual dysfunction, and dose-related hypertension. One meta-analysis indicated that venlafaxine did not adversely affect the control of blood pressure for patients with preexisting hypertension (Thase 1998), but more extensive studies involving patients with cardiovascular disease are still needed.

Mirtazapine has a dual mode of action that differs from venlafaxine and the SSRIs. It increases noradrenergic and serotonergic activity by antagonizing the α_2 autoreceptors and α_2 heteroreceptors. This direct enhancement of noradrenergic-mediated and 5-HT_1 α-receptor-mediated serotonergic neurotransmission is likely responsible for the antidepressant activity of mirtazapine. Mirtazapine also potently blocks postsynaptic 5-HT_2 and 5-HT_3 receptors, which may account for its anxiolytic, sleep-improving properties and fewer gastrointestinal side effects (Thompson 1999). Its mechanism of action does not include reuptake inhibition. Mirtazapine's side effects include dry mouth, sedation, increased appetite, and weight gain. In premarketing trials, 2 of 2,796 patients taking mirtazapine developed agranulocytosis, and one-third developed neutropenia. All patients recovered after discontinuation of the drug. Reboxetine is a selective noradrenergic reuptake inhibitor. It is free of the side effects associated with TCAs (i.e., reboxetine is not cardiotoxic), lacks affinity for serotonin and dopamine uptake sites, and is devoid of affinity for α-adrenergic, histaminergic, and muscarinic receptors (Burrows et al. 1998). Side effects include constipation, nausea, increased sweating, blurred vision, headache, insomnia, and dry mouth.

Overdose

TCAs carry substantial risk of death in overdose. The greatest danger comes from cardiac conduction delays that cause malignant ventricular arrhythmias. Risk of cardiac toxicity is particularly high if the Q-R-S interval is at least 0.1 seconds (Boehnert and Lovejoy 1985); if given a TCA, such patients should receive cardiac monitoring in an intensive care unit for 48 hours. A blood level of at least 1,000 ng/mL is also a risk factor for cardiac problems (Foulke and Albertson 1987). Levels greater than 2,500 ng/mL are often fatal. Severe hyperpyrexia from anticholinergic effects also can occur. Multiple-dose-activated charcoal therapy is useful, with appropriate caution regarding the risk of aspiration, bowel obstruction, and electrolyte disturbances (Harris and Kingston 1992; Jawary et al. 1992; Palatnick and Tenebein 1992). Because TCAs are highly protein bound, they are not removed by dialysis. The risk of death from overdose is substantially reduced by antidepressants that do not have quinidine-like properties, such as the SSRIs, trazodone, bupropion, venlafaxine, nefazodone, mirtazapine, and reboxetine.

Withdrawal and Rebound

A withdrawal syndrome can occur when TCAs are discontinued, especially if it is done rapidly. Many symptoms of this syndrome are those associated with anticholinergic rebound, including gastrointestinal upset, nausea, vomiting, diarrhea, excessive salivation, increased perspiration, anxiety, restlessness, piloerection, and sometimes delirium (Dilsaver and Greden 1984). Dizziness, headache, malaise, and nightmares are also reported. After long-term use, TCAs should be tapered slowly (e.g., decreased by 25–50 mg every 2–3 days).

A significant withdrawal phenomenon can occur with other antidepressant drugs, particularly those with shorter half-lives (i.e., paroxetine, sertraline, citalopram, and venlafaxine). Symptoms can include vertigo, dizziness, light-headedness, nausea, fainting, myalgias, and paresthesias. A slow taper of the antidepressants with shorter half-lives helps minimize withdrawal symptoms. Although fluoxetine is unlikely to produce these symptoms acutely after discontinuation, a similar syndrome may exist weeks later, when its metabolite is finally cleared.

Drug Interactions

Inhibitors of the CYP system can increase antidepressant blood levels, whereas smoking and certain medications, such as barbiturates, can increase hepatic metabolism and reduce antidepressant levels (see Table 42–6). Adding an SSRI, especially fluoxetine, to a TCA regimen often increases blood levels of the tricyclic (Preskorn et al. 1992).

Anticholinergic effects of TCAs add to the anticholinergic burden of other drugs such as antiparkinsonian agents and low-potency neuroleptics. Sedation is increased when antidepressants are combined with benzodiazepines or alcohol. When given together, the levels and effects of antidepressants and neuroleptics are increased. Thiazide diuretics and acetazolamide can worsen an antidepressant's hypotensive effects. The use of TCAs with medications that contain epinephrine, norepinephrine, or phenylephrine can produce hypertension or arrhythmias. The combination of TCAs with stimulants and sympathomimetic amines can also produce arrhythmias, particularly in predisposed patients. TCAs prolong and magnify the effects of other class IA antiarrhythmic agents such as quinidine and procainamide. Because TCAs block the uptake of guanethidine and guanadrel, the antihypertensive mechanism of these drugs is interrupted. Tricyclics can also block the effects of clonidine and methyldopa.

Concurrent use of MAOIs with antidepressants that enhance serotonergic activity can produce a serotonin syndrome, with symptoms of mental status changes, restlessness, myoclonus, hyperreflexia, fever, diaphoresis, shivering, tremor, seizures, and death. If a treatment-resistant depression requires a trial of combination therapy with TCAs and an MAOI, the medications should be started simultaneously to decrease the chances of serotonin syndrome (Lader 1983; White and Simpson 1981). Clomipramine is particularly problematic and should not be given with MAOIs. A severe serotonin syndrome occurs when MAOIs are given concomitantly with SSRIs or venlafaxine. This interaction is particularly problematic with fluoxetine because of its long-lasting active metabolite (see Table 42–8). Fluoxetine should be stopped at least 6 weeks before an MAOI is started. After prolonged treatment with fluoxetine, blood levels of fluoxetine and norfluoxetine should be obtained to ensure that levels are zero before MAOI treatment is started (Coplan and Gorman 1993), especially in patients with hepatic disease or in elderly patients who are taking multiple medications. Antidepressants (other than venlafaxine) are tightly protein bound and can displace other protein-bound drugs. As with the TCAs, simultaneous use of SSRIs and neuroleptics can increase the levels and effects of both.

Monoamine Oxidase Inhibitors

Types

Because of the potential side effects and life-threatening interactions with drugs and foods associated with MAOIs, psychiatrists rarely prescribe them to patients who are medically ill. The available MAOIs are the hydrazine agent phenelzine (Nardil) and the nonhydrazine agent tranylcypromine (Parnate) (Table 42–11). Moclobemide is a reversible MAOI not currently available in the United States (Amrein et al. 1992). Selegiline is a selective inhibitor of monoamine oxidase (MAO) type B at low doses (i.e., 10 mg/day). It is typically used in combination with L-dopa/carbidopa for Parkinson's disease; it may also have antidepressant properties, especially at higher doses. However, at higher doses, selegiline

becomes a nonspecific MAOI that can interact with SSRIs and other medications.

Mechanism of Action

There are two forms of MAO: 1) MAO type A, which degrades serotonin, norepinephrine, and epinephrine; and 2) MAO type B, which degrades dopamine and phenylalanine. Tyramine, an exogenous amino acid, is also degraded by the MAO type A system. If tyramine is ingested in large amounts, such as that found in some aged cheeses, it can cause a massive release of norepinephrine from nerve terminals precipitating a hypertensive crisis. For this reason, patients are instructed to avoid foods high in tyramine when taking MAOIs. Phenelzine and tranylcypromine both bind irreversibly to MAO type A and MAO type B throughout the body and inactivate them. Even after an irreversibly bound MAOI is discontinued, inhibition continues for approximately 2 weeks, until the body regenerates new MAO. In addition to its MAOI activity, tranylcypromine is structurally similar to amphetamine and is believed to exert stimulant-like action in the brain (Krishnan 1995).

Pharmacokinetics

MAOIs are rapidly absorbed. They are hepatically inactivated and are excreted primarily via the intestinal tract. Patients who are so-called slow acetylators may experience a prolonged effect.

Indications

The MAOIs may have advantages in the treatment of atypical depressions (i.e., depression characterized by anxiety, hypersomnia, increased appetite, and rejection sensitivity) in relatively healthy patients. Studies also indicate effectiveness for panic disorder, social phobia, posttraumatic stress disorder (PTSD), premenstrual dysphoria, and atypical facial pain (Krishnan 1995).

TABLE 42–11.   Monoamine oxidase (MAO) inhibitors

Generic name	Trade name	MAO inhibition	Initial dose (mg)[a]	Usual therapeutic dose range (mg)[a]
Phenelzine	Nardil	MAO-A and -B	15 bid/tid	45–90
Tranylcypromine	Parnate	MAO-A and -B	10–20 every morning	30–60
Moclobemide[b]	Manerix	Reversible MAO-A	300	300–600
Selegiline[c]	Eldepryl	MAO-B selective below 10 mg/day, can inhibit both MAO-A and -B at higher doses	5 bid	10

Note.   bid = twice daily; tid = three times daily.
[a]Doses for elderly and medically ill patients are often lower; caution is advised because of drug interactions.
[b]Not available in the United States.
[c]Used for Parkinson's disease in combination with L-dopa/carbidopa.

Side Effects

MAOIs are generally activating, and side effects frequently include CNS hyperactivity with restlessness, restless sleep, and insomnia. Daytime sleepiness can occur, particularly with phenelzine, and orthostatic hypotension often occurs with both MAOIs (Teicher et al. 1988).

Drug Interactions

Hypertensive crises are produced by the "cheese effect," when a patient consumes food containing large amounts of tyramine or other pressors. Symptoms include headache, flushing, palpitations, nausea and vomiting, photophobia, and retroorbital pain. Similar reactions occur in patients taking MAOIs with simultaneous use of a number of medications, including sympathomimetic amines and bronchodilators, psychostimulants, L-dopa, and buspirone. High doses of caffeine and chocolate can also stimulate the sympathetic nervous system and raise blood pressure. Chlorpromazine and, more recently, nifedipine are given as temporary acute treatment until the patient reaches an emergency room. Once there, patients with severe reactions are given 5 mg of phentolamine. Selegiline is less likely than other MAOIs to induce a hypertensive reaction, unless higher doses are used. Several common over-the-counter cold preparations contain ingredients (e.g., pseudoephedrine, dextromethorphan, phenylephrine, and phenlylpropanolamine) contraindicated for patients receiving MAOI therapy because of their sympathomimetic activity. These compounds can produce a hypertensive crisis when combined with MAOIs, as can illicit amphetamine and cocaine use (Stoudemire et al. 1990).

Interaction with agents that enhance serotonergic transmission, such as SSRIs and TCAs, can produce a serotonin syndrome. A potentially fatal interaction also occurs with meperidine, which has activity as a serotonin reuptake inhibitor. Patients taking MAOIs should be urged to immediately disclose this information to doctors and pharmacists to avoid these potentially dangerous drug interactions.

Patients taking TCAs or SSRIs with shorter half-lives should have a 1-week drug-free period before beginning MAOI therapy; patients switching from an MAOI to a tricyclic or an SSRI should have a 2-week drug-free interval between medications. Because of its long-lasting metabolites, fluoxetine should be stopped for at least 6 weeks before MAOI therapy begins. In patients with refractory depression in whom both TCAs and an MAOI are to be used concomitantly, the medications should be started simultaneously. The sedative effects of benzodiazepines and other sedative-hypnotics are enhanced by MAOIs, especially phenelzine. MAOIs can sometimes augment blood pressure reduction in patients already taking antihypertensive medications, such as high-dose β-blockers, clonidine, diuretics, guanethidine, guanadrel, methyldopa, and reserpine. This hypotensive reaction is especially prominent with phenothiazines. The effects of insulin and oral hypoglycemic medications are also increased. Concurrent use of succinylcholine during anesthesia can cause prolonged apnea and paralysis. Given the potential for these interactions, the discontinuation of MAOIs at least 2 weeks before surgery is often recommended. This is certainly preferable, but successful surgery is possible if the anesthesiologist and other physicians are informed about the MAOI.

Psychostimulants

Types

The commonly used psychostimulants are methylphenidate, a piperidine derivative related to amphetamine; dextroamphetamine; and pemoline, which is similar in structure to methylphenidate (Table 42–12). Modafinil is a novel psychostimulant that may have lower abuse potential than the others; it is approved for the treatment of excessive daytime sleepiness.

Mechanism of Action

Psychostimulant medications are structural analogues of catecholamines. They increase dopamine release and block its reuptake. They also increase norepinephrine's effect. Modafinil has a different, although unclear, mode of action. It increases extracellular dopamine but does not increase dopamine release.

Pharmacokinetics

Psychostimulants are readily absorbed and are not tightly protein bound. Excretion is essentially via the kidneys; acidification of the urine increases excretion. Pemoline has a longer half-life and a more delayed onset of action than the more commonly used psychostimulants.

Indications

The use of psychostimulants has been limited by real and perceived risks of abuse. In patients who have primary depression, lack of clear scientific evidence of efficacy has limited the use of these agents. Stimulant use for secondary depression (i.e., depression secondary to medical illness, such as poststroke depression) appears more promising. The stimulants provide specific advantages for

TABLE 42–12. Psychostimulants

Generic name	Trade name	Starting dose range (mg)	Usual dose range (mg)	Half-life (hours)
Dextroamphetamine	Dexedrine	5–10	5–30	8–12
	Adderall[a]	5–10	5–10	8–12
Methylphenidate				
Immediate release	Ritalin	5–10	5–60	1–3[b]
Sustained release	Ritalin-SR	20	20–60	4–5[b]
Extended release	Concerta	18	18–54	3.5[b]
Modafinil	Provigil	100–200	100–400	15
Pemoline	Cylert	37.5	18.75–75	12

[a]This is a combination of two amphetamine and two dextroamphetamine compounds.
[b]Represents plasma half-life; concentrations in the brain exceed those of plasma.

medically ill patients with anergic depressions (Kraus 1995; Wallace et al. 1995) and may also aid some patients who are demoralized or apathetic (Satel and Nelson 1989). The psychostimulants are also used effectively in patients with acquired immunodeficiency syndrome (AIDS), either with or without cognitive impairment (Fernandez and Levy 1990). Contrary to expectation, psychostimulants are associated with increased appetite in medically ill patients who are depressed.

Dosage and Administration

Dextroamphetamine is usually started at 5–10 mg/day and is taken in the morning. Immediate-release methylphenidate is usually started at a dosage of 2.5–5 mg twice daily (Frierson et al. 1991). Sustained-release methylphenidate is usually started at 20 mg/day. To prevent insomnia, doses of these drugs are typically not given after 3:00 P.M. The usual maximum daily dosage of dextroamphetamine is 30 mg and of immediate-release methylphenidate, 60 mg. Sustained-release methylphenidate can be given in dosages up to 60 mg/day. Pemoline is usually started at 37.5 mg/day and is taken in the morning; the dosage is either reduced to 18.75 mg/day or increased to a maximum of 75 mg/day, depending on response and side effects.

Response

Response to an appropriate dosage of a psychostimulant usually appears within 1–2 days but can take longer, especially with pemoline. The rapid response of patients to psychostimulants has led to an evaluation of their effectiveness in predicting antidepressant response to TCAs and other antidepressants. Some evidence indicates that dextroamphetamine predicts antidepressant efficacy (Little 1988) and that methylphenidate may

predict efficacy of antidepressants with more noradrenergic properties (Gwirtsman and Guze 1989); however, the use of psychostimulants in this context is controversial (Joyce and Paykel 1989). Modafinil and other stimulants are also used to augment other antidepressant treatments (Menza et al. 2000). Tolerance to the effects of psychostimulants sometimes develops with extended use.

Side Effects

Side effects are infrequent at the relatively low dosages used to treat depression in patients who are medically ill. Appetite suppression and insomnia can occur with psychostimulants, but anorexia caused by depression (along with other neurovegetative symptoms) is reversed by psychostimulants, if an antidepressant effect occurs. Possible CNS side effects are activation, exacerbation of anxiety, and exacerbation of confusion. Other reported side effects are nausea, tremor, headache, exacerbation of spasticity, blurred vision, dry mouth, constipation, dizziness, and fatigue. Cardiovascular effects may include palpitations, dysrhythmias, tachycardia, and blood pressure changes. Dystonias rarely occur. A delayed hepatic hypersensitivity reaction is reported with pemoline (Elitsur 1990; Patterson 1984; Pratt and Dubois 1990; Tolman et al. 1973). The effects of psychostimulants during pregnancy are not well known. With maternal use during the first trimester, they can cause birth defects and premature births (Bays 1991; Gilbody 1991). Neonatal withdrawal can occur.

Overdose and Toxicity

A toxic syndrome occurs at high doses of psychostimulants. These agents can produce paranoid delusions and visual, auditory, or tactile hallucinations at high dosages or in predisposed patients. A relatively small dose of a neuroleptic, such as haloperidol, 2–5 mg intramuscularly, usually resolves stimulant-induced psychosis. Also occurring in overdose are palpitations, arrhythmias, hypertension, perspiration, dizziness, tremor, hyperreflexia, headache, confusion, and euphoria. Seizures and coma can occur in severe cases.

Withdrawal

Abstinence symptoms following long-term use of psychostimulants may include drug craving, somnolence, rebound depression, and fatigue as well as nausea, vomiting, hyperphagia, and tremor.

Drug Interactions

Psychostimulants have additive effects with other drugs that produce CNS stimulation, such as caffeine. They also have additive cardioacceleratory effects with TCAs and interfere with the hypotensive effects of guanethidine and similar drugs (Table 42–13). Potentially dangerous interactions with MAOIs are described in the MAOI section of this chapter. The blood levels of imipramine and desipramine can be increased when combined with methylphenidate. Hepatic enzyme inhibition is the hypothesized cause, although the specific isoenzymes that are affected have not been identified (Markowitz et al. 1999).

Lithium as an Antidepressant

Lithium is used to treat unipolar or bipolar depression. Its usefulness in treating bipolar disorder with depressive symptoms is better documented than its efficacy in the treatment of unipolar depression.

Lithium has also been used to augment the antidepressant effect of cyclic antidepressants. Study results indicate that lithium augmentation should be used for a minimum of 7 days at doses that are sufficient to reach lithium serum levels of greater than or equal to 0.5 mEq/L (Bauer and Dopfmer1999). Adding lithium to a regimen of drugs that induce strong serotonin reuptake inhibition requires caution because of the possibility of serotonin syndrome (Kojima et al. 1993; Ohman and Spigset 1993).

Other Medications

Adding triiodothyronine, 25–50 μg/day, to a TCA regimen can speed or induce a response in some patients (Joffe et al. 1993).

The benzodiazepine alprazolam is approved by the Food and Drug Administration (FDA) for use in patients with mild depression. Although its use in patients with

TABLE 42–13. Reported drug interactions with psychostimulants

Medication	Interactive effect
Guanethidine	Decreased antihypertensive effect
Vasopressors	Increased pressor effect
Oral anticoagulants	Increased prothrombin time
Anticonvulsants	Increased levels of phenobarbital, primidone, and phenytoin
Tricyclic antidepressants	Increased blood levels of antidepressant
Monoamine oxidase inhibitors	Hypertension

Source. Reprinted from Stoudemire A, Moran MG, Fogel BS: "Psychotropic Drug Use in the Medically Ill, Part II." *Psychosomatics* 32:38, 1991. Copyright 1991, Academy of Psychosomatic Medicine. Used with permission.

mild depression with prominent anxiety is theoretically desirable, the availability of alternative agents without addictive and other problems eliminates this advantage.

When depressive symptoms are associated with inadequately treated pain, analgesics are effective as antidepressants. Pain can produce depressed mood, lack of motivation, poor sleep, reduced appetite, and lack of energy. These symptoms are eliminated with adequate analgesia.

MOOD-STABILIZING MEDICATIONS

Basic Concepts

In the not-so-distant past, lithium was the mainstay for mood stabilization in patients with primary bipolar disorder. It is now joined by several anticonvulsants including carbamazepine, valproic acid, gabapentin, and lamotrigine (Table 42–14). Compliance, or adherence as it is often now called, is a particular problem in patients with bipolar disorder. Patients who are in a manic or hypomanic phase resist treatment because they do not perceive a problem exists; they enjoy the euphoria and are reluctant to give it up.

Indications

Mood stabilizers are also used to treat secondary mania (e.g., in patients taking high-dose steroids immediately after organ transplant) and schizoaffective disorder and to calm agitated and violent patients with CNS disorders and other conditions.

TABLE 42–14.   Antimanic/mood-stabilizing medications

Generic name	Trade name	Starting dose (mg)[a]	Usual therapeutic dose range (mg)[a]
Lithium	Lithium, Lithobid	300 bid	600–1,200
Carbamazepine	Tegretol	200 bid	600–1,600
Valproic acid	Depakote, others	250 bid	625–3,800
Gabapentin	Neurontin	300 qd	900–1,800
Lamotrigine	Lamictal	50 qd[b]	300–500[b]
Topiramate	Topamax	25–50 qd	200–400

Note.   bid = twice daily; qd = once daily.
[a]Doses for elderly and medically ill patients are often lower.
[b]If patient is also taking valproic acid, starting dose is 25 mg every other day and maximum dose is 150 mg/day.
Source.   Reprinted from Rundell JR, Wise MG: *Concise Guide to Consultation Psychiatry*, 3rd Edition. Washington, DC, American Psychiatric Press, 2000, p. 87. Used with permission.

Lithium

Mechanism of Action

Explanations for lithium's effectiveness are diverse. Hypotheses include effects on neurotransmission, circadian rhythm slowing, inhibition of endocrine systems, membrane stabilization, and ion transmission changes. None of these hypotheses has clearly explained lithium's effects.

Pharmacokinetics

Lithium is a cation, like sodium, which helps explain its behavior in the kidney. Lithium is administered as a salt, in tablet or capsule form, as lithium carbonate (an alternative extended-release form exists), or in liquid form, as lithium citrate. The single-dose elimination half-life of lithium is 5–8 hours; at maintenance dosage levels, lithium's half-life is about 1 day. Its half-life is longer in patients with reduced renal clearance (e.g., in patients with renal disease and most elderly patients). Steady state is achieved in 3–8 days.

Lithium is not metabolized and is directly eliminated via excretion from the kidneys. In the kidney, lithium is reabsorbed in the proximal tubule, along with water and sodium, but undergoes minimal reabsorption in the distal tubule. In patients who are sodium deficient, both sodium and lithium are reabsorbed; this can produce lithium toxicity. Conversely, high lithium levels can cause more sodium excretion. Lithium levels are also sensitive to the body's fluid balance. Dehydration will increase lithium concentration, especially if sodium intake is not maintained. However, when dehydration is induced by increases in ambient temperature accompanied by sweating, lithium concentration can decrease because sweat can contain high concentrations of lithium (Jefferson et al. 1982). Conversely, marked polydipsia, often induced by the lithium, can reduce lithium blood levels.

Dosage and Administration

Lithium has a narrow therapeutic window (i.e., the therapeutic level of lithium is very close to toxic levels). Despite this, it is possible to reach and continue a stable maintenance level without major difficulty, even in hospitalized medically ill patients. Serum concentrations must be monitored closely, especially when initiating treatment. Lithium levels should be measured 10–12 hours after the last dose. The therapeutic level for patients with acute mania is 0.8–1.5 mEq/L. For long-term maintenance or prophylaxis in most patients with bipolar illness, the optimal therapeutic level is 0.8–1.0 mEq/L (Gelenberg et al. 1989). Prophylactic levels are higher for some patients. As with all drug levels, certain patients require a modification of guidelines. When lithium treatment is started, levels should be obtained weekly. Once a steady state is achieved, frequency of monitoring can be reduced to monthly and then quarterly. More frequent monitoring is often needed in patients who are at increased risk for toxicity, such as elderly patients, patients who are taking another medication known to interact with lithium, and patients with dementia or impaired renal function.

Response

An optimal therapeutic response in patients with acute mania may take 5–14 days. Before this response occurs, patients who are highly agitated or those who have psychosis usually require adjunctive treatment with a benzodiazepine such as clonazepam or with a neuroleptic medication.

Side Effects

The most frequent side effects of lithium are gastric irritation, mild diarrhea, polydipsia, and polyuria (DasGupta and Jefferson 1990). Fine tremors often occur and are treated by reducing the lithium dosage or adding a β-blocking medication. Tremors are more likely to occur in patients with underlying CNS disorders. Nausea and fatigue usually resolve after the first weeks of lithium treatment but can reemerge and be accompanied by vomiting if blood levels climb abruptly. Weight gain and edema are sometimes persistent. Lithium may also cause mild leukocytosis; this side effect has been used to advantage in patients who have conditions with problematic leukopenia, such as in patients with AIDS or in patients who have received bone marrow transplants. Other reported side effects include a metallic taste and a decreased sense of creativity.

A number of organs are potentially affected by lithium. Renal effects include tubular lesions, interstitial fibrosis, decreased creatinine clearance, nephrogenic diabetes insipidus, and renal tubular acidosis. A progressive decrease in renal function is rare, and irreversible renal failure with chronic lithium therapy has not been reported (Marangell et al. 1999). Lithium depletes intracellular potassium, which can cause cardiac effects. ST segment and T-wave changes, such as T-wave flattening or inversion, are common. T-wave changes are potentially useful as an indirect indicator of compliance. Cardiac arrhythmias are rare and are usually atrial in origin; they include atrial fibrillation and flutter, sick sinus syndrome, atrioventricular block, and premature ventricular contractions, especially in predisposed patients. Thyroid effects include goiter and hypothyroidism, especially in women. Hyperthyroidism is unusual, as are other endocrine effects such as hypoglycemia and hyperparathyroidism. Dermatological side effects include severe acne, psoriasis, folliculitis, and hair loss. In unusual cases, patients can experience persistent nausea and vomiting, parkinsonian symptoms, exophthalmos, Raynaud's phenomenon, or pseudotumor cerebri.

Because of side effects, lithium use demands special monitoring in elderly patients and in patients with dementia. Impaired renal function, cardiac disease, extracellular volume depletion, and use of potentially interacting medications increase the risk of toxicity. Caution is also needed in patients with impaired fluid balance, decreased sodium intake, or increased sodium loss. Because problems can develop quickly among hospitalized medically ill patients, close monitoring is important. Pretreatment screening should include an ECG, serum creatinine level, urinalysis, and thyroid function tests, including thyroid-stimulating hormone. In elderly patients or chronically ill medical patients, serum creatinine is often artificially low because of reduced muscle mass; 24-hour creatinine clearance for evaluation of kidney function is sometimes required in older patients and in patients with renal dysfunction.

Lithium use should be avoided during early pregnancy, if possible. It can cause cardiovascular birth defects, particularly Ebstein's anomaly. This defect consists of right ventricular hypoplasia, patent ductus arteriosus, and tricuspid valve insufficiency. Data from recent studies indicate that the risk for Ebstein's anomaly is not as high as was originally thought (L. S. Cohen et al. 1994). Initial information regarding the teratogenic risk of lithium treatment was derived from biased retrospective studies. The best estimate of the risk of major congenital anomalies among the children of women taking lithium during early pregnancy is on the order of 4%–12% as observed by several cohort studies (Jacobson 1995; Kallen and Tandberg 1983). In contrast, the prevalence of congenital anomalies in the untreated comparison groups in these studies was 2%–4%. Clinicians should consider discontinuing lithium use in pregnant patients during their first trimester, although discontinuation must be weighed against the risk of morbidity due to a relapse of a mood disorder. Reproductive risk counseling should occur as early in the pregnancy as possible. Prenatal diagnosis using fetal echocardiography and high-resolution ultrasound can be offered at 16–18 weeks' gestation. Pregnancy also increases glomerular filtration and can decrease lithium levels. Once a patient has delivered, her glomerular filtration rate will return to baseline levels and lithium dosage should be adjusted. Lithium is generally found in breast milk at a level one-third to one-half that of the mother's serum level (Wise et al. 1990).

Overdose

Lithium levels greater than 1.5 mEq/L are usually problematic, and levels greater than 2.0 mEq/L are considered toxic. Lower levels can produce troublesome side effects in severely ill, elderly, or predisposed patients. Symptoms include ataxia, muscle weakness, confusion, lethargy, slurred speech, vomiting, diarrhea, increased urination, tinnitus, blurred vision, and nystagmus. These effects can progress to stupor, coma, convulsions, and permanent neurological impairment (Reed 1989). Treatment consists of hydration and supportive treatment. Hemodialysis is indicated if the lithium level is greater than 3.0 mEq/L and signs of toxicity are severe, or if there is poor urine output or renal failure (Hyman et al. 1995).

Withdrawal

Relapse in patients with bipolar disorder is the primary concern with lithium discontinuation. Following abrupt lithium discontinuation, patients with precarious fluid or electrolyte balance should be monitored closely. Infrequently, patients who have stopped taking lithium will experience temporary anxiety or irritability.

Drug Interactions

Most diuretics, especially thiazides, decrease lithium clearance and increase the lithium level. However, furosemide, osmotic diuretics, and carbonic anhydrase inhibitors have the opposite effect. Nonsteroidal anti-inflammatory drugs (NSAIDs) reduce lithium clearance and can increase levels. Spectinomycin and tetracycline also decrease lithium excretion, whereas aminophylline and theophylline increase it. Prolongation of succinylcholine's effects is also reported. Because lithium has variable effects on glucose and insulin, patients may require adjustment of insulin doses. Cyclosporine inhibits renal excretion of lithium, and lithium toxicity can occur quickly (Wise et al. 1988). This can be an issue particularly in patients who develop mania secondary to high-dose steroids after organ transplantation. Mood stabilization with valproic acid is recommended in such cases.

Concerns have been posed about the potential for neurotoxicity with concurrent use of lithium and neuroleptics (especially haloperidol) and the use of lithium in neurologically predisposed patients (W. Cohen and Cohen 1974). The cases that prompted these concerns probably represent variants of NMS. A number of case reports involving haloperidol and other neuroleptics have been published. Patients taking neuroleptics and lithium should be monitored for symptoms of NMS; however, there is no evidence of frequent, consistent, or predictable problems with this drug combination. The combination of lithium and TCAs may worsen symptoms of lithium toxicity, especially tremor. Preexisting extrapyramidal symptoms from medications or movement disorder are sometimes exacerbated by lithium (Addonizio et al. 1988; Sachdev 1986). Increased sedation can occur with concurrent sedative use. Lithium neurotoxicity is also more likely with concurrent carbamazepine use (Chaudhry and Waters 1983; Shukla et al. 1984).

Anticonvulsants

Types

The use of anticonvulsants is a relatively recent pharmacological approach to mood stabilization. The primary anticonvulsants used are carbamazepine (a tricyclic medication) and valproic acid (a branched-chain carboxylic acid) (see Table 42–14). These medications have produced data showing clear-cut efficacy (Bowden et al. 1994; Pope

et al. 1991). Gabapentin, lamotrigine, and topiramate have received attention as treatments for bipolar disorder. Further studies are needed to establish roles for these medications in the treatment of bipolar disorder, but preliminary observations appear promising (Cabras et al. 1999; Calabrese et al. 1998; Frye et al. 2000).

Anticonvulsant medications are especially useful for patients who are resistant to or cannot tolerate treatment with lithium and for patients who have rapid-cycling bipolar disorder (i.e., more than four major mood swings during the previous 12-month period) (McElroy et al. 1989). Some consultation-liaison psychiatrists believe that an anticonvulsant is a better treatment than lithium for secondary mania, although data beyond anecdotal reports are lacking. Cases have been reported in which drug interactions involving lithium preclude its use (Wise et al. 1990). Anticonvulsants are also preferred when mania is associated with a seizure disorder or for patients with atypical or mixed mania (commonly seen in consultation-liaison settings).

Mechanism of Action

Carbamazepine is known to decrease noradrenergic release and reuptake. Valproic acid increases brain γ-aminobutyric acid (GABA) neurotransmission by increasing its synthesis, inhibiting its breakdown, and enhancing its postsynaptic effects. Gabapentin exerts its effects on the GABAergic system as well, although its exact mechanism of action is unclear. Lamotrigine blocks type 2 sodium channels and decreases the release of excitatory amino acids. The relationship of these effects to clinical efficacy is unknown.

Pharmacokinetics

Carbamazepine is well absorbed, but drug levels that produce therapeutic effects vary widely among patients. It is both a substrate and an inducer of its own metabolism; therefore, a predictable decrease in carbamazepine blood levels occurs about 3–4 weeks after initiation of treatment. Carbamazepine is metabolized by the CYP3A3/4 isoenzymes. Care should be taken when combining carbamazepine with other drugs metabolized by this isoenzyme (see Table 42–6). Valproic acid is rapidly absorbed and is highly protein bound. It is metabolized primarily by conjugation in the liver and does not induce its own metabolism; it may inhibit it.

Gabapentin is excreted in the kidneys and has few drug interactions. Because of its relatively benign side-effect profile and lack of drug interactions, it may be particularly useful as an adjunctive therapy, if it proves useful in further clinical trials (Post et al. 1998). One of the authors (MGW) has seen three cases of severe agitation and violent behavior when gabapentin was given to patients who had long-standing brain injury. Lamotrigine is rapidly and completely absorbed after oral administration and has negligible first-pass metabolism. Its principal route of elimination is glucuronidation followed by renal excretion. Lamotrigine is more rapidly eliminated in patients taking other hepatically metabolized anticonvulsants, such as carbamazepine, phenytoin, phenobarbital, or primidone. Paradoxically, valproic acid decreases the clearance of lamotrigine, more than doubling its elimination half-life.

Indications

Carbamazepine is used for acute treatment of primary and secondary mania, as prophylaxis in patients with bipolar disorder, and to control patients who are agitated or violent. In medically ill patients, concerns about reliability of response and potential hematological side effects have limited its use. Valproic acid is effective for mood stabilization in a number of disorders, including bipolar disorder, schizoaffective disorder, and secondary mood disorders. The appropriate role of gabapentin and lamotrigine in treating psychiatric disorders has not been determined.

Dosage and Administration

Although the effective range of carbamazepine blood levels for patients with psychiatric disorders has not been established, suggested levels for treatment are 6–12 μg/mL. These levels are usually achieved by starting with a dosage of 200 mg twice daily and then increasing the dosage to 200 mg three times daily in 3–5 days. The maintenance dosage of carbamazepine ranges from 600 to 1,600 mg/day, provided no complications occur.

Valproic acid is usually started at 250 mg twice daily and then increased by 250 mg every 3–4 days. Maintenance dosages range from 600 to 3,800 mg/day, with an average of 1,200 mg/day. The target blood level is 50–100 μg/mL.

Blood monitoring is not required for gabapentin or lamotrigine. A typical starting dosage for gabapentin is 300–900 mg/day; the therapeutic dosage range appears to be 600–5,000 mg/day. Lamotrigine should be started at a low dosage (i.e., 25–50 mg/day) and increased biweekly to help reduce the potential for rashes and neurological side effects. If given concomitantly with valproic acid, lamotrigine should be started at 12.5 mg/day for 2 weeks and then increased by 25 mg/week, as tolerated (Ketter et al. 1999). The maximum recommended dosage is 500 mg/day in adults.

Response

As with lithium, response to anticonvulsants is usually delayed 7–14 days in patients with acute mania.

Side Effects

Transient leukopenia is typically seen with initiation of carbamazepine treatment. The major concern with carbamazepine is aplastic anemia, a rare and sometimes fatal hematological condition. Patients should be monitored for any sign of petechiae, infection, or anemia. A complete blood count is recommended weekly for 1 month and then every 3 months thereafter, although some clinicians have argued that only a baseline hematological evaluation is needed in otherwise healthy and asymptomatic patients (Pellock and Willmore 1991). Medically ill patients may require more frequent monitoring. Carbamazepine produces a skin rash in 10%–15% of patients. The medication should be discontinued if a rash occurs. Rapid dosage increases can cause incoordination, ataxia, drowsiness, dizziness, and slurred speech. Asterixis and hyponatremia have also been reported. There have been reports of spina bifida occurring in babies exposed to carbamazepine in utero (Rosa 1991).

Valproic acid's most common side effect is sedation. Also common are nausea, vomiting, and anorexia. Enteric coating, available with some preparations, helps to prevent these side effects. Valproic acid can cause an idiosyncratic, fatal hepatotoxicity (Brown 1989). Healthy patients can tolerate increases of up to two or, less comfortably, three times the normal levels of serum glutamic-oxaloacetic transaminase or serum glutamic-pyruvic transaminase, but valproic acid treatment is usually discontinued if increased elevations persist or if higher elevations occur (Pellock and Willmore 1991; Stoudemire et al. 1991). Weight gain, hair-thinning, or a fine hand tremor also may occur. A daily multivitamin containing 25 mg of selenium and 50 mg of zinc may prevent hair brittleness. Thrombocytopenia is a rare event. Neural tube defects have been reported after use during the first trimester of pregnancy.

Gabapentin is generally well tolerated but can cause sedation, dizziness, ataxia, fatigue, and weight gain (Goa and Sorkin 1993). Lamotrigine can cause dizziness, ataxia, headache, sedation, tremor, and nausea. Serious rashes requiring hospitalization and treatment discontinuation have been reported with lamotrigine. The incidence of these rashes, which have included Stevens-Johnson syndrome, is approximately 1% in pediatric populations (age < 16 years) and 0.3% in adults (*Physicians' Desk Reference* 2000). A less severe rash can occur in approximately 10% of patients taking lamotrigine (Post et al. 1998). Slow titration may reduce the incidence of these phenomena.

Overdose

Coma and death can occur with overdoses of carbamazepine or valproic acid. Because valproic acid is highly protein bound at therapeutic concentrations, it is not dialyzable. However, higher concentrations may result in free valproic acid, which can be cleared by hemodialysis (Kandrotas et al. 1990; Tank and Palmer 1993). Carbamazepine is bound by charcoal. Overdoses involving up to 15 g have been reported for lamotrigine; some were fatal. Overdose has resulted in ataxia, nystagmus, seizures, decreased level of consciousness, coma, and intraventricular conduction delay. Overdoses of gabapentin involving up to 49 g have been reported. In these cases, double vision, slurred speech, drowsiness, lethargy, and diarrhea were observed. All patients recovered with supportive care (Fischer et al. 1994). Gabapentin is subject to hemodialysis, although it has not been performed in the few overdose cases reported. Hemodialysis may be indicated by the patient's clinical state or renal impairment.

Drug Interactions

Carbamazepine's induction of hepatic enzymes produces several drug interactions (see Tables 42–4 and 42–6). These interactions can decrease the effectiveness of anticoagulants, neuroleptics, oral contraceptives (Rapport and Calabrese 1989), and theophylline. Also, carbamazepine toxicity is increased by medications that decrease hepatic metabolism, such as calcium antagonists and cimetidine. Conversely, carbamazepine's therapeutic effect is inhibited by medications that induce metabolism (see Table 42–6).

Valproic acid levels are also lowered by enzyme-inducing drugs, including carbamazepine, and are increased by inhibitors of hepatic metabolism. Valproic acid itself does not increase hepatic metabolism and appears to inhibit it. Gabapentin is excreted via the kidneys and has minimal effects on the CYP microsomal enzyme system. Lamotrigine is metabolized to a glucuronide form and is then excreted via the kidneys.

Other Mood Stabilizers

Data suggest that the benzodiazepine clonazepam has antimanic properties, although any benzodiazepine can potentially decrease anxiety and promote sleep. The sedative effects of benzodiazepines such as clonazepam or lorazepam are useful for the treatment of acute agitation. Compared with other drugs used to treat mania (see Table 42–14), benzodiazepines have a rapid onset of action. Clonazepam is used in dosages of 4–20 mg/day for acute mania. Lorazepam is typically used in dosages of 1–6 mg/day, although higher dosages have been reported.

NEUROLEPTICS

Basic Concepts

Neuroleptics are powerful medications that have the potential to relieve intensely disturbing symptoms. They can also cause significant side effects. Neuroleptics are helpful in the treatment of psychosis, delirium, and dementia in which agitation, paranoia, and confusion are often troublesome symptoms.

Indications

The target symptoms for neuroleptic use include the classic psychotic symptoms of hallucinations and delusions as well as more general symptoms of suspiciousness, confusion, belligerence, psychomotor agitation, and assaultiveness. In the past, it was believed that antipsychotic medications were less helpful against the negative symptoms of schizophrenia, such as impaired judgment, flat affect, and lack of motivation. However, data indicate that negative symptoms improve with adequate traditional neuroleptic treatment (Serban et al. 1992; Tandon et al. 1993) and with treatment with atypical agents. Neuroleptics are the drugs of choice for treatment of schizophrenia. In patients with primary or secondary mania, neuroleptics are often used to suppress the symptoms of excitement and psychosis until lithium or an anticonvulsant takes effect. Occasionally, neuroleptics are also needed to treat recurrent mania. In patients with psychotic depression, the combination of an antidepressant and a neuroleptic is more effective than either drug alone, although ECT is considered the treatment of choice. In patients with dementia or delirium, neuroleptics are used to control specific psychotic symptoms and general symptoms of agitation. Neuroleptics are also prescribed by consultation-liaison psychiatrists for patients with acute severe panic or extreme anxiety. The use of neuroleptic drugs for simple primary anxiety is not warranted, given the availability of alternative medications with less serious long-term side effects. Patients with Tourette's syndrome also respond to neuroleptics, particularly haloperidol and pimozide. Neuroleptics, especially pimozide, are widely used to treat delusional disorder, especially the somatic subtype.

Types

Neuroleptics are typically divided into two major groups, typical and atypical agents. The typical neuroleptics include traditional low-, medium-, and high-potency agents with a high affinity for dopamine type 2 (D_2) receptors, whereas the atypicals include clozapine, risperidone, olanzapine, quetiapine, and ziprasidone. Agents are called atypical if they have a lower incidence of extrapyramidal symptoms owing to a decreased affinity for D_2 receptors, and they also commonly exert effects on serotonin receptors (Casey 1996). Because all neuroleptics have similar efficacy at equivalent doses, the selection of a particular medication is based on side effects. The typical neuroleptics are ranked from low to high potency, a spectrum that helps predict side effects. Antipsychotic equivalencies are generally measured relative to chlorpromazine, the first antipsychotic developed (Table 42–15).

Mechanism of Action

Typical neuroleptics block the postsynaptic dopamine receptor, particularly the D_2 subtype. Blockage occurs in the mesolimbic and mesocortical dopamine pathways, as well as in the nigrostriatal pathway; the latter is the likely site for parkinsonian side effects. The tuberoinfundibular dopamine system is also affected, elevating prolactin levels and producing neuroendocrine side effects. Neuroleptics, especially low-potency antipsychotics, also block α-noradrenergic receptors, producing hypotensive symptoms; low-potency neuroleptics also block muscarinic acetylcholine receptors, resulting in anticholinergic side effects. In addition, some neuroleptics block histaminic and serotoninergic receptors.

Among the atypical neuroleptics, clozapine is a unique medication that blocks dopamine at limbic sites but has substantially less effect on the extrapyramidal and neuroendocrine systems; however, it also antagonizes adrenergic, cholinergic, histaminergic, and serotonergic receptors. Risperidone's antipsychotic activity is mediated through a combination of D_2 and 5-HT_{2A} antagonism. Olanzapine blocks 5-HT_2 receptors and D_1–D_4 receptors. It also has significant muscarinic, histaminic, and α_1-adrenergic receptor blockade. Quetiapine affects serotonin 5-HT_{1A} and 5-HT_2 receptors as well as D_1 and D_2, histaminic, and adrenergic receptors. Quetiapine has no appreciable affinity for muscarinic receptor sites. Ziprasidone has high 5-HT_{2A} and moderate D_2 antagonism. It also exerts antagonism at other serotonergic receptor sites. It is a moderately potent α_1 and H_1 blocker.

Pharmacokinetics

Neuroleptics have variable oral absorption. They are highly lipophilic and protein bound. Half-lives range from about 10 hours to 1 day. There are depot forms (two for fluphenazine and one for haloperidol), which are typically given every 1–4 weeks. The duration of action in the brain after long-term administration can be months or even more than a year with the decanoate forms.

Other Indications

In addition to being used to treat psychosis and agitation, neuroleptics are sometimes used for their antiemetic effect. Prochlorperazine and droperidol are often used for this purpose, as is metoclopramide, another dopamine antagonist. Both prochlorperazine (Lapierre et al. 1969) and droperidol can provide antipsychotic effects at doses higher than those generally given for nausea. Metoclopramide and prochlorperazine can produce, at any dose, the side effects seen with neuroleptics, especially dystonic reactions. One exception to the general rule of using neuroleptics as the primary medications to treat psychotic symptoms is in patients with CNS sedative withdrawal, including alcohol (delirium tremens) and benzodiazepine withdrawal. In such situations, benzodiazepines are preferred because they more directly treat the withdrawal syndrome. Neuroleptics are also used for acute control of mania; for acute management of delirium symptoms; and in cases of severe panic, which can occur when weaning a patient off a ventilator.

Dosage and Administration

Doses equivalent to 300–600 mg of chlorpromazine are generally adequate for treating an acute antipsychotic effect. Doses greater than 20 mg of haloperidol are thought to produce little additional benefit (and possibly less effect). However, much higher doses are often used to treat delirium. Patients who have neuropsychiatric syndromes associated with dementia generally show symptom relief with much lower doses, as low as 0.25–2.0 mg of haloperidol. Unlike the psychotic symptoms associated with schizophrenia, those associated with dementia and delirium may respond within hours to relatively low doses of neuroleptics.

Atypical agents are at least as effective as typical agents, with reasonable target dosages of 6 mg/day of risperidone, 20 mg/day of olanzapine, 300 mg/day of quetiapine, 300–600 mg/day of clozapine, and 40–80 mg/day of ziprasidone (see Table 42–15).

One model previously used in the treatment of psychosis was rapid neuroleptization. This regimen consists of administering doses of a neuroleptic medication—for example, 5–10 mg of haloperidol—intramuscularly every 30–60 minutes until psychosis clears. Outcome studies of patients who were given rapid treatment show that they fared no better than patients who were given more conservative doses. Moreover, patients given rapid treat-

TABLE 42–15. Neuroleptic agents

Generic name	Trade name	Class	Dose equivalent	Usual therapeutic dose range (mg)[b]	Parenteral form	Effect[a]			
						Sedation	Extrapyramidal symptoms	Anticholinergic	Orthostatic blood pressure
Chlorpromazine	Thorazine	Phenothiazines, aliphatic	100	30–1,500	Yes	4	2	3	4
Thioridazine	Mellaril	Phenothiazines, piperidine	100	50–800	No	4	1	4	4
Clozapine	Clozaril	Dibenzodiazepine	50	300–900	No	3	0	4	1
Prochlorperazine	Compazine	Phenothiazines, piperazine	15	50–150	Yes	3	2	2	3
Loxapine	Loxitane	Dibenzoxazepine	15	25–100	Yes	3	3	2	2
Perphenazine	Trilafon	Phenothiazines, piperazine	10	4–64	Yes	3	3	2	3
Molindone	Moban	Dihydroindolone	10	25–100	No	1	3	2	2
Trifluoperazine	Stelazine	Phenothiazines, piperazine	5	2–40	Yes	1	3	2	2
Thiothixene	Navane	Thioxanthene, piperazine	4	6–60	Yes	2	4	2	2
Haloperidol	Haldol	Butyrophenone	2	5–40	Yes	1	4	1	1
Fluphenazine	Prolixin	Phenothiazines, piperazine	2	1–40	Yes	2	4	2	2
Risperidone	Risperdal	Benzisoxazole derivative	2	4–16	No	2	1	2	3
Pimozide	Orap	Diphenylbutylpiperidine	1	1–10	No	3	4	2	3
Olanzapine	Zyprexa	Thienobenzodiazepine	2	5–20	No	4[c]	0–1	3	1
Quetiapine	Seroquel	Dibenzothiazepine	25	150–750	No	2	0–1	2	2
Ziprasidone	Geodon	3-Benzisothiazolylpiperazine	40	80–160	No	3	0–1	2	4

[a] 0 = least effect; 4 = most effect.

[b] Doses for elderly and medically ill patients may be lower.

[c] Most potent H_1 antagonist known.

Source. Some information in this table has been extracted from Richelson E: "Receptor Pharmacology of Neuroleptics: Relation to Clinical Effects." *Journal of Clinical Psychiatry* 60 (suppl 10):5–14, 1999.

ment were exposed to greater risk of extrapyramidal symptoms and possibly NMS. Rapid tranquilization is a related technique aimed at calming a patient who has acute psychotic agitation rather than at alleviating psychosis. Rapid tranquilization is often used for hospitalized patients who become delirious, especially in ICUs. Rapid tranquilization with a neuroleptic is usually accomplished with haloperidol, 5–10 mg given orally, intramuscularly, or intravenously every 20–30 minutes until the patient is calm. Intravenous haloperidol is typically used in ICU settings at doses of 0.5–2.0 mg for patients with mild agitation, 5–10 mg for those with moderate agitation, and 10 mg or more for patients who are severely agitated (Tesar and Stern 1986; see also Chapter 15 in this volume). Much higher doses are used in some cases, but recent evidence links prolongation of Q-Tc and torsade de pointes ventricular tachycardia with very-high-dose therapy (Metzger and Friedman 1993). Droperidol is also used for delirium-associated agitation (Frye et al. 1995; see also Chapter 15 in this volume). The benzodiazepine lorazepam (which, in contrast to diazepam and chlordiazepoxide, is effectively absorbed intramuscularly) is also used for rapid tranquilization, alone or in conjunction with neuroleptics, especially haloperidol.

Side Effects

Low- and high-potency neuroleptic medications have significantly different side-effect profiles. Low-potency medications, such as thioridazine, are more sedating and have more orthostatic effects. High-potency medications, such as haloperidol and piperazine phenothiazines, produce more extrapyramidal symptoms. Atypical agents generally have a lower incidence of such symptoms when compared with typical agents, although they can still occur.

Extrapyramidal effects include dystonic reactions, parkinsonian symptoms, akathisia, and tardive phenomena. Dystonia usually appears within 1–5 days of the start of treatment. Dystonic symptoms include opisthotonos, torticollis, and oculogyric crises. Laryngeal and diaphragmatic dystonias occur, although rarely. Young men, very ill patients, and patients with neurological disorders are particularly vulnerable to extrapyramidal symptoms. Acute treatment for dystonia requires benztropine, 1 or 2 mg given intramuscularly or intravenously, or diphenhydramine, 25–50 mg.

Parkinsonian signs are masked facies, cogwheel rigidity, tremor, and parkinsonian gait. Akinesia and bradykinesia also occur. These extrapyramidal signs can appear from a few days to several weeks after initiating or increasing the dose of an antipsychotic. Anticholinergic medications are usually effective in counteracting most

side effects; these agents include benztropine, biperiden, procyclidine, and trihexyphenidyl. The antihistaminic medication diphenhydramine and the dopamine agonist amantadine are also used. A typical dosage of benztropine in general psychiatric settings is 0.5–2.0 mg three times daily; lower dosages are typically used in consultation-liaison settings because patients are older or medically frail, they have cognitive deficits, or they are already taking other medications with anticholinergic effects. Amantadine is excreted by the kidneys and can reach toxic levels in patients with impaired renal function. Arrhythmias and hypotension can occur in amantadine overdose; a 2- or 3-g dose is sometimes fatal, an amount that a patient may be able to obtain by filling a 30-day prescription.

Akathisia is an internal sense of restlessness that is usually manifest by outward restlessness, especially leg movements. Because akathisia can resemble agitation secondary to psychosis, the clinician may increase the dosage of an antipsychotic, further worsening the akathisia. Akathisia can also increase the risk of suicide in a suicide-prone patient. Akathisia does not usually abate, but lowering the dosage or changing to a low-potency neuroleptic often reduces this side effect. Propranolol, 20–60 mg/day, is often used to reduce this symptom, as are benzodiazepines. Sedation from antihistaminic effect can occur with neuroleptics but is most prominent with the low-potency medications such as chlorpromazine. Tolerance often develops to sedative effects. Anticholinergic effects are more prominent with the low-potency aliphatic and piperidine phenothiazines.

Orthostatic hypotension also occurs more frequently with low-potency aliphatic and piperidine phenothiazines. Cardiac effects are rare but can include prolonged ventricular repolarization and quinidine-like effects, especially with the low-potency medications, particularly thioridazine. Torsade de pointes and other ventricular arrhythmias can occur with thioridazine and high-dose intravenous haloperidol (Hunt and Stern 1995). ECG changes, including ST segment depression and prolonged T waves, are seen, especially with aliphatic and piperazine phenothiazines.

All neuroleptics, with the exception of clozapine and quetiapine, increase prolactin release and occasionally induce galactorrhea and menstrual changes. Impotence, decreased libido, and inhibition of ejaculation and orgasm can also occur. The syndrome of inappropriate antidiuretic hormone secretion is reported in patients taking neuroleptics, but this syndrome also occurs among patients with psychosis who are not taking neuroleptics. Low-potency phenothiazines can interfere with temperature regulation.

Any neuroleptic can lower the seizure threshold. Especially at higher doses, low-potency medications, such as chlorpromazine, tend to do so more often. Neurotoxicity in patients with hyperthyroidism occurs on occasion with butyrophenone use. Neuroleptics, especially chlorpromazine, can produce cholestatic jaundice. Low-potency medications have more of a tendency to cause cholestatic jaundice as well as hepatitis. Weight gain can occur with neuroleptic use, more often with phenothiazines than butyrophenones. Excessive salivation occurs more often with the high-potency medications. Clozapine, although it is a low-potency neuroleptic, is particularly problematic in this regard.

Skin abnormalities, including rashes and photosensitivity, occur more often with low-potency medications. Skin pigmentation and blue-gray discoloration are rare reactions to low-potency phenothiazines. A lupus-like syndrome is a rare side effect of aliphatic phenothiazines. Anticholinergic effects include visual blurring and impaired memory. Aliphatic and piperazine phenothiazines can, in rare instances, produce lenticular deposits and opacities. The upper limit for thioridazine dosages, 800 mg/day, is based on the high incidence of pigmentary retinopathy at dosages above this level. Quetiapine produced cataracts when administered to dogs, although it is unclear how this observation translates to human use. FDA labeling recommends baseline and interval examination of the eyes with long-term use of quetiapine. Drug-induced cataracts have not been reported in humans (Stip and Boisjoly 1999). All neuroleptics, especially the butyrophenones, occasionally cause blood dyscrasias. Agranulocytosis is rare, except with clozapine. It has not been established which neuroleptics are safest in patients with bone marrow suppression; clozapine is contraindicated in patients with myeloproliferative disorders.

Clozapine's common side effects are sedation, excessive salivation, anticholinergic effects, weight gain, and postural hypotension. Extrapyramidal symptoms are rare and can improve with this medication. Constipation, ECG changes, hypertension, increase in body temperature, priapism, pancreatitis, eosinophilia, and dose-dependent decreases in seizure threshold also occur. The most serious side effect is potentially fatal granulocytopenia or agranulocytosis, which is estimated to occur in about 1% of patients. Weekly blood counts are required initially to monitor for decreases in white blood cell count. After 6 months of treatment, biweekly counts may be drawn if there are no indications of agranulocytosis. More than 95% of cases of agranulocytosis occur in the first 6 months; most cases occur during weeks 4–18.

Although neuroleptic use is weakly linked to fetal limb abnormalities, several large-scale studies failed to show an increased risk of congenital malformations associated with exposure during pregnancy (L. S. Cohen et al. 1991). Effects from prenatal exposure, reported in neonates and infants, are extrapyramidal symptoms, sedation, hyperbilirubinemia, neonatal jaundice, and induction of hepatic enzymes (Hauser 1985; Robinson et al. 1986).

Tardive Phenomena

Tardive phenomena include tardive dystonia, tardive akathisia, and especially tardive dyskinesia. Tardive dyskinesia can occur with any neuroleptic. These involuntary buccolingual and choreoathetoid movements disappear during sleep. The Abnormal Involuntary Movement Scale (Guy 1976; Lane et al. 1985) is used to rate these movements (Table 42–16). Estimates of the prevalence of tardive dyskinesia vary widely, but the average estimate is 20%–30% of patients exposed to neuroleptics. Tardive dyskinesia usually does not develop unless a patient is exposed to neuroleptics for at least 3 months (Glazer et al. 1993), but tardive dyskinesia has been reported after shorter periods of exposure, particularly in elderly patients (Harris and Kingston 1992; Yassa et al. 1992). However, it is also estimated that 5% of geriatric patients never taking neuroleptic medications have signs of tardive dyskinesia (Yassa et al. 1992). Risk factors for tardive dyskinesia include increased age, exposure to antipsychotics for 3 months or more, higher cumulative dose, and concurrent presence of a mood disorder or diabetes mellitus.

Not surprisingly, tardive dyskinesia is probably a disorder in the dopamine system. One etiological model for the disorder postulates that it is an acquired dopamine supersensitivity. However, the lack of uniform response to pharmacological manipulation of the dopamine system suggests that this theory does not completely explain the phenomenon. Cholinergic, noradrenergic, and GABA involvement have all been postulated. Stopping the neuroleptic is the primary intervention. Symptoms are usually worse at the time of withdrawal and gradually improve in 3–6 months. If the symptoms do not remit by then, the condition often is permanent. At that point, treatment has only a limited chance of success. Medications used to treat tardive dyskinesia include baclofen, benzodiazepines, reserpine, tetrabenazine, calcium channel blockers, and vitamin E (Szymanski et al. 1993). Botulin toxin injections every few months can alleviate the sustained spasms in tardive dystonia, such as blepharospasm and torticollis. It is believed that clozapine does not cause tardive dyskinesia and, in fact, may help it. Other atypical neuroleptics are probably less likely to produce tardive

TABLE 42–16. Abnormal Involuntary Movement Scale (AIMS)

Movements are rated from 0 to 4, based on the highest severity observed.

Movements seen on activation are rated one less than those seen spontaneously.

Code

0 = None

1 = Minimal, may be extreme normal (not clearly a TD movement)

2 = Mild

3 = Moderate

4 = Severe

Facial and oral movements

1. Muscles of facial expression (e.g., movements of forehead, eyebrows, periorbital area, cheeks; include frowning, blinking, smiling, grimacing)
2. Lips and perioral areas (e.g., puckering, pouting, smacking)
3. Jaw (e.g., biting, clenching, chewing, mouth-opening, lateral movements)
4. Tongue (rate only increase in movement both in and out of mouth, not inability to sustain movement)

Extremity movements

5. Upper extremities—arms, wrists, hands, fingers (include choreic movements [i.e., rapid, objectively purposeless, irregular, complex, serpentine]); do not include tremor (i.e., repetitive, regular, rhythmic)
6. Lower extremities—legs, knees, ankles, toes (e.g., lateral knee movement, foot tapping, heel dropping, foot squirming, inversion and eversion of foot)

Trunk movements

7. Neck, shoulders, hips (e.g., rocking, twisting, squirming, pelvic gyrations)

Global judgments

8. Severity of abnormal movements
9. Incapacitation due to abnormal movements
10. Awareness of abnormal movements (rate only patient's report)

(*Severity scale here refers to degree of distress.*)

Dental status

11. Current problems with teeth and/or dentures?   (Yes/No)
12. Does patient usually wear dentures?   (Yes/No)

Instructions	Applies to AIMS item #
Unobtrusively observe the patient at rest before the examination	All
Use a hard, firm chair without arms	All
Ask the patient to remove anything in his or her mouth (e.g., gum)	1–4
Ask the patient about the current state of his or her teeth and/or dentures and whether they are bothersome now	11–12
Ask the patient if he or she notices any movements and if they bother or interfere with the patient's activities	9–10
Have the patient sit in chair with hands on knees, legs slightly apart, and feet flat on floor	All
Ask patient to sit with hands hanging unsupported	All, especially 5
Ask patient to protrude tongue; repeat	4
Ask patient to tap thumb, with each finger, as rapidly as possible for 10–15 seconds, first with the right, and then with the left hand (activation)	1–4, 6
Flex and extend each of the patient's arms separately, examining for rigidity	5
Ask patient to stand up	All
Ask patient to extend both arms outstretched in front with palms turned down (activation)	1–4, 6–7
Have patient walk a few paces, turn, and walk back to chair; repeat	Gait, 5

Note. TD = tardive dyskinesia.

Source. Reprinted from Guy W: *ECDEU Assessment Manual for Psychopharmacology,* Revised 1976. Washington, DC, United States Department of Health, Education and Welfare, 1976.

dyskinesia than typical agents, but use of atypicals does not completely eliminate this risk. The physician should discuss the risk of tardive dyskinesia with the patient before initiating a prolonged course of neuroleptic treatment, even in medical and surgical settings.

Neuroleptic Malignant Syndrome

NMS is a rare but serious and potentially fatal complication of treatment with neuroleptics. NMS is reported in other situations, such as rapid discontinuation of L-dopa/carbidopa (Wise and Rundell 1994) and combination treatment with amitriptyline and lithium (Fava and Galizia 1995). Knowledge about NMS is especially important for the consulting psychiatrist. In the medically ill patient the differential diagnosis of NMS is extensive and includes catatonia, lethal catatonia, heat stroke, malignant hyperthermia, serotonin syndrome, anticholinergic toxicity, meningitis, viral encephalitis, Parkinson's disease, Wilson's disease, collagen vascular diseases, cerebrovascular disease, head trauma, epilepsy, myotonia, akinetic mutism, general paresis, diabetic ketoacidosis, hepatic encephalopathy, acute intermittent porphyria, pellagra, hypocalcemia, tetanus, botulism, and the effects of strychnine, curare, phencyclidine, and sedative withdrawal.

The primary signs of NMS are hyperthermia, tremor, marked increase in muscle tone (usually lead-pipe rigidity), other extrapyramidal symptoms, altered consciousness (from confusion to coma), and autonomic instability. Autonomic instability usually manifests as changes in blood pressure and heart rate, dysrhythmias, diaphoresis, pallor, and sialorrhea. Patients may also have oculogyric crises, opisthotonos, trismus, Babinski sign, and seizures. Laboratory findings include dehydration; white blood cell count of 15,000–30,000 (with or without a left shift); elevated levels of serum glutamic-oxaloacetic transaminase, serum glutamic-pyruvic transaminase, lactic dehydrogenase, and alkaline phosphatase; elevated creatine phosphokinase (possibly exceeding 16,000); and myoglobinuria. The elevated creatine phosphokinase is believed to occur in 40%–50% of patients (Janicak et al. 1987). Electroencephalogram and lumbar puncture findings are nonspecific.

NMS generally develops over a 1- to 3-day period and lasts for 5–10 days after a nondepot neuroleptic is discontinued. Mortality is high, most often quoted as 20%–30% (Gelenberg et al. 1988). Mortality is higher if rhabdomyolysis develops. Prospective studies place the incidence of NMS in patients exposed to neuroleptics between 0.02% and 1.8% (Adityanjee et al. 1999). NMS can occur at any age, but it occurs most often in patients younger than age 40 years and may occur more frequently in men. Patients who receive neuroleptics for any disorder or condition can develop NMS. In consultation-liaison settings, the clinician should not overlook the possible contribution of metoclopramide and prochlorperazine to NMS. Case reports suggest that a similar disorder can develop in patients who have received medications other than neuroleptics—essentially, a neuroleptic malignant disorder without the neuroleptic (Gelenberg et al. 1988). NMS has occurred in patients who have discontinued using anticholinergic medications and dopamine agonists such as amantadine and L-dopa. NMS-like reactions have also been reported with tricyclics, MAOIs, and the combination of lithium and haloperidol.

The precise mechanism for the development of NMS is uncertain. It may be the result of a rapid decrease in dopamine activity in the nigrostriatal pathways, along with effects on preoptic anterior hypothalamic temperature regulatory centers. Nothing is certain about precipitating or contributing factors. Several such factors are suspected, including dehydration, high-potency neuroleptics, high doses of neuroleptics, rapid dose increases of neuroleptics, exhaustion, organic brain disease, and mood disorders.

The main intervention in NMS is to discontinue the neuroleptic. All other treatments are dictated by the patient's condition (e.g., supportive care, such as respiratory support and cooling the body core temperature). Medication interventions include dopaminergic medications to decrease the effects of dopamine receptor blockade, β-adrenergic blockers to decrease the heart rate, and calcium channel blockers or muscle relaxants to decrease rigidity.

Bromocriptine is a dopamine agonist used in dosages of 2.5–10 mg orally three times daily. Amantadine, another dopamine agonist, is used in dosages of 100 mg orally two to four times daily. Dantrolene acts as a direct muscle relaxant; daily dosages are 8–10 mg/kg body weight intravenously or 50–200 mg orally. The use of dantrolene is limited by hepatic toxicity. Other interventions include antiparkinsonian medications, L-dopa, lorazepam, propranolol, curare, and ECT. Rechallenge with a neuroleptic after NMS is a controversial topic. It is estimated that the recurrence rate is 30% with rechallenge (Rosebush et al. 1989). At least 2 weeks should elapse before neuroleptic treatment is restarted; then a different, low-potency medication should be used. The dosage should be increased slowly, and the clinician should carefully monitor the patient's body temperature and mental status and look for the occurrence of muscle rigidity or cogwheeling and increases in creatine phosphokinase levels.

Overdose

Although neuroleptics are usually not lethal in overdose, life-threatening hypotension and cardiac arrhythmias occur with overdoses of low-potency medications.

Withdrawal

In rare cases, phenothiazines produce dizziness and tremulousness following cessation of high-dose therapy. Sudden discontinuation of high doses of neuroleptics can cause a short-lived flulike syndrome and withdrawal-related dyskinesias. Of course, recurrence of the psychotic illness is the most worrisome consequence of discontinuing neuroleptics. The time delay before the return of psychotic symptoms is quite variable. Premature discontinuation of haloperidol in patients receiving treatment for delirium can lead to rapid relapse (see Chapter 15 in this volume).

Drug Interactions

Anticholinergic effects are especially problematic when neuroleptics are added to other medications with anticholinergic potency (see Table 42–5). Alcohol causes additive sedative effects. The use of low-potency neuroleptics with TCAs or other class IA antiarrhythmic medications (e.g., quinidine) can delay cardiac conduction and precipitate arrhythmias. When used concomitantly with neuroleptics, NSAIDs can cause extreme drowsiness, especially the combination of haloperidol and indomethacin. β-Blockers can worsen the orthostatic side effects of neuroleptic drugs. Anesthetics can produce severe hypotension in patients taking phenothiazines. Chlorpromazine, thioridazine, and mesoridazine are potent α-adrenergic blockers and can induce hypotension in combination with vasodilators. Haloperidol has virtually no α-adrenergic-blocking properties. A decreased antihypertensive effect can occur, however, with guanethidine and related drugs. Because of its mixed α and β effects, epinephrine can lower the blood pressure of persons taking phenothiazines (i.e., unopposed β effect); as a result, phenylephrine or levarterenol should be used to treat marked hypotension in these patients.

As hepatically degraded drugs, the neuroleptics are susceptible to decreased effects resulting from concomitant use of medications, such as anticonvulsants, that induce metabolism. Antacids can delay absorption. Because of the ability of neuroleptics to block dopamine receptors, antiparkinsonian medications are antagonized. Neurotoxic interactions with lithium have also been reported. The reasons for the initial report of severe reactions between haloperidol and lithium (Turpin and Schuller 1978) have

been debated, but case reports continue, including interactions of lithium with thioridazine (Spring 1979) and clozapine (Blake et al. 1992; McElroy et al. 1991).

ANTIANXIETY AND SEDATIVE MEDICATIONS

Basic Concepts

Antianxiety agents are quite effective and are safe when used properly. Unfortunately, the perceived potential for abuse has limited the use of benzodiazepines in patients who could benefit from them. Antidepressants are also effective in the treatment of anxiety and anxiety disorders. Antidepressants are FDA approved for generalized anxiety disorder (venlafaxine), obsessive-compulsive disorder (clomipramine, fluvoxamine, sertraline, fluoxetine, and paroxetine), PTSD (sertraline), panic disorder (sertraline and paroxetine), and social phobia (paroxetine). (For further discussion of anxiety and anxiety disorders, see Chapter 20 in this volume.)

Indications

Most anxiety disorders are amenable to treatment with antianxiety or antidepressant medications. Antidepressants are considered mainstays in the treatment of most anxiety disorders (Schatzberg 2000). Antidepressants are often used in conjunction with benzodiazepines, especially during the initiation of treatment. Benzodiazepines are usually tapered once the antidepressant has had time to take full effect.

Before using sedative-hypnotic agents, the patient should be evaluated for insomnia. Is the patient really not sleeping? Patient self-reports about sleep are notoriously inaccurate, because they are not aware during at least a portion of the period of data collection. Does the problem represent normal changes in sleep architecture that occur with age? Is the insomnia acute or chronic? Does the patient experience excessive daytime somnolence? Are contributing factors present, such as pain, sleep apnea, or a noisy hospital environment? The old joke about awakening patients to give them a sleeping pill is sometimes an accurate depiction of the source of the patient's sleep problem.

Benzodiazepines

Types

Benzodiazepines are subdivided into several groups (Table 42–17). The 2-ketobenzodiazepines include diazepam and chlordiazepoxide. Oxazepam, lorazepam, and

TABLE 42–17. Benzodiazepines

Generic name	Trade name	Onset	Duration of action	Usual therapeutic dose range (mg)[a]	Approximately equivalent antianxiety dose (mg)	Approximately equivalent hypnotic dose (mg)
Alprazolam	Xanax	Intermediate	Short	2–8	0.5	1
Clonazepam	Klonopin	Intermediate	Short	1–3	1	1
Chlordiazepoxide	Librium	Intermediate	Long	15–150	10	25
Clorazepate	Tranxene	Rapid	Long	15–60	7.5	15
Diazepam	Valium	Rapid	Long	5–40	5	10
Estazolam	ProSom	Rapid	Intermediate	1–2	—	1
Flurazepam	Dalmane	Rapid to intermediate	Long	15–30	—	30
Lorazepam	Ativan	Intermediate	Intermediate	1–6	1	2
Midazolam	Versed	Rapid	Very short	0.1 mg/kg body weight	2	2
Oxazepam	Serax	Intermediate to slow	Intermediate	30–120	15	30
Prazepam	Centrax	Slow	Long	20–60	10	20
Quazepam	Doral	Rapid	Long	7.5–15	—	15
Temazepam	Restoril	Intermediate to slow	Short	15–30	15	30
Triazolam	Halcion	Intermediate	Short	0.125–0.5	—	0.5

[a]Doses for elderly and medically ill patients are often lower.

temazepam are 3-hydroxybenzodiazepines. Alprazolam and triazolam are triazolobenzodiazepines. Clonazepam is a 7-nitrobenzodiazepine. Midazolam is an imidazobenzodiazepine derivative.

Mechanism of Action

Benzodiazepines induce binding of GABA, an inhibitory neurotransmitter.

Pharmacokinetics

The benzodiazepines are rapidly absorbed in the gastrointestinal tract. Intramuscular absorption is quite variable, except with lorazepam and midazolam. The absorption of diazepam and chlordiazepoxide administered intramuscularly is particularly erratic. There are significant differences in the half-lives and kinetics among the benzodiazepines. Benzodiazepines are lipophilic and have a relatively rapid onset of action. Most are degraded by hepatic oxidation, and some have several active metabolites. Benzodiazepine metabolism slows with age, medication interactions (i.e., inhibition of the CYP isoenzymes), and hepatic insults such as cirrhosis. Lorazepam, oxazepam, and temazepam are degraded primarily by glucuronide conjugation and are without active metabolites; as a result, these three benzodiazepines have a distinct advantage for older or seriously ill patients.

Indications

Benzodiazepines are widely prescribed for their antianxiety and hypnotic effects. Alprazolam is the only benzodi-

azepine currently approved by the FDA for panic disorder, but further studies have shown that other benzodiazepines, especially clonazepam, are also effective for this purpose if used in adequate doses (Charney and Woods 1989; Tesar et al. 1991). Benzodiazepines are also used for patients who are withdrawing from alcohol (delirium tremens) and from benzodiazepines. Because of their duration of action, chlordiazepoxide and diazepam are frequently used for this purpose. Lorazepam is also used for patients undergoing withdrawal in situations in which close monitoring is possible; its shorter duration of action allows finer response to symptoms, and it is not metabolized to active compounds. The latter is an especially important benefit for individuals who have severe liver damage from chronic alcohol use. Lorazepam's advantage over oxazepam is the availability of a parenteral form. (For further details on substance-related disorders, see Chapter 21 in this volume.)

Midazolam is an ultra-short-acting benzodiazepine commonly administered parenterally in surgical, imaging, and intensive care settings. It typically produces amnesia during use. It is three to four times more potent than diazepam. Although it is expensive (about $1,500/day), a continuous midazolam drip is occasionally effective in an agitated patient. When this drug is properly tapered, rebound anxiety or withdrawal is not observed (Reeves et al. 1985); however, caution is advised, especially when giving midazolam to patients with impaired renal function, because conjugated, biologically active metabolites of the drug can accumulate and cause prolonged sedation (Bauer et al. 1995).

Dosage and Administration

Benzodiazepines are given in as-needed or regularly scheduled doses. A daily maximum of 40 mg of diazepam or its equivalent is usually sufficient, although higher doses are occasionally needed in patients who are undergoing detoxification. The dosage of alprazolam for the treatment of panic disorder can be approximately 2–8 mg/day; most patients require 4–8 mg (see Table 42–17). Concomitant use of antidepressants decreases benzodiazepine requirements in many patients.

Response

The onset of anxiolysis with benzodiazepines is usually rapid. Maximum benefit is usually reached by 6 weeks (Rickels and Schweizer 1987).

Side Effects

Sedation and drowsiness are the most common acute effects of the benzodiazepines. These effects are often more pronounced in elderly patients and in patients who are medically ill. Other cognitive effects include transient anterograde amnesia. Rarely, patients who are receiving treatment for anxiety or insomnia experience amnesia for a few hours after taking a benzodiazepine; however, these drugs are used regularly, with good effects, in patients who are undergoing surgical procedures and in those receiving treatment in ICUs. There are occasional problems with confusion, impaired attention, impaired psychomotor skills, and dizziness. Ataxia also occurs frequently. Benzodiazepines can rarely cause behavioral disinhibition resulting in aggressive behavior, particularly in the elderly and in patients with brain injuries (Kales et al. 1987). Paradoxical excitement, paradoxical rage reactions, and paradoxical anxiety have also been reported (Lion et al. 1975). Depression can occur. Although the benzodiazepines provide a hypnotic effect, they also decrease sleep latency and the amount of delta sleep. Benzodiazepines are contraindicated in patients with sleep apnea because the decrease in central respiratory response to elevated CO_2 levels caused by benzodiazepines is potentially fatal (Dolly and Block 1982).

Dependence develops with chronic benzodiazepine use. This includes both psychological and physical dependence (e.g., tolerance and withdrawal symptoms). Because benzodiazepines are also used as recreational drugs, the clinician must weigh the risks of dependence against the substantial benefits accrued from treatment of a primary or secondary anxiety disorder.

Benzodiazepines have a respiratory depressant effect that is potentially dangerous in patients with compromised respiration. In hospitals, flumazenil is available as an antidote in cases of intentional, accidental, or iatrogenic toxicity. Because benzodiazepines suppress the respiratory response to hypoxia, they are contraindicated in patients who retain CO_2. Rare side effects include hypotension, blood dyscrasias, jaundice, and allergic reactions. Stuttering is an unusual sign associated with alprazolam. A range of abnormalities, including cleft palate, have been temporally associated with benzodiazepine use during pregnancy; however, recent evidence suggests that benzodiazepines are not teratogenic (Gelenberg 1992a).

Overdose

Benzodiazepines are considered relatively safe and, if taken alone in overdose, are rarely lethal. Of concern to consultation-liaison psychiatrists, however, is that an overdose can produce respiratory depression requiring intubation and respiratory support. In cases of benzodiazepine overdose, flumazenil, a benzodiazepine antagonist, is administered intravenously in doses of 0.1 mg. Doses are repeated every few minutes up to 3 mg in 0.5–3 hours. Additional doses are often needed as flumazenil wears off and sedation reappears.

Withdrawal

Benzodiazepines can cause a clinically significant withdrawal syndrome. The likelihood of symptoms increases with higher daily dosage, duration of treatment, and speed of discontinuance. Benzodiazepine withdrawal symptoms include dizziness, sweating, shakiness, headache, blurred vision, and tinnitus. Also possible are hypotension, nausea and vomiting, twitching, muscle cramps, paresthesias, and irritability. Hallucinations sometimes occur. The most serious withdrawal effect is seizure. In addition to return of pretreatment anxiety, some patients develop rebound withdrawal anxiety or insomnia. The withdrawal syndrome is worse with benzodiazepines that have short half-lives; the gradual clearance of benzodiazepines that have a long half-life results in a gradual tapering, although withdrawal symptoms from drugs such as diazepam have been reported. Clinicians report that withdrawal from alprazolam is especially difficult (Albeck 1987; Risse et al. 1990). Seizures have been documented in patients rapidly withdrawn from alprazolam, even though they received other benzodiazepines normally considered adequate for cross-coverage (Browne and Hauge 1986; Warner et al. 1990). Although this is not clearly documented, it suggests that clinicians must administer at least an equivalent dose of other benzodiazepines during withdrawal (see Table 42–17; see also Chapter 21 in this volume).

Drug Interactions

An additive effect occurs when alcohol is combined with other CNS depressants. Prolonged neuromuscular blockade with succinylcholine can occur with concomitant benzodiazepine use. Benzodiazepines can induce digoxin toxicity by reducing its excretion (Castillo-Fernando et al. 1980; Guven et al. 1993; Tollefson et al. 1984). Alprazolam's metabolism is significantly decreased by other drugs that affect the CYP3A3/4 isoenzyme (e.g., nefazodone). As with other drugs that are metabolized by oxidation, the long-acting benzodiazepines are vulnerable to medications that inhibit hepatic enzymes, such as cimetidine.

Buspirone

Buspirone is an azaspirodecanedione. It has moderate affinity for D_2 receptors and appears to have mixed agonist/antagonist activity for $5-HT_{1A}$ receptors but no significant antipsychotic effect. It does not affect benzodiazepine or GABA receptors to any significant degree (Sussman 1994).

Buspirone is a lipophilic drug that is well absorbed, but much of the drug is lost to first-pass effect. It is metabolized by hepatic oxidation and has a half-life of 2–11 hours.

Buspirone has a number of clinical advantages, especially in consultation-liaison settings. It does not cause the sedation or functional impairment that occurs with the benzodiazepines. It does not change the seizure threshold and has no known abuse potential. It is associated with fewer drug interactions than are the benzodiazepines. In particular, it does not interact with alcohol. Because it stimulates respiration in animals and is not known to suppress respiration in humans, buspirone is particularly useful in patients with anxiety whose respiratory status is compromised. Because of these features, buspirone is recommended for the treatment of chronic anxiety, particularly in patients who are older, in those who are sicker, and in those in whom substance abuse or dependence is a potential complication. For acute treatment of anxiety, buspirone has a significant disadvantage: it usually takes 1–4 weeks for its anxiolytic properties to take effect. In addition, buspirone is sometimes less effective—or may be seemingly ineffective—in patients who previously took a benzodiazepine. Buspirone is not effective against panic attacks, and it does not have cross-tolerance with benzodiazepines. As a result, if the benzodiazepine is tapered too quickly, withdrawal anxiety will occur. If a patient has been taking a benzodiazepine for years, an appropriate taper often takes several months to avoid withdrawal anxiety.

An initial buspirone dosage is 5 mg twice daily, which can be increased by 5 mg/day every 3 or 4 days. Symptoms usually resolve at a dosage of 30 mg daily (15 mg twice daily). Dosages as high as 60 mg/day are required in some patients. A delay of 1–4 weeks usually occurs before anxiolytic effects are seen. Buspirone's most frequent side effects are dizziness and headache. Less frequent effects are nausea, diarrhea, nervousness, and paresthesias.

After rapid or abrupt discontinuation of buspirone, a patient may experience drowsiness, insomnia, nervousness, dizziness, headache, or gastrointestinal upset, although such reports are rare.

Buspirone can produce a serotonin syndrome when taken with MAOIs or with other drug combinations that overly enhance serotonin activity. It also can displace less firmly protein-bound drugs such as digoxin.

Antidepressants

As stated earlier in this chapter, antidepressants are effective in treating anxiety disorders and they are not abused. When used to treat obsessive-compulsive disorder, dosages are often higher than those required for treating depression. When antidepressants are used to treat panic disorder, generalized anxiety disorder, social phobia, or PTSD, dosages are similar to those used to treat depression. It is necessary to start antidepressants at low doses in patients with prominent anxiety, because such patients are more sensitive to medication side effects, particularly activation. Trazodone, 25–100 mg, is often used to treat insomnia or SSRI-induced sleep problems.

Other Medications

Zolpidem is the only imidazopyridine currently available in the United States for the treatment of insomnia. It is associated with a favorable safety profile, although occasional transient sensory distortions and hallucinations have been reported in some female patients (Markowitz and Brewerton 1996). Zolpidem is likely preferred over benzodiazepines for patients with chronic obstructive pulmonary disease, because it does not impair nocturnal respiratory and sleep architecture (Girault et al. 1996). Zolpidem also has a low potential for tolerance and a lack of withdrawal effects, which further supports its use over the benzodiazepine hypnotics (Scharf et al. 1994).

Zaleplon is a relatively new nonbenzodiazepine hypnotic agent. It is of the pyrazolopyrimidine class and interacts with the GABA-benzodiazepine receptor complex (Henney 1999). Its half-life is only 1 hour, making it particularly useful in patients who have difficulty falling asleep. The drug did not demonstrate efficacy in patients with frequent awakening or total shortened sleep times (Henney 1999). Like zolpidem, it also has a favorable profile, with no tolerance or withdrawal symptoms reported to date (Elie et al. 1999).

For sedation in medical-surgical patients, antihistamines, including diphenhydramine and hydroxyzine, are frequently used, although these medications are less reliable in inducing sleep when compared with other hypnotics (Kupfer and Reynolds 1997). Because of their significant anticholinergic effects, they should not be used in patients with delirium, cardiac problems, or prostatic hypertrophy. Chloral hydrate is an effective hypnotic for patients with brief episodes of insomnia. It is effective for 1–3 nights but loses its effectiveness within 2 weeks; continued use leads to physical dependence. The usual hypnotic dose of chloral hydrate is 0.5–1.0 g. Chloral hydrate is highly toxic for medical patients who are seriously ill and in overdose; death can occur after overdoses of as little as 4 g. The drug is especially harmful to children who have ingested it accidentally. Drug interaction occurs with warfarin-like anticoagulants; chloral hydrate displaces these drugs from plasma protein-binding sites.

The β-blockers, especially propranolol and metoprolol, are used to reduce anxiety symptoms. They are effective in controlling the somatic sensations of anxiety. This effect is particularly beneficial for patients with performance anxiety. β-Blockers are contraindicated for patients with asthma or diabetes. Narcotics are sometimes used to provide a brief sedative effect before medical or surgical procedures and when agitation occurs during emergency agitation situations; the fact that the effects of narcotics are reversed by naloxone increases their safety.

Neuroleptics are major tranquilizing medications, but their use for patients with mild anxiety is not appropriate; neuroleptics are reserved for the treatment of anxiety that occurs with other disorders such as acute psychosis. They are also indicated for extreme anxiety in patients who cannot tolerate the decreased respiratory drive associated with benzodiazepines (e.g., patients with intra-aortic balloon pumps or those being weaned from respirators). For patients with delirium who have significant anxiety or agitation, high-potency neuroleptics are used to provide a calming effect without added sedation and increased confusion. When sedation is desirable, low dosages of more sedating neuroleptics (e.g., perphenazine, 4 mg at bedtime, or thioridazine, 10 mg four times daily) have proven effective.

HERBAL MEDICINALS

Patients seen by consultation-liaison psychiatrists frequently are or will take herbal medicinals. As Crone and Wise (1998) suggest, "Patients struggling with the physical and emotional effects of acute and chronic disease…may be prone to use alternative approaches, including herbal medicines, to regain a sense of control or hope regarding their illness" (pp. 3–4). Because most patients taking herbal medicinals do not reveal this use to their physicians, the clinician must ask the patient directly about over-the-counter medications (i.e., both herbal and nonherbal preparations). Failure to know that a patient is taking an herbal medicinal can have life-threatening consequences. For example, concomitant use of St. John's wort, which apparently induces CYP3A3/4, can render antiviral AIDS treatment ineffective (Piscitelli et al. 2000) and cyclosporine ineffective in transplant patients (Ruschitzka et al. 2000).

In any discussion about herbal medicinals, several caveats are necessary. Many benefits and few, if any, side effects are claimed. Little regulation exists, and naming systems vary, as do methods of cultivation and processing. The concentration of the advertised active ingredient varies. For example, wide variation exists among ginseng products; in fact, assays found that only 25% of these products contained any ginseng at all (Miller 1998). Adulteration with unadvertised biologically active compounds is not uncommon and is often intentional. Adulterants found include anti-inflammatory agents, steroids, diuretics, antihistamines, tranquilizers, hormones, and heavy metals (Crone and Wise 1998). These elements make it difficult, if not impossible, to make predictions about drug interactions or a patient's response to a particular herb. Despite these limitations, Table 42–18 attempts to summarize some of this information. For patients taking herbal medicinals, potentially toxic drugs with narrow therapeutic windows deserve special attention; these include digoxin, phenobarbital, phenytoin, and warfarin (Miller 1998).

SPECIFIC MEDICAL-SURGICAL POPULATIONS

Until now, the material presented in this chapter was organized according to class of psychotropic medication, with specific organ effects mentioned, when pertinent. In the real world, however, the consultation-liaison psychiatrist is asked to see patients who have diseases and are taking

TABLE 42–18.   Effects of herbal medicinals

Herbal medicinals	Purported use(s)	Possible issues/interactions
Chamomile	Mild sedative, antispasmodic, antiseptic	Allergic reactions common; contains coumarin (monitor closely if patient is taking warfarin or other anticoagulants).
Echinacea (three kinds)	Immunostimulant	Hepatotoxicity with continued use; use with caution with other hepatotoxic drugs such as anabolic steroids, amiodarone, methotrexate, and ketoconazole.
Feverfew	Antimigraine; suppresses prostaglandin production	Allergic reactions common; NSAIDs may reduce effectiveness; inhibits platelet activity (caution with warfarin or other anticoagulants); withdrawal syndrome may occur.
Garlic	Antispasmodic, antiseptic, antiviral, antihypertensive, anticholesterol; promotes leukocytosis	Inhibits platelet aggregation activity (caution with warfarin or other anticoagulants).
Ginger	Antispasmodic, antinausea, antivertigo; used to treat hyperemesis gravidarum	Possible mutagenesis; prolonged bleeding time (caution with warfarin or other anticoagulants, avoid during pregnancy).
Ginkgo biloba	Antidementia, free radical scavenger	Inhibits platelet activation (caution with warfarin or other anticoagulants); may decrease seizure threshold and diminish effectiveness of anticonvulsants.
Ginseng	"Adaptogenic," helps patients with type 2 diabetes; immunostimulant; mood enhancer	May interfere with determination of digoxin; side effects include hypertension, headache, and epistaxis; inhibits platelet function (caution with warfarin or other anticoagulants); interacts with MAOIs; avoid use in patients with bipolar disorder.
Saw palmetto	Diuretic, antiseptic, anabolic; reduces prostatic hypertrophy	Antiandrogen, estrogenic (therefore, additive effect to hormonal therapy in women).
St. John's wort	Antidepressant, anxiolytic, sedative	Doubtful MAOI activity; photosensitivity (do not combine with tetracycline or piroxicam); induces CYP3A3/4 (decreases cyclosporine in transplant patients and antiviral levels in AIDS treatment, reduces warfarin effects, may reduce effectiveness of oral contraceptives and digoxin); do not combine with MAOIs; avoid combining with SSRIs.
Valerian	Hypnotic	Prolongs barbiturate sedation.

Note.   AIDS = acquired immunodeficiency syndrome; MAOIs = monoamine oxidase inhibitors; NSAIDS = nonsteroidal anti-inflammatory drugs; SSRIs = selective serotonin reuptake inhibitors.

medications that interact with organ systems. Therefore, it is useful to know which psychotropic agents are least harmful and most useful for a particular patient. In this section, information is organized according to patient population. Table 42–19 summarizes specific considerations by organ system. This discussion is abbreviated and should be used as an introduction to a more in-depth review.

Patients With Cardiac Disease

A common side effect of some psychotropic medications is orthostatic hypotension; this is a serious problem for debilitated patients, given the potential for significant injuries from falls, such as hip fractures or subdural hematomas. The propensity of many antidepressants and neuroleptics to cause orthostatic hypotension via α_1 blockade is shown in Tables 42–7 and 42–15, respectively. MAOIs also commonly cause orthostasis, whereas anxi-

olytics, lithium, psychostimulants, and anticonvulsants typically do not. Patients with CHF are at high risk for developing orthostatic hypotension. Roose et al. (1991b) reported that the occurrence of orthostatic hypotension in patients who took imipramine was 50% if they had CHF and 8% if they did not.

Patients with preexisting intraventricular conduction delays are at increased risk for complete heart block when given medications with quinidine-like properties (e.g., TCAs). The SSRIs are safer in such patients than are TCAs (Glassman 1998). Bupropion and ECT also have established records of safety in this context. MAOIs and psychostimulants do not have quinidine-like properties and are usually safe when given to patients with arrhythmias or conduction delays.

Among the neuroleptics, high-potency agents, such as haloperidol, are typically safe when given orally, intramuscularly, or intravenously, although caution is needed

TABLE 42–19. Psychoactive medications and organ systems

System	Antidepressant	MAOIs	Psychostimulants	Lithium	Anticonvulsants	Antipsychotics	Anxiolytics
Cardiovascular	Orthostatic hypotension is common with TCAs, not SSRIs Among TCAs, nortriptyline causes least orthostatic hypotension TCAs are quinidine-like Antiarrhythmics can cause slow conduction Tachycardia (usually benign) Flattening/inversion of T-wave and ST segment depression	Orthostatic hypotension is common No quinidine-like effects Interactions with drugs and food can cause hypertensive reactions SSRIs can cause potentially fatal serotonin syndrome	Relatively benign in patients with conduction delays, arrhythmias, CHF	Flattening, inversion of T-wave Sinoatrial node dysfunction Does not typically aggravate arrhythmias at therapeutic levels	Carbamazepine has quinidine-like effects	Low-potency agents have quinidine-like effects and can cause orthostatic hypotension	
Pulmonary	Drying of pulmonary secretions (anticholinergic effect)					Acute dystonia and TD can (rarely) affect respiratory muscles	Avoid benzodiazepines if pCO_2 is increased Lorazepam is preferred benzodiazepine in patients with respiratory disease Benzodiazepines are contraindicated in patients with sleep apnea Benzodiazepines may "induce" sleep apnea Buspirone stimulates respiration in animals Trazodone (as hypnotic) does not suppress respiration
Hepatic/gastrointestinal	Decreased protein synthesis can result in more unbound drug active at receptors Severe liver disease slows metabolism and can result in longer half-life Anticholinergic effect can cause decreased gastrointestinal motility, increased absorption, and increased blood levels SSRIs can inhibit cytochrome P450 and displace other protein-bound drugs Venlafaxine is the least protein-bound antidepressant	Phenelzine can cause hepatotoxicity	Methylphenidate inhibits hepatic enzymes Delayed hepatic hypersensitivity reaction with pemoline use	Gastric irritation, nausea, mild diarrhea, thirst with polydipsia Ascites can cause decreased lithium level	Carbamazepine and phenytoin are strong inducers of hepatic enzymes Valproic acid inhibits hepatic enzymes; can elevate liver function tests	Inhibit hepatic enzymes Preexisting liver disease not typically a contraindication	Oxidation decreased by hepatic disease Conjugation pathway (short-half-life benzodiazepines) less affected by hepatic disease. Therefore, lorazepam, oxazepam, and temazepam are preferred in patients with hepatic disease

TABLE 42–19. Psychoactive medications and organ systems (continued)

System	Antidepressant	MAOIs	Psychostimulants	Lithium	Anticonvulsants	Antipsychotics	Anxiolytics
Renal	Patients with renal failure may have higher levels of unmeasured hydroxylated metabolites. Anticholinergic effect can cause urinary retention			Dialyzable. Most diuretics increase levels. Can cause glomerular nephritis; progressive decrease in renal function rare and not clearly demonstrated	Carbamazepine inhibits lithium-induced polyuria. Carbamazepine can decrease serum sodium	Anticholinergic effect with low-potency agents can cause urinary retention	
Endocrine				Hypothyroidism in 10%–15% of patients, especially women	Carbamazepine increases thyroid metabolism and decreases TSH secretion	Amenorrhea, gynecomastia, galactorrhea (reversible with discontinuation)	
Hematopoietic	Agranulocytosis rarer than with neuroleptics; incidence peaks at 3–4 weeks			Benign leukocytosis common	Carbamazepine can cause benign decreased white blood count during first 4 months. Carbamazepine: agranulocytosis (rare but serious). Valproic acid can cause decreased platelets	Leukopenia a relative contraindication. Clozapine causes agranulocytosis in 1%–2% of patients	
Central nervous system	Anticholinergic effect a common cause of delirium. Maprotiline, bupropion, and clomipramine may increase seizure risk	Restlessness and insomnia. Lowers seizure threshold less than TCAs	Insomnia, exacerbation of anxiety	Overdose can cause ataxia, weakness, confusion, lethargy, slurred speech, nystagmus; then coma, convulsions	Sedation from valproic acid	May be contraindicated in patients with acute brain injury. Clozapine induces seizures in 1%–5% of patients. Molindone least affects seizure threshold	Benzodiazepines can cause sedation and drowsiness; amnesia, confusion, disinhibition, and paradoxical effects; and increased seizure threshold

Note. A cell is left blank if the organ system in question is not affected in a clinically significant way by the drug class. CHF = congestive heart failure; MAOIs = monoamine oxidase inhibitors; SSRIs = selective serotonin reuptake inhibitors; TCAs = tricyclic antidepressants; TD = tardive dyskinesia; TSH = thyroid-stimulating hormone.

when using the intravenous route because of the potential risk of Q-T prolongation and ventricular arrhythmias. Not only are anxiolytics safe for use in patients with cardiac disease, but reduction in anxiety offers significant benefits in patients after myocardial infarction. At therapeutic levels, lithium is also generally safe; rare cases of atrial arrhythmias have been reported. Anticonvulsants are typically safe, with the exception of carbamazepine, which is tricyclic in structure and has quinidine-like properties.

Patients With Pulmonary Disease

The psychopharmacological class of greatest concern in patients with pulmonary disease is the anxiolytics because of their respiratory-depressant properties. As noted earlier in this chapter, this is of particular concern in patients who retain CO_2. For short-term treatment of acute anxiety, the shorter-acting benzodiazepines are preferred. Lorazepam, because of its metabolism, many routes of administration, and reliable absorption, is the agent of choice for patients in this population. In addition, the availability of flumazenil, a benzodiazepine antagonist, adds a margin of safety when a benzodiazepine is prescribed to a hospitalized patient with respiratory compromise.

For the treatment of chronic anxiety, antidepressants or buspirone are recommended over benzodiazepines. Trazodone is an option for patients who have pulmonary disease because it is hypnotic and anxiolytic and does not suppress respiratory drive. To date, no fatal overdoses have been associated with trazodone when taken alone. Buspirone stimulates respiration in animals and should be considered for long-term management of anxiety in patients with respiratory disease. Antipsychotics and antidepressants with anticholinergic properties chiefly affect the pulmonary system by drying secretions. MAOIs, lithium, psychostimulants, and anticonvulsants typically do not alter respiratory drive. Patients using sympathomimetic bronchodilators or decongestants should avoid taking MAOIs.

Patients With Hepatic or Gastrointestinal Disease

Almost all psychotropic medications are metabolized by the liver and are highly protein bound; the exceptions are lithium, which is excreted by the kidneys, and venlafaxine, which is not highly protein bound. Hepatic insufficiency can increase the blood levels and half-lives of all drugs, except lithium, through several mechanisms: 1) decrease in phase I (oxidative) metabolism through cytochrome and other oxidative enzymes; 2) possible reduction of phase II (conjugation) pathways for drugs that predominantly undergo glucuronidation, such as oxazepam; 3) decrease in hepatic blood flow because of portacaval shunting and cytoarchitectural abnormalities associated with hepatocellular disease; 4) decrease in quantities and affinity of plasma proteins, especially albumin, thereby increasing free-drug levels; and 5) increase in volume of distribution in patients with ascites (Leipzig 1990).

As a general rule, when psychotropic medications are given to patients who have liver insufficiency, the clinician should prescribe lower doses at greater intervals and increase the dosage more slowly. Because parenteral administration avoids first-pass effects, the time to onset and peak levels are similar to those observed in patients with normal hepatic function. This is in contrast to the first-pass effects observed with oral medications in patients with or without severe liver disease.

Among antidepressants, TCAs usually have less inhibitory effects on CYP enzymes than do SSRIs. Among the currently available SSRIs (fluoxetine, fluvoxamine, paroxetine, sertraline, and citalopram), the comparative rankings are debated, although paroxetine appears to exert the greatest inhibitory effect on CYP2D6 (Crewe et al. 1992; see also Table 42–8). Antidepressants, including SSRIs and TCAs, are over 90% protein bound, except for venlafaxine, which is 27% protein bound. Among the benzodiazepines, it makes sense to use agents that do not undergo oxidative metabolism, such as lorazepam and oxazepam, for patients who have severe liver disease or for those taking multiple medications. Among the neuroleptics, the higher-potency agents are better tolerated because they present the liver with the fewest milligrams of substrate to metabolize. Among the anticonvulsants, carbamazepine and phenytoin induce hepatic enzymes, whereas valproic acid can inhibit hepatic enzymes.

Psychotropics with anticholinergic effects decrease gastric acid secretion and may also decrease absorption of drugs in the small intestine. Patients with duodenal ulcers may benefit from the H_2-blocking activity of certain psychotropic drugs (see Table 42–7). Patients at risk for confusion, however, can develop delirium from medications with anticholinergic potency. Delayed gastric emptying can postpone the onset of action of some psychotropic medications. Patients taking prochlorperazine or metoclopramide are at risk for side effects associated with antipsychotic drug treatment (Leipzig 1990).

Patients With Renal Disease

In patients with renal failure, protein binding is reduced because of 1) decreased albumin levels in patients with the nephrotic syndrome and 2) the presence of unexcreted metabolites that compete for protein-binding sites. Thus, drugs that are highly protein bound have a greater bioavailability of free, active drug in the presence of renal failure.

Many medications require dosage reduction in patients with renal failure (Aronoff et al. 1999). Although the dosing guideline for psychotropic medications indicates only gabapentin, dosage reductions according to the patient's glomerular filtration rate are required for primidone, topiramate, venlafaxine, phenobarbital, chlordiazepoxide, midazolam, lithium, ethchlorvynol, meprobamate, and paroxetine (Aronoff et al. 1999). Most clinicians start patients who have renal disease at a lower-than-usual dosage and monitor side effects closely; however, a usual adult dosage may be required for a therapeutic response. Blood levels should be obtained when available, especially after dosage changes. However, blood levels are sometimes misleading in patients with renal failure because most assays do not distinguish between active (not protein-bound) and nonactive (protein-bound) drugs. High, unmeasured levels of active hydroxylated metabolites may be present.

Medications with a molecular weight of 500 daltons or less are generally dialyzable, unless they are highly protein bound. Almost all psychotropic medications are fat soluble and are not dialyzable; lithium is an exception. The glucuronidated metabolites of some antidepressants are removed by dialysis (Lieberman et al. 1985). For patients receiving dialysis and lithium therapy, the lithium should be replaced after each dialysis session; typical doses are 300–600 mg. The patient's lithium level should be checked 2–3 hours after the dose. Patients taking lithium sometimes have polyuria, which may be inhibited by carbamazepine (Levy 1990) or amiloride (Gelenberg 1985). Because orthostatic hypotension is common immediately after dialysis, psychotropic medications that minimize this side effect are desirable.

Patients With Endocrine Disease

Lithium induces hypothyroidism in 10%–15% of patients; the rate in women is nine times that in men (Jefferson et al. 1987). However, hypothyroidism is not a contraindication to lithium therapy, as long as exogenous thyroid hormone is prescribed and lithium levels and thyroid function are monitored. Carbamazepine can increase the metabolism of thyroid hormone and inhibit thyroid-stimulating hormone secretion.

Because neuroleptic medications block dopamine receptors, they can increase prolactin levels, which can produce amenorrhea, gynecomastia, or galactorrhea. The clinician should consult with an endocrinologist before medicating a patient with psychosis who has hyperprolactinemia.

Patients With Hematopoietic Disease

Consultation-liaison psychiatrists perform consultations on patients who have leukopenia, on those who have more global immunocompromise (e.g., human immunodeficiency virus [HIV] infection), or on those who are undergoing bone marrow transplantation (Balon and Berchou 1986). In these patients, the possibility of bone marrow suppression secondary to psychotropic agents is an important consideration. Agranulocytosis is a rare but significant risk with neuroleptics and TCAs. The peak incidence is 3–4 weeks after initiation of therapy. TCAs induce agranulocytosis less frequently than neuroleptics. Clozapine is associated with a higher risk of bone marrow suppression than are the other neuroleptics. With the exception of clozapine, the incidence is so low with psychotropics that it is not yet possible to determine which agents within a given class are preferred (Grohmann et al. 1989).

Lithium can cause a benign leukocytosis, which is sometimes used to therapeutic advantage. Carbamazepine can induce a benign decrease in the white blood cell count, typically during the first 4 months of treatment; agranulocytosis or aplastic anemia occurs rarely. Valproic acid reportedly induces thrombocytopenia on rare occasions (Brichard et al. 1994; May and Sunder 1993).

Patients With Neurological Disease

Patients who have had a stroke are at increased risk for depression; antidepressants are effective in treating poststroke depression. The safest antidepressants are those with little tendency to induce orthostatic hypotension (e.g., SSRIs and bupropion). The TCAs are more likely to induce orthostatic hypotension than are the SSRIs. If a tricyclic is used, nortriptyline is the safest choice for most patients with neurological disease.

A major concern when psychotropic medications are used in any patient with structural brain disease is the possibility of seizures. TCAs and neuroleptics lower seizure threshold and are, therefore, used with caution. Because maprotiline and bupropion are associated with seizures, they should be avoided. MAOIs lower the seizure threshold less frequently than do TCAs. The relative tendency of SSRIs to induce seizures is not known. Among neuroleptics, clozapine induces seizures more commonly than do other neuroleptics, whereas molindone and fluphenazine affect seizure threshold the least. For depressed patients with a seizure disorder, the threshold for using anticonvulsants as antidepressants is reduced. Benzodiazepines have anticonvulsant properties and are an attractive option for patients in this population who have a benzodiazepine-responsive anxiety disorder (e.g., panic disorder).

Patients with delirium or dementia are particularly sensitive to anticholinergic side effects. For these patients, drugs with minimal or no significant anticholinergic effects should be used. Sedative medications can also worsen confusion. Low-dose, high-potency neuroleptics should be used for patients with confusion and agitation; medications such as haloperidol produce less sedation and orthostasis than do low-potency neuroleptics.

Psychotic symptoms in patients with Parkinson's disease who are taking dopaminergic medications pose a serious dilemma. Treatment of the psychosis with a neuroleptic usually worsens parkinsonian symptoms; treatment of Parkinson's disease with dopaminergic drugs usually worsens the psychosis. A reasonable approach is to treat the most problematic disorder. If the hallucinations or delusions do not cause much difficulty, neuroleptic use should be avoided. If the psychotic symptoms are severe, neuroleptics should be introduced with great caution. The lack of extrapyramidal side effects associated with clozapine makes this drug a useful intervention for Parkinson's disease (Wolk and Douglas 1992). If clozapine use is not possible, a low dose of a low-potency neuroleptic, such as thioridazine, can be tried. The anticholinergic properties of the low-potency antipsychotics tend to lessen extrapyramidal symptoms. ECT has beneficial effects on both the psychosis and the rigidity associated with Parkinson's disease (Moellentine et al. 1998), although improvement is usually transient.

Neuroleptics should not be given, if at all possible, to patients who have acute traumatic brain injuries because deficits in dopaminergic neurotransmitters are implicated in the pathophysiology of traumatic brain injury (Feeny et al. 1982). Psychostimulants are useful in lessening distractibility and apathy in such patients. Propranolol, trazodone, buspirone, and anticonvulsants are sometimes useful in treating aggression in individuals with brain injuries.

Patients with HIV disease (Janicak 1995) often have CNS involvement and psychiatric symptoms as well as psychopathological reactions to their medications and other treatments. These patients are especially sensitive to the side effects of medications, especially neuroleptics; therefore, low doses should be used whenever possible. If the patient's cognitive status permits, depression and energy are sometimes improved with antidepressant treatment. Psychostimulant treatment is often of benefit to patients with subcortical dementia and to those with mood syndromes associated with HIV disease, especially in later stages of the disease (Fernandez and Levy 1990).

Pregnant Patients

During their childbearing years, women frequently experience psychiatric disorders, making psychotropic drug use during pregnancy a common and important issue (see Chapter 31 in this volume). Risks associated with drug therapy during pregnancy include teratogenic effects, direct neonatal toxicity, perinatal effects, and the potential for long-term neurobehavioral sequelae. Against these risks, the patient and the clinician must weigh the consequences of treatment without medication. Table 42–20 lists general guidelines for the use of psychotropic medications in pregnant and breast-feeding women.

A recent meta-analysis reports a higher-than-normal rate of fetal malformation after first trimester exposure to low-potency neuroleptic agents (Altshuler et al. 1996). Exposure to other typical and atypical neuroleptic agents reveals no clear pattern of teratogenicity (Arana and Rosenbaum 2000). Perinatal effects of neuroleptic agents include extrapyramidal side effects such as tremors, hypertonicity, and dyskinesias (Auerbach et al. 1992). Given the relative paucity of data, it is best to avoid giving antipsychotics, particularly low-potency agents, to pregnant patients whenever possible. However, failure to provide treatment to a mother who is psychotic typically poses a greater risk to the fetus than the risk associated with exposure to an antipsychotic drug. ECT is probably the treatment of choice for a pregnant woman who has a psychotic depression (Wise et al. 1984).

The TCAs are relatively safe to prescribe during pregnancy (Altschuler et al. 1996), although withdrawal syndromes are described in newborns when exposure occurs close to the time of delivery. Symptoms include jitteriness, irritability, and seizures (Webster 1973). Fluoxetine is not associated with major congenital malformations, although minor malformations were noted in one study (Chambers et al. 1996). These authors also found more admissions to special care nurseries when women took fluoxetine during the later stages of pregnancy. This study had methodological problems, however, which make interpretation of the data difficult (L. S. Cohen and Rosenbaum 1997). Pregnancy outcomes following maternal use of the SSRIs fluvoxamine, paroxetine, and sertraline show no increased risk in major malformations and no higher rates of miscarriage, stillbirth, or prematurity (Kulin et al. 1998). Data regarding the

TABLE 42–20.   Recommendations for medication use during pregnancy or while breast-feeding

Perform a risk-benefit analysis. Document problems in daily living and the ability of the mother to care for the fetus or infant, target symptoms, and the rationale for medication use.

Ask about and record all drug exposures (prescribed, over-the-counter, herbal, and illicit) during pregnancy and during postpartum period, if the patient is breast-feeding. Be sure to ask about alcohol consumption during pregnancy.

Obtain informed consent. Discuss with the mother the risks and unknown aspects of taking psychotropic medication while pregnant or breast-feeding, to include the remote possibility of long-term effects on the child. Document this discussion, and have the patient sign the informed consent, especially if the patient insists on taking medications despite recommendations to the contrary (e.g., patient has a severe chronic psychotic illness that responds only to clozapine and insists on breast-feeding despite recommendations against breast-feeding while taking clozapine). If the patient's capacity to make an informed decision is influenced by the illness, have the spouse participate in the decision-making process and have him also sign the informed consent.

Use a medication that has worked in the past, unless contraindicated.

Choose medication that has some supporting data versus a novel compound with no supporting data.

Attempt monotherapy. Data on combination pharmacotherapy do not exist. Do not forget that electroconvulsive therapy is the treatment of choice when a woman has a psychotic depression.

While the patient is breast-feeding, try to avoid prescribing medications that require invasive monitoring (e.g., clozapine).

Use the minimum effective dose.

Urge patient who is breast-feeding to take doses so that medication level in breast milk is minimized at the time the baby nurses (i.e., take medication immediately after the baby nurses or take dose immediately prior to baby's long afternoon nap).

Source.   Adapted from recommendations found in Llewellyn A, Stowe ZN: "Psychotropic Medications in Lactation." *Journal of Clinical Psychiatry* 59 (suppl 2):41–52, 1998.

safety of the MAOIs and newer antidepressants are lacking. Therefore, these drugs should be avoided, whenever possible, in pregnant women.

Lithium can cause cardiovascular defects, particularly when taken during the first trimester, although this risk is significantly lower than previously believed (L. S. Cohen et al. 1994; Gelenberg 1992b). When lithium is used during the first trimester, fetal echocardiography and ultrasonography are recommended. Carbamazepine and valproic acid are known to cause fetal neural tube defects (Lammer et al. 1987; Rosa 1991); these medications should be avoided, if possible, especially during the first trimester.

Diazepam was initially thought to increase the incidence of fetal oral clefts (Saxen 1975), but no increased risk was subsequently found in large cohort and case-control studies (Rosenberg et al. 1983).

Patients Who Are Breast-Feeding

Unfortunately, for some women the postpartum period is complicated by depression, mania, or psychosis. For women predisposed to major psychiatric disorders or who develop such disorders postpartum, treatment with psychotropic medications is usually necessary. Breast-feeding has many advantages and few drawbacks for the newborn and the mother. More than 60% of women breast-feed

during puerperium (Llewellyn and Stowe 1998). The benefits of breast-feeding and the desire to breast-feed lead to the question of whether it is safe for the newborn to breast-feed while the mother is taking psychotropic medications. The information available to the clinician and the mother to try to answer this question is limited. Adverse effects attributed to psychotropic medications are found only in case reports. In addition, the pharmacokinetics of a medication's passage into breast milk and then into the infant is quite complicated. Variables include the mother (e.g., metabolism, volume of distribution, amount taken, and timing of dose), the breast milk (e.g., breast-feeding schedule in relation to the time of ingestion, pH, composition), and the infant (e.g., absorption, metabolism, volume of distribution, excretion), "each of which changes and matures independently" (Llewellyn and Stowe 1998, p. 42). The American Academy of Pediatrics (1994) published a policy statement that classifies medications according to their risk to the breast-fed infant (Table 42–21). This information is presented with the caveat that these recommendations have limitations and clinical judgment must prevail. For example, valproic acid is considered compatible with breast-feeding; however, some investigators recommend against its use because of the potential risk of hepatotoxicity in children (Chaudron and Jefferson 2000). Carbamazepine is considered compatible with breast-feeding; however,

TABLE 42–21. Medications and breast-feeding

Medication	Classification	Reason (if listed)
Mood stabilizers		
Carbamazepine	Compatible with breast-feeding	
Lithium	Contraindicated	Infant's levels one-third to one-half of mother's level
Valproic acid	Compatible with breast-feeding	
Anxiolytics		
Diazepam	Unknown but may be of concern	
Lorazepam	Unknown but may be of concern	
Midazolam	Unknown but may be of concern	
Prazepam[a]	Unknown but may be of concern	
Quazepam	Unknown but may be of concern	
Temazepam	Unknown but may be of concern	
Antipsychotics		
Chlorpromazine	Unknown but may be of concern	Drowsiness and lethargy in infants
Haloperidol	Unknown but may be of concern	
Perphenazine	Unknown but may be of concern	
Antidepressants		
Amitriptyline	Unknown but may be of concern	
Amoxapine	Unknown but may be of concern	
Desipramine	Unknown but may be of concern	
Doxepin	Unknown but may be of concern	
Fluoxetine	Unknown but may be of concern	
Fluvoxamine	Unknown but may be of concern	
Imipramine	Unknown but may be of concern	
Trazodone	Unknown but may be of concern	
Hypnotics		
Chloral hydrate	Compatible with breast-feeding	
Zolpidem	Compatible with breast-feeding	

[a]Accumulates in breast milk.
Source. From American Academy of Pediatrics Policy Statement: "The Transfer of Drugs and Other Chemicals into Human Milk (RE9403)." *Pediatrics* 93:137–150, 1994. Used with permission.

there are case reports of poor feeding and hepatic dysfunction (Chaudron and Jefferson 2000). Lithium is contraindicated for women who breast-feed; however, there is insufficient negative information to support such a strong recommendation (Chaudron and Jefferson 2000).

SUMMARY

Many psychotropic medications are available for use by medically ill patients who have psychiatric symptoms. With careful diagnosis, target symptom identification, and the use of other treatment modalities, these medications can relieve the psychic suffering of patients and improve the chances that their physical illnesses will heal. Further research is needed to help define the causes of secondary psychiatric disorders. Further knowledge about mechanisms of action of psychotropic medications,

especially in patients who are medically ill, will facilitate the development of new drugs that are more effective and safer than those currently available. Meanwhile, education about the current psychiatric pharmacopoeia and the psychoactive effects of nonpsychiatric medications will help the consultation-liaison psychiatrist to improve treatment. Consultation-liaison psychiatrists must also educate patients, so that, in partnership with them, the principles outlined in this chapter can be used to tailor treatment to individual patient needs.

REFERENCES

Ackerman AD, Lyons JS, Hammer JS, et al: The impact of coexisting depression and timing of psychiatric consultation on medical patients' length of stay. Hospital and Community Psychiatry 39:173–176, 1988

Addonizio G, Roth SD, Stokes PE, et al: Increased extrapyramidal symptoms with addition of lithium to neuroleptics. J Nerv Ment Dis 176:682–685, 1988

Adityanjee, Aderibigbe YA, Mathews T: Epidemiology of neuroleptic malignant syndrome. Clin Neuropharmacol 22:151–158, 1999

Albeck JH: Withdrawal and detoxification from benzodiazepine dependence: a potential role for clonazepam. J Clin Psychiatry 48 (suppl):43–49, 1987

Altman DF: Changes in gastrointestinal, pancreatic, biliary, and hepatic function with aging. Gastroenterol Clin North Am 19:227–234, 1990

Altshuler LL, Cohen LS, Szuba MP, et al: Pharmacological management of psychiatric illness in pregnancy: dilemmas and guidelines. Am J Psychiatry 153:592–606, 1996

American Academy of Pediatrics: Policy statement: the transfer of drugs and other chemicals into human milk (RE9403). Pediatrics 93:137–150, 1994

Amrein R, Hetzel W, Stabl M, et al: RIMA: a safe concept in the treatment of depression with moclobemide. Can J Psychiatry 37 (suppl 1):7–11, 1992

Anderson IM, Tomenson BM: The efficacy of selective serotonin re-uptake inhibitors in depression: a meta-analysis of studies against tricyclic antidepressants. J Psychopharmacol 8:238–249, 1994

Arana GW, Rosenbaum JF: Handbook of Psychiatric Drug Therapy, 4th Edition. Philadelphia, PA, Lippincott Williams & Wilkins, 2000, pp 37–38

Aronoff GR, Berns JS, Brier ME, et al: Drug Prescribing in Renal Failure, 4th Edition. Philadelphia, PA, American College of Physicians, 1999

Auerbach JG, Hans SL, Marcus J, et al: Maternal psychotropic medication and neonatal behavior. Neurotoxicol Teratol 14:399–406, 1992

Ayd FJ: Paroxetine, a new selective serotonin reuptake inhibitor. International Drug Therapy Newsletter 28:5–12, 1993

Balon R, Berchou R: Hematologic side effects of psychotropic drugs. Psychosomatics 27:119–127, 1986

Bauer M, Dopfmer S: Lithium augmentation in treatment-resistant depression: meta-analysis of placebo-controlled studies. J Clin Psychopharmacol 19:427–434, 1999

Bauer TM, Ritz R, Haberthur C, et al: Prolonged sedation due to accumulation of conjugated metabolites of midazolam. Lancet 346:145–147, 1995

Bays J: Fetal vascular disruption with prenatal exposure to cocaine or methamphetamine. Pediatrics 87:416–418, 1991

Blake LM, Marks RC, Luchins DJ: Reversible neurologic symptoms with clozapine and lithium. J Clin Psychopharmacol 12:297–299, 1992

Boehnert MT, Lovejoy FH: Value of the QRS duration versus the serum drug level in predicting seizures and ventricular arrhythmias after an acute overdose of tricyclic antidepressants. N Engl J Med 313:474–479, 1985

Bowden CL, Brugger AM, Swann AC, et al: Efficacy of divalproex vs lithium and placebo in the treatment of mania: the Depakote Mania Study Group. JAMA 271:918–924, 1994

Brichard B, Vermylen C, Scheiff JM, et al: Haematological disturbances during long-term valproate therapy. Eur J Pediatr 153:378–380, 1994

Brodie-Meijer CC, Diemont WL, Buijs PJ: Nefazodone-induced clitoral priapism. Int Clin Psychopharmacol 14:257–258, 1999

Brown R: U.S. experience with valproate in manic depressive illness: a multicenter trial. J Clin Psychiatry 50:13–16, 1989

Browne JL, Hauge KJ: A review of alprazolam withdrawal. Drug Intelligence and Clinical Pharmacy 20:837–841, 1986

Burrows GD, Maguire KP, Norman TR: Antidepressant efficacy and tolerability of the selective norepinephrine reuptake inhibitor reboxetine: a review. J Clin Psychiatry 59 (suppl 14):4–7, 1998

Cabras PL, Hardoy MJ, Hardoy MC, et al: Clinical experience with gabapentin in patients with bipolar or schizoaffective disorder: results of an open-label study. J Clin Psychiatry 60:245–248, 1999

Calabrese JR, Rapport DJ, Shelton MD, et al: Clinical studies on the use of lamotrigine in bipolar disorder. Neuropsychobiology 38:185–191, 1998

Casey DE: Side effect profiles of new antipsychotic agents. J Clin Psychiatry 57 (suppl 11):40–45, 1996

Castillo-Fernando JR, Garcia M, Carmona J, et al: Digoxin levels and diazepam (letter). Lancet 2:368, 1980

Chambers C, Johnson K, Dick L, et al: Birth outcomes in pregnant women taking fluoxetine. N Engl J Med 335:1010–1015, 1996

Charney DS, Woods SW: Benzodiazepine treatment of panic disorder: a comparison of alprazolam and lorazepam. J Clin Psychiatry 50:418–423, 1989

Chaudhry RP, Waters BG: Lithium and carbamazepine interaction: possible neurotoxicity. J Clin Psychiatry 44:30–31, 1983

Chaudron LH, Jefferson JW: Mood stabilizers during breast-feeding: a review. J Clin Psychiatry 61:79–90, 2000

Cohen LS, Rosenbaum JF: Birth outcomes in pregnant women taking fluoxetine (letter). N Engl J Med 336:872, 1997

Cohen LS, Rosenbaum JF, Heller VL: Psychotropic drug use in pregnancy, in The Practitioner's Guide to Psychoactive Drugs, 3rd Edition. Edited by Gelenberg AJ, Bassuk EL, Schoonover SC. New York, Plenum, 1991, pp 389–405

Cohen LS, Friedman JM, Jefferson JW, et al: A reevaluation of risk of in utero exposure to lithium. JAMA 271:146–150, 1994

Cohen W, Cohen N: Lithium carbonate, haloperidol and irreversible brain damage. JAMA 230:1283–1287, 1974

Coplan JD, Gorman JM: Detectable levels of fluoxetine metabolites after discontinuation: an unexpected serotonin syndrome (letter). Am J Psychiatry 150:837, 1993

Crewe HK, Lennard MS, Tucker GT, et al: The effect of selective serotonin re-uptake inhibitors on cytochrome P4502D6 (CYP2D6) activity in human liver microsomes. Br J Clin Pharmacol 34:262–265, 1992

Crone CC, Wise TN: Use of herbal medicines among consultation-liaison populations. Psychosomatics 39:3–13, 1998

DasGupta K, Jefferson JW: The use of lithium in the medically ill. Gen Hosp Psychiatry 12:83–97, 1990

DeVane CL: Pharmacogenetics and drug metabolism of newer antidepressant agents. J Clin Psychiatry 55 (suppl 12):38–45, 1994

DeVane CL: Differential pharmacology of newer antidepressants. J Clin Psychiatry 59 (suppl 20):85–93, 1998

Dew MA, Reynolds CF, Houck PR, et al: Temporal profiles of the course of depression during treatment: predictors of pathways toward recovery in the elderly. Arch Gen Psychiatry 54:1016–1024, 1997

Dilsaver SC, Greden JF: Antidepressant withdrawal phenomena. Biol Psychiatry 19:237–256, 1984

Dolly FR, Block AJ: Effect of flurazepam on sleep-disordered breathing and nocturnal oxygen desaturation in asymptomatic subjects. Am J Med 73:239–243, 1982

Dubovsky SL, Buzan R: Mood disorders, in Textbook of Psychiatry, 3rd Edition. Edited by Hales RE, Yudofsky SC, Talbott JA. Washington, DC, American Psychiatric Press, 1999, pp 479–566

Elie R, Ruther E, Farr I, et al: Sleep latency is shortened during 4 weeks of treatment with zaleplon, a novel nonbenzodiazepine hypnotic. J Clin Psychiatry 60:536–544, 1999

Elitsur Y: Pemoline (Cylert)-induced hepatotoxicity. J Pediatr Gastroenterol Nutr 11:143–144, 1990

Fann JR: The epidemiology of delirium: a review of studies and methodological issues. Seminars in Clinical Neuropsychiatry 5:64–74, 2000

Fava M: Weight gain and antidepressants. J Clin Psychiatry 61 (suppl 11):37–41, 2000

Fava S, Galizia AC: Neuroleptic malignant syndrome and lithium carbonate. J Psychiatry Neurosci 20:305–306, 1995

Fawcett J: Compliance: definitions and key issues. J Clin Psychiatry 56 (suppl 1):4–8; discussion 9–10, 1995

Feeny DM, Gonzalez A, Law WA: Amphetamine, haloperidol, and experience interact to affect rate of recovery after motor cortex injury. Science 217:855–857, 1982

Feighner J: Overview of antidepressants currently used to treat anxiety disorders. J Clin Psychiatry 60 (suppl 22):18–22, 1999

Fernandez F, Levy JK: Psychiatric diagnosis and pharmacotherapy of patients with HIV infection, in American Psychiatric Press Review of Psychiatry, Vol 9. Edited by Tasman A, Goldfinger SM, Kaufmann CA. Washington, DC, American Psychiatric Press, 1990, pp 614–630

Fischer JH, Barr AN, Rogers SL, et al: Lack of serious toxicity following gabapentin overdose. Neurology 44:982–983, 1994

Foulke GE, Albertson TE: QRS interval in tricyclic antidepressant overdose: inaccuracy as a toxicity indicator in emergency setting. Ann Emerg Med 16:160–163, 1987

Frances AJ, Kahn DA, Carpenter D, et al: The Expert Consensus Guidelines for treating depression in bipolar disorder. J Clin Psychiatry 59 (suppl 4):73–79, 1998

Frierson RL, Wey JJ, Tabler JB: Psychostimulants for depression in the medically ill. Am Fam Physician 43:163–170, 1991

Frye MA, Coudreaut MF, Hakeman SM, et al: Continuous droperidol infusion for management of agitated delirium in an intensive care unit. Psychosomatics 36:301–305, 1995

Frye MA, Ketter TA, Kimbrell TA, et al: A placebo-controlled study of lamotrigine and gabapentin monotherapy in refractory mood disorders. J Clin Psychopharmacol 20:607–614, 2000

Fulop G, Strain JJ, Vita J, et al: Impact of psychiatric comorbidity on length of hospital stay for medical/surgical patients: a preliminary report. Am J Psychiatry 144:878–882, 1987

Gelenberg AJ: Amiloride (Midamor) for lithium-induced polyuria (letter). Biological Therapies in Psychiatry 8:23, 1985

Gelenberg AJ: Benzodiazepines: not teratogenic? Biological Therapies in Psychiatry 16:2–3, 1992a

Gelenberg AJ: Lithium teratogenesis revisited. Biological Therapies in Psychiatry 15:25–26, 1992b

Gelenberg AJ: Fluoxetine and bradycardia. Biological Therapies in Psychiatry 18:41, 1995

Gelenberg AJ, Bellinghausen B, Wojcik JD, et al: A prospective survey of neuroleptic malignant syndrome in a short-term psychiatric hospital. Am J Psychiatry 145:517–518, 1988

Gelenberg AJ, Kane JM, Keller MB, et al: Comparison of standard and low serum levels of lithium for maintenance treatment of bipolar disorder. N Engl J Med 321:1489–1493, 1989

Gilbody JS: Effects of maternal drug addiction on the fetus. Adverse Drug React Toxicol Rev 10:77–88, 1991

Girault C, Muir JF, Mihaltan F, et al: Effects of repeated administration of zolpidem on sleep, diurnal and nocturnal respiratory function, vigilance and physical performance in patients with COPD. Chest 110:1203–1211, 1996

Glassman AH: Cardiovascular effects of antidepressant drugs: updated. Int Clin Psychopharmacol 13 (suppl 5):S25–S30, 1998

Glassman AH, Roose SP, Bigger JT: The safety of tricyclic antidepressants in cardiac patients. JAMA 269:2673–2675, 1993

Glazer WM, Morgenstern H, Doucette JT: Predicting the long-term risk of tardive dyskinesia in outpatients maintained on neuroleptic medications. J Clin Psychiatry 54:133–139, 1993

Goa KL, Sorkin EM: Gabapentin: a review of its pharmacological properties and clinical potential in epilepsy. Drugs 46:409–427, 1993

Grohmann R, Schmidt LG, Spiess-Kiefer C, et al: Agranulocytosis and significant leucopenia with neuroleptic drugs: results from the AMÜP program. Psychopharmacology 99:S109–S112, 1989

Guven H, Tuncok Y, Guneri S, et al: Age-related digoxin-alprazolam interaction. Clin Pharmacol Ther 54:42–44, 1993

Guy W: ECDEU Assessment Manual for Psychopharmacology, Revised. Washington, DC, United States Department of Health, Education and Welfare, 1976

Gwirtsman HE, Guze BH: Amphetamine, but not methylphenidate, predicts antidepressant response. J Clin Psychopharmacol 9:453–454, 1989

Hall RC, Wise MG: The clinical and financial burden of mood disorders: cost and outcome. Psychosomatics 36:S11–S18, 1995

Harris CR, Kingston R: Gastrointestinal decontamination: which method is best? Postgrad Med 92:116–122, 125, 128, 1992

Hauser LA: Pregnancy and psychiatric drugs. Hospital and Community Psychiatry 36:817–818, 1985

Henney JE: From the Food and Drug Administration: new drug for sleeplessness. JAMA 282:1218, 1999

Hunt N, Stern TA: The association between intravenous haloperidol and torsades de pointes. Psychosomatics 36:541–549, 1995

Hurt RD, Sachs DPL, Glover ED, et al: A comparison of sustained-release bupropion and placebo for smoking cessation. N Engl J Med 337:1195–1202, 1997

Hussein S, Kaufman BM: Bradycardia associated with fluoxetine in an elderly patient with sick sinus syndrome (letter). Postgrad Med J 70:819, 1994

Hyman SE, Arana GW, Rosenbaum JF: Handbook of Psychiatric Drug Therapy, 3rd Edition. Boston, Little, Brown, 1995

Jacobson SJ, Jones K, Johnson X, et al: Prospective multi-center study of pregnancy outcome after lithium exposure during first trimester. Lancet 339:530–533, 1995

Janicak PG: Psychopharmacotherapy in the HIV-infected patient. Psychiatric Annals 25:609–613, 1995

Janicak PG, Bresnahan DB, Comaty JE: The neuroleptic malignant syndrome: a clinical update. Psychiatric Annals 17:551–555, 1987

Jawary D, Cameron PA, Dziukas L, et al: Drug overdose—reducing the load. Med J Aust 156:343–346, 1992

Jefferson JW: Cardiovascular effects and toxicity of anxiolytics and antidepressants. J Clin Psychiatry 50:368–378, 1989

Jefferson JW, Greist JH, Clagnaz PJ, et al: Effect of strenuous exercise on serum lithium level in man. Am J Psychiatry 139:1593–1595, 1982

Jefferson JW, Greist JH, Ackerman DL, et al: Lithium Encyclopedia for Clinical Practice, 2nd Edition. Washington, DC, American Psychiatric Press, 1987

Joffe RT, Singer W, Levitt AJ, et al: A placebo-controlled comparison of lithium and triiodothyronine augmentation of tricyclic antidepressants in unipolar refractory depression. Arch Gen Psychiatry 50:387–393, 1993

Joyce PR, Paykel ES: Predictors of drug response in depression. Arch Gen Psychiatry 46:89–99, 1989

Kales A, Bixler EO, Vela-Bueno A, et al: Alprazolam: effects on sleep and withdrawal phenomena. J Clin Pharmacol 27:508–515, 1987

Kallen B, Tandberg A: Lithium and pregnancy: a cohort study on manic-depressive women. Acta Psychiatr Scand 68:134–139, 1983

Kamlet MS, Paul N, Greenhouse J, et al: Cost utility analysis of maintenance treatment for recurrent depression. Control Clin Trials 16:17–40, 1995

Kandrotas RJ, Love JM, Gal P, et al: The effect of hemodialysis and hemoperfusion on serum valproic acid concentration. Neurology 40:1456–1458, 1990

Ketter TA, Frye MA, Cora-Locatelli G, et al: Metabolism and excretion of mood stabilizers and new anticonvulsants. Cell Mol Neurobiol 19(4):511–532, 1999

Kiev A: A double-blind, placebo-controlled study of paroxetine in depressed outpatients. J Clin Psychiatry 52 (suppl):27–29, 1992

Kojima H, Terao T, Yoshimura R: Serotonin syndrome during clomipramine and lithium treatment (letter). Am J Psychiatry 150:1897, 1993

Kraus MF: Neuropsychiatric sequelae of stroke and traumatic brain injury: the role of psychostimulants. Int J Psychiatry Med 25:39–51, 1995

Krishnan KRR: Monoamine oxidase inhibitors, in Textbook of Psychopharmacology. Edited by Schatzberg AF, Nemeroff CB. Washington, DC, American Psychiatric Press, 1995, pp 183–193

Kulin NA, Pastuszak A, Sage SR, et al: Pregnancy outcome following maternal use of the new selective serotonin reuptake inhibitors. JAMA 279:609–610, 1998

Kupfer DJ, Reynolds CF III: Management of insomnia. N Engl J Med 336:341–346, 1997

Lader M: Combined use of tricyclic antidepressants and monoamine oxidase inhibitors. J Clin Psychiatry 44 (part 2):20–24, 1983

Lammer EJ, Sever LE, Oakley GP Jr: Teratogen update: valproic acid. Teratology 35:465–473, 1987

Lane R, Glazer W, Hansen T, et al: Assessment of tardive dyskinesia using the Abnormal Involuntary Movement Scale. J Nerv Ment Dis 173:353–357, 1985

Lapierre J, Amin M, Hattangadi S: Prochlorperazine—a review of the literature since 1956. Can J Psychiatry 14:267–274, 1969

Leipzig RM: Psychopharmacology in patients with hepatic and gastrointestinal disease. Int J Psychiatry Med 20:109–139, 1990

Leo RJ, David GL, Hershey LA: Parkinsonism associated with fluoxetine and cimetidine: a case report. J Geriatr Psychiatry Neurol 8:231–233, 1995

Levy NB: Psychopharmacology in patients with renal failure. Int J Psychiatry Med 20:325–334, 1990

Lieberman JA, Cooper TB, Suckow RF, et al: Tricyclic antidepressant and metabolite levels in chronic renal failure. Clin Pharmacol Ther 37:301–307, 1985

Lin EH, Von Korff M, Katon W, et al: The role of the primary care physician in patients' adherence to antidepressant therapy. Med Care 33:67–74, 1995

Lion JR, Azcarate CL, Koepke HH: Paradoxical rage reactions during psychotropic medication. Diseases of the Nervous System 36:557–558, 1975

Little KY: Amphetamine, but not methylphenidate, predicts antidepressant efficacy. J Clin Psychopharmacol 8:177–183, 1988

Llewellyn A, Stowe ZN: Psychotropic medications in lactation. J Clin Psychiatry 59 (suppl 2):41–52, 1998

Marangell LB, Yudofsky SC, Silver JM: Psychopharmacology and electroconvulsive therapy, in Textbook of Psychiatry, 3rd Edition. Edited by Hales RE, Yudofsky SC, Talbott JA. Washington, DC, American Psychiatric Press, 1999, pp 1025–1132

Markowitz JS, Brewerton TD: Zolpidem-induced psychosis. Ann Clin Psychiatry 8:89–91, 1996

Markowitz JS, Morrison SD, DeVane CL: Drug interactions with psychostimulants. Int Clin Psychopharmacol 14:1–18, 1999

May RB, Sunder TR: Hematologic manifestations of long-term valproate therapy. Epilepsia 34:1098–1101, 1993

McElroy SL, Keck PE Jr, Pope HG Jr, et al: Valproate in psychiatric disorders: literature review and clinical guidelines. J Clin Psychiatry 50 (suppl):23–29, 1989

McElroy SL, Dessain EC, Pope HG, et al: Clozapine in the treatment of psychotic mood disorders, schizoaffective disorder, and schizophrenia. J Clin Psychiatry 52:411–414, 1991

Menza MA, Kaufman KR, Castellanos A: Modafinil augmentation of antidepressant treatment in depression. J Clin Psychiatry 61:378–381, 2000

Metzger E, Friedman R: Prolongation of the corrected QT and torsade de pointes cardiac arrhythmia associated with intravenous haloperidol in the medically ill. J Clin Psychopharmacol 13:128–132, 1993

Michelson D, Amsterdam JD, Quitkin FM, et al: Changes in weight during a 1-year trial of fluoxetine. Am J Psychiatry 156:1170–1176, 1999

Miller LG: Herbal medicinals: selected clinical considerations focusing on known or potential drug-herb interactions. Arch Intern Med 158:2200–2211, 1998

Moellentine C, Rummans T, Ahlskog JE, et al: Effectiveness of ECT in patients with parkinsonism. Journal of Neuropsychiatry and Clinical Neurosciences 10:187–193, 1998

Ohman R, Spigset O: Serotonin syndrome induced by fluvoxamine-lithium interaction (letter). Pharmacopsychiatry 26:263–264, 1993

Ouslander JG: Drug therapy in the elderly. Ann Intern Med 95:711–722, 1981

Palatnick W, Tenebein M: Activated charcoal in the treatment of drug overdose: an update. Drug Saf 7:3–7, 1992

Patterson JF: Hepatitis associated with pemoline (letter). South Med J 77:938, 1984

Pellock JM, Willmore LJ: A rational guide to routine blood monitoring in patients receiving antiepileptic drugs. Neurology 41:961–964, 1991

Physicians' Desk Reference, 54th Edition. Montvale, NJ, Medical Economics Company, 2000

Piscitelli SC, Burstein AH, Chaitt D, et al: Indinavir concentrations and St John's wort (letter). Lancet 355:547–548, 2000

Pope HG, McElroy SL, Keck PE Jr, et al: A placebo-controlled study of valproate in mania. Arch Gen Psychiatry 48:62–68, 1991

Post RM, Frye MA, Denicoff KD, et al.: Beyond lithium in the treatment of bipolar illness. Neuropsychopharmacology 19:206–219, 1998

Pratt DS, Dubois RS: Hepatotoxicity due to pemoline (Cylert): a report of two cases. J Pediatr Gastroenterol Nutr 10:239–241, 1990

Preskorn SH, Alderman J, Kaufman BM, et al: Desipramine levels after sertraline or fluoxetine. Poster presented at the annual meeting of the American Psychiatric Association, Washington, DC, May 1992

Rapport DJ, Calabrese JR: Interactions between carbamazepine and birth control pills. Psychosomatics 30:462–464, 1989

Ray WA, Griffin MR, Schaffner W, et al: Psychotropic drug use and the risk of hip fracture. N Engl J Med 316:363–369, 1987

Reed SM, Wise MG, Timmerman I: Choreoathetosis: a sign of lithium toxicity. J Neuropsychiatry Clin Neurosci 1:57–60, 1989

Reeves JG, Fragen RJ, Gillette PC, et al: Midazolam: pharmacology and uses. Anesthesia 62:310–324, 1985

Richelson ER: The pharmacology of antidepressants at the synapse: focus on newer compounds. J Clin Psych 55 (suppl A):34–39; discussion 40–41, 98–100, 1994

Rickels K, Schweizer EE: Current pharmacotherapy of anxiety and panic, in Psychopharmacology: The Third Generation of Progress. Edited by Meltzer HY. New York, Raven, 1987, pp 1193–1203

Risse SC, Whitters A, Burke J, et al: Severe withdrawal symptoms after discontinuation of alprazolam in eight patients with combat-induced posttraumatic stress disorder. J Clin Psychiatry 51:206–209, 1990

Robinson GE, Stewart DE, Flak E: The rational use of psychotropic drugs in pregnancy and postpartum. Can J Psychiatry 31:183–190, 1986

Roose SP, Glassman AH: Antidepressant choice in the patient with cardiac disease: lessons from the Cardiac Arrhythmia Suppression Trial (CAST) studies. J Clin Psychiatry 55:83–100, 1994

Roose SP, Spatz E: Treating depression in patients with ischemic heart disease: which agents are best to use and to avoid. Drug Saf 20:459–465, 1999

Roose SP, Dalack GW, Glassman AH, et al: Cardiovascular effects of bupropion in depressed patients with heart disease. Am J Psychiatry 148:512–516, 1991a

Roose SP, Dalack GW, Woodring S: Death, depression and heart disease. J Clin Psychiatry 52 (suppl 6):34–39, 1991b

Roose SP, Laghrissi-Thode F, Kennedy JS, et al: Comparison of paroxetine and nortriptyline in depressed patients with ischemic heart disease. JAMA 279:287–291, 1998

Rosa FW: Spina bifida in infants of women treated with carbamazepine during pregnancy. N Engl J Med 324:674–677, 1991

Rosebush PI, Stewart TD, Gelenberg AJ: Twenty neuroleptic rechallenges after neuroleptic malignant syndrome in 15 patients. J Clin Psychiatry 50:295–298, 1989

Rosenberg L, Mitchell AA, Parsells JL, et al: Lack of relation of oral clefts to diazepam use during pregnancy. N Engl J Med 309:1282–1285, 1983

Ruschitzka F, Meler PJ, Turina M, et al: Acute heart transplant rejection due to St John's Wort (letter). Lancet 355:548, 2000

Sachdev PS: Lithium potentiation of neuroleptic-related extrapyramidal side effects (letter). Am J Psychiatry 143: 942, 1986

Saravay SM, Strain JJ: APM Task Force on Funding Implications of Consultation-Liaison Outcome Studies: special series introduction: a review of outcome studies. Psychosomatics 35:227–232, 1994

Satel SL, Nelson, JC: Stimulants in the treatment of depression: a critical overview. J Clin Psychiatry 50:241–249, 1989

Saxen I: Associations between oral clefts and drugs taken during pregnancy. Int J Epidemiol 4:37–44, 1975

Scharf M, Roth T, Vogel GW, et al: A multicenter, placebo-controlled study evaluating zolpidem in the treatment of chronic insomnia. J Clin Psychiatry 55:192–199, 1994

Schatzberg AF: New indications for antidepressants. J Clin Psychiatry 61 (suppl 11):9–17, 2000

Schmucker DL: Aging and drug disposition: an update. Pharmacol Rev 37:133–148, 1985

Serban G, Siegel S, Gaffney M: Response of negative symptoms of schizophrenia to neuroleptic treatment. J Clin Psychiatry 53:229–234, 1992

Shader RI, von Moltke LL, Schmider J, et al: The clinician and drug interactions—an update. J Clin Psychopharmacol 16:197–201, 1996

Shukla S, Godwin CD, Long LE, et al: Lithium-carbamazepine neurotoxicity and risk factors. Am J Psychiatry 141:1604–1606, 1984

Siris SG, Rifkin A: The problem of psychopharmacotherapy in the medically ill. Psychiatr Clin North Am 4:379–390, 1981

Spencer MJ: Fluoxetine hydrochloride (Prozac) toxicity in a neonate. Pediatrics 92:721–722, 1993

Spiller HA, Ramoska EA, Krenzelok EP, et al: Bupropion overdose: a 3-year multi-center retrospective analysis. Am J Emerg Med 12:43–45, 1994

Spring GK: Neurotoxicity with combined use of lithium and thioridazine. J Clin Psychiatry 40:135–138, 1979

Stip E, Boisjoly H: Quetiapine: are we overreacting in our concern about cataracts (the beagle effect)? Can J Psychiatry 44:503, 1999

Stoudemire A, Moran MG, Fogel BS: Psychotropic drug use in the medically ill, part I. Psychosomatics 31:377–391, 1990

Stoudemire A, Moran MG, Fogel BS: Psychotropic drug use in the medically ill, part II. Psychosomatics 32:34–46, 1991

Sussman N: The uses of buspirone in psychiatry. J Clin Psychiatry Monograph 129:3–19, 1994

Szymanski S, Munne R, Safferman A, et al: A selective review of recent advances in the management of tardive dyskinesia. Psychiatric Annals 23:209–215, 1993

Tandon R, Ribeiro SCM, DeQuardo JR, et al: Covariance of positive and negative symptoms during neuroleptic treatment in schizophrenia: a replication. Biol Psychiatry 34: 495–497, 1993

Tank JE, Palmer BF: Simultaneous "in series" hemodialysis and hemoperfusion in the management of valproic acid overdose. Am J Kidney Dis 22:341–344, 1993

Teicher MH, Cohen BM, Baldessarini RJ, et al: Severe daytime somnolence in patients treated with an MAOI. Am J Psychiatry 145:1552–1556, 1988

Tesar GE, Stern TA: Evaluation and treatment of agitation in the intensive care unit. Journal of Intensive Care Medicine 1:137–148, 1986

Tesar GE, Rosenbaum JF, Pollack MH, et al: Double-blind, placebo-controlled comparison of clonazepam and alprazolam for panic disorder. J Clin Psychiatry 52:69–76, 1991

Thapa PB, Gideon P, Fought RL, et al: Psychotropic drugs and risk of recurrent falls in ambulatory nursing home residents. Am J Epidemiol 142:202–211, 1995

Thase M: Effects of venlafaxine on blood pressure: a meta-analysis of original data from 3744 depressed patients. J Clin Psychiatry 59:502–508, 1998

Thompson C: Mirtazapine versus selective serotonin reuptake inhibitors. J Clin Psychiatry 60 (suppl 17):18–22; discussion 46–48, 1999

Tollefson G, Lesar T, Grothe D, et al: Alprazolam-related digoxin toxicity. Am J Psychiatry 141:1612–1613, 1984

Tolman KG, Freston JW, Berenson MM, et al: Hepatotoxicity due to pemoline: report of two cases. Digestion 9:532–539, 1973

Turpin JP, Schuller AB: Lithium and haloperidol incompatibility reviewed. Psychiatric Journal of the University of Ottawa 3:245–251, 1978

Verbosky LA, Franco K, Zrull JP: The relationship between depression and length of stay in the general hospital patient. J Clin Psychiatry 54:177–181, 1993

Wallace A, Kofoed LL, West AN: Double-blind, placebo-controlled trial of methylphenidate in older, depressed, medically ill patients. Am J Psychiatry 152:929–931, 1995

Warner MD, Peabody CA, Boutros NN, et al: Alprazolam and withdrawal seizures. J Nerv Ment Dis 178:208–209, 1990

Warrington SJ, Padgham C, Lader M: The cardiovascular effects of antidepressants. Psychol Med 16 (monograph suppl):1–40, 1989

Webster PAC: Withdrawal symptoms in neonates associated with maternal antidepressant therapy. Lancet 2:318–319, 1973

White K, Simpson G: Combined monoamine oxidase inhibitors–tricyclic antidepressant treatment: a reevaluation. J Clin Psychopharmacol 1:264–282, 1981

Wise MG, Rundell JR: Concise Guide to Consultation Psychiatry, 2nd Edition. Washington, DC, American Psychiatric Press, 1994

Wise MG, Tierney J: Psychopharmacology in the elderly. Journal of the Louisiana State Medical Society 144:471–476, 1992

Wise MG, Ward SC, Townsend-Parchman W, et al: Case report of ECT during a high risk pregnancy. Am J Psychiatry 141:99–101, 1984

Wise MG, Brannan SK, Shanfield SB, et al: Psychiatric aspects of organ transplantation (letter). JAMA 260:3437, 1988

Wise MG, Javors MA, Funderburg LG, et al: Lithium levels in bodily fluids of a nursing mother and infant. Lithium 1:189–191, 1990

Wolk SI, Douglas CJ: Clozapine treatment of psychosis in Parkinson's disease: a report of five consecutive cases. J Clin Psychiatry 53:373–376, 1992

Yassa R, Nastase C, DuPont D, et al: Tardive dyskinesia in elderly psychiatric patients: a 5-year study. Am J Psychiatry 149:1206–1211, 1992

43

Pain Management

Anna Holmgren, M.D.

Michael G. Wise, M.D.

Anthony J. Bouckoms, M.D.[†]

As the field of pain medicine has grown since the early 1990s, so has the demand for psychiatrists well versed in the treatment of pain syndromes. Pain teams are increasingly multidisciplinary, providing an opportunity for consultation-liaison psychiatrists to join neurologists, anesthesiologists, and physiatrists in evaluating patients.

Unfortunately, training in pain management during medical school and residency has lagged behind the need for knowledge in clinical practice. As a result, physicians often feel uncomfortable or incapable of helping patients in pain, particularly chronic pain. This situation is compounded by the difficulty of studying a subjective symptom such as pain. Although the overlap and comorbidity between pain and psychiatric syndromes are well known, it is often forgotten that every class of psychiatric medication is used in the management of pain (Table 43–1) and that many pain syndromes are responsive to psychiatric medications (Table 43–2). This chapter highlights important areas of this overlap and provides a guide and references for the physician interested in this growing and interesting field. Although the assessment and treatment of chronic pain is usually complicated, it also can be quite rewarding.

TABLE 43–1. Psychiatric medications used in the treatment of pain disorders

Class of medication	Specific medications	Dosage instructions	Clinical use/efficacy
Antidepressants	Primarily tricyclics	Often need to titrate to full antidepressant dose; allow 2 months for full effect	Neuropathic pain, migraine, failed back syndrome
Antianxiety	Clonazepam and other benzodiazepines	Usual doses	Neuropathic pain, migraine, failed back syndrome
Mood stabilizers (anticonvulsants)	Valproic acid, carbamazepine (lithium does not seem to be effective)	Usual doses and blood levels	Neuropathic pain, migraine, failed back syndrome
Antipsychotics	Haloperidol (including intravenous), perphenazine	Generally low doses; particularly helpful when patient is extremely fearful	Decreases associated fear; augments opioid analgesic effect
Stimulants	Dextroamphetamine, methylphenidate	Immediate effect, can titrate as patient tolerates (e.g., on daily basis in inpatient setting)	Augments opioid analgesic effect; decreases opioid side effects (e.g., sedation, anorexia)

†Deceased.

TABLE 43–2. Pain syndromes often responsive to psychiatric medications

Migraine headaches
Chronic tension headaches
Reflex sympathetic dystrophy
Phantom limb pain
Neuropathic pain following injury
Postherpetic neuralgia
Dysmenorrhea
Central pain
Diabetic neuropathy
Polyneuropathies

TABLE 43–3. Barriers to effective pain management

System- and physician-related barriers
  Inadequate physician training and education in assessment and treatment of pain
  Fear of regulatory board investigation
  Concerns that patient will become addicted to opioid medications
  Concerns about malingering
  Concerns about diversion of medications

Patient-related barriers
  Fear of becoming addicted
  Concerns about being seen as weak, drug seeking, or ungrateful
  Assumption that residual pain is due to limitations in medications or pain management
  Denial of pain equals denial of illness or illness progression

Source. Data from Haddox JD, Joranson D, Angarola RT, et al: "The Use of Opioids for the Treatment of Chronic Pain." Consensus statement from the American Academy of Pain Medicine and American Pain Society, 1996.

INTRODUCTORY ISSUES

The Tragedy of Needless Pain

Despite the increased awareness among physicians and the public about the need for and ability to treat pain, adequate pain management remains a problem. As articles in the lay press and professional journals attest, the problem of needless pain persists. Journals of virtually every clinical specialty have featured articles on the problem. Yet, even when severe pain is expected and the use of opioid medication is accepted, pain is often undertreated. In a study of burn inpatients receiving pain medication on an as-needed (prn) basis, 23% reported severe ("horrible") pain and 30% reported extremely severe ("excruciating") pain during débridement and physiotherapy. When pain was evaluated at rest, 13% of patients endorsed severe pain, and 20% endorsed extremely severe pain (Melzack 1990). In a study of patients with metastatic cancer treated at a cancer center, 42% of patients received inadequate pain management, and physicians tended to underestimate the amount of pain their patients endured even though opioid treatment of terminal cancer pain is widely accepted (Cleeland et al. 1994). In a survey of 1,300 physicians, 30% endorsed occasionally or frequently underdosing outpatients who had cancer pain out of fear of regulatory investigation. In the same study, 50% of physicians endorsed occasionally or frequently prescribing a lower quantity of medication, and over 50% acknowledged occasionally or frequently prescribing fewer refills (Guglielmo 2000). In legislatures and within public policies, attempts are ongoing to reduce some of the barriers to treatment (Table 43–3), including excessive regulatory oversight. For example, efforts are under way to decrease regulations such as special multiple-copy prescriptions. These forms are used in some states to monitor physician prescribing practice and often leave well-intentioned physicians reluctant to prescribe opioid medications (Guglielmo 2000).

With regard to inadequate pain control, in 1999 a medical board for the first time disciplined an Oregon physician for undertreating patients' pain. As of 2001, the Joint Commission on Accreditation of Healthcare Organizations mandated assessment of pain at every clinical encounter as part of a directive to improve pain management.

Contrary to popular belief and clinical lore, patients are more likely to underreport than overendorse pain. It is true that a few patients malinger or amplify pain complaints in order to receive medication and that significant numbers of patients report pain when, in fact, they are experiencing anxiety, fear, or depression. However, patients often do not report pain out of fear of being seen as weak, bad, ungrateful, or—worse yet—an addict. Patients may deny pain because "if the pain isn't there, the disease isn't progressing." Patients also often assume that pain is maximally treated and that any residual pain is the result of limitations in medical science (Rich 2000).

Role of the Consultation-Liaison Psychiatrist in Pain Management

Clearly, pain has both mental and physical components. Attempts to split pain into two categories, one exclusively mental ("it's all in your head") and the other exclusively physical ("real") pain, confuses clinicians and patients and derails treatment efforts. When the psychiatrist is called for consultation, too often it is as a last resort. The patient's interpretation of the consultation is that he or she is not believed. A more successful approach to consultation is to include the psychiatrist as a member of the pain team. The psychiatrist is then introduced as a physician routinely involved in treating difficult types of pain. This approach also acknowledges the intimate and complicated relationships among pain, depression, anxiety, and other psychiatric symptoms. With this relatively simple organizational change, most patients can begin to address the toll pain has taken on their lives and begin to form an alliance with the psychiatrist.

The consultation-liaison psychiatrist's tasks in the assessment of patients with pain include looking for pain syndromes that are responsive to psychotropic medications and assessing the patient for comorbid psychiatric conditions and psychological factors that amplify pain symptoms. Additionally, the evaluation includes examination for complications from pain medications (e.g., side effects, drug interactions, misuse, abuse). Each of these tasks is discussed in this chapter.

DEFINING PAIN

Pain can be a symptom of illness or an illness in its own right. Cancer, trauma, and sickle-cell crises are examples of illnesses in which pain is a symptom. Phantom pain, neuropathic pain, and migraine pain are examples of disorders in which pain is the illness. Pain is best thought of as a disorder with distinct diagnostic features, epidemiology, and a chemical and neurological pathology.

Pain is also a subjective experience. It is affected by context and emotional state. Attempts to study or objectify pain include applying irritating substances or stimuli to a mouse's foot or heat to a person's skin. Pain threshold is established when the affected limb is withdrawn or when the person asks that the experiment stop. In clinical practice, pain is obviously much more complicated. For example, if a 50-year-old man whose father died at age 50 from an acute myocardial infarction begins to experience chest pain, fear and anxiety are likely to magnify the perceived pain. Similarly, a person who is depressed or irritable will also have a lowered pain tolerance. The International Association for the Study of Pain (1994) (IASP) recognized the importance of psychological factors when it defined pain as "always a psychological state" (p. 210). Therefore, the assessment of pain in clinical situations must always include the context in which the pain occurs and the patient's associated emotional state.

Difficulties often arise when trying to define pain and describe its characteristics to other clinicians. These seemingly simple tasks are further complicated by the diversity of pain. For example, defining pain as that which occurs as the result of ongoing noxious or damaging stimuli omits pain due to absent or nonnoxious stimuli (e.g., phantom limb pain). To facilitate discussion and treatment of pain, the consultation-liaison psychiatrist must have a working knowledge of common pain terms. A discussion of common clinical definitions follows.

- *Pain* is an unpleasant sensory and emotional experience that is associated with actual or potential tissue damage or is described as such.
- A *nociceptor* is a receptor that is preferentially sensitive to a noxious stimulus or to a stimulus that would become noxious if prolonged. "One should avoid terms such as pain receptor, pain pathway, and the like because they reflect anachronistic concepts and can mislead. Pain is a complex perception that takes place at higher levels of the central nervous system" (International Association 1994, classification of chronic pain).
- *Acute pain* is a term used for a nociceptive stimulus, acute in onset, waxing and waning in intensity, that resolves within days to weeks. It generally follows a defined pathophysiological process and pattern (e.g., postoperative pain, anginal chest pain) (Bonica 1990).
- *Chronic pain* refers to pain that is prolonged beyond the expected recovery time for a particular disease process or, somewhat arbitrarily, as pain persisting beyond 3 months. Chronic pain is often further subcategorized as malignant or nonmalignant chronic pain.
- *Allesthesia* is a condition in which a sensation is referred to a site distant from where the stimulus is applied.
- *Allodynia* is pain caused by a nonnoxious stimulus (i.e., stimuli that normally would not cause pain) such as cold, vibration, or light touch.
- *Hypoesthesia* is a decreased sensitivity to *any* stimulation. *Hypoalgesia* is diminished sensitivity to *noxious* stimulation; it is a subtype of hypoesthesia.
- *Hyperesthesia* is an increased sensitivity to noxious or nonnociceptive stimuli such as touch or temperature. *Hyperalgesia* is an increased sensitivity to noxious stimulation.
- *Hyperpathia* is a form of hyperesthesia that is typically delayed after the offending stimulus is removed, continues to worsen for minutes or hours, and is sometimes felt at a site distant from the original stimulus (*allesthesia*).
- *Neuropathic pain* is initiated or caused by damage or dysfunction of the peripheral or central nervous system (CNS). Typically, it is described as stabbing, burning, shooting, or searing pain. *Central pain*, a subset of neuropathic pain, is pain initiated or caused by damage to or dysfunction of the CNS (e.g., thalamic pain following stroke, phantom limb pain).

- *Reflex sympathetic dystrophy* (technically encompassed by the term *complex regional pain syndrome*, or CRPS) is a clinical term used to define pain, following an injury, that appears regionally and has a distal predominance of abnormal findings. Commonly associated symptoms are a burning pain with allodynia, vasomotor symptoms, sweating, and late trophic changes; atrophy of skin and nails and loss of hair over the affected area; and muscle and bone wasting that ultimately produces a swollen, painful, discolored, and dysfunctional appendage.
- *Sympathetically mediated pain* is defined as "pain that is maintained by sympathetic efferent innervation or by circulating catecholamines" (International Association 1994). Sympathetic blockade removes the pain, which is the defining characteristic. There may be a component of CRPS and other pain syndromes, but that is not essential.
- The *placebo effect* is a combination of expectation and neurochemical and conditioned responses that transforms an anticipated effect into a real effect. The placebo effect can positively or negatively affect pain, swelling, the patient's mental state, and the side effects of treatment.

Pain and the Placebo Effect

The placebo effect and true effects are *not* independent, consistent within an individual, or related to personality. Prior conditioning, active versus inactive placebo, and expectation can all vary the placebo response within and among individuals. Unfortunately, the placebo effect is often tested in a patient who has pain by surreptitious substitution of saline for a strong analgesic. The intention is to test whether the patient's pain is "real" by deceiving him or her. This is not helpful, and it usually destroys the doctor-patient relationship by establishing the physician as an agent of deception. A positive placebo response (i.e., analgesia with saline) does not prove that the pain is bogus, that the person is an addict or a malingerer, or that the patient would not benefit from an active medication. A significant percentage of healthy individuals have a positive placebo response because everyone is subject to conditioning and expectation. The more effective the previous medication, the more effective a subsequent placebo is likely to be; this is an expected, typical conditioned response. Placebo trials should be performed only with the cooperation of informed patients (Wall 1992). In fact, in 2000, the World Medical Association declared that the use of placebo medications in nearly all clinical trials is unethical when a treatment exists for the disease being studied (*Psychiatric News* 2000).

Measurement of Pain

In the end, the only tool to assess the patient's pain is often the patient's own report of the pain. The visual analogue scale (VAS) is the commonly used scale (Figure 43–1). Patients mark a spot on the line to rate the degree of their pain, or, on a numbered VAS, rate their pain on a scale of 0 to 10, with 0 being no pain and 10 being "extreme pain" or "the worst pain you've ever experienced." A commonly used measurement of significant pain reduction in research studies is a 50% reduction in a patient's report of pain on the VAS.

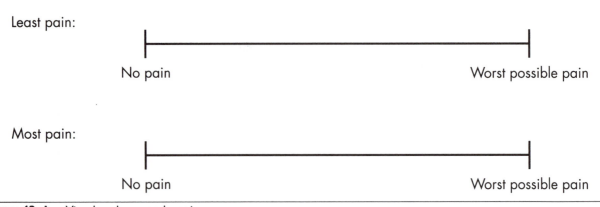

Name:

Please mark the line below with a cross to give a measure of your pain when it was least severe, and when it was most severe, over the past month.

Least pain:

No pain   Worst possible pain

Most pain:

No pain   Worst possible pain

FIGURE 43–1.   Visual analogue scale: pain.

THE USE OF OPIOIDS IN PAIN MANAGEMENT

Prior to a detailed examination of the use of opioids and other analgesics in the management of acute, malignant (continuous), and chronic nonmalignant pain, a basic discussion of terminology, pharmacology, equivalence, and common problems and solutions is necessary. *Opiates* are strictly defined as medications derived from opium (e.g., morphine, codeine). *Opioid* is a more inclusive term denoting both natural and synthetic drugs that mediate pharmacological effects similar to morphine (e.g., fentanyl, meperidine). *Narcotic* originated as a legal term that encompassed many psychoactive drugs, including marijuana and cocaine. The term was defined in *Dorland's Illustrated Medical Dictionary* (1985) as "pertaining to or producing narcosis or an agent that produces insensibility or stupor" (p. 868). In a later edition, that definition was modified to include "applied especially to the opioids, i.e., to any natural or synthetic drug that has morphine-like actions" (*Dorland's Illustrated Medical Dictionary* 2000). The term *narcotic* is now often used interchangeably with the term *opioid*.

The consultation-liaison psychiatrist should be familiar with commonly used opioid medications and their half-lives, bioavailability by route of administration, and common side effects. Opioids are available in oral, rectal, intravenous, intramuscular, intrathecal, and even transmucosal and nasal preparations (Table 43–4).

When a pure opioid agonist is prescribed, there is no set maximum dose. Dosing limitations are based on opioid side effects; during acute administration of opioids, respiratory depression, sedation, and delirium are the more common limiting side effects. With chronic opioid use, constipation is a universal phenomenon. Table 43–5 lists common narcotic-related problems and possible solutions.

Opioid medications follow first-order kinetics, are conjugated by the liver, and are excreted by the kidneys. They reach their peak plasma concentration approximately 60–90 minutes after oral or rectal dosing and 30 minutes after subcutaneous injection. Peak plasma concentration occurs approximately 6 minutes after intravenous injection. The half-life of each opioid depends on its rate of renal clearance. Opioid agonist-antagonists have a ceiling effect that limits their usefulness (Emanuel et al. 1999). Opioid medications are used differently in the management of acute pain, cancer pain, and nonmalignant pain.

ACUTE PAIN MANAGEMENT

An internist or surgeon typically manages acute pain in the general hospital. Objective signs, such as elevated pulse or blood pressure, diaphoresis, and dilated pupils are often present. However, the absence of these signs does not exclude the presence of pain. Treatment of acute pain usually follows a hierarchy with opioid analgesics at the apex (Table 43–6). Psychiatry is generally consulted only when behavioral problems arise.

TABLE 43–4. Comparison of opiate potency and dosage

Drug (trade name)	Equal analgesic dose (mg/IM)	Oral equivalent dose (mg)	Duration of analgesia (hrs)
Opioid agonists			
Morphine	10	30–60	4–5
Codeine	120	200	4–6
Heroin	4	60	3–5
Hydromorphone (Dilaudid)	1.5	7.5	4–5
Levorphanol (Levo-Dromoran)	2	4	4–5
Meperidine (Demerol)	75–100	300	2–5
Methadone (Dolophine)	10	20	3–8
Morphine sustained release (MS-Contin)	—	[a]	8–12
Opioid agonists-antagonists[b]			
Butorphanol (Stadol)	2	—	2.5–3.5
Nalbuphine (Nubain)	12	—	4–6
Pentazocine (Talwin)	60	180	2–3

[a]Take total morphine use for 24 hours, then divide this by 2 or 3 and give that number of milligrams of MS-Contin two or three times daily, respectively.
[b]May precipitate withdrawal symptoms if patient has used pure opioid agonists extensively. Abuse possible, but the potential for it is less.
Source. Modified from Bouckoms 1988; Cassem 1989; Jaffe and Martin 1990.

TABLE 43–5.   Common narcotics-related problems and their solutions

Problem	Effects of problem	Solutions
As-needed (prn) dosing	Steep dose-response curve makes pain relief erratic (e.g., if one dose is missed, it can take 24 hours to return to therapeutic analgesia).	Avoid prn dosing.
Large individual variations in kinetics: Variation in release 5× variation in absorption 8× variation in volume of distribution 8× variation in elimination half-life	Failure to reach steady state.	Sample solutions: MS Contin does not release morphine evenly, so 12-hour dosing intervals will have more peaks and troughs than oral morphine given every 4 hours; hence, supplemental oral morphine doses should be given until steady state is reached. Do not break, chew, or crush MS Contin tablets because release becomes more erratic if tablets are not ingested intact.
Underdosing	Ignorance and fear cause underdosing; safe administration of 450 mg/hour of iv morphine and 800 mg/day of oral morphine have been reported.	Dose adequately; avoid the three most common errors of underdosing when 1) switching from parenteral to oral forms of a narcotic, 2) beginning MS Contin, or 3) beginning fentanyl patches.
Active metabolites	Morphine-6-glucuronide (M6G), the most potent analgesic morphine sulfate metabolite, has a duration of action of 38–103 hours; M6G:MS ratio is 2:1 following a single dose of morphine and up to 20:1 during chronic use; the ratio reaches 45:1 during intrathecal administration.	Prescribe doses according to individual response. M6G levels may be more important in the spinal cord than in the brain. Measure M6G if possible.
Toxicity	Confusion, disorientation, hypomania, paranoia, hallucinations, seizures, muscle twitches, and agitation can occur with narcotics, especially meperidine, even at normal doses; normeperidine toxicity should be expected when meperidine is given intravenously, when renal function is impaired, or when dosage exceeds 300 mg/day for more than 4 days.[a,b] Hydromorphone can produce myoclonus, even when other evidence of toxicity, such as sedation, is not evident. When GFR is poor and hydromorphone doses are high, toxicity may occur, even when equivalent doses of morphine were previously used without signs of toxicity.[c] Methadone doses necessary for analgesia on day 2 can accumulate and cause significant respiratory depression by day 5.	Morphine does not often cause toxicity; hence, it is the analgesic of choice for severe pain.
Errors in conversion from one route of administration to another (e.g., im to oral)	Lack of pain relief when switching from parenteral to oral (e.g., failure to triple the dose of morphine when switching from im to oral).	Transdermal fentanyl takes 24 hours to reach steady state; hence, augmentation with narcotics is necessary during the first 24 hours. Because methadone's analgesic half-life is 6 hours, methadone for analgesic effect is given more frequently than when used to treat drug addiction.
Renal impairment	Decreased renal clearance that occurs with aging may increase narcotics level 2–3 times in a 70-year-old compared with a 20-year-old patient.	Decrease dose of narcotic in elderly patients. Morphine, despite increased levels of morphine sulfate and its metabolites in elderly patients, is generally well tolerated. Hydromorphone and metabolites accumulate less than morphine in patients with decreased GFR.
Opiate-insensitive pain	Neuropathic pain, especially with low doses of narcotics, does not respond.	Perform single-blind test giving morphine, 10 mg iv bolus; positive result is relief of ongoing pain or > 3 cm decrease on VAS; if no result, give morphine, 20 mg iv bolus; if no result, give naloxone, 0.4 mg iv bolus, to confirm lack of opiate effect.
Delivery of drug is not consistent or adequate	Erratic clinical response.	Consider alternative methods of delivery: iv, intrathecal, epidural, ventricular, or transdermal.[d]
Tolerance or excessive sedation	Efficacy decreases or side effects make narcotic intolerable.	Narcotic adjuvants (e.g., methylphenidate or antidepressants).[e,f]

Note.   CNS = central nervous system; GFR = glomerular filtration rate; im = intramuscular; iv = intravenous; VAS = visual analogue scale.
Source.   [a]Bruera et al. 1992; [b]Jellema 1987; [c]Babul and Darke 1992; [d]Portenoy et al. 1990; [e]Bouckoms 1981; [f]Bruera et al. 1989b.

TABLE 43–6. Medications used in treatment of acute pain (World Health Organization analgesic ladder)

Mild pain	Aspirin, acetaminophen, NSAIDs, COX-2 agents, ± adjuvants[a]
Moderate pain	Codeine, hydrocodone, oxycodone, dihydrocodeine, tramadol, ± adjuvants[a]
Severe pain	Morphine or equivalent ± nonopioid analgesics ± adjuvants[a]

Note. NSAIDs = nonsteroidal anti-inflammatory drugs.
[a]Adjuvants are medications used concurrently with another medication to enhance analgesia or to counteract side effects of opioid medications.
Source. Reprinted from World Health Organization: Cancer Pain Relief: Palliative Care: Report of a WHO Expert Committee. (Technical Report 804.) Geneva, World Health Organization, 1990.

Opioid Analgesics in Acute Pain Management

In general, the earlier acute pain is treated, the better. Current theories of CNS neuroplasticity argue for aggressive and early treatment of acute pain symptoms. In fact, preemptive analgesia is being studied in surgical settings. This form of analgesia involves administering analgesic medication, such as nonsteroidal anti-inflammatory drugs (NSAIDs), opioids, or local anesthetics, in anticipation of pain. Intriguing protocols have been tried, including preincisional administration of analgesics (Woolf 1993). Patients premedicated with opioids appear to require less postoperative analgesia and may have better long-term outcomes.

The following principles apply to the use of opioid medications in the management of acute severe and unremitting pain:

1. Regularly scheduled opioid medication helps prevent reemergence of pain. Opioid medications should not be prescribed on an as-needed basis. Such dosing requires the patient to ask for more medication. Some patients don't want to bother busy staff, fear addiction, don't want to be seen as drug seeking, or try to tough it out. Alternatively, patients may be afraid that pain indicates disease progression and become very anxious or may try to deny the pain. Alternatively, a busy staff may label a patient's repeated requests for medication as drug-seeking behavior. "That patient is on the buzzer constantly!" is a common refrain. A patient who receives as-needed meperidine may need to call for a dose every 3–4 hours, which equals eight calls to an overworked nursing staff during a 24-hour period. Although as-needed dosing may make some sense to a staff who fears the patient will become addicted, the end result is usually a staff that resents the additional work.

2. Prevention of pain (versus treatment of emergent pain) usually leads to *lower* total doses of medication (Reuler et al. 1980).
3. Cognitively limited patients, such as the frail elderly with delirium or dementia, or the very young, often have difficulty requesting as-needed pain medications.
4. A trial of opioid medications should not be undertaken in place of an appropriate and full assessment of the patient's pain symptoms.
5. In general, patient preferences about route of administration and medication options should be considered.

For a patient who is cognitively intact, the treatment of choice for severe pain is often patient-controlled analgesia (PCA). Patients are given a base rate of opioid use with a set dose and interval. The patient self-administers medication by pressing a button. The patient is "locked out" if the button is pressed outside these parameters. If the patient is sedated and falls asleep, less medication is obviously needed. The family should be instructed not to push the button for the patient. The PCA computer tracks how often the patient self-administers medication, how often the patient requests medication, and the total dosage administered. With PCA, patients tend to use smaller doses of opioids, experience fewer side effects, and have less sedation (Graves 1983). Additionally, the computer provides the treatment team with important feedback that helps guide dose and interval changes (e.g., whether the patient has seldom used the PCA or has continuously pressed the button).

Psychiatric Consultation in Acute Pain Management

In acute pain management, psychiatric consultation is typically requested when a patient is not responding to usual doses of pain medications, has a history of substance abuse, or is considered to be a behavioral problem (e.g., is drug seeking or belligerent). This section addresses common clinical questions and dilemmas presented to the consultation-liaison psychiatrist.

"The patient is not responding to pain medication."

When assessing a patient who is not responding as expected to a pain medicine regimen, the physician should first look at the current opioid dose and interval compared with the medication's expected effective half-life. Inadequate pain management commonly results from underestimating the dose (Sriwatanakul et al. 1983), use of as-needed dosing, or a dosing interval longer than the medication's effective half-life. The usual dose of an opioid is an estimation; effectiveness varies and is related to an individual's tolerance, metabolism, distribution, and pain threshold. Although a good starting point, usual opioid doses are often inadequate.

An unexpected response to medication can also occur when a patient who is already receiving a pure opioid agonist (e.g., morphine, oxycodone) is given a mixed opioid agonist-antagonist (e.g., nalbuphine, pentazocine). This combination may inadequately treat pain that was previously well controlled and may even precipitate a withdrawal syndrome (Emanuel et al. 1999).

Finally, an unanticipated exacerbation of pain can occur when a patient is changed from a parenteral form of medication to the oral dose. A careful review of the patient's medication history, including a comparison of oral and parenteral medication equivalence and duration of action (see Table 43–4), is essential to understanding and correcting the situation. An initial overlap of the oral with the parenteral medication is usually necessary.

"The patient is drug seeking."

Patients in acute pain who are labeled drug seeking because of repeated requests for opioid medications are rarely dependent or addicted. Undertreatment is far more common in such patients (Melzack 1990); this behavior has been called pseudoaddiction. The patient appears to be drug seeking and, in fact, is drug seeking. However, the medication is sought to relieve pain rather than craved or sought for its euphoric effect (Table 43–7). In some cases, patients do use opioids unknowingly, to help control anxiety or fear. At other times, nurses may give opioids for those purposes as well, because an as-needed prescription for narcotics is ordered for the patient and therefore convenient to use. In such cases, identifying symptoms that respond to a nonopioid medication (i.e.,

a benzodiazepine for anxiety) often allows a lower dose of an opioid to be a more effective analgesic.

"The patient has a history of substance abuse and has acute pain."

The treatment of acute pain in a patient who has a history of substance abuse seems complicated. The situation commonly occurs postoperatively or following trauma. In general, patients with a history of substance abuse are at risk of becoming addicted to opioid medication. Those most at risk have a history of opioid misuse or abuse. For that reason, it is prudent to monitor these patients' opioid usage carefully; however, appropriate pain management and opioid medication should not be withheld.

In the case of the patient who has both active opioid addiction and acute pain at the time of admission, the opioid addiction and acute pain should be treated separately. Patients with active opioid addiction have increased tolerance and report less analgesia from opioids. They typically require higher than usual doses, up to 50% higher, even with concurrent methadone treatment. (At higher doses, patients should be observed for respiratory depression.) If a patient has a recent history of opioid dependence but is not actively using at the time of admission, that patient may also have residual tolerance to the analgesic effects of usual doses of pain medication. Long-term treatment for the opioid addiction is best arranged as part of discharge planning.

Although opiate withdrawal is not life threatening, it is very uncomfortable, can amplify pain symptoms, and should be avoided. The psychiatrist should monitor the patient for objective symptoms of opioid withdrawal (i.e., tachycardia, hypertension, dilated pupils, gooseflesh, rhinorrhea, and lacrimation) and treat these symptoms promptly. Two medications are appropriately used to prevent and treat opioid withdrawal: clonidine and methadone.

TABLE 43–7.   Differential diagnosis of drug-seeking behavior

Differential	Hallmark	Effect on functioning
Physical dependence	Expected in patients chronically treated with opioid medications. Discontinuation of medication leads to withdrawal syndrome or symptoms: increased pain, rhinorrhea, lacrimation, increased pulse.	Dependency does not in and of itself interfere with patient functioning.
Addiction	A behavioral pattern of compulsive preoccupation with opioid; escalating dose. Although physical dependence may be present, it is not essential.	Functioning decreases; continued use despite negative consequences.
Pseudoaddiction	Patient appears preoccupied with medications; may be demanding; underlying problem is untreated pain.	Functioning improves with increased opioid dosing.

Although clonidine controls many of the objective symptoms of opioid withdrawal, it is much less effective in controlling the associated cravings and has no cross-reactivity with opiate receptors. The typical starting dose is 0.1 mg, with increases as needed to doses of 0.3 mg three times daily (Arana and Rosenbaum 2000). Methadone, by contrast, is a long-acting opiate agonist that more successfully treats the subjective symptoms, particularly the drug craving. It has good analgesic effect but little associated euphoria. Unless the patient has an established dose because of recent treatment with methadone, the dose is best determined by monitoring objective criteria of opioid withdrawal. A general guideline is to begin with a dose of 10 mg and repeat this dose every 4 hours if two objective signs of withdrawal emerge (Arana and Rosenbaum 2000).

Fear and Acute Pain

Uncontrolled anxiety, fear, or terror greatly amplifies pain and leads to escalating requests for analgesic medication. Although benzodiazepines can help the anxious patient, a patient who is "scared to death" will usually respond to a short course of neuroleptic medication. Small doses of a sedating neuroleptic, such as perphenazine, 2 mg three or four times daily, or risperidone, 0.5 mg three or four times daily, are usually quite effective and break the pain-fear cycle. If parenteral dosing is needed, intravenous haloperidol, 0.5–1 mg two to four times daily, is a good choice.

CHRONIC (CONTINUOUS) MALIGNANT PAIN MANAGEMENT

Chronic pain, sometimes also called continuous pain, is generally divided into malignant and nonmalignant categories. The treatment of chronic cancer-related pain and pain in the terminally ill follows many of the same rules as the treatment of acute pain. The goal of treatment is comfort and relief of pain. Physiological dependence on opioids is expected and occurs within 3–4 weeks. After this time, the patient is at risk of withdrawal if opioids are abruptly discontinued. Tolerance to the analgesic effects of the medication can occur. However, in cases of cancer, an increase in pain on a stable dose of medication often indicates disease progression and should be investigated. Tolerance develops to some side effects of opioids but not to the constipation and miosis, which occur nearly universally in patients receiving treatment on a regular basis. Side effects such as sedation and constipa-

tion should be treated aggressively. Associated depressive and anxiety symptoms should also be treated promptly. See Chapter 29, this volume, for a full discussion of psychiatric issues in oncology patients.

CHRONIC NONMALIGNANT PAIN MANAGEMENT

Epidemiology

Chronic pain is common and costly. Pain can exhaust the chronic sufferer, impair the immune system, promote tumor growth, impair respiratory function and mobility, and encourage drug and alcohol overuse (Liebeskind 1991). Back and muscle pain, head and face pain, posttraumatic pain, and secondary psychiatric problems account for the bulk of pain-related cost and disability. Chronic nonmalignant pain costs the U.S. economy $40 billion a year (Sheehan et al. 1996).

A definitive physical diagnosis is reached in only 5%–10% of individuals with low back pain, the most common reason for disability (Osterweis et al. 1987). A population survey (Taylor and Curran 1985) showed that 9% of the population had back or joint pain for more than 100 days during the preceding 5 months. Muscle pain from fibromyalgia afflicts as many as 6 million people in the United States and accounts for 5% of people coming to a general medical clinic. Headache is a problem for 73% of the general population, with 7% reporting more than 100 days with a headache per year (Taylor and Curran 1985). The estimated annual cost in lost productivity in the United States because of migraine headaches is $5.6 to $17.2 billion (Osterhaus et al. 1992).

Mechanism

The exact ways in which chronic nonmalignant pain continues are not well understood. The phenomena are complex and involve neuroplasticity. Pain is a perception of the CNS, and nociceptive input is only one factor in pain threshold, intensity, quality, time course, and location. Although a relationship exists between nociception and perception, it is not direct or linear (Wall 1988). One explanation for neuroplasticity is that acute pain from nerve trauma results in a rewiring of cortical and subcortical neurons. Within days of the injury, disconnected nerve cells receive input from other parts of the body. For example, cells previously responsive to the pinprick of a finger may now respond to light touch of a hair on the forehead. Consequently, touching a hair may trigger a burst of pain at a site distant from the injury (allodynia and allesthesia). Prevention of chronic pain caused by neuroplasticity includes early aggressive treatment of acute pain. A major goal for research is to better understand the pathophysiology of neuroplasticity in order to prevent the transition from acute to chronic pain (Baringa 1992; Coderre et al. 1993).

Traumatic injury well illustrates three puzzling facts about pain: 1) up to 40% of injured patients admitted to hospitals initially have no pain complaints; 2) 90% of patients with brachial plexus root avulsions have pain, even though afferent pain fibers are absent; and 3) hyperalgesia at the site of injury is associated with an increased flexion withdrawal reflex, even after a local anesthetic is used to numb the site of tissue injury. Apparently, posttraumatic pain is associated with excitability in the spinal cord even without afferent input (Sweet 1984; Tverskoy et al. 1990).

Psychiatric Comorbidity

The cause-and-effect relationship between comorbid physical pain and psychiatric disorders is often unresolvable. The psychiatric morbidity associated with chronic pain is often a consequence of rather than an antecedent to pain. Chronic pain can precipitate psychiatric conditions (most commonly depression). In addition, depression, anxiety, fatigue, and worry amplify pain symptoms and decrease pain tolerance.

When psychiatry is consulted regarding a patient who has a pain syndrome, the patient usually has chronic pain. Keep in mind that chronic pain is not a diagnosis; it subsumes a variety of divergent conditions. It includes pain persisting longer than expected for a particular condition and pain that is intermittent but persists for months or years (Bonica 1990). Somewhat more simplistically, chronic pain is usually defined by its temporal course (i.e., pain persists beyond 3–6 months).

In chronic pain syndromes, acute signs of distress (e.g., elevated pulse or blood pressure) have long since resolved. In addition, the patient typically has a complex medication regimen. Clinicians often raise questions about the patient's misuse of medication, or, less frequently, the patient may raise questions about addiction. A significant number of patients with chronic pain have comorbid psychiatric symptoms or disorders. Insomnia, depression, anxiety, or posttraumatic stress disorder symptoms can amplify pain symptoms, decrease a patient's pain tolerance, and thwart the effects of analgesic medications. The consultation-liaison psychiatrist must, therefore, ensure the thorough assessment and appropriate treatment of psychiatric disorders in patients with pain syndromes.

PSYCHIATRIC EXAMINATION AND DIFFERENTIAL DIAGNOSIS IN PATIENTS WHO HAVE CHRONIC PAIN

The role of the consultation-liaison psychiatrist is to ensure that both physical and psychiatric aspects of pain are appropriately evaluated and treated. Unfortunately, when the consultation-liaison psychiatrist introduces himself or herself to the patient who has chronic pain, the patient's interpretation is, "My doctors must believe that the pain is all in my head." Even if the psychiatrist and patient agree that a comorbid psychiatric disorder exists (i.e., the pain is real and a complicating psychiatric diagnosis exists), many others—insurance companies, managed care organizations, disability providers, legal and social agencies, and some physicians—may not. For these reasons, diagnostic precision is particularly important because of its long-term implications.

The evaluation of patients who have chronic pain requires an expanded focus (Table 43–8). Although assessment for psychiatric comorbidity is essential, the psychiatrist must also assess the patient for pain conditions that might respond to treatment with psychiatric medications. The pain team may have specific questions for the psychiatrist (e.g., whether the patient is appropriate for treatment with chronic opioids or whether the psychiatrist can help in managing a particularly difficult patient or pain syndrome).

Although assessment is individualized, it is helpful to begin by reviewing the patient's pain symptoms. This allows the psychiatrist to assess pain symptoms typically responsive to psychotropic medications and personality style (e.g., dramatic, emotionless). Focusing initially on the complaint also helps put at ease the patient who is concerned about being rejected as "crazy" or "just depressed."

The onset, duration, and nature of the pain as well as factors that cause exacerbations or improvements should be reviewed. During the early part of the interview, it often helps if the psychiatrist educates and reassures the patient about psychiatric symptoms. The psychiatrist should explain the importance of treating both pain and associated psychiatric symptoms. This approach often increases the physician's alliance with a reticent patient. Early on, pain symptoms are usually associated with anxiety (e.g., fear that something bad will happen, anticipation about what to expect). Later, symptoms of demoralization and depression are more common in chronic pain (e.g., something bad has happened; the patient knows

TABLE 43–8. Components of psychiatric evaluation in patients who have chronic pain

Determine reason for referral and patient's understanding of referral

Obtain history of pain onset, course, and factors that improve pain or worsen pain

Educate patient; assess for normalization around comorbidity of pain and psychiatric symptoms, especially depression and anxiety

Obtain history of prepain psychiatric symptoms and disorders and of current psychiatric symptoms

Determine current medications, including usual dose, maximum dose ("on a really bad day of pain how many pills would you need/take?"), effectiveness, and side effects

Assess for medication-induced psychiatric side effects

Assess for interactions or potential interactions between psychiatric and pain medications

Determine current functional level (i.e., social, occupational, and financial) and previous functional level

Ask about current and past substance use or abuse

Ask about support system

Obtain psychiatric history and history of trauma (including sexual abuse history)

Obtain medical history, including past response to analgesic medications and procedures

more or less what to expect, and it's not good). The normalization of mood or anxiety symptoms may allow the patient to reveal information otherwise kept secret. Given this opening, many patients describe feelings of depression, despair, demoralization, and hopelessness, which then can be explored further.

The psychiatrist should pay particular attention to the patient's current and past medication usage. An integrative approach is essential in this area. Many patients who have chronic pain are prescribed opioid medications, and some of these patients will contact more than one physician for opioid prescriptions. Even though the psychiatrist is not usually the prescribing physician, he or she must review the patient's opioid use. The patient should be asked, "How many tablets do you need to take on a really bad pain day?" Attention should be paid to whether the opioid medications have short- or long-acting half-lives and how they are used. In general, short-acting opioids are best used for breakthrough pain, whereas longer-acting opioids are used for chronic, enduring pain.

POTENTIAL PROBLEMS WITH PAIN MEDICATIONS

The psychiatrist should carefully assess the patient for psychiatric complications of pain and review analgesic medications with particular attention to drug interactions and other potential medication problems (Table 43–9). For example, agonist-antagonist opioids can precipitate withdrawal when administered to a patient already receiving a pure opioid agonist, and toxic metabolites can build up with propoxyphene (Emanuel et al. 1999). Meperidine is well known for its potentially toxic active metabolite, normeperidine, which has a long half-life and can cause CNS toxicity, including seizures. Risk is increased with a dose of 300 mg/day given for 4 days. One study reported side effects in 38% of patients who were given meperidine (Demerol) parentally. Risk of toxicity is also increased if renal dysfunction is present (Shochet and Murray 1988). The psychiatrist should be vigilant about these issues.

The psychiatrist should examine the patient closely for psychiatric disorders. Psychiatric disorders increase the perception of pain and the patient's suffering. Table 43–10 lists the most common psychiatric disorders and their relationships with pain. These are discussed in more detail in the sections that follow.

TABLE 43–9. Significant analgesic and psychiatric medication interactions

Analgesic	Psychiatric medication	Possible consequence
Meperidine	MAOI	Serotonin syndrome (hypertensive crisis)
NSAID, including COX-2 inhibitors	Lithium	Lithium toxicity
Tramadol	TCA	Seizure
	SSRI	Serotonin syndrome
	Opioid	
	Neuroleptic	
TCA	SSRI	Serotonin syndrome
		TCA toxicity possible if SSRI inhibits TCA's metabolism
Codeine	Fluoxetine, paroxetine	Possible decrease in analgesia for codeine, hydrocodone (Hycodan), and oxycodone (Percodan) through inhibition of CYP450 2D6

Note. MAOI = monoamine oxidase inhibitor; NSAID = nonsteroidal anti-inflammatory drug; SSRI = selective serotonin reuptake inhibitor; TCA = tricyclic antidepressant.

TABLE 43–10.   Fifteen psychiatric conditions that can coexist with, cause, or exacerbate pain

Key diagnostic features	Psychiatric diagnosis in patient with pain
Depression	Anhedonia, sadness, and early morning awakening
Anxiety disorders	Panic or generalized anxiety not fully relieved by analgesics
Somatoform disorders (six disorders—see Table 43–11)	Physical complaints unexplained by physical diagnoses that are associated with psychological factors
Factitious disorder with physical symptoms	Deception of the physician in order to maintain a sick role
Malingering	Withholds information deliberately
	Antisocial
	Somatic findings are changeable
	Treatment compliance is erratic
	External gains
Dissociative states	Amnesia (partial), anxiety, nightmares, flashbacks, conflicted avoidance of close relationships
Sexual pain disorders	Dyspareunia or vaginismus
Psychosis	Bizarre, illogical thought; disordered attributions of cause and effect
Personality disorders	Diminished ability to cope with pain
Chronic pain syndrome	Physical disability is emphasized while the importance of interpersonal factors in the suffering is both demonstrated and denied

Depression

Major depression commonly occurs in patients who have chronic pain. Geisser et al. (1997) found that one-third (33%) of chronic pain patients met DSM-IV (American Psychiatric Association 1994) criteria for major depression. This is an important finding because depression magnifies pain, it can decrease a patient's compliance with prescribed treatments, and it increases the likelihood that a patient will misuse pain medications. Denial, masking of depressive symptoms with narcotics or benzodiazepines, and other comorbid psychiatric diagnoses can obscure depression in patients who have chronic pain (Bouckoms et al. 1985; Holmes et al. 1986).

Neurovegetative symptoms are often difficult to assess in patients who have chronic pain; a patient with pain is likely to sleep poorly and feel lethargic during the day. Psychological symptoms can help differentiate a depression from physical symptoms related to pain (Cavanaugh 1995). The presence of depressed mood, irritability, mood reactivity, crying spells, and anhedonia often helps make the diagnosis. Even though depression is an understandable and common response to chronic pain, it should be treated aggressively. Also, patients with subthreshold mood disorders should receive treatment to maximize their comfort and the control of pain.

When selecting an antidepressant for a patient who has chronic pain, the psychiatrist should apply the usual considerations (i.e., prior response to medications, family members' response to medications, associated psychiatric symptoms, and a medication's side-effect profile). In addition, the psychiatrist should keep in mind that tricyclic antidepressants (TCAs) are effective in treating a variety of chronic pain syndromes, independent of depressive or other psychiatric symptoms. The use of TCAs is discussed in more detail in the pharmacotherapy section of this chapter.

Anxiety Disorders

Anxiety symptoms sufficient to meet DSM-IV-TR criteria (American Psychiatric Association 2000) for an anxiety disorder (usually generalized anxiety or panic disorder) occur in approximately 30% of patients who have intractable pain. More than half of patients with anxiety disorders have other psychiatric disorders; major depression and substance abuse or dependence are the psychiatric disorders most commonly associated with anxiety (Bouckoms and Hackett 1991). Treatment of comorbid conditions often reduces anxiety and pain complaints. A combination of clonazepam and a TCA are particularly helpful for the patient with pain who has anxiety. These medications decrease panic, anxiety, and depression as well as neuropathic and muscle pain.

Somatoform Disorders

In somatoform disorders, physical symptoms are a manifestation of psychopathology (Table 43–11). Somatization disorder is the flagship somatoform disorder, derived historically from Briquet's syndrome; the diagnostic criteria are quite specific and reliably predict an individual's future illness behavior. Unfortunately, most people with physical complaints and no physical findings do not fit

TABLE 43–11. Diagnostic features of somatoform disorders

Somatoform disorders	Key diagnostic features
Somatization disorder	Years of physical complaints, beginning before age 30; complaints lead to treatment or impairment in function. The patient must have had four pain symptoms, two gastrointestinal symptoms, one sexual symptom, and one pseudoneurological symptom other than pain.
Conversion disorder	Motor or sensory symptoms, other than just pain or sexual symptoms, that cannot be explained medically or culturally but are associated with psychological factors.
Hypochondriasis	Persistent preoccupation for at least 6 months with fear or the idea of illness, despite negative test results and reassurance.
Pain disorder	Pain is the predominant focus, causes distress or impairment, and is related to psychological factors.
Undifferentiated somatoform disorder	One or more physical complaints that either cannot be explained medically or are in gross excess of what is expected and cause distress or impairment for at least 6 months.
Somatoform disorder, not otherwise specified	Somatoform symptoms that do not meet somatoform disorder criteria (e.g., brief symptoms of fatigue or hypochondriasis).

into this neatly defined diagnosis. The other somatoform disorders have less stringent criteria; therefore, clinicians should have a great deal of knowledge about the psychology of illness and must exercise good judgment. The diagnosis of a somatoform disorder in a patient who has chronic pain is confounded by five problems:

1. Central pain can mimic a somatoform disorder.
2. Symptoms from an unrecognized medical condition can lead the clinician to diagnose the pain as psychiatric in origin.
3. Judging whether pain is excessive for a particular individual or medical condition is almost always an impossible task.
4. Pain can decrease when psychotropic drugs or psychological techniques are used. Such a decrease does not prove that a psychiatric diagnosis is present.
5. Deciding which came first, the psychopathology or the pain, is often impossible in a patient who has chronic pain.

Patients with somatoform disorders exhibit exaggerated physical complaints, irrational fears, and anxiety about physical illness. In a study of 210 patients with chronic pain who were involved in litigation, Weintraub (1992) found that 63% had so-called psychogenic symptoms, meaning nonanatomical or nonphysiological sensory and motor examination findings—that is, somatoform findings. Weintraub stated that strict reliance on subjective complaints of pain is often misleading and is potentially harmful. Unfortunately, objective findings do not always reflect pain-producing pathology either. For example, 20%–30% of patients who have myelograms for

reasons other than pain have disk bulges (Deyo et al. 1992). Even though 20%–80% of all pain complaints to physicians do not have well-defined etiologies, these complaints do not always warrant a somatoform or psychiatric diagnosis. For example, patients with pain have about the same prevalence of psychiatric diagnoses as other medically ill patient populations (Bouckoms 1989). However, somatizing patients may account for as many as 36% of individuals with psychiatric disability and 48% of individuals on sick leave (Sigvardsson and von Knorring 1984). Prevalence studies of somatoform disorders report a rate of 5%–15% among patients receiving treatment for chronic pain (Bouckoms and Hackett 1991). Comorbidity and variation within population samples make these studies of somatoform disorders in patients with chronic pain problematic.

Four pragmatic tactics can improve the clinician's diagnostic accuracy. First, the clinician should perform a physical examination. The physical examination often unmasks illness behavior and helps decrease the patient's antipsychiatry bias. It also allows a neurological examination for central pain and myofascial pain. Second, the clinician should search for positive criteria for a psychiatric illness so that a somatoform disorder is not diagnosed by default. Third, if a somatoform diagnosis is present, the clinician should look for additional Axis I disorders using DSM-IV-TR criteria. The two conditions most commonly comorbid with somatoform disorders are major depression and an anxiety disorder; the odds are 3:1 that the patient also has depression and are similarly high for an anxiety disorder. Fourth, the clinician should perform objective tests to reduce reliance on subjective impressions. For example, he or she could use computerized motion analysis to reliably and reproducibly compare degrees of flexion, extension, and torque with national normative statistics.

Conversion Disorder

The diagnosis of conversion disorder requires one or more symptoms, or deficits affecting voluntary motor or sensory function, that suggest a neurological or medical condition. The symptoms must cause significant distress or must impair function. If pain or sexual dysfunction is the only complaint, a diagnosis of conversion disorder is not made; the correct diagnosis in these cases is pain disorder or sexual pain disorder, respectively. If the symptom is initiated, exacerbated, or preceded by conflicts or other stressors, psychological factors are judged to be associated with the symptom. The diagnosis also requires that the symptom cannot be fully explained by a neurological or medical condition. From a study of patients seen in a pain clinic, Weintraub (1988) observed that the triad of pain, numbness, and weakness represents a common conversion syndrome. The presence of primary gain increases diagnostic certainty, whereas *la belle indifférence* and histrionic personality traits do not. Although not diagnostic, a conversion V on the Minnesota Multiphasic Personality Inventory (MMPI) denotes hypochondriacal traits and a relative absence of depression. This pattern is consistent with conversion disorder. Electromyograms, electroencephalograms, and repeated physical examinations often help to identify the approximately 50% of patients who have a medical disorder but are erroneously diagnosed as hysterical (Reed 1975).

Hypochondriasis

Hypochondriasis is preoccupation with fears of having, or the idea that one has, a serious disease, based on the misinterpretation of bodily symptoms. Head and orofacial pains; cardiac pain; dyspeptic pain; or tingling, burning, or numbing pains are common foci of hypochondriacal concern. "Yes, doctor, but..." is a statement that typifies the defiant and help-rejecting complaints of the hypochondriac. No test, reassurance, discussion, or explanation is enough. The person interprets every physical sensation as evidence of physical illness, is significantly distressed or impaired by the symptoms, yet is not delusional, nor does he or she have an anxiety disorder or major depression. Patients with pain who have hypochondriasis frequently see nonpsychiatrists because these patients firmly believe that the pain is not "in their head." The consultation-liaison psychiatrist must also be on the lookout for patients with pseudohypochondriasis, in which the perception of illness foretells an early cancer, multiple sclerosis, or a central pain syndrome. Transient hypochondriasis some-

times occurs in elderly patients. These hypochondriacal symptoms often persist over a period of at least 2 years, although these individuals are not likely to develop hypochondriasis that satisfies DSM-IV-TR criteria.

Separation of hypochondriasis from psychosis, major depression, somatic symptoms of panic or generalized anxiety disorder, obsessive-compulsive disorder, and somatization disorder is important because the treatments for these disorders are quite different. Severe hypochondriasis can mask psychosis or major depression. Therefore, two important tests for the hypochondriacal patient are a pain drawing (Figure 43–2), which can demonstrate psychotic somatic beliefs, and a review of symptoms for a mood disorder. The consulting psychiatrist must rule out diseases with persistent symptoms, reassure and not reject the patient, label maladaptive dangerous behaviors, and allay the patient's fears by open discussion.

Pain Disorder

Pain disorder is defined in DSM-IV-TR as a syndrome in which pain is the focus of clinical presentation. Physical pathology, if present, does not adequately explain the pain. Psychological factors must play an important role in the onset, severity, exacerbation, or maintenance of the pain.

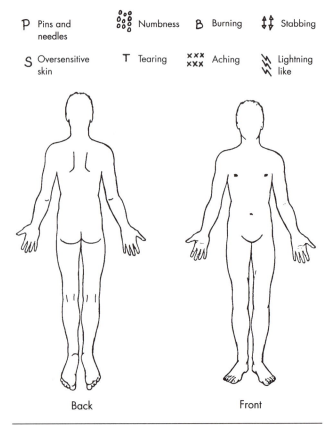

FIGURE 43–2. Pain drawing.

Factitious Disorder With Physical Symptoms

Intentional production or feigning of pain to achieve the sick role is diagnosed as a factitious disorder. Renal colic, orofacial pains, and abdominal pain are three commonly feigned pain complaints. Common stories include multiple, never-seen renal stones; an absent dentist or physician who "usually" treats the toothache or trigeminal neuralgia; or abdominal pain with multiple scars from past surgeries. These individuals are not psychotic, despite the vague, meandering nature of their stories. The onset of factitious disorder is usually in early adulthood, and a lifelong pattern of repeated hospitalizations is typical. Pain is often reported in such elaborate, exaggerated detail that it intrigues the listener (e.g., pseudologia fantastica). Other characteristics are narcotics-seeking behavior, multiple hospitalizations under different names in different cities, nondiagnostic invasive investigations and surgeries, nonexistent family members, and truculence. Assiduous, detailed inquiry into the exact circumstances of previous admissions and discharges will often lead to a sudden demand for discharge from the hospital. (For a detailed discussion of factitious disorders and malingering, see Chapter 25, this volume.)

Malingering

A patient who is malingering intentionally produces false physical or psychological symptoms and is motivated by secondary gain (e.g., avoiding work, obtaining financial compensation, evading criminal prosecution, obtaining drugs). Lack of external gain or evidence of an intrapsychic need to maintain a sick role suggests factitious disorder rather than malingering. A patient who is malingering is unlikely to present with symptoms of an emotional conflict; the last thing such a patient wants is a psychiatric consultation. A clever patient who is malingering can skew MMPI results toward normality, evade accountability (e.g., old medical records are missing or altered), and defeat attempts to uncover data via an interview using intravenous lorazepam or hypnosis. Three examination findings help the clinician to make the diagnosis of malingering in the patient who complains of pain (these are also found in patients who have somatoform disorders): lateral anesthesia to pinprick that ends sharply at the midline; sharp cutoffs for vibratory sensation; and astasia-abasia, with the upper body lurching first.

Dissociative States

According to DSM-IV-TR, dissociation is a disturbance or alteration in the normally integrative functions of iden-tity, memory, or consciousness. A history of childhood abuse is quite common in individuals who develop chronic pain; abused children are prone to dissociative disorders. Pelvic pain, sexual pain disorders, headache, and abdominal pain are the most common pain complaints in developmentally traumatized individuals (Barsky et al. 1994). Walker et al. (1992) noted that in 22 women with chronic pelvic pain, 18 reported childhood abuse. Of the 21 women selected as control subjects (i.e., women who had no pelvic pain), 9 reported childhood abuse ($P < 0.0005$). Dissociation, somatic distress, and general disability were more frequent in the group with pain. Denial is also common in patients with pain, just as amnesia or partial recall is common in patients with dissociative disorders. Disconnection from important events, emotionally or by amnesia, is characteristic of patients with dissociative disorders. Denial makes the diagnosis of dissociative disorders in patients with pain a longitudinal process, because truth is shared slowly with the physician and then only as the patient can tolerate it. Clues to an underlying dissociative disorder are periods of full or partial amnesia, nightmares, flashbacks, or panic anxiety, as well as avoidance of sexual intimacy or a history of conflicted relationships.

Personality Disorders

No single personality type or pathology is uniquely associated with chronic pain. Even in individuals with frequent migraine headaches, who are often fastidious and have obsessive traits, no characterological differences were found between control subjects and patients who had migraines (Kohler and Kosnaic 1992). However, clinicians who work with patients longitudinally might disagree. The patient's attachments to others, such as doctors and family, are problematic. Typically, the psychodynamics are a mixture of regression, ambivalence over care and getting well, shame, and reexperiencing of old conflicts about nurturance. Ambivalence over getting well is manifested by noncompliance, loss of autonomy, and regression to an anxious state of dependency (Genova 1992). Two aspects of adaptive coping are threatened by chronic pain. First, an idealized protective figure (the doctor) becomes ambivalently viewed and is a target for anger when cure does not occur. Second, the patient's sense of self-respect and value, based on the caregiver's behavior, is not validated if care is fragmented and driven by unrealistic expectations. This is exacerbated if peer and family support decreases. The resulting conflicts in the doctor-patient relationship, fragile sense of self, and decreasing psychosocial supports challenge the patient's ability to cope.

Psychosis

Failure to physically examine patients who are psychotic is the reason that acute abdomens, ischemic heart disease, and traumatic injuries are overlooked in these patients. Physical examination may reveal evidence of injury obscured by the psychiatric presentation. Psychosis is easy to recognize when it occurs in the context of active schizophrenic symptoms, a delusional idea of persecution, a depressive illness, substance-induced psychosis, or dementia. However, when pain is the only complaint, denial is prominent, and some physical findings are present, teasing out a psychotic process is not easy. The psychiatrist can ask the patient to draw a picture of the pain in his or her body (see Figure 43–2). This exercise can illustrate a thought disorder that is otherwise obscured by denial and rationalization. The answer to the question "What have you learned from the other doctors?" may also help to uncover a thought disorder.

Chronic pain syndrome is a term sometimes used to describe pain behaviors and interpersonal and affective features that merge into a pattern that emphasizes physical disability, suffering, and the need for attention from others. Treatment typically addresses self-defeating behavioral patterns as well as the affective dysfunction and psychodynamic conflicts inherent in the behavior (Table 43–12).

PHYSICAL EXAMINATION OF THE PATIENT WHO HAS CHRONIC PAIN

Physical examination (Tables 43–13 and 43–14) of patients who have chronic pain or central pain is essential in order to make a correct diagnosis (Deyo et al. 1992). Psychiatrists who believe they should not touch patients during an evaluation cannot properly evaluate pain. The physical examination involves a traditional neurological examination, during which the clinician looks for abnormal pain behavior, inconsistencies, and vague or changeable findings. A physical examination should also include examination for features of central pain (see Table 43–14).

PHARMACOTHERAPY AND ADJUNCTIVE TREATMENTS FOR CHRONIC PAIN

Treatment Planning

An integrative approach to treatment planning is essential. Therefore, the consultation-liaison psychiatrist must communicate directly with the patient and with other treating clinicians. The psychiatrist should focus with the patient on modulating pain and increasing function rather than on a cure. It is beyond the scope of this chapter to review the diverse medications used in chronic pain treatment (e.g., steroids, NSAIDs, dextromethorphan, mexiletine, muscle relaxants, clonidine, calcium-channel blockers, antihistamines, topical medications). The focus in the following sections is on the application of psychotropic medication to pain management. The use of opioids in chronic nonmalignant pain is also discussed.

Antidepressants

TCAs are effective for a range of pain disorders. Classically, they are used as first-line treatments in phantom limb pain, postherpetic neuralgia, and other peripheral neuropathic pain syndromes (Galer 1995). TCAs are also useful in less common syndromes such as ankylosing spondylitis (Koh et al. 1997) and chronic orofacial pain (Pettengill and Reisner-Keller 1997). A review article comparing TCAs to lorazepam, acyclovir, capsaicin, and acupuncture found that only the TCAs had proven benefit for the treatment of postherpetic neuralgia (Volmink 1996).

Results with antidepressants outside the TCA family have been disappointing. Studies of the selective serotonin reuptake inhibitors (SSRIs) fluoxetine (Max 1992), trazodone (Davidoff et al. 1987), paroxetine (Atkinson et al. 1999; Dickens et al. 2000), sertraline (Engel et al. 1998), and citalopram (Bendtsen et al. 1996; Norregaard et al. 1995) have failed to show effectiveness in treating pain syndromes in nondepressed individuals. Clinical studies of venlafaxine, nefazadone, buproprion, and mirtazapine are currently lacking. Therefore, serotonin reuptake blockade does not appear essential for pain relief. There are also doubts about the effectiveness of SSRIs for treatment of neuropathic pain (Gourlay et al. 1986; Max 1992; Watson and Evans 1985).

All effective antidepressants (i.e., amitriptyline, desipramine, nortriptyline, imipramine, maprotiline) in placebo-controlled trials for neuropathic pain are associated with some inhibition of norepinephrine reuptake (Watson et al. 1992). In a depressed or anxious individual who has chronic pain, any antidepressant that successfully treats depression or anxiety may decrease pain; however, only the TCAs provide analgesic effect in nondepressed, nonanxious individuals.

Among the TCAs, amitriptyline's analgesic effect is the best documented. Clinically, the tetracyclics (i.e., maprotiline), other tertiary amines (i.e., imipramine), and the secondary amines (i.e., nortriptyline, desipramine)

TABLE 43–12. Characteristics of chronic pain syndrome

Behavior[a]	Interpersonal[b]	Affective features[c]
Physical display of disability maximized	"Nothing helps"	Sour, angry resentment for others
Suffering emphasized (verbally)	Authenticity of complaint emphasized	Sweet, endearing, denying, passive
Suffering dramatized (nonverbally)	High anxiety expressed and denied	Strong moods, dysphoria, and irritability
Disability prolonged by avoidance and noncompliance	"Only you can help; I can't do anything"	Weak, low self-esteem, counterdependent

Source. Adapted from [a]Fordyce 1976; [b]Bouckoms and Hackett 1991; [c]Bouckoms 1989.

TABLE 43–13. Psychiatrists' physical examination for patients who have chronic pain

Findings	Diagnostic considerations
Abnormal motor movements	Functional paresis, ataxia, or involuntary movements suggest a somatoform disorder.
Trigger points in the muscles	Are any of the 18 common myofascial trigger points present, and what relation do they have to the pain complaint?
Abnormal pain behavior	Look for emphasis on authenticity of pain, extreme suffering (in words and disability), and nature of the examination.
Sympathetic or vascular dysfunction	Look for swelling, skin dysfunction, discoloration, and changes in sweating or temperature that suggest a vascular or sympathetic element to the pain.

TABLE 43–14. Physical examination for central pain

Clinical feature	Examination findings
Nondermatomal distribution of pain	Pinprick or light touch examination of the distribution of pain is nondermatomal.
Increased sensory threshold	Pinprick is not felt as sharp but rather as light touch.
Decreased pain threshold; patient perceives pain from nonnoxious stimulation	Allodynia is present (i.e., painful response to vibration, minimal movement of a few body hairs, or contact with a cold metallic object or ice cube).
Hyperpathia	Delay, summation, and prolonged after-sensation to nonnoxious stimulation; allesthesia may be present.
Paroxysmal attacks of pain	Pain is paroxysmal, either occurring spontaneously or induced by light touch.

are also effective. More important, they are often better tolerated than amitriptyline (Atkinson et al. 1998; Max 1992; McQuay et al. 1996; Watson et al. 1998). Nortriptyline has the additional advantage of having reliable blood levels. TCAs are usually sedating, a particularly useful side effect for the patient with chronic pain who also has insomnia.

Previously, it was thought that low-dose TCAs were effective in producing analgesia. This is the case for some patients, but clinical experience has shown that antidepressant-level dosing is often needed (e.g., nortriptyline, 75 mg daily for several weeks to obtain full analgesic effect).

In an effort to clarify data from pain-antidepressant studies, Onghena and Van Houdenhove (1992) conducted a meta-analysis of 39 controlled trials of antidepressants for nonmalignant pain. Of these, 28 studies showed a statistically significant difference between drug and placebo. Overall, the average patient with chronic pain who received an antidepressant had less pain than

74% of those who received placebo. The review also showed an antidepressant treatment response for central pain, pain in the head or face, and pain caused by tension, compared with other pain types and locations. Rheumatological pain, a commonly studied type of pain, showed very small benefit from antidepressant treatment. For neuropathic pain, imipramine, amitriptyline, clomipramine, desipramine, and nortriptyline were effective (Gomez-Perez et al. 1985; Kvinesdal et al. 1984; Lynch et al. 1990; Max et al. 1987, 1988, 1991, 1992; Sindrup et al. 1989; Watson and Evans 1992; Watson et al. 1982). Sedation was not significantly correlated with analgesic effect; even so, the antihistaminic profile of the antidepressant correlated with analgesic effect (Onghena and Van Houdenhove 1992).

Despite the proven clinical effectiveness of TCAs, a study in 1997 of 1,145 patients referred to a large multidisciplinary pain center found that only 25% of the patients were prescribed TCAs. Further, 75% of those patients were given low to intermediate doses of the TCA, even when the dose was not limited by side effects or there was a suboptimal clinical response (Richeimer et al. 1997).

Analgesic effects are at least partly independent of antidepressant effects. The degree of the analgesic effect is not significantly different in the presence or absence of depression. Therefore, a trial of a TCA in any chronic pain condition is warranted, regardless of whether the patient is depressed. The usual precautions regarding TCAs apply (e.g., check electrocardiogram before prescribing).

Anticonvulsants/Mood-Stabilizing Agents

Like the TCAs, anticonvulsant medications have become first-line treatments for neuropathic pain. Carbamazepine, a tricyclic, is often used in clinical and research situations. Its effectiveness overlaps that of the TCAs. Specifically, it has been used successfully to treat trigeminal neuralgia, postherpetic neuralgia, diabetic neuropathy, phantom limb pain, and reflex sympathy dystrophy (Bartusch et al. 1996). Interestingly, the first anticonvulsant, phenytoin, does not have significant analgesic effect in treating neuropathic or chronic pain syndromes (Backonja 2000).

The newer anticonvulsants, including valproic acid, gabapentin, and lamotrigine, have shown good results in treating neuropathic pain syndromes, idiopathic pain syndromes associated with multiple sclerosis, and neuralgias (Backonja 2000; Maciewicz et al. 1985). Dosing, side effects, and monitoring of these medications are discussed in Chapter 42, this volume.

One of the more promising newer medications is gabapentin. It is generally well tolerated, does not require blood level monitoring, appears to lack significant drug interactions, and seems to have good analgesic effect in treating neuropathic pain (Laird and Gidal 2000), neuropathic cancer pain (Caraceni 1999), pain associated with multiple sclerosis (Houtchens et al. 1997; Samkoff et al. 1997), and neuropathic head and neck pain (Sist et al. 1997). It also has an antianxiety effect. Physicians should keep in mind, however, that gabapentin costs significantly more than the older agents, especially the TCAs. Lithium has not been shown to be effective in the treatment of pain syndromes.

Benzodiazepines

Benzodiazepines, in particular clonazepam, are also routinely used in the treatment of neuropathic pain and chronic pain syndromes. Although the exact mechanism is not known, it is thought to be similar to the anticonvulsants (i.e., possibly via membrane stabilization). Although clonazepam is often used, other benzodiazepines

are also effective. For example, Serrao et al. (1992) reported that intrathecal midazolam is effective for chronic low mechanical back pain. Intravenous lorazepam was superior to morphine, lidocaine, and placebo in a single-blind study of neuropathic pain (Bouckoms 1987). However, clonazepam has emerged as the oral drug of choice. It decreases allodynia, and it binds more to central than to peripheral benzodiazepine receptors. It is synergistic with serotonergic pain mechanisms, which distinguishes it from other benzodiazepines. Numerous publications cite the value of clonazepam in treating neuralgias and neuropathic pain syndromes (Bouckoms and Litman 1985). For maximum clinical effect, benzodiazepines are often combined with TCAs or opiates.

A useful diagnostic test for benzodiazepine-sensitive pain is to administer lorazepam, in a 2-mg intravenous bolus, in a single-blind manner with the response evaluated by VAS monitoring. Positive results (a VAS decrease >3 cm) signify relief of ongoing pain. If positive results are achieved, the pain cycle in patients with severe pain may be broken with sequential intravenous doses of lorazepam or oral clonazepam, 1 mg twice a day and doses up to 2–4 mg at bedtime.

Opiates in Chronic Pain Management

The use of opiates in management of chronic nonmalignant pain is generally reserved for patients who have not responded to other analgesics and physiotherapy interventions. These patients must be selected and monitored carefully. In one study, long-term oral narcotics provided effective pain relief in about two-thirds of patients with chronic nonmalignant pain; however, even when patients were carefully selected (i.e., they lacked previous substance dependency or severe personality disorder), one-third developed abuse, tolerance, or dependency over a 3-year period (Bouckoms et al. 1992). Nociceptive pain and absence of depression and drug abuse were all significantly associated with long-term narcotic treatment efficacy. Patients with neuropathic pain and major depression did particularly poorly: these patients were four times more likely to experience minimal or no pain relief than to experience marked to complete pain relief. The effectiveness of opioid medications in neuropathic pain management remains controversial (Arner and Meyerson 1988).

The following eight recommendations apply to maintenance therapy with narcotic analgesics in patients with chronic pain:

1. Do not prescribe narcotics for patients who previously used, abused, or were addicted to illicit drugs,

unless there is a new major medical illness with severe pain (e.g., cancer, trauma). In such cases, a second opinion from another physician is suggested for narcotics prescribed longer than 1 month.

2. Consider maintenance narcotics only after other methods of pain control fail. Other methods typically include NSAIDs, epidural opiates and nonopiates, anticonvulsant medications, TCAs, benzodiazepines, nerve blocks and nerve stimulation, and physical therapy.

3. Designate one pharmacy and one prescriber as the exclusive agent for opiate treatment.

4. Define narcotic dosage and consequences if deviations occur. For example, the development of abuse should lead to rapid tapering of the drug and a detoxification program, if necessary. Leave the patient with no doubt that the drug will be discontinued if use becomes inappropriate.

5. Document informed consent to include the rationale for use, risks, benefits, and alternative treatments.

6. Document the treatment course, including response to treatment, changes in the disease process, medication efficacy and abuse, tolerance, or the appearance of addictive behaviors.

7. Obtain a second opinion from a physician who is familiar with pain management if narcotics are prescribed for longer than 3 months and a follow-up consultation at least once a year if narcotics are continued.

8. Do not place pregnant opiate users at risk for withdrawal. Therefore, any pregnant woman with opiate dependency should receive methadone, about 20 mg/day, to prevent withdrawal effects on the fetus (Allen 1991).

The Opioid Paradox

Increased sensitivity to pain (i.e., hyperalgesia) caused by narcotics presents an apparent paradox. Nevertheless, clinicians describe patients who experience more pain when taking, rather than not taking, narcotics. This paradox is partially explained by narcotic-sensitive "on" and "off" cells in the medulla (Kaplan and Fields 1991). Pain-enhancing "on" cells in the rostral ventromedial medulla have increased activity when narcotic levels decline. Therefore, as narcotic levels fall, painful hyperalgesia occurs. Pain-inhibiting "off" cells have increased activity when narcotic levels are steady. This model helps explain heightened pain sensitivity as narcotic levels fall. Therefore, when treating chronic pain, the clinician must consider the possibility that fluctuations in narcotic levels can increase pain. For this reason, the clinician should consider a trial without narcotics, not because of fear of addiction but because pain sometimes decreases without narcotics.

Stimulants

Stimulants, namely methylphenidate and amphetamine, are effective analgesic adjuncts. They also decrease sedation produced by opiates. These benefits occur rapidly (6–48 hours), tolerance is not usually a problem, and side effects disappear quickly when the medication is stopped or dosage decreased. Patients with postoperative pain and patients with cancer-related pain respond well to analgesic-stimulant combinations. One of the most quoted studies is Forrest et al.'s (1977) double-blind administration of 5–10 mg of intramuscular dextroamphetamine with morphine. The combination doubled the acute postoperative pain relief achieved by morphine alone and also improved cognition and lessened sedation. Yee and Berde (1994) studied 11 children and found that oral amphetamines safely counteracted opiate-induced sedation. A series of studies by Bruera et al. (1986, 1987, 1989a, 1989b) showed that cancer pain also decreased with stimulants. Methylphenidate significantly decreased pain and sedation and increased activity in a 3-day double-blind, crossover study; 70% of patients chose methylphenidate as more effective than placebo (Bruera et al. 1987, 1989a, 1989b). Joshi et al. (1982) conducted an open, uncontrolled study giving dextroamphetamine, 10 mg/day, to 18 patients with cancer-related pain; amphetamines improved pain control, activity, and appetite in these patients. At this point in time, no research exists on the use of modafinil, a sympathomimetic, as an analgesic or analgesic adjunct.

Methylphenidate has a 2- to 7-hour half-life, compared with dextroamphetamine's less predictable 4- to 21-hour half-life (Frierson et al. 1991). This finding may explain the clinical perception that methylphenidate is better tolerated than dextroamphetamine (Katon and Roskind 1980).

Neuroleptics

Neuroleptics are usually not thought of as analgesics. However, analgesic effects are reported for some neuroleptics such as haloperidol. The most interesting potential explanation for this analgesic effect is that haloperidol binds to sigma opiate receptors. Levopromazine, 15 mg, compared favorably with morphine, 10 mg, in a double-blind study by Bloomfield et al. (1964). Methotrimeprazine, which has some analgesic effect, is about half as potent as morphine. Flupentixol helped to ease cancer pain, although its addition to amitriptyline added nothing to the analgesic effects of amitriptyline alone (Zitman et al. 1991). Phenothiazines and butyrophenones all have some pain-relieving effects (Farber and Burks 1974; Nathan 1978).

The genesis of clinical interest in neuroleptics as analgesics came from the finding that a combination of amitriptyline and fluphenazine relieved one of the most resistant pain syndromes, postherpetic neuralgia (Taub 1973). Diabetic neuropathy also responded to the amitriptyline-fluphenazine combination (Davis et al. 1977). It is common clinical lore, unproven by rigorous study, that a neuroleptic combined with an antidepressant is more potent for pain relief than either medication used alone (Zitman et al. 1991).

REHABILITATION

Rehabilitation of patients who have chronic pain syndromes typically combines the disciplines of physiatry, physical therapy, psychiatry, behavioral psychology, and neurology. Successful rehabilitation requires an integrated approach to mind-body issues. A consultation-liaison psychiatrist is in a good position to help with this integration, both by sharing information and by applying the general principles of pain therapy (Table 43–15). Psychiatrists can prescribe neuropsychopharmacological agents, transcutaneous electrical nerve stimulation (TENS), cognitive and behavioral therapies, and psychotherapy.

Nonmedication Treatment Modalities

Hypnosis, relaxation techniques (discussed in Chapter 46, this volume), massage and behavioral programs, and yoga are quite helpful for many patients and can help them regain a sense of control. Lifestyle modification, exercise, and physical reconditioning are important parts of any pain management program, whether inpatient or outpatient. These treatments are aimed at helping patients adapt to the pain and eliminating maladaptive behaviors. Cure of the pain is not the goal. These techniques are meant to supplement, not substitute for, psychopharmacological interventions.

For patients who have chronic pain, bibliotherapy can be quite helpful. *Managing Pain Before It Manages You* (Caudill 1995) and *Mastering Pain: A Twelve-Step Program for Coping With Chronic Pain* (Sternbach 1995) are educational books that can help reduce the isolation that patients with chronic pain often feel.

Many patients have learned intuitively the power of distraction, for example, finding that pain symptoms are more tolerable or even forgotten while absorbed in a movie. A patient who reports chronic pain but is observed appearing comfortable while engaged in conversation or while watching television is not automatically a malingerer. Physicians, like everyone else, learn about pain from personal experience, usually injuries or minor trauma, and from observing patients with dramatic acute pain, such as a patient with renal colic. Patients with chronic pain do not obey the rules learned from life's experience with acute pain. Unless this is understood, physicians and medical personnel are destined to doubt everyone who complains of chronic pain but appears composed and even laughs occasionally. Distraction can be therapeutically utilized through hypnosis or relaxation techniques.

Transcutaneous Electrical Nerve Stimulation

TENS is no panacea, and it has received criticism as a pain treatment. However, this criticism is partially the result of errors in its use. A common mistake made with TENS is the use of continuous or nonintermittent, nonpulsed stimulation, which rapidly leads to tolerance. Burst intermittent stimulation is generally more helpful. Another error is in prescribing TENS for central pain disorders, which it can exacerbate. Neuralgia without a central component responds quite well to TENS, however. Also, the use of excessively strong stimulation leads to muscle contractions that exacerbate the pain. TENS should use a subsensory threshold stimulus. Used judiciously, it is often quite effective. When used appropriately, half of long-term TENS users had pain reduced by more than one-half. TENS can help restore the patient's sense of self-control and avoids medication side effects.

Cognitive and Behavioral Therapies

Fernandez and Turk (1992) performed a meta-analysis on the use of cognitive strategies for the alteration of pain perception. Imagery methods were the most effective, whereas positive expectancy was equivalent to no treatment. The reality is that patients often use cognitive imagery methods themselves, typically in combination with other methods of pain control. Combined therapies are in wide use but have not been assiduously studied. In their extensive review, Turner and Chapman (1982a, 1982b) examined relaxation training, biofeedback, operant conditioning, hypnosis, and cognitive-behavioral therapy and concluded that biofeedback and relaxation training were probably equally effective for headache and that evidence for the efficacy of the other therapies was inconclusive. Malone et al. (1988) performed a meta-analysis of 109 studies of nonmedical therapies for chronic pain—only 48 provided sufficient information to calculate effect. They concluded that the data necessary

TABLE 43–15. General principles of pain therapy

Goal	Method
Integration of diagnostic, pharmacological, behavioral, and psychodynamic aspects of care	Multidisciplinary team routinely works together and consults one another as often as they consult on patients.
Display of patient's pain on a rating scale to make it visible to patient and caregivers	Patient completes visual analogue scales, categorical rating scales, or similar simple pain rating at least daily.
Prompt feedback at each visit utilizing the pain rating information	At each visit, discuss with patient how pain ratings are useful diagnostically, pharmacologically, and psychologically.
Continuous improvement in quality of care at a programmatic and individual level	Routinely measure unrelieved pain, untreated psychiatric illness, drug toxicity, and other measures of morbidity as variances requiring changes in evaluation or treatment.

Source. Adapted from Max MB: "Improving Outcomes of Analgesic Treatment: Is Education Enough?" *International Association for the Study of Pain Newsletter*, November–December 1992, pp 2–6. Used with permission.

for evaluation of long-term benefits do not exist in the published literature. The most effective short-term treatments were autogenic relaxation, hypnosis, and placebo. Cognitive therapy and operant conditioning were the least effective.

Psychotherapy

Coping is a word used to describe the sum of many things such as attachment behavior and intrapsychic defenses (Jensen and Romano 1991). In a randomized, controlled study, Keefe and Williams (1990) showed that helping the patient to develop cognitive-behavioral coping skills is more effective in decreasing pain and psychological disability than education alone. Coping is also context dependent, which means that coping skills are most effective when the focus includes the patient and his or her partner or family (Manne and Zautra 1990). Therefore, efforts to improve a patient's ability to cope must include more than education and counseling. The psychological aspects of coping involve conflicts over autonomy and care. To help the patient cope, the psychiatrist must be a teacher, doctor, soothsayer, and wise friend with the right mixture of palliative care, hope, denial, catharsis, family counseling, relaxation, exercise, physical rehabilitation, pharmacotherapy, and sensitivity to the unconscious.

Multidisciplinary Pain Clinics

In one study, comprehensive multidisciplinary treatment returned 48% of 42 patients to work and an additional 28% to vocational rehabilitation; none of the 15 control subjects improved (Deardorff et al. 1991). Aranoff's (1985) review of follow-up studies of pain clinics suggested that at least 50% of patients achieved some benefit from this multidisciplinary approach. Multidisciplinary pain clinics are successful because they work at

the interface of psychiatry, neurology, psychology, and physical therapy. Recognition and treatment of psychiatric illness in patients with chronic pain are also cost-effective. For example, proper treatment of hypochondriasis reduces dollar costs by 53%; recognition and treatment of somatization disorder save an average of $5,000 per year per patient (Bouckoms and Hackett 1991; Smith et al. 1986). Multidisciplinary pain clinics are useful for some patients with chronic pain (Gach 1983; Manniche et al. 1991; Schatz 1991).

There is danger in overemphasizing behavioral explanations for chronic pain because most pain is driven not by behavioral maladaptation but rather by intransigent physical pathology. There is also a danger in claiming that behavioral methods relieve pain. Behavioral treatments are not intended to relieve pain but rather to extinguish the behaviors associated with it (Fordyce 1985). Quality-control guidelines developed by the Commission on Accreditation of Rehabilitation Facilities and the Joint Commission on Accreditation of Healthcare Organizations led to nationwide certification of multidisciplinary pain management programs. The following are recommendations for situations in which patients should be considered for referral to a multidisciplinary pain clinic:

- When a patient with chronic nonmalignant pain is under consideration for chronic opioid medication
- When evaluation of the physical and psychiatric pathology is complete, or the diagnosis is so obscured that intensive observation is necessary (e.g., when malingering is suspected)
- When consultation from an independent physician, who is an expert in the treatment of chronic pain, confirms that no single modality of outpatient treatment is likely to work
- When the patient reports maximum benefit from outpatient treatments (e.g., NSAIDs, nerve blocks, anti-

TABLE 43–16.   Medication contract

Pain-relieving medications, muscle relaxants, antianxiety agents, and some sleep medications can lead to addiction and abuse. It is therefore important that we agree on the specific guidelines outlined below:

1. You will obtain potentially addictive medications, such as analgesics, tranquilizers, and muscle relaxants, only from the Pain Management Center while you are under our care.
2. You will obtain these medications only from the pharmacy listed below.
3. You will not drink alcohol, because the medication you receive from us is dangerous when combined with alcohol or any other potentially sedating or addicting substances. If you are using these substances, it is your responsibility to discuss it with us.
4. You are responsible for your medication. Do not leave medications where they are available to minors or where they may be easily stolen. Do not leave medication in a locked car. Have medications delivered by Federal Express or handed directly to you in a pharmacy. We will not replace medications that are lost, even by accident (dropped in the sink, eaten by the dog, left in clothes that are then put in the washing machine). We will not replace unfilled prescriptions that are lost, stolen, or destroyed.
5. Abuse behaviors—including (but not limited to) obtaining potentially addictive medications from friends, relatives, or other doctors, as well as purchasing them illicitly, hoarding them for future use, or increasing the dose without authorization—are both illegal and unacceptable. We view such behaviors as evidence that you cannot manage medications responsibly, and we will discontinue these medications.
6. You will take medications based on a schedule that is mutually agreed on. This will minimize the risk of abuse and provide you with greater control of your medication use. In addition, during the course of treatment, it is expected that you will gradually eliminate your dependence on these agents, because most people can successfully manage without them.

Patient: _____

Date: _____

Medical director: _____

Source.   James F. Brodey, M.D., Pain Management and Behavioral Medicine Center, Inc., Farmington, CT, 1992. Used with permission.

depressants, simple physical and behavioral rehabilitation)
- When intensive daily interventions are required, usually with multiple concurrent types of therapy such as nerve blocks, physical therapy, and behavior modification
- When the patient exhibits abnormal pain behavior and behavior modification is the focus of the clinic
- When medications for the pain are so complex or compliance so problematic that direct supervision of medical therapy is necessary (e.g., when high-dose narcotics are needed or drug abuse is a problem)

Table 43–16 shows a medication contract between a patient and a pain treatment center.

CONCLUSION

The consultation-liaison psychiatrist is a key person in the evaluation, management, and treatment of chronic pain because no other physician is as prepared to examine the patient psychiatrically and physically; to prescribe neuropsychopharmacological, psychological, and adjunctive therapies; and to integrate these therapies into a rehabilitation program for the patient (Bouckoms 1988).

The psychiatrist can assume all these responsibilities as a pain expert or can provide consultation to a team of caregivers.

The complex issues surrounding the diagnosis, management, and treatment of chronic pain syndromes are increasing as we learn more about CNS dysfunction in chronic pain and while health care administrators simultaneously insist on using the least costly treatments. Still, effective pain management rests on the judicious selection of medical, psychiatric, and rehabilitation modalities tailored to an individual patient's needs.

REFERENCES

Allen MH: Detoxification considerations in the medical management of substance abuse in pregnancy. Bulletin of the New York Academy of Medicine 67:270–276, 1991

American Psychiatric Association: Diagnostic and Statistical Manual of Mental Disorders, 4th Edition. Washington, DC, American Psychiatric Association, 1994

American Psychiatric Association: Diagnostic and Statistical Manual of Mental Disorders, 4th Edition, Text Revision. Washington, DC, American Psychiatric Association, 2000

Arana GW, Rosenbaum JF: Handbook of Psychiatric Drug Therapy, 4th Edition. Philadelphia, PA, Lippincott Williams & Wilkins, 2000

Aranoff GM: Evaluation and Treatment of Chronic Pain. Baltimore, MD, Urban & Schwarzenberg, 1985

Arner S, Meyerson BA: Lack of analgesic effect of opioids on neuropathic and idiopathic forms of pain. Pain 33:11–23, 1988

Atkinson JH, Slater MA, Williams RA, et al: A placebo-controlled randomized clinical trail of nortriptyline for chronic lower back pain. Pain 76:287–296, 1998

Atkinson JH, Slater MA, Wahlgren DR, et al: Effects of noradrenergic and serotonergic antidepressants on chronic low back pain intensity. Pain 83:137–145, 1999

Babul N, Darke AC: Putative role of hydromorphone metabolites in myoclonus (letter). Pain 51:260–261, 1992

Backonja MM: Anticonvulsants (antineuropathics) for neuropathic pain syndromes. Clin J Pain 16 (suppl):S67–S72, 2000

Baringa M: The brain remaps its own contours. Science 258:216–218, 1992

Barsky A, Wool C, Barnett M, et al: Histories of childhood trauma in adult hypochondriacal patients. Am J Psychiatry 151:397–401, 1994

Bartusch SL, Sanders BJ, D'Alessio, et al: Clonazepam for the treatment of lancinating phantom limb pain. Clin J Pain 12:59–62, 1996

Bendtsen L, Jensen R, Olesen J: A non-selective (amitriptyline), but not a selective (citalopram), serotonin reuptake inhibitor is effective in the prophylactic treatment of chronic tension-type headache. J Neurol Neurosurg Psychiatry 61:285–290, 1996

Bloomfield S, Simard-Savoie S, Bernier J, et al: Comparative analgesic activity of levopromazine and morphine in patients with chronic pain. Can Med Assoc J 90:1156–1159, 1964

Bonica JJ: The Management of Pain, 2nd Edition. Philadelphia PA, Lea & Febiger, 1990

Bouckoms AJ: The role of psychotropics, anticonvulsants, and prostaglandin inhibitors. Drug Therapy 6(11):41–48, 1981

Bouckoms AJ: Intravenous lorazepam for pain relief of intractable neuralgia. Pain 32 (suppl 4):S347–S472, 1987

Bouckoms AJ: Pharmacological treatment of severe pain and suffering in the critically ill. Problems in Critical Care 2:47–62, 1988

Bouckoms AJ: Pain Outpatient Psychiatry, Diagnosis and Treatment, 2nd Edition. Baltimore, MD, Williams & Wilkins, 1989

Bouckoms AJ, Hackett TP: The pain patient: evaluation and treatment, in Massachusetts General Hospital Handbook of General Hospital Psychiatry, 3rd Edition. Edited by Cassem NH. St. Louis, MO, CV Mosby, 1991, pp 39–68

Bouckoms AJ, Litman RE: Clonazepam in the treatment of neuralgic pain syndromes. Psychosomatics 26:933–936, 1985

Bouckoms AJ, Litman RE, Baer L: Denial in the depressive and pain-prone disorders of chronic pain. Clin J Pain 1:165–169, 1985

Bouckoms AJ, Masand PS, Murray GB, et al: Non-malignant pain treated with long term oral narcotics. Ann Clin Psychiatry 4:185–192, 1992

Bruera E, Carraro S, Roca E, et al: Double-blind evaluation of the effects of mazindol on pain, depression, anxiety, appetite and activity in terminal cancer patients. Cancer Treat Reports 70(2):295–298, 1986

Bruera E, Brenneis C, Chadwick C, et al: Methylphenidate associated with narcotics for the treatment of cancer pain. Cancer Treat Reports 71(1):67–70, 1987

Bruera E, Macmillan K, Hanson J, et al: The cognitive effects of the administration of narcotic analgesics in patients with cancer pain. Pain 39:13–16, 1989a

Bruera E, Brenneis C, Paterson AHG, et al: Use of methylphenidate as an adjuvant to narcotic analgesics in patients with advanced cancer. J Pain Symptom Manage 4:3–6, 1989b

Bruera E, Schoeller T, Montejo G: Organic hallucinosis in patients receiving high doses of opiates for cancer pain. Pain 48:397–399, 1992

Cassem NH: Pain (Current Topics in Medicine, Chapter 2), in Scientific American Medicine. Edited by Rubenstein E, Federman DD. New York, Scientific American, 1989

Caraceni A, Zecca E, Martini C, et al: Gabapentin as an adjuvant to opioid analgesia for neuropathic cancer pain. J Pain Symptom Manage 17:441–445, 1999

Caudill MA: Managing Pain Before It Manages You. New York, Guilford, 1995

Cavanaugh SA: Depression in the medically ill: critical issues in diagnostic assessment. Psychosomatics 36:48–59, 1995

Cleeland CS, Gonin R, Hatfield AK, et al: Pain and its treatment in outpatients with metastatic cancer. N Engl J Med 330:592–596, 1994

Coderre TJ, Katz J, Vaccarino AL, et al: Contribution of central neuroplasticity to pathological pain: review of clinical and experimental evidence. Pain 52:259–285, 1993

Davidoff G, Guarracini M, Roth E, et al: Trazodone hydrochloride in the treatment of dysesthetic pain in traumatic myelopathy: a randomized, double-blind, placebo-controlled study. Pain 29:151–161, 1987

Davis JL, Gerich JE, Schultz TA: Peripheral diabetic neuropathy treated with amitriptyline and fluphenazine. JAMA 238:2291–2292, 1977

Deardorff W, Rubin H, Scott D: Comprehensive multidisciplinary treatment of chronic pain: a follow-up study of treated and non-treated groups. Pain 45:35–44, 1991

Deyo RA, Rainville J, Kent DL: What can the history and physical examination tell us about low back pain? JAMA 268:760–765, 1992

Dickens C, Jayson M, Sutton C, et al: The relationship between pain and depression in a trial using paroxetine in sufferers of chronic lower back pain. Psychosomatics 41:490–499, 2000

Dorland's Illustrated Medical Dictionary, 26th Edition. Philadelphia, PA, WB Saunders, 1985

Dorland's Illustrated Medical Dictionary, 29th Edition. Philadelphia, PA, WB Saunders, 2000

Emanuel LL, von Gunten CF, Ferris FD: The education for physicians on end-of-life care curriculum. The Robert Wood Johnson Foundation 4:1–13, 1999

Engel CC, Walker EA, Engel Al, et al: A randomized, double-blind crossover trial of sertraline in women with chronic pelvic pain. J Psychosom Res 44:203–207, 1998

Farber GA, Burks JW: Chlorprothixene therapy for herpes zoster neuralgia. South Med J 67:808–812, 1974

Fernandez E, Turk DC: The utility of cognitive coping strategies for altering pain perception: a meta analysis. Pain 38:123–135, 1992

Fordyce W: Behavioral Methods for Chronic Pain and Illness. St. Louis, MO, CV Mosby, 1976

Fordyce W: The behavioral management of chronic pain: a response to critics. Pain 22:113–125, 1985

Forrest W, Brown B, Brown C: Dextroamphetamine with morphine for treatment of postoperative pain. N Engl J Med 296:712–715, 1977

Frierson RL, Wey JJ, Tabler JB: Psychostimulants for depression in the medically ill. Am Fam Physician 43:163–170, 1991

Gach MR: The Bum Back Book. Berkeley, CA, Acu Press, 1983

Galer BS: Neuropathic pain of peripheral origin: advances in pharmacological treatment. Neurology 45:S17–S25, S35–S36, 1995

Geisser ME, Roth RS, Robinson ME: Assessing depression among persons with chronic pain using the Center for Epidemiology Studies–Depression Scale and the Beck Depression Inventory: a comparative analysis. Clin J Pain 13(2):163–170, 1997

Genova P: Rebellion in the body. The Main Scholar 5:67–83, 1992

Gomez-Perez FJ, Rull JA, Dies H, et al: Nortriptyline and fluphenazine in the symptomatic treatment of diabetic neuropathy: a double blind cross-over study. Pain 23:395–400, 1985

Gourlay GK, Cherry DA, Cousins MJ, et al: A controlled study of a serotonin reuptake blocker, zimelidine, in the treatment of chronic pain. Pain 25:35–52, 1986

Graves DA, Foster TS, Batenhorst RL, et al: Patient-controlled analgesia. Ann Intern Med 99:360–366, 1983

Guglielmo WJ: Treating pain: can doctors put their fears to rest? Medical Economics 77(4):46–48, 53–54, 57–58, 2000

Holmes V, Rafuls W, Bouckoms AJ: Covert psychopathology in chronic pain. Clinical Diagnosis 2(2):79–85, 1986

Houtchens MK, Richert JR, Sami A, et al: Open label gabapentin treatment for pain in multiple sclerosis. Multiple Sclerosis 3:250–253, 1997

Jaffe JH, Martin WR: Opioid analgesics and antagonists, in The Pharmacological Basis of Therapeutics. Edited by Gilman AG et al. New York, Pergamon, 1990

Jellema JG: Hallucinations during sustained-release morphine and methadone administration (letter). Lancet 2:392, 1987

Jensen MP, Romano JA: Coping with chronic pain: a critical review of the literature. Pain 47:249–283, 1991

Joshi J, DeJongh C, Schnepper N: Amphetamine therapy for enhancing the comfort of terminally ill cancer patients (Abstract C-213). Proceedings of the 18th annual meeting of the American Society of Clinical Oncology. Baltimore, MD, Waverly Press, 1982, p 55

Kaplan H, Fields HL: Hyperalgesia during acute opioid abstinence: evidence for a nociceptive facilitating function of the rostral ventromedial medulla. J Neurosci 11:1433–1439, 1991

Katon W, Roskind M: Treatment of depression in medically ill elderly with methylphenidate. Am J Psychol 137:963–965, 1980

Keefe FJ, Williams DA: A comparison of coping strategies in chronic pain patients in different age groups. J Gerontol 45:161–165, 1990

Koh WH, Pande I, Samuels A, et al: Low dose amitriptyline in ankylosing spondylitis: a short term, double blind, placebo controlled study. J Rheumatol 24:2158–2161, 1997

Kohler T, Kosnaic S: Are persons with migraine characterized by a high degree of ambition, orderliness, and rigidity? Pain 48:321–323, 1992

Kvinesdal B, Molin J, Froland A, et al: Imipramine treatment of painful diabetic neuropathy. JAMA 251:1727–1730, 1984

Laird MA, Gidal BE: Use of gabapentin in the treatment of neuropathic pain. Ann Pharmacother 34:802–807, 2000

Liebeskind JC: Pain can kill. Pain 44:3–4, 1991

Lynch S, Max MB, Muir J, et al: Efficacy of antidepressants in relieving diabetic neuropathy pain: amitriptyline vs desipramine, and fluoxetine vs placebo. Neurology 40 (suppl 1): 437, 1990

Maciewicz R, Bouckoms AJ, Martin J: Drug therapy of neuropathic pain. Clin J Pain 1:39–49, 1985

Malone MD, Strube MJ, Scogin FR: Meta-analysis of non-medical treatments for chronic pain. Pain 34:231–244, 1988

Manne SL, Zautra AJ: Couples coping with chronic illness: women with rheumatoid arthritis and their healthy husbands. J Behav Med 13:327–342, 1990

Manniche C, Lundberg E, Christensen I, et al: Intensive dynamic back exercises for chronic low back pain: a clinical trial. Pain 47:53–63, 1991

Max MB: Improving outcomes of analgesic treatment: is education enough? International Association for the Study of Pain Newsletter, November–December 1992, pp 2–6

Max MB, Culnane M, Schafer SC: Amitriptyline relieves diabetic neuropathy pain in patients with normal or depressed mood. Neurology 37:589–596, 1987

Max MB, Schafer SC, Culnane M, et al: Amitriptyline, but not lorazepam, relieves postherpetic neuralgia. Neurology 38:1427–1432, 1988

Max MB, Kishore-Kumar R, Schafer SC, et al: Efficacy of desipramine in painful diabetic neuropathy: a placebo controlled trial. Pain 45:3–9, 1991

Max MB, Lynch SA, Muir J, et al: Effects of desipramine, amitriptyline, and fluoxetine on pain in diabetic neuropathy. N Engl J Med 326:1250–1256, 1992

McQuay HJ, Mramaer M, Mye BA, et al: A systematic review of antidepressants in neuropathic pain. Pain 68:217–227, 1996

Melzack R: The tragedy of needless pain. Sci Am 262:27–33, 1990

Nathan PW: Chlorprothixene (Taractan) in postherpetic neuralgia and other severe chronic pains. Pain 5:367–371, 1978

Norregaard J, Volkmann H, Danneskiold-Samsoe B: A randomized controlled trial of citalopram in the treatment of fibromyalgia. Pain 61:445–449, 1995

Onghena P, Van Houdenhove B: Antidepressant-induced analgesia in chronic non-malignant pain: a meta-analysis of 39 placebo-controlled studies. Pain 49:205–219, 1992

Osterhaus JT, Gutterman DL, Plachetka JR: Healthcare resource and lost labor costs of migraine headache in the US. PharmacoEconomics 2(1):67–76, 1992

Osterweis M, Kleinman A, Mechanic D: Institute of Medicine's Committee on Pain, Disability, and Chronic Illness Behavior. Washington, DC, National Academy Press, 1987

Pettengill CA, Reisner-Keller L: The use of tricyclic antidepressants for control of chronic orofacial pain. Cranio 15:53–56, 1997

Portenoy R, Foley K, Inturrisi R: The nature of opioid responsiveness and its implications for neuropathic pain: new hypothesis derived from studies of opioids infusions. Pain 43:273–286, 1990

Psychiatric News: Group rejects placebos in most clinical trials. November 17, 2000, p. 20

Reed JL: The diagnosis of "hysteria." Psychol Med 5(1);13–17, 1975

Reuler JB, Girard DE, Nardone DA: The chronic pain syndrome: misconceptions and management. Ann Intern Med 93:588–596, 1980

Rich BA: An ethical analysis of the barriers to effective pain management. Cambridge Quarterly of Healthcare Ethics 9:54–70, 2000

Richeimer SH, Bajwa ZH, Kahraman SS, et al: Utilization patterns of tricyclic antidepressants in a multidisciplinary pain clinic: a survey. Clin J Pain 13:324–329, 1997

Samkoff LM, Daras M, Tuchman AJ, et al: Amelioration of refractory dysesthetic limb pain in multiple sclerosis by gabapentin. Multiple Sclerosis 3:250–253, 1997

Schatz MP: Back Care Basics. Berkeley, CA, Rodmell Press, 1991

Serrao JM, Marks RL, Morley SJ, et al: Intrathecal midazolam for the treatment of chronic mechanical low back pain. Pain 48:5–12, 1992

Sheehan J, McKay J, Ryan M, et al: What cost chronic pain? Ir Med J 89(6):218–219, 1996

Shochet RB, Murray GB: Neuropsychiatric toxicity of meperidine. Journal of Intensive Care Medicine 3:246–252, 1988

Sigvardsson S, von Knorring A: An adoption study of somatoform disorders, I: the relationship of somatization to psychiatric disability. Arch Gen Psychiatry 41:853–862, 1984

Sindrup SH, Ejertsen B, Froland A, et al: Imipramine treatment in diabetic neuropathy: relief of subjective symptoms without changes in peripheral and autonomic nerve function. Eur J Clin Pharmacol 37:151–153, 1989

Sist TC, Filadora VA, Miner M, et al: Experience with gabapentin in neuropathic pain in the head and neck: report of ten cases. Regional Anesthesia 22:473–478, 1997

Smith JR, Monson RA, Ray DC: Psychiatric consultation in somatization disorder. N Engl J Med 314:1407–1413, 1986

Sternbach RA: Mastering Pain: A Twelve-Step Program for Coping With Chronic Pain. New York, Ballentine Books, 1995

Sweet WH: Deafferentation pain after posterior rhizotomy, trauma to a limb, and herpes zoster. Neurosurgery 15:928–932, 1984

Taub A: Relief of postherpetic neuralgia with psychotropic drugs. J Neurosurg 39:235–239, 1973

Taylor H, Curran NM (eds): Nuprin Pain Report. New York, Louis Harris & Associates, September 1985

Turner JA, Chapman CR: Psychological interventions for chronic pain: a critical review, I: relaxation training and biofeedback. Pain 12:1–21, 1982a

Turner JA, Chapman CR: Psychological interventions for chronic pain: a critical review, II: operant conditioning, hypnosis, and cognitive behavioral therapy. Pain 12:23–46, 1982b

Tverskoy M, Cozavoc C, Ayache M, et al: Postoperative pain after inguinal herniorrhaphy with different types of anesthesia. Anesth Analg 70:29–35, 1990

Volmink J, Lancaster T, Gray S, et al: Treatment for postherpetic neuralgia—a systematic review of randomized controlled trials. Family Practice 13:84–91, 1996

Walker EA, Katon WJ, Neraas K, et al: Dissociation in woman with chronic pelvic pain. Am J Psychiatry 149:534–536, 1992

Wall PD: The prevention of postoperative pain (editorial). Pain 33:289–290, 1988

Wall PD: The placebo effect: an unpopular topic. Pain 51:1–3, 1992

Watson CPN, Evans RJ: A comparative trial of amitriptyline and zimelidine in postherpetic neuralgia. Pain 23:387–394, 1985

Watson CPN, Evans RJ: The postmastectomy pain syndrome and topical capsaicin: a randomized trial. Pain 51:375–379, 1992

Watson CP, Evans RJ, Reed K, et al: Amitriptyline versus placebo in postherpetic neuralgia. Neurology 32:671–673, 1982

Watson CPN, Chipman M, Reed K, et al: Amitriptyline versus maprotiline in postherpetic neuralgia: a randomized, double blind, crossover trial. Pain 48:29–36, 1992

Watson CP, Vernich L, Chipman M, et al: Nortriptyline versus amitriptyline in postherpetic neuralgia: a randomized trial. Neurology 51:1166–1171, 1998

Weintraub MI: Regional pain is usually hysterical. Arch Neurol 45:914–915, 1988

Weintraub MI: Litigation chronic pain syndrome—a distinct entity: analysis of 210 cases. American Journal of Pain Management 2:198–204, 1992

Woolf CJ, Chong MS: Preemptive analgesia—treating postoperative pain but preventing the establishment of central sensitization. Anesth Analg 77:362–379, 1993

Yee JD, Berde CB: Dextroamphetamine or methylphenidate as adjuvants to opioid analgesia for adolescents with cancer. J Pain Symptom Manage 9:122–125, 1994

Zitman FG, Linseen ACG, Edelbroek PM, et al: Does addition of low-dose flupentixol enhance the analgesic effects of low-dose amitriptyline in somatoform pain disorder? Pain 47:25–30, 1991

44

Electroconvulsive Therapy

An Overview

Charles H. Kellner, M.D.

Mark D. Beale, M.D.

Electroconvulsive therapy (ECT) has been in continuous use as a treatment for severe psychiatric illness since its introduction in 1938 (Cerletti and Bini 1938). As a result of recent research and refinements in technique, ECT is now, more than ever, an integral and effective part of the psychiatric armamentarium. Studies have shown that patients' attitudes about ECT are positive after receiving it, and over 80% would agree to have it again if necessary (Bernstein et al. 1998; Freeman and Kendell 1986). The consultation-liaison psychiatrist must be well informed about all aspects of ECT and comfortable presenting it as a treatment option to patients and their families. In this chapter, we review those aspects of ECT that are most relevant to the consultation-liaison psychiatrist, with an emphasis on indications, recent advances in technique, and administration of ECT to medically ill patients. Additional valuable information on the application of ECT to medically ill patients is available in other references (American Psychiatric Association Task Force on Electroconvulsive Therapy 2001; Abrams 1997; Kellner et al. 1997; Knos and Sung 1993; Weiner and Coffey 1993).

INDICATIONS

ECT is most commonly used in cases of severe depression, both bipolar and unipolar. It is also used for patients in the manic phase of bipolar illness and for those in mixed affective states (American Psychiatric Association Task Force on Electroconvulsive Therapy 2001). Additionally, ECT is indicated for schizoaffective disorder; for the treatment of depressive, manic, or acute psychotic episodes in schizophrenia with catatonic or prominent affective features; or when the patient has a history of favorable response to ECT (American Psychiatric Association Task Force on Electroconvulsive Therapy 2001) (Table 44–1).

ECT is typically prescribed only after a patient fails to respond adequately to psychotropic medications; however, it is used as a first-line treatment in several specific instances (Table 44–2), including the following: 1) when there is a need for rapid improvement in depression for medical or psychiatric reasons (e.g., malnutrition, catatonia, or suicidality); 2) when the risks of other treatments outweigh the risks of ECT; 3) when the patient has a history of favorable response to ECT; or 4) when the patient prefers to proceed directly to ECT (American Psychiatric Association Task Force on Electroconvulsive Therapy 1990). ECT is also indicated when a patient cannot tolerate the side effects of psychotropic medications or when his or her condition deteriorates to the point at which a more rapid and definitive treatment is required.

TABLE 44–1. Indications for electroconvulsive therapy

Major depressive episode (unipolar and bipolar)
Mania
Mixed affective state
Catatonia
Schizophrenia (with prominent affective symptoms or acute psychosis)
Schizoaffective disorder

Source. Adapted from American Psychiatric Association Task Force on Electroconvulsive Therapy 2001. Used with permission.

TABLE 44–2. Indications for electroconvulsive therapy as a first-line treatment

When there is a need for rapid improvement
    Suicidality
    Malnutrition
    Catatonia
    Severe psychosis with agitation

When other treatments are considered more risky
    Elderly patients
    Pregnancy

When the patient prefers electroconvulsive therapy

SITUATIONS OF INCREASED RISK

There are no absolute contraindications and few relative contraindications to ECT. With the lifetime suicide rate of major affective illness approaching 15% (Kaplan and Saddock 1990), the psychiatrist will sometimes choose ECT despite the presence of medical risk factors. Situations that increase risk are listed in Table 44–3. Other more common medical conditions slightly increase the risk of adverse events during ECT (Table 44–4), and modifications in technique that allow patients with such conditions to receive ECT safely are discussed later in this chapter (see "Electroconvulsive Therapy in Patients With Medical Illness" section).

TABLE 44–3. Situations of increased risk

Space-occupying cerebral lesion
Increased intracranial pressure
Recent myocardial infarction
Recent hemorrhagic cerebrovascular accident
Unstable aneurysm
Retinal detachment
Pheochromocytoma

Source. Adapted from American Psychiatric Association Task Force on Electroconvulsive Therapy 1990. Used with permission.

TABLE 44–4. Common medical conditions that may necessitate modifications in electroconvulsive therapy techniques

Chronic obstructive pulmonary disease
Asthma
Hypertension
Coronary artery disease
Remote history of myocardial infarction
Cardiac arrhythmia
Remote history of cerebrovascular accident

CONSENT AND PRETREATMENT EVALUATION

Informed consent should be obtained from the patient and, if possible, from the patient's family before ECT is begun. In cases in which informed consent cannot be given by the patient, it should be obtained from whoever is legally responsible for the patient's care, be it the patient's family, a guardian, or the court system. The legal process of substituted consent varies from state to state (see Chapter 11, this volume). Information about ECT should be presented in such a way that it does not frighten the patient. Depressed patients often have difficulty processing new information and making decisions, and the psychiatrist should be sensitive to this difficulty during the consent process.

The pretreatment evaluation (Table 44–5) must include a medical history, physical examination, psychiatric history, and mental status examination. Complete blood count, electrolyte measurements, and electrocardiogram are recommended in patients over age 40 years or when the patient's medical history indicates further investigations are needed. Computed tomography or magnetic resonance imaging of the brain may be necessary for patients in consultation-liaison settings to rule out space-occupying lesions or increased intracranial pressure. If no brain image is obtained, particular attention should be paid to the funduscopic examination to rule out papilledema. An electroencephalogram may be helpful in detecting previously undiagnosed organic brain disease (e.g., delirium or toxic-metabolic encephalopathy). Anesthesia consultation is an important part of the evaluation before ECT, and cooperation between the consultation-liaison and anesthesia teams is essential. Other consultations may be obtained (e.g., neurology, cardiology) if history, physical examination, or laboratory findings suggest the need for further evaluation.

Because no additive benefit has been demonstrated, we advise tapering and discontinuation of most psychotropic medications before a course of ECT (Beale and Kellner 1996). Neuroleptics may be given during ECT, with the dosage decreased as the patient's agitation and psychosis subside over the course of several ECT treatments. It is especially important to discontinue lithium because delirium has been reported in patients given ECT and lithium (Weiner et al. 1980). Other possible adverse interactions include a risk of prolonged seizures and status epilepticus in patients with high serum theophylline levels, impaired efficacy in patients taking benzodiazepines (Pettinati et al. 1990), prolonged apnea in

TABLE 44–5. Evaluation before electroconvulsive therapy

Medical and psychiatric history
Physical examination
Mental status examination
Complete blood count
Serum electrolytes
Liver function tests
Electrocardiogram
Anesthesia consultation
Consider
    Computed tomography or magnetic resonance imaging of
      the head
    Electroencephalogram
    Chest X ray

TABLE 44–6. Orders before electroconvulsive therapy

Patient should take nothing by mouth after midnight.
Patient should void before transport to electroconvulsive therapy session.
If cardiac drugs or medications for gastric reflux are prescribed, these should be taken with a sip of water about 2 hours before treatment.

TABLE 44–7. Electroconvulsive therapy technique

Place intravenous catheter.
Give glycopyrrolate (0.2–0.4 mg intravenously).
Give methohexital (0.75–1.0 mg/kg intravenously).
Inflate blood pressure cuff on right ankle.
Give succinylcholine (0.5–1.0 mg/kg intravenously).
Ventilate with 100% oxygen by Ambu bag and mask.
Deliver stimulus when muscle relaxation is achieved and bite block is in place.

patients taking cholinesterase inhibitors, and increased seizure threshold in patients taking anticonvulsants (including benzodiazepines).

ELECTROCONVULSIVE THERAPY TECHNIQUE

ECT continues to be refined, with the result that it is better tolerated today than ever before. A typical treatment sequence is described in Tables 44–6 and 44–7. Before ECT, the patient should receive nothing by mouth for 6–8 hours other than cardiac drugs and medications for gastric reflux. An intravenous catheter is placed in the patient's arm, and the patient is given either intravenous atropine, 0.4–1.0 mg, or intravenous glycopyrrolate, 0.2–0.4 mg, to reduce the risk of vagally mediated brady-arrhythmias (American Psychiatric Association Task Force on Electroconvulsive Therapy 1990). Light general anesthesia is then induced with intravenous methohexital, 0.75–1.0 mg/kg (American Psychiatric Association Task Force on Electroconvulsive Therapy 2001). Intravenous succinylcholine, 0.5–1.0 mg/kg, is administered to produce muscle relaxation (American Psychiatric Association Task Force on Electroconvulsive Therapy 2001). A blood pressure cuff is inflated on the right ankle before injection of the succinylcholine (cuffed-limb method). This is done so that the clinician can observe motor activity associated with the seizure. While the patient is unconscious, 100% oxygen is administered by Ambu bag and mask.

Stimulus electrodes are placed on the head, and once neuromuscular block is complete—about 100 seconds after injection of succinylcholine (Beale et al. 1994a)—the electrical stimulus is delivered and the seizure, measured by both motor and electroencephalographic evidence,

is timed and recorded. If a seizure does not occur, or if motor activity lasts for less than 20 seconds, restimulation is performed at a higher stimulus intensity. A seizure is terminated if it lasts longer than 3 minutes (American Psychiatric Association Task Force on Electroconvulsive Therapy 2001). Commonly, seizures are terminated by administration of 50%–100% of the original dose of methohexital. If this drug does not terminate the seizure, intravenous midazolam, 1–3 mg, or diazepam, 5–10 mg, may be used (Abrams 1997).

Electrode Placement

Two types of stimulus electrode placement are commonly used in ECT—bilateral (bifrontotemporal) and nondominant-unilateral (d'Elia 1970). A third electrode placement, bifrontal, has recently received considerable attention as a possible alternative with the potential for high efficacy and fewer cognitive effects (Bailine et al. 2000; Kellner and McCall 1999; Letemendia et al. 1993). Much controversy exists regarding selection of laterality of electrode placement. Bilateral electrode placement is associated with a more robust and rapid therapeutic response, but it also causes more cognitive impairment (Abrams 1997). Nondominant-unilateral ECT causes less cognitive impairment, but some patients may not respond to it and may need to be switched to bilateral treatments after several sessions (Abrams 1997). We recommend that the choice of electrode placement be based on severity of illness. Patients with severe illness, those who are suicidal, or those with psychosis should receive bilateral ECT; patients without psychosis who are less severely ill should initially receive nondominant-unilateral ECT. In addition, the clinician may change electrode placement during a course of treatment, depending on the patient's response. For example, if a patient's condition has not improved after four to six nondominant-unilateral ECT treatments, then bilateral ECT should be administered. Alternatively, if a patient develops severe cognitive impairment with bilateral ECT, then nondominant-unilateral ECT should be given for the remainder of the ECT course.

Currently available ECT devices (e.g., MECTA and THYMATRON) deliver a constant-current, brief-pulse, square-wave stimulus. This type of stimulus, when compared with the sine-wave current generated by older ECT machines, causes less cognitive impairment (Weiner et al. 1986), presumably because the overall electrical dose delivered to the brain is much lower with the newer devices.

Stimulus Dosing

Several methods for selecting the stimulus dose in ECT have been proposed (Beale 1998). For example, it has been recommended that the dose be selected based on the patient's age (e.g., 50 years equals 50% stimulus intensity on the THYMATRON DGX machine) (Swartz and Abrams 1994). Others estimate the dose based on a combination of patient characteristics (e.g., age, gender) (MECTA Corporation 1986). A third method is the administration of a relatively high, fixed dose to all patients (Abrams et al. 1991).

There may be up to a 40-fold variation in seizure threshold among patients (Sackeim et al. 1993). Although seizure threshold estimates may be valid in some cases, the inherent variability of this individual characteristic may lead to excessively high doses being administered to patients whose seizure threshold does not fall within the estimated range (Beale et al. 1994b). Excessively high stimulus doses contribute to cognitive impairment in patients receiving ECT (Ottoson 1960; Weiner et al. 1986). Therefore, we recommend tailoring the stimulus dose to individual patients using the technique of stimulus dose titration first reported by Sackeim et al. (1987). This technique involves giving successive, incremental stimuli at the first session until a seizure is produced—for example, 12, 20, 40, 80 static joules (J) on MECTA devices or 10%, 20%, 40%, 80% energy on THYMATRON devices. The seizure threshold is then estimated to be the midpoint between the stimulus producing a seizure and the previous stimulus that did not cause a seizure (e.g., if a patient does not have a seizure after a 12-J or 20-J stimulus but does have a seizure at 40 J, the threshold is considered to be 30 J) (Beale et al. 1994b).

At the second treatment, the patient is given a stimulus dose slightly above seizure threshold for bilateral ECT or between 2.5 and 6 times the threshold for nondominant-unilateral ECT (McCall et al. 2000; Sackeim et al. 1987, 2000). Stimulus doses are then increased by about 5 J (25 mC) for each subsequent treatment in order to remain above the threshold. Other variations of the dose titration method have been published (Sackeim et al. 1987), and the practitioner should consult the instruction manual that accompanies his or her ECT device.

Treatments are usually given three times per week on alternate days in a course of 6–12 treatments. This number may vary depending on patient response. Treatments are usually discontinued when the patient has reached his or her best achievable baseline. The Mini-Mental State Exam (Folstein et al. 1975) and the Hamilton Rating Scale for Depression (Hamilton 1960) are used to monitor cognitive effects and clinical improvement, respectively.

ADVERSE EFFECTS

The most bothersome, commonly observed effect of ECT is transient cognitive impairment, usually in verbal memory (American Psychiatric Association Task Force on Electroconvulsive Therapy 2001). If a patient experiences significant cognitive impairment during a course of ECT, the physician should review medications, spacing of treatments, and ECT technique (i.e., laterality of electrode placement, stimulus dosing) (American Psychiatric Association Task Force on Electroconvulsive Therapy 2001) (Table 44–8). If bilateral electrode placement is being used, switching to nondominant-unilateral placement minimizes cognitive effects and may allow continuation of the ECT course. If treatments are being administered thrice weekly, reducing the frequency to twice or once weekly should be considered. The physician should also consider decreasing the stimulus dose, especially if bilateral electrode placement is used. If modifications in technique do not solve the problem, interruption or discontinuation of ECT should be considered. In the vast majority of cases, severe cognitive impairment does not occur, and, in fact, improved cognitive functioning is often observed as the patient's psychiatric condition improves (Abrams 1997). There are rare reports of patients claiming extensive, permanent memory loss after ECT; however, the explanation for such unusual claims is unclear.

Other complications, including unusually prolonged apnea, persistent cardiovascular dysfunction, and between-

TABLE 44–8. Measures to take if severe cognitive dysfunction develops

Switch from bilateral to unilateral electrode placement

Decrease treatment frequency (from thrice to twice or once weekly)

Decrease stimulus dose

Review concurrent medications for contribution to cognitive dysfunction

treatment seizure activity, are rare. Transient benign cardiac arrhythmias frequently occur during and immediately after the seizure but usually do not require any intervention. Myalgias, headache, and nausea are common reactions, are usually self-limited, and respond to symptomatic treatment.

MAINTENANCE ELECTROCONVULSIVE THERAPY

Continuation or maintenance ECT is used to sustain remission in some patients following response to acute ECT. Systematic studies are under way to better define the use of ECT as a maintenance therapy. Currently, however, practice patterns vary with ECT maintenance treatments being given on various schedules. A typical schedule involves weekly ECT for 4 weeks, followed by biweekly ECT for 8 weeks, then monthly ECT for a total of 6–12 months of treatment. Some practitioners combine maintenance ECT and psychotropic agents; however, this practice has not been adequately studied to provide firm recommendation. The American Psychiatric Association Task Force on Electroconvulsive Therapy (2001) recommends maintenance ECT for those patients who fail to remain well on medications alone following an initial positive ECT response.

ELECTROCONVULSIVE THERAPY IN PATIENTS WITH MEDICAL ILLNESS

Because the consultation-liaison psychiatrist sees many patients who have concurrent, serious medical illnesses, he or she may sometimes need to make modifications in ECT technique. In the following sections, we discuss a number of specific medical conditions encountered in the consultation-liaison setting that require special consideration in relation to the administration of ECT.

Central Nervous System Diseases

Parkinson's Disease

It has been estimated that up to 40%–60% of patients with Parkinson's disease experience major depression (Brown and Wilson 1972; Oh et al. 1992). ECT is effective in such patients not only for the psychiatric illness but also for the motor symptoms of the disease. A growing body of literature supports the efficacy of ECT for patients with Parkinson's disease (Andersen et al. 1987). The mechanism of action is probably related to ECT's dopamine-enhancing effects (Fochtmann 1988). Fink (1988) suggested that patients with Parkinson's disease that is refractory to medication be given a trial of ECT, particularly before surgery is considered (e.g., fetal tissue transplantation into the basal ganglia). ECT may be indicated as a primary treatment for Parkinson's disease that has become refractory to antiparkinsonian medications or for patients who cannot tolerate the side effects of such medications (Kellner et al. 1994). However, giving patients ECT earlier in the course of their illness may allow lower doses of antiparkinsonian medications to be used, thereby reducing the medication-related side effects that are so common in these patients (Rasmussen and Abrams 1991).

Dementia

When cognitive impairment is the result of depression (i.e., dementia syndrome of depression or pseudodementia), it is likely to improve as the depression improves. When dementia coexists with depression, cognitive function may improve as depression remits (Weiner and Coffey 1987). When patients with dementia experience cognitive worsening with ECT, the treatment frequency should be decreased from thrice to once or twice weekly and, if bilateral electrode placement is being used, a change to nondominant-unilateral placement should be considered (American Psychiatric Association Task Force on Electroconvulsive Therapy 2001).

Delirium

Although not a primary treatment for delirium, ECT has been reported to benefit patients with several specific causes of delirium. These include alcohol withdrawal delirium (Dudley and Williams 1972), delirium induced by withdrawal from phencyclidine (Dinwiddie et al. 1988; Rosen et al. 1984), and delirium caused by lupus erythematosus (Allen and Pitts 1978; Guze 1967) or enteric (typhoid) fever (Hafeiz 1987). The use of ECT in such cases is rare and should be reserved for patients with delirium refractory to other, more conventional treatments or for patients who require an urgent response (American Psychiatric Association Task Force on Electroconvulsive Therapy 2001).

Central Nervous System Tumor

ECT causes a transient increase in intracranial pressure, probably the result of increased cerebral blood flow during the seizure (Weiner and Coffey 1987). Increased intracranial pressure puts patients with space-occupying lesions at risk for brain herniation during ECT (Savitsky and Kavlinger 1953). However, modifications in technique can allow such patients to receive ECT successfully. These modifications include the use of antihypertensives, steroids, osmotic diuretics (e.g., mannitol), and hyperventilation. Zwil et al. (1990) prescribed oral dexamethasone, 40 mg/day, several days before beginning a course of ECT in a patient with an intracranial mass; no clinical signs of increased intracranial pressure were noted before or after treatment with ECT. Abrams (1997) recommended beginning parenteral steroids 24–48 hours before the first ECT treatment and continuing an oral dose during the ECT course. Not all brain tumors present the same risk. Small, slow-growing, or calcified tumors are less dangerous than large malignant tumors of more recent onset (Abrams 1997). For example, small meningiomas probably pose relatively little risk (Goldstein and Richardson 1988; Hsiao and Evans 1984; Kellner et al. 1991a; McKinney et al. 1998). Thus, the presence of a brain tumor, once considered an absolute contraindication to ECT, no longer automatically precludes a patient from receiving ECT (Abrams 1997), but the presence of a brain tumor remains one of the most serious risks (Maltbie et al. 1980).

Subdural Hematoma

A subdural hematoma is also a potential cause of increased intracranial pressure and, whenever possible, should be evacuated before ECT. There is at least one report of the successful use of ECT in a patient with a chronic subdural hematoma (Malek-Ahmadi et al. 1990).

Cerebrovascular Accident

There are no specific guidelines regarding how long one should delay ECT in a patient with a recent cerebrovascular accident (American Psychiatric Association Task Force on Electroconvulsive Therapy 2001). Generally, waiting weeks to months following a cerebrovascular accident is recommended before proceeding with ECT. The waiting period is particularly important following a hemorrhagic stroke because such patients are at risk for recurrent bleeding during the seizure (Weiner and Coffey 1993). However, if the waiting period is believed to

be dangerous itself (because of the severity of the psychiatric illness), ECT may be carried out sooner (Weiner and Coffey 1993). Longer waiting periods are advised if the cerebrovascular accident is large or is associated with significant edema or increased intracranial pressure (American Psychiatric Association Task Force on Electroconvulsive Therapy 2001).

Patients who have had a stroke and whose symptoms include spastic paralysis can become hyperkalemic because of the depolarizing effect of succinylcholine at the neuromuscular junction (this also occurs in patients with spinal cord injury). The use of a defasciculating agent (e.g., curare) is recommended in such cases (Weiner and Coffey 1987). In patients with ischemic cerebrovascular disease, intravenous antihypertensives must be used with caution in order to avoid hypotension. Control of hypertension is also important in patients with cerebrovascular disease (Weiner and Coffey 1987). ECT has been used safely in patients with cerebrovascular aneurysms, with attention to strict blood pressure control (Husum et al. 1983).

Epilepsy

The increase in seizure threshold during a course of ECT may reduce the frequency of spontaneous seizures in patients with epilepsy. ECT has rarely been used in patients with intractable epilepsy and status epilepticus (Dubovsky et al. 1985; Greisemer et al. 1997; Hsiao et al. 1987; Sackeim et al. 1983; Schnur et al. 1989). Patients with concurrent psychiatric illness and epilepsy can be given ECT safely. It is recommended that patients with epilepsy continue to receive their anticonvulsant medications during a course of ECT, although higher stimulus settings are typically necessary to produce adequate seizures (Abrams 1997). Continuing regularly prescribed anticonvulsants protects against the theoretical risk of spontaneous seizures during the course of ECT.

Brain Injury or Craniotomy

In patients with a skull fracture or craniotomy, the practitioner should not place ECT stimulus electrodes directly over a skull defect. This is to avoid unusually high current densities in the brain tissue underlying the defect (Everman et al. 1999; Weiner and Coffey 1987). Patients with recent brain trauma can have prolonged or spontaneous seizures and may need treatment with anticonvulsants (e.g., carbamazepine) while receiving ECT.

Intraventricular Shunts

Patients with intraventricular shunts may be given ECT safely; however, shunt patency must be established before beginning ECT, because shunt blockage may lead to increased intracranial pressure (Coffey et al. 1987). Patients should undergo brain imaging and funduscopic examination to rule out increased intracranial pressure before ECT begins.

Central Nervous System Infection

Patients with central nervous system infection should be given aggressive treatment for the infection before beginning ECT. Theoretically, because of the temporary disruption of the blood-brain barrier that accompanies electrically induced seizures, patients with such infections may be at risk for disseminated infection or sepsis if given ECT (Weiner and Coffey 1993). However, they can receive ECT successfully after the infection has resolved.

Chronic Pain

ECT may be of some benefit for patients with chronic pain, possibly through endorphin release (Mandel 1975). It is not yet clear whether ECT is beneficial only in patients with chronic pain and concomitant depression or if ECT is useful as a treatment for chronic pain alone.

Cardiovascular Disease

Myocardial Infarction and Ischemic Heart Disease

Serious cardiac complications are rare in patients who receive ECT; however, such complications represent the most common cause of death associated with ECT (American Psychiatric Association Task Force on Electroconvulsive Therapy 2001). In patients who have had a recent myocardial infarction, it is prudent to wait as long as possible (e.g., 1 month) before beginning ECT. This is not always feasible if a patient's psychiatric condition demands immediate treatment. In order to decrease the risk of cardiac ischemia, the use of nitrates and intravenous administration of β-blockers and careful attention to maximal oxygenation are all important measures. We recommend liberal use of intravenous labetalol, 5–20 mg, or intravenous esmolol, 5–60 mg, for patients with hypertension or tachycardia, and nitroglycerine paste or sublingual aerosol for patients with coronary artery disease. Also, regularly prescribed cardiac medications (e.g., antihypertensives or digoxin) should be given with a small sip of water the morning of each ECT session in order to optimize cardiovascular status before treatment.

Arrhythmias

Patients at risk for bradycardia (including those receiving sympathetic blocking agents) should receive an anticho-

linergic medication (e.g., glycopyrrolate or atropine) before each ECT session to protect against worsening bradycardia or asystole (American Psychiatric Association Task Force on Electroconvulsive Therapy 2001). Some practitioners recommend routine use of anticholinergics for all patients receiving ECT, particularly if the stimulus dose titration method is used at the first treatment (Beale et al. 1994a). Patients with tachyarrhythmias (as well as those with hypertension) may be given intravenous β-blockers. However, it is common for transient, inconsequential arrhythmias, tachycardia, and hypertension to persist for several minutes after ECT and to resolve spontaneously (Weiner and Coffey 1993). Therefore, unless life-threatening arrhythmias occur, it may be prudent to adopt a do-no-harm approach during the immediate postictal period. Patients who have other arrhythmias present before ECT may need further evaluation by a cardiologist who can provide recommendations for optimal hemodynamic management during ECT.

Cardiac Pacemakers

Many patients with cardiac pacemakers have safely received ECT (Alexopoulos and Frances 1980; Gibson et al. 1973; Tchou et al. 1989). Because the electrical stimulus itself does not reach the heart, there is little risk of interfering with pacemaker function. The cardiovascular effects of the increase in sympathetic tone can be modified with cardioactive agents (e.g., β-blockers), as in patients without pacemakers. If there is any doubt about the functioning of the pacemaker, a cardiologist should be consulted.

Other Medical Conditions

Pulmonary Disease

Patients with chronic obstructive pulmonary disease or asthma should have these conditions medically optimized before ECT. This may involve obtaining pulmonary function tests and consultation with an internist or pulmonary specialist (Knos and Sung 1993). For patients with reactive airway disease, inhalant bronchodilators (e.g., albuterol, two puffs) are recommended before each ECT session (Knos and Sung 1993). Theophylline (and aminophylline) should be avoided or kept in the low therapeutic range (e.g., <15 μg/mL) to prevent prolonged seizures or status epilepticus (Weiner and Coffey 1993).

Cancer

Petty and Noyes (1981) reported that depression is found in up to 25% of hospitalized patients with cancer. Levine et al. (1978) and others have found that it is often unrecognized in this population (see Chapter 29, this volume). Furthermore, particularly in patients with cancer, depression is inadequately treated once diagnosed (Derogatis et al. 1979). This may be the result of the mistaken notion that it is normal or expected for one to be depressed if he or she has cancer. Evans et al. (1988) found that nearly half of all patients with gynecological cancer had major or minor depression. These researchers also found that improved psychosocial adjustment and better life adaptation occurred in 12 patients with cancer after treatment of their depression (Evans et al. 1988). Many consultation-liaison psychiatrists urge that all patients with cancer receive a systematic assessment for depression (Bukberg et al. 1984; Evans et al. 1988).

Limited data exist on the use of ECT in depressed cancer patients. Goldfarb et al. (1967) reported on three patients with advanced carcinomatosis and depression who responded well to cancer chemotherapy and ECT. These authors and others have hypothesized that ECT may have some beneficial effect on immune function, thereby working synergistically with cancer chemotherapy in the treatment of the malignancy. Beale et al. (1997) reported the successful use of ECT in three patients with depression and cancer. As mentioned earlier, patients with intracranial tumors who require emergent treatment may receive ECT successfully, after careful consideration of the risk-benefit ratio.

Human Immunodeficiency Virus Disease and Acquired Immunodeficiency Syndrome

Much has been written about the neuropsychiatric manifestations of acquired immunodeficiency syndrome (AIDS) (see Chapter 36, this volume). Depressive syndromes are common among patients with human immunodeficiency virus (HIV) disease and AIDS (Dilley et al. 1985; Frierson and Lippman 1987; Perry and Tross 1984). Schaerf et al. (1989) reported successful treatment of depression using ECT in three HIV-seropositive men and one man with AIDS. None of the four patients had signs of increased intracranial pressure at the time of ECT. Kessing et al. (1994) reported the successful treatment of HIV-related catatonia with ECT.

Systemic Lupus Erythematosus

In a study of 101 patients with systemic lupus erythematosus (SLE), Guze (1967) found that psychiatric disorders were more prevalent among patients with SLE than in the general medical population. Psychiatric disorders were not attributable solely to steroid use (common in patients with SLE) because many who did not receive steroid therapy developed severe psychiatric disorders. SLE is known to be associated with catatonia in some patients with central nervous system manifestations. Case reports suggest that some patients who are unresponsive to traditional therapies may respond dramatically to ECT (Allen and Pitts 1978; Douglas and Schwartz 1982; Fricchione et al. 1990; Mac and Pardo 1983). While such patients are undergoing ECT, aggressive treatment of active SLE with concurrent immunosuppressive therapy is recommended (Fricchione et al. 1990).

Catatonia

Catatonia, a motor syndrome associated with both schizophrenia and mood disorders (Abrams and Taylor 1976), is a life-threatening neuropsychiatric condition. It is often refractory to pharmacotherapy but is dramatically responsive to bilateral ECT (Francis and Fink 1992; Mann et al. 1990; Pataki et al. 1992). Catatonia may also be associated with systemic medical disorders, and ECT is effective in these instances (Pataki et al. 1992). As noted earlier, ECT may be used as a first-line treatment in patients with catatonia and should be considered a treatment of choice once the diagnosis of catatonia is made (American Psychiatric Association Task Force on Electroconvulsive Therapy 2001).

Pregnancy

ECT has been used during all trimesters of pregnancy without adverse effects (Weiner and Coffey 1987). In fact, ECT may be preferred over pharmacotherapy during pregnancy and the nursing period because of concerns of teratogenicity from psychotropic medications (Abrams 1997). Fetal monitoring during ECT is recommended only in cases of high-risk pregnancy (Abrams 1997; Weiner and Coffey 1987). It is clinically prudent to have an obstetric consultant readily available when a pregnant woman undergoes ECT.

Organ Transplantation

Few data exist regarding organ transplantation and ECT. The teams of Kellner et al. (1991b) and Block et al. (1992) have each reported successful use of ECT without special modifications in a patient with depression who had undergone cardiac transplantation. Showalter et al. (1993) reported similar experience with a patient with depression who had had a liver transplant. Although we know of no reported cases of ECT in patients with renal or lung transplants, ECT would likely be useful in appropriately selected cases.

Neuroleptic Malignant Syndrome

ECT is an effective treatment for patients with neuroleptic malignant syndrome (NMS) (Casey 1987; Greenberg and Gujavarty 1985; Pearlman 1990). Davis et al. (1991) reported that 60% of patients with NMS respond, and the mortality rate is reduced by about one-half. Furthermore, the response rate in patients receiving ECT is equal to that of patients receiving pharmacological treatment (Davis et al. 1991). Abrams (1997) condemned the concurrent use of ECT and neuroleptics in the presence of NMS because this combination has resulted in death from cardiac arrest (Davis et al. 1991; Hughes 1986; Regestein et al. 1971). In our opinion, ECT is indicated as a treatment for NMS when patients do not respond to pharmacological treatment.

Electroconvulsive Therapy in Children and Adolescents

ECT is rarely used in children but is more commonly used in adolescents. Case report literature supports its use for well-selected cases of mania, psychotic mood disorders, and catatonia (Kellner et al. 1998).

Electroconvulsive Therapy in Elderly Patients

Increasing age has been associated with a favorable response to ECT (Carney et al. 1965; Mendels 1965; Roberts 1959). Abrams (1997) stated that "some of the most rewarding results with convulsive therapy are obtained in elderly, debilitated patients whose primary affective disorder masquerades as senile dementia" (p. 105). Modification in technique should include careful attention to cardiovascular status. Also, in patients with osteoporosis, avoidance of the cuffed limb method (see "Electroconvulsive Therapy Technique" section, earlier in this chapter) is advised (Abrams 1997).

CONCLUSION

ECT is a safe and effective treatment for a well-defined set of psychiatric conditions. Consultation-liaison psychiatrists should be familiar with modern methods of ECT delivery, particularly for patients who are medically ill. As we learn more about the mechanisms of action of ECT and as ECT becomes further refined, consultation-liaison psychiatrists will be increasingly able to provide this treatment to patients with concomitant serious medical and psychiatric illness.

REFERENCES

Abrams R: Electroconvulsive Therapy, 3rd Edition. New York, Oxford University Press, 1997

Abrams R, Taylor MA: Catatonia: a prospective study. Arch Gen Psychiatry 33:579–581, 1976

Abrams R, Swartz CM, Vedak C: Antidepressant effects of high-dose right unilateral electroconvulsive therapy. Arch Gen Psychiatry 48:746–748, 1991

Alexopoulos GS, Frances RJ: ECT and cardiac patients with pacemakers. Am J Psychiatry 137:111–112, 1980

Allen RE, Pitts FN: ECT for depression in patients with lupus erythematosus. Am J Psychiatry 135:367–368, 1978

American Psychiatric Association Task Force on Electroconvulsive Therapy: The Practice of Electroconvulsive Therapy: Recommendations for Treatment, Training, and Privileging. Washington, DC, American Psychiatric Association, 1990

American Psychiatric Association Task Force on Electroconvulsive Therapy [Weiner RD, Coffey CE, Fochtmann L, et al]: The Practice of Electroconvulsive Therapy: Recommendations for Treatment, Training, and Privileging, 2nd Edition. Washington, DC, American Psychiatric Association, 2001

Andersen K, Balldin J, Gottfries CG, et al: A double-blind evaluation of electroconvulsive therapy in Parkinson's disease with "on-off" phenomena. Acta Neurol Scand 76:191–199, 1987

Bailine SH, Rifkin A, Kayne E, et al: Comparison of bifrontal and bitemporal ECT for major depression. Am J Psychiatry 157:121–123, 2000

Beale MD: Stimulus dosing methods in ECT. Psychiatric Annals 28:510–512, 1998

Beale MD, Kellner CH: Electroconvulsive therapy and drug interactions, in Psychiatric Clinics of North America Annual of Drug Therapy: Treatment Resistance. Edited by Jefferson JW, Griest JH. Philadelphia, PA, WB Saunders, 1996

Beale MD, Kellner CH, Lemert R, et al: Skeletal muscle relaxation in patients undergoing electroconvulsive therapy (letter). Anesthesiology 80:957, 1994a

Beale MD, Kellner CH, Pritchett JT, et al: Stimulus dose-titration in ECT: a 2-year clinical experience. Convulsive Therapy 10:171–176, 1994b

Beale MD, Kellner CH, Parsons PJ: ECT for the treatment of mood disorders in cancer patients. Convulsive Therapy 13:222–226, 1997

Bernstein HJ, Beale MD, Burne CM, et al: Patient attitudes about ECT after treatment. Psychiatric Annals 28:524–527, 1998

Block M, Admon D, Bonne O, et al: Electroconvulsive therapy in a depressed heart transplant patient. Convulsive Therapy 8:290–293, 1992

Brown GL, Wilson WP: Parkinsonism and depression. South Med J 65:540–545, 1972

Bukberg J, Penman D, Holland JC: Depression in hospitalized cancer patients. Psychosom Med 46:199–212, 1984

Carney MWP, Roth M, Garside RF: The diagnosis of depressive syndromes and the prediction of ECT response. Br J Psychiatry 111:659–674, 1965

Casey DA: Electroconvulsive therapy in the neuroleptic malignant syndrome. Convulsive Therapy 3:278–283, 1987

Cerletti U, Bini L: Un nuevo metodo di shockterapie "L'elettroshock" [A new method of shock therapy]. Bollettino Accademia Medica Roma 64:136–138, 1938

Coffey CE, Hoffman G, Weiner RD: Electroconvulsive therapy in a depressed patient with a functioning ventriculo-atrial shunt. Convulsive Therapy 3:302–306, 1987

Davis JM, Janicak PG, Sakkus P, et al: Electroconvulsive therapy in the treatment of the neuroleptic malignant syndrome. Convulsive Therapy 7:111–120, 1991

d'Elia G: Comparison of electroconvulsive therapy with unilateral and bilateral stimulation, II: therapeutic efficiency in endogenous depression. Acta Psychiatr Scand Suppl 215:30–43, 1970

Derogatis LR, Feldstein M, Morrow G, et al: A survey of psychotropic drug prescriptions in an oncology population. Cancer 44:1919–1929, 1979

Dilley JW, Ochitill HN, Perl M, et al: Findings in psychiatric consultations with patients with acquired immune deficiency syndrome. Am J Psychiatry 142:82–86, 1985

Dinwiddie SH, Drevets WC, Smith DR: Treatment of phencyclidine-associated psychosis with ECT. Convulsive Therapy 4:230–235, 1988

Douglas CJ, Schwartz HI: ECT for depression caused by lupus cerebritis: a case report. Am J Psychiatry 139:1631–1632, 1982

Dubovsky SL, Gay M, Franks RD, et al: ECT in the presence of increased intracranial pressure and respiratory failure: case report. J Clin Psychiatry 46:489–491, 1985

Dudley WH Jr, Williams JG: Electroconvulsive therapy in delirium tremens. Compr Psychiatry 13:357–360, 1972

Evans DL, McCartney CF, Haggerty JJ: Treatment of depression in cancer patients is associated with better life adaptation: a pilot study. Psychosom Med 50:72–76, 1988

Everman PO, Kellner CH, Beale MD: Modified electrode placement in patients with neurosurgical skull defects. J ECT 15:237–239, 1999

Fink M: ECT for Parkinson's disease? Convulsive Therapy 4:189–191, 1988

Fochtmann L: A mechanism for the efficacy of ECT in Parkinson's disease. Convulsive Therapy 4:321–327, 1988

Folstein MF, Folstein SE, McHugh PR: Mini-Mental State: a practical method for grading the cognitive state of patients for the clinician. J Psychiatr Res 12:189–198, 1975

Francis A, Fink M: ECT response in catatonia (letter). Am J Psychiatry 149:581–582, 1992

Freeman CP, Kendell RE: Patients' experiences of and attitudes to electroconvulsive therapy. Ann N Y Acad Sci 462:341–352, 1986

Fricchione GL, Kaufman LD, Gruber BL, et al: Electroconvulsive therapy and cyclophosphamide in combination for severe neuropsychiatric lupus with catatonia. Am J Med 88:442–443, 1990

Frierson RL, Lippman SB: Psychological implications of AIDS. Am Fam Physician 35:109–116, 1987

Gibson TC, Leaman DM, Devors J, et al: Pacemaker function in relation to electroconvulsive therapy. Chest 63:1025–1027, 1973

Goldfarb C, Driesen J, Cole D: Psychophysiologic aspects of malignancy. Am J Psychiatry 123:1545–1552, 1967

Goldstein MZ, Richardson C: Meningioma with depression: ECT risk or benefit? Psychosomatics 29:349–351, 1988

Greenberg LB, Gujavarty K: The neuroleptic malignant syndrome: review and report of three cases. Compr Psychiatry 26:63–70, 1985

Greisemer DA, Kellner CH, Beale MD, et al: Electroconvulsive therapy for treatment of intractable seizures: initial findings in two children. Neurology 49:1389–1392, 1997

Guze SB: The occurrence of psychiatric illness in systemic lupus erythematosus. Am J Psychiatry 123:1562–1570, 1967

Hafeiz HB: Psychiatric manifestations of enteric fever. Acta Psychiatr Scand 75:69–73, 1987

Hamilton M: A rating scale for depression. J Neurol Neurosurg Psychiatry 23:56–62, 1960

Hsiao JK, Evans DL: ECT in a depressed patient after craniotomy. Am J Psychiatry 141:442–444, 1984

Hsiao JK, Messenheimer JH, Evans DL: ECT and neurological disorders. Convulsive Therapy 3:121–136, 1987

Hughes JR: ECT during and after the neuroleptic malignant syndrome: case report. J Clin Psychiatry 47:42–43, 1986

Husum B, Vester-Andersen T, Buchmann G, et al: Electroconvulsive therapy and intracranial aneurysm: prevention of blood pressure elevation in a normotensive patient by hydralazine and propranolol. Anesthesia 38:1205–1207, 1983

Kaplan HI, Saddock BJ: Pocket Handbook of Clinical Psychiatry. Baltimore, MD, Williams & Wilkins, 1990

Kellner CH, McCall WV: Novel electrode placements: time to reassess (editorial). J ECT 15:115–117, 1999

Kellner CH, Burns CM, Bernstein JH, et al: Safe administration of ECT in a patient with a calcified frontal mass (letter). J Neuropsychiatry Clin Neurosci 3:353–354, 1991a

Kellner CH, Monroe RR, Burns CM, et al: Electroconvulsive therapy in a patient with a heart transplant (letter). N Engl J Med 325:669, 1991b

Kellner CH, Beale MD, Pritchett JT, et al: Parkinson's disease and ECT: the case for further study. Psychopharmacol Bull 30:495–500, 1994

Kellner CH, Pritchett JM, Beale MD, et al: Handbook of ECT. Washington, DC, American Psychiatric Press, 1997

Kellner CH, Beale MD, Bernstein HJ: ECT in children and adolescents, in Handbook of Child and Adolescent Psychiatry. Edited by Noshpitz JD. New York, Wiley, 1998, pp 269–272

Kessing L, LaBianca JH, Bolwig TG: HIV-induced stupor treated with ECT. Convulsive Therapy 10:232–235, 1994

Knos GB, Sung YF: ECT anesthesia strategies in the high risk medical patient, in Psychiatric Care of the Medical Patient, 2nd Edition. Edited by Stoudemire A, Fogel B. New York, Oxford University Press, 1993, pp 225–240

Letemendia FJ, Delva NJ, Rodenburg M, et al: Therapeutic advantage of bifrontal electrode placement in ECT. Psychol Med 23:349–360, 1993

Levine PM, Siwerfarb PM, Lipowski ZJ: Mental disorders in cancer patients. Cancer 42:1385–1391, 1978

Mac DS, Pardo MP: Systemic lupus erythematosus and catatonia: a case report. J Clin Psychiatry 44:155–156, 1983

Malek-Ahmadi P, Beceiro JR, McNeil BW, et al: Electroconvulsive therapy and chronic subdural hematoma. Convulsive Therapy 6:38–41, 1990

Maltbie AA, Wingfield MS, Volow MR, et al: Electroconvulsive therapy in the presence of brain tumor: case reports and an evaluation risk. J Nerv Ment Dis 168:400–405, 1980

Mandel MR: Electroconvulsive therapy for chronic pain associated with depression. Am J Psychiatry 132:632–636, 1975

Mann SC, Caroff SN, Bleier HR, et al: Electroconvulsive therapy of the lethal catatonia syndrome. Convulsive Therapy 6:239–247, 1990

McCall WV, Reboussin DM, Weiner RD, et al: Titrated, moderately suprathreshold versus fixed, high-dose RUL ECT: acute antidepressant and cognitive effects. Arch Gen Psychiatry 57:438–444, 2000

McKinney PA, Beale MD, Kellner CH: Electroconvulsive therapy in a patient with a cerebellar meningioma. J ECT 14:49–52, 1998

MECTA Corporation: Instruction Manual, SR and JR Models. Portland, OR, 1986

Mendels J: Electroconvulsive therapy and depression, I: the prognostic significance of clinical factors. Br J Psychiatry 111:675–681, 1965

Oh JJ, Rummans TA, O'Conner MK, et al: Cognitive impairment after ECT in patients with Parkinson's disease and psychiatric illness (letter). Am J Psychiatry 149:271, 1992

Ottoson JO: Experimental studies of the mode of action of electroconvulsive therapy. Acta Psychiatr Scand Suppl 145:1–141, 1960

Pataki J, Zervas I, Jandorf L: Catatonia in a university inpatient service (1985–1990). Convulsive Therapy 8:167–173, 1992

Pearlman C: Neuroleptic malignant syndrome and electroconvulsive therapy. Convulsive Therapy 6:251–254, 1990

Perry SW, Tross S: Psychiatric problems of AIDS inpatients at the New York Hospital: preliminary report. Public Health Rep 99:200–205, 1984

Pettinati HM, Stephens SM, Willie KM, et al: Evidence for less improvement in depression in patients taking benzodiazepines during unilateral ECT. Am J Psychiatry 147:1029–1036, 1990

Petty R, Noyes R Jr: Depression in cancer. Biol Psychiatry 16:1203–1221, 1981

Rasmussen K, Abrams R: Treatment of Parkinson's disease with electroconvulsive therapy. Psychiatr Clin North Am 14:925–933, 1991

Regestein QR, Kahn CB, Siegel AJ, et al: A case of catatonia occurring simultaneously with severe urinary retention. J Nerv Ment Dis 152:432–435, 1971

Roberts JM: Prognostic factors in the electroshock treatment of depressive states, I: clinical features from history and examination. Journal of Mental Science 105:693–702, 1959

Rosen AM, Mukherjee S, Shinbach K: The efficacy of ECT in phencyclidine-induced psychosis. J Clin Psychiatry 45:220–222, 1984

Sackeim HA, Decina P, Prohovnik I, et al: Anticonvulsant and antidepressant properties of electroconvulsive therapy: a proposed mechanism of action. Biol Psychiatry 18:1302–1310, 1983

Sackeim H[A], Decina P, Prohovnik I, et al: Seizure threshold in electroconvulsive therapy. Arch Gen Psychiatry 44:355–360, 1987

Sackeim H[A], Prudic J, Devanand DP, et al: Effects of stimulus intensity and electrode placement on the efficacy and cognitive side-effects of electroconvulsive therapy. N Engl J Med 328:839–846, 1993

Sackeim HA, Prudic J, Devanand DP, et al: A prospective double-blind comparison of bilateral and right unilateral ECT at different stimulus intensities. Arch Gen Psychiatry 57:425–434, 2000

Savitsky N, Kavlinger W: Electroshock in the presence of organic disease of the nervous system. Journal of Hillside Hospital 2:3–22, 1953

Schaerf FW, Miller RR, Lipsey JR, et al: ECT for major depression in four patients infected with human immunodeficiency virus. Am J Psychiatry 146:782–784, 1989

Schnur D, Mukherjee S, Silver J, et al: ECT in the treatment of episodic aggressive dyscontrol in psychotic patients. Convulsive Therapy 5:353–361, 1989

Showalter PE, Young SA, Bilello JF, et al: Electroconvulsive therapy for depression in a liver transplant patient (letter). Psychosomatics 34:537, 1993

Swartz CM, Abrams R: ECT Instruction Manual, 5th Edition. Lake Bluff, IL, Somatics Inc., 1994

Tchou PT, Piasecki E, Gutmann M, et al: Psychological support and psychiatric management of patients with automatic implantable cardioverter defibrillators. Int J Psychiatry Med 19:393–407, 1989

Weiner RD, Coffey CE: Electroconvulsive therapy in the medically ill, in Principles of Medical Psychiatry. Edited by Stoudemire A, Fogel BS. New York, Grune & Stratton, 1987, pp 113–134

Weiner RD, Coffey CE: Electroconvulsive therapy in the medical and neurologic patient, in Psychiatric Care of the Medical Patient, 2nd Edition. Edited by Stoudemire A, Fogel BS. New York, Oxford University Press, 1993, pp 207–224

Weiner RD, Whanger AB, Erwin CW, et al: Prolonged confusional state and EEG seizure activity following concurrent ECT and lithium use. Am J Psychiatry 137:1452–1453, 1980

Weiner RD, Rogers HJ, Davidson JR, et al: Effects of stimulus parameters on cognitive side effects. Ann N Y Acad Sci 462:315–325, 1986

Zwil AS, Bowring MA, Price TRP, et al: Prospective electroconvulsive therapy in the presence of intracranial tumor. Convulsive Therapy 6:299–307, 1990

45

Psychotherapy

Don R. Lipsitt, M.D.

In 1904, Freud acknowledged that "psychotherapy is in no way a modern method of healing" (p. 250). "On the contrary," he wrote, "it is the most ancient form of therapy in medicine" (Freud 1904/1959, p. 250). Although psychoanalysis drifted from its medical roots, Freud nonetheless continued to link psychotherapy to medicine. Believing that physicians must recognize the psychotherapeutic effects of their ministrations, Freud (1904/1959) lectured the College of Physicians in Vienna that all physicians were "continuously practicing psychotherapy" even without intent (p. 251). It was, Freud said, "disadvantageous...to leave entirely in the hands of the patient what the mental factor in your treatment of him shall be" (p. 251). With these cautionary words, Freud urged his listeners to "exert a mental influence" on patients whose conditions warranted it. These words, in effect, proclaimed the useful application of psychoanalytic principles and understanding to the more or less routine practice of medicine and, in so doing, underscored their importance to future developments in consultation-liaison psychiatry.

Despite such early intimations of the relevance of psychotherapy to patients in medical settings, surprisingly little has been written or researched on psychotherapy in patients who are medically ill. Until recently, techniques for research and data analysis on medical inpatients have been inadequate to the task. Patients seen in psychiatric consultation on inpatient medical-surgical services have a multiplicity of medical and psychiatric diagnoses, hospital stay is brief, assessment is often abbreviated, and upon discharge patients are often lost to follow-up. Such handicaps have limited the opportunities for outcome and efficacy studies of medical psychotherapy on inpatient settings. But a number of good outpatient studies have begun to appear, especially of the treatment of depression in medically ill patients (Black et al. 1998; Koenig 1998; Moynihan et al. 1998; Spiegel 1997; Speckens et al. 1995; Von Korff et al. 1998; Walker et al. 2000; Ward et al. 2000). Grourep treatment has been particularly useful in long-term outcome studies, especially of patients with cancer (Fawzy and Fawzy 1994; Spiegel et al. 1989).

Some psychoanalytic accounts (Alexander 1950) of the treatment of psychosomatic diseases in the 1940s and 1950s are highly instructive but have relatively limited application to clinical situations encountered by the consultation-liaison psychiatrist in contemporary medical settings. The more circumscribed psychosomatic approach of earlier decades has been further elaborated—based on scientific progress and greater understanding of the complex determinants of illness—into an integrated biopsychosocial matrix (Engel 1977; Yamada et al. 2000). In this setting, psychodynamic principles of working with patients who are medically ill continue, nonetheless, to have selective utility and to enhance the consultation-liaison psychiatrist's versatility.

Systematic application of early findings, however, has occurred only since about 1940 (Lipowski 1986). At a time when most psychiatrists in the United States confined their interest and attention to the treatment of mental illness in large remote institutions, a small number of psychoanalyst-psychiatrists became interested in studying patients with psychosomatic diseases such as hypertension, peptic ulcer disease, and neurodermatitis. Attempts to understand the "mysterious leap from the mind to the body" (Deutsch 1959, p. 101) generated hypotheses about mind-body interrelations that could be studied systematically in medical settings. These endeavors coincided with the evolution of general hospital psychiatry, which burgeoned during and after World War II (Lipsitt 2000).

Consultation-liaison psychiatry became the beneficiary of these trends in psychoanalysis, psychosomatic medicine, and general hospital psychiatry. From these early foundations have emerged a variety of psychotherapeutic approaches to the broad spectrum of illness and disease encountered in medical settings today.

In this chapter, I 1) define medical psychotherapy as it is similar to and differs from psychoanalytic and psychodynamic interventions, 2) describe the unique aspects of psychotherapy in the general hospital and the specialized skills and tasks of the consultation-liaison psychiatrist, 3) enumerate and describe varieties of psychotherapy used in the medical setting, 4) illustrate psychotherapeutic applications of consultation-liaison psychiatry, and 5) demonstrate a specialized model of outpatient medical psychotherapy.

DEFINITION OF MEDICAL PSYCHOTHERAPY

Although many mental health professionals work with patients in a variety of medical settings, I focus on medical psychotherapy based on the medical model. Psychotherapeutic intervention is defined here as that which is intentionally (as contrasted with coincidentally) exercised on patients with medical illness by physicians with psychiatric training. This should not, however, obscure other practitioners' considerable psychotherapeutic effects on the state of health or illness of individuals who are medically ill.

It is well known that many nonpsychiatrist physicians are skilled in creating a psychotherapeutic experience for their patients (Adler 1997). As Marmor (1979a) stated, "The very fact that the patient is able to discuss a personal problem in an ambiance of hope and positive expectancy is the beginning of a therapeutic experience" (p. 523). Indeed, the initial interview, skillfully negotiated, is "a therapeutic transaction, although neither the physician nor the patient may consciously regard it as such" (p. 523). Consider the following brief case example:

Case Example 1

A recalcitrant, angry male patient in his 40s, with chronic obstructive lung disease, had been refusing all treatments from the staff. In their frustration, the staff requested a psychiatric consultation. The patient, facing toward the wall and mostly mute, at first refused to acknowledge the psychiatrist. When he was asked why a psychiatrist was called, he furiously—with expletives—said he didn't know and told the psychiatrist to leave. A comment from the psychiatrist that he would also be mad as hell if someone called a psychiatrist without explaining it to him elic-

ited a gesture of acquiescence from the patient as he turned to face the psychiatrist and vociferously began listing a series of complaints against the staff (some of which were not unfounded).

In this case, a potentially futile interaction was converted to a useful intervention through a tactful interview technique.

What the psychiatrist does is very different from what the primary care physician does, although the various elements of medical care, when sensitively attended to, can carry incidental emotional benefit for the patient via the physician-patient relationship, the placebo effect, tactful history-taking, and physical examination. Many nonpsychiatrist physicians have honed their interview and counseling skills to a high degree of sophistication, but they generally are not capable of practicing medical psychotherapy without the intense case supervision and special training of the psychiatrist (Balint 1964; Greenhill 1981).

Other nonpsychiatrist mental health practitioners include psychiatric nurse clinicians, social workers, and psychologists, who may indeed be part of the consultation-liaison team. Although they contribute an invaluable dimension to comprehensive patient care, they do not practice medical psychotherapy as herein defined. I refer here essentially to psychiatrists who identify themselves as consultation-liaison practitioners and who apply the principles of that special domain of psychiatry and medicine to a great spectrum of situations, conditions, systems, and settings related to the general practice of medicine. This definition does, however, exempt psychiatrists who—by choice or chance—have excluded patients with significant medical disease from their practices.

Commonalities in Psychotherapies

A noted psychiatrist has written that "present-day theories about how people become emotionally ill are exceeded in number only by the available remedies for making them well again" (Wolberg 1972, p. xi). Some investigators now believe that there are at least 400 forms of psychotherapy (Waldinger 1990). Virtually all these forms, including the rituals and incantations of shamans, have been accorded their share of cures. Some forms have attributed cures to the transference relationship between healer and patient (Gitelson 1973), and others have suggested the power of persuasion (Frank 1973), the placebo effect (Shapiro 1959), or merely empathic listening (Jackson 1992) as the preeminent therapeutic ingredient.

Psychotherapy, as described and practiced today in all its forms and by all its practitioners, has no unanimity of definition. Outcome studies are a recent invention, and the methodologies, data, and results often are controversial (Wallerstein 1975, 1996). Not all psychotherapies (e.g., psychoanalysis) readily lend themselves to methodological scrutiny, although some progress has been made in that direction (Bachrach et al. 1991; Jones et al. 1992; Marshall et al. 1996; Vaughan et al. 2000). Whatever the theoretical underpinnings and psychotherapeutic techniques, however, most psychotherapies are believed to share some commonalities (Barber et al. 2001).

So plentiful are the variables that influence the outcome of illness that a single satisfactory definition of psychotherapy is untenable. But the usual requisites of virtually all forms of successful psychotherapy include a socially sanctioned healer, professionally trained and accepted by the patient and his or her immediate social group; an individual who seeks relief from suffering; and a more-or-less structured situation in which improvement in the patient's condition is offered and expected (Frank 1973). The coloration of the treatment by the therapist's personality, the setting in which therapy takes place, the chemistry or alliance between the participants, and the theoretical assumptions undoubtedly influence the process and the result.

Whatever the differences in these features, all psychotherapeutic interventions rely on some form of communication and a sharing of interest and expectation on the part of patient and therapist. One attempt at a comprehensive definition (Polatin 1966, p. 41) suggested that "psychotherapy is a form of treatment in psychiatry relying essentially on the verbal communication between therapist and patient and on the interaction between the personalities of therapist and patient in a dynamic interpersonal relationship, whereby maladaptive behavior is altered toward a more effective adaptation, relief of symptoms occurs, and insights are developed."

Bibring (1954) suggested that virtually all psychotherapies make use of five major psychotherapeutic principles: suggestion, abreaction, manipulation (related to furthering the aims of effective therapy), clarification, and interpretation. In Bibring's exposition, interpretation is the "supreme agent" of psychoanalysis, whereas psychodynamic and other psychotherapies are constructed around various selections and combinations of all five techniques. The unique aspects of psychotherapy in the general hospital (discussed later in this chapter in the sections "Unique Aspects of Psychotherapy With Medically Ill Patients" and "Illustrations of Psychotherapeutic Applications in Consultation-Liaison Psychiatry") lend themselves more to techniques other than interpretation, although opportunities for use of this technique are not entirely absent.

Psychoanalytic Foundations

Although psychoanalysis was utilized in medical settings during the heyday of psychosomatic medicine, this is no longer the case in its orthodox form (Lazarus 2000). Nonetheless, basic concepts on which this psychotherapy rests, such as transference, resistance, the unconscious, and repression, remain as significant aspects of many other psychotherapeutic approaches. Opportunities abound in inpatient medical situations to recognize management problems that are caused by maladaptive transferences (Groves 1975), by unconscious meanings of symptoms or procedures (Abram 1970), and by fantasies or complications related to neuropsychiatric syndromes. Furthermore, the developmental aspects of psychoanalytic theory are relevant to all of medicine; they help the physician to understand time-related changes in each individual's life cycle, thus permitting illness to be viewed in relation to normal growth. A physician would realize, for example, that the psychological tasks confronting a woman with abnormal menstruation at menarche (i.e., in adolescence) are very different from those confronting a woman with the same symptom at menopause (i.e., in adulthood). Because of the importance of the phase in the life cycle, all case presentations in medicine begin with the age of the patient as a backdrop for all else about the individual.

Other derivatives of psychoanalysis that are relevant to consultation-liaison psychiatry include "working through," "grief work," and "object identification" (O'Dowd and Gomez 2001). An example in which these concepts apply might be the woman whose physically painful left arm improves only after discussion (with tears) of her intense dependency on a mother who died after a stroke that affected the same limb as the patient's. Furthermore, the psychoanalytic model of depression as anger directed inward is widely subscribed to in treating all varieties and degrees of depression in medical-surgical patients (Jarvik et al. 1982; Klerman et al. 1984). Many interpretive leaps made in the medical setting by consultation-liaison psychiatrists are based on much cumulative psychoanalytic wisdom even when sufficient time for "working through" is unavailable.

Psychoanalytic knowledge has also contributed greatly to the need to recognize the uniqueness of each individual in personality structure; in specific patterns of response to stress (Horowitz 1973); in use of defense mechanisms; and in production of memories, fantasies, wishes, dreams, thoughts, and feelings. Whether dealing with patients' adjustment disorders, coping skills, anxiety, depression, psychosis, or personality disorders, psychoanalytic insights contribute significantly to medical psychotherapy. However, psychoanalysis, in its full application, is reserved for outpatient settings with carefully selected candidates for treatment.

Psychodynamic Foundations

Psychodynamic psychotherapy draws heavily on the theories and techniques of psychoanalysis but differs in several important respects (Wallerstein 1975). Dynamic psychotherapy is more focused on symptoms and their relief than on restructuring of personality. It utilizes a more or less free interview method rather than free association to generate data under limited regressive conditions. Its goals are more modest, seeking stabilization rather than reformation. It focuses more on the patient's life situation and environmental circumstances in the therapeutic relationship, whereas psychoanalysis puts a higher premium on intrapsychic conflict and the transference neurosis. By lifting repression and making the unconscious conscious, psychodynamic psychotherapy aims to alleviate symptoms in the context of a corrective experience.

Many authors who have written of medical psychotherapy suggest that a psychodynamic orientation is the sine qua non of consultation-liaison psychiatry on which foundation other psychotherapeutic interventions rest (Gabbard 1990; Green 1993; Greenhill 1981; Hackett and Weisman 1960a, 1960b; Horowitz 1990; Levenson and Hales 1993; Luborsky 1990; Perry et al. 1987; Ursano and Hales 1986; Wolberg 1972). According to Gabbard (1990),

> dynamic psychiatry...provides a coherent conceptual framework within which all treatments are prescribed. Regardless of whether the treatment is dynamic psychotherapy, behavior therapy, or pharmacotherapy, it is *dynamically informed*.... [A] crucial component of the dynamic psychiatrist's expertise is knowing when to avoid exploratory psychotherapy in favor of treatments that do not threaten the patient's psychic equilibrium. (p. 4)

For example, in negotiating psychopharmacologic treatment for a young woman who was fearful of addiction, it was important to know that her father was an alcohol abuser and her depressed mother, with whom she was negatively identified, had overdosed on pills; significant related fears and fantasies needed to be addressed before she would agree to try medication.

Expanding on Gabbard's remarks, Levenson and Hales (1993) suggested that

> mental health professionals should focus their initial interview on a psychodynamic understanding of patients and their situation, whereas subsequent treatments may include a variety of specialized techniques such as cognitive restructuring, hypnosis, psychopharmacology, or more traditionally recognizable psychodynamic interventions. (p. 4)

UNIQUE ASPECTS OF PSYCHOTHERAPY WITH MEDICALLY ILL PATIENTS

Variations From Traditional Psychotherapy

The experience of the consultation-liaison psychiatrist informs him or her that standard definitions of psychotherapy do not fully represent the interaction between the psychiatrist and the patient who is medically ill. Most psychotherapies encompass specific theories, selection criteria, and techniques and may be prescribed in much the way medications are for specific symptoms or syndromes. Psychotherapeutic intervention in the consultation-liaison context, however, relies more on a potpourri of eclecticism required to understand patients and their often unspoken problems, the relationships of staff to patients and to each other, the dynamics of interviewing (both medical and psychiatric), and the systems structure of the hospital setting. To date, however, there is no systematized theory of consultation-liaison intervention that parallels that of psychotherapy as traditionally defined (Greenhill 1981).

Referral

Although psychotherapy in the consultation-liaison setting encompasses essential components of the therapeutic experience such as consultation, evaluation, diagnosis, formulation, intervention, and education, the referral process differs significantly from that of traditional outpatient psychotherapy cases. All patients who are referred to the consultation-liaison psychiatrist are usually seen, unless the patient refuses the consultation, but not all referrals will be appropriate for every phase of the psychotherapeutic process. Even with a reluctant patient, a satisfactory encounter with a psychiatrist may ameliorate fantasies, distortions, and fears and thus facilitate future receptivity to psychiatric consultation or evaluation, if needed.

Traditional selection criteria do not apply in the inpatient medical setting. The consultation-liaison psychiatrist usually goes to the patient rather than having the patient seek him or her out. The psychiatrist's patients usually have not identified a particular problem of an emotional nature for which they seek help; it is more often the attending physician, house officer, or nurse who requests consultation. This would appear to violate those definitions of psychotherapy that require a patient to seek the help of the therapist and to have expectations of outcome that match those of the psychiatrist. Patients in the consultation-liaison setting, therefore, seldom have the motivation for or receptivity to psychotherapy in its purer sense; some would consider this orientation as a dilution or an alloying of the more refined definition of psychotherapy.

Setting

Although consultation-liaison psychiatrists provide their services in a variety of outpatient facilities, the setting of the medical psychotherapist is often the bedside, a hospital conference room, an intensive care unit (ICU), or—in special circumstances—even a hallway, not a well-furnished consulting office. Hospitalized patients wear hospital garb and are exposed to an extraordinary lack of privacy. The stereotypical 50-minute hour is nowhere more challenged than in these environs, where encounters may last anywhere from a few minutes to more than an hour. Initial consultations may have to be performed in installments, depending on the patient's and the staff members' schedules.

Patients are often ill prepared for receiving the psychiatrist, and part of the initial encounter may be spent clarifying the purpose of the visit and dealing with distortions, befuddlement, anger, or resistance. The consultation-liaison psychiatrist may also have to address negative attitudes toward psychiatry among the staff as well as in the patient and his or her family.

In this atypical patient assessment context, it is impressive that medically hospitalized patients are so frequently receptive to psychiatric attention. An alliance often develops within minutes, and effective psychotherapeutic intervention can be achieved during a single bedside visit (Lipsitt 1985). Consider the following brief case example:

Case Example 2

House physicians were called for a consultation on a 42-year-old obese woman with asthma who remained "excessively long" in the hospital after her asthma was considered quite ameliorated. Because she cried when they wanted to discharge her, they assumed she was depressed. A 15-minute interview revealed that she was not depressed but was afraid to return home where her husband was very sick. She feared he might worsen and felt guilty for not being able to care for him. She explained she was too embarrassed and proud to be able to reveal this to her doctors. Social Services was enlisted, arrangements were made for help at home, and the patient readily accepted discharge to home.

With such brief contacts, the consultation-liaison psychiatrist is frequently called on to diagnose and treat emotional idiosyncrasies as well as a variety of anxiety reactions and depressive disorders, acute grief, delirium, conversion, adjustment disorders, psychosis, and atypical pain reactions to acute physical illness. These interventions, tailored to individual personality styles and defenses, selectively involve the psychotherapeutic principles mentioned in Table 45–1 to alleviate symptoms, clarify distortions, and minimize the negative effects of the patient's dysfunctional relationships with staff that may compromise medical care.

Psychotherapeutic Range and Limitations

An essential skill of the consultation-liaison psychiatrist in the consultative role is the ability to apply a variety of brief psychotherapeutic techniques (Groves and Kucharski 1991). He or she may enlist a broad range of applications from brief (Budman and Stone 1983; Horowitz and Kaltreider 1979; Malan 1963; Mann 1973; Marmor 1979b; Sifneos 1972; Strupp and Binder 1984) to very brief (Liberzon et al. 1992) to single session (Bloom 1981) to briefest (Blacher 1984), as well as to crisis intervention as practiced during wartime and other emergencies.

This array has been classified as supportive-suppressive-directive or exploratory-expressive-ventilative, according to the general aim and mode of treatment (Harrison and Carek 1966). Psychotherapies are further characterized according to the therapist's stance in any particular situation as interpretive, suggestive, persuasive, or educative. Furthermore, depending on the depth of psychic exploration, they may be said to be superficial or deep. The duration of time varies from brief to prolonged, and psychotherapy may be applied to an individual, a group, or a family. It is not unusual to include staff in joint meetings with patients and/or their families in order to improve understanding, communication, and knowledge, as for example in working with borderline patients or clarifying the wishes and needs of terminally ill patients.

TABLE 45–1.   Common psychotherapeutic principles

		Use in type of therapy	
Principle	Description	Expressive	Supportive
Suggestion	Induction of mental processes by therapist	+	+++
Abreaction	Emotional discharge, catharsis	+	++
Manipulation	Use of patient's existing emotional systems to achieve therapeutic change	+	++++
Clarification	Helping patient "to see more clearly"	+++	+
Interpretation	Attempt to change attitudes by explaining unconscious thoughts	++++	+

Note.   + = least use; + + + + = most use.

Source.   Adapted from Bibring E: "Psychoanalysis and the Dynamic Psychotherapies." *Journal of the American Psychoanalytic Association* 2:745–770, 1954.

The more exploratory techniques are rarely used in the hospital setting. They are more likely to be utilized in outpatient settings with patients discharged from the hospital or in need of more protracted treatment for chronic conditions. Even when hospitalized patients appear suitable for more insight-oriented psychotherapy, abbreviated hospital stays in today's medical care system often preclude such treatment.

Consultation-liaison psychiatrists and liaison teams have found treatment in groups to be useful for patients who tend to express affects through somatic representation. Such groups tend to facilitate communication with several people (rather than one person), who may share similar diagnoses, characteristics, interests, anxieties, and misperceptions about illness. Patients in groups learn from one another, depend less on the therapist, maintain a focus on purpose, share stressful experiences, and sometimes model behavior after the therapist or other group members. Such groups may be psychoeducational, supportive, expressive, homogeneous or heterogeneous (regarding illness), closed or open ended, and inpatient or outpatient, although reduced hospital stays have made the former less practical.

Groups have been useful for a wide range of physical conditions, including human immunodeficiency virus (HIV) disease and acquired immunodeficiency syndrome (AIDS), Parkinson's disease, multiple sclerosis, rheumatoid arthritis, cancer, post–myocardial infarction, organ transplantation, respiratory diseases, gastrointestinal (GI) disorders, and chronic somatization (Cunningham et al. 1978; Spira and Spiegel 1993; Stein and Weiner 1978; Yalom 1975). Patients who are sometimes thought to have alexithymia (Sifneos 1973) are found to become more communicative in group settings and to relinquish denial that has previously hampered relationships with others. For example, a woman with an avoidant lifestyle developed hypertension in her early 60s, and although she said that group psychotherapy was not her "thing," she reluctantly accepted referral to a relaxation group for people with hypertension. She not only lowered her pressure but also became an enthusiast of the group, developed social relationships, signed up for another group course, and extolled its virtues to all who would listen.

Brevity, the Soul of Consultation-Liaison Psychiatry

Because of the time-limited nature of episodic acute illness, the consultation-liaison therapist's orientation is, of necessity, one of brevity. Psychotherapy in the consultation-liaison setting cannot take on the quality of specificity that is defined by the models of brief psychotherapy identified with psychotherapists such as Sifneos (1984), Mann (1973), Davanloo (1978), Malan (1963), Marmor (1979b), and others. These models, all basically psychoanalytic focal techniques utilizing stringent selection criteria, represent a carefully elaborated set of interventionist techniques not easily adapted to the needs of the consultation-liaison psychiatrist in the general hospital. An evaluation of the hospitalized medical patient typically includes criteria for brief or short-term psychotherapy (Table 45–2). Although many patients meet several of these criteria, it is rare that patients in this setting would be able to participate in formal psychotherapy while hospitalized because of logistical constraints described previously and because they are physically ill.

TABLE 45–2.   Selection criteria for brief psychotherapy

Presence of intact attention, cognition, and concentration
Evidence of ego strength
At least one meaningful interpersonal relationship
Ability to interact in the first session
Psychological-mindedness or capacity for insight
Ability to experience feelings
Experience and identification of focal conflict
Motivation to change

Source.   Adapted from Marmor 1979a.

Many patients in the general hospital have illnesses that have compromised their ability to maintain attention, concentration, and orientation (e.g., brain disorders such as delirium or dementia, toxicities, severe pain). For these and other reasons, the consultation-liaison psychiatrist's therapeutic interventions more often consist of shoring up rather than challenging intact defenses (Despland et al. 2001). Consider the following brief case example:

Case Example 3

A psychiatric consultation was requested by an oncology fellow for a 50-year-old single man with terminal lung cancer who was visibly depressed and agitated. The fellow, a recent convert to the theories of Elisabeth Kübler-Ross, was concerned that "the patient has only a short time to live and he has not yet dealt with his denial and anger phases." He asked that the psychiatrist help the patient to confront his denial "so that he may die at peace." In interviewing the patient, the psychiatrist discovered that the patient's father had been a military man and had wanted his son to join the army. The patient was regretful that he had not pleased his father and would die a failure in his own eyes (his father knew full well about his lung cancer). The psychiatrist suggested to the patient that he seemed to have a kind of strength of his own and that, in battling his cancer, he was being every bit a soldier fighting the good fight. The patient's spirits lifted, and he became calm, was comforted by staff, and succumbed peacefully to his cancer 3 days later.

Although most medical-surgical patients who are seen by the consultation-liaison psychiatrist do have "the ability to interact in the first session" (Marmor 1979a, p. 153), this easy receptivity may be the result of 1) the regression accompanying sickness and hospitalization, 2) fulfillment of the sick role (Parsons 1951) through increased dependency and passivity, or 3) feelings of isolation and alienation that heighten the desire to speak to virtually anyone who will listen. Supporting this hypothesis is the observation that many patients who would not otherwise seek psychiatric attention on an outpatient basis will accept and benefit from such attention in the hospital. Evidence of ego strength is almost always possible to find in most patients, even if only in their capacity to cope more or less successfully with the stressful and sometimes strange experience of hospitalization. Sometimes the patient's distraction by physical illness or discomfort is inappropriately perceived by staff as a willful failure of the patient to communicate.

The gulf between the theory of brief psychotherapy and clinical practicality prompted one group of authors to comment that "it is safe to assume at this point (the short-term theorists') selection criteria are more theoretically elegant than practically useful" (W.P. Henry et al. 1986, p. 28). Nonetheless, as long ago as 1954, a prominent psychoanalyst of the day, Fenichel (1954), noting that "brief psychotherapy is the child of bitter practical necessity," advocated its use in traumatic neuroses and acute conflicts, immature personalities who need reeducation, hysterical types with a readiness for dramatic transference, and patients "suggestible to magical influences" (p. 255). Even earlier, with some prescience, if not smugness, Freud (1919/1955) anticipated that "it is very probable that we shall be compelled to alloy the pure gold of analysis with the copper of other therapeutic measures" (p. 163).

These historical footnotes are cogent reminders of the caution not to throw the baby out with the bathwater. Indeed, the requirement of versatility in the consultation-liaison psychiatrist determines that his or her therapeutic interventions will fall typically between uncomplicated consultation or evaluation and more formal psychotherapy. Knowledge, if not unmodified use, of the varieties of psychotherapy is an essential part of the consultation-liaison psychiatrist's armamentarium. Some psychotherapies from which the consultation-liaison psychiatrist may choose are listed in Table 45–3.

TASKS OF THE CONSULTATION-LIAISON PSYCHIATRIST

The consulting psychiatrist in the medical setting is called on to provide assistance in circumstances covering the spectrum from an immediate crisis (e.g., in emergent situations wherever they occur in the hospital) to a chronic condition requiring protracted outpatient follow-up. Outpatient treatment may be brief, extended, or, as is described later in this chapter, attenuated. In each instance, assessment follows evaluation of the situation, whether patient, staff, or system centered. Whatever the setting and focus, appraisal includes a psychodynamic assessment in addition to a review of reasons (medical or surgical) for the patient's illness and reactions and reasons for the consultee's concerns. The latter may range from the primary physician's puzzlement over a diagnostic dilemma to concern about psychological risks in a patient with schizophrenia who is scheduled for major surgery. In order to be of maximal assistance to the consulter, the psychiatrist must understand the medical circumstances of the case, know the medication regimens and their effects, and glean as much as possible from the patient's chart. Early in the encounter, a decision is made whether active crisis intervention or a more extended and methodical approach is indicated. Ultimately, a plan

TABLE 45–3. Types and characteristics of psychotherapies

Characterized by	Description	Consultation-liaison example	Reference
Time			
Brief	Limited (<12–20) sessions	Unresolved grief exacerbating physical disease	Davanloo 1978; Malan 1963; Mann 1973; Marmor 1979b; Sifneos 1972
	Focus on specific problem		
	Exploratory or supportive		
	Stringent selection criteria		
	Motivated or receptive patient		
		Single-session evaluation of depressive response to illness	Bloom 1981
		Briefest—acute postsurgical reactions	Blacher 1984
		Attenuated treatment of somatization disorder in outpatient setting	Lipsitt 1986
Extensive	Protracted treatment	Only in cases in which initial brief intervention leads to discovery of long-standing conflicts amenable to treatment	Gabbard 1990; Gitelson 1973
	Exploratory		
	Reconstructive		
	Deals with transference and development of insight		
Format			
Individual	Patient seen alone	Patient with unremitting abdominal pain with no physical findings	Harrison and Carek 1966; Ursano and Hales 1986
	Others usually (but not always) not involved		
Couples	Usually for interpersonal problems between two related people (not necessarily married)	Young married executive with myocardial infarction who aggravates and frightens wife by denying seriousness of illness; she requests appointment	Melges 1985
Family	Related groups with usually one identified patient	20-year-old woman with anorexia seen with family to explore stresses	Jacobs 1993
	Explores family dynamics as contributor to problem		
Group	Heterogeneous or homogeneous assembly of 8–10 patients with sense of shared stress, symptoms, interests, conflicts	Group of women with breast cancer; also Alcoholics Anonymous groups	Spira and Spiegel 1993; Stein and Weiner 1978; Yalom 1975
	Provides modeling, sharing, learning		
	Time limited or open		

TABLE 45–3. Types and characteristics of psychotherapies (continued)

Characterized by	Description	Consultation-liaison example	Reference
Goals			
Supportive	Strengthen defenses and coping skills to reduce anxiety and to enhance well-being and social function Here-and-now orientation	Patient with asthma who is afraid to return home because of spouse who has cardiac disease and smokes	Barber et al. 2001; Green 1993; Hackett and Weisman 1960a, 1960b; Viederman 1983
Reconstructive	Bring about changes in adaptation, behavior, and personality to alter lifelong patterns Intensive, insight-oriented; deals with transference neurosis, early developmental problems Psychoanalysis, dynamic psychotherapy	After nearly dying in automobile accident, college professor decides to examine his life, relationships, and goals	Gitelson 1973
Reeducational	Remove symptoms by direct intervention, guidance, persuasion, and relearning Correct misperceptions and misattributions Here-and-now orientation No exploration of early events; no transference or insight Behavioral and cognitive approaches Symptom removal is goal	Patient becomes acutely anxious in magnetic resonance imaging machine; responds to systematic desensitization	Hamburg and Adams 1967; Horowitz et al. 1984
Techniques			
Suppressive	Reassure, support strengths, bolster ego-syntonic defenses Use suggestion, clarification, and manipulation to enhance self-control	Management of patient with labile hypertension who has difficulty in following diet and taking medications	Green 1993; Viederman 1984, 1985
Exploratory	Encourage self-discovery and insight through interpretation of behavior, conflict, and transference Make unconscious conscious Examine early life	Help patient to understand persistent smoking in face of recently diagnosed pulmonary disease	Davanloo 1978; Malan 1963; Mann 1973; Sifneos 1972, 1973
Directive	Retrain or reframe ways of thinking, feeling, and behaving through direct intervention, guidance, and persuasion	Redirect thinking of patient with diabetes who feels guilt and depression about difficulty in controlling brittle diabetes	Hersen and Bellack 1982; Klerman et al. 1984; Zeiss et al. 1979

will derive from a formulation of the case. Consider the following case example:

Case Example 4

An emergency psychiatric consultation was requested for a 67-year-old scientist who became severely agitated as he was being anesthetized for gallbladder surgery. The psychiatrist learned that the patient had been in a concentration camp as an adolescent when he had been a non-Jewish member of the underground in Scandinavia. Being anesthetized by a physician with a German accent had mobilized old vulnerabilities and fears that caused him to fight the administration of anesthesia. The elective surgery was postponed, a different anesthetist assigned, and in the intervening day and a half, discussion was held with the patient about his earlier adolescent experience. He underwent surgery without complication.

According to Greenhill (1981), a major task of the consultation-liaison psychiatrist is dealing with psychosocial influences in medical illness. In that regard, "he or she works over an extended period of time on the various nonpsychiatric services of a general hospital" (p. 674). The tasks required to make a psychiatric consultation therapeutic are delineated in Table 45–4. These tasks culminate in selection of an appropriate psychotherapeutic approach based on formulation of the case (Hackett and Weisman 1960b).

Establishing the Alliance

The term *therapeutic alliance* as it applies to psychotherapy refers to the readiness and motivation of a patient to work with energy and commitment with a willing psychotherapist. Deriving primarily from psychoanalytic writings, the term has not commonly been applied to the type of brief consultative encounter experienced by consultation-liaison psychiatrists in hospital settings. Nonetheless, insofar as the consulting psychiatrist fosters hope and expectation in patients seen in that context, however brief the contact, the relationship (the alliance) has the capacity to promote maturation and well-being in any patient, whether in the psychiatrist's office or in a family practice clinic. The power of the alliance is illustrated by an anecdote told about himself by the late Dr. Hermann Blumgart, professor of medicine at Harvard Medical School and physician-in-chief at the Beth Israel Hospital in Boston. Dr. Blumgart had been on rounds with his house officers and, stopping by a woman's bedside, discussed her illness with her and rendered a suggestion for treatment. In asking what she thought about his suggestion, she said she would have to discuss it with her doctor and see what he said. Dr. Blumgart discovered the next day that her "doctor" was a second-year medical student.

TABLE 45–4. Psychotherapeutic tasks of the consultation-liaison psychiatrist

Identify most relevant problem as expressed by primary care physician

Establish alliance with patient

Take history through associative interviewing

Assess personality structure and defenses

Understand, empathize, translate, inform, communicate, and educate, based on historical data

Derive psychodynamic formulation

Enhance self-esteem of patient

Selectively gratify transference wishes

Decrease intensity of painful affects

Normalize (universalize) reactions

Enhance healing environment

Propose practical management plan

Define psychiatrist's and other staff's participation

As I have written elsewhere (Lipsitt 1986), "The psychiatric consultant makes use of all the principles of good psychotherapy, although they are often modified to accommodate the realities of the hospital setting and the unusual way in which psychiatrist and patient are brought together" (p. 8). Although transferential reactions can occur in any setting, that which accompanies the alliance in the medical setting is not addressed as it would be in extended psychodynamic therapies. Rather, it is acknowledged in terms of empathic understanding, reassurance, supportive interaction, and meaningful communication. Because the psychiatrist in the medical setting does not undertake reconstructive therapy of long-standing problems, he or she usually has no sustained working relationship that relies on a so-called working alliance and analysis of transference reactions. Awareness of their existence, however, permits them to be utilized in the manipulative aspects of psychotherapeutic interventions (Andrusyna et al. 2001; Bibring 1954) in even the briefest encounters. Blacher (1984), for example, described how to use the principles of psychotherapy effectively in a single session to provide treatment to patients in medical crises that "evoke old conflicts and problems about the self and family relationships" (p. 226). It is only necessary, according to Blacher, that the consulting psychiatrist have a dynamic understanding of the meaning of emerging conflicts behind the anxiety and fear of the patient's response to medical predicaments. Although the therapeutic alliance does not exist in the psychoanalytic sense, the acceptance by the patient of the psychiatrist's investment creates a holding environment in which the clinical improvement occurs, often without adjunctive psychopharmacological treatment.

Making a Personality Diagnosis

Because medical psychotherapy is often of the briefest sort and because it lacks a specific organizing theoretical structure of its own, a useful foundation for consultation-liaison work has been the personality typology developed by Kahana and Bibring (1964) for application in the general hospital setting. *Personality diagnosis* is based on normal character development and is not to be misconstrued as personality disorder or other psychopathology. Based on the psychoanalytic theory of character structure and development, it facilitates description of the meaning of illness to patients of different personality types, permitting some degree of matching of therapeutic interventions with more or less predictable patient responses. To delineate nonpathological behaviors as they are influenced by developmental differences in individuals, Kahana and Bibring identified seven types (Table 45–5).

Defensive and adaptive coping approaches that are fairly characteristic of each personality type are called into play in the face of threatening situations such as medical illness, surgery, or hospitalization. Rarely do types exist in pure form; clinical experience suggests that there is considerable overlap. (For further discussion about the relation between personality and response to illness, see Chapter 8, this volume.) A few case examples will illustrate the relevance and application of personality diagnosis.

Case Example 5

A 23-year-old graduate student in physics was admitted to the hospital because of unremitting hematemesis. A large gastric ulcer was discovered; it was unresponsive to conservative medical treatment. Surgery was advised. Postoperatively, the patient became markedly anxious and fearful, but the cause was not readily recognized by either the patient or the staff. Psychiatric consultation was requested. The patient was noted to be hyperventilating and complaining of severe pain in his abdomen. He held a pillow over the incision site on which he exerted pressure to provide himself some relief. At the very outset of the interview, he indicated that he had been given instructions by the physical therapist about the importance of deep breathing in order to avoid serious complications such as pneumonia or embolism.

The consultation-liaison psychiatrist explained to him that this did not mean he must constantly hyperventilate to the point of exhaustion. The patient expressed surprise that this was not specifically said to him. He immediately relaxed, breathed fairly normally, and continued with the interview. He was extremely bright and articulate and explained that he had grown up in a family in which high achievement

was expected and in which his father was a dominating presence whose "word was law." He revealed a pattern of marked compliance, with an outstanding academic record from a very young age. He indicated his desire to be a "good patient" so that he could recover quickly and return to his studies.

This patient reveals the characteristics of a compulsive personality in a startling way, although there was no other evidence of psychopathology. The consultation-liaison psychiatrist recognized the meaning of illness in this patient's life; he feared losing control and needed to understand in great detail the nature of all interventions. These compulsive characteristics had served him well in the past. He had been academically successful, and his adaptation to the demands of everyday life was satisfactory. However, the stress of hospitalization and surgery fostered transient regression that rendered these traits maladaptive under the circumstances. Discussion and understanding of his problem resulted in rapid resolution, with accompanying amelioration of hyperventilation, anxiety, and fear. Follow-up revealed an anxiety-free patient breathing normally, with occasional deep breaths. Staff were advised to be thorough in their communications with the patient, to inquire whether he had any questions, and to review all recommended behaviors with him.

Case Example 6

A very attractive 32-year-old woman underwent a right mastectomy for cancer. Postoperatively, she puzzled the surgical team on rounds by her "extremely good response" to such serious, disfiguring surgery. She would tell jokes to the physicians on rounds and on one occasion called attention to a small blemish on her skin for which she requested a dermatology consultation. She was always carefully made up and wore attractive nightgowns rather than those provided by the hospital.

Psychiatric assessment was requested to evaluate this patient's behavior. She described herself as her father's favorite child and a person who was always praised for her self-confidence, attractiveness, and poise. She had many friends who enjoyed her sense of humor and fun. When asked why she felt she had to entertain the doctors, she said they worked hard and did not want to hear patients complain. When asked what she would do if she didn't smile, she burst into tears and began talking about her worries about how she would look, how her husband might no longer be interested in her, and how she could not wear nice bathing suits at the beach.

This patient's responses were typical of the dramatizing, histrionic personality type. Her original indifference to the meaning of surgery and her attempt to distract others (and herself) from the effect this had on her

TABLE 45–5.   Personality types in medical management

Personality type	Psychodynamic descriptor	Illness behavior	Treatment approach
Dependent, overdemanding	Oral, needy	Urgent requests	Show signs of caring but with clear limit setting
Orderly, controlled	Compulsive	Self-disciplined	Use "scientific" approach; share information
Dramatizing, emotional	Hysterical	Flighty, teasing	Use calm professional approach
Long-suffering, self-sacrificing	Masochistic	Help-rejecting	Avoid excessive reassurance; acknowledge pain
Guarded, querulous	Paranoid	Suspicious, wary	Acknowledge, but do not reinforce, perceptions; do not argue or withhold information
Superior, grandiose	Narcissistic	Exaggerated self-confidence	Do not challenge patient's "expert" status
Uninvolved, aloof	Schizoid	Seeks isolation	Accept unsociability but avoid complete withdrawal

Source. Originally adapted from Kahana RJ, Bibring GL: "Personality Types in Medical Management," in *Psychiatry and Medical Practice in a General Hospital.* Edited by Zinberg NE. New York, International Universities Press, 1964, pp. 108–123. Reprinted from Waldinger RJ: *Psychiatry for Medical Students,* 2nd Edition. Washington, DC, American Psychiatric Press, 1990. Used with permission.

gave surgeons the sense that she was emotionally disturbed. However, understanding how this personality type responds to illness facilitated a more appropriate interaction with her physicians and acceptance by the patient of the recommendation to work with a psychiatric nurse in adjusting to a change in her body image. She needed to work through (normal) feelings of loss and grief. This case shows characteristics of a stress response syndrome (Horowitz and Kaltreider 1979) that was partially addressed by the consultation-liaison psychiatrist through a combination of psychodynamic and cognitive psychotherapeutic techniques. In so doing, "the disturbing role relationships or self-images (were) once again subordinated to more adaptive, mature self-images and role relationships" (p. 370). According to Horowitz and Kaltreider (1979) "intensive work in a brief therapy model may both alter the symptomatic response to a stressful life event and facilitate further progress along developmental lines" (p. 371).

Responses to critical events are experienced and processed through the unique defense structure of individual personality styles (Horowitz et al. 1984). This influences the disposition of affective and cognitive responses to trauma. Normal resolution of symptoms results in reintegration of the ego, whereas failure to accomplish this by successful working through can result in prolonged symptoms. Numbing, dissociative states, vivid dreams, depression, anxiety, and panic may define a stress response syndrome or chronic posttraumatic stress disorder (PTSD). DSM-IV-TR (American Psychiatric Association 2000) distinguishes acute stress disorder (less than 4 weeks) from the more intense chronic PTSD (3 months or more). Recognition of early acute symptoms permits therapeutic and preventive work through brief psycho-

therapy, in groups or individually (e.g., debriefing groups, crisis intervention, supportive psychotherapy, psychoeducation). Personality diagnosis is, by itself, insufficient to serve psychotherapeutic purposes but is a valuable adjunct to all medical psychotherapy. It must also be kept in mind that an individual's personality may be altered in appearance, either transiently or more permanently, under conditions of marked emotional stress or physical disease.

ESSENTIAL SKILLS OF THE CONSULTATION-LIAISON PSYCHIATRIST

Even if the consultation-liaison psychiatrist is not using a specific model of brief psychodynamic intervention, knowledge of psychodynamic theory and application enhances his or her skill and versatility. In company with other skills and knowledge, psychodynamic thinking offers the eclecticism and flexibility required of an effective psychiatrist in outpatient or inpatient general medical settings. The repertoire of the consultation-liaison psychiatrist calls on psychiatry's roots in psychoanalysis, psychosomatic medicine, stress theory about the relevance of critical life events and trauma, biopsychosocial concepts of illness and illness behavior, as well as general medicine, neurology, and psychopharmacology.

Versatility

The activities of the consultation-liaison psychiatrist are always potentially psychotherapeutic. They range from a single skillful interview to crisis intervention, to comprehensive evaluation, to follow-up during hospitalization, and to continued involvement following hospital discharge, at which time additional psychotherapy may include a range of approaches from behavioral therapy to insight-oriented psychotherapy. The skills of the consultation-liaison psychiatrist are those of the most proficient full-time psychotherapist, with perhaps a greater versatility born of necessity. Consultation-liaison psychiatrists who interact on a daily basis with patients who are medically ill and their caregivers should be adept at the skills listed in Table 45–6.

Associative Anamnesis

One interview technique especially suited to consultation-liaison work is that described as *associative anamnesis* (Deutsch 1939; Deutsch and Murphy 1955), derived in part from the psychoanalytic free associative process. Deutsch and Murphy found that it was possible to obtain both physiological and psychological data by allowing the patient considerable latitude in speaking of his or her symptoms. They noted that the patient "drifts into a communication in which he inattentively mixes emotional and symptom material" (p. 20). In this way, they said, "it is possible to observe the somatic and the psychic components more nearly simultaneously" (p. 19). Empathic concern for the patient's physical distress strengthened the alliance, whereas through repetition of key somatic or affective words (i.e., the interviewer is not passive), "the patient is stimulated to give the needed information…without being made aware of a psychological background in his illness" (p. 20).

This process of data gathering informs the interviewer of the patient's personality structure, salient defenses, style of interacting with others (including the patient's physician), patterns of adapting to and coping with stresses, personal and family psychodynamics, physical symptoms, and social skills. These kaleidoscopic observations fulfill, as much as any technique, the requirements of a biopsychosocial portrait of the patient. Viederman's (1984) *active dynamic interview* has characteristics similar to the associative anamnesis.

The interview process, performed properly, is as psychotherapeutic as it is diagnostic. The techniques delineated by Bibring (1954) are common to both and are "considered to be applicable to all methods of psychotherapy independent of their respective ideologies" (p. 760).

Consultation-liaison psychiatrists offer crisis intervention, supportive assistance to nonpsychiatric staff in the care of the patient, and psychologically sophisticated recommendations for treatment and management of

TABLE 45–6. Psychotherapeutic skills of the consultation-liaison psychiatrist

Knowing about psychoanalytic and psychodynamic concepts, biopsychosocial approach, stress theory, general medicine, neurology, and psychopharmacology

Knowing how to conduct medical-psychiatric interviewing (e.g., associative anamnesis)

Knowing how to extrapolate meaning from casual talk and empathic listening

Knowing when and how to confront a patient's worries

Knowing how and when to neutralize negative emotional conflicts with psychopharmacological agents[a]

Knowing how to create a supportive holding environment

Knowing how to select and apply tailored psychotherapeutic approach

Knowing how and when to appropriately use interventions such as reassurance, support, limit setting, guidance, and management

Knowing how to relate comfortably to nonpsychiatrist professionals and to work with liaison team members

Knowing how to curb inappropriate therapeutic zeal, especially outside one's field of expertise

Knowing how to combine psychotherapy and psychopharmacotherapy

[a]After Fenichel 1954.

patients who are medically ill. Being able to respond in an integrated way to a host of psychosocial, psychiatric, and behavioral nuances enhances the consultation-liaison psychiatrist's expertise considerably. Differences in setting, motivation, affect tolerance, and forms of request for help all differ markedly from the usual characteristics of a traditional psychotherapeutic enterprise.

Preassessment

Before any psychotherapeutic intervention can begin, the consultation-liaison psychiatrist sizes up the situation. This preassessment may include as much exploration as necessary to grasp the precipitating reason for the consultation request. The attending physician's perception of the need for psychiatric assessment, a fairly detailed review of the patient's medical record, and the primary care nurse's impressions of the patient usually constitute the desirable minimum. When available, family members offer valuable contributions to the total assessment and are often involved in the follow-up, treatment, and care of the patient (Jacobs 1993; Lipsitt and Lipsitt 1991; Melges 1985). This systemic appraisal before face-to-face interaction with the patient facilitates a focused approach to the core problem during the actual interview with the patient and may well enter into the subsequent formulation of the problem.

Therapeutic Examination

The examination or interview itself can carry a high psychotherapeutic valence. A skillful interview may include any or all of the following elements of therapeutic effectiveness: trust, alliance, abreaction, insight, attitude change, correction of perceptual distortion, suggestion, clarification, manipulation, education, and even interpretation. Unlike the interview of the self-referred patient that might take place in an outpatient setting, the interview of the hospitalized patient must avoid testing for motivation or heightening anxiety through uncovering techniques. Questions that too quickly attempt to assay feelings or even details of interpersonal relationships often bring forth only quizzical expressions from the patient (Lipsitt 1977). Although the psychiatrist is usually accustomed to exploring broadly beyond the chief complaint, the consultant's exploration is usually limited initially to only those aspects of the history that are absolutely necessary to address the question posed by the primary physician.

Special Considerations in the General Hospital Setting

The consultation-liaison psychiatrist must be able to adapt to the realities of the general hospital environment. Because of time limitations, consultation-liaison psychiatrists will sometimes have to be comfortable with a degree of incompleteness of the anamnesis as well as with the tendency of many patients to want to sustain a medical or physical focus during much of the interview. The consultation-liaison psychiatrist who cannot tolerate the patient's attachment to pain may be inclined erroneously to interpret this as a "negative therapeutic reaction" (Valenstein 1973).

Successful alliance and therapeutic effectiveness depend on the consultation-liaison psychiatrist's capacity for empathic resonance to "where the patient lives" at any particular moment, whether during a mental status examination or associatively following self-disclosures considered by the patient to be relevant to the problem. Positive alliances (Lipsitt 1985) can develop quickly, even in patients who are initially resistant to psychiatric assessment, and can allow the patient to comfortably disclose abundant personal data in a short time. Occasionally, more expanded inquiry may be useful to assess the patient's suitability for outpatient follow-up with more intensive psychotherapy (whether brief or extended). These transitions must be accomplished with finesse, utilizing effective communication with future or ongoing therapists as well as with the patient's primary care physician.

Physicians often create barriers to psychiatric consultation when they say something like "I would like to have a psychiatrist see this patient, but I am afraid it would be too upsetting." Usually they either misunderstand the nature of psychiatry as practiced in the medical setting or they misunderstand the patient. It is not unusual for patients to acknowledge an improved sense of well-being after a good cry, which may be interpreted erroneously by skeptical staff as psychiatrist-induced distress. Some patients even express relief with "I'm glad you came" and some actually request psychiatric consultation on their own when they realize their physician is unlikely to do so. When patients enter a hospital for medical or surgical treatment, they often experience some degree of regression. In this predicament, professional contact that provides comfort, compassion, honesty, and empathy fosters a high degree of receptivity in the patient, with alliance following soon after engagement (Nadelson 1980).

Defenses that are weakened by the experience of sickness and hospitalization must be not only respected but also bolstered because they are often useful in adapting to the current crisis. Part of the consultation-liaison psychiatrist's task is to assess the patient's personality and defense structure during the first examination. The patient's adaptation to illness will confirm the old-time medical dictum that "it is as important to know what kind of patient has the disease as to know what disease the patient has," as illustrated by the important aspect of medical psychotherapy that addresses personality diagnosis in the patient (Kahana and Bibring 1964), described earlier in this chapter.

Formulation

Utilizing data from a variety of sources, the consultation-liaison psychiatrist must derive a formulation. Before standardized DSM classification, traditional psychiatric diagnoses had little utility in consultation-liaison psychiatry. Most patients seen in the general medical hospital did not have schizophrenia or mania, for instance. The formulation, more than the diagnostic label, remains the road map to further intervention. Based on the data obtained from the patient and other sources, the formulation includes features listed in Table 45–7. Such formulation, although it need not include all these elements in every case, can lead quite naturally to recommendations for treatment.

Selecting and Implementing Treatment

After arriving at a formulation, the consultation-liaison psychiatrist has a range of psychotherapeutic interventions from which to choose. These generally embrace the

TABLE 45–7.   Elements of formulation

Character structure (personality diagnosis)

Presenting problem (reason for request of consultation)

Patient's narrative (life story), including perceptions and attributions of current illness

Identified life event(s) or crisis that precipitated response

Defenses used by patient to negotiate stresses of medical illness, surgery, and hospitalization

Patterns of engagement from past as predictors of patient's response to caregivers and treatment interventions

Leads to guidelines for
  Psychotherapeutic intervention
  Physicians and other staff about
    Doctor-patient relationship
    Relevance of patient's behavior to current illness
    Consultation-liaison psychiatrist's role in care of the patient

TABLE 45–8.   Common psychotherapeutic activities of the consultation-liaison psychiatrist in the general hospital

Helping patients endure or overcome pain, fear, and denial

Helping patients' families cope with disruption by illness

Facilitating medical-surgical treatment

Helping patients grieve losses or face dying and death

Enhancing patients' capacity to bear dependency, isolation, rumination, sleep disturbance, and other perturbations of illness

Helping patients adapt to the sick role

Helping patients to effect changes in self-representation, object representation, and ideal self-representation[a]

Helping caregiving staff to recognize and utilize psychosocial factors in patient care planning

[a] Adapted from Mohl and Burstein 1982; Viederman 1985.

TABLE 45–9.   Threats and fears that accompany illness

Threat to narcissistic integrity and the sources of self-esteem

Regressive fear of strangers on whom patient must rely

Separation anxiety, reflecting regressive activation of childhood fears of loss of nurturing and protective objects

Regressive activation of fears of loss of love and approval

Regressive fears of loss of control of developmentally acquired functions (e.g., bowel and bladder control, motor functions, speech, emotional regulation)

Guilt and fear of retaliation, reflecting unconscious view that illness is a punishment for past unacceptable behavior

Source.   Adapted from Strain JJ, Grossman S: *Psychological Care of the Medically Ill.* New York, Appleton-Century-Crofts, 1975.

five basic principles elaborated by Bibring (1954), and referred to earlier (see Table 45–1), as essential to all forms of therapy, although not necessarily all in every instance. The first three basic principles—suggestion, abreaction, and manipulation—characterize less insight-oriented approaches, and the last two—clarification and interpretation—characterize more insight-oriented approaches. The consultant applies these techniques when indicated in commonly encountered situations in the general hospital calling for psychotherapeutic intervention (Table 45–8).

Viederman's (1985) *life narrative approach* elicits the patient's personal fears and the meanings of symptoms as experienced by the patient and revealed through his or her individualized attributions of illness. The psychiatrist then formulates a jargon-free statement that psychodynamically helps to explain the meaning of the illness to the patient at this particular moment in his or her life. According to Viederman (1985), the life narrative formulated by the consultation-liaison psychiatrist summarizes the patient's response to illness and describes it to him or her as a disturbance that is a natural product of his or her personal psychology. This technique lessens the emotional disequilibrium that has been aroused by the crisis of illness by giving it a rational foundation.

The life narrative approach is an excellent example of the synthesis of psychoanalytic, experiential, cognitive, supportive, and brief approaches to the acute emotional needs of the patient (Viederman and Perry 1980). This technique is intended to help the patient place the physical illness "in the context of the patient's life trajectory" and acknowledges the threats and fears of the person confronted with serious physical disease, as described by Strain and Grossman (1975, p. 26) (Table 45–9).

According to Viederman (1985), the life narrative approach is applicable at the bedside even in relatively brief contacts. However, when extended interpretation may be required and usable by the patient, full intervention may have to await treatment in an outpatient setting. The choice of psychotherapy often determines which member(s) of the consultation-liaison team will most actively work with the patient and, as appropriate, with his or her family. The psychiatric examination by the consultation-liaison psychiatrist may itself constitute a psychotherapeutic intervention, and follow-up visits may be utilized to consolidate the benefits of the intervention or to assess its durability. At other times, for example, in helping a patient work through acute or delayed grief, a psychiatric nurse, social worker, or psychologist on the team may undertake the therapeutic work while the psychiatrist provides a bridge with staff involved with the patient's care. In still other instances, the consultation-liaison psychiatrist may provide psychopharmacological oversight while psychotherapy is administered by another member of the team. At times the recommendation may be "no intervention at all"

(Frances and Clarkin 1981, p. 925). At other times, behavioral or cognitive approaches, including hypnosis, stress reduction, or other interventions, are used. Some programs are able to provide brief inpatient group experiences.

The consultation-liaison psychiatrist selects the approach—or, more commonly, the combination of approaches—that most parsimoniously addresses the patient's conditions or symptoms. Consideration of many factors will determine whether the approach will be primarily supportive or exploratory in its application (Table 45–10).

Seldom is the issue that of frank mental illness but rather "illnesses requiring modification in patterns of life adjustment and...attitudes" (Whitehorn 1952, p. 330). The task of adaptation "may strain the personality resources of many patients or arouse definite and obstinate noncooperation" (p. 330); today we speak of adherence to or compliance with medical recommendations. If these issues will pose a problem for the patient beyond discharge from inpatient status, then therapeutic maintenance will require outpatient follow-up that is acceptable to the reluctant patient. Modification in therapeutic expectation and treatment setting may be required.

The psychotherapeutic approach selected depends on not only the needs of the patient but also the training and theoretical predilection of the therapist. Because, as mentioned earlier in this chapter, all therapies contain certain common denominators and there is a nondetectable difference in outcome among different treatments (Jarvik et al. 1982; Zeiss et al. 1979), the efficacy of the treatment relies heavily on a combination of the therapist's skill and the patient's expectant faith in the treatment. However, others (Hersen and Bellack 1982) found that behavioral approaches were superior to insight approaches in patients with some types of depression. Fortunately, for most consultation-liaison psychiatrists, theoretical orthodoxy does not pose a significant problem. The ultimate aim of medical psychotherapy is to systematically apply biopsychosocial interventions toward psychotherapeutic change.

Helping the patient to develop or resume adequate coping mechanisms partially fulfills this aim. Hamburg and Adams (1967) described several psychotherapeutic goals of successful coping (Table 45–11), especially in long-term illness. These goals parallel the objectives of psychotherapy with patients who are medically ill.

The magnitude of this challenge is heightened in the medical setting, where the psychiatrist often encounters a prominent mind-body dualism that is detrimental to effective health care. Maintenance of a biopsychosocial mindset is further compromised by the current trend to

TABLE 45–10. Factors determining selection of therapeutic approach

	Supportive	Exploratory
Level of cognitive function	Low	High
Psychosis	Yes	No
Suicidality	Yes	No
Life-threatening behavior	Yes	No
Time available for consultation-liaison care	Short	Long
Level of sexual development	Low	High
Setting	Inpatient	Outpatient
Educational level	Low, variable	High, variable
Interpersonal patterns (ability to interact with others)	Uneasy	Comfortable
Degree of autonomy	Low	High
Ability to assume responsibility	Low	High
Ability to tolerate affect	Low	High
Ability to express feelings	Low	High
Level of motivation to change	Low	High
Ability to maintain focus on conflict	Low	High
Capacity for insight	Low	High
Ability to trust	Low	High
Ability to identify stressors	Low	High
External support system	Poor	Good

TABLE 45–11. Goals of successful coping

Keeping distress limited

Maintaining self-esteem

Maintaining relationships with significant others

Maximizing chances for physical recovery by addressing mood, motivation, and compliance

Setting the stage for longer-term psychotherapeutic interventions

Source. Adapted from Hamburg and Adams 1967.

abbreviate hospital stays and to focus strictly on symptom amelioration. Sometimes, for example, a patient complaining of chest pain may be medically discharged immediately after myocardial infarction is ruled out, even though other emotional explanations for chest pain (e.g., somatization) have not been fully explored.

The transition of consultation-liaison activities to outpatient settings offers an opportunity to apply more standard therapeutic modalities. The consultation-liaison psychiatrist who consults on patients in the hospital may continue work begun there in the outpatient setting. Making this bridge requires some degree of assessment of the patient's motivation to continue and some therapeutic sensitivity and skill in helping the patient to make this transition successfully.

ILLUSTRATIONS OF PSYCHOTHERAPEUTIC APPLICATIONS IN CONSULTATION-LIAISON PSYCHIATRY

Treatment strategies include engaging and shoring up successful defenses that bolster self-esteem, promoting restoration of adaptive strategies and patterns that have been effective under previous stress, and facilitating effective medical management by reducing dysphoric affects. The case examples in this section more fully illustrate these strategies and the process of psychotherapeutic intervention by a consultation-liaison psychiatrist.

Utilizing the skills of the consultation-liaison psychiatrist enumerated in Table 45–6, the clinician is able to produce a portrait of the patient based on their encounter. This portrait emerges not in a standardized sequential manner but in the style of the artist who puts a dab of paint here and another there to round out the picture. The portrait is complete when it has made use of only those ingredients—no more or less—that are essential to the total picture in each instance. Each encounter is a unique production in a special setting. All elements of the consultation are seamlessly interwoven.

Case Example 7

Emergency psychiatric consultation was requested early in the morning by the assigned house officer because an elderly man, Mr. A, had "become psychotic during the night" and was "putting on his clothes and saying he is leaving." Mr. A had refused implorings of the nursing staff to stay and was determined to get dressed. He was half-dressed, sitting on the edge of his bed, when the psychiatrist arrived. He was angry, yelling in a difficult-to-understand voice, in what sounded like a middle-European accent. He insisted on leaving the hospital because he had been so "poorly treated." Several young student nurses and their supervisors stood apprehensively near the bedside and explained that Mr. A had become "uncooperative" when advised that "doctor's orders had insisted that he remain at bed rest for treatment of a deep vein thrombophlebitis."

The treatment required bed rest and leg elevation. Mr. A had to call for a nurse when he required a urinal or a bedpan. He was considered a "good patient" for 2 days and nights but lost this designation on the third night when he climbed out of bed intending to go to the bathroom a very short distance from his bed. He was reminded of the treatment plan and reprimanded by a nurse during the night. Urged back to bed, he became "belligerent" and threw a urinal on

the floor. He was placed in bed in Posey restraints and, following a visit from a male house officer, was administered 1 mg of lorazepam intramuscularly. He slept the rest of the night only to become "belligerent" again in the morning and attempted to get dressed. Mr. A was forcefully returned to bed by several nurses, and the request was made for psychiatric intervention. The nursing staff described him as a "management problem" and perhaps "psychotic."

With no time to examine Mr. A's medical record, the consultation-liaison psychiatrist quietly asked Mr. A to tell him what had happened and why he was in the hospital. His story revealed that he was a 78-year-old Russian-born Jewish tailor with a first-time admission to this hospital. He had customarily gone to another hospital, where he recently had undergone a prostatectomy and bilateral orchiectomy, unrecorded in his history and physical examination. Mr. A indicated that he had decided not to return to his previous hospital because he had become disgruntled with his surgeon. "I was treated like an animal," he said but seemed not to want to provide details and hardly alluded to the nature of his surgery.

As he spoke to the consultation-liaison psychiatrist, Mr. A gradually returned to a reclining position in his bed and spoke quite spontaneously. He explained that he came to the United States when he was young and earned his living as a tailor, a skill he learned in Europe. He expressed pride at having achieved success in his work, citing several notables among his clientele. He described how it had become increasingly difficult for him to ply his art as he had become more arthritic and visually impaired by cataracts over the past several years. Nonetheless, he avidly recounted a recent experience when he chased a hoodlum who had attempted to snatch the purse of a woman passing by his shop and took great pride in his ability to hold the thief until police arrived. The psychiatrist expressed admiration for what a strong and active man Mr. A was despite some current physical difficulties.

This brought forth from Mr. A more anecdotes of physical prowess throughout his life. But now he felt useless, unable to care for himself—at which point he alluded to the "little girls" who had physically returned him to bed during the night. Discussion ensued about his current illness. He was given a basic explanation of the need for bed rest to help restore his strength and to stop the possibility of further physical compromise. As Mr. A became more relaxed and comfortable with the discussion, his voice was less high pitched and easier to understand. His demeanor shifted to cooperation rather than antagonism. He recounted his behavior, as well as that of the nurses, and expressed a sense of shame and humiliation. The psychiatrist said that he understood Mr. A's behavior and that he believed Mr. A would have behaved differently if he had understood the staff's concern for him.

Formulation of this case described the patient as a nonpsychotic self-made man who survived by his wits after losing his parents in Europe. He had found pride, self-esteem, and acceptance in his work and now felt deprived of this gratification. Furthermore, his sense of self had now been further compromised by recent surgical castration, a condition that caused shame and humiliation. He failed to report this surgery during an initial admission workup. After a couple of days of compliance with recommendations, he ventured toward the bathroom (after delayed responses to his bell call for a nurse) in what he regarded as minimal self-assertion. He was reminded abruptly and authoritatively that he must follow the doctor's orders. This caused him to rebel in an attempt to regain a sense of control and mastery. In addition to the immediate crisis, he had unresolved grief about his surgical loss, which may have further revived more protracted grief over his loss of family and work. Although this formulation focuses on the psychodynamics of the case, it does not overlook the possibility that a transient delirium, as observed in sundowning, may have contributed to a lessening of ego control, increased regression, and heightened dependency. Because these features were addressed, the need for additional medication was avoided.

Recommendations for management were to

- Assign a male nurse in this instance who could interact "man-to-man" with the patient to restore self-esteem.
- Avoid psychopharmacological control that would risk stirring up further feelings of lack of control, dependence, and passivity.
- Try to communicate more clearly and explain all interventions to convey respect for the patient's status, intelligence, and dignity. Sufficient time is required to understand his accented, high-pitched speech.
- Express interest in the patient's past life, especially his work.
- Begin short-term psychotherapy to work through residual grief; this process should be continued after eventual discharge to the outpatient consultation-liaison psychiatry clinic.
- Look for and avoid potential causes of delirium.

The patient remained for the requisite time for effective treatment of his thrombophlebitis, without further incident. The consultation-liaison psychiatrist saw him every other day, with a focus on his surgical experience (for cancer of the prostate). Interventions included education about the medical-surgical aspects of the operation; facilitation of expressions of anger, shame, and diminished self-esteem; reinforcement of old useful defenses to restore pride, self-esteem, accomplishment, and physical competence; and encouragement to recall his positive experiences whenever he felt down in the dumps.

This psychotherapeutic encounter included prompt alleviation of the crisis. Brief, psychodynamically informed psychotherapy utilized supportive, cognitive, interpersonal, and behavioral techniques after establishment of a mutually respectful alliance that contributed to restoration of the patient's self-image and self-esteem. Enlightenment and education of staff and assistance to the primary care physician in the successful completion of the medical treatment also constituted an important part of the intervention. Little is gained by attempting a procrustean fit of this example of medical psychotherapy into one or another theoretical mold.

Case Example 8

Mrs. B, a 72-year-old widowed woman, was found unconscious by her son on the floor of her apartment with significant amounts of blood in evidence. The blood was fresh, and she had, he thought, not been long in that condition. He made emergency arrangements for her hospital admission.

In the hospital, Mrs. B was given supportive measures, including intravenous fluids and blood replacement. When she was revived (rather promptly), she advised attending physicians that she wanted no further medical intervention. Because she was a rather young elderly person, members of the hospital staff were astounded at her negativity about further diagnostic workup. She was not opposed to remaining in the hospital, but she rejected the need for upper-GI radiograms and endoscopy to make a definitive diagnosis. As house officers became more insistent, Mrs. B revealed that she had a living will, which she kept at home, specifying her wish to have no heroic measures taken to keep her alive in the event of serious illness. Her son, an attorney, verified this and seemed impatient with, but otherwise tolerant and understanding of, his mother.

A psychiatric consultation was requested for assessment of Mrs. B's competence. Assessment revealed a thin, perky woman who was very receptive to talking but insistent on retaining her position about further studies. She described her past life, the death of her husband many years ago, and her long work history as a librarian-researcher in a university setting. She described her voracious reading appetite, her pleasures in retirement, and a lifelong appreciation of nature and its beauty. Although Mrs. B's cognitive function was not compromised, she could not describe any aspect of life on which she put any negative coloration. She had no symptoms of depression, suicidal ideation, or other apparent psychopathology.

In an attempt to appeal to rational thinking, the consultation-liaison psychiatrist pointed out to Mrs. B that her living will required that she know the diagnosis before making a decision to adhere to its intent.

At this point in her medical evaluation, the disease she had was still unknown. Was it cancer, as she implicitly assumed, or some more benign condition? She was steadfast in her resolve. She did not want to know whether it was cancer. The psychiatrist reported to the medical staff that she understood the situation and that there was no reason that her wishes should not be respected. House officers were overtly angry, stating she "should be kicked the hell out of that bed." There was no indication for active psychotherapeutic intervention with Mrs. B, but the members of the house staff were able to explore their own strong feelings about the physician's wish to control, their need for certainty, and their sense of being denied the exercise of their knowledge and skill.

The intensity of affect diminished in the staff. Mrs. B was discharged to home when her symptoms and abnormal laboratory findings improved. Mrs. B accepted no other follow-up, but, quite spontaneously, she wrote a lengthy letter of appreciation to the consultation-liaison psychiatrist for his interest and acceptance of her attitudes. About a year later, when the psychiatrist was to discuss living wills with a group of medical students, Mrs. B responded to a telephone request to teach them something about the topic. She gladly appeared, gave a "little lecture," and revealed little more about herself than she had during her hospitalization. No further follow-up was available.

In this case, the formulation was that a struggle for control between physician and patient resulted in the patient being feared incompetent. The consulter wanted psychiatric corroboration in order to carry out a well-established diagnostic protocol for hematemesis. The consultation-liaison psychiatrist could do little more than describe the patient as able to make her own decisions and to render a (nonpathological) personality diagnosis of narcissistic type, or eccentric individual, with no need for further psychotherapeutic intervention. It was hoped that her satisfactory experience with a consultation-liaison psychiatrist would facilitate an appeal for later assistance if the time and circumstances warranted it.

Case Example 9

An urgent call for psychiatric consultation was received from the ICU when Mr. C, a 76-year-old man, climbed over his bedrails, removed his intravenous pole, and smashed an outer window, threatening to jump. This stocky, robust man, described as psychotic by the ICU staff, was restrained in bed and given a mild sedative. The staff reported that Mr. C underwent open heart surgery for replacement of a defective valve and that, under rather heavy sedation, he appeared to be progressing very well. However, shortly after extubation and lightening of sedation, he became quite agitated and hypervigilant. He repeatedly asked nurses for water and was repeatedly (and

increasingly emphatically) told that he was not allowed to have liquids. Shortly thereafter, he climbed over his bedrails.

Mr. C's relative calm when the psychiatrist arrived permitted a review of his chart. The chart contained detailed notes about Mr. C's surgery and anesthesia but little personal, social, or family history. When approached by the consultation-liaison psychiatrist, Mr. C was lying quietly in bed with a cold cloth across his forehead and a Posey restraint on his torso. He was quite receptive, rational, and cooperative. There was no evidence of psychosis, poor reality-testing, or suicidal intent. He recounted what happened with bewilderment and shame. He gave a chronological account of his physical condition that had warranted surgery and was forthcoming about his early personal history.

He was a Polish immigrant to the United States shortly after World War II and had lived through the experience of labor camps where he and his future wife were forced to toil for 10–11 hours a day without water. He recalled that experience as he became more alert following surgery; he cried as he recounted it. He described a life in which he had adapted to cruel behavior, many losses, impoverished circumstances, and other hardships. He expressed his gratitude at being able to live in the United States, to own his own home, to have a good and steady job in a bakery, and to raise a son who was now in a United States medical school. Again with tears, he expressed puzzlement that "anything like this" could occur because it would seem that he had "everything to live for," especially with the success of his surgery.

In this case, the formulation, after one consultation visit, was that the patient, who had evidence of considerable ego strength and good patterns of adaptation to stress in the past, was compromised by medications and the physiological stress of surgery (with possible mild cerebral hypoxia). In this twilight zone of perception, he reexperienced the labor camps of his youth, which he had survived without impulsive self-defeating behavior. Now, at age 76, while confused, he experienced panic—most likely triggered by the refusal of water—and was overcome with the need to escape.

Recommendations included the use of ice chips in acceptable moderation; avoidance of sedating drugs, although small doses of haloperidol were recommended in the face of further psychotic behavior; transport of the patient to a less hectic and stressful environment as soon as appropriate to normalize behavior; avoidance of the exploration of early history at this time; an increase in communication with the patient; and assignment of tasks that could be performed in bed to instill a greater sense of activity, freedom, and mastery.

On follow-up visits, the consultation-liaison psychiatrist found that no further episodes occurred and the patient was soon moved to a ward bed; he continued to recover from surgery without medical, surgical, or psychiatric complications. He did express feelings of depression, intense shame, and embarrassment over his experience in the ICU. Visits from the ICU head nurse, who explained her understanding and acceptance of the event, did much to allay his concerns. The patient was seen in follow-up after discharge when he returned to the hospital for postsurgical evaluation. At that time, he requested continued outpatient visits with the consultation-liaison psychiatrist because of difficulty sleeping, poor appetite, and anxiety. Monthly visits and small doses of thioridazine continued until his dysphoria improved.

ATTENUATED BRIEF PSYCHOTHERAPY: A MODEL OF OUTPATIENT PSYCHOTHERAPY

Although in this chapter I deal primarily with medical psychotherapy as applied to medical inpatients in the general hospital, I call the reader's attention to an approach that was used successfully in an outpatient clinic of a general hospital in the early 1960s. Referred to here as brief, intermittent, attenuated therapy (BIAT), the brevity of this treatment was the length of visits (no more than 30 minutes) and the interval of time between visits (almost always monthly). This translates to 12 sessions (6 hours) or fewer in 1 year, or 24 sessions (12 hours) or fewer in 2 years. This is less total time than most models of brief psychotherapy. Because none of the classical models of brief psychotherapy were derived from experience in a medical setting, this summary is offered to shed light on the special requirements of an outpatient *medical* population. Indeed, the selection criteria in Mann's (1973) model specifically exclude patients with psychosomatic disorders who do not tolerate loss well.

BIAT was found to be appropriate and effective for patients referred to a special (integration) clinic (Lipsitt 1964) for the evaluation and management of patients with chronic medical diseases who used somatization as a major defense. Earliest referrals were in response to the request for "problem patients to be sent to the clinic." The approach developed in working with these patients utilized some of the principles of brief psychotherapy, psychodynamic formulation, personality diagnosis, and supportive psychotherapy. It did not, however, develop selection criteria, in that every patient referred or who wanted to attend was seen, and a termination date was never set. In fact, it was the policy of the clinic that once

registered, patients were never discharged and were informed that they could make use of the clinic on an as-needed basis after they were not required to attend any longer, a policy that, in today's managed care climate, is not easily maintained.

These patients were high utilizers of medical services, including emergency room and inpatient hospitalization, and were generally not amenable to psychiatric referral. A pilot study (Lipsitt 1964) showed that many of those previously referred to the department of psychiatry were no-shows, but they did accept subsequent appointments to the integration clinic. It was hypothesized that these patients could accept a setting in the medical outpatient area that did not threaten their need to retain a physical definition of illness. The nondescript name of the clinic reinforced their denial of emotional problems.

A first visit usually began with "tell me about your problems." This almost invariably elicited from patients an "organ recital" of complaints, customarily ending in the expectation that now, finally, someone would fulfill their unrealistic expectation that all would be made well. From this very moment, such expectations and dependent idealizations of the physician were aborted with a comment such as "I don't know why Dr. X thought I would be able to help," or "Why would you think I had any medicine that Dr. X had not already tried," and so on. Those who questioned this response were informed by the psychiatrist that he needed more time to get to know them, that they had already had a lot of treatment and nothing seemed to help very much. Those who urged the therapist to read their chart were told that it would be more useful to hear their story from themselves than to read what someone else had written about them. The objective was to establish a relationship these patients could tolerate without needing to use barriers of medications and unfulfilled promises as a way of perpetuating their complaints and somatizations. Their histories were punctuated with projections shared with their physicians that "those pills didn't work, we'll try something else" or "maybe something was missed" (often a metaphor for "the doctor didn't listen to me, didn't understand, or wasn't interested").

It was the psychiatrist's intent to have the patients perceive him or her as having no investment in the presence or absence of symptoms but only in what the patients had to say. Only in rare instances were requests for additional appointments granted on the basis of intensification of symptoms, and virtually never was a symptom that was present one month but absent the next inquired about. The psychiatrist also exercised special restraint to never express pleasure at the disappearance of a symptom. It was anticipated that patients who were so dependent would need an approach that simultaneously permitted dependency but encouraged independence, a technique that often requires the consultation-liaison psychiatrist to walk a fine line. Often, neediness took the form of the terminal comment, which, delivered with hand on doorknob, was designed to extend the session by at least a few more minutes. For the most part, these patients needed to be able to trust, to experience an honest relationship, and to be assured that they would not be abandoned. Efforts to provide these reassurances more often took the form of actions than of words, with indications that patients could make telephone calls that would, at some point, be answered and that they would never be refused access to the clinic. Testing by patients of this kind of intervention usually occurred earlier in treatment but eventually diminished when they assured themselves of the availability of doctors and the clinic.

Improvement was measured by decreased telephone calls, by decreased visits to medical facilities, and ultimately by decreased visits to the integration clinic. Because initial requests from patients were a test of the outpatient consultation-liaison psychiatrist's interest, the psychiatrist would question the patient about his or her wish to increase the intervals between visits and register initial resistance to the idea, lest the patient interpret swift acquiescence as the doctor's wish to be rid of the patient. If a patient eventually wanted to stop clinic visits "unless something comes up," he or she was given an appointment for a "checkup whether you have symptoms or not" to diminish the connection between visits and symptoms. Other evidence of change appeared in the patients' eventual shift away from the organ recital to conversation about family, activities, or interests. This shift usually occurred without prompting by the outpatient consultation-liaison psychiatrist when the relationship was acceptable and tolerable without the presence of physical complaints (Lipsitt 2001). Although this was not labeled for the patients, it would appear that an unspoken insight occurred, just as transference and alliance elements were incorporated therapeutically without their being expressly identified.

Month-long intervals between appointments diminished the potential for regression while fulfilling patients' needs for attachment. Demands for medications or changes in appointment frequency (most often increases) were perceived by the therapist as reflections of neediness, dependency, uncertainty, and a compulsive need for patients to check out their feelings of self-worth and acceptability. Although reconstructive objectives were not part of the technique, this did occur in some patients seen over protracted periods of time. Unfortunately, this attenuated form of treatment, although requiring small expense of time and money, is not understood or readily accepted by the new approach promoted by insurance companies, managed programs, and health maintenance organizations. This approach clearly has economic and preventive value but requires further controlled research to measure its apparent efficacy on somatizing high utilizers of health care services. It encompasses elements of a variety of approaches, including interpersonal, psychodynamic, cognitive, behavioral, supportive, and reconstructive and, as such, is a gratifying example of the eclecticism and versatility required of the consultation-liaison psychiatrist in general medical settings. Most outpatient liaison clinics have found broad applicability of both the structural and the therapeutic principles of the integration clinic approach (Dickson et al. 1992; Dolinar 1993; Kaplan 1981).

CONCLUSION

The concept of the consultation-liaison psychiatrist as psychotherapist is relatively recent. The first paper on liaison psychiatry was published in 1929. It described functions of the liaison psychiatrist, which included virtually all those embraced today except for that of psychotherapist (G.W. Henry 1929–1930). Indeed, even in the 1930s, when psychosomatic medicine and psychoanalysis held sway in the general hospital psychiatrist's orientation, there was minimal description of exactly what the liaison psychiatrist did that was considered psychotherapeutic. Not until well after World War II did descriptions of actual therapeutic interventions begin to appear. Even into the 1980s, as noted by Cohen-Cole et al. (1986), specific psychosocial and other psychotherapeutic interventions had been poorly described and researched, although there had been some efforts at controlled trials using "psychoeducational therapy, supportive therapy, psychodynamic therapy, focal short-term therapy, rational emotive therapy, and stress monitoring and management" (p. 327). This review of research does not make clear which studies involved inpatients and which involved outpatients.

Because of the broad array of patients seen by the consultation-liaison psychiatrist, especially in the inpatient general medical setting, strict adherence to one intervention approach is untenable. A consultation-liaison psychiatrist is a generalist as well as a subspecialist who has familiarity with a spectrum of therapeutic tools. Psychotherapy should be prescribed cafeteria style, according to the needs of the patient rather than in an ideologically orthodox manner. The consultation-liaison psychiatrist is thus challenged to synthesize both evaluative and therapeutic dimensions of the consultative opportunity and to apply, most flexibly, those therapeutic models (or aspects of them) that most usefully fit the time and circumstances as they exist.

In this chapter, I have reviewed the challenges that the consultation-liaison psychiatrist encounters in the rich milieu of the general hospital, whether in inpatient or outpatient settings. The needs and demands that confront him or her offer countless opportunities to be helpful to patients, to educate other caregivers in the biopsychosocial approach, and to be personally and professionally gratified.

POSTSCRIPT ON MANAGED CARE

In this chapter on psychotherapy in medical settings, I have elaborated on the principles of good clinical practice with only modest acknowledgment of the potential impact of managed care on their thoughtful application. Although the literature is replete with both pros and cons of managed care (Goldman et al. 1998) as they relate to the quality and cost of health care, little has been written specifically about the impact on consultation-liaison services, both inpatient and outpatient. Most states have had no provision for coverage of psychiatric services for patients with concomitant medical illness (Alter et al. 1997), and rarely will managed care organizations understand or reimburse the potential cost-offset benefits of an integration clinic approach, described in the preceding section. Some managed care organizations have disallowed repeated follow-up visits to medical inpatients after an initial consultation, requiring that a new referral be made for such monitoring (e.g., of psychopharmacotherapy) and continuity of care. And the need for documentation becomes ever more demanding (Keefe and Hall 1999; Kunkel et al. 1999). The evidence for cost-effectiveness of psychotherapy (Lazar and Gabbard 1997) seems not to have penetrated policies of managed care organizations to date (Olfson et al. 1999). Although attentiveness to excess costs is imperative, the extent to which this focus may compromise access to comprehensive health care is uneconomical in the long run. Consultation-liaison psychiatrists, in bringing the benefits of mental health care to primary health care, can enhance the opportunities for achieving this integration (deGruy 2000). As Meyer and Sotsky (1995) propose, psychiatrists will need to extend their collaborations with other disciplines, especially primary care. In so doing, it is possible to gain recognition that "psychiatry augments efforts to reduce lengths-of-stay and uncompensated care, permits treatment of difficult behavioral management cases, and collaborates with the complex, costly cases of combined physical and mental illness" (p. 73).

REFERENCES

Abram HS: Survival by machine: the psychological stress of chronic hemodialysis. Psychiatry in Medicine 1:37–51, 1970

Adler HM: The history of the present illness as treatment: who's listening, and why does it matter? J Am Board Fam Pract 10:28–35, 1997

Alexander F: Psychosomatic Medicine: Its Principles and Applications. New York, WW Norton, 1950

Alter CL, Schindler BA, Hails K, et al: Funding for consultation-liaison services in public sector-managed care plans; the experience of the Consultation-Liaison Association of Philadelphia. Psychosomatics 38:93–97, 1997

American Psychiatric Association: Diagnostic and Statistical Manual of Mental Disorders, 4th Edition, Text Revision. Washington, DC, American Psychiatric Association, 2000

Andrusyna TP, Tang TZ, DeRubeis RJ, et al : The factor structure of the working alliance inventory in cognitive-behavioral therapy. J Psychother Pract Res 10:173–178, 2001

Bachrach HM, Galatzer-Levy R, Skolnikoff, et al: On the efficacy of psychoanalysis. J Am Psychoanal Assoc 39:871–916, 1991

Balint M: The Doctor, His Patient and the Illness. London, Pitman, 1964

Barber JP, Stratt R, Halperin G, et al: Supportive techniques: are they found in different therapies? J Psychother Pract Res 10:165–172, 2001

Bibring E: Psychoanalysis and the dynamic psychotherapies. J Am Psychoanal Assoc 2:745–770, 1954

Blacher RS: The briefest encounter: psychotherapy for medical and surgical patients. Gen Hosp Psychiatry 6:226–232, 1984

Black JL, Allison TG, Williams DE, et al: Effect of intervention for psychological distress on rehospitalization rates in cardiac rehabilitation patients. Psychosomatics 39:134–143, 1998

Bloom BL: Focused single-session therapy: initial development and evaluation, in Forms of Brief Therapy. Edited by Budman S. New York, Guilford, 1981, pp 131–175

Budman SH, Stone J: Advances in brief psychotherapy: a review of recent literature. Hospital and Community Psychiatry 34:939–946, 1983

Cohen-Cole SA, Pincus HA, Stoudemire A, et al: Recent research developments in consultation-liaison psychiatry. Gen Hosp Psychiatry 8:326–329, 1986

Cunningham J, Strassburg D, Roback H: Group psychotherapy for medical patients. Compr Psychiatry 19:135–140, 1978

Davanloo H: Basic Principles and Techniques in Short-Term Dynamic Psychotherapy. New York, Spectrum, 1978 deGruy FV 3rd: Mental health diagnoses and the costs of primary care. J Fam Pract 49:311–313, 2000

Despland JN, de Roten Y, Despars J, et al: Contribution of patient defense mechanisms and therapist interventions to the development of early therapeutic alliance in a brief psychodynamic investigation. J Psychother Pract Res 10:155–164, 2001

Deutsch F: The associative anamnesis. Psychoanal Q 8:354–381, 1939

Deutsch F: The Mysterious Leap From the Mind to the Body. New York, International Universities Press, 1959

Deutsch F, Murphy W: The Clinical Interview. New York, International Universities Press, 1955

Dickson LR, Hays LR, Kaplan C, et al: Psychological profile of somatizing patients attending the integrative clinic. Int J Psychiatry Med 22:141–153, 1992

Dolinar LJ: A historical review of outpatient consultation-liaison psychiatry. Gen Hosp Psychiatry 15:363–368, 1993

Engel G: The need for a new medical model: a challenge for biomedicine. Science 196:129–135, 1977

Fawzy FI, Fawzy NW: A structured psychoeducational intervention for cancer patients. Gen Hosp Psychiatry 16:149–192, 1994

Fenichel O: Brief psychotherapy, in The Collected Papers of Otto Fenichel, Second Series. New York, WW Norton, 1954, pp 243–259

Frances AJ, Clarkin JF: No treatment as the prescription of choice. Arch Gen Psychiatry 142:922–926, 1981

Frank J: Persuasion and Healing. Baltimore, MD, Johns Hopkins University Press, 1973

Freud S: On psychotherapy (1904), in Collected Papers, Vol 1. Edited by Jones E. New York, Basic Books, 1959, pp 249–271

Freud S: Lines in the advance of psychoanalytic therapy (1919), in The Standard Edition of the Complete Psychological Works of Sigmund Freud, Vol 17. Translated and edited by Strachey J. London, Hogarth Press, 1955, pp 157–168

Gabbard GO: Psychodynamic Psychiatry in Clinical Practice. Washington, DC, American Psychiatric Press, 1990

Gitelson M: On the curative factors in the first phase of analysis, in Psychoanalysis: Science and Profession. Edited by Gitelson M. New York, International Universities Press, 1973, pp 311–341

Goldman W, McCulloch J, Sturm R: Costs and use of mental health services before and after managed care. Health Affairs 17:40–53, 1998

Green SA: Principles of medical psychotherapy, in Psychiatric Care of the Medical Patient. Edited by Stoudemire A, Fogel BS. New York, Oxford University Press, 1993, pp 1–18

Greenhill MH: Liaison psychiatry, in American Handbook of Psychiatry, 2nd Edition, Vol 7. Advances and New Directions. Edited by Arieti S, Brodie HKH. New York, Basic Books, 1981, pp 672–702

Groves JE: Management of the borderline patient on a medical or surgical ward: the psychiatric consultant's role. Int J Psychiatry Med 6:337–348, 1975

Groves JE, Kurcharski A: Brief psychotherapy, in Massachusetts General Hospital Handbook of General Hospital Psychiatry, 3rd Edition. Edited by Cassem NH. St Louis, MO, CV Mosby, 1991, pp 321–341

Hackett TP, Weisman AD: Psychiatric management of operative syndromes, I: the therapeutic consultation and the effect of noninterpretive intervention. Psychosom Med 22:267–282, 1960a

Hackett TP, Weisman AD: Psychiatric management of operative syndromes, II: psychodynamic factors in formulation and management. Psychosom Med 22:356–372, 1960b

Hamburg D, Adams JE: A perspective on coping behavior. Arch Gen Psychiatry 17:277–284, 1967

Harrison SI, Carek DJ: A Guide to Psychotherapy. Boston, MA, Little, Brown, 1966

Henry GW: Some modern aspects of psychiatry in general hospital practice. Am J Psychiatry 9:481–499, 1929–1930

Henry WP, Schact TE, Strupp HH: Structural analysis of social behavior: application to a study of interpersonal process in differential psychotherapeutic outcome. J Consult Clin Psychol 54:27–31, 1986

Hersen M, Bellack AS: Perspectives in the behavioral treatment of depression. Behav Modif 6:95–106, 1982

Horowitz MJ: Phase oriented treatment of stress response syndromes. Am J Psychother 27:506–515, 1973

Horowitz MJ: A model of mourning: change in schemas of self and others. J Am Psychoanal Assoc 38:297–324, 1990

Horowitz MJ, Kaltreider NB: Brief therapy for the stress response syndrome. Psychiatr Clin North Am 2:365–377, 1979

Horowitz MJ, Marmar C, Krupnick J, et al: Personality Styles and Brief Psychotherapy. New York, Basic Books, 1984

Jackson SW: The listening healer in the history of psychological healing. Am J Psychiatry 149:1623–1632, 1992

Jacobs J: Family therapy in the context of chronic medical illness, in Psychiatric Care of the Medical Patient. Edited by Stoudemire A, Fogel BS. New York, Oxford University Press, 1993, pp 19–30

Jarvik LF, Mintz J, Steuer J: Treating geriatric depression: a 26-week interim analysis. J Am Geriatr Soc 30:713–717, 1982

Jones EE, Caston J, Skolnikoff A: Research on the efficacy of psychoanalysis. J Am Psychoanal Assoc 40:625–630, 1992

Kahana RJ, Bibring GL: Personality types in medical management, in Psychiatry and Medical Practice in a General Hospital. Edited by Zinberg NE. New York, International Universities Press, 1964, pp 108–123

Kaplan KH: Development and function of a psychiatric liaison clinic. Psychosomatics 22:502–512, 1981

Keefe RH, Hall ML: Private practitioners' documentation of outpatient psychiatric treatment: questioning managed care. J Behav Health Serv Res 26:151–170, 1999

Klerman GL, Weissman MM, Rounsaville BR, et al: Interpersonal Psychotherapy of Depression. New York, Basic Books, 1984

Koenig HG: Depression in hospitalized older patients with congestive heart failure. Gen Hosp Psychiatry 20:29–43, 1998

Kunkel EJ, Worley LL, Monti DA, et al: Follow-up consultation billing and documentation. Gen Hosp Psychiatry 21:197–208, 1999

Lazar SG, Gabbard GO: The cost-effectiveness of psychotherapy. J Psychother Pract Res 6:307–314, 1997

Lazarus AA: Will reason prevail? from classic psychoanalysis to new age therapy. Am J Psychother 54:152–155, 2000

Levenson H, Hales RE: Brief psychodynamically informed therapy for medically ill patients, in Medical-Psychiatric Practice, Vol 2. Edited by Stoudemire A, Fogel BS. Washington, DC, American Psychiatric Press, 1993, pp 3–37

Liberzon I, Goldman RS, Hendrickson WJ: Very brief psychotherapy in the psychiatric consultation setting. Int J Psychiatry Med 22:65–75, 1992

Lipowski ZJ: Consultation-liaison psychiatry: the first half century. Gen Hosp Psychiatry 8:305–315, 1986

Lipsitt DR: Integration clinic: an approach to the teaching and practice of medical psychology in an outpatient setting, in Psychiatry and Medical Practice in a General Hospital. Edited by Zinberg NE. New York, International Universities Press, 1964, pp 231–249

Lipsitt DR: Some problems in the teaching of psychosomatic medicine, in Psychosomatic Medicine: Current Trends and Clinical Applications. Edited by Lipowski ZJ, Lipsitt DR, Whybrow PC. New York, Oxford University Press, 1977, pp 599–611

Lipsitt DR: Therapeutic alliance in psychiatric consultation, in Psychiatry, Vol 2. Edited by Michels R, Cavenar JO Jr, Brodie HKH, et al. Philadelphia, PA, JB Lippincott, 1986, pp 1–10

Lipsitt DR: Psyche and soma in postwar psychiatry: struggles to close the gap, in American Psychiatry After World War II (1944–1994). Edited by Menninger RW, Nemiah JC. Washington, DC, American Psychiatric Press, 2000, pp 152–186

Lipsitt DR: The patient-physician relationship in the treatment of hypochondriasis, in Hypochondriasis: Modern Perspectives on an Ancient Malady. Edited by Starcevic V, Lipsitt DR. New York, Oxford University Press, 2001, pp 265–290

Lipsitt DR, Lipsitt MP: Guidelines for working with families in consultation-liaison psychiatry, in Handbook of Studies on General Hospital Psychiatry. Edited by Judd FK, Burrows GD, Lipsitt DR. Amsterdam, The Netherlands, Elsevier, 1991, pp 179–194

Luborsky L: Theory and technique in dynamic psychotherapy—curative factors and training therapists to maximize them. Psychother Psychosom 53:50–57, 1990

Malan DH: A Study of Brief Psychotherapy. London, Tavistock, 1963

Mann J: Time-Limited Psychotherapy. Cambridge, MA, Harvard University Press, 1973

Marmor J: The physician as psychotherapist, in Psychiatry in General Medical Practice. Edited by Usdin G, Lewis JM. New York, McGraw-Hill, 1979a

Marmor J: Short-term dynamic psychotherapy. Am J Psychiatry 136:149–155, 1979b

Marshall RD, Vaughan SC, MacKinnon RA, et al: Assessing outcome in psychoanalysis and long-term dynamic psychotherapy. J Am Acad Psychoanal 24:575–604, 1996

Melges FT: Family approaches to health and disease, in Psychiatry, Vol 2. Edited by Michels R, Cavenar JO Jr, Brodie HKH, et al. Philadelphia, PA, JB Lippincott, 1985, pp 1–9

Meyer RE, Sotsky SM: Managed care and the role and training of psychiatrists. Health Affairs 14:65–77, 1995

Mohl PC, Burstein AG: The application of Kohutian self-psychology to consultation-liaison psychiatry. Gen Hosp Psychiatry 4:113–119, 1982

Moynihan C, Bliss JM, Davidson J, et al. Evaluation of adjuvant psychological therapy in patients with testicular cancer: randomised controlled trial. British Medical Journal 316:429–435, 1998

Nadelson T: Engagement before alliance. Psychother Psychosom 33:76–86, 1980

O'Dowd MA, Gomez MF: Psychotherapy in consultation-liaison psychiatry. Am J Psychother 55:122–132, 2001

Olfson M, Sing M, Schlesinger HJ: Mental health/medical care cost offsets: opportunities for managed care. Health Affairs 18:79–90, 1999

Parsons T: The Social System. Glencoe, IL, Free Press, 1951

Perry S, Cooper AM, Michels R: The psychodynamic formulation: its purpose, structure and clinical application. Am J Psychiatry 144:543–551, 1987

Polatin P: A Guide to Treatment in Psychiatry. Philadelphia, PA, JB Lippincott, 1966

Shapiro AK: The placebo effect in the history of medical treatment: implications for psychiatry. Am J Psychiatry 116:298–304, 1959

Sifneos P: Short-Term Psychotherapy and Emotional Crisis. Cambridge, MA, Harvard University Press, 1972

Sifneos PE: The prevalence of "alexithymic" characteristics in psychosomatic patients. Psychother Psychosom 22:255–262, 1973

Sifneos PE: Short-term dynamic psychotherapy for patients with physical symptomatology. Psychother Psychosom 42:48–51, 1984

Speckens AE, van Hemert AM, Spinhoven P, et al: Cognitive behavioural therapy for medically unexplained physical symptoms: a randomised controlled trial. British Medical Journal 311:1328–1332, 1995

Spiegel D: Psychosocial aspects of breast cancer treatment. Semin Oncol 24:(S1)36–47, 1997

Spiegel D, Bloom J, Kraemer HC, et al: Effect of psychosocial treatment on survival of patients with metastatic breast cancer. Lancet 2:888–891, 1989

Spira JL, Spiegel D: Group psychotherapy of the medically ill, in Psychiatric Care of the Medical Patient. Edited by Stoudemire A, Fogel BS. New York, Oxford University Press, 1993, pp 31–50

Stein A, Weiner S: Group therapy with medically ill patients, in Psychotherapeutic Approaches to Medicine. Edited by Karasu TB, Steinmuller RI. New York, Grune & Stratton, 1978, pp 223–242

Strain JJ, Grossman S: Psychological Care of the Medically Ill. New York, Appleton-Century-Crofts, 1975

Strupp HH, Binder JL: Psychotherapy in a New Key: A Guide to Time-Limited Dynamic Psychotherapy. New York, Basic Books, 1984

Ursano RJ, Hales RE: A review of brief individual psychotherapies. Am J Psychiatry 143:1507–1517, 1986

Valenstein AF: On attachment to painful feelings and the negative therapeutic reaction. Psychoanal Study Child 28:365–391, 1973

Vaughan SC, Marshall RD, Mackinnon RA, et al: Can we do psychoanalytic outcome research? A feasibility study. Int J Psychoanal 81:513–527, 2000

Viederman M: The psychodynamic life narrative: a psychotherapeutic intervention useful in crisis situations. Psychiatry 46:236–246, 1983

Viederman M: The active dynamic interview and the supportive relationship. Compr Psychiatry 25:147–157, 1984

Viederman M: Psychotherapeutic approaches in the medically ill, in Psychiatry, Vol 2. Edited by Michels R, Cavenar JO Jr, Brodie HKH, et al. Philadelphia, PA, JB Lippincott, 1985, pp 1–12

Viederman M, Perry S: Use of psychodynamic life narrative in the treatment of depression in the physically ill. Gen Hosp Psychiatry 2:177–185, 1980

Von Korff M, Katon W, Bush T, et al. Treatment costs, cost offset, and cost-effectiveness of collaborative management of depression. Psychosom Med 60:143–149, 1998

Waldinger RJ: Psychiatry for Medical Students, 2nd Edition. Washington, DC, American Psychiatric Press, 1990

Walker EA, Katon WJ, Russo J, et al: Predictors of outcome in a primary care depression trial. J Gen Intern Med 15:859–867, 2000

Wallerstein R: Psychotherapy and Psychoanalysis: Theory, Practice, Research. New York, International Universities Press, 1975

Wallerstein R: Research in psychodynamic psychotherapy. Mt Sinai J Med 63:167–177, 1996

Ward E, King M, Lloyd M, et al: Randomised controlled trial of non-directive counselling, cognitive-behavior therapy, and usual general practitioner care for patients with depression, I: clinical effectiveness. BMJ 321:1383–1388, 2000

Whitehorn JC: Basic psychiatry in medical practice. JAMA 148:329–334, 1952

Wolberg LR: Introduction, in Inside Psychotherapy. Edited by Bry A. New York, Basic Books, 1972, pp xi–xxvii

Yalom ID: Theory and Practice of Group Psychotherapy. New York, Basic Books, 1975

Yamada S, Greene G, Bauman K, et al: A biopsychosocial approach to finding common ground in the clinical encounter. Acad Med 75:643–648, 2000

Zeiss AM, Lewinsohn PM, Munoz RF: Nonspecific improvement effects in depression using interpersonal, cognitive and pleasant events focused treatments. J Consult Clin Psychol 47:427–439, 1979

46

Behavioral Medicine

Andrew B. Littman, M.D.

Mark W. Ketterer, Ph.D.

The Russians have a proverb: "The brain is capable of holding a conversation with the body that ends in death" (Eliot and Breo 1984, p. 15).

"Small disconnected facts, if you take note of them, have a way of becoming connected" (Percy 1987, p. 67).

Behavioral medicine is a field that was initially inspired by the potential application of classical and operant learning theory to behavioral problems in medical patients (G. E. Schwartz and Weiss 1978) and that was historically applied to outpatients with psychophysiological or somatoform disorders. While behavioral medicine evolves into a theoretically and therapeutically more eclectic arena, practitioners of the field continue to find behavioral techniques (e.g., relaxation and hypnosis, environmental modification, biofeedback, cognitive-behavioral therapy) useful and effective. Studies on the underdiagnosis and inadequate treatment of psychiatric disorders and subsyndromal conditions in nonpsychiatric medical settings (Katon 1987; Katon et al. 1992; Von Korff et al. 1992; Wells et al. 1989) now complement the observation that patients undergoing psychotherapy make less use of the medical system (Borus et al. 1985; Budman et al. 1984; Rosen and Wiens 1979).

Somatization and denial confound patient reporting of symptoms and physician recognition of behavioral syndromes (Barsky 1992; Ford and Smith 1987; Kellner 1985; Miranda et al. 1991). In addition, the relative neglect of teaching behavioral syndromes during medical education and training (Badger and Rand 1988; Blackwell 1985; Eisenberg 1992) results in the potential contributions of a patient's behavior being, to a large extent, unrealized (Ormel et al. 1991). Such findings support the need for greater integration of behavioral science in routine medical care. Not only are such contributions potential improvements in the quality of care, but they may also represent a source of cost savings (Connelly et al. 1991).

Much research in behavioral medicine is conducted in an attempt to elucidate psychopathophysiological mechanisms, or the means by which psychological events (i.e., cognitions, emotions, behavior, and psychosocial environments) affect physiological events in a pathogenic manner. Researchers apply the scientific method to test the validity of hypothesized relationships between psychosocial variables and physical disease end points. A growing body of literature demonstrates the efficacy of treatment in reducing morbidity or mortality in the so-called psychophysiological disorders—medical conditions that are initiated or aggravated by psychological events. Because such treatment studies are the only true experiments in validating risk factor research, they are the gold standard for establishing causality. Although there are numerous data evaluating many physical diseases cross-sectionally for psychosocial correlates, relatively few prospective analyses and even fewer treatment trials have been conducted.

The goals of behavioral medicine encompass reduction in emotional and somatic distress and disability as well as decrease in physical morbidity and mortality, alteration of unhealthy behaviors, alleviation of medication side effects, and reduction in inappropriate utilization of medical resources by patients who somatize (Muldoon et al. 1990; Smith and Pekkanen 1992).

Central to the behavioral medicine approach is a belief that the arousal of emotion fosters disease end points in the psychophysiological disorders—or symptoms, in the case of the somatoform disorders—by way of either psychoneuroendocrine or psychobehavioral pathways. Psychoneuroendocrine pathways encompass the downstream neural or endocrine effects of chronic or acute emotional arousal (Chrousos and Gold 1992). Psychobehavioral pathways are mediated by the impact of exogenous substances, such as alcohol, caffeine, and nicotine, or behaviors, such as noncompliance. Psychopathophysiological arousal may be the result of genetic-constitutional factors, early life experiences that subsequently shape interpersonal beliefs and coping, or environments that are sometimes universally and sometimes idiosyncratically stressful. Intervention can be instituted in an attempt to influence any or all of these modifiable elements. Quantification of the psychopathophysiological contribution to illness is hampered by uncertainties of measuring emotional arousal. For example, interpersonal factors often inhibit overt expressive behavior and subjective reports of distress. Furthermore, chronic arousal appears to result in either a loss of the subjective experience of emotion or a resetting of normative expectations regarding one's own mood (Ketterer, in press). Chronic arousal may then manifest clinically as alexithymia (Lesser 1985) or denial.

In an early approach to psychosomatic disorders, several investigators attempted to demonstrate specificity of relationships between personality characteristics and medical conditions (Alexander 1950; Dunbar 1947). Behavioral medicine has taken a less theoretically constrained, and more empirically driven, approach to understanding psyche-soma relationships. Some of the psychological phenomena investigated are probably subclinical psychiatric disorders, whereas others seem to call for an entirely new way of conceptualizing psychopathology in this arena. For example, it is striking that the DSM-IV-TR (American Psychiatric Association 2000) system contains large sections on depressive and anxiety disorders but no focused discussion of anger, a central concern in the behavioral treatment of ischemic heart disease (IHD), as discussed later in this chapter (see "Cardiovascular Diseases" section). Other examples of phenomena that are difficult to categorize within the DSM-IV-TR nosology include the impact of high-demand or low-control jobs, low social support, and vital exhaustion, each of which is associated with physical disease outcomes. The currently used DSM-IV-TR (American Psychiatric Association 2000) diagnostic entity "316—psychological factor affecting medical condition" is unsatisfying because each of the entities listed above potentially implies a different theoretical conceptual paradigm, pathophysiology, set of outcome measures, and treatment strategy. A new categorization of these behav-

ioral factors must be developed. We have based the material in this chapter on an empirical, outcome-based approach to evaluating the clinical significance of a behavioral approach and treatment in various medical conditions.

CARDIOVASCULAR DISEASES[1]

There is increased focus on primary and secondary prevention of IHD, including modification of cardiovascular risk factors and other negative health behaviors (Public Health Service 1991). Unfortunately, it is notoriously difficult to modify risk factors, such as cigarette smoking, physical inactivity, high serum cholesterol levels, elevated dietary fat intake, depression, and excessive stress and hostility.

Numerous studies have been performed demonstrating the influence of psychosocial and behavioral risk factors in the etiology of IHD (Blumenthal and Kamarck 1987). The most well known of these factors is type A behavior, the chronic and habitual response of the individual to perceived demands with time urgency and/or easily provoked annoyance, anger, and aggression (Friedman and Ulmer 1984). The initial enthusiasm for the global type A concept, including elements such as perfectionism, mistrust, competitiveness, arrogance, practicality, and controlling nature or hyper-responsibility, waned in the middle to late 1980s as hostility was found to be the "toxic" element of the syndrome (Dembroski et al. 1989; Shekelle et al. 1985). Whereas global type A behavior is not always predictive of IHD risk, hostility is (Dimsdale 1988). Hostility is pathophysiologically related to IHD by numerous mechanisms (Table 46–1).

Depressive symptoms are fairly ubiquitous in patients after a myocardial infarction and have been traditionally been considered to be reactive in etiology, self-limited, and of minimal importance (Wishnie et al. 1971). Klerman (1989) pointed out that, traditionally, depressive symptoms are minimized in clinical settings as demoralization, expectable reactions, and neurotic depression. However, 18% of patients with IHD have major depressive disorder that predates the diagnosis of IHD or myocardial infarction (Cay et al. 1972; Lloyd and Cawley 1978). In addition to the 20% of IHD patients with major depressive disorder, another 20%–30% of IHD patients have depressive symptoms not meeting criteria for major depressive disorder. These studies confirm the

---

[1] Portions of this section are reprinted from Littman AB: "A Review of Psychosomatic Aspects of Cardiovascular Disease." *Psychotherapy and Psychosomatics* 60:148–167, 1993. Used with permission.

TABLE 46–1. Associations between hostility and ischemic heart disease

Association	Reference
Increased atherosclerosis	Clarkson 1987
Precipitation of myocardial ischemia	Rozanski et al. 1988; Yeung et al. 1989
Precipitation of coronary vasospasm	Verrier et al. 1987
Mental workload induction of parasympathetic-sympathetic autonomic imbalance	Kamada et al. 1992
Sudden death by ventricular arrhythmia	Frank and Smith 1990
Caffeine use	Ketterer and Maercklein 1991
Persistent cigarette smoking after diagnosis of ischemic heart disease	Ketterer and Maercklein 1992

clinical impression that depressive symptoms are common among patients with IHD before the onset of symptomatic IHD. The Medical Outcome Study demonstrated the significant morbidity of depressive symptoms, especially in comorbid medical conditions, including the powerful negative impact of depressive symptoms on patients' functional status and quality of life (Wells et al. 1989).

Increasingly abundant literature demonstrates that depressive symptoms significantly affect health outcomes beyond the considerable influence of depressive symptoms on functional status and quality of life. For instance, adherence to treatment is lower in patients with IHD who have depressive symptoms (Blumenthal et al. 1982; Finnegan and Suler 1985). Depressive symptoms predict lack of improvement of exercise functioning in patients with IHD who are undergoing cardiac rehabilitation (Downing et al. 1992; Milani et al. 1993; A.B. Littman, unpublished data, 1993). A prospective study in Dutch men of "vital exhaustion" (e.g., feelings of hopelessness, inability to cope with problems, and wanting to give up) showed increased risk of myocardial infarction in those affected (Appels and Mulder 1988). In a population-based study of 2,800 American adults (Anda et al. 1993), the investigators found, after controlling for demographic and risk factors, that individuals with depressed mood and hopelessness had higher IHD morbidity and mortality. Thus, in patients with IHD with depressive symptoms and/or hopelessness, in the absence of major depressive disorder, evidence suggests that this affective state is clinically relevant. No controlled psychopharmacological or psychotherapeutic treatment trials of patients with IHD with depressive symptoms are currently available, but anecdotal evidence suggests that treatment with selective serotonin reuptake inhibitors (SSRIs) is highly effective. In addition, evidence suggests that treatment of the type A behavior pattern by cognitive-behavioral group therapy is associated with significant reductions in levels of anxiety and depressive symptoms (Fava et al. 1991). The ENRICHD trial, sponsored by the National Institutes of Health, is evaluating the efficacy of cognitive-behavioral therapy and, if needed, psychopharmacologic treatment with post–myocardial infarction patients with depressive symptoms and social isolation. The trial is in its last year, and shortly we will have data on cognitive-behavioral treatment of depressive symptoms and social isolation in IHD patients and its effect on morbidity and mortality.

Several studies demonstrate that patients with major depressive disorder have higher mortality from IHD than those who are not depressed (Murphy et al. 1987; Rubins et al. 1985). In addition, studies report that major depressive disorder is present in about 20% of patients just before IHD diagnosis and that only 10%–20% of these patients with depression receive a clinical diagnosis or treatment (Carney et al. 1988a, 1988b; Schleifer et al. 1989). Studies also show that, after traditional cardiac risk factors are controlled, untreated major depressive disorder predicts major cardiac events, including death, after diagnosis of IHD (Ahern et al. 1990; Carney et al. 1988a; Ladwig et al. 1991). In one study, 18% of patients hospitalized for myocardial infarction had major depressive disorder, and depression predicted mortality at 6 months, with a relative risk of 4.3 after other risk factors were controlled (Frasure-Smith et al. 1993). The impact of major depressive disorder on cardiovascular mortality is at least equivalent to that of left ventricular dysfunction and history of previous myocardial infarction, among the most potent known indicators of prognosis (Frasure-Smith et al. 1993). Despite all this evidence, and one study showing a marked increase in myocardial infarction in patients receiving inadequate treatment for depression compared with those receiving adequate treatment (Avery and Winokur 1976), no current study has evaluated the effect of treatment for major depressive disorder on IHD end points. SADHART is a study evaluating the efficacy of sertraline in treating major depressive disorder in IHD patients. It is hoped that this study will evaluate the impact of sertraline treatment of depression on cardiac morbidity and mortality.

Along with hostility, depressive symptoms, and major depressive disorder, a number of other psychosocial factors have been implicated as risk factors for IHD (Table 46–2). The specific interrelations among these factors and their mediating pathophysiologies have not been established (Frank and Smith 1990; Kamarck and Jennings 1991; Lown 1987). Musselman et al. (2000) demonstrated that patients with IHD and depression have stickier platelets and that SSRI treatment of depression and reduction of depressive symptoms appeared to be related to reversal of the platelet abnormality. It has been proposed that, because of their associations with depression itself, these social and environmental factors may relate to clinical outcomes in patients with cardiac disease (Dohrenwend et al. 1992). Finally, research demonstrates that emotional distress among post–myocardial infarction patients quadruples rehospitalization costs. Controlling for other potential mediating factors did not reduce the strength of the association of psychological distress and increased costs in this study (Allison et al. 1995).

The term *denial* has at least two presumably correlated meanings as applied to populations of patients with cardiac disease. First, patients sometimes deny their emotions during the initial phases of cardiac illness (Ketterer 1992). Second, patients sometimes deny acute cardiac symptoms themselves. Denial independently predicts better medical outcomes during acute hospitalization for unstable angina (Levenson et al. 1989). During hospitalization for myocardial infarction or bypass surgery, deniers spend fewer days in the intensive care unit (Levine et al. 1987). However, these benefits are short lived. Over the subsequent year, these same deniers are more noncompliant with medical recommendations and require more days of rehospitalization compared with other patients. Similarly, denying emotional distress during the acute phase of a myocardial infarction is associated with increased likelihood of returning to work and being sexually active at 1 year follow-up but also with resumption of smoking (Stern et al. 1976). Thus, it appears that emotional denial during acutely stressful medical events, such as myocardial infarction or cardiac surgery, is adaptive in the short run but deleterious over the long haul (Suls and Fletcher 1985).

A study examining the relationship between emotional and symptomatic denial found that 60% of all myocardial infarctions result in death before hospital admission (American Heart Association 1991). At least 25% of all nonfatal myocardial infarctions are unrecognized on their occurrence (Bertolet and Hill 1989). Up to 80% of all patients with diagnosed myocardial infarctions arrive at an emergency facility too late to benefit fully from modern thrombolytic therapy or emergency revascularization. Several investigations have been unable to identify factors that can account for this widespread failure in

TABLE 46–2. Psychosocial factors implicated as risk factors for ischemic heart disease

Risk factor	Reference
Lack of social support	Tyroler et al. 1987
Social isolation and alienation	Ruberman et al. 1984
Low socioeconomic status	Williams et al. 1992
Low-control/high-demand jobs	Karasek et al. 1981
Phobic anxiety	Haines et al. 1987
Anxiety disorders	Coryell et al. 1986
Depressive symptoms	Anda et al. 1993
Vital exhaustion	Appels and Mulder 1988
Major depressive disorder	Frasure-Smith et al. 1993
Hostility	Dembroski et al. 1989

symptom perception and response, including age, gender, socioeconomic status, prior cardiac diagnosis, and insurance status. Patient interviews reveal that many patients spend most of the time before admission deciding if they are ill, or ill enough, to warrant immediate care. Thus, reality-based cognitive processing of anginal symptoms appears to be the primary determinant of delay of treatment-seeking behavior. Measures of somatic nonawareness and alexithymia are strongly associated with prolonged treatment-seeking delay during acute myocardial infarction (Kenyon et al. 1991). Thus, a relationship appears to exist between lack of somatic and emotional awareness. Patients who score highly on somatic awareness measurement report more salient symptoms (e.g., more rapid onset, sharp as opposed to dull pain) and are more likely to believe they are experiencing a myocardial infarction. Thus, their more rapid treatment seeking is understandable. Patients who scored highly on the alexithymia measure, controlling for level of myocardial damage, had more cardiac symptoms yet were less likely to arrive at an emergency facility quickly. There are no studies on effective treatments for alexithymia or delay of treatment-seeking behavior, despite its obvious powerful contribution to poor health outcome.

A variety of behavioral and psychological interventions can reduce type A behavior in both healthy individuals (Gill et al. 1985) and patients with IHD (Friedman et al. 1984). A meta-analysis of the type A treatment literature revealed that a variety of interventions are effective, including yoga, emotional support, community-wide public health efforts, and more standard group therapy (Nunes et al. 1987). The therapies that were most successful in reducing type A behavior were incorporated into a multimodal comprehensive treatment plan, including an educational focus and coping methods using relaxation or cognitive and behavioral techniques (Nunes et al. 1987; L. H. Powell and Thoreson 1987).

Case History of a Patient With Stress and IHD

Mr. A, a 47-year-old man, developed unstable angina and subsequently had an uncomplicated myocardial infarction. His risk factors for IHD included a family history of IHD in his father and paternal uncles, elevated serum cholesterol (250 mg/dL) with low high-density lipoprotein level (29 mg/dL) and elevated low-density lipoprotein level (130 mg/dL), physical inactivity for more than 5 years, mild obesity (25 pounds over his ideal body weight), cigarette smoking, and long-standing stress. He entered a preventive cardiology program designed to modify his risk factors for IHD. During the multidisciplinary evaluation, it became clearer that Mr. A's pattern of coping with a range of work and personal demands was to react excessively with a great deal of worry, irritation, impatience, and anger. He was increasingly frustrated by a difficult work situation that did not afford him any advancement or recognition, and he felt inappropriately trapped by his circumstances. Whenever he attempted to quit smoking, Mr. A developed persistent, intolerable shortening of his "fuse," without depressive disorder, and found that the return to smoking lengthened his fuse to a more tolerable level.

Psychiatric examination revealed that Mr. A had no current or past Axis I or II psychiatric diagnoses except nicotine dependence. He and his wife recognized the health and quality-of-life benefits of reducing his hostility and began a behavioral treatment plan. Initially, this treatment consisted of reading about the affective, behavioral, and cognitive signs of hostility and beginning to recognize these manifestations when expressed in everyday life. Mr. A took notes about these events so that he could report them at the next session. He received training in behavioral skills so that he could truncate these episodes. Skills that were taught as part of his treatment plan included early recognition of the signs of stress, relaxation training, and cognitive restructuring so that the aggravating event is not personalized. With these skills in place, the frequency and intensity of Mr. A's behavioral and cognitive symptoms diminished, and the intensity of the stressors needed to stimulate the signs and symptoms increased.

With these changes in episode intensity and frequency, it became clear that several identifiable themes triggered the stress response. These themes paralleled issues surrounding Mr. A's early experience of his father's repeated extended absences and an overly critical and punitive mother. Mr. A had initially vehemently denied that these early experiences had any effect on his current behavior but recognized their impact in the later phases of treatment. Mr. A's anger, tension, irritability, worry, and inability to relax diminished and his ability to be content, relaxed, and serene improved with the treatment. His work and family relationships also improved.

A meta-analysis of type A–reduction treatment studies in patients with IHD demonstrated a 3-year reduction of 50% for combined mortality and recurrent myocardial infarction (Nunes et al. 1987). A recent comparison of the efficacy of behavioral with medical and surgical interventions to reduce the risk of nonfatal myocardial infarction and cardiac death showed behavioral therapies to be superior to all methods of treatment, except the use of aspirin in patients with unstable angina and bypass surgery in patients who were classified as high risk (Ketterer 1993). The largest single project to date to evaluate the effects of group treatment of type A behavior is the Recurrent Coronary Prevention Project, involving 862 post–myocardial infarction patients (Friedman et al. 1987). Four and one-half years after the start of the study, 35% of the treatment group, compared with 10% of the placebo care group, markedly reduced their type A behavior. The rate of recurrence of myocardial infarction was significantly lower in the type A treatment group than in the placebo care group (13% versus 21%, respectively). The type A treatment group showed a significant reduction in cardiac death (2.7% versus 6.7%) when patients with preexisting severe heart damage were excluded from the analysis.

A total of 461 post–myocardial infarction men participated in a 1-year, randomized, controlled trial of stress reduction (Frasure-Smith 1991). Study subjects were monitored monthly for psychological distress, and patients identified by the monitoring procedure as stressed received counseling visits by nurses. Highly stressed patients who did not undergo any stress reduction had a threefold increase in risk of cardiac mortality compared with nonstressed patients who underwent stress reduction over a 5-year follow-up period. In addition, those who were highly stressed who received the 1-year program of stress monitoring and intervention did not experience any significant long-term increase in risk. Low-stress patients did not experience any benefit from the stress-monitoring program.

Blumenthal et al. (1997) evaluated the effect of stress management and exercise training on cardiac patients with stress-induced or ambulatory myocardial ischemia. Stress management (cognitive-behavioral therapy) produced a statistically significant relative risk reduction (0.26) in cardiac events, whereas exercise did not produce a significant reduction. Only stress management was associated with reduced stress-induced and ambulatory myocardial ischemia.

Ornish et al. (1990) used a multifaceted treatment of comprehensive lifestyle change, including low-fat vegetarian diet (8% of calories as dietary fat), stress management training (yoga, meditation, and group therapy), and moderate exercise, in an attempt to reduce coronary atherosclerosis without the use of lipid-lowering agents. Over a

1-year period, the coronary lesions in the treatment group regressed in 82% of the subjects, whereas the lesions progressed in the usual care group. Overall adherence to the treatment intervention was the best predictor of the extent of atherosclerotic regression (Ornish et al. 1990). Four-year follow-up data showed a highly significant difference in outcomes between the two groups, with continued regression (39.7%–43.6% in average percentage diameter of coronary artery stenosis) in the comprehensive lifestyle change group and continued progression (41.6%–51.4%) in the usual care group (Ornish et al. 1993).

Pharmacotherapy for Type A Behavior, Hostility, and Anger

The specific effects of pharmacological treatments on type A behaviors and associated clinical outcomes are not well studied in controlled settings. β-Blockers have had inconsistent and modest effects on type A behavior (Schmiedler et al. 1983). Benzodiazepines reduce catecholamines, cortisol, and blood pressure responses to acute mental stress in patients with type A behavior (Williams et al. 1986) and significantly reduce duration of silent ischemia in a small sample ($n = 8$) of patients with coronary disease (Shell and Swan 1986). However, benzodiazepines do not alter type A behavior or hostility. Investigators have hypothesized the presence of lowered central serotonergic function in patients with hostility associated with elevated risk for IHD (Littman et al. 1993). Individuals with low levels of central nervous system (CNS) serotonin have a lowered threshold for aggressive responses to noxious stimuli and appear to have a strong "urge to act out hostility" (Coccaro 1989; A. Roy et al. 1989). Elevating CNS serotonin activity may inhibit flow of arrhythmogenic sympathetic activity from the brain to the heart (Rabinowitz and Lown 1978). Anger attacks are common (44%) in individuals with major depressive disorder, and treatment with fluoxetine, an SSRI, reduces the presence of these anger outbursts by 70% (Fava et al. 1993). In patients with IHD with hostility and type A behavior but no Axis I psychiatric disorder, a clinical trial demonstrated that buspirone, a central serotonin$_{1A}$ partial agonist, significantly reduced hostility and type A behavior (Littman et al. 1993).

Lipids and Behavior

A clear association exists between elevated serum cholesterol and risk for IHD. Lower serum cholesterol reduces IHD events and IHD mortality in both primary and secondary prevention trials yet is not associated with improvement in overall survival (Jacobs et al. 1992). A

meta-analysis of these trials showed that counterbalancing the reduction in IHD mortality was an increase in deaths due to accidents, suicide, and violence (Muldoon et al. 1990). One study demonstrated that lowering dietary fat intake produced increased contact aggression and diminished central levels of serotonin in monkeys (Muldoon et al. 1991). The most recent meta-analysis of lipid-lowering trials showed an increased risk of death from violence and suicide only for subjects using medications to lower their cholesterol. This finding is consistent with another study that showed that patients with IHD who were receiving medical treatment for hypercholesterolemia reported significantly more symptoms of depression than those who were not receiving treatment (Ketterer et al. 1993). Intermittent case reports of the depressogenic effects of cholesterol-lowering agents, especially HMG-CoA inhibitors, also suggests that cholesterol-lowering agents may have behavioral effects.

The lipid and behavior story has become more complicated with the recognition that omega-3 fatty acids, the primary fat substituents found in the Mediterranean diet, appear to be cardioprotective by protecting against cardiac events and ventricular arrhythmia (Leaf 1999). These compounds have been found to stabilize mood, reduce anger, and reduce stress both in psychiatric patients (Stoll et al. 1999) and in nonpsychiatric populations (Hamazaki 1996; Stevens et al. 1996). Fats have now begun to be classified as "good" (i.e., polyunsaturated fats and monounsaturated fats, or more specifically omega-3 unsaturated fats) or "bad" (i.e., saturated fats) in terms of cardiac risk. Similarly, there may now be a difference between good and bad fats in terms of their effect on behavior.

In the Lyon Heart Study (deLorgeril et al. 1999), a diet rich in the good fats, the so-called Mediterranean diet, was given to cardiac patients and compared with a diet following American Heart Association dietary standards. In this study, the use of monounsaturated fat (from olive oil) and omega-3 fatty acids (from fish, canola, and flaxseed oil) reduced cardiac morbidity and mortality by over 85%.

Physical Activity

Physical activity appears to have numerous beneficial effects in individuals who are healthy and in those who have already developed IHD. Cardiac rehabilitation programs, primarily exercise programs, reduce mortality by 25% from all causes, including cardiovascular (Oldridge et al. 1988). The Multiple Risk Factor Intervention Trial (Leon et al. 1987) classified individuals at high risk for IHD according to levels of leisure-time physical activity (i.e., low, moderate, or high). Moderate levels of leisure-time physical activity were associated with 63% fewer cardiovascular deaths and 70% fewer total deaths compared with low leisure-time physical activity. Interestingly, mortality rates for the high leisure-time physical activity group were similar to those of the moderate leisure-time physical activity group. The study showed that 30–60 minutes of predominately light- to moderate-intensity activities on a daily basis reduces cardiovascular risk (Leon et al. 1987). In addition, the Centers for Disease Control and Prevention reviewed existing observational studies of healthy individuals and found a significant and graded relationship between physical inactivity and risk of coronary artery disease (K.E. Powell et al. 1987). A study from the Cooper Clinic with more than 13,000 subjects showed a strong, stepwise, and consistent inverse relationship between physical fitness and mortality, with the major burden for morbidity and mortality in the lowest quintile of fitness (Blair et al. 1989).

Attempts to validate or quantify the impact of an exercise-training program on psychosocial functioning in patients with IHD or in healthy subjects are fraught with uninterpretable or contradictory results because of variations in medical severity, levels of psychosocial distress, and psychiatric diagnoses among the heterogeneous populations studied (Greist et al. 1979; Hughes 1984; Taylor et al. 1986). Exercise, strength, and flexibility programs reduced type A behavior in healthy middle-aged men, but only exercise reduced the cardiovascular and sympathoadrenal responses to mental stress (Blumenthal et al. 1990). Other physiological and psychological benefits of exercise are summarized in Table 46–3.

Exercise and dieting appear to have equal efficacy in reducing plasma lipids in overweight sedentary men (Wood et al. 1988). Adherence to a regular exercise routine appears to be difficult, with about half of those enrolled in a well-equipped and well-staffed program dropping out within the first several months, and many of the remainder dropping out within 2 years. Surveys suggest that despite the cultural fascination with fitness, two-thirds of Americans do not exercise on a regular basis, and between 30% and 45% do not exercise at all (Martin and Dubbert 1985).

Obesity and Weight Loss

Weight loss is often urged for patients with cardiac disease because of the adverse effects of excess weight on hypertension, diabetes mellitus, lipid abnormalities, and physical inactivity. This encouragement occurs, unfortunately, despite strong evidence that weight loss is a futile goal for the majority of people. Although about one-third

TABLE 46–3. Physiological and psychological benefits of exercise

More regulated eating patterns
Longer and more restful sleep
Decreased anxiety and depression
Improved sexual adjustment
Greater ease in handling daily stress
Improvement in glucose tolerance
Enhancement of fibrinolysis
Reduction in systolic blood pressure and heart rate at rest and at comparable levels of submaximal work
Increases in peak oxygen uptake
Decreases in myocardial work at rest and submaximal work
Decrease in body weight
Reduction in body fat and increase in muscle mass
Changes in the central and peripheral circulation comparable with those observed in otherwise physically active subjects
Improvements in lipid parameters

Source. Adapted from Naughton JP: "Physical Activity and Coronary Artery Disease," in *Adult Fitness and Cardiac Rehabilitation.* Edited by Wilson PK. Baltimore, MD, University Park Press, 1975, pp 200–218.

of individuals seem to be able to lose weight and maintain the loss (Schachter 1982), relapse is inevitable for a large majority of people (NIH Technology Assessment Conference Panel 1992; Stunkard 1980). *Consumer Reports* confirmed these findings in a report titled "Losing Weight: What Works, What Doesn't," an evaluation of the differential effectiveness of the various commercial diet plans available ("Losing Weight" 1993). There is some suggestion in the literature that work-site behavioral weight reduction programs are as effective as self-help and commercial groups at one-third the cost (Brownell et al. 1985). Because genetic factors play a strong role in obesity (Stunkard et al. 1990), it is possible that urging patients to lose weight as a goal is merely setting them up for frustration, demoralization, and so-called weight-cycling, in which worse outcomes result than the initial problem (Garner and Wooley 1991). If a patient is mildly or moderately overweight and not hypertensive or diabetic, or these two conditions are present but controlled, and if the patient exercises regularly, it may be most productive to encourage weight maintenance, most preferably at an 8%–15% weight reduction level. There is evidence that the health risks of obesity may be ameliorated by this approach. Although studies have demonstrated the impact of obesity on risk for IHD (Manson et al. 1990), no studies are currently available to demonstrate that induced weight loss lowers the risk for cardiac end points.

Depression has been shown to play a substantial role in the complex patterns of sex-, age-, and education-related weight change among adults (DiPietro et al. 1992). These patterns of weight change may contribute to the adverse health effects associated with depression. Pharmacological interventions to reduce weight have not been of interest since the use of amphetamines for that purpose in the 1970s and before. The findings of efficacy of weight loss with the use of drugs such as dexfenfluramine (Turner 1992) and the evaluation of fluoxetine for that purpose have begun to shift the view of some investigators and clinicians to considering the chronic pharmacological treatment of obesity (Bjorntorp 1992). However, findings of heart valve abnormalities and possible increased incidence of symptomatic pulmonary hypertension in obese patients given the combination of fenfluramine and phentermine, commonly called fen-phen, chilled enthusiasm for these treatments, and the product was removed from the United States market. At the same time and working counter to this reaction is the enormous interest in a host of specific anorexigenic agents; specific anorexic properties of serotonin$_{1C}$ agonists (Silverstone 1992), leptin, and various other neuroregulatory compounds of appetite.

Systemic Arterial Hypertension

Numerous studies have demonstrated that social factors, such as social stress and conflict, and low degrees of social support are associated with elevated blood pressure (Dressler et al. 1986, 1988). The nonpharmacological approaches to the treatment of hypertension are relaxation training, biofeedback, weight loss, exercise, dietary sodium restriction, and nutritional supplementation (i.e., with calcium, magnesium, potassium, and fish oil) (Chesney et al. 1987). Biofeedback methods are effective in reducing blood pressure, and this effect on blood pressure has been shown to generalize from practice sessions to daily life and sleep periods with some degree of persistence (Chesney et al. 1987).

Only one study (Patel et al. 1985), with 192 hypertensive patients, showed the efficacy of multimodal stress management in reducing blood pressure at 8 weeks and 4 years. A meta-analysis of nine other controlled studies of stress management with 733 subjects found a significant effect (2 mm Hg) only in diastolic blood pressure in nonmedicated patients and no effect in patients who were already taking medication (Kaufman et al. 1988). A study of 2,200 subjects comparing four nonpharmacological interventions (weight reduction, dietary sodium restriction, stress management, and nutritional supplementation) on blood pressure in individuals with high baseline blood pressure demonstrated significant effects on blood pressure only from weight reduction and

sodium restriction (Trials of Hypertension Prevention Collaborative Research Group 1992). The DASH diet is a further evolution in the dietary treatment of hypertension. To a degree not seen with previous nonpharmacological treatments (Svetkey et al. 1999), there is evidence that diet can significantly affect hypertension. The DASH diet includes sodium restriction with a diet that emphasizes fruits, vegetables, and low-fat dairy foods; includes whole grains, poultry, fish, and nuts; and is reduced in fats, red meat, sweets, and sugar-containing beverages.

Despite conventional wisdom and hopes to the contrary, recent studies cast serious doubt on whether relaxation therapies significantly reduce blood pressure. Ongoing studies may shed light on whether a definable subgroup of patients, such as those with elevated urinary catecholamine or cortisol excretion, may benefit from relaxation treatments. Focus on weight reduction in patients with hypertension appears to be an effective nonpharmacological method to reduce blood pressure, although subsequent weight maintenance will be a significant problem. In addition, medication compliance is one of the most critical elements in the successful treatment of hypertension. Adherence remains a sizable problem despite antihypertensive medications' having less negative impact on patients' quality of life (Haynes et al. 1979).

Smoking Cessation

Cigarette smoking is the single most avoidable cause of death (Shopland 1984). Studies indicate that the mortality rate is lower among patients with coronary artery disease who stop smoking than among those who continue to smoke (Vlietstra et al. 1986). In addition, passive cigarette smoking also poses an increased risk to those in smoky environments (L'Enfant and Liu 1980). There are clearly delineated short-term economic and health benefits of reducing adult smoking (Lightwood and Glantz 1997).

Public awareness of the health benefits of stopping smoking has motivated many individuals to quit. Although the percentage of adults who smoke has declined dramatically in the United States since 1960 (J.L. Schwartz 1987), a larger proportion of smokers cannot quit, continue to smoke heavily, and are addicted to nicotine (Shopland 1984). Despite the major public health initiative marshaled against tobacco usage (Iglehart 1986), smoking prevention and cessation are not given any major priority by organized medicine and the health insurance industry (Ginzel 1985). This lack of prioritization may change with the boon of payments states are now receiving in the settlement of tobacco industry litigation.

Historically, most organized treatments designed to assist in smoking cessation have been behaviorally or psychologically based. Long-term quit rates associated with these programs have averaged 30% (J. L. Schwartz 1987). Pharmacological approaches have been developed to provide adjunctive means to help smokers quit. Randomized trials, including double-blind, placebo-controlled studies with nicotine chewing gum—the most widely used pharmacological agent for smoking cessation—indicate that the use of nicotine gum improves long-term quit rates (Hughes and Miller 1984). The efficacy of the chewing gum seems to be attributable to its ability to relieve symptoms of nicotine withdrawal, including irritability, anxiety, difficulty concentrating, and restlessness (Hughes and Hatsukami 1986).

The effectiveness of nicotine gum in smoking cessation depends on several factors. First, when nicotine gum is used to stop smoking independent of specialized smoking cessation services, it appears to have minimal effect (Hughes et al. 1989). Other factors that may adversely affect successful smoking cessation without a formal program include lack of personal support and lack of instructions on the correct use of the nicotine gum. Finally, nicotine gum with specialized smoking cessation treatment appears to significantly increase treatment efficacy. This treatment efficacy with nicotine gum is maximized when combined with specific behavioral skills training rather than a standard didactic approach (Goldstein et al. 1989).

Transdermal nicotine patches are now available for smoking cessation (Abelin et al. 1989). This constant delivery system offers nicotine to an individual without the regular reinforcing behaviors of cigarette smoking and nicotine gum use. Patients with cardiac disease should not smoke while using the nicotine patch and should not use the highest-dosage patch. In addition, two new nicotine delivery systems are now available: nicotine nasal spray and nicotine inhalation. Clonidine has been used in smoking cessation efforts but is not in current clinical usage. In one study, at 6-month follow-up, clonidine offered a significant effect compared with placebo in women only (Glassman et al. 1988). In the course of this study, Glassman and colleagues found a 61% prevalence of past major depressive disorder among subjects in the study sample. In addition, those with a history of regular smoking more frequently had a history of major depressive disorder. Another study in patients with coronary arteriosclerosis showed significantly higher smoking rates among those patients with depressive disorder than among those without a mood disorder (Carney et al. 1988a, 1988b).

Other studies demonstrate that many patients who have difficulty quitting smoking have a history of major depressive disorder (Glassman et al. 1990). These researchers also noted that when a patient with a history of depression quits smoking, depressive symptoms or major depressive symptoms may recur. Further analysis of this study population demonstrated that during the first week of smoking cessation, subjects who were ultimately unsuccessful at quitting experienced cravings, depressed mood, and difficulty concentrating more intensely than those who were successful at quitting smoking (Covey et al. 1990). The successful double-blind treatment trial of doxepin in smoking cessation (Edwards et al. 1989) suggested that drug therapies specifically tailored to treating depressive symptoms present either while smoking or during smoking cessation may be a useful adjunct to treatment (Glassman and Covey 1990).

Other mood states aside from depression may have a role in continuation of smoking and poor ability to stop smoking. Symptoms such as anger, poor frustration tolerance, and tension predict greater difficulty in quitting smoking (Pomerleau et al. 1978). Smokers with baseline elevated levels of these symptoms, or those smokers who develop these symptoms in the midst of a quit attempt, may benefit from treatment. Two studies—one open (Gawin et al. 1989) and one placebo-controlled (Hillerman et al. 1992) with buspirone, a serotonergic antianxiety agent—have shown reductions in craving, anxiety, irritability, restlessness, and sadness during withdrawal from nicotine. Bupropion is now the first non-nicotine agent approved by the FDA to assist in smoking cessation. Several studies demonstrate the efficacy of bupropion, sustained-release 150 mg twice daily. There are no current studies demonstrating improved quit rates specifically in depressed smokers taking bupropion. However, a study of fluoxetine shows that depressed smokers taking fluoxetine quit smoking at the same rate as nondepressed smokers. Hughes et al. (1999) have reviewed recent advances in the pharmacotherapy of smoking cessation.

Return to Work and Work Disability

Although many patients with IHD return to work after acute events, a sizable number who become disabled do not. One study showed that 25% of 814 men younger than age 60 years with IHD were disabled from work (Hlatky et al. 1986). Time off from work was predicted, in decreasing order of importance, by low education level, number of previous myocardial infarctions, and degree of depression. The best predictor of actual job loss (16%) 1 year after an initial evaluation was the patient's level of depression. These data confirm the importance of attending to psychosocial factors in patients with IHD.

Currently, there are no psychosocial intervention trials to evaluate this problem in more detail, despite the profound personal and societal costs of disability among large numbers of patients with IHD (Littman 1993).

Spouses of patients with IHD commonly experience a host of symptoms, including anxiety and depression (Shanfield 1990). Serious marital conflict is common in the immediate convalescence period after a myocardial infarction (Wishnie et al. 1971). Most patients with IHD experience a decline in quantity and quality of sexual activity. A majority of patients with IHD continue to have reduced frequency of sexual activity, and decreased sexual desire and impotence are commonly reported (Hlatky et al. 1986). A randomized trial of counseling of the wives of men with myocardial infarction resulted in significantly less anxiety among the wives at 6 months posthospitalization than among control subjects (Thompson and Meddis 1990). It is critical to provide patients with unambiguous information about when it is safe to resume sexual activity. A patient's physiological readiness to resume sexual activity is frequently evaluated by observing his or her capacity to climb two flights of stairs at a brisk pace (McLane et al. 1980). For those patients who experience angina during sex, positioning and prophylactic use of nitro compounds is helpful (Blaustein et al. 1984). Both patient and spousal beliefs and fears about the likelihood of having a myocardial infarction during sexual activity should be explored and corrected. It is also critical to keep in mind that patients with IHD frequently have vascular, medication-related, or neurogenic causes for impotence or lack of vaginal responsiveness during sex (see also Chapter 22, this volume). For example, β-blockers can decrease libido and cause impotence (Kolodny et al. 1979).

Many patients who are seen in cardiology and general medical practices complain of chest pain or discomfort that is not associated with objectively verifiable cardiac conditions. When no medical condition is found to explain the chest discomfort, these patients have historically received a diagnosis of cardiac neurosis, neurocirculatory asthenia, or hyperventilation syndrome (Mayou 1989). Among cardiologists, a term that is sometimes heard is *syndrome X* (Cannon et al. 1992). Of all patients who are seen in cardiology clinics who have nonanginal or atypical chest pain, 59% have panic disorder (Beitman et al. 1987). Other studies have found a high incidence of psychiatric symptoms, such as anxiety, depression, and hypochondriasis, among patients who complain of nonorganic chest pain. Panic disorder is characteristically responsive to antidepressant medication and to behavioral therapy. A well-controlled trial of cognitive-behavioral therapy for patients with atypical noncardiac chest pain

demonstrated a reduction in chest pain, activity limitations, disruption of daily routines, autonomic symptoms, distress, and psychiatric morbidity that persisted for at least 6 months after treatment (Klimes et al. 1990). Imipramine has been shown to improve the symptoms of chest pain occurring in patients despite the presence of a normal coronary angiogram. The response to imipramine was not dependent on cardiac, esophageal, or psychiatric testing at baseline or change in psychiatric profile (Cannon et al. 1994).

GASTROINTESTINAL DISEASES

Whitehead and Bosmajian (1982), after reviewing several studies, concluded that psychological stress exacerbates esophageal motility disorders. However, no clear-cut data have demonstrated that treatment of psychological stress can reduce symptoms of these esophageal disorders.

Although emotional factors play a role in the pathogenesis of peptic ulcer disease, the development of highly cost-effective histamine-receptor antagonists and new antibiotic treatments places behavioral therapies in a secondary role. However, despite histamine-antagonist therapy, recurrence of peptic ulcer disease is frequent. The role for behavioral therapies in the treatment of recurrent peptic ulcer disease requires elucidation. Behavioral treatment may improve medication compliance or affect emotional factors that are operative in the initiation or aggravation of peptic ulcer disease (Whitehead and Bosmajian 1982).

As many as 50%–90% of patients suspected of having peptic ulcer disease do not, on examination, have evidence of an ulcer. Functional (nonulcer) dyspepsia is characterized by chronic or recurrent upper abdominal pain or discomfort for at least 3 months without endoscopic evidence of other disease (Drossman et al. 1990a). The community prevalence of dyspepsia is estimated at 30% (Krag 1982). Psychiatric comorbidity among patients with dyspepsia is high—87% of patients with functional (nonulcer) dyspepsia have one or more anxiety disorders as compared with 25% of those with dyspepsia associated with endoscopic evidence of gastrointestinal disease (Magni et al. 1987). Functional (nonulcer) dyspepsia and irritable bowel syndrome overlap a great deal diagnostically. No studies have evaluated the efficacy of behavioral or psychopharmacological interventions in patients with functional (nonulcer) dyspepsia (Whitehead 1992).

Irritable bowel syndrome is a disturbance characterized by at least 3 months' duration of abdominal discomfort, relieved with defecation or associated with a change in frequency or consistency of stool. In addition, there is an irregular pattern of defecation at least 25% of the time that includes two or more of the following: altered stool frequency, altered stool form, passage of mucus, and bloating, without the presence of demonstrable gastrointestinal pathology (Drossman et al. 1990a). A reported 10% of patients seen by gastroenterologists have irritable bowel syndrome (Everhart and Renault 1991); 70%–80% of individuals with symptoms consistent with irritable bowel syndrome do not seek medical care and score normally on psychometric testing compared with those individuals who seek medical care and have psychological symptoms. Thus, it appears that among patients with irritable bowel syndrome, physician contact and not gastrointestinal distress predicts psychological symptoms (Drossman et al. 1988). In addition, trauma during childhood, such as loss of a parent through marital separation or death (Lowman et al. 1987) and sexual abuse (Drossman et al. 1990b), was found to be more frequent among patients with irritable bowel syndrome who go to physicians than among control subjects. Patients with irritable bowel syndrome have increased pain sensitivity compared with control subjects (Kullman and Fielding 1981) and no altered colonic motility as had been commonly thought (Snape et al. 1977).

Since the early 1980s, there have been numerous studies of psychological treatment for irritable bowel syndrome, with investigators examining the efficacy of behavioral therapies alone or in combination with standard medical therapies. Brief, insight-oriented psychotherapy in combination with medical therapy has been shown to be superior to medications alone in reducing abdominal pain and diarrhea (Guthrie et al. 1991; Svedlund et al. 1983). Relaxation and stress management (Bennett and Wilkinson 1985) or hypnotherapy alone (Whorell et al. 1984) has been found to reduce abdominal pain and diarrhea. Biofeedback, in contrast, has equivocal results in symptom alteration (Radnitz and Blanchard 1988).

There is no objective evidence that emotional stress produces or worsens the symptoms of inflammatory bowel disease, Crohn's disease, or ulcerative colitis (Whitehead and Bosmajian 1982). Patients with Crohn's disease have more psychological symptoms than do patients with ulcerative colitis, but this difference is not present when controlling for severity of physical symptoms (Drossman et al. 1991). Reviews of psychological treatment studies in patients with inflammatory bowel disease (Schwarz and Blanchard 1990, 1991) demonstrated both better and worse outcomes with behavioral treatment. Thus, there are no current convincing data that the physical symptoms of inflammatory bowel disease can be reduced by psychological treatment.

As many as 50% of patients who complain of chronic constipation have pelvic floor dyssynergia (Loening-Baucke 1989). This is caused by the paradoxical contraction of the anal sphincter and pelvic floor musculature during defecation (Preston and Leonard-Jones 1985). Biofeedback appears to be an effective treatment for patients with this disorder (Wald et al. 1987). In addition, patients with chronic rectal pain, in the absence of any medical diagnosis or irritable bowel syndrome, may have similar pelvic floor dyssynergia and may respond to biofeedback relaxation of the pelvic floor musculature (Grimaud et al. 1991).

IMMUNE-RELATED ILLNESSES

Psychoneuroimmunology refers to the field of investigation directed at understanding how behavior and mental states affect immune function (Ader et al. 1991). Although it has long been suspected that host resistance is influenced by emotional well-being, only with the availability of increasingly precise technology for measuring immune cell activity has it become possible to conduct in vitro tests of the potential association between various psychosocial factors and immune activity. Most persuasive among these tests were Ader's early studies of classical conditioning of hemagglutinating antibody titers by pairing of specific titers with the nausea caused by an immunosuppressant. By carefully controlling all possible alternative explanations for the conditioned response, Ader incontrovertibly demonstrated a CNS influence on the immune system, an effect that has been replicated in humans (Buske-Kirschbaum et al. 1992).

The behavioral states listed in Table 46–4 are associated with suppression of markers of immune function, usually measured by lymphocyte response to antigens and natural killer cell activity (Cohen and Williamson 1991; O'Leary 1990; Weisse 1992). Such studies are correlational in nature and do not directly imply direction of causality. Findings might also be explained by immune influences on the CNS or by currently unknown direct or indirect psychobehavioral mechanisms. It is possible, for example, that distress-related variables such as smoking, alcohol use, or nutritional changes associated with depression mediate these observed relationships instead of being CNS responses to the stress itself. In addition, the uncertain relation of absolute immune level to disease susceptibility limits the conclusions of such studies (Stein et al. 1991). Only randomly assigned, controlled treatment studies can demonstrate experimentally that a true causal relationship exists between external events and internal immune function (Kiecolt-Glaser and Glaser 1992). Three studies attempting to utilize this paradigm have been published. The first of these studies involved nursing home residents who were randomly assigned to receive relaxation training. The treatment group had increased in vitro natural killer cell activity and decreased herpes simplex virus antibody titers compared with those who received only social contact or no intervention (Kiecolt-Glaser et al. 1985). The other two studies were performed on young and healthy subjects. In healthy medical students who participated in a stress management program, the percentage of helper T cells was positively related to the amount of practice of relaxation (Kiecolt-Glaser et al. 1986). Healthy undergraduates who wrote essays about traumatic events displayed better mitogen response to phytohemagglutinin than those who wrote about emotionally neutral topics (Pennebaker et al. 1988). It is unclear from the studies summarized in Table 46–4 whether the treatment effect is of sufficient magnitude or duration to influence disease onset or course.

CANCER

A large body of literature has established the existence of a relationship between psychosocial events and cancer. Some correlational studies have suggested that cancer onset or survival is partially associated with life stressors (Geyer 1991) or personality (Dean and Surtees 1989; Derogatis et al. 1979; Greer et al. 1979). This relationship may also be explained by indirect behavioral-lifestyle factors associated with the psychosocial variables. As discussed earlier in this chapter, treatment studies remain the acid test in establishing causality. Such studies can significantly reduce the possibility that the effect is mediated by behavioral-lifestyle factors by concomitantly observing changes in such factors in the treatment and control groups and then controlling for them in analyses.

Inadequate randomization of baseline staging of illness can easily distort the findings of intervention studies that attempt to influence the course of illness in cancer patients (Morganstern et al. 1984). Spiegel et al. (1989) found significantly increased survival in patients with breast cancer who were randomized to participate in an emotional support group in contrast to those receiving standard care alone (Spiegel et al. 1989). This finding provides a compelling case for considering emotional support as a potentially important intervention that influences the course of disease as well as quality of life. Although this result has evinced much skepticism, equivalent results from a drug or surgery trial would be greeted much more enthusiastically. One line of argu-

TABLE 46–4. Behavioral states associated with suppression of immune function

Behavioral state	Reference
Experimentally induced acute negative emotion	Knapp et al. 1992
Disturbed sleep function	Irwin et al. 1992; Palmblad et al. 1979
Life stressors	Kiecolt-Glaser et al. 1984; Laudenslager et al. 1983; Locke et al. 1984
Clinical anxiety	Schlesinger and Yodfat 1991
Major depression	Maes et al. 1991; Schleifer et al. 1984, 1985
Loneliness	Kiecolt-Glaser et al. 1984
Emotional distress	Cohen et al. 1991
Recent divorce	Kiecolt-Glaser et al. 1987
Bereavement	Bartrop et al. 1977; Schleifer et al. 1983

ment that limits the interpretability of these results derives from the observation that the overall survival rate was low, with the treatment group's survival approximating that seen nationally in patients with breast cancer (Fox 1992). Such an argument implies that the randomization procedures failed in Spiegel's study. The staging of illness was the only variable associated with prognosis that marginally favored ($P < .07$) the treatment group, and analysis of treatment efficacy controlled for this finding. To control for the variability of site-specific survival, a study using site-specific, matched comparison data from nationally gathered breast cancer data is under way (B.H. Fox, personal communication, May 1993). Several replication studies are also currently under way (Cunningham and Lockwood 1992; LeShan 1991; Spiegel 1992).

Another group has demonstrated improved immune function in patients with malignant melanoma who received a 6-week structured psychiatric group treatment intervention (Fawzy et al. 1990). The follow-up report from Fawzy et al. (1993) on this group of patients evaluated the effects of this intervention, provided early after diagnosis, and of initial surgical treatment for malignant melanoma. Fawzy and colleagues assessed the therapy's effect on coping, affective state, tumor recurrence, and survival 6 years after diagnosis. Low levels of baseline distress were significantly associated with recurrence and death, and active coping was associated with improved outcomes. In addition, those who received the group therapy intervention had a significantly reduced recurrence and death rate, a rate that remained significant after the investigators controlled for all significant physiological prognostic factors.

Anticipatory nausea and vomiting are common side effects of chemotherapy. Patients with heightened autonomic reactivity, measured by slower autonomic habituation, appear to be most susceptible to this phenomenon (Andrykowski 1990; Kvale et al. 1991). In severe instances, patients report nausea elicited simply by their driving on the side of town where they receive treatment. Approximately 25% of patients receiving chemotherapy discontinue treatment because of the impact of nausea and vomiting on their quality of life. Morrow and Dobkin (1988) reported the first effort at controlling anticipatory nausea and vomiting via relaxation procedures. A significant reduction in nausea and vomiting was observed, a result that has since been replicated several times (Andrykowski 1990). It is unclear whether new antiemetic medications are sufficiently effective to eliminate the need for behavioral treatment.

Pain control remains a major problem in cancer patients. Frequently, clinicians are forced to choose between having patients who are somnolent and having patients awake and suffering. As for other patients with chronic pain (Lynch and Vasudevan 1988), relaxation procedures can be useful adjuncts to pharmacotherapy.

INFECTIOUS DISEASES

Stress has also been found to co-vary with infectious diseases (Cohen and Williamson 1991). Herpes titers and visible sores, upper respiratory infections, tuberculosis, pyorrhea, and tularemia are more common, or more virulent, in individuals with high stress levels (Antoni et al. 1990). Manipulation of infectious agent exposure in three studies also confirmed an associative relationship and supported the notion of a causal role for stress (Cantor 1972; Glaser et al. 1992; Meyer and Haggerty 1962). For example, the clinical expression of deliberate exposure to cold viruses relates to emotional distress in a dose-response relationship (Cohen et al. 1991). As with all psychophysiological disorders, both psychoneuroendocrine and psychobehavioral pathways may help to explain some of these results, and only treatment studies provide true experimental evidence for a possible causal role. At least one treatment study in a geriatric population undergoing relaxation training indicated a reduction in herpes simplex virus titers and an increase in natural killer cell activity above their pretreatment baselines (Kiecolt-Glaser et al. 1985).

Behavior change remains the only known means of altering disease susceptibility in acquired immunodeficiency syndrome (AIDS) (Kelly and Murphy 1992). There is a perception that high-risk populations such as individuals who abuse substances, members of some ethnic minority groups, women, and adolescents are unaffected by educational programs. However, a number of psychoeducational programs directed at these populations now indicate some response to treatment (Jemmott et al. 1992; Kelly and St. Lawrence 1990; Kelly et al. 1989, 1990; Rotherman-Borus and Koopman 1991; Schilling et al. 1991; Sorenson et al. 1988; Valdiserri et al. 1989). Interventions directed at subgroup opinion leaders have had a wider effect on risk behavior within a gay community than just the leadership group that is trained (Kelly et al. 1991). Although these programs are not a panacea, they remain the only current possibility for prevention until a vaccine is ready for general use.

Although CD4 T-cell counts, per se, are not associated with emotional distress within a population of persons with AIDS (Rabkin et al. 1991), disease progression is associated with emotional distress (Cecchi 1984; Coates et al. 1984; Donlau et al. 1985; Solomon and Temoshok 1987). Studies to date that show this association have not addressed the question of psychological impact of knowledge of disease progression and deteriorating prognosis. Neither have they addressed specific psychiatric predispositions of individuals who were infected by the virus in early years of the epidemic as opposed to later years. Preliminary evidence demonstrates that cognitive-behavioral stress management may be associated with improved CD4 counts, natural killer cell counts, and in vitro lymphocyte response in a randomly assigned, controlled treatment study of patients who had positive tests for infection with the human immunodeficiency virus (HIV) (Antoni et al. 1991). However, another group did not find a similar effect (Coates et al. 1989). No studies using hard clinical end points, such as mortality or length of survival, have been published (Kelly and Murphy 1992). The degree to which HIV disease progression causes distress and the degree to which distress causes progression remain undefined for HIV disease and other immune-related disorders.

The treatment of hepatitis C with interferon has been found to produce negative serum assays in 30%–50% of patients. However, interferon can cause depression, anxiety, or irritability (Johnson et al. 1998; Nozaki et al. 1997; Pavol et al. 1995; Valentine et al. 1998; VanThiel et al. 1995). Psychiatric intervention may be needed in this group to prevent relationship conflict, compliance problems, and suicide (Levenson and Fallon 1993).

HYPERIMMUNE DISORDERS

The prevalence of hay fever in shy and inhibited children and their parents is approximately double that observed in more socially outgoing children (Bell et al. 1990; Kagan et al. 1991). It is unclear whether the traits of shyness and inhibition, when present, are fostered by the allergic condition or treatment regimens or whether they are simply manifestations of an underlying biochemical phenomenon. Treatment studies have not yet been undertaken to test the viability of behavioral approaches to managing allergic conditions (Marshall 1993).

Several dermatological conditions are responsive to behavioral treatments. Two different behavioral therapies are successful in treating psychogenic pruritus (Daniels 1973; Dobes 1977). Chronic hyperhidrosis, or excessive sweating, is related to psychological stress or psychopharmacologic agents, such as SSRIs, in many patients. Biofeedback therapies reduce sweating and associated stress symptoms (Duller and Gentry 1980). In patients with atopic dermatitis, behavioral factors play a part in precipitating and maintaining the condition by influencing the itch-scratch cycle (Schoenberg and Carr 1963). Interventions such as behavioral deconditioning can influence the scratching behavior, which aggravates and maintains the dermatitis. Patients with psoriasis may sometimes have stress-induced relapses and progression. Unfortunately, there is no clear evidence for the effectiveness of behavioral techniques in the treatment of this disorder (Van Moffaert 1992).

The morbidity and mortality associated with asthma have increased in recent decades, quite possibly because of soaring levels of environmental pollutants and adverse effects of chronic bronchodilator use (Sly 1988). The chronic use of theophylline is also a frequent cause of delirium and secondary anxiety syndrome in middle-aged to elderly urban dwellers. Although chronic use of anti-inflammatory therapy is becoming the treatment of choice for patients with asthma and many types of allergies, the long-term effects of these regimens are unknown. Studies indicate a large segment of those with chronic respiratory illnesses, such as asthma, have concomitant anxiety disorders (Bussing et al. 1996; Smoller et al. 1996).

Psychoeducational programs directed at improving self-management of asthma and its therapies increase accuracy of medication and peak flow meter use, improve the patient's sense of control, and decrease outpatient medical system use (Klingelhofer and Gershwin 1988). The effect of relaxation, particularly facial muscle relaxation, or biofeedback on pulmonary function seems to indicate increased bronchiolar smooth muscle relaxation, decreased frequency of attacks, and decreased medication use (Lehrer et al. 1992). Family therapy designed to diminish excessive involvement and interpersonal rigidity and to resolve latent conflict improves clinical asthmatic

rating scores, peak expiratory flow, medication use, and functional impairment (Lehrer et al. 1992). Studies directed at quantifying the reduction in frequency of asthma attacks, if properly designed, could answer questions about mechanisms. For instance, are these reductions in asthma attack frequency solely attributable to more appropriate use of medications on an as-needed basis, or might this reduction be due to decreased emotional distress? What is the role of anxiety disorder treatment in lowering overall treatment costs, medical utilization, and the level of pulmonary symptomatology? Estimates of the cost savings per child as a result of decreased outpatient and emergency room utilization remain unquantified.

AUTOIMMUNE DISORDERS

Suspicion that emotional stress may trigger exacerbations of autoimmune conditions is long standing. In addition, the relatively high prevalence of emotional distress among patients with autoimmune disorders is commonly attributed to reactions to such disorders. For example, one group found that patients with multiple sclerosis who had depression or anxiety had higher levels of T4 cells than did patients who were not distressed (Foley et al. 1988). Currently, no treatment studies have been done involving such patients that would begin to clarify these relationships.

Although the so-called arthritic personality (i.e., passive, conscientious, "catastrophizing," perfectionistic, and emotionally constricted) was initially dismissed as a reaction to the illness rather than a premorbidly existent character style (Anderson et al. 1985), patients with postmorbid coping characterized by these traits clearly have poorer psychosocial functioning (Young 1992). The role of poor coping and emotional distress in determining functional outcome for such patients is strong. For example, anxiety and depression are stronger correlates of increased pain in patients with rheumatoid arthritis than are physical indices of disease severity such as erythrocyte sedimentation rate and number of swollen joints (Hagglund et al. 1989). Thus, functional disability strongly relates to intensity of suffering and emotional well-being. However, electromyogram activity is also higher in affected joints in patients with rheumatoid arthritis than in nonaffected joints or than in subjects in control groups. This observation suggests the presence of guarding behavior (i.e., site-specific muscle tension to achieve immobilization and decrease anticipated movement-related pain), which is believed to aggravate chronic pain conditions as a result of chronic tendon stretch.

Rheumatoid arthritis is a condition widely believed to be aggravated by psychological stress. Most studies indicate that acute stressors (e.g., life events, marital conflict) may occur more frequently before rheumatoid arthritis flare-ups than during quiescent periods (Anderson et al. 1985). At least nine controlled treatment studies have been done in patients with rheumatoid arthritis. Studies designed to decrease pain or pain behaviors were consistently successful in decreasing reported pain and constriction of activities of daily living, whereas those directed at traditional mental health targets alone (depression and anxiety) were not (Young 1992). Several of these studies have found evidence of reduced disease activity. For example, one group found that a cognitive-behavioral treatment regimen improved pain behavior and was associated with lower levels of rheumatoid factor (Bradley et al. 1985, 1987). A second group found that a similar treatment program improved joint function as rated by blinded rheumatologists, although T-cell subsets or lymphocyte responsiveness did not change (O'Leary et al. 1988). A third group reported lower erythrocyte sedimentation rates and improved joint function in patients with rheumatoid arthritis who were undergoing psychological treatment (Achterberg et al. 1981). Thus, the utility of stress management in improving pain-related dysfunction and distress seems well established. The impact on disease mechanisms is more tentative. The role of such treatment in objective disease progression is entirely unknown.

There is much speculation, based on cross-sectional or retrospective studies, that psychosocial stress initiates the autoimmune attack of β cells, thus causing diabetes mellitus or further alterations in glucose metabolism in brittle diabetic patients (McClelland et al. 1991; Robinson and Fuller 1986). No prospective studies exist to test this hypothesis. Some cross-sectional studies suggest an association between higher glucose levels and emotional distress, but these studies are intrinsically confounded by behavioral factors such as diet, exercise, alcohol use, and, in clinical samples, insulin compliance. Some studies have suggested that a subgroup of diabetic patients may have acute glucose excursions (difference between pre-meal and post-meal glucose levels) associated with acute emotional distress (Gonder-Frederick et al. 1990). However, it is not clear that this phenomenon is valid as a stable characteristic of clinically relevant intensity and duration. Less controversial, and better established, is the association between emotional distress and poor control of glucose levels. Some studies have demonstrated consistent associations between poor glucose control and anxiety, depression, familial conflict and dysfunction, loss of social contacts, social alienation,

and impulsivity (Lustman et al. 1991; Mazze et al. 1984; McClelland et al. 1991; Nagasawa et al. 1990). Such correlational observations may be the result of indirect mechanisms such as noncompliance but also may be neuropsychiatric outcomes of poor control and systemic hyperglycemia (C. S. Holmes et al. 1983). There is clear evidence of the acute and long-term effects of diabetes on diminished cognitive functioning (Cox and Gonder-Frederick 1992). The cognitive dysfunction is generally of subclinical intensity—creating interpersonal problems at times because of misconstrual by others. A meta-analysis of available prospective studies that test the effects of induced alterations of psychosocial distress on improvement of glucose control indicated significant benefits to patients who have diabetes (Padgett et al. 1988).

CHRONIC PAIN CONDITIONS

Most chronic pain conditions exact a heavy toll on patients' levels of psychosocial functioning (Turk and Flor 1987). Patients who have chronic pain conditions may benefit from behavioral therapies regardless of whether the etiology of the pain is clearly the result of known pathophysiologies. Many patients with arthritis, neuropathies, sickle-cell disease, Crohn's disease, reflex sympathetic dystrophy, temporomandibular joint syndrome, and cancer-related pain may minimize analgesic use or increase the activities of daily living in which they are able to engage if exposed to cognitive-behavioral treatment (Hendler 1981). The increased sense of control and increased sense of usefulness are important in improving mood and quality of life. Even for patients with somatoform pain disorders, it is this loss of control and the development of dependency and helplessness that seem to foster depression. In one national survey, 14% of the general population reported having chronic pain. However, depression occurred in less than one-fourth of those reporting chronic pain (Magni et al. 1990). The depression observed in patients with chronic pain usually occurs temporally with pain exacerbations (Atkinson et al. 1988; Brown 1990; Gamsa 1990; Goldberg et al. 1991; R. Roy et al. 1984; Rudy et al. 1988). Treatment of the chronic pain seems to resolve most cases of depression among patients with chronic pain (Kramlinger et al. 1983; Maruta et al. 1989). It is important to note, however, that patients with chronic pain often have a strong family history of depression (Magni 1987). Although antidepressant medication will often improve mood and reported pain in a patient with depression and chronic pain, it is also necessary to alter the pain behavior and cognition, with its self-debilitating impact, to achieve a relatively stable long-term outcome (Keefe et al. 1992; Pilowsky and Barrow 1990; Workman 1991; Zitman et al. 1990).

Perhaps the best studied of chronic pain conditions is low back pain. Fordyce et al. (1973) and Turk et al. (1987) recognized that the well-intended solicitousness of the interpersonal environment fosters distress and disability. When combined with the sole use of mood-modulating chronic analgesic or psychotropic therapies, there is a risk that this reinforcement fosters pain behavior (Table 46–5).

Fordyce used operant principles to extinguish pain behavior in an inpatient program and found that he could increase activity levels, decrease analgesic use, and decrease ruminative preoccupation with pain (Fordyce 1976; Fordyce et al. 1986). These insights have focused clinicians on the primary role of the patient's cognition and interpersonal environment, particularly the spouse, in maintaining pain behavior (Flor et al. 1987a, 1987b; Kerns et al. 1990). For example, increased faith in one's capacity to cope and control are associated with decreased pain intensity, lower degree of disability, and higher endorphin levels (Bandura et al. 1987; Toomey et al. 1991). In addition, attention to rather than distraction from chronic pain seems to foster healthy adaptation (J.A. Holmes and Stevenson 1990). Cognitive-behavioral treatment also decreases medical clinic utilization (Caudill et al. 1991).

Other psychosocial processes may also contribute to maintaining chronic pain. Guarding behavior results in pain from chronic tendon stretch and becomes indistinguishable from the original pain source to the patient over time (Ahern et al. 1988). Relaxation alone can acutely diminish this source of discomfort (Phillips 1988). Some evidence also exists that interpersonal conflict increases site-specific muscle tension (Flor et al. 1985; Slater et al. 1991). The role of secondary gain is clearly important, too, with patients actively involved in litigation being less likely to respond to treatment. In clinical settings, patients with premorbid personality dysfunction, patients who perceive that their jobs are emotionally unrewarding, and patients who have several traits suggested by Hackett and Bouckoms's (1987) MADISON scale are prone to prolonged, disabling pain (Table 46–6). Other important aspects of the treatment of chronic pain include monitoring of the patient's propensity for doctor shopping and analgesic or psychotropic dependence. Many patients with chronic pain need detoxification before treatment can begin in earnest.

Compared with no treatment, cognitive-behavioral treatment of chronic low back pain decreases physical in-

TABLE 46–5. Pain behavior

Dependency
Passivity
"Catastrophizing"
Attentional diversion
Guarding
Avoidance of activity
Nonverbal expressiveness
Belief that the intensity of the pain is entirely uncontrollable by the patient
Anticipatory analgesic use

activity, pain, depression, hospitalizations, and analgesic and psychotropic use and increases the likelihood of return to employment (Guck et al. 1985). Compared with control subjects on waiting lists or those who were randomly assigned to control groups, patients in cognitive-behavioral programs exhibited improved mood and decreased pain-related distress, disability, passivity, and analgesic and psychotropic use and increased exercise tolerance, with maintenance up to 12 months (Basler and Rehfisch 1991; Peters and Large 1990; Phillips 1987). Comparison of a similar program with placebo medication or placebo psychological treatment favored the program in outcome measures for pain and perceived control (Engstrom 1983; Nicholas et al. 1992). Compared with physical therapy alone, behavioral treatment alone decreased distress (Heinrich et al. 1985). Both pain and physical disability improved with a cognitive-behavioral treatment group compared with an educational treatment group (Keefe et al. 1990). Other preventive cognitive-behavioral programs for patients with acute back injury appeared to decrease pain behavior, distress, fatigue, and subsequent absenteeism from work (Linton et al. 1989).

Most patients with headache do not have life-threatening conditions. Although such patients commonly receive classification of their headaches as vascular or tension in origin, it remains unclear whether the majority of these patients truly follow different courses or merely have clinical variations of a common ailment (Bakal 1982). Cognitive-behavioral techniques represent well-established and well-studied treatment for headaches (Blanchard 1992). When compared with medication therapies (generally amitriptyline, propranolol, diazepam, or ergotamine), behavioral therapies demonstrate a roughly equivalent reduction in headache load along with reduced analgesic use and adverse effects. Even more important is that patients who undergo behavioral therapy maintain these gains for up to 3 years longer than do patients receiving standard medication therapies. Surveys of patients exposed to such treatment, consisting of

TABLE 46–6. MADISON scale

Multiplicity	The pain occurs in more than one place or is of more than one variety. Successful treatment leads to new pain.
Authenticity	The patient is at least as interested in your accepting the pain as real as he or she is in a cure.
Denial	The patient denies emotional problems or the impact of emotional state on pain.
Interpersonal relationships	Pain is consistently exacerbated by physical or mental presence of a significant other.
Singularity	The patient insists that his or her pain is unique in some way.
Only you	The patient treats the current physician as omniscient and omnipotent, at least initially.
Nothing helps/No change	The pain does not vary from hour to hour, day to day, or year to year, or it only gets worse.

Source. Adapted from Hackett TP, Bouckoms A: "The Pain Patient: Evaluation and Treatment," in *Massachusetts General Hospital Handbook of General Hospital Psychiatry,* 2nd Edition. Edited by Hackett TP, Cassem NH. Littleton, MA, PSG Publishing, 1987, pp 42–68.

relaxation and cognitive self-modification, indicate the spontaneous use of the cognitive-behavioral skills on an as-needed basis when headaches begin to increase. The mechanisms that account for these effects are as yet unclear. The most sophisticated examination of various psychophysiological pathways (e.g., muscle tension, thermal biofeedback, vascular relaxation and contraction) seems to imply that the effect is at least partly due to attributional processes—patients who believe they are doing well at their relaxation exercises, even if incorrect, also report reduction in their headaches (Holroyd et al. 1984). Most studies to date have not concomitantly examined lifestyle factors, such as reduced alcohol or caffeine use, which might also help account for positive aspects of cognitive-behavioral therapy. As with all chronic pain conditions, medication misuse, whether iatrogenic, intentional, or accidental, may be a problem and become a necessary part of treatment planning (Blanchard 1992).

Case History of a Patient With Headache

Ms. B, a middle-aged, white, married, college-educated woman and the mother of two grown children, was referred for intractable headaches following a thorough neurological workup. Ms. B reported a 4-month history of tension-type headaches unaccompanied by migrainous phenomena. Although she had had headaches three or four times a year before this period, the frequency now approximated three times a week, with each episode lasting several hours and occasionally becoming severe enough to interfere with routine domestic duties. Initial use of several over-the-counter analgesics according to her physician's recommendation resulted in some relief but soon became ineffective. Before considering potentially dependence-forming analgesics, her primary care physician believed that an evaluation for stress counseling was in order.

On initial examination, Ms. B's cognitive status was unremarkable, and no clear evidence of psychotic, anxiety, substance abuse, or depressive disorders was obvious, although she described increasingly disturbed sleep during the same 4-month period. Her caffeine use was nominal (two to three cups of coffee a day). Premarin was her only prescription medication. She consumed alcohol socially and averaged about 2–3 ounces a week. She wore corrective lenses but had her vision checked once a year; there were no recent changes. She denied grinding or clenching of her teeth.

During her psychosocial history, it became apparent that Ms. B grew up in a very religious home and was highly traditional about gender role expectations. However, the most remarkable response came when the interviewer sought to discuss her love life. She became defensive and annoyed, protested its irrelevance, and, in a surprisingly uncharacteristic move, walked out. The interviewer followed Ms. B and was able to persuade her to return. He then explained that sexual activity can be very important to one's emotional well-being and that she might have to choose between talking about this subject and continuing with the headaches. After some hesitancy, Ms. B cooperated with a review of coital frequency and functioning. Apparently, it was this couple's pattern for the husband to always initiate lovemaking, and they had a normative frequency of twice a month until 6 months previously. His interest then disappeared. Ms. B reported relatively constant preoccupation with this but was avoiding discussing it with her husband for fear of precipitating a confrontation or even a divorce. At various times, she worried that she was getting old and unattractive or that her husband had a new lover.

The therapist suggested that the husband should have an individual evaluation (nothing notable was discovered except for severe business problems of about a year's duration). At the end of this evaluation, when asked why their lovemaking frequency had changed, the husband appeared puzzled for a moment and then asked, "Has it really been that long?" His wife rejoined the interview, and when the husband's perspective was communicated to her, she cried briefly and relaxed visibly. After two more visits, the headaches had diminished to a frequency of one every other month. Relaxation therapy was effective "most of the time" in relieving Ms. B's headaches. The couple's coital frequency had returned to its old pattern.

The motivation behind Ms. B's not discussing her situation with her husband was fear of catastrophic outcomes such as abandonment. His obliviousness to her distress and lack of attention to lovemaking appeared to be motivated by preoccupation with his company's problems. He did not want "to take home" these matters because he believed he could isolate their effects on him to his work hours. Ms. B's chronic anxiety and worry eventually resulted in the headaches.

Fibromyalgia has been found to respond positively to exercise and cognitive-behavioral therapy (Mason et al. 1998), presumably because of the high prevalence rate of depression, anxiety, and posttraumatic stress disorder in these patients (Belfer et al. 1991; Boisset-Pioro et al. 1995; Nicassio et al. 1995). However, no controlled studies of psychopharmacological treatment of fibromyalgia exist.

A history of sexual abuse is common in patients with chronic pelvic pain (Toomey et al. 1993). Other psychological characteristics found in patients with chronic pelvic pain include vocational and social dysfunction, medical disability, somatic amplification, and emotional distress (Walker et al. 1992). Combining behavioral and medical treatment decreases pain, anxiety, and depression and improves psychosocial, occupational, and sexual functioning (Kames et al. 1990).

MISCELLANEOUS CONDITIONS

Other conditions, such as some of the sleep disorders (Kryger et al. 1989) and the sexual dysfunction disorders (Kolodny et al. 1979; LoPiccolo and LoPiccolo 1978), respond so well to behavioral therapies that they are now first-line treatment choices. Relaxation training and cognitive-behavioral treatment can minimize tinnitus (Andersson et al. 1995). Neuropsychology is a behavioral medicine endeavor, and the effectiveness of cognitive rehabilitation of traumatic and other brain injuries improves with behavioral techniques (Schmitt and Farber 1987).

SUMMARY

The field of behavioral medicine is growing rapidly. Research in behavioral medicine interventions demonstrates that specific behavioral techniques are useful for various chronic, intractable conditions. Treatments are effective in the modification of deleterious behavior patterns, reduction in morbidity and mortality in individuals

with comorbid medical conditions, and enhancement of quality of life. The integration of behavioral medicine research with psychiatric diagnostic phenomenology is a recent one. For example, psychiatry has generally ignored the importance of hostility and depressive symptoms in the treatment of comorbid medical illnesses. Similarly, behavioral medicine has, until recently, tended to ignore the evaluation of the effect of psychiatric conditions on psychosomatic processes. Research in the area of behavioral medicine practice is needed to assess the potential effect of psychosocial interventions on offsetting the cost of medical care.

REFERENCES

Abelin T, Buehler A, Muller P, et al: Controlled trial of transdermal nicotine patch in tobacco withdrawal. Lancet 1:7–10, 1989

Achterberg J, McGaw P, Lawlis GF: Rheumatoid arthritis: a study of relaxation and temperature biofeedback training as an adjunctive therapy. Biofeedback and Self-Regulation 6:207–223, 1981

Ader R, Felton DL, Cohen N (eds): Psychoneuroimmunology. New York, Academic Press, 1991

Ahern DK, Follick MJ, Council JR, et al: Comparison of lumbar paravertebral EMG patterns in chronic low back pain patients and nonpatient controls. Pain 34:153–160, 1988

Ahern DK, Gorkin L, Anderson JL, et al: Biobehavioral variables and mortality or cardiac arrest in the Cardiac Arrhythmia Pilot Study (CAPS). Am J Cardiol 66:59–62, 1990

Alexander F: Psychosomatic Medicine. New York, WW Norton, 1950

Allison TG, Williams DE, Miller TD, et al: Medical and economic costs of psychologic distress in patients with coronary artery disease. Mayo Clin Proc 70:734–742, 1995

American Heart Association: Heart and Stroke Facts. Dallas, TX, American Heart Association, 1991

American Psychiatric Association: Diagnostic and Statistical Manual of Mental Disorders, 4th Edition, Text Revision. Washington, DC, American Psychiatric Association, 2000

Anda R, Williamson D, Jones D, et al: Depressed affect, hopelessness, and the risk of ischemic heart disease in a cohort of U.S. adults. Epidemiology 4:285–294, 1993

Anderson KO, Bradley LA, Young LD, et al: Rheumatoid arthritis: review of psychological factors related to etiology, effects and treatment. Psychol Bull 98:358–387, 1985

Andersson G, Melin L, Hagnebo C, et al: A review of psychological treatment approaches for patients suffering from tinnitus. Ann Behav Med 17:357–366, 1995

Andrykowski MA: The role of anxiety in the development of anticipatory nausea in cancer chemotherapy: a review and synthesis. Psychosom Med 52:458–475, 1990

Antoni MH, Schneiderman N, Fletcher MA, et al: Psycho-neuroimmunology and HIV-1. J Consult Clin Psychol 58:38–49, 1990

Antoni MH, Bagget L, Ironson G, et al: Cognitive-behavioral stress management intervention buffers distress responses and immunologic changes following notification of HIV-1 seropositivity. J Consult Clin Psychol 59:906–915, 1991

Appels A, Mulder P: Excess fatigue as a precursor of myocardial infarction. Eur Heart J 9:758–764, 1988

Atkinson JH, Slater MA, Grant I, et al: Depression and stressful life events in chronic pain. Psychosom Med 50:198–204, 1988

Avery D, Winokur G: Mortality in depressed patients treated with electroconvulsive therapy and anticonvulsants. Arch Gen Psychiatry 33:1029–1037, 1976

Badger LW, Rand EH: Unlearning psychiatry: a cohort effect in the training environment. Int J Psychiatry Med 18:123–129, 1988

Bakal DA: The Psychobiology of Chronic Headache. New York, Springer, 1982

Bandura A, O'Leary A, Taylor CB, et al: Perceived self-efficacy and pain control: opioid and nonopioid mechanisms. J Pers Soc Psychol 53:563–571, 1987

Barsky AJ: Amplification, somatization and the somatoform disorders. Psychosomatics 33:28–34, 1992

Bartrop RW, Luckhurst E, Lazarus L, et al: Depressed lymphocyte function after bereavement. Lancet 1:834–836, 1977

Basler HD, Rehfisch HP: Cognitive/behavioral therapy in patients with ankylosing spondylitis in a German self-help organization. J Psychosom Res 35:345–354, 1991

Beitman BD, Basha I, Flaker G, et al: Atypical or nonanginal chest pain, panic disorder or coronary artery disease? Arch Intern Med 147:1548–1552, 1987

Belfer P, Robbins M, Goldenberg D: Fibromyalgia: psychological characteristics of individuals seeking group pain management treatment (abstract). Proceedings of the Society of Behavioral Medicine XII:141, 1991

Bell IR, Jasnoski ML, Kagan J, et al: Is allergic rhinitis more frequent in young adults with extreme shyness? Psychosom Med 52:517–525, 1990

Bennett P, Wilkinson S: A comparison of psychological and medical treatment of the irritable bowel syndrome. Br J Clin Psychol 24:215–216, 1985

Bertolet BD, Hill JA: Unrecognized myocardial infarction, in Acute Myocardial Infarction. Edited by Pepine CJ. Philadelphia, PA, FA Davis, 1989

Bjorntorp P: Treatment of obesity. Int J Obes Relat Metab Disord 16 (suppl 3):S81–S84, 1992

Blackwell B: Medical education and modest expectations. Gen Hosp Psychiatry 7:1–3, 1985

Blair SN, Kohl HW, Paffenberger RS, et al: Physical fitness and all-cause mortality: a prospective study. JAMA 262:2395–2401, 1989

Blanchard EB: Psychological treatment of benign headache disorders. J Consult Clin Psychol 60:537–551, 1992

Blaustein AS, Heller GV, Kolman BS: Adjunctive nifedipine therapy in high-risk, medically refractory, unstable angina pectoris. Am J Cardiol 52:950–954, 1984

Blumenthal JA, Kamarck T: Assessment of the type A behavior pattern, in Applications in Behavioral Medicine and Health Psychology: A Clinician's Source Book. Edited by Blumenthal JA, McKee DC. Sarasota, FL, Professional Resource Exchange, 1987, pp 3–39

Blumenthal JA, Williams RS, Wallace AG, et al: Physiological and psychological variables predict compliance to prescribed exercise therapy for inpatients recovering from myocardial infarction. Psychosom Med 44:519–527, 1982

Blumenthal JA, Fredrickson M, Kuhn CM, et al: Aerobic exercise reduces levels of cardiovascular and sympathoadrenal responses to mental stress in subjects without prior evidence of myocardial ischemia. Am J Cardiol 65:93–98, 1990

Blumenthal JA, Jiang W, Babyak MA, et al: Stress management and exercise training in cardiac patients with myocardial ischemia. Arch Int Med 157:2213–2223, 1997

Boisset-Pioro MH, Esdaile JM, Fitzcharles MA: Sexual and physical abuse in women with fibromyalgia syndrome. J Behav Med 38:235–241, 1995

Borus JF, Olendzki MC, Kessler L, et al: The "offset effect" of mental health treatment on ambulatory medical care utilization and charges. Arch Gen Psychiatry 42:573–578, 1985

Bradley LA, Turner RA, Young LD, et al: Effects of cognitive-behavioral therapy on pain behavior in rheumatoid arthritis patients: preliminary outcomes. Scandinavian Journal of Behavior Therapy 14:51–64, 1985

Bradley LA, Young LD, Anderson KO, et al: Effects of psychological therapy on pain behavior of rheumatoid arthritis patients: treatment outcome and six month followup. Arthritis Rheum 30:1105–1114, 1987

Brown GK: A causal analysis of chronic pain and depression. J Abnorm Psychol 99:121–137, 1990

Brownell KD, Stunkard AJ, McKeon PE: Weight reduction at the work site: a promise partially fulfilled. Am J Psychiatry 142:47–52, 1985

Budman SH, Demby A, Feldstein ML: Insight into reduced use of medical services after psychotherapy. Professional Psychology: Research and Practice 15:353–361, 1984

Buske-Kirschbaum A, Kirschbaum C, Stierle H, et al: Conditioned increase of natural killer cell activity (NKCA) in humans. Psychosom Med 54:123–132, 1992

Bussing R, Burket RC, Kelleher ET: Prevalence of anxiety disorders in a clinic-based sample of pediatric asthma patients. Psychosomatics 37:108–115, 1996

Cannon RO, Camici RG, Epstein SE: Pathophysiological dilemma of syndrome X. Circulation 85:883–892, 1992

Cannon RO, Quyyumi AA, Mincemoyer R, et al: Imipramine in patients with chest pain despite normal coronary angiograms. N Engl J Med 350:1411–1447, 1994

Cantor A: Changes in mood during incubation of acute febrile disease and the effects of pre-exposure psychologic status. Psychosom Med 34:424–430, 1972

Carney RM, Rich MW, Friedland KE: Major depressive disorder predicts cardiac events in patients with coronary artery disease. Psychosom Med 50:627–633, 1988a

Carney RM, Rich MW, TeVelde A, et al: The relationship between heart rate, heart rate variability, and depression in patients with coronary artery disease. J Psychosom Res 31:4981–4988, 1988b

Caudill M, Zuttermeister P, Benson H, et al: Decreased clinic utilization by chronic pain patients after behavioral medicine intervention (abstract). Proceedings of the Society of Behavioral Medicine XII:133, 1991

Cay EL, Vetter N, Philip AE, et al: Psychological status during recovery from an acute heart attack. J Psychosom Res 16:425–435, 1972

Cecchi RL: Stress: prodrome to immune deficiency. Ann N Y Acad Sci 437:286–289, 1984

Chesney MA, Agras WS, Benson H, et al: Nonpharmacologic approaches to the treatment of hypertension. Circulation 76 (suppl I):104–109, 1987

Chrousos GP, Gold PW: The concepts of stress and stress system disorders. JAMA 267:1244–1252, 1992

Clarkson TB: Personality, gender and coronary artery atherosclerosis of monkeys. Atherosclerosis 7:16–23, 1987

Coates TJ, Temoshok L, Mandel J: Psychosocial research is essential to understanding and treating AIDS. Am Psychol 39:1309–1314, 1984

Coates TJ, McKusick L, Kuno R, et al: Stress reduction training changed number of sexual partners but not immune function in men with HIV. Am J Public Health 79:885–887, 1989

Coccaro E: Central serotonin and impulsive aggression. Br J Psychiatry 155:52–62, 1989

Cohen S, Williamson GM: Stress and infectious disease in humans. Psychol Bull 109:5–24, 1991

Cohen S, Tyrrell DAJ, Smith AP: Psychological stress and susceptibility to the common cold. N Engl J Med 325:606–612, 1991

Connelly JE, Smith GR, Philbrick JT, et al: Healthy patients who perceive poor health and their use of primary care services. J Gen Intern Med 6:47–51, 1991

Coryell W, Noyes R, House DJ: Mortality among outpatients with anxiety disorders. Am J Psychiatry 143:508–510, 1986

Covey LS, Glassman AH, Stetner F: Depression and depressive symptoms in smoking cessation. Compr Psychiatry 31:350–354, 1990

Cox DJ, Gonder-Frederick L: Major developments in behavioral diabetes research. J Consult Clin Psychol 60:628–638, 1992

Cunningham AJ, Lockwood GA: There is simply no valid methodological alternative to randomization of subjects. Adv Cancer Res 8(2):80–82, 1992

Daniels LK: Treatment of urticaria and severe headache by behavior therapy. Psychosomatics 14:347–351, 1973

Dean C, Surtees PG: Do psychological factors predict survival in breast cancer? J Psychosom Res 33:561–569, 1989

deLorgeril M, Salem P, Martin JL, et al: Mediterranean diet, traditional risk factors and the rate of cardiovascular complications after myocardial infarction: final report of the Lyon Heart Study. Circulation 99:779–785, 1999

Dembroski TM, MacDougall JM, Costa PT, et al: Components of hostility as predictors of sudden death and myocardial infarction in the Multiple Risk Factor Intervention Trial. Psychosom Med 51:514–522, 1989

Derogatis LR, Abeloff MD, Melisaratos N: Psychological coping mechanisms and survival time in metastatic breast cancer. JAMA 242:1504–1508, 1979

Dimsdale JE: A perspective on type A behavior and coronary artery disease. N Engl J Med 318:110–112, 1988

DiPietro L, Anda RF, Williamson DF, et al: Depressive symptoms and weight change in a national cohort of adults. Int J Obes Relat Metab Disord 16:745–753, 1992

Dobes RW: Amelioration of psychosomatic dermatitis by reinforced inhibition of scratching. J Behav Ther Exp Psychiatry 8:185–187, 1977

Dohrenwend BP, Levav I, Shrout PE, et al: Socioeconomic status and psychiatric disorders: the causation-selection issue. Science 255:946–952, 1992

Donlau JN, Wolcott MS, Gottlieb MS, et al: Psychosocial aspects of AIDS and AIDS-related complex: a pilot study. Journal of Psychosocial Oncology 3:39–55, 1985

Downing J, Littman A, Scheer J, et al: Depressive symptoms in cardiac rehabilitation patients correlates with blunted training effect (abstract). J Am Coll Cardiol 19:257A, 1992

Dressler WW, Mata A, Chavez A, et al: Social support and arterial pressure in a Central Mexican community. Psychosom Med 48:338–349, 1986

Dressler WW, Grell GA, Gallagher PN, et al: Blood pressure and social class in a Jamaican community. Am J Public Health 78:714–716, 1988

Drossman DA, McKee DC, Sandler RS, et al: Psychosocial factors in the irritable bowel syndrome. Gastroenterology 95:701–708, 1988

Drossman DA, Thompson WG, Talley NJ, et al: Identification of subgroups of functional gastrointestinal disorders. Gastroenterology International 3:159–172, 1990a

Drossman DA, Leserman J, Nachman G, et al: Sexual and physical abuse in women with functional or organic gastrointestinal disorders. Ann Intern Med 113:828–833, 1990b

Drossman DA, Leserman J, Mitchell CM, et al: Health status and health care use in persons with inflammatory bowel disease: a national sample. Dig Dis Sci 36:1746–1755, 1991

Duller P, Gentry WD: Use of biofeedback in treating chronic hyperhydrosis. Br J Dermatol 103:143–146, 1980

Dunbar F: Mind and Body: Psychosomatic Medicine. New York, Random House, 1947

Edwards WB, Murphy JK, Downs AD, et al: Doxepin as an adjunct to smoking cessation: a double-blind pilot study. Am J Psychiatry 146:373–376, 1989

Eisenberg L: Treating depression and anxiety in primary care. N Engl J Med 326:1080–1084, 1992

Eliot RS, Breo DL: Is It Worth Dying For? New York, Bantam Books, 1984, p 15

Engstrom D: Cognitive behavioral therapy methods in chronic pain treatment, in Advances in Pain Research and Therapy, Vol 5. Edited by Bonic JJ. New York, Raven, 1983, pp 829–838

Everhart JE, Renault PF: Irritable bowel syndrome in office-based practice in the United States. Gastroenterology 100:998–1005, 1991

Fava M, Littman A, Halperin P, et al: Psychological and behavioral benefits of a stress/type A reduction program for healthy middle-aged army officers. Psychosomatics 32: 337–342, 1991

Fava M, Rosenbaum JF, Pava JA, et al: Anger attacks in unipolar depression, part 1: clinical correlates and response to fluoxetine treatment. Am J Psychiatry 150:1158–1163, 1993

Fawzy FI, Kemeny ME, Fawzy NW, et al: A structured psychiatric intervention for cancer patients, II: changes over time in immunological measures. Arch Gen Psychiatry 47:729–735, 1990

Fawzy FI, Fawzy NW, Hyun CS, et al: Malignant melanoma: effects of an early structured psychiatric intervention, coping, and affective state on recurrence and survival 6 years later. Arch Gen Psychiatry 50:681–689, 1993

Finnegan DL, Suler JR: Psychological factors with maintenance of improved health behaviors in postcoronary patients. J Psychol 119:81–94, 1985

Flor H, Turk DC, Birbaumer N: Assessment of stress related psychophysiological reactions in chronic back pain patients. J Consult Clin Psychol 53:354–364, 1985

Flor H, Turk DC, Scholz OB: Impact of chronic pain on the spouse: marital, emotional and physical consequences. J Psychosom Res 31:63–71, 1987a

Flor H, Kerns RD, Turk DC: The role of spouse reinforcement, perceived pain and activity levels of chronic pain patients. J Psychosom Res 31:251–259, 1987b

Foley FW, Miller AH, Traugott U, et al: Psychoimmunological dysregulation in multiple sclerosis. Psychosomatics 29:398–403, 1988

Ford CV, Smith GR: Somatoform disorders, factitious disorders and disability syndromes, in Principles of Medical Psychiatry. Edited by Stoudemire A, Fogel BS. New York, Harcourt Brace Jovanovich, 1987, pp 389–401

Fordyce WE: Behavioral Methods for Chronic Pain and Illness. St. Louis, MO, CV Mosby, 1976

Fordyce WE, Fowler RS, Lehmann JF, et al: Operant conditioning in the treatment of chronic pain. Arch Phys Med Rehabil 54:399–408, 1973

Fordyce WE, Brockway JA, Bergman JA, et al: Acute back pain: a control-group comparison of behavioral versus traditional management methods. J Behav Med 9:127–140, 1986

Fox BH: LeShan's hypothesis is provocative, but is it plausible? Adv Cancer Res 8(2):82–84, 1992

Frank C, Smith S: Stress and the heart: biobehavioral aspects of sudden cardiac death. Psychosomatics 31:255–264, 1990

Frasure-Smith N: In hospital symptoms of psychological stress as predictors of long term outcome after acute myocardial infarction in men. Am J Cardiol 67:121–127, 1991

Frasure-Smith N, Lesperance F, Talajic M: Depression following myocardial infarction: impact on 6-month survival. JAMA 270:1819–1825, 1993

Friedman M, Ulmer D: Treating Type A Behavior and Your Heart. New York, Fawcett-Crest, 1984

Friedman M, Thoreson CE, Gill JJ, et al: Alteration of type A behavior and reduction in cardiac recurrences in post-myocardial infarction patients. Am Heart J 108:237–248, 1984

Friedman M, Thoreson CE, Gill JJ, et al: Alteration of type A behavior and its effect on cardiac recurrences in postmyocardial infarction patients: summary results of the Recurrent Coronary Prevention Project. Am Heart J 114:483–490, 1987

Gamsa A: Is emotional disturbance a precipitator or a consequence of chronic pain? Pain 42:183–195, 1990

Garner DM, Wooley SC: Confronting the failure of behavioral and dietary treatments for obesity. Clin Psychol Rev 11:729–780, 1991

Gawin F, Compton M, Byck R: Potential use of buspirone as treatment for smoking cessation: a preliminary trial. Family Practice Recertification 11:74–78, 1989

Geyer S: Life events prior to manifestation of breast cancer: a limited prospective study covering eight years before diagnosis. J Psychosom Res 35:355–363, 1991

Gill JJ, Price VA, Friedman M, et al: Reduction in type A behavior in healthy middle-aged American military officers. Am Heart J 110:503–514, 1985

Ginzel KH: The underemphasis on smoking in medical education. New York State Journal of Medicine 85:299–301, 1985

Glaser R, Kiecolt-Glaser JK, Bonneau RH, et al: Stress-induced modulation of the immune response to recombinant hepatitis B vaccine. Psychosom Med 54:22–29, 1992

Glassman AH, Covey LS: Future trends in the pharmacologic treatment of smoking cessation. Drugs 40:1–5, 1990

Glassman AH, Stetner F, Walsh BT, et al: Heavy smokers, smoking cessation, and clonidine. JAMA 259:2863–2866, 1988

Glassman AH, Helzer JE, Covey LS, et al: Smoking, smoking cessation, and major depression. JAMA 264:1546–1549, 1990

Goldberg GM, Kerns RD, Rosenberg R, et al: Activities, marital support and depression in chronic pain patients (abstract). Proceedings of the Society of Behavioral Medicine XII: 130, 1991

Goldstein MG, Niaura R, Follick MJ, et al: Effects of behavioral skills training and schedule of nicotine gum administration on smoking cessation. Am J Psychiatry 146:56–60, 1989

Gonder-Frederick LA, Carter WR, Cox DJ, et al: Environmental stress and blood glucose change in insulin-dependent diabetes mellitus. Health Psychol 9:503–515, 1990

Greer S, Morris T, Pettingale KW: Psychological response to breast cancer: effect on outcome. Lancet 2:785–787, 1979

Greist JH, Klein MH, Eischens RR, et al: Running as treatment for depression. Compr Psychiatry 20:41–54, 1979

Grimaud JC, Bouvier M, Naudy B, et al: Manometric and radiologic investigations and biofeedback treatment of chronic idiopathic anal pain. Dis Colon Rectum 34:690–695, 1991

Guck TP, Skultety FM, Meilman PW, et al: Multidisciplinary pain center followup study: evaluation with a nontreatment control group. Pain 21:295–306, 1985

Guthrie E, Creed F, Dawson D, et al: A controlled trial of psychological treatment for the irritable bowel syndrome. Gastroenterology 100:450–457, 1991

Hackett TP, Bouckoms A: The pain patient: evaluation and treatment, in Massachusetts General Hospital Handbook of General Hospital Psychiatry, 2nd Edition. Edited by Hackett TP, Cassem NH. Littleton, MA, PSG Publishing, 1987, pp 42–68

Hagglund KJ, Haley WE, Reveille JD, et al: Predicting individual differences in pain and functional impairment among patients with rheumatoid arthritis. Arthritis Rheum 32:851–858, 1989

Haines AP, Imeson JD, Meade TW: Phobic anxiety and ischemic heart disease. BMJ 295:297–299, 1987

Hamazaki T: The effect of docosahexaenoic acid on aggression in young adults. J Clin Investigation 97:1129–1133, 1996

Haynes RB, Taylor DW, Sackett DL: Compliance in Health Care. Baltimore, MD, Johns Hopkins University Press, 1979

Heinrich RL, Cohen MJ, Naliboff BD, et al: Comparing physical and behavior therapy for chronic low back pain on physical disabilities, psychological distress and patients' perceptions. J Behav Med 8:61–78, 1985

Hendler N: Diagnosis and Nonsurgical Management of Chronic Pain. New York, Raven, 1981

Hillerman DE, Mohuiddin SM, Del Core MG, et al: Effect of buspirone on withdrawal symptoms associated with smoking cessation. Arch Intern Med 152:350–352, 1992

Hlatky MA, Haney T, Barefoot JC, et al: Medical, psychological and social correlates of work disability among men with coronary artery disease. Am J Cardiol 58:911–915, 1986

Holmes CS, Hayford JT, Gonzalez JL, et al: A survey of cognitive functioning at different levels in diabetic persons. Diabetes Care 6(2):180–185, 1983

Holmes JA, Stevenson CAZ: Differential effects of avoidant and attentional coping strategies on adaptation to chronic recent onset pain. Health Psychol 9:577–584, 1990

Holroyd KA, Penzien DB, Hursey KG, et al: Change mechanisms in EMG biofeedback training: cognitive changes underlying improvements in tension headache. J Consult Clin Psychol 52:1039–1053, 1984

Hughes JR: Psychological effects of habitual aerobic exercise: a critical review. Prev Med 13:66–78, 1984

Hughes JR, Hatsukami D: Signs and symptoms of tobacco withdrawal. Arch Gen Psychiatry 43:289–294, 1986

Hughes JR, Miller SA: Nicotine gum to help stop smoking. JAMA 252:2855–2858, 1984

Hughes JR, Gust SW, Keenan RM, et al: Nicotine versus placebo gum in general medical practice. JAMA 261:1300–1305, 1989

Hughes JR, Goldstein MG, Hurt RD, et al: Recent advances in the pharmacotherapy of smoking. JAMA 281:72–76, 1999

Iglehart JK: The campaign against smoking gains momentum. N Engl J Med 314:1059–1064, 1986

Irwin M, Smith TL, Gillin JC: Electroencephalographic sleep and natural killer activity in depressed patients and control subjects. Psychosom Med 54:10–21, 1992

Jacobs D, Blackburn H, Higgins M, et al: Report of the conference on low cholesterol: mortality associations. Circulation 86:1046–1060, 1992

Jemmott JB, Jemmott LS, Fong GT: Reductions in HIV risk-associated sexual behaviors among black male adolescents: effects of an AIDS prevention intervention. Am J Public Health 82:372–377, 1992

Johnson ME, Fisher PG, Fenaughty A, et al: Hepatitis C virus and depression in drug users. Am J Gastroenterol 93:785–789, 1998

Kagan J, Snidman N, Julia-Sellers M, et al: Temperament and allergic symptoms. Psychosom Med 53:332–340, 1991

Kamada T, Miyake S, Kumashiro M, et al: Power spectral analysis of heart rate variability in type As and type Bs during mental workload. Psychosom Med 54:462–470, 1992

Kamarck T, Jennings JR: Biobehavioral factors in sudden cardiac death. Psychol Bull 109:42–75, 1991

Kames LD, Rapkin AJ, Naliboff BD, et al: Effectiveness of an interdisciplinary pain management program for the treatment of chronic pelvic pain. Pain 41:41–46, 1990

Karasek R, Baker D, Marxer F, et al: Job decision, latitude, job demands and cardiovascular disease: a prospective study of Swedish men. Am J Public Health 71:694–705, 1981

Katon W: The epidemiology of depression in medical care. Int J Psychiatry Med 17:93–112, 1987

Katon W, Von Korff M, Lin E, et al: Adequacy and duration of antidepressant treatment in primary care. Med Care 30:67–76, 1992

Kaufman PG, Jacob RG, Ewart CK: Hypertension intervention pooling project. Health Psychol 7 (suppl):209–224, 1988

Keefe FJ, Caldwaell DS, Williams DA, et al: Pain coping skills training in the management of osteoarthritic knee pain: a comparative study. Behavior Therapy 21:49–62, 1990

Keefe FJ, Dunsmore J, Burnett R: Behavioral and cognitive-behavioral approaches to chronic pain: recent advances and future directions. J Consult Clin Psychol 60:528–536, 1992

Kellner R: Functional somatic symptoms and hypochondriasis. Arch Gen Psychiatry 42:321–329, 1985

Kelly JA, Murphy DA: Psychological interventions with AIDS and HIV: prevention and treatment. J Consult Clin Psychol 60:576–585, 1992

Kelly JA, St. Lawrence JS: The impact of community-based groups to help persons reduce behaviors that create risk for HIV infection. AIDS Care 2:25–36, 1990

Kelly JA, St. Lawrence JS, Hood HV, et al: Behavioral interventions to reduce AIDS risk activities. J Consult Clin Psychol 57:60–67, 1989

Kelly JA, St. Lawrence JS, Betts RA, et al: A skills training group intervention model to assist persons in reducing risk behaviors for HIV infection. AIDS Educ Prev 2:25–35, 1990

Kelly JA, St. Lawrence JS, Diaz YE, et al: HIV risk behavior reduction following intervention with key opinion leaders of a population: an experimental community-level analysis. Am J Public Health 81:168–171, 1991

Kenyon LW, Ketterer MW, Gheorgiade M, et al: Psychological factors related to prehospital delay during acute myocardial infarction. Circulation 84:1969–1976, 1991

Kerns RD, Haythornthwaite J, Southwick S, et al: The role of marital interaction in chronic pain and depressive symptom severity. J Psychosom Res 34:401–408, 1990

Ketterer MW: Denial specific to Friedman's pathogenic emotions in Jenkins activity survey of type A and angiography-referred males. Psychosomatics 33:72–80, 1992

Ketterer MW: Secondary prevention of ischemic heart disease: the case for aggressive behavioral monitoring and intervention. Psychosomatics 34:478–484, 1993

Ketterer MW: Cognizance of chronic negative emotion and stressors: the phenomenological imperative in the treatment of the psychophysiological disorders. Journal of Integrative and Eclectic Psychotherapy (in press)

Ketterer MW, Maercklein GH: Caffeinated beverage use among type A male patients suspected of CAD/CHD: a mechanism for increased risk? Stress Medicine 7:119–124, 1991

Ketterer MW, Maercklein GH: The association of Friedman's pathogenic emotions (AIAI) with current smoking, but not smoking history, in males suspected of coronary artery disease. Stress Medicine 8:99–103, 1992

Ketterer MW, Brymer J, Rhoads K, et al: Lipid-lowering therapy and violent death: is depression a culprit? Proceedings of the Academy of Psychosomatic Medicine 40:28–29, 1993

Kiecolt-Glaser JK, Glaser R: Psychoneuroimmunology: can psychological interventions moderate immunity? J Consult Clin Psychol 60:569–575, 1992

Kiecolt-Glaser JK, Ricker D, George J, et al: Urinary cortisol levels, cellular immunocompetency, and loneliness in psychiatric inpatients. Psychosom Med 46:15–21, 1984

Kiecolt-Glaser JK, Glaser R, Williger D, et al: Psychosocial enhancement of immunocompetence in a geriatric population. Health Psychol 4:25–41, 1985

Kiecolt-Glaser JK, Glaser R, Strain E, et al: Modulation of cellular immunity in medical students. J Behav Med 9:5–21, 1986

Kiecolt-Glaser JK, Fisher LD, Ogrocki P, et al: Marital quality, marital disruption and immune function. Psychosom Med 49:13–34, 1987

Klerman GL: Depressive disorders—further evidence of increased medical morbidity and impairment of social functioning. Arch Gen Psychiatry 46:856–858, 1989

Klimes SI, Mayou RA, Pearce MJ, et al: Psychological treatment for atypical noncardiac chest pain: a controlled trial. Psychol Med 20:605–611, 1990

Klingelhofer EL, Gershwin KD: Asthma self management programs: premises, not promises. J Asthma 25:89–101, 1988

Knapp PH, Levy EM, Giorgi RG, et al: Short-term immunological effects of induced emotion. Psychosom Med 54:133–148, 1992

Kolodny RC, Masters WH, Johnson VE: Textbook of Sexual Medicine. Boston, MA, Little, Brown, 1979

Krag E: Nonulcer dyspepsia: epidemiological data. Scand J Gastroenterol 17 (suppl 79):6–8, 1982

Kramlinger KG, Swanson DW, Maruta T: Are patients with chronic pain depressed? Am J Psychiatry 140:747–749, 1983

Kryger MH, Roth T, Dement WC (eds): Principles and Practices of Sleep Medicine. Philadelphia, PA, WB Saunders, 1989

Kullman G, Fielding JF: Rectal distensibility in the irritable bowel syndrome. Ir Med J 74:140–142, 1981

Kvale G, Hugdahl K, Asbjornsen A: Anticipatory nausea and vomiting in cancer patients. J Consult Clin Psychol 59:894–898, 1991

Ladwig KH, Kieserm M, Konig J, et al: Affective disorder and survival after acute myocardial infarction: results from the post infarction late potential study. Eur Heart J 12:959–964, 1991

Laudenslager ML, Ryan SM, Drugan RC, et al: Coping and immunosuppression: inescapable but not escapable shock suppresses lymphocyte proliferation. Science 221:568–570, 1983

Leaf A: n-3 fatty acids in the prevention of cardiac arrhythmias. Lipids 34:S187–S189, 1999

Lehrer PM, Sargunaraj D, Hochron S: Psychological approaches to the treatment of asthma. J Consult Clin Psychol 60:639–643, 1992

L'Enfant C, Liu BM: (Passive) smokers versus (voluntary) smokers (editorial). N Engl J Med 302:742–743, 1980

Leon AS, Connett J, Jacobs DR, et al: Leisure-time physical activity levels and risk of coronary heart disease and death: the Multiple Risk Factor Intervention Trial. JAMA 258:2388–2395, 1987

LeShan L: A new question in studying psychosocial interventions and cancer. Adv Cancer Res 7:69–71, 1991

Lesser IM: Current concepts in psychiatry: alexithymia. N Engl J Med 312:690–692, 1985

Levenson JL, Mishra A, Hamer RM, et al: Denial and medical outcome in unstable angina. Psychosom Med 51:27–35, 1989

Levenson J, Fallon H: Fluoxetine treatment of depression caused by interferon-alpha. Am J Gastroenterol 88:760–761, 1993

Levine J, Warrenburg S, Kerns R, et al: The role of denial in recovering from coronary heart disease. Psychosom Med 49:109–117, 1987

Lightwood JM, Glantz SA: Short-term economic and health benefits of smoking cessation. Circulation 96:1089–1096, 1997

Linton SJ, Bradley LA, Jensen I, et al: The secondary prevention of low back pain: a controlled study with followup. Pain 43:299–307, 1989

Littman AB: Prevention of disability due to cardiovascular diseases. Heart Disease and Stroke 2:274–277, 1993

Littman AB, Fava M, McKool K, et al: The use of buspirone in the treatment of stress, hostility and type A behavior in cardiac patients: an open trial. Psychother Psychosom 59:107–110, 1993

Lloyd GG, Cawley RH: Psychiatric morbidity in men one week after first acute myocardial infarction. BMJ 2:1453–1454, 1978

Locke SE, Kraus L, Leserman J, et al: Life change stress, psychiatric symptoms and natural killer cell activity. Psychosom Med 46:441–448, 1984

Loening-Baucke V: Factors determining outcome in children with chronic constipation and fecal soiling. Gut 30:999–1006, 1989

LoPiccolo J, LoPiccolo L (eds): Handbook of Sex Therapy. New York, Plenum, 1978

Losing weight: what works, what doesn't. Consumer Reports, June 1993, pp 347–357

Lowman BC, Drossman DA, Cramer EM, et al: Recollection of childhood events in adults with irritable bowel syndrome. J Clin Gastroenterol 9:324–330, 1987

Lown B: Sudden cardiac death: biobehavioral perspective. Circulation 76 (suppl I):186–196, 1987

Lustman PJ, Frank BL, McGill JB: Relationship of personality characteristics to glucose regulation in adults with diabetes. Psychosom Med 53:305–312, 1991

Lynch NT, Vasudevan SV: Persistent Pain. Boston, MA, Kluwer Academic, 1988

Maes M, Bosmans E, Suy E, et al: A further exploration of the relationships between immune parameters and the HPA-axis activity in depressed patients. Psychol Med 21:313–320, 1991

Magni G: On the relationship between chronic pain and depression when there is no organic lesion. Pain 31:1–21, 1987

Magni G, di Mario F, Bernasconi G, et al: DSM-III diagnoses associated with dyspepsia of unknown cause. Am J Psychiatry 144:1222–1223, 1987

Magni G, Caldieron C, Rigatti-Luchini S, et al: Chronic musculoskeletal pain and depressive symptoms in the general population: an analysis of the first national health and nutrition examination survey data. Pain 43:299–307, 1990

Manson JE, Colditz GA, Stampfer MJ, et al: A prospective study of obesity and risk of coronary heart disease in women. N Engl J Med 322:882–889, 1990

Marshall PS: Allergy and depression: a neurochemical threshold model of the relation between the illnesses. Psychol Bull 113:23–43, 1993

Martin JE, Dubbert PM: Adherence to exercise, in Exercise and Sport Sciences Reviews, Vol 13. Edited by Terjung RL. New York, Macmillan, 1985, pp 137–167

Maruta T, Vatterott MK, McHardy MJ: Pain management as an antidepressant: long-term resolution of pain-associated depression. Pain 36:335–337, 1989

Mason LW, Godkasian P, McCain GA: Evaluation of a multimodal treatment program for fibromyalgia. J Behav Med 21:163–174, 1998

Mayou R: Atypical chest pain. J Psychosom Res 33:393–406, 1989

Mazze RS, Lucido D, Shamoon H: Psychological and social correlates of glycemic control. Diabetes Care 7:360–366, 1984

McClelland DC, Patel V, Brown D, et al: The role of affiliative loss in the recruitment of helper cells among insulin dependent diabetics. Behav Med 17:5–14, 1991

McLane M, Krop H, Mehta J: Psychosexual adjustment and counseling after myocardial infarction. Ann Intern Med 92:514–519, 1980

Meyer RJ, Haggerty RJ: Streptococcal infections in families. Pediatrics 29:539–549, 1962

Milani R, Littman A, Lavie C: Depressive symptoms predict functional improvement following cardiac rehabilitation and exercise program. J Cardiopulm Rehabil 13:406–411, 1993

Miranda J, Perez-Stable EJ, Munoz RF, et al: Somatization, psychiatric disorder and stress in utilization of ambulatory medical services. Health Psychol 10:46–51, 1991

Morganstern H, Gellert GA, Walter SD, et al: The impact of a psychosocial support program on survival with breast cancer: the importance of selection bias in program evaluation. Journal of Chronic Diseases 37:273–276, 1984

Morrow GR, Dobkin PL: Anticipatory nausea and vomiting in cancer patients undergoing chemotherapy treatment: prevalence, etiology and behavioral interventions. Clin Psychol Rev 8:517–556, 1988

Muldoon MF, Manuck SB, Matthews KA: Lowering cholesterol concentrations and mortality: a quantitative review of primary prevention trials. BMJ 301:309–314, 1990

Muldoon MF, Kaplan JR, Manuck SB, et al: Effects of dietary fat on central nervous system serotonergic activity. Psychosom Med 53:216–221, 1991

Murphy JM, Monson RR, Oliver DC, et al: Affective disorders and mortality. Arch Gen Psychiatry 44:473–480, 1987

Musselman DL, Marzec UM, Manatunga A, et al: Platelet reactivity in depressed patients treated with paroxetine: preliminary findings. Arch Gen Psychiatry 57:875–882, 2000

Nagasawa M, Smith MC, Barnes JH, et al: Meta-analysis of correlates of diabetes patients' compliance with prescribed medications. Diabetes Educator 16:192–200, 1990

Nicassio PM, Rodojevic V, Schoenfeld-Smith K, et al: The contribution of family cohesion and the pain-coping process to depressive symptoms in fibromyalgia. Ann Behav Med 17:349–356, 1995

Nicholas MK, Wilson PH, Goyen J: Comparison of cognitive/behavioral group treatment and an alternative nonpsychological treatment for chronic low back pain. Pain 48:339–347, 1992

NIH Technology Assessment Conference Panel: Methods for voluntary weight loss and control. Ann Intern Med 116: 942–949, 1992

Nozaki O, Takagi C, Takaoka K, et al: Psychiatric manifestations accompanying interferon therapy for patients with chronic hepatitis C: an overview of cases in Japan. Psychiatry Clin Neurosci 51:175–180, 1997

Nunes EV, Frank KA, Kornfeld DS: Psychologic treatment for the type A behavior pattern and coronary artery disease: a meta-analysis of the literature. Psychosom Med 48:159–173, 1987

Oldridge NB, Guyett GH, Fischer ME, et al: Cardiac rehabilitation after myocardial infarction: combined experience of randomized clinical trials. JAMA 260:945–950, 1988

O'Leary A: Stress, emotion and human immune function. Psychol Bull 108:363–382, 1990

O'Leary A, Shoor S, Lorig K, et al: A cognitive-behavioral treatment for rheumatoid arthritis. Health Psychol 7:527–544, 1988

Ormel J, Koeter MWJ, van den Brink W, et al: Recognition, management and course of anxiety and depression in general practice. Arch Gen Psychiatry 48:700–710, 1991

Ornish D, Brown SE, Scherwitz LW, et al: Can lifestyle changes reverse coronary heart disease? Lancet 336:129–133, 1990

Ornish D, Brown SE, Billings JH, et al: Can lifestyle changes reverse coronary atherosclerosis? Four-year results of the Lifestyle Heart Trial (abstract). Abstracts from the 66th Scientific Sessions of the American Heart Association, November 1993. Circulation 88:1–385, 1993

Padgett D, Mumford E, Haynes M: Meta-analysis of the effects of educational and psychosocial interventions on management of diabetes mellitus. J Clin Epidemiol 41:1007–1030, 1988

Palmblad J, Petrini B, Wasserman J, et al: Lymphocyte and granulocyte reactions during sleep deprivation. Psychosom Med 41:273–279, 1979

Patel C, Marmot MG, Terry DJ, et al: Trial of relaxation in reducing coronary risk: four year followup. BMJ 290:1103–1106, 1985

Pavol MA, Meyers CA, Rexer JL, et al: Pattern of neurobehavioral deficits associated with interferon alpha therapy for leukemia. Neurology 45:947–950, 1995

Pennebaker JW, Kiecolt-Glaser JK, Glaser R: Disclosure of traumas and immune function: health implications for psychotherapy. J Consult Clin Psychol 56:239–245, 1988

Percy W: The Thanatos Syndrome. New York, Farrar, Straus and Giroux, 1987, p 67

Peters JL, Large RG: A randomized control trial evaluating in and outpatient pain management programmes. Pain 41:283–293, 1990

Phillips HC: The effects of behavioral treatment on chronic pain. Behav Res Ther 25:365–377, 1987

Phillips HC: Changing chronic pain experience. Pain 32:165–172, 1988

Pilowsky I, Barrow CG: A controlled study of psychotherapy and amitriptyline used individually and in combination in the treatment of chronic intractable, "psychogenic" pain. Pain 40:3–19, 1990

Pomerleau OF, Adkins DM, Pertschuk M: Predictors of outcome and recidivism in smoking-cessation treatment. Addict Behav 3:65–70, 1978

Powell KE, Thompson PD, Casperson CJ, et al: Physical activity and the incidence of coronary artery disease. Annu Rev Public Health 8:253–287, 1987

Powell LH, Thoreson CE: Modifying the type A behavior pattern: a small group treatment approach, in Applications in Behavioral Medicine and Health Psychology: A Clinician's Source Book. Edited by Blumenthal JA, McKee DC. Sarasota, FL, Professional Resource Exchange, 1987, pp 171–207

Preston DM, Leonard-Jones JE: Anismus in chronic constipation. Dig Dis Sci 34:1168–1172, 1985

Public Health Service: Healthy People 2000. Rockville, MD, Department of Health and Human Services, 1991

Rabinowitz S, Lown B: Central neurochemical factors related to serotonin metabolism and cardiac ventricular vulnerability for repetitive electrical activity. Am J Cardiol 41:516–522, 1978

Rabkin JG, Williams JBW, Remien RH: Depression, distress, lymphocyte subsets and human immunodeficiency virus symptoms on two occasions in HIV-positive homosexual men. Arch Gen Psychiatry 48:111–119, 1991

Radnitz CL, Blanchard EB: Bowel sound biofeedback as a treatment for irritable bowel syndrome. Biofeedback and Self-Regulation 13:169–179, 1988

Robinson N, Fuller JH: Severe life events and their relationship to the etiology of insulin-dependent (type I) diabetes mellitus. Pediatric Adolescent Endocrinology 15:129–133, 1986

Rosen JC, Wiens AN: Changes in medical problems and use of medical services following psychological intervention. Am Psychol 34:420–431, 1979

Rotherman-Borus MJ, Koopman C: Sexual risk behaviors, AIDS knowledge and beliefs about AIDS among runaways. Am J Public Health 81:208–210, 1991

Roy A, Adinoff B, Linnolla M: Acting out hostility in normal volunteers: negative correlation with levels of 5-HIAA in cerebrospinal fluid. Psychiatry Res 24:187–194, 1989

Roy R, Thomas M, Matas M: Chronic pain and depression: a review. Compr Psychiatry 25:96–103, 1984

Rozanski A, Bairey CN, Krantz DS, et al: Mental stress and the induction of silent myocardial ischemia in patients with coronary artery disease. N Engl J Med 318:1005–1012, 1988

Ruberman W, Weinblatt E, Goldberg JD: Psychosocial influences on mortality after myocardial infarction. N Engl J Med 311:552–559, 1984

Rubins PV, Harris K, Koven S: High fatality rates of late life depression associated with cardiovascular disease. J Affect Disord 9:165–167, 1985

Rudy TE, Kerns RD, Turk DC: Chronic pain and depression: toward a cognitive-behavioral mediation model. Pain 34:53–60, 1988

Schachter S: Recidivism and self-cure of smoking and obesity. Am Psychol 37:436–444, 1982

Schilling RF, El-Bassel N, Schinke SP, et al: Building skills of recovering women drug users to reduce heterosexual AIDS transmission. Public Health Rep 106:297–304, 1991

Schleifer SJ, Keller SE, Camerino M, et al: Suppression of lymphocyte stimulation following bereavement. JAMA 250:374–377, 1983

Schleifer SJ, Keller SE, Meyerson AT, et al: Lymphocyte function in major depressive disorder. Arch Gen Psychiatry 41:484–486, 1984

Schleifer SJ, Keller SE, Siris SG, et al: Depression and immunity: lymphocyte function in ambulatory depressed patients, hospitalized schizophrenic patients and patients hospitalized for herniorrhaphy. Arch Gen Psychiatry 42:129–133, 1985

Schleifer SJ, Macari-Hinson MM, Coyle DA: The nature and course of depression following myocardial infarction. Arch Intern Med 149:1785–1789, 1989

Schlesinger M, Yodfat Y: The impact of stressful life events on natural killer cells. Stress Medicine 7:53–60, 1991

Schmiedler R, Freidrich G, Neus H, et al: The influence of beta blockers on cardiovascular reactivity and type A behavior pattern in hypertensives. Psychosom Med 45:417–423, 1983

Schmitt FA, Farber J: Perspectives on memory retraining of persons with cognitive deficits, in Applications in Behavioral Medicine and Health Psychology: A Clinician's Source Book. Edited by Blumenthal JA, McKee DC. Sarasota, FL, Professional Resource Exchange, 1987, pp 209–236

Schoenberg B, Carr AC: An investigation of criteria for brief psychotherapy of neurodermatitis. Psychosom Med 25:253–263, 1963

Schwartz GE, Weiss SM: Behavioral medicine revisited: an amended definition. J Behav Med 1:249–251, 1978

Schwartz JL: Review and evaluation of smoking cessation methods: the United States and Canada, 1978–1985. U.S. DHHS Public Health Service, NIH Publication No 87–2940, U.S. Government Printing Office, Washington, DC, 1987

Schwarz SP, Blanchard EB: Inflammatory bowel disease: a review of the psychological assessment and treatment literature. Ann Behav Med 12:95–105, 1990

Schwarz SP, Blanchard EB: Evaluation of a psychological treatment for inflammatory bowel disease. Behav Res Ther 29:167–177, 1991

Shanfield SB: Myocardial infarction and patients' wives. Psychosomatics 31:138–145, 1990

Shekelle RB, Hulley SB, Neaton JD, et al: The MRFIT behavior pattern study. Am J Epidemiol 122:559–570, 1985

Shell WE, Swan HJC: Treatment of silent myocardial ischemia with transdermal nitroglycerine added to beta-blockers and alprazolam. Cardiol Clin 4:697–704, 1986

Shopland D: The Health Consequences of Smoking: Chronic Obstructive Lung Disease: A Report of the Surgeon General. USDHEW Publication PHS–84–50205. Washington, DC, U.S. Government Printing Office, 1984

Silverstone T: Drugs, appetite, and obesity: a personal odyssey. Int J Obes Relat Metab Disord 16 (suppl 2):S49–S52, 1992

Slater MA, Good AB, Atkinson JH: An evaluation of psychophysiologic responses to stress in chronic low back pain patients. Psychosom Med 53:211–245, 1991

Sly RM: Mortality from asthma: 1979–1984. J Allergy Clin Immunol 82:705–717, 1988

Smith GD, Pekkanen J: Should there be a moratorium on the use of cholesterol lowering drugs? BMJ 304:431–434, 1992

Smoller JW, Pollack MH, Otto MW, et al: Panic anxiety, dyspnea, and respiratory disease. Am J Respir Crit Care Med 154:6–17, 1996

Snape WJ, Carlson GM, Matarazzo SA, et al: Evidence that abnormal myoelectric activity produces colonic motor dysfunction in the irritable bowel syndrome. Gastroenterology 72:383–387, 1977

Solomon GF, Temoshok L: A psychoneuroimmunologic perspective on AIDS research: questions, preliminary findings and suggestions. Journal of Applied Social Psychology 17:286–308, 1987

Sorenson JL, Gibson DR, Heitzman C, et al: AIDS prevention with drug abusers in residential treatment: preliminary results. Pharmacol Biochem Behav 30:548–549, 1988

Spiegel D: Our goal is to see to it that every cancer patient who wants it has access to supportive/expressive therapy. Adv Cancer Res 8:85–86, 1992

Spiegel D, Bloom JR, Kraemer HC, et al: Effect of psychosocial treatment on survival of patients with metastatic breast cancer. Lancet 2:888–891, 1989

Stein M, Miller AH, Trestman RL: Depression, the immune system and health and illness. Arch Gen Psychiatry 48:171–177, 1991

Stern M, Pascale L, McLoone J: Psychosocial adaptation following an acute myocardial infarction. Journal of Chronic Diseases 29:513–526, 1976

Stevens LJ, Zentall SS, Abate ML, et al: O-3 fatty acids in boys with behavior, learning and health problems. Physiol Behav 54:915–920, 1996

Stoll A, Severus WE, Freeman MP, et al: O-3 fatty acids in bipolar disorder: a preliminary double-blind placebo-controlled trial. Arch Gen Psychiatry 56:407–412, 1999

Stunkard AJ (ed): Obesity. Philadelphia, PA, WB Saunders, 1980

Stunkard AJ, Harris JR, Pederson NL, et al: The body mass index of twins who have been reared apart. N Engl J Med 322:1483–1487, 1990

Suls J, Fletcher B: The relative efficacy of avoidant and non-avoidant coping strategies: a meta-analysis. Health Psychol 4:249–288, 1985

Svedlund J, Sjodin I, Ottosson JO, et al: Controlled study of psychotherapy in irritable bowel syndrome. Lancet 2:589–592, 1983

Svetkey LP, Sacks FM, Obarzarek F, et al: The DASH diet; sodium intake and blood pressure trial (DASH-sodium) rationale and design. DASH-Sodium Collaborative Research Group. Journal of the American Dietary Association 99:S96–S104, 1999

Taylor CB, Houston-Miller N, Ahn DK, et al: The effects of exercise training programs on psychosocial improvement in uncomplicated postmyocardial infarction patients. J Psychosom Res 30:581–587, 1986

Thompson DR, Meddis R: Wives' responses to counselling early after myocardial infarction. J Psychosom Res 34:249–258, 1990

Toomey TC, Mann JD, Abashian S, et al: Relationship between perceived self-control of pain, pain description and functioning. Pain 45:129–133, 1991

Toomey TC, Hernandez JT, Gittelman DF, et al: Relationship of sexual and physical abuse to pain and psychological assessment variables in chronic pelvic pain patients. Pain 53:105–109, 1993 [comment in Pain 56:361, 1994]

Trials of Hypertension Prevention Collaborative Research Group: The effects of nonpharmacologic interventions on blood pressure of persons with high normal levels. JAMA 267:1213–1220, 1992

Turk DC, Flor H: Pain and pain behaviors: the utility and limitations of the pain behavior construct. Pain 31:277–295, 1987

Turk DC, Flor H, Rudy TE: Pain and families, I: etiology, maintenance and psychosocial impact. Pain 30:3–27, 1987

Turner P: Benefit:risk consideration in long-term therapy with dexfenfluramine. Int J Obes Relat Metab Disord 16 (suppl 3):S15–S17, 1992

Tyroler HA, Haynes SG, Cobb LA, et al: Environmental risk factors in coronary artery disease. Circulation 76 (suppl I):139–144, 1987

Valdiserri R, Lyte D, Leviton L, et al: AIDS prevention in homosexual and bisexual men: results of a randomized trial evaluating two risk reduction intervention. AIDS 3:21–26, 1989

Valentine AD, Meyers CA, Kling MA, et al: Mood and cognitive side-effects of interferon therapy. Semin Oncol 25:39–47, 1998

Van Moffaert M: Psychodermatology: an overview. Psychother Psychosom 58:125–136, 1992

VanThiel DH, Friedlander L, Molloy PJ, et al: Interferon alpha can be used successfully in patients with hepatitis-C virus-positive chronic hepatitis who have psychiatric illness. Eur J Gastroenterol Hepatol 7:165–168, 1995

Verrier RL, Hagestad EL, Lown B: Delayed myocardial ischemia by anger. Circulation 75:249–254, 1987

Vlietstra RE, Kronmal RA, Oberman A, et al: Effect of cigarette smoking on survival of patients with angiographically documented coronary artery disease. JAMA 255:1023–1027, 1986

Von Korff M, Ormel J, Katon W, et al: Disability and depression among distressed high utilizers of healthcare. Arch Gen Psychiatry 49:91–100, 1992

Wald A, Chandra R, Gabel S, et al: Evaluation of biofeedback in childhood encopresis. J Pediatr Gastroenterol Nutr 6:554–558, 1987

Walker EA, Katon WJ, Neraas K, et al: Dissociation in women with chronic pelvic pain. Am J Psychiatry 149:534–537, 1992

Weisse CS: Depression and immunocompetence: a review of the literature. Psychol Bull 111:475–489, 1992

Wells KB, Stewart A, Hays RD, et al: The functioning and well-being of depressed patients: results from the Medical Outcome Study. JAMA 262:914–919, 1989

Whitehead WE: Behavioral medicine approaches to gastrointestinal disorders. J Consult Clin Psychol 60:605–612, 1992

Whitehead WE, Bosmajian LS: Behavioral medicine approaches to gastrointestinal disorders. J Consult Clin Psychol 50:672–683, 1982

Whorell PJ, Prior A, Faragher EB: Controlled trial of hypnotherapy in the treatment of severe refractory irritable bowel syndrome. Lancet 2:1232–1234, 1984

Williams RB, Schanberg SM, Kuhn CM, et al: Influence of alprazolam on neuroendocrine and cardiovascular response to stress in type A men. Paper presented at the annual meeting of the American College of Neuropsychopharmacology, Washington, DC, September 1986

Williams RB, Barefoot JC, Califf RM, et al: Prognostic importance of social and economic resources among medically treated patients with angiographically documented coronary artery disease. JAMA 267:520–524, 1992

Wishnie HA, Hackett TP, Cassem NH: Psychological hazards of convalescence following myocardial infarction. JAMA 215:1292–1296, 1971

Wood PD, Stefanick ML, Dreon DM, et al: Changes in plasma lipids and lipoproteins in overweight men during weight loss through dieting as compared with exercise. N Engl J Med 319:1173–1179, 1988

Workman EA: Multimodal treatment of chronic pain: combining medical and behavioral interventions (abstract). Proceedings of the Society of Behavioral Medicine XII:132, 1991

Yeung AC, Vekshtein VI, Vita JA, et al: Vasomotor response of coronary arteries to mental stress. Circulation 80 (suppl II):591–596, 1989

Young LD: Psychological factors in rheumatoid arthritis. J Consult Clin Psychol 60:619–627, 1992

Zitman FG, Linssen ACG, Edelbroek PM, et al: Low dose amitriptyline in chronic pain: the gain is modest. Pain 42:35–42, 1990

Index

*Page numbers printed in **boldface** type refer to tables or figures.*

AA (Alcoholics Anonymous), 420–421
A Test for Vigilance, 66, 72
Abacavir, **811, 818,** 823, 834
Abdominal pain, 552
   psychostimulant-induced, 723
Abnormal Involuntary Movement Scale,
   966, **967**
Abortion, 706
ABPP (American Board of Professional
   Psychology), 98–99
Absorption of drug, 941
   aging and, 861, **862,** 941
Abstracting abilities
   assessment of, 65
   in delirium, 261
Abulia, 73
Abuse
   dissociation and, 1003
   domestic violence and child abuse,
      711–712, 908–909
   of drugs (*See* Substance-related
      disorders)
   of elderly persons, 859, **860,** 909
   emergency department screening for,
      908
   gastrointestinal disease and,
      114–115, 552
   Munchausen syndrome by proxy,
      521, 523–526
   reporting suspected cases of, 909
   sexual
      anorexia nervosa and, 479
      chronic pelvic pain and, 1070
      of elderly persons, 859, **860**
      factitious, 519, 523
      flunitrazepam incapacitation for,
         434
      rape and domestic violence,
         711–712
   somatization and, 369

Academy of Psychosomatic Medicine, 7,
   18, 206
   position statement on Psychiatric
      Aspects of Excellent End-of-Life
      Care, 805–806
Acalculia, 73
Acamprosate, 432
Accreditation Council for Graduate
   Medical Education, 18
ACE (angiotensin-converting enzyme)
   inhibitors, 322, **944**
Acetaminophen, **943, 995**
   interaction with alcohol, 427
   overdose of, 129, 724–725
Acetazolamide, **349, 461,** 953
Acetylcholine, aggression and, 155
L-α-Acetylmethadol (LAAM), 418, 438
Achalasia, 553
Acid-base balance, 546
Acitretin, **461**
Acne, lithium-induced, 959
Acoustic neuromas, **681**
Acquired immunodeficiency syndrome
   (AIDS). *See* Human
   immunodeficiency virus infection
   and acquired immunodeficiency
   syndrome
Acromegaly, **564,** 567, 682
Acrylamide, **284**
ACTG-76 (AIDS Clinical Trials Group-
   76), 459
ACTH. *See* Adrenocorticotropic hormone
Active dynamic interview, 1039
Activities of daily living (ADLs), 854
Acupuncture, 834, 836
Acute intermittent porphyria, **680,** 688
Acute stress disorder, 403–404, 1038
   cancer and, 660–661
   diagnosis of, 394
   HIV/AIDS and, 833

Acyclovir, 688, **818**
Adderall. *See* Dextroamphetamine
Addiction Severity Index, 428
Addiction specialists, 417. *See also*
   Substance-related disorders
Addison's disease, 566, **816**
   depression and, 308, **311,** 732
   prevalence of psychiatric comorbidity
      with, **564**
Adenylate cyclase, 436
ADHD. *See* Attention-deficit/
   hyperactivity disorder
Adjustment disorders, 41
   with anxiety, 397
      in dying patients, 780, **781**
   assessment for, 95–96
   cancer and, 245, 397, 661, 780
   definition of, 397
   with depressed mood, 312
   after head and neck surgery, 615
   heart transplantation and, 627
   HIV/AIDS and, 831–833
   insomnia and, 500
   liver transplantation and, 628
   with mixed features, 397
   prevalence in medically ill patients,
      241, 397
   in rehabilitation settings, 732, 734
   somatization and, **362**
ADLs (activities of daily living), 854
Administration of consultation-liaison
   service, 17–21
   keys to establishing effective service,
      21, **21**
   liaison with other specialties, 20, **20**
   models for organization of service,
      18–20
   optimizing financial viability of
      service, **27,** 27–31
   in pediatrics, 722

Adolescents. *See* Children and
    adolescents
Adrenal insufficiency, 572
Adrenocorticotropic hormone (ACTH),
    346, 539
Advance directives, 169, **174,** 175–176.
    See also End-of-life decisions
    definition of, 168
    health care proxy form, 187–189
    right to die, 174, 790
Advanced Research Projects Agency
    Network (ARPANET), 934
Aerophagia, 552
Affect, 62–63
    appropriateness of, 63
    assessment of, 62–63
    definition of, 62
    intensity of, 62
    lability of, 63, 262
    range of, 62
Age at onset of psychiatric disorders, **63**
Ageism, 859
Agency for Health Care Policy and
    Research, 40, 558
Agency for Health Care Research and
    Quality, 558
Agenerase. *See* Amprenavir
Aggression, 149–163
    active vs. passive, 736
    assault of physicians by patients, 149
    diagnosis of, **150,** 150–152, **151**
    differential diagnosis of, 151–152,
        156, 156–157, **157**
    documentation of, 152
    DSM-IV diagnoses associated with,
        156
    among elderly patients, 149–150
    episodic dyscontrol syndrome, 684
    history taking for, 156–157
    intermittent explosive disorder, 150,
        150
    involuntary hospitalization for, 179
    legal liability for treatment of patients
        exhibiting, 167
    management of, 157–163
        for acute aggression, 158–160,
            159, 160
        for chronic aggression, 160–162,
            161, 162
        four D's for, **157**
        multifaceted approach to, 157
        nonpharmacological, 157–158
        pharmacological, 158–163, 171
        violent patients in emergency
            department, 890, 898–900
    neuropathology of, 150, **151**

neuropsychiatric disorders associated
    with, 149, **156**
    Alzheimer's disease, 149, 150
    brain injury, 149, 156
neurotransmitters and, 155–156
among nursing home residents, 149
Overt Aggression Scale for, 149, 151,
    152, **153, 155**
rape and domestic violence, 711–712
    (*See also* Sexual abuse/assault)
rating scales for, 151
in rehabilitation settings, 736
self-directed, 150 (*See also*
    Suicidality)
substance-induced, **156**
    benzodiazepines, 971
    inhalants, 446
    phencyclidine, 443
in type A behavior pattern, 113
in Wilson's disease, 279
Aging, 853–866. *See also* Elderly persons
    dementia and, 9, **63,** 273, 275, 295
    memory impairment and, 253, 854
    normal, 273, 853–854
    pharmacodynamics and, 862
    pharmacokinetics and, 861, **862**
    suicide and, 241
Agitation, 108
    in Alzheimer's disease, 149, 277
    brain injury and, 149
    among cardiothoracic surgery
        patients, 603–605
    among critically ill patients, 761–762,
        762
    delirium and, 258, 267
    in delirium tremens, 901
    differential diagnosis of, 152, **156,**
        156–157, **157**
    documentation of, 152–155
    among elderly patients, 149–150
    history taking for, 156–157
    neurotransmitters and, 155–156
    nocturnal, 504
    among nursing home residents,
        149
    Overt Agitation Severity Scale for,
        151–155, **154**
    substance-induced, **156**
        antiemetic drugs, 604
        bupropion, 952
        cocaine, 441
        psychostimulants, 442, 761
    terminal, 792
    treatment of, 157–163
        for acute agitation, 158–160,
            159, 160

    for chronic agitation, 160–162,
        161, 162
    nonpharmacological, 157
    pharmacological, 157–163
Agnosia, 73, 273
    in Alzheimer's disease, 277, **278**
    in vascular dementia, **280**
Agonist drugs, 944
β_2-Agonists, **502**
Agoraphobia, 395, 404
    asthma and, 399
    behavioral treatment of, 546–547
    definition of, 404
    among elderly persons, 858
    gastrointestinal disease and, 245
    irritable bowel syndrome and, 555,
        555
    panic disorder with, 394
    prevalence of, **396**
Agranulocytosis, drug-induced
    antipsychotics, 978
    carbamazepine, 351, 978
    clozapine, 966, 978
    mirtazapine, 327, 953
    tricyclic antidepressants, 951, 978
Agraphia, 73
Agreeableness, **116**
AICD (automatic implantable
    cardioverter-defibrillator), 608,
    627
AIDS. *See* Human immunodeficiency
    virus infection and acquired
    immunodeficiency syndrome
AIDS Clinical Trials Group-76
    (ACTG-76), 459
Air hunger, 547
Akathisia
    antiemetic-induced, 604
    antipsychotic-induced, **156,** 158,
        691, 965
    in cancer patients, 660
    differentiation from aggression, 152
    differentiation from anxiety, 660
    tardive, 966
    treatment of, 965
Alanine aminotransferase. *See* Hepatic
    disease
Alcohol dehydrogenase, 426, 427
Alcohol use disorders, 242–243,
    422–433. *See also* Substance-
    related disorders
    age at onset of, 422
    alcohol-attributable fractions for
        medical disorders, 243, **243**
    alcohol-drug interactions, 427, **428**
        antidepressants, 953

antipsychotics, 969
benzodiazepines, **349**
cocaine, 440
cytochrome P450–related, 427, **428**
alcohol-induced persisting amnestic disorder, 86, 265, 283, 426
alcohol-induced psychotic disorder, 426
treatment of, 432, **433**
behavioral complications of, 242
benzodiazepine abuse and, 902–903
brain injury and, 685
among burn patients, **239,** 612
cancer and, 660
cirrhosis and, 239, 242, **243**
course and outcome in medically ill patients, 251
criminal behavior and, 423
definition of alcoholism, 422
diagnosis of, 422–423
duration of ethanol detectability in urine, **895**
laboratory testing, 427–428, **428**
physical examination, 427
screening tests, 428, **429, 430**
in elderly persons, 859
epidemiology of, 422–423
gender and, 422, 424
genetic factors and, 423
health care expenditures related to, 423
Huntington's disease and, 686
insomnia and, **502**
intoxication, **156,** 423–424
blood alcohol concentration, 418, 424
development of tolerance, 424
emergency department management of, 890, 900
management of, 430, **433**
rate of alcohol metabolism, 424
management of, 430–433, **433**
acamprosate, 432
acute, 430–432
Alcoholics Anonymous, 420–421
disulfiram, 432
inpatient medical-psychiatric treatment, 875
intoxication, 430
long-term, 432
naltrexone, 432, 875
outcome of, 432–433
outpatient psychiatric consultation, 923–924

Wernicke's encephalopathy, 432, **433**
withdrawal symptoms, 430–432, **430–432**
medical complications of, 423
Korsakoff's psychosis, 86, 265, 283, 426
liver disease, 426
neurological disease, 426
traumatic injury, 423
Wernicke's encephalopathy, 263, 265, 283, 296, 426, **433**
mortality from, 242
neuroimaging in, 293
neurological and neurosurgical disorders and, 679
nomenclature for, 422
predisposition and risk factors for, 423
in pregnancy, 243
prevalence in medically ill patients, 241–243, 422
psychiatric comorbidity with, 422, 423
anxiety disorders, 423
dementia, 276, 277, 283, **284,** 288
depression, **311,** 323–324
mania, **345**
personality disorders, 423
schizophrenia, 423
somatization, **362,** 367, 423
in rehabilitation settings, 737–738
sexual dysfunction and, **461**
smoking and, 445
suicide and, 128, 129, **133,** 133–134, **134, 136,** 142–143, **243,** 423
transplantation for patients with, 427, 629–630
liver transplantation, 427, 628
psychiatric evaluation for, 427
underrecognition of, 242–243
Alcohol withdrawal, **156,** 263, 265, 424–426, **433**
anxiety due to, **781**
benzodiazepines for, 268, 430–432, **431,** 970
clinical features of, 901
Clinical Institute Withdrawal Assessment for Alcohol–Revised for, 424, **425–426**
delirium due to, 258, 259, 262–263, 424–426, **433,** 901
detoxification for, 430–432, **430–432,** 901

differentiation from postsurgical complications, 424
emergency department management of, 900–901
hypothalamic-pituitary-adrenal dysfunction during, 424
inpatient vs. outpatient management of, 430–431
magnesium sulfate for, 432
seizures due to, 424, 901
treatment of, 432, **432, 433**
thiamine for, 432
uncomplicated, 424
Alcoholics Anonymous (AA), 420–421
Aldehyde dehydrogenase, 426
Alexander, Franz, 4
Alexia, 73
Alexithymia, 117, 118, **118,** 122, 369, 907, 1032
Allergic conditions, 1066
Allesthesia, 991
Allocation of medical resources, 167, 207
Allodynia, 991
Allopurinol, **943**
Alopecia, drug-induced
lithium, 959
selective serotonin reuptake inhibitors, 952
valproate, 961
Alprazolam, **903,** 970, **970**
abuse of, 902–903, 907
dosage of, **407, 434, 903, 970,** 971
drug interactions with, 972
cytochrome P450 metabolism and, **945**
nefazodone, 327
ritonavir, 814, **815,** 834
half-life of, **407, 903**
indications for
anxiety, 782, **782**
depression, **785,** 787, 957
psychiatric aspects of, **669**
side effects of
mania, **345**
sexual dysfunction, **461**
use in specific patient groups or medical conditions
chemotherapy patients, 659
dying patients, 782, **782, 785,** 787
elderly persons, **863**
withdrawal from, 434, 904, 971
Alprostadil, 466
ALS. *See* Amyotrophic lateral sclerosis
Aluminum poisoning, **284**

Alzheimer Association, 298
Alzheimer's disease, 273. *See also*
    Dementia
    aggression and agitation in, 149,
        150
        β–blockers for, 150
    aging and, **63**, 275, 276, 295
    apolipoprotein E4 allele and, 276
    "catastrophic reactions" in, 295
    clinical features of, 277, **279**
    computerized
        electroencephalography in, 57
    course and prognosis for, 295
    depression and, 316, 857
    diagnostic criteria for, **278**
    familial, 277
    genetic factors and, 276, 277
    guardianship of patients with,
        176–177
    insomnia and, 504
    neuroimaging in, 293
        functional, 56
        structural, 53
    neurotransmitter deficits in, 297
    Parkinson's disease and, 275, 279
    pathophysiology of, 286
    pharmacotherapy for, 296–297
    prevalence of, 275, **680**
    psychosis and, 858–859
    risk factors for, 276
    sexual behavior and, 468
    sleep disorders and, 512
    stages of, **279**
    vascular dementia and, 275
Amantadine
    indications for
        aggression, 159
        neuroleptic malignant syndrome,
            968
        parkinsonism, 965
    mania induced by, **345**
    overdose of, 965
    for patients undergoing
        rehabilitation, **742**
Amblyopia, nutritional, 426
Amenorrhea
    in anorexia nervosa, 480, 483, 486,
        705
    antipsychotic-induced, 978
American Board of Professional
    Psychology (ABPP), 98–99
American Board of Psychiatry and
    Neurology, 9, 417
American Journal of Health-System
    Pharmacy, 45
American Journal of Insanity, 4

American Psychiatric Association
    guidelines
    collaborative, consultative, and
        supervisory relationships with
        nonmedical therapists, 181–182
    proper uses of seclusion and restraint,
        180
American Psychological Association, 98,
    99, **99**
American Society of Addiction
    Medicine, 417, 420, 422
Americans Against Human Suffering,
    790
Americans With Disabilities Act of 1990
    (P.L. 101-336), 87, 631
Amiloride, 349, **461**
γ–Aminobutyric acid (GABA), 400
    aggression and, 155
    in alcohol intoxication, 423–424
    carbamazepine effects on, 351
    GABA-benzodiazepine complex,
        400–401, **401**, 902
    mania and, 344
    receptors for, 400
    role in anxiety, 400–401
    role in ventilation, 547
Aminocaproic acid, **461**
Aminoglutethimide, **667**
Aminophylline, **349**, 960
Amiodarone, **461**
Amitriptyline, 325, **948**
    cytochrome P450 metabolism and,
        945
    dosage of, **948**
    indications for
        agitation and aggression, 161
        fibromyalgia or chronic pain, 571,
            1004–1005
        headache, 1068
        hypochondriasis, 384
        pathological laughing and crying,
            693, **693**
    injectable, 601
    receptor site activity of, **948**
    side effects of
        cardiac effects, 543
        sexual dysfunction, **461**
    use in specific patient groups or
        medical conditions
        breast-feeding women, **981**
        chronic pain syndrome, 693, **693**
        dying patients, 785, **785**
        migraine, 693, **693**
        patients undergoing rehabilitation,
            742
        pregnancy, **708**

Ammonium chloride, 905
Amnesia. *See* Memory impairment
Amobarbital, **434**, 895, 904, **904**
Amotivational syndrome, cannabis-
    induced, 444
Amoxapine, 325, 947, **948**
    dosage of, **948**
    for dying patients, **785**
    interaction with dopamine blockers,
        786
    receptor site affinity of, **948**
    side effects of
        extrapyramidal symptoms, 693,
            951
        insomnia, **502**
        sexual dysfunction, **461**
    use during breast-feeding, **981**
Amphetamines. *See also*
    Dextroamphetamine
    abuse of, **156**, 243, 442
        in anorexia nervosa, 479
        in bulimia nervosa, 481
        management of, 442
    duration of detectability in urine, **895**
    interaction with monoamine oxidase
        inhibitors, 955
    management of emergencies related
        to, 901
    mechanism of action of, 442
    sexual dysfunction induced by, **461**
    side effects of, 442
        depression, **311**
        mania, 345
        sleep disorders, **502**
    suicidality and, 243
Amphotericin B, **311**, 323, **818**
Amprenavir, **811**
Amputation, 65, **733**, 735, 991
Amygdala, role in emotional responses,
    401–402
Amyl nitrite, **461**
Amyloid angiopathy, 286
Amyloidosis, 513
Amyotrophic lateral sclerosis (ALS),
    319, 687
Amytal. *See* Amobarbital
Anabolic steroids, **311**, 324, **345**,
    345–346
Anadamide, 444
Anafranil. *See* Clomipramine
Analgesics, 989, **989**, 1004–1008. *See*
    also Pain management
    for acute pain, 995–997
    anticonvulsants, 315, **989**, 1006
    antidepressants, 314, 693, **693**, 950,
        989, 1004–1006, 1067

antipsychotics, **989,** 1007–1008
anxiety induced by, **400**
benzodiazepines, **989,** 1006
for burn patients, 612
for children, 724, **724**
for chronic pain, 435, 1006–1007
delirium induced by, **156, 762,** 793
for depression, 957
drug interactions with, 999, **999**
     alcohol, 427, **428**
     ritonavir, 815
drug-seeking behavior and, 996, **996**
for dying patients, 782–783, 796, **797**
lack of response to, 995–996
medication contract for, **1010**
nonsteroidal anti-inflammatory
     drugs, 995, **995**
opioids, 435, 796, **797,** 993, **993,**
     994, 1006–1007
overdose of, 129
placebo effect and, 992
psychostimulants, **989,** 1007
somatization and, **362**
for somatoform pain disorder, 384
use in rehabilitation settings, 741,
     742
World Health Organization analgesic
     ladder, **995**
Anemia, **816**
aplastic, carbamazepine-induced,
     351, 961, 978
eating disorders and, 482
megaloblastic, 569
pernicious, 288, 569
sexual dysfunction and, 458
Anesthetics. *See also* specific drugs
anxiety induced by, **400**
drug interactions with, 596,
     597–598, 944
     antipsychotics, 969
     monoamine oxidase inhibitors,
          955
Angel dust. *See* Phencyclidine-related
     disorders
"Angels of death," 519
Anger, 108, 1054
amphetamine-induced, 442
delirium and, 262
after disfiguring head and neck
     surgery, 616
episodic dyscontrol syndrome, 684
ischemic heart disease and, 539, 543,
     1054, **1055**
pharmacotherapy for, 1058
type A behavior pattern and,
     113, 1054

Angina pectoris
insomnia and, 502–503
nocturnal, 502, 511
panic disorder and, 242
sexual dysfunction and, 456
     sildenafil for, 460
stress and, 538, 1057
Angioplasty, 456
Angiotensin-converting enzyme (ACE)
     inhibitors, 322, **944**
Anisotropine, **461**
Ankylosing spondylitis, 1004
Annals of Pharmacotherapy, 45
Anorexia, drug-induced. *See* Appetite
     changes
Anorexia nervosa, 477–480
age at onset of, 477–479
clinical features of, 479–480
course of, 479
definition of, 477
diagnostic criteria for, **478**
epidemiology of, 477–479
medical complications of, **483,**
     483–487
     amenorrhea and infertility, 480,
          483, 486, 705
     cardiac abnormalities, 482,
          484–485
     edema, 486
     electrolyte abnormalities, 485
     endocrine abnormalities, 480,
          483, 486–487
     hematological abnormalities, 483,
          486
     in hospitalized patients, **482,**
          482–483
     osteoporosis, **239,** 483
     related to substance use, 479, 481,
          481, 484
     renal abnormalities, 485
outcome of, 479
predisposing factors for, 479
psychiatric comorbidity and, 479
treatment of, 487–488
Anorgasmia. *See also* Sexual dysfunction
after cardiac transplantation, 457
selective serotonin reuptake
     inhibitor–induced, 465
spinal cord injury and, 466
Anoxia, **284**
Antabuse. *See* Disulfiram
Antacid interactions with
     antipsychotics, **944,** 969
Antagonist drugs, 944
Antiandrogen drugs
for aggression, 162

for paraphilias, 470–471
for sexual acting-out, 468
Antiarrhythmic agents
delirium induced by, **762**
drug interactions with
     antidepressants, **943,** 953
     antipsychotics, **944**
     carbamazepine, **349**
     cytochrome P450 metabolism
          and, **945**
for electroconvulsive therapy, 329
tricyclic antidepressants, 543, 951
Anticholinergic drugs
abuse of, 905
for agitation, 604
interaction with antidepressants, **943**
overdose of, 129, 905
to prevent neuroleptic-induced
     dystonia, 897
side effects of
     anxiety, **400**
     delirium, 150, **156,** 239, **239,**
          259, 325, **762,** 785, 905
     dementia, **284**
     for ophthalmic preparations, 611
Anticholinergic effects
of antihistamines, 973
of antipsychotics, 409, **964,** 965,
     966, 969
in elderly persons, 325
in patients with delirium or
     dementia, 979
of tricyclic antidepressants, 325, 408,
     543, 761, 950, 951
in children, 723
Anticoagulant interactions
with alcohol, 427, **428**
with carbamazepine, 962
with chloral hydrate, 973
with psychostimulants, **957**
Anticonvulsants, **958,** 960–962. *See also*
     specific drugs
dosage and administration of, **958,**
     961
drug interactions with, 962
     antipsychotics, 969
     psychostimulants, **957**
electroconvulsive therapy and, 1017
indications for, 961
     agitation and aggression, 160–161,
          161, 171
     mania, **347,** 350–353, 960–962
     pain syndromes, **989,** 1006
     rapid-cycling bipolar disorder, 960
mechanism of action of, 960
pharmacokinetics of, 960–961

Anticonvulsants *(continued)*
  response to, 961
  side effects of, 961–962, **975–976**
    dementia, **284**
  types of, 960
  use in specific patient groups or
     medical conditions, **975–976**
    brain injury, 979
    HIV/AIDS, 826–827, 839
    neurological disorders, 693–694
    patients undergoing rehabilitation,
     742
    systemic lupus erythematosus,
     568
Antidepressants, 325–327, 944–957,
  948, 972. *See also* specific drugs
  and classes
  adequate trial of, 946, 950
  alprazolam, 957
  analgesics, 957
  augmentation of, 328, 957
    lithium, 328, 957
    thyroid hormone, 328, 957
  bupropion, 326
  classes of, 947
  combined with benzodiazepines,
    969
  compliance with, 941
  dosage and administration of, 946,
    948, 950
  drug interactions with, **943,** 953–954
    chemotherapy agents, 663
    cytochrome P450 metabolism
     and, **945,** 953
    immunosuppressants, 643
    ritonavir, 814, **815**
    tramadol, **999**
  duration of treatment with, 946
  emergency department initiation of,
    906
  indications for, 944, 946–950
    agitation and aggression, **161,**
     161–162
    anorexia nervosa, 488
    anxiety disorders, 408, 947, **950,**
     969, 972
    bulimia nervosa, 489, 950
    depression, 325–328, 946–947
    narcolepsy, 509–510
    pain syndromes, 950, **989,**
     1004–1006, 1067
    somatoform disorders, 384
    systemic lupus erythematosus,
     568
    urinary incontinence, 950
  lithium, 328, 957

mechanism of action of, 947, **948,**
  949
mirtazapine, 327
monoamine oxidase inhibitors, 327,
  954, 954–955
nefazodone, 327
onset of action of, 950
overdose of, 129, 953
pharmacokinetics of, 947
predictors of good response to, 946
psychostimulants, 327, 955–957,
  956
response to, 950
sedating, 505
selective serotonin reuptake
  inhibitors, 326
side effects of, 307, 950–953,
  975–976
  anxiety, **400**
  delirium, **156**
  insomnia, **502**
  mania, **346**
St. John's wort, 973, **974**
structures of, 947
suicide risk after initiation of, 946
switching between, 947, 955
use in specific patient groups or
  medical conditions
  breast-feeding women, **981**
  cancer, 660, 662–663
  cardiac disease, 408, 537,
    542–543, 634, 974, **975**
  children, 723, **723**
  chronic pain or fibromyalgia, 314,
    693, **693,** 1000
  critically ill patients, 760–761
  dialysis patients, 561
  dying patients, 784–787, **785**
  elderly persons, **863,** 863–864,
    946, 950
  epilepsy, 318
  hepatic/gastrointestinal disease,
    977
  HIV/AIDS, 320, 828–830
  Huntington's disease, 318, 693,
    693
  hyperthyroidism, 320
  irritable bowel syndrome,
    555–556
  neurological disorders, 692–693,
    693, 741, **976**
  Parkinson's disease, 317, 693, **693**
  patients undergoing rehabilitation,
    742
  pregnancy, 708, **708,** 979–980
  pulmonary disease, 977

surgical patients, **597,** 601
transplant candidates, 634–638,
  636–637
vascular dementia, 297
venlafaxine, 326–327
withdrawal from, 953
Antidepressants, tricyclics (TCAs) and
  related agents, 325–326, **943,** 947,
  948
  discontinuation of, 953
  dosage and administration of, 950
  drug interactions with, 953
    antipsychotics, **944,** 969
    cytochrome P450 metabolism
     and, **945**
    lithium, 960
    monoamine oxidase inhibitors,
     327, 954, 955
    psychostimulants, 957, **957**
    selective serotonin reuptake
     inhibitors, **999**
    tramadol, **999**
  mechanism of action of, 947
  overdose of, 953
  parenteral, 601, 785
  rectal, 785
  serum level of, 947
  side effects of, 325, 408, 543,
    760–761, 950–951
  for specific disorders
    anxiety disorders, **950**
    bulimia nervosa, 489
    depression, 325–326
    fibromyalgia and chronic pain,
     384, 571, 1000, 1004–1006
  structure of, 947
  use in specific patient groups or
    medical conditions
    cancer, 662, 785
    cardiac disease, 543, 974, **975**
    children, 723
    dying patients, 782, 785, **785**
    HIV/AIDS, 829
    pregnancy, 979
    surgical patients, **597**
    transplant candidates, 634, **636**
  withdrawal from, 953
Antiemetics
  agitation induced by, 604
  antipsychotics as, 963
  anxiety induced by, 781, **781**
  for cancer patients, 659, 660
  psychiatric aspects of, **669**
Antihistamines, 973
  contraindications to, 973
  for insomnia, 505

interaction with alcohol, 427, **428**
overdose of, 129
side effects of
  anxiety, **400**
  delirium, **762**
Antihypertensive agents
  drug interactions with
    antidepressants, **943,** 953
    antipsychotics, 989
    monoamine oxidase inhibitors, 955
  electroconvulsive therapy and, 1021
  side effects of
    anxiety, **400**
    dementia, **284**
    depression, **311,** 321–322
    insomnia, **502**
Antimicrobial agents, **284, 400,** 762
Antiphospholipid antibodies, 568
Antipsychotics, 962–969, **964.** *See also*
  specific drugs
  atypical, 962–963
    for Alzheimer's disease, 296
    for anxiety, 409
    for delirium, 268
    dosage of, 963, **964**
    for mania, 354
    mechanism of action of, 963
    side effects of, 409
  benzodiazepines combined with, 408
  dosage and administration of, 963–965, **964**
    for rapid neuroleptization, 963
    for rapid tranquilization, 965
  drug interactions with, **944,** 969
    antidepressants, 953
    carbamazepine, 962
    cytochrome P450 metabolism and, **945**
    lithium, 694, 960
    ritonavir, 814
    tramadol, **999**
  indications for, 962
    acute psychosis, 896–897
    aggression and agitation, 151, 171, **763**
      acute, 158–159, **159,** 965
      chronic, 160, **161**
    Alzheimer's disease, 296, 297
    anorexia nervosa, 488
    anxiety, 408–409, 782, **782,** 962, 973
    delirium, 267–268, 408, **763**
    insomnia, 505
    mania, 353–354, 962
    nausea/vomiting, 963

pain syndromes, **989,** 1007–1008
psychotic depression, 947, 962
schizophrenia, 962
suicidality, 141
Tourette's syndrome, 962
mechanism of action of, 963
overdose of, 969
pharmacokinetics of, 963
side effects of, **156,** 158, 263, 353, 408, 691, **964,** 965–968, **975–976**
  anxiety, **400**
  extrapyramidal symptoms, 158, 686, 691, 965–968
  neuroleptic malignant syndrome, 968
  oculogyric crisis, 611
  seizures, 966, 978–979
  sleep disorders, **502**
  tardive phenomena, 966–968
typical, 962–963
use in specific patient groups or medical conditions
  brain injury, 692, 979
  breast-feeding women, **981**
  cardiac disease, 544, 974, **975,** 977
  children, 723–724
  chronic obstructive pulmonary disease, 549
  critically ill patients, 759–763, **760, 763**
  dialysis patients, 561
  dying patients, 782, **782,** 793–795, **794**
  elderly persons, **863,** 864
  epilepsy, 692
  hepatic disease, 977
  HIV/AIDS, 409, 825, 839
  Huntington's disease, 692
  Parkinson's disease, 691–692, 979
  patients undergoing rehabilitation, **743**
  pregnancy, **708,** 966, 979
  surgical patients, **597–598**
  systemic lupus erythematosus, 568
  transplant patients, **636,** 641
withdrawal from, 969
Antiretroviral therapy, 810–815. *See also*
  specific drugs
  cerebrospinal fluid penetration by, 823
  compliance with, 813–814
  drug interactions with, 814–815, **815,** 834, 835

efficacy of, 811–812
highly active (HAART), 810–813, 823–824
for HIV-associated neurocognitive impairment, 823–824
limitations of, 813
in pregnancy, 809
reduction in central nervous system opportunistic conditions by, 815
resistance to, 813
side effects of, 807, **812,** 812–813
  neuropsychiatric disorders, 815–817, **818**
  sexual dysfunction, 835
  sleep disorders, 834
Antisocial personality disorder, **116,** 117
  countertransference and, 122
  Huntington's disease and, 686
  prevalence of, 119, **120**
  psychiatric emergencies in patients with, 907–908
  psychopathy checklist for, 908, **909**
  somatization disorder and, 375
  substance-related disorders and, 908
Anxiety, 393–410. *See also* Fear; Panic attacks
  assessment of, 405–406
  biology of, 399–402
    anatomic substrate, 401–402
    neurotransmitters, 399–401, **401**
  costs of care for, **872**
  in critically ill patients, 759–760
  definition of, 394
  delirium and, 262
  differential diagnosis of, 393, **393,** 405–406
  fatigue and, 570
  fibromyalgia and, 571
  hospital environmental factors associated with, **405**
  laboratory evaluation of, 406
  limbic encephalopathy and, 280
  mechanical ventilation and, 606, 765
  nicotine withdrawal, 445
  opioid abuse and, 437
  pain and, 997
  perioperative, 595
    cardiothoracic surgery, 603
    cosmetic surgery, 613
    head and neck surgery, 615, **615**
  physical signs and symptoms of, 394, **394**
  in postconcussion syndrome, 685
  poststroke, 250–251, 398
  pregnancy-related, 707
  primary (pathological), 393

Anxiety *(continued)*
   rating scales for, 93, **371**, 406, **407**
   somatization and, **362**, 365, 367, 376
   thyroid disorders and, **239**, 242, 398
   during transplant waiting period, 633
   about voluntary sterilization, 704
Anxiety disorders, **394**. *See also* specific disorders
   acute stress disorder, 394, 403–404
   course and outcome in medically ill patients, 250–251
   depression and, 242, 399
   due to general medical condition, 395, 402–403
   in dying patients, 780–783, **781, 782**
   in elderly persons, 858
   generalized anxiety disorder, 395, 403
   hypochondriasis and, 378
   insomnia and, 500–501
   medical conditions associated with
      cancer, 245, 398, 659–661, 780, 781
      cardiac disease, 396, 402, 536, 544–545, 627
      chronic pain, 997, 1000, **1000**
      Cushing's syndrome, **564**
      diabetes mellitus, 397, **564**
      esophageal motility disorders, 553–554
      HIV/AIDS, 398–399, 712, 781–782, 833–834
      hyperparathyroidism, **564**
      hyperthyroidism, **564**
      hypothyroidism, **564**
      irritable bowel syndrome, 554–555, **555**
      lung disease, 627
      neurological disorders, 63, 736
      pain, 997, 1000, **1000**
      pheochromocytoma, **564**, 566–657
   medical and toxic etiologies of, 397–399, **398**, 405
   not otherwise specified, 395
   obsessive-compulsive disorder, 395, 404–405
   outpatient psychiatric consultation for, 923
   panic disorder, 394, 403
   phobias, 404
   posttraumatic stress disorder, 394, 403–404
   prevalence of, 25, 241, 242, 395–397, **396**

psychiatric emergencies in patients with, 907
   in rehabilitation settings, 736–737
   respiration in, 547–548
   social phobia, 395
   somatization and, **362, 365**, 367, 376
   specific phobias, 395
   substance-induced, 395, 399, **400**, 405, 423, 441, 780–781, **781**
   in surgical patients, 596
   in transplant recipients, 642–643
   treatment of, 406–410
      antidepressants, 408, 947, 950, **950**, 954, 969, 972
      antipsychotics, 408–409, 782, **782**, 962
      benzodiazepines, hypnotics, and barbiturates, **407**, 407–408, 433, 969–972, **970**
      β–blockers, 409
      in cardiac disease, 544–545
      in dying patients, **782**, 782–783
      in intensive care setting, 759, **760**
      nonbenzodiazepine anxiolytics, 409, 972–973
Anxiety Status Inventory (ASI), 406, **407**
Anxiolytics, 969–973
   for agitation and aggression, 159–160
      acute, 159, **160**
      chronic, 160
   benzodiazepines, **407**, 407–408, 782, **782**, 969–972, **970**
   for children, **723**, 724
   disinhibition induced by, **156**
   for elderly persons, **863**, 864
   indications for, 969
   nonbenzodiazepine, 409, 972–973
      antihistamines, 973
      antipsychotics, 973
      barbiturates, 408
      β–blockers, 973
      buspirone, 972
      chloral hydrate, 973
      narcotics, 973
      zaleplon, 972–973
      zolpidem, 972
   side effects of, **975–976**
   use in specific patient groups or medical conditions
      breast-feeding women, **981**
      critically ill patients, 759, **760**
      dying patients, **782**, 782–783
      HIV/AIDS, 833, 834
      pulmonary disease, 977
      transplant candidates, **635**, 638

Apathy
   in Alzheimer's disease, 277
   delirium and, 262
   HIV-associated, 282, 818–819
   in Huntington's disease, 278
   in Korsakoff's psychosis, 283
Aphasia, 273. *See also* Language and speech disturbances
   in Alzheimer's disease, 277, **278**
   anomic, **67**
   assessment for, 67, 289, **290**
   Broca's, **67**
   clinical characteristics of, **67**
   conduction, **67**
   in frontotemporal dementia, 278
   global, **67**
   posttraumatic, 281
   in vascular dementia, **280**, 281
   Wernicke's, **67**
Aplastic anemia, carbamazepine-induced, 351, 961, 978
Apolipoprotein E4 allele, 276
Appearance assessment, 62
Appetite changes
   cancer-related anorexia, 666
   drug-induced
      bupropion, 952
      mirtazapine, 327, 953
      psychostimulants, 723, 761, 956
      valproate, 961
      venlafaxine, 326
Approach to consultation, 14–17
   consultation process, 15–17
      in pediatrics, 719–720
   elements of initial consultation note, **16**
   examination style, 14–15
   tools used for, 15
Apraxia, 73, 273
   in Alzheimer's disease, 277, **278**
   constructional, in delirium, 261, **261**
   in vascular dementia, **280**, 281
Aprosodia, poststroke, 681
Argyll Robertson pupils, 576
ARPANET (Advanced Research Projects Agency Network), 934
Arrhythmias
   anorexia nervosa and, 479, 482–485
   automatic implantable cardioverter-defibrillator for, 608, 627
   depression and, 307–308
   drug-induced
      cocaine, 243, 441
      ipecac, 484
      lithium, 350, 959
      MDMA, 443

monoamine oxidase inhibitors, 544
in neuroleptic malignant syndrome, 968
psychostimulants, 544, 761, 956, 957
risperidone, 354
trazodone, 952
tricyclic antidepressants, 325–326, 408, 543, 761, 950–951
electroconvulsive therapy–induced, 329, 544, 1019, 1021
fight-or-flight response and, 536
sleep disorders and, 508, 510–511
ventricular
effect of meditation on, 542
sudden cardiac death and, 537
Arsenic poisoning, **284, 502**
Arthralgia, selective serotonin reuptake inhibitor–induced, 952
"Arthritic personality," 1066
Arthritis
anxiety and, 736
depression, suicidality and, **733**
in Lyme disease, 575
prevalence of psychiatric comorbidity with, 240
sexual dysfunction and, 738
sleep disorders and, 504
use of Beck Depression Inventory in, 92, **93**
use of Minnesota Multiphasic Personality Inventory in, 89, **90**
Artificial organs, 633
heart, 604
Ascites, lithium and, 427
Ascorbic acid, 906
Asendin. *See* Amoxapine
ASI (Anxiety Status Inventory), 406, **407**
Ask-a-Doc program, 934
L-Asparaginase, **311, 323, 667,** 793
Aspartame, **345**
Aspartate aminotransferase. *See* Hepatic disease
Asphyxiophilia, 470
Aspirin, **943, 995**
Alzheimer's disease and, 297
for angina, 1057
interaction with valproate, **349**
for vascular dementia, 296
Assault. *See also* Aggression
domestic violence, 711–712, 908–909
of physicians by patients, 149

Assertiveness training, for somatization, 373
Assessment instruments. *See also* specific instruments
for aggression and agitation, 151, **153–155**
for alcoholism, 428, **429, 430**
for anxiety, 93, **371,** 406, **407**
cognitive function tests, 72–73 (*See also* Mental status examination)
for delirium, 263, 792
for dementia, 294
for depression, 92–93, **93, 371**
distortion by malingering patients, 527–528
of general distress and life-event scales, 93
for health-related quality of life, 93–94, **95**
neuropsychological tests, 80–83
pain measures, **371,** 992, **992**
for pediatric patients, **720,** 720–721
personality measures, 89–92, **371**
for schizophrenia, 929
for somatization, 371, **371**
for suicidality, 135, **135**
for transplantation candidates, 625–626
use in Nordic countries, 209
Assisted suicide and euthanasia, 144–146, 175, 789–791, **790,** 831
Associative anamnesis, 1039
Astemizole, 327, **946**
Asterixis, 689
carbamazepine-induced, 961
delirium and, 262–263
Asthenia
antiretroviral drug–induced, 812
neurocirculatory, 1062
Asthma, 4, 115, 546, 549–550, 1066
depression and, 550
factitious, 550
insomnia and, 503–504
nocturnal attacks of, 503
panic disorder and, 245, 399, 402, 550
psychiatric comorbidity with, 244–245
psychoeducational programs for, 1066
psychological management of, 550
as psychosomatic disease, 549–550
side effects of medications for, 550, **550**
Astrocytomas, **681**
Ataxia, 73

drug-induced
alcohol, 424
benzodiazepines, 353, 407
carbamazepine, 961
gabapentin, 961
inhalants, 446
lamotrigine, 353, 961
lithium, 350
phencyclidine, 443
Friedreich's, 687
in Lyme disease, 575
in neurosyphilis, 576
in transplant recipients, 643
in Wernicke's encephalopathy, 265, 283
Atenolol, 350, **461**
Atherosclerosis, 538–541. *See also* Coronary artery disease
stroke due to, 679
Ativan. *See* Lorazepam
Atopic dermatitis, 1066
Atorvastatin calcium, **461**
Atropine, **461,** 762
Attachment behavior, somatization and, 368
Attention bias in research, **199**
Attention-deficit/hyperactivity disorder (ADHD)
bupropion for, 326
cocaine dependence and, 442
diagnosis of, 98
computerized continuous performance tests, 98
neuropsychological testing of adults, 87–88
stimulants for, 722–723
traumatic brain injury and, 86
Attentional deficits
assessment for, 66–67, 289
delirium and, 260
after head injury, 281
HIV-associated, 282, 818
Attenuated brief psychotherapy, 1046–1047
AUDIT, 428
Australia, consultation-liaison psychiatry in, 217–218
background of, 217–218
in general hospital, 218
official status and training, 218
research, 218
telepsychiatry programs, 929, 930
Austria, consultation-liaison psychiatry in, 209–212
Autocastration, 468
Autoimmune disorders, 1066–1067

Automatic implantable cardioverter-
 defibrillator (AICD), 608, 627
Autonomic dysfunction, 394
 during alcohol withdrawal, 424
 in neuroleptic malignant syndrome,
  968
 in systemic lupus erythematosus,
  568
Autonomy of patient, 167
 advance directives, 175–176
 do-not-resuscitate orders, 175, 778
 refusal of treatment and, 169
 right to die, 174–175, 790
Avoidant personality disorder, **116**
 prevalence of, **120**
 somatization disorder and, 120,
  375
AZT. *See* Zidovudine

Babinski reflex, 73, 346, 968
"Baby blues," 710
BAC (blood alcohol concentration), 418,
 424
Baclofen
 side effects of
  mania, **345**
  sexual dysfunction, **461**
  sleep disorders, **502**
 for tardive dyskinesia, 966
"Bad trip," 443
BAI (Beck Anxiety Inventory), 93, 406,
 407
Balint groups, 217
Barbiturates, **904, 943**
 abuse potential of, 902
 dosage of, **434**
 drug interactions with
  antipsychotics, **944**
  antiretroviral drugs, 814
  cytochrome P450 metabolism
   and, **945**
 duration of detectability in urine,
  895
 half-lives of, **904**
 indications for
  anxiety, 408
  insomnia, 505
 overdose of, 129, 902
 side effects of, 408
  sexual dysfunction, **461**
  sleep disorders, **502**
 withdrawal from, 902–904
Basic science research, 191–193
 behavioral science, 193
 neuroimaging, 193
 neuroscience, 192–193

Battery-based approaches to
 neuropsychological assessment,
 82–83
BDD. *See* Body dysmorphic disorder
BDI (Beck Depression Inventory),
 92–93, **93, 371,** 527, 556, 607,
 626, 661
Beck Anxiety Inventory (BAI), 93, 406,
 407
Beck Depression Inventory (BDI),
 92–93, **93, 371,** 527, 556, 607,
 626, 661
Behavior
 aggression and agitation, 149–163
 assessment of, 62
 of critically ill patients, 763–765, **764**
 drug-seeking, 996, **996**
 lipids and, 1058
 management in patient with
  delirium, **266**
 patient's response to illness, 108–111
 problems in rehabilitation settings,
  736, **736**
 type A, 113–114, 117, **118,** 539–540,
  1054, 1058
 view of future as organizer of, 107
Behavioral disinhibition
 anxiolytic-induced
  benzodiazepines, 759, 971
 in children, 724
 in frontotemporal dementia, 277
 HIV-associated, 818
 in Wilson's disease, 279
Behavioral management
 of agitation and aggression, 157–158
 of anticipatory nausea and vomiting in
  chemotherapy patients,
  659–660
 of anxiety, 409–410, 923
 of globus sensation, 553
 of HIV-associated symptoms, 824,
  834
 of insomnia, 504–505
 of mania, 355
 of medically ill children, 725–726
 of pain syndromes, 1008–1009
 of peptic ulcer disease, 1062
 in rehabilitation settings, 744
 of somatoform disorders, 385, 922
 of surgical patients, 601
 of type A behavior, 1056
Behavioral medicine, 1053–1070
 autoimmune disorders and,
  1066–1067
 background of, 1053
 cancer and, 1064–1065

cardiovascular disease and,
 1054–1062, **1055**
chronic pain and, 1067–1070
gastrointestinal disease and,
 1062–1063
goals of, 1053
hyperimmune disorders and,
 1065–1066
immune-related illness and,
 1063–1064, **1064**
infectious disease and, 1065
other conditions and, 1070
relation of consultation-liaison
 psychiatry to, 204–206
research in, 1053–1054
Behavioral science research, **192,** 193
Bender Gestalt Test, 72
Bendroflumethiazide, **461**
Beneficence, 167
Benzodiazepine antagonists, 400
Benzodiazepine inverse agonists, 400
Benzodiazepine receptors, 400–402,
 401
Benzodiazepines, **903,** 969–972, **970**
 abuse/dependence on, 158, 433–435,
  971
  acute management of, **434,**
   434–435, **435**
  categories of abusers, 433
  complications of, 433–434
  drug seeking and, 907
  emergency department
   management of, 902–903
  opioid dependence and, 902
  prevention of, 434
  recognition of, 433, 545
  relapses of, 433
  risk factors for, 433, 902
 γ-aminobutyric acid–benzodiazepine
  complex, 400–401, **401**
 antidepressants combined with, 969
 antipsychotics combined with, 408
 classification of, 969–970
 development of tolerance to, 353
 dosage and administration of, **407,**
  434, 763, 903, 970, 971
 drug interactions with, **349,** 971
  antidepressants, 953
  antiretroviral drugs, 814, **815,** 834
  cytochrome P450 metabolism
   and, 505, **945**
  methadone, 440
  monoamine oxidase inhibitors,
   955
  valproate, 351
 duration of detectability in urine, **895**

electroconvulsive therapy and, 1016–1017
flumazenil reversal of, 400, 435, 971
half-lives of, 407, **407**, 433, **903**, 970
indications for, 970
  aggression and agitation, 158, 159, **160, 161,** 171, 407, **763,** 899
  akathisia, 965
  alcohol withdrawal, 268, 430–432, **431, 433,** 970
  Alzheimer's disease, 296
  anxiety, 407–408, 433, 970
  chemical restraint of suicidal patient, 141
  cocaine intoxication, 441
  insomnia, 505, **506**
  mania, **347,** 353, 962
  narcolepsy, 510
  pain syndromes, **989,** 1006
  periodic leg movements of sleep, 510
  restless legs syndrome, 510
  snoring, 504
  tardive dyskinesia, 966
intramuscular, 407
mechanism of action of, 970
onset of action of, 962
overdose of, 129, 971
pharmacokinetics of, 970
  active metabolites, 407, **407**
prophylactic, 940–941
response to, 971
side effects of, 158, 353, 407–408, 545, 971
  depression, **311,** 323
  hip fracture risk among long-term users, 399
  memory impairment, 158, 288
  sleep disorders, **502**
use in specific patient groups or medical conditions
  cardiac disease, 510, 544–545
  chemotherapy patients, 659, 660
  chronic obstructive pulmonary disease, 503, 505, 511, 548
  critically ill patients, 759, 761–763, **763**
  delirium, **266,** 268
  dialysis patients, 561
  dying patients, 782, **782, 785,** 787
  elderly persons, **863,** 864, 970
  hepatic disease, 977
  HIV/AIDS, 825, 834
  irritable bowel syndrome, 555
  liver disease, 407, 504, 641

patients undergoing rehabilitation, **743**
  sleep apnea, 971
  stroke, 741
  surgical patients, **598**
  transplant patients, **635,** 638, 641
  withdrawal from, 158, 353, 408, 433–435, **435,** 505, 545, 902, 971
    anxiety due to, **781**
    emergency department management of, 903–904
Benzoylecgonine, 440
Benztropine mesylate
  for agitation, 604
  for neuroleptic-induced extrapyramidal symptoms, 897, 965
  for patients undergoing rehabilitation, **742**
  sexual dysfunction induced by, **461**
Bereavement. *See also* Grief
  feigned, 523
  HIV/AIDS and, 828
Betaxolol, 611
Bezoars, 481
Biases in research, 198–200, **199**
BIAT (brief, intermittent, attenuated therapy), 1046–1047
Bibliotherapy, for pain syndromes, 1008
Billing for consultation-liaison services, 28–29
Billings, Edward G., 5
Binswanger's disease, 53, 281
Biofeedback
  for anxiety, 410
  for asthma, 1066
  for esophageal motility disorders, 554
  for globus sensation, 553
  for headache, 1069
  for hypertension, 1060
  for patients with HIV/AIDS, 834
  for pelvic floor dyssynergia, 1063
  in rehabilitation settings, 744
  for somatoform disorders, 385
Biogenic amine hypothesis
  of depression, 947
  of mania, 344
Biological markers
  for alcoholism, 427–428
  for depression, 313
Bipolar disorder. *See also* Mania
  age at onset of, **63,** 341, 344
  agitation and, 161
  alcoholism and, 423
  cancer and, 663

  definition of, 339
  genetic factors in, 341–342
  irritable bowel syndrome and, **555**
  lifetime number of affective episodes in, 341, 342
  mood stabilizers for, 347–354, 957–962, **958**
    anticonvulsants, **347,** 350–353, 693–694, 960–962
    lithium, **347–349,** 347–350, 858–960
    other medications, 354, 962
  postoperative management of, 601
  postpartum recurrence of, 341
  prevalence of, 339–340, **680**
  psychosocial factors and, 342
  rapid cycling, 339
  seasonal, 339
  suicide and, 133
  thyroid disease and, 245, 320
  treatment compliance in, 957
Bismuth poisoning, **284**
Bladder cancer, 457
Bleomycin, 793
Blessed Dementia Scale, 72
Blindness. *See* Vision loss
Bloating, postprandial, 552
α-Blockers
  interaction with antidepressants, **943**
  use in stroke patients, 741
β-Blockers. *See also* specific drugs
  alcohol or sedative withdrawal masked by concomitant use of, 901
  contraindications to, 973
  drug interactions with, 611–612
    antipsychotics, 969
    cytochrome P450 metabolism and, **945**
    monoamine oxidase inhibitors, 955
    selective serotonin reuptake inhibitors, 543
  indications for
    agitation and aggression, 150, **161,** 162, **162,** 171
    anxiety, 409, 973
    before electroconvulsive therapy, 329, 1021
    glaucoma, 611
    lithium-induced tremor, 350, 959
    neuroleptic malignant syndrome, 968
  ophthalmic, 611–612
  side effects of, 611
    delirium, **762**

β-Blockers (continued)
    side effects of (continued)
        dementia, **284**
        depression, 162, **311**, 322, 611
    use in specific patient groups or
        medical conditions
        cardiothoracic surgery patients,
            604
        neurological disease, 694
        patients undergoing rehabilitation,
            743
Blood alcohol concentration (BAC),
    418, 424
Blunting, as coping strategy, 111
Body dysmorphic disorder (BDD), 373,
    380–381
    age at onset of, 381
    clinical course and prognosis for, 381
    clinical features of, 381
    among cosmetic surgery patients, 613
    definition of, 380
    delusional, 381
    diagnostic criteria for, **380**
    differential diagnosis of, 381
    epidemiology of, 381
    management of, 383–387
    as obsessive-compulsive disorder
        spectrum disorder, 380
    psychiatric comorbidity with, 381
    somatization and, **362**
Body image changes, 734–735
Boerhaave's syndrome, 487
Bone marrow transplantation, 978
Bone tumors, 671
Borderline personality disorder, **116**
    comorbidity with other personality
        disorders, 119
    among cosmetic surgery patients, 614
    countertransference and, 122
    dialectical behavior therapy for, 911
    factitious disorders and, 523
    prevalence of, **120**
    psychiatric emergencies in patients
        with, 907–908
    substance-related disorders and, 423,
        902
Borrelia burgdorferi infection, 575
Boston Diagnostic Aphasia Examination,
    82
Boston Naming Test–Third Edition, 82
Boston Process Approach to
    neuropsychological assessment,
    80–82
Botulin toxin, for tardive dyskinesia,
    966
Boxers' dementia, 281

BPRS (Brief Psychiatric Rating Scale),
    929
Bradycardia
    in anorexia nervosa, 484, 485
    drug-induced
        phenelzine, 544
        selective serotonin reuptake
            inhibitors, 542, 952
    sleep apnea and, 510
Bradykinesia, 685
Brain
    aging effects on, 259
    anatomic substrate of anxiety,
        401–402
    imaging of (*See* Neuroimaging)
    receptor site activity of psychotropic
        drugs in, 943–944
        antidepressants, 947, **948, 949**
    respiratory center of, 547
"Brain death," 167
Brain injury, 281–282, 685
    aggression, agitation and, 149, 156,
        159
    alcohol intoxication and, 685
    anxiety and, 736
    cognitive rehabilitation and retraining
        after, 744–745, 1070
    delirium and, 259
    dementia and, **274**, 276, 281–282,
        287
    electroconvulsive therapy for patients
        with, 1020
    Luria's model of brain functioning
        and, 78–80, **79**
    malingering and, 97
    mood disorders and, 685
        depression, **733**
        mania, 342–344, **343, 345**, 346,
            685
    neuropsychiatric sequelae of, 685
    neuropsychological testing in, 86
    pathophysiology of, 287
    personality changes after, 685
    postconcussion syndrome, 281, **680,**
        685
    prevalence of, **680**, 685
    psychiatric comorbidity with, 244
    psychotropic drug use in patients
        with, 741, 979
        antidepressants, 693, **693**
        antipsychotics, 692, 979
        β-blockers, 692
        lithium, 161
        psychostimulants, 979
    seizures after, 281, 685
    sleep disorders and, 504, 512

spinal cord injury and, 734
suicide and, 129
Brain mapping
    cortical mapping of brain
        dysfunction, **74**
    topographical, 77
        applications of, 56–57
        basic science of, 52
Brain tumors, 681–683
    anxiety and, 398
    dementia and, **274**, 283, **284**
    electroconvulsive therapy for patients
        with, 1020
    frequency of, **681**
    mania and, **345, 346**, 663
    metastatic, 664, **664, 681**
    neuropsychiatric symptoms of,
        681–682
    paraneoplastic syndromes and, 682
    prevalence of, **680**
    psychotropic drug use in patients
        with
        antidepressants, **693**
        lithium, 347
    sites of, 681
Brazil, consultation-liaison psychiatry in,
    220–221
    background of, 220
    future development, 220–221
    in general hospital, 220
    research, 220
Breast cancer, **594**, 670
    behavioral medicine and, 1064
    brain metastases from, 664, **664, 681**
    central nervous system paraneoplastic
        syndromes and, 682
    depression and, 314
    psychotherapy for patients with,
        663–664, 1064
    sexual dysfunction and, 457
    suicidality and, 129
Breast-feeding
    benefits of, 980
    HIV transmission via, 809
    psychotropic drug use during, 710,
        980, 980–981, **981**
Breathing. *See* Lung disease; Respiration
Breathing-related sleep disorder, **496,**
    501. *See also* Sleep apnea
Brief Psychiatric Rating Scale (BPRS),
    929
Brief psychotherapy, 1032–1033, **1034.**
    See also Psychotherapy
    brief, intermittent, attenuated
        therapy (BIAT), 1046–1047
    patient selection criteria for, **1032**

Brief Symptom Inventory, 93, 661
Briquet's syndrome, 374, 1000. *See also*
  Somatization disorder
Bromide, **345**
Bromocriptine
  for cocaine craving, 901
  for neuroleptic malignant syndrome,
    968
  for Parkinson's disease, 686
  for patients undergoing
    rehabilitation, **743**
  for patients with neurological disease,
    692
  sexual dysfunction induced by, **461**
  sleep disorders induced by, 513
[^{76}Br]Bromolisuride, 55
Bronchitis, 546
Bronchodilators
  drug interactions with
    lithium, **349,** 960
    monoamine oxidase inhibitors,
      955
  side effects of, **550,** 1066
    anxiety, **400,** 781, **781**
    insomnia, **502**
    mania, 346
Brudzinski sign, 73
Bulimia nervosa, 480–481
  age at onset of, 477
  binge eating in, 477, 480, 481
  clinical features of, 481
  course of, 480
  definition of, 477
  diagnostic criteria for, **478**
  epidemiology of, 480
  medical complications of, 487
    dental problems, 487
    hematological abnormalities, 486
    in hospitalized patients, **482,**
      482–483
    related to laxative or diuretic
      abuse, 481, **481**
  predisposing factors for, 480
  psychiatric comorbidity with, 480
  relapse rates for, 489
  treatment of, 488–489
    selective serotonin reuptake
      inhibitors, 171, 489, 950
Bulletin of the Royal College, 213
Buprenorphine, 438
Bupropion, 326, **948**
  contraindications to, 326
  dosage of, **948**
  drug interactions with
    levodopa, 693
    ritonavir, 814, **815,** 829

indications for
  attention-deficit/hyperactivity
    disorder, 326
  bulimia nervosa, 489
  smoking cessation, 446, 549, 950,
    1061
mechanism of action of, 326, **948**
overdose of, 952
side effects of, 326, 952
  anxiety, **400**
  seizures, 326, 408, 951
  sexual dysfunction, **461**
structure of, 947
use in specific patient groups or
    medical conditions
  cardiac disease, 543, 951, 974
  dialysis patients, 561
  dying patients, **785,** 785–786
  elderly persons, **863,** 864
  HIV/AIDS, 829
  neurogenic bladder with
    retention, 693, **693**
  Parkinson's disease, 693, **693**
  surgical patients, **597**
  transplant candidates, **636**
Burn patients, 612–613
  in acute phase, 612
  delirium among, 259, 612
  denial among, 612
  depression among, 612
  long-term adjustment of, 613
  pain control for, 612, 990
  posttraumatic stress disorder among,
    613
  predisposing factors for injury among,
    612
  in reconstructive phase, 612–613
  with self-inflicted burns, 612
  sleep disorders among, 613
  substance-related disorders among,
    417, 612
    alcoholism, **239**
Buserelin, **461**
Buspirone, 972
  discontinuation of, 972
  dosage of, 972
  drug interactions with, 972
    monoamine oxidase inhibitors,
      955, 972
  indications for
    agitation and aggression, 160, **161**
    Alzheimer's disease, 296
    anxiety, 409, 434, 972
    delirium, 268
    smoking cessation, 1061
  mechanism of action of, 401, 972

pharmacokinetics of, 972
response to, 409, 972
side effects of, 409
  mania, **345**
  sexual dysfunction, **461**
use in specific patient groups or
    medical conditions
  brain injury, 979
  cardiac disease, 545
  dying patients, 783
  elderly persons, **863**
  HIV/AIDS, 834
  irritable bowel syndrome, 555
  patients undergoing rehabilitation,
    743
  pulmonary disease, 977
  transplant candidates, **635,** 638
Busulfan, **461**
Butabarbital, **895**
Butalbital, **434, 895, 904, 904**
Butaperazine, **461**
Butorphanol, **993**
Butyrophenones, **964.** *See also*
  Antipsychotics
  for pain syndromes, 1007
  sleep disorders induced by, **502**
  use in specific patient groups or
    medical conditions
  surgical patients, **597**
  transplant candidates, **636**

CA (Cocaine Anonymous), 421
CABG. *See* Coronary artery bypass graft
  patients
CAD. *See* Coronary artery disease
Cadmium poisoning, **284**
Caffeine
  abuse of, in anorexia nervosa, 479,
    484
  drug interactions with
    cytochrome P450 metabolism
      and, **945**
    monoamine oxidase inhibitors,
      955
    psychostimulants, 957
  intoxication with, 484
  side effects of
    anxiety, **400**
    insomnia, **502,** 505
CAGE Questionnaire, 428, **430,** 859
Calcium acetylhomotaurinate, 432
Calcium-channel blockers
  drug interactions with
    carbamazepine, 351, 962
    cytochrome P450 metabolism
      and, **946**

Calcium-channel blockers *(continued)*
    drug interactions with *(continued)*
        lithium, **349**, 694
        ophthalmic β-blockers, 612
        selective serotonin reuptake
            inhibitors, 543
    indications for
        esophageal motility disorders, 554
        mania, 354
        neuroleptic malignant syndrome,
            968
        tardive dyskinesia, 966
    side effects of
        anxiety, **400**
        depression, 322
California Verbal Learning Test—Second
    Edition, 82
CAM (Confusion Assessment Method),
    263
Cambridge Examination for Mental
    Disorders of the Elderly, 96
Cambridge Neuropsychological Test
    Automated Battery, 98
Cancer, 8, 63, 657–673. *See also* specific
    types
    adjustment disorder and, 245, 397,
        661, 780
    anxiety and, 245, 398, 659–661, 780,
        781
        acute and posttraumatic stress
            disorder, 660–661
        alcoholism and, 660
        anticipatory nausea and vomiting,
            659–660
        claustrophobia, 660
        complex partial seizures and, 660
        differentiation from akathisia,
            660
        pulmonary embolus or edema and,
            660
    behavioral medicine and, 1064–1065
    of bone, 671
    brain tumors, **681**, 681–683
    of breast, 670
    in children and adolescents, 672
    of colon and rectum, 670
    complications of treatment for,
        665–669
        anorexia, 666
        antiemetic drugs, **669**
        chemotherapy, 666, **667–668**
        dementia, 666
        radiation therapy, 665–666
        sexual dysfunction and infertility,
            666–669
    delirium and, **259**, 663, 665, 780

dementia and, **274**, 283, **284**, 666,
    780
depression and, 241, **310**, **311**, 314,
    661–663
    assessment of, 783–784, **784**
    correlates of vulnerability to, 661,
        662
    diagnosis of, 661
    electroconvulsive therapy for,
        1021–1022
    etiological links between, 661
    pharmacological treatment of,
        662–663
    prevalence of, 661, **733**, 779–780,
        783
    suicidality, 129, 131, **132**,
        661–662, **662**, **733**, 788–789
families of patients with, 671–672
gynecological, 713
of head and neck, 670
    surgery for, 614–617
HIV-associated, 815, **816**
insomnia and, 504
of lung, 669–670
lymphoma and leukemia, 671
mania and, 663
memory impairment and, 780
mortality from, 772
neurological complications of,
    664–665
    brain metastases, 664, **664**
    complex partial seizures, 665
    leptomeningeal disease, 665
    limbic encephalopathy, 280
    other causes of delirium, 665
    paraneoplastic syndromes, 280,
        665, 682–683
    progressive multifocal
        leukoencephalopathy, 282
pain control for, 435, 796, **797**, 997,
    1065
of pancreas, 670
pediatric, 724
of prostate, 670–671
psychiatric illness in patients with,
    245, 659, 779–780
psychological responses during phases
    of, 657–659, **658**
psychooncology, 657
psychotherapy for patients with, 329,
    663–664, 1032
quality-of-life scales for patients
    with, 94
recurrence of, **658**, 659
sexual dysfunction and, 457,
    666–669, 713

spirituality and, 658, 776–777
staff issues related to, 672–673, **673**
of testes, 670
Cancer chemotherapy
    complications of, 658–659
    drug interactions with
        antidepressants, 663
        cytochrome P450 metabolism
            and, **946**
    nausea and vomiting induced by
        anticipatory, 659–660, 1065
        antiemetics for, 659, 660, **669**
        relaxation training for, 1065
        Δ⁹-tetrahydrocannabinol for, 444
    neuropsychiatric side effects of, 666,
        667–668
        delirium, 793
        dementia, **284**
        depression, **311**, 323
    psychological reactions to, **658**
    sexual dysfunction and infertility
        induced by, 666–669
Cannabinoid receptors, 444
Cannabis
    abuse of, 444
        acute management of, 444, 906
        consultation requests for, 444
        genetic factors and, 444
        intoxication, 444
        laboratory testing for, 444, **895**
        long-term management of, 444
        physical signs of, 444
    for chemotherapy-induced nausea
        and vomiting, 444
    sexual dysfunction and, **461**
    withdrawal from, 444
Canterbury v. Spence, 170
Capgras' syndrome, 295
Captopril, **345**, **461**, **944**
Carbamazepine, **943**, **958**, 960–962
    dosage and administration of, **347**,
        958, 961
    drug interactions with, **349**, 352,
        596, 962
        antidepressants, **943**
        antiretroviral drugs, 814, **815**,
            839
        cytochrome P450 metabolism
            and, **945**, 960
        lithium, 694, 960
        methadone, 438
        nefazodone, 694
        selective serotonin reuptake
            inhibitors, 694
    half-life and serum level of, **347**
    indications for, 961

agitation and aggression, 160–161, **161,** 694

benzodiazepine withdrawal, 435

delirium, 268

mania, **347,** 351–352, 693–694, 961

pain syndromes, 315, **989,** 1006

mechanism of action of, 351, 960

overdose of, 962

pharmacokinetics of, 960

side effects of, 351–352, 961, **975–976**

mania, **345**

sexual dysfunction, **461**

use in specific patient groups or medical conditions

Alzheimer's disease, 296

breast-feeding women, 980–981, **981**

cardiac disease, 544

chronic pain, 315

elderly persons, **863**

hepatic disease, 351

HIV/AIDS, 826, 839

neurological disease, 693–694

patients undergoing rehabilitation, **742**

pregnancy, 352, 707, 961, 980

surgical patients, **598**

transplant candidates, **635**

Carbidopa-levodopa, **461.** *See also* Levodopa

β-Carboline derivatives, 400

Carbon dioxide

partial pressure of (pCO_2), 546

in anxiety disorders, 547–548

in depression, 547

regulation of blood and lung levels of, 547

Carbon disulfide, **284**

Carbon monoxide poisoning, 263, 265, **284**

Carbon tetrachloride, **284**

Carcinoid tumor, **345**

Cardiac Arrhythmia Suppression Trial, 951

Cardiac assist devices, 604, 605

Cardiac disease, 8, 536–545

acquired and congenital, 602, **603,** 626–627

anxiety disorders and, 396, 402, 536, 627

panic disorder, 403, 536, 541

treatment of, 544–545

behavioral medicine and, 536, 1054–1062, **1055**

denial among patients with, 540, 1056

depression and, 39, 113, 241, 249–250, 307–308, 536, 540–541, 627, 1054–1055

effect on health outcomes, 1055

electroconvulsive therapy for, 544, 1021

pharmacotherapy for, 542–544

underdiagnosis of, 542

fight-or-flight response and, 536–537

mortality from, 772

nervous system and, 537–541

direct effect of stress on myocardium, 538

stress and hypertension, 537–538

stress and pathogenesis of coronary artery disease, 538–541

stress-induced ischemia, 538

ventricular arrhythmias and sudden cardiac death, 537

obesity and, 1059–1060

prevalence of psychiatric comorbidity with, 240

psychological treatment of patients with, 541–542

psychotropic drug use in patients with, 974, **975,** 977

anticonvulsants, 977

antipsychotics, 974, 977

anxiolytics, 977

bupropion, 543, 952, 974

lithium, 350

selective serotonin reuptake inhibitors, 408, 537, 974

tricyclic antidepressants, 325–326, 951, 974

risk factors for ischemic heart disease, 1055–1056, **1056**

sexual dysfunction and, **456,** 456–457, **457,** 1062

sleep disorders and, 502–503, 510–511

somatic treatment for patients with, 542–545

anxiety, 544–545

delirium, 544

depression, 542–544

suicide and, 129

type A behavior and, 113–114, 539–540, 1054

behavioral and psychological interventions for, 1056

effect of treatment on risk of recurrent myocardial infarction, 1057

pharmacotherapy for, 1058

Cardiac effects, 327, 543–544

of amphetamines, 442

of anorexia nervosa, 482, 484–485

of antipsychotics, 158, 409, 544, 723, 757, **964,** 965

of bupropion, 543

of cannabis, 444

of carbamazepine, 351, 352, 544

of cocaine, 243, 441

combined with alcohol, 440

of droperidol, 544

of electroconvulsive therapy, 329, 544, 1019

of haloperidol, 267, 544, 897, 965

of hormone replacement therapy, 703

of lithium, 350, 544, 959

of MDMA, 443

of monoamine oxidase inhibitors, 327, 543–544

of nefazodone combined with terfenadine or astemizole, 327

of phencyclidine, 443

of pimozide, 488

of propofol, 762

of psychostimulants, 327, 544, 956, 957

of risperidone, 354

of selective serotonin reuptake inhibitors, 542, 952

of trazodone, 543

of tricyclic antidepressants, 325, 408, 542, 543, 757, 760–761, **943,** 950–951

in children, 723

of valproic acid, 544

Cardiac neurosis, 1062

Cardiac pacemakers, 510, 1021

Cardiac rehabilitation, 542, 607, 1058–1059

Cardiac transplantation. *See also* Transplantation

for acquired or congenital defects, 626–627

for alcohol-related cardiomyopathy, 629

electroconvulsive therapy and, 1022

movement disorders after, 643

psychiatric disorders in candidates for, 626–627

adjustment disorders, 627

anxiety and panic disorder, 403, 627

depression, 627

psychopharmacological considerations and, **635–637**

Cardiac transplantation *(continued)*
  return to employment after, 646
  sexual dysfunction after, 457, **457**
  waiting period for, 633–638
Cardiopulmonary resuscitation (CPR), 175
Cardiothoracic surgery, 602–608
  for acquired and congenital conditions, 602, **603**
  insomnia and, 503
  patients' fear of, 541, 604
  perioperative issues related to, 604–606
    cardiac assist devices, 605
    confusion and agitation, 604–605
    family support, 606
    pain control, 605, **605**
    substance withdrawal, 605
    ventilator weaning, 606
  postoperative issues related to, 606–608
    automatic implantable cardioverter-defibrillator, 608, 627
    delirium, 38, 257, 259, 765–766, **767**
    depression and return to function, 607
    neuropsychological changes, 606–607
    valve replacement, 607–608
  preoperative issues related to, 602–604
    agitation, 603–604
    anxiety, 603, 737
    cardiac assist devices, 604
    competency and compliance, 602–603
  psychiatric clearance of patients undergoing, 42
  psychiatric interviews before, 38
  sexual dysfunction and, 456
Caregivers. *See also* Family therapy and support
  for disabled patients, 739, 745
  for elderly persons, 865
  for patients with HIV/AIDS, 833
CARF (Certified Acute Rehabilitation Facility), 734
Carisoprodol, **434**
Carmustine, 793
Carvedilol, **461**
Case-control studies, **192, 195,** 195–196
Case detection, 39
Case managers, 30

Case studies, **192,** 193–194, **194**
Cataplexy, 509, 513
Catapres. *See* Clonidine
Cataracts, drug-induced
  chlorpromazine, 611
  quetiapine, 611, 966
Catatonia, 328, 905, 1022
CBF. *See* Cerebral blood flow studies
CCSE (Cognitive Capacity Screening Examination), 66, 83
CCU. *See* Coronary care unit
CD4$^+$ lymphocyte count, 807, 810, **810,** 815, 1065
CDP-choline, **743**
CDR (Clinical Dementia Rating) scale, 294
Celexa. *See* Citalopram
Cellulitis, cocaine-related, 243
Center for Substance Abuse Treatment, 428
Central nervous system (CNS)
  infection, 265
  cerebrospinal fluid findings in, 689–690
  electroconvulsive therapy for patients with, 1021
  encephalitis, 688
  human immunodeficiency virus, 687
  meningitis, 688
  neurosyphilis, 282, **345,** 398, 576, 687–688
Central pontine myelinolysis, 426, 643
Centrax. *See* Prazepam
Cephaeline toxicity, 484
Cerebellar abnormalities
  in degenerative diseases, 687
  in Wilson's disease, 279
Cerebral blood flow (CBF), 50, 51, 55, 546
  anxiety-induced hyperventilation and, 547
  in delirium tremens, 258
Cerebral embolism, 679
Cerebral metabolic rate of glucose (CMRG), 55–56, 402
Cerebrospinal fluid (CSF)
  antiretroviral drug penetration of, 823
  examination of, 689–690
    in delirium, 264
    in elderly persons, 861
    in HIV-associated neurocognitive impairment, 821
Cerebrovascular accident (CVA). *See* Stroke

Certified Acute Rehabilitation Facility (CARF), 734
Certified Outpatient Rehabilitation Facility (CORF), 734
Ceruloplasmin defect, 279. *See also* Wilson's disease
Cervical cancer, 457
Cesarean delivery, 701, 707
Cetirizine, **461**
CFS. *See* Chronic fatigue syndrome
Chamomile, **974**
"Cheese effect," 955
Chest pain
  anxiety and, 403, 406, 907
  esophageal dysmotility and, 554
  noncardiac, **365,** 1062
    panic disorder and, 1062
Cheyne-Stokes respiration, 502, 511
CHF. *See* Congestive heart failure
Child Behavior Checklist, **720**
Child psychiatry, 717–718
Child Somatization Inventory, **720**
Childbirth, 702, 707–709
Children and adolescents, 717–726. *See also* Pediatrics
  abuse of, 908–909
    dissociation and, 1003
    Munchausen syndrome by proxy, 521, 523–526
    somatization and, 369
  adolescent pregnancy, 709
  assessment of, **720,** 720–721, **721**
  cancer in, 672, 724
  causes of death among, 772
  delirium in, 257–259
  eating disorders in, 477
  electroconvulsive therapy for, 1023
  factitious disorders among, 521
  HIV/AIDS in, 712–713, 808–809
  hospital units for, 719
    child life services of, 719
  inhalant abuse among, 446
  orthopedic surgery in, 608
  postpartum custody issues, 711
  psychotropic drug use in, 722–724, **723, 724**
  renal transplantation in, 557–558
  reporting abuse of, **168,** 169
  suicidality among, 128, 724–725
  survival of premature infants, 724
  vision loss in, 610
Children's Depression Inventory, **720**
Chloral hydrate, **904, 943,** 973
  for agitation and aggression, 159
  dosage of, **434**
  drug interactions with, 973

alcohol, 427
 for insomnia, 505
 overdose of, 973
 use during breast-feeding, **981**
Chlorambucil, **461**
Chloramphenicol, **943**
Chlordiazepoxide, **903, 970**
 for alcohol withdrawal, 430–431,
  431, 901
 dosage of, **407, 434, 903, 970**
 half-life of, **407, 903**
 pharmacokinetics of, 970
 sexual dysfunction induced by, **461**
Chlorothiazide, **461**
Chlorpromazine, **763, 964**
 for delirium, 267–268
  in burn patients, 612
  in terminally ill patients, **794**
 dosage of, 159, **763, 964**
 drug interactions with
  alcohol, 427, **428**
  propranolol, 611–612
  vasodilators, 969
 for monoamine oxidase inhibitor–
  induced hypertensive crisis, 955
 for schizophrenia, 159
 side effects of, **964**
  cataracts, 611
  seizures, 966
  sexual dysfunction, **461**
 use in specific patient groups or
  medical conditions
  breast-feeding women, **981**
  dying patients, 782, **782, 794**
  HIV/AIDS, 825
  pregnancy, **708**
Chlorpropamide, 427
Chlorprothixene, **461**
Chlorthalidone, **461**
Cholecystokinin, 401
Cholesterol, 1058
Cholesterol-lowering drugs, 1057, 1058
Cholinesterase inhibitors
 for Alzheimer's disease, 297
 electroconvulsive therapy and, 1017
 for HIV-associated neurocognitive
  impairment, 824
Chorea
 in Huntington's disease, 278
 in Lyme disease, 575
 Sydenham's, 398
 in systemic lupus erythematosus, 568
Chromosome abnormalities
 in Alzheimer's disease, 277
 in frontotemporal dementias, 286
 in Huntington's disease, 277, 286

in Wilson's disease, 277, 286
Chronic fatigue syndrome (CFS),
  571–576
 adrenal insufficiency and, 572
 depression and, **310,** 321, 570
 diagnostic criteria for, 571
 Epstein-Barr virus and, 321, 571, 574
 evaluation and classification of, **573**
 postinfectious syndromes associated
  with, 574–576
  acute hepatitis, 575
  acute mononucleosis, 574
  cytomegalovirus infection, 574
  human herpesvirus-6 infection,
   575
  Lyme disease, 575
  neurosyphilis, 576
  postviral syndrome, 574
  toxoplasmosis, 575
 prognostic factors in, 574
 psychiatric comorbidity with, 571–
  572
 treatment of, 572–574
Chronic obstructive pulmonary disease
  (COPD), 548–549
 cognitive impairment in, 548
 marijuana use and, 444
 oxygen therapy for, 548
 psychiatric comorbidity with,
  244–245
  anxiety, 397, 399, 402
  depression, 548
  panic disorder, 245, 399, 548
 psychotropic drug use in, 548–549
  benzodiazepines, 503, 505, 511,
   548
  clonazepam, 353
  sertraline, 408
  zolpidem, 972
 respiratory dyskinesia and, 551
 sleep disorders and, 503, 511
 smoking and, 445
Chronic pain syndrome, **1000,** 1004,
  1005. *See also* Pain, chronic
Cimetidine, **943**
 drug interactions with
  alcohol, 427
  benzodiazepines, **349,** 505
  carbamazepine, 962
  cytochrome P450 metabolism
   and, **945, 946**
  immunosuppressants, 643
 side effects of
  delirium, **762**
  depression, **311,** 323
  mania, **345**

sexual dysfunction, **461**
 sleep disorders, **502**
Ciprofloxacin, **945**
Circadian rhythm, 495
Circadian rhythm sleep disorders,
  496–498, **497**
Cirrhosis
 alcoholic, 239, 242, **243,** 426
  liver transplantation for, 427
 suicide and, 129
Cisapride, 326, **946**
Cisplatin, 793
Citalopram, 326, **948**
 cytochrome P450 metabolism and,
  326, **949,** 952
 dosage of, **948**
 half-life of, **949**
 receptor site affinity of, **948**
 sexual dysfunction induced by, **461**
 structure of, 947
 use in specific patient groups or
  medical conditions
  children, **723**
  dying patients, **785**
  elderly persons, 863, **863**
  HIV/AIDS, 829
 withdrawal from, 953
CIWA-Ar (Clinical Institute Withdrawal
  Assessment for Alcohol–Revised),
  424, **425–426,** 431
Claustrophobia
 magnetic resonance imaging and, 395,
  404, 660
 in rehabilitation settings, 737
Clidinium, **461**
Clinical Dementia Rating (CDR) scale,
  294
Clinical Institute Withdrawal
  Assessment for Alcohol–Revised
  (CIWA-Ar), 424, **425–426,** 431
Clinical intervention studies, 197
*Clinical Pharmacology and
  Therapeutics,* 45
Clitoral engorgement, trazodone-
  induced, 950, 952
Clock drawing task, 72, 261, **261,** 290,
  291, 929
Clofibrate, **461**
Clomipramine, 325, **948**
 dosage of, **948**
 indications for
  narcolepsy, 510
  obsessive-compulsive disorder,
   969
  pain syndromes, 1005
 injectable, 601

Clomipramine *(continued)*
  interaction with monoamine oxidase
      inhibitors, 954
  receptor site affinity of, **948**
  side effects of
      seizures, 951
      sexual dysfunction, **461**
  use in specific patient groups or
      medical conditions
      cardiac disease, 543
      dying patients, 785, **785**
      pregnancy, **708**
Clonazepam, **903**, 970, **970**
  dosage of, **347, 407, 434, 903**, 962,
      970
  drug interactions with, **349**
      lithium, 694
      ritonavir, 814, **815**
  half-life of, **347, 353, 407, 903**
  indications for
      agitation and aggression, 160
      alprazolam withdrawal, 434, **904**
      Alzheimer's disease, 296
      insomnia, 505, **506**
      mania, **347,** 353, 962
      pain syndromes, 1006
      periodic leg movements of sleep,
          510
  side effects of, 353
  use in specific patient groups or
      medical conditions
      chronic obstructive pulmonary
          disease, 353
      dialysis patients, 561
      dying patients, 782, **782**
      HIV/AIDS, 834
      neurological disease, 694
      pain syndromes, 1000
      patients undergoing rehabilitation,
          743
  withdrawal from, 353
Clonidine
  alcohol or sedative withdrawal
      masked by concomitant use of,
      901
  drug interactions with
      antidepressants, **943,** 953
      antipsychotics, **944**
      monoamine oxidase inhibitors,
          955
  indications for
      cocaine abuse, 901
      hallucinogen-related flashbacks,
          443
      opioid detoxification, 436, 439,
          439, 905, 996–997

  smoking cessation, 1061
  side effects of, 439
      depression, 322
      mania, **345**
      sexual dysfunction, **461**
      sleep disorders, **502**
  use in rehabilitation settings, **743**
Clopidogrel, 296
Clorazepate, **903, 970**
  dosage of, **407, 434, 903, 970**
  half-life of, **407, 903**
  interaction with ritonavir, **815**
Clorgyline, 787
CLOX, 294
Clozapine, 963, **964**
  contraindicated in patients with
      myeloproliferative disorders,
      966
  dosage of, 159, **964**
  drug interactions with
      cytochrome P450 metabolism
          and, **945**
      ritonavir, 814, **815**
  indications for
      agitation and aggression, 160
      mania, 354
      schizoaffective disorder, 354
      schizophrenia, 159
  mechanism of action of, 963
  side effects of, **964,** 966
      agranulocytosis, 966
      hypersalivation, 966
      sexual dysfunction, **461**
  use in specific patient groups or
      medical conditions
      dialysis patients, 561
      elderly persons, **863**
      HIV/AIDS, 839
      Parkinson's disease, 691–692, 979
      surgical patients, **598**
      transplant candidates, **636**
Clozaril. *See* Clozapine
Cluster headache, 504, 512
CMRG (cerebral metabolic rate of
      glucose), 55–56, 402
CMV (cytomegalovirus) infection, 574
Co-trimoxazole, **818**
Coagulation disorders
  in anorexia nervosa, 486
  valproate-induced, 350, 351
Cobalamin deficiency, **284,** 288, **345,**
      569
Cocaethylene, 440
Cocaine Anonymous (CA), 421
Cocaine-related disorders, 243,
      440–442

  anorexia nervosa and, 479
  binges, 441
  bulimia nervosa and, 481
  cocaine–monoamine oxidase
      inhibitor interaction, 955
  complications of, 243, 441
  crack cocaine, 440
  depression, **311,** 324
  DSM-IV classification of, 440
  epidemiology of, 440, 901
  "freebasing," 440
  intoxication, **156,** 440–441
  management of, 441–442
      Cocaine Anonymous, 421
      in emergency department, 440,
          901–902
      inpatient vs. outpatient, 442
      outcome of, 442
  mania, **345**
  mortality from, 441
  paranoia, **156**
  pharmacology of, 440
  physical signs of, 441
  in pregnancy, 243, 441
  relapses of, 442
  sexual dysfunction and, **461**
  sleep disorders and, **502**
  "speedballing," 435
  tolerance, 440, 441
  urine testing for, 440, **895,** 901
  withdrawal or abstinence, 441
      phases of, 441
      suicidality during, 441
Codecs, 928, 929
Codeine, **995**
  for children, **724**
  detoxification from, 437, 438
  dosage of, **437, 993**
  drug interactions with
      cytochrome P450 metabolism
          and, **945**
      selective serotonin reuptake
          inhibitors, 326, **999**
  duration of action of, **993**
  duration of detectability in urine,
      895
  indications for
      opioid detoxification, 438, **439**
      periodic leg movements of sleep
          and restless legs syndrome,
          510
Coding procedures, 28, 29, 41
COGNISTAT, 83
Cognitive-behavioral therapy
  for anorexia nervosa, 488
  for anxiety disorders, 410

for borderline personality disorder, 911
for bulimia nervosa, 489
for cancer patients, 664
for critically ill patients, 760
for depression, 329
for dying patients, 783
for nicotine dependence, 445
for noncardiac chest pain, 1062
for pain syndromes, 314, 1008–1009, 1067–1070
    fibromyalgia, 1070
    headache, 1068–1069
for patients with HIV/AIDS, 834
in rehabilitation settings, 744
for somatoform disorders, 385, **386**
for tinnitus, 1070
for type A behavior, 1056
Cognitive Capacity Screening Examination (CCSE), 66, 83
Cognitive impairment
in Alzheimer's disease, 277, **278**
assessment for
    computerized, 97–98
    in intensive care unit, 754
    mental status examination, **62,** 65–73
    neuropsychological and psychological testing, 77–100
after cardiothoracic surgery, 606–607
in chronic obstructive pulmonary disease, 548
delirium, 257–269
dementia, 273–298
among dying patients, **259,** 792–796
in elderly persons, 257–259, 856–857
electroconvulsive therapy–induced, 1018, **1019**
after head trauma, 685
HIV-associated, 259, 276, 282, 795–796, 817–824
in Huntington's disease, 278
in hyperparathyroidism, **564**
in hypothyroidism, 564, **564**
legal competence and, 172–174
length of stay and, 35–36
in meningitis, 688
mild, 277
in multiple sclerosis, 686
nondetection by nonpsychiatric medical providers, 61
nonverbal, 61
in Parkinson's disease, 279, 686
posttraumatic, 281–282
in rehabilitation settings, 733–734

renal failure and, 560
systemic lupus erythematosus and, 568
in Wilson's disease, 279
Cognitive rehabilitation and retraining, 744–745, 1070
CogScreen, 98
Coherence, sense of, 111
Cohort studies, **192, 195,** 196–197
Colitis, 504, 552, 556, 1063
Colombia, consultation-liaison psychiatry in, 221
Colorectal cancer, 457, **664,** 670, 682
Coma, drug-induced
    alcohol, 424
    benzodiazepines, 435
    opioids, 437
    phencyclidine, 443
    psychostimulants, 957
Commission on Accreditation of Rehabilitation Facilities, 1009
Commitment statutes, 178–179
Comorbid psychiatric and medical conditions, 9
    detection and diagnosis of, 39
    economic effects of, 251–252, 871, **872**
    effect of consultation-liaison services on outcome and costs of, 26–27
    effect on medical outcome and costs, 25–26
    among elderly persons, 241
    epidemiology of, 237–252 (*See also* Epidemiology)
    hospital length of stay for, 9, 25–26, 35–36, 876, **876**
    limitations of traditional approaches to, 875–876
    models of, 238–240, **239**
    prevalence of, 9, 25, 35–36, 61, 871, **872**
    suicidality and, 129–133, **130, 132,** 141
    underdetection by nonpsychiatric physicians, 13, 34–35
Compazine. *See* Prochlorperazine
Competency
    definition of, 168, 172
    determination of, 167, 172–174
        legal contexts for, **172,** 173
        standards for, 173
    to give informed consent, 170, 172
    for surgery, 596, **599,** 600, 602–603
    incompetent person
        consent options for, **174**

definition of, 172, 173, 177
denial of illness by, 172–173
differentiation from incapacitated person, 172
guardianship of, 176–177
substituted judgment for, 177–178
of medically ill patients, 174
of mentally ill persons, 172, 173
of minors, 173
of patients in rehabilitation settings, 739–740
recovery of, 177–178
right to die and, 174–175, 790
Complex regional pain syndrome (CRPS), 992
Complexity Prediction Instrument (COMPRI), 222–223, **224**
Compliance with treatment
    antiretroviral therapy, 813–814
    for bipolar disorder, 957
    after cardiac valve replacement surgery, 603
    doctor-patient relationship and, 111
    impact of personality disorders on, 121
    after organ transplantation, 558, 603, 632, 644–645
    of pediatric patients, 725
    pharmacotherapy, 941
    during pregnancy, 706–707
    in rehabilitation settings, 735
    serum drug levels and, 942–943
Composite International Diagnostic Interview, 251
COMPRI (Complexity Prediction Instrument), 222–223, **224**
Compulsions, 404. *See also* Obsessive-compulsive disorder
Computed tomography (CT)
    in Alzheimer's disease, **279**
    applications of, 52–53
    basic science of, 49, 50
    for brain injury, 281
    cost and utilization review of, 52
    in delirium, 264, **264**
    in dementia, 54, 292–294
    in depression, 313
    in elderly persons, 861
    before electroconvulsive therapy, 1016, **1017**
    in emergency department, 891, 894
    of head, 53, 690
        to identify brain metastases, 664
        neuropsychiatric indications for, **691**

Computed tomography (CT) *(continued)*
  of head *(continued)*
    subdural hematoma on, 891
    in HIV-associated neurocognitive
        impairment, 821
    in mania, 346
Computerized psychological testing,
    97–98
Concentration problems
  HIV-associated, 818
  in postconcussion syndrome, 685
Concerta. *See* Methylphenidate
Concrete thinking, 261
Conduct disorder, 686
Confidentiality, 15, 168–169
  breaching of, 168–169
    liability for, 169
  definition of, 168
  maintenance in hospital, 168–169
  related to management of factitious
      disorders, 525
  statutory exceptions to, **168**
  testimonial privilege and, 169
  in treatment of pediatric patients,
      722
Confounding bias in research, **199**
Confusion. *See also* Delirium
  acute confusional state, 258, 259
  after cardiothoracic surgery, 604–605
  among critically ill patients, 761–762,
      762
  differential diagnosis of, 263–264
  drug-induced
    benzodiazepines, 158, 353, 407,
        971
    in neuroleptic malignant
        syndrome, 968
    neuroleptics, 158
    nicotine, 445
    phencyclidine, 443
    psychostimulants, 442, 761, 956,
        957
    tricyclic antidepressants, 951
  mechanical ventilation and, 765
  in Wernicke's encephalopathy, 265,
      283
Confusion Assessment Method (CAM),
    263
Congestive heart failure (CHF), 542.
    See also Cardiac disease
  depression and, 241, 627
  electroconvulsive therapy–induced,
      329
  sleep disorders and, 502, 511
  use of tricyclic antidepressants in,
      543, 951, 974

Conjunctivitis, cannabis-induced, 444
Conscientiousness, **116**
Consent for treatment. *See* Informed
    consent
Consolidated Omnibus Budget
    Reconciliation Act, 891
Constipation
  drug-induced, 552
    clozapine, 966
    methadone, 438
    nefazodone, 327
    opioids, 993
    psychostimulants, 956
    reboxetine, 953
    tricyclic antidepressants, 325,
        761, 950, 951
  due to pelvic floor dyssynergia, 1063
Constructional tasks, 290
Consultation-liaison psychiatry
  approach to consultation, 14–17
  areas of, 8–9
  cost-effectiveness of service for,
      25–31
  definition of, 4
  economic support for, 7–9
  educational function of, 4
  effective psychiatric consultant,
      13–14, **14**
  functions of, 4
  future trends in, 9
  history of, 3–9
  international perspectives on,
      203–226
  journals devoted to, 7
  liaison psychiatry, 5, 6, 8, 20, 33–46
  models for, 5–6, **6**
  need for development of, 4
  neuroimaging and, 49–57
  organization of service for, 17–21
  organizations devoted to, 7
  pediatric, 717
  as psychiatric subspecialty, 7, 21
  psychosomatic medicine and, 3–5,
      204–206
  research in, 4, 8–9, 191–200
  telepsychiatry, 927–935
  tracking patterns of use of, 41
  training in, 4, 7–9
Consultee-oriented consultation, **6**
Consumption, 483. *See also* Anorexia
    nervosa
Continuous performance tests (CPTs),
    computerized, 98
Continuous positive airway pressure
    (CPAP), 508, 509, 511, 551
Control, lack of, 110–111

Conversion disorder, 373, 378–380, **520**
  age at onset of, 380
  clinical course and prognosis for, 380
  clinical features of, 379–380
  definition of, 378
  diagnosis of, 378–379, 1002
  diagnostic criteria for, **379**
  differential diagnosis of, 380, 688–689
    delirium, 689
    "focal" findings, 689
    malingering, 380, 527
    movement disorders, 689
    seizures, 689
    stupor, 689
    syncope, 689
  epidemiology of, 379
  factitious, 523
  management of, 383–387
    in neurology and neurosurgery
        settings, **690**
  multiple sclerosis and, 687
  pain and, **1001**, 1002
  prevalence in general hospital
      patients, 373
  psychiatric comorbidity with, 380
    dementia, 285
    somatization, **362,** 365
  secondary gain and, 379–380
Coordination, problems with. *See*
    Incoordination
COPD. *See* Chronic obstructive
    pulmonary disease
Coping strategies, 108–110, **109,** 406,
    1037–1038. *See also* Adjustment
    disorders
  in adaptation to HIV disease,
      831–832
  in adaptation to terminal illness and
      death, 779
  goals of successful coping, 1042,
      1042
  of patients with pain, 1009
  problems in rehabilitation settings,
      734
  during transplant waiting period, 633
Copper metabolism disorder, 286. *See
    also* Wilson's disease
Copper poisoning, **502**
CORF (Certified Outpatient
    Rehabilitation Facility), 734
Coronary artery bypass graft (CABG)
    patients
  anxiety among, 737
  delirium among, 257, 641
  depression and return to function
      of, 607

neuropsychological impairment among, 606
psychological treatment of, 541
sexual dysfunction among, 456
Coronary artery disease (CAD). *See also* Ischemic heart disease; Myocardial infarction
depression and, 241, 307–308, **310,** 314, 325, 540–542
fight-or-flight response and, 536
lifestyle change strategies for patients with, 1057–1058
schizophrenia and, **239**
sleep disorders and, 511
stress and pathogenesis of, 538–541
animal studies, 538–539
denial, 540
depression, 540–541
panic disorder, 541
psychological factors affecting medical condition, 541
social support, 540
type A behavior, 113–114, 539–540, 1054
stress-induced ischemia, 538, 1057–1058
Coronary Artery Surgery Study, 607
Coronary care unit (CCU). *See also* Intensive care unit
anxiety disorders in, 396
treatment of, 544–545
denial in, 540
use of tricyclic antidepressants in, 951
Cortical dementia, 273, **274, 276,** 277–278
Corticosteroids
for chronic obstructive pulmonary disease, 549
cytochrome P450 metabolism and, **946**
side effects of, **550**
anxiety, **400,** 780–781, **781**
delirium, **156,** 641, 793
dementia, **284**
depression, **311,** 323
mania, 64, **156,** 345, **345, 346**
neuropsychiatric effects, 323, 549, **667,** 793, **818**
sexual dysfunction, **464**
sleep disorders, **502**
for systemic lupus erythematosus, 568
Corticotropin-releasing hormone (CRH)
in chronic fatigue syndrome, 572
in panic disorder, 401
test for Cushing's syndrome, 566

Cortisol
Cushing's syndrome and, 566
fight-or-flight response and, 536
type A behavior and, 539
Cosmetic surgery patients, 613–614
body dysmorphic disorder among, 613
borderline personality disorder among, 614
delirium among, 614
depression among, 613
in immediate postoperative period, 614
initial psychiatric consultation with, 613
"insatiable," 614
in long-term postoperative period, 614
personality of, 595
in preoperative and intraoperative periods, 613–614
Cost-effectiveness studies, 25–31, 37–38, 197–198. *See also* Economic issues
Countertransference reactions, 7, 112–113
gender dysphoria and, 469
hate, 139
personality disorders and, 122
somatization and, 373
suicidality and, 139
vision loss and, 611
Couples therapy, **1034**
for agitation and aggression, 157
for HIV/AIDS, 833, 835
for somatoform disorders, 387
COX-2 inhibitors, **995, 999**
CPA (cyproterone acetate), **461,** 470
CPAP (continuous positive airway pressure), 508, 509, 551
CPK (creatine phosphokinase), 894
CPR (cardiopulmonary resuscitation), 175
CPT (Current Procedural Terminology) codes, 41
CPTs (continuous performance tests), computerized, 98
Crack cocaine, 440, 901. *See also* Cocaine-related disorders
Cranial nerve palsies, 263, 576, 688
Cranial nerve testing, 73
Craniopharyngioma, 682
Craniotomy, 1020
Creatine phosphokinase (CPK), 894
Creutzfeldt-Jakob disease, 282, 687
course and prognosis for, 296

electroencephalography in, 56, 294, 691
pathophysiology of, 287–288
sleep disorders and, 512
CRH. *See* Corticotropin-releasing hormone
Criminal behavior, 423, 446
Crisis-oriented therapeutic consultation, **6**
Critical care. *See* Intensive care unit
Crixivan. *See* Indinavir
Crohn's & Colitis Foundation of America, 556
Crohn's disease, 556, 1063
Cross-sectional population descriptive studies, **192,** 194–195
CRPS (complex regional pain syndrome), 992
Cruzan v. Director, Missouri Department of Health, 174–175
Cryptococcal meningoencephalitis, **345,** 688, 815
CT. *See* Computed tomography
Culture/ethnicity
HIV disease and, 808
perspectives on dying, 775–776, 778–779
pica and, 477
rehabilitation medicine and, 731
somatization and, 369
Curare, 968
Current Procedural Terminology (CPT) codes, 41
Cushing's syndrome, **565, 566, 594**
causes of, 321
depression and, 241, 308, **310, 311,** 321, 566
differentiation from Cushing's disease, 321
due to pituitary adenoma, 682
mania and, **345,** 563
psychiatric comorbidity with, **564**
suicide and, 129, 563
testing for, 566
CVA (cerebrovascular accident). *See* Stroke
Cyclic adenosine monophosphate (cAMP), 436
Cyclobenzaprine, **345,** 571
Cyclophosphamide, **461**
Cycloserine, **550**
Cyclosporine
drug interactions with antidepressants, 642
cytochrome P450 metabolism and, **946**

Cyclosporine *(continued)*
  drug interactions with *(continued)*
    lithium, 960
    St. John's wort, 973
  holidays from, 640, 642
  side effects of
    movement disorders, 643
    neurotoxicity, 640–641
    psychotic symptoms, 642
    seizures, 642
Cyclothymia, 117, **118**
  definition of, 339
  irritable bowel syndrome and, **555**
  thyroid disease and, 245
Cylert. *See* Pemoline
Cyproheptadine, **345,** 505
Cyproterone acetate (CPA), **461,** 470
Cystic fibrosis, 504, 627
Cytochrome P450–related drug
    interactions, 596, 942, **945–946**
  with alcohol, 427, **428**
  with antiretroviral drugs, 814
  with benzodiazepines, 505
  with carbamazepine, 352, 596
  with nefazodone, 327, 427
  with selective serotonin reuptake
    inhibitors, 326, 427, 543, 761
  in surgical patients, 596
Cytomegalovirus (CMV) infection, 574
Cytosine arabinoside, **461, 667**

Dalmane. *See* Flurazepam
Danazol, **349, 461**
Dantrolene, 968
Day treatment programs, 839
ddC. *See* Zalcitabine
DDI. *See* Didanosine
Death. *See* Dying patients; Mortality
Deception syndrome, 519
Defense mechanisms, 108–110, **109.**
    See also Coping strategies
Defensive Functioning Scale, 108
Degenerative neurological diseases,
    685–687
Delavirdine, **461, 811,** 814
Delinquent bills, 28–29
Delirium, 9, 257–269
  affective lability and, 262
  age at onset of, **63**
  aggressive behavior and, 149
  agitation and, 258, 267
  in Alzheimer's disease, 257
  anxiety and, 780, **781**
  assessment for, 263, 264, **264**
  burn trauma and, 259, 612
  cancer and, **259,** 663, 665, 780, 793

cardiac disease and, 544
  intra-aortic balloon pumps, 604,
    765
  postcardiotomy delirium, 38, 259,
    268, 605, 765–766, **767**
causes of, 54, 258, 264
in children, 257–259
clinical features of, 260–263, 792
costs of care for, **872**
in critically ill patients, 756,
    761–762, **762**
delusions and, 262
dementia and, 257, 259
diagnosis of, 263
diagnostic criteria for, 257–258, **258**
differential diagnosis of, 257,
    263–265
  conversion disorder, 689
  critical items (I WATCH
    DEATH), 265, **265**
  depression, 262
  emergent items (WHHHHIMP),
    141, 264–265, 756, **756,** 895
  laboratory tests, 264, **264**
diffuse cognitive impairment in,
    260–262, 267
  attentional deficits, 260
  disorientation, 68, 261
  memory impairment, 260
  prefrontal executive functions,
    261
  visuoconstructional impairment,
    261, **261**
due to general medical condition, 258
effect on hospital length of stay, 257,
    269
in elderly persons, 9, 54, 257–259,
    262, 856
electroencephalography in, **261,** 263,
    691, 895
in encephalitis, 688
endocrine disorders and, **564**
epidemiology of, 258–260, **259**
HIV-associated, 259, **259,** 793,
    795–795, 824–825, **825**
hypoalbuminemia and, 259
hypoxia and, 546, 548
language disturbances and, 262
magnetic resonance imaging in, 54
management of, **266,** 266–268
  electroconvulsive therapy,
    1019–1020
  environmental interventions, 268
  medications, 267–268, 761–762,
    763
  psychological support, 268

in terminally ill patients, 793–795,
    794
  morbidity associated with, 269
  mortality associated with, 257, 269
  neurological disorders and, 259,
    262–263, 265
  nocturnal, 512
  perceptual disturbances and, 262
  postoperative, 36, 259, **259**
    cardiothoracic surgery, 38, 257,
      259, 268, 605, 765–766, **767**
    cosmetic surgery, 614
    head and neck surgery, 616
    orthopedic surgery, 257, 259, 269,
      609
    transplant surgery, 259, 638, 640–
      641
  prevalence in general hospital
    patients, 257, 258–260, **260**
  prevention of, 266
  prodrome for, 260
  prognosis for, 268–269
  psychomotor disturbances and, 257,
    258, 262
  in rehabilitation settings, 734
  restraint of patient with, 179
  seizures and, 268–269
  sleep disturbances and, 259–260,
    262, 502
  structural brain disease and, 259
  substance-induced, **156,** 258, 265,
    762, 793
    anticholinergics, 150, 239, **239,**
      259, 325, 785, 905
    hallucinogens, 905
    tricyclic antidepressants, 408,
      761, 785, 951
  during substance withdrawal, 259
  systemic lupus erythematosus and,
    568
  temporal course of, 260, 268
  among terminally ill patients,
    792–796
  thought disturbances and, 262
Delirium Rating Scale (DRS), 263,
    792–793
Delirium tremens (DT), 258, 262–263,
    424–426, 901
  clinical course of, 424
  propofol for, 268
  risk factors for, 424–426
  signs and symptoms of, 424
Delis-Kaplan Executive Function
    Sequence, 82
Delusions
  in Alzheimer's disease, 858

antipsychotics for, 962
assessment for, 64
delirium and, 262
in Huntington's disease, 278
mania and, 342
in Parkinson's disease, 279
somatic type, **362**, 376, 381
in vascular dementia, 281
Dementia, 273–298
aggressive behavior and, 149
alcohol-related, 276, 277, 283, 288,
426
of Alzheimer's type (*See* Alzheimer's
disease)
associated with psychiatric disorders,
275, 283–286
acute psychosis, 285
conversion disorder, 285
depression, 275, 277, 283–285,
293–294, 297, **310**, 316
malingering, 285–286
cancer and, **274,** 283, **284,** 666, 780
causes of, 273, **274**
clinical course and prognosis for,
295–296
cobalamin deficiency and, 569
compared with normal aging, 273
computerized
electroencephalography in,
56–57
cortical, 273, **274, 276,** 277–278
definition of, 273
delirium and, 257, 259
depression and, 275, 277, 283–285,
293–294, **310, 311**
dialysis, **284,** 561
differential diagnosis of, 273,
289–294, 294
dementia rating scales, 83, 294
depression, 86–87, 316
laboratory tests, 291, **293**
longitudinal history, 291
mental status examination,
289–290, **289–292**
neuroimaging, 53–54, 56, 281,
292–294, **293**
neurological examination, 290
neuropsychological testing,
84–85, 278, 294
reversible etiologies, 273, 275,
291
due to general medical condition, 283
in elderly persons, 9, 273, 856–857
epidemiology of, 275–277, **680**
family studies of, 277
frontotemporal, 273, 275, 286

guardianship of patients with,
176–177
head trauma and, **274,** 276, 281–282,
287
Huntington's disease, 278, 286,
686
hydrocephalic, **274,** 282
"hysterical," 285
incidence/prevalence of, 275–276
infection-related, **274,** 282
Creutzfeldt-Jakob disease, 282,
287–288
herpes simplex encephalitis, 282
HIV/AIDS, 259, 276, 282, 287,
795–796, 817–824
Lyme disease, 575
meningitis, 282
neurosyphilis, 282, 576
progressive multifocal
leukoencephalopathy, 282
with Lewy bodies, 273, 275, 279,
286, 297
limbic encephalopathy, 280
management of, 296–298
electroconvulsive therapy, 1019
family therapy/support, 298
medical therapy, 296
pharmacotherapy, 296–297
ward management, 297–298
in medically ill patients, 276
mixed, 275, 280–283
mortality associated with, 257
multi-infarct, 56, 280
neoplastic, **274,** 283, 288–289
nocturnal agitation in, 504
Parkinson's disease, 275, 276, 279,
286, 685–686
pathophysiology of, 286–289
Pick's disease, 273
postanoxic, **284**
predisposition and risk factors for,
276–277
progressive supranuclear palsy,
279–280, 287
pugilistica, 281
restraint of patient with, 179
reversible, 273, 275, 291
sexual behavior and, 468
sleep disorders and, 512
strategic infarct, 280
subcortical, **274,** 274–275, **276,**
278–280, 796
substance-induced persisting, 283,
285
suicide and, 129
in terminally ill patients, 792–793

toxic-metabolic, **274,** 282–283, **284,**
288
transplantation for patients with, 631
use of β-blockers in, 692
vascular, **274,** 275, **280,** 280–281,
287
Wilson's disease, 279, 286
Dementia Rating Scale, 83
Demerol. *See* Meperidine
Denervation hypersensitivity, 944
Denial, 108, 110, 1053
among burn patients, 612
cancer and, 657
among cardiac disease patients, 540,
1056
competency to make treatment
decisions and, 172–173
end-stage renal disease and, 560
in patients with pain, 990, 1003
in rehabilitation settings, 735, **735**
Denmark, consultation-liaison
psychiatry in, 207–209
Dental problems, 487
Depakene, Depakote. *See* Valproate
Dependent patients, 109, 112
Dependent personality disorder, **116,
120**
Deprenyl, 327
Depression, 307–330
age at onset of, **63**
anorexia nervosa and, 480
anxiety disorders and, 242, 399
atypical, 947, 954
biogenic amine hypothesis of, 947
blindness and, 610
body dysmorphic disorder and, 381
bulimia nervosa and, 481
cardiothoracic surgery and, 607
character spectrum disorder, 310,
311
chronic, 310
cosmetic surgery and, 613
course and outcome of, 249–250,
324–325
in critically ill patients, 760–761
dementia syndrome of (DSD), 275,
277, 283–285, 857
electroconvulsive therapy for, 297
neuroimaging in, 293–294
diagnosis of, 312–313, 946
biological markers, 313
in dying patients, 783–784, **784**
family history, 312
history of present illness, 312
laboratory tests, 313
mental status examination, 312

Depression *(continued)*
diagnosis of *(continued)*
by nonpsychiatrists, 40, 46
past history, 312
physical examination, 313
underdiagnosis, 307, **307**, 944
diagnostic criteria for, 309, **309**
Endicott's substitutive criteria,
309–310
differential diagnosis of
delirium, 262
dementia, 86–87, 316
somatization disorder, 376
in dying patients, 783–787
economic impact of, 308
in elderly persons, 9, 54, 241, 854,
857–858
electroconvulsive therapy for, 241,
297, 328, 947, 1015
etiologies of, 732–733, 946
factitious, 523
head and neck surgery and, 615
hypochondriasis and, 367, 378
immune dysfunction and, 238
as initial manifestation of physical
illness, 308
insomnia and, 501
legal competency of persons with,
172
masked, 367
mechanical ventilation and, 765
medical conditions associated with,
311, 313–321
acromegaly and, **564**
Addison's disease, 308, **564**, 733
burn injuries, 612
cancer, 241, 245, **310**, 314,
661–663, **733**, 779–780,
783–784, **784**, 1021–1022
cardiac disease, 241, 307–308,
310, 314, 325, 540–544,
627, 1054–1055
chronic fatigue syndrome, **310**,
321
chronic obstructive pulmonary
disease, 548
chronic pain, **310**, 314–315, 367,
383, **733**, 998, 1000, **1000**,
1067
cobalamin deficiency, 569
Cushing's syndrome, 241, 308,
310, 321, **564**, 566
dementia, 275, 277, 283–285,
293–294, 297, **310**, 316
diabetes mellitus, 245, 250, **310**,
320–321, 563, **564**

end-stage renal disease and
dialysis, 308, **310**, 313–314,
561, 628
epilepsy, 241, **310**, 318, **319**, 683
esophageal motility disorders, 553
fibromyalgia, 571
gastrointestinal disease, 245
head trauma, 685
HIV/AIDS, **310**, 319–320, **827**,
827–830, 1022
Huntington's disease, 238, 241,
278, 308, **310**, 317–318
hyperparathyroidism, 320, **564**,
566
irritable bowel syndrome, **555**,
555–556
limbic encephalopathy, 280
lung disease, 627
Lyme disease, 575
multiple sclerosis, **310**, 318–319,
686–687, **733**
myocardial infarction, 39, 113,
249–250, 307–308, 537,
541, 627, 1054–1055
neurological and neurosurgical
disorders, 679
neurosyphilis, 576
nicotine dependence, 240
Parkinson's disease, 241, 279,
310, 316–317, 685, 686, 858
pheochromocytoma and, **564**
progressive supranuclear palsy,
280
stroke, 63, 238, 244, 281, 308,
310, 315–316, 679–681,
732, **733**, 741, 857–858, 978
systemic lupus erythematosus,
568
thyroid disorders, 63, 245, 308,
310, 320, 564, **564**
traumatic brain injury, 281
Wilson's disease, 279
in medically ill patients, 241, 310,
858, 946
characteristics compared with
primary major depression,
310
economic cost of, **872**
effect on hospital length of stay,
35–36
prevalence of, 25, 241, 307, **310**,
872
menopause and, 703
morbidity and mortality associated
with, 307–308
nicotine dependence and, 445

outpatient psychiatric consultation
for, 922–923
pathophysiology of, 693
positron-emission tomography in, 55
postpartum, 710
presentations and definitions of,
308–312
adjustment disorder with
depressed mood, 312
dysthymic disorder and minor
depression, 310–311, **311**
major depressive episode, 308–
310, **309**, **310**
mood disorder due to general
medical condition, **311**,
311–312
substance-induced mood disorder,
311, **311**
prevalence of, 307, **680**
psychiatric emergencies in patients
with, 906
psychotic, 141, 328, 947
rating scales for, 92–93, **93**, **371**
in rehabilitation settings, 732–733,
733
respiration in, 547
sleep apnea and, 509
smoking and, 445, 549, 1061
somatization and, **362**, 367
somatization disorder and, 375
substance-induced, 63–64, **239**, 311,
311, 321–324, 732
alcohol, 323–324
amphetamine, 323
anabolic steroids, 324
antihypertensive agents, 321–322
benzodiazepines, 323
cancer chemotherapy agents, 323
cimetidine, 323
cocaine withdrawal, 324
contraceptives, 322–323
corticosteroids, 323
efavirenz, 816
interferon, 239, **239**
methyldopa, 322
opiates, 324, 436–437
progesterone, 703
propranolol and other β-blockers,
162, 322
ranitidine, 323
reserpine, 63, 321–322
suicide and, 128, 129, **133**, 133–134,
134, 136
in transplant recipients, 642
treatment of, 325–330, 944–957 (*See
also* Antidepressants)

electroconvulsive therapy, 141, **328,** 328–329
family therapy, 329–330
monoamine oxidase inhibitors, 327
other antidepressants, 326–327
in patients with cardiac disease, 542–544
psychostimulants, 327
psychotherapy, 329
selective serotonin reuptake inhibitors, 326
transcranial magnetic stimulation, 329
for treatment-resistant depression (TRD), 328
tricyclic and related antidepressants, 325–326
for underlying medical conditions, 325
undertreatment, 307, **307**
treatment-resistant, 946
weight changes and, 1059–1060
Depression in Primary Care, 40
Depressive equivalents, 367
Depressive personality disorder, **118**
Dermatological disorders
behavioral management of, 1066
drug-induced
antipsychotics, 966
antiretroviral drugs, 812
carbamazepine, 961
lamotrigine, 353, 961
selective serotonin reuptake inhibitors, 952
tricyclic antidepressants, 951
in Lyme disease, 575
personality disorders and, 121
Desensitization, 410
of anticipatory nausea and vomiting in chemotherapy patients, 659–660
after head and neck surgery, 615
Desipramine, 325, **948**
dosage of, **948**
drug interactions with
carbamazepine, 352
cytochrome P450 metabolism and, **945**
methadone, 438
for pain syndromes, 1004–1005
receptor site affinity of, **948**
serum level of, 947
side effects of
insomnia, **502,** 505
sexual dysfunction, **461**

use in specific patient groups or medical conditions
breast-feeding women, **981**
chronic pain syndrome, **693**
dying patients, 785, **785**
elderly persons, **863,** 864
HIV/AIDS, 829
patients undergoing rehabilitation, **742**
Desyrel. *See* Trazodone
Detoxification, 420. *See also* Substance-related disorders
from alcohol, 430–432, **430–432,** 901
from opioids, 437–440, **439**
from sedative-hypnotics, 433–435, **435**
Developmental perspective, 718
Dexamethasone
anxiety induced by, **781**
for chemotherapy patients, 660
cytochrome P450 metabolism and, **946**
insomnia and agitation induced by, 666
psychiatric aspects of, **669**
Dexamethasone suppression test (DST), 313
conditions associated with positive response to, 313
for depression, 313
poststroke, 680
in eating disorders, 486
Dexedrine. *See* Dextroamphetamine
Dextroamphetamine, 955–957, **956**
cardiac effects of, 544
dosage of, 956, **956**
half-life of, **956,** 1007
indications for
depression, 327
narcolepsy, 509
pain syndromes, **989,** 1007
use in specific patient groups or medical conditions
cancer patients, 662
critically ill patients, 761
dying patients, **785,** 786–787
HIV/AIDS, 824, 829–830
neurological disease, 692
transplant candidates, **637**
Dextromethorphan, **345,** 955
Diabetes insipidus, lithium-induced, 348
Diabetes mellitus, 288, 564, **565**
antidepressants for patients with, 951
anxiety disorders and, 397, **564**
behavioral medicine and, 1067

depression and, 245, 250, **310,** 320–321, 563
eating disorders and, 564
outpatient medical-psychiatric treatment for, 874
prevalence of psychiatric comorbidity with, 245, **564**
psychiatric disorders in candidates for transplantation, 628
sexual dysfunction and, 458–459
sleep disorders and, 504, 511
suicidality and, 245
Diagnosis
case detection and, 39
diagnostic groups in rehabilitation medicine, 730, **730**
in elderly persons, 859–861
formulation of, 939–940, 1040, **1041**
in intensive care unit, 754–756, **755**
mental status examination, 61–75
via telepsychiatry, 929
Diagnosis-related groups (DRGs), 26–29, **27, 29**
Diagnostic access bias in research, **199**
Diagnostic criteria, 29
Alzheimer's disease, 278
amnestic disorders due to general medical condition, **86**
anorexia nervosa, **478**
body dysmorphic disorder, **380**
bulimia nervosa, **478**
chronic fatigue syndrome, 571
conversion disorder, **379**
delirium, 257–258, **258**
fibromyalgia, 571
hypochondriasis, **377**
intermittent explosive disorder, **150**
irritable bowel syndrome, 554, **554**
major depressive episode, **309,** 309–310
manic episode, **340**
mood disorder due to general medical condition, **340**
neuroaggressive disorder (proposed), **151**
pain disorder, **382**
panic attack, **395**
personality change due to general medical condition, **151**
pica, **478**
psychological factor affecting medical condition, 363–364, **364**
somatization disorder, 374, **375**
substance dependence, **419**
substance-induced mood disorder, **341**

Diagnostic criteria *(continued)*
  substance-induced persisting
    dementia, **285**
  undifferentiated somatoform
    disorder, **376**
  vascular dementia, **280**
Diagnostic Interview Schedule (DIS),
  243, 249, 397, 628
Diagnostic Interview Schedule for
  Children, 249
Diagnostic purity bias in research, **199**
Dialectical behavior therapy, 911
Dialysis patients, 558–561. *See also*
  Renal failure
  electroconvulsive therapy for, 561
  ethical issues and discontinuing
    dialysis, 559–560
  medical expenditures for, 558
  neuropsychiatric syndromes among,
    560–561
    depression, 308, **310,** 313–314,
      628
    dialysis dementia, **284,** 561
    mania, **345**
    renal transplant candidates, 628
    suicidality, 131–132
  psychotropic medications for, 561, 978
    antidepressants, 561
    antipsychotics, 561
    anxiolytics, 561
    mood stabilizers, 348, 561
  quality of life of, 559
  sexual dysfunction among, 458, 559
Diaphoresis. *See* Sweating
Diarrhea, drug-induced
  antiretroviral drugs, 812
  lithium, 350, 958
  nicotine, 445
  opioid withdrawal, 438
  risperidone, 354
Diazepam, **763, 903, 970**
  abuse of, 902, 907
  dosage of, **407, 434, 763, 903, 970,**
    971
  drug interactions with
    alcohol, 427, **428**
    cytochrome P450 metabolism
      and, **945**
    ritonavir, 814, **815,** 834
  half-life of, **407, 903**
  indications for
    aggressive behavior, 899, 902
    alcohol withdrawal, 430–432,
      431, 433, 901
    benzodiazepine withdrawal,
      434–435, **435**

cocaine intoxication, 441
  hallucinogen intoxication, 443,
    905
  headache, 1068
  phencyclidine intoxication, 443,
    906
  sedative-hypnotic withdrawal,
    434–435, **435,** 904
  seizures, 432, **433**
  intramuscular, 941
  pharmacokinetics of, 970
  side effects of
    depression, 323
    sexual dysfunction, **461**
  use in specific patient groups or
    medical conditions
    breast-feeding women, **981**
    dialysis patients, 561
    dying patients, 782, **782**
    patients undergoing rehabilitation,
      743
    pregnancy, 707–708, **708,**
      980
    withdrawal from, 903–904
Diazepam challenge test, 434
Dichlorphenamide, **461**
Dicyclomine, 438, **462**
DID (dissociative identity disorder),
  118, 121, 523
Didanosine, **811, 818,** 834
Diet
  cobalamin deficiency, 288, 569
  DASH, 1060
  high-protein liquid diets, 484
  for hypertension, 1060
  low-fat, 1057, 1058
  low-sodium, 1060
  Mediterranean, 1058
  omega-3 fatty acids in, 1058
  thiamine deficiency, 426
  tyramine–monoamine oxidase
    inhibitor interaction, 327,
      543–544, 954, 955
Diet pills, 479, 481
Diethylpropion, **462**
Digitalis, **400**
Digitoxin, **943**
Digoxin, **284, 462,** 543, 1021
Dihydrocodeine, **995**
Dilaudid. *See* Hydromorphone
Diltiazem
  drug interactions with
    carbamazepine, **349,** 351
    cytochrome P450 metabolism
      and, **946**
  for mania, 354

Diphenhydramine, 973
  abuse of, 905
  for agitation and aggression, 159
  for children, **723**
  delirium induced by, **762**
  for insomnia, 505, **506**
  for neuroleptic-induced
    extrapyramidal symptoms, 965
  psychiatric aspects of, **669**
  sexual dysfunction induced by, **462**
Diplopia, lamotrigine-induced, 353
DIS (Diagnostic Interview Schedule),
  243, 249, 397, 628
Disability, 735
  definition of, 729
  of patients with ischemic heart
    disease, 1061–1062
Disclosure of patient information,
  168–169
Disease vs. illness, 363
Disopyramide, **462**
Disorientation
  in Alzheimer's disease, 277
  assessment for, 68
  delirium and, 68, 261
  efavirenz-induced, 816
  in limbic encephalopathy, 280
  during manic episode, 344
  to self, 68
  spatial, 68
Displacement, 108
Dissociative disorders
  childhood abuse and, 1003
  differentiation from conversion
    disorder, 380
  pain and, **1000,** 1003
Dissociative identity disorder (DID),
  118, 121, 523
Distractibility
  in Alzheimer's disease, 277
  delirium and, 261
Distraction techniques, for pain
  syndromes, 1008
Distribution of drug, 941–942
Disulfiram, **943**
  for alcoholism, 432
  contraindications to, 432
  drug interactions with, 432
    alcohol, **428**
    benzodiazepines, 349, 505
  sexual dysfunction induced by, **462**
Diuretics
  abuse of
    in anorexia nervosa, 479
    in bulimia nervosa, 481
    medical complications of, 481, **481**

drug interactions with
    antidepressants, 953
    lithium, 348, **349,** 960
    monoamine oxidase inhibitors, 955
for lithium-induced polyuria, 349, 350
side effects of, 322
    insomnia, **502**
    sexual dysfunction, **464**
Divalproex sodium. *See* Valproate
Dizziness
    drug-induced
        buspirone, 409
        carbamazepine, 961
        gabapentin, 961
        lamotrigine, 353, 961
        nefazodone, 327
        nicotine, 445
        psychostimulants, 956, 957
        venlafaxine, 326
    in neurosyphilis, 576
    in postconcussion syndrome, 685
Do-not-resuscitate (DNR) orders, 175, 778
Doctor-patient relationship, 14–17, 111–113
    in caring for dying patients, 775
    confidentiality in, 15, **168,** 168–169
    establishing therapeutic alliance, 15, 111–113, 1036
        with pediatric patients, 720
    fiduciary nature of, 169
    impact on treatment compliance, 111
    implied contractual arrangement, 178
    influence of patient's defense mechanisms on, 108–110
    moral-ethical foundation for, 167
    obtaining patient's psychodynamic life narrative, 112, 1041
    patient suicide and, 131
    patients who stir dislike in doctors, 109–110
    with somatizing patient, 370, 373
    via telepsychiatry, 927–935
    transference and countertransference, 112–113
"Doctor shopping," 122
Documentation, 15
    of aggression, 152, **153, 155**
    of agitation, 152–155, **154**
    elements of initial consultation note, **16**
    by medical students, 18
    Medicare guidelines for, 15

Dolphine. *See* Methadone
Domestic violence, 711–712, 908–909. *See also* Aggression
Donepezil
    for Alzheimer's disease, 297
    for HIV-associated neurocognitive impairment, 824
    sexual dysfunction induced by, **462**
    side effects of, 297
L-Dopa. *See* Levodopa
Dopamine
    aggression and, 155–156
    mania and, 344
    neuroleptic malignant syndrome and, 968
    Parkinson's disease and, 286
    tardive dyskinesia and, 966
Dopaminergic agents
    for neuroleptic malignant syndrome, 968
    for Parkinson's disease, 295, 686
    for periodic leg movements of sleep and restless legs syndrome, 510
Doral. *See* Quazepam
Doriden. *See* Glutethimide
Down's syndrome, 276
Doxepin, 325, **948**
    dosage of, **948**
    for insomnia, 505
    receptor site affinity of, **948**
    sexual dysfunction induced by, **462**
    use in specific patient groups or medical conditions
        breast-feeding women, **981**
        chronic pain syndrome, 693, **693**
        dying patients, 785, **785**
        migraine, **693**
        patients undergoing rehabilitation, **742**
Draw-a-Person Test, 760
DRGs (diagnosis-related groups), 26–29, **27, 29**
Dronabinol, **345**
Droperidol, **763**
    antiemetic effects of, 963
    for delirium, 267, **794,** 965
    dosage of, **669**
    psychiatric aspects of, **669**
    use in specific patient groups or medical conditions
        cardiac disease, 544
        surgical patients, **597**
        terminally ill patients, **794**
        transplant recipients, 641
Drowsiness, drug-induced
    benzodiazepines, 971

carbamazepine, 961
DRS (Delirium Rating Scale), 263, 792–793
Drug Abuse Warning Network, 440
Drug holidays, postoperative, 601
Drug interactions, 33, 45, 757, 944
    with alcohol, 427, **428**
    with analgesics, 999, **999**
    with anticonvulsants, 962
    with antidepressants, **943,** 953–954
    with antipsychotics, **944**
    with antiretroviral agents, 814–815, **815**
    with benzodiazepines, **349,** 505, 972
    with carbamazepine, **349,** 352, 438, 596, 694
    with chloral hydrate, 973
    cytochrome P450–related, 596, 942, **945–946**
        with alcohol, 427, **428**
        with benzodiazepines, 505
        with carbamazepine, 352, 596
        with nefazodone, 327, 427
        with selective serotonin reuptake inhibitors, 326, 427, 543, 761
        in surgical patients, 596
    delirium due to, 265
    with electroconvulsive therapy, 354, 1016–1017
    with herbal medicinals, 973
    with immunosuppressants, 643
    with lamotrigine, 353
    with lithium, 348, **349,** 694, 864, 960
    with methadone, 438
    with monoamine oxidase inhibitors, 327, 787
    with nefazodone, 327, 427
    with nicotine, 445
    obtaining drug history to minimize risk of, 944
    with ophthalmic β-blockers, 611–612
    pharmacodynamic, 944
    pharmacokinetic, 944
    with selective serotonin reuptake inhibitors, 326, 427, 543, 761
    sources of information on, 45
    in surgical patients, 596, **597–598**
    between thioridazine and propranolol, 162
    with valproate, **349,** 351
    with venlafaxine, 327
Drug overdose. *See also* Substance-related disorders
    acetaminophen, 129, 724–725

Drug overdose (continued)
  amantadine, 965
  amphetamine, 442
  analgesics, 129
  anticholinergic drugs, 129, 905
  anticonvulsants, 962
  antidepressants, 129, 953
  antihistamines, 129
  antipsychotics, 969
  barbiturates, 129, 902
  benzodiazepines, 129, 158, 971
  bupropion, 952
  chloral hydrate, 973
  lithium, 959, **976**
  presenting in emergency department,
    417
  psychiatric clearance of patients after,
    41
  psychostimulants, 956–957
  suicide attempts from, 127, 129
Drug Safety, 45
Drug-seeking behavior, 996, **996**
Drug therapy. See Pharmacotherapy
Drugs, 45
Dry mouth, drug-induced
  cannabis, 444
  mirtazapine, 953
  nefazodone, 327
  psychostimulants, 956
  reboxetine, 953
  selective serotonin reuptake
    inhibitors, 829
  tricyclic antidepressants, 325, 950,
    951
  venlafaxine, 326
DSD (dementia syndrome of
    depression), 275, 277, 283–285,
    293–294
DST. See Dexamethasone suppression
    test
d4T. See Stavudine
Dunbar, Helen Flanders, 5
Durable power of attorney, 168,
    174–176, 596
Dust. See Phencyclidine-related
    disorders
Dutch consultation-liaison psychiatry,
    214–215
  background of, 214
  future development, 215
  in general hospital, 214
  official status and training, 214–215
  research, 215
Dutch Federation for General Hospital
    Psychiatry, 215
Dutch Psychiatric Association, 215

Dying patients, 771–798. See also
    Mortality
  achieving a good death, 772–773
  advance directives for, 175–176
  advocacy for, 778
  in America, 772
  anxiety disorders in, 780–783
    causes of, 780–781, **781**
    pharmacotherapy for, **782,**
      782–783
    prevalence of, 781–782
    psychotherapy for, 783
  with cancer, **658,** 659
  causes of death among, 772
  cognitive impairment among, **259,**
    792–796
  complexity of caring for, 771
  criteria for "appropriate death," 773
  cultural perspectives on dying,
    775–776
  depression in, 783–787
    assessment of, 783–784, **784**
    electroconvulsive therapy for, 787
    management of, 784
    pastoral counseling for, 787
    pharmacotherapy for, 784–787,
      785
      benzodiazepines, 787
      bupropion, 785–786
      heterocyclic antidepressants,
        786
      lithium, 787
      monoamine oxidase inhibitors,
        787
      psychostimulants, 786–787
      selective serotonin reuptake
        inhibitors, 786
      trazodone, 785
      tricyclic antidepressants, 785
    prevalence of, 783
    psychotherapy for, 787
  do-not-resuscitate orders for, 175,
    778
  doctor-patient communication in
    caring for, 775
  education in treatment of, 771, 772
  factors affecting adaptation to
    terminal illness and death, **778,**
    778–779
    medical factors, 779
    personal factors, 779
    sociocultural factors, 778–779
  fear of, 771
  with HIV/AIDS, 836
  holistic treatment of, 771
  home care for, 772, 777

  incidence of psychiatric disorders
    among, 779–780
  pain management for, 773–774, 796,
    797
  palliative care for, **773,** 773–775, **774**
  place of death of, 772
  psychiatric aspects of excellent end-
    of-life care for, 805–806
  psychiatric management strategies
    for, 780
  psychological issues and management
    of, 779
  psychotherapy for, 778, 779, 783,
    784, 787
  quality of life of, 776
  role of consultation-liaison
    psychiatrist with, **777,** 777–778
  spirituality and, 776–777
  staff issues in care of, 796–798
  suicidality of, 129–130, 778,
    788–792
    AIDS patients, 129, **132,**
      132–133, 144, **144,** 319, 791
    euthanasia and physician-assisted
      suicide, 144–146, 175,
      789–791, **790,** 831
    evaluation and management, 791
    right to die, 174–175, 790
    risk factors, **788,** 788–789
  view of future, 107
Dysarthria, 73
  drug-induced, tricyclic
    antidepressants, 951
  in progressive supranuclear palsy, 280
  in transplant recipients, 643
  in Wilson's disease, 279
Dyskinesia
  orofacial, after liver transplantation,
    643
  psychostimulant-induced, 787
  respiratory, 551
  tardive, 158, 160, **239,** 408, 691
Dyslexia, 73, **680**
Dyslipidemia, 536
Dysphagia
  benzodiazepine-induced, 407
  differentiation from globus sensation,
    553
  functional, 552
Dysphasia, 73
Dyspnea, 245, 546
  causes of, 546
  due to chronic obstructive pulmonary
    disease, 548
  paroxysmal nocturnal, 502
  patient's perception of severity of, 546

psychiatric disorders associated with, 627
suicidality and, 548
Dysprosody, 73
Dyssomnias, **496, 497,** 499–500. *See also* Sleep disorders
Dysthymic disorder, 117, **118**
among cardiac transplant candidates, 627
diagnosis of, 310–311
hypochondriasis and, 378
insomnia and, 501
irritable bowel syndrome and, 555, **555**
in postconcussion syndrome, 685
poststroke, 679–680
in rehabilitation settings, 732
somatization and, **362**
somatization disorder and, 375
subaffective, 310, **311**
suicide and, **133**
Dystonia
anticholinergics for prevention of, 897
drug-induced
neuroleptics, 158, 691, 965
psychostimulants, 956
tardive, 691, 966
treatment of, 965
in Wilson's disease, 279

E-mail consultation, 934
EACLPP (European Association for Consultation-Liaison Psychiatry and Psychosomatics), 206
Eating Attitudes Test, **720**
Eating disorders, 477–489
anorexia nervosa, 477–480
brain tumors and, 682
bulimia nervosa, 480–481
definitions of, 477
diabetes mellitus and, 564
laboratory evaluation of, 482, **482**
medical complications of, 477, 482–487
hospitalized patients, **482,** 482–483
patients with anorexia, **483,** 483–487
patients with bulimia, 487
medical complications of laxative or diuretic abuse in, 481, **481**
pica, 481
presenting in obstetrics and gynecology settings, 713
treatment of, 487–489

anorexia, 487–488
bulimia, 488–489
types of, 477
Eaton, James, 7
Eaton-Lambert myasthenic syndrome, 682
Ebstein's anomaly, lithium-induced, 959
EBV (Epstein-Barr virus) infection, 321, 571, 574
ECA (Epidemiologic Catchment Area) study, 134, 195, 240, 339, 369, 395, 396, 422, 907, 908
ECG. *See* Electrocardiography
Echinacea, **974**
ECLW (European Consultation-Liaison Workgroup) Collaborative Study, 206, 208, 214, 216, 221–222, **223**
Economic issues, 25–31
cost-effectiveness studies, 197–198
cost of neuroimaging studies, 52
cost of suicide attempts, 127
"cost-offset" of psychiatric care, 37–38, **872**
depression and medical resource utilization, 308
economic effects of comorbid psychiatric and medical illness, 25–26, 251–252, 871, **872**
effect of consultation-liaison services on costs, 26–27, 37
financial support for consultation-liaison psychiatry, 7–9
financing of outpatient consultation-liaison services, 921
integrated medical-psychiatry services, 882–883
managed care, 182–183
psychotherapy and, 1048
optimizing financial viability of consultation-liaison service, **27,** 27–31
psychiatric comorbidity and length of stay, 9, 25–26, 35–36
psychiatric treatment costs in general medical vs. specialty mental health settings, 27
"Ecstasy," 443, 905
ECT. *See* Electroconvulsive therapy
ED. *See* Emergency department
Edema
in anorexia nervosa, 486
lithium-induced, 959
pulmonary
in cancer patients, 660
in opioid-addicted patients, 905
Edronax. *See* Reboxetine

EDS. *See* Excessive daytime somnolence
Education. *See* Teaching consultation-liaison psychiatry
EEG. *See* Electroencephalography
Efavirenz, **811**
cerebrospinal fluid penetration by, 823
drug interactions with
methadone, 838
psychotropic drugs, 814
neuropsychiatric side effects of, 816–817, **818**
sleep disorders induced by, 834
Effexor, Effexor XR. *See* Venlafaxine
Elavil. *See* Amitriptyline
Elderly persons, 9, 853–866
abuse of, 859, **860,** 909
agitation and aggression in, 149–150
anxiety in, 858
causes of death among, 772
challenges to psychiatric diagnosis in, 854
chronic medical illnesses among, 853
cohort effects and ageism in treatment of, 859
delirium in, 9, 54, 257–259, 262, 856
dementia in, 9, **63,** 273, 275, 856–857 (*See also* Alzheimer's disease)
demographic trends related to, 854
depression in, 9, 54, 241, 854, 857–858, 946
diagnostic evaluation of, 859–861
clinical examination, 859
electroencephalography, 861
laboratory findings, 860–861
mental status examination, 860
neuroimaging, 861
physical examination, 860
differences in psychiatric diagnoses between younger patients and, 854, **855**
electroconvulsive therapy for, 864, 1023
environmental modifications for, 865
hip fracture in, 26, 37, 257, 259, 269, 399, 608, 855
insomnia in, 244, 854
late-life psychosis in, 858–859
memory impairment among, 253, 854
mental disorders among hospitalized patients, 853, 854, **855**
models of consultation-liaison psychiatry for, 855–856

Elderly persons *(continued)*
  normal aging and quality of life of, 853–854
  psychiatric consultation requests for, 854–855
  psychotherapy for, 864–865
  psychotropic drug use in, 861–864, **863**
    age-related pharmacodynamics, 862
    age-related pharmacokinetics, 861, **862**
    antidepressants, 863–864, 946, 950
    antipsychotics, 864, 966
    benzodiazepines, 864, 970
    guidelines for, 865–866
    lithium, 861, 864, 959
    mood stabilizers, 864
    plasma drug levels, 863
    polypharmacy and drug interactions with, 862, 865
    psychostimulants, 864
    side effects of, **863**, 866
  screening for psychiatric disorders in, 241
  side effects of over-the-counter medications in, 859
  sleep physiology in, 495
  strategies for psychiatric consultation with, **865**, 865–866
  substance-related disorders in, 859
  suicidality among, 241, 858
  treating medical problems of, 861
  young-old and old-old, 853
Electrocardiography (ECG). *See also* Arrhythmias
  in anorexia nervosa, 484–485
  in anxiety, 406
  drug effects on
    carbamazepine, 352
    clozapine, 966
    lithium, 350, 544
    tricyclic antidepressants, 543, 723, 950–951
  in mania, 347
Electroconvulsive therapy (ECT), 328, 1015–1023
  adverse effects of, 1018–1019, **1019**
  discontinuing medications before, 1016–1017
    lithium, 354, 1016
  as first-line treatment, 328, **328**, 1015, **1016**
  frequency and duration of, 1018
  indications for, 1015, **1015–1016**

catatonia, 328, 1022
chronic pain, 1021
dementia syndrome of depression, 297
depression, 241, 328, 1015
mania, 354–355, 1015
neuroleptic malignant syndrome, 968, 1023
psychotic depression, 328, 947
schizoaffective disorder, 1015
schizophrenia, 1015
suicidality, 141, 328
informed consent for, 1016
mechanism of action of, 693
mortality associated with, 329
orders before, **1017**
patients' attitudes about, 1015
pretreatment evaluation for, 1016–1017, **1017**
situations of increased risk of, 328–329, 1016, **1016**
technique for, **1017**, 1017–1018
  electrode placement, 1017–1018
  stimulus dosing, 1018
use in specific patient groups or medical conditions, 1016, **1016**, 1019–1022
  arrhythmias, 1021
  brain injury or craniotomy, 1020
  brain tumor, 1020
  cancer, 1021–1022
  cardiac disease, 329, 544, 974, 1021
  cardiac pacemakers, 1021
  central nervous system infection, 1021
  Cushing's syndrome, 566
  delirium, 1019–1020
  dementia, 1019
  dialysis patients, 561
  dying patients, 787
  elderly persons, 864, 1023
  epilepsy, 1020
  HIV/AIDS, 320, 830, 1022
  Huntington's disease, 318
  intraventricular shunts, 1020–1021
  Parkinson's disease, 874, 979, 1019
  pediatric patients, 1023
  poststroke depression, 315, 694
  pregnancy, 1022
  pulmonary disease, 1021
  stroke, 1020
  subdural hematoma, 1020

systemic lupus erythematosus, 568, 1022
transplant patients, 1022
Electroencephalography (EEG), 49, 691
  in Alzheimer's disease, 57, **279**
  in anxiety, 406
  computed tomography findings and abnormalities on, 53
  computerized (CEEG), 52, 56–57, 77
  constructional apraxia, mental status and, **261**
  in Creutzfeldt-Jakob disease, 56, 294, 691
  in delirium, **261**, 263, 691, 895
    pediatric, 259
  in delirium tremens, 258
  in dementia, 56–57
    dialysis dementia, 561
  in elderly persons, 861
  before electroconvulsive therapy, 1016, **1017**
  in emergency department, 894–895
  in encephalopathies, 56
  in epilepsy, 683, 691
  in fibromyalgia, 571
  in immunosuppressant neurotoxicity, 640
  in mania, 347
  patterns during sleep, 495
Electromagnetic (EM) radiation, 49–52. *See also* Neuroimaging
Electronic mail consultation, 934
Elimination of drug, 942
  aging and, 861, **862**, 942
EM (electromagnetic) radiation, 49–52. *See also* Neuroimaging
Emancipated minor, 173
Embolism
  cerebral, 679
  pulmonary, 550–551, 780
    in cancer patients, 660
    cocaine-related, 243, 441
Emergency department (ED), 889–913
  cocaine-related disorders in, 440
  common psychiatric emergencies, 906–911
    domestic violence and child abuse, 908–909
    in homeless persons, 909–910
    in patients with anxiety and phobic disorders, 907
    in patients with borderline or antisocial personality disorder, 907–908, **909**

in patients with mood disorders, 906–907

psychiatric emergency repeaters, 910–911

continuous observation of psychiatric patients in, 890

disposition of patients presenting in, 911–912

do-not-resuscitate orders and, 175, 778

drug overdoses seen in, 417

informed consent in, 170

life-endangering psychiatric emergencies, 895–906

acute psychosis, 895–897, **896**

substance-related, 417, 440, 900–906

suicide risk, 136–138, 897–898, **898**

violent patients, 890, 898–900

managing patient belongings in, 890

mobile crisis programs and, 912

patients' reasons for seeking help in, 892

prevalence of delirium among patients in, 258

psychiatric consultation in, 889

psychiatric emergency services in, 889

safety issues in, 889–891

case examples of, 889–890

seclusion and mechanical restraint, 890–891

violent patients, 890, 898–900

weapons screening, 890

staff-patient contractual relationship in, 178

treatment of myocardial infarction in, 540

triage and evaluation in, 891–895

case example of, 891

interview and mental status examination, 892–893

laboratory evaluation, 893–894, **894, 895**

neuroimaging, 894–895

patient transfers, 891–892

physical examination, 893

Emetine toxicity, 484

Emotions

airway reactivity to, 550

breathing and, 546

delirium and, 262

disease and, 1053–1054

Emphysema, 546, 627

Employee assistance programs, 871

Employment

behavioral weight reduction programs in places of, 1059

after cardiac transplantation, 646

of patients' caregivers, 739

of patients with ischemic heart disease, 1061–1062

vocational rehabilitation, 731, 732

Enalapril, **349, 944**

Encainide, 951

Encephalitis, 688

anxiety and, 398

delirium and, 265

dementia and, 265

herpes simplex, 265, 688

sleep apnea and, 513

St. Louis type A, **345**

Encephalomyelitis

in Lyme disease, 575

paraneoplastic sensory neuropathy, 682

Encephalopathy

computerized electroencephalography in, 56

hepatic, 258, 263, 627–628, 640

HIV, **345**

hypertensive, 265

hypoxic, **816**

limbic, 280, 682–683

pancreatic, **284**

portosystemic, **284**

posttraumatic, **345**

progressive multifocal leukoencephalopathy, 282

subcortical arteriosclerotic, 53

uremic, **284,** 560–561

Wernicke's, 263, 265, 283, 296, 426, 901

End-of-life decisions, 167. *See also* Dying patients

advance directives for, 169, **174,** 175–176, 187–189

discontinuing dialysis, 559–560

do-not-resuscitate orders, 175, 778

ethics of, 778

palliative care, **173,** 173–175, **174**

physician-assisted suicide and euthanasia, 144–146, 175, 789–791, **790,** 831

psychiatric aspects of excellent end-of-life care, 805–806

right to die, 174–175, 790

End-stage renal disease (ESRD). *See* Dialysis patients; Renal failure

Endicott Substitution Criteria, 784, **784**

Endocarditis

cocaine-related, 243, 441

opioid-related, 436

Endocrine disorders, 563–567

acromegaly, 567

Addison's disease, 566

anxiety disorders and, 397–398, 563

Cushing's syndrome, 566

dementia and, **284,** 288

depression and, **310, 311,** 320–321, 563

diabetes mellitus, 564

differential diagnosis of, 563

eating disorders and, 486–487

hyperparathyroidism, 566

hyperthyroidism, 564

hypothyroidism, 564

mania and, 563

pheochromocytoma, 566–567

pituitary tumors and, 682

psychiatric comorbidity with, 245, 563–564, **564**

psychosis due to, **896**

psychotropic drug use and, **976**

sexual dysfunction and, 457–458

sleep disorders and, 504, 511

Endometrial cancer, 457

Endotracheal intubation, 765

Enflurane, **944**

Engel, George, 6

Entitled demanders, 109–110

Environmental interventions

to decrease suicide in hospitals, 130, 131

for delirium, **266,** 268

for dementia, 297–298

for elderly persons, 865

in intensive care unit, 757–758

Eosinophilia, clozapine-induced, 966

Epidemiologic Catchment Area (ECA) study, 134, 195, 240, 339, 369, 395, 396, 422, 907, 908

Epidemiologic studies

cross-sectional, **192,** 194–195

longitudinal, **192, 195,** 195–197

case-control studies, 195–196

cohort studies, 196–197

of series of patients referred for psychiatric consultation, 245–249

MICRO-CARES database studies, 41, 206, 218, 221, 246, **247**

University of Iowa study, 246–249, **247–249**

Epidemiology

of alcohol use disorders, 422–423

of anorexia nervosa, 477–479

Epidemiology *(continued)*
of anxiety disorders, 395–397, **396**
of body dysmorphic disorder, 381
of bulimia nervosa, 480
of chronic pain, 997
of cocaine-related disorders, 440
of conversion disorder, 379
of delirium, 258–260, **259**
of dementia, 275–277
of factitious disorders, 521
of gastrointestinal disorders, 552
of HIV/AIDS, 808–809
of hypochondriasis, 377
of malingering, 526
of mania, 339–342
of neurological and neurosurgical
disorders, 679, **680**
of opioid-related disorders, 436
of pain disorder, 382
of personality disorders, 119–120,
243
of psychiatric disorders in medically
ill patients, 237–252
anxiety disorders, 242
clinical population studies of,
240–241
mood disorders, 241
multiple psychiatric disorders,
240–241
course and outcome, 249–251
of anxiety disorders, 250–251
of depression, 249–250
of medical illnesses, 251
of personality disorders, 251
of substance use disorders, 251
economic effects of psychiatric
illness in primary care,
251–252
general population studies of, 240
methodological issues in, **237,**
237–238
models of medical-psychiatric
comorbidity, 238–240, **239**
other psychiatric disorders, 244
personality disorders, 243
risk factors, 249
somatoform disorders, 243–244
specific medical populations,
244–245
cancer, 245
diabetes and endocrine
disorders, 245
gastrointestinal disease, 245
respiratory disease, 244–245
seizure disorders, 244
stroke, 244

traumatic brain injury, 244
studies of series of patients
referred for psychiatric
consultation, 245–249
MICRO-CARES database
studies, 41, 206, 218,
221, 246, **247**
University of Iowa study,
246–249, **247–249**
substance use disorders, 242–243,
243
summary of, 252
of psychiatric disorders in primary
care, 917–918
of seizures, 683
of somatization disorder, 374
of suicidality, 127–131, **128–130**
of undifferentiated somatoform
disorder, 376
Epilepsy, 683–685. *See also* Seizures
definition of, 683
depression and, 241, **310, 311,** 318,
319, 683
electroencephalography in, 683, 691
episodic dyscontrol syndrome and,
684
generalized, 511
interictal behavioral syndrome, 685
Lafora's myoclonic, 687
morpheic, 511
partial, 512
prevalence of, **680,** 683
psychotropic drug use in patients
with
antidepressants, 693, **693**
antipsychotics, 692
β-blockers, 692
lithium, 694
rolandic, 512
schizophreniform psychosis of,
683–684
sleep disorders and, 504, 511–512
suicide and, 129
Epinephrine
drug interactions with
antidepressants, **943,** 953
antipsychotics, **944,** 969
in fight-or-flight response, 536
Episodic dyscontrol syndrome, 684
EPQ (Eysenck Personality
Questionnaire), 209
EPS. *See* Extrapyramidal symptoms
Epstein-Barr virus (EBV) infection, 321,
571, 574
Erectile dysfunction. *See* Sexual
dysfunction

Ergoloid mesylates, for Alzheimer's
disease, 297
Ergotamine, 1068
Erythema migrans, 575
Erythromycin interactions, **943**
with benzodiazepines, 505
with carbamazepine, **349**
cytochrome P450 metabolism and,
946
with immunosuppressants, 643
Esmolol, 1021
Esophageal disorders, 114
alcohol-related cancer, **243**
eating disorders and, 482, 483
motility disorders, 553–554
stress and, 1062
psychiatric complications of, **594**
ESRD (end-stage renal disease). *See*
Dialysis patients; Renal failure
Estazolam, **970**
dosage of, **407, 434, 970**
half-life of, **407**
for insomnia, 505, **506**
interaction with ritonavir, **815**
Estrogen
for Alzheimer's disease, 296
changes at menopause, 702, **703**
effect on mood, 703
in hormone replacement therapy, 703
interaction with benzodiazepines,
505
for sexual disorders, 471
side effects of, 471
anxiety, **400**
sexual dysfunction, **462**
Ethchlorvynol, **434, 904**
Ethical issues, 9, 167–168. *See also* Legal
issues
discontinuing dialysis, 559–560
end-of-life decisions, 778
fetal vs. maternal rights, 707
in management of factitious
disorders, 525
physician-assisted suicide and
euthanasia, 144–146, 175,
789–791, **790,** 831
in research, 200
in transplantation surgery, 626, 631
Ethosuximide, **400, 462**
Ethoxzolamide, **462**
Ethylene oxide, **284**
Etretinate, **462**
Euphoria
delirium and, 262
drug-induced
alcohol, 424

cannabis, 444
cocaine, 440
inhalants, 446
methadone, 438
nicotine, 445
phencyclidine, 443
psychostimulants, 442, 957
mania and, 339, 342
European Association for Consultation-
Liaison Psychiatry and
Psychosomatics (EACLPP), 206
European consultation-liaison
psychiatry, 207–217
German-speaking countries, 204,
209–212
Netherlands, 214–215
Nordic countries, 207–209
southern European and
Mediterranean countries,
215–217
United Kingdom, 212–213
European studies, 221–225
European Consultation-Liaison
Workgroup (ECLW)
Collaborative Study, 206, 208,
214, 216, 221–222, **223**
INTERMED, 223–225, **225**
quality management study, 225
risk factor study, 222–223, **224**
Euthanasia and physician-assisted
suicide, 144–146, 175, 789–791,
790, 831
Euthyroid sick syndrome, 485, 487
Evidence-based telepsychiatry,
929–930. *See also* Telepsychiatry
Evoked potentials, 56–57, 77
Ewing's sarcoma, 671
Examination style, 14–15
Excessive daytime somnolence (EDS),
507, **507.** *See also* Narcolepsy
Executive function deficits. *See also*
Cognitive impairment
in Alzheimer's disease, 277, **278**
assessment for, 290
in delirium, 261
in frontotemporal dementia, 278
in Huntington's disease, 278
in vascular dementia, **280**
Executive Interview (EXIT), 294
Exercise
for hypertension, 1060
for ischemic heart disease,
1058–1059
for nicotine dependence, 445
physiological and psychological
benefits of, 1059

for somatoform disorders, 384
EXIT (Executive Interview), 294
Exophthalmos, lithium-induced, 959
Expanded psychiatric consultation, **6**
Expectation bias in research, **199**
Exploitation of elderly persons, 859, **860**
Extracorporeal membrane oxygenation,
604
Extrapyramidal symptoms (EPS), drug-
induced, 408, 686, 691
amoxapine, 951
antiemetics, 604
antipsychotics, **964,** 965–968
intravenous haloperidol, 267
risperidone, 354
clozapine for, 966
neuroleptic malignant syndrome, 968
in patients with HIV/AIDS, 825
rating scale for, 966, **967**
selective serotonin reuptake
inhibitors, 952
tardive phenomena, 966–968
Extroversion, **116**
Eysenck Personality Questionnaire
(EPQ), 209

Facial pain, 954, 1004
Factitious disorders, 4, 115–116,
519–526
by adult proxy, **520**
asthma, 550
with combined physical and
psychological symptoms, 523
compared with malingering, 519, **520**
diagnosis and differential diagnosis of,
524, **524**
differentiation from somatoform
disorders, 373
conversion disorder, 380
pain disorder, 383
somatization disorder, 376
undifferentiated somatoform
disorder, 377
DSM-IV classification of, 519
epidemiology of, 521
etiology of, 524, **524**
extreme variants of, **520**
genital manipulation and, 469
literature on, 519
management of, 525–526
confrontation, 525–526
ethical and legal issues, 525, **525**
psychotherapy, 526
not otherwise specified, 523–524
personality disorders and,
120–121, 523

with predominantly physical
symptoms, 521–523, **522, 1000,**
1003
with predominantly psychological
symptoms, 523
prognosis for, 526
by proxy, **520,** 521, 523–526
psychodynamic explanations for,
524
somatization and, 115, **362,** 365
in surgical patients, 596
systemic lupus erythematosus, 521
Family studies. *See also* Genetic factors
of alcoholism, 423
of dementia, 277
of smoking behavior, 445
of somatization, 368
Family therapy and support, **1034**
for agitation and aggression, 157
for anxiety, 410
for asthma, 1066
for bulimia nervosa, 489
for cancer, 671–672
for cardiothoracic surgery, 606
for dementia, 298
for depression, 329–330
for disfiguring head and neck surgery,
617
for elderly persons, 865
for HIV/AIDS, 833
in hospital pediatric units, 719
for neurological disease, 695
in rehabilitation settings, 739, **740,**
745
for somatoform disorders, 387
for substance-related disorders, 420
for terminal illness and death, 779
Family violence, 711–712, 908–909
Famotidine, **462**
Fat, dietary, 1058
Fat emulsion, **462**
Fatigue, 570–576
anxiety and, 570
causes of, 570, **571**
chronic fatigue syndrome, 571–576
depression and, **310,** 321, 570
drug-induced
gabapentin, 961
lithium, 959
psychostimulants, 956
risperidone, 354
dyspnea and, 546
fibromyalgia and, 570–571
high-tension, 570
laboratory evaluation of, 570, **571**
in postconcussion syndrome, 685

Fatigue *(continued)*
    radiation therapy–associated,
        665–666
    suicidality and, 788
FDA (Food and Drug Administration),
    170–171
Fear. *See also* Anxiety; Panic attacks
    acute pain and, 997
    of critically ill patients, 759
    of death, 771, 781
    delirium and, 262
    of disease, 377–378, 1041, **1041** (*See
        also* Hypochondriasis)
    after disfiguring head and neck
        surgery, 616
    of dyspnea, 546
    of impending surgery, 541, 593, 604
    phobias, 404
Fellowships, 18–19, **19**, 30
Fenfluramine
    mania induced by, **345**
    sexual dysfunction induced by, **462**
Fenofibrate, sexual dysfunction induced
    by, **462**
Fentanyl
    abuse of, 435
    for burn patients, 612
    delirium due to, 265
    interaction with ritonavir, **815**
    for terminally ill patients, **797**
Fertility, 705–706
    cancer and, 666–669
    eating disorders and, 705
    prevalence of problems with, 705
Fever
    in delirium tremens, 901
    drug-induced
        clozapine, 966
        MDMA, 443
        in neuroleptic malignant
            syndrome, 692, 968
        opioid withdrawal, 437
        phencyclidine, 443
        selective serotonin reuptake
            inhibitors, 952
        in serotonin syndrome, 953
    in encephalitis, 688
    malignant hyperthermia, **597**
    in meningitis, 688
Feverfew, **974**
Fibromyalgia, 570–571
    anxiety and, 571
    cognitive-behavioral therapy for,
        1070
    definition of, 570, 571
    depression and, 571

diagnostic criteria for, 571
    fatigue and, 571
    irritable bowel syndrome and, 571
    pharmacotherapy for, 571
        antidepressants, 693
    prevalence of, 997
    sleep disorders and, 504, 513, 571
    trigger point locations in, 571, **572**
Fibrositis syndrome, 513
Fight-or-flight response, 394, 536–537,
    547
Financial support for consultation-liaison
    psychiatry, 7–9
Financial viability of consultation-liaison
    service, **27**, 27–31
Finasteride, **462**
Finland, consultation-liaison psychiatry
    in, 207–209
Fioricet, Fiorinal, **904**. *See also* Butalbital
Fire deaths, alcohol-related, **243**
FK-506, 641–643
Flashbacks, drug-induced
    hallucinogens, 443, 905
    phencyclidine, 443
Flecainide, **945**, 951
Fluconazole, 643, 815, **946**
Flumazenil, 400, 435, 971
Flunitrazepam, 434
Fluorescent treponemal antibody (FTA)
    test, 576
5-Fluorouracil, **667**, 793
Fluoxetine, 948
    active metabolite of, 326, 786, **945**,
        949
    dosage and administration of, **948**,
        950
    drug interactions with, 786
        benzodiazepines, 505
        codeine, **999**
        cytochrome P450 metabolism
            and, 326, **945**, **949**, 952
        digitoxin, **943**
        monoamine oxidase inhibitors,
            954
        ritonavir, 814
    half-life of, 326, 786, **949**
    indications for, 171
        agitation and aggression, 161–162
        Alzheimer's disease, 296
        hypochondriasis, 384
        paraphilias, 471
        smoking cessation, 1061
    receptor site affinity of, **948**
    side effects of, 786
        insomnia, **502**, 505
        parkinsonism, 686

sexual dysfunction, **462**
    structure of, 947
    suicidality and, 141, 952
    use in specific patient groups or
        medical conditions
        breast-feeding women, **981**
        cancer, 663
        cardiac disease, 408, 542, 951
        children, **723**, 952
        critically ill patients, 761
        dialysis patients, 561
        dying patients, **785**, 786
        elderly persons, 863, **863**
        HIV/AIDS, 828–829
        irritable bowel syndrome, 556
        neurogenic bladder with
            retention, 693
        Parkinson's disease, 693
        pregnancy, **708**, 979
        stroke, 741
        transplant patients, **636**, 643
    withdrawal from, 953
Fluoxymesterone, **667**
Flupentixol, 1007
Fluphenazine, **964**
    cytochrome P450 metabolism and,
        945
    dosage of, **964**
    for pain syndromes, 1008
    side effects of, **964**
        sexual dysfunction, **462**
    use in specific patient groups or
        medical conditions
        epilepsy, 692
        Parkinson's disease, 691
Fluphenazine decanoate, 963
Flurazepam, 407, **903**, **970**
    dosage of, **407**, **434**, **903**, **970**
    half-life of, **407**, **903**
    for insomnia, **506**
    interaction with ritonavir, **815**
Fluvoxamine
    for bulimia nervosa, 489
    drug interactions with
        cytochrome P450 metabolism
            and, **945**, **949**, 952
        ritonavir, 814, **815**
    for elderly persons, 863, **863**
    half-life of, **949**
    for obsessive-compulsive disorder,
        969
    sexual dysfunction induced by, **462**
    structure of, 947
    use in specific patient groups or
        medical conditions
        breast-feeding women, **981**

dying patients, **785,** 786
hepatic disease, 427
pregnancy, 979
Folate deficiency, **284**
Follicle-stimulating hormone (FSH), 471
Folliculitis, lithium-induced, 959
Follow-up visits
billing for, 29
in intensive care unit, 758–759
in primary care clinics, 920
with somatizing patients, 372
with suicidal patients, 141–142
Food and Drug Administration (FDA), 170–171
Food-drug interactions
cytochrome P450 metabolism and, **945**
grapefruit juice, **945**
tyramine and monoamine oxidase inhibitors, 327, 543–544, 954, 955
Formaldehyde, **284**
Fortovase. *See* Saquinavir
Forward Digit Span test, 66
Foster care, 711
France, consultation-liaison psychiatry in, 215–217
Frank Jones story, 72
"Freebasing," 440
Freud, Sigmund, 1027
Friedreich's ataxia, 687
Frontal Assessment Battery, 294
Frontal convexity syndrome, 682
Frontal lobe syndromes, 685, 688
Frontotemporal dementia, 273, 275
clinical features of, 277–278
genetic factors in, 277
neuroimaging in, 293
pathophysiology of, 286
FSH (follicle-stimulating hormone), 471
FTA (fluorescent treponemal antibody) test, 576
Functional Assessment of Cancer Therapy Scale, 94
Functional Assessment of Chronic Illness Therapy-Spiritual Well-Being scale, 776
Functional capacity assessment, 731–732
Furosemide, 348
Future of consultation-liaison psychiatry, 9
in Brazil, 220–221
in German-speaking countries, 211–212

in Japan, 220
in Netherlands, 215
in Nordic countries, 209
in southern European and Mediterranean countries, 217
in United Kingdom, 213

G proteins, 436
GABA. *See* γ-Aminobutyric acid
Gabapentin, **958,** 960–962
dosage and administration of, **347,** 352, **958,** 961
half-life of, **347,** 352
indications for
Alzheimer's disease, 296
insomnia, 505
mania, **347,** 352
pain syndromes, 1006
mechanism of action of, 352, 960
overdose of, 962
pharmacokinetics of, 352, 960, 962
side effects of, 352, 961
use in specific patient groups or medical conditions
brain injury, 961
chronic pain syndrome, 693, **693**
HIV/AIDS, 839
neurological disease, 694
patients undergoing rehabilitation, **742**
transplant candidates, **635**
Gait abnormalities
in Parkinson's disease, 685
in progressive supranuclear palsy, 280
in vascular dementia, **280**
in Wilson's disease, 279
Galactorrhea, 965, 978
Galantamine, 297
Gallstones, medroxyprogesterone acetate–induced, 471
Gamma rays, 51
Ganciclovir, **818**
Gangliosides, **743**
Ganser's "syndrome of approximate answers," 275, 285, 523
Garlic, **974**
Gas exchange, 546
Gastrointestinal disorders, 552–556, 1062–1063
behavioral medicine and, 1062–1063
bulimia nervosa and, 487
cancer
brain metastases from, **681**
central nervous system paraneoplastic syndromes and, 682

suicidality and, 131
chronic gastritis, 552
diagnostic criteria for, 552
epidemiology of, 552
esophageal dysfunction, 553–554, 1062
functional dyspepsia, 1062
gastroesophageal reflux, 504, 513
gender distribution of, 552
globus sensation, 553
history of abuse and, 114–115, 552
inflammatory bowel disease, 556, 1063
irritable bowel syndrome, **554,** 554–556, **555,** 1062–1063
mucous colitis, 552
personality and, 114–115
psychopathology and, 245, 552–553, **594,** 1062–1063
psychotherapy for patients with, 1032
psychotropic drug use in, 601, **975,** 977
sleep disorders and, 504, 513
spastic colon, 552
Gastrointestinal effects, **975,** 977
of buspirone, 409
of lamotrigine, 353
of lithium, 350, 958
of methadone, 438
of nefazodone, 327
of nicotine, 445
of opioid withdrawal, 438
of risperidone, 354
of selective serotonin reuptake inhibitors, 326, 829
of tricyclic antidepressants, 325
of valproate, 350
of venlafaxine, 326
Gemfibrozil, **462**
Gender
alcoholism and, 422, 424
gastrointestinal disorders and, 552
seizures and, 683
somatization and, 369
Gender identity, 702
Gender identity disorders, 468–469
countertransference reactions to patients with, 469
depression and, 469
differential diagnosis of, **469**
medical and surgical treatments for, **470**
General Health Questionnaire (GHQ), 209, 244, 251, 406, **407**
General Hospital Psychiatry, 7
General paresis, 345

Generalized anxiety disorder, 403
    age at onset of, **63**, 403
    antidepressants for, **950**, 969, 972
    cancer and, 780
    clinical course of, 403
    clinical features of, 403
    diabetes mellitus and, 397, 403
    diagnosis of, 395
    differentiation from somatization
        disorder, 376
    among dying patients, 781
    esophageal motility disorders and, 553
    hyperthyroidism and, 398, 403
    insomnia and, 500
    irritable bowel syndrome and, 555,
        555
    migraine headache and, 398
    poststroke, 250–251, 398, 681
    prevalence of, **396**
    somatization and, **362**
Generic drugs, 941
Genetic factors
    alcoholism and, 423
    Alzheimer's disease and, 276, 277
    bipolar disorder and, 341–342
    cannabis dependence and, 444
    frontotemporal dementias and, 277,
        286
    heroin abuse and, 436
    Huntington's disease and, 277, 286,
        686
    obesity and, 1059
    Parkinson's disease and, 277
    smoking and, 445
    somatization and, 368
    stress, hypertension and, 538
    suicide and, 134, **136**
    Wilson's disease and, 277, 279
Genitalia
    female, 702
        injuries due to rape, 712
    manipulations and injuries of,
        468–470
Geodon. See Ziprasidone
Geriatric Depression Scale, 93, 733
Geriatric medicine, 853–866. See also
    Elderly persons
German Association of Psychologists,
    210
German College of Psychosomatic
    Medicine, 210
German Psychiatric Association, 210
German-speaking countries,
    consultation-liaison psychiatry in,
    204–206, 209–212
    background of, 209

future development, 211–212
    official status and training, 210–211
    psychological medicine in general
        hospital, 209–210
    research, 211
GHQ (General Health Questionnaire),
    209, 244, 251, 406, **407**
Giessener symptom distress checklist,
    209
Ginger, **974**
Ginkgo biloba, **974**
Ginseng, 973, **974**
Glaucoma, 611, 951
Glioblastomas, **681**
Gliomas, **345, 346, 681**
Global Assessment of Functioning Scale,
    929
Globus sensation, 552, 553
L-Glutamine, **345**
Glutethimide, **434, 462, 904**
Glycopyrrolate, **462**
Goiter, 511, 959
Gold poisoning, **284**
Gonadotropin-releasing hormone
    agents, 471
Good Samaritan standards, 596
Goserelin, **462**, 471
Granisetron, **669**
Granulovacuolar degeneration, 286
Grapefruit juice–drug interactions,
    945–946
Graves' disease, 403. See also
    Hyperthyroidism
Greece, consultation-liaison psychiatry
    in, 215–217
Grepafloxacin, **462**
Grief
    anticipatory, of dying patients, 778, 779
    due to pregnancy loss, 710–711
    HIV/AIDS and, 828
    in intensive care settings, 760
    in rehabilitation settings, 735
Griseofulvin, 427, **428, 943**
Group practice in consultation-liaison
    psychiatry, 20
Group therapy, 1032, **1034**
    for bulimia nervosa, 489
    for cancer patients, 329, 664
    for cocaine dependence, 442
    indications for, 1032
    for patients with cardiac disease, 540,
        542
    for patients with HIV/AIDS, 329,
        833, 1032
    for patients with ischemic heart
        disease, 1057

in rehabilitation settings, 745
    for somatization, 373
    for somatoform disorders, 386
Growth hormone
    in anorexia nervosa, 487
    type A behavior and, 539
Guanabenz, **462**
Guanadrel, **462**, 955
Guanethidine
    drug interactions with
        antidepressants, **943**
        antipsychotics, **944**, 969
        monoamine oxidase inhibitors,
            955
        psychostimulants, 957, **957**
    side effects of
        depression, 322
        sexual dysfunction, **462**
Guanfacine, **462**
Guardianship, 176–177
Guided imagery
    for dying patients, 783
    after head and neck surgery, 615
    for insomnia, 504
    for surgical patients, 601
Guillain-Barré syndrome, 568, 690, 737
Guilt, 111, 113
Gynecology. See Obstetrics and
    gynecology
Gynecomastia, 978

HAART (highly active antiretroviral
    therapy), 810–813, 823–824. See
    also Antiretroviral therapy
Hachinski Ischemia Score, **281**
HAD (Hospital Anxiety Depression
    Questionnaire), 209
Hair loss, drug-induced
    lithium, 959
    selective serotonin reuptake
        inhibitors, 952
    valproate, 961
Halazepam, **407**
Halcion. See Triazolam
Haldol. See Haloperidol
Half-life of drug, 942
Hallervorden-Spatz disease, 687
Hallucinations
    in alcohol-induced psychotic
        disorder, 426
    in Alzheimer's disease, 858
    in amphetamine psychosis, 442
    in amyotrophic lateral sclerosis, 319
    antipsychotics for, 962
    assessment for, 64
    auditory, 64–65

benzodiazepine-withdrawal, 971
cocaine-induced, 441
in delirium tremens, 424, 901
hypnagogic, 509
limbic encephalopathy and, 280
mania and, 342
other types of, 65
in Parkinson's disease, 279
in schizophrenia, 64–65
suicide and, 133, 138
tactile, 65
in vascular dementia, 281
visual, 65
    brain tumors and, 682
    in transplant recipients, 642
    in visually impaired patients, 610
Hallucinogen-related disorders, **345,**
    443, 905
Haloperidol, **763, 964**
    benzodiazepines combined with, 408
    discontinuation of, 969
    dosage of, 159, **763,** 963, **964**
    drug interactions with
        cytochrome P450 metabolism
            and, **945**
        lithium, 960
    indications for
        acute psychosis, 896–897
        agitation and aggression, 159, **160,**
            408, 899
        alcohol withdrawal symptoms,
            431, 432, **433**
        Alzheimer's disease, 296
        cocaine psychosis, 441
        delirium, **266,** 267, 268,
            793–794, **794**
        pain syndromes, **989,** 1007
        phencyclidine intoxication, 906
        rapid tranquilization, 965
        schizophrenia, 159
        stimulant-induced psychosis, 957
    intramuscular, 897
    intravenous, **266,** 267, 268, 794
        contraindications to, 897
        for delirium, **266,** 267, 268
        in emergency department, 896–
            897
        extrapyramidal symptoms and,
            267
    psychiatric aspects of, **669**
    side effects of, **964**
        sexual dysfunction, **462**
    subcutaneous, 794
    use in specific patient groups or
        medical conditions
        breast-feeding women, **981**

burn patients, 612
cardiac disease, 544
children, **723**
critically ill patients, 761–762,
    965
dying patients, 782, **782,**
    793–794, **794**
elderly persons, **863**
HIV/AIDS, 825, 826
Parkinson's disease, 691
patients undergoing rehabilitation,
    743
patients with cardiac assist
    devices, 604
pregnancy, **708**
stroke, 741
surgical patients, **597**
transplant recipients, 641
Haloperidol decanoate, 963
Halstead-Reitan Neuropsychological
    Test Battery (HRNTB), 80, **81,** 82,
    157
Hamilton Anxiety Scale (HAS), **371,**
    406, **407**
Hamilton Rating Scale for Depression,
    93, **371,** 1018
Handicapping conditions
    definition of handicap, 730
    prevalence of psychiatric comorbidity
        with, 240
HAS (Hamilton Anxiety Scale), **371,**
    406, **407**
Hashish, 444, 906
Hawthorne effect, **199**
Hay fever, 1065–1066
HCFA (Health Care Financing
    Administration), 18, 40
Head and neck cancer, 670
Head and neck surgery, 614–617
    family problems and, 617
    for patients with primary psychiatric
        disorders, 614–615
    preparing patients for, 614
    psychiatric contraindications to, 614
    psychiatric disorders secondary to,
        615–616
        anxiety, 615, **615**
        delirium, 616
        depression, 615
    reactions to loss and body image
        problems after, 616–617
    staff issues related to, 617
    substance withdrawal and, 617
Head trauma. *See* Brain injury
Headache, 362
    behavioral medicine and, 1068–1070

cognitive-behavioral therapy for,
    1068–1069
drug-induced
    antiretroviral drugs, 812
    buspirone, 409
    lamotrigine, 353, 961
    naltrexone, 432
    nefazodone, 327
    nicotine, 445
    psychostimulants, 956, 957
    selective serotonin reuptake
        inhibitors, 761, 829, 951
    sildenafil, 460
hypercapnia and, 546
in meningitis, 688
in neurosyphilis, 576
outpatient medical-psychiatric
    treatment for, 874
pharmacotherapy for, 1068
in postconcussion syndrome, 685
prevalence of, 997
systemic lupus erythematosus and,
    568
among transplant recipients, 642
vascular
    anxiety and, 397, 398
    sleep disorders and, 504, 512
Health care costs. *See also* Economic issues
    "cost-offset" of psychiatric care,
        37–38, **872**
    effect of consultation-liaison services
        on, 26–27, 37
    effect of psychiatric illness on, 25–26,
        251–252, 871, **872**
    for neuroimaging studies, 52
    psychiatric treatment costs in general
        medical vs. specialty mental
        health settings, 27
Health Care Financing Administration
    (HCFA), 18, 40
Health Care for the Homeless, 910
Health care professionals. *See also*
    Psychiatric consultant
    "angels of death," 519
    factitious disorders among, 521
    opioid dependence among, 435
    psychiatric nurse practitioners, 1028
    psychotherapeutic skills of, 1028
    triage nurses, 891
Health care proxy, 168, 175–176,
    187–189. *See also* Substituted
    judgment
Health maintenance organizations
    (HMOs), 182
Health-related quality-of-life scales,
    93–94, **95**

Health Resources Services
  Administration, 42
Heart disease. *See* Cardiac disease
Heavy metal toxicity, **284, 400, 502**
Heldt, Thomas J., 4
Helicobacter pylori infection, 569
Helplessness, 110–111, 537, 616
Hematological disorders, 978
  in anorexia nervosa, 483, 486
  drug-induced, **976,** 978
    antipsychotics, 966, 978
    carbamazepine, 351, 961, 978
    clozapine, 966, 978
    lithium, 959
    mirtazapine, 327, 953
    tricyclic antidepressants, 951,
      978
    valproate, 350, 351, 978
  hyperviscosity syndrome, 665
Hematoma
  epidural, 679
  subdural, 265, 281, 679, 891
Hemineglect, 735
Hemiplegia
  in Lyme disease, 575
  psychogenic, 689
Hemodialysis. *See* Dialysis patients
Hemophilia, 809
Hemorrhage
  intraparenchymal, 265
  stroke due to, 679
  subarachnoid, 265, 441, **680,** 690
  vascular dementia and, 280
Henry, George W., 5
"Hepatic dialysis," 633
Hepatic disease
  alcohol-related, 239, 242, **243,** 426
    liver transplantation for, 427
  cocaine-related, 243, 441
  delirium and, 258, 259
  dementia and, **284**
  insomnia and, 504
  intravenous opioid abuse and, 436
  psychotropic drug use in, 757, **975,**
    977
    benzodiazepines, 407, 504
    carbamazepine, 351
    fluvoxamine, 427
    lithium, 427
    methadone, 438
    nefazodone, 427
    pemoline, 787
    sildenafil, 460
    valproate, 351
Hepatic drug metabolism, 942
  aging and, 861, **862**

Hepatic effects, **975,** 977
  of antipsychotics, 966
  of carbamazepine, 351
  of dantrolene, 968
  of pemoline, 956
  of selective serotonin reuptake
    inhibitors, 952
  of tricyclic antidepressants, 951
  of valproate, 350–351, 961
Hepatic encephalopathy, 258, 263
  insomnia and, 504
  before and after liver transplantation,
    627–628, 640
  use of benzodiazepines in, 641
Hepatitis B
  cocaine-related, 243, 441
  fatigue and, 575
Hepatitis C
  alcoholism and, 426
  cocaine-related, 243, 441
  interferon for, 1065
  intravenous opioid abuse and, 436
Hepatocerebral degeneration, **284**
Herbal medicinals, 973, **974**
Heroin, 435–438, **437, 462, 895,** 904,
  993. *See also* Opioid-related
  disorders
Herpes simplex virus infection
  encephalitis, 265, 688
  postherpetic neuralgia, 1004, 1006,
    1008
Hexamethonium, **462**
Hexocyclium, **462**
HHV-6 (human herpesvirus-6)
  infection, 575
5-HIAA (5-hydroxyindoleacetic acid),
  489, 858
Hiatal hernia, 504
Highly active antiretroviral therapy
  (HAART), 810–813, 823–824. *See
  also* Antiretroviral therapy
Hip fracture, 26, 37, 608, 974
  benefits of psychiatric consultation
    after, 855
  delirium after surgery for, 257, 259,
    269
  long-term benzodiazepine use and
    risk of, 399
  prevalence of psychiatric morbidity
    after, 608
Hippocratic oath, 167
Histamine H$_2$ receptor antagonists, **284,**
  311, 323, **762**
History of consultation-liaison
  psychiatry, 3–9
  conceptual-development phase of, 6–7

international perspectives, 203–204
  organizational phase of, 5–6
  rapid-growth phase of, 7–8
History taking, 15
  for agitation and aggression, 156–157
  for dementia, 291
  for depression, 312
  in intensive care unit, 754
  for substance-related disorders,
    419–420, **420**
  for suicidality, 134
Histrionic personality disorder, **116**
  comorbidity with other personality
    disorders, 119
  prevalence of, **120**
  somatization and, 120, 375
HIV infection. *See* Human
  immunodeficiency virus infection
  and acquired immunodeficiency
  syndrome
HLCS (Multi Dimensional Health
  Locus of Control Scale), 209
HMOs (health maintenance
  organizations), 182
Hodgkin's disease, 671
Homatropine, **462**
Homeless persons, 909–910
  HIV disease among, 809, 838
  substance abuse among, 909, 910
Homicide, 150, **243.** *See also* Aggression
Hoover's test, 371
Hopelessness, 138–140, 784, 1055
Horizontally integrated medical-
  psychiatry services, 873
Hormone replacement therapy, 703
Hospice care, 777
Hospital Anxiety Depression
  Questionnaire (HAD), 209
Hospital Anxiety/Depression Scale, 398
Hospitalization, psychiatric
  for factitious disorders, 525
  involuntary, 168, 179
  leaving against medical advice, 179
  as risk factor for suicide, 133, **133,**
    134
  of suicidal patients, 140–142, **142,**
    144
  dying patients, 791
  voluntary, 168, 178–179
Hospitals, general
  aggression among patients in, 149
  development of psychiatric units in,
    3–4, 7
  effecting structural changes in, 41–42
  emergency department of, 889–913
  length of stay in

delirium and, 257, 269
effect of consultation-liaison
services on, 26, 36–37
hypnotic drug use and, 500
psychiatric comorbidity and, 9,
25–26, 35–36, 876, **876**
limitations of traditional approaches
to comorbid medical and
psychiatric illness in, 876
maintaining patient confidentiality in,
168–169
management of dementia in,
297–298
medical-psychiatric units in, 41, 871
(*See also* Integrated medical-
psychiatry services)
mental disorders among elderly
persons in, 853, 854, **855**
mental status testing in, 62
organization of consultation-liaison
service in teaching hospitals,
18–20
pediatric units in, 719
prevalence of psychiatric comorbidity
among patients in, 9, 25, 871,
872
psychiatric interventions in, 36–38
psychiatric treatment costs in, 27
psychosocial factors associated with
admission to, 36
psychotherapy in, 1040, **1041**
suicidality among patients in,
130–131
value of consultation-liaison service
to, 25–27
Hostility. *See* Anger
"Hot flashes," 471, 702
HRNTB (Halstead-Reitan
Neuropsychological Test Battery),
80, **81,** 82, 157
Human herpesvirus-6 (HHV-6)
infection, 575
Human immunodeficiency virus (HIV)
infection and acquired
immunodeficiency syndrome
(AIDS), 687, 807–840
access to care for, 840
adjustment disorders and, 831–833,
832
anxiolytics for, 833
coping styles and, 832
couples therapy for, 833
factors contributing to,
831–832
family and caregiver support
for, 833

group therapy and support groups
for, 833
psychoeducation for, 832
psychotherapy for, 832–833
aggressive behavior and, 149
anxiety disorders and, 398–399, 712,
781–782, 833–834
pharmacotherapy for, 834
prevalence of, 834
psychotherapy for, 834
behavioral medicine and, 807, 1065
chronic and persistent mental illness
and, 838–839
day treatment programs for, 839
pharmacotherapy for, 839
clinical course and progression of,
807, 809–810
acute seroconversion, 809
CD4$^+$ lymphocyte count, 807,
810, **810**
immune response and viral load,
809–810, **811**
considerations in psychiatric
management of, 807–808
depression and, 63, **310,** 319–320,
827–830
bereavement, unresolved grief
and, 828
diagnosis of, 828
differential diagnosis of, 827, **827**
drug-induced, **818**
electroconvulsive therapy for,
320, 830, 1022
factors contributing to, 827–828
laboratory evaluation in, 828
pharmacotherapy for, 320,
828–830
prevalence of, 827
psychotherapy for, 830
dying patients with, 771
epidemiology of, 808–809
factitious enactment of, 521
group therapy for persons with, 329
health care delivery for, 839–840
in hemophiliac patients, 809
in homeless persons, 809, 838
in infants and children, 712–713,
808–809
mania and, 343, 819, 825–827
drug-induced, **818**
etiologies of, 825–826
prevalence of, 826
treatment of, 826–827
medical management of, 807,
810–815
adherence to, 813–814

antiretroviral therapy, 810–812,
811
drug interactions with, 814–815,
815
drug resistance and, 813
in pregnancy, 809
principles of, 810
side effects of, 807, 812, **812,**
815–817, **818**
neurocognitive impairment in, 276,
282, 795–796, 817–824
behavior therapy for, 824
brain imaging in, 821, **822**
cerebrospinal fluid examination
and, 821
course and prognosis for, 296, 795
diagnosis of, 795–796, 820
HIV-1–associated dementia
complex, 282, 817–820
HIV-1–associated minor
cognitive/motor disorder,
282, 817, 820
morbidity associated with, 820
neuroimaging in, 293
neuropathophysiology of, 287,
822
neuropsychological testing for,
820–821
nomenclature for, 282, 817
pharmacotherapy for, 823–824
prevalence of, **680,** 795, 817
psychotherapy for, 824
risk factors for, 818
staging system for, 817–818, **819**
symptoms of, 795, 818
neuropsychiatric syndromes in, **594,**
815–817
CD4$^+$ lymphocyte count and, 815
central nervous system
dysfunction, **680,** 815
delirium, 259, **259,** 793, 795,
824–825, **825**
differential diagnosis of, 815, **816**
due to drug side effects, 815–817,
818
management of, 817
opportunistic infections in, 807, 810
central nervous system, 815, **817**
meningitis, 688
opportunistic infections and
syphilis, 576
pain syndromes in, 835–836, **836**
assessment of, 835–836
peripheral neuropathy, 836
in terminal stage of disease, 836
personality and, 114

Human immunodeficiency virus (HIV)
   infection and acquired
   immunodeficiency syndrome
   (AIDS) (continued)
in pregnancy, 712–713, 809
primary prevention of, 807, 1065
psychological distress associated
   with, 807, 1065
psychosis and, 838–839
   pharmacotherapy for, 839
psychotherapy for persons with, 808,
   824, 830, 832–834, 1032
psychotropic drug use in, 796, 807,
   823–824, 979
   anticonvulsants, 826–827, 839
   antidepressants, 320, 828–830
   antipsychotics, 409, 825, 839, 979
   anxiolytics, 833, 834
   drug interactions and, 814–815,
      815
   lithium, 826
   psychostimulants, 824, 829–830,
      956, 979
screening rape victims for, 712
sexual dysfunction and, 459–460,
   835
sleep disorders and, 834–835
   diagnosis of, 834
   primary disorders, 834
   secondary disorders, 834
   treatment of, 834–835
substance-related disorders and, 417,
   808, 809, 837–838
   cocaine, 243, 441, 837
   harm reduction prevention
      programs for, 837
   intravenous opioids, 436, 837–838
   management of, 837–838
   methadone maintenance for, 838
   prevalence of, 837
suicidality and, 129, **132**, 132–133,
   144, **144**, 319, 792, 830–831
   epidemiology of, 830
   euthanasia and physician-assisted
      suicide, 831
   management of, 831
   risk assessment for, 830–831, **831**
transmission of, 713
   blood transfusion, 809
   breast-feeding, 809
   injection drug use, 808
   perinatal, 712–713, 809
virology of, 809
in women, 712–713, 808
Humane and Dignified Death Act, 790
Huntingtin, 286

Huntington's disease, 278, 686
age at onset of, 295
anxiety and, 398
clinical features of, 278, 686
course and prognosis for, 295
depression and, 238, 241, 278, 308,
   310, 311, 317–318
genetic factors and, 277, 286, 686
juvenile, 688
mania and, **345**
neuroimaging in, 294
pathophysiology of, 286
prevalence of, **680**
psychiatric comorbidity with, 686
psychotropic drug use in patients with
   antidepressants, 318, 693, **693**
   β-blockers, 692
   neuroleptics, 692
sleep disorders and, 504, 512
suicidality and, 129, 278, 686
Hydergine, 297
Hydralazine, **400, 462**
Hydrocephalus
dementia and, **274,** 282
normal-pressure, 282
   neuroimaging in, 293
   shunting for, 296
sleep disorders and, 512
Hydrochlorothiazide, 349, **462**
Hydrocodone, 326, 438–439, **895, 995**
Hydrogen sulfide, **284**
Hydromorphone
abuse of, 904
dosage of, **437, 993**
duration of action of, **993**
duration of detectability in urine, **895**
for terminally ill patients, **797**
toxicity of, **994**
Hydroxybupropion, 326
Hydroxycodone, 326
5-Hydroxyindoleacetic acid (5-HIAA),
   489, 858
Hydroxyzine, **462,** 505, **506,** 973
Hyperactivity. See also Attention-
   deficit/hyperactivity disorder
delirium and, 257, 258, 262
Hyperammonemia, valproate-induced,
   351
Hyperamylasemia, 487
Hypercalcemia, 665
Hypercapnia, 546
Hypercortisolemia, 566
Hyperemesis gravidarum, 706
Hyperhidrosis, 1066. See also Sweating
Hypericum, **345,** 346
Hyperimmune disorders, 1065–1066

Hyperlipidemia, 536, 762
Hypernatremia, **284**
Hyperparathyroidism, **565,** 566
depression and, **311,** 320
lithium-induced, 959
prevalence of psychiatric comorbidity
   with, **564**
Hyperpathia, 991
Hyperprolactinemia, 965, 978
Hypersalivation, drug-induced
antipsychotics, 966
nicotine, 445
phencyclidine, 443
Hypersomnia, **496, 497,** 499, 682. See
   also Sleep disorders
Hypertension, 4, 537–538, 1060
drug-induced
   bupropion, 543, 952
   clozapine, 966
   cocaine, 441
   monoamine oxidase inhibitors,
      327, 543–544, 761, 954
   opioid withdrawal, 437
   phencyclidine, 443, 905
   psychostimulants, 442, 544, 761,
      787, 957
   venlafaxine, 326, 952
fight-or-flight response and, 536
genetic factors and, 538
ischemic heart disease and, 1060
nonpharmacological interventions
   for, 1060
sleep apnea and, 508
smoking and, 445
stress and, 537–538
Hypertensive encephalopathy, 265
Hyperthermia. See Fever
Hyperthyroidism, 564, **565**
anxiety and, **239,** 398, 403, 564
cerebrospinal fluid protein level in,
   690
depression and, 63, 308, **310, 311,**
   320, 564
lithium-induced, 959
mania and, **345, 346**
prevalence of psychiatric comorbidity
   with, **564**
sleep disorders and, 504, 511
Hyperventilation, anxiety-induced, 547
Hyperventilation syndrome, 1062
hypervigilance, 394
to bodily sensations, 363, 377
delirium and, 262
drug-induced
   amphetamines, 442
   cocaine, 440–441

Hyperviscosity syndrome, 665
Hypnotherapy
    for anxiety, 410
    for critically ill patients, 760
    for insomnia, 504
    for irritable bowel syndrome, 1063
    for pain syndromes, 1008
    for somatoform disorders, 385
Hypoactivity, delirium and, 257, 258, 262
Hypoalbuminemia, 259
Hypoalgesia, 991
Hypocapnia, 547
Hypochondriasis, 243–244, 373, 377–378
    age at onset of, 377
    clinical course and prognosis for, 378
    clinical features of, 377–378
    cognitive model of, **386**
    definition of, 377
    diagnostic criteria for, **377**
    differential diagnosis of, 378, 1002, **1002**
    epidemiology of, 377
    irritable bowel syndrome and, **555**
    management of, 383–387
    pain and, **1001,** 1002
    primary vs. secondary, 377
    psychiatric comorbidity with, 378
        depression, 367
        panic disorder, 242
        personality disorders, 120, 121, 378
    somatization and, 362, **362,** 367, 378
Hypoesthesia, 991
Hypoglycemia, 265
    anxiety due to, 780, **781**
    delirium and, 258, 756
    dementia and, 288
    lithium-induced, 959
    recurrent, **284**
Hypoglycemic agent interactions
    with alcohol, 427
    with monoamine oxidase inhibitors, 955
Hypokalemia, 482, 485
Hypomagnesemia, 482–484, 665
Hypomania, 342
    cyclothymia, 339
    definition of, 339
    fatigue and, 570
    HIV-associated, 819
    psychiatric emergencies in patients with, 906–907

Hyponatremia
    dementia and, 284
    drug-induced
        carbamazepine, 352, 961
        MDMA, 443
        selective serotonin reuptake inhibitors, 952
Hypoperfusion, 265
Hypopituitarism, **284**
Hypoproteinemia, 482, 486
Hypotension. *See* Orthostatic hypotension
Hypothermia
    in anorexia nervosa, 480
    cocaine-induced, 441
Hypothyroidism, 563, 564, **565, 816**
    anxiety and, 398, 564
    cognitive impairment in, 564
    depression and, 308, **310, 311,** 320, 564, 733
    lithium-induced, 959, 978
    mania and, 563–564
    prevalence of psychiatric comorbidity with, **564**
    sleep disorders and, 504, 511
    subclinical, 320
Hypoxemia, 265
Hypoxia, 546, 756
    anxiety due to, 780, **781**
    benzodiazepine-induced, 408
    in chronic obstructive pulmonary disease, 548
    in sleep apnea, 508
    ventilatory support for, 765
Hypoxyphilia, 470
Hysterectomy, 701

I WATCH DEATH mnemonic for delirium, 265, **265**
IABP (intra-aortic balloon pump), 602, 604, 765
IASP (International Association for the Study of Pain), 991
IBD (inflammatory bowel disease), 556, 1063
IBS. *See* Irritable bowel syndrome
Ibuprofen, **349,** 438
ICD (International Statistical Classification of Diseases and Related Health Problems), 33, 121, 242
Iceland, consultation-liaison psychiatry in, 207–209
ICU. *See* Intensive care unit
Ideas of reference, 64
Ifosfamide, **668**

IHD. *See* Ischemic heart disease
Ileus, tricyclic antidepressant–induced, 325
Illness Attitudes Scale, **371**
Illness behavior, 363, **520**
    abnormal, 363
    definition of, 363
    factors affecting, 363
Illness Behaviour Questionnaire, **371**
Illness vs. disease, 363
Illusions, 64
Imaging. *See* Neuroimaging
Imipramine, 325, **948**
    cytochrome P450 metabolism and, **945**
    dosage of, **948**
    injectable, 601
    for pain syndromes, 1004–1005
        noncardiac chest pain, 1062
    platelet binding of, 313
    receptor site affinity of, **948**
    serum level of, 947
    side effects of
        insomnia, **502,** 505
        sexual dysfunction, **462**
    use in specific patient groups or medical conditions
        brain injury, 741
        breast-feeding women, **981**
        children, 723, **723**
        dying patients, 785, **785**
        HIV/AIDS, 828, 829
        irritable bowel syndrome, 555
        Parkinson's disease, 693, **693**
        patients undergoing rehabilitation, **742**
        pregnancy, **708**
Immune dysfunction
    autoimmune disorders, 1066–1067
    behavioral medicine and, 1063–1064
    behavioral states associated with, 1063, **1064**
    depression and, 238
    HIV/AIDS, 687, 807–840
    hyperimmune disorders, 1065–1066
    psychoneuroimmunology, 661, 664, 1063
Immunosuppressants
    drug interactions with
        antidepressants, 643
        tremor due to, 643
    effects on quality of life, 646
    mood symptoms due to, 642
    movement disorders due to, 643
    neurotoxicity of, 640–641
    psychotic symptoms due to, 642
    seizures induced by, 642

Impairment, defined, 729
Impostureship, 519
Impotence. *See* Sexual dysfunction
Impulsivity, 130, 138, 277
In re Certification of William R, 178
In re Conroy, 174
In re Quinlan, 145
In the Guardianship of John Roe, 172–173
Incapacity, 172
Incomplete sentences test, 92
Incoordination, drug-induced
    alcohol, 424
    benzodiazepines, 158, 407
    carbamazepine, 961
    phencyclidine, 905
Indapamide, **462**
Independent practice associations (IPAs), 182
Indinavir, **811**, 823
Indomethacin, **349**, **462**, 969
Industrial agents and pollutants, **284**
Infections
    anxiety and, 780, **781**
    behavioral medicine and, 1065
    central nervous system, 687–688
        electroconvulsive therapy for patients with, 1021
    cocaine-related septicemia, 243, 441
    delirium and, 265
    dementia and, **274**, 282
    HIV/AIDS, 687, 807–840
    neurosyphilis, 282, **345**, 576, 687–688
    opioid-related septicemia, 436
    opportunistic, in HIV/AIDS, 807, 810
        neuropsychiatric syndromes due to, 815, **817**
    postinfectious syndromes associated with chronic fatigue, 574–576
        acute hepatitis, 575
        cytomegalovirus infection, 574
        Epstein-Barr virus infection, 574
        human herpesvirus-6 infection, 575
        Lyme disease, 575
        neurosyphilis, 576
        postviral syndrome, 574
        toxoplasmosis, 575
    sexually transmitted, 712–713
Infertility, 705–706
    among cancer patients, 666–669
    eating disorders and, 705
    prevalence of, 705
Inflammatory bowel disease (IBD), 556, 1063

Information bias in research, **199**
Information management system, 287
Informed consent, 167, 169–172
    competency to give, 170, 172–174, **174**
    definition of, 168
    for electroconvulsive therapy, 1016
    essential components of, 170
    exceptions to requirement for, 170, **170**
        emergencies, 170
        incompetency, 170
        therapeutic privilege, 170
        waiver, 170
    for factitious disorders, management of, 525
    Good Samaritan standards and, 596
    information to be disclosed for, 170, **170**
    legal doctrine of, 169
    liability for not obtaining, 170
    for participation in research, 171–172, 200
    for prescribing medication for unapproved uses, 170–171
    right to die and, 174–175, 790
    for surgery, 596, **599**, 600
    voluntariness of, 170
    withholding of, 169 (*See also* Refusal of treatment)
Inhalant-related disorders, 446, 906
Insight assessment, 65
Insomnia. *See also* Sleep disorders
    approach to patient with, 500–502
    classifications of, **496**, **497**
    definition of, 500
    due to general medical condition, **496**, 502–504, **503**, 510–513
    in elderly persons, 244, 854
    evaluation of, 969
    among medical and surgical inpatients, 499–500
    personality disorders and, 243
    in postconcussion syndrome, 685
    psychiatric comorbidity with, 244
    psychophysiological, 501
    secondary to mental disorder, 500–501
    sleep state misperception, 501–502
    substance-induced, 502, **502**
        antiretroviral drugs, 812, 816
        bupropion, 952
        monoamine oxidase inhibitors, 955
        psychostimulants, 723, 761, 956
        reboxetine, 953
        selective serotonin reuptake inhibitors, 326, 761, 951

    tricyclic antidepressants, 951
    treatment of, 504–505, **506**
        trazodone, 505, 972
        zolpidem, 505, 972
Instrument bias in research, **199**
Insulin
    anxiety induced by, **400**
    drug interactions with
        lithium, 960
        monoamine oxidase inhibitors, 955
    type A behavior and, 539
Insulinoma, **284**
Insurance reimbursement, 27–31. *See also* Economic issues
Integrated Auditory and Visual Continuous Performance Test, 98
Integrated medical-psychiatry services, 3–4, 871–884
    biopsychosocial model for, 873
    case examples of, 873–875
        inpatient, 874–875
        outpatient, 874
    components of, 884
    economics of, 882–884
        inpatient services, 883–884
        outpatient services, 882–883
    horizontal integration, 873
    improvement in patient outcomes with, 877–882
        critical components for, 873, **873**
        inpatient programs, 880–881
            admission criteria of, 880–881
            unit organization of, 881, **881**
        outpatient programs, 877–880
            mental health team model, **878**, 878–879
            stand-alone psychiatric clinics, 879–880
    intangible benefits of, 884
    limitations of traditional approaches to comorbid medical and psychiatric illness, 875–876
        inpatient, 876
        outpatient, 875–876
    vertical integration, 873, 882
Integrated Services Digital Network (ISDN), 928
Intelligence tests, 294
Intensive care unit (ICU), 753–768
    agitation in, 159–160
        haloperidol for, 965
        midazolam for, 407
    anxiety in, 759–760, **760**
    clinical situations unique to, 765–766

intra-aortic balloon pumps and
cardiac surgery, 604,
765–766, **767**
respirators, 765
confusion/delirium in, 756, 761–762,
762
delirium tremens in, 901
depression in, 760–761
personality traits and behavioral
problems in, 763–765, **764, 766**
psychiatric evaluation of patient in,
753–756
cognitive assessment, 754
general approach, 753–754
history gathering, 754
making diagnosis, 754–756, **755**
patient examination, 754
psychiatric treatment of patient in,
756–759
changes in medical-surgical
management, 756
follow-up visits, 758–759
involuntary treatment, 758
nonpharmacological measures,
757–758
pharmacotherapy, 756–757, **757**
psychotherapy, 758
restraints, 758
ward management, 758
psychosis in, 264, 498–499,
757–758, 762–763, **763**
reasons for psychiatric consultation
in, 753
sedation in, 267, 758
sleep patterns of patients in, 496–499
clinical consequences of sleep
changes, 498–499
decreased total sleep time, 496
disrupted day/night circadian
cycles, 496–498
disrupted sleep architecture, 498
staff stress in, 766–767
related to transplant surgery, 644
waiting for transplant in, 633
Interact, 45
Interactive television, 927–928. *See also*
Telepsychiatry
Interferon
for hepatitis C, 1065
side effects of
depression, 239, **239, 311,** 323
neuropsychiatric effects, 323,
668, 818, 1065
sexual dysfunction, **462**
Interleukin-2, **668**
INTERMED, 223–225, **225**

Intermittent explosive disorder, 150,
150
Internal medicine, 535–577
cardiac disease, 536–545
cobalamin deficiency, 569
endocrine disorders, 563–567
fatigue, 570–576
gastrointestinal disorders, 552–556
lung disease, 546–551
renal disease, 557–562
systemic lupus erythematosus, 568
International Association for the Study
of Pain (IASP), 991
International College of Psychosomatic
Medicine, 219
International consultation-liaison
psychiatry, 203–226
Australia and New Zealand, 217–218
Europe, 207–217
German-speaking countries,
204–206, 209–212
Netherlands, 214–215
Nordic countries, 207–209
southern European and
Mediterranean countries,
215–217
United Kingdom, 212–213
European studies, 221–225
ECLW Collaborative Study,
221–222, **223**
INTERMED, 223–225, **225**
quality management study, 225
risk factor study, 222–223, **224**
history of, 203–204
international networking, 206
Japan, 218–220
Latin America, 220–221
Brazil, 220–221
Colombia, 221
Mexico, 221
Uruguay, 221
relation to psychosomatics and
behavioral medicine, 204–206
institutions and professions,
205–206
traditions and concepts, 205
trends, 206
resource allocation and, 206
summary of, 225–226
International Organization for
Consultation-Liaison Psychiatry, 206
*International Statistical Classification of
Diseases and Related Health
Problems* (ICD), 33, 121, 242
Internet
consultation via, 934

creation of fictional identities and
diseases on, 519
Interpersonal therapy, 320
Interstitial lung disease, 504
Intoxication. *See also* Substance-related
disorders
alcohol, 423–424
management of, 430
caffeine, 484
cannabis, 444
cocaine, 440–441
hallucinogen, 443
inhalants, 446
opioid, 437, 905
psychosis due to, **896**
Intra-aortic balloon pump (IABP), 602,
604, 765
Intramuscular drug administration, 941
Intravenous drug administration, 941
Invirase. *See* Saquinavir
Involuntary psychiatric treatment
hospitalization, 168, 179
in intensive care unit, 758
IPAs (independent practice
associations), 182
Ipecac, 484
Ipratropium bromide, **550**
Iproniazid, **345**
Irritability
drug-related
amphetamines, 442
nicotine withdrawal, 445
stimulants, 723
in frontotemporal dementia, 277
HIV-associated, 282
in Huntington's disease, 278
in mania, 339
in postconcussion syndrome, 685
in type A behavior pattern, 113
in Wilson's disease, 279
Irritable bowel syndrome (IBS), 114,
115, 552, 554–556, 1062–1063
anxiety disorders and, 402, 555
approach to patient with, 554
behavioral medicine and, 1062–1063
childhood trauma and, 1063
diagnostic criteria for, 554, **554,**
1062–1063
epidemiology of, 554
fibromyalgia and, 571
mood disorders and, 555–556
with no psychiatric disorders, 556
nonpharmacological management of,
554, 1063
psychiatric comorbidity with, 245,
554–555, **555, 594**

Ischemia
    Hachinski Ischemia Score, **281**
    stroke due to, 679
    vascular dementia due to, 280
Ischemic heart disease (IHD),
        1054–1062. *See also* Coronary
        artery disease; Myocardial infarction
    depression and, 1054–1055
    effects on spouses of patients with,
        1062
    hypertension and, 1060
    physical activity and, 1058–1059
    risk factors for, 1055–1056, **1056**
    serum cholesterol and, 1058
    sexual dysfunction and, **456,**
        456–457, **457,** 1062
    smoking cessation and, 1060–1061
    stress and, 538, 1057–1058
    type A behavior and, 113–114,
        539–540, 1054
        behavioral and psychological
            interventions for, 1056
        effect of treatment on risk of
            recurrent myocardial
            infarction, 1057
        pharmacotherapy for, 1058
        weight loss for, 1059–1060
        work for patients with, 1061–1062
ISDN (Integrated Services Digital
        Network), 928
Isocarboxazid, 327, **462, 785**
Isoflurane, **944**
Isoniazid, **943**
    drug interactions with
        benzodiazepines, **349,** 505
        disulfiram, 432
    side effects of, **550**
        mania, **345**
        neuropsychiatric effects, **818**
Italy, consultation-liaison psychiatry in,
        215–217
Itraconazole, **943, 946**

Japan, consultation-liaison psychiatry in,
        218–220
    background of, 218–219
    future development, 220
    in general hospital, 219
    official status and training, 219
    research, 219–220
*Japanese Journal of General Hospital
    Psychiatry, The,* 219
Japanese Society of General Hospital
        Psychiatry, 219–220
Jaundice, antipsychotic-induced, 966
Jet fuels, **284**

Joint Commission on Accreditation of
        Healthcare Organizations, 180,
        990, 1009
Journal of Psychosomatic Research, 7
Journals
    on consultation-liaison psychiatry, 7
        international, 217, 219
    on pharmacology and drug
        interactions, 45
Judgment
    assessment of, 65
    cocaine-induced impairment of, 440
    in delirium, 261
    in frontotemporal dementia, 277
Juvenile justice system, 717

Kaopectate, 438
Kaplan Baycrest Neurocognitive
        Assessment, 82
Kaposi's sarcoma, **816**
Karnofsky scale, 25
Kaufman, M. R., 5
Kernig sign, 73
Ketamine abuse, 442
Ketoconazole, **943**
    drug interactions with
        antiretroviral drugs, 815
        cytochrome P450 metabolism
            and, **946**
        immunosuppressants, 643
        nefazodone, 327
    sexual dysfunction induced by, **462**
Kevorkian, Jack, 790
Kidcope, **720**
Kleine-Levin syndrome, **345,** 512, 513
Klinefelter's syndrome, 129, **345**
Klonopin. *See* Clonazepam
Klüver-Bucy syndrome, 278, 468
Knee replacement surgery, 856
Knowledge base for liaison psychiatry,
        33, 40–41
Korsakoff's psychosis, 86, 265, 283,
        426

La belle indifférence, 1002
LAAM (L-α-acetylmethadol), 418, 438
Labetalol, **462,** 1021
Labor, psychiatric consultation during,
        709, **709**
Laboratory evaluation. *See also* specific
        diagnostic tests
    of alcoholism, 427–428, **428**
    of anxiety, 406
    of cannabis abuse, 444
    of delirium, 264, **264**
    of dementia, 291, **293**

of depression, 313
of eating disorders, 482, **482**
    anorexia nervosa, 485, **485**
of elderly persons, 860–861
    before electroconvulsive therapy,
        1016–1017, **1017**
    in emergency department, 893–895,
        894, 895
of fatigue, 570, **571**
of hepatitis B virus infection, 575
in HIV infection
    before antidepressant initiation,
        828
    for neurocognitive impairment,
        820, 821
    before lithium treatment, 348, **348,**
        959
of Lyme disease, 575
of mania, 346, **346**
of neuroleptic malignant syndrome,
        968
of neurological disorders, 689–690
of syphilis, 576
of toxoplasmosis, 575
Lactation, psychotropic drug use during,
        710, **980,** 980–981, **981**
Lacunar strokes and infarcts, 681
Lafora's myoclonic epilepsy, 687
Lamictal. *See* Lamotrigine
Lamivudine, **811,** 813, **818,** 823
Lamotrigine, **958,** 960–962
    dosage and administration of, **347,**
        353, **958,** 961
    drug interactions with, 353
        other anticonvulsants, 961
    indications for
        mania, **347,** 352–353
        pain syndromes, 1006
    mechanism of action of, 353, 960
    pharmacokinetics of, 353, 961, 962
    side effects of, 353, 961
    use in specific patient groups or
        medical conditions
        neurological disease, 694
        transplant candidates, **635**
Language and speech disturbances. *See
    also* Aphasia
    in Alzheimer's disease, 277
    assessment for, 67, 289
    delirium and, 262
    drug-induced
        carbamazepine, 961
        lithium, 350
        tricyclic antidepressants, 951
    in pediatric patients, 721
    poststroke aprosodia, 681

Latin America, consultation-liaison psychiatry in, 220–221
  Brazil, 220–221
  Colombia, 221
  Mexico, 221
  Uruguay, 221
Laxative abuse, 479, 481, **481**, 484
Lead poisoning, **284,** 481, **502**
Learning, somatization and, 368
Learning disabilities
  neuropsychological testing of adults for, 87–88
  traumatic brain injury and, 86
Least restrictive environment, 891
Left ventricular assist device, 604
Legal issues
  advance directives, 169, **174,** 175–176
  competency determination, 167, **172,** 172–174
  confidentiality, **168,** 168–169
  definitions related to, 168
  duty to warn of patient's homicidal intent, 900
  guardianship, 176–177
  importance of being knowledgeable about, 167
  informed consent and right to refuse treatment, 169–172
  involuntary hospitalization, 168, 179
  litigation trend, 183–184
  malingering, 526–528
  managed care, 182–183
  "patient dumping" and interhospital transfers, 891
  physician-assisted suicide and euthanasia, 144–146, 175, 789–791, **790,** 831
  psychiatric malpractice, 183, **184**
  rape, 711–712
  related to factitious disorders, 525, **525**
  related to malingering, 527, 528
  reporting suspected cases of abuse, 909
  right to die, 174–175, 790
  risk management, 183–184
  seclusion and restraint, 179–181, **180,** 890–891
  substituted judgment, 177–178
  voluntary hospitalization, 168, 178–179
  weapons screening in emergency department, 890
Length of stay (LOS) in hospital
  delirium and, 257, 269

effect of consultation-liaison services on, 26, 36–37
  hypnotic drug use and, 500
  psychiatric comorbidity and, 9, 25–26, 35–36, 876, **876**
Leptomeningeal disease, 665
Leriche's syndrome, 182
Lesch-Nyhan syndrome, **680**
Leukemia, 671
Leuko-ariosis, 53
Leukocytosis, drug-induced
  lithium, 959, 978
  selective serotonin reuptake inhibitors, 952
  tricyclic antidepressants, 951
Leukoencephalopathy
  disseminated necrotizing, 666
  progressive multifocal, 282, 815
Leukopenia
  drug-induced
    carbamazepine, 351, 961, 978
    tricyclic antidepressants, 951
  in eating disorders, 483, 486
Leuprolide
  for aggression, 162
  for Alzheimer's disease, 296
  for prostate cancer, 471
  for sexual disorders, 471
  side effects of, 471
    sexual dysfunction, **462**
Levarterenol, 969
Level of consciousness, 66
Levo-Dromoran. *See* Levorphanol
Levodopa
  drug interactions with
    bupropion, 693
    monoamine oxidase inhibitors, 955
  indications for
    neuroleptic malignant syndrome, 968
    Parkinson's disease, 686
    periodic leg movements of sleep and restless legs syndrome, 510
  side effects of
    anxiety, **400**
    mania, **345, 346**
    sexual dysfunction, **462**
    sleep disorders, 501, **502,** 504, 513
Levopromazine, 1007
Levorphanol, **437,** 793, **993**
  for terminally ill patients, **797**
Lewy body dementia, 273, 275, 279, 286, 297

LH (luteinizing hormone), 471
Liaison psychiatry, 5, 6, 8, 20, 33–46
  computer-assisted physician management system for, 33, **34**
  conceptual framework of, 38, 46
  definition of, 34
  distinction from consultation psychiatry, 33–35, 38
  functions of, 33, 38–42
    assessing medical care providers, 39–40
    detection and diagnosis, 39
    developing autonomy in nonpsychiatric staff, 40, **40**
    developing new knowledge, 40–41
    effecting structural changes in medical setting, 41–42
    primary, secondary, and tertiary prevention, 38–39
  knowledge base for, 33
    drug interactions, 45
  models of psychiatric training for primary care physicians, **42,** 42–45
  psychiatric interventions in inpatient medical setting, 36–38
  tailoring to achieve maximum effect, 38
Librium. *See* Chlordiazepoxide
Lidocaine, **762, 946**
Life expectancy, 772
Life narrative approach, 112, 1041
Life-sustaining treatment. *See also* Dying patients; End-of-life decisions
  advance directives and, 175–176
  physician liability related to, 174
  right to die, 174–175, 790
  withholding or withdrawal of, 145, 146, 167, 174
Limbic encephalopathy, 280, 682–683
Limbic system, role in emotional responses, 401–402
Lipodystrophy, antiretroviral drug-induced, 812, **812**
Lipophilic drugs, 941, 942
Lithium, **958,** 958–960
  dosage and administration of, **347,** 958, **958**
  drug interactions with, 348, **349,** 694, 864, 960
    antipsychotics, 969
    diuretics, 348, 349, 960
    nonsteroidal anti-inflammatory drugs, 349, 960, **999**
  electroconvulsive therapy and, 354, 1016

Lithium *(continued)*
  half-life and serum level of, **347,** 348, 958
  indications for
    agitation and aggression, 161, **161,** 171
    depression, 328, 957
    hypoxyphilia, 470
    mania, **347–349,** 347–350, 958–960
  mechanism of action of, 958
  overdose and toxicity of, 959, **976**
  pharmacokinetics of, 958
  pretreatment evaluation for, 348, **348,** 959
  response to, 958
  side effects of, 263, 349–350, 958–959, **975–976**
    cardiac effects, 350, 544, 959
    central nervous system toxicity, 350
    insomnia, 505
    nystagmus, 350, 611
    parkinsonism, 686
    polydipsia and polyuria, 350, 958, **975**
    renal effects, **239,** 959
    sexual dysfunction, **462**
  slow-release formulations of, 350
  use in specific patient groups or medical conditions
    brain injury, 161
    breast-feeding women, 981, **981**
    cancer, 663
    cardiac disease, 350, 544, **975**
    dialysis patients, 348, 561
    dying patients, 787
    elderly persons, 861, **863,** 864, 959
    hepatic disease, 427
    HIV/AIDS, 826
    neurological disease, 694
    patients undergoing rehabilitation, **743**
    pregnancy, 350, 707, **708,** 959, 980
    surgical patients, **598**
    transplant candidates, **635**
  withdrawal from, 959–960
Lithobid. *See* Lithium
Litigation trend, 183–184
Liver flap. *See* Asterixis
Liver transplantation, 35, 42, 417. *See also* Transplantation
  for alcoholic patients, 427, 629–630
  electroconvulsive therapy and, 1022

evaluation of living donors for, 625
movement disorders after, 643
psychiatric disorders in candidates for, 627–628, 640
psychopharmacological considerations and, **635–637**
  neuroleptics, 641
in psychotic patients, 630–631
psychotropic drug use and, 427
return to employment after, 645
transient paranoid psychosis after, 642
waiting period for, 633–638
Living will, 168, 174, 175–176
LNNB (Luria-Nebraska Neuropsychological Battery), **81,** 82–83, 157
Locus coeruleus
  opioid receptors in, 436
  role in anxiety, 400, 401
Longitudinal population descriptive studies, **192, 195,** 195–197
  case-control studies, 195–196
  cohort studies, 196–197
Lorazepam, **763, 903,** 969, **970**
  abuse of, 902, 907
  antipsychotics combined with, 408, 897
  dosage of, **407, 434, 763, 903,** 962, **970**
  half-life of, **407, 903**
  indications for
    acute psychosis, 897
    agitation and aggression, 159, **160,** 899, 902
    alcohol withdrawal, 430–431, **431**
    Alzheimer's disease, 296
    anxiety, 267
    cocaine intoxication, 441
    delirium, 268, 794, **794**
    insomnia, 505, **506**
    mania, 353, 962
    neuroleptic malignant syndrome, 968
    pain syndromes, 1006
    rapid tranquilization, 965
  intramuscular, 407, 897
  pharmacokinetics of, 970
  psychiatric aspects of, **669**
  side effects of
    mania, **345**
    sexual dysfunction, **462**
  use in specific patient groups or medical conditions
    breast-feeding women, **981**
    chemotherapy patients, 659, 660

    children, **723**
    critically ill patients, 759
    dialysis patients, 561
    dying patients, 782, **782,** 794, **794**
    elderly persons, **863**
    hepatic disease, 977
    HIV/AIDS, 825
    neurological disease, 694
    patients undergoing rehabilitation, **743**
    transplant candidates, 638
  withdrawal from, 904
LOS. *See* Length of stay in hospital
Loss. *See also* Grief
  in rehabilitation settings, 735
  somatization and, 362
  suicide and, 134–135
Low back pain, 1068
Loxapine, **964**
Loxitane. *See* Loxapine
LSD (lysergic acid diethylamide), 443, **462,** 905
Ludiomil. *See* Maprotiline
Lumbar puncture, 291, 690
Luminal. *See* Phenobarbital
Lung cancer, 669–670
  brain metastases from, 664, **664, 681**
  limbic encephalopathy and, 280
  marijuana use and, 444
  paraneoplastic syndromes and, 682–683
    Eaton-Lambert myasthenic syndrome, 682
    limbic encephalitis, 682–683
  smoking and, 445
  suicidality and, 131
Lung disease, 546–551
  anxiety and, 245, 397, 399, 402
  asthma, 549–550, 1066
  chronic obstructive pulmonary disease, 548–549
  depression and, 547
  electroconvulsive therapy and, 1021
  insomnia and, 503–504
  marijuana use and, 444
  opioid dependence and, 905
  psychiatric comorbidity with, 244–245
  psychotherapy for patients with, 1032
  psychotropic drug use in, **975,** 977
  pulmonary embolus, 550–551, 780
    in cancer patients, 660
    cocaine-related, 243, 441
  respiratory dyskinesia, 551
  sleep apnea, 507–509, **508, 509,** 551

sleep disorders and, 503, 511
smoking and, 445, 549
use of benzodiazepines in, 407–408
Lung transplantation. *See also*
    Transplantation
    psychiatric disorders in candidates
        for, 627
    psychopharmacological
        considerations and, **635–637**
    return to employment after, 646
Luria, A. R.
    approach to neuropsychological
        assessment, 81
    model of brain functioning, 78–80,
        79
Luria hand sequence test, **292**
Luria-Nebraska Neuropsychological
    Battery (LNNB), **81**, 82–83, 157
Luteinizing hormone (LH), 471
Luvox. *See* Fluvoxamine
Lyme disease, 575
Lymphokine-activated killer cells, **668**
Lymphoma, 671
    central nervous system, 815, **816**
    sexual dysfunction and, 457
Lyon Heart Study, 1058
Lysergic acid diethylamide (LSD), 443,
    462, 905

MADISON scale, 1068, **1069**
Magnetic resonance angiography, 50
Magnetic resonance imaging (MRI), 77
    in Alzheimer's disease, **279**
    applications of, **53**, 53–54, **54**
    basic science of, 49, 50
    for brain injury, 281
    in cerebral toxoplasmosis, 815, **817**
    claustrophobia and, 395, 404, 660
    cost and utilization review of, 52
    in delirium, 54, 264, **264**
    in dementia, 54, 292–294, **293**
    in depression, 313
    in elderly persons, 861
    before electroconvulsive therapy,
        1016, **1017**
    in emergency department, 894
    functional, 77
    of head, 690–691
    in HIV-associated neurocognitive
        impairment, 821, **822**
    in immunosuppressant neurotoxicity,
        640
    in Lyme disease, 575
    in mania, 346
    in multiple sclerosis, 398
    in vascular dementia, 281

Magnetic resonance spectroscopy, 50
    in HIV-associated neurocognitive
        impairment, 821
Malabsorption syndromes, 602
Malignant hyperthermia, **597**
Malignant melanoma, 664, **664, 681,**
    1064
Malingering, 519, 526–528
    assessment for, 97
    clinical features of, 526–527, **527**
    compared with factitious disorders,
        519, **520**
    diagnosis and differential diagnosis of,
        527–528
        dementia, 285–286
        psychological testing, 527
    differentiation from somatoform
        disorders, 373, 527
        conversion disorder, 380, 527
        pain disorder, 383
        somatization disorder, 376
    DSM-IV classification of, 519
    epidemiology of, 526
    etiology of, 527
    management of, 528
    morality of some cases of, 528
    motivations for, 526
    pain complaints due to, 990, **1000,**
        1003
    prognosis for, 528
    somatization and, **362**
Mallory-Weiss tears, 487
Malnutrition, 259
Malpractice, 183–184, **184.** *See also*
    Legal issues
Managed care, 182–183
    definition of, 168
    psychotherapy and, 1048
Manganese poisoning, **284**
Mania, 339–355. *See also* Bipolar
    disorder
    age at onset of, 341, 344
    agitation in, 161
    atypical, 960
    clinical features of, **340,** 342
    definitions related to, 339
    differential diagnosis of, 344–347
    epidemiology of, 339–342
    evaluation of, **346,** 346–347
    hypomania, 339
    legal competency of persons with, 172
    manic episode, 339, **340**
        stages of progression to, 342
    medical conditions associated with,
        344, **345, 346**
        cancer, 663

endocrine disorders, 563–564
head trauma, 281, 685
HIV/AIDS, 343, 819, 825–827
Huntington's disease, 278
multiple sclerosis, 686
neurosyphilis, 576
stroke, 346, 681
mental status examination for, 346
mixed, 960
neurochemical theories of, 343–344
neuroimaging in, **346,** 346–347
neurological examination for, 346
pathophysiology of, 342–344, **343**
primary vs. secondary, 339, 342–344,
    343, 345, 346
psychiatric emergencies in patients
    with, 906–907
in rehabilitation settings, 733
substance-induced, 63–64, 339, **341,**
    345, 346
    risperidone, 354
in transplant recipients, 642
treatment of, 347–355, 957–962
    anticonvulsants, **347,** 350–353,
        693–694, **958,** 960–962
    antipsychotics, 353–354, 962
    behavioral management, 355
    benzodiazepines, **347,** 353
    electroconvulsive therapy,
        354–355, 1015
    lithium, **347–349,** 347–350, **958,**
        958–960
    other medications, 354, **958,** 962
    psychotherapy, 355
Manipulative help rejecters, 110
MAO (monoamine oxidase), 954
Maprotiline, **948**
    dosage of, **948**
    for dying patients, **785,** 786
    for pain syndromes, 1004–1005
    receptor site affinity of, **948**
    side effects of
        seizures, 786, 951
        sexual dysfunction, **462**
Marchiafava-Bignami disease, 283, 426
Marie Three Paper Test, 72
Marijuana, 444, 906. *See also* Cannabis
Marital therapy. *See* Couples therapy
Marlowe-Crowne Social Desirability
    Scale, 115
Massage therapy, 1008
MAST (Michigan Alcoholism Screening
    Test), 428, **429**
Mazindol, **462**
MBHI (Millon Behavioral Health
    Inventory), 91

McGill Pain Questionnaire, **371**

MCMI (Millon Clinical Multiaxial Inventory), 91, **371**

MDA (3,4-methylenedioxyamphetamine), 443, **463**

MDMA (3,4-methylenedioxymethamphetamine), 443, 905

Mebaral. *See* Mephobarbital

Mecamylamine, **462**

Mechanical ventilation, 765
  panic and, 399
  weaning from, 606

Medial frontal syndrome, 682

Medical-psychiatric units, 41, 871. *See also* Integrated medical-psychiatry services

Medical student training, 15, 18

Medically unexplained symptoms, 362

Medication Event Monitoring Systems (MEMSCaps), 813–814

Medications. *See* Pharmacotherapy

Medicolegal competence determination, 96–97

Meditation
  for anxiety, 410
  for patients with cardiac disease, 542, 1057
  for patients with somatoform disorders, 385

Mediterranean countries, consultation-liaison psychiatry in, 215–217
  background of, 215–216
  future development, 217
  in general hospital, 216–217
  official status and training, 217
  research, 217

Medroxyprogesterone acetate (MPA)
  for aggression, 162
  for Alzheimer's disease, 296
  for paraphilias, 470–471
  for sexual acting-out, 468
  side effects of, 471
  for sleep apnea, 551

Medulloblastomas, **681**

Megaloblastic anemia, 569

Megestrol acetate, **667**

Mellaril. *See* Thioridazine

Melphalan, **462**

Memantine, 824

Memory impairment
  age-related, 273, 854
  in Alzheimer's disease, 277, **278**
  assessment for, 68–69, 289
    neuropsychological testing, 86
  in cancer, 780
  in delirium, 260

in dementia, 273
  frontotemporal, 278
  vascular, **280**, 281

diagnostic criteria for amnestic disorders due to general medical condition, **86**

due to cobalamin deficiency, 569

electroconvulsive therapy–induced, 1018, **1019**

factitious, 523

HIV-associated, 282, 818

in Huntington's disease, 278

in limbic encephalopathy, 280

in Lyme disease, 575

in postconcussion syndrome, 685

posttraumatic amnesia, 281

in progressive supranuclear palsy, 280

substance-induced, 86
  alcohol-induced persisting amnestic disorder, 86, 265, 283, 426
  antipsychotics, 966
  benzodiazepines, 158, 288, 408, 971

MEMSCaps (Medication Event Monitoring Systems), 813–814

Menarche, 702

Meningeal carcinoma, 690

Meningiomas, **345, 346, 681**

Meningismus, 690

Meningitis, 688
  cerebrospinal fluid findings in, 690
  chronic, 688
    dementia and, 282
    Mycobacterium tuberculosis, 688
  delirium and, 265
  in Lyme disease, 575
  in systemic lupus erythematosus, 568

Meningoencephalitis, 688
  cryptococcal, **345,** 688, 815
  viral, **345**

Menopause, 702–703, **703**
  cancer- or chemotherapy-related, 666, 668
  depression and, 703

Menstrual cycle, 702
  in anorexia nervosa, 480, 483, 486

Mental health team model in outpatient setting, **878,** 878–879

Mental retardation, 421, 631

Mental status examination (MSE), 15, 61–75, **62, 81**
  cognitive components of, **62,** 65–69
    attention, 66–67
    level of consciousness, 66
    memory, 68–69

orientation, 68
    speech and language, 67, **67**

cognitive function tests, 72–73
  A Test for Vigilance, 72
  Bender Gestalt Test, 72
  Blessed Dementia Scale, 72
  draw a clock face, 72
  Frank Jones story, 72
  Marie Three Paper Test, 72
  Reitan-Indiana Aphasia Screening Test, 72
  Set Test, 72
  Taylor Equivalent Test, 72, **73**
  Trail Making Test, 72

for delirium, **261**

for dementia, 289–290, **289–292**

for depression, 312

difficulty of performing in general hospital, 62

of elderly persons, 860

in emergency department, 892–893

extended, 83

integration with patient's history, 61

for mania, 346

neurological examination, 73, **74**

noncognitive components of, **62,** 62–65
  abstracting abilities, 65
  affect and mood, 62–64
  appearance and behavior, 62
  insight, 65
  judgment, 65
  perceptions, 64–65
  thought processes and content, 64

of pediatric patients, 721, **721**

screening examinations, **69,** 69–72, 83
  advantages and disadvantages of, 69, **69, 81**
  Mini-Mental State Exam, 69–71, **70, 71**
  Neurobehavioral Cognitive Status Examination, 71–72

for somatization, 370, **370**

for suicidality, 140

via telepsychiatry, 929

Mental Status Questionnaire, 83

Mepenzolate bromide, **463**

Meperidine
  for burn patients, 612
  for children, **724**
  delirium induced by, 265, **762,** 793
  detoxification from, 437, 438
  dosage of, **437, 993**
  drug interactions with
    monoamine oxidase inhibitors, 327, 787, **999**

ritonavir, **815**
duration of action of, **993**
for terminally ill patients, **797**
toxicity of, **994,** 999
Mephobarbital, **904**
Meprobamate, **434, 904**
Mercury poisoning, **284, 502**
Mercy killing, 144–146
Mescaline, 443
Mesoridazine, **463,** 969
Metabolic disorders
anxiety due to, 780, **781**
cocaine use and, 441
dementia and, **274,** 282–283, 288
psychosis due to, **896**
Metabolism of drugs, 942
aging and, 861, **862**
inhibitors and inducers of, **943**
Metachromatic leukodystrophy, **680**
Methadone
benzodiazepines to potentiate
euphoria induced by, 433
detoxification from, 438
dosage and administration of, **437,**
438, **993**
drug interactions with, 438
antiretroviral drugs, **815,** 838
benzodiazepines, 440
zidovudine, 814
duration of action of, **993**
duration of detectability in urine, **895**
half-life of, 438
maintenance treatment with,
437–438, 905
for patients with HIV/AIDS, 838
neonatal withdrawal from, 437
for opioid detoxification, 997
side effects of, 438
sexual dysfunction, **463**
use in specific patient groups or
medical conditions
liver disease, 438
pregnancy, 437, 1007
rehabilitation settings, **742**
terminally ill patients, **797**
Methamphetamine abuse, 442
Methandrostenolone, **463**
Methantheline bromide, **463**
Methaqualone, **434, 463,** 895
Methazolamide, **463**
Methotrexate, **463,** 667, 793
Methotrimeprazine, 794, **794,** 1007
3-Methoxy-4-hydroxyphenylglycol
(MHPG)
aggression and, 155
in anorexia nervosa, 487

opioid withdrawal and, 436
Methscopolamine, **463**
Methyl chloride, **284**
N-Methyl-D-aspartate (NMDA)
receptors
in alcohol intoxication/withdrawal,
423–424
in opioid-related disorders, 436
Methyldopa
drug interactions with
monoamine oxidase inhibitors,
955
tricyclic antidepressants, 953
side effects of
depression, 63, **311,** 322
insomnia, **502**
sexual dysfunction, **463**
3,4-Methylenedioxyamphetamine
(MDA), 443, **462**
3,4-Methylenedioxymethamphetamine
(MDMA), 443, 905
Methylphenidate, **943,** 955–957, **956**
dosage of, 956, **956**
drug interactions with, 957
cytochrome P450 metabolism
and, **945**
half-life of, **956,** 1007
indications for
depression, 327
narcolepsy, 509
pain syndromes, **989,** 1007
side effects of
cardiac effects, 544
mania, **345**
sleep disorders, **502**
use in specific patient groups or
medical conditions
cancer patients, 662
children, **723**
critically ill patients, 761
dying patients, **785,** 786–787
HIV/AIDS, 824, 829–830
neurogenic bladder with
retention, 693, **693**
neurological disease, 692
stroke, **693**
transplant candidates, **637**
Methylprednisolone, 643
[^{11}C]-*N*-Methylspiperone, 55
[^{18}F]-*N*-Methylspiperone, 55
Methyprylon, **434, 904**
Methysergide, **502**
Metoclopramide
antiemetic effects of, 963
psychiatric aspects of, **669**
side effects of

anxiety, 781, **781**
depression, 733
mania, 345
parkinsonism, 686
sexual dysfunction, **463**
Metocurine, **763**
Metoprolol
for anxiety, 973
interaction with selective serotonin
reuptake inhibitors, 543
sexual dysfunction induced by, **463**
use in patients with neurological
disease, 694
Metrizamide, **345**
Metronidazole, **349,** 427
Metyrosine, **463**
Mexico, consultation-liaison psychiatry
in, 221
Mexiletine, **463,** 762
Meyer, Adolf, 4, 5
MHPG. *See* 3-Methoxy-4-
hydroxyphenylglycol
MI. *See* Myocardial infarction
Mianserin, 786
Michigan Alcoholism Screening Test
(MAST), 428, **429**
Miconazole, **946**
MICRO-CARES database studies, 41,
206, 218, 221, 246, **247**
MicroCog, 98
MID. *See* Multi-infarct dementia
Midazolam, 407, **763, 903,** 970, **970**
cost of, 970
dosage of, **763, 903, 970**
drug interactions with
cytochrome P450 metabolism
and, **945**
ritonavir, 814, **815**
for dying patients, 782, **782,** 794,
794
half-life of, **407, 903**
indications for, 970
agitation in intensive care unit,
407, 970
pain syndromes, 1006
sedation, 267, 407
intramuscular, 407
pharmacokinetics of, 970
side effects of, 407
sexual dysfunction, **463**
use during breast-feeding, **981**
Midodrine, **463**
Migraine headache, 997
antidepressants for, 693, **693**
anxiety and, 397, 398
sleep disorders and, 504, 512

Millon Behavioral Health Inventory
(MBHI), 91
Millon Clinical Multiaxial Inventory
(MCMI), 91, **371**
Miltown. *See* Meprobamate
Mini-Mental State Exam (MMSE), 15,
25, 66, 69–71, **70, 71,** 83, 260, 263,
294, 616, 754, 793, 860, 893, 929,
1018
Minnesota Multiphasic Personality
Inventory (MMPI), 89–91, **90,** 94,
95, 97, 157, 371, **371,** 527, 607,
625–626, 661, 1002, 1003
Mirtazapine, 327, **948**
for anxiety disorders, **950**
dosage of, **948**
drug interactions with, 596
mechanism of action of, 327, **948,** 953
side effects of, 327, 953
sexual dysfunction, **463**
structure of, 947
use in specific patient groups or
medical conditions
cardiac disease, 543
chronic pain and fibromyalgia, 693
dying patients, **785**
elderly persons, **863,** 864
migraine, 693
surgical patients, **597**
transplant candidates, **637**
Missing data bias in research, **199**
Mixed dementia, 275, 280–283
MMPI (Minnesota Multiphasic
Personality Inventory), 89–91, **90,**
94, 95, 97, 157, 371, **371,** 527, 607,
625–626, 661, 1002, 1003
MMSE (Mini-Mental State Exam), 15,
25, 66, 69–71, **70, 71,** 83, 260, 263,
294, 616, 754, 793, 860, 893, 929,
1018
Moban. *See* Molindone
Mobile crisis programs, 912
Moclobemide, 954, **954**
for dying patients, **785,** 787
Modafinil, 955–956, **956**
for dying patients, 787
for narcolepsy, 509
Modified Somatic Perception
Questionnaire (MSPQ), **371**
Modified WORLD test, 294
Molindone, **964**
dosage of, **964**
for epileptic patients, 692
side effects of, **964**
sexual dysfunction, **463**
for terminally ill patients, **794**

Monitoring
as coping strategy, 111
of serum drug levels, 942–943
Monoamine oxidase (MAO), 954
Monoamine oxidase inhibitors (MAOIs),
327, **943, 954,** 954–955
drug interactions with, 327, 787,
953–955
alcohol, 427, **428**
buspirone, 955, 972
meperidine, 327, 787, **999**
methadone, 438
psychostimulants, 957, **957**
selective serotonin reuptake
inhibitors, 327, 954,
955
serotonin syndrome due to, 327,
953–955
tricyclic antidepressants, 327,
954, 955
venlafaxine, 327, 954
indications for, 954
anxiety disorders, **950,** 954
atypical depression, 947, 954
bulimia nervosa, 489
narcolepsy, 510
mechanism of action of, 954
pharmacokinetics of, 954
reversible, 954
side effects of, 761, 955, **975–976**
insomnia, 505
orthostatic hypotension, 327,
544
tyramine-induced hypertensive
crisis, 327, 543–544, 954,
955
types of, 954
use in specific patient groups or
medical conditions
cardiac disease, 543–544, **975**
critically ill patients, 760–761
dying patients, **785,** 787
elderly persons, 864
epilepsy, **693**
patients undergoing rehabilitation,
742
pregnancy, 980
surgical patients, **597**
transplant candidates, **636**
Mononucleosis, 345, 574
Mood
assessment of, 62–63
definition of, 62
descriptive terms for, 62
effects of hormone replacement
therapy on, 703

Mood disorders. *See also* Bipolar
disorder; Depression; Dysthymic
disorder; Mania
assessment for, 63–64
after brain injury, 685
clinical population studies of, 241
cocaine dependence and, 442
depression, 307–330
due to general medical condition, 63,
339, **340**
Huntington's disease and, 686
insomnia and, 501
mania, 339–355
multiple sclerosis and, 686
psychiatric emergencies in patients
with, 906–907
somatization and, **362,** 365
substance-induced, 63–64, **239,** 311,
311, 341
suicide and, **133,** 133–134, **134**
in surgical patients, 595
treatment in patients who can
take nothing by mouth,
601–602
in transplant recipients, 642–643
Mood stabilizers, 347–354, 957–962,
958. *See also* specific drugs
anticonvulsants, **347,** 350–353,
693–694, **958,** 960–962
compliance with, 957
indications for, 957–958
agitation and aggression, 160–161,
161, 957
mania, **347–349,** 347–354,
957–962
pain syndromes, **989**
schizoaffective disorder, 957
lithium, **958,** 958–960
other medications, 354, **958,** 962
use in specific patient groups or
medical conditions
breast-feeding women, **981**
cardiac disease, 544
dialysis patients, 561
elderly persons, **863,** 864
HIV/AIDS, 826–827
neurological and neurosurgical
disease, 693–694
pregnancy, 980
surgical patients, **598,** 601
transplant candidates, **635**
Moricizine, 951
Morphine, **763, 995**
abuse of, 904
for burn patients, 612
for children, **724**

cytochrome P450 metabolism and, **945**

delirium induced by, **762,** 793

detoxification from, 438

dosage of, **437, 763, 993**

duration of action of, **993**

duration of detectability in urine, **895**

sexual dysfunction induced by, **463**

sustained-release, **993, 994**

for terminally ill patients, 783, **797**

use in rehabilitation settings, 741, **742**

Morphine-6-glucuronide, **994**

Mortality. *See also* Dying patients

anorexia nervosa and, 479

delirium and, 257, 269, 856

dementia and, 257

depression and, 307–308

electroconvulsive therapy and, 329

Munchausen syndrome by proxy and, 524

from myocardial infarction, 1056

substance-related disorders and

alcoholism, 242

cocaine, 441

heroin, 435

nicotine, 445, 1060

sudden cardiac death, 537

Mosher, George, 4

Motor programming tasks, 290, **292**

Motor vehicle crashes, alcohol-related, **243**

Mourning. *See also* Bereavement; Grief

in rehabilitation settings, 735

Movement disorders. *See also* Extrapyramidal symptoms; Parkinson's disease

differentiation from conversion disorder, 689

periodic leg movements of sleep, **497,** 502, **502,** 504, 510

restless legs syndrome, **497,** 510

in transplant recipients, 643

MPA. *See* Medroxyprogesterone acetate

MRI. *See* Magnetic resonance imaging

MS. *See* Multiple sclerosis

MS-Contin. *See* Morphine

MSE. *See* Mental status examination

MSLT (Multiple Sleep Latency Test), 507

MSPQ (Modified Somatic Perception Questionnaire), **371**

Multi Dimensional Health Locus of Control Scale (HLCS), 209

Multi-infarct dementia (MID), 56, 280

depression and, 316, 857

sleep disorders and, 512

Multidisciplinary pain clinics, 1009–1010

Multiple Risk Factor Intervention Trial, 539, 1058

Multiple sclerosis (MS), 63, 686–687

age at onset of, 466, 686

antidepressants for patients with, 693, **693**

anxiety and, 398

assessing emotional sequelae of, 96

clinical features of, 686

conversion symptoms and, 687

depression and, **310, 311,** 318–319, 686–687, **733**

etiology of, 686

intellectual decline in, 686

lesion on magnetic resonance imaging and psychiatric presentations of, 398

mania and, **345, 346,** 686, 733

neuropsychiatric symptoms of, 686–687

personality changes in, 686

prevalence of, 318, **680**

psychotherapy for persons with, 1032

sexual dysfunction and, 466–467, 738

sleep disorders and, 513

suicidality and, 129, **733**

Multiple Sleep Latency Test (MSLT), 507

Multiple system atrophy, 513

Munchausen syndrome, 115, **520,** 520–522. *See also* Factitious disorders

etiology of, 524, **524**

features of, 521, **522**

by proxy, 521, 523–526

in surgical patients, 596

Muscle relaxants, **400**

Muscular dystrophy, 686

Musculoskeletal disease, sleep disorders and, 504, 513

Mutism

akinetic, after liver transplantation, 643

in neuroleptic malignant syndrome, 692

Myasthenia gravis, 398

Mycobacterium tuberculosis meningitis, 688

Myelinoclastic disorders, **274**

Myelosuppression, tricyclic antidepressant-induced, 951

Myocardial infarction (MI). *See also* Coronary artery disease; Ischemic heart disease

anxiety disorders and, 396

depression and, 39, 113, 249–250, 307–308, 537, 541, 627, 1054–1055

drug-related

cocaine, 243, 441

MDMA, 443

electroconvulsive therapy and, 329, 1021

emergency department treatment of, 540

fight-or-flight response and, 536

insomnia and, 503

marital conflict after, 1062

mortality from, 1056

psychiatric clearance of patients after, 42

psychological distress and rehospitalization costs after, 1056

psychological treatment after, 541–542, 1032

sexual dysfunction and, 456, 1062

social support and, 540

type A behavior and, 539–540

behavioral and psychological interventions for, 1056

effect of treatment on risk of recurrent myocardial infarction, 1057

pharmacotherapy for, 1058

use of antidepressants after, 951

Myocardial ischemia, 538

Myocardial necrosis, 538

Myoclonus

delirium and, 262–263

differentiation from conversion movement disorder, 689

drug-induced

hydromorphone, **994**

in serotonin syndrome, 953

tricyclic antidepressants, 951

Myofascial trigger points, 571, **572**

Myotonic dystrophy, **680**

Myxedema, 263, 288

NA (Narcotics Anonymous), 421

Nadolol, 162, **463,** 694

Nafarelin, **463**

Nalbuphine, **993**

Naloxone challenge test, 437, **437,** 905

Naltrexone
  for alcoholism, 432, 875
  for hallucinogen-related flashbacks,
    443
  for opioid detoxification, 439, **439**
  side effects of, 432
    sexual dysfunction, **463**
Naproxen
  for fibromyalgia, 571
  sexual dysfunction induced by, **463**
Naratriptan, **463**
Narcissistic personality disorder, **116,
  120**
Narcolepsy, 501, 509–510
  age at onset of, 509
  classifications of, **496, 497**
  prevalence of, **680**
  symptoms of, 509
  treatment of, 509–510
Narcotics, defined, 993. *See also* Opioid
  analgesics
Narcotics Anonymous (NA), 421
Nasal effects
  of cocaine, 441
  of sildenafil, 460
Natanson v. Kline, 170
National Comorbidity Survey (NCS),
  340, 395
National Council on Alcoholism and
  Drug Dependence, 422
National Health Service (United
  Kingdom), 212
National Hemlock Society, 790
National Hospital Discharge Survey, 52
National Household Survey on Drug
  Abuse, 440
National Institute of Mental Health
  (NIMH), 7–8, 42
Nausea/vomiting
  antipsychotics for, 963
  in cancer patients
    anticipatory, 659–660, 1065
    antiemetics for, 659, 660, **669**
    relaxation training for, 1065
    Δ^9-tetrahydrocannabinol for, 444
  drug-induced
    antiretroviral drugs, 812
    bupropion, 952
    cancer chemotherapy, 659
    cocaine, 441
    fluoxetine, 786
    lamotrigine, 353, 961
    lithium, 350, 959
    naltrexone, 432
    nefazodone, 327
    nicotine, 445

opioid withdrawal, 437
psychostimulants, 956
reboxetine, 953
risperidone, 354
selective serotonin reuptake
  inhibitors, 761, 951
valproate, 350, 961
venlafaxine, 326, 829, 952
hyperemesis gravidarum, 706
Navane. *See* Thiothixene
NCS (National Comorbidity Survey),
  340, 395
NCSE (Neurobehavioral Cognitive
  Status Examination), 71–72, 83
Neck stiffness, 688
Necrotizing leukoencephalopathy,
  disseminated, 666
Nefazodone, 327, **948**
  for agitation and aggression, **161,** 162
  for anxiety disorders, **950**
  dosage of, **948**
  drug interactions with, 327
    antiretroviral drugs, 814, **815,** 829
    carbamazepine, 694
    cytochrome P450 metabolism
      and, **945**
  mechanism of action of, 327, **948,**
    952
  side effects of, 327, 950, 952
    sexual dysfunction, **463**
  structure of, 947
  use in specific patient groups or
    medical conditions
    cardiac disease, 543
    chronic pain, 693
    elderly persons, **863,** 864
    hepatic disease, 427
    HIV/AIDS, 829
    migraine, 693
    surgical patients, **597**
    transplant patients, **637,** 643
Negativistic personality disorder, **118**
Neglect of elderly persons, 859, **860**
Nelfinavir, **811**
Nembutal. *See* Pentobarbital
Nephrotic syndrome, 259, 978. *See also*
  Renal failure
Nervousness, drug-induced
  buspirone, 409
  psychostimulants, 787
  selective serotonin reuptake
    inhibitors, 326, 951
  venlafaxine, 326
Netherlands, consultation-liaison
  psychiatry in, 214–215
  background of, 214

future development, 215
in general hospital, 214
official status and training, 214–215
research, 215
Neurilemmomas, **681**
Neuritic plaques, 286, 858
Neurobehavioral Cognitive Status
  Examination (NCSE), 71–72, 83
Neurocirculatory asthenia, 1062
Neurofibrillary tangles, 286, 858
Neurogenic bladder, 693, **693**
Neuroimaging, 49–57, 77. *See also*
  specific imaging modalities
  in alcohol abusers, 293
  in Alzheimer's disease, **279**
  in amyotrophic lateral sclerosis, 319
  in anxiety, 406
  background of, 49–50
  for brain injury, 281
  in delirium, 264, **264**
  in delirium tremens, 258
  in dementia, 53–54, 56, 281,
    292–294, **293**
  in depression, 313
  before electroconvulsive therapy,
    1016, **1017**
  in emergency department, 894–895
  functional, 50–52
    applications of, 55–57
    in elderly persons, 861
    positron-emission tomography,
      51–52
    single photon emission computed
      tomography, 50–51
    topographical brain mapping, 52
  in HIV-associated neurocognitive
    impairment, 821, **822**
  limitations of, 77
  in mania, **346,** 346–347
  in panic disorder, 402
  research in, **192,** 193
  structural, 50
    applications of, 52–54, **53, 54**
    computed tomography, 50, 690,
      691
    in elderly persons, 861
    magnetic resonance imaging, 50,
      690–691
    utilization review of, 52
Neuroleptic malignant syndrome
  (NMS), 158, 263, 353, 408, 691,
    692, 968
  clinical features of, 968
  course and prognosis for, 968
  among dialysis patients, 561
  differential diagnosis of, 968

malignant hyperthermia, **597**
drugs associated with, 968
amoxapine, 951
etiology of, 968
laboratory findings in, 968
among patients with HIV/AIDS, 839
prevalence of, 968
rapid neuroleptization and, 965
treatment of, 968
electroconvulsive therapy, 968, 1023
Neuroleptics. *See* Antipsychotics
Neurological effects, **976**, 978–979
of antipsychotics, 966, 979
of bupropion, 326, 952, 978
of lithium, 350, 960
of psychostimulants, 787, 956
of tricyclic antidepressants, 951, 978
Neurological examination, 73, **74**, 290
Neurological and neurosurgical disorders. *See also* specific disorders
alcohol-related, 426
assessing emotional sequelae of, 96
brain injury, 281–282, 685
brain tumors, **681**, 681–683
central nervous system infections, 687–688
cerebrovascular disease, 679–681
cobalamin deficiency and, 569
degenerative diseases, 685–687
differential diagnosis of, 688–691
computed tomography of head, 690, **691**
electroencephalography, 691
etiologies of neuropsychiatric disorders, 688
examination for conversion disorder and somatoform pain disorder, 688–689, **690**
laboratory evaluation, 689–690
magnetic resonance imaging, **53**, 53–54, 690–691
neuropsychological testing, 691
electroconvulsive therapy for patients with, 1019–1020
epidemiology of, 679, **680**
psychiatric comorbidity with, 240, 679
anxiety, 398
delirium, 259, 262–263, 265
depression, 241, **310, 311,** 315–320
mania, **345, 346,** 733
psychosis, **896**
psychiatric management of patients with, 691–695, 978–979

anticonvulsants, 693–694
antidepressants, 692–693, **693**
β-blockers, 694
cognitive rehabilitation and retraining, 744–745
dopaminergics, 692
electroconvulsive therapy, 694
lithium, 694
neuroleptics, 691–692
psychostimulants, 692
psychotherapy, 694–695
ward management, 695
seizures, 683–685, **684**
sexual dysfunction and, 465–468
sleep disorders and, **497,** 504, 511–513
Neurological terminology, 73
Neurontin. *See* Gabapentin
Neuropathology
of alcoholic dementia, 288
of Alzheimer's disease, 286
of Creutzfeldt-Jakob disease, 287–288
of HIV-associated dementia, 287
of Huntington's disease, 286
of Parkinson's disease, 286
of Pick's disease, 286
of progressive supranuclear palsy, 287
of traumatic brain injury, 287
of vascular dementia, 287
Neuropeptide Y, 401
Neuroprotectants, 297
Neuropsychiatric Inventory (NPI), 294
Neuropsychological assessment, 15, 77–88. *See also* Psychological assessment
advantages and disadvantages of methods for, **81**
applications of, **84,** 84–88
agitation and aggression, 157
amnestic syndromes, 86, **86**
cerebrovascular accident, 85–86
dementia, 84–85, 278, 294
depression vs. dementia, 86–87
developmental learning disorders in adults, 87–88
HIV-associated neurocognitive impairment, 820–821
medicolegal competence determination, 96–97
traumatic brain injury, 86
battery-based approaches to, 82–83
Halstead-Reitan Neuropsychological Test Battery, 82

Luria-Nebraska Neuropsychological Battery, 82–83
bedside screening and extended mental status examinations, 83 (*See also* Mental status examination)
computerized, 97–98
functions of, 77–78
goals of, 80
Luria's model of brain functioning, 78–80, **79**
patient-centered and process-oriented approaches to, 80–82
Boston Process Approach, 81–82
flexible battery approach, 81
Luria's methods, 81
referral for, 98–100
preparing patient for evaluation, 99–100
selecting neuropsychologist, 98–99, **99**
writing referral, 99, **100**
summary of methods for, 83–84
Neuropsychologist, 30, 98–100, **99**
Neuroscience research, **192,** 192–193
Neurosyphilis, 282, **345,** 398, 576, 687–688
Neuroticism, **116**
Neurotransmitters. *See also* specific neurotransmitters
aggression, agitation and, 155–156
aging and, 862
alcohol intoxication and, 423–424
Alzheimer's disease and, 297
anxiety and, 399–401, **401**
depression and, 947
fight-or-flight response and, 536
mania and, 344
personality and, 116
psychotropic drug action and, 944
role in ventilation, 547
smoking and, 549
Nevirapine, **811**
cerebrospinal fluid penetration by, 823
drug interactions with
methadone, 838
psychotropic drugs, 814
in pregnancy, 809
"New Age healing," 363
New Zealand, consultation-liaison psychiatry in, 217–218
background of, 217–218
in general hospital, 218
official status and training, 218
research, 218

Niacin deficiency, **284, 345**
Nickel poisoning, **284**
Nicotine-related disorders, 239–240, 445–446, 1060. *See also* Smoking
  alcoholism and, 445, 549
  depression and, 445, 549, 1061
  effects of, 445
  genetic factors in, 445
  management of, 445–446, 1060–1061
    bupropion, 446
    clonidine, 1061
    factors associated with poor outcome of, 445
    fluoxetine, 171
    nicotine replacement therapy, 446, 549, 1061
    nortriptyline, 446
  nicotine-drug interactions, 445
  predisposition to, 445
  prevalence of, 445
  risk factors for, 445
  sleep disorders and, **502**
  symptoms of acute nicotine poisoning, 445
  tolerance, 445
  withdrawal, 445
    postsurgical, 600
Nicotine replacement therapy, 446, 549, 1061
  gum, 446, 1061
  inhaler, 446, 1061
  intranasal spray, 446, 1061
  transdermal patch, 446, 1061
Nifedipine
  for esophageal motility disorders, 554
  for monoamine oxidase inhibitor–induced hypertensive crisis, 955
  sexual dysfunction induced by, **463**
Nightmare disorder, **496**
Nilutamide, **463**
NIMH (National Institute of Mental Health), 7–8, 42
Nimodipine, 824
Nisoldipine, **463**
Nitrates, interaction with sildenafil, 460
Nitric oxide, 460
Nitroglycerin, 1021
Nitrous oxide abuse, 446
Nizatidine, **463**
NMDA receptors. *See* N-Methyl-D-aspartate receptors
NMS. *See* Neuroleptic malignant syndrome
NNRTIs. *See* Nonnucleoside reverse transcriptase inhibitors

Nociceptors, 991
Noctec. *See* Chloral hydrate
Noludar. *See* Methyprylon
Non-Hodgkin's lymphoma, 671
Non-rapid eye movement (NREM) sleep, 495
Noncontemporaneous control bias in research, **199**
Nonmaleficence, 167
Nonnucleoside reverse transcriptase inhibitors (NNRTIs), 810–811, **811**
  psychotropic drug interactions with, 814
  resistance to, 813
Nonresponse bias in research, **199**
Nonsteroidal anti-inflammatory drugs (NSAIDs)
  for acute pain, 995, **995**
  Alzheimer's disease and, 297
  anxiety induced by, **400**
  dementia induced by, **284**
  drug interactions with
    antipsychotics, 969
    cytochrome P450 metabolism and, **945**
    lithium, **349**, 960, **999**
  use in rehabilitation settings, 741, **742**
Nordiazepam, 904
Nordic countries, consultation-liaison psychiatry in, 207–209
  background of, 207
  future development, 209
  official status and training, 208
  psychiatry and general hospital patients, 207–208
  psychobiological approach, 209
  psychometric assessments, 209
  research, 208–209
  types of patients seen and specific services, 208
Norepinephrine
  aggression and, 155
  Alzheimer's disease and, 297
  depression and, 947
  fight-or-flight response and, 536
  interaction with antidepressants, **943**, 953
  mania and, 344
  platelet aggregation and, 536
Norethandrolone, **463**
Norfluoxetine, 326, 786, **945, 949**
Normal-pressure hydrocephalus (NPH), 282, 293, 296
Normeperidine, 999
Norplant, 323

Norpramin. *See* Desipramine
Nortriptyline, 325, **948**
  cytochrome P450 metabolism and, **945**
  dosage of, **948,** 950
  indications for
    pain syndromes, 1004–1005
    smoking cessation, 446, 549
  receptor site affinity of, **948**
  serum level of, 947
  side effects of
    cardiac effects, 542, 543
    sexual dysfunction, **463**
  use in specific patient groups or medical conditions
    chronic obstructive pulmonary disease, 549
    dying patients, 785, **785**
    elderly persons, **863,** 864
    Parkinson's disease, 693, **693**
    pathological laughing and crying, 693, **693**
    patients undergoing rehabilitation, **742**
    stroke, **693,** 741
    tinnitus, 693, **693**
Norvir. *See* Ritonavir
Norway, consultation-liaison psychiatry in, 207–209
NPH (normal-pressure hydrocephalus), 282, 293, 296
NPI (Neuropsychiatric Inventory), 294
NREM (non-rapid eye movement) sleep, 495
NRTIs (nucleoside reverse transcriptase inhibitors), 810–811, **811**
NSAIDs. *See* Nonsteroidal anti-inflammatory drugs
Nubain. *See* Nalbuphine
Nuclear magnetic resonance, 50. *See also* Magnetic resonance imaging
Nucleoside reverse transcriptase inhibitors (NRTIs), 810–811, **811**
Numorphan. *See* Oxymorphone
Nurses
  psychiatric nurse practitioners, 1028
  triage, 891
"Nutcracker esophagus," 114, 553
Nystagmus
  drug-induced
    lithium, 350, 611
    phencyclidine, 443, 905
  in transplant recipients, 643

OAS (Overt Aggression Scale), 149, 151, 152, **153, 155,** 159

OASS (Overt Agitation Severity Scale), 151–155, **154,** 159
Obesity, **594**
    cardiac disease and, 1059–1060
    genetic factors and, 1059
Obesity-hyperventilation syndrome, 507
Obsessive-compulsive disorder (OCD), 395, 404–405
    anorexia nervosa and, 479, 480
    antidepressants for, **950,** 969
    body dysmorphic disorder and, 381
    bulimia nervosa and, 480
    definition of, 404
    fluoxetine for, 171
    HIV/AIDS and, 833
    irritable bowel syndrome and, 555, **555**
    migraine headache and, 398
    "poor insight" type, 404
    positron-emission tomography in, 55
    somatization and, **362**
    thyroid disease and, 245
Obsessive-compulsive personality disorder, **116,** 117
    prevalence of, **120**
    somatization disorder and, 120, 375
Obstetrics and gynecology, 701–713. *See also* Pregnancy
    abortion, 706
    adolescent pregnancy, 709
    child custody issues, 711
    eating disorders, 713
    gynecological cancers, 713
        suicidality and, 129
    HIV/AIDS and other sexually transmitted diseases, 712–713
    menopause, 702–703, **703**
    other reasons for psychiatric consultation, 711
    postpartum patient, 709–710
    pregnancy loss, 710–711
    psychiatric complications of pregnancy, 706–709
        acute psychiatric decompensation, 707–709, **709**
        hyperemesis gravidarum, 706
        morbid anxiety, 707
        noncompliance with obstetric advice, 706–707
        pseudocyesis, 706
        unacknowledged pregnancy, 709
    psychiatric consultation during labor, 709, **709**
    psychiatric presentations related to, 704

psychotropic drug use in pregnancy, 707–708, **708**
    rape and domestic violence, 711–712
    reproductive physiology and psychology through life cycle, 701–703, **702**
    sterility, fertility, and infertility, 704–706
        infertility and its treatment, 705–706
        voluntary sterilization, 704–705
    training in, 701
    women's health and health care, 701, 703–704
Occupational therapists, 731, 732
Occupational therapy, for agitation and aggression, 157
OCD. *See* Obsessive-compulsive disorder
Ocular effects. *See also* Ophthalmology
    of chlorpromazine, 611
    neuroleptic-induced oculogyric crisis, 611
    of quetiapine, 611, 966
    of thioridazine, 966
OKT3, 641–643
Olanzapine, 963, **964**
    cytochrome P450 metabolism and, **945**
    dosage of, **964**
    indications for
        Alzheimer's disease, 296
        delirium, 268, **794**
        mania, 354
        schizophrenia, 354
    mechanism of action of, 963
    side effects of, 354, **964**
        sexual dysfunction, **463**
    use in specific patient groups or medical conditions
        dying patients, 782, **782, 794**
        elderly persons, **863**
        HIV/AIDS, 825, 839
        surgical patients, **598**
        transplant patients, **636,** 641
Olivopontocerebellar atrophy, 512, 687
Omega-3 fatty acids, 1058
Omeprazole, **463, 945**
Oncology, 657–673. *See also* Cancer
Ondansetron, 268, 660, **669**
Openness to experience, **116**
Operative syndromes, 593–594
Ophthalmology, 610–612. *See also* Ocular effects
    acute vision loss in adults, 610–611

neuropsychiatric aspects of blindness, 611–612
    ophthalmic-psychotropic drug interactions, 611–612
    "psychosomatic," 610
    vision loss in children, 610
Ophthalmoplegia, 265, 283
Opiates, defined, 993
Opioid agonists, 438–439
Opioid analgesics, 993, **993**
    for acute pain, 995, **995**
    administration routes for, 993
    agonists and agonist-antagonists, **993**
    for chronic pain, 435, 1006–1007
    development of tolerance to, **994**
    dosage of, **993**
        potency conversion, **437**
        prn dosing, **994**
        underdosing, 990, **994**
    drug interactions with
        alcohol, 427, **428**
        antipsychotics, **944**
    duration of action of, **993**
    opioid paradox, 1007
    for patient-controlled analgesia, 995
    pharmacokinetics of, 993, **994**
    principles of use of, 995
    problems associated with use of, **994**
    side effects of, **994,** 999
        delirium, **762,** 793
        sleep disorders, **502**
    somatization and, **362**
    for somatoform pain disorder, 384
    use in specific patient groups or medical conditions
        cancer, 435
        children, 724, **724**
        dying patients, 782–783, 796, **797**
        patients undergoing rehabilitation, 741, **742**
        patients with history of substance abuse, 440, 996–997
        renal dysfunction, **994**
Opioid receptors, 436
Opioid-related disorders, 435–440
    clinical cues to, 435, **436**
    duration of opioid detectability in urine, **895**
    emergency department management of, 904–905
    epidemiology of, 436
    genetic factors in, 436
    among health care professionals, 435
    intoxication, 437, 905
    medical complications of, 436, 905
    mortality from, 435

Opioid-related disorders *(continued)*
  naloxone challenge test for, 437, 905
  pain management in persons with,
      440, 996–997
  pathophysiology of, 436
  polysubstance abuse and, 435
    benzodiazepines, 902
  psychiatric comorbidity with,
      436–437
    depression, **311,** 324, 436–437
  "speedballing," 435
  suicide and, 134
  treatment of, 437–440
    L-α-acetylmethadol maintenance,
        418, 438
    buprenorphine maintenance, 438
    detoxification from combinations
        of opioids and other
        substances, 440
    detoxification from heroin and
        other opiates, 438–439
    detoxification from methadone,
        438
    detoxification using clonidine,
        436, 439, **439,** 905
    detoxification using clonidine and
        naltrexone, 439, **439**
    methadone maintenance,
        437–438, **439,** 905
    Narcotics Anonymous, 421
  withdrawal, 436, 437, **437, 781,** 905,
      996–997
Oral contraceptives, **943**
  depression induced by, **311,** 322–323
  drug interactions with
    carbamazepine, 352, 962
    immunosuppressants, 643
  sleep disorders induced by, **502**
Oral drug administration, 941
Orap. *See* Pimozide
Orbitofrontal syndrome, 682
Organ transplant psychiatry (OTP),
    623–624, 646, **647.** *See also*
    Transplantation
Organic mental disorders, 41, 792
  anorexia nervosa and, 480
  cancer and, 245
  HIV infection and, 259
Organization of consultation-liaison
    service, 17–21
  administrative concerns, 17
  general medical-surgical hospitals
      with teaching programs, 18–20
    fellows, 18–19, **19,** 30
    medical students, 18
    other staff, 20, **20**

residents, 18
group practice, 20
information needed for, 17, **17**
keys to establishing effective service,
    21, **21**
liaison with other specialties, 20
private practice, 20
Organochlorine pesticides, **284**
Organophosphate insecticides, **284**
Orientation assessment, 68. *See also*
    Disorientation
Orientation-Memory-Concentration
    test, 294
Oropharyngeal cancer, 314, 445
Orthopedic surgery, 37, 608–610
  benefits of psychiatric consultation
      for, 608
  categories of, 608
  in children, 608
  chronic pain and, 609
  delirium after, 257, 259, 269, 609,
      856
  substance abuse and, 609–610
Orthostatic hypotension, drug-induced,
    974
  antipsychotics, 158, 409, 544, 723,
      964, 965
  clozapine, 966
  methotrimeprazine, 794
  monoamine oxidase inhibitors, 327,
      544, 864
  risperidone, 354
  trazodone, 543, 952
  tricyclic antidepressants, 325, 408,
      543, 950, 951
Osteoporosis, **239,** 483, 703
Osteosarcoma, 671
Ostomy patients, 457
OTP (organ transplant psychiatry),
    623–624, 646, **647.** *See also*
    Transplantation
Outcome studies, 25–27
  for telepsychiatry, 929–930
Outpatient consultation-liaison
    psychiatry services, 30, 41
  clinical disorders presenting to,
      922–924
    anxiety disorders, 923
    depression, 922–923
    functional somatic symptoms, 922
    substance use disorders, 923–924
  effectiveness of, 918
  integrated medical-psychiatry
      services, 871–884 (*See also*
      Integrated medical-psychiatry
      services)

liaison activities of, 922
limitations of, 875–876
rehabilitation and, 746
roles and expectations for, 921–922
  consultant, 921
  patient, 922
  primary care physician, 921–922
settings for, 918–919
  medical specialty clinics, 918–919
  primary care group practices, 918
  training clinics, 918
structure of, 919–921
  communication following
      consultation, 920
  consultation visit, 919–920
  continuity, 920
  financing, 921
  follow-up, 920
  location, 919
  referral, 919
  service planning, 920–921
Ovarian cancer, 457
Overdose. *See* Drug overdose
Overt Aggression Scale (OAS), 149,
    151, 152, **153, 155,** 159
Overt Agitation Severity Scale (OASS),
    151–155, **154,** 159
Oxazepam, **903,** 969, **970**
  for alcohol withdrawal, 430–431, **431**
  for Alzheimer's disease, 296
  dosage of, **407, 434, 903, 970**
  half-life of, **407, 903**
  pharmacokinetics of, 970
  use in specific patient groups or
      medical conditions
    dialysis patients, 561
    elderly persons, **863**
    hepatic disease, 977
    HIV/AIDS, 834
    transplant candidates, 638
Oxybutynin, **463**
Oxycodone, **995**
  abuse of, 904
  for children, **724**
  detoxification from, 437, 438–439
  dosage of, **437**
  drug interactions with
    ritonavir, **815**
    selective serotonin reuptake
        inhibitors, 326
  duration of detectability in urine, **895**
  for periodic leg movements of sleep
      and restless legs syndrome, 510
Oxygen therapy, 548
Oxyhemoglobin desaturation, 508
Oxymetholone, **463**

Oxymorphone, **437**
Oxyphencyclimine, **463**

P300, 57, 77
Pacemakers, 510, 1021
PACT (Psychosocial Assessment of Candidates for Transplant), 625–626
PAI (Personality Assessment Inventory), 91, 94, 95, 97
Pain
  abdominal, 552
    psychostimulant-induced, 723
  acute, 991
    drug-seeking behavior and, 996, **996**
    fear and, 997
    objective signs of, 993
  biliary, 552
  cancer and, 435, **796,** 797, 997
  central, 991, **1005**
  chest, 991
    anxiety and, 403, 406
    esophageal dysmotility and, 554
    noncardiac, **365,** 1062
  child's exaggerated complaints of, 725
  chronic, 991, 997–999
    behavioral medicine and, 1067–1070, **1068**
    cancer-related, 997
    chronic pain syndrome, **1000,** 1004, **1005**
    differential diagnosis of, 998–999
    economic cost of, 997
    epidemiology of, 997
    "guarding" behavior and, 1068
    MADISON scale for, 1068, **1069**
    mechanism of, 997–998
    physical examination for, 1004, **1005**
    prevalence of, 997
    psychiatric evaluation of patients with, 998, **999**
  complex regional pain syndrome, 992
  definitions related to, 991–992
  denial in patients with, 990, 1003
  drawing a picture of, 1002, **1002,** 1004
  fibromyalgia, 570–571, 997
  HIV/AIDS and, 835–836, **836**
  low back, 1068
  management of (*See* Pain management)
  measurement of, **371,** 992, **992**

  mental and physical components of, 990
  neuropathic, 991, 1004–1006
  opiate-insensitive, **994**
  orthopedic, 609
  patient complaints of, 990
  pelvic, 1070
  phantom limb, 65, 735, 991
  placebo effect in persons with, 992
  postherpetic neuralgia, 1004, 1006, 1008
  posttraumatic, 998
  psychiatric comorbidity with, 383, 998, **1000,** 1000–1004
    anxiety disorders, 1000
    conversion disorder, **1001,** 1002
    depression, **310,** 314–315, 367, 383, **733,** 998, 1000, 1067
    dissociative states, 1003
    factitious disorder with physical symptoms, 1003
    hypochondriasis, **1001,** 1002, **1002**
    malingering, 1003
    pain disorder, 381–383, **382, 1001,** 1002
    personality disorders, 1003
    psychosis, 1004
    somatoform disorders, **362,** 365, 1000–1002, **1001**
  rectal, 1063
  rehabilitation of persons with, 1008
  in rehabilitation settings, 738
  sexual pain disorders, **1000**
  sympathetically mediated, 992
  tolerance for, 991
  unnecessary, 990
Pain disorder, 373, 381–383, **1001,** 1002
  chronic, 8
  clinical course and prognosis for, 383
  clinical features of, 382–383
  definition of, 381, 1002
  diagnostic criteria for, 381–382, **382**
  differential diagnosis of, 383
  epidemiology of, 382
  management of, 383–387
  psychiatric comorbidity with, 383
  somatization and, **362,** 365
Pain management, 383–387, 989–1010.
    See also Analgesics
  for acute pain, 993–997
    medications, **995,** 995–997
    psychiatric consultation, 995–997
  barriers to, 990, **990**
  for burn patients, 612, 990
  for cancer patients, 435, 796, **797,** 997, 1065

  for children, 724, **724**
  for chronic pain, 435
  for dying patients, 773–774, 782–783, 796, **797**
  inadequate, 990
  multidisciplinary pain clinics for, 1009–1010
  nonpharmacological, 1008–1009
    cognitive and behavioral therapies, 314, 1008–1009, 1067–1070
    electroconvulsive therapy, 1021
    psychotherapy, 1009
    transcutaneous electrical nerve stimulation, 1008
  in opioid-addicted patients, 440, 996–997
  pharmacological, 989, **989,** 1004–1008
    for acute pain, **995,** 995–997
    anticonvulsants, 315, **989,** 1006
    antidepressants, 314, 693, **693,** 950, **989,** 1004–1006, 1067
    antipsychotics, **989,** 1007–1008
    benzodiazepines, **989,** 1006
    drug interactions with, 999, **999**
    drug-seeking behavior and, 996, **996**
    lack of response to, 995–996
    medication contract, **1010**
    opioid analgesics, 435, 796, **797,** 993, **993, 994,** 1006–1007
    pain syndromes responsive to psychiatric medications, 990
    placebo effect and, 992
    psychostimulants, **989,** 1007
    World Health Organization analgesic ladder, **995**
  postoperative, 602
    after cardiothoracic surgery, 605, **605**
  principles of, **1009**
  in rehabilitation settings, 741, **742**
  role of consultation-liaison psychiatrist in, 990–991, 995–997
  for somatoform pain disorder, 384
  team approach to, 989, 991
  training in, 989
  treatment planning for, 1004
Pain measures, **371,** 992, **992**
Pain-prone disorder, **118,** 122
Palliative care, 773–775. *See also* Dying patients
  definition of, 773
  early concept of, 773, **773**
  goals of, 774
  growing need for, 774
  progressive concept of, 773, **774**

Palliative Care Foundation, 773
Pamelor. *See* Nortriptyline
Pancreas transplantation. *See also*
     Transplantation
     psychiatric disorders among
          candidates for, 628
          anxiety disorders, 397, 403
     in psychotic patients, 630–631
Pancreatic disease
     cancer, 670
          depression and, 245, 314, 661
          clozapine-induced, 966
          dementia and, **284**
Pancuronium, **763**
Panhypopituitarism, **284**
Panic attacks, 394. *See also* Anxiety; Fear
     before cosmetic surgery, 613
     diagnostic criteria for, **395**
     drug seeking for, 907
     mechanical ventilation–associated,
          399
     nocturnal, 501
          sleep apnea and, 399
     outpatient psychiatric consultation
          for, 923
     pharmacological provocation of, 400
     in surgical patients, 595, 596
Panic disorder, 394, 403
     age at onset of, **63**
     alcoholism and, 423
     atypical chest pain and, 1062
     cardiac disease and, 403, 536, 541,
          627
     chronic obstructive pulmonary
          disease and, 245, 399, 548
     delirium and, 262
     diagnosis of, 394, **395**
     among dying patients, 781
     esophageal motility disorders and,
          554
     fatigue and, 570
     gastrointestinal disease and, 245
     HIV/AIDS and, 833
     hypochondriasis and, 378
     insomnia and, 500–501
     irritable bowel syndrome and,
          554–555, **555**
     migraine headache and, 398
     neurophysiology of, 400–401
     positron-emission tomography in,
          402, 403
     prevalence of, 242, **396, 680, 872**
     psychiatric emergencies in patients
          with, 907
     respiration in, 547–548
     sleep deprivation and, 403

somatization and, 242, **362**, 375, 376
suicide and, 134
thyroid disease and, 245
in transplant recipients, 642
treatment of
     antidepressants, **950**, 954, 969,
          972
     benzodiazepines, 970
Papaverine, **463**, 466
Paraldehyde, 159, 505
Paralytic agents, 761, 762, **763**
Paraneoplastic syndromes, 280, 665,
     682–683
Paranoia, drug-induced
     amphetamines, **156**
     cocaine, **156**, 441
     hallucinogens, 443
Paranoid personality disorder, **116**, 121
     countertransference and, 122
     prevalence of, **120**
     somatization disorder and, 120, 375
Paraphilias, 469–470
     treatment of, 470–471
Parasomnias, **496, 497**, 499. *See also*
     Sleep disorders
Parathyroid disorders
     dementia and, **284**
     hyperparathyroidism, **565**, 566
          depression and, **311**, 320
          prevalence of psychiatric
               comorbidity with, **564**
Parenteral drugs, 941
Pargyline, **463**
Parkinsonism, 279
     drug-induced, 686
          amoxapine, 686
          fluoxetine, 686
          lithium, 686, 959
          MDMA, 443
          metoclopramide, 686
          neuroleptics, 158, 686, 691, 965
          treatment of, 965
     postencephalopathic, **345**
Parkinson's–amyotrophic lateral
     sclerosis–dementia complex, 513
Parkinson's disease, 279, 685–686
     Alzheimer's disease and, 275, 279
     anxiety disorders and, 398
     clinical features of, 279, 685–686
     course and prognosis for, 295
     dementia and, 275, 276, 513
     depression and, 279, **310, 311**,
          316–317, 685, 686, 858
     genetic factors in, 277
     inpatient medical-psychiatric
          treatment for, 874

mood disorders and, 62, 63, 241
neuroimaging in, 294
pathophysiology of, 286
prevalence of, **680**
psychiatric comorbidity with, 150
psychotherapy for persons with,
     1032
psychotropic drug use in
     antidepressants, 317, 693, **693**
     antipsychotics, 691–692, 979
sleep disorders and, 501, 504, 513
treatment of, 686
     dopaminergic agents, 295, 686
     electroconvulsive therapy, 874,
          979, 1019
     selegiline, 686, 693
Parotid gland enlargement, 487
Paroxetine, 326, **948**
     dosage of, **948**
     drug interactions with
          codeine, **999**
          cytochrome P450 metabolism
               and, 326, **945, 949, 952**
     half-life of, **949**
     indications for
          agitation and aggression, 161–162
          anxiety disorders, 969
          neuropathic pain, 786
     receptor site affinity of, **948**
     side effects of
          sedation, 951
          sexual dysfunction, **463**
     structure of, 947
     use in specific patient groups or
          medical conditions
          cancer, 663
          cardiac disease, 408, 542, 951
          children, **723**
          critically ill patients, 761
          dying patients, **785**, 786
          elderly persons, 863, **863**
          HIV/AIDS, 828–829
          neurogenic bladder with
               retention, 693
          Parkinson's disease, 693
          pregnancy, 979
          transplant recipients, 643
     withdrawal from, 953
Paroxysmal limbic disorder, 688
Partial pressure of carbon dioxide
     (pCO$_2$), 546
     in anxiety disorders, 547–548
     in depression, 547
PAS (physician-assisted suicide) and
     euthanasia, 144–146, 175,
          789–791, **790**, 831

Passive-aggressive personality disorder, **118,** 121, 122
    prevalence of, **120**
Pastoral counseling, 787
Pathological laughing and crying, 693,
    693
Patient-controlled analgesia (PCA), 995
"Patient dumping," 891
Patient-oriented consultation, **6**
Patient Self-Determination Act, 175
Paxil. *See* Paroxetine
PCA (patient-controlled analgesia), 995
PCD (postcardiotomy delirium), 38,
    259, 268, 605, 765–766, **767**
pCO₂. *See* Partial pressure of carbon
    dioxide
PCP. *See* Phencyclidine-related disorders
PDR *(Physicians' Desk Reference)*, 171
PDRT (Portland Digit Recognition Test),
    97
Pediatrics, 717–726. *See also* Children
    and adolescents
    administrative issues in, 722
    characteristics of consultation in, **726**
    child psychiatric assessment, **720,**
        720–721, **721**
    clinical issues in consultation,
        724–726
        behavioral intervention in
            medically ill patient,
            725–726
        compliance with medical regimen,
            725
        exaggerated pain, 725
        suicide attempt, 724–725
    developmental and behavioral, 718
    developmental perspective of, 718
    evolution of consultation-liaison
        psychiatry in, 717
    family focus of, 719
    hospital pediatric units, 719
    preventive emphasis of, 718
    process of consultation in, 719–720,
        726
    psychotropic drug use in, 722–724,
        723, 724
    relationship with child psychiatry,
        717
    specialty of, 718
Pelvic floor dyssynergia, 1063
Pelvic inflammatory disease, 712
Pelvic pain, 1070
Pemoline, 955–956, **956**
    for cancer patients, 662
    chewable form of, 662
    dosage of, 956, **956**

for dying patients, **785,** 786–787
sleep disorders induced by, **502**
use in liver disease, 662
Penicillamine, 295
Penicillin, **762**
Pennebaker Inventory of Limbic
    Languidness (PILL), **371**
Pentamidine, **818**
Pentazocine, **762, 993**
Pentobarbital, **434, 895, 904, 904**
Pentobarbital challenge test, 434, **435,**
    904
Pentothal. *See* Thiopental
Peptic ulcer disease, 4, 1062
    behavioral therapies for, 1062
    differentiation from functional
        dyspepsia, 1062
    eating disorders and, 482, 487
    panic disorder and, 242
    sleep disorders and, 504, 513
    suicide and, 129
Peptide T, 824
Perceived Competence Scale for
    Children, **720**
Perceptual disturbances
    assessment for, 64–65
    delirium and, 262
    drug-induced
        bupropion, 326
        hallucinogens, 443
        inhalants, 446
        phencyclidine, 443
    due to vision loss, 610–612
    in postconcussion syndrome, 685
Perchloroethylene, **284**
Percocet. *See* Oxycodone
Peregrination, 522
Pergolide
    for Parkinson's disease, 686
    for periodic leg movements of sleep
        and restless legs syndrome, 510
    sexual dysfunction induced by, **463**
Periodic leg movements of sleep
    (PLMS), **497,** 502, **502,** 504, 510
Peripheral neuropathy
    HIV/AIDS and, 836
    systemic lupus erythematosus and,
        568
    tricyclic antidepressant–induced, 951
Pernicious anemia, 288, 569
Perphenazine, **964**
    dosage of, **964**
    for organic mental disorder, 480
    for pain syndromes, **989**
    psychiatric aspects of, **669**
    side effects of, **964**

sexual dysfunction, **463**
use during breast-feeding, **981**
Perseveration, 261
Personality, 107–116
    "arthritic," 1066
    definition of, 107, 116, 123
    dynamic nature of, 107
    effect on interactions with treatment
        team, 107
    five-factor model of, 116, **116**
    impact on doctor-patient
        relationship, 111–113
    impact on patient's response to
        illness, 108–111
        defense mechanisms, 108–110, **109**
        helplessness and control, 110–111
        in intensive care unit, 763–765,
            764, 766
        shame and guilt, 111
    of intensive care unit patient,
        763–765
    making a personality diagnosis,
        1037–1038
    somatization and, 368
    specific illness, behavior, and, 113–116
        AIDS, 114
        cardiac disease, 113–114
        gastrointestinal disease, 114–115
        somatization and somatization
            disorder, 115–116
    suicide and, 129
    type A, 113–114, 117, **118,** 1054
        behavioral and psychological
            interventions for, 1056
        cardiac disease and, 113–114,
            539–540, 1054, 1058
        effect on risk of recurrent
            myocardial infarction, 1057
        pharmacotherapy for, 1058
        sympathoadrenal system and,
            539, 1059
    types of, 1037–1038, **1038**
Personality Assessment Inventory (PAI),
    91, 94, 95, 97
Personality changes
    in amyotrophic lateral sclerosis, 687
    after brain injury, 685
    due to general medical condition,
        150, **151**
    in frontotemporal dementia, 277
    in herpes simplex encephalitis, 688
    in HIV/AIDS, 282
    in Huntington's disease, 278
    in multiple sclerosis, 686
    posttraumatic, 281
    in Wilson's disease, 279

Personality disorders, 116–123
anorexia nervosa and, 479
bulimia nervosa and, 480
cancer and, 245
character spectrum disorder and, 310
classification of, 116–117, **116–117**
combinations of, 119
comorbidity with Axis I disorders, 119
conversion disorder and, 380
course and outcome in medically ill patients, 251
defense mechanisms and, 108
definition of, 116, 123
dermatological conditions and, 121
diagnosis of, 118–119
disorders not included in list of Axis II disorders, 117–118, **118**
epidemiology of, 119–120
factitious disorder and, 120–121, 523
Huntington's disease and, 686
hypochondriasis and, 120, 121, 378
impact on medication use, 121
interaction with somatic illness, 120–122
in medically ill patients, 243
neurological and neurosurgical disorders and, 679
pain and, **1000**, 1003
prevalence of, 119, **120**, 243
psychiatric emergencies in patients with, 907–908
somatization and, 115–116, 120, 368
somatization disorder and, 375
substance-related disorders and, 423
suicide and, 133, **134**
in surgical patients, 595
transference reactions and, 120
transplantation for patients with, 632
treatment compliance and, 121
Personality measures, 89–92, **371**
objective, 89–91
advantages and disadvantages of, **95**
cautions about use in medical patients, 89
Millon Behavioral Health Inventory, 91
Millon Clinical Multiaxial Inventory, 91
Minnesota Multiphasic Personality Inventory, 89–91, **90**
Personality Assessment Inventory, 91
projective, 91–92

advantages and disadvantages of, **95**
Rorschach inkblot test, 92
Rotter Incomplete Sentences Blank, 92
Thematic Apperception Test, 92
PET. *See* Positron-emission tomography
Phantom limb pain, 65, 735, 991
Pharmacodynamics, 943–944
aging and, 862
Pharmacokinetics, 941–942
aging and, 861, **862**
of anticonvulsants, 353, 960–961
of antidepressants, 947
monoamine oxidase inhibitors, 954
of antipsychotics, 963
of benzodiazepines, 970
drug absorption, 941
drug distribution, 941–942
drug elimination, 942
drug metabolism, 942
of lithium, 958
of opioids, 993, **994**
of psychostimulants, 955
Pharmacotherapy, 939–981, **942**. *See also* specific drugs and classes
administration routes for, 941
cautions about use in medically ill patients, 940
choice of drug, 941
compliance with, 941 (*See also* Compliance with treatment)
discontinuing before electroconvulsive therapy, 1016–1017
dosage for, 940–941
avoiding prn dosing, 940
drug combinations for, 940–941
drug interactions with, **943–946,** 944 (*See also* Drug interactions)
for elderly persons, 861–864, **863,** 940
formulating diagnosis for, 939–940, 1040, **1041**
generic drugs, 941
initiation of, 939–940
medications for, 944–973
anticonvulsants, 960–962
antidepressants, 325–327, 944–957, 972
antipsychotics, 962–969, **964**
anxiolytics and sedatives, 969–973
benzodiazepines, 969–972, **970**
buspirone, 972

herbal medicinals, 973, **974**
lithium, 957–960
mood stabilizers, 957–962
psychostimulants, 955–957, **956**
patient education about, 941, **942**
for pediatric patients, 722–724, **723, 724**
pharmacodynamics and receptor site activity, 943–944
pharmacokinetics and, 941–942 (*See also* Pharmacokinetics)
poor response to, 941
during pregnancy and lactation, 979–981, **980, 981**
prescribing medication for unapproved uses, 170–171
principles of, **940,** 940–941
prophylactic, 940–941
serum drug level monitoring, 942–943
side effects of, 239, 940 (*See also* Substance-induced disorders)
for specific disorders
agitation and aggression, 157–163, **159–162**
Alzheimer's disease, 296–297
anxiety disorders, 406–409
bulimia nervosa, 489
delirium, **266,** 267–268
depression, 325–327
erectile dysfunction, 460
HIV-associated neurocognitive impairment, 823–824
insomnia, 505, **506**
mania, **347–349,** 347–354
narcolepsy, 509–510
opioid dependence, 438–439, **439**
pain syndromes, 989, **989,** 1004–1008
Parkinson's disease, 295
periodic leg movements of sleep, 510
restless legs syndrome, 510
somatoform disorders, 384
type A behavior, hostility, and anger, 1058
vascular dementia, 296, 297
Wilson's disease, 295
for specific patient groups or medical conditions, 973–981, **975–976**
cancer, 662–663
cardiac disease, 542–545, 974, 977
critically ill patients, 756–757, **757**
dying patients, **782,** 782–787, **785**

endocrine disease, 978
gastrointestinal disease, 977
hematopoietic disease, 978
hepatic disease, 757, 977
HIV/AIDS, 823–824, 828–830,
833, 834
irritable bowel syndrome,
555–556
malabsorption syndromes, 602
neurological disease, 978–979
patients undergoing rehabilitation,
740–741, **742–743**
patients who can take nothing by
mouth, 601–602
pregnancy and lactation, 707–708,
708, 710
pulmonary disease, 548–549, 977
renal disease, 757, 977–978
surgical patients, 596, **597–598,**
601–602
transplant patients, 634–638,
635–637
switching between drugs, 940
Pharmacotherapy, 45
Phenacetin, **945**
Phencyclidine (PCP)-related disorders,
442–443
acute management of, 443, 905–906
complications of, 443, 905
psychiatric comorbidity with, 443
mania, **345**
sexual dysfunction and, **463**
symptoms of, 443
urine testing for, 443, **895**
Phenelzine, 327, 954, **954**
side effects of
cardiac effects, 544
insomnia, **502**
sexual dysfunction, **463**
use in dying patients, **785**
use in pregnancy, **708**
Phenmetrazine, **463**
Phenobarbital, **904**
for benzodiazepine withdrawal, 435
dosage of, **434**
drug interactions with
cytochrome P450 metabolism
and, **945, 946**
methadone, 438
valproate, **349,** 351
duration of detectability in urine, **895**
Phenothiazines, **943, 964.** *See also*
Antipsychotics
drug interactions with
antidepressants, **943**

cytochrome P450 metabolism
and, **945**
monoamine oxidase inhibitors,
955
ophthalmic β-blockers, 611
for pain syndromes, 1007
sleep disorders induced by, **502**
use in specific patient groups or
medical conditions
surgical patients, **598**
transplant candidates, **636**
withdrawal from, 969
Phenoxybenzamine, **463**
Phentermine, **345**
Phentolamine, **463,** 466, 955
Phenylbutazone, **349, 943**
Phenylephrine, 969
insomnia and, **502**
interaction with antidepressants,
943, 953, 955
mania induced by, **346**
Phenylpropanolamine, 479, 481, 955
Phenytoin, **943**
for alcohol withdrawal seizures, 432,
433
drug interactions with
alcohol, 427, **428**
antiretroviral drugs, 814, 839
cytochrome P450 metabolism
and, **945, 946**
disulfiram, 432
methadone, 438
for patients undergoing
rehabilitation, **742**
sexual dysfunction induced by, **463**
Pheochromocytoma, **565,** 566–567, **594**
anxiety and, 402, 566–567
psychiatric comorbidity with, **564**
Phobias, 404
diabetes mellitus and, 397
among dying patients, 781
among elderly persons, 858
prevalence of, **396**
psychiatric emergencies in patients
with, 907
somatization disorder and, 375
thyroid disease and, 245
Photosensitivity, drug-induced
antipsychotics, 966
tricyclic antidepressants, 951
Physical examination
for chronic pain, 1004, **1005**
for depression, 313
of elderly persons, 860
in emergency department, 893
for somatization, 370–371

Physical medicine and rehabilitation,
729–747
cardiac rehabilitation, 542, 607,
1058–1059
competency issues in, 739–740
consultation-liaison psychiatry
training in, 746–747
context of, 730–732
comprehensive evaluation, 731
cultural sensitivity, 731
diagnostic groups and problems,
730, **730**
functional assessment, 731–732
management protocols, 731
multidisciplinary focus, 732
referring source, 730
rehabilitation teams, 731
rehabilitation vs. acute medicine
and surgery, 730
three-hour rule, 730–731
time and patient stability, 730
definitions related to, 729–730
increasing use of, 729
management of problems related to,
740–746
behavioral and cognitive therapies,
744
brief and supportive
psychotherapy, 744
cognitive rehabilitation and
retraining, 744–745
family treatment, 745, **745**
group psychotherapy, 745
medical interventions, 740
pharmacotherapy, 740–741,
742–743
ward management, 745–746
outpatient consultation-liaison
psychiatry and, 746
problems among families and
caregivers, 739, **740**
reasons for psychiatric consultation
related to, 732–739
adjustment and coping problems,
734
anxiety, 736–737
behavior problems, 736, **736**
body image changes, 734–735
cognitive and neurobehavioral
problems, 733–734
depression and suicidality,
732–733, **733,** 746
loss and mourning, 735, **735**
mania, 733
nonadherence to treatment, 735
pain, 738

Physical medicine and rehabilitation *(continued)*
　reasons for psychiatric consultation related to *(continued)*
　　sexual dysfunction, 738–739
　　sleep problems, 738
　　substance-related problems, 737–738
　role of psychiatry in, 729
　staff problems related to, 740
Physical reactivation, for somatoform disorders, 384
Physical therapists, 731
Physical therapy, for somatoform disorders, 384
Physician-assisted suicide (PAS) and euthanasia, 144–146, 175, 789–791, **790,** 831
Physicians, nonpsychiatric
　assessment of, 39–40
　developing autonomy of, 40, **40**
　expectations of psychiatric consultant, 14
　missed diagnosis of cognitive impairment by, 61
　models of psychiatric training for, **42,** 42–45
　pedagogical relationship between psychiatrists and, 46
　primary care, 921–922
　psychotherapeutic skills of, 1028
Physicians' Desk Reference (PDR), 171
Physicians Online, 934
Physostigmine, **743**
Pica, 477, **478,** 481
Pick bodies, 286
Pick cells, 286
Pick's disease, 273, 277–278
　clinical features of, 277–278
　mania and, **345**
　pathophysiology of, 286
　prevalence of, **680**
　sleep disorders and, 512
Pickwickian syndrome, 507
Pigmentary retinopathy, thioridazine-induced, 966
PILL (Pennebaker Inventory of Limbic Languidness), **371**
Pimozide, **964**
　for delusional disorder, 962
　dosage of, **964**
　drug interactions with
　　cytochrome P450 metabolism and, **945**
　　ritonavir, 814, **815**
　side effects of, **964**

sexual dysfunction, **463**
　for Tourette's syndrome, **945**
Pindolol, 162, **463,** 694
Pinealomas, **681**
Piracetam, 297
Piroxicam, **349**
PIs. *See* Protease inhibitors
Pituitary tumors, **681,** 682
Placebo effect, 992, 1028
Placidyl. *See* Ethchlorvynol
Platelet aggregation, 536
Play therapy, 720
PLMS (periodic leg movements of sleep), **497,** 502, 504
PML (progressive multifocal leukoencephalopathy), 282, 815
Poisoning, 265
Poliomyelitis, 398
Polycystic ovary disease, 483
Polydipsia, lithium-induced, 350, 958
Polypharmacy in elderly persons, 862, 865
Polysomnography, 502, 508, 513
Polyuria, lithium-induced, 348, 350, 958
Population studies
　clinical, 240–241
　　of mood disorders, 241
　　of multiple psychiatric disorders, 240–241
　cross-sectional, **192,** 194–195
　general, 240
　longitudinal, **192, 195,** 195–197
　　case-control studies, 195–196
　　cohort studies, 196–197
Porphyria
　acute intermittent, **680,** 688
　anxiety and, 398
　dementia and, **284**
　suicide and, 129
Portland Digit Recognition Test (PDRT), 97
Portugal, consultation-liaison psychiatry in, 215–217
Positron-emission tomography (PET), 77
　during alcohol withdrawal, 424
　in Alzheimer's disease, **279**
　in amyotrophic lateral sclerosis, 319
　applications of, 55–56
　basic science of, 51–52
　in dementia, 56
　in elderly persons, 861
　in HIV-associated neurocognitive impairment, 821
　in mood disorders, 55
　in obsessive-compulsive disorder, 55

　in panic disorder, 402, 403
　in schizophrenia, 55
　in stress-induced myocardial ischemia, 538
Postcardiotomy delirium (PCD), 38, 259, 268, 605, 765–766, **767**
Postconcussion syndrome, 281, **680,** 685
Postherpetic neuralgia, 1004, 1006, 1008
Postpolio syndrome, 513
Poststroke depression (PSD), 63, 238, 244, 281, 308, **310, 311,** 315–316, 679–681, 692
　electroconvulsive therapy for, 315, 694
Posttraumatic amnesia, 281
Posttraumatic stress disorder (PTSD), 403–404, 1038
　antidepressants for, **950,** 954, 969, 972
　burn trauma and, 613
　cancer and, 660–661
　diagnosis of, 394
　among dying patients, 781
　factitious, 523
　HIV/AIDS and, 833
　insomnia and, 501
　prevalence of, 242, 396
　in rehabilitation settings, 737
　somatization and, **362,** 367
　among Vietnam War veterans, 396
Postural disturbances
　in Parkinson's disease, 686
　in progressive supranuclear palsy, 280
　in Wilson's disease, 279
Postural hypotension. *See* Orthostatic hypotension
Postviral syndrome, 574
PPOs (preferred provider organizations), 182
Practice guidelines, 40, 417
Pramipexole, **463,** 510
Pramiracetam, **743**
Prazepam, **407, 903, 970, 981**
Prazosin, **463, 943, 944**
Prednisone, 323, **781**
Preferred provider organizations (PPOs), 182
Pregnancy, 702. *See also* Obstetrics and gynecology
　domestic violence during, 712
　drug use in, 707–708, **708,** 979–980, **980**
　　antidepressants, 979–980
　　antipsychotics, 966, 979

antiretroviral drugs, 809
carbamazepine, 352, 707, 961
diazepam, 707–708
lithium, 350, 707, 959
methadone, 437, 1007
psychostimulants, 956
valproate, 351, 961
electroconvulsive therapy in, 1022
HIV transmission to fetus during, 712–713, 809
induced abortion of, 706
infertility and its treatment, 705–706
loss of, 710–711
postpartum custody issues and, 711
postpartum psychiatric disorders, 709–710
psychiatric complications of, 706–709
acute psychiatric decompensation, 707–709, **709**
hyperemesis gravidarum, 706
morbid anxiety, 707
noncompliance with obstetric advice, 706–707
pseudocyesis, 706
unacknowledged pregnancy, 709
psychiatric consultation during labor, 709, **709**
sleep disorders in, 511
substance abuse in, 243
cocaine, 441
smoking, 445
voluntary sterilization for prevention of, 704–705
Premenstrual dysphoria
fluoxetine for, 171
monoamine oxidase inhibitors for, 954
postpartum depression and, 710
Presuicidal syndrome, 138
Prevalence-incidence bias in research, **199**
Prevention
of delirium, 266
of falls, 179
primary, secondary, and tertiary, 38–39
of sedative-hypnotic abuse, 434
of suicide, 142–144, **143**
Priapism, drug-induced
clozapine, 966
nefazodone, 952
trazodone, 950, 952

Primary care clinics, 917–924. *See also* Outpatient consultation-liaison psychiatry services
clinical disorders presenting in, 922–924
anxiety disorders, 923
depression, 922–923
functional somatic symptoms, 922
substance use disorders, 923–924
effectiveness of consultation-liaison programs in, 918
epidemiology of psychiatric disorders in, 917–918
liaison activities in, 922
roles and expectations in, 921–922
settings for outpatient consultation-liaison services, 918–919
structure of outpatient consultation-liaison program in, 919–921
Primary Care Evaluation of Mental Disorders (PRIME-MD), 39
Primary prevention, 38
Prime-MD, 856
PRIME-MD (Primary Care Evaluation of Mental Disorders), 39
Primidone, **463, 946**
Prions, 287–288. *See also* Creutzfeldt-Jakob disease
Private psychiatric practitioners, 20
Probucol, **463**
Procainamide, **345, 762, 943**
Procaine, **400**
Procarbazine
for cancer patients, 663
interaction with monoamine oxidase inhibitors, 787
side effects of
anxiety, **400**
delirium, 793
depression, **311**, 323
mania, **345**
neuropsychiatric effects, **667**
sexual dysfunction, **464**
Process of consultation, 15–17
in pediatrics, 719–720, **726**
Prochlorperazine, **964**
antiemetic effects of, 963
dosage of, **964**
psychiatric aspects of, **669**
side effects of, **964**
anxiety, 781, **781**
Procyclidine, **345**
Profile of Mood States, 93

Progesterone
in hormone replacement therapy, 703
role in ventilation, 547
Progestins, **464**
Progressive multifocal leukoencephalopathy (PML), 282, 815
Progressive supranuclear palsy (PSP), 279–280, 287, 296, 512
Prolactin
in anorexia nervosa, 487
antipsychotic-induced elevation of, 965, 978
Prolixin. *See* Fluphenazine
Promethazine, **762**
Propafenone, **345, 945**
Propantheline bromide, **464**
Propofol, **763**
for akathisia, 965
for delirium tremens, 268
for sedation, 267
side effects of, 762
sexual dysfunction, **464**
for terminal delirium, **794**
use in intensive care setting, 762
Propoxyphene, **815, 895**
Propranolol
drug interactions with
chlorpromazine, 611–612
cytochrome P450 metabolism and, **945**
thioridazine, 162, 611–612
indications for
agitation and aggression, **161**, 162, **162**
anxiety, 973
benzodiazepine withdrawal, 435
cocaine intoxication, 441
headache, 1068
neuroleptic malignant syndrome, 968
side effects of
delirium, **762**
depression, 162, 322, 733
sexual dysfunction, **464**
use in specific patient groups or medical conditions
brain injury, 979
cardiothoracic surgery patients, 604
neurological disease, 694
ProSom. *See* Estazolam
Prostate cancer, 670–671
leuprolide for, 471
nerve-sparing surgery for, 457
sexual dysfunction and, 457
Prostatic hypertrophy, 129

Protease inhibitors (PIs), 810, 811, **811**
drug interactions with, 814–815, **815**
cytochrome P450 metabolism and, **946**
for HIV-associated neurocognitive impairment, 823
neuropsychiatric side effects of, **818**
resistance to, 813
Protein binding of drug, 942, **943**
aging and, 861, **862**
Protriptyline, 325, **948**
dosage of, **948,** 950
indications for
chronic obstructive pulmonary disease, 549
narcolepsy, 510
sleep apnea, 549, 551
receptor site affinity of, **948**
side effects of
insomnia, **502,** 505
sexual dysfunction, **464**
Provigil. *See* Modafinil
Prozac. *See* Fluoxetine
Pruritus, psychogenic, 1066
PSD. *See* Poststroke depression
Pseudobulbar palsy, 281, 643
Pseudocholinesterase deficiency, 441
Pseudocyesis, 706
Pseudodementia, 275, 523, 857
Pseudoephedrine, **502,** 955
Pseudologia fantastica, 519, 522, 523.
See also Factitious disorders
"Pseudomalingering," 527
Pseudoseizures, 683, 689
Pseudotumor cerebri, 568, 959
Psilocybin, 905
Psoriasis, 1066
lithium-induced, 959
PSP (progressive supranuclear palsy), 279–280, 287, 296
Psychedelic drugs, 443
Psychiatric clinics, stand-alone, 879–880
Psychiatric consultant, 13–14
collaborative, consultative, and supervisory relationships with nonmedical therapists, 181–182
in general medical-surgical hospitals with teaching programs, 18–20
in group practice, 20
liaison with other specialties, 20, **20**
other physicians' expectations of, 14
outpatient consultation performed by, 921
for pediatric patients, 717–718
in private practice, 20
qualities of, 13–14, **14**

reimbursement for services of, 27–30
as subspecialist, 21
Psychiatric Side Effects of Prescription and Over the Counter Medications, 45
Psychiatry in Medicine, 7
Psychoanalysis, 4, 1029–1030
Psychodynamic psychotherapy, 1030.
See also Psychotherapy
for agitation and aggression, 157
for anxiety, 409
Psychological abuse of elderly persons, 859, **860**
Psychological assessment, 78, 88–98. *See also* Neuropsychological assessment
advantages and disadvantages of methods for, **95**
applications of, 94–97, **95**
adjustment to medical illness, 95–96
differential diagnosis of psychiatric disorder, 94
emotional factors and physical symptoms, 94–95
emotional sequelae of neurological disorders, 96
malingering, 97
medicolegal competence determination, 96–97
computerized, 97–98
functions of, 88
objective personality measures, 89–91
cautions about use in medical patients, 89
Millon Behavioral Health Inventory, 91
Millon Clinical Multiaxial Inventory, 91
Minnesota Multiphasic Personality Inventory, 89–91, **90**
Personality Assessment Inventory, 91
projective personality measures, 91–92
Rorschach inkblot test, 92
Rotter Incomplete Sentences Blank, 92
Thematic Apperception Test, 92
reliability of, 89
self-rating scales, 92–94
anxiety scales, 93
depression scales, 92–93, **93**
general distress and life-event scales, 93

health-related quality-of-life and well-being scales, 93–94
standardized tests for, 89
summary of instruments for, 94
validity of, 89
Psychological factors affecting medical condition, 363–364, **364,** 541, 1054
Psychologists, 1028
Psychomotor disturbances
delirium and, 257, 258, 262
drug-induced
benzodiazepines, 158
bupropion, 952
cocaine, 441
HIV-associated, 282, 819, 820
Psychoneuroendocrine pathways, 1053–1054
Psychoneuroimmunology, 661, 664, 1063
Psychooncology, 657–673. *See also* Cancer
Psychophysiological disorders, 1053–1054
Psychosis
acute, 895–897
causes of, 895, **896**
emergency department management of, 895–897
Alzheimer's disease and, 858–859
antipsychotics for, 962
"black patch," 610
brain tumors and, 681, 682
differentiation from dementia, 285
differentiation from hypochondriasis, 378
endocrine disorders and, **564**
in epilepsy, 683–684
factitious, 523
in herpes simplex encephalitis, 688
HIV disease and, 838–839
Huntington's disease and, 686
insomnia and, 501
in intensive care unit, 264, 498–499, 757–758, 762–763
late-life, 858–859
neurological and neurosurgical disorders and, 679
pain and, **1000,** 1004
in Parkinson's disease, 279
posttraumatic, 281
premenstrual, **345**
puerperal, **345**
somatization and, **362,** 367
substance-induced
alcohol, 86, 265, 283, 426

treatment of, 432, **433**
amphetamines, 442
cocaine, 441
inhalants, 446
tricyclic antidepressants, 951
systemic lupus erythematosus and,
568
transplantation for patients with,
630–631
in vascular dementia, 281
Psychosocial Assessment of Candidates
for Transplant (PACT), 625–626
Psychosocial factors. *See also* Stress
bipolar disorder and, 342
cardiac disease and, 536
hypertension, 538
myocardial infarction, 540
reactions to illness and injury, 4, 9
suicide and, 134–135
transplantation and, 624
Psychosomatic medicine, 3–5, 204–206.
See also Somatization
Psychosomatic Medicine, 7
Psychosomatics, 7
Psychostimulants, 955–957, **956**. *See
also* specific drugs
abuse of
in anorexia nervosa, 479, 484
in bulimia nervosa, 480
emergency department
management of, 901–902
development of tolerance to, 956
dosage and administration of, 956,
956
drug interactions with, 957, **957**
alcohol, 427
monoamine oxidase inhibitors, 955
tricyclic antidepressants, 953
half-lives of, **956**
indications for, 955–956
Alzheimer's disease, 297
attention-deficit/hyperactivity
disorder, 722
depression, 327, 955–956
narcolepsy, 509
pain syndromes, **989**, 1007
vascular dementia, 297
legal regulation of, 442
mechanism of action of, 955
overdose and toxicity of, 956–957
pharmacokinetics of, 955
response to, 956
side effects of, 442, 723, 761, 787,
956, **975–976**
sleep disorders, **502**
types of, 955

use in specific patient groups or
medical conditions
brain injury, 979
cancer, 662
cardiac disease, 327, 544, **975**
children, 722–723, **723**
critically ill patients, 760, 761
dying patients, **785**, 786–787
elderly persons, 864
HIV/AIDS, 824, 829–830, 956,
979
neurological disease, 692, **976**
patients undergoing rehabilitation,
743
pregnancy, 956
transplant patients, **637, 638**, 644
withdrawal from, 957
Psychotherapy, 1027–1048
case examples of, 1043–1046
countertransference reactions in, 7,
112–113
to gender dysphoric patients, 469
hate, 139
personality disorders and, 122
somatization and, 373
suicidality and, 139
vision loss and, 611
definition of, 1028, 1029
duration of, **1034**
essential skills of consultation-liaison
psychiatrist, 1038–1042, **1039**
associative anamnesis, 1039
formulation, 1040, **1041**
preassessment, 1039
selecting and implementing
treatment, 1040–1042,
1041, 1042
special considerations in general
hospital setting, 1040, **1041**
therapeutic examination, 1040
versatility, 1038–1039
forms of, **1034–1035**
commonalities in, 1028–1029
factors determining selection of
approach, 1042, **1042**
goals of, **1035**
in groups, 1032 (*See also* Group
therapy)
historical background of, 1027–1028
psychoanalytic foundations,
1029–1030
psychodynamic foundations, 1030
indications for
agitation and aggression, 157
anorexia nervosa, 488
anxiety disorders, 409–410

bulimia nervosa, 488–489
cocaine dependence, 442
depression, 329–330
European uses, 206
factitious disorders, 526
hyperemesis gravidarum, 706
mania, 355
pain syndromes, 1009
somatoform disorders, 386
suicidality, 141
life narrative approach to, 112, 1041
managed care and, 1048
outpatient
brief, intermittent, attenuated
therapy, 1046–1047
transition to, 1042
principles of, 1031, **1032**, 1041
tasks of consultation-liaison
psychiatrist, 1033–1038, **1036**
establishing therapeutic alliance,
15, 111–113, 1036
making personality diagnosis,
1037–1038, **1038**
techniques for, 1028, **1034,**
1040–1042
transference reactions in, 112–113,
1028, 1036
personality disorders and, 120
vision loss and, 611
unique aspects with medically ill
patients, 1030–1033
brevity, **1032**, 1032–1033
psychotherapeutic range and
limitations, 1031–1032
referral, 1030–1031
setting, 1031
use in specific patient groups or
medical conditions
cancer, 663–664
cardiac disease, 541–542
critically ill patients, 758
dying patients, 778, 779, 783,
784, 787
elderly persons, 864–865
HIV/AIDS, 808, 824, 830,
832–834
irritable bowel syndrome, 1063
neurological disease, 694–695
patients undergoing rehabilitation,
741, 744, **744**
rape victims, 712
surgical patients, 600–601
transplant patients, **634**
Psychotherapy and Psychosomatics, 7
Psychotropic drugs. *See*
Pharmacotherapy

PTSD. *See* Posttraumatic stress disorder

Public Law 101-336 (Americans With Disabilities Act of 1990), 87

Pulmonary artery pressure, 546

Pulmonary disease. *See* Lung disease

Pulmonary edema

in cancer patients, 660

in opioid-addicted patients, 905

Pulmonary embolus, 550–551, 780

in cancer patients, 660

cocaine-related, 243, 441

Pulmonary fibrosis, 627

Pupils

Argyll Robertson, 576

responses to drugs

amphetamines, 442

cannabis, 443

cocaine, 441

hallucinogens, 443

opioids, 437

Purpura, tricyclic antidepressant–induced, 951

Q-T interval prolongation

in anorexia nervosa, 484, 485

drug-induced

haloperidol, 267, 544, 897, 965

ipecac metabolites, 484

tricyclic antidepressants, 325–326, 543, 723, **943**

Quaalude. *See* Methaqualone

Quality of care, 871

Quality of Life Inventory, 94

Quazepam, 407, **903, 970**

dosage of, **434, 903, 970**

for insomnia, **506**

use during breast-feeding, **981**

Quetiapine, 963, **964**

for Alzheimer's disease, 296

dosage of, **964**

drug interactions with

antiretroviral drugs, 814, 839

cytochrome P450 metabolism and, **945**

mechanism of action of, 963

side effects of, **964**

cataracts, 611

sexual dysfunction, **464**

use in surgical patients, **598**

Quill, Timothy, 790

Quinacrine, 427

Quinidine, **943**

delirium induced by, **762**

drug interactions with

antidepressants, **943**

antipsychotics, 969

cytochrome P450 metabolism and, **945, 946**

[^{11}C]Raclopride, 55

Radiation therapy

complications of, 665–666

dementia and, 666

lithium and, 663

psychological reactions to, **658**

Radiopharmaceuticals, 51–52, 55

Rage. *See also* Aggression; Anger

delirium and, 262

episodic dyscontrol syndrome, 684

intermittent explosive disorder, 150, **150**

Ranitidine, **311,** 323, **762**

Rape, 711–712. *See also* Sexual abuse/assault

Rapid eye movement (REM) sleep, 495

in depression, 313

Rapid neuroleptization, 963

Rapid tranquilization, 965

Rash, drug-induced

antipsychotics, 966

antiretroviral drugs, 812

carbamazepine, 961

lamotrigine, 353, 961

selective serotonin reuptake inhibitors, 952

tricyclic antidepressants, 951

Raynaud's phenomenon, 959

RCPP (Recurrent Coronary Prevention Project), 539–540, 1057

RDC (Research Diagnostic Criteria), 311, 314, 540, 783

Reboxetine, **948**

for anxiety disorders, **950**

dosage of, **948**

receptor site affinity of, **948,** 953

side effects of, 953

structure of, 947

Recall bias in research, **199**

Receptor site activity of drugs, 943–944

antidepressants, 947, **948, 949**

Recreation therapists, 731, 732

Rectal drug administration, 941

Rectal pain, 1063

Recurrent Coronary Prevention Project (RCPP), 539–540, 1057

Referral

for neuropsychological evaluation, 98–100, **100**

for outpatient consultation-liaison services, 919

for psychotherapy, 1030–1031

Referral filter bias in research, **199**

Reflex sympathetic dystrophy, 992

Reflex testing, 73

Refusal of treatment, 167, 169. *See also* Informed consent

advance directives, 175–176

definition of, 168

do-not-resuscitate orders, 175, 778

right to die, 174–175, 790

surgery, 595, 596, **599,** 600

transplant refusal, 631

Regression, 108, 112

Reichsman, Franz, 6

Reimbursement

for consultation-liaison services, 27–30

managed care and, 182–183

for neuroimaging studies, 52

for transplantation surgery, 623

Reitan-Indiana Aphasia Screening Test, 67, 72

Relaxation training

for anxiety, 410, 923

for asthma, 1066

for critically ill patients, 760

for dying patients, 783

for esophageal motility disorders, 554

after head and neck surgery, 615

for headache, 1069

for hyperemesis gravidarum, 706

for hypertension, 1060

for insomnia, 504

for irritable bowel syndrome, 1063

for pain syndromes, 1008, 1068

for patients with cardiac disease, 542

for patients with HIV/AIDS, 834

in rehabilitation settings, 744

for somatoform disorders, 385, 922

for surgical patients, 595, 600

for tinnitus, 1070

Reliability of test, 89

Religion. *See* Spirituality and religion

REM sleep. *See* Rapid eye movement sleep

Remeron. *See* Mirtazapine

Renal cancer, **664, 681,** 682

Renal drug excretion, 942

aging and, 861, **862,** 942

Renal effects, **976,** 977–978

of lithium, **239,** 959

of phencyclidine, 443

of tricyclic antidepressants, 951

Renal failure, 63, 557–562

anorexia nervosa and, 479, 485

dementia and, **284**

depression and, 313–314

dialysis for, 558–561 (*See also* Dialysis patients)

neuropsychiatric syndromes and, 560–561, **594**

psychotropic drug use in, 757, **976,** 977–978

opioids, **994**

quality of life and, 559

sexual dysfunction and, 457–458, 559

sleep disorders and, 513

suicidality and, 129, 131–132, **132**

Renal transplantation, 417, 557–558. *See also* Transplantation

in children and adolescents, 557–558

evaluation of living donors for, 625

noncompliance after, 558

psychiatric disorders in candidates for, 628

psychiatric participation on transplant team, 558

psychopharmacological considerations and, **635–637**

in psychotic patients, 631

quality of life after, 557, 559

return to employment after, 646

sexual function after, 458

suicide and, 132

survival after, 557

waiting period for, 633–638

Repeatable Battery for the Assessment of Neuropsychological Status, 83

Reproduction. *See also* Pregnancy

cancer and, 666–669

infertility and its treatment, 705–706

physiology and psychology through life cycle, 701–703, **702**

Rescriptor. *See* Delavirdine

Research in consultation-liaison psychiatry, 4, 8–9, 191–200

biases in, 198–200, **199**

clinical settings for, 8

difficulties in, 191

ethical issues in, 200

historical perspective and context for, 191

importance of, 191

informed consent for participation in, 171–172, 200

international

Australia and New Zealand, 218

Brazil, 220

German-speaking countries, 211

Japan, 219–220

Netherlands, 215

Nordic countries, 208–209

southern European and Mediterranean countries, 217

United Kingdom, 213

methodologies for, 191–198, **192**

basic science research, 191–193

behavioral science, 193

neuroimaging, 193

neuroscience, 192–193

case studies, 193–194, **194**

clinical intervention studies, 197

cost-effectiveness studies, 197–198

cross-sectional population descriptive studies, 194–195

longitudinal population descriptive studies, **195,** 195–197

case-control studies, 195–196

cohort studies, 196–197

monies for, 30

regulation of, 171

Research Diagnostic Criteria (RDC), 311, 314, 540, 783

Reserpine

depression induced by, 63, **311,** 321–322, 733

insomnia induced by, **502**

interaction with antidepressants, **943,** 955

for tardive dyskinesia, 966

Residency training, 18

Resource allocation, 167, 207

Respect, 167

Respiration, 546. *See also* Lung disease

in anxiety disorders, 547–548, 923

awareness of breathing, 546–547

in depression, 547

drug effects on

benzodiazepines, 407–408, 545, 971

buspirone, 409

phencyclidine, 905

selective serotonin reuptake inhibitors, 952

neurophysiology of, 547

Respirators, 765

weaning from, 606

Respiratory acidosis, 441

Restless legs syndrome (RLS), **497,** 504, 510

Restlessness. *See also* Akathisia

monoamine oxidase inhibitor–induced, 955

in serotonin syndrome, 953

terminal, 792

Restoril. *See* Temazepam

Restraint of patient, 179–181

for aggressive behavior, 158

contraindications to, 179, **180**

definition of, 168

for delirium or dementia, 179

in emergency department, 890–891

guidelines for proper use of, 180–181

indications for, **180**

in intensive care unit, 758

legal regulation of, 180

before naloxone administration, 905

to prevent falls, 179

for suicidal behavior, 141

Retrovir. *See* Zidovudine

Reverse transcriptase inhibitors, 810–811

Revised Children's Manifest Anxiety Scale, **720**

Rhabdomyolysis, drug-induced

cocaine, 441

phencyclidine, 443

Rheumatoid arthritis, 1067

anxiety and, 736

behavioral medicine and, 1067

depression, suicidality and, **733**

psychotherapy for persons with, 1032

sexual dysfunction and, 738

use of Beck Depression Inventory in, 92, **93**

use of Minnesota Multiphasic Personality Inventory in, 89, **90**

Rhinitis, 354

Rifabutin, **946**

Rifampin, **943**

drug interactions with

antiretroviral drugs, 815

benzodiazepines, **349**

cytochrome P450 metabolism and, **945, 946**

methadone, 438, 838

side effects of, **550**

delirium, **762**

Right to die, 174–175, 790

competent patients, 174–175

do-not-resuscitate orders, 175, 778

euthanasia and physician-assisted suicide, 144–146, 175, 789–791, **790,** 831

incompetent patients, 174

Right ventricular assist device, 604

Rigidity

in neuroleptic malignant syndrome, 692

in Parkinson's disease, 685

phencyclidine-induced, 443

in progressive supranuclear palsy, 279

in Wilson's disease, 279

Riluzole, 464
Risk factors, 249
    for alcohol use disorders, 423
    for bipolar disorder, 341–342
    for delirium, 258–260
    for delirium tremens, 424–426
    for dementia, 276–277
    European study of, 222–223, **224**
    for ischemic heart disease,
        1055–1056, **1056**
    models of medical-psychiatric
        comorbidity, 238–240, **239**
    for nicotine-related disorders, 445
    for sedative-hypnotic abuse, 433
    for sleep apnea, **509**
    for somatization disorder, 115
    for suicide, 127, **128,** 131–135
        among emergency department
            patients, 898, **898**
        among terminally ill patients, **788,**
            788–789
Risk management, 168, 183–184
Risperdal. *See* Risperidone
Risperidone, 963, **964**
    antidepressant properties of, 354
    cytochrome P450 metabolism and,
        945
    dosage of, **964**
    indications for
        agitation and aggression, 160
        Alzheimer's disease, 296
        delirium, 268, **794**
        mania, 354
    mechanism of action of, 354, 963
    side effects of, 354, **964**
        sexual dysfunction, **464**
    use in specific patient groups or
        medical conditions
        dying patients, **794**
        elderly persons, **863**
        HIV/AIDS, 839
        Parkinson's disease, 692
        surgical patients, **598**
        transplant candidates, **636**
Ritalin, Ritalin-SR. *See*
    Methylphenidate
Ritonavir, **811**
    drug interactions with
        psychotropic drugs, 814, **815,**
            829
        sildenafil, 835
    for HIV-associated neurocognitive
        impairment, 823
    sexual dysfunction induced by, **464**
Rivastigmine, 297
RLS (restless legs syndrome), **497,** 510

Romano, John, 6
Ronald McDonald Houses, 719
Rorschach inkblot test, 92, 94
Rotter Incomplete Sentences Blank, 92
Royal Australian and New Zealand
    College of Psychiatrists, 218
Royal College of Psychiatrists, 212–213
Rubeola, 575
Rumination disorder of infancy, 477
Rush, Benjamin, 3
Russell's sign, 483

"Sad Heart" study, 542
SAD PERSONS Scale, 135, **135**
Sadistic personality disorder, 117
Safety issues in emergency department,
    889–891
Salicylates, 427, **428**
SANS (Scale for the Assessment of
    Negative Symptoms), 929
SAPS (Scale for the Assessment of
    Positive Symptoms), 929
Saquinavir, **464, 811,** 823
SAR (Sexuality Attitude Reassessment),
    739
Sarcoma, **664**
Saw palmetto, **974**
Scale for the Assessment of Negative
    Symptoms (SANS), 929
Scale for the Assessment of Positive
    Symptoms (SAPS), 929
Scandinavian countries, consultation-
    liaison psychiatry in, 207–209
Schedule of Attitudes Toward Hastened
    Death, 791
Schedule of Recent Experience, 93
Schizoaffective disorder
    clozapine for, 354
    electroconvulsive therapy for, 1015
    mood stabilizers for, 957, 961
    risperidone-induced mania in, 354
Schizoid personality disorder, **116,** 119,
    120, 121
Schizophrenia
    age at onset of, **63**
    alcohol use and, 423
    antipsychotics for, 962
        for agitation and aggression,
            158–159
        olanzapine, 354
    coronary artery disease and, **239**
    differentiation from dementia, 285
    differentiation from somatization
        disorder, 376
    electroconvulsive therapy for, 1015
    hallucinations in, 64–65

    legal competency of persons with,
        172, 173
    neurological and neurosurgical
        disorders and, 679
    positron-emission tomography in, 55
    prevalence of, **680**
    psychiatric comorbidity with,
        150–151
    rating scales for, 929
    smoking and, 549
    somatization and, **362,** 367
    suicide and, 133, **133,** 134, **134**
    tardive dyskinesia in, **239**
    telepsychiatry for assessment of, 929
    transplantation for patients with,
        630–631
Schizotypal personality disorder, **116,**
    120, 631
*Schloendorff v. Society of New York
    Hospital,* 167
SCL-90 (Symptom Checklist—90), 25,
    36, 371, **371,** 508
SCL-90-R (Symptom Checklist—90—
    Revised), 93, 399, 406, **407**
Scopolamine, **464, 669, 943**
Seclusion of patient, 179–180
    for aggressive behavior, 158
    contraindications to, **180**
    definition of, 168
    in emergency department, 890–891
    guidelines for proper use of, 180
    indications for, **180**
    legal regulation of, 180
Secobarbital, **434, 895, 904**
Seconal. *See* Secobarbital
Secondary prevention, 38
Sedation
    drug-induced
        antipsychotics, 408, 409, **964,**
            965
        benzodiazepines, 158, 353, 971
        clonidine, 439
        clozapine, 966
        gabapentin, 961
        lamotrigine, 961
        methadone, 438
        methotrimeprazine, 794
        mirtazapine, 327, 953
        nefazodone, 327
        selective serotonin reuptake
            inhibitors, 761, 951
        trazodone, 952
        tricyclic antidepressants, 325,
            950, 951
        valproate, 961
    in intensive care unit, 267, 758

terminal, 145
of violent patients in emergency
department, 899
Sedative-hypnotics, 969–973. *See also*
Anxiolytics; specific drugs and classes
abuse/dependence on, 433–435
acute management of, **434,**
434–435, **435**
categories of abusers, 433
complications of, 433–434
detection of, 433
detoxification from opioid abuse
and, 440
emergency department
management of, 902–903
prevention of, 434
relapses of, 433
risk factors for, 433
antihistamines, 973
benzodiazepines, 969–972, **970**
chloral hydrate, 973
dosage of, **407, 434**
for elderly persons, **863**
indications for, 969
insomnia, 505, **506**
patients with HIV/AIDS, 835
terminal delirium, **794**
prescription for general hospital
patients, 500
side effects of
anxiety, **400**
disinhibition, **156**
sleep disorders, **502**
use during breast-feeding, **981**
withdrawal from, 903–904
zaleplon, 972–973
zolpidem, 972
Seizures
alcohol withdrawal, 424, 901
management of, 432, **433**
anorexia nervosa and, 479, 484
after brain injury, 281, 685
in cancer patients, 660, 665
classification of, 683, **684**
conversion, 689
in delirium, 268–269
drug-induced, 978–979
alprazolam, 971
antipsychotics, 966, 978–979
bupropion, 326, 408, 952, 978
clozapine, 966, 978
cocaine, 243, 441
maprotiline, 786, 978
MDMA, 443
in neuroleptic malignant
syndrome, 968

phencyclidine, 905
psychostimulants, 957
selective serotonin reuptake
inhibitors, 952
tricyclic antidepressants, 951,
978
epidemiology of, 683
epilepsy, 683–685
factitious, 523
in herpes simplex encephalitis, 688
in limbic encephalopathy, 280
in Lyme disease, 575
management in patients with HIV/
AIDS, 839
mania and, **345, 346**
in meningitis, 688
in neurosyphilis, 576
nocturnal, 511–512
pseudoseizures, 683, 689
psychiatric comorbidity with, 244
"psychogenic fits," 689
radiation therapy–induced, 666
systemic lupus erythematosus and,
568
in transplant recipients, 641–642
Selection bias in research, **199**
Selective serotonin reuptake inhibitors
(SSRIs), 326, **943, 949.** *See also*
specific drugs
dosage of, **948**
drug interactions with
antiretroviral drugs, 814, 828–829
carbamazepine, 694
codeine, 326, **999**
cytochrome P450 metabolism
and, 326, 427, 543, 761, **945,**
947, **949,** 952
monoamine oxidase inhibitors,
327, 954, 955
tramadol, **999**
tricyclic antidepressants, **999**
half-lives of, **949**
indications for
agitation and aggression, **161,**
161–162
anorexia nervosa, 488
anxiety disorders, 408, **950,** 969
body dysmorphic disorder, 384
bulimia nervosa, 171, 489, 950
narcolepsy, 510
pain syndromes, 1004
lack of response to, 328
mechanism of action of, 542, **948**
side effects of, 326, 663, 761, 829,
951–952
anxiety, **400**

sexual dysfunction, 326, 465, 829,
835
sleep disorders, **502**
structure of, 947
use in specific patient groups or
medical conditions
brain tumors, **693**
cancer, 662–663
cardiac disease, 408, 537,
542–543, 545, 951, 974
children, 723, **723**
chronic obstructive pulmonary
disease, 549
chronic pain, 693, **693**
critically ill patients, 760–761
dialysis patients, 561
dying patients, **785,** 786
elderly persons, **863,** 863–864
epilepsy, 318, **693**
hepatic disease, 977
HIV/AIDS, 320, 828–829, 834
Huntington's disease, **693**
multiple sclerosis, **693**
neurogenic bladder with
retention, 693, **693**
neurological disorders, 692–693,
741
Parkinson's disease, 693, **693**
pathological laughing and crying,
693
patients undergoing rehabilitation,
742
pregnancy and lactation, 708, **708,**
710, 979
stroke, **693**
surgical patients, 597
transplant patients, 634, **636,** 643
withdrawal from, 953
Selegiline, 954, **954**
for Parkinson's disease, 686, 693
sexual dysfunction induced by, **464**
Self-defeating personality disorder, 117,
120–122, 375
Self-destructive deniers, 110
Self-determination, 167, 169, 175. *See
also* Autonomy of patient
Self-mutilation
genital, 468
self-inflicted burns, 612
Self-Rating Anxiety Scale (SRAS), **407**
Self-regulation and health, 110–111
Sensory deprivation, 259
Septicemia, drug-related. *See also*
Infections
cocaine, 243, 441
opioids, 436

Serax. *See* Oxazepam
Seroquel. *See* Quetiapine
Serotonin
    aggression and, 155
    Alzheimer's disease and, 297
    anxiety and, 401
    depression and, 947
    mania and, 344
    suicidality and, 134
    ventricular arrhythmias and, 537
Serotonin syndrome
    clinical features of, 953–954
    due to concurrent use of sertraline
        and anesthetics, **597**
    due to concurrent use of venlafaxine
        and monoamine oxidase
        inhibitor, 327
    due to drug interactions with
        analgesics, **999**
    due to drug interactions with
        monoamine oxidase inhibitors,
        327, 953–955, **999**
Sertindole, **464**
Sertraline, 326, **948**
    dosage of, **948**
    drug interactions with
        cytochrome P450 metabolism
            and, 326, **945, 949,** 952
        ritonavir, 814
    half-life of, **949**
    indications for
        agitation and aggression, 162
        anxiety disorders, 969
        hallucinogen-related flashbacks,
            443
    receptor site affinity of, **948**
    sexual dysfunction induced by, **464**
    structure of, 947
    use in specific patient groups or
        medical conditions
        cardiac disease, 408, 542, 951
        children, **723**
        chronic obstructive pulmonary
            disease, 408
        critically ill patients, 761
        dying patients, **785,** 786
        elderly persons, 863, **863**
        HIV/AIDS, 828–829
        neurogenic bladder with
            retention, 693
        Parkinson's disease, 693
        pregnancy, 979
        transplant recipients, 643
    withdrawal from, 953
Serum drug levels, 942–943
    of antidepressants, 947

    of carbamazepine, **347**
    of lithium, **347,** 348, 958
    of valproate, **347,** 961
Serzone. *See* Nefazodone
Set Test, 72
[^{18}F]Setoperone, 55
7-Minute screen, 294
Sex and Love Addicts Anonymous, 471
Sexual abuse/assault
    anorexia nervosa and, 479
    chronic pelvic pain and, 1070
    of elderly persons, 859, **860**
    factitious, 519, 523
    flunitrazepam incapacitation for, 434
    rape and domestic violence, 711–712
    somatization and, 369
Sexual behavior problems, 736
Sexual dysfunction, 455–471
    anorexia nervosa and, 480
    behavioral medicine and, 1070
    cancer and, 457, 666–669, 713
    cardiac disease and, **456,** 456–457,
        457, 1062
    dementia and, 468
    diabetes mellitus and, 458–459
    after disfiguring head and neck
        surgery, 616
    drug-induced, 460, **461–464**
        antipsychotics, 965
        nefazodone, 952
        risperidone, 354
        selective serotonin reuptake
            inhibitors, 326, 465, 829,
            835, 951
        trazodone, 835, 950, 952
        tricyclic antidepressants, 951
    due to general medical condition, 456
    factors indicating psychological
        source of, 455
    gender identity disorders, 468–469,
        469, 470
    HIV infection and, 459–460, 835
    multiple sclerosis and, 466–467, 738
    other disorders presenting in hospital
        setting, 469–470, **470**
        treatment of, 470–471
    in rehabilitation settings, 738–739
    related to disease acceptance, 456
    renal failure and, 457–458, 559
    self-referral for, 469
    sildenafil citrate for, 460, 835
    spinal cord injury and, 466, 738
        pharmacological erection
            programs for, 466
    stroke and, **467,** 467–468, 738–739
    among transplant recipients, 643

Sexual health, 455
Sexual pain disorders, **1000**
Sexual response cycle, 455, **455**
Sexuality Attitude Reassessment (SAR),
    739
Sexually transmitted diseases
    HIV/AIDS, 807–840
    screening rape victims for, 712
    syphilis, 282
        anxiety and, 398
        HIV infection and, 576
        neurosyphilis, 282, **345,** 576,
            687–688
    in women, 712–713
"Shadowing," 295
Shame, 111
Shedler-Western Assessment Procedure
    (SWAP-200), 117
Short Blessed test, 294
Short-gut syndrome, 602, 628
Short Portable Mental Status
    Questionnaire, 83
Shy-Drager syndrome, 513
SIADH (syndrome of inappropriate
    antidiuretic hormone secretion),
    965
Sickle-cell disease, 423
Sildenafil citrate, 460, 835
    interaction with antiretroviral drugs,
        835
    sexual dysfunction induced by, **464**
    side effects of, 460
    for spinal cord-injured patients,
        466
    for women, 460
Simulation of disease, 519, **520.** *See also*
    Factitious disorders; Malingering
Simultaneous Video Reliability
    Interview, 929
Sinequan. *See* Doxepin
Single photon emission computed
    tomography (SPECT), 77
    in Alzheimer's disease, **279**
    applications of, 55–56
    basic science of, 50–51
    in delirium tremens, 258
    in elderly persons, 861
    in HIV-associated neurocognitive
        impairment, 821
    radiopharmaceuticals for, 51
Situation-oriented consultation, **6**
Sjögren's syndrome, 54
SLE. *See* Systemic lupus erythematosus
Sleep apnea, 495, **497,** 499, 502,
    507–509, 551
    arrhythmias and, 508, 510–511

benzodiazepines contraindicated in, 971
central, 508
classification of, 507
definition of, 508
dementia and, 512
depression and, 509
headache and, 512
in obesity-hyperventilation syndrome, 507
obstructive, 507, 508
    in amyloidosis, 513
    signs and symptoms of, **508**
panic attacks and, 399
pathophysiology of, 508
during postpolio syndrome, 513
prevalence of, 508
risk factors for, **509**
sleep laboratory evaluation of, 508
snoring due to, 504
treatment of, 508–509
    continuous positive airway pressure, 508, 509, 551
    medroxyprogesterone, 551
    protriptyline, 549, 551
    tracheostomy, 507
    uvulopalatopharyngoplasty, 509
Sleep disorders, 495–513
    approach to patient with insomnia, 500–502
    behavioral medicine and, 1070
    classifications of, 495, **496, 497**
    due to general medical condition, **496,** 502–504, **503,** 510–513
        amyloidosis, 513
        burn injuries, 613
        cancer, 504
        cardiac disease, 502–503, 510–511
        diagnosis of, 501
        endocrine disease, 504, 511
        gastrointestinal disease, 504, 513
        HIV/AIDS, 834–835
        musculoskeletal disease, 504, 513
        neurological disease, 504, 511–513
        pregnancy, 511
        pulmonary disease, 503–504, 511
        renal failure, 513
    evaluation of, 969
    excessive daytime somnolence (EDS), 507
        causes of, **507**
        evaluation of, 507
    fibromyalgia and, 504, 513, 571

among intensive care unit patients, 496–499
    clinical consequences of sleep changes, 498–499
    decreased total sleep time, 496
    disrupted day/night circadian cycles, 496–498
    disrupted sleep architecture, 498
among medical and surgical inpatients, 499–500
    effects of hypnotic drug use for, 500
narcolepsy, 509–510
periodic leg movements of sleep, 510
physiology of normal sleep, 495–496
psychiatric comorbidity with, 244
    delirium, 259–260, 262, 502
    mania, 342, 344
    personality disorders, 243
in rehabilitation settings, 738
related to another mental disorder, **496**
restless legs syndrome, 510
sleep apnea, 495, **497,** 499, 502, 507–509, **508, 509,** 551
substance-induced, **496, 502, 502**
    antidepressants, 505
    bupropion, 326
    levodopa, 501, 504, 513
    monoamine oxidase inhibitors, 955
    nicotine withdrawal, 445
    opioid withdrawal, 437, 438
    psychostimulants, 327, 442, 956
    selective serotonin reuptake inhibitors, 326, 761
subtypes in hospitalized patients, 500
treatment of insomnia, 504–505, **506**
weight loss and, 496
Sleep paralysis, 509
Sleep-related neurogenic tachypnea, 513
Sleep state misperception, 501–502
Sleep terror disorder, **496,** 499
Sleepwalking disorder, **496,** 499
Small bowel transplantation, 628. *See also* Transplantation
Smoking, 239–240. *See also* Nicotine-related disorders
    age at onset of, 445
    alcoholism and, 445, 549
    depression and, 445, 549, 1061
    drug interactions with, 445
        benzodiazepines, **349**
    lung disease and, 445, 549
    mortality from, 445, 1060

nicotine-related disorders, 239–240, 445–446
    passive, 1060
    in pregnancy, 445
    prevalence of, 445
    schizophrenia and, 549
    sleep disorders and, **502**
    twin studies of, 445
Smoking cessation, 445–446, 549, 1060–1061
    bupropion for, 446, 549, 950, 1061
    buspirone for, 1061
    clonidine for, 1061
    counseling for, 549
    fluoxetine for, 171
    health benefits of, 1060
    nicotine replacement therapy for, 446, 549, 1061
    nortriptyline for, 446, 549
    psychological approaches to, 1061
Snoring, 504, 507
Social justice, 167
Social phobia, 395, 404
    alcoholism and, 423
    antidepressants for, **950,** 954, 969, 972
    body dysmorphic disorder and, 381
    esophageal motility disorders and, 554
    irritable bowel syndrome and, **555**
    migraine headache and, 398
    prevalence of, **396**
Social Readjustment Rating Scale, 93
Social skills training, 373, 744
Social support
    for cardiac disease patients, 540
    after disfiguring surgery, 616–617
    homelessness and lack of, 909–910
    for patients with anxiety disorders, 410
Social withdrawal
    body dysmorphic disorder and, 381
    frontotemporal dementia and, 277
    HIV-associated, 818–819
Social workers, 30, 36, 732, 1028
Soma. *See* Carisoprodol
Somatization, 361–373, 1053
    acute vs. persistent, 365
    as amplifying personal perceptual style, 365
    clinical implications of components of, 362, **362**
    clinical management of, 371–373
        avoiding confrontation, 372
        directive approach, 371–372
        doctor-patient relationship, 373

Somatization *(continued)*
  clinical management of *(continued)*
    explanation of symptoms, 372
    minimization of polypharmacy,
        372–373
    negative reactions and
        countertransference, 373
    principles of, **372,** 372–373
    psychotherapeutic approach,
        371–372
    reattribution approach, 371–372
    regular follow-up, 372
    social dynamics, 373
    specific therapy when indicated,
        373
    treatment of mood or anxiety
        disorders, 372
  as clinical problem, 364–365
  costs of care for, **872**
  definition of, 361–362
  diagnostic process for, 369–371
    alliance with patient, 370
    collaboration with family and
        friends, 370
    collaboration with referral
        sources, 369–370
    mental status examination, 370,
        370
    physical examination, 370–371
    psychometric tests, 371, **371**
    review of medical records, 370
  economic burden of, 365
  etiological factors in, 368–369
    development and social learning
        and attachment behavior, 368
    gender, 369
    genetic factors, 368
    iatrogenesis, 369
    pathophysiologic mechanisms,
        368, **368**
    personality characteristics, 368
    psychodynamics, 368–369
    sexual and physical abuse, 369
    sociocultural factors, 369
  factitious disorder and, 115
  hypochondriacal, 362
  as masked presentation of psychiatric
      illness, 365
  outpatient psychiatric consultation
      for, 922
  patterns of, 362
  as process, 362–364
    defining new diagnoses at
        borderline of psychiatry and
        medicine, 364, **365**
    illness behavior, 363

    medically unexplained symptoms,
        362
    psychological factors affecting
        medical condition, 363–364,
        364
    somatosensory amplification, 363
  psychiatric conditions associated
      with, **362,** 365, 367
    anxiety, 365, 367
    depression, 365, 367
    personality disorders, 115–116,
        120, 368
    posttraumatic stress disorder, 367
    psychosis, 367
    substance abuse, 367, 423
  psychotherapy for, 1032
  relation between psychiatric
      disorders and, 365–367, **366**
  research on, 9
  as response to incentives of health
      care system, 367
  as response to loss, 362
  as tendency to seek care for common
      symptoms, 367
Somatization disorder, 374–376
  age at onset of, **63,** 374
  clinical course of, 375–376
  clinical features of, 374
  definition of, 374
  diagnostic criteria for, 374, **375**
  differential diagnosis of, 376
  epidemiology of, 374
  esophageal motility disorders and,
      553
  hypochondriasis and, 378
  irritable bowel syndrome and, **555**
  long-term stability of diagnosis of,
      374
  management of, 383–387
  pain and, 1000–1001, **1001**
  prevalence in medically ill patients,
      243–244, 374, **872**
  psychiatric comorbidity with,
      374–375
    personality disorders, 115–116,
        120, 375
  risk factors for, 115
Somatoform disorders, 4, **362,** 373–387
  body dysmorphic disorder, **380,** 380–
      381
  clinical presentation of, 373
  conversion disorder, 378–380, **379,**
      1001
  criticisms of diagnostic category of,
      373–374
  definition of, 373

  differential diagnosis of
    factitious disorder or malingering,
        373
    neurological disorders, 688–689
    in patients with chronic pain,
        1001
  etiological factors in, 368–369
    development and social learning
        and attachment behavior, 368
    gender, 369
    genetic factors, 368
    iatrogenesis, 369
    pathophysiologic mechanisms,
        368, **368**
    personality characteristics, 368
    psychodynamics, 368–369
    sexual and physical abuse, 369
    sociocultural factors, 369
  hypochondriasis, **377,** 377–378,
      1001
  management of, 383–387
    approach to patient, 383–384
    behavioral treatment, 385
    cognitive therapy, 385, **386**
    group psychotherapy, 386
    individual psychotherapy, 386
    marital and family therapy, 387
    pharmacotherapy, 384
    physical reactivation and physical
        therapy, 384
    relaxation therapies, meditation,
        and hypnotherapy, 385
    suggestion, 385
    therapeutic role of psychiatric
        consultation, 383, **384**
  not otherwise specified, 373, 383,
      1001
  pain and, **1000,** 1000–1002, **1001**
    pain disorder, 381–383, **382,**
        1001, 1002
  personality disorders and, 115–116
  prevalence in medically ill patients,
      243–244
  somatization disorder, 374–376, **375,**
      1001
  undifferentiated, 373, 376–377,
      1001
    clinical and associated features of,
        377
    clinical course and prognosis for,
        377
    definition of, 376
    diagnostic criteria for, **376**
    differential diagnosis of, 377
    epidemiology of, 376
    multisomatoform disorder, 376

Somatosensory amplification, 363
Somatosensory Amplification Scale, **371**
Somatostatin, 401
Somatothymia, 362
Somnolence
    excessive daytime, 507, **507**
    selective serotonin reuptake
        inhibitor–induced, 952
Spain, consultation-liaison psychiatry in,
    215–217
Spanish Society of Psychosomatic
    Medicine, 217
Spastic colon, 552
SPECT. *See* Single photon emission
    computed tomography
Spectinomycin, 960
Spectral analysis, 77
Speech assessment, 67, 289. *See also*
    Aphasia; Language and speech
    disturbances
Speech therapists, 731, 732
"Speed," 442. *See also* Amphetamines
"Speedballing," 435
Spinal cord injury
    alcohol use disorder and, 737
    anxiety and, 736
    depression, suicidality and, **733**
    occult head injury and, 734
    sexual dysfunction and, 466, 738
        pharmacological erection
            programs for, 466
Spinocerebellar degeneration, 512
[^{76}Br]Spiperone, 55
Spirituality and religion
    Alcoholics Anonymous and, 421
    cancer and, 658, 776–777
    counseling for agitation and
        aggression, 157
    dying and, 776–777
Spironolactone, 348, **349, 464**
Split treatment, 181
SRAS (Self-Rating Anxiety Scale), **407**
SSAD (summer seasonal affective
    disorder), 55
SSRIs. *See* Selective serotonin reuptake
    inhibitors
St. John's wort, **974**
    drug interactions with
        antiretroviral drugs, 814, 973
        cyclosporine, 973
    mania induced by, **345,** 346
St. Louis type A encephalitis, **345**
Stadol. *See* Butorphanol
Staff issues, 731, 732
    in intensive care settings, **764,**
        766–767

in rehabilitation settings, 740
    multidisciplinary rehabilitation
        teams, 731, 732
    related to cancer, 672–673, **673**
    related to disfiguring surgery, 617
    related to dying patients, 796–798
    related to neurological disease, 695
    related to transplant surgery, 644
    safety in emergency department,
        889–891
STAI (State-Trait Anxiety Inventory),
    93, 94, **371,** 406, **407**
State-Trait Anxiety Inventory (STAI),
    93, 94, **371,** 406, **407**
Status epilepticus, 642, 683, **684.** *See*
    also Seizures
Stavudine, **818,** 823
Steele-Richardson-Olszewski syndrome,
    687
Stelazine. *See* Trifluoperazine
Stereotypical behavior
    in Alzheimer's disease, 277
    cocaine-induced, 441
    phencyclidine-induced, 443
Sterilization, voluntary female,
    704–705
Stevens-Johnson syndrome, 353, 961
Stomachache, 362
Strain, James, 246
Stress. *See also* Anxiety; Behavioral
    medicine
    acute stress disorder, 394, 403–404,
        1038
    of acute vision loss, 610
    autoimmune disorders and, 1066
    cancer and, 660–661
    cardiac disease and, 537–541,
        1057–1058
        coronary artery disease, 538–541
        hypertension, 537–538
        ischemia, 538
        myocardial effects, 538
        ventricular arrhythmias and
            sudden cardiac death, 537
    esophageal motility disorders and,
        1062
    flight-or-fight response to, 394
    HIV disease progression and, 1065
    Horowitz's stress response model,
        403–404
    infectious disease and, 1065
    physiologic concomitants of, 400
    posttraumatic stress disorder,
        403–404, 1038 (*See also*
            Posttraumatic stress disorder)
    staff (*See* Staff issues)

stress-diathesis model of suicidality,
    135, **136**
Stress management training
    for HIV/AIDS, 1065
    for hypertension, 1060
    for irritable bowel syndrome, 1063
    for ischemic heart disease, 1057
    in rehabilitation settings, 744
Stress response, 394, 536
Striatonigral degeneration, 513
Stroke, 679–681
    alcohol-related, **243**
    anxiety and, 250–251, 398, 681, 736
    dementia and (*See* Vascular
        dementia)
    hemorrhagic, 679
    ischemic, 679
    lacunar, 681
    mortality from, 772
    neuropsychological testing in, 85–86
        medicolegal competence, 96–97
    poststroke depression (PSD), 63,
        238, 244, 281, 308, **310, 311,**
        315–316, 679–681, 692, 694,
        732, **733,** 741, 857–858, 978
    poststroke mania, **345,** 346, **346,**
        681
    prevalence of, **680**
    psychiatric comorbidity with, 244
    psychotropic drug use in patients
        with, 741
        antidepressants, **693**
    sexual dysfunction and, **467,**
        467–468, 738–739
    sleep disorders and, 512
    systemic lupus erythematosus and,
        568
Structured Clinical Interview for
    DSM-III, 780, 835
Structured Interview of Reported
    Symptoms, 97
Stupor
    clonazepam-induced, 353
    differentiation from conversion
        stupor, 689
    in encephalitis, 688
Subarachnoid hemorrhage, 265, 441,
    680, 690
Subcortical arteriosclerotic
    encephalopathy, 53
Subcortical dementia, **274,** 274–275,
    276, 278–280, 796
Subcutaneous drug administration, 941
Subdural hematoma, 265, 281, 679,
    891
Sublingual drug administration, 941

Substance-induced disorders, **975–976**
  agitation and aggression, **156**
  anxiety, 395, 399, **400**, 405, 423,
      780–781, **781**
  delirium, 150, **156**, 239, **239**, 258,
      259, 265, 325, **762**, 793
  dementia, 283, **284, 285**, 288
  DSM-IV classification of, 418
  medical morbidity, 239, **239**
  mood disorders, 63–64, **239**, 311,
      311, 341
      depression, 63–64, **239**, 311, **311**,
          321–324
      fluoxetine and suicidality, 141
      mania, 63–64, 339, **341, 345, 346**
  persisting amnestic disorder, 86
      alcohol-induced, 86, 265, 283,
          426
  psychosis, **896**
  seizures, 978–979
  sexual dysfunction, 460, **461–464**
  sleep disorders, 326, 502, **502**
  vision loss, 611
Substance-related disorders, 417–446.
      See also specific disorders
  acute assessment of, 419–420, **420**
  alcohol use disorders, 242–243,
      422–433
  amphetamine-related disorders, 442
  body dysmorphic disorder and, 381
  among burn patients, **239**, 417, 612
  cannabis-related disorders, 444
  characteristics of persons with, 903
  cocaine-related disorders, 440–442
  consultation problems related to,
      417–419
  costs of care for, **872**
  course and outcome in medically ill
      patients, 251, 421–422
  Cushing's syndrome and, **564**
  definitions related to, 418
  dependence, 418
      on benzodiazepines/sedative-
          hypnotics, 158, 433–435
      chronicity of, 420
      diagnostic criteria for, 418, **419**
  diabetes mellitus and, **564**
  diagnosis of, 418
  DSM-IV classification of, 418
  in elderly persons, 859
  emergency department management
      of, 900–906
      toxicology screening, 893–894,
          894, 895
  esophageal motility disorders and,
      553–554
  extent of, 417
  factitious, 523
  hallucinogen-related disorders, 443
  HIV infection and, 417, 808, 809,
      837–838
  in homeless persons, 909–910
  hyperthyroidism and, **564**
  inhalant-related disorders, 446
  medical education about, 417
  mental retardation and, 421
  neurological and neurosurgical
      disorders and, 679
  nicotine-related disorders, 239–240,
      445–446
  opioid-related disorders, 435–440
  among orthopedic surgery patients,
      609–610
  outpatient psychiatric consultation
      for, 923–924
  pain management in patients with,
      440, 996–997
  personality disorders and, 243
  phencyclidine-related disorders,
      442–443
  prevalence in medically ill patients,
      242–243, **243, 872**
  principles of consultation for,
      418–419, **419**
  in rehabilitation settings, 737–738
  sedative-, hypnotic-, and anxiolytic-
      related disorders, 433–435
  somatization and, **362**, 367, 375
  suicide and, 128, 129, **133**, 133–134,
      134, 136, 142–143, 421
  tolerance, 418
      to alcohol, 424
      to benzodiazepines, 353
      definition of, 418
  transplantation for patients with,
      629, 629–630
      liver transplant, 628
      lung transplant, 627
  traumatic brain injury and, 86
  treatment of, 420–421
      community resources for, 420
      detoxification, 420
      education and motivational
          approach to, 420
      including family in, 420
      insurance coverage for, 420
      multidisciplinary approach to, 417
      outcome of, 421–422
      patients with comorbid
          psychiatric conditions, 421
      patients with concomitant
          medical illness, 421
      relapse prevention, 422
      stages of, 420
      suicidal patients, 421
      12-step programs, 420–421
  tuberculosis and, 417
  violence due to, 899
Substance withdrawal, 141, 418
  from alcohol, 263, 265, 424–426
  anxiety due to, 781
  from benzodiazepines and sedative-
      hypnotics, 158, 263, 353, 408,
      433–435, **435**, 505, 545,
      903–904
  after cardiothoracic surgery, 605
  among critically ill patients, 761
  definition of, 418
  delirium due to, 259, 265
  from opioids, 436, 437, **437, 781**,
      905, 996–997
  protracted withdrawal syndrome,
      418
  among surgical patients, 596, 600
Substituted judgment, 177–178
Succinylcholine
  for agitation in intensive care unit,
      159–160
  drug interactions with
      benzodiazepines, 972
      lithium, 354, 960
      monoamine oxidase inhibitors,
          955
Sudden cardiac death, 537
"Suggestion of cure," 385
Suicidality, 127–146
  amphetamines and, 243
  antidepressants and, 946
      fluoxetine, 141, 952
  assessment for, 127, 136–139, 150
      in emergency department,
          136–138
      fundamentals of, **139**
      matrix approach to, 136, **137**
      presuicidal syndrome, 138
      psychodynamic formulation for,
          138
      purpose of, 136
      ten commonalities of suicide, 138,
          139
      time perspective profiles,
          138–139, **139**
      variables of focus for, 136, **137**
  body dysmorphic disorder and, 381
  diabetes and, 245
  of dying patients, 129–130, 778,
      788–792
  dyspnea and, 548

economic cost of suicide attempts, 127

among elderly persons, 241, 858

epidemiology of, 127–131

in general population, 127–129, **128, 129**

in hospitalized medical-surgical patients, 130–131

in medically ill patients, 129–130, **130**

factitious, 523

family history of, 134

Huntington's disease and, 129, 278, 686

management of, 139–142

based on identified risk level, 139–140

contracting for safety, 142

electroconvulsive therapy, 141, 328

in emergency department, 136–138, 897–898, **898**

follow-up, 141–142

outpatient, 142

psychiatric hospitalization, 140–142, **142,** 144

psychotherapy, 141

restraint, 141

treating underlying medical problems, 141

neurological disorders and, 679, **733**

among pediatric patients, 128, 724–725

personality and, 129

physician-assisted suicide and euthanasia, 144–146, 175, 789–791, **790,** 831

prevention of, 142–144, **143**

in rehabilitation settings, 733, **733,** 746

risk factor scales for, 135, **135**

risk factors for, 127, **128,** 131–135, 898, **898**

alcoholism, 128, 129, 133–134, 142–143, **243**

biological and genetic factors, 134

cancer, 129, 131, **132,** 661–662, **662, 733,** 788–789

chronic renal failure, 131–132, **132**

HIV/AIDS, **132,** 132–133, 144, **144,** 319, 830–831, **831**

physical illness, 129, **733**

psychiatric factors, 128, 129, **133,** 133–134, **134,** 239

psychological and psychosocial factors, 134–135

terminal illness, **788,** 788–789

self-inflicted burns, 612

stress-diathesis model of, 135, **136**

substance-related disorders and, 421

alcoholism, 128, 129, **133,** 133–134, **134, 136,** 142–143, **243,** 423

cocaine, 441

transplantation and, 132, 631

Sulfasalazine, **464**

Summer seasonal affective disorder (SSAD), 55

Sundowning, 512

Surgery, 593–617

burn units, 612–613

cardiothoracic, 602–608

changes in practice of, 593

cosmetic, 613–614

head and neck, 614–617

ophthalmology, 610–612

orthopedic, 608–610

preoperative issues, 595–600

anxiety and transient treatment refusal, 595

competency and informed consent, 596, **599,** 600

context of consultation, 595

psychiatric illness in surgical patients, 595–596

psychotropic medications, 596, **597–598**

psychiatric complications of, 593–594, **594,** 600

delirium, 257, 259, **259,** 600

differentiation from alcohol withdrawal, 424

operative syndromes, 593–594

substance withdrawal, 596, 600

psychiatric treatment considerations related to, 600–602

pain management, 602

pharmacotherapy for patients who can take nothing by mouth, 601–602

pharmacotherapy for patients with malabsorption syndromes, 602

reducing fear and stress associated with, 593

role of surgeons in patient's life, 593

roles of psychiatric consultation for, 594

same-day, 593, 595

sleep disturbances and, 499–500

Sustiva. *See* Efavirenz

SWAP-200 (Shedler-Western Assessment Procedure), 117

Sweating

chronic hyperhidrosis, 1066

drug-induced

cocaine, 441

hallucinogens, 443

in neuroleptic malignant syndrome, 968

nicotine, 445

opioid withdrawal, 437

psychostimulants, 957

reboxetine, 953

in serotonin syndrome, 953

tricyclic antidepressants, 951

venlafaxine, 326

methadone-induced reduction in, 438

Sweden, consultation-liaison psychiatry in, 207–209

Swiss Medical Association, 211

Switzerland, consultation-liaison psychiatry in, 209–212

Sympathomimetic agents

anxiety induced by, **400**

interaction with antidepressants, **943**

monoamine oxidase inhibitors, 327, 955

tricyclics, 953

mania induced by, **345, 346**

Symptom Checklist—90 (SCL-90), 25, 36, 371, **371,** 508

Symptom Checklist—90—Revised (SCL-90-R), 93, 399, 406, **407**

Symptom-Driven Diagnostic System, 39

Symptom validity testing, 97

Syncope, vs. conversion disorder, 689

Syndrome of inappropriate antidiuretic hormone secretion (SIADH), 965

Syndrome X, 1062

Syphilis, 282

anxiety and, 398

HIV infection and, 576

neurosyphilis, 282, **345,** 576, 687–688

Systemic lupus erythematosus (SLE), 54, 568

electroconvulsive therapy for patients with, 568, 1022

factitious, 521

lupus cerebritis, 688, 690

neuropsychiatric, 568

Systems of Belief Inventory, 776

T$_4$ (thyroxine)
in anorexia nervosa, 485, 486
role in ventilation, 547
sleep disorders induced by, **502**
T$_3$ (triiodothyronine)
in anorexia nervosa, 485, 487
for antidepressant augmentation, 320, 328, 957
Tachycardia, drug-induced
cannabis, 444
cocaine, 441
haloperidol, 267, 544, 965
nicotine, 445
opioid withdrawal, 437
psychostimulants, 442, 544, 761, 956
risperidone, 354
tricyclic antidepressants, 950
Tachykinins, 547
Tacrine, **945**
Tacrolimus, 641–643
Talwin. *See* Pentazocine
Tamoxifen, **464, 667**
Tamsulosin, **464**
Tarasoff v. Regents of the University of California, 900
Tardive dyskinesia, 158, **239**, 408, 691, 966–968
amoxapine-induced, 951
atypical antipsychotics and, 160, 966–968
in elderly persons, 966
etiology of, 966
medications for, 966
prevalence of, 966
rating scale for, 966, **967**
Tardive dystonia, 691, 966
Targeting consultation-liaison services, 28, 30
TAS (Toronto Alexithymia Scale), 122, 209
TAT (Thematic Apperception Test), 92
Tax Equity and Fiscal Responsibility Act (TEFRA), 883
Tax issues, 30
Taylor Equivalent Test, 15, 72, **73**
TBM. *See* Topographical brain mapping
TCAs. *See* Antidepressants, tricyclics and related agents
Teaching consultation-liaison psychiatry, 4, 7–9, 18–20, 33
to fellows, 18–19, **19**, 30
international
Australia and New Zealand, 218
German-speaking countries, 210–211
Japan, 219

Netherlands, 214–215
Nordic countries, 208
southern European and Mediterranean countries, 217
United Kingdom, 213
to medical students, 15, 18
models of training for primary care physicians, **42**, 42–45
autonomous, psychiatric model, 43
biological model, 44
bridge model, 43
consultation model, 43
critical care model, 44
double-board training model, 43
hybrid model, 43
integral model, 44–45
liaison model, 43, 44
milieu model, 44
postgraduate specialty training model, 43
by nonpsychiatrists, 45
to other hospital staff, 20, **20**
in rehabilitation settings, 746–747
to residents, 18
telepsychiatry, 933
Technetium 99m, 51
TEFRA (Tax Equity and Fiscal Responsibility Act), 883
Tegretol. *See* Carbamazepine
Telephone consultation, 933–934
Telepsychiatry, 927–935
conducting a session, 933
considerations in implementation of, **931**, 931–932
access, 932
accountability, 932
alliance, 931, **931**
anticipation, 932
apprehension, 932
approach, 932
assessment, 932
electronic mail consultation, 934
history and development of, 927–930
period 1: interactive television, 927–928
period 2: affordable videoconferencing, 928–929
period 3: evidence-based telepsychiatry, 929–930
Internet consultation, 934
number of programs, 928–929
preparing for session, 932–933
telephone consultation, 933–934
training in, 933

utilization patterns and acceptance of, 930–931
in Australia, 930
in United States, 930
Temazepam, 407, **903**, 970, **970**
dosage of, **407, 434, 903, 970**
half-life of, **407, 903**
indications for
insomnia, 505, **506**
opioid withdrawal symptoms, 438
periodic leg movements of sleep, 510
pharmacokinetics of, 970
use in specific patient groups or medical conditions
breast-feeding women, **981**
dialysis patients, 561
elderly persons, **863**
HIV/AIDS, 834
transplant candidates, 638
Teratogenic effects, 979–980
of antipsychotics, 979
of carbamazepine, 352, 961, 980
of lithium, 350, 959, 980
of valproate, 351, 980
Terazosin, **464**
Terfenadine, 327
Terminal illness. *See* Dying patients
TERS (Transplantation Evaluation Rating Scale), 625–626
Tertiary prevention, 38–39
Test of Variables of Attention, 98
Testicular cancer, 457, 670, 682
Testimonial privilege, 168, 169
Testosterone
for HIV-associated depression, 830
sexual dysfunction induced by, **464**
type A behavior and, 539
Tetrabenazine, 966
Tetracycline
interaction with lithium, **349,** 960
sleep disorders induced by, **502**
Δ^9-Tetrahydrocannabinol (Δ^9-THC), 444, 906. *See also* Cannabis
Texas Functional Living Scale, 294
Thalamic metastases, **345, 346**
Thalamotomy, **345**
Thalidomide, 707
Thallium poisoning, **284**
Δ^9-THC (Δ^9-tetrahydrocannabinol), 444, 906. *See also* Cannabis
Thematic Apperception Test (TAT), 92
Theophylline
drug interactions with carbamazepine, 962

cytochrome P450 metabolism and, **945**
lithium, **349,** 960
electroconvulsive therapy and, 1016
side effects of, **550**
anxiety, **400**
Therapeutic alliance, 15, 111–113, 1036. *See also* Doctor-patient relationship
definition of, 1036
with pediatric patients, 720
Therapeutic drug levels, 942–943
of antidepressants, 947
of carbamazepine, **347**
of lithium, **347,** 348, 958
of valproate, **347,** 961
Therapeutic examination, 1040
Therapeutic privilege, 170
Thiabendazole, sexual dysfunction induced by, **464**
Thiamine
for anorexia nervosa, 480, 488
deficiency of, **284,** 426
for Wernicke's encephalopathy, 263, 265, 296, 432, **433**
Thiopental, **904**
Thioridazine, 267, **964**
dosage of, **964**
drug interactions with
lithium, 969
propranolol, 162, 611–612
vasodilators, 969
side effects of, **964**
ocular effects, 611, 966
sexual dysfunction, **464**
use in specific patient groups or medical conditions
dying patients, 782, **782,** 794, **794**
elderly persons, **863**
Parkinson's disease, 691, 979
patients undergoing rehabilitation, **743**
Thiothixene, **964**
dosage of, **964**
for elderly persons, **863**
side effects of, **964**
sexual dysfunction, **464**
Thoracic surgery, 602, **603.** *See also* Cardiothoracic surgery
Thorazine. *See* Chlorpromazine
Thought disorders
assessment for, 64
delirium and, 262
primary vs. secondary, 64
in transplant recipients, 642

3TC. *See* Lamivudine
Thrombocytopenia
in anorexia nervosa, 486
valproate-induced, 961, 978
Thrombolytic therapy, 540
Thyroid disorders, 564, **565, 594**
anorexia nervosa and, 485, 487
anxiety disorders and, **239,** 242, 398, 403
cancer, 682
dementia and, **284**
depression and, 63, 245, 308, **310, 311,** 320
lithium-induced, 959
panic disorder and, 242
prevalence of psychiatric comorbidity with, 245, **564**
screening for, 313
sleep disorders and, 504, 511
Thyroid preparations
for antidepressant augmentation, 320, 328, 957
anxiety induced by, **400**
mania induced by, **345**
Thyroid-releasing hormone (TRH), 313, 320
Thyroid-stimulating hormone (TSH), 313, 320, 328
Thyroxine (T_4)
in anorexia nervosa, 485, 486
role in ventilation, 547
sleep disorders induced by, **502**
Tiagabine, **464**
Tiapride, 160
Ticlopidine, 296
Tics, psychostimulant-induced, 787
Time and Change Test, 294
Timolol, **464,** 611
Tin poisoning, **284**
Tinnitus
behavioral management of, 1070
nortriptyline for, 693, **693**
tricyclic antidepressant–induced, 951
TMS (transcranial magnetic stimulation), 329
Tofranil. *See* Imipramine
Token economy, 157
Tolbutamide, 427, **945**
Tolcapone, **464**
Tolmetin, **345**
Toluene, **284**
Topamax. *See* Topiramate
Topiramate, **958,** 960
Topographical brain mapping (TBM), 77
applications of, 56–57
basic science of, 52

Toronto Alexithymia Scale (TAS), 122, 209
Torsades de pointes, 267, 544, 965
Torsion dystonia, 512
Tourette's syndrome, **680,** 688
antipsychotics for, 962
sleep disorders and, 512
"Touring," 295
Toxic-metabolic dementias, **274, 282–283, 284,** 288
Toxicology screening, 893–894, **894, 895**
Toxoplasmosis, 575, 815, **817**
Tracheostomy, 507
Trail Making Test, 72, 261
Training. *See* Teaching consultation-liaison psychiatry
Tramadol, **995, 999**
Trandolapril, **464**
Transcranial magnetic stimulation (TMS), 329
Transfer of patient, 891–892
Transference reactions, 112–113, 1028, 1036
personality disorders and, 120
vision loss and, 611
Transplant Recipient International Organization (TRIO), 633–634
Transplantation, 9, 35, 167, 623–647
in alcoholic patients, 427
liver transplantation, 427
psychiatric evaluation for, 427
biopsychosocial assessment of candidates and living related donors for, 624–626
living donors, 625
rating scales for candidate assessment, 625–626
team concept, 624
bone marrow, 623, 630
contraindications to, **626,** 628–629
electroconvulsive therapy and, 1022
ethical issues and, 626, 631
liver, 35, 42, 417, 427
organ allocation and distribution for, 623
organ transplant psychiatry, 623–624, 646, **647**
perioperative issues related to, 638–640
adjustment to medical complications or retransplantation, 639–640
donor information, 638
isolation procedures, 638
medication regimen, 638–639
rejection, 639

Transplantation *(continued)*
  perioperative neuropsychiatric
     problems related to, 640–644,
     641
     delirium and disorders of
       consciousness, 259, 638,
       640–641
     headache and visual symptoms,
       642
     movement disorders, 643
     other constitutional symptoms,
       643–644
     secondary mood, anxiety, and
       thought disorders, 642–643
     seizures, 641–642
     staff stress, 644
  postoperative course and life after,
     644–646
     adherence, 644–645
     adjustment, 645–646
     return to employment, 645–646
  psychiatric disorders in candidates
     for, 626–628
     patients with cardiac disease,
       626–627
     patients with chronic intestinal
       dysfunction, 628
     patients with diabetes, 628
     patients with liver disease,
       627–628
     patients with pulmonary disease,
       627
     patients with renal disease, 628
  psychiatric pathology and, **594**
  psychosocial selection criteria and
     predicting outcome of, 628–632
     compliance, 558, 603, 632
     dementia and mental retardation,
       631
     lack of consensus about, 629, **629**
     psychotic illness, 630–631
     substance-related disorders, 629–
       630
     suicidal ideation and/or transplant
       refusal, 631
     treatment-refractory psychiatric
       illness, 631–632
  psychotherapy and, **634**, 1032
  reimbursement for, 623
  renal, 557–558
  role of selection committee for,
     632–633
  suicide and, 132
  technical advances in, 623
  treatment compliance after, 603
  waiting period for, 623, 633–638

  anxiety and coping, 633–634
  artificial organs, 604, 633
  psychiatric treatment issues, 634
  psychopharmacological
     considerations, 634–638,
     635–637
  support groups, 633–634
Transplantation Evaluation Rating Scale
  (TERS), 625–626
Transverse myelitis, 568, 575
Tranxene. *See* Clorazepate
Tranylcypromine, 327, 954, **954**
  for dying patients, **785**
  side effects of
     cardiac effects, 544
     insomnia, **502**
     sexual dysfunction, **464**
Traumatic brain injury. *See* Brain injury
Trazodone, 325, **948**
  dosage of, **948**
  indications for
     agitation and aggression, 161, **161**
     Alzheimer's disease, 296
     bulimia nervosa, 489
     esophageal motility disorders, 554
     insomnia, 505, 972
  interaction with ritonavir, **815**
  receptor site affinity of, **948**
  response to, 950
  side effects of, 950, 952
     sexual dysfunction, **464**, 835,
      950, 952
  structure of, 947
  use in specific patient groups or
     medical conditions
     brain injury, 693, **693**, 979
     brain tumors, **693**
     breast-feeding women, **981**
     cancer, 662
     cardiac disease, 543
     dying patients, 785, **785**
     elderly persons, **863**
     epilepsy, **693**
     HIV/AIDS, 835
     irritable bowel syndrome, 556
     multiple sclerosis, **693**
     neurogenic bladder with
      retention, 693, **693**
     neurological disease, 692
     Parkinson's disease, 693, **693**
     patients undergoing rehabilitation,
      742
     pulmonary disease, 977
     stroke, **693**
     surgical patients, **597**
     transplant candidates, **637**

Treatment. *See also* specific treatments
  behavioral medicine, 1053–1070
  electroconvulsive therapy,
     1015–1023
  of pain, 383–387, 989–1010
  pharmacotherapy, 939–981
  psychotherapy, 1027–1048
Tremor
  alcohol withdrawal, 424
  delirium and, 262–263
  drug-induced
     bupropion, 326, 952
     lamotrigine, 961
     lithium, 350, 959
     in neuroleptic malignant
      syndrome, 968
     psychostimulants, 787, 956, 957
     in serotonin syndrome, 954
     tricyclic antidepressants, 951
     valproate, 961
  perioral, 691
  in transplant recipients, 643
  in Wilson's disease, 279
TRH (thyroid-releasing hormone), 313,
  320
Triamterene, 348, **349**
Triazolam, 407, **903**, 970, **970**
  dosage of, **407, 434, 903, 970**
  drug interactions with
     cytochrome P450 metabolism
      and, **945**
     nefazodone, 327
     ritonavir, 814, **815**
  for elderly persons, **863**
  half-life of, **407, 903**
  for insomnia, 505, **506**
     in chronic obstructive pulmonary
      disease, 503
  mania induced by, **345**
  for periodic leg movements of sleep,
     510
Trichloroethane, **284**
Trichloroethylene, **284**
Tridihexethyl chloride, **464**
Trifluoperazine, **464, 964**
Trihexyphenidyl, **464**
Triiodothyronine (T$_3$)
  in anorexia nervosa, 485, 487
  for antidepressant augmentation,
     320, 328, 957
Trilafon. *See* Perphenazine
Trimethaphan, **464**
Trimipramine, **464**
TRIO (Transplant Recipient
  International Organization),
  633–634

Triptorelin, **464,** 471
Trovafloxacin, **464**
TSH (thyroid-stimulating hormone), 313, 320, 328
Tubal ligation, 704–705
Tuberculosis, 417, 436
Tumors. *See* Cancer
Turner's syndrome, 480
TWEAK, 428
12-step programs, 420–421
Type A behavior, 117, **118**
    cardiac disease and, 113–114, 539–540, 1054
    sympathoadrenal system and, 539, 1059
    treatment of
        behavioral and psychological interventions, 1056
        effect on risk of recurrent myocardial infarction, 1057
        pharmacotherapy, 1058
Tyramine–monoamine oxidase inhibitor interaction, 327, 543–544, 954, 955

UGPPA (Uniform Guardianship and Protective Proceeding Act), 177
Ulcerative colitis, 556, 1063
"Ulysses Contract," 176
Unacceptability bias in research, **199**
Uniform Guardianship and Protective Proceeding Act (UGPPA), 177
Uniform Probate Code (UPC), 177
United Kingdom, consultation-liaison psychiatry in, 212–213
    background of, 212
    future development, 213
    in general hospital, 212–213
    official status and training, 213
    research, 213
UPC (Uniform Probate Code), 177
Uremia, 345. *See also* Renal failure
Uremic encephalopathy, **284,** 560–561
Urethral manipulation, 469
Urinary retention, tricyclic antidepressant–induced, 325, 950, 951
Urine acidification
    for amphetamine overdose, 442
    for phencyclidine intoxication, 443, 905
Urine toxicology screening, 893–894, **894, 895**
Uruguay, consultation-liaison psychiatry in, 221

Vacuum erection devices, 466
Valerian, **974**
Validity of test, 89
Valium. *See* Diazepam
Valproate, **943, 958,** 960–962
    dosage and administration of, **347, 958,** 961
    drug interactions with, **349,** 351, 962
        lamotrigine, 961
    half-life and serum level of, **347,** 961
    indications for, 961
        agitation and aggression, 161, **161**
        mania, **347,** 350–351, 694, 961
        pain syndromes, **989,** 1006
    intravenous, 601–602
    mechanism of action of, 960
    overdose of, 962
    pharmacokinetics of, 960
    side effects of, 350–351, 961
    use in specific patient groups and medical conditions
        Alzheimer's disease, 296
        breast-feeding women, **981**
        cancer, 663
        cardiac disease, 544
        dialysis patients, 561
        elderly persons, **863**
        HIV/AIDS, 826–827
        neurological disease, 694
        patients undergoing rehabilitation, **742**
        pregnancy, 351, 961, 980
        surgical patients, **598**
        transplant candidates, **635**
Valsartan, **464**
Valve replacement surgery, 607–608
VAS (visual analogue scale) for pain, 992, **992**
Vascular dementia, **274,** 275, 280–281
    age and gender distribution of, 276
    Alzheimer's disease and, 275
    causes of, 280
    clinical presentation of, 281
    course and prognosis for, 296
    diagnostic criteria for, **280**
    Hachinski Ischemia Score in, 281, **281**
    in medically ill patients, 276
    neuroimaging in, 293–294
    pathophysiology of, 287
    pharmacotherapy for, 296, 297
    risk factors for, 276–277
Vasculitis, 243, 441
Vasodilators, 969
Vasopressin, 487
Venlafaxine, 326–327, **948**

for anxiety disorders, **950,** 969
dosage of, **948**
drug interactions with, 327, 596
    cytochrome P450 metabolism and, **945**
    monoamine oxidase inhibitors, 327, 954
mechanism of action of, 326, **948,** 952
side effects of, 326, 786, 829, 952
    sexual dysfunction, **464**
structure of, 947
use in specific patient groups or medical conditions
    cardiac disease, 543
    dying patients, 786
    elderly persons, **863,** 864
    HIV/AIDS, 829
    surgical patients, **597**
    transplant candidates, **637**
withdrawal from, 953
Ventilation. *See* Lung disease; Respiration
Ventilatory support, 765
    weaning from, 606
Verapamil
    drug interactions with
        carbamazepine, **349,** 351
        cytochrome P450 metabolism and, **945**
        immunosuppressants, 643
    for mania, 354
    sexual dysfunction induced by, **464**
    use in dialysis patients, 561
Versed. *See* Midazolam
Vertically integrated medical-psychiatry services, 873, 882
Veterans Affairs Cooperative Study, 607
Viagra. *See* Sildenafil citrate
Videoconferencing, 928–929. *See also* Telepsychiatry
Videx. *See* Didanosine
Vinblastine, **311,** 323, **464, 668,** 793, **818**
Vincristine, **311,** 323, **668,** 793, **818**
Violent patients, 890, 898–900. *See also* Aggression
Viracept. *See* Nelfinavir
Viramune. *See* Nevirapine
Vision loss, 610–612
    acute, in adults, 610–611
    adaptation to, 610, 611
    in children, 610
    drug-induced, 611
    neuropsychiatric aspects of, 611–612
    transference and countertransference responses to, 611

Visual analogue scale (VAS) for pain, 992, **992**
Visual disturbances
  in delirium, 261, **261**
  drug-induced
    antipsychotics, 966
    inhalants, 446
    lamotrigine, 353
    psychostimulants, 956
    reboxetine, 953
    tricyclic antidepressants, 325, 951
  in transplant recipients, 642
Vitamin deficiency
  B$_{12}$, **284**, 288, **345**, 569
  dementia and, **284**, 288
  K, 486
  niacin, **284**, **345**
  psychosis due to, **896**
  thiamine, **284**, 426
Vitamin E
  for Alzheimer's disease, 297
  for tardive dyskinesia, 966
Vivactil. *See* Protriptyline
Vocational rehabilitation counselors, 731, 732
Volume of distribution of drug, 942
Volunteer bias in research, **199**
Vomiting. *See* Nausea/vomiting
Vorbeireden, 523
Vulvar cancer, 457

WAIS (Wechsler Adult Intelligence Scale), 81, 82, 560
Wandering, in frontotemporal dementia, 277
Ward management
  of critically ill patients, 758
  of patients with dementia, 297–298
  of patients with neurological disease, 695
  in rehabilitation settings, 745–746
Warfarin interactions
  with chloral hydrate, 973
  cytochrome P450 metabolism and, **945**
  with selective serotonin reuptake inhibitors, 543
Weakness
  antiretroviral drug–induced, 812
  in transplant recipients, 643
Weapons screening in emergency department, 890
Wechsler Adult Intelligence Scale (WAIS), 81, 82, 560

Weight gain
  drug-induced
    antipsychotics, 966
    clozapine, 966
    gabapentin, 961
    lithium, 959
    medroxyprogesterone acetate, 471
    mirtazapine, 327, 953
    nicotine withdrawal, 445
    risperidone, 354
    selective serotonin reuptake inhibitors, 951–952
    tricyclic antidepressants, 950
    valproate, 961
  during treatment of anorexia nervosa, 487–488
Weight loss
  amphetamine abuse and treatment for, 442
  in anorexia nervosa, 479
  cocaine-related, 243, 441
  due to opioid withdrawal, 437
  for hypertension, 1060
  for ischemic heart disease, 1059–1060
  sleep pattern and, 496
  work-site behavioral programs for, 1059
Wellbutrin, Wellbutrin SR. *See* Bupropion
Wernicke's encephalopathy, 263, 265, 283, 296, 426, 901
  thiamine therapy for, 263, 265, 296, 432, **433**
West Haven–Yale Multidimensional Pain Inventory (WHYMPI), **371**
Western Collaborative Group Study, 539
WHHHHIMP mnemonic for delirium, 141, 264–265, 756, **756**, 895
White matter brain lesions, 53–54
WHYMPI (West Haven–Yale Multidimensional Pain Inventory), **371**
Wickline v. California, 182–183
Wilson v. Blue Cross of Southern California et al., 182–183
Wilson's disease, 279
  anxiety and, 398
  clinical features of, 279
  course and prognosis for, 295
  genetic factors in, 277, 279
  mania and, **345**

pathophysiology of, 286
  penicillamine for, 295
  prevalence of, **680**
  psychotropic drug use in patients with, β-blockers, 692
Wise, T. N., 17
Women's health care, 701, 703–704. *See also* Obstetrics and gynecology
Work-site behavioral weight reduction programs, 1059
"Workaholism," 113, 122
Working alliance, 1036

Xanax. *See* Alprazolam
Xenon, 51

Yoga, 546–547, 1057
Yohimbine, **345**, 400
Youngberg v. Romeo, 180

Zalcitabine, **811**
Zaleplon, 505, **506**, 972–973
Ziagen. *See* Abacavir
Zidovudine (AZT), 810, **811**
  cerebrospinal fluid penetration by, 823
  for HIV-associated neurocognitive impairment, 823
  interaction with methadone, 814
  resistance to, 813
  side effects of
    mania, **345**
    neuropsychiatric disorders, **818**
    sleep disorders, 834
  use in pregnancy, 809
Zinc
  for anorexia nervosa, 480, 488
  propofol-induced deficiency of, 762
Zinermon v. Burch, 178–179
Ziprasidone, 963, **964**
Zoloft. *See* Sertraline
Zolpidem, 972
  for elderly persons, **863**
  for insomnia, 505, **506**, 972
    in chronic obstructive pulmonary disease, 503
  interaction with ritonavir, 814, **815**
  sexual dysfunction induced by, **464**
  use during breast-feeding, **981**
Zung Self-Rating Depression Scale, 25, 93, 661
Zyprexa. *See* Olanzapine